The Comparative Guide to American Hospitals

Volume 3

Second Edition

The Comparative Guide to American Hospitals

Volume 3: Central Region

4,383 Hospitals with Key Personnel and
24 Quality Measures in Treating Heart Attack, Heart Failure,
Pneumonia, Pregnancy and Surgical Infection Prevention

A SEDGWICK PRESS Book

Grey House Publishing

PUBLISHER . . . . Leslie Mackenzie
EDITOR. . . . . David Garoogian
EDITORIAL DIRECTOR. . . . . Laura Mars-Proietti
PRODUCTION MANAGER . . . . Karen Stevens
MARKETING DIRECTOR . . . . Jessica Moody

A Sedgewick Press Book
Grey House Publishing, Inc.
185 Millerton Road
Millerton, NY 12546
518.789.8700
FAX 518.789.0545
www.greyhouse.com
e-mail: books @greyhouse.com

10 9 8 7 6 5 4 3 2

Comparative guide to American hospitals. Vol. 1, Eastern region; [ed. David Garoogian]. -- 2nd ed. (2007)

v. ; cm.

Includes index.
"4,383 hospitals with key personnel and 24 quality measures in treating heart attack, heart failure, pneumonia, pregnancy and surgical infection prevention."

1. Hospitals--United States--Directories. 2. Hospitals--United States--Periodicals. 3. Hospitals--Ratings--United States--Statistics--Periodicals. 4. Myocardial infarction--Hospitals--United States--Directories. 5. Heart failure--Hospitals--United States--Directories. 6. Pneumonia--Hospitals--United States--Directories. I. Garoogian, David.

RA977 .C66
610/.025

4-Volume Set ISBN: 978-1-59237-182-2
Volume 1 ISBN: 978-1-59237-280-5
Volume 2 ISBN: 978-1-59237-281-2
Volume 3 ISBN: 978-1-59237-282-9
Volume 4 ISBN: 978-1-59237-283-6

Table of Contents

Introduction

Welcome to the second edition of *The Comparative Guide to American Hospitals*. It reports on how 4,383 hospitals in America measure up when caring for patients with a number of specific conditions. The first edition reported on **Heart Attacks, Heart Failure** and **Pneumonia**. In this second edition, each hospital profile includes additional data on **Pregnancy Care** and **Surgical Infection Prevention.** Also new are two Appendixes - **30-Day Mortality Data** and **Glossary of Terms**.

The content of this work is based on a Federal study (Hospital Compare) in which short-term acute care and critical access hospitals around the country voluntarily reported on quality measures in order to receive an incentive payment established by the Medicare Prescription Drug, Improvement and Modernization Act of 2003. Each hospital is rated on 24 recognized quality measures - **Seven More Than Last Edition** -- and is compared to both state and national averages, and to the top hospitals in the country (best practices).

Due to the increased data, and the regional use of such data, this edition is comprised of four regional volumes - **Eastern, Southern, Central** and **Western**. In addition to comprehensive hospital profiles for all states in the region, each volume includes a **State-by-State Statistical Summary**.

Each hospital profile in *The Comparative Guide to American Hospitals* is comprised of data from Hospital Compare (the Medicare sponsored web site) and The Joint Commission plus value-added data from Grey House's *Directory of Hospital Personnel*. You will find **20,700 key contact names** managing the care at 4,383 hospitals - that's 5,509 more names at 180 more hospitals than last edition. In addition, each state chapter includes **State Rankings**.

Section One: Hospital Rankings & State Profiles

The first section of each regional volume of *The Comparative Guide to American Hospitals* is arranged alphabetically by state. Each state starts with a ranking section that rates hospitals in that state on how often they meet the accepted quality protocols. Following the ranking section, hospital profiles are listed first by city, then alpha within city. Profiles include name, address, phone, fax, web site and number of licensed beds. Further, each profile includes an average of 10 key medical contacts -- **Five More Than Last Edition** -- including hospital administration, patients, and those who provide products and services to the industry -- representing not only the facility's top administration but also the physicians specifically responsible for the care of heart, pneumonia, and pregnant patients, as well as surgical infection prevention.

The first section of *The Comparative Guide to American Hospitals*:

- **Evaluates 24 Quality Measures:** The quality measures rated in *The Comparative Guide to American Hospitals* are based on accepted, effective treatments supported by the Centers for Medicare & Medical Services of the US Department of Health & Human Services and the Hospital Quality Alliance (HQA) - a public/private collaboration established to promote on hospital quality of care. HQA represents consumers, hospitals, doctors, employers, accrediting organizations and Federal agencies.
- **Examines Critical Conditions: Heart Attack Care** measures include aspirin at arrival and discharge, beta blockers at arrival and discharge, use of ACE/ARB inhibitors, and PCI administration and fibrinolytic medication timing. **Heart Failure Care** measures include LVF assessment, use of ACE/ARB inhibitors, discharge instructions and smoking cessation advice. **Pneumonia Care** measures include use of initial antibiotics and pneumococcal vaccine, use of oxygenation and blood culture results, smoking cessation advice, and administration of influenza vaccine. **Surgical Infection Prevention** measures ***(NEW)*** include use of prophylactic antibiotics. **Pregnancy Care** measures ***(NEW)*** include inpatient neonatal mortality, and degree of vaginal lacerations.

Section Two: Statistical Summary, Appendixes & Index

The second section of *The Comparative Guide to American Hospitals includes:*

- **Regional State-by-State Statistical Summary Tables** show at a glance how hospitals in the same state score and compare with each other. They are arranged alphabetically by state in easy-to-read landscape format.
- **Appendix A: 30-Day Mortality Chart** ***(NEW)*** lists hospitals nationwide that are "better" or "worse" than the national average, plus a State Summary of Hospital Mortality.
- **Appendix B: Glossary of Terms** ***(NEW)*** provides a list of 60 medical terms to make the best use possible of the data in this edition.
- **Regional Hospital Profile Index** lists hospitals alphabetically, including city and state.

This completely revised second edition of *The Comparative Guide to American Hospitals,* **now in four regional volumes**, is a valuable guide for the entire medical community, with more hospitals, more criteria measures and more key executives than the first edition. It offers an indispensable snapshot of how hospitals measure up, not only to established "best practices," but also to each other.

We welcome your comments to this edition.

User's Guide

Shown below is a fictitious listing illustrating the kind of information that is or might be included in a Hospital Profile. Each numbered item of information is described in the paragraphs following the example.

❶ Bowling Green Medical Center

250 Park Street — Phone: 270-745-1255
Bowling Green, KY 42101 — Fax: 270-745-1253
E-mail: SKWebb@mcbg.org
URL: www.mcbg.org
Ownership: Voluntary non-profit - Private — Accredited: Yes
Emergency Services: Yes — Licensed Beds: 330

❷ **Key Personnel:**

CEO/President. . . . . Wayne Bush, MD
Emergency Room Director. . . . . Pliois Prerost
Director Medical/Surgical Nursing . . . . Kathleen Riley, RN
Chief OB/GYN . . . . Joseph Gass, MD
Surgery Chair. . . . . James Bergin, MD
Chief Radiology . . . . Ken Bartholomew, MD

	Measure	Cases	This Hospital	State Average	U.S. Average	Top Hospital
❸						
❹	**Heart Attack Care**					
	ACE Inhibitor or ARB for LVSD	63	73%	75%	82%	100%
	Aspirin at Arrival	191	95%	89%	92%	100%
	Aspirin at Discharge	243	96%	86%	90%	100%
	Beta Blocker at Arrival	140	91%	82%	87%	100%
	Beta Blocker at Discharge	274	97%	86%	90%	100%
	Fibrinolytic Medication Timing[1]	10	10%	31%	31%	100%
	PCI Within 90 Minutes of Arrival[1]	6	17%	44%	54%	95%
	Smoking Cessation Advice	147	100%	84%	88%	100%
❺	**Heart Failure Care**					
	ACE Inhibitor or ARB for LVSD	162	84%	78%	82%	100%
	Discharge Instructions	394	50%	59%	61%	93%
	Evaluation of LVS Function	466	90%	79%	83%	99%
	Smoking Cessation Advice	123	100%	82%	82%	100%
❻	**Pneumonia Care**					
	Appropriate Initial Antibiotic	277	84%	82%	83%	94%
	Blood Culture Timing	225	92%	89%	90%	100%
	Influenza Vaccine	87	84%	76%	70%	100%
	Initial Antibiotic Timing	382	69%	82%	80%	93%
	Oxygenation Assessment	483	100%	99%	99%	100%
	Pneumococcal Vaccine	284	87%	75%	69%	94%
	Smoking Cessation Advice	170	100%	84%	80%	100%
❼	**Surgical Infection Prevention**					
	Prophylactic Antibiotic Given[3]	427	89%	74%	77%	95%
	Prophylactic Antibiotic Selection	245	87%	85%	90%	100%
	Prophylactic Antibiotic Stopped[3]	424	91%	69%	72%	95%
❽	**Pregnancy Care**					
	Inpatient Neonatal Mortality	1,979	0.25%	-	-	-
	Third or Fourth Degree Laceration	1,283	4.36%	3.25%	3.63%	3.27%

➊ **Hospital Name and Record Header:** hospital name; alternate name (if applicable); street address; phone; fax; e-mail; URL; ownership; accredited (Yes/No); emergency services (Yes/No); and number of licensed beds. *Source: Directory of Hospital Personnel, 2007, Grey House Publishing; www.hospitalcompare.hhs.gov, Centers for Medicare & Medicaid Services (CMS), an agency of the U.S. Department of Health and Human Services (DHHS) along with the Hospital Quality Alliance (HQA).*

➋ **Key Personnel:** includes the names of key personnel primarily related to the five conditions covered in this publication. *Source: Directory of Hospital Personnel, 2007, Grey House Publishing*

➌ **Hospital Compare Data:** each table contains data covering the five conditions and twenty-four associated measures contained in the Hospital Compare database. There are six columns:

Measure: the twenty-four quality measures reported.

There are five possible footnotes:

1. *The number of cases is too small (n<25) for purposes of reliably predicting hospital performance.*
   For each measure, the rate is displayed as a percent of the number of patients for whom the measured treatment is appropriate. For hospitals with small numbers of patients for whom the measured treatment is appropriate during the reporting period (fewer than 25 patients), the calculated rate may not be predictive of the hospital's future performance. As the quality data base is expanded to a full rolling four quarters of data for each measure, the number of cases used to determine hospitals' rates will likely increase, thereby increasing the reliability and stability of the rates. Note: This footnote does not necessarily reflect hospital size or overall patient volume.

2. *Measure reflects the hospital's indication that its submission was based upon a sample of its relevant discharges.*
   Rates are based on the cases reported by hospitals. A rate may be based upon the total number of cases treated by a hospital, or for a facility with a large caseload, a rate may be based on a random sample of the cases the hospital treated. This footnote indicates that a hospital chose to submit data for a sample of its total cases (following specific rules for how to the select the cases).

3. *Rate reflects fewer than the maximum possible quarters of data for the measure.*
   Each rate reflects the care provided over a specific time period, up to a maximum of four quarters. The number of quarters of data available is determined by when hospitals first began to report data using a specific measure. For example, for the ten measures in the "Starter Set", the maximum number of quarters for which a hospital could have provided data is four quarters. For measures added more recently, the maximum will be fewer than four quarters. This footnote indicates that the hospital's rate was based on data from fewer than the maximum possible number of quarters that the measure was generally collected.

4. *Inaccurate information submitted and suppressed for one or more quarters.*
   Hospitals are required to submit accurate, reportable data to the Centers for Medicare and Medicaid Services (CMS). The rates for these measures were calculated by excluding data that had been suppressed for one or more quarters because they were identified as inaccurate.

5. *No data is available from the hospital for this measure.*
   Hospitals volunteer to provide data for reporting on Hospital Compare. This footnote is applied when the hospital did not submit any cases for a measure.

Cases: the size of the data sample (number of patients) for each hospital and quality measure. In addition, the notation "0" is applied when a hospital provided care to patients with a condition, such as pneumonia, but the cases that the hospital submitted did not meet the specific criteria for being included in the calculation of the measure.

This Hospital: the performance rate that the hospital achieved for each quality measure. This value is expressed as a percentage of the sample size that was measured.

State Average: the average rate for all hospitals reporting data in the state the hospital is located in.

U.S. Average: the average rate for all hospitals reporting nationwide.

Top Hospital: the average rate for the 90th percentile (or top 10%) of hospitals reporting data.

Note: A two-step process was used to calculate the national and state comparison group rates. The national and state comparison rates for each measure were calculated using all of the data submitted to the QIO Clinical Data Warehouse for hospitals with at least one case that met the measure's inclusion criteria (that is, for which the denominator was greater than zero).

First, the individual hospital performance rates were calculated using the method described above for all hospitals. Next, hospitals with "0 patients" were excluded from the calculation. For the determination of the 90th percentile (or top 10%) of hospitals on a national basis, the individual rates were then rank ordered and the top 10th percentile score identified. For the national and state averages, a simple average was constructed where the numerator was the sum of all non-excluded hospitals' scores and the denominator was the total number of hospitals, each calculated at either the national or individual state level.

❹ Heart Attack Care

Every year, about one million people suffer a heart attack (acute myocardial infarction or AMI). AMI is among the leading causes of hospital admission for Medicare beneficiaries, age 65 and older.

Scientific evidence indicates that the following process of care measures represent the best practices for the treatment of AMI. Higher scores are better.

- **ACE Inhibitor or ARB for LVSD** - AMI patients with left ventricular systolic dysfunction (LVSD) and without angiotensin converting enzyme inhibitor (ACE inhibitor) contraindications or angiotensin receptor blocker (ARB) contraindications who are prescribed an ACE inhibitor or an ARB at hospital discharge.
- **Aspirin at Arrival** - Acute myocardial infarction (AMI) patients without aspirin contraindications who received aspirin within 24 hours before or after hospital arrival.
- **Aspirin at Discharge** - AMI patients without aspirin contraindications who were prescribed aspirin at hospital discharge.
- **Beta Blocker at Arrival** - AMI patients without beta-blocker contraindications who received a beta-blocker within 24 hours after hospital arrival.
- **Beta Blocker at Discharge** - AMI patients without beta-blocker contraindications who were prescribed a beta-blocker at hospital discharge.
- **Fibrinolytic Medication Timing** - AMI patients receiving fibrinolytic therapy during the hospital stay and having a time from hospital arrival to fibrinolysis of 30 minutes or less.
- **PCI Within 90 Minutes of Arrival** - AMI patients receiving Percutaneous Coronary Intervention (PCI) during the hospital stay with a time from hospital arrival to PCI of 90 minutes or less.
- **Smoking Cessation Advice** - AMI patients with a history of smoking cigarettes, who are given smoking cessation advice or counseling during a hospital stay.

❺ Heart Failure Care

Heart failure is the most common hospital admission diagnosis in patients age 65 or older, accounting for more than 700,000 hospitalizations among Medicare beneficiaries every year. It is associated with severe functional impairments and high rates of mortality and morbidity.

Substantial scientific evidence indicates that the following process of care measures represent the best practices for the treatment of heart failure. Higher scores are better.

- **ACE Inhibitor or ARB for LVSD** - Heart failure patients with left ventricular systolic dysfunction (LVSD) and without angiotensin converting enzyme inhibitor (ACE inhibitor) contraindications or angiotensin receptor blocker (ARB) contraindications who are prescribed an ACE inhibitor or an ARB at hospital discharge.
- **Discharge Instructions** - Heart failure patients discharged home with written instructions or educational material given to patient or care giver at discharge or during the hospital stay addressing all of the following: activity level, diet, discharge medications, follow-up appointment, weight monitoring, and what to do if symptoms worsen.
- **Evaluation of LVS Function** - Heart failure patients with documentation in the hospital record that an evaluation of the left ventricular systolic (LVS) function was performed before arrival, during hospitalization, or is planned for after discharge.
- **Smoking Cessation Advice** - Heart failure patients with a history of smoking cigarettes, who are given smoking cessation advice or counseling during a hospital stay.

❻ Pneumonia Care

Community acquired pneumonia is a major contributor to illness and mortality in the United States, causing four million episodes of illness and nearly one million hospital admissions each year.

Scientific evidence indicates that the following process of care measures represent the best practices for the treatment of community-acquired pneumonia. Higher scores are better.

- **Appropriate Initial Antibiotic** - Immunocompetent patients with pneumonia who receive an initial antibiotic regimen that is consistent with current guidelines.
- **Blood Culture Timing** - Pneumonia patients whose initial emergency room blood culture specimen was collected prior to first hospital dose of antibiotics.
- **Influenza Vaccination** - Pneumonia patients age 50 years and older, hospitalized during October, November, December, January, or February who were screened for influenza vaccine status and were vaccinated prior to discharge, if indicated.
- **Initial Antibiotic Timing** - Pneumonia inpatients who receive antibiotics within 4 hours of hospital arrival. Evidence shows better outcomes for administration times less than four hours.
- **Oxygenation Assessment** - Pneumonia inpatients who receive an oxygenation assessment, arterial blood gas (ABG), or pulse oximetry within 24 hours of hospital arrival.
- **Pneumococcal Vaccination** - Pneumonia inpatients age 65 and older who were screened for pneumococcal vaccine status and were administered the vaccine prior to discharge, if indicated.
- **Smoking Cessation Advice** - Pneumonia patients with a history of smoking cigarettes, who are given smoking cessation advice or counseling during a hospital stay.

❼ Surgical Infection Prevention

Hospitals can reduce the risk of wound infection after surgery by providing the right medicines at the right time on the day of surgery. Studies show a strong association of reduced incidence of post-operative infection with administration of antibiotics within the one hour prior to surgery. After the incision is closed, however, studies show that prolonged administration of prophylaxis with antibiotics may increase the risk of certain other infections at no additional benefit to the surgical patient.

Scientific evidence indicates that the following process of care measures represent the best practices for the prevention of infections after selected surgeries (colon surgery, hip and knee arthroplasty, abdominal and vaginal hysterectomy, cardiac surgery (including coronary artery bypass grafts (CABG)) and vascular surgery). Higher scores are better.

- **Prophylactic Antibiotic Given** - Surgical patients who received prophylactic antibiotics within 1 hour prior to surgical incision.
- **Prophylactic Antibiotic Selection** - Surgical patients who received the recommended antibiotics for their particular type of surgery.
- **Prophylactic Antibiotic Stopped** - Surgical patients whose prophylactic antibiotics were discontinued within 24 hours after surgery end time.

❽ Pregnancy Care

- **Inpatient Neonatal Mortality** - This measure reports how often infants died before 28 days of birth; it is adjusted to reflect the fact that some babies are sicker than others at or shortly after birth.
- **Third or Fourth Degree Laceration** - This measure reports how often patients have significant tears between the vagina and anus while having a baby. These types of tears can lead to other medical complications.

Information about Hospital Performance

Hospital performance rates tell you the proportion of cases where a hospital provided the recommended process of care. Only patients meeting the inclusion criteria for a measure are included in the calculation of the rate for a measure. A rate of 88% means that the hospital provided the recommended process of care 88% of the time. For example, the rates for initial antibiotic timing tell you the percentage of patients who received their first dose of antibiotics within four hours of arrival to the hospital. The ultimate goal for all measures listed (except Pregnancy Care) is 100%. With the two measures under Pregnancy Care, lower numbers are preferable. Hospitals with effective quality improvement programs are continually working toward this goal.

Confidence Intervals

The table below enables the user to calculate confidence intervals for each reported measure.

Confidence intervals can be used to estimate the precision of the calculated rates for an individual hospital. A confidence interval is the range of values, within which an estimated value or rate is likely to fall. A confidence interval is a statistical determination of the degree of certainty associated with an estimated value. As can be seen in the table of estimated values (below), large differences between individual hospitals' rates may be significant, and small differences between hospitals are usually not significant.

The smaller the sample size, the greater the difference in rates must be order for that difference to be statistically meaningful. Also, as sample size varies between hospitals, it is difficult to precisely compare their rates, without considering the confidence intervals.

Over time, as the quality data base is expanded, a full four quarters of data will ultimately be available, so the number of cases used to determine hospitals' rates will likely increase, thereby increasing the reliability and stability of the rates.

Estimating Confidence Intervals for the Quality Measures: Estimated Values for Proportion Data

Sample Size	Observed Rate								
	10%	20%	30%	40%	50%	60%	70%	80%	90%
< 25	*	*	24.9	26.6	27.2	26.6	24.9	*	*
25 - 75	8.3	11.1	12.7	13.6	13.9	13.6	12.7	11.1	8.3
76 - 125	5.9	7.8	9.0	9.6	9.8	9.6	9.0	7.8	5.9
126 - 175	4.8	6.4	7.3	7.8	8.0	7.8	7.3	6.4	4.8
176 - 225	4.2	5.5	6.4	6.8	6.9	6.8	6.4	5.5	4.2
226 -275	3.7	5.0	5.7	6.1	6.2	6.1	5.7	5.0	3.7
276+	2.9	3.9	4.5	4.8	4.9	4.8	4.5	3.9	2.9

Source: CMS/OCSQ/QIG. The values in the table are the approximate amount to add and subtract from the observed rate to estimate a 95 percent confidence interval for the given sample size. (Interpolation between the values in the table is appropriate.)
** Estimates of an interval in these cells exceed the natural limits for proportions.*

Source of Data

The information in this book comes from the quality data submitted by hospitals to the QIO Clinical Data Warehouse for inpatient discharges. Heart Attack Care, Heart Failure Care, Pneumonia Care, Pregnancy Care and Surgical Infection Prevention data is from www.hospitalcompare.hhs.gov, a website tool developed by the Centers for Medicare & Medicaid Services (CMS). Data covers October 2005 through September 2006. Hospital Mortality data is also from www.hospitalcompare.hhs.gov. Data covers July 2005 through June 2006.

Pregnancy Care data is from www.qualitycheck.org, a service of The Joint Commission. The Joint Commission (formerly the Joint Commission on Accreditation of Healthcare Organizations (JCAHO)), is a US-based non-profit organization formed in 1951 with a mission to maintain and elevate the standards of healthcare delivery through evaluation and accreditation of healthcare organizations. Data covers January 2006 through December 2006.

Heart Attack Care

1. ACE Inhibitor or ARB for LVSD

Hospital Name	City	Rate	Cases
Edward Hospital	Naperville	100%	58
Good Samaritan Regional Health Center	Mount Vernon	100%	42
Hinsdale Hospital	Hinsdale	100%	26
Proctor Hospital	Peoria	100%	27
Rush-Copley Medical Center	Aurora	100%	30
Advocate Good Samaritan Hospital	Downers Grove	98%	64
Northwestern Memorial Hospital	Chicago	98%	46
Gottlieb Memorial Hospital	Melrose Park	97%	29
Saint Joseph Medical Center	Bloomington	97%	34
Elmhurst Memorial Hospital	Elmhurst	96%	49
Evanston Hospital	Evanston	96%	89
Methodist Medical Center of Illinois	Peoria	96%	49
Northwest Community Hospital	Arlington Heights	96%	46
Provena Covenant Medical Center	Urbana	96%	45
Memorial Medical Center	Springfield	95%	128
Silver Cross Hospital	Joliet	95%	41
Saint Anthony Medical Center	Rockford	94%	69
Swedish American Hospital	Rockford	94%	80
Advocate Lutheran General Children's Hospital	Park Ridge	92%	77
University of Chicago Hospitals	Chicago	91%	55
Advocate Christ Med Ctr/Hope Children's	Oak Lawn	90%	83
Alexian Brothers Medical Center	Elk Grove Village	90%	59
Saint Francis Medical Center	Peoria	90%	155
Decatur Memorial Hospital	Decatur	88%	76
Our Lady of the Resurrection Medical Center	Chicago	88%	43
Saint John's Hospital	Springfield	87%	237
Trinity Medical Center	Rock Island	87%	82
Advocate Good Shephard Hospital	Barrington	86%	42
Advocate South Suburban Hospital	Hazel Crest	86%	43
Mercy Hospital	Chicago	86%	44
Blessing Hospital	Quincy	85%	54
Holy Cross Hospital	Chicago	85%	33
Rockford Memorial Hospital	Rockford	85%	54
Loyola University Health System	Maywood	84%	37
MacNeal Hospital	Berwyn	84%	102
Saint Alexius Medical Center	Hoffman Estates	84%	44
Saint James Hospital and Health Center	Olympia Fields	84%	56
Saint Elizabeth's Hospital	Belleville	82%	55
Advocate Illinois Masonic Medical Center	Chicago	81%	48
Palos Community Hospital	Palos Heights	81%	32
Sherman Hospital	Elgin	80%	46
Genesis Medical Center-Illini Campus	Silvis	79%	66
Saint Francis Hospital & Health Center	Blue Island	79%	33
Weiss Memorial Hospital	Chicago	79%	29
John H Stroger Jr Hospital of Cook County	Chicago	78%	40
Advocate Trinity Hospital	Chicago	77%	30
Saint Joseph Medical Center	Joliet	77%	73
Adventist LaGrange Memorial Hospital	La Grange	76%	41
Central DuPage Hospital	Winfield	76%	34
Ingalls Memorial Hospital	Harvey	76%	46
Memorial Hospital Carbondale	Carbondale	76%	70
Condell Medical Center	Libertyville	75%	63
Provena Saint Joseph Hospital	Elgin	74%	31
West Suburban Medical Center	Oak Park	72%	25
Carle Foundation Hospital	Urbana	69%	49
Memorial Hospital	Belleville	69%	36
Provena Mercy Center	Aurora	68%	41
Resurrection Medical Center	Chicago	62%	73

2. Aspirin at Arrival

Hospital Name	City	Rate	Cases
Advocate Illinois Masonic Medical Center	Chicago	100%	107
Advocate Lutheran General Children's Hospital	Park Ridge	100%	268
Edward Hospital	Naperville	100%	263
Loyola University Health System	Maywood	100%	169
MacNeal Hospital	Berwyn	100%	246
Northwestern Memorial Hospital	Chicago	100%	215
Palos Community Hospital	Palos Heights	100%	264
Riverside Medical Center	Kankakee	100%	93
Rush University Medical Center	Chicago	100%	112
Saint Bernard Hospital and Health Care Center	Chicago	100%	32
Saint Joseph Medical Center	Bloomington	100%	90
Saint Mary's Good Samaritan	Centralia	100%	52
Saints Mary & Elizabeth Medical Center	Chicago	100%	63
Sarah Bush Lincoln Health Center	Mattoon	100%	36
Swedish Covenant Hospital	Chicago	100%	199
University of Illinois at Chicago Med Ctr	Chicago	100%	56
Advocate Christ Med Ctr/Hope Children's	Oak Lawn	99%	190
Advocate Good Samaritan Hospital	Downers Grove	99%	215
Carle Foundation Hospital	Urbana	99%	158
Decatur Memorial Hospital	Decatur	99%	164
Delnor Community Hospital	Geneva	99%	98
Elmhurst Memorial Hospital	Elmhurst	99%	225
Evanston Hospital	Evanston	99%	515
Memorial Hospital	Belleville	99%	151
Memorial Hospital Carbondale	Carbondale	99%	87
Provena Mercy Center	Aurora	99%	166
Rush-Copley Medical Center	Aurora	99%	154
Saint Anthony Medical Center	Rockford	99%	228
Saint John's Hospital	Springfield	99%	180
Swedish American Hospital	Rockford	99%	234
Advocate Good Shephard Hospital	Barrington	98%	179
Alexian Brothers Medical Center	Elk Grove Village	98%	214
Anderson Hospital	Maryville	98%	66
Blessing Hospital	Quincy	98%	206
Bromenn Healthcare	Normal	98%	132
Good Samaritan Regional Health Center	Mount Vernon	98%	98
Hinsdale Hospital	Hinsdale	98%	132
Iroquois Memorial Hospital & Resident Home	Watseka	98%	40
Katherine Shaw Bethea Hospital	Dixon	98%	48
Memorial Medical Center	Springfield	98%	295
Morris Hospital	Morris	98%	40
Northwest Community Hospital	Arlington Heights	98%	389
Proctor Hospital	Peoria	98%	88
Rockford Memorial Hospital	Rockford	98%	196
Saint Francis Hospital	Evanston	98%	121
Saint Francis Medical Center	Peoria	98%	246
Saint Joseph Hospital	Chicago	98%	56
Westlake Community Hospital	Melrose Park	98%	80
Central DuPage Hospital	Winfield	97%	180
FHN Memorial Hospital	Freeport	97%	34
Heartland Regional Medical Center	Marion	97%	63
Methodist Medical Center of Illinois	Peoria	97%	114
Our Lady of the Resurrection Medical Center	Chicago	97%	238
Pekin Hospital	Pekin	97%	29
Provena Covenant Medical Center	Urbana	97%	107
Resurrection Medical Center	Chicago	97%	343
Saint Alexius Medical Center	Hoffman Estates	97%	152
West Suburban Medical Center	Oak Park	97%	120
Alton Memorial Hospital	Alton	96%	106
CGH Medical Center	Sterling	96%	72
John H Stroger Jr Hospital of Cook County	Chicago	96%	144
Lake Forest Hospital	Lake Forest	96%	26
Little Company of Mary Hospital	Evergreen Park	96%	154
Provena United Samaritans Medical Center	Danville	96%	74
Rush North Shore Medical Center	Skokie	96%	106
Rush Oak Park Hospital	Oak Park	96%	53
Saint Anthony Hospital	Chicago	96%	28
Saint Francis Hospital & Health Center	Blue Island	96%	122
Trinity Medical Center	Rock Island	96%	291
University of Chicago Hospitals	Chicago	96%	141
Centegra Northern Illinois Medical Center	McHenry	95%	124
Gottlieb Memorial Hospital	Melrose Park	95%	114
Mount Sinai Hospital	Chicago	95%	125
Saint Elizabeth's Hospital	Belleville	95%	174
Sherman Hospital	Elgin	95%	199
Adventist LaGrange Memorial Hospital	La Grange	94%	134
Advocate South Suburban Hospital	Hazel Crest	94%	188
Genesis Medical Center-Illini Campus	Silvis	94%	99
Holy Cross Hospital	Chicago	94%	200
Ingalls Memorial Hospital	Harvey	94%	175
Memorial Medical Center	Woodstock	94%	35
Provident Hospital	Chicago	94%	53
Silver Cross Hospital	Joliet	94%	170
Condell Medical Center	Libertyville	93%	216
Provena Saint Joseph Hospital	Elgin	93%	106
Advocate Trinity Hospital	Chicago	92%	159
Saint Elizabeth's Hospital	Chicago	92%	38
Saint Joseph Medical Center	Joliet	92%	280
Vista Medical Center East	Waukegan	92%	137
Weiss Memorial Hospital	Chicago	92%	85
Gateway Regional Medical Center	Granite City	91%	112
Mercy Hospital	Chicago	91%	129
Saint Anthony's Health Center	Alton	91%	79
Saint James Hospital and Health Center	Olympia Fields	91%	246
Saint Mary's Hospital	Decatur	91%	33
Norwegian-American Hospital	Chicago	90%	42
Saint Mary's Hospital of Kankakee	Kankakee	90%	83
Loretto Hospital	Chicago	89%	28
OSF Saint Mary Medical Center	Galesburg	89%	38
Saint Anthony's Memorial Hospital	Effingham	89%	38
Michael Reese Hospital	Chicago	88%	48
Galesburg Cottage Hospital	Galesburg	81%	31
South Shore Hospital	Chicago	81%	48
Jersey Community Hospital	Jerseyville	74%	68

NOTE: Hospital profiles are in alphabetical order by state, then city, then hospital within the city; Rankings are sorted by rate in descending order and exclude hospitals with less than 25 cases; (1) The number of cases is too small (n<25) for purposes of reliably predicting hospital performance; (2) Measure reflects the hospital's indication that its submission was based upon a sample of its relevant discharges; (3) Rate reflects fewer than the maximum possible quarters of data for the measure; (4) Inaccurate information submitted and suppressed for one or more quarters; (5) No data is available from the hospital for this measure; Please refer to the User's Guide for a full explanation of data

3. Aspirin at Discharge

Hospital Name	City	Rate	Cases
Advocate Christ Med Ctr/Hope Children's	Oak Lawn	100%	214
Edward Hospital	Naperville	100%	268
Elmhurst Memorial Hospital	Elmhurst	100%	229
Good Samaritan Regional Health Center	Mount Vernon	100%	202
Hinsdale Hospital	Hinsdale	100%	148
Loyola University Health System	Maywood	100%	188
Northwestern Memorial Hospital	Chicago	100%	232
Riverside Medical Center	Kankakee	100%	100
Rush University Medical Center	Chicago	100%	148
Swedish American Hospital	Rockford	100%	290
Advocate Good Samaritan Hospital	Downers Grove	99%	192
Advocate Good Shephard Hospital	Barrington	99%	201
Advocate Lutheran General Children's Hospital	Park Ridge	99%	244
Bromenn Healthcare	Normal	99%	143
Carle Foundation Hospital	Urbana	99%	249
Decatur Memorial Hospital	Decatur	99%	197
Delnor Community Hospital	Geneva	99%	81
Evanston Hospital	Evanston	99%	518
John H Stroger Jr Hospital of Cook County	Chicago	99%	199
Memorial Medical Center	Springfield	99%	507
Methodist Medical Center of Illinois	Peoria	99%	183
Northwest Community Hospital	Arlington Heights	99%	337
Proctor Hospital	Peoria	99%	93
Provena Covenant Medical Center	Urbana	99%	249
Saint Anthony Medical Center	Rockford	99%	321
Saint John's Hospital	Springfield	99%	553
Saint Joseph Medical Center	Bloomington	99%	104
Swedish Covenant Hospital	Chicago	99%	176
Westlake Community Hospital	Melrose Park	99%	68
Advocate South Suburban Hospital	Hazel Crest	98%	125
Alexian Brothers Medical Center	Elk Grove Village	98%	218
Memorial Hospital	Belleville	98%	130
Provena Saint Joseph Hospital	Elgin	98%	95
Saint Francis Medical Center	Peoria	98%	511
Saint Joseph Hospital	Chicago	98%	62
University of Chicago Hospitals	Chicago	98%	219
Blessing Hospital	Quincy	97%	211
Palos Community Hospital	Palos Heights	97%	213
Provena Mercy Center	Aurora	97%	184
Rockford Memorial Hospital	Rockford	97%	272
Rush North Shore Medical Center	Skokie	97%	95
Rush-Copley Medical Center	Aurora	97%	153
Saints Mary & Elizabeth Medical Center	Chicago	97%	99
Centegra Northern Illinois Medical Center	McHenry	96%	123
Central DuPage Hospital	Winfield	96%	167
Gateway Regional Medical Center	Granite City	96%	91
MacNeal Hospital	Berwyn	96%	223
Michael Reese Hospital	Chicago	96%	54
Our Lady of the Resurrection Medical Center	Chicago	96%	192
Saint Elizabeth's Hospital	Belleville	96%	253
Alton Memorial Hospital	Alton	95%	87
Gottlieb Memorial Hospital	Melrose Park	95%	103
Heartland Regional Medical Center	Marion	95%	83
Little Company of Mary Hospital	Evergreen Park	95%	82
Memorial Hospital Carbondale	Carbondale	95%	175
Saint James Hospital and Health Center	Olympia Fields	95%	197
Saint Joseph Medical Center	Joliet	95%	290
Sherman Hospital	Elgin	95%	232
University of Illinois at Chicago Med Ctr	Chicago	95%	59
Mount Sinai Hospital	Chicago	94%	111
Saint Anthony's Health Center	Alton	94%	64
Saint Francis Hospital	Evanston	94%	110
Trinity Medical Center	Rock Island	94%	394
Condell Medical Center	Libertyville	93%	191
Mercy Hospital	Chicago	93%	135
Resurrection Medical Center	Chicago	93%	316
Saint Alexius Medical Center	Hoffman Estates	93%	123
Saint Francis Hospital & Health Center	Blue Island	93%	138
Silver Cross Hospital	Joliet	93%	143
Weiss Memorial Hospital	Chicago	93%	71
Katherine Shaw Bethea Hospital	Dixon	92%	26
Adventist LaGrange Memorial Hospital	La Grange	91%	112
Advocate Illinois Masonic Medical Center	Chicago	91%	136
Anderson Hospital	Maryville	91%	35
Provena United Samaritans Medical Center	Danville	91%	44
Saint Mary's Hospital of Kankakee	Kankakee	90%	61
Rush Oak Park Hospital	Oak Park	89%	38
Vista Medical Center East	Waukegan	89%	112
Genesis Medical Center-Illini Campus	Silvis	86%	103
Ingalls Memorial Hospital	Harvey	85%	177
Jersey Community Hospital	Jerseyville	84%	51
West Suburban Medical Center	Oak Park	83%	98
Advocate Trinity Hospital	Chicago	80%	90
CGH Medical Center	Sterling	80%	55
Holy Cross Hospital	Chicago	77%	118

4. Beta Blocker at Arrival

Hospital Name	City	Rate	Cases
Edward Hospital	Naperville	100%	229
Northwestern Memorial Hospital	Chicago	100%	212
Pekin Hospital	Pekin	100%	31
Rush University Medical Center	Chicago	100%	95
Saint Joseph Hospital	Chicago	100%	45
Sarah Bush Lincoln Health Center	Mattoon	100%	32
Advocate Good Shephard Hospital	Barrington	99%	152
Advocate Lutheran General Children's Hospital	Park Ridge	99%	225
Delnor Community Hospital	Geneva	99%	91
Elmhurst Memorial Hospital	Elmhurst	99%	189
Evanston Hospital	Evanston	99%	477
Northwest Community Hospital	Arlington Heights	99%	327
Proctor Hospital	Peoria	99%	90
Rush-Copley Medical Center	Aurora	99%	118
Saint Joseph Medical Center	Bloomington	99%	81
Advocate Christ Med Ctr/Hope Children's	Oak Lawn	98%	147
Alton Memorial Hospital	Alton	98%	103
Loyola University Health System	Maywood	98%	160
MacNeal Hospital	Berwyn	98%	205
Palos Community Hospital	Palos Heights	98%	217
Riverside Medical Center	Kankakee	98%	53
Saint John's Hospital	Springfield	98%	138
Swedish Covenant Hospital	Chicago	98%	183
Advocate Good Samaritan Hospital	Downers Grove	97%	190
Anderson Hospital	Maryville	97%	58
Hinsdale Hospital	Hinsdale	97%	120
Katherine Shaw Bethea Hospital	Dixon	97%	29
Provena Mercy Center	Aurora	97%	159
Saint Anthony Medical Center	Rockford	97%	205
Advocate Illinois Masonic Medical Center	Chicago	96%	81
Decatur Memorial Hospital	Decatur	96%	132
John H Stroger Jr Hospital of Cook County	Chicago	96%	101
Loretto Hospital	Chicago	96%	25
Our Lady of the Resurrection Medical Center	Chicago	96%	222
Provena United Samaritans Medical Center	Danville	96%	73
Silver Cross Hospital	Joliet	96%	106
University of Illinois at Chicago Med Ctr	Chicago	96%	48
Weiss Memorial Hospital	Chicago	96%	76
West Suburban Medical Center	Oak Park	96%	127
Westlake Community Hospital	Melrose Park	96%	70
Alexian Brothers Medical Center	Elk Grove Village	95%	168
Blessing Hospital	Quincy	95%	152
Good Samaritan Regional Health Center	Mount Vernon	95%	77
Heartland Regional Medical Center	Marion	95%	65
Mercy Hospital	Chicago	95%	111
Rockford Memorial Hospital	Rockford	95%	189
Rush Oak Park Hospital	Oak Park	95%	40
Saint Francis Medical Center	Peoria	95%	228
Sherman Hospital	Elgin	95%	188
Swedish American Hospital	Rockford	95%	135
Trinity Medical Center	Rock Island	95%	260
Carle Foundation Hospital	Urbana	94%	140
FHN Memorial Hospital	Freeport	94%	35
Gottlieb Memorial Hospital	Melrose Park	94%	104
Memorial Medical Center	Springfield	94%	255
Methodist Medical Center of Illinois	Peoria	94%	96
Saint Mary's Hospital of Kankakee	Kankakee	94%	71
Advocate South Suburban Hospital	Hazel Crest	93%	149
CGH Medical Center	Sterling	93%	71
Central DuPage Hospital	Winfield	93%	146
Memorial Hospital	Belleville	93%	146
Little Company of Mary Hospital	Evergreen Park	92%	111
Rush North Shore Medical Center	Skokie	92%	86
Saint Alexius Medical Center	Hoffman Estates	92%	106
Saint Francis Hospital & Health Center	Blue Island	92%	107
Centegra Northern Illinois Medical Center	McHenry	91%	93
Genesis Medical Center-Illini Campus	Silvis	91%	90
Memorial Hospital Carbondale	Carbondale	91%	75
Norwegian-American Hospital	Chicago	91%	35
Provena Saint Joseph Hospital	Elgin	91%	85
University of Chicago Hospitals	Chicago	91%	125
Adventist LaGrange Memorial Hospital	La Grange	90%	104
Bromenn Healthcare	Normal	90%	99
Michael Reese Hospital	Chicago	90%	41
Saint Bernard Hospital and Health Care Center	Chicago	90%	30
Saint Elizabeth's Hospital	Belleville	90%	153
Saints Mary & Elizabeth Medical Center	Chicago	90%	61
Gateway Regional Medical Center	Granite City	89%	87

NOTE: Hospital profiles are in alphabetical order by state, then city, then hospital within the city; Rankings are sorted by rate in descending order and exclude hospitals with less than 25 cases; (1) The number of cases is too small (n<25) for purposes of reliably predicting hospital performance; (2) Measure reflects the hospital's indication that its submission was based upon a sample of its relevant discharges; (3) Rate reflects fewer than the maximum possible quarters of data for the measure; (4) Inaccurate information submitted and suppressed for one or more quarters; (5) No data is available from the hospital for this measure; Please refer to the User's Guide for a full explanation of data

Hospital Name	City	Rate	Cases
Memorial Medical Center	Woodstock	89%	27
Provena Covenant Medical Center	Urbana	89%	56
Resurrection Medical Center	Chicago	89%	199
Advocate Trinity Hospital	Chicago	88%	138
Holy Cross Hospital	Chicago	88%	152
Mount Sinai Hospital	Chicago	87%	110
Provident Hospital	Chicago	87%	54
Saint Anthony's Health Center	Alton	86%	72
Saint Elizabeth's Hospital	Chicago	86%	35
Saint Francis Hospital	Evanston	86%	86
Ingalls Memorial Hospital	Harvey	85%	157
Saint Anthony's Memorial Hospital	Effingham	85%	34
Saint James Hospital and Health Center	Olympia Fields	85%	160
Saint Joseph Medical Center	Joliet	85%	255
Saint Mary's Good Samaritan	Centralia	84%	32
Saint Mary's Hospital	Decatur	84%	25
Iroquois Memorial Hospital & Resident Home	Watseka	83%	30
OSF Saint Mary Medical Center	Galesburg	83%	30
Vista Medical Center East	Waukegan	83%	123
Condell Medical Center	Libertyville	82%	182
South Shore Hospital	Chicago	79%	42
Jersey Community Hospital	Jerseyville	74%	57

5. Beta Blocker at Discharge

Hospital Name	City	Rate	Cases
Advocate Good Samaritan Hospital	Downers Grove	100%	214
Alton Memorial Hospital	Alton	100%	92
Edward Hospital	Naperville	100%	264
Elmhurst Memorial Hospital	Elmhurst	100%	219
Good Samaritan Regional Health Center	Mount Vernon	100%	221
Loyola University Health System	Maywood	100%	201
Proctor Hospital	Peoria	100%	111
Rockford Memorial Hospital	Rockford	100%	284
Rush University Medical Center	Chicago	100%	147
Saint Alexius Medical Center	Hoffman Estates	100%	129
Saint Joseph Medical Center	Bloomington	100%	126
Advocate Christ Med Ctr/Hope Children's	Oak Lawn	99%	239
Bromenn Healthcare	Normal	99%	141
Decatur Memorial Hospital	Decatur	99%	209
Heartland Regional Medical Center	Marion	99%	86
Little Company of Mary Hospital	Evergreen Park	99%	81
Memorial Medical Center	Springfield	99%	539
Northwest Community Hospital	Arlington Heights	99%	382
Northwestern Memorial Hospital	Chicago	99%	252
Provena Covenant Medical Center	Urbana	99%	227
Rush-Copley Medical Center	Aurora	99%	161
Saint Francis Medical Center	Peoria	99%	595
Swedish American Hospital	Rockford	99%	327
Swedish Covenant Hospital	Chicago	99%	171
Advocate Good Shephard Hospital	Barrington	98%	252
Advocate Lutheran General Children's Hospital	Park Ridge	98%	259
Blessing Hospital	Quincy	98%	234
Delnor Community Hospital	Geneva	98%	86
Evanston Hospital	Evanston	98%	523
Gateway Regional Medical Center	Granite City	98%	87
Hinsdale Hospital	Hinsdale	98%	141
Memorial Hospital	Belleville	98%	150
Mercy Hospital	Chicago	98%	142
Methodist Medical Center of Illinois	Peoria	98%	213
Provena Mercy Center	Aurora	98%	183
Riverside Medical Center	Kankakee	98%	97
Saint John's Hospital	Springfield	98%	639
Alexian Brothers Medical Center	Elk Grove Village	97%	236
Anderson Hospital	Maryville	97%	33
Centegra Northern Illinois Medical Center	McHenry	97%	137
Gottlieb Memorial Hospital	Melrose Park	97%	101
John H Stroger Jr Hospital of Cook County	Chicago	97%	182
Saint Anthony Medical Center	Rockford	97%	306
Central DuPage Hospital	Winfield	96%	168
FHN Memorial Hospital	Freeport	96%	27
MacNeal Hospital	Berwyn	96%	229
Michael Reese Hospital	Chicago	96%	53
Our Lady of the Resurrection Medical Center	Chicago	96%	198
Provena Saint Joseph Hospital	Elgin	96%	111
Saint Elizabeth's Hospital	Belleville	96%	251
Saint Francis Hospital & Health Center	Blue Island	96%	140
Sherman Hospital	Elgin	96%	234
University of Chicago Hospitals	Chicago	96%	210
Advocate South Suburban Hospital	Hazel Crest	95%	142
Memorial Hospital Carbondale	Carbondale	95%	219
Saint Mary's Hospital of Kankakee	Kankakee	95%	60
Silver Cross Hospital	Joliet	95%	151
Trinity Medical Center	Rock Island	95%	371
Weiss Memorial Hospital	Chicago	95%	78

Hospital Name	City	Rate	Cases
Adventist LaGrange Memorial Hospital	La Grange	94%	133
Carle Foundation Hospital	Urbana	94%	256
Katherine Shaw Bethea Hospital	Dixon	94%	31
Mount Sinai Hospital	Chicago	94%	109
Westlake Community Hospital	Melrose Park	94%	65
CGH Medical Center	Sterling	93%	55
Palos Community Hospital	Palos Heights	93%	211
Provena United Samaritans Medical Center	Danville	93%	55
Saint James Hospital and Health Center	Olympia Fields	93%	198
Advocate Illinois Masonic Medical Center	Chicago	92%	159
Rush North Shore Medical Center	Skokie	92%	99
Rush Oak Park Hospital	Oak Park	92%	39
University of Illinois at Chicago Med Ctr	Chicago	92%	59
Condell Medical Center	Libertyville	91%	217
Morris Hospital	Morris	91%	32
Saint Joseph Medical Center	Joliet	91%	292
Vista Medical Center East	Waukegan	91%	115
Saints Mary & Elizabeth Medical Center	Chicago	90%	99
Genesis Medical Center-Illini Campus	Silvis	89%	101
Saint Joseph Hospital	Chicago	89%	65
OSF Saint Mary Medical Center	Galesburg	88%	25
Resurrection Medical Center	Chicago	88%	316
South Shore Hospital	Chicago	88%	25
Ingalls Memorial Hospital	Harvey	87%	189
Saint Anthony's Health Center	Alton	87%	71
Saint Francis Hospital	Evanston	84%	96
Advocate Trinity Hospital	Chicago	82%	95
West Suburban Medical Center	Oak Park	81%	113
Holy Cross Hospital	Chicago	77%	117
Jersey Community Hospital	Jerseyville	73%	52

8. Smoking Cessation Advice

Hospital Name	City	Rate	Cases
Advocate Good Samaritan Hospital	Downers Grove	100%	59
Advocate South Suburban Hospital	Hazel Crest	100%	51
Alton Memorial Hospital	Alton	100%	36
Bromenn Healthcare	Normal	100%	49
Centegra Northern Illinois Medical Center	McHenry	100%	56
Central DuPage Hospital	Winfield	100%	53
Decatur Memorial Hospital	Decatur	100%	86
Edward Hospital	Naperville	100%	71
Elmhurst Memorial Hospital	Elmhurst	100%	52
Gottlieb Memorial Hospital	Melrose Park	100%	34
Hinsdale Hospital	Hinsdale	100%	37
Loyola University Health System	Maywood	100%	60
Memorial Medical Center	Springfield	100%	201
Northwestern Memorial Hospital	Chicago	100%	56
Proctor Hospital	Peoria	100%	29
Riverside Medical Center	Kankakee	100%	43
Rush University Medical Center	Chicago	100%	51
Rush-Copley Medical Center	Aurora	100%	52
Saint Alexius Medical Center	Hoffman Estates	100%	48
Saint Francis Medical Center	Peoria	100%	212
Saint Mary's Hospital of Kankakee	Kankakee	100%	25
Swedish Covenant Hospital	Chicago	100%	53
Trinity Medical Center	Rock Island	100%	117
Vista Medical Center East	Waukegan	100%	43
Advocate Good Shephard Hospital	Barrington	99%	74
Alexian Brothers Medical Center	Elk Grove Village	99%	79
Methodist Medical Center of Illinois	Peoria	99%	92
Northwest Community Hospital	Arlington Heights	99%	84
Saint John's Hospital	Springfield	99%	275
Advocate Lutheran General Children's Hospital	Park Ridge	98%	66
Ingalls Memorial Hospital	Harvey	98%	53
Memorial Hospital	Belleville	98%	48
Memorial Hospital Carbondale	Carbondale	98%	101
Saint Anthony Medical Center	Rockford	98%	104
Saint Joseph Medical Center	Bloomington	98%	50
Silver Cross Hospital	Joliet	98%	55
West Suburban Medical Center	Oak Park	98%	54
Gateway Regional Medical Center	Granite City	97%	31
Heartland Regional Medical Center	Marion	97%	34
Provena Covenant Medical Center	Urbana	97%	100
Saint Francis Hospital & Health Center	Blue Island	97%	58
Saint James Hospital and Health Center	Olympia Fields	97%	79
Swedish American Hospital	Rockford	97%	146
Blessing Hospital	Quincy	96%	90
Condell Medical Center	Libertyville	96%	70
Good Samaritan Regional Health Center	Mount Vernon	96%	92
Our Lady of the Resurrection Medical Center	Chicago	96%	53
Palos Community Hospital	Palos Heights	96%	68
Advocate Christ Med Ctr/Hope Children's	Oak Lawn	94%	86
Evanston Hospital	Evanston	94%	80
MacNeal Hospital	Berwyn	93%	73

NOTE: Hospital profiles are in alphabetical order by state, then city, then hospital within the city; Rankings are sorted by rate in descending order and exclude hospitals with less than 25 cases; (1) The number of cases is too small (n<25) for purposes of reliably predicting hospital performance; (2) Measure reflects the hospital's indication that its submission was based upon a sample of its relevant discharges; (3) Rate reflects fewer than the maximum possible quarters of data for the measure; (4) Inaccurate information submitted and suppressed for one or more quarters; (5) No data is available from the hospital for this measure; Please refer to the User's Guide for a full explanation of data

Hospital Name	City	Rate	Cases
Mount Sinai Hospital	Chicago	93%	43
Rockford Memorial Hospital	Rockford	93%	98
Saints Mary & Elizabeth Medical Center	Chicago	92%	40
Holy Cross Hospital	Chicago	91%	35
Mercy Hospital	Chicago	91%	67
Adventist LaGrange Memorial Hospital	La Grange	90%	39
Resurrection Medical Center	Chicago	90%	87
Saint Joseph Medical Center	Joliet	90%	101
Sherman Hospital	Elgin	90%	81
University of Chicago Hospitals	Chicago	90%	88
Carle Foundation Hospital	Urbana	89%	93
Saint Elizabeth's Hospital	Belleville	89%	87
John H Stroger Jr Hospital of Cook County	Chicago	84%	112
Advocate Illinois Masonic Medical Center	Chicago	83%	82
Little Company of Mary Hospital	Evergreen Park	83%	30
Genesis Medical Center-Illini Campus	Silvis	81%	43
Weiss Memorial Hospital	Chicago	32%	34

Heart Failure Care

9. ACE Inhibitor or ARB for LVSD

Hospital Name	City	Rate	Cases
Alton Memorial Hospital	Alton	100%	49
Anderson Hospital	Maryville	100%	53
Herrin Hospital	Herrin	100%	28
Rush-Copley Medical Center	Aurora	100%	76
Sarah Bush Lincoln Health Center	Mattoon	100%	74
Thorek Hospital and Medical Center	Chicago	100%	27
Proctor Hospital	Peoria	99%	71
Advocate Good Shephard Hospital	Barrington	98%	92
Kishwaukee Community Hospital	De Kalb	98%	51
Provena Covenant Medical Center	Urbana	98%	120
Gottlieb Memorial Hospital	Melrose Park	97%	118
Loretto Hospital	Chicago	96%	49
Methodist Medical Center of Illinois	Peoria	96%	156
Northwestern Memorial Hospital	Chicago	96%	307
Rush University Medical Center	Chicago	96%	139
Bromenn Healthcare	Normal	95%	93
Elmhurst Memorial Hospital	Elmhurst	95%	222
Memorial Medical Center	Springfield	95%	207
John H Stroger Jr Hospital of Cook County	Chicago	94%	144
Riverside Medical Center	Kankakee	94%	145
Saint Mary's Good Samaritan	Centralia	94%	96
Swedish American Hospital	Rockford	94%	209
Advocate Lutheran General Children's Hospital	Park Ridge	93%	228
Clay County Hospital	Flora	93%	30
Edward Hospital	Naperville	93%	215
Oak Forest Hospital of Cook County	Oak Forest	93%	73
Saint Joseph Medical Center	Bloomington	93%	72
Saint Mary's Hospital	Streator	93%	42
Silver Cross Hospital	Joliet	93%	179
FHN Memorial Hospital	Freeport	92%	62
Provident Hospital	Chicago	92%	163
Saint Alexius Medical Center	Hoffman Estates	92%	120
University of Illinois at Chicago Med Ctr	Chicago	92%	142
Advocate Good Samaritan Hospital	Downers Grove	91%	155
Gateway Regional Medical Center	Granite City	91%	81
Loyola University Health System	Maywood	91%	408
Provena United Samaritans Medical Center	Danville	91%	151
Rockford Memorial Hospital	Rockford	91%	108
Taylorville Memorial Hospital	Taylorville	91%	35
Katherine Shaw Bethea Hospital	Dixon	90%	42
Morris Hospital	Morris	90%	50
Our Lady of the Resurrection Medical Center	Chicago	90%	202
Pekin Hospital	Pekin	90%	50
Saint Anthony Medical Center	Rockford	90%	146
CGH Medical Center	Sterling	89%	55
Decatur Memorial Hospital	Decatur	89%	219
Michael Reese Hospital	Chicago	89%	167
University of Chicago Hospitals	Chicago	89%	170
Advocate Christ Med Ctr/Hope Children's	Oak Lawn	88%	154
Advocate Illinois Masonic Medical Center	Chicago	88%	178
Blessing Hospital	Quincy	88%	88
Carle Foundation Hospital	Urbana	88%	96
Good Samaritan Regional Health Center	Mount Vernon	88%	94
Little Company of Mary Hospital	Evergreen Park	88%	125
Mercy Hospital	Chicago	88%	278
Saint Elizabeth's Hospital	Belleville	88%	173
Saint Francis Medical Center	Peoria	88%	272
Delnor Community Hospital	Geneva	87%	62
Evanston Hospital	Evanston	87%	252
Lake Forest Hospital	Lake Forest	87%	45
Advocate South Suburban Hospital	Hazel Crest	86%	146
Harrisburg Medical Center	Harrisburg	86%	29
OSF Saint Mary Medical Center	Galesburg	86%	59
Roseland Community Hospital	Chicago	86%	97
Saint Mary's Hospital	Decatur	86%	72
Saint James Hospital and Health Center	Olympia Fields	85%	106
Saint Mary's Hospital of Kankakee	Kankakee	85%	96
Centegra Northern Illinois Medical Center	McHenry	84%	116
Memorial Hospital	Belleville	84%	218
Mount Sinai Hospital	Chicago	84%	189
Saint Elizabeth's Hospital	Chicago	84%	75
Swedish Covenant Hospital	Chicago	84%	173
Touchette Regional Hospital	Centreville	84%	31
Alexian Brothers Medical Center	Elk Grove Village	83%	161
Galesburg Cottage Hospital	Galesburg	83%	48
Saint Anthony's Memorial Hospital	Effingham	83%	30
Saint Bernard Hospital and Health Care Center	Chicago	83%	109
Saints Mary & Elizabeth Medical Center	Chicago	83%	117
Advocate Trinity Hospital	Chicago	82%	256
Illinois Valley Community Hospital	Peru	82%	28
Lincoln Park Hospital	Chicago	82%	66
Passavant Memorial Area Hospital	Jacksonville	82%	34
Heartland Regional Medical Center	Marion	81%	42
Kenneth Hall Regional Hospital	East Saint Louis	81%	57
Trinity Medical Center	Rock Island	81%	173
Genesis Medical Center-Illini Campus	Silvis	80%	59
Jackson Park Hospital & Medical Center	Chicago	80%	71
Saint Joseph Hospital	Chicago	80%	128
Northwest Community Hospital	Arlington Heights	79%	91
Rush North Shore Medical Center	Skokie	79%	146
South Shore Hospital	Chicago	79%	62
MacNeal Hospital	Berwyn	78%	243
Saint Francis Hospital & Health Center	Blue Island	78%	423
Saint John's Hospital	Springfield	78%	274
Saint Joseph Medical Center	Joliet	78%	287
Vista Medical Center East	Waukegan	78%	123
Weiss Memorial Hospital	Chicago	78%	100
West Suburban Medical Center	Oak Park	78%	195
Westlake Community Hospital	Melrose Park	78%	92
Holy Cross Hospital	Chicago	77%	123
Adventist LaGrange Memorial Hospital	La Grange	76%	85
Ingalls Memorial Hospital	Harvey	76%	90
Provena Mercy Center	Aurora	76%	117
Richland Memorial Hospital	Olney	76%	25
Rush Oak Park Hospital	Oak Park	76%	62
Saint Anthony's Health Center	Alton	76%	62
Saint James OSF	Pontiac	76%	25
Hinsdale Hospital	Hinsdale	74%	93
Central DuPage Hospital	Winfield	73%	152
McDonough District Hospital	Macomb	73%	33
Memorial Medical Center	Woodstock	73%	64
Saint Francis Hospital	Evanston	72%	163
Sherman Hospital	Elgin	71%	127
Condell Medical Center	Libertyville	70%	129
Graham Hospital	Canton	69%	42
Provena Saint Joseph Hospital	Elgin	69%	67
Resurrection Medical Center	Chicago	63%	258
Norwegian-American Hospital	Chicago	62%	76
Memorial Hospital Carbondale	Carbondale	61%	113
Saint Anthony Hospital	Chicago	60%	60
Palos Community Hospital	Palos Heights	58%	64
Jersey Community Hospital	Jerseyville	56%	34

10. Discharge Instructions

Hospital Name	City	Rate	Cases
Hardin County General Hospital	Rosiclare	100%	38
Loretto Hospital	Chicago	100%	102
Silver Cross Hospital	Joliet	100%	450
Riverside Medical Center	Kankakee	99%	305
Thorek Hospital and Medical Center	Chicago	99%	100
Rush-Copley Medical Center	Aurora	98%	189
Taylorville Memorial Hospital	Taylorville	98%	81
CGH Medical Center	Sterling	97%	154
Fairfield Memorial Hospital	Fairfield	97%	36
Lawrence County Memorial Hospital	Lawrenceville	97%	34
Proctor Hospital	Peoria	97%	145
Saint Bernard Hospital and Health Care Center	Chicago	97%	275
Swedish American Hospital	Rockford	97%	367
Decatur Memorial Hospital	Decatur	96%	354
Elmhurst Memorial Hospital	Elmhurst	96%	453
Saint Joseph Medical Center	Joliet	95%	663
Clay County Hospital	Flora	94%	65
Hamilton Memorial Hospital	McLeansboro	94%	32
Alton Memorial Hospital	Alton	92%	140
Edward Hospital	Naperville	91%	402
Lake Forest Hospital	Lake Forest	90%	107

NOTE: Hospital profiles are in alphabetical order by state, then city, then hospital within the city; Rankings are sorted by rate in descending order and exclude hospitals with less than 25 cases; (1) The number of cases is too small (n<25) for purposes of reliably predicting hospital performance; (2) Measure reflects the hospital's indication that its submission was based upon a sample of its relevant discharges; (3) Rate reflects fewer than the maximum possible quarters of data for the measure; (4) Inaccurate information submitted and suppressed for one or more quarters; (5) No data is available from the hospital for this measure; Please refer to the User's Guide for a full explanation of data

Memorial Hospital	Belleville	90%	474
Memorial Medical Center	Springfield	90%	400
Morris Hospital	Morris	90%	130
Rockford Memorial Hospital	Rockford	90%	239
Community Hospital of Ottawa	Ottawa	89%	74
Trinity Medical Center	Rock Island	89%	429
Abraham Lincoln Memorial Hospital	Lincoln	88%	26
Genesis Medical Center-Illini Campus	Silvis	88%	150
Saint Anthony Medical Center	Rockford	88%	302
Delnor Community Hospital	Geneva	87%	164
Ingalls Memorial Hospital	Harvey	87%	271
Red Bud Regional Hospital	Red Bud	87%	30
Saint Mary's Hospital	Decatur	87%	122
Roseland Community Hospital	Chicago	86%	279
Anderson Hospital	Maryville	85%	113
Mercy Hospital	Chicago	85%	521
OSF Saint Mary Medical Center	Galesburg	85%	122
Perry Memorial Hospital	Princeton	85%	55
Saint Elizabeth's Hospital	Chicago	85%	145
Saint Joseph Medical Center	Bloomington	85%	115
FHN Memorial Hospital	Freeport	84%	128
Advocate Good Shephard Hospital	Barrington	83%	278
Provena Covenant Medical Center	Urbana	83%	292
Saint Alexius Medical Center	Hoffman Estates	82%	238
Sarah Bush Lincoln Health Center	Mattoon	82%	181
Galesburg Cottage Hospital	Galesburg	81%	91
Kewanee Hospital	Kewanee	81%	58
Michael Reese Hospital	Chicago	81%	242
Saint Joseph's Hospital	Breese	81%	48
Alexian Brothers Medical Center	Elk Grove Village	80%	413
Hinsdale Hospital	Hinsdale	80%	200
Katherine Shaw Bethea Hospital	Dixon	80%	87
Oak Forest Hospital of Cook County	Oak Forest	80%	137
Saint Mary's Hospital	Streator	80%	79
Salem Township Hospital	Salem	80%	30
West Suburban Medical Center	Oak Park	80%	522
Advocate Lutheran General Children's Hospital	Park Ridge	79%	455
Bromenn Healthcare	Normal	79%	151
Herrin Hospital	Herrin	79%	141
Memorial Medical Center	Woodstock	78%	171
Rush University Medical Center	Chicago	78%	311
Advocate Good Samaritan Hospital	Downers Grove	77%	298
Harrisburg Medical Center	Harrisburg	77%	88
Heartland Regional Medical Center	Marion	77%	125
Kishwaukee Community Hospital	De Kalb	77%	111
Northwestern Memorial Hospital	Chicago	77%	666
Saint James OSF	Pontiac	77%	35
Passavant Memorial Area Hospital	Jacksonville	76%	96
Advocate South Suburban Hospital	Hazel Crest	75%	296
Methodist Medical Center of Illinois	Peoria	75%	294
MacNeal Hospital	Berwyn	74%	384
Saint Anthony's Memorial Hospital	Effingham	74%	176
Saint Joseph Memorial Hospital	Murphysboro	74%	50
Saint Joseph's Hospital	Highland	74%	31
Provident Hospital	Chicago	73%	402
Sparta Community Hospital	Sparta	73%	26
McDonough District Hospital	Macomb	72%	58
Saint Mary's Good Samaritan	Centralia	72%	198
Centegra Northern Illinois Medical Center	McHenry	71%	250
Our Lady of the Resurrection Medical Center	Chicago	71%	380
Pekin Hospital	Pekin	71%	86
Wabash General Hospital	Mount Carmel	71%	34
Adventist GlenOaks Hospital	Glendale Heights	70%	43
Advocate Christ Med Ctr/Hope Children's	Oak Lawn	69%	263
Saint Anthony's Health Center	Alton	69%	146
Advocate Illinois Masonic Medical Center	Chicago	68%	268
Gottlieb Memorial Hospital	Melrose Park	68%	285
Illinois Valley Community Hospital	Peru	68%	74
Saint Margaret's Hospital	Spring Valley	68%	74
Loyola University Health System	Maywood	66%	693
Rush Oak Park Hospital	Oak Park	65%	203
Union County Hospital District	Anna	65%	34
Blessing Hospital	Quincy	64%	226
South Shore Hospital	Chicago	64%	205
Good Samaritan Regional Health Center	Mount Vernon	63%	238
Saint Elizabeth's Hospital	Belleville	63%	465
Central DuPage Hospital	Winfield	62%	309
Crossroads Community Hospital	Mount Vernon	62%	26
Mount Sinai Hospital	Chicago	62%	340
Adventist LaGrange Memorial Hospital	La Grange	61%	293
Memorial Hospital	Chester	61%	44
Palos Community Hospital	Palos Heights	61%	211
Saint Mary's Hospital of Kankakee	Kankakee	60%	187
Saint Francis Hospital	Evanston	59%	290
Saint Joseph Hospital	Chicago	59%	330
Lincoln Park Hospital	Chicago	58%	139
Saint Francis Hospital & Health Center	Blue Island	57%	821
Carle Foundation Hospital	Urbana	56%	205
Iroquois Memorial Hospital & Resident Home	Watseka	56%	80
Pana Community Hospital	Pana	56%	27
Saint Francis Medical Center	Peoria	56%	455
Shelby Memorial Hospital	Shelbyville	56%	25
Evanston Hospital	Evanston	55%	609
Richland Memorial Hospital	Olney	54%	48
Saint Francis Hospital	Litchfield	54%	61
Saint John's Hospital	Springfield	54%	437
Westlake Community Hospital	Melrose Park	54%	221
Greenville Regional Hospital	Greenville	52%	29
Graham Hospital	Canton	51%	59
Northwest Community Hospital	Arlington Heights	51%	213
Provena Mercy Center	Aurora	50%	32
Provena United Samaritans Medical Center	Danville	50%	359
Sherman Hospital	Elgin	50%	289
Saints Mary & Elizabeth Medical Center	Chicago	48%	307
University of Chicago Hospitals	Chicago	46%	298
Resurrection Medical Center	Chicago	45%	613
Rush North Shore Medical Center	Skokie	45%	285
Kenneth Hall Regional Hospital	East Saint Louis	44%	174
Memorial Hospital Carbondale	Carbondale	43%	215
Jersey Community Hospital	Jerseyville	42%	76
Saint Anthony Hospital	Chicago	42%	162
Saint James Hospital and Health Center	Olympia Fields	40%	292
Condell Medical Center	Libertyville	37%	314
Advocate Trinity Hospital	Chicago	35%	583
Weiss Memorial Hospital	Chicago	34%	180
Gateway Regional Medical Center	Granite City	33%	223
Swedish Covenant Hospital	Chicago	31%	348
Vista Medical Center East	Waukegan	28%	269
Little Company of Mary Hospital	Evergreen Park	26%	279
University of Illinois at Chicago Med Ctr.	Chicago	24%	71
Norwegian-American Hospital	Chicago	23%	202
Holy Cross Hospital	Chicago	12%	265
John H Stroger Jr Hospital of Cook County	Chicago	11%	283
Jackson Park Hospital & Medical Center	Chicago	6%	200
Hoopeston Community Memorial Hospital	Hoopeston	4%	28
Sacred Heart Hospital	Chicago	4%	152
Doctor John Warner Hospital	Clinton	0%	30

11. Evaluation of LVS Function

Hospital Name	City	Rate	Cases
Hardin County General Hospital	Rosiclare	100%	51
Kishwaukee Community Hospital	De Kalb	100%	130
Memorial Medical Center	Springfield	100%	504
Mount Sinai Hospital	Chicago	100%	374
Northwestern Memorial Hospital	Chicago	100%	745
Our Lady of the Resurrection Medical Center	Chicago	100%	608
Proctor Hospital	Peoria	100%	201
Rush University Medical Center	Chicago	100%	338
Advocate Good Shephard Hospital	Barrington	99%	340
Decatur Memorial Hospital	Decatur	99%	449
Evanston Hospital	Evanston	99%	836
Loyola University Health System	Maywood	99%	754
Memorial Hospital	Belleville	99%	576
Memorial Medical Center	Woodstock	99%	230
Morris Hospital	Morris	99%	168
Provena Covenant Medical Center	Urbana	99%	373
Provena United Samaritans Medical Center	Danville	99%	421
Riverside Medical Center	Kankakee	99%	365
Rush-Copley Medical Center	Aurora	99%	234
Saint Anthony Medical Center	Rockford	99%	406
Saint Mary's Good Samaritan	Centralia	99%	279
Sarah Bush Lincoln Health Center	Mattoon	99%	249
Silver Cross Hospital	Joliet	99%	549
Advocate Illinois Masonic Medical Center	Chicago	98%	317
Clay County Hospital	Flora	98%	101
Edward Hospital	Naperville	98%	517
FHN Memorial Hospital	Freeport	98%	179
Hamilton Memorial Hospital	McLeansboro	98%	46
Mercy Hospital	Chicago	98%	563
Michael Reese Hospital	Chicago	98%	313
Rockford Memorial Hospital	Rockford	98%	320
Saint John's Hospital	Springfield	98%	528
Saint Joseph Medical Center	Bloomington	98%	156
Swedish American Hospital	Rockford	98%	470
University of Chicago Hospitals	Chicago	98%	326
West Suburban Medical Center	Oak Park	98%	568
Advocate Good Samaritan Hospital	Downers Grove	97%	405
Advocate Lutheran General Children's Hospital	Park Ridge	97%	624
Carlinville Area Hospital	Carlinville	97%	37

NOTE: Hospital profiles are in alphabetical order by state, then city, then hospital within the city; Rankings are sorted by rate in descending order and exclude hospitals with less than 25 cases; (1) The number of cases is too small (n<25) for purposes of reliably predicting hospital performance; (2) Measure reflects the hospital's indication that its submission was based upon a sample of its relevant discharges; (3) Rate reflects fewer than the maximum possible quarters of data for the measure; (4) Inaccurate information submitted and suppressed for one or more quarters; (5) No data is available from the hospital for this measure; Please refer to the User's Guide for a full explanation of data

Centegra Northern Illinois Medical Center	McHenry	97%	324
Delnor Community Hospital	Geneva	97%	236
Elmhurst Memorial Hospital	Elmhurst	97%	546
Good Samaritan Regional Health Center	Mount Vernon	97%	273
Memorial Hospital	Chester	97%	64
Methodist Medical Center of Illinois	Peoria	97%	370
Northwest Community Hospital	Arlington Heights	97%	313
Oak Forest Hospital of Cook County	Oak Forest	97%	145
Saint Alexius Medical Center	Hoffman Estates	97%	315
Saint Bernard Hospital and Health Care Center	Chicago	97%	326
Saint James OSF	Pontiac	97%	63
Saint Mary's Hospital	Decatur	97%	182
Thorek Hospital and Medical Center	Chicago	97%	118
Abraham Lincoln Memorial Hospital	Lincoln	96%	54
Advocate Christ Med Ctr/Hope Children's	Oak Lawn	96%	340
Alexian Brothers Medical Center	Elk Grove Village	96%	511
Alton Memorial Hospital	Alton	96%	183
Bromenn Healthcare	Normal	96%	202
Central DuPage Hospital	Winfield	96%	421
Gottlieb Memorial Hospital	Melrose Park	96%	348
Hinsdale Hospital	Hinsdale	96%	273
John H Stroger Jr Hospital of Cook County	Chicago	96%	294
Katherine Shaw Bethea Hospital	Dixon	96%	113
Mercy Harvard Hospital	Harvard	96%	26
OSF Saint Mary Medical Center	Galesburg	96%	166
Rush North Shore Medical Center	Skokie	96%	418
Saint Joseph Medical Center	Joliet	96%	808
Trinity Medical Center	Rock Island	96%	559
University of Illinois at Chicago Med Ctr	Chicago	96%	310
Advocate South Suburban Hospital	Hazel Crest	95%	366
Anderson Hospital	Maryville	95%	152
Galesburg Cottage Hospital	Galesburg	95%	142
Holy Cross Hospital	Chicago	95%	313
Lake Forest Hospital	Lake Forest	95%	128
Loretto Hospital	Chicago	95%	131
Passavant Memorial Area Hospital	Jacksonville	95%	153
Saint Elizabeth's Hospital	Chicago	95%	186
Culbertson Memorial Hospital	Rushville	94%	34
Graham Hospital	Canton	94%	96
Lawrence County Memorial Hospital	Lawrenceville	94%	53
Sacred Heart Hospital	Chicago	94%	160
Saint James Hospital and Health Center	Olympia Fields	94%	353
Saint Joseph Hospital	Chicago	94%	421
Saint Mary's Hospital	Streator	94%	124
Little Company of Mary Hospital	Evergreen Park	93%	351
Memorial Hospital Carbondale	Carbondale	93%	242
Palos Community Hospital	Palos Heights	93%	290
Pekin Hospital	Pekin	93%	128
Saint Margaret's Hospital	Spring Valley	93%	98
Illini Community Hospital	Pittsfield	92%	25
Provena Mercy Center	Aurora	92%	273
Saint Francis Hospital	Evanston	92%	401
South Shore Hospital	Chicago	92%	247
Swedish Covenant Hospital	Chicago	92%	504
Westlake Community Hospital	Melrose Park	92%	288
Community Hospital of Ottawa	Ottawa	91%	98
MacNeal Hospital	Berwyn	91%	507
Saint Francis Medical Center	Peoria	91%	574
Saint Mary's Hospital of Kankakee	Kankakee	91%	238
Shelby Memorial Hospital	Shelbyville	91%	104
Taylorville Memorial Hospital	Taylorville	91%	110
Vista Medical Center East	Waukegan	91%	347
Advocate Trinity Hospital	Chicago	90%	634
Heartland Regional Medical Center	Marion	90%	167
Provena Saint Joseph Hospital	Elgin	90%	162
Resurrection Medical Center	Chicago	90%	868
Saint Francis Hospital & Health Center	Blue Island	90%	902
Weiss Memorial Hospital	Chicago	90%	250
Herrin Hospital	Herrin	89%	173
Richland Memorial Hospital	Olney	89%	73
Saint Anthony's Memorial Hospital	Effingham	89%	202
Valley West Community Hospital	Sandwich	89%	27
Adventist GlenOaks Hospital	Glendale Heights	88%	73
Condell Medical Center	Libertyville	88%	406
Genesis Medical Center-Illini Campus	Silvis	88%	207
Gibson Community Hospital	Gibson City	88%	25
Mason District Hospital	Havana	88%	26
Provident Hospital	Chicago	88%	382
Saint Joseph's Hospital	Breese	88%	64
Saints Mary & Elizabeth Medical Center	Chicago	88%	336
Wabash General Hospital	Mount Carmel	88%	49
Carle Foundation Hospital	Urbana	87%	283
Gateway Regional Medical Center	Granite City	87%	269
Red Bud Regional Hospital	Red Bud	87%	61
Rush Oak Park Hospital	Oak Park	87%	255
Saint Anthony Hospital	Chicago	87%	179
Lincoln Park Hospital	Chicago	86%	174
Sherman Hospital	Elgin	86%	366
Adventist LaGrange Memorial Hospital	La Grange	85%	385
Harrisburg Medical Center	Harrisburg	85%	119
Perry Memorial Hospital	Princeton	85%	88
Saint Elizabeth's Hospital	Belleville	85%	585
Blessing Hospital	Quincy	84%	325
Iroquois Memorial Hospital & Resident Home	Watseka	84%	125
Greenville Regional Hospital	Greenville	83%	47
Ingalls Memorial Hospital	Harvey	83%	303
Union County Hospital District	Anna	83%	42
Norwegian-American Hospital	Chicago	82%	242
Sparta Community Hospital	Sparta	82%	39
CGH Medical Center	Sterling	81%	197
Illinois Valley Community Hospital	Peru	80%	113
Kewanee Hospital	Kewanee	80%	96
Methodist Hospital of Chicago	Chicago	79%	48
Pinckneyville Community Hospital	Pinckneyville	79%	28
Crossroads Community Hospital	Mount Vernon	78%	45
Fairfield Memorial Hospital	Fairfield	78%	55
Mendota Community Hospital	Mendota	78%	32
Roseland Community Hospital	Chicago	78%	295
Doctor John Warner Hospital	Clinton	76%	38
McDonough District Hospital	Macomb	76%	95
Saint Joseph Memorial Hospital	Murphysboro	74%	57
Crawford Memorial Hospital	Robinson	73%	30
Community Medical Center	Monmouth	72%	39
Jackson Park Hospital & Medical Center	Chicago	71%	217
Saint Anthony's Health Center	Alton	71%	212
Jersey Community Hospital	Jerseyville	69%	114
Ferrell Hospital	Eldorado	66%	29
Touchette Regional Hospital	Centreville	66%	98
Saint Francis Hospital	Litchfield	64%	91
Saint Joseph's Hospital	Highland	64%	50
Community Memorial Hospital	Staunton	63%	27
Kenneth Hall Regional Hospital	East Saint Louis	60%	192
Pana Community Hospital	Pana	56%	41
Salem Township Hospital	Salem	34%	47
Hoopeston Community Memorial Hospital	Hoopeston	4%	27

12. Smoking Cessation Advice

Hospital Name	City	Rate	Cases
Advocate Good Shephard Hospital	Barrington	100%	41
Advocate South Suburban Hospital	Hazel Crest	100%	65
Bromenn Healthcare	Normal	100%	25
Decatur Memorial Hospital	Decatur	100%	56
Gottlieb Memorial Hospital	Melrose Park	100%	46
Loretto Hospital	Chicago	100%	44
Memorial Hospital	Belleville	100%	83
Memorial Medical Center	Springfield	100%	84
Morris Hospital	Morris	100%	25
Provena United Samaritans Medical Center	Danville	100%	63
Riverside Medical Center	Kankakee	100%	66
Rush-Copley Medical Center	Aurora	100%	48
Saint James Hospital and Health Center	Olympia Fields	100%	59
Saint Joseph Medical Center	Bloomington	100%	43
Saint Mary's Hospital of Kankakee	Kankakee	100%	63
Sarah Bush Lincoln Health Center	Mattoon	100%	26
Silver Cross Hospital	Joliet	100%	112
Thorek Hospital and Medical Center	Chicago	100%	29
Edward Hospital	Naperville	99%	68
Oak Forest Hospital of Cook County	Oak Forest	99%	68
Saint Joseph Medical Center	Joliet	99%	77
Trinity Medical Center	Rock Island	99%	113
Vista Medical Center East	Waukegan	99%	82
Central DuPage Hospital	Winfield	98%	55
MacNeal Hospital	Berwyn	98%	85
Rockford Memorial Hospital	Rockford	98%	62
Saint Alexius Medical Center	Hoffman Estates	98%	51
Saint Bernard Hospital and Health Care Center	Chicago	98%	129
West Suburban Medical Center	Oak Park	98%	131
Delnor Community Hospital	Geneva	97%	31
Rush University Medical Center	Chicago	97%	71
Saint Elizabeth's Hospital	Chicago	97%	32
Alexian Brothers Medical Center	Elk Grove Village	96%	72
Elmhurst Memorial Hospital	Elmhurst	96%	73
Our Lady of the Resurrection Medical Center	Chicago	96%	82
Saint Anthony Medical Center	Rockford	96%	56
Saint Francis Hospital & Health Center	Blue Island	96%	202
Saint John's Hospital	Springfield	96%	110
Saint Mary's Good Samaritan	Centralia	96%	26
Holy Cross Hospital	Chicago	95%	82
Northwestern Memorial Hospital	Chicago	95%	155

NOTE: Hospital profiles are in alphabetical order by state, then city, then hospital within the city; Rankings are sorted by rate in descending order and exclude hospitals with less than 25 cases; (1) The number of cases is too small (n<25) for purposes of reliably predicting hospital performance; (2) Measure reflects the hospital's indication that its submission was based upon a sample of its relevant discharges; (3) Rate reflects fewer than the maximum possible quarters of data for the measure; (4) Inaccurate information submitted and suppressed for one or more quarters; (5) No data is available from the hospital for this measure; Please refer to the User's Guide for a full explanation of data

Provident Hospital	Chicago	95%	185
Advocate Christ Med Ctr/Hope Children's	Oak Lawn	94%	50
Mercy Hospital	Chicago	94%	128
Methodist Medical Center of Illinois	Peoria	94%	93
Saint Francis Medical Center	Peoria	94%	146
Saint Mary's Hospital	Decatur	93%	29
Swedish American Hospital	Rockford	93%	88
Advocate Good Samaritan Hospital	Downers Grove	92%	37
Advocate Trinity Hospital	Chicago	92%	131
Iroquois Memorial Hospital & Resident Home	Watseka	92%	25
Saint Anthony Hospital	Chicago	92%	51
Adventist LaGrange Memorial Hospital	La Grange	91%	33
Blessing Hospital	Quincy	91%	54
Good Samaritan Regional Health Center	Mount Vernon	91%	46
Advocate Illinois Masonic Medical Center	Chicago	90%	58
Genesis Medical Center-Illini Campus	Silvis	90%	39
Loyola University Health System	Maywood	90%	155
Rush Oak Park Hospital	Oak Park	90%	52
Centegra Northern Illinois Medical Center	McHenry	89%	47
Memorial Hospital Carbondale	Carbondale	89%	54
Heartland Regional Medical Center	Marion	88%	25
Ingalls Memorial Hospital	Harvey	88%	58
Little Company of Mary Hospital	Evergreen Park	88%	69
Westlake Community Hospital	Melrose Park	88%	57
Advocate Lutheran General Children's Hospital	Park Ridge	87%	47
Gateway Regional Medical Center	Granite City	87%	47
Mount Sinai Hospital	Chicago	87%	127
Palos Community Hospital	Palos Heights	86%	29
Provena Covenant Medical Center	Urbana	85%	59
Evanston Hospital	Evanston	83%	82
Saint Joseph Hospital	Chicago	83%	60
Sherman Hospital	Elgin	83%	59
University of Chicago Hospitals	Chicago	83%	82
South Shore Hospital	Chicago	82%	60
Condell Medical Center	Libertyville	80%	60
Memorial Medical Center	Woodstock	80%	41
Saint Anthony's Health Center	Alton	78%	41
Saint Elizabeth's Hospital	Belleville	78%	72
Carle Foundation Hospital	Urbana	76%	33
Michael Reese Hospital	Chicago	75%	79
Saint Francis Hospital	Evanston	74%	70
University of Illinois at Chicago Med Ctr	Chicago	74%	81
John H Stroger Jr Hospital of Cook County	Chicago	73%	126
Resurrection Medical Center	Chicago	73%	77
Saints Mary & Elizabeth Medical Center	Chicago	72%	68
Swedish Covenant Hospital	Chicago	71%	38
Roseland Community Hospital	Chicago	70%	124
Kenneth Hall Regional Hospital	East Saint Louis	68%	97
Lincoln Park Hospital	Chicago	53%	36
Weiss Memorial Hospital	Chicago	35%	68
Norwegian-American Hospital	Chicago	21%	68
Jackson Park Hospital & Medical Center	Chicago	4%	90

Pneumonia Care

13. Appropriate Initial Antibiotic

Hospital Name	City	Rate	Cases
Illini Community Hospital	Pittsfield	100%	33
Memorial Hospital	Chester	100%	33
Red Bud Regional Hospital	Red Bud	98%	42
FHN Memorial Hospital	Freeport	97%	120
Katherine Shaw Bethea Hospital	Dixon	97%	78
Kewanee Hospital	Kewanee	95%	66
Rush-Copley Medical Center	Aurora	95%	132
Blessing Hospital	Quincy	94%	290
Gibson Community Hospital	Gibson City	94%	32
McDonough District Hospital	Macomb	93%	110
Methodist Medical Center of Illinois	Peoria	93%	159
Palos Community Hospital	Palos Heights	93%	120
Rush University Medical Center	Chicago	93%	58
Anderson Hospital	Maryville	92%	181
Delnor Community Hospital	Geneva	92%	128
Evanston Hospital	Evanston	92%	375
Mason District Hospital	Havana	92%	26
Rockford Memorial Hospital	Rockford	92%	103
Saint Francis Medical Center	Peoria	92%	273
Edward Hospital	Naperville	91%	271
Memorial Medical Center	Springfield	91%	261
Passavant Memorial Area Hospital	Jacksonville	91%	117
Provena Covenant Medical Center	Urbana	91%	119
Saint Bernard Hospital and Health Care Center	Chicago	91%	149
Saint Mary's Hospital	Streator	91%	94
Silver Cross Hospital	Joliet	91%	250
Swedish American Hospital	Rockford	91%	174
Advocate South Suburban Hospital	Hazel Crest	90%	105
Central DuPage Hospital	Winfield	90%	192
Galena-Stauss Hospital & Healthcare Center	Galena	90%	30
Good Samaritan Regional Health Center	Mount Vernon	90%	150
Kishwaukee Community Hospital	De Kalb	90%	107
Michael Reese Hospital	Chicago	90%	31
Provena United Samaritans Medical Center	Danville	90%	264
Saint Anthony's Health Center	Alton	90%	140
Saint John's Hospital	Springfield	90%	151
Westlake Community Hospital	Melrose Park	90%	58
Adventist GlenOaks Hospital	Glendale Heights	89%	35
Bromenn Healthcare	Normal	89%	106
Lake Forest Hospital	Lake Forest	89%	150
Morris Hospital	Morris	89%	118
Community Hospital of Ottawa	Ottawa	88%	93
Gottlieb Memorial Hospital	Melrose Park	88%	104
Little Company of Mary Hospital	Evergreen Park	88%	105
Memorial Hospital Carbondale	Carbondale	88%	67
Pekin Hospital	Pekin	88%	99
Proctor Hospital	Peoria	88%	147
Provident Hospital	Chicago	88%	253
Saint Anthony Hospital	Chicago	88%	69
Sarah Bush Lincoln Health Center	Mattoon	88%	168
Abraham Lincoln Memorial Hospital	Lincoln	87%	67
Carle Foundation Hospital	Urbana	87%	91
Clay County Hospital	Flora	87%	46
Hinsdale Hospital	Hinsdale	87%	156
Memorial Medical Center	Woodstock	87%	139
Oak Forest Hospital of Cook County	Oak Forest	87%	54
Saint Francis Hospital & Health Center	Blue Island	87%	369
Saint Joseph Hospital	Chicago	87%	117
Saint Mary's Good Samaritan	Centralia	87%	188
MacNeal Hospital	Berwyn	86%	258
Northwest Community Hospital	Arlington Heights	86%	85
Northwestern Memorial Hospital	Chicago	86%	207
OSF Saint Mary Medical Center	Galesburg	86%	131
Rush Oak Park Hospital	Oak Park	86%	96
Saint Joseph Medical Center	Bloomington	86%	92
Saint Joseph's Hospital	Breese	86%	72
Advocate Christ Med Ctr/Hope Children's	Oak Lawn	85%	85
Advocate Lutheran General Children's Hospital	Park Ridge	85%	206
Centegra Northern Illinois Medical Center	McHenry	85%	146
Holy Cross Hospital	Chicago	85%	142
Hoopeston Community Memorial Hospital	Hoopeston	85%	52
Loyola University Health System	Maywood	85%	120
Perry Memorial Hospital	Princeton	85%	46
Riverside Medical Center	Kankakee	85%	124
Saint Alexius Medical Center	Hoffman Estates	85%	156
Saint Elizabeth's Hospital	Belleville	85%	245
Saint Francis Hospital	Evanston	85%	261
Saints Mary & Elizabeth Medical Center	Chicago	85%	158
Advocate Illinois Masonic Medical Center	Chicago	84%	103
Advocate Trinity Hospital	Chicago	84%	197
Alexian Brothers Medical Center	Elk Grove Village	84%	212
Alton Memorial Hospital	Alton	84%	165
Community Medical Center	Monmouth	84%	43
Provena Saint Joseph Hospital	Elgin	84%	25
Saint Anthony Medical Center	Rockford	84%	195
Saint James OSF	Pontiac	84%	50
Advocate Good Samaritan Hospital	Downers Grove	83%	111
Decatur Memorial Hospital	Decatur	83%	258
Saint Joseph Memorial Hospital	Murphysboro	83%	41
Sherman Hospital	Elgin	83%	146
Trinity Medical Center	Rock Island	83%	96
Wabash General Hospital	Mount Carmel	83%	42
Weiss Memorial Hospital	Chicago	83%	63
Adventist LaGrange Memorial Hospital	La Grange	82%	214
CGH Medical Center	Sterling	82%	146
Heartland Regional Medical Center	Marion	82%	101
Mercy Hospital	Chicago	82%	127
Our Lady of the Resurrection Medical Center	Chicago	82%	142
Resurrection Medical Center	Chicago	82%	260
Saint James Hospital and Health Center	Olympia Fields	82%	131
Saint Mary's Hospital	Decatur	82%	87
Taylorville Memorial Hospital	Taylorville	82%	44
West Suburban Medical Center	Oak Park	82%	178
Advocate Good Shephard Hospital	Barrington	81%	70
Hammond-Henry Hospital	Geneseo	81%	26
Hardin County General Hospital	Rosiclare	81%	26
Ingalls Memorial Hospital	Harvey	81%	123
Iroquois Memorial Hospital & Resident Home	Watseka	81%	122
Mount Sinai Hospital	Chicago	81%	69
Richland Memorial Hospital	Olney	81%	58
Roseland Community Hospital	Chicago	81%	109
Gateway Regional Medical Center	Granite City	80%	142

NOTE: Hospital profiles are in alphabetical order by state, then city, then hospital within the city; Rankings are sorted by rate in descending order and exclude hospitals with less than 25 cases; (1) The number of cases is too small (n<25) for purposes of reliably predicting hospital performance; (2) Measure reflects the hospital's indication that its submission was based upon a sample of its relevant discharges; (3) Rate reflects fewer than the maximum possible quarters of data for the measure; (4) Inaccurate information submitted and suppressed for one or more quarters; (5) No data is available from the hospital for this measure; Please refer to the User's Guide for a full explanation of data

Memorial Hospital	Belleville	80%	186
Rush North Shore Medical Center	Skokie	80%	138
Saint Anthony's Memorial Hospital	Effingham	80%	176
Valley West Community Hospital	Sandwich	80%	46
Elmhurst Memorial Hospital	Elmhurst	79%	243
Illinois Valley Community Hospital	Peru	79%	101
Jackson Park Hospital & Medical Center	Chicago	79%	66
Jersey Community Hospital	Jerseyville	79%	96
Saint Joseph Medical Center	Joliet	79%	420
Thorek Hospital and Medical Center	Chicago	79%	48
University of Illinois at Chicago Med Ctr	Chicago	79%	82
Pinckneyville Community Hospital	Pinckneyville	78%	41
Provena Mercy Center	Aurora	78%	37
Doctor John Warner Hospital	Clinton	77%	26
Saint Margaret's Hospital	Spring Valley	77%	70
Salem Township Hospital	Salem	77%	60
Herrin Hospital	Herrin	76%	116
Saint Mary's Hospital of Kankakee	Kankakee	76%	210
University of Chicago Hospitals	Chicago	76%	93
Vista Medical Center East	Waukegan	76%	156
Crossroads Community Hospital	Mount Vernon	75%	106
Galesburg Cottage Hospital	Galesburg	75%	91
Graham Hospital	Canton	75%	61
John & Mary Kirby Hospital	Monticello	75%	28
Sparta Community Hospital	Sparta	75%	28
Union County Hospital District	Anna	75%	40
Fairfield Memorial Hospital	Fairfield	74%	70
Norwegian-American Hospital	Chicago	74%	61
Greenville Regional Hospital	Greenville	73%	63
Saint Joseph's Hospital	Highland	73%	41
South Shore Hospital	Chicago	73%	62
Condell Medical Center	Libertyville	72%	161
Genesis Medical Center-Illini Campus	Silvis	72%	90
Hamilton Memorial Hospital	McLeansboro	72%	25
Saint Elizabeth's Hospital	Chicago	72%	106
Shelby Memorial Hospital	Shelbyville	72%	36
Lincoln Park Hospital	Chicago	68%	57
Marshall Browning Hospital	DuQuoin	68%	31
Swedish Covenant Hospital	Chicago	65%	223
Harrisburg Medical Center	Harrisburg	60%	87
Loretto Hospital	Chicago	59%	54
Kenneth Hall Regional Hospital	East Saint Louis	57%	51
Carlinville Area Hospital	Carlinville	53%	66
Saint Francis Hospital	Litchfield	53%	98
John H Stroger Jr Hospital of Cook County	Chicago	50%	187
Ferrell Hospital	Eldorado	42%	36

14. Blood Culture Timing

Hospital Name	City	Rate	Cases
Clay County Hospital	Flora	100%	58
Hardin County General Hospital	Rosiclare	100%	34
FHN Memorial Hospital	Freeport	99%	120
Gottlieb Memorial Hospital	Melrose Park	99%	128
Saint Alexius Medical Center	Hoffman Estates	99%	205
Saint Anthony's Memorial Hospital	Effingham	99%	124
Adventist GlenOaks Hospital	Glendale Heights	98%	63
Palos Community Hospital	Palos Heights	98%	127
Red Bud Regional Hospital	Red Bud	98%	52
Richland Memorial Hospital	Olney	98%	46
Saint Anthony's Health Center	Alton	98%	154
Alexian Brothers Medical Center	Elk Grove Village	97%	267
Kewanee Hospital	Kewanee	97%	58
MacNeal Hospital	Berwyn	97%	256
McDonough District Hospital	Macomb	97%	59
Provena Covenant Medical Center	Urbana	97%	155
Riverside Medical Center	Kankakee	97%	177
Rockford Memorial Hospital	Rockford	97%	158
Saint Elizabeth's Hospital	Chicago	97%	119
Saint Joseph's Hospital	Highland	97%	38
Saint Mary's Good Samaritan	Centralia	97%	178
Wabash General Hospital	Mount Carmel	97%	35
Advocate Good Samaritan Hospital	Downers Grove	96%	131
Anderson Hospital	Maryville	96%	224
Crossroads Community Hospital	Mount Vernon	96%	56
Edward Hospital	Naperville	96%	370
Graham Hospital	Canton	96%	51
Hinsdale Hospital	Hinsdale	96%	252
Kenneth Hall Regional Hospital	East Saint Louis	96%	28
Marshall Browning Hospital	DuQuoin	96%	27
Memorial Medical Center	Woodstock	96%	164
Methodist Medical Center of Illinois	Peoria	96%	147
Oak Forest Hospital of Cook County	Oak Forest	96%	49
Resurrection Medical Center	Chicago	96%	308
Rush North Shore Medical Center	Skokie	96%	156
Saint John's Hospital	Springfield	96%	157
Thorek Hospital and Medical Center	Chicago	96%	57
Advocate Lutheran General Children's Hospital	Park Ridge	95%	242
Alton Memorial Hospital	Alton	95%	184
Condell Medical Center	Libertyville	95%	140
Jersey Community Hospital	Jerseyville	95%	78
Kishwaukee Community Hospital	De Kalb	95%	83
Proctor Hospital	Peoria	95%	181
Saint Anthony Hospital	Chicago	95%	73
Saint Joseph Medical Center	Joliet	95%	74
Taylorville Memorial Hospital	Taylorville	95%	66
Trinity Medical Center	Rock Island	95%	91
Advocate Good Shephard Hospital	Barrington	94%	49
Centegra Northern Illinois Medical Center	McHenry	94%	186
Decatur Memorial Hospital	Decatur	94%	243
Elmhurst Memorial Hospital	Elmhurst	94%	204
Heartland Regional Medical Center	Marion	94%	98
Loyola University Health System	Maywood	94%	145
Pekin Hospital	Pekin	94%	106
Rush Oak Park Hospital	Oak Park	94%	129
Saint Anthony Medical Center	Rockford	94%	193
Saint Francis Medical Center	Peoria	94%	199
Saint James Hospital and Health Center	Olympia Fields	94%	131
Saint James OSF	Pontiac	94%	34
Saint Joseph Hospital	Chicago	94%	143
Saint Margaret's Hospital	Spring Valley	94%	81
Saints Mary & Elizabeth Medical Center	Chicago	94%	142
West Suburban Medical Center	Oak Park	94%	169
Abraham Lincoln Memorial Hospital	Lincoln	93%	55
Adventist LaGrange Memorial Hospital	La Grange	93%	231
CGH Medical Center	Sterling	93%	87
Central DuPage Hospital	Winfield	93%	226
Gateway Regional Medical Center	Granite City	93%	103
Greenville Regional Hospital	Greenville	93%	60
Herrin Hospital	Herrin	93%	107
Loretto Hospital	Chicago	93%	97
Saint Francis Hospital	Evanston	93%	424
Saint Joseph's Hospital	Breese	93%	46
Swedish American Hospital	Rockford	93%	142
Valley West Community Hospital	Sandwich	93%	28
Advocate Trinity Hospital	Chicago	92%	189
Blessing Hospital	Quincy	92%	449
Community Hospital of Ottawa	Ottawa	92%	74
Evanston Hospital	Evanston	92%	504
Good Samaritan Regional Health Center	Mount Vernon	92%	151
Holy Cross Hospital	Chicago	92%	150
Iroquois Memorial Hospital & Resident Home	Watseka	92%	146
Northwest Community Hospital	Arlington Heights	92%	111
Northwestern Memorial Hospital	Chicago	92%	190
OSF Saint Mary Medical Center	Galesburg	92%	116
Rush-Copley Medical Center	Aurora	92%	91
Saint Francis Hospital	Litchfield	92%	48
Saint Mary's Hospital	Decatur	92%	105
Galesburg Cottage Hospital	Galesburg	91%	103
Saint Elizabeth's Hospital	Belleville	91%	195
Saint Mary's Hospital	Streator	91%	111
Advocate Christ Med Ctr/Hope Children's	Oak Lawn	90%	93
Katherine Shaw Bethea Hospital	Dixon	90%	79
Memorial Hospital	Belleville	90%	193
Provena Mercy Center	Aurora	90%	59
Rush University Medical Center	Chicago	90%	71
Saint Joseph Memorial Hospital	Murphysboro	90%	29
Vista Medical Center East	Waukegan	90%	235
Delnor Community Hospital	Geneva	89%	114
Morris Hospital	Morris	89%	118
Provena United Samaritans Medical Center	Danville	89%	246
Weiss Memorial Hospital	Chicago	89%	82
Westlake Community Hospital	Melrose Park	89%	73
Our Lady of the Resurrection Medical Center	Chicago	88%	180
Saint Bernard Hospital and Health Care Center	Chicago	88%	183
Saint Joseph Medical Center	Bloomington	88%	98
Silver Cross Hospital	Joliet	88%	257
Advocate South Suburban Hospital	Hazel Crest	87%	86
Fairfield Memorial Hospital	Fairfield	87%	30
Lake Forest Hospital	Lake Forest	87%	120
Michael Reese Hospital	Chicago	87%	52
Norwegian-American Hospital	Chicago	87%	46
Little Company of Mary Hospital	Evergreen Park	86%	118
Mount Sinai Hospital	Chicago	86%	83
Provena Saint Joseph Hospital	Elgin	86%	29
Saint Mary's Hospital of Kankakee	Kankakee	86%	217
Carle Foundation Hospital	Urbana	85%	95
Saint Francis Hospital & Health Center	Blue Island	85%	412
Swedish Covenant Hospital	Chicago	85%	142
Advocate Illinois Masonic Medical Center	Chicago	84%	95

NOTE: Hospital profiles are in alphabetical order by state, then city, then hospital within the city; Rankings are sorted by rate in descending order and exclude hospitals with less than 25 cases; (1) The number of cases is too small (n<25) for purposes of reliably predicting hospital performance; (2) Measure reflects the hospital's indication that its submission was based upon a sample of its relevant discharges; (3) Rate reflects fewer than the maximum possible quarters of data for the measure; (4) Inaccurate information submitted and suppressed for one or more quarters; (5) No data is available from the hospital for this measure; Please refer to the User's Guide for a full explanation of data

Genesis Medical Center-Illini Campus	Silvis	84%	69
Memorial Medical Center	Springfield	84%	331
Sparta Community Hospital	Sparta	84%	25
Bromenn Healthcare	Normal	83%	145
Illinois Valley Community Hospital	Peru	82%	98
Memorial Hospital Carbondale	Carbondale	82%	79
South Shore Hospital	Chicago	82%	76
Mercy Hospital	Chicago	81%	187
Harrisburg Medical Center	Harrisburg	80%	49
Passavant Memorial Area Hospital	Jacksonville	80%	134
Provident Hospital	Chicago	80%	231
Sarah Bush Lincoln Health Center	Mattoon	80%	124
Sherman Hospital	Elgin	79%	136
Lincoln Park Hospital	Chicago	78%	37
John H Stroger Jr Hospital of Cook County	Chicago	77%	109
Methodist Hospital of Chicago	Chicago	76%	83
Union County Hospital District	Anna	76%	29
University of Chicago Hospitals	Chicago	76%	59
University of Illinois at Chicago Med Ctr	Chicago	76%	124
Ingalls Memorial Hospital	Harvey	73%	99
Roseland Community Hospital	Chicago	64%	99

15. Influenza Vaccine

Hospital Name	City	Rate	Cases
Delnor Community Hospital	Geneva	100%	44
Proctor Hospital	Peoria	97%	38
Saint Mary's Hospital	Decatur	97%	29
Crossroads Community Hospital	Mount Vernon	96%	27
Methodist Medical Center of Illinois	Peoria	96%	51
Decatur Memorial Hospital	Decatur	95%	73
McDonough District Hospital	Macomb	94%	31
OSF Saint Mary Medical Center	Galesburg	94%	50
Heartland Regional Medical Center	Marion	93%	27
Trinity Medical Center	Rock Island	93%	28
Bromenn Healthcare	Normal	92%	51
Hinsdale Hospital	Hinsdale	90%	62
Passavant Memorial Area Hospital	Jacksonville	90%	41
Alton Memorial Hospital	Alton	89%	44
Saint Anthony Medical Center	Rockford	89%	47
Gottlieb Memorial Hospital	Melrose Park	88%	26
Taylorville Memorial Hospital	Taylorville	88%	26
Blessing Hospital	Quincy	87%	117
Saint Mary's Hospital	Streator	87%	31
Herrin Hospital	Herrin	86%	29
Jersey Community Hospital	Jerseyville	86%	28
Saint Francis Medical Center	Peoria	85%	80
Saint Mary's Good Samaritan	Centralia	84%	61
Lake Forest Hospital	Lake Forest	83%	35
Saint Joseph Medical Center	Bloomington	82%	28
Sarah Bush Lincoln Health Center	Mattoon	82%	45
Galesburg Cottage Hospital	Galesburg	81%	27
Northwestern Memorial Hospital	Chicago	81%	42
FHN Memorial Hospital	Freeport	80%	41
Loyola University Health System	Maywood	80%	35
Memorial Medical Center	Springfield	78%	81
Rockford Memorial Hospital	Rockford	77%	31
Community Hospital of Ottawa	Ottawa	76%	25
Advocate Lutheran General Children's Hospital	Park Ridge	74%	66
Condell Medical Center	Libertyville	74%	34
MacNeal Hospital	Berwyn	73%	60
Good Samaritan Regional Health Center	Mount Vernon	72%	60
Our Lady of the Resurrection Medical Center	Chicago	72%	40
Rush Oak Park Hospital	Oak Park	71%	35
Saint Mary's Hospital of Kankakee	Kankakee	71%	51
Saint James Hospital and Health Center	Olympia Fields	70%	33
Swedish American Hospital	Rockford	69%	35
Sherman Hospital	Elgin	68%	41
Saint Alexius Medical Center	Hoffman Estates	64%	47
Saint Joseph's Hospital	Breese	64%	28
Central DuPage Hospital	Winfield	62%	45
Elmhurst Memorial Hospital	Elmhurst	62%	58
Genesis Medical Center-Illini Campus	Silvis	62%	26
Saint Francis Hospital & Health Center	Blue Island	62%	93
Palos Community Hospital	Palos Heights	61%	31
Saint Anthony's Health Center	Alton	61%	38
Memorial Medical Center	Woodstock	60%	43
Rush North Shore Medical Center	Skokie	60%	47
University of Chicago Hospitals	Chicago	60%	25
Provena United Samaritans Medical Center	Danville	59%	46
Saint Joseph Hospital	Chicago	58%	45
Adventist LaGrange Memorial Hospital	La Grange	57%	53
CGH Medical Center	Sterling	54%	26
Gateway Regional Medical Center	Granite City	54%	28
Little Company of Mary Hospital	Evergreen Park	52%	29

Morris Hospital	Morris	52%	44
Centegra Northern Illinois Medical Center	McHenry	51%	35
Advocate Good Shephard Hospital	Barrington	50%	26
Provena Covenant Medical Center	Urbana	48%	46
Riverside Medical Center	Kankakee	44%	52
Saint John's Hospital	Springfield	43%	49
Saint Joseph Medical Center	Joliet	41%	117
Silver Cross Hospital	Joliet	39%	77
Vista Medical Center East	Waukegan	38%	64
Saint Francis Hospital	Evanston	35%	99
Illinois Valley Community Hospital	Peru	34%	35
Mercy Hospital	Chicago	34%	29
Saint Elizabeth's Hospital	Belleville	34%	100
Evanston Hospital	Evanston	24%	122
Saint Bernard Hospital and Health Care Center	Chicago	22%	32
Swedish Covenant Hospital	Chicago	21%	84
John H Stroger Jr Hospital of Cook County	Chicago	15%	26
Provident Hospital	Chicago	15%	33
Advocate Trinity Hospital	Chicago	14%	35
Pekin Hospital	Pekin	12%	33

16. Initial Antibiotic Timing

Hospital Name	City	Rate	Cases
Mercy Harvard Hospital	Harvard	100%	25
Hoopeston Community Memorial Hospital	Hoopeston	98%	51
Perry Memorial Hospital	Princeton	97%	59
Adventist GlenOaks Hospital	Glendale Heights	95%	76
Clay County Hospital	Flora	95%	75
Katherine Shaw Bethea Hospital	Dixon	95%	96
Passavant Memorial Area Hospital	Jacksonville	95%	205
Proctor Hospital	Peoria	95%	214
Rush-Copley Medical Center	Aurora	95%	175
Abraham Lincoln Memorial Hospital	Lincoln	94%	77
Memorial Hospital	Chester	94%	47
Pinckneyville Community Hospital	Pinckneyville	94%	33
Sarah Bush Lincoln Health Center	Mattoon	94%	210
Community Hospital of Ottawa	Ottawa	93%	138
Hardin County General Hospital	Rosiclare	93%	46
Saint Elizabeth's Hospital	Chicago	93%	151
Taylorville Memorial Hospital	Taylorville	93%	98
Evanston Hospital	Evanston	92%	683
Hamilton Memorial Hospital	McLeansboro	92%	38
Saint James OSF	Pontiac	92%	49
Saint Mary's Hospital	Streator	92%	182
Alton Memorial Hospital	Alton	91%	243
Decatur Memorial Hospital	Decatur	91%	332
Delnor Community Hospital	Geneva	91%	207
Illinois Valley Community Hospital	Peru	91%	160
Saint Joseph's Hospital	Breese	91%	79
Saint Margaret's Hospital	Spring Valley	91%	128
Trinity Medical Center	Rock Island	91%	123
Lawrence County Memorial Hospital	Lawrenceville	90%	42
MacNeal Hospital	Berwyn	90%	337
Memorial Medical Center	Woodstock	90%	205
Morris Hospital	Morris	90%	212
FHN Memorial Hospital	Freeport	89%	192
Iroquois Memorial Hospital & Resident Home	Watseka	89%	217
OSF Saint Mary Medical Center	Galesburg	89%	164
Red Bud Regional Hospital	Red Bud	89%	63
Saint Alexius Medical Center	Hoffman Estates	89%	274
Alexian Brothers Medical Center	Elk Grove Village	88%	312
Galena-Stauss Hospital & Healthcare Center	Galena	88%	25
Good Samaritan Regional Health Center	Mount Vernon	88%	238
Jersey Community Hospital	Jerseyville	88%	113
Kishwaukee Community Hospital	De Kalb	88%	145
Northwest Community Hospital	Arlington Heights	88%	173
Richland Memorial Hospital	Olney	88%	83
Saint John's Hospital	Springfield	88%	262
Saint Joseph Memorial Hospital	Murphysboro	88%	50
Saint Mary's Good Samaritan	Centralia	88%	312
Saints Mary & Elizabeth Medical Center	Chicago	88%	199
Shelby Memorial Hospital	Shelbyville	88%	42
Union County Hospital District	Anna	88%	73
Wabash General Hospital	Mount Carmel	88%	67
Blessing Hospital	Quincy	87%	519
Centegra Northern Illinois Medical Center	McHenry	87%	210
Memorial Hospital Carbondale	Carbondale	87%	114
Mendota Community Hospital	Mendota	87%	31
Resurrection Medical Center	Chicago	87%	422
Silver Cross Hospital	Joliet	87%	431
Advocate Lutheran General Children's Hospital	Park Ridge	86%	328
Gibson Community Hospital	Gibson City	86%	42
Gottlieb Memorial Hospital	Melrose Park	86%	153
Pekin Hospital	Pekin	86%	187

NOTE: Hospital profiles are in alphabetical order by state, then city, then hospital within the city; Rankings are sorted by rate in descending order and exclude hospitals with less than 25 cases; (1) The number of cases is too small (n<25) for purposes of reliably predicting hospital performance; (2) Measure reflects the hospital's indication that its submission was based upon a sample of its relevant discharges; (3) Rate reflects fewer than the maximum possible quarters of data for the measure; (4) Inaccurate information submitted and suppressed for one or more quarters; (5) No data is available from the hospital for this measure; Please refer to the User's Guide for a full explanation of data

Saint Joseph Hospital	Chicago	86%	199
Advocate Good Samaritan Hospital	Downers Grove	85%	171
Elmhurst Memorial Hospital	Elmhurst	85%	334
Lake Forest Hospital	Lake Forest	85%	159
Marshall Browning Hospital	DuQuoin	85%	34
Our Lady of the Resurrection Medical Center	Chicago	85%	247
Rush North Shore Medical Center	Skokie	85%	233
Saint Anthony Hospital	Chicago	85%	93
Saint Anthony's Memorial Hospital	Effingham	85%	209
Saint Mary's Hospital	Decatur	85%	157
Advocate Good Shephard Hospital	Barrington	84%	132
CGH Medical Center	Sterling	84%	159
Culbertson Memorial Hospital	Rushville	84%	38
Kewanee Hospital	Kewanee	84%	108
Saint Francis Hospital	Evanston	84%	518
Swedish American Hospital	Rockford	84%	226
Harrisburg Medical Center	Harrisburg	83%	143
Memorial Medical Center	Springfield	83%	433
Saint Joseph's Hospital	Highland	83%	71
Sherman Hospital	Elgin	83%	224
Central DuPage Hospital	Winfield	82%	277
Mason District Hospital	Havana	82%	44
Riverside Medical Center	Kankakee	82%	262
Saint Anthony's Health Center	Alton	82%	221
Saint Francis Hospital	Litchfield	82%	159
Saint Francis Medical Center	Peoria	82%	409
Edward Hospital	Naperville	81%	439
Galesburg Cottage Hospital	Galesburg	81%	151
Hinsdale Hospital	Hinsdale	81%	278
McDonough District Hospital	Macomb	81%	142
Methodist Medical Center of Illinois	Peoria	81%	237
Rush Oak Park Hospital	Oak Park	81%	155
Bromenn Healthcare	Normal	80%	182
Heartland Regional Medical Center	Marion	80%	152
Herrin Hospital	Herrin	80%	168
Illini Community Hospital	Pittsfield	80%	45
Pana Community Hospital	Pana	80%	30
Rockford Memorial Hospital	Rockford	80%	192
Saint Elizabeth's Hospital	Belleville	80%	410
Anderson Hospital	Maryville	79%	249
Provena Saint Joseph Hospital	Elgin	79%	189
Rochelle Community Hospital	Rochelle	79%	33
Rush University Medical Center	Chicago	79%	96
Saint Anthony Medical Center	Rockford	79%	290
Saint Mary's Hospital of Kankakee	Kankakee	79%	310
Weiss Memorial Hospital	Chicago	79%	131
Adventist LaGrange Memorial Hospital	La Grange	78%	307
Advocate Christ Med Ctr/Hope Children's	Oak Lawn	78%	161
Doctor John Warner Hospital	Clinton	78%	27
Loretto Hospital	Chicago	78%	119
Northwestern Memorial Hospital	Chicago	78%	282
Norwegian-American Hospital	Chicago	78%	79
Fairfield Memorial Hospital	Fairfield	77%	82
Ferrell Hospital	Eldorado	77%	52
Gateway Regional Medical Center	Granite City	77%	186
Greenville Regional Hospital	Greenville	77%	98
Methodist Hospital of Chicago	Chicago	77%	139
Michael Reese Hospital	Chicago	77%	82
Salem Township Hospital	Salem	77%	87
Carle Foundation Hospital	Urbana	76%	116
Community Medical Center	Monmouth	76%	49
Crossroads Community Hospital	Mount Vernon	76%	136
Graham Hospital	Canton	76%	104
Lincoln Park Hospital	Chicago	76%	63
Swedish Covenant Hospital	Chicago	76%	367
Provena Mercy Center	Aurora	75%	309
West Suburban Medical Center	Oak Park	75%	250
South Shore Hospital	Chicago	74%	118
Westlake Community Hospital	Melrose Park	74%	124
Condell Medical Center	Libertyville	73%	200
Holy Cross Hospital	Chicago	73%	218
Saint Francis Hospital & Health Center	Blue Island	73%	529
Saint Joseph Medical Center	Bloomington	73%	118
Sparta Community Hospital	Sparta	73%	45
Advocate Illinois Masonic Medical Center	Chicago	72%	167
Saint Bernard Hospital and Health Care Center	Chicago	72%	232
Genesis Medical Center-Illini Campus	Silvis	71%	127
Oak Forest Hospital of Cook County	Oak Forest	71%	63
Provena United Samaritans Medical Center	Danville	71%	385
Kenneth Hall Regional Hospital	East Saint Louis	70%	66
Provena Covenant Medical Center	Urbana	70%	230
Jackson Park Hospital & Medical Center	Chicago	69%	52
University of Chicago Hospitals	Chicago	69%	123
Advocate South Suburban Hospital	Hazel Crest	68%	164
Memorial Hospital	Belleville	68%	301
Saint James Hospital and Health Center	Olympia Fields	68%	221
Ingalls Memorial Hospital	Harvey	67%	183
Vista Medical Center East	Waukegan	66%	398
Palos Community Hospital	Palos Heights	65%	153
Saint Joseph Medical Center	Joliet	65%	609
John & Mary Kirby Hospital	Monticello	64%	50
University of Illinois at Chicago Med Ctr	Chicago	64%	183
Mercy Hospital	Chicago	63%	230
Advocate Trinity Hospital	Chicago	62%	257
Little Company of Mary Hospital	Evergreen Park	62%	169
Loyola University Health System	Maywood	62%	176
Carlinville Area Hospital	Carlinville	61%	61
Thorek Hospital and Medical Center	Chicago	61%	125
Midwestern Regional Medical Center	Zion	60%	50
Touchette Regional Hospital	Centreville	60%	25
Mount Sinai Hospital	Chicago	58%	130
Crawford Memorial Hospital	Robinson	57%	30
Roseland Community Hospital	Chicago	56%	154
Provident Hospital	Chicago	52%	292
John H Stroger Jr Hospital of Cook County	Chicago	33%	210

17. Oxygenation Assessment

Hospital Name	City	Rate	Cases
Abraham Lincoln Memorial Hospital	Lincoln	100%	100
Adventist GlenOaks Hospital	Glendale Heights	100%	99
Advocate Christ Med Ctr/Hope Children's	Oak Lawn	100%	171
Advocate Good Samaritan Hospital	Downers Grove	100%	210
Advocate Good Shephard Hospital	Barrington	100%	158
Advocate Illinois Masonic Medical Center	Chicago	100%	200
Advocate Lutheran General Children's Hospital	Park Ridge	100%	436
Alexian Brothers Medical Center	Elk Grove Village	100%	445
Alton Memorial Hospital	Alton	100%	283
Anderson Hospital	Maryville	100%	328
Blessing Hospital	Quincy	100%	688
Bromenn Healthcare	Normal	100%	236
Carle Foundation Hospital	Urbana	100%	142
Carlinville Area Hospital	Carlinville	100%	81
Centegra Northern Illinois Medical Center	McHenry	100%	261
Central DuPage Hospital	Winfield	100%	348
Clay County Hospital	Flora	100%	89
Community Medical Center	Monmouth	100%	65
Community Memorial Hospital	Staunton	100%	32
Condell Medical Center	Libertyville	100%	264
Crossroads Community Hospital	Mount Vernon	100%	161
Culbertson Memorial Hospital	Rushville	100%	51
Decatur Memorial Hospital	Decatur	100%	411
Delnor Community Hospital	Geneva	100%	243
Edward Hospital	Naperville	100%	577
Elmhurst Memorial Hospital	Elmhurst	100%	384
Evanston Hospital	Evanston	100%	777
FHN Memorial Hospital	Freeport	100%	234
Fairfield Memorial Hospital	Fairfield	100%	105
Galena-Stauss Hospital & Healthcare Center	Galena	100%	30
Genesis Medical Center-Illini Campus	Silvis	100%	149
Gibson Community Hospital	Gibson City	100%	57
Gottlieb Memorial Hospital	Melrose Park	100%	186
Greenville Regional Hospital	Greenville	100%	127
Hammond-Henry Hospital	Geneseo	100%	32
Heartland Regional Medical Center	Marion	100%	181
Herrin Hospital	Herrin	100%	210
Hinsdale Hospital	Hinsdale	100%	375
Holy Cross Hospital	Chicago	100%	233
Hoopeston Community Memorial Hospital	Hoopeston	100%	60
Ingalls Memorial Hospital	Harvey	100%	203
Iroquois Memorial Hospital & Resident Home	Watseka	100%	275
John H Stroger Jr Hospital of Cook County	Chicago	100%	243
Katherine Shaw Bethea Hospital	Dixon	100%	120
Kewanee Hospital	Kewanee	100%	123
Kishwaukee Community Hospital	De Kalb	100%	175
Lake Forest Hospital	Lake Forest	100%	193
Lawrence County Memorial Hospital	Lawrenceville	100%	48
Loretto Hospital	Chicago	100%	129
Loyola University Health System	Maywood	100%	254
MacNeal Hospital	Berwyn	100%	391
Marshall Browning Hospital	DuQuoin	100%	44
McDonough District Hospital	Macomb	100%	191
Memorial Hospital	Belleville	100%	345
Memorial Hospital	Chester	100%	61
Memorial Hospital Carbondale	Carbondale	100%	152
Memorial Medical Center	Springfield	100%	561
Memorial Medical Center	Woodstock	100%	251
Mercy Harvard Hospital	Harvard	100%	28
Mercy Hospital	Chicago	100%	261
Methodist Medical Center of Illinois	Peoria	100%	327

NOTE: Hospital profiles are in alphabetical order by state, then city, then hospital within the city; Rankings are sorted by rate in descending order and exclude hospitals with less than 25 cases; (1) The number of cases is too small (n<25) for purposes of reliably predicting hospital performance; (2) Measure reflects the hospital's indication that its submission was based upon a sample of its relevant discharges; (3) Rate reflects fewer than the maximum possible quarters of data for the measure; (4) Inaccurate information submitted and suppressed for one or more quarters; (5) No data is available from the hospital for this measure; Please refer to the User's Guide for a full explanation of data

Midwestern Regional Medical Center	Zion	100%	62
Morris Hospital	Morris	100%	228
Northwest Community Hospital	Arlington Heights	100%	189
Northwestern Memorial Hospital	Chicago	100%	365
Norwegian-American Hospital	Chicago	100%	81
OSF Saint Mary Medical Center	Galesburg	100%	214
Oak Forest Hospital of Cook County	Oak Forest	100%	72
Our Lady of the Resurrection Medical Center	Chicago	100%	301
Palos Community Hospital	Palos Heights	100%	203
Pana Community Hospital	Pana	100%	37
Passavant Memorial Area Hospital	Jacksonville	100%	252
Perry Memorial Hospital	Princeton	100%	81
Proctor Hospital	Peoria	100%	267
Provena Covenant Medical Center	Urbana	100%	283
Provena Mercy Center	Aurora	100%	379
Provena Saint Joseph Hospital	Elgin	100%	240
Provident Hospital	Chicago	100%	308
Red Bud Regional Hospital	Red Bud	100%	88
Richland Memorial Hospital	Olney	100%	108
Riverside Medical Center	Kankakee	100%	304
Rochelle Community Hospital	Rochelle	100%	38
Rockford Memorial Hospital	Rockford	100%	238
Roseland Community Hospital	Chicago	100%	164
Rush North Shore Medical Center	Skokie	100%	278
Rush Oak Park Hospital	Oak Park	100%	193
Rush University Medical Center	Chicago	100%	145
Rush-Copley Medical Center	Aurora	100%	230
Saint Alexius Medical Center	Hoffman Estates	100%	315
Saint Anthony Hospital	Chicago	100%	115
Saint Anthony's Health Center	Alton	100%	270
Saint Anthony's Memorial Hospital	Effingham	100%	258
Saint Bernard Hospital and Health Care Center	Chicago	100%	260
Saint Elizabeth's Hospital	Chicago	100%	178
Saint Francis Hospital	Evanston	100%	622
Saint Francis Hospital	Litchfield	100%	176
Saint Francis Hospital & Health Center	Blue Island	100%	593
Saint Francis Medical Center	Peoria	100%	460
Saint James OSF	Pontiac	100%	65
Saint John's Hospital	Springfield	100%	302
Saint Joseph Hospital	Chicago	100%	252
Saint Joseph Medical Center	Bloomington	100%	156
Saint Joseph Medical Center	Joliet	100%	673
Saint Joseph Memorial Hospital	Murphysboro	100%	59
Saint Joseph's Hospital	Breese	100%	103
Saint Joseph's Hospital	Highland	100%	81
Saint Margaret's Hospital	Spring Valley	100%	168
Saint Mary's Good Samaritan	Centralia	100%	371
Saint Mary's Hospital	Streator	100%	217
Saint Mary's Hospital of Kankakee	Kankakee	100%	362
Sarah Bush Lincoln Health Center	Mattoon	100%	272
Shelby Memorial Hospital	Shelbyville	100%	72
Sherman Hospital	Elgin	100%	262
Silver Cross Hospital	Joliet	100%	468
Sparta Community Hospital	Sparta	100%	52
Swedish American Hospital	Rockford	100%	275
Swedish Covenant Hospital	Chicago	100%	439
Taylorville Memorial Hospital	Taylorville	100%	136
Touchette Regional Hospital	Centreville	100%	25
Union County Hospital District	Anna	100%	85
University of Chicago Hospitals	Chicago	100%	165
Valley West Community Hospital	Sandwich	100%	63
Wabash General Hospital	Mount Carmel	100%	90
Weiss Memorial Hospital	Chicago	100%	166
West Suburban Medical Center	Oak Park	100%	285
Westlake Community Hospital	Melrose Park	100%	153
Adventist LaGrange Memorial Hospital	La Grange	99%	358
Advocate Trinity Hospital	Chicago	99%	295
Community Hospital of Ottawa	Ottawa	99%	173
Galesburg Cottage Hospital	Galesburg	99%	177
Gateway Regional Medical Center	Granite City	99%	198
Good Samaritan Regional Health Center	Mount Vernon	99%	272
Graham Hospital	Canton	99%	126
Illinois Valley Community Hospital	Peru	99%	178
Jackson Park Hospital & Medical Center	Chicago	99%	67
Jersey Community Hospital	Jerseyville	99%	154
Little Company of Mary Hospital	Evergreen Park	99%	212
Michael Reese Hospital	Chicago	99%	94
Pekin Hospital	Pekin	99%	224
Provena United Samaritans Medical Center	Danville	99%	432
Saint Anthony Medical Center	Rockford	99%	347
Saint Elizabeth's Hospital	Belleville	99%	501
Saint James Hospital and Health Center	Olympia Fields	99%	280
Saint Mary's Hospital	Decatur	99%	186
Trinity Medical Center	Rock Island	99%	156
University of Illinois at Chicago Med Ctr	Chicago	99%	196
Vista Medical Center East	Waukegan	99%	428
Advocate South Suburban Hospital	Hazel Crest	98%	187
Hamilton Memorial Hospital	McLeansboro	98%	41
Harrisburg Medical Center	Harrisburg	98%	171
Illini Community Hospital	Pittsfield	98%	60
John & Mary Kirby Hospital	Monticello	98%	60
Mendota Community Hospital	Mendota	98%	44
Resurrection Medical Center	Chicago	98%	466
Saints Mary & Elizabeth Medical Center	Chicago	98%	215
Thorek Hospital and Medical Center	Chicago	98%	141
Doctor John Warner Hospital	Clinton	97%	36
Mount Sinai Hospital	Chicago	97%	136
CGH Medical Center	Sterling	96%	191
Ferrell Hospital	Eldorado	96%	67
Hardin County General Hospital	Rosiclare	96%	55
Mason District Hospital	Havana	96%	52
Pinckneyville Community Hospital	Pinckneyville	96%	46
South Shore Hospital	Chicago	95%	147
Crawford Memorial Hospital	Robinson	94%	35
Lincoln Park Hospital	Chicago	93%	84
Methodist Hospital of Chicago	Chicago	93%	169
Kenneth Hall Regional Hospital	East Saint Louis	91%	67
Salem Township Hospital	Salem	90%	90

18. Pneumococcal Vaccine

Hospital Name	City	Rate	Cases
Hardin County General Hospital	Rosiclare	100%	34
Delnor Community Hospital	Geneva	99%	176
Methodist Medical Center of Illinois	Peoria	98%	204
OSF Saint Mary Medical Center	Galesburg	98%	134
Proctor Hospital	Peoria	98%	205
Culbertson Memorial Hospital	Rushville	97%	35
Saint Mary's Hospital	Decatur	97%	116
Clay County Hospital	Flora	96%	51
Memorial Hospital	Chester	95%	44
Taylorville Memorial Hospital	Taylorville	95%	103
Sarah Bush Lincoln Health Center	Mattoon	94%	183
Decatur Memorial Hospital	Decatur	93%	287
Saint John's Hospital	Springfield	93%	190
Alton Memorial Hospital	Alton	92%	186
Gottlieb Memorial Hospital	Melrose Park	92%	110
Kishwaukee Community Hospital	De Kalb	91%	113
Crossroads Community Hospital	Mount Vernon	88%	83
Saint James OSF	Pontiac	88%	42
Abraham Lincoln Memorial Hospital	Lincoln	87%	69
Blessing Hospital	Quincy	87%	479
Bromenn Healthcare	Normal	87%	167
Heartland Regional Medical Center	Marion	87%	106
Northwest Community Hospital	Arlington Heights	87%	140
Passavant Memorial Area Hospital	Jacksonville	87%	176
Saint Mary's Good Samaritan	Centralia	86%	226
Katherine Shaw Bethea Hospital	Dixon	85%	81
Saint Joseph Medical Center	Bloomington	85%	101
Community Hospital of Ottawa	Ottawa	84%	127
FHN Memorial Hospital	Freeport	84%	169
Galesburg Cottage Hospital	Galesburg	84%	120
Saint Elizabeth's Hospital	Chicago	84%	89
Hinsdale Hospital	Hinsdale	83%	266
Saint Mary's Hospital	Streator	83%	170
Trinity Medical Center	Rock Island	83%	112
Valley West Community Hospital	Sandwich	83%	35
Gibson Community Hospital	Gibson City	82%	33
Illini Community Hospital	Pittsfield	82%	49
Loyola University Health System	Maywood	82%	125
Mendota Community Hospital	Mendota	82%	40
Advocate Lutheran General Children's Hospital	Park Ridge	81%	321
Galena-Stauss Hospital & Healthcare Center	Galena	81%	26
Sparta Community Hospital	Sparta	81%	32
Advocate Good Samaritan Hospital	Downers Grove	80%	142
Northwestern Memorial Hospital	Chicago	80%	169
Saint Anthony Medical Center	Rockford	80%	239
Alexian Brothers Medical Center	Elk Grove Village	79%	305
Rush-Copley Medical Center	Aurora	79%	130
Saint Francis Medical Center	Peoria	79%	282
Saint Joseph's Hospital	Highland	79%	57
Anderson Hospital	Maryville	78%	221
Lake Forest Hospital	Lake Forest	78%	135
Red Bud Regional Hospital	Red Bud	78%	51
Sherman Hospital	Elgin	78%	121
Adventist GlenOaks Hospital	Glendale Heights	77%	57
Memorial Medical Center	Springfield	77%	358
Union County Hospital District	Anna	77%	48
Saint Anthony's Health Center	Alton	76%	168
Saint Anthony's Memorial Hospital	Effingham	76%	180

NOTE: Hospital profiles are in alphabetical order by state, then city, then hospital within the city; Rankings are sorted by rate in descending order and exclude hospitals with less than 25 cases; (1) The number of cases is too small (n<25) for purposes of reliably predicting hospital performance; (2) Measure reflects the hospital's indication that its submission was based upon a sample of its relevant discharges; (3) Rate reflects fewer than the maximum possible quarters of data for the measure; (4) Inaccurate information submitted and suppressed for one or more quarters; (5) No data is available from the hospital for this measure; Please refer to the User's Guide for a full explanation of data

Swedish American Hospital	Rockford	76%	169
Advocate South Suburban Hospital	Hazel Crest	75%	118
Fairfield Memorial Hospital	Fairfield	75%	69
Rush University Medical Center	Chicago	75%	63
Saint Alexius Medical Center	Hoffman Estates	75%	193
Saint Joseph's Hospital	Breese	75%	64
Mason District Hospital	Havana	74%	42
McDonough District Hospital	Macomb	74%	152
Michael Reese Hospital	Chicago	74%	39
Carle Foundation Hospital	Urbana	73%	108
Herrin Hospital	Herrin	73%	134
Iroquois Memorial Hospital & Resident Home	Watseka	73%	198
Genesis Medical Center-Illini Campus	Silvis	72%	100
Edward Hospital	Naperville	70%	395
Pinckneyville Community Hospital	Pinckneyville	70%	40
Rush Oak Park Hospital	Oak Park	70%	108
Wabash General Hospital	Mount Carmel	70%	67
Good Samaritan Regional Health Center	Mount Vernon	69%	188
Ingalls Memorial Hospital	Harvey	68%	98
MacNeal Hospital	Berwyn	68%	256
Memorial Medical Center	Woodstock	68%	157
Our Lady of the Resurrection Medical Center	Chicago	68%	193
Condell Medical Center	Libertyville	67%	151
Kewanee Hospital	Kewanee	67%	82
Rockford Memorial Hospital	Rockford	67%	159
Advocate Christ Med Ctr/Hope Children's	Oak Lawn	65%	106
Shelby Memorial Hospital	Shelbyville	65%	52
Lawrence County Memorial Hospital	Lawrenceville	64%	39
Saint Francis Hospital & Health Center	Blue Island	64%	313
Centegra Northern Illinois Medical Center	McHenry	63%	150
Central DuPage Hospital	Winfield	63%	225
Memorial Hospital Carbondale	Carbondale	63%	100
Provena United Samaritans Medical Center	Danville	63%	220
Jersey Community Hospital	Jerseyville	62%	112
Community Medical Center	Monmouth	61%	41
Palos Community Hospital	Palos Heights	61%	142
Saint James Hospital and Health Center	Olympia Fields	60%	146
Advocate Good Shephard Hospital	Barrington	59%	119
Advocate Illinois Masonic Medical Center	Chicago	59%	86
Gateway Regional Medical Center	Granite City	59%	96
Carlinville Area Hospital	Carlinville	58%	62
Rush North Shore Medical Center	Skokie	58%	213
Morris Hospital	Morris	57%	163
Saints Mary & Elizabeth Medical Center	Chicago	57%	109
CGH Medical Center	Sterling	56%	121
Graham Hospital	Canton	56%	84
Provena Covenant Medical Center	Urbana	56%	183
Harrisburg Medical Center	Harrisburg	55%	108
Illinois Valley Community Hospital	Peru	54%	131
University of Chicago Hospitals	Chicago	54%	84
Adventist LaGrange Memorial Hospital	La Grange	52%	228
Crawford Memorial Hospital	Robinson	52%	25
John & Mary Kirby Hospital	Monticello	52%	50
Richland Memorial Hospital	Olney	51%	72
Elmhurst Memorial Hospital	Elmhurst	50%	266
Marshall Browning Hospital	DuQuoin	50%	28
Saint Joseph Memorial Hospital	Murphysboro	50%	40
Little Company of Mary Hospital	Evergreen Park	49%	128
Riverside Medical Center	Kankakee	49%	202
Saint Mary's Hospital of Kankakee	Kankakee	49%	156
University of Illinois at Chicago Med Ctr	Chicago	49%	65
West Suburban Medical Center	Oak Park	48%	122
Memorial Hospital	Belleville	46%	217
Saint Joseph Hospital	Chicago	46%	151
Saint Francis Hospital	Litchfield	45%	121
Silver Cross Hospital	Joliet	45%	256
Saint Francis Hospital	Evanston	44%	382
Saint Anthony Hospital	Chicago	43%	44
Pekin Hospital	Pekin	41%	157
Vista Medical Center East	Waukegan	39%	225
Norwegian-American Hospital	Chicago	37%	30
Saint Joseph Medical Center	Joliet	37%	399
Thorek Hospital and Medical Center	Chicago	36%	69
Greenville Regional Hospital	Greenville	35%	85
Mercy Hospital	Chicago	35%	128
Evanston Hospital	Evanston	34%	545
Mount Sinai Hospital	Chicago	34%	44
Provena Mercy Center	Aurora	34%	220
Provena Saint Joseph Hospital	Elgin	34%	142
Holy Cross Hospital	Chicago	33%	93
Swedish Covenant Hospital	Chicago	33%	293
Saint Margaret's Hospital	Spring Valley	32%	108
Advocate Trinity Hospital	Chicago	31%	134
Roseland Community Hospital	Chicago	31%	48
Lincoln Park Hospital	Chicago	28%	36
Saint Elizabeth's Hospital	Belleville	28%	323
Resurrection Medical Center	Chicago	27%	322
Westlake Community Hospital	Melrose Park	27%	81
Ferrell Hospital	Eldorado	25%	32
Provident Hospital	Chicago	25%	69
Perry Memorial Hospital	Princeton	24%	58
Weiss Memorial Hospital	Chicago	20%	98
Loretto Hospital	Chicago	18%	44
Saint Bernard Hospital and Health Care Center	Chicago	16%	86
Hoopeston Community Memorial Hospital	Hoopeston	14%	50
John H Stroger Jr Hospital of Cook County	Chicago	12%	52
Methodist Hospital of Chicago	Chicago	8%	99
Salem Township Hospital	Salem	3%	71
South Shore Hospital	Chicago	3%	66

19. Smoking Cessation Advice

Hospital Name	City	Rate	Cases
Advocate South Suburban Hospital	Hazel Crest	100%	50
CGH Medical Center	Sterling	100%	34
Gottlieb Memorial Hospital	Melrose Park	100%	41
Loretto Hospital	Chicago	100%	37
Memorial Medical Center	Springfield	100%	144
Morris Hospital	Morris	100%	43
Provena United Samaritans Medical Center	Danville	100%	110
Riverside Medical Center	Kankakee	100%	63
Rush-Copley Medical Center	Aurora	100%	60
Saint Alexius Medical Center	Hoffman Estates	100%	62
Saint Elizabeth's Hospital	Chicago	100%	43
Saint Mary's Hospital	Streator	100%	31
Saint Mary's Hospital of Kankakee	Kankakee	100%	90
Thorek Hospital and Medical Center	Chicago	100%	36
Decatur Memorial Hospital	Decatur	99%	77
Saint Bernard Hospital and Health Care Center	Chicago	99%	92
Alton Memorial Hospital	Alton	98%	58
Bromenn Healthcare	Normal	98%	53
Heartland Regional Medical Center	Marion	98%	44
OSF Saint Mary Medical Center	Galesburg	98%	51
Rush Oak Park Hospital	Oak Park	98%	40
Saint Joseph Medical Center	Bloomington	98%	43
Saint Mary's Hospital	Decatur	98%	45
Vista Medical Center East	Waukegan	98%	89
Central DuPage Hospital	Winfield	97%	64
Our Lady of the Resurrection Medical Center	Chicago	97%	58
Saint Anthony Hospital	Chicago	97%	39
Saint Francis Medical Center	Peoria	97%	136
Silver Cross Hospital	Joliet	97%	120
Swedish American Hospital	Rockford	97%	75
Methodist Medical Center of Illinois	Peoria	96%	96
Taylorville Memorial Hospital	Taylorville	96%	26
Trinity Medical Center	Rock Island	96%	47
Hinsdale Hospital	Hinsdale	95%	60
Oak Forest Hospital of Cook County	Oak Forest	95%	43
Provena Covenant Medical Center	Urbana	95%	64
Provident Hospital	Chicago	95%	154
Rush University Medical Center	Chicago	95%	41
Saint James Hospital and Health Center	Olympia Fields	95%	66
Centegra Northern Illinois Medical Center	McHenry	94%	67
Memorial Hospital	Belleville	94%	81
Sarah Bush Lincoln Health Center	Mattoon	94%	62
West Suburban Medical Center	Oak Park	94%	93
FHN Memorial Hospital	Freeport	93%	45
Ingalls Memorial Hospital	Harvey	93%	57
MacNeal Hospital	Berwyn	93%	81
Saint Francis Hospital & Health Center	Blue Island	93%	159
McDonough District Hospital	Macomb	92%	25
Saint Anthony Medical Center	Rockford	92%	53
Anderson Hospital	Maryville	91%	69
Edward Hospital	Naperville	91%	80
Alexian Brothers Medical Center	Elk Grove Village	90%	77
Condell Medical Center	Libertyville	90%	58
Herrin Hospital	Herrin	90%	50
Mount Sinai Hospital	Chicago	90%	48
Proctor Hospital	Peoria	90%	50
Adventist LaGrange Memorial Hospital	La Grange	89%	55
Advocate Trinity Hospital	Chicago	89%	88
Kishwaukee Community Hospital	De Kalb	89%	38
Crossroads Community Hospital	Mount Vernon	88%	50
Lake Forest Hospital	Lake Forest	88%	26
Memorial Hospital Carbondale	Carbondale	88%	34
Rockford Memorial Hospital	Rockford	88%	51
Blessing Hospital	Quincy	87%	149
Holy Cross Hospital	Chicago	87%	61
Little Company of Mary Hospital	Evergreen Park	87%	38
Memorial Medical Center	Woodstock	87%	39

NOTE: Hospital profiles are in alphabetical order by state, then city, then hospital within the city; Rankings are sorted by rate in descending order and exclude hospitals with less than 25 cases; (1) The number of cases is too small (n<25) for purposes of reliably predicting hospital performance; (2) Measure reflects the hospital's indication that its submission was based upon a sample of its relevant discharges; (3) Rate reflects fewer than the maximum possible quarters of data for the measure; (4) Inaccurate information submitted and suppressed for one or more quarters; (5) No data is available from the hospital for this measure; Please refer to the User's Guide for a full explanation of data

Hospital Name	City	Rate	Cases
Northwestern Memorial Hospital	Chicago	87%	91
Saint Anthony's Health Center	Alton	87%	61
Iroquois Memorial Hospital & Resident Home	Watseka	86%	50
Advocate Illinois Masonic Medical Center	Chicago	85%	41
Elmhurst Memorial Hospital	Elmhurst	85%	53
Palos Community Hospital	Palos Heights	85%	40
Saint John's Hospital	Springfield	85%	98
Advocate Good Samaritan Hospital	Downers Grove	84%	37
Carle Foundation Hospital	Urbana	84%	37
Good Samaritan Regional Health Center	Mount Vernon	84%	57
Passavant Memorial Area Hospital	Jacksonville	83%	54
Advocate Lutheran General Children's Hospital	Park Ridge	82%	68
Gateway Regional Medical Center	Granite City	82%	67
Saint Elizabeth's Hospital	Belleville	82%	115
Saint Joseph Hospital	Chicago	82%	51
Saint Anthony's Memorial Hospital	Effingham	81%	47
Saints Mary & Elizabeth Medical Center	Chicago	81%	57
Michael Reese Hospital	Chicago	80%	35
Saint Joseph Medical Center	Joliet	80%	124
Harrisburg Medical Center	Harrisburg	79%	28
Mercy Hospital	Chicago	79%	76
Galesburg Cottage Hospital	Galesburg	78%	32
Resurrection Medical Center	Chicago	78%	54
Roseland Community Hospital	Chicago	78%	69
Loyola University Health System	Maywood	77%	48
Illinois Valley Community Hospital	Peru	76%	25
Saint Mary's Good Samaritan	Centralia	76%	98
University of Chicago Hospitals	Chicago	76%	41
Saint Francis Hospital	Evanston	73%	103
Pekin Hospital	Pekin	72%	50
South Shore Hospital	Chicago	71%	31
Evanston Hospital	Evanston	70%	74
Genesis Medical Center-Illini Campus	Silvis	70%	37
Sherman Hospital	Elgin	69%	59
Graham Hospital	Canton	68%	28
Saint Margaret's Hospital	Spring Valley	68%	25
Swedish Covenant Hospital	Chicago	68%	47
University of Illinois at Chicago Med Ctr	Chicago	65%	60
Methodist Hospital of Chicago	Chicago	62%	66
Richland Memorial Hospital	Olney	61%	28
Rush North Shore Medical Center	Skokie	60%	25
Westlake Community Hospital	Melrose Park	58%	31
Jersey Community Hospital	Jerseyville	56%	25
John H Stroger Jr Hospital of Cook County	Chicago	56%	131
Kenneth Hall Regional Hospital	East Saint Louis	54%	28
Norwegian-American Hospital	Chicago	24%	34
Weiss Memorial Hospital	Chicago	17%	29

Surgical Infection Prevention

20. Prophylactic Antibiotic Given

Hospital Name	City	Rate	Cases
Abraham Lincoln Memorial Hospital	Lincoln	98%	52
Neurologic and Orthopedic Insitute of Chicago	Chicago	97%	33
OSF Saint Mary Medical Center	Galesburg	97%	374
Genesis Medical Center-Illini Campus	Silvis	96%	92
Memorial Hospital	Chester	96%	28
Rush North Shore Medical Center	Skokie	96%	194
Silver Cross Hospital	Joliet	96%	499
Elmhurst Memorial Hospital	Elmhurst	95%	659
FHN Memorial Hospital	Freeport	95%	406
Loyola University Health System	Maywood	95%	283
Passavant Memorial Area Hospital	Jacksonville	95%	170
Saint Joseph Medical Center	Bloomington	95%	553
Advocate Lutheran General Children's Hospital	Park Ridge	94%	559
Alton Memorial Hospital	Alton	94%	275
Katherine Shaw Bethea Hospital	Dixon	94%	154
Memorial Medical Center	Springfield	94%	1496
Provena United Samaritans Medical Center	Danville	94%	270
Swedish American Hospital	Rockford	94%	1114
Advocate Good Samaritan Hospital	Downers Grove	93%	339
Alexian Brothers Medical Center	Elk Grove Village	93%	592
Anderson Hospital	Maryville	93%	568
CGH Medical Center	Sterling	93%	311
Mercy Harvard Hospital	Harvard	93%	41
Mercy Hospital	Chicago	93%	404
Rush-Copley Medical Center	Aurora	93%	456
Saint James OSF	Pontiac	93%	116
Sarah Bush Lincoln Health Center	Mattoon	93%	374
Trinity Medical Center	Rock Island	93%	281
Adventist LaGrange Memorial Hospital	La Grange	92%	151
Advocate Christ Med Ctr/Hope Children's	Oak Lawn	92%	345
MacNeal Hospital	Berwyn	92%	613
Northwestern Memorial Hospital	Chicago	92%	2347
Saint Alexius Medical Center	Hoffman Estates	92%	287
Saint Anthony Medical Center	Rockford	92%	1107
Saint Francis Hospital & Health Center	Blue Island	92%	391
Hammond-Henry Hospital	Geneseo	91%	35
Holy Cross Hospital	Chicago	91%	170
McDonough District Hospital	Macomb	91%	161
Methodist Medical Center of Illinois	Peoria	91%	681
Northwest Community Hospital	Arlington Heights	91%	339
Advocate Good Shephard Hospital	Barrington	90%	320
Advocate Illinois Masonic Medical Center	Chicago	90%	305
Memorial Medical Center	Woodstock	90%	326
Rush University Medical Center	Chicago	90%	425
Saint Francis Medical Center	Peoria	90%	1730
Evanston Hospital	Evanston	89%	2015
Gottlieb Memorial Hospital	Melrose Park	89%	167
Rockford Memorial Hospital	Rockford	89%	506
Saint Elizabeth's Hospital	Chicago	89%	121
Saint Margaret's Hospital	Spring Valley	89%	244
Saint Mary's Hospital	Decatur	89%	284
Sherman Hospital	Elgin	89%	696
Westlake Community Hospital	Melrose Park	89%	197
Ingalls Memorial Hospital	Harvey	88%	407
Saint John's Hospital	Springfield	88%	359
Herrin Hospital	Herrin	87%	170
John H Stroger Jr Hospital of Cook County	Chicago	87%	147
Saint Mary's Good Samaritan	Centralia	87%	196
Adventist GlenOaks Hospital	Glendale Heights	86%	37
Advocate Trinity Hospital	Chicago	86%	229
Bromenn Healthcare	Normal	86%	1056
Good Samaritan Regional Health Center	Mount Vernon	86%	442
Richland Memorial Hospital	Olney	86%	85
Saint Mary's Hospital of Kankakee	Kankakee	86%	336
Saints Mary & Elizabeth Medical Center	Chicago	86%	233
Advocate South Suburban Hospital	Hazel Crest	85%	236
Blessing Hospital	Quincy	85%	226
Galesburg Cottage Hospital	Galesburg	85%	177
Proctor Hospital	Peoria	85%	634
Saint Joseph Hospital	Chicago	85%	345
University of Chicago Hospitals	Chicago	85%	337
Gibson Community Hospital	Gibson City	84%	31
Saint James Hospital and Health Center	Olympia Fields	84%	379
Edward Hospital	Naperville	83%	983
Lake Forest Hospital	Lake Forest	83%	511
Provena Mercy Center	Aurora	83%	128
Valley West Community Hospital	Sandwich	83%	35
West Suburban Medical Center	Oak Park	83%	468
Decatur Memorial Hospital	Decatur	82%	448
Oak Forest Hospital of Cook County	Oak Forest	82%	28
Provena Covenant Medical Center	Urbana	82%	603
Provena Saint Joseph Hospital	Elgin	82%	77
Centegra Northern Illinois Medical Center	McHenry	81%	544
Palos Community Hospital	Palos Heights	81%	221
Saint Anthony's Memorial Hospital	Effingham	81%	661
Saint Elizabeth's Hospital	Belleville	81%	361
Thorek Hospital and Medical Center	Chicago	81%	59
Rush Oak Park Hospital	Oak Park	80%	80
Weiss Memorial Hospital	Chicago	80%	228
Hinsdale Hospital	Hinsdale	79%	175
Morris Hospital	Morris	79%	216
Riverside Medical Center	Kankakee	79%	402
Condell Medical Center	Libertyville	78%	503
Pekin Hospital	Pekin	78%	299
Michael Reese Hospital	Chicago	75%	96
Resurrection Medical Center	Chicago	75%	60
Saint Joseph Medical Center	Joliet	75%	989
Saint Mary's Hospital	Streator	75%	154
Kewanee Hospital	Kewanee	74%	34
Memorial Hospital	Belleville	74%	175
Vista Medical Center East	Waukegan	74%	263
Swedish Covenant Hospital	Chicago	73%	60
Crawford Memorial Hospital	Robinson	72%	67
Kishwaukee Community Hospital	De Kalb	72%	157
University of Illinois at Chicago Med Ctr	Chicago	72%	275
Central DuPage Hospital	Winfield	71%	297
Delnor Community Hospital	Geneva	71%	368
Saint Anthony Hospital	Chicago	70%	33
Saint Francis Hospital	Evanston	70%	310
Carle Foundation Hospital	Urbana	66%	215
Taylorville Memorial Hospital	Taylorville	66%	44
Our Lady of the Resurrection Medical Center	Chicago	63%	153
Saint Anthony's Health Center	Alton	63%	273
Red Bud Regional Hospital	Red Bud	62%	29
Saint Joseph's Hospital	Breese	60%	25
Mount Sinai Hospital	Chicago	59%	177
Little Company of Mary Hospital	Evergreen Park	58%	179

NOTE: Hospital profiles are in alphabetical order by state, then city, then hospital within the city; Rankings are sorted by rate in descending order and exclude hospitals with less than 25 cases; (1) The number of cases is too small (n<25) for purposes of reliably predicting hospital performance; (2) Measure reflects the hospital's indication that its submission was based upon a sample of its relevant discharges; (3) Rate reflects fewer than the maximum possible quarters of data for the measure; (4) Inaccurate information submitted and suppressed for one or more quarters; (5) No data is available from the hospital for this measure; Please refer to the User's Guide for a full explanation of data

Hospital Name	City	Rate	Cases
Illinois Valley Community Hospital	Peru	48%	184
Saint Francis Hospital	Litchfield	42%	40
Memorial Hospital Carbondale	Carbondale	40%	226
Graham Hospital	Canton	36%	143
Heartland Regional Medical Center	Marion	34%	260
Gateway Regional Medical Center	Granite City	30%	177
Crossroads Community Hospital	Mount Vernon	25%	113

21. Prophylactic Antibiotic Selection

Hospital Name	City	Rate	Cases
Advocate South Suburban Hospital	Hazel Crest	100%	62
Advocate Trinity Hospital	Chicago	100%	53
CGH Medical Center	Sterling	100%	73
Central DuPage Hospital	Winfield	100%	77
Herrin Hospital	Herrin	100%	41
Rush North Shore Medical Center	Skokie	100%	68
Rush Oak Park Hospital	Oak Park	100%	26
Saint James OSF	Pontiac	100%	31
Saint Mary's Hospital	Streator	100%	34
Advocate Good Samaritan Hospital	Downers Grove	99%	82
Alton Memorial Hospital	Alton	99%	70
Edward Hospital	Naperville	99%	335
Genesis Medical Center-Illini Campus	Silvis	99%	92
Northwest Community Hospital	Arlington Heights	99%	85
Saint Anthony Medical Center	Rockford	99%	280
Saint Anthony's Memorial Hospital	Effingham	99%	170
Adventist LaGrange Memorial Hospital	La Grange	98%	56
Advocate Lutheran General Children's Hospital	Park Ridge	98%	81
Alexian Brothers Medical Center	Elk Grove Village	98%	147
Ingalls Memorial Hospital	Harvey	98%	81
Kishwaukee Community Hospital	De Kalb	98%	62
Mercy Hospital	Chicago	98%	110
Northwestern Memorial Hospital	Chicago	98%	513
Resurrection Medical Center	Chicago	98%	60
Rush University Medical Center	Chicago	98%	102
Saint Joseph Medical Center	Bloomington	98%	121
Saint Margaret's Hospital	Spring Valley	98%	53
Swedish Covenant Hospital	Chicago	98%	62
Bromenn Healthcare	Normal	97%	241
Crossroads Community Hospital	Mount Vernon	97%	30
Katherine Shaw Bethea Hospital	Dixon	97%	35
Little Company of Mary Hospital	Evergreen Park	97%	61
Rockford Memorial Hospital	Rockford	97%	106
Advocate Illinois Masonic Medical Center	Chicago	96%	71
Galesburg Cottage Hospital	Galesburg	96%	52
Graham Hospital	Canton	96%	53
Illinois Valley Community Hospital	Peru	96%	46
Lake Forest Hospital	Lake Forest	96%	169
MacNeal Hospital	Berwyn	96%	136
Proctor Hospital	Peoria	96%	164
Saint Mary's Hospital	Decatur	96%	70
Saint Mary's Hospital of Kankakee	Kankakee	96%	78
Swedish American Hospital	Rockford	96%	247
Westlake Community Hospital	Melrose Park	96%	49
Anderson Hospital	Maryville	95%	118
Holy Cross Hospital	Chicago	95%	38
Morris Hospital	Morris	95%	42
OSF Saint Mary Medical Center	Galesburg	95%	100
Passavant Memorial Area Hospital	Jacksonville	95%	62
Sherman Hospital	Elgin	95%	174
Trinity Medical Center	Rock Island	95%	66
FHN Memorial Hospital	Freeport	94%	80
Riverside Medical Center	Kankakee	94%	94
Rush-Copley Medical Center	Aurora	94%	86
Saint Francis Hospital	Evanston	94%	111
Saint Joseph Hospital	Chicago	94%	90
West Suburban Medical Center	Oak Park	94%	105
Condell Medical Center	Libertyville	93%	82
Decatur Memorial Hospital	Decatur	93%	132
Elmhurst Memorial Hospital	Elmhurst	93%	59
Advocate Good Shephard Hospital	Barrington	92%	77
Good Samaritan Regional Health Center	Mount Vernon	92%	102
Hinsdale Hospital	Hinsdale	92%	59
Pekin Hospital	Pekin	92%	77
Saint Elizabeth's Hospital	Chicago	92%	26
Saint Francis Hospital & Health Center	Blue Island	92%	130
McDonough District Hospital	Macomb	91%	33
Memorial Hospital	Belleville	91%	58
Methodist Medical Center of Illinois	Peoria	91%	243
Evanston Hospital	Evanston	90%	520
Saint John's Hospital	Springfield	90%	86
Saint Joseph Medical Center	Joliet	90%	228
Silver Cross Hospital	Joliet	90%	124
Weiss Memorial Hospital	Chicago	90%	62
Centegra Northern Illinois Medical Center	McHenry	89%	121
Gateway Regional Medical Center	Granite City	89%	47
Heartland Regional Medical Center	Marion	89%	75
Memorial Hospital Carbondale	Carbondale	89%	72
Provena United Samaritans Medical Center	Danville	89%	64
Saint James Hospital and Health Center	Olympia Fields	89%	93
University of Illinois at Chicago Med Ctr	Chicago	89%	57
Loyola University Health System	Maywood	88%	74
Memorial Medical Center	Springfield	88%	84
Saint Alexius Medical Center	Hoffman Estates	87%	61
Saint Francis Medical Center	Peoria	87%	406
Mount Sinai Hospital	Chicago	86%	49
Provena Covenant Medical Center	Urbana	86%	153
Memorial Medical Center	Woodstock	85%	74
Carle Foundation Hospital	Urbana	82%	71
Gottlieb Memorial Hospital	Melrose Park	82%	55
Saint Anthony's Health Center	Alton	82%	61
Saints Mary & Elizabeth Medical Center	Chicago	82%	60
Richland Memorial Hospital	Olney	81%	27
Saint Elizabeth's Hospital	Belleville	80%	84
Saint Joseph's Hospital	Breese	80%	25
Delnor Community Hospital	Geneva	79%	89
Palos Community Hospital	Palos Heights	78%	73
Blessing Hospital	Quincy	77%	112
Saint Mary's Good Samaritan	Centralia	77%	30
Advocate Christ Med Ctr/Hope Children's	Oak Lawn	72%	88
Sarah Bush Lincoln Health Center	Mattoon	71%	91
Michael Reese Hospital	Chicago	69%	26
University of Chicago Hospitals	Chicago	65%	69
Vista Medical Center East	Waukegan	65%	72
John H Stroger Jr Hospital of Cook County	Chicago	50%	44

22. Prophylactic Antibiotic Stopped

Hospital Name	City	Rate	Cases
Swedish Covenant Hospital	Chicago	100%	57
Saint Francis Hospital	Litchfield	97%	37
Abraham Lincoln Memorial Hospital	Lincoln	96%	47
Michael Reese Hospital	Chicago	96%	93
Katherine Shaw Bethea Hospital	Dixon	93%	139
Memorial Medical Center	Springfield	93%	1456
Passavant Memorial Area Hospital	Jacksonville	93%	161
Saint John's Hospital	Springfield	92%	354
Crossroads Community Hospital	Mount Vernon	90%	112
OSF Saint Mary Medical Center	Galesburg	90%	363
Advocate Christ Med Ctr/Hope Children's	Oak Lawn	89%	337
Methodist Medical Center of Illinois	Peoria	89%	650
Evanston Hospital	Evanston	88%	1962
Graham Hospital	Canton	88%	137
Loyola University Health System	Maywood	88%	276
Northwestern Memorial Hospital	Chicago	88%	2308
Rush North Shore Medical Center	Skokie	88%	192
Anderson Hospital	Maryville	87%	548
Saint Anthony's Memorial Hospital	Effingham	87%	653
Saint Francis Medical Center	Peoria	87%	1707
Proctor Hospital	Peoria	86%	623
Rush University Medical Center	Chicago	86%	417
Rockford Memorial Hospital	Rockford	85%	498
Saint Anthony Medical Center	Rockford	85%	1077
Adventist GlenOaks Hospital	Glendale Heights	83%	35
Advocate Good Shephard Hospital	Barrington	83%	314
McDonough District Hospital	Macomb	82%	154
Neurologic and Orthopedic Insitute of Chicago	Chicago	82%	33
Adventist LaGrange Memorial Hospital	La Grange	81%	146
Advocate Good Samaritan Hospital	Downers Grove	81%	323
Red Bud Regional Hospital	Red Bud	81%	27
FHN Memorial Hospital	Freeport	80%	388
Mercy Hospital	Chicago	80%	391
Saint Francis Hospital	Evanston	80%	290
Saint Joseph's Hospital	Breese	80%	25
Sherman Hospital	Elgin	80%	681
Taylorville Memorial Hospital	Taylorville	80%	41
University of Illinois at Chicago Med Ctr	Chicago	80%	268
Centegra Northern Illinois Medical Center	McHenry	79%	525
Galesburg Cottage Hospital	Galesburg	79%	174
Herrin Hospital	Herrin	79%	151
John H Stroger Jr Hospital of Cook County	Chicago	79%	141
MacNeal Hospital	Berwyn	79%	563
Saint Joseph Medical Center	Bloomington	79%	542
Carle Foundation Hospital	Urbana	78%	205
Alexian Brothers Medical Center	Elk Grove Village	77%	554
Kishwaukee Community Hospital	De Kalb	77%	149
Memorial Medical Center	Woodstock	77%	311
Saint Alexius Medical Center	Hoffman Estates	77%	277
Saint Elizabeth's Hospital	Chicago	76%	105

NOTE: Hospital profiles are in alphabetical order by state, then city, then hospital within the city; Rankings are sorted by rate in descending order and exclude hospitals with less than 25 cases; (1) The number of cases is too small (n<25) for purposes of reliably predicting hospital performance; (2) Measure reflects the hospital's indication that its submission was based upon a sample of its relevant discharges; (3) Rate reflects fewer than the maximum possible quarters of data for the measure; (4) Inaccurate information submitted and suppressed for one or more quarters; (5) No data is available from the hospital for this measure; Please refer to the User's Guide for a full explanation of data

Saint Mary's Hospital	Decatur	76%	272
Silver Cross Hospital	Joliet	75%	463
University of Chicago Hospitals	Chicago	75%	338
Northwest Community Hospital	Arlington Heights	74%	323
Provena United Samaritans Medical Center	Danville	74%	249
Trinity Medical Center	Rock Island	74%	269
Genesis Medical Center-Illini Campus	Silvis	73%	91
Good Samaritan Regional Health Center	Mount Vernon	73%	426
Saint Mary's Hospital	Streator	73%	134
Saint Elizabeth's Hospital	Belleville	72%	350
Saint Mary's Good Samaritan	Centralia	72%	184
Ingalls Memorial Hospital	Harvey	71%	404
Provena Saint Joseph Hospital	Elgin	71%	76
Advocate Illinois Masonic Medical Center	Chicago	70%	293
CGH Medical Center	Sterling	70%	298
Kewanee Hospital	Kewanee	70%	33
Advocate South Suburban Hospital	Hazel Crest	69%	225
Provena Mercy Center	Aurora	69%	127
Saint Joseph Hospital	Chicago	69%	332
Central DuPage Hospital	Winfield	68%	289
Riverside Medical Center	Kankakee	68%	380
Swedish American Hospital	Rockford	68%	1100
Bromenn Healthcare	Normal	67%	1022
Memorial Hospital	Belleville	67%	163
Gateway Regional Medical Center	Granite City	66%	176
Provena Covenant Medical Center	Urbana	66%	585
Advocate Lutheran General Children's Hospital	Park Ridge	65%	528
Advocate Trinity Hospital	Chicago	65%	220
Alton Memorial Hospital	Alton	65%	263
Delnor Community Hospital	Geneva	65%	353
Holy Cross Hospital	Chicago	65%	153
Rush-Copley Medical Center	Aurora	64%	439
Saint Mary's Hospital of Kankakee	Kankakee	64%	328
Saints Mary & Elizabeth Medical Center	Chicago	64%	219
Vista Medical Center East	Waukegan	64%	259
Blessing Hospital	Quincy	63%	214
Sarah Bush Lincoln Health Center	Mattoon	63%	365
Lake Forest Hospital	Lake Forest	62%	498
Decatur Memorial Hospital	Decatur	61%	432
Elmhurst Memorial Hospital	Elmhurst	61%	628
Morris Hospital	Morris	61%	207
Resurrection Medical Center	Chicago	61%	51
Condell Medical Center	Libertyville	59%	494
Illinois Valley Community Hospital	Peru	57%	181
Memorial Hospital Carbondale	Carbondale	57%	218
Richland Memorial Hospital	Olney	57%	82
Mercy Harvard Hospital	Harvard	56%	41
Palos Community Hospital	Palos Heights	56%	213
Pekin Hospital	Pekin	56%	287
Saint James Hospital and Health Center	Olympia Fields	55%	365
Westlake Community Hospital	Melrose Park	55%	185
Little Company of Mary Hospital	Evergreen Park	52%	163
Crawford Memorial Hospital	Robinson	51%	63
Saint Francis Hospital & Health Center	Blue Island	51%	363
West Suburban Medical Center	Oak Park	50%	448
Hinsdale Hospital	Hinsdale	48%	162
Saint Joseph Medical Center	Joliet	47%	959
Gottlieb Memorial Hospital	Melrose Park	46%	162
Saint James OSF	Pontiac	46%	112
Hammond-Henry Hospital	Geneseo	45%	33
Mount Sinai Hospital	Chicago	45%	156
Saint Anthony Hospital	Chicago	45%	31
Saint Anthony's Health Center	Alton	45%	260
Heartland Regional Medical Center	Marion	44%	239
Edward Hospital	Naperville	42%	954
Our Lady of the Resurrection Medical Center	Chicago	42%	133
Weiss Memorial Hospital	Chicago	38%	209
Oak Forest Hospital of Cook County	Oak Forest	36%	25
Rush Oak Park Hospital	Oak Park	36%	77
Saint Margaret's Hospital	Spring Valley	31%	239
Thorek Hospital and Medical Center	Chicago	31%	58
Gibson Community Hospital	Gibson City	29%	31
Valley West Community Hospital	Sandwich	26%	34

Pregnancy Care

23. Inpatient Neonatal Mortality

Hospital Name	City	Rate	Cases
Advocate South Suburban Hospital	Hazel Crest	0.00%	255
Genesis Medical Center-Illini Campus	Silvis	0.00%	780
Good Samaritan Regional Health Center	Mount Vernon	0.00%	739
Greenville Regional Hospital	Greenville	0.00%	130
McDonough District Hospital	Macomb	0.00%	391
Saint Elizabeth's Hospital	Belleville	0.00%	1255
Saint Mary's Hospital	Streator	0.00%	215
Saint Mary's Hospital of Kankakee	Kankakee	0.00%	553
Delnor Community Hospital	Geneva	0.06%	1587
Swedish American Hospital	Rockford	0.17%	2300
Advocate Trinity Hospital	Chicago	0.18%	1697
Northwest Community Hospital	Arlington Heights	0.18%	3398
Provena Mercy Center	Aurora	0.19%	1580
Little Company of Mary Hospital	Evergreen Park	0.21%	1436
Memorial Hospital Carbondale	Carbondale	0.21%	1436
Saint Joseph Medical Center	Joliet	0.21%	1926
Provena United Samaritans Medical Center	Danville	0.22%	896
Saint Mary's Good Samaritan	Centralia	0.22%	459
Saint Joseph's Hospital	Breese	0.23%	427
Elmhurst Memorial Hospital	Elmhurst	0.25%	1570
Touchette Regional Hospital	Centreville	0.31%	652
Provena Covenant Medical Center	Urbana	0.32%	1236
Sherman Hospital	Elgin	0.34%	891
Alton Memorial Hospital	Alton	0.35%	566
Saint Mary's Hospital	Decatur	0.35%	567
Evanston Hospital	Evanston	0.36%	4959
Decatur Memorial Hospital	Decatur	0.37%	1088
Provident Hospital	Chicago	0.38%	526
Silver Cross Hospital	Joliet	0.39%	2076
Jackson Park Hospital & Medical Center	Chicago	0.40%	251
Riverside Medical Center	Kankakee	0.40%	1238
Saint James OSF	Pontiac	0.44%	226
Northwestern Memorial Hospital	Chicago	0.46%	10299
Rush-Copley Medical Center	Aurora	0.54%	3717
Advocate Good Shephard Hospital	Barrington	0.55%	363
Edward Hospital	Naperville	0.55%	3972
Ingalls Memorial Hospital	Harvey	0.55%	1461
Advocate Illinois Masonic Medical Center	Chicago	0.61%	657
Provena Saint Joseph Hospital	Elgin	0.66%	607
Mount Sinai Hospital	Chicago	0.71%	3951
Advocate Good Samaritan Hospital	Downers Grove	0.73%	1770
Advocate Christ Med Ctr/Hope Children's	Oak Lawn	1.03%	871
Community Hospital of Ottawa	Ottawa	1.04%	288
Advocate Lutheran General Children's Hospital	Park Ridge	1.09%	822
John H Stroger Jr Hospital of Cook County	Chicago	1.91%	1254
Loyola University Health System	Maywood	2.27%	1895

24. Third or Fourth Degree Laceration

Hospital Name	City	Rate	Cases
Mount Sinai Hospital	Chicago	0.98%	2660
Jackson Park Hospital & Medical Center	Chicago	1.08%	186
Touchette Regional Hospital	Centreville	1.31%	459
Advocate Illinois Masonic Medical Center	Chicago	1.41%	707
Saint Mary's Hospital	Decatur	1.45%	414
Provena United Samaritans Medical Center	Danville	1.58%	634
Advocate South Suburban Hospital	Hazel Crest	1.75%	343
Advocate Trinity Hospital	Chicago	1.92%	1301
John H Stroger Jr Hospital of Cook County	Chicago	1.95%	768
Ingalls Memorial Hospital	Harvey	2.06%	1067
Riverside Medical Center	Kankakee	2.23%	852
Community Hospital of Ottawa	Ottawa	2.27%	220
Silver Cross Hospital	Joliet	2.28%	1446
Saint Elizabeth's Hospital	Belleville	2.34%	942
Little Company of Mary Hospital	Evergreen Park	2.36%	932
Loyola University Health System	Maywood	2.41%	997
Saint Joseph's Hospital	Breese	2.43%	329
Saint Mary's Hospital	Streator	2.47%	162
Provident Hospital	Chicago	2.49%	401
Memorial Hospital Carbondale	Carbondale	2.59%	1002
Sherman Hospital	Elgin	2.70%	667
McDonough District Hospital	Macomb	2.80%	286
Saint Mary's Good Samaritan	Centralia	2.90%	310
Advocate Good Shephard Hospital	Barrington	3.03%	462
Provena Covenant Medical Center	Urbana	3.15%	890
Rush-Copley Medical Center	Aurora	3.28%	2503
Good Samaritan Regional Health Center	Mount Vernon	3.36%	476
Genesis Medical Center-Illini Campus	Silvis	3.49%	545
Alton Memorial Hospital	Alton	3.52%	398
Saint James OSF	Pontiac	3.57%	140
Elmhurst Memorial Hospital	Elmhurst	3.68%	1168
Advocate Good Samaritan Hospital	Downers Grove	3.74%	1070
Swedish American Hospital	Rockford	3.82%	1572
Saint Mary's Hospital of Kankakee	Kankakee	3.88%	387
Advocate Christ Med Ctr/Hope Children's	Oak Lawn	4.05%	642
Saint Joseph Medical Center	Joliet	4.16%	1202
Evanston Hospital	Evanston	4.51%	3393
Provena Mercy Center	Aurora	4.60%	999
Advocate Lutheran General Children's Hospital	Park Ridge	4.76%	630
Provena Saint Joseph Hospital	Elgin	4.94%	445
Decatur Memorial Hospital	Decatur	5.03%	656

NOTE: Hospital profiles are in alphabetical order by state, then city, then hospital within the city; Rankings are sorted by rate in descending order and exclude hospitals with less than 25 cases; (1) The number of cases is too small (n<25) for purposes of reliably predicting hospital performance; (2) Measure reflects the hospital's indication that its submission was based upon a sample of its relevant discharges; (3) Rate reflects fewer than the maximum possible quarters of data for the measure; (4) Inaccurate information submitted and suppressed for one or more quarters; (5) No data is available from the hospital for this measure; Please refer to the User's Guide for a full explanation of data

Northwest Community Hospital	Arlington Heights	5.29%	2099
Northwestern Memorial Hospital	Chicago	6.35%	7198
Edward Hospital	Naperville	6.58%	2506
Delnor Community Hospital	Geneva	8.33%	984
Greenville Regional Hospital	Greenville	10.53%	76

NOTE: Hospital profiles are in alphabetical order by state, then city, then hospital within the city; Rankings are sorted by rate in descending order and exclude hospitals with less than 25 cases; (1) The number of cases is too small (n<25) for purposes of reliably predicting hospital performance; (2) Measure reflects the hospital's indication that its submission was based upon a sample of its relevant discharges; (3) Rate reflects fewer than the maximum possible quarters of data for the measure; (4) Inaccurate information submitted and suppressed for one or more quarters; (5) No data is available from the hospital for this measure; Please refer to the User's Guide for a full explanation of data

Alton Memorial Hospital

One Memorial Drive
Alton, IL 62002
Ownership: Voluntary non-profit - Private
Emergency Services: Yes
Phone: 618-463-7311
Fax: 618-463-7850
Accredited: Yes
Licensed Beds: 222

Key Personnel:

CEO. . . . . Ronald B McMullen
Chief of Medical Staff. . . . . David Burnside
Director Medical/Surgical Nursing . . . . Karen Barnett
OB/GYN Womens Health. . . . . Alicia Jayboush

Measure	Cases	This Hospital	State Average	U.S. Average	Top Hospital
Heart Attack Care					
ACE Inhibitor or ARB for LVSD[1]	12	92%	79%	82%	100%
Aspirin at Arrival	106	96%	93%	92%	100%
Aspirin at Discharge	87	95%	90%	90%	100%
Beta Blocker at Arrival	103	98%	87%	87%	100%
Beta Blocker at Discharge	92	100%	88%	90%	100%
Fibrinolytic Medication Timing	0	-	21%	31%	100%
PCI Within 90 Minutes of Arrival	0	-	47%	54%	95%
Smoking Cessation Advice	36	100%	84%	88%	100%
Heart Failure Care					
ACE Inhibitor or ARB for LVSD	49	100%	83%	82%	100%
Discharge Instructions	140	92%	67%	61%	93%
Evaluation of LVS Function	183	96%	88%	83%	99%
Smoking Cessation Advice[1]	19	100%	83%	82%	100%
Pneumonia Care					
Appropriate Initial Antibiotic	165	84%	83%	83%	94%
Blood Culture Timing	184	95%	91%	90%	100%
Influenza Vaccine	44	89%	63%	70%	100%
Initial Antibiotic Timing	243	91%	81%	80%	93%
Oxygenation Assessment	283	100%	99%	99%	100%
Pneumococcal Vaccine	186	92%	62%	69%	94%
Smoking Cessation Advice	58	98%	80%	80%	100%
Surgical Infection Prevention					
Prophylactic Antibiotic Given	275	94%	74%	77%	95%
Prophylactic Antibiotic Selection	70	99%	91%	90%	100%
Prophylactic Antibiotic Stopped	263	65%	67%	72%	95%
Pregnancy Care					
Inpatient Neonatal Mortality	566	0.35%	-	-	-
Third or Fourth Degree Laceration	398	3.52%	3.89%	3.63%	3.27%

Saint Anthony's Health Center

1 Saint Anthony's Way
PO Box 340
Alton, IL 62002
URL: www.sahc.org
Ownership: Voluntary non-profit - Church
Emergency Services: Yes
Phone: 618-465-2571
Fax: 618-474-4860
Accredited: Yes
Licensed Beds: 292

Key Personnel:

Administrator/President . . . . William E Kessler
Chief Medical Staff. . . . . Joesph Paone, MD
Director Cardiology . . . . Joe Lombardo
Emergency Room . . . . Erick Falconer, MD

Measure	Cases	This Hospital	State Average	U.S. Average	Top Hospital
Heart Attack Care					
ACE Inhibitor or ARB for LVSD[1]	14	71%	79%	82%	100%
Aspirin at Arrival	79	91%	93%	92%	100%
Aspirin at Discharge	64	94%	90%	90%	100%
Beta Blocker at Arrival	72	86%	87%	87%	100%
Beta Blocker at Discharge	71	87%	88%	90%	100%
Fibrinolytic Medication Timing[1]	4	50%	21%	31%	100%
PCI Within 90 Minutes of Arrival[1]	3	0%	47%	54%	95%
Smoking Cessation Advice[1]	18	89%	84%	88%	100%
Heart Failure Care					
ACE Inhibitor or ARB for LVSD	62	76%	83%	82%	100%
Discharge Instructions	146	69%	67%	61%	93%
Evaluation of LVS Function	212	71%	88%	83%	99%
Smoking Cessation Advice	41	78%	83%	82%	100%
Pneumonia Care					
Appropriate Initial Antibiotic	140	90%	83%	83%	94%
Blood Culture Timing	154	98%	91%	90%	100%
Influenza Vaccine	38	61%	63%	70%	100%
Initial Antibiotic Timing	221	82%	81%	80%	93%
Oxygenation Assessment	270	100%	99%	99%	100%
Pneumococcal Vaccine	168	76%	62%	69%	94%
Smoking Cessation Advice	61	87%	80%	80%	100%
Surgical Infection Prevention					
Prophylactic Antibiotic Given	273	63%	74%	77%	95%
Prophylactic Antibiotic Selection	61	82%	91%	90%	100%
Prophylactic Antibiotic Stopped	260	45%	67%	72%	95%
Pregnancy Care					
Inpatient Neonatal Mortality	-	-	-	-	-
Third or Fourth Degree Laceration	-	-	3.89%	3.63%	3.27%

Union County Hospital District

517 N Main Street
Anna, IL 62906
Ownership: Govt - Hospital District or Authority
Emergency Services: Yes
Phone: 618-833-4511
Fax: 618-833-4183
Accredited: No
Licensed Beds: 58

Key Personnel:

CEO. . . . . James R Farris
Chief Medical Staff. . . . . Deanna St Germain, DO
Emergency Room . . . . Judy Lewis, RN
Chief Radiology . . . . Peter Wories

Measure	Cases	This Hospital	State Average	U.S. Average	Top Hospital
Heart Attack Care					
ACE Inhibitor or ARB for LVSD[3]	0	-	79%	82%	100%
Aspirin at Arrival[1,3]	4	100%	93%	92%	100%
Aspirin at Discharge[1,3]	3	67%	90%	90%	100%
Beta Blocker at Arrival[1,3]	3	100%	87%	87%	100%
Beta Blocker at Discharge[1,3]	3	100%	88%	90%	100%
Fibrinolytic Medication Timing[3]	0	-	21%	31%	100%
PCI Within 90 Minutes of Arrival[5]	-	-	47%	54%	95%
Smoking Cessation Advice[3]	0	-	84%	88%	100%
Heart Failure Care					
ACE Inhibitor or ARB for LVSD[1]	7	100%	83%	82%	100%
Discharge Instructions	34	65%	67%	61%	93%
Evaluation of LVS Function	42	83%	88%	83%	99%
Smoking Cessation Advice[1]	2	50%	83%	82%	100%
Pneumonia Care					
Appropriate Initial Antibiotic	40	75%	83%	83%	94%
Blood Culture Timing	29	76%	91%	90%	100%
Influenza Vaccine[1]	9	67%	63%	70%	100%
Initial Antibiotic Timing	73	88%	81%	80%	93%
Oxygenation Assessment	85	100%	99%	99%	100%
Pneumococcal Vaccine	48	77%	62%	69%	94%
Smoking Cessation Advice[1]	24	79%	80%	80%	100%
Surgical Infection Prevention					
Prophylactic Antibiotic Given[2,3]	0	-	74%	77%	95%
Prophylactic Antibiotic Selection[2]	0	-	91%	90%	100%
Prophylactic Antibiotic Stopped[2,3]	0	-	67%	72%	95%
Pregnancy Care					
Inpatient Neonatal Mortality	-	-	-	-	-
Third or Fourth Degree Laceration	-	-	3.89%	3.63%	3.27%

Northwest Community Hospital

800 W Central Road
Arlington Heights, IL 60005
URL: www.nch.org
Ownership: Voluntary non-profit - Other
Emergency Services: Yes
Phone: 847-618-1000
Fax: 847-618-5509
Accredited: Yes
Licensed Beds: 400

Key Personnel:

Administrator/President . . . . Bruce Crowther
Chief Medical Staff. . . . . Donald E Pochly
Emergency Room . . . . Nancy Ryan, MD
Director Infection/Disease Control . . . . Karen Gormen
CCU Spvg. Nurse . . . . Phyllis Cerone
OB/GYN Womens Health. . . . . Roger Leavy, MD
Chief Radiology . . . . Lee A Malmed, MD
Director Respiratory Therapy . . . . Bobbi Lawrence

Measure	Cases	This Hospital	State Average	U.S. Average	Top Hospital

NOTE: Hospital profiles are in alphabetical order by state, then city, then hospital within the city; Rankings are sorted by rate in descending order and exclude hospitals with less than 25 cases; (1) The number of cases is too small (n<25) for purposes of reliably predicting hospital performance; (2) Measure reflects the hospital's indication that its submission was based upon a sample of its relevant discharges; (3) Rate reflects fewer than the maximum possible quarters of data for the measure; (4) Inaccurate information submitted and suppressed for one or more quarters; (5) No data is available from the hospital for this measure; Please refer to the User's Guide for a full explanation of data

Heart Attack Care					
ACE Inhibitor or ARB for LVSD	46	96%	79%	82%	100%
Aspirin at Arrival	389	98%	93%	92%	100%
Aspirin at Discharge	337	99%	90%	90%	100%
Beta Blocker at Arrival	327	99%	87%	87%	100%
Beta Blocker at Discharge	382	99%	88%	90%	100%
Fibrinolytic Medication Timing	0	-	21%	31%	100%
PCI Within 90 Minutes of Arrival[1]	15	27%	47%	54%	95%
Smoking Cessation Advice	84	99%	84%	88%	100%
Heart Failure Care					
ACE Inhibitor or ARB for LVSD[2]	91	79%	83%	82%	100%
Discharge Instructions[2]	213	51%	67%	61%	93%
Evaluation of LVS Function[2]	313	97%	88%	83%	99%
Smoking Cessation Advice[1,2]	24	96%	83%	82%	100%
Pneumonia Care					
Appropriate Initial Antibiotic[2]	85	86%	83%	83%	94%
Blood Culture Timing[2]	111	92%	91%	90%	100%
Influenza Vaccine[1,2]	22	95%	63%	70%	100%
Initial Antibiotic Timing[2]	173	88%	81%	80%	93%
Oxygenation Assessment[2]	189	100%	99%	99%	100%
Pneumococcal Vaccine[2]	140	87%	62%	69%	94%
Smoking Cessation Advice[1,2]	23	78%	80%	80%	100%
Surgical Infection Prevention					
Prophylactic Antibiotic Given[2]	339	91%	74%	77%	95%
Prophylactic Antibiotic Selection[2]	85	99%	91%	90%	100%
Prophylactic Antibiotic Stopped[2]	323	74%	67%	72%	95%
Pregnancy Care					
Inpatient Neonatal Mortality	3,398	0.18%	-	-	-
Third or Fourth Degree Laceration	2,099	5.29%	3.89%	3.63%	3.27%

Provena Mercy Center

Alternate Name: Mercy Center for Health Care Services
1325 N Highland Avenue — Phone: 630-859-2222
Aurora, IL 60506 — Fax: 630-801-2608
URL: www.provenamercy.com
Ownership: Voluntary non-profit - Church — Accredited: Yes
Emergency Services: Yes — Licensed Beds: 356

Key Personnel:

President/CEO. . . . . Jack Barto
Chief Medical Staff. . . . . Michael Loebach, MD
Emergency Room . . . . James Kolka, MD
Director Infection/Disease Control . . . . Kathy Hettinger
CCU Spvg. Nurse . . . . Beth Martinez, RN
Director Medical/Surgical Nursing . . . . Beth Martinez, RN
Chief Radiology . . . . EH Dolin, MD

Measure	Cases	This Hospital	State Average	U.S. Average	Top Hospital
Heart Attack Care					
ACE Inhibitor or ARB for LVSD	41	68%	79%	82%	100%
Aspirin at Arrival	166	99%	93%	92%	100%
Aspirin at Discharge	184	97%	90%	90%	100%
Beta Blocker at Arrival	159	97%	87%	87%	100%
Beta Blocker at Discharge	183	98%	88%	90%	100%
Fibrinolytic Medication Timing[3]	0	-	21%	31%	100%
PCI Within 90 Minutes of Arrival[1]	9	33%	47%	54%	95%
Smoking Cessation Advice[1,3]	12	92%	84%	88%	100%
Heart Failure Care					
ACE Inhibitor or ARB for LVSD	117	76%	83%	82%	100%
Discharge Instructions[3]	32	50%	67%	61%	93%
Evaluation of LVS Function	273	92%	88%	83%	99%
Smoking Cessation Advice[1,3]	3	33%	83%	82%	100%
Pneumonia Care					
Appropriate Initial Antibiotic[3]	37	78%	83%	83%	94%
Blood Culture Timing[3]	59	90%	91%	90%	100%
Influenza Vaccine[5]	-	-	63%	70%	100%
Initial Antibiotic Timing	309	75%	81%	80%	93%
Oxygenation Assessment	379	100%	99%	99%	100%
Pneumococcal Vaccine	220	34%	62%	69%	94%
Smoking Cessation Advice[1,3]	23	4%	80%	80%	100%
Surgical Infection Prevention					
Prophylactic Antibiotic Given[2,3]	128	83%	74%	77%	95%
Prophylactic Antibiotic Selection[5]	-	-	91%	90%	100%
Prophylactic Antibiotic Stopped[2,3]	127	69%	67%	72%	95%
Pregnancy Care					
Inpatient Neonatal Mortality	1,580	0.19%	-	-	-
Third or Fourth Degree Laceration	999	4.60%	3.89%	3.63%	3.27%

Rush-Copley Medical Center

Alternate Name: Copley Memorial Hospital
2000 Ogden Avenue — Phone: 630-978-6200
Aurora, IL 60504 — Fax: 630-978-6888
URL: www.rushcopley.com
Ownership: Voluntary non-profit - Private — Accredited: Yes
Emergency Services: Yes — Licensed Beds: 150

Key Personnel:

President/CEO. . . . . Barry Finn
Cardiac Lab Manager. . . . . Sharon Domurat, RN
Chief Medical Staff. . . . . James Ferlmann, MD
Emergency Room . . . . Nancy Wilson, RN
Infection Control. . . . . Maria Montero
ICU . . . . Brenda Carlevato, RN
Manager Medical Surgery . . . . Janet Smith, RN
Respiratory/Cardiopulmonary. . . . . Ruth Karales

Measure	Cases	This Hospital	State Average	U.S. Average	Top Hospital
Heart Attack Care					
ACE Inhibitor or ARB for LVSD	30	100%	79%	82%	100%
Aspirin at Arrival	154	99%	93%	92%	100%
Aspirin at Discharge	153	97%	90%	90%	100%
Beta Blocker at Arrival	118	99%	87%	87%	100%
Beta Blocker at Discharge	161	99%	88%	90%	100%
Fibrinolytic Medication Timing[1]	2	50%	21%	31%	100%
PCI Within 90 Minutes of Arrival[1]	2	100%	47%	54%	95%
Smoking Cessation Advice	52	100%	84%	88%	100%
Heart Failure Care					
ACE Inhibitor or ARB for LVSD	76	100%	83%	82%	100%
Discharge Instructions	189	98%	67%	61%	93%
Evaluation of LVS Function	234	99%	88%	83%	99%
Smoking Cessation Advice	48	100%	83%	82%	100%
Pneumonia Care					
Appropriate Initial Antibiotic	132	95%	83%	83%	94%
Blood Culture Timing	91	92%	91%	90%	100%
Influenza Vaccine[4,5]	-	-	63%	70%	100%
Initial Antibiotic Timing	175	95%	81%	80%	93%
Oxygenation Assessment	230	100%	99%	99%	100%
Pneumococcal Vaccine	130	79%	62%	69%	94%
Smoking Cessation Advice	60	100%	80%	80%	100%
Surgical Infection Prevention					
Prophylactic Antibiotic Given[2]	456	93%	74%	77%	95%
Prophylactic Antibiotic Selection[2]	86	94%	91%	90%	100%
Prophylactic Antibiotic Stopped[2]	439	64%	67%	72%	95%
Pregnancy Care					
Inpatient Neonatal Mortality	3,717	0.54%	-	-	-
Third or Fourth Degree Laceration	2,503	3.28%	3.89%	3.63%	3.27%

Advocate Good Shephard Hospital

450 W Highway 22 — Toll-Free: 847-381-9600
Barrington, IL 60010 — Phone: 847-381-0123
Fax: 847-842-4060
URL: www.advocatehealth.com
Ownership: Voluntary non-profit - Church — Accredited: Yes
Emergency Services: Yes — Licensed Beds: 154

Key Personnel:

CEO. . . . . Karen Lambert
Director Medical/Surgical Nursing . . . . Anne Rychlik
OB/GYN Womens Health. . . . . Daniel Pesavento, MD
Chief Radiology . . . . George Cassidy, MD
Director Respiratory Therapy . . . . Tim McDonnell

Measure	Cases	This Hospital	State Average	U.S. Average	Top Hospital
Heart Attack Care					
ACE Inhibitor or ARB for LVSD	42	86%	79%	82%	100%
Aspirin at Arrival	179	98%	93%	92%	100%
Aspirin at Discharge	201	99%	90%	90%	100%
Beta Blocker at Arrival	152	99%	87%	87%	100%

NOTE: Hospital profiles are in alphabetical order by state, then city, then hospital within the city; Rankings are sorted by rate in descending order and exclude hospitals with less than 25 cases; (1) The number of cases is too small (n<25) for purposes of reliably predicting hospital performance; (2) Measure reflects the hospital's indication that its submission was based upon a sample of its relevant discharges; (3) Rate reflects fewer than the maximum possible quarters of data for the measure; (4) Inaccurate information submitted and suppressed for one or more quarters; (5) No data is available from the hospital for this measure; Please refer to the User's Guide for a full explanation of data

Beta Blocker at Discharge	252	98%	88%	90%	100%
Fibrinolytic Medication Timing	0	-	21%	31%	100%
PCI Within 90 Minutes of Arrival[1]	5	80%	47%	54%	95%
Smoking Cessation Advice	74	99%	84%	88%	100%
Heart Failure Care					
ACE Inhibitor or ARB for LVSD[2]	92	98%	83%	82%	100%
Discharge Instructions[2]	278	83%	67%	61%	93%
Evaluation of LVS Function[2]	340	99%	88%	83%	99%
Smoking Cessation Advice[2]	41	100%	83%	82%	100%
Pneumonia Care					
Appropriate Initial Antibiotic[2]	70	81%	83%	83%	94%
Blood Culture Timing[2]	49	94%	91%	90%	100%
Influenza Vaccine	26	50%	63%	70%	100%
Initial Antibiotic Timing[2]	132	84%	81%	80%	93%
Oxygenation Assessment[2]	158	100%	99%	99%	100%
Pneumococcal Vaccine[2]	119	59%	62%	69%	94%
Smoking Cessation Advice[1,2]	19	63%	80%	80%	100%
Surgical Infection Prevention					
Prophylactic Antibiotic Given[2]	320	90%	74%	77%	95%
Prophylactic Antibiotic Selection[2]	77	92%	91%	90%	100%
Prophylactic Antibiotic Stopped[2]	314	83%	67%	72%	95%
Pregnancy Care					
Inpatient Neonatal Mortality[2]	363	0.55%	-	-	-
Third or Fourth Degree Laceration[2]	462	3.03%	3.89%	3.63%	3.27%

Memorial Hospital

4500 Memorial Drive
Belleville, IL 62226
Phone: 618-233-7750
Fax: 618-257-6911
E-mail: bschneider@memhosp.com
URL: www.memhosp.com
Ownership: Voluntary non-profit - Private
Accredited: Yes
Emergency Services: Yes
Licensed Beds: 391

Key Personnel:

Administrator/President . . . . Harry R Maier
Chief Medical Staff. . . . . Thomas Cahill, MD
Chief Catheterization Laboratory . . . . B Dincer, MD
Emergency Room . . . . Thomas Byrne, MD
Director Infection/Disease Control . . . . Kathy Harms
OB/GYN Womens Health. . . . . William Chadwick, MD
Director Respiratory Therapy . . . . Micheal Urban

Measure	Cases	This Hospital	State Average	U.S. Average	Top Hospital
Heart Attack Care					
ACE Inhibitor or ARB for LVSD	36	69%	79%	82%	100%
Aspirin at Arrival	151	99%	93%	92%	100%
Aspirin at Discharge	130	98%	90%	90%	100%
Beta Blocker at Arrival	146	93%	87%	87%	100%
Beta Blocker at Discharge	150	98%	88%	90%	100%
Fibrinolytic Medication Timing	0	-	21%	31%	100%
PCI Within 90 Minutes of Arrival[1]	4	75%	47%	54%	95%
Smoking Cessation Advice	48	98%	84%	88%	100%
Heart Failure Care					
ACE Inhibitor or ARB for LVSD	218	84%	83%	82%	100%
Discharge Instructions	474	90%	67%	61%	93%
Evaluation of LVS Function	576	99%	88%	83%	99%
Smoking Cessation Advice	83	100%	83%	82%	100%
Pneumonia Care					
Appropriate Initial Antibiotic	186	80%	83%	83%	94%
Blood Culture Timing	193	90%	91%	90%	100%
Influenza Vaccine[4,5]	-	-	63%	70%	100%
Initial Antibiotic Timing	301	68%	81%	80%	93%
Oxygenation Assessment	345	100%	99%	99%	100%
Pneumococcal Vaccine	217	46%	62%	69%	94%
Smoking Cessation Advice	81	94%	80%	80%	100%
Surgical Infection Prevention					
Prophylactic Antibiotic Given[3]	175	74%	74%	77%	95%
Prophylactic Antibiotic Selection	58	91%	91%	90%	100%
Prophylactic Antibiotic Stopped[3]	163	67%	67%	72%	95%
Pregnancy Care					
Inpatient Neonatal Mortality	-	-	-	-	-
Third or Fourth Degree Laceration	-	-	3.89%	3.63%	3.27%

Saint Elizabeth's Hospital

211 S Third Street
Belleville, IL 62220
Phone: 618-234-2120
Fax: 618-222-4650
URL: www.steliz.org
Ownership: Voluntary non-profit - Church
Accredited: Yes
Emergency Services: Yes
Licensed Beds: 498

Key Personnel:

Administrator . . . . Tim Brady
Emergency Room . . . . Bill Cruzen, DO
Director Infection/Disease Control . . . . Adrienne Garcia
Director Medical/Surgical Nursing . . . . Lucy Beaver
Chief Radiology . . . . Greg Holdemer, MD
Director Respiratory Therapy . . . . John Ancy

Measure	Cases	This Hospital	State Average	U.S. Average	Top Hospital
Heart Attack Care					
ACE Inhibitor or ARB for LVSD	55	82%	79%	82%	100%
Aspirin at Arrival	174	95%	93%	92%	100%
Aspirin at Discharge	253	96%	90%	90%	100%
Beta Blocker at Arrival	153	90%	87%	87%	100%
Beta Blocker at Discharge	251	96%	88%	90%	100%
Fibrinolytic Medication Timing	0	-	21%	31%	100%
PCI Within 90 Minutes of Arrival[1]	5	60%	47%	54%	95%
Smoking Cessation Advice	87	89%	84%	88%	100%
Heart Failure Care					
ACE Inhibitor or ARB for LVSD	173	88%	83%	82%	100%
Discharge Instructions	465	63%	67%	61%	93%
Evaluation of LVS Function	585	85%	88%	83%	99%
Smoking Cessation Advice	72	78%	83%	82%	100%
Pneumonia Care					
Appropriate Initial Antibiotic[2]	245	85%	83%	83%	94%
Blood Culture Timing[2]	195	91%	91%	90%	100%
Influenza Vaccine[2]	100	34%	63%	70%	100%
Initial Antibiotic Timing[2]	410	80%	81%	80%	93%
Oxygenation Assessment[2]	501	99%	99%	99%	100%
Pneumococcal Vaccine[2]	323	28%	62%	69%	94%
Smoking Cessation Advice[2]	115	82%	80%	80%	100%
Surgical Infection Prevention					
Prophylactic Antibiotic Given[2]	361	81%	74%	77%	95%
Prophylactic Antibiotic Selection[2]	84	80%	91%	90%	100%
Prophylactic Antibiotic Stopped[2]	350	72%	67%	72%	95%
Pregnancy Care					
Inpatient Neonatal Mortality	1,255	0.00%	-	-	-
Third or Fourth Degree Laceration	942	2.34%	3.89%	3.63%	3.27%

MacNeal Hospital

3249 S Oak Park Avenue
Berwyn, IL 60402
Phone: 708-783-9100
Fax: 708-783-3489
URL: www.macneal.com
Ownership: Voluntary non-profit - Private
Accredited: Yes
Emergency Services: Yes
Licensed Beds: 427

Key Personnel:

President/CEO . . . . Brooks Turkel
Chief of Medical Staff. . . . . Gary Wainer
Emergency Room . . . . Brian Fchurgin
Director of Pulmonary/Respiratory Care. . . . . . . Roger Jones

Measure	Cases	This Hospital	State Average	U.S. Average	Top Hospital
Heart Attack Care					
ACE Inhibitor or ARB for LVSD	102	84%	79%	82%	100%
Aspirin at Arrival	246	100%	93%	92%	100%
Aspirin at Discharge	223	96%	90%	90%	100%
Beta Blocker at Arrival	205	98%	87%	87%	100%
Beta Blocker at Discharge	229	96%	88%	90%	100%
Fibrinolytic Medication Timing	0	-	21%	31%	100%
PCI Within 90 Minutes of Arrival[1]	11	45%	47%	54%	95%
Smoking Cessation Advice	73	93%	84%	88%	100%
Heart Failure Care					
ACE Inhibitor or ARB for LVSD	243	78%	83%	82%	100%
Discharge Instructions	384	74%	67%	61%	93%
Evaluation of LVS Function	507	91%	88%	83%	99%
Smoking Cessation Advice	85	98%	83%	82%	100%
Pneumonia Care					

NOTE: Hospital profiles are in alphabetical order by state, then city, then hospital within the city; Rankings are sorted by rate in descending order and exclude hospitals with less than 25 cases; (1) The number of cases is too small (n<25) for purposes of reliably predicting hospital performance; (2) Measure reflects the hospital's indication that its submission was based upon a sample of its relevant discharges; (3) Rate reflects fewer than the maximum possible quarters of data for the measure; (4) Inaccurate information submitted and suppressed for one or more quarters; (5) No data is available from the hospital for this measure; Please refer to the User's Guide for a full explanation of data

Measure	Cases	This Hospital	State Average	U.S. Average	Top Hospital
Appropriate Initial Antibiotic	258	86%	83%	83%	94%
Blood Culture Timing	256	97%	91%	90%	100%
Influenza Vaccine	60	73%	63%	70%	100%
Initial Antibiotic Timing	337	90%	81%	80%	93%
Oxygenation Assessment	391	100%	99%	99%	100%
Pneumococcal Vaccine	256	68%	62%	69%	94%
Smoking Cessation Advice	81	93%	80%	80%	100%
Surgical Infection Prevention					
Prophylactic Antibiotic Given[2]	613	92%	74%	77%	95%
Prophylactic Antibiotic Selection[2]	136	96%	91%	90%	100%
Prophylactic Antibiotic Stopped[2]	563	79%	67%	72%	95%
Pregnancy Care					
Inpatient Neonatal Mortality	-	-	-	-	-
Third or Fourth Degree Laceration	-	-	3.89%	3.63%	3.27%

Saint Joseph Medical Center

2200 East Washington Street — Phone: 309-662-3311
Bloomington, IL 61701 — Fax: 309-662-7665
Ownership: Voluntary non-profit - Church — Accredited: Yes
Emergency Services: Yes — Licensed Beds: 182

Key Personnel:

CEO. . . . . Kenneth Natzke
Chief Medical Staff. . . . . Herbert Weiser, MD
Director Medical/Surgical Nursing . . . . Sandra Scheidenhelm
OB/GYN Womens Health. . . . . Dan Nord, MD
Chief Radiology . . . . James Peng, MD

Measure	Cases	This Hospital	State Average	U.S. Average	Top Hospital
Heart Attack Care					
ACE Inhibitor or ARB for LVSD	34	97%	79%	82%	100%
Aspirin at Arrival	90	100%	93%	92%	100%
Aspirin at Discharge	104	99%	90%	90%	100%
Beta Blocker at Arrival	81	99%	87%	87%	100%
Beta Blocker at Discharge	126	100%	88%	90%	100%
Fibrinolytic Medication Timing	0	-	21%	31%	100%
PCI Within 90 Minutes of Arrival[1]	6	67%	47%	54%	95%
Smoking Cessation Advice	50	98%	84%	88%	100%
Heart Failure Care					
ACE Inhibitor or ARB for LVSD	72	93%	83%	82%	100%
Discharge Instructions	115	85%	67%	61%	93%
Evaluation of LVS Function	156	98%	88%	83%	99%
Smoking Cessation Advice	43	100%	83%	82%	100%
Pneumonia Care					
Appropriate Initial Antibiotic	92	86%	83%	83%	94%
Blood Culture Timing	98	88%	91%	90%	100%
Influenza Vaccine	28	82%	63%	70%	100%
Initial Antibiotic Timing	118	73%	81%	80%	93%
Oxygenation Assessment	156	100%	99%	99%	100%
Pneumococcal Vaccine	101	85%	62%	69%	94%
Smoking Cessation Advice	43	98%	80%	80%	100%
Surgical Infection Prevention					
Prophylactic Antibiotic Given	553	95%	74%	77%	95%
Prophylactic Antibiotic Selection	121	98%	91%	90%	100%
Prophylactic Antibiotic Stopped	542	79%	67%	72%	95%
Pregnancy Care					
Inpatient Neonatal Mortality	-	-	-	-	-
Third or Fourth Degree Laceration	-	-	3.89%	3.63%	3.27%

Saint Francis Hospital & Health Center

12935 S Gregory Street — Phone: 708-597-2000
Blue Island, IL 60406 — Fax: 708-389-9480
URL: www.stfrancisblueisland.com
Ownership: Voluntary non-profit - Church — Accredited: Yes
Emergency Services: Yes — Licensed Beds: 410

Key Personnel:

President/CEO. . . . . Colleen Kannaday
Chief Medical Staff. . . . . Kurt Erickson, MD
Director Catheterization Lab. . . . . Robert Iaffaldano, MD
Emergency Room . . . . Daniel Kowalzyk, MD
Medical Director Infection/Disease. . . . . Robert Fliegelman, MD
Director Radiology . . . . Vicki McFarlane

Measure	Cases	This Hospital	State Average	U.S. Average	Top Hospital
Heart Attack Care					
ACE Inhibitor or ARB for LVSD	33	79%	79%	82%	100%
Aspirin at Arrival	122	96%	93%	92%	100%
Aspirin at Discharge	138	93%	90%	90%	100%
Beta Blocker at Arrival	107	92%	87%	87%	100%
Beta Blocker at Discharge	140	96%	88%	90%	100%
Fibrinolytic Medication Timing[1]	1	0%	21%	31%	100%
PCI Within 90 Minutes of Arrival[1]	4	25%	47%	54%	95%
Smoking Cessation Advice	58	97%	84%	88%	100%
Heart Failure Care					
ACE Inhibitor or ARB for LVSD	423	78%	83%	82%	100%
Discharge Instructions	821	57%	67%	61%	93%
Evaluation of LVS Function	902	90%	88%	83%	99%
Smoking Cessation Advice	202	96%	83%	82%	100%
Pneumonia Care					
Appropriate Initial Antibiotic	369	87%	83%	83%	94%
Blood Culture Timing	412	85%	91%	90%	100%
Influenza Vaccine	93	62%	63%	70%	100%
Initial Antibiotic Timing	529	73%	81%	80%	93%
Oxygenation Assessment	593	100%	99%	99%	100%
Pneumococcal Vaccine	313	64%	62%	69%	94%
Smoking Cessation Advice	159	93%	80%	80%	100%
Surgical Infection Prevention					
Prophylactic Antibiotic Given[3]	391	92%	74%	77%	95%
Prophylactic Antibiotic Selection	130	92%	91%	90%	100%
Prophylactic Antibiotic Stopped[3]	363	51%	67%	72%	95%
Pregnancy Care					
Inpatient Neonatal Mortality	-	-	-	-	-
Third or Fourth Degree Laceration	-	-	3.89%	3.63%	3.27%

Saint Joseph's Hospital

9515 Holy Cross Lane — Phone: 618-526-4511
Breese, IL 62230 — Fax: 618-526-8022
E-mail: phinton@sjh.hshs.org
URL: www.stjoebreese.com
Ownership: Voluntary non-profit - Church — Accredited: Yes
Emergency Services: Yes — Licensed Beds: 85

Key Personnel:

CEO. . . . . Jacolyn Schlautman
Director Medical/Surgical Nursing . . . . Janet Schweirjohn
OB/GYN Womens Health. . . . . R Dermody
Chief Radiology . . . . Karon Whitlatch
Director Respiratory Therapy . . . . Tim Toennies

Measure	Cases	This Hospital	State Average	U.S. Average	Top Hospital
Heart Attack Care					
ACE Inhibitor or ARB for LVSD	0	-	79%	82%	100%
Aspirin at Arrival[1]	9	100%	93%	92%	100%
Aspirin at Discharge[1]	4	75%	90%	90%	100%
Beta Blocker at Arrival[1]	9	78%	87%	87%	100%
Beta Blocker at Discharge[1]	6	100%	88%	90%	100%
Fibrinolytic Medication Timing[1]	1	0%	21%	31%	100%
PCI Within 90 Minutes of Arrival	0	-	47%	54%	95%
Smoking Cessation Advice	0	-	84%	88%	100%
Heart Failure Care					
ACE Inhibitor or ARB for LVSD[1]	10	70%	83%	82%	100%
Discharge Instructions	48	81%	67%	61%	93%
Evaluation of LVS Function	64	88%	88%	83%	99%
Smoking Cessation Advice[1]	5	80%	83%	82%	100%
Pneumonia Care					
Appropriate Initial Antibiotic	72	86%	83%	83%	94%
Blood Culture Timing	46	93%	91%	90%	100%
Influenza Vaccine	28	64%	63%	70%	100%
Initial Antibiotic Timing	79	91%	81%	80%	93%
Oxygenation Assessment	103	100%	99%	99%	100%
Pneumococcal Vaccine	64	75%	62%	69%	94%
Smoking Cessation Advice[1]	12	92%	80%	80%	100%
Surgical Infection Prevention					
Prophylactic Antibiotic Given[3]	25	60%	74%	77%	95%
Prophylactic Antibiotic Selection	25	80%	91%	90%	100%
Prophylactic Antibiotic Stopped[3]	25	80%	67%	72%	95%

NOTE: Hospital profiles are in alphabetical order by state, then city, then hospital within the city; Rankings are sorted by rate in descending order and exclude hospitals with less than 25 cases; (1) The number of cases is too small (n<25) for purposes of reliably predicting hospital performance; (2) Measure reflects the hospital's indication that its submission was based upon a sample of its relevant discharges; (3) Rate reflects fewer than the maximum possible quarters of data for the measure; (4) Inaccurate information submitted and suppressed for one or more quarters; (5) No data is available from the hospital for this measure; Please refer to the User's Guide for a full explanation of data

Pregnancy Care					
Inpatient Neonatal Mortality	427	0.23%	-	-	-
Third or Fourth Degree Laceration	329	2.43%	3.89%	3.63%	3.27%

Graham Hospital

210 W Walnut Street
Canton, IL 61520
URL: www.grahamhospital.org
Ownership: Voluntary non-profit - Other
Emergency Services: Yes
Phone: 309-647-5240
Fax: 309-649-5197
Accredited: Yes
Licensed Beds: 124

Key Personnel:
President . . . . D Ray Slaubaugh
Chief Medical Staff. . . . . Shirley Frantz, MD

Measure	Cases	This Hospital	State Average	U.S. Average	Top Hospital
Heart Attack Care					
ACE Inhibitor or ARB for LVSD[1]	4	75%	79%	82%	100%
Aspirin at Arrival[1]	6	67%	93%	92%	100%
Aspirin at Discharge[1]	7	57%	90%	90%	100%
Beta Blocker at Arrival[1]	6	50%	87%	87%	100%
Beta Blocker at Discharge[1]	6	50%	88%	90%	100%
Fibrinolytic Medication Timing	0	-	21%	31%	100%
PCI Within 90 Minutes of Arrival	0	-	47%	54%	95%
Smoking Cessation Advice[1]	2	100%	84%	88%	100%
Heart Failure Care					
ACE Inhibitor or ARB for LVSD	42	69%	83%	82%	100%
Discharge Instructions	59	51%	67%	61%	93%
Evaluation of LVS Function	96	94%	88%	83%	99%
Smoking Cessation Advice[1]	13	92%	83%	82%	100%
Pneumonia Care					
Appropriate Initial Antibiotic	61	75%	83%	83%	94%
Blood Culture Timing	51	96%	91%	90%	100%
Influenza Vaccine[1]	21	76%	63%	70%	100%
Initial Antibiotic Timing	104	76%	81%	80%	93%
Oxygenation Assessment	126	99%	99%	99%	100%
Pneumococcal Vaccine	84	56%	62%	69%	94%
Smoking Cessation Advice	28	68%	80%	80%	100%
Surgical Infection Prevention					
Prophylactic Antibiotic Given[3]	143	36%	74%	77%	95%
Prophylactic Antibiotic Selection	53	96%	91%	90%	100%
Prophylactic Antibiotic Stopped[3]	137	88%	67%	72%	95%
Pregnancy Care					
Inpatient Neonatal Mortality	-	-	-	-	-
Third or Fourth Degree Laceration	-	-	3.89%	3.63%	3.27%

Memorial Hospital Carbondale

405 West Jackson Street
PO Box 10000
Carbondale, IL 62902
URL: www.sih.net
Ownership: Voluntary non-profit - Other
Emergency Services: Yes
Phone: 618-549-0721
Fax: 618-529-0449
Accredited: Yes
Licensed Beds: 150

Key Personnel:
President/CEO. . . . . George Maroney
Chief of Medical Staff. . . . . Marshall Ryan
Emergency Room . . . . Cindy Pribelle
OB/GYN Womens Health. . . . . Lewis Gueinellen, MD
Respiratory . . . . Darell Bryant

Measure	Cases	This Hospital	State Average	U.S. Average	Top Hospital
Heart Attack Care					
ACE Inhibitor or ARB for LVSD	70	76%	79%	82%	100%
Aspirin at Arrival	87	99%	93%	92%	100%
Aspirin at Discharge	175	95%	90%	90%	100%
Beta Blocker at Arrival	75	91%	87%	87%	100%
Beta Blocker at Discharge	219	95%	88%	90%	100%
Fibrinolytic Medication Timing[1]	3	67%	21%	31%	100%
PCI Within 90 Minutes of Arrival[1]	2	0%	47%	54%	95%
Smoking Cessation Advice	101	98%	84%	88%	100%
Heart Failure Care					
ACE Inhibitor or ARB for LVSD	113	61%	83%	82%	100%
Discharge Instructions	215	43%	67%	61%	93%
Evaluation of LVS Function	242	93%	88%	83%	99%
Smoking Cessation Advice	54	89%	83%	82%	100%
Pneumonia Care					
Appropriate Initial Antibiotic[2]	67	88%	83%	83%	94%
Blood Culture Timing[2]	79	82%	91%	90%	100%
Influenza Vaccine[1,2]	18	56%	63%	70%	100%
Initial Antibiotic Timing[2]	114	87%	81%	80%	93%
Oxygenation Assessment[2]	152	100%	99%	99%	100%
Pneumococcal Vaccine[2]	100	63%	62%	69%	94%
Smoking Cessation Advice[2]	34	88%	80%	80%	100%
Surgical Infection Prevention					
Prophylactic Antibiotic Given[2,3]	226	40%	74%	77%	95%
Prophylactic Antibiotic Selection[2]	72	89%	91%	90%	100%
Prophylactic Antibiotic Stopped[2,3]	218	57%	67%	72%	95%
Pregnancy Care					
Inpatient Neonatal Mortality	1,436	0.21%	-	-	-
Third or Fourth Degree Laceration	1,002	2.59%	3.89%	3.63%	3.27%

Carlinville Area Hospital

1001 E Morgan
Carlinville, IL 62626
Ownership: Voluntary non-profit - Private
Emergency Services: Yes
Toll-Free: 800-828-9923
Phone: 217-854-3141
Fax: 217-854-7861
Accredited: No
Licensed Beds: 33

Key Personnel:
CEO. . . . . Steve Hannah
Emergency Room . . . . Winston Townsend
Emergency Room . . . . Robert England, MD
Director Medical/Surgical Nursing . . . . Sharon Young, RN

Measure	Cases	This Hospital	State Average	U.S. Average	Top Hospital
Heart Attack Care					
ACE Inhibitor or ARB for LVSD[1,3]	4	100%	79%	82%	100%
Aspirin at Arrival[1,3]	13	100%	93%	92%	100%
Aspirin at Discharge[1,3]	9	100%	90%	90%	100%
Beta Blocker at Arrival[1,3]	14	93%	87%	87%	100%
Beta Blocker at Discharge[1,3]	9	89%	88%	90%	100%
Fibrinolytic Medication Timing[1,3]	1	0%	21%	31%	100%
PCI Within 90 Minutes of Arrival	0	-	47%	54%	95%
Smoking Cessation Advice[1,3]	1	0%	84%	88%	100%
Heart Failure Care					
ACE Inhibitor or ARB for LVSD[1]	6	100%	83%	82%	100%
Discharge Instructions[1]	20	65%	67%	61%	93%
Evaluation of LVS Function	37	97%	88%	83%	99%
Smoking Cessation Advice[1]	2	0%	83%	82%	100%
Pneumonia Care					
Appropriate Initial Antibiotic	66	53%	83%	83%	94%
Blood Culture Timing[1]	3	100%	91%	90%	100%
Influenza Vaccine[1]	16	69%	63%	70%	100%
Initial Antibiotic Timing	61	61%	81%	80%	93%
Oxygenation Assessment	81	100%	99%	99%	100%
Pneumococcal Vaccine	62	58%	62%	69%	94%
Smoking Cessation Advice[1]	8	62%	80%	80%	100%
Surgical Infection Prevention					
Prophylactic Antibiotic Given[5]	-	-	74%	77%	95%
Prophylactic Antibiotic Selection[5]	-	-	91%	90%	100%
Prophylactic Antibiotic Stopped[5]	-	-	67%	72%	95%
Pregnancy Care					
Inpatient Neonatal Mortality	-	-	-	-	-
Third or Fourth Degree Laceration	-	-	3.89%	3.63%	3.27%

Thomas H Boyd Memorial Hospital

800 School Street
Carrollton, IL 62016
Ownership: Voluntary non-profit - Other
Emergency Services: Yes
Phone: 217-942-6946
Fax: 217-942-6091
Accredited: No
Licensed Beds: 65

Key Personnel:
CEO. . . . . Deborah Campbell
Chief Medical Staff. . . . . Jude Caselfen
Chief Medical Staff. . . . . August Adams
Emergency Room . . . . Renan Mapue
Chief Radiology . . . . Edward Ragsdale, MD

NOTE: Hospital profiles are in alphabetical order by state, then city, then hospital within the city; Rankings are sorted by rate in descending order and exclude hospitals with less than 25 cases; (1) The number of cases is too small (n<25) for purposes of reliably predicting hospital performance; (2) Measure reflects the hospital's indication that its submission was based upon a sample of its relevant discharges; (3) Rate reflects fewer than the maximum possible quarters of data for the measure; (4) Inaccurate information submitted and suppressed for one or more quarters; (5) No data is available from the hospital for this measure; Please refer to the User's Guide for a full explanation of data

Measure	Cases	This Hospital	State Average	U.S. Average	Top Hospital
Heart Attack Care					
ACE Inhibitor or ARB for LVSD[3]	0	-	79%	82%	100%
Aspirin at Arrival[1,3]	1	100%	93%	92%	100%
Aspirin at Discharge[1,3]	1	100%	90%	90%	100%
Beta Blocker at Arrival[1,3]	1	100%	87%	87%	100%
Beta Blocker at Discharge[1,3]	1	100%	88%	90%	100%
Fibrinolytic Medication Timing[3]	0	-	21%	31%	100%
PCI Within 90 Minutes of Arrival[5]	-	-	47%	54%	95%
Smoking Cessation Advice[3]	0	-	84%	88%	100%
Heart Failure Care					
ACE Inhibitor or ARB for LVSD[3]	0	-	83%	82%	100%
Discharge Instructions[1,3]	2	50%	67%	61%	93%
Evaluation of LVS Function[1,3]	3	0%	88%	83%	99%
Smoking Cessation Advice[3]	0	-	83%	82%	100%
Pneumonia Care					
Appropriate Initial Antibiotic[1,3]	6	67%	83%	83%	94%
Blood Culture Timing[1,3]	1	100%	91%	90%	100%
Influenza Vaccine[1]	1	100%	63%	70%	100%
Initial Antibiotic Timing[1,3]	12	92%	81%	80%	93%
Oxygenation Assessment[1,3]	16	100%	99%	99%	100%
Pneumococcal Vaccine[1,3]	15	47%	62%	69%	94%
Smoking Cessation Advice[1,3]	1	0%	80%	80%	100%
Surgical Infection Prevention					
Prophylactic Antibiotic Given[5]	-	-	74%	77%	95%
Prophylactic Antibiotic Selection[5]	-	-	91%	90%	100%
Prophylactic Antibiotic Stopped[5]	-	-	67%	72%	95%
Pregnancy Care					
Inpatient Neonatal Mortality	-	-	-	-	-
Third or Fourth Degree Laceration	-	-	3.89%	3.63%	3.27%

Saint Mary's Good Samaritan

Alternate Name: Saint Mary's Hospital
400 N Pleasant Avenue
Centralia, IL 62801
Phone: 618-532-6731
Fax: 618-436-8046
URL: www.stmarys-goodsamaritan.com
Ownership: Voluntary non-profit - Church
Accredited: Yes
Emergency Services: No
Licensed Beds: 276

Key Personnel:
CEO. . . . . James W Sanger
Chief Medical Staff. . . . . Tom Martin, MD
OB/GYN Womens Health. . . . . John Griffith, MD
Chief Radiology . . . . Richard Rudman, MD

Measure	Cases	This Hospital	State Average	U.S. Average	Top Hospital
Heart Attack Care					
ACE Inhibitor or ARB for LVSD[1]	6	100%	79%	82%	100%
Aspirin at Arrival	52	100%	93%	92%	100%
Aspirin at Discharge[1]	21	95%	90%	90%	100%
Beta Blocker at Arrival	32	84%	87%	87%	100%
Beta Blocker at Discharge[1]	18	94%	88%	90%	100%
Fibrinolytic Medication Timing	0	-	21%	31%	100%
PCI Within 90 Minutes of Arrival	0	-	47%	54%	95%
Smoking Cessation Advice[1]	6	83%	84%	88%	100%
Heart Failure Care					
ACE Inhibitor or ARB for LVSD	96	94%	83%	82%	100%
Discharge Instructions	198	72%	67%	61%	93%
Evaluation of LVS Function	279	99%	88%	83%	99%
Smoking Cessation Advice	26	96%	83%	82%	100%
Pneumonia Care					
Appropriate Initial Antibiotic	188	87%	83%	83%	94%
Blood Culture Timing	178	97%	91%	90%	100%
Influenza Vaccine	61	84%	63%	70%	100%
Initial Antibiotic Timing	312	88%	81%	80%	93%
Oxygenation Assessment	371	100%	99%	99%	100%
Pneumococcal Vaccine	226	86%	62%	69%	94%
Smoking Cessation Advice	98	76%	80%	80%	100%
Surgical Infection Prevention					
Prophylactic Antibiotic Given	196	87%	74%	77%	95%
Prophylactic Antibiotic Selection	30	77%	91%	90%	100%
Prophylactic Antibiotic Stopped	184	72%	67%	72%	95%
Pregnancy Care					
Inpatient Neonatal Mortality	459	0.22%	-	-	-
Third or Fourth Degree Laceration	310	2.90%	3.89%	3.63%	3.27%

Touchette Regional Hospital

5900 Bond Avenue
Centreville, IL 62207
Phone: 618-332-3060
Fax: 618-332-5256
E-mail: sihfhro@apci.net
URL: www.touchette.org
Ownership: Voluntary non-profit - Private
Accredited: Yes
Emergency Services: Yes
Licensed Beds: 114

Key Personnel:
CEO. . . . . Robert Klutts
Chief Medical Staff. . . . . Jose Ramon
Emergency Room . . . . Louis Gary
Director Infection/Disease Control . . . . Pat Giacin
OB/GYN Womens Health. . . . . Cheryl Fielden
Chief Radiology . . . . Ray Teliczan
Director Respiratory Therapy . . . . Addie Randolph

Measure	Cases	This Hospital	State Average	U.S. Average	Top Hospital
Heart Attack Care					
ACE Inhibitor or ARB for LVSD[1]	2	100%	79%	82%	100%
Aspirin at Arrival[1]	15	80%	93%	92%	100%
Aspirin at Discharge[1]	10	80%	90%	90%	100%
Beta Blocker at Arrival[1]	16	81%	87%	87%	100%
Beta Blocker at Discharge[1]	10	90%	88%	90%	100%
Fibrinolytic Medication Timing[3]	0	-	21%	31%	100%
PCI Within 90 Minutes of Arrival	0	-	47%	54%	95%
Smoking Cessation Advice[1,3]	1	0%	84%	88%	100%
Heart Failure Care					
ACE Inhibitor or ARB for LVSD	31	84%	83%	82%	100%
Discharge Instructions[1,3]	14	36%	67%	61%	93%
Evaluation of LVS Function	98	66%	88%	83%	99%
Smoking Cessation Advice[1,3]	9	67%	83%	82%	100%
Pneumonia Care					
Appropriate Initial Antibiotic[1,3]	2	100%	83%	83%	94%
Blood Culture Timing[1,3]	1	100%	91%	90%	100%
Influenza Vaccine[5]	-	-	63%	70%	100%
Initial Antibiotic Timing	25	60%	81%	80%	93%
Oxygenation Assessment	25	100%	99%	99%	100%
Pneumococcal Vaccine[1]	11	9%	62%	69%	94%
Smoking Cessation Advice[1,3]	1	0%	80%	80%	100%
Surgical Infection Prevention					
Prophylactic Antibiotic Given[1,3]	15	53%	74%	77%	95%
Prophylactic Antibiotic Selection[5]	-	-	91%	90%	100%
Prophylactic Antibiotic Stopped[1,3]	13	69%	67%	72%	95%
Pregnancy Care					
Inpatient Neonatal Mortality	652	0.31%	-	-	-
Third or Fourth Degree Laceration	459	1.31%	3.89%	3.63%	3.27%

Memorial Hospital

1900 State Street
Chester, IL 62233
Phone: 618-826-4581
Fax: 618-826-4813
URL: www.mhchester.com
Ownership: Govt - Hospital District or Authority
Accredited: Yes
Emergency Services: Yes
Licensed Beds: 25

Key Personnel:
CEO. . . . . Eric Freeburg
Chief Medical Staff. . . . . Allen Liefer, MD
Emergency Room . . . . Mary Rosendohl, RN
Infection Control. . . . . Machelle Kureker
Infection Control. . . . . Sharon Lambert
Respiratory/Cardiopulmonary. . . . . Brett Bollman
Director Cardiopulmonary Services . . . . Brett Bollmann

Measure	Cases	This Hospital	State Average	U.S. Average	Top Hospital
Heart Attack Care					
ACE Inhibitor or ARB for LVSD[1]	1	100%	79%	82%	100%
Aspirin at Arrival[1]	4	100%	93%	92%	100%
Aspirin at Discharge[1]	1	100%	90%	90%	100%
Beta Blocker at Arrival[1]	4	100%	87%	87%	100%
Beta Blocker at Discharge[1]	2	100%	88%	90%	100%
Fibrinolytic Medication Timing[1]	1	0%	21%	31%	100%

NOTE: Hospital profiles are in alphabetical order by state, then city, then hospital within the city; Rankings are sorted by rate in descending order and exclude hospitals with less than 25 cases; (1) The number of cases is too small (n<25) for purposes of reliably predicting hospital performance; (2) Measure reflects the hospital's indication that its submission was based upon a sample of its relevant discharges; (3) Rate reflects fewer than the maximum possible quarters of data for the measure; (4) Inaccurate information submitted and suppressed for one or more quarters; (5) No data is available from the hospital for this measure; Please refer to the User's Guide for a full explanation of data

PCI Within 90 Minutes of Arrival	0	-	47%	54%	95%
Smoking Cessation Advice	0	-	84%	88%	100%
Heart Failure Care					
ACE Inhibitor or ARB for LVSD[1]	6	50%	83%	82%	100%
Discharge Instructions	44	61%	67%	61%	93%
Evaluation of LVS Function	64	97%	88%	83%	99%
Smoking Cessation Advice[1]	5	100%	83%	82%	100%
Pneumonia Care					
Appropriate Initial Antibiotic	33	100%	83%	83%	94%
Blood Culture Timing[1]	16	100%	91%	90%	100%
Influenza Vaccine[1]	14	100%	63%	70%	100%
Initial Antibiotic Timing	47	94%	81%	80%	93%
Oxygenation Assessment	61	100%	99%	99%	100%
Pneumococcal Vaccine	44	95%	62%	69%	94%
Smoking Cessation Advice[1]	9	100%	80%	80%	100%
Surgical Infection Prevention					
Prophylactic Antibiotic Given	28	96%	74%	77%	95%
Prophylactic Antibiotic Selection[1]	6	83%	91%	90%	100%
Prophylactic Antibiotic Stopped[1]	24	100%	67%	72%	95%
Pregnancy Care					
Inpatient Neonatal Mortality	-	-	-	-	-
Third or Fourth Degree Laceration	-	-	3.89%	3.63%	3.27%

Advocate Illinois Masonic Medical Center

836 West Wellington Avenue
Chicago, IL 60657
URL: www.advocatehealth.com
Ownership: Voluntary non-profit - Church
Emergency Services: Yes
Phone: 773-975-1600
Fax: 773-296-8119
Accredited: Yes
Licensed Beds: 551

Key Personnel:

CEO. . . . . Susan Lopez

Measure	Cases	This Hospital	State Average	U.S. Average	Top Hospital
Heart Attack Care					
ACE Inhibitor or ARB for LVSD	48	81%	79%	82%	100%
Aspirin at Arrival	107	100%	93%	92%	100%
Aspirin at Discharge	136	91%	90%	90%	100%
Beta Blocker at Arrival	81	96%	87%	87%	100%
Beta Blocker at Discharge	159	92%	88%	90%	100%
Fibrinolytic Medication Timing	0	-	21%	31%	100%
PCI Within 90 Minutes of Arrival[1]	5	40%	47%	54%	95%
Smoking Cessation Advice	82	83%	84%	88%	100%
Heart Failure Care					
ACE Inhibitor or ARB for LVSD[2]	178	88%	83%	82%	100%
Discharge Instructions[2]	268	68%	67%	61%	93%
Evaluation of LVS Function[2]	317	98%	88%	83%	99%
Smoking Cessation Advice[2]	58	90%	83%	82%	100%
Pneumonia Care					
Appropriate Initial Antibiotic[2]	103	84%	83%	83%	94%
Blood Culture Timing[2]	95	84%	91%	90%	100%
Influenza Vaccine[1]	21	81%	63%	70%	100%
Initial Antibiotic Timing[2]	167	72%	81%	80%	93%
Oxygenation Assessment[2]	200	100%	99%	99%	100%
Pneumococcal Vaccine[2]	86	59%	62%	69%	94%
Smoking Cessation Advice[2]	41	85%	80%	80%	100%
Surgical Infection Prevention					
Prophylactic Antibiotic Given[2]	305	90%	74%	77%	95%
Prophylactic Antibiotic Selection[2]	71	96%	91%	90%	100%
Prophylactic Antibiotic Stopped[2]	293	70%	67%	72%	95%
Pregnancy Care					
Inpatient Neonatal Mortality[2]	657	0.61%	-	-	-
Third or Fourth Degree Laceration[2]	707	1.41%	3.89%	3.63%	3.27%

Advocate Trinity Hospital

2320 E 93rd Street
Chicago, IL 60617
URL: www.advocatehealth.com/trin
Ownership: Voluntary non-profit - Church
Emergency Services: Yes
Phone: 773-967-2000
Fax: 773-967-4209
Accredited: Yes

Measure	Cases	This Hospital	State Average	U.S. Average	Top Hospital
Heart Attack Care					
ACE Inhibitor or ARB for LVSD	30	77%	79%	82%	100%
Aspirin at Arrival	159	92%	93%	92%	100%
Aspirin at Discharge	90	80%	90%	90%	100%
Beta Blocker at Arrival	138	88%	87%	87%	100%
Beta Blocker at Discharge	95	82%	88%	90%	100%
Fibrinolytic Medication Timing[1]	6	0%	21%	31%	100%
PCI Within 90 Minutes of Arrival	0	-	47%	54%	95%
Smoking Cessation Advice[1]	24	92%	84%	88%	100%
Heart Failure Care					
ACE Inhibitor or ARB for LVSD	256	82%	83%	82%	100%
Discharge Instructions	583	35%	67%	61%	93%
Evaluation of LVS Function	634	90%	88%	83%	99%
Smoking Cessation Advice	131	92%	83%	82%	100%
Pneumonia Care					
Appropriate Initial Antibiotic	197	84%	83%	83%	94%
Blood Culture Timing	189	92%	91%	90%	100%
Influenza Vaccine	35	14%	63%	70%	100%
Initial Antibiotic Timing	257	62%	81%	80%	93%
Oxygenation Assessment	295	99%	99%	99%	100%
Pneumococcal Vaccine	134	31%	62%	69%	94%
Smoking Cessation Advice	88	89%	80%	80%	100%
Surgical Infection Prevention					
Prophylactic Antibiotic Given[2]	229	86%	74%	77%	95%
Prophylactic Antibiotic Selection[2]	53	100%	91%	90%	100%
Prophylactic Antibiotic Stopped[2]	220	65%	67%	72%	95%
Pregnancy Care					
Inpatient Neonatal Mortality	1,697	0.18%	-	-	-
Third or Fourth Degree Laceration	1,301	1.92%	3.89%	3.63%	3.27%

Holy Cross Hospital

2701 W 68th Street
Chicago, IL 60629
URL: www.holycrosshospital.org
Ownership: Voluntary non-profit - Church
Emergency Services: Yes
Phone: 773-884-9000
Fax: 773-884-8013
Accredited: Yes
Licensed Beds: 331

Key Personnel:

CEO. . . . . Brian Lemon
Chief of Medical Staff. . . . . Chin Waung
Emergency Room . . . . G Cholewa
Emergency Room . . . . Ann Reninger, RN
Chief Radiology . . . . Ron Shimonas
Respiratory Director . . . . Caroline Elick

Measure	Cases	This Hospital	State Average	U.S. Average	Top Hospital
Heart Attack Care					
ACE Inhibitor or ARB for LVSD[2]	33	85%	79%	82%	100%
Aspirin at Arrival[2]	200	94%	93%	92%	100%
Aspirin at Discharge[2]	118	77%	90%	90%	100%
Beta Blocker at Arrival[2]	152	88%	87%	87%	100%
Beta Blocker at Discharge[2]	117	77%	88%	90%	100%
Fibrinolytic Medication Timing[1,2]	8	38%	21%	31%	100%
PCI Within 90 Minutes of Arrival[1,2]	3	0%	47%	54%	95%
Smoking Cessation Advice[2]	35	91%	84%	88%	100%
Heart Failure Care					
ACE Inhibitor or ARB for LVSD[2]	123	77%	83%	82%	100%
Discharge Instructions[2]	265	12%	67%	61%	93%
Evaluation of LVS Function[2]	313	95%	88%	83%	99%
Smoking Cessation Advice[2]	82	95%	83%	82%	100%
Pneumonia Care					
Appropriate Initial Antibiotic[2]	142	85%	83%	83%	94%
Blood Culture Timing[2]	150	92%	91%	90%	100%
Influenza Vaccine[1,2]	24	25%	63%	70%	100%
Initial Antibiotic Timing[2]	218	73%	81%	80%	93%
Oxygenation Assessment[2]	233	100%	99%	99%	100%
Pneumococcal Vaccine[2]	93	33%	62%	69%	94%
Smoking Cessation Advice[2]	61	87%	80%	80%	100%
Surgical Infection Prevention					
Prophylactic Antibiotic Given[2]	170	91%	74%	77%	95%
Prophylactic Antibiotic Selection[2]	38	95%	91%	90%	100%
Prophylactic Antibiotic Stopped[2]	153	65%	67%	72%	95%
Pregnancy Care					

NOTE: Hospital profiles are in alphabetical order by state, then city, then hospital within the city; Rankings are sorted by rate in descending order and exclude hospitals with less than 25 cases; (1) The number of cases is too small (n<25) for purposes of reliably predicting hospital performance; (2) Measure reflects the hospital's indication that its submission was based upon a sample of its relevant discharges; (3) Rate reflects fewer than the maximum possible quarters of data for the measure; (4) Inaccurate information submitted and suppressed for one or more quarters; (5) No data is available from the hospital for this measure; Please refer to the User's Guide for a full explanation of data

Measure	Cases	This Hospital	State Average	U.S. Average	Top Hospital
Inpatient Neonatal Mortality	-	-	-	-	-
Third or Fourth Degree Laceration	-	-	3.89%	3.63%	3.27%

Jackson Park Hospital & Medical Center

7531 S Stony Island Avenue
Chicago, IL 60649
Ownership: Voluntary non-profit - Other
Emergency Services: Yes

Phone: 773-947-7500
Fax: 773-947-7791
Accredited: Yes
Licensed Beds: 326

Key Personnel:

President/CEO . . . . Merritt J Hasbrouck
Chief Medical Staff . . . . Bangalore Murthy, MD
Director of Cardiac Lab . . . . D Kumar, MD
Infection Control . . . . Martha Lyons, RN
ICU . . . . Produb David, RN
Director Radiology . . . . M Louise Holden
Director Respiratory Therapy . . . . Jarmel Barnett

Measure	Cases	This Hospital	State Average	U.S. Average	Top Hospital
Heart Attack Care					
ACE Inhibitor or ARB for LVSD[1]	2	50%	79%	82%	100%
Aspirin at Arrival[1]	18	89%	93%	92%	100%
Aspirin at Discharge[1]	7	71%	90%	90%	100%
Beta Blocker at Arrival[1]	20	65%	87%	87%	100%
Beta Blocker at Discharge[1]	7	14%	88%	90%	100%
Fibrinolytic Medication Timing[1]	4	25%	21%	31%	100%
PCI Within 90 Minutes of Arrival	0	-	47%	54%	95%
Smoking Cessation Advice[1]	3	0%	84%	88%	100%
Heart Failure Care					
ACE Inhibitor or ARB for LVSD	71	80%	83%	82%	100%
Discharge Instructions	200	6%	67%	61%	93%
Evaluation of LVS Function	217	71%	88%	83%	99%
Smoking Cessation Advice	90	4%	83%	82%	100%
Pneumonia Care					
Appropriate Initial Antibiotic	66	79%	83%	83%	94%
Blood Culture Timing[1]	16	62%	91%	90%	100%
Influenza Vaccine	0	-	63%	70%	100%
Initial Antibiotic Timing	52	69%	81%	80%	93%
Oxygenation Assessment	67	99%	99%	99%	100%
Pneumococcal Vaccine[1]	16	0%	62%	69%	94%
Smoking Cessation Advice[1]	20	0%	80%	80%	100%
Surgical Infection Prevention					
Prophylactic Antibiotic Given[1,3]	3	33%	74%	77%	95%
Prophylactic Antibiotic Selection[1]	2	100%	91%	90%	100%
Prophylactic Antibiotic Stopped[1,3]	3	33%	67%	72%	95%
Pregnancy Care					
Inpatient Neonatal Mortality	251	0.40%	-	-	-
Third or Fourth Degree Laceration	186	1.08%	3.89%	3.63%	3.27%

John H Stroger Jr Hospital of Cook County

1901 W Harrison St
Chicago, IL 60612
URL: www.cchil.org
Ownership: Government - Local
Emergency Services: Yes

Phone: 312-864-6000
Accredited: Yes
Licensed Beds: 464

Key Personnel:

President/CEO . . . . Lacy L Thomas
Chief Medical Staff . . . . Stephen Hamburger, MD
Director Infection/Disease Control . . . . Robert Weinstein, MD
CCU Spvg. Nurse . . . . Mary O'Flaherty
Director Medical/Surgical Nursing . . . . Joyce Archie
Director Respiratory Therapy . . . . Frank Brown

Measure	Cases	This Hospital	State Average	U.S. Average	Top Hospital
Heart Attack Care					
ACE Inhibitor or ARB for LVSD[2]	40	78%	79%	82%	100%
Aspirin at Arrival[2]	144	96%	93%	92%	100%
Aspirin at Discharge[2]	199	99%	90%	90%	100%
Beta Blocker at Arrival[2]	101	96%	87%	87%	100%
Beta Blocker at Discharge[2]	182	97%	88%	90%	100%
Fibrinolytic Medication Timing[2]	0	-	21%	31%	100%
PCI Within 90 Minutes of Arrival[1,2]	1	0%	47%	54%	95%
Smoking Cessation Advice[2]	112	84%	84%	88%	100%
Heart Failure Care					
ACE Inhibitor or ARB for LVSD[2]	144	94%	83%	82%	100%
Discharge Instructions[2]	283	11%	67%	61%	93%
Evaluation of LVS Function[2]	294	96%	88%	83%	99%
Smoking Cessation Advice[2]	126	73%	83%	82%	100%
Pneumonia Care					
Appropriate Initial Antibiotic[2]	187	50%	83%	83%	94%
Blood Culture Timing[2]	109	77%	91%	90%	100%
Influenza Vaccine[2]	26	15%	63%	70%	100%
Initial Antibiotic Timing[2]	210	33%	81%	80%	93%
Oxygenation Assessment[2]	243	100%	99%	99%	100%
Pneumococcal Vaccine[2]	52	12%	62%	69%	94%
Smoking Cessation Advice[2]	131	56%	80%	80%	100%
Surgical Infection Prevention					
Prophylactic Antibiotic Given[2,3]	147	87%	74%	77%	95%
Prophylactic Antibiotic Selection[2]	44	50%	91%	90%	100%
Prophylactic Antibiotic Stopped[2,3]	141	79%	67%	72%	95%
Pregnancy Care					
Inpatient Neonatal Mortality	1,254	1.91%	-	-	-
Third or Fourth Degree Laceration	768	1.95%	3.89%	3.63%	3.27%

Lincoln Park Hospital

550 W Webster Avenue
Chicago, IL 60614
Ownership: Proprietary
Emergency Services: Yes

Phone: 773-883-2000
Fax: 773-883-5168
Accredited: Yes
Licensed Beds: 465

Key Personnel:

CEO . . . . Greg Cierlik
CNO . . . . Virginia Friesen
Chief Medical Staff . . . . William Markey
Director Cardiology . . . . Danilo Deano
Director Pulmonary . . . . Venkata Buddheraju

Measure	Cases	This Hospital	State Average	U.S. Average	Top Hospital
Heart Attack Care					
ACE Inhibitor or ARB for LVSD[1]	5	40%	79%	82%	100%
Aspirin at Arrival[1]	12	100%	93%	92%	100%
Aspirin at Discharge[1]	13	77%	90%	90%	100%
Beta Blocker at Arrival[1]	12	58%	87%	87%	100%
Beta Blocker at Discharge[1]	13	62%	88%	90%	100%
Fibrinolytic Medication Timing	0	-	21%	31%	100%
PCI Within 90 Minutes of Arrival	0	-	47%	54%	95%
Smoking Cessation Advice[1]	4	25%	84%	88%	100%
Heart Failure Care					
ACE Inhibitor or ARB for LVSD	66	82%	83%	82%	100%
Discharge Instructions	139	58%	67%	61%	93%
Evaluation of LVS Function	174	86%	88%	83%	99%
Smoking Cessation Advice	36	53%	83%	82%	100%
Pneumonia Care					
Appropriate Initial Antibiotic	57	68%	83%	83%	94%
Blood Culture Timing	37	78%	91%	90%	100%
Influenza Vaccine[1]	4	25%	63%	70%	100%
Initial Antibiotic Timing	63	76%	81%	80%	93%
Oxygenation Assessment	84	93%	99%	99%	100%
Pneumococcal Vaccine	36	28%	62%	69%	94%
Smoking Cessation Advice[1]	16	44%	80%	80%	100%
Surgical Infection Prevention					
Prophylactic Antibiotic Given[1,3]	22	64%	74%	77%	95%
Prophylactic Antibiotic Selection[1]	22	91%	91%	90%	100%
Prophylactic Antibiotic Stopped[1,3]	21	86%	67%	72%	95%
Pregnancy Care					
Inpatient Neonatal Mortality	-	-	-	-	-
Third or Fourth Degree Laceration	-	-	3.89%	3.63%	3.27%

Loretto Hospital

645 S Central Avenue
Chicago, IL 60644
Ownership: Voluntary non-profit - Other
Emergency Services: Yes

Phone: 773-626-4300
Fax: 773-626-2613
Accredited: Yes
Licensed Beds: 223

Key Personnel:

CEO . . . . Steve Drucker
Chief Medical Staff . . . . Dr. Humid M Humayum, MD
Emergency Room . . . . Patricia Lindeman
Infection Control . . . . Omar Jrab

NOTE: Hospital profiles are in alphabetical order by state, then city, then hospital within the city; Rankings are sorted by rate in descending order and exclude hospitals with less than 25 cases; (1) The number of cases is too small (n<25) for purposes of reliably predicting hospital performance; (2) Measure reflects the hospital's indication that its submission was based upon a sample of its relevant discharges; (3) Rate reflects fewer than the maximum possible quarters of data for the measure; (4) Inaccurate information submitted and suppressed for one or more quarters; (5) No data is available from the hospital for this measure; Please refer to the User's Guide for a full explanation of data

President/CEO . . . . Steven Druker
Chief Radiology . . . . Raymond Deak, MD
Director Respiratory/Cardiopulmonary . . . . Katherine McGrath

Measure	Cases	This Hospital	State Average	U.S. Average	Top Hospital
Heart Attack Care					
ACE Inhibitor or ARB for LVSD[1]	4	75%	79%	82%	100%
Aspirin at Arrival	28	89%	93%	92%	100%
Aspirin at Discharge[1]	14	100%	90%	90%	100%
Beta Blocker at Arrival	25	96%	87%	87%	100%
Beta Blocker at Discharge[1]	16	94%	88%	90%	100%
Fibrinolytic Medication Timing[1]	3	67%	21%	31%	100%
PCI Within 90 Minutes of Arrival	0	-	47%	54%	95%
Smoking Cessation Advice[1]	7	100%	84%	88%	100%
Heart Failure Care					
ACE Inhibitor or ARB for LVSD[2]	49	96%	83%	82%	100%
Discharge Instructions[2]	102	100%	67%	61%	93%
Evaluation of LVS Function[2]	131	95%	88%	83%	99%
Smoking Cessation Advice[2]	44	100%	83%	82%	100%
Pneumonia Care					
Appropriate Initial Antibiotic	54	59%	83%	83%	94%
Blood Culture Timing	97	93%	91%	90%	100%
Influenza Vaccine[4,5]	-	-	63%	70%	100%
Initial Antibiotic Timing	119	78%	81%	80%	93%
Oxygenation Assessment	129	100%	99%	99%	100%
Pneumococcal Vaccine	44	18%	62%	69%	94%
Smoking Cessation Advice	37	100%	80%	80%	100%
Surgical Infection Prevention					
Prophylactic Antibiotic Given[1,3]	8	88%	74%	77%	95%
Prophylactic Antibiotic Selection[1]	3	100%	91%	90%	100%
Prophylactic Antibiotic Stopped[1,3]	8	0%	67%	72%	95%
Pregnancy Care					
Inpatient Neonatal Mortality	-	-	-	-	-
Third or Fourth Degree Laceration	-	-	3.89%	3.63%	3.27%

Mercy Hospital

2525 S Michigan Avenue
Chicago, IL 60616
E-mail: mercy@mercy-chicago.org
URL: www.mercy-chicago.org
Phone: 312-567-2000
Fax: 312-567-5562
Ownership: Voluntary non-profit - Church
Emergency Services: Yes
Accredited: Yes
Licensed Beds: 507

Key Personnel:
President . . . . Sheila Lynn, RSM
Manager Cardiac Services . . . . Toni Fields
Manager Catheterization Laboratory . . . . David Nichols
Chairperson Emergency Room . . . . Helene Reidy, MD
Manager Emergency Room . . . . Jo Reidy, RN
Infection Control Nurse . . . . Jean Kirk, RN
Director Medical/Surgical Nursing . . . . Sandra Rose, RN
OB/GYN Womens Health . . . . Donna Kirz, MD
Manager Respiratory Therapy . . . . Yuriy Kozel

Measure	Cases	This Hospital	State Average	U.S. Average	Top Hospital
Heart Attack Care					
ACE Inhibitor or ARB for LVSD	44	86%	79%	82%	100%
Aspirin at Arrival	129	91%	93%	92%	100%
Aspirin at Discharge	135	93%	90%	90%	100%
Beta Blocker at Arrival	111	95%	87%	87%	100%
Beta Blocker at Discharge	142	98%	88%	90%	100%
Fibrinolytic Medication Timing[1]	5	20%	21%	31%	100%
PCI Within 90 Minutes of Arrival[1]	5	20%	47%	54%	95%
Smoking Cessation Advice	67	91%	84%	88%	100%
Heart Failure Care					
ACE Inhibitor or ARB for LVSD	278	88%	83%	82%	100%
Discharge Instructions	521	85%	67%	61%	93%
Evaluation of LVS Function	563	98%	88%	83%	99%
Smoking Cessation Advice	128	94%	83%	82%	100%
Pneumonia Care					
Appropriate Initial Antibiotic	127	82%	83%	83%	94%
Blood Culture Timing	187	81%	91%	90%	100%
Influenza Vaccine	29	34%	63%	70%	100%
Initial Antibiotic Timing	230	63%	81%	80%	93%
Oxygenation Assessment	261	100%	99%	99%	100%
Pneumococcal Vaccine	128	35%	62%	69%	94%
Smoking Cessation Advice	76	79%	80%	80%	100%
Surgical Infection Prevention					
Prophylactic Antibiotic Given[2]	404	93%	74%	77%	95%
Prophylactic Antibiotic Selection[2]	110	98%	91%	90%	100%
Prophylactic Antibiotic Stopped[2]	391	80%	67%	72%	95%
Pregnancy Care					
Inpatient Neonatal Mortality	-	-	-	-	-
Third or Fourth Degree Laceration	-	-	3.89%	3.63%	3.27%

Methodist Hospital of Chicago

5025 N Paulina Street
Chicago, IL 60640
URL: www.bethanymethodist.org
Phone: 773-271-9040
Fax: 773-989-1348
Ownership: Voluntary non-profit - Church
Emergency Services: Yes
Accredited: Yes
Licensed Beds: 245

Key Personnel:
CEO . . . . Steven Dahl
Chief Medical Staff . . . . Irzing Tracer, MD
Director Respiratory Therapy . . . . Joseph Chandy

Measure	Cases	This Hospital	State Average	U.S. Average	Top Hospital
Heart Attack Care					
ACE Inhibitor or ARB for LVSD[1,3]	2	50%	79%	82%	100%
Aspirin at Arrival[1,3]	7	100%	93%	92%	100%
Aspirin at Discharge[1,3]	5	60%	90%	90%	100%
Beta Blocker at Arrival[1,3]	8	75%	87%	87%	100%
Beta Blocker at Discharge[1,3]	5	40%	88%	90%	100%
Fibrinolytic Medication Timing[3]	0	-	21%	31%	100%
PCI Within 90 Minutes of Arrival	0	-	47%	54%	95%
Smoking Cessation Advice[1,3]	1	100%	84%	88%	100%
Heart Failure Care					
ACE Inhibitor or ARB for LVSD[1]	10	30%	83%	82%	100%
Discharge Instructions[1]	15	100%	67%	61%	93%
Evaluation of LVS Function	48	79%	88%	83%	99%
Smoking Cessation Advice[1]	17	35%	83%	82%	100%
Pneumonia Care					
Appropriate Initial Antibiotic[1]	12	67%	83%	83%	94%
Blood Culture Timing	83	76%	91%	90%	100%
Influenza Vaccine[1]	13	23%	63%	70%	100%
Initial Antibiotic Timing	139	77%	81%	80%	93%
Oxygenation Assessment	169	93%	99%	99%	100%
Pneumococcal Vaccine	99	8%	62%	69%	94%
Smoking Cessation Advice	66	62%	80%	80%	100%
Surgical Infection Prevention					
Prophylactic Antibiotic Given[1]	7	57%	74%	77%	95%
Prophylactic Antibiotic Selection[1]	1	100%	91%	90%	100%
Prophylactic Antibiotic Stopped[1]	7	100%	67%	72%	95%
Pregnancy Care					
Inpatient Neonatal Mortality	-	-	-	-	-
Third or Fourth Degree Laceration	-	-	3.89%	3.63%	3.27%

Michael Reese Hospital

2929 S Ellis Avenue
Chicago, IL 60616
URL: michaelreesehospital.com
Phone: 312-791-2000
Fax: 312-791-2299
Ownership: Proprietary
Emergency Services: Yes
Accredited: Yes
Licensed Beds: 565

Key Personnel:
Chief Medical Staff . . . . Kathy Neely, RN,MSN
Cardiac Lab . . . . Charles Beaver
Emergency Room . . . . Michelle Caskill, RN
Emergency Room . . . . Diane Hanes
Infection Control . . . . Vanida Komutanon, RN
Medical/Surgical Nursing . . . . Clarice Glenn, RN
OB/GYN Womens Health . . . . Lewis Blumenthal, MD
Manager Respiratory Therapy . . . . Charles Beaver

Measure	Cases	This Hospital	State Average	U.S. Average	Top Hospital
Heart Attack Care					
ACE Inhibitor or ARB for LVSD[1]	20	95%	79%	82%	100%
Aspirin at Arrival	48	88%	93%	92%	100%

NOTE: Hospital profiles are in alphabetical order by state, then city, then hospital within the city; Rankings are sorted by rate in descending order and exclude hospitals with less than 25 cases; (1) The number of cases is too small (n<25) for purposes of reliably predicting hospital performance; (2) Measure reflects the hospital's indication that its submission was based upon a sample of its relevant discharges; (3) Rate reflects fewer than the maximum possible quarters of data for the measure; (4) Inaccurate information submitted and suppressed for one or more quarters; (5) No data is available from the hospital for this measure; Please refer to the User's Guide for a full explanation of data

Measure	Cases	This Hospital	State Average	U.S. Average	Top Hospital
Aspirin at Discharge	54	96%	90%	90%	100%
Beta Blocker at Arrival	41	90%	87%	87%	100%
Beta Blocker at Discharge	53	96%	88%	90%	100%
Fibrinolytic Medication Timing	0	-	21%	31%	100%
PCI Within 90 Minutes of Arrival[1]	2	0%	47%	54%	95%
Smoking Cessation Advice[1]	22	86%	84%	88%	100%
Heart Failure Care					
ACE Inhibitor or ARB for LVSD[2]	167	89%	83%	82%	100%
Discharge Instructions[2]	242	81%	67%	61%	93%
Evaluation of LVS Function[2]	313	98%	88%	83%	99%
Smoking Cessation Advice[2]	79	75%	83%	82%	100%
Pneumonia Care					
Appropriate Initial Antibiotic	31	90%	83%	83%	94%
Blood Culture Timing	52	87%	91%	90%	100%
Influenza Vaccine[1]	15	67%	63%	70%	100%
Initial Antibiotic Timing	82	77%	81%	80%	93%
Oxygenation Assessment	94	99%	99%	99%	100%
Pneumococcal Vaccine	39	74%	62%	69%	94%
Smoking Cessation Advice	35	80%	80%	80%	100%
Surgical Infection Prevention					
Prophylactic Antibiotic Given[2,3]	96	75%	74%	77%	95%
Prophylactic Antibiotic Selection[2]	26	69%	91%	90%	100%
Prophylactic Antibiotic Stopped[2,3]	93	96%	67%	72%	95%
Pregnancy Care					
Inpatient Neonatal Mortality	-	-	-	-	-
Third or Fourth Degree Laceration	-	-	3.89%	3.63%	3.27%

Mount Sinai Hospital

California Avenue at 15th Street — Phone: 773-542-2000
Chicago, IL 60608 — Fax: 773-257-6208
URL: www.sinai.org
Ownership: Voluntary non-profit - Private — Accredited: Yes
Emergency Services: Yes — Licensed Beds: 431

Key Personnel:
Administrator/President . . . . Larry Volkmar
Chief Medical Staff . . . . Peter Bell, MD
Chief Catheterization Laboratory . . . . Sandeep Kowsla, MD
Emergency Room . . . . Leslie Zun, MD
Director Infection/Disease Control . . . . Susan Hosty
Director Radiology . . . . Mike Cvengros

Measure	Cases	This Hospital	State Average	U.S. Average	Top Hospital
Heart Attack Care					
ACE Inhibitor or ARB for LVSD[1]	24	75%	79%	82%	100%
Aspirin at Arrival	125	95%	93%	92%	100%
Aspirin at Discharge	111	94%	90%	90%	100%
Beta Blocker at Arrival	110	87%	87%	87%	100%
Beta Blocker at Discharge	109	94%	88%	90%	100%
Fibrinolytic Medication Timing[1]	2	0%	21%	31%	100%
PCI Within 90 Minutes of Arrival[1]	3	0%	47%	54%	95%
Smoking Cessation Advice	43	93%	84%	88%	100%
Heart Failure Care					
ACE Inhibitor or ARB for LVSD	189	84%	83%	82%	100%
Discharge Instructions	340	62%	67%	61%	93%
Evaluation of LVS Function	374	100%	88%	83%	99%
Smoking Cessation Advice	127	87%	83%	82%	100%
Pneumonia Care					
Appropriate Initial Antibiotic[2]	69	81%	83%	83%	94%
Blood Culture Timing[2]	83	86%	91%	90%	100%
Influenza Vaccine[1,2]	16	31%	63%	70%	100%
Initial Antibiotic Timing[2]	130	58%	81%	80%	93%
Oxygenation Assessment[2]	136	97%	99%	99%	100%
Pneumococcal Vaccine[2]	44	34%	62%	69%	94%
Smoking Cessation Advice[2]	48	90%	80%	80%	100%
Surgical Infection Prevention					
Prophylactic Antibiotic Given[2,3]	177	59%	74%	77%	95%
Prophylactic Antibiotic Selection[2]	49	86%	91%	90%	100%
Prophylactic Antibiotic Stopped[2,3]	156	45%	67%	72%	95%
Pregnancy Care					
Inpatient Neonatal Mortality	3,951	0.71%	-	-	-
Third or Fourth Degree Laceration	2,660	0.98%	3.89%	3.63%	3.27%

Neurologic and Orthopedic Insitute of Chicago

4501 N Winchester Avenue — Phone: 773-250-0000
Chicago, IL 60640 — Fax: 312-494-4556
E-mail: info@neuro-ortho.org
URL: www.neuro-ortho.org
Ownership: Proprietary — Accredited: Yes
Emergency Services: Yes — Licensed Beds: 78

Key Personnel:
President/CEO . . . . Stephanie Spiegel

Measure	Cases	This Hospital	State Average	U.S. Average	Top Hospital
Heart Attack Care					
ACE Inhibitor or ARB for LVSD[5]	-	-	79%	82%	100%
Aspirin at Arrival[5]	-	-	93%	92%	100%
Aspirin at Discharge[5]	-	-	90%	90%	100%
Beta Blocker at Arrival[5]	-	-	87%	87%	100%
Beta Blocker at Discharge[5]	-	-	88%	90%	100%
Fibrinolytic Medication Timing[5]	-	-	21%	31%	100%
PCI Within 90 Minutes of Arrival[5]	-	-	47%	54%	95%
Smoking Cessation Advice[5]	-	-	84%	88%	100%
Heart Failure Care					
ACE Inhibitor or ARB for LVSD[5]	-	-	83%	82%	100%
Discharge Instructions[5]	-	-	67%	61%	93%
Evaluation of LVS Function[5]	-	-	88%	83%	99%
Smoking Cessation Advice[5]	-	-	83%	82%	100%
Pneumonia Care					
Appropriate Initial Antibiotic[5]	-	-	83%	83%	94%
Blood Culture Timing[5]	-	-	91%	90%	100%
Influenza Vaccine[5]	-	-	63%	70%	100%
Initial Antibiotic Timing[5]	-	-	81%	80%	93%
Oxygenation Assessment[5]	-	-	99%	99%	100%
Pneumococcal Vaccine[5]	-	-	62%	69%	94%
Smoking Cessation Advice[5]	-	-	80%	80%	100%
Surgical Infection Prevention					
Prophylactic Antibiotic Given	33	97%	74%	77%	95%
Prophylactic Antibiotic Selection[1]	21	95%	91%	90%	100%
Prophylactic Antibiotic Stopped	33	82%	67%	72%	95%
Pregnancy Care					
Inpatient Neonatal Mortality	-	-	-	-	-
Third or Fourth Degree Laceration	-	-	3.89%	3.63%	3.27%

Northwestern Memorial Hospital

Alternate Name: NMH
251 E Huron Street — Phone: 312-926-2000
Chicago, IL 60611 — Fax: 312-926-3858
URL: www.nmh.org
Ownership: Voluntary non-profit - Private — Accredited: Yes
Emergency Services: Yes — Licensed Beds: 720

Key Personnel:
President/CEO . . . . Dean M Harrison
Chief Medical Staff . . . . John Clarke, MD
Cardiac Lab . . . . Alan Kadish, MD
Catheterization Lab . . . . Charles Davidson, MD
Emergency Room . . . . James Adams, MD
Infection Control . . . . Steve Wolinsky, MD
Chief CCU . . . . Richard Davison, MD
Medical/Surgical Nursing . . . . Jill Stemmerman, RN
Sr VP Womens Health . . . . Anne Bolger
Chief Radiology . . . . Eric Russell, MD
Respiratory/Cardiopulmonary . . . . Brian Smith

Measure	Cases	This Hospital	State Average	U.S. Average	Top Hospital
Heart Attack Care					
ACE Inhibitor or ARB for LVSD	46	98%	79%	82%	100%
Aspirin at Arrival	215	100%	93%	92%	100%
Aspirin at Discharge	232	100%	90%	90%	100%
Beta Blocker at Arrival	212	100%	87%	87%	100%
Beta Blocker at Discharge	252	99%	88%	90%	100%
Fibrinolytic Medication Timing	0	-	21%	31%	100%
PCI Within 90 Minutes of Arrival[1]	12	25%	47%	54%	95%
Smoking Cessation Advice	56	100%	84%	88%	100%
Heart Failure Care					
ACE Inhibitor or ARB for LVSD	307	96%	83%	82%	100%

NOTE: Hospital profiles are in alphabetical order by state, then city, then hospital within the city; Rankings are sorted by rate in descending order and exclude hospitals with less than 25 cases; (1) The number of cases is too small (n<25) for purposes of reliably predicting hospital performance; (2) Measure reflects the hospital's indication that its submission was based upon a sample of its relevant discharges; (3) Rate reflects fewer than the maximum possible quarters of data for the measure; (4) Inaccurate information submitted and suppressed for one or more quarters; (5) No data is available from the hospital for this measure; Please refer to the User's Guide for a full explanation of data

Discharge Instructions	666	77%	67%	61%	93%
Evaluation of LVS Function	745	100%	88%	83%	99%
Smoking Cessation Advice	155	95%	83%	82%	100%
Pneumonia Care					
Appropriate Initial Antibiotic	207	86%	83%	83%	94%
Blood Culture Timing	190	92%	91%	90%	100%
Influenza Vaccine	42	81%	63%	70%	100%
Initial Antibiotic Timing	282	78%	81%	80%	93%
Oxygenation Assessment	365	100%	99%	99%	100%
Pneumococcal Vaccine	169	80%	62%	69%	94%
Smoking Cessation Advice	91	87%	80%	80%	100%
Surgical Infection Prevention					
Prophylactic Antibiotic Given[2]	2,347	92%	74%	77%	95%
Prophylactic Antibiotic Selection[2]	513	98%	91%	90%	100%
Prophylactic Antibiotic Stopped[2]	2,308	88%	67%	72%	95%
Pregnancy Care					
Inpatient Neonatal Mortality	10,299	0.46%	-	-	-
Third or Fourth Degree Laceration	7,198	6.35%	3.89%	3.63%	3.27%

Norwegian-American Hospital

1044 N Francisco Avenue
Chicago, IL 60622
URL: www.n-ahs.org
Ownership: Voluntary non-profit - Private
Emergency Services: Yes
Phone: 773-292-8200
Fax: 773-278-3531
Accredited: Yes
Licensed Beds: 220

Key Personnel:

President/CEO. . . . . Michael E Haley
Chief Medical Staff. . . . . Jose De Leon, MD
Emergency Room . . . . Lilia Charpe, RN
OB/GYN Womens Health. . . . . Eduardo Barriuso, MD
Chief Radiology . . . . Howard Lopata, MD
Director Respiratory Therapy . . . . Diego Lopez

Measure	Cases	This Hospital	State Average	U.S. Average	Top Hospital
Heart Attack Care					
ACE Inhibitor or ARB for LVSD[1]	4	25%	79%	82%	100%
Aspirin at Arrival	42	90%	93%	92%	100%
Aspirin at Discharge[1]	21	76%	90%	90%	100%
Beta Blocker at Arrival	35	91%	87%	87%	100%
Beta Blocker at Discharge[1]	22	77%	88%	90%	100%
Fibrinolytic Medication Timing[1]	4	0%	21%	31%	100%
PCI Within 90 Minutes of Arrival	0	-	47%	54%	95%
Smoking Cessation Advice[1]	10	10%	84%	88%	100%
Heart Failure Care					
ACE Inhibitor or ARB for LVSD	76	62%	83%	82%	100%
Discharge Instructions	202	23%	67%	61%	93%
Evaluation of LVS Function	242	82%	88%	83%	99%
Smoking Cessation Advice	68	21%	83%	82%	100%
Pneumonia Care					
Appropriate Initial Antibiotic	61	74%	83%	83%	94%
Blood Culture Timing	46	87%	91%	90%	100%
Influenza Vaccine[4,5]	-	-	63%	70%	100%
Initial Antibiotic Timing	79	78%	81%	80%	93%
Oxygenation Assessment	81	100%	99%	99%	100%
Pneumococcal Vaccine	30	37%	62%	69%	94%
Smoking Cessation Advice	34	24%	80%	80%	100%
Surgical Infection Prevention					
Prophylactic Antibiotic Given[1,3]	18	50%	74%	77%	95%
Prophylactic Antibiotic Selection[1]	19	84%	91%	90%	100%
Prophylactic Antibiotic Stopped[1,3]	18	28%	67%	72%	95%
Pregnancy Care					
Inpatient Neonatal Mortality	-	-	-	-	-
Third or Fourth Degree Laceration	-	-	3.89%	3.63%	3.27%

Our Lady of the Resurrection Medical Center

5645 W Addison Street
Chicago, IL 60634
URL: www.reshealth.org
Ownership: Voluntary non-profit - Church
Emergency Services: Yes
Phone: 773-282-7000
Fax: 773-794-8353
Accredited: Yes
Licensed Beds: 407

Key Personnel:

President/CEO. . . . . Ivette Estrada
President Medical Staff . . . . Shirish Shah, MD
Catheterization Lab Manager. . . . . Karen Conoboy, RN
Coordinator Infection Control . . . . Ann Marie Ogle, RN
ICU Supervising Nurse. Kathleen Wians, RN
Manager Medical Staff. Linda Smith
Surgical Services . . . . Crystal Mobley, RN
Director Respiratory/Cardiopulmonary . . . . Sue Victor

Measure	Cases	This Hospital	State Average	U.S. Average	Top Hospital
Heart Attack Care					
ACE Inhibitor or ARB for LVSD	43	88%	79%	82%	100%
Aspirin at Arrival	238	97%	93%	92%	100%
Aspirin at Discharge	192	96%	90%	90%	100%
Beta Blocker at Arrival	222	96%	87%	87%	100%
Beta Blocker at Discharge	198	96%	88%	90%	100%
Fibrinolytic Medication Timing	0	-	21%	31%	100%
PCI Within 90 Minutes of Arrival[1]	4	50%	47%	54%	95%
Smoking Cessation Advice	53	96%	84%	88%	100%
Heart Failure Care					
ACE Inhibitor or ARB for LVSD	202	90%	83%	82%	100%
Discharge Instructions	380	71%	67%	61%	93%
Evaluation of LVS Function	608	100%	88%	83%	99%
Smoking Cessation Advice	82	96%	83%	82%	100%
Pneumonia Care					
Appropriate Initial Antibiotic	142	82%	83%	83%	94%
Blood Culture Timing	180	88%	91%	90%	100%
Influenza Vaccine	40	72%	63%	70%	100%
Initial Antibiotic Timing	247	85%	81%	80%	93%
Oxygenation Assessment	301	100%	99%	99%	100%
Pneumococcal Vaccine	193	68%	62%	69%	94%
Smoking Cessation Advice	58	97%	80%	80%	100%
Surgical Infection Prevention					
Prophylactic Antibiotic Given[3]	153	63%	74%	77%	95%
Prophylactic Antibiotic Selection[5]	-	-	91%	90%	100%
Prophylactic Antibiotic Stopped[3]	133	42%	67%	72%	95%
Pregnancy Care					
Inpatient Neonatal Mortality	-	-	-	-	-
Third or Fourth Degree Laceration	-	-	3.89%	3.63%	3.27%

Provident Hospital

500 E 51st Street
Chicago, IL 60615
URL: www.providentfoundation.org
Ownership: Government - Local
Emergency Services: Yes
Phone: 312-572-2000
Fax: 312-572-2796
Accredited: Yes
Licensed Beds: 243

Key Personnel:

Administrator . . . . Stephanie Brigh Griggs
Chief Medical Staff. . . . . James Myles

Measure	Cases	This Hospital	State Average	U.S. Average	Top Hospital
Heart Attack Care					
ACE Inhibitor or ARB for LVSD[1]	2	100%	79%	82%	100%
Aspirin at Arrival	53	94%	93%	92%	100%
Aspirin at Discharge[1]	22	77%	90%	90%	100%
Beta Blocker at Arrival	54	87%	87%	87%	100%
Beta Blocker at Discharge[1]	24	62%	88%	90%	100%
Fibrinolytic Medication Timing	0	-	21%	31%	100%
PCI Within 90 Minutes of Arrival	0	-	47%	54%	95%
Smoking Cessation Advice[1]	11	64%	84%	88%	100%
Heart Failure Care					
ACE Inhibitor or ARB for LVSD[2]	163	92%	83%	82%	100%
Discharge Instructions[2]	402	73%	67%	61%	93%
Evaluation of LVS Function[2]	382	88%	88%	83%	99%
Smoking Cessation Advice[2]	185	95%	83%	82%	100%
Pneumonia Care					
Appropriate Initial Antibiotic	253	88%	83%	83%	94%
Blood Culture Timing	231	80%	91%	90%	100%
Influenza Vaccine	33	15%	63%	70%	100%
Initial Antibiotic Timing	292	52%	81%	80%	93%
Oxygenation Assessment	308	100%	99%	99%	100%
Pneumococcal Vaccine	69	25%	62%	69%	94%
Smoking Cessation Advice	154	95%	80%	80%	100%
Surgical Infection Prevention					

NOTE: Hospital profiles are in alphabetical order by state, then city, then hospital within the city; Rankings are sorted by rate in descending order and exclude hospitals with less than 25 cases; (1) The number of cases is too small (n<25) for purposes of reliably predicting hospital performance; (2) Measure reflects the hospital's indication that its submission was based upon a sample of its relevant discharges; (3) Rate reflects fewer than the maximum possible quarters of data for the measure; (4) Inaccurate information submitted and suppressed for one or more quarters; (5) No data is available from the hospital for this measure; Please refer to the User's Guide for a full explanation of data

Measure	Cases	This Hospital	State Average	U.S. Average	Top Hospital
Prophylactic Antibiotic Given[1,3]	17	29%	74%	77%	95%
Prophylactic Antibiotic Selection[1]	14	86%	91%	90%	100%
Prophylactic Antibiotic Stopped[1,3]	16	44%	67%	72%	95%
Pregnancy Care					
Inpatient Neonatal Mortality	526	0.38%	-	-	-
Third or Fourth Degree Laceration	401	2.49%	3.89%	3.63%	3.27%

Resurrection Medical Center

7435 West Talcott Avenue
Chicago, IL 60631
URL: www.reshealthcare.org
Ownership: Voluntary non-profit - Church
Emergency Services: Yes
Phone: 773-774-8000
Fax: 773-792-9926
Accredited: Yes
Licensed Beds: 434

Key Personnel:

Manager Catheterization Laboratory . . . . Debbie Serwa
Catheterization Lab . . . . Patricia Nedved
Medical Director Emergency Room . . . . M Rosemberg, MD
Director Infection/Disease Control . . . . Marcia Beckerdite
Director Medical/Surgical Nursing . . . . Cathy Holden
OB/GYN Womens Health. . . . . Mary Hillard, RN
Director Radiology . . . . John McGreevy

Measure	Cases	This Hospital	State Average	U.S. Average	Top Hospital
Heart Attack Care					
ACE Inhibitor or ARB for LVSD	73	62%	79%	82%	100%
Aspirin at Arrival	343	97%	93%	92%	100%
Aspirin at Discharge	316	93%	90%	90%	100%
Beta Blocker at Arrival	199	89%	87%	87%	100%
Beta Blocker at Discharge	316	88%	88%	90%	100%
Fibrinolytic Medication Timing[1]	2	0%	21%	31%	100%
PCI Within 90 Minutes of Arrival[1]	21	5%	47%	54%	95%
Smoking Cessation Advice	87	90%	84%	88%	100%
Heart Failure Care					
ACE Inhibitor or ARB for LVSD	258	63%	83%	82%	100%
Discharge Instructions	613	45%	67%	61%	93%
Evaluation of LVS Function	868	90%	88%	83%	99%
Smoking Cessation Advice	77	73%	83%	82%	100%
Pneumonia Care					
Appropriate Initial Antibiotic	260	82%	83%	83%	94%
Blood Culture Timing	308	96%	91%	90%	100%
Influenza Vaccine[4,5]	-	-	63%	70%	100%
Initial Antibiotic Timing	422	87%	81%	80%	93%
Oxygenation Assessment	466	98%	99%	99%	100%
Pneumococcal Vaccine	322	27%	62%	69%	94%
Smoking Cessation Advice	54	78%	80%	80%	100%
Surgical Infection Prevention					
Prophylactic Antibiotic Given[3]	60	75%	74%	77%	95%
Prophylactic Antibiotic Selection	60	98%	91%	90%	100%
Prophylactic Antibiotic Stopped[3]	51	61%	67%	72%	95%
Pregnancy Care					
Inpatient Neonatal Mortality	-	-	-	-	-
Third or Fourth Degree Laceration	-	-	3.89%	3.63%	3.27%

Roseland Community Hospital

45 W 111th Street
Chicago, IL 60628
URL: www.roselandhospital.org
Ownership: Voluntary non-profit - Other
Emergency Services: Yes
Phone: 773-995-3000
Fax: 773-995-1052
Accredited: Yes
Licensed Beds: 162

Key Personnel:

President/CEO. . . . . Donald C Sibery

Measure	Cases	This Hospital	State Average	U.S. Average	Top Hospital
Heart Attack Care					
ACE Inhibitor or ARB for LVSD[1]	3	100%	79%	82%	100%
Aspirin at Arrival[1]	24	96%	93%	92%	100%
Aspirin at Discharge[1]	11	91%	90%	90%	100%
Beta Blocker at Arrival[1]	24	92%	87%	87%	100%
Beta Blocker at Discharge[1]	11	91%	88%	90%	100%
Fibrinolytic Medication Timing[1]	4	25%	21%	31%	100%
PCI Within 90 Minutes of Arrival	0	-	47%	54%	95%
Smoking Cessation Advice[1]	5	60%	84%	88%	100%
Heart Failure Care					
ACE Inhibitor or ARB for LVSD[2]	97	86%	83%	82%	100%
Discharge Instructions[2]	279	86%	67%	61%	93%
Evaluation of LVS Function[2]	295	78%	88%	83%	99%
Smoking Cessation Advice[2]	124	70%	83%	82%	100%
Pneumonia Care					
Appropriate Initial Antibiotic	109	81%	83%	83%	94%
Blood Culture Timing	99	64%	91%	90%	100%
Influenza Vaccine[4,5]	-	-	63%	70%	100%
Initial Antibiotic Timing	154	56%	81%	80%	93%
Oxygenation Assessment	164	100%	99%	99%	100%
Pneumococcal Vaccine	48	31%	62%	69%	94%
Smoking Cessation Advice	69	78%	80%	80%	100%
Surgical Infection Prevention					
Prophylactic Antibiotic Given[1,3]	10	30%	74%	77%	95%
Prophylactic Antibiotic Selection[1]	2	100%	91%	90%	100%
Prophylactic Antibiotic Stopped[1,3]	8	25%	67%	72%	95%
Pregnancy Care					
Inpatient Neonatal Mortality	-	-	-	-	-
Third or Fourth Degree Laceration	-	-	3.89%	3.63%	3.27%

Rush University Medical Center

1653 W Congress Parkway
Chicago, IL 60612
URL: www.rush.edu
Ownership: Voluntary non-profit - Private
Emergency Services: Yes
Phone: 312-942-5000
Fax: 312-942-8021
Accredited: Yes
Licensed Beds: 809

Key Personnel:

Administrator/President . . . . Leo M Henikoff, MD
Chief Medical Staff. . . . . Erich Bruescke, MD
Director Catheterization Laboratory . . . . Gary Schaer, MD
Emergency Room . . . . Paul K Hanashiro, MD
Director Infection/Disease Control . . . . Gorden Trenholme, MD
CCU Spvg. Nurse . . . . Joan Mathien, RN
OB/GYN Womens Health. . . . . Thomas A Deutsch
Chief Radiology . . . . Jerry Petasnick, MD
Director Respiratory Therapy . . . . Grant Larson

Measure	Cases	This Hospital	State Average	U.S. Average	Top Hospital
Heart Attack Care					
ACE Inhibitor or ARB for LVSD[1]	24	96%	79%	82%	100%
Aspirin at Arrival	112	100%	93%	92%	100%
Aspirin at Discharge	148	100%	90%	90%	100%
Beta Blocker at Arrival	95	100%	87%	87%	100%
Beta Blocker at Discharge	147	100%	88%	90%	100%
Fibrinolytic Medication Timing	0	-	21%	31%	100%
PCI Within 90 Minutes of Arrival[1]	4	50%	47%	54%	95%
Smoking Cessation Advice	51	100%	84%	88%	100%
Heart Failure Care					
ACE Inhibitor or ARB for LVSD[2]	139	96%	83%	82%	100%
Discharge Instructions[2]	311	78%	67%	61%	93%
Evaluation of LVS Function[2]	338	100%	88%	83%	99%
Smoking Cessation Advice[2]	71	97%	83%	82%	100%
Pneumonia Care					
Appropriate Initial Antibiotic[2]	58	93%	83%	83%	94%
Blood Culture Timing[2]	71	90%	91%	90%	100%
Influenza Vaccine[1,2]	24	67%	63%	70%	100%
Initial Antibiotic Timing[2]	96	79%	81%	80%	93%
Oxygenation Assessment[2]	145	100%	99%	99%	100%
Pneumococcal Vaccine[2]	63	75%	62%	69%	94%
Smoking Cessation Advice[2]	41	95%	80%	80%	100%
Surgical Infection Prevention					
Prophylactic Antibiotic Given[2,3]	425	90%	74%	77%	95%
Prophylactic Antibiotic Selection[2]	102	98%	91%	90%	100%
Prophylactic Antibiotic Stopped[2,3]	417	86%	67%	72%	95%
Pregnancy Care					
Inpatient Neonatal Mortality	-	-	-	-	-
Third or Fourth Degree Laceration	-	-	3.89%	3.63%	3.27%

NOTE: Hospital profiles are in alphabetical order by state, then city, then hospital within the city; Rankings are sorted by rate in descending order and exclude hospitals with less than 25 cases; (1) The number of cases is too small (n<25) for purposes of reliably predicting hospital performance; (2) Measure reflects the hospital's indication that its submission was based upon a sample of its relevant discharges; (3) Rate reflects fewer than the maximum possible quarters of data for the measure; (4) Inaccurate information submitted and suppressed for one or more quarters; (5) No data is available from the hospital for this measure; Please refer to the User's Guide for a full explanation of data

Sacred Heart Hospital

3240 W Franklin Boulevard
Chicago, IL 60624
URL: www.sacredheartchicago.com
Ownership: Proprietary
Emergency Services: Yes
Phone: 773-722-3020
Fax: 773-722-5535
Accredited: Yes
Licensed Beds: 119

Key Personnel:
CEO. . . . . Edward J Novak
Infection Control. . . . . Helen Sethurama

Measure	Cases	This Hospital	State Average	U.S. Average	Top Hospital
Heart Attack Care					
ACE Inhibitor or ARB for LVSD[1,3]	1	0%	79%	82%	100%
Aspirin at Arrival[1,3]	2	100%	93%	92%	100%
Aspirin at Discharge[3]	0	-	90%	90%	100%
Beta Blocker at Arrival[1,3]	1	0%	87%	87%	100%
Beta Blocker at Discharge[1,3]	1	0%	88%	90%	100%
Fibrinolytic Medication Timing[3]	0	-	21%	31%	100%
PCI Within 90 Minutes of Arrival	0	-	47%	54%	95%
Smoking Cessation Advice[3]	0	-	84%	88%	100%
Heart Failure Care					
ACE Inhibitor or ARB for LVSD[1]	20	50%	83%	82%	100%
Discharge Instructions	152	4%	67%	61%	93%
Evaluation of LVS Function	160	94%	88%	83%	99%
Smoking Cessation Advice[1]	20	25%	83%	82%	100%
Pneumonia Care					
Appropriate Initial Antibiotic[1]	9	89%	83%	83%	94%
Blood Culture Timing[1]	3	33%	91%	90%	100%
Influenza Vaccine[1]	3	0%	63%	70%	100%
Initial Antibiotic Timing[1]	15	33%	81%	80%	93%
Oxygenation Assessment[1]	16	94%	99%	99%	100%
Pneumococcal Vaccine[1]	5	0%	62%	69%	94%
Smoking Cessation Advice[1]	6	17%	80%	80%	100%
Surgical Infection Prevention					
Prophylactic Antibiotic Given[1,2,3]	1	0%	74%	77%	95%
Prophylactic Antibiotic Selection[2]	0	-	91%	90%	100%
Prophylactic Antibiotic Stopped[1,2,3]	1	0%	67%	72%	95%
Pregnancy Care					
Inpatient Neonatal Mortality	-	-	-	-	-
Third or Fourth Degree Laceration	-	-	3.89%	3.63%	3.27%

Saint Anthony Hospital

2875 W 19th Street
Chicago, IL 60623
URL: www.cath-health.org
Ownership: Voluntary non-profit - Church
Emergency Services: Yes
Phone: 773-484-1000
Fax: 773-521-7902
Accredited: Yes
Licensed Beds: 183

Key Personnel:
CEO. . . . . Kathleen K DeVine
Director Emergency Room. . . . . Nancy Badruv
Infection Control Nurse. Julie Sammarco

Measure	Cases	This Hospital	State Average	U.S. Average	Top Hospital
Heart Attack Care					
ACE Inhibitor or ARB for LVSD[1]	2	50%	79%	82%	100%
Aspirin at Arrival	28	96%	93%	92%	100%
Aspirin at Discharge[1]	9	78%	90%	90%	100%
Beta Blocker at Arrival[1]	14	100%	87%	87%	100%
Beta Blocker at Discharge[1]	6	83%	88%	90%	100%
Fibrinolytic Medication Timing[1]	1	100%	21%	31%	100%
PCI Within 90 Minutes of Arrival	0	-	47%	54%	95%
Smoking Cessation Advice[1]	3	67%	84%	88%	100%
Heart Failure Care					
ACE Inhibitor or ARB for LVSD	60	60%	83%	82%	100%
Discharge Instructions	162	42%	67%	61%	93%
Evaluation of LVS Function	179	87%	88%	83%	99%
Smoking Cessation Advice	51	92%	83%	82%	100%
Pneumonia Care					
Appropriate Initial Antibiotic	69	88%	83%	83%	94%
Blood Culture Timing	73	95%	91%	90%	100%
Influenza Vaccine[1]	12	58%	63%	70%	100%
Initial Antibiotic Timing	93	85%	81%	80%	93%
Oxygenation Assessment	115	100%	99%	99%	100%
Pneumococcal Vaccine	44	43%	62%	69%	94%
Smoking Cessation Advice	39	97%	80%	80%	100%
Surgical Infection Prevention					
Prophylactic Antibiotic Given[3]	33	70%	74%	77%	95%
Prophylactic Antibiotic Selection[1]	16	75%	91%	90%	100%
Prophylactic Antibiotic Stopped[3]	31	45%	67%	72%	95%
Pregnancy Care					
Inpatient Neonatal Mortality	-	-	-	-	-
Third or Fourth Degree Laceration	-	-	3.89%	3.63%	3.27%

Saint Bernard Hospital and Health Care Center

326 West 64th Street
Chicago, IL 60621
E-mail: info@stbh.org
URL: www.stbh.org
Ownership: Voluntary non-profit - Church
Emergency Services: Yes
Phone: 773-962-3900
Fax: 773-962-0034
Accredited: Yes
Licensed Beds: 143

Key Personnel:
President/CEO. . . . . Sr Elizabeth Van Straten, RHSJ

Measure	Cases	This Hospital	State Average	U.S. Average	Top Hospital
Heart Attack Care					
ACE Inhibitor or ARB for LVSD[1]	3	67%	79%	82%	100%
Aspirin at Arrival	32	100%	93%	92%	100%
Aspirin at Discharge[1]	16	75%	90%	90%	100%
Beta Blocker at Arrival	30	90%	87%	87%	100%
Beta Blocker at Discharge[1]	16	62%	88%	90%	100%
Fibrinolytic Medication Timing	0	-	21%	31%	100%
PCI Within 90 Minutes of Arrival	0	-	47%	54%	95%
Smoking Cessation Advice[1]	3	100%	84%	88%	100%
Heart Failure Care					
ACE Inhibitor or ARB for LVSD[2]	109	83%	83%	82%	100%
Discharge Instructions[2]	275	97%	67%	61%	93%
Evaluation of LVS Function[2]	326	97%	88%	83%	99%
Smoking Cessation Advice[2]	129	98%	83%	82%	100%
Pneumonia Care					
Appropriate Initial Antibiotic[2]	149	91%	83%	83%	94%
Blood Culture Timing[2]	183	88%	91%	90%	100%
Influenza Vaccine[2]	32	22%	63%	70%	100%
Initial Antibiotic Timing[2]	232	72%	81%	80%	93%
Oxygenation Assessment[2]	260	100%	99%	99%	100%
Pneumococcal Vaccine[2]	86	16%	62%	69%	94%
Smoking Cessation Advice[2]	92	99%	80%	80%	100%
Surgical Infection Prevention					
Prophylactic Antibiotic Given[1,2,3]	21	29%	74%	77%	95%
Prophylactic Antibiotic Selection[1,2]	5	100%	91%	90%	100%
Prophylactic Antibiotic Stopped[1,2,3]	20	5%	67%	72%	95%
Pregnancy Care					
Inpatient Neonatal Mortality	-	-	-	-	-
Third or Fourth Degree Laceration	-	-	3.89%	3.63%	3.27%

Saint Elizabeth's Hospital

1431 N Claremont Avenue
Chicago, IL 60622
URL: www.ancilla.org
Ownership: Voluntary non-profit - Church
Emergency Services: Yes
Phone: 312-491-5000
Fax: 312-633-5932
Accredited: Yes
Licensed Beds: 276

Key Personnel:
CEO. . . . . Margaret McDermot
Chief of Medical Staff. . . . . H Velarde, MD
Director of Cardiology/Cardiac Lab. . . . . John Fedivy
Emergency Room . . . . Geraldine Kentgen
Director Medical/Surgical Nursing . . . . Betty Bayona
OB/GYN Womens Health. . . . . Pamela White
Chief Radiology . . . . Marian Demus
Director Respiratory Therapy . . . . Caeser Troya

Measure	Cases	This Hospital	State Average	U.S. Average	Top Hospital
Heart Attack Care					
ACE Inhibitor or ARB for LVSD[1]	4	50%	79%	82%	100%
Aspirin at Arrival	38	92%	93%	92%	100%

Measure	Cases	This Hospital	State Average	U.S. Average	Top Hospital
Aspirin at Discharge[1]	21	95%	90%	90%	100%
Beta Blocker at Arrival	35	86%	87%	87%	100%
Beta Blocker at Discharge[1]	22	91%	88%	90%	100%
Fibrinolytic Medication Timing[1]	6	33%	21%	31%	100%
PCI Within 90 Minutes of Arrival	0	-	47%	54%	95%
Smoking Cessation Advice[1]	8	100%	84%	88%	100%
Heart Failure Care					
ACE Inhibitor or ARB for LVSD	75	84%	83%	82%	100%
Discharge Instructions	145	85%	67%	61%	93%
Evaluation of LVS Function	186	95%	88%	83%	99%
Smoking Cessation Advice	32	97%	83%	82%	100%
Pneumonia Care					
Appropriate Initial Antibiotic	106	72%	83%	83%	94%
Blood Culture Timing	119	97%	91%	90%	100%
Influenza Vaccine[1]	24	50%	63%	70%	100%
Initial Antibiotic Timing	151	93%	81%	80%	93%
Oxygenation Assessment	178	100%	99%	99%	100%
Pneumococcal Vaccine	89	84%	62%	69%	94%
Smoking Cessation Advice	43	100%	80%	80%	100%
Surgical Infection Prevention					
Prophylactic Antibiotic Given	121	89%	74%	77%	95%
Prophylactic Antibiotic Selection	26	92%	91%	90%	100%
Prophylactic Antibiotic Stopped	105	76%	67%	72%	95%
Pregnancy Care					
Inpatient Neonatal Mortality	-	-	-	-	-
Third or Fourth Degree Laceration	-	-	3.89%	3.63%	3.27%

Saint Joseph Hospital

2900 N Lake Shore Drive | Phone: 773-665-3000
Chicago, IL 60657 | Fax: 773-665-6502
URL: www.res-health.org
Ownership: Voluntary non-profit - Church | Accredited: Yes
Emergency Services: Yes | Licensed Beds: 492

Key Personnel:
CEO . . . . Ronald Struxness
Chief Medical Staff . . . . Andrew Gorchynky
Emergency Room . . . . Geoffery Grassle
Respiratory Care . . . . Bill Hayakawa

Measure	Cases	This Hospital	State Average	U.S. Average	Top Hospital
Heart Attack Care					
ACE Inhibitor or ARB for LVSD[1]	22	77%	79%	82%	100%
Aspirin at Arrival	56	98%	93%	92%	100%
Aspirin at Discharge	62	98%	90%	90%	100%
Beta Blocker at Arrival	45	100%	87%	87%	100%
Beta Blocker at Discharge	65	89%	88%	90%	100%
Fibrinolytic Medication Timing	0	-	21%	31%	100%
PCI Within 90 Minutes of Arrival[1]	2	50%	47%	54%	95%
Smoking Cessation Advice[1]	17	88%	84%	88%	100%
Heart Failure Care					
ACE Inhibitor or ARB for LVSD	128	80%	83%	82%	100%
Discharge Instructions	330	59%	67%	61%	93%
Evaluation of LVS Function	421	94%	88%	83%	99%
Smoking Cessation Advice	60	83%	83%	82%	100%
Pneumonia Care					
Appropriate Initial Antibiotic	117	87%	83%	83%	94%
Blood Culture Timing	143	94%	91%	90%	100%
Influenza Vaccine	45	58%	63%	70%	100%
Initial Antibiotic Timing	199	86%	81%	80%	93%
Oxygenation Assessment	252	100%	99%	99%	100%
Pneumococcal Vaccine	151	46%	62%	69%	94%
Smoking Cessation Advice	51	82%	80%	80%	100%
Surgical Infection Prevention					
Prophylactic Antibiotic Given[3]	345	85%	74%	77%	95%
Prophylactic Antibiotic Selection	90	94%	91%	90%	100%
Prophylactic Antibiotic Stopped[3]	332	69%	67%	72%	95%
Pregnancy Care					
Inpatient Neonatal Mortality	-	-	-	-	-
Third or Fourth Degree Laceration	-	-	3.89%	3.63%	3.27%

Saints Mary & Elizabeth Medical Center

2233 W Division Street | Phone: 312-770-2000
Chicago, IL 60622 | Fax: 312-770-2392
URL: www.reshealth.org
Ownership: Voluntary non-profit - Church | Accredited: Yes
Emergency Services: Yes | Licensed Beds: 387

Key Personnel:
CEO . . . . Margaret McDermott
Chief Medical Staff . . . . Hugo Velrade, MD
Director Cardiac Lab . . . . John Sedivy
Medical Director Catheterization Lab . . . . Danilo A Deano, MD
Director Emergency Room . . . . Beverly Weaver, RN MS
Emergency Room . . . . Scott Betzelos, MD
Coordinator Infection Control . . . . Pat Alexander, RN
Director Medical/Surgical Nursing . . . . Maria Schwartz, RN
Director Respiratory Therapy . . . . Cesar Troya, RT

Measure	Cases	This Hospital	State Average	U.S. Average	Top Hospital
Heart Attack Care					
ACE Inhibitor or ARB for LVSD[1]	24	79%	79%	82%	100%
Aspirin at Arrival	63	100%	93%	92%	100%
Aspirin at Discharge	99	97%	90%	90%	100%
Beta Blocker at Arrival	61	90%	87%	87%	100%
Beta Blocker at Discharge	99	90%	88%	90%	100%
Fibrinolytic Medication Timing[1]	5	20%	21%	31%	100%
PCI Within 90 Minutes of Arrival	0	-	47%	54%	95%
Smoking Cessation Advice	40	92%	84%	88%	100%
Heart Failure Care					
ACE Inhibitor or ARB for LVSD	117	83%	83%	82%	100%
Discharge Instructions	307	48%	67%	61%	93%
Evaluation of LVS Function	336	88%	88%	83%	99%
Smoking Cessation Advice	68	72%	83%	82%	100%
Pneumonia Care					
Appropriate Initial Antibiotic	158	85%	83%	83%	94%
Blood Culture Timing	142	94%	91%	90%	100%
Influenza Vaccine[4,5]	-	-	63%	70%	100%
Initial Antibiotic Timing	199	88%	81%	80%	93%
Oxygenation Assessment	215	98%	99%	99%	100%
Pneumococcal Vaccine	109	57%	62%	69%	94%
Smoking Cessation Advice	57	81%	80%	80%	100%
Surgical Infection Prevention					
Prophylactic Antibiotic Given	233	86%	74%	77%	95%
Prophylactic Antibiotic Selection	60	82%	91%	90%	100%
Prophylactic Antibiotic Stopped	219	64%	67%	72%	95%
Pregnancy Care					
Inpatient Neonatal Mortality	-	-	-	-	-
Third or Fourth Degree Laceration	-	-	3.89%	3.63%	3.27%

South Shore Hospital

8012 S Crandon Avenue | Phone: 773-768-0810
Chicago, IL 60617 | Fax: 773-768-8154
URL: www.southshorehospital.com
Ownership: Voluntary non-profit - Other | Accredited: Yes
Emergency Services: Yes | Licensed Beds: 170

Key Personnel:
President/CEO . . . . Jesus M Ong
Chief Medical Staff . . . . Surinder Parmar
Emergency Room . . . . Issac Plamoohil, MD
Emergency Room . . . . Jackie Levandowski, RN
Director Radiology . . . . Rayeon Lamp Kir

Measure	Cases	This Hospital	State Average	U.S. Average	Top Hospital
Heart Attack Care					
ACE Inhibitor or ARB for LVSD[1]	8	62%	79%	82%	100%
Aspirin at Arrival	48	81%	93%	92%	100%
Aspirin at Discharge[1]	19	79%	90%	90%	100%
Beta Blocker at Arrival	42	79%	87%	87%	100%
Beta Blocker at Discharge	25	88%	88%	90%	100%
Fibrinolytic Medication Timing[1]	2	0%	21%	31%	100%
PCI Within 90 Minutes of Arrival	0	-	47%	54%	95%
Smoking Cessation Advice[1]	4	50%	84%	88%	100%
Heart Failure Care					
ACE Inhibitor or ARB for LVSD	62	79%	83%	82%	100%

NOTE: Hospital profiles are in alphabetical order by state, then city, then hospital within the city; Rankings are sorted by rate in descending order and exclude hospitals with less than 25 cases; (1) The number of cases is too small (n<25) for purposes of reliably predicting hospital performance; (2) Measure reflects the hospital's indication that its submission was based upon a sample of its relevant discharges; (3) Rate reflects fewer than the maximum possible quarters of data for the measure; (4) Inaccurate information submitted and suppressed for one or more quarters; (5) No data is available from the hospital for this measure; Please refer to the User's Guide for a full explanation of data

Discharge Instructions	205	64%	67%	61%	93%
Evaluation of LVS Function	247	92%	88%	83%	99%
Smoking Cessation Advice	60	82%	83%	82%	100%
Pneumonia Care					
Appropriate Initial Antibiotic	62	73%	83%	83%	94%
Blood Culture Timing	76	82%	91%	90%	100%
Influenza Vaccine[1]	20	15%	63%	70%	100%
Initial Antibiotic Timing	118	74%	81%	80%	93%
Oxygenation Assessment	147	95%	99%	99%	100%
Pneumococcal Vaccine	66	3%	62%	69%	94%
Smoking Cessation Advice	31	71%	80%	80%	100%
Surgical Infection Prevention					
Prophylactic Antibiotic Given[1,3]	15	20%	74%	77%	95%
Prophylactic Antibiotic Selection[1]	15	67%	91%	90%	100%
Prophylactic Antibiotic Stopped[1,3]	14	100%	67%	72%	95%
Pregnancy Care					
Inpatient Neonatal Mortality	-	-	-	-	-
Third or Fourth Degree Laceration	-	-	3.89%	3.63%	3.27%

Swedish Covenant Hospital

5145 N California Avenue
Chicago, IL 60625
Ownership: Voluntary non-profit - Church
Emergency Services: Yes
Phone: 773-878-8200
Fax: 773-878-6152
Accredited: Yes
Licensed Beds: 330

Key Personnel:

CEO . . . . Mark Newton
Chief Medical Staff . . . . Albert Saporta, MD
Emergency Room . . . . William Lauth
Emergency Room . . . . Sun Be Lee, RN
OB/GYN Womens Health . . . . Peter Delneky, MD
Chief Radiology . . . . Bruce Silver, MD
Chief Pulmonary Services . . . . Claude Vanetti

Measure	Cases	This Hospital	State Average	U.S. Average	Top Hospital
Heart Attack Care					
ACE Inhibitor or ARB for LVSD[1]	17	94%	79%	82%	100%
Aspirin at Arrival	199	100%	93%	92%	100%
Aspirin at Discharge	176	99%	90%	90%	100%
Beta Blocker at Arrival	183	98%	87%	87%	100%
Beta Blocker at Discharge	171	99%	88%	90%	100%
Fibrinolytic Medication Timing	0	-	21%	31%	100%
PCI Within 90 Minutes of Arrival	0	-	47%	54%	95%
Smoking Cessation Advice	53	100%	84%	88%	100%
Heart Failure Care					
ACE Inhibitor or ARB for LVSD	173	84%	83%	82%	100%
Discharge Instructions	348	31%	67%	61%	93%
Evaluation of LVS Function	504	92%	88%	83%	99%
Smoking Cessation Advice	38	71%	83%	82%	100%
Pneumonia Care					
Appropriate Initial Antibiotic	223	65%	83%	83%	94%
Blood Culture Timing	142	85%	91%	90%	100%
Influenza Vaccine	84	21%	63%	70%	100%
Initial Antibiotic Timing	367	76%	81%	80%	93%
Oxygenation Assessment	439	100%	99%	99%	100%
Pneumococcal Vaccine	293	33%	62%	69%	94%
Smoking Cessation Advice	47	68%	80%	80%	100%
Surgical Infection Prevention					
Prophylactic Antibiotic Given[2,3]	60	73%	74%	77%	95%
Prophylactic Antibiotic Selection[2]	62	98%	91%	90%	100%
Prophylactic Antibiotic Stopped[2,3]	57	100%	67%	72%	95%
Pregnancy Care					
Inpatient Neonatal Mortality	-	-	-	-	-
Third or Fourth Degree Laceration	-	-	3.89%	3.63%	3.27%

Thorek Hospital and Medical Center

850 W Irving Park
Chicago, IL 60613
URL: www.thorek.org
Ownership: Voluntary non-profit - Other
Emergency Services: Yes
Phone: 773-525-6780
Fax: 773-975-6703
Accredited: Yes
Licensed Beds: 218

Key Personnel:

Chairman/CEO . . . . Frank A Solare
Chief Medical Staff . . . . Jagan Mohan, MD
Emergency Room . . . . Effie Heale
OB/GYN Womens Health . . . . Farhad Saed, MD
Chief Radiology . . . . Gustavo Espinosa, MD
Director Respiratory Therapy . . . . Nestor Ferreria

Measure	Cases	This Hospital	State Average	U.S. Average	Top Hospital
Heart Attack Care					
ACE Inhibitor or ARB for LVSD[1,2]	4	100%	79%	82%	100%
Aspirin at Arrival[1,2]	22	100%	93%	92%	100%
Aspirin at Discharge[1,2]	15	100%	90%	90%	100%
Beta Blocker at Arrival[1,2]	21	95%	87%	87%	100%
Beta Blocker at Discharge[1,2]	18	94%	88%	90%	100%
Fibrinolytic Medication Timing[1,2]	2	0%	21%	31%	100%
PCI Within 90 Minutes of Arrival[2]	0	-	47%	54%	95%
Smoking Cessation Advice[1,2]	3	100%	84%	88%	100%
Heart Failure Care					
ACE Inhibitor or ARB for LVSD[2]	27	100%	83%	82%	100%
Discharge Instructions[2]	100	99%	67%	61%	93%
Evaluation of LVS Function[2]	118	97%	88%	83%	99%
Smoking Cessation Advice[2]	29	100%	83%	82%	100%
Pneumonia Care					
Appropriate Initial Antibiotic[2]	48	79%	83%	83%	94%
Blood Culture Timing[2]	57	96%	91%	90%	100%
Influenza Vaccine[1]	13	8%	63%	70%	100%
Initial Antibiotic Timing[2]	125	61%	81%	80%	93%
Oxygenation Assessment[2]	141	98%	99%	99%	100%
Pneumococcal Vaccine[2]	69	36%	62%	69%	94%
Smoking Cessation Advice[2]	36	100%	80%	80%	100%
Surgical Infection Prevention					
Prophylactic Antibiotic Given[2]	59	81%	74%	77%	95%
Prophylactic Antibiotic Selection[1,2]	13	92%	91%	90%	100%
Prophylactic Antibiotic Stopped[2]	58	31%	67%	72%	95%
Pregnancy Care					
Inpatient Neonatal Mortality	-	-	-	-	-
Third or Fourth Degree Laceration	-	-	3.89%	3.63%	3.27%

University of Chicago Hospitals

5841 S Maryland
Chicago, IL 60637
URL: www.uchospitals.edu
Ownership: Voluntary non-profit - Private
Emergency Services: Yes
Phone: 773-702-1000
Fax: 773-702-9005
Accredited: Yes
Licensed Beds: 662

Key Personnel:

President/CEO . . . . Ralph Muller
Chief Medical Staff . . . . Jofar Al-Sadir, MD
Director Catheterization Laboratory . . . . David Faxon, MD
Chief Catheterization Laboratory . . . . David Faxon, MD
Emergency Room . . . . James Walter, MD
Director Infection/Disease Control . . . . Paul Arnow, MD
Director Medical/Surgical Nursing . . . . Diane Smith
OB/GYN Womens Health . . . . Arthur Herbst, MD
Director Respiratory Therapy . . . . Jesse Hall, MD

Measure	Cases	This Hospital	State Average	U.S. Average	Top Hospital
Heart Attack Care					
ACE Inhibitor or ARB for LVSD[2]	55	91%	79%	82%	100%
Aspirin at Arrival[2]	141	96%	93%	92%	100%
Aspirin at Discharge[2]	219	98%	90%	90%	100%
Beta Blocker at Arrival[2]	125	91%	87%	87%	100%
Beta Blocker at Discharge[2]	210	96%	88%	90%	100%
Fibrinolytic Medication Timing[2]	0	-	21%	31%	100%
PCI Within 90 Minutes of Arrival[1,2]	6	33%	47%	54%	95%
Smoking Cessation Advice[2]	88	90%	84%	88%	100%
Heart Failure Care					
ACE Inhibitor or ARB for LVSD[2]	170	89%	83%	82%	100%
Discharge Instructions[2]	298	46%	67%	61%	93%
Evaluation of LVS Function[2]	326	98%	88%	83%	99%
Smoking Cessation Advice[2]	82	83%	83%	82%	100%
Pneumonia Care					
Appropriate Initial Antibiotic[2]	93	76%	83%	83%	94%
Blood Culture Timing[2]	59	76%	91%	90%	100%
Influenza Vaccine[2]	25	60%	63%	70%	100%

NOTE: Hospital profiles are in alphabetical order by state, then city, then hospital within the city; Rankings are sorted by rate in descending order and exclude hospitals with less than 25 cases; (1) The number of cases is too small (n<25) for purposes of reliably predicting hospital performance; (2) Measure reflects the hospital's indication that its submission was based upon a sample of its relevant discharges; (3) Rate reflects fewer than the maximum possible quarters of data for the measure; (4) Inaccurate information submitted and suppressed for one or more quarters; (5) No data is available from the hospital for this measure; Please refer to the User's Guide for a full explanation of data

Initial Antibiotic Timing[2]	123	69%	81%	80%	93%
Oxygenation Assessment[2]	165	100%	99%	99%	100%
Pneumococcal Vaccine[2]	84	54%	62%	69%	94%
Smoking Cessation Advice[2]	41	76%	80%	80%	100%
Surgical Infection Prevention					
Prophylactic Antibiotic Given[2,3]	337	85%	74%	77%	95%
Prophylactic Antibiotic Selection[2]	69	65%	91%	90%	100%
Prophylactic Antibiotic Stopped[2,3]	338	75%	67%	72%	95%
Pregnancy Care					
Inpatient Neonatal Mortality	-	-	-	-	-
Third or Fourth Degree Laceration	-	-	3.89%	3.63%	3.27%

University of Illinois at Chicago Med Ctr

Alternate Name: University of Illinois Hospital
1740 W Taylor Street
Suite 1400
Chicago, IL 60612
Phone: 312-996-7000
Fax: 312-996-7049
URL: www.uic.edu
Ownership: Government - State
Accredited: Yes
Emergency Services: Yes
Licensed Beds: 570

Key Personnel:

Administrator/CEO . . . . John DeNardo
Chief Medical Staff. . . . . Lawrence Frohman, MD
Chief Catheterization Laboratory . . . . George Kondos, MD
Emergency Room . . . . Gary Strange, MD
Director Infection/Disease Control . . . . James L Cook, MD
OB/GYN Womens Health. . . . . Sherman Elias, MD
Chief Radiology . . . . Mahmood Mafee, MD
Director Respiratory Therapy . . . . Wade Jones

Measure	Cases	This Hospital	State Average	U.S. Average	Top Hospital
Heart Attack Care					
ACE Inhibitor or ARB for LVSD[1]	24	79%	79%	82%	100%
Aspirin at Arrival	56	100%	93%	92%	100%
Aspirin at Discharge	59	95%	90%	90%	100%
Beta Blocker at Arrival	48	96%	87%	87%	100%
Beta Blocker at Discharge	59	92%	88%	90%	100%
Fibrinolytic Medication Timing	0	-	21%	31%	100%
PCI Within 90 Minutes of Arrival[1]	4	25%	47%	54%	95%
Smoking Cessation Advice[1]	18	61%	84%	88%	100%
Heart Failure Care					
ACE Inhibitor or ARB for LVSD[2]	142	92%	83%	82%	100%
Discharge Instructions[2,3]	71	24%	67%	61%	93%
Evaluation of LVS Function[2]	310	96%	88%	83%	99%
Smoking Cessation Advice[2]	81	74%	83%	82%	100%
Pneumonia Care					
Appropriate Initial Antibiotic[2]	82	79%	83%	83%	94%
Blood Culture Timing[2]	124	76%	91%	90%	100%
Influenza Vaccine[5]	-	-	63%	70%	100%
Initial Antibiotic Timing[2]	183	64%	81%	80%	93%
Oxygenation Assessment[2]	196	99%	99%	99%	100%
Pneumococcal Vaccine[2]	65	49%	62%	69%	94%
Smoking Cessation Advice[2]	60	65%	80%	80%	100%
Surgical Infection Prevention					
Prophylactic Antibiotic Given[2,3]	275	72%	74%	77%	95%
Prophylactic Antibiotic Selection[2]	57	89%	91%	90%	100%
Prophylactic Antibiotic Stopped[2,3]	268	80%	67%	72%	95%
Pregnancy Care					
Inpatient Neonatal Mortality	-	-	-	-	-
Third or Fourth Degree Laceration	-	-	3.89%	3.63%	3.27%

Weiss Memorial Hospital

4646 N Marine Drive
Chicago, IL 60640
Phone: 773-878-8700
Fax: 773-564-5359
E-mail: cboykin@weisshospital.org
URL: www.weisshospital.org
Ownership: Voluntary non-profit - Other
Accredited: Yes
Emergency Services: Yes
Licensed Beds: 357

Key Personnel:

CEO. . . . . Tracey Rogers
Chief Medical Staff. . . . . Stuart Kraussn, MD
Emergency Room . . . . Khalid Malik, MD
Infection Control. . . . . David Balling, MD
Medical/Surgical Nursing . . . . Anne Solak, RN
OB/GYN Womens Health. . . . . Harrith Hasson, MD
Respiratory/Cardiopulmonary. . . . . Nelson Kanter, MD

Measure	Cases	This Hospital	State Average	U.S. Average	Top Hospital
Heart Attack Care					
ACE Inhibitor or ARB for LVSD	29	79%	79%	82%	100%
Aspirin at Arrival	85	92%	93%	92%	100%
Aspirin at Discharge	71	93%	90%	90%	100%
Beta Blocker at Arrival	76	96%	87%	87%	100%
Beta Blocker at Discharge	78	95%	88%	90%	100%
Fibrinolytic Medication Timing	0	-	21%	31%	100%
PCI Within 90 Minutes of Arrival[1]	1	0%	47%	54%	95%
Smoking Cessation Advice	34	32%	84%	88%	100%
Heart Failure Care					
ACE Inhibitor or ARB for LVSD	100	78%	83%	82%	100%
Discharge Instructions	180	34%	67%	61%	93%
Evaluation of LVS Function	250	90%	88%	83%	99%
Smoking Cessation Advice	68	35%	83%	82%	100%
Pneumonia Care					
Appropriate Initial Antibiotic[2]	63	83%	83%	83%	94%
Blood Culture Timing[2]	82	89%	91%	90%	100%
Influenza Vaccine[1,2]	18	22%	63%	70%	100%
Initial Antibiotic Timing[2]	131	79%	81%	80%	93%
Oxygenation Assessment[2]	166	100%	99%	99%	100%
Pneumococcal Vaccine[2]	98	20%	62%	69%	94%
Smoking Cessation Advice[2]	29	17%	80%	80%	100%
Surgical Infection Prevention					
Prophylactic Antibiotic Given[2]	228	80%	74%	77%	95%
Prophylactic Antibiotic Selection[2]	62	90%	91%	90%	100%
Prophylactic Antibiotic Stopped[2]	209	38%	67%	72%	95%
Pregnancy Care					
Inpatient Neonatal Mortality	-	-	-	-	-
Third or Fourth Degree Laceration	-	-	3.89%	3.63%	3.27%

Doctor John Warner Hospital

422 West White Street
Clinton, IL 61727
Phone: 217-935-9571
Fax: 217-935-4928
URL: www.djwhospital.org
Ownership: Government - Local
Accredited: No
Emergency Services: Yes
Licensed Beds: 43

Key Personnel:

Administrator/CEO . . . . Patty Luker
Chief of Medical Staff. J Powell
Emergency Room . . . . Sally Waite
ICU . . . . Brenda Lehman

Measure	Cases	This Hospital	State Average	U.S. Average	Top Hospital
Heart Attack Care					
ACE Inhibitor or ARB for LVSD[1,3]	1	100%	79%	82%	100%
Aspirin at Arrival[1,3]	7	71%	93%	92%	100%
Aspirin at Discharge[1,3]	5	80%	90%	90%	100%
Beta Blocker at Arrival[1,3]	5	80%	87%	87%	100%
Beta Blocker at Discharge[1,3]	5	60%	88%	90%	100%
Fibrinolytic Medication Timing[3]	0	-	21%	31%	100%
PCI Within 90 Minutes of Arrival	0	-	47%	54%	95%
Smoking Cessation Advice[1,3]	2	0%	84%	88%	100%
Heart Failure Care					
ACE Inhibitor or ARB for LVSD[1]	5	40%	83%	82%	100%
Discharge Instructions	30	0%	67%	61%	93%
Evaluation of LVS Function	38	76%	88%	83%	99%
Smoking Cessation Advice[1]	1	0%	83%	82%	100%
Pneumonia Care					
Appropriate Initial Antibiotic	26	77%	83%	83%	94%
Blood Culture Timing[1]	18	100%	91%	90%	100%
Influenza Vaccine[1]	7	29%	63%	70%	100%
Initial Antibiotic Timing	27	78%	81%	80%	93%
Oxygenation Assessment	36	97%	99%	99%	100%
Pneumococcal Vaccine[1]	24	38%	62%	69%	94%
Smoking Cessation Advice[1]	9	22%	80%	80%	100%
Surgical Infection Prevention					
Prophylactic Antibiotic Given[5]	-	-	74%	77%	95%

NOTE: Hospital profiles are in alphabetical order by state, then city, then hospital within the city; Rankings are sorted by rate in descending order and exclude hospitals with less than 25 cases; (1) The number of cases is too small (n<25) for purposes of reliably predicting hospital performance; (2) Measure reflects the hospital's indication that its submission was based upon a sample of its relevant discharges; (3) Rate reflects fewer than the maximum possible quarters of data for the measure; (4) Inaccurate information submitted and suppressed for one or more quarters; (5) No data is available from the hospital for this measure; Please refer to the User's Guide for a full explanation of data

Prophylactic Antibiotic Selection[5]	-	-	91%	90%	100%
Prophylactic Antibiotic Stopped[5]	-	-	67%	72%	95%
Pregnancy Care					
Inpatient Neonatal Mortality	-	-	-	-	-
Third or Fourth Degree Laceration	-	-	3.89%	3.63%	3.27%

Provena United Samaritans Medical Center

812 N Logan Avenue
Danville, IL 61832
URL: www.provenausmc.com
Ownership: Voluntary non-profit - Church
Emergency Services: Yes

Phone: 217-443-5000
Fax: 217-443-1965
Accredited: Yes
Licensed Beds: 308

Key Personnel:

CEO. . . . . Mark Wiener
Chief of Medical Staff. . . . . Charanjit Rakalla, MD
Director of Emergency Room. . . . . Nichol Boose
Emergency Room . . . . Mary Miller, RN
Infection Control. . . . . JoAnne Guyman, RN
ICU . . . . Sharon Tuggle
Director Medical/Surgical Nursing . . . . Norma Taylor
OB/GYN Womens Health. . . . . Roy McClintock, MD
Director of Pulmonary . . . . Angie Fielder

Measure	Cases	This Hospital	State Average	U.S. Average	Top Hospital
Heart Attack Care					
ACE Inhibitor or ARB for LVSD[1]	20	85%	79%	82%	100%
Aspirin at Arrival	74	96%	93%	92%	100%
Aspirin at Discharge	44	91%	90%	90%	100%
Beta Blocker at Arrival	73	96%	87%	87%	100%
Beta Blocker at Discharge	55	93%	88%	90%	100%
Fibrinolytic Medication Timing	0	-	21%	31%	100%
PCI Within 90 Minutes of Arrival	0	-	47%	54%	95%
Smoking Cessation Advice[1]	19	100%	84%	88%	100%
Heart Failure Care					
ACE Inhibitor or ARB for LVSD	151	91%	83%	82%	100%
Discharge Instructions	359	50%	67%	61%	93%
Evaluation of LVS Function	421	99%	88%	83%	99%
Smoking Cessation Advice	63	100%	83%	82%	100%
Pneumonia Care					
Appropriate Initial Antibiotic	264	90%	83%	83%	94%
Blood Culture Timing	246	89%	91%	90%	100%
Influenza Vaccine	46	59%	63%	70%	100%
Initial Antibiotic Timing	385	71%	81%	80%	93%
Oxygenation Assessment	432	99%	99%	99%	100%
Pneumococcal Vaccine	220	63%	62%	69%	94%
Smoking Cessation Advice	110	100%	80%	80%	100%
Surgical Infection Prevention					
Prophylactic Antibiotic Given[2]	270	94%	74%	77%	95%
Prophylactic Antibiotic Selection[2]	64	89%	91%	90%	100%
Prophylactic Antibiotic Stopped[2]	249	74%	67%	72%	95%
Pregnancy Care					
Inpatient Neonatal Mortality	896	0.22%	-	-	-
Third or Fourth Degree Laceration	634	1.58%	3.89%	3.63%	3.27%

Decatur Memorial Hospital

2300 N Edward Street
Decatur, IL 62526
URL: www.dmhcares.org
Ownership: Voluntary non-profit - Other
Emergency Services: Yes

Phone: 217-876-8121
Fax: 217-876-6118
Accredited: Yes
Licensed Beds: 401

Key Personnel:

President/CEO. . . . . Ken Smithmier
Chief Medical Staff. . . . . Jame L Wade, MD
Chief Surgery. . . . . Tim Bailey, MD
Emergency Room . . . . Gerald Snyder, MD
Director Infection/Disease Control . . . . Alma Miller, RN
Director Medical/Surgical Nursing . . . . Kathy Sleavin
OB/GYN Womens Health. . . . . Derin Rominger, MD
Chief Radiology . . . . G Richard Locke, MD

Measure	Cases	This Hospital	State Average	U.S. Average	Top Hospital
Heart Attack Care					
ACE Inhibitor or ARB for LVSD	76	88%	79%	82%	100%
Aspirin at Arrival	164	99%	93%	92%	100%
Aspirin at Discharge	197	99%	90%	90%	100%
Beta Blocker at Arrival	132	96%	87%	87%	100%
Beta Blocker at Discharge	209	99%	88%	90%	100%
Fibrinolytic Medication Timing	0	-	21%	31%	100%
PCI Within 90 Minutes of Arrival[1]	7	43%	47%	54%	95%
Smoking Cessation Advice	86	100%	84%	88%	100%
Heart Failure Care					
ACE Inhibitor or ARB for LVSD	219	89%	83%	82%	100%
Discharge Instructions	354	96%	67%	61%	93%
Evaluation of LVS Function	449	99%	88%	83%	99%
Smoking Cessation Advice	56	100%	83%	82%	100%
Pneumonia Care					
Appropriate Initial Antibiotic	258	83%	83%	83%	94%
Blood Culture Timing	243	94%	91%	90%	100%
Influenza Vaccine	73	95%	63%	70%	100%
Initial Antibiotic Timing	332	91%	81%	80%	93%
Oxygenation Assessment	411	100%	99%	99%	100%
Pneumococcal Vaccine	287	93%	62%	69%	94%
Smoking Cessation Advice	77	99%	80%	80%	100%
Surgical Infection Prevention					
Prophylactic Antibiotic Given[2,3]	448	82%	74%	77%	95%
Prophylactic Antibiotic Selection[2]	132	93%	91%	90%	100%
Prophylactic Antibiotic Stopped[2,3]	432	61%	67%	72%	95%
Pregnancy Care					
Inpatient Neonatal Mortality	1,088	0.37%	-	-	-
Third or Fourth Degree Laceration	656	5.03%	3.89%	3.63%	3.27%

Saint Mary's Hospital

1800 E Lake Shore Drive
Decatur, IL 62521
URL: www.stmarys-hospital.com
Ownership: Voluntary non-profit - Church
Emergency Services: Yes

Phone: 217-464-2966
Fax: 217-464-1616
Accredited: Yes
Licensed Beds: 371

Key Personnel:

President/CEO. . . . . Anthony D Pfitzer
Chief Medical Staff. . . . . D Patel, MD
Emergency Room . . . . Phillip Barnell, MD
Intensive/Coronary Care . . . . Glen Griesheim, RN
Medical/Surgical Nursing . . . . Ed Yundt
OB/GYN Womens Health. . . . . S Apachi, MD
Chief Radiology . . . . J Agee, MD
Director Respiratory Therapy . . . . Amy Grandone

Measure	Cases	This Hospital	State Average	U.S. Average	Top Hospital
Heart Attack Care					
ACE Inhibitor or ARB for LVSD[1]	8	88%	79%	82%	100%
Aspirin at Arrival	33	91%	93%	92%	100%
Aspirin at Discharge[1]	19	84%	90%	90%	100%
Beta Blocker at Arrival	25	84%	87%	87%	100%
Beta Blocker at Discharge[1]	19	100%	88%	90%	100%
Fibrinolytic Medication Timing[1]	1	0%	21%	31%	100%
PCI Within 90 Minutes of Arrival	0	-	47%	54%	95%
Smoking Cessation Advice[1]	5	100%	84%	88%	100%
Heart Failure Care					
ACE Inhibitor or ARB for LVSD	72	86%	83%	82%	100%
Discharge Instructions	122	87%	67%	61%	93%
Evaluation of LVS Function	182	97%	88%	83%	99%
Smoking Cessation Advice	29	93%	83%	82%	100%
Pneumonia Care					
Appropriate Initial Antibiotic	87	82%	83%	83%	94%
Blood Culture Timing	105	92%	91%	90%	100%
Influenza Vaccine	29	97%	63%	70%	100%
Initial Antibiotic Timing	157	85%	81%	80%	93%
Oxygenation Assessment	186	99%	99%	99%	100%
Pneumococcal Vaccine	116	97%	62%	69%	94%
Smoking Cessation Advice	45	98%	80%	80%	100%
Surgical Infection Prevention					
Prophylactic Antibiotic Given	284	89%	74%	77%	95%
Prophylactic Antibiotic Selection	70	96%	91%	90%	100%
Prophylactic Antibiotic Stopped	272	76%	67%	72%	95%
Pregnancy Care					

NOTE: Hospital profiles are in alphabetical order by state, then city, then hospital within the city; Rankings are sorted by rate in descending order and exclude hospitals with less than 25 cases; (1) The number of cases is too small (n<25) for purposes of reliably predicting hospital performance; (2) Measure reflects the hospital's indication that its submission was based upon a sample of its relevant discharges; (3) Rate reflects fewer than the maximum possible quarters of data for the measure; (4) Inaccurate information submitted and suppressed for one or more quarters; (5) No data is available from the hospital for this measure; Please refer to the User's Guide for a full explanation of data

Inpatient Neonatal Mortality	567	0.35%	-	-	-
Third or Fourth Degree Laceration	414	1.45%	3.89%	3.63%	3.27%

Kishwaukee Community Hospital

626 Bethany Road
De Kalb, IL 60115

Toll-Free: 800-397-1521
Phone: 815-756-1521
Fax: 815-756-7665

URL: www.kishhospital.org
Ownership: Voluntary non-profit - Other
Emergency Services: Yes

Accredited: Yes
Licensed Beds: 172

Key Personnel:
President/CEO . . . . Kevin Poorten
Chief Medical Staff . . . . Bhagavatlal Morker, MD
Emergency Room . . . . Chris Jones
OB/GYN Womens Health . . . . Frank Luedtke, MD
Chief Radiology . . . . Paresh Dixit, MD
Director Respiratory Therapy . . . . Mike Kokott

Measure	Cases	This Hospital	State Average	U.S. Average	Top Hospital
Heart Attack Care					
ACE Inhibitor or ARB for LVSD[1]	3	67%	79%	82%	100%
Aspirin at Arrival[1]	17	100%	93%	92%	100%
Aspirin at Discharge[1]	8	100%	90%	90%	100%
Beta Blocker at Arrival[1]	8	88%	87%	87%	100%
Beta Blocker at Discharge[1]	7	100%	88%	90%	100%
Fibrinolytic Medication Timing	0	-	21%	31%	100%
PCI Within 90 Minutes of Arrival	0	-	47%	54%	95%
Smoking Cessation Advice	0	-	84%	88%	100%
Heart Failure Care					
ACE Inhibitor or ARB for LVSD	51	98%	83%	82%	100%
Discharge Instructions	111	77%	67%	61%	93%
Evaluation of LVS Function	130	100%	88%	83%	99%
Smoking Cessation Advice[1]	8	100%	83%	82%	100%
Pneumonia Care					
Appropriate Initial Antibiotic	107	90%	83%	83%	94%
Blood Culture Timing	83	95%	91%	90%	100%
Influenza Vaccine[1]	24	67%	63%	70%	100%
Initial Antibiotic Timing	145	88%	81%	80%	93%
Oxygenation Assessment	175	100%	99%	99%	100%
Pneumococcal Vaccine	113	91%	62%	69%	94%
Smoking Cessation Advice	38	89%	80%	80%	100%
Surgical Infection Prevention					
Prophylactic Antibiotic Given[3]	157	72%	74%	77%	95%
Prophylactic Antibiotic Selection	62	98%	91%	90%	100%
Prophylactic Antibiotic Stopped[3]	149	77%	67%	72%	95%
Pregnancy Care					
Inpatient Neonatal Mortality	-	-	-	-	-
Third or Fourth Degree Laceration	-	-	3.89%	3.63%	3.27%

Katherine Shaw Bethea Hospital

403 E 1st St
Dixon, IL 61021
Ownership: Voluntary non-profit - Other
Emergency Services: Yes

Phone: 815-288-5531
Accredited: No

Measure	Cases	This Hospital	State Average	U.S. Average	Top Hospital
Heart Attack Care					
ACE Inhibitor or ARB for LVSD[1]	6	83%	79%	82%	100%
Aspirin at Arrival	48	98%	93%	92%	100%
Aspirin at Discharge	26	92%	90%	90%	100%
Beta Blocker at Arrival	29	97%	87%	87%	100%
Beta Blocker at Discharge	31	94%	88%	90%	100%
Fibrinolytic Medication Timing[1]	1	0%	21%	31%	100%
PCI Within 90 Minutes of Arrival	0	-	47%	54%	95%
Smoking Cessation Advice[1]	4	100%	84%	88%	100%
Heart Failure Care					
ACE Inhibitor or ARB for LVSD	42	90%	83%	82%	100%
Discharge Instructions	87	80%	67%	61%	93%
Evaluation of LVS Function	113	96%	88%	83%	99%
Smoking Cessation Advice[1]	12	92%	83%	82%	100%
Pneumonia Care					
Appropriate Initial Antibiotic	78	97%	83%	83%	94%
Blood Culture Timing	79	90%	91%	90%	100%
Influenza Vaccine[1]	18	67%	63%	70%	100%
Initial Antibiotic Timing	96	95%	81%	80%	93%
Oxygenation Assessment	120	100%	99%	99%	100%
Pneumococcal Vaccine	81	85%	62%	69%	94%
Smoking Cessation Advice[1]	23	100%	80%	80%	100%
Surgical Infection Prevention					
Prophylactic Antibiotic Given	154	94%	74%	77%	95%
Prophylactic Antibiotic Selection	35	97%	91%	90%	100%
Prophylactic Antibiotic Stopped	139	93%	67%	72%	95%
Pregnancy Care					
Inpatient Neonatal Mortality	-	-	-	-	-
Third or Fourth Degree Laceration	-	-	3.89%	3.63%	3.27%

Advocate Good Samaritan Hospital

3815 Highland Avenue
Downers Grove, IL 60515
URL: www.advocatehealth.com/gsam
Ownership: Voluntary non-profit - Church
Emergency Services: Yes

Phone: 630-275-5880
Fax: 630-963-8605

Accredited: Yes
Licensed Beds: 302

Key Personnel:
CEO . . . . Jon Bruss

Measure	Cases	This Hospital	State Average	U.S. Average	Top Hospital
Heart Attack Care					
ACE Inhibitor or ARB for LVSD	64	98%	79%	82%	100%
Aspirin at Arrival	215	99%	93%	92%	100%
Aspirin at Discharge	192	99%	90%	90%	100%
Beta Blocker at Arrival	190	97%	87%	87%	100%
Beta Blocker at Discharge	214	100%	88%	90%	100%
Fibrinolytic Medication Timing	0	-	21%	31%	100%
PCI Within 90 Minutes of Arrival[1]	17	100%	47%	54%	95%
Smoking Cessation Advice	59	100%	84%	88%	100%
Heart Failure Care					
ACE Inhibitor or ARB for LVSD	155	91%	83%	82%	100%
Discharge Instructions	298	77%	67%	61%	93%
Evaluation of LVS Function	405	97%	88%	83%	99%
Smoking Cessation Advice	37	92%	83%	82%	100%
Pneumonia Care					
Appropriate Initial Antibiotic[2]	111	83%	83%	83%	94%
Blood Culture Timing[2]	131	96%	91%	90%	100%
Influenza Vaccine[1]	23	87%	63%	70%	100%
Initial Antibiotic Timing[2]	171	85%	81%	80%	93%
Oxygenation Assessment[2]	210	100%	99%	99%	100%
Pneumococcal Vaccine[2]	142	80%	62%	69%	94%
Smoking Cessation Advice[2]	37	84%	80%	80%	100%
Surgical Infection Prevention					
Prophylactic Antibiotic Given[2]	339	93%	74%	77%	95%
Prophylactic Antibiotic Selection[2]	82	99%	91%	90%	100%
Prophylactic Antibiotic Stopped[2]	323	81%	67%	72%	95%
Pregnancy Care					
Inpatient Neonatal Mortality	1,770	0.73%	-	-	-
Third or Fourth Degree Laceration	1,070	3.74%	3.89%	3.63%	3.27%

Marshall Browning Hospital

900 N Washington Street
DuQuoin, IL 62832
URL: www.marshallbrowninghospital.com
Ownership: Voluntary non-profit - Private
Emergency Services: Yes

Phone: 618-542-2146
Fax: 618-542-4756

Accredited: Yes
Licensed Beds: 25

Key Personnel:
CEO/Administrator . . . . William J Huff

Measure	Cases	This Hospital	State Average	U.S. Average	Top Hospital
Heart Attack Care					
ACE Inhibitor or ARB for LVSD	0	-	79%	82%	100%
Aspirin at Arrival[1]	7	100%	93%	92%	100%
Aspirin at Discharge[1]	5	60%	90%	90%	100%
Beta Blocker at Arrival[1]	7	43%	87%	87%	100%
Beta Blocker at Discharge[1]	5	60%	88%	90%	100%
Fibrinolytic Medication Timing	0	-	21%	31%	100%
PCI Within 90 Minutes of Arrival	0	-	47%	54%	95%

NOTE: Hospital profiles are in alphabetical order by state, then city, then hospital within the city; Rankings are sorted by rate in descending order and exclude hospitals with less than 25 cases; (1) The number of cases is too small (n<25) for purposes of reliably predicting hospital performance; (2) Measure reflects the hospital's indication that its submission was based upon a sample of its relevant discharges; (3) Rate reflects fewer than the maximum possible quarters of data for the measure; (4) Inaccurate information submitted and suppressed for one or more quarters; (5) No data is available from the hospital for this measure; Please refer to the User's Guide for a full explanation of data

Smoking Cessation Advice[1]	1	0%	84%	88%	100%
Heart Failure Care					
ACE Inhibitor or ARB for LVSD[1]	4	75%	83%	82%	100%
Discharge Instructions[1]	20	40%	67%	61%	93%
Evaluation of LVS Function[1]	24	54%	88%	83%	99%
Smoking Cessation Advice	0	-	83%	82%	100%
Pneumonia Care					
Appropriate Initial Antibiotic	31	68%	83%	83%	94%
Blood Culture Timing	27	96%	91%	90%	100%
Influenza Vaccine[1]	8	12%	63%	70%	100%
Initial Antibiotic Timing	34	85%	81%	80%	93%
Oxygenation Assessment	44	100%	99%	99%	100%
Pneumococcal Vaccine	28	50%	62%	69%	94%
Smoking Cessation Advice[1]	5	20%	80%	80%	100%
Surgical Infection Prevention					
Prophylactic Antibiotic Given[5]	-	-	74%	77%	95%
Prophylactic Antibiotic Selection[5]	-	-	91%	90%	100%
Prophylactic Antibiotic Stopped[5]	-	-	67%	72%	95%
Pregnancy Care					
Inpatient Neonatal Mortality	-	-	-	-	-
Third or Fourth Degree Laceration	-	-	3.89%	3.63%	3.27%

Kenneth Hall Regional Hospital

129 N 8th Street
East Saint Louis, IL 62201
E-mail: bmiller@ancilla.org
Phone: 618-274-1900
Fax: 618-482-7095
Ownership: Voluntary non-profit - Church
Emergency Services: Yes
Accredited: Yes
Licensed Beds: 169

Key Personnel:

CEO. . . . . Robert Klutts
Chief Medical Staff. . . . . Poten Jacob, MD
Emergency Room . . . . Linda Brown
Emergency Room . . . . Glenda Robinson
Chief Radiology . . . . Joseph Dugan, MD
Pulmonary Chief . . . . Charles Ampadu

Measure	Cases	This Hospital	State Average	U.S. Average	Top Hospital
Heart Attack Care					
ACE Inhibitor or ARB for LVSD[1]	1	100%	79%	82%	100%
Aspirin at Arrival[1]	6	100%	93%	92%	100%
Aspirin at Discharge[1]	2	100%	90%	90%	100%
Beta Blocker at Arrival[1]	8	88%	87%	87%	100%
Beta Blocker at Discharge[1]	3	100%	88%	90%	100%
Fibrinolytic Medication Timing	0	-	21%	31%	100%
PCI Within 90 Minutes of Arrival	0	-	47%	54%	95%
Smoking Cessation Advice[1]	2	100%	84%	88%	100%
Heart Failure Care					
ACE Inhibitor or ARB for LVSD	57	81%	83%	82%	100%
Discharge Instructions	174	44%	67%	61%	93%
Evaluation of LVS Function	192	60%	88%	83%	99%
Smoking Cessation Advice	97	68%	83%	82%	100%
Pneumonia Care					
Appropriate Initial Antibiotic	51	57%	83%	83%	94%
Blood Culture Timing	28	96%	91%	90%	100%
Influenza Vaccine[1]	7	0%	63%	70%	100%
Initial Antibiotic Timing	66	70%	81%	80%	93%
Oxygenation Assessment	67	91%	99%	99%	100%
Pneumococcal Vaccine[1]	24	17%	62%	69%	94%
Smoking Cessation Advice	28	54%	80%	80%	100%
Surgical Infection Prevention					
Prophylactic Antibiotic Given[1,3]	10	20%	74%	77%	95%
Prophylactic Antibiotic Selection[1]	10	80%	91%	90%	100%
Prophylactic Antibiotic Stopped[1,3]	10	20%	67%	72%	95%
Pregnancy Care					
Inpatient Neonatal Mortality	-	-	-	-	-
Third or Fourth Degree Laceration	-	-	3.89%	3.63%	3.27%

Saint Anthony's Memorial Hospital

503 N Maple Street
Effingham, IL 62401
E-mail: hospital@effingtham.net
URL: www.stanthonyshospital.org
Phone: 217-342-2121
Fax: 217-347-1563
Ownership: Voluntary non-profit - Church
Emergency Services: Yes
Accredited: Yes
Licensed Beds: 146

Key Personnel:

President/CEO. . . . . Daneial J Woods
Emergency Room . . . . Kate Weber
Infection Control. . . . . Kim Howell
ICU . . . . Sharyn Phillips
Intensive/Coronary Care . . . . Sharyn Phillips
Medical/Surgical Nursing . . . . Tammy Lett
Respiratory/Cardiopulmonary. . . . . Jim Whitehair

Measure	Cases	This Hospital	State Average	U.S. Average	Top Hospital
Heart Attack Care					
ACE Inhibitor or ARB for LVSD[1]	6	83%	79%	82%	100%
Aspirin at Arrival	38	89%	93%	92%	100%
Aspirin at Discharge[1]	20	95%	90%	90%	100%
Beta Blocker at Arrival	34	85%	87%	87%	100%
Beta Blocker at Discharge[1]	19	95%	88%	90%	100%
Fibrinolytic Medication Timing	0	-	21%	31%	100%
PCI Within 90 Minutes of Arrival	0	-	47%	54%	95%
Smoking Cessation Advice[1]	3	67%	84%	88%	100%
Heart Failure Care					
ACE Inhibitor or ARB for LVSD	30	83%	83%	82%	100%
Discharge Instructions	176	74%	67%	61%	93%
Evaluation of LVS Function	202	89%	88%	83%	99%
Smoking Cessation Advice[1]	24	92%	83%	82%	100%
Pneumonia Care					
Appropriate Initial Antibiotic	176	80%	83%	83%	94%
Blood Culture Timing	124	99%	91%	90%	100%
Influenza Vaccine[4,5]	-	-	63%	70%	100%
Initial Antibiotic Timing	209	85%	81%	80%	93%
Oxygenation Assessment	258	100%	99%	99%	100%
Pneumococcal Vaccine	180	76%	62%	69%	94%
Smoking Cessation Advice	47	81%	80%	80%	100%
Surgical Infection Prevention					
Prophylactic Antibiotic Given	661	81%	74%	77%	95%
Prophylactic Antibiotic Selection	170	99%	91%	90%	100%
Prophylactic Antibiotic Stopped	653	87%	67%	72%	95%
Pregnancy Care					
Inpatient Neonatal Mortality	-	-	-	-	-
Third or Fourth Degree Laceration	-	-	3.89%	3.63%	3.27%

Ferrell Hospital

1201 Pine Street
Eldorado, IL 62930
Phone: 618-273-3361
Fax: 618-273-2571
Ownership: Government - State
Emergency Services: Yes
Accredited: No
Licensed Beds: 51

Key Personnel:

CEO. . . . . William Hartley
Chief of Medical Staff. Eliott Partirdge
Emergency Room . . . . Jackie Tripp
Manager of Respiratory Care. . . . . Beth Castell

Measure	Cases	This Hospital	State Average	U.S. Average	Top Hospital
Heart Attack Care					
ACE Inhibitor or ARB for LVSD[1]	2	0%	79%	82%	100%
Aspirin at Arrival[1]	12	33%	93%	92%	100%
Aspirin at Discharge[1]	10	50%	90%	90%	100%
Beta Blocker at Arrival[1]	11	55%	87%	87%	100%
Beta Blocker at Discharge[1]	11	18%	88%	90%	100%
Fibrinolytic Medication Timing[1]	1	0%	21%	31%	100%
PCI Within 90 Minutes of Arrival	0	-	47%	54%	95%
Smoking Cessation Advice[1]	6	0%	84%	88%	100%
Heart Failure Care					
ACE Inhibitor or ARB for LVSD[1]	8	25%	83%	82%	100%
Discharge Instructions[1]	18	0%	67%	61%	93%
Evaluation of LVS Function	29	66%	88%	83%	99%
Smoking Cessation Advice[1]	7	57%	83%	82%	100%

NOTE: Hospital profiles are in alphabetical order by state, then city, then hospital within the city; Rankings are sorted by rate in descending order and exclude hospitals with less than 25 cases; (1) The number of cases is too small (n<25) for purposes of reliably predicting hospital performance; (2) Measure reflects the hospital's indication that its submission was based upon a sample of its relevant discharges; (3) Rate reflects fewer than the maximum possible quarters of data for the measure; (4) Inaccurate information submitted and suppressed for one or more quarters; (5) No data is available from the hospital for this measure; Please refer to the User's Guide for a full explanation of data

Pneumonia Care					
Appropriate Initial Antibiotic[2]	36	42%	83%	83%	94%
Blood Culture Timing[1,2]	6	83%	91%	90%	100%
Influenza Vaccine[1]	10	50%	63%	70%	100%
Initial Antibiotic Timing[2]	52	77%	81%	80%	93%
Oxygenation Assessment[2]	67	96%	99%	99%	100%
Pneumococcal Vaccine[2]	32	25%	62%	69%	94%
Smoking Cessation Advice[1,2]	24	54%	80%	80%	100%
Surgical Infection Prevention					
Prophylactic Antibiotic Given[1]	11	18%	74%	77%	95%
Prophylactic Antibiotic Selection[1]	2	50%	91%	90%	100%
Prophylactic Antibiotic Stopped[1]	4	100%	67%	72%	95%
Pregnancy Care					
Inpatient Neonatal Mortality	-	-	-	-	-
Third or Fourth Degree Laceration	-	-	3.89%	3.63%	3.27%

Provena Saint Joseph Hospital

Alternate Name: Saint Joseph Hospital
77 N Airlite Street
Elgin, IL 60123
URL: www.provenasaintjoeph.com
Ownership: Voluntary non-profit - Church
Emergency Services: Yes
Phone: 847-695-3200
Fax: 847-622-2070
Accredited: Yes
Licensed Beds: 260

Key Personnel:
CEO. . . . . William McDonald
Chief Medical Staff. . . . . Charles Carallo, MD
Director Cardiac Laboratory . . . . Jeff Berchner
Director Catheterization Laboratory . . . . Jeff Beichner
Coordinator Emergency Room. . . . . Wendy Seleen
Coordinator Infection Control . . . . Kathy Hogan
Manager Medical Surgical Nursing. . . . . Sandy Meana
Director OB/GYN Womens Health . . . . Laurel Ann Peterson
Director Radiology . . . . Laurie Schachtner
Respiratory Therapy. . . . . Nancy Tribby

Measure	Cases	This Hospital	State Average	U.S. Average	Top Hospital
Heart Attack Care					
ACE Inhibitor or ARB for LVSD	31	74%	79%	82%	100%
Aspirin at Arrival	106	93%	93%	92%	100%
Aspirin at Discharge	95	98%	90%	90%	100%
Beta Blocker at Arrival	85	91%	87%	87%	100%
Beta Blocker at Discharge	111	96%	88%	90%	100%
Fibrinolytic Medication Timing[3]	0	-	21%	31%	100%
PCI Within 90 Minutes of Arrival[1]	9	44%	47%	54%	95%
Smoking Cessation Advice[1,3]	11	100%	84%	88%	100%
Heart Failure Care					
ACE Inhibitor or ARB for LVSD	67	69%	83%	82%	100%
Discharge Instructions[1,3]	17	76%	67%	61%	93%
Evaluation of LVS Function	162	90%	88%	83%	99%
Smoking Cessation Advice[1,3]	9	100%	83%	82%	100%
Pneumonia Care					
Appropriate Initial Antibiotic[3]	25	84%	83%	83%	94%
Blood Culture Timing[3]	29	86%	91%	90%	100%
Influenza Vaccine[5]	-	-	63%	70%	100%
Initial Antibiotic Timing	189	79%	81%	80%	93%
Oxygenation Assessment	240	100%	99%	99%	100%
Pneumococcal Vaccine	142	34%	62%	69%	94%
Smoking Cessation Advice[1,3]	6	67%	80%	80%	100%
Surgical Infection Prevention					
Prophylactic Antibiotic Given[2,3]	77	82%	74%	77%	95%
Prophylactic Antibiotic Selection[5]	-	-	91%	90%	100%
Prophylactic Antibiotic Stopped[2,3]	76	71%	67%	72%	95%
Pregnancy Care					
Inpatient Neonatal Mortality	607	0.66%	-	-	-
Third or Fourth Degree Laceration	445	4.94%	3.89%	3.63%	3.27%

Sherman Hospital

934 Center Street
Elgin, IL 60120
URL: www.shermanhealth.com
Ownership: Voluntary non-profit - Other
Emergency Services: Yes
Phone: 847-742-9800
Fax: 847-429-2035
Accredited: Yes
Licensed Beds: 353

Key Personnel:
President/CEO. . . . . Richard B Floyd, FACHE
Chief Medical Staff. . . . . Edgar Feldman, MD, FACS
Catheterization Lab . . . . Bonnie DeGrande
Emergency Room . . . . Betty Mortensen, RN
Director Infection/Disease Control . . . . Sallie Rivera, RN
CCU Spvg. Nurse . . . . Mary Fran Mc Nally
Director Medical/Surgical Nursing . . . . Debbie Camacho
Director Medical/Surgical Nursing . . . . Edgar Feldman, MD, FACS
OB/GYN Womens Health. . . . . Mary Ann Schaefer, RN
Director Respiratory Therapy. . . . . Ron Dorushka

Measure	Cases	This Hospital	State Average	U.S. Average	Top Hospital
Heart Attack Care					
ACE Inhibitor or ARB for LVSD	46	80%	79%	82%	100%
Aspirin at Arrival	199	95%	93%	92%	100%
Aspirin at Discharge	232	95%	90%	90%	100%
Beta Blocker at Arrival	188	95%	87%	87%	100%
Beta Blocker at Discharge	234	96%	88%	90%	100%
Fibrinolytic Medication Timing	0	-	21%	31%	100%
PCI Within 90 Minutes of Arrival[1]	17	88%	47%	54%	95%
Smoking Cessation Advice	81	90%	84%	88%	100%
Heart Failure Care					
ACE Inhibitor or ARB for LVSD	127	71%	83%	82%	100%
Discharge Instructions	289	50%	67%	61%	93%
Evaluation of LVS Function	366	86%	88%	83%	99%
Smoking Cessation Advice	59	83%	83%	82%	100%
Pneumonia Care					
Appropriate Initial Antibiotic	146	83%	83%	83%	94%
Blood Culture Timing	136	79%	91%	90%	100%
Influenza Vaccine	41	68%	63%	70%	100%
Initial Antibiotic Timing	224	83%	81%	80%	93%
Oxygenation Assessment	262	100%	99%	99%	100%
Pneumococcal Vaccine	121	78%	62%	69%	94%
Smoking Cessation Advice	59	69%	80%	80%	100%
Surgical Infection Prevention					
Prophylactic Antibiotic Given	696	89%	74%	77%	95%
Prophylactic Antibiotic Selection	174	95%	91%	90%	100%
Prophylactic Antibiotic Stopped	681	80%	67%	72%	95%
Pregnancy Care					
Inpatient Neonatal Mortality[2]	891	0.34%	-	-	-
Third or Fourth Degree Laceration[2]	667	2.70%	3.89%	3.63%	3.27%

Alexian Brothers Medical Center

800 Biesterfield Road
Elk Grove Village, IL 60007
URL: www.alexian.org
Ownership: Voluntary non-profit - Church
Emergency Services: Yes
Phone: 847-437-5500
Fax: 847-981-5766
Accredited: Yes
Licensed Beds: 473

Key Personnel:
President/CEO. . . . . Roger W Johnson

Measure	Cases	This Hospital	State Average	U.S. Average	Top Hospital
Heart Attack Care					
ACE Inhibitor or ARB for LVSD	59	90%	79%	82%	100%
Aspirin at Arrival	214	98%	93%	92%	100%
Aspirin at Discharge	218	98%	90%	90%	100%
Beta Blocker at Arrival	168	95%	87%	87%	100%
Beta Blocker at Discharge	236	97%	88%	90%	100%
Fibrinolytic Medication Timing	0	-	21%	31%	100%
PCI Within 90 Minutes of Arrival[1]	15	73%	47%	54%	95%
Smoking Cessation Advice	79	99%	84%	88%	100%
Heart Failure Care					
ACE Inhibitor or ARB for LVSD	161	83%	83%	82%	100%
Discharge Instructions	413	80%	67%	61%	93%
Evaluation of LVS Function	511	96%	88%	83%	99%

NOTE: Hospital profiles are in alphabetical order by state, then city, then hospital within the city; Rankings are sorted by rate in descending order and exclude hospitals with less than 25 cases; (1) The number of cases is too small (n<25) for purposes of reliably predicting hospital performance; (2) Measure reflects the hospital's indication that its submission was based upon a sample of its relevant discharges; (3) Rate reflects fewer than the maximum possible quarters of data for the measure; (4) Inaccurate information submitted and suppressed for one or more quarters; (5) No data is available from the hospital for this measure; Please refer to the User's Guide for a full explanation of data

Smoking Cessation Advice	72	96%	83%	82%	100%
Pneumonia Care					
Appropriate Initial Antibiotic	212	84%	83%	83%	94%
Blood Culture Timing	267	97%	91%	90%	100%
Influenza Vaccine[4,5]	-	-	63%	70%	100%
Initial Antibiotic Timing	312	88%	81%	80%	93%
Oxygenation Assessment	445	100%	99%	99%	100%
Pneumococcal Vaccine	305	79%	62%	69%	94%
Smoking Cessation Advice	77	90%	80%	80%	100%
Surgical Infection Prevention					
Prophylactic Antibiotic Given[2]	592	93%	74%	77%	95%
Prophylactic Antibiotic Selection[2]	147	98%	91%	90%	100%
Prophylactic Antibiotic Stopped[2]	554	77%	67%	72%	95%
Pregnancy Care					
Inpatient Neonatal Mortality	-	-	-	-	-
Third or Fourth Degree Laceration	-	-	3.89%	3.63%	3.27%

Elmhurst Memorial Hospital

200 Berteau Avenue
Elmhurst, IL 60126
URL: www.emhs.com
Ownership: Voluntary non-profit - Other
Emergency Services: Yes

Phone: 630-833-1400
Fax: 630-782-7844

Accredited: Yes
Licensed Beds: 427

Key Personnel:

President/CEO . . . . Leo F Fronza, Jr
Chief Medical Staff . . . . Ronald F Cheff, MD
Emergency Room . . . . Fred Jacobs, MD
Director Infection/Disease Control . . . . Patricia Funderburk
Director Medical/Surgical Nursing . . . . Bonnie Michaels
OB/GYN Womens Health . . . . James S Watts, MD
Chief Radiology . . . . Jerold Weinberg, MD
Director Respiratory Therapy . . . . Nabil Migala

Measure	Cases	This Hospital	State Average	U.S. Average	Top Hospital
Heart Attack Care					
ACE Inhibitor or ARB for LVSD	49	96%	79%	82%	100%
Aspirin at Arrival	225	99%	93%	92%	100%
Aspirin at Discharge	229	100%	90%	90%	100%
Beta Blocker at Arrival	189	99%	87%	87%	100%
Beta Blocker at Discharge	219	100%	88%	90%	100%
Fibrinolytic Medication Timing	0	-	21%	31%	100%
PCI Within 90 Minutes of Arrival[1]	5	80%	47%	54%	95%
Smoking Cessation Advice	52	100%	84%	88%	100%
Heart Failure Care					
ACE Inhibitor or ARB for LVSD	222	95%	83%	82%	100%
Discharge Instructions	453	96%	67%	61%	93%
Evaluation of LVS Function	546	97%	88%	83%	99%
Smoking Cessation Advice	73	96%	83%	82%	100%
Pneumonia Care					
Appropriate Initial Antibiotic	243	79%	83%	83%	94%
Blood Culture Timing	204	94%	91%	90%	100%
Influenza Vaccine	58	62%	63%	70%	100%
Initial Antibiotic Timing	334	85%	81%	80%	93%
Oxygenation Assessment	384	100%	99%	99%	100%
Pneumococcal Vaccine	266	50%	62%	69%	94%
Smoking Cessation Advice	53	85%	80%	80%	100%
Surgical Infection Prevention					
Prophylactic Antibiotic Given[2]	659	95%	74%	77%	95%
Prophylactic Antibiotic Selection[2]	59	93%	91%	90%	100%
Prophylactic Antibiotic Stopped[2]	628	61%	67%	72%	95%
Pregnancy Care					
Inpatient Neonatal Mortality	1,570	0.25%	-	-	-
Third or Fourth Degree Laceration	1,168	3.68%	3.89%	3.63%	3.27%

Evanston Hospital

2650 Ridge Avenue
Evanston, IL 60201

URL: www.hphosp.org
Ownership: Voluntary non-profit - Other
Emergency Services: Yes

Toll-Free: 888-364-6400
Phone: 309-949-2286
Fax: 847-570-5243

Accredited: Yes

Key Personnel:

Administrator/President . . . . Raymond Grady
Chief Medical Staff . . . . Arnold Wagner
Emergency Room . . . . Jeffrey Graff, MD
Infection Control . . . . Kay O'Connor, RN
Medical/Surgical Nursing . . . . Mary Lon Powell, RN
OB/GYN Womens Health . . . . Ginger Beavers

Measure	Cases	This Hospital	State Average	U.S. Average	Top Hospital
Heart Attack Care					
ACE Inhibitor or ARB for LVSD	89	96%	79%	82%	100%
Aspirin at Arrival	515	99%	93%	92%	100%
Aspirin at Discharge	518	99%	90%	90%	100%
Beta Blocker at Arrival	477	99%	87%	87%	100%
Beta Blocker at Discharge	523	98%	88%	90%	100%
Fibrinolytic Medication Timing[1]	1	0%	21%	31%	100%
PCI Within 90 Minutes of Arrival[1]	19	37%	47%	54%	95%
Smoking Cessation Advice	80	94%	84%	88%	100%
Heart Failure Care					
ACE Inhibitor or ARB for LVSD[2]	252	87%	83%	82%	100%
Discharge Instructions[2]	609	55%	67%	61%	93%
Evaluation of LVS Function[2]	836	99%	88%	83%	99%
Smoking Cessation Advice[2]	82	83%	83%	82%	100%
Pneumonia Care					
Appropriate Initial Antibiotic	375	92%	83%	83%	94%
Blood Culture Timing	504	92%	91%	90%	100%
Influenza Vaccine	122	24%	63%	70%	100%
Initial Antibiotic Timing	683	92%	81%	80%	93%
Oxygenation Assessment	777	100%	99%	99%	100%
Pneumococcal Vaccine	545	34%	62%	69%	94%
Smoking Cessation Advice	74	70%	80%	80%	100%
Surgical Infection Prevention					
Prophylactic Antibiotic Given[2]	2,015	89%	74%	77%	95%
Prophylactic Antibiotic Selection[2]	520	90%	91%	90%	100%
Prophylactic Antibiotic Stopped[2]	1,962	88%	67%	72%	95%
Pregnancy Care					
Inpatient Neonatal Mortality	4,959	0.36%	-	-	-
Third or Fourth Degree Laceration	3,393	4.51%	3.89%	3.63%	3.27%

Saint Francis Hospital

355 Ridge Avenue
Evanston, IL 60202
URL: www.reshealth.org
Ownership: Voluntary non-profit - Church
Emergency Services: Yes

Phone: 847-316-4000
Fax: 847-316-4500

Accredited: Yes
Licensed Beds: 445

Key Personnel:

President/CEO . . . . Jeffrey Murphy
Chief Medical Staff . . . . Ann Kinnealey, MD
Chief Catheterization Laboratory . . . . Alberto E Foschi, MD
Emergency Room . . . . Glen Aldinger, MD
Director Infection/Disease Control . . . . Chris Costas, MD
ICU Supervising Nurse . . . . Pamela Malone, RN
Director Medical/Surgical Nursing . . . . Denice Tudor
OB/GYN Womens Health . . . . John Knaus, DO
Surgical Services . . . . Pamela Bemaung, RN
Chief Radiology . . . . Thomas Cronin, MD
Director Respiratory Therapy . . . . Thomas Lynch

Measure	Cases	This Hospital	State Average	U.S. Average	Top Hospital
Heart Attack Care					
ACE Inhibitor or ARB for LVSD[1]	20	50%	79%	82%	100%
Aspirin at Arrival	121	98%	93%	92%	100%
Aspirin at Discharge	110	94%	90%	90%	100%
Beta Blocker at Arrival	86	86%	87%	87%	100%
Beta Blocker at Discharge	96	84%	88%	90%	100%
Fibrinolytic Medication Timing[1]	1	0%	21%	31%	100%
PCI Within 90 Minutes of Arrival[1]	4	0%	47%	54%	95%
Smoking Cessation Advice[1]	23	91%	84%	88%	100%
Heart Failure Care					
ACE Inhibitor or ARB for LVSD	163	72%	83%	82%	100%
Discharge Instructions	290	59%	67%	61%	93%
Evaluation of LVS Function	401	92%	88%	83%	99%
Smoking Cessation Advice	70	74%	83%	82%	100%
Pneumonia Care					
Appropriate Initial Antibiotic	261	85%	83%	83%	94%

NOTE: Hospital profiles are in alphabetical order by state, then city, then hospital within the city; Rankings are sorted by rate in descending order and exclude hospitals with less than 25 cases; (1) The number of cases is too small (n<25) for purposes of reliably predicting hospital performance; (2) Measure reflects the hospital's indication that its submission was based upon a sample of its relevant discharges; (3) Rate reflects fewer than the maximum possible quarters of data for the measure; (4) Inaccurate information submitted and suppressed for one or more quarters; (5) No data is available from the hospital for this measure; Please refer to the User's Guide for a full explanation of data

Blood Culture Timing	424	93%	91%	90%	100%
Influenza Vaccine	99	35%	63%	70%	100%
Initial Antibiotic Timing	518	84%	81%	80%	93%
Oxygenation Assessment	622	100%	99%	99%	100%
Pneumococcal Vaccine	382	44%	62%	69%	94%
Smoking Cessation Advice	103	73%	80%	80%	100%
Surgical Infection Prevention					
Prophylactic Antibiotic Given[3]	310	70%	74%	77%	95%
Prophylactic Antibiotic Selection	111	94%	91%	90%	100%
Prophylactic Antibiotic Stopped[3]	290	80%	67%	72%	95%
Pregnancy Care					
Inpatient Neonatal Mortality	-	-	-	-	-
Third or Fourth Degree Laceration	-	-	3.89%	3.63%	3.27%

Little Company of Mary Hospital

2800 W 95th Street
Evergreen Park, IL 60805
Toll-Free: 866-540-5264
Phone: 708-422-6200
Fax: 708-229-6733
URL: www.lcmh.org
Ownership: Voluntary non-profit - Church
Accredited: Yes
Emergency Services: Yes
Licensed Beds: 477

Key Personnel:

Administrator/President . . . . Dennis Reilly
Chief Medical Staff. . . . . Kent Armruster, MD
Emergency Room . . . . Michael O'Mara, DO
ICU . . . . Andrea Klatt, RN
Surgical Services . . . . Madonna Halicki
Respiratory Therapy. . . . . Mary Silder

Measure	Cases	This Hospital	State Average	U.S. Average	Top Hospital
Heart Attack Care					
ACE Inhibitor or ARB for LVSD[1]	23	96%	79%	82%	100%
Aspirin at Arrival	154	96%	93%	92%	100%
Aspirin at Discharge	82	95%	90%	90%	100%
Beta Blocker at Arrival	111	92%	87%	87%	100%
Beta Blocker at Discharge	81	99%	88%	90%	100%
Fibrinolytic Medication Timing[1]	1	0%	21%	31%	100%
PCI Within 90 Minutes of Arrival[1]	3	0%	47%	54%	95%
Smoking Cessation Advice	30	83%	84%	88%	100%
Heart Failure Care					
ACE Inhibitor or ARB for LVSD[2]	125	88%	83%	82%	100%
Discharge Instructions[2]	279	26%	67%	61%	93%
Evaluation of LVS Function[2]	351	93%	88%	83%	99%
Smoking Cessation Advice[2]	69	88%	83%	82%	100%
Pneumonia Care					
Appropriate Initial Antibiotic[2]	105	88%	83%	83%	94%
Blood Culture Timing[2]	118	86%	91%	90%	100%
Influenza Vaccine[2]	29	52%	63%	70%	100%
Initial Antibiotic Timing[2]	169	62%	81%	80%	93%
Oxygenation Assessment[2]	212	99%	99%	99%	100%
Pneumococcal Vaccine[2]	128	49%	62%	69%	94%
Smoking Cessation Advice[2]	38	87%	80%	80%	100%
Surgical Infection Prevention					
Prophylactic Antibiotic Given[2,3]	179	58%	74%	77%	95%
Prophylactic Antibiotic Selection[2]	61	97%	91%	90%	100%
Prophylactic Antibiotic Stopped[2,3]	163	52%	67%	72%	95%
Pregnancy Care					
Inpatient Neonatal Mortality	1,436	0.21%	-	-	-
Third or Fourth Degree Laceration	932	2.36%	3.89%	3.63%	3.27%

Fairfield Memorial Hospital

303 NW 11th Street
Fairfield, IL 62837
Phone: 618-842-2611
Fax: 618-842-2011
URL: www.fairfieldob.com
Ownership: Voluntary non-profit - Private
Accredited: Yes
Emergency Services: Yes
Licensed Beds: 80

Key Personnel:

CEO/President. . . . . Michale Brown
Chief Medical Staff. . . . . Patrick Molt
Emergency Room . . . . Andrew Britt
Emergency Room . . . . Bo Schneider, MD
Director Infection/Disease Control . . . . Hazel Best, RN
Director Medical/Surgical Nursing . . . . Vicki Wagner
OB/GYN Womens Health. . . . . Steven Scott, MD
Director Respiratory Therapy . . . . Kathy Draper

Measure	Cases	This Hospital	State Average	U.S. Average	Top Hospital
Heart Attack Care					
ACE Inhibitor or ARB for LVSD[1,3]	2	50%	79%	82%	100%
Aspirin at Arrival[1,3]	3	100%	93%	92%	100%
Aspirin at Discharge[1,3]	3	67%	90%	90%	100%
Beta Blocker at Arrival[1,3]	3	67%	87%	87%	100%
Beta Blocker at Discharge[1,3]	3	100%	88%	90%	100%
Fibrinolytic Medication Timing[3]	0	-	21%	31%	100%
PCI Within 90 Minutes of Arrival[5]	-	-	47%	54%	95%
Smoking Cessation Advice[1,3]	1	100%	84%	88%	100%
Heart Failure Care					
ACE Inhibitor or ARB for LVSD[1]	16	75%	83%	82%	100%
Discharge Instructions	36	97%	67%	61%	93%
Evaluation of LVS Function	55	78%	88%	83%	99%
Smoking Cessation Advice[1]	2	100%	83%	82%	100%
Pneumonia Care					
Appropriate Initial Antibiotic	70	74%	83%	83%	94%
Blood Culture Timing	30	87%	91%	90%	100%
Influenza Vaccine[4,5]	-	-	63%	70%	100%
Initial Antibiotic Timing	82	77%	81%	80%	93%
Oxygenation Assessment	105	100%	99%	99%	100%
Pneumococcal Vaccine	69	75%	62%	69%	94%
Smoking Cessation Advice[1]	19	74%	80%	80%	100%
Surgical Infection Prevention					
Prophylactic Antibiotic Given[1]	11	91%	74%	77%	95%
Prophylactic Antibiotic Selection[1]	1	100%	91%	90%	100%
Prophylactic Antibiotic Stopped[1]	11	91%	67%	72%	95%
Pregnancy Care					
Inpatient Neonatal Mortality	-	-	-	-	-
Third or Fourth Degree Laceration	-	-	3.89%	3.63%	3.27%

Clay County Hospital

911 Stacy Burk Drive
PO Box 280
Flora, IL 62839
Phone: 618-662-2131
Fax: 618-662-1486
E-mail: cchdas@wabash.net
URL: www.claycountyhospital.org
Ownership: Voluntary non-profit - Other
Accredited: No
Emergency Services: Yes
Licensed Beds: 18

Key Personnel:

Administrator . . . . Linda U Jordan
Chief Medical Staff. . . . . Bradley Reynolds, MD
Emergency Room . . . . Eileen Enlow, RN

Measure	Cases	This Hospital	State Average	U.S. Average	Top Hospital
Heart Attack Care					
ACE Inhibitor or ARB for LVSD	0	-	79%	82%	100%
Aspirin at Arrival[1]	6	100%	93%	92%	100%
Aspirin at Discharge[1]	2	100%	90%	90%	100%
Beta Blocker at Arrival[1]	7	100%	87%	87%	100%
Beta Blocker at Discharge[1]	5	100%	88%	90%	100%
Fibrinolytic Medication Timing	0	-	21%	31%	100%
PCI Within 90 Minutes of Arrival	0	-	47%	54%	95%
Smoking Cessation Advice	0	-	84%	88%	100%
Heart Failure Care					
ACE Inhibitor or ARB for LVSD	30	93%	83%	82%	100%
Discharge Instructions	65	94%	67%	61%	93%
Evaluation of LVS Function	101	98%	88%	83%	99%
Smoking Cessation Advice[1]	11	91%	83%	82%	100%
Pneumonia Care					
Appropriate Initial Antibiotic	46	87%	83%	83%	94%
Blood Culture Timing	58	100%	91%	90%	100%
Influenza Vaccine[1]	19	100%	63%	70%	100%
Initial Antibiotic Timing	75	95%	81%	80%	93%
Oxygenation Assessment	89	100%	99%	99%	100%
Pneumococcal Vaccine	51	96%	62%	69%	94%
Smoking Cessation Advice[1]	24	100%	80%	80%	100%
Surgical Infection Prevention					
Prophylactic Antibiotic Given[1,3]	9	89%	74%	77%	95%

NOTE: Hospital profiles are in alphabetical order by state, then city, then hospital within the city; Rankings are sorted by rate in descending order and exclude hospitals with less than 25 cases; (1) The number of cases is too small (n<25) for purposes of reliably predicting hospital performance; (2) Measure reflects the hospital's indication that its submission was based upon a sample of its relevant discharges; (3) Rate reflects fewer than the maximum possible quarters of data for the measure; (4) Inaccurate information submitted and suppressed for one or more quarters; (5) No data is available from the hospital for this measure; Please refer to the User's Guide for a full explanation of data

Measure	Cases	This Hospital	State Average	U.S. Average	Top Hospital
Prophylactic Antibiotic Selection[1]	1	100%	91%	90%	100%
Prophylactic Antibiotic Stopped[1,3]	7	71%	67%	72%	95%
Pregnancy Care					
Inpatient Neonatal Mortality	-	-	-	-	-
Third or Fourth Degree Laceration	-	-	3.89%	3.63%	3.27%

FHN Memorial Hospital

1045 West Stephenson Street
Freeport, IL 61032
URL: www.fhn.org
Ownership: Voluntary non-profit - Private
Emergency Services: Yes
Phone: 815-599-6000
Fax: 815-599-6311
Accredited: Yes
Licensed Beds: 183

Key Personnel:
CEO. . . . . Dennis L Hamilton

Measure	Cases	This Hospital	State Average	U.S. Average	Top Hospital
Heart Attack Care					
ACE Inhibitor or ARB for LVSD[1]	8	100%	79%	82%	100%
Aspirin at Arrival	34	97%	93%	92%	100%
Aspirin at Discharge[1]	24	100%	90%	90%	100%
Beta Blocker at Arrival	35	94%	87%	87%	100%
Beta Blocker at Discharge	27	96%	88%	90%	100%
Fibrinolytic Medication Timing[1]	2	50%	21%	31%	100%
PCI Within 90 Minutes of Arrival	0	-	47%	54%	95%
Smoking Cessation Advice[1]	3	100%	84%	88%	100%
Heart Failure Care					
ACE Inhibitor or ARB for LVSD	62	92%	83%	82%	100%
Discharge Instructions	128	84%	67%	61%	93%
Evaluation of LVS Function	179	98%	88%	83%	99%
Smoking Cessation Advice[1]	15	100%	83%	82%	100%
Pneumonia Care					
Appropriate Initial Antibiotic	120	97%	83%	83%	94%
Blood Culture Timing	120	99%	91%	90%	100%
Influenza Vaccine	41	80%	63%	70%	100%
Initial Antibiotic Timing	192	89%	81%	80%	93%
Oxygenation Assessment	234	100%	99%	99%	100%
Pneumococcal Vaccine	169	84%	62%	69%	94%
Smoking Cessation Advice	45	93%	80%	80%	100%
Surgical Infection Prevention					
Prophylactic Antibiotic Given[2]	406	95%	74%	77%	95%
Prophylactic Antibiotic Selection[2]	80	94%	91%	90%	100%
Prophylactic Antibiotic Stopped[2]	388	80%	67%	72%	95%
Pregnancy Care					
Inpatient Neonatal Mortality	-	-	-	-	-
Third or Fourth Degree Laceration	-	-	3.89%	3.63%	3.27%

Galena-Stauss Hospital & Healthcare Center

215 Summit St
Galena, IL 61036
Ownership: Govt - Hospital District or Authority
Emergency Services: Yes
Phone: 815-777-1340
Accredited: No

Measure	Cases	This Hospital	State Average	U.S. Average	Top Hospital
Heart Attack Care					
ACE Inhibitor or ARB for LVSD[3]	0	-	79%	82%	100%
Aspirin at Arrival[3]	0	-	93%	92%	100%
Aspirin at Discharge[3]	0	-	90%	90%	100%
Beta Blocker at Arrival[3]	0	-	87%	87%	100%
Beta Blocker at Discharge[3]	0	-	88%	90%	100%
Fibrinolytic Medication Timing[3]	0	-	21%	31%	100%
PCI Within 90 Minutes of Arrival	0	-	47%	54%	95%
Smoking Cessation Advice[3]	0	-	84%	88%	100%
Heart Failure Care					
ACE Inhibitor or ARB for LVSD[1,3]	1	100%	83%	82%	100%
Discharge Instructions[1,3]	7	29%	67%	61%	93%
Evaluation of LVS Function[1,3]	12	50%	88%	83%	99%
Smoking Cessation Advice[1,3]	2	50%	83%	82%	100%
Pneumonia Care					
Appropriate Initial Antibiotic	30	90%	83%	83%	94%
Blood Culture Timing	0	-	91%	90%	100%
Influenza Vaccine[1]	5	100%	63%	70%	100%
Initial Antibiotic Timing	25	88%	81%	80%	93%
Oxygenation Assessment	30	100%	99%	99%	100%
Pneumococcal Vaccine	26	81%	62%	69%	94%
Smoking Cessation Advice[1]	4	25%	80%	80%	100%
Surgical Infection Prevention					
Prophylactic Antibiotic Given[5]	-	-	74%	77%	95%
Prophylactic Antibiotic Selection[5]	-	-	91%	90%	100%
Prophylactic Antibiotic Stopped[5]	-	-	67%	72%	95%
Pregnancy Care					
Inpatient Neonatal Mortality	-	-	-	-	-
Third or Fourth Degree Laceration	-	-	3.89%	3.63%	3.27%

Galesburg Cottage Hospital

695 N Kellogg Street
Galesburg, IL 61402
URL: www.cottagehospital.com
Ownership: Proprietary
Emergency Services: Yes
Phone: 309-343-8131
Fax: 309-343-2393
Accredited: Yes
Licensed Beds: 170

Key Personnel:
CEO. . . . . Kenneth Hutchennider
Chief Medical Staff. . . . . Mark Daus, MD
Cardiac Lab . . . . Johanna Steller
Emergency Room . . . . Theresa Rutherford
Infection Control. . . . . Linda Newcomb
ICU . . . . Deb Rickard
Intensive/Coronary Care . . . . Deb Rickard
Medical Surgical Nursing . . . . Theresa Rutherford
OB/GYN Womens Health. . . . . Marva Spencer
Respiratory/Cardiopulmonary. . . . . Johanna Steller

Measure	Cases	This Hospital	State Average	U.S. Average	Top Hospital
Heart Attack Care					
ACE Inhibitor or ARB for LVSD[1]	4	75%	79%	82%	100%
Aspirin at Arrival	31	81%	93%	92%	100%
Aspirin at Discharge[1]	19	58%	90%	90%	100%
Beta Blocker at Arrival[1]	20	70%	87%	87%	100%
Beta Blocker at Discharge[1]	20	85%	88%	90%	100%
Fibrinolytic Medication Timing	0	-	21%	31%	100%
PCI Within 90 Minutes of Arrival	0	-	47%	54%	95%
Smoking Cessation Advice[1]	6	100%	84%	88%	100%
Heart Failure Care					
ACE Inhibitor or ARB for LVSD	48	83%	83%	82%	100%
Discharge Instructions	91	81%	67%	61%	93%
Evaluation of LVS Function	142	95%	88%	83%	99%
Smoking Cessation Advice[1]	19	84%	83%	82%	100%
Pneumonia Care					
Appropriate Initial Antibiotic[2]	91	75%	83%	83%	94%
Blood Culture Timing[2]	103	91%	91%	90%	100%
Influenza Vaccine[2]	27	81%	63%	70%	100%
Initial Antibiotic Timing[2]	151	81%	81%	80%	93%
Oxygenation Assessment[2]	177	99%	99%	99%	100%
Pneumococcal Vaccine[2]	120	84%	62%	69%	94%
Smoking Cessation Advice[2]	32	78%	80%	80%	100%
Surgical Infection Prevention					
Prophylactic Antibiotic Given[2,3]	177	85%	74%	77%	95%
Prophylactic Antibiotic Selection[2]	52	96%	91%	90%	100%
Prophylactic Antibiotic Stopped[2,3]	174	79%	67%	72%	95%
Pregnancy Care					
Inpatient Neonatal Mortality	-	-	-	-	-
Third or Fourth Degree Laceration	-	-	3.89%	3.63%	3.27%

OSF Saint Mary Medical Center

Alternate Name: Saint Mary Medical Center
3333 N Seminary Street
Galesburg, IL 61401
URL: www.osfhealthcare.org
Ownership: Voluntary non-profit - Church
Emergency Services: Yes
Phone: 309-344-3161
Fax: 309-344-9494
Accredited: Yes
Licensed Beds: 156

Key Personnel:
CEO. . . . . Richard Kowalski
Emergency Room . . . . Cathy Anderson
Infection Control. . . . . Bonnie Fransene
ICU . . . . Rosie Friend
Intensive/Coronary Care . . . . Rosie Friend

NOTE: Hospital profiles are in alphabetical order by state, then city, then hospital within the city; Rankings are sorted by rate in descending order and exclude hospitals with less than 25 cases; (1) The number of cases is too small (n<25) for purposes of reliably predicting hospital performance; (2) Measure reflects the hospital's indication that its submission was based upon a sample of its relevant discharges; (3) Rate reflects fewer than the maximum possible quarters of data for the measure; (4) Inaccurate information submitted and suppressed for one or more quarters; (5) No data is available from the hospital for this measure; Please refer to the User's Guide for a full explanation of data

Medical Surgical Nursing . . . . Carrie Hagen
OB/GYN/Women's Health . . . . Sharon Clevenger
Respiratory/Cardiopulmonary. . . . . Steve Hogan

Measure	Cases	This Hospital	State Average	U.S. Average	Top Hospital
Heart Attack Care					
ACE Inhibitor or ARB for LVSD[1]	5	60%	79%	82%	100%
Aspirin at Arrival	38	89%	93%	92%	100%
Aspirin at Discharge[1]	18	100%	90%	90%	100%
Beta Blocker at Arrival	30	83%	87%	87%	100%
Beta Blocker at Discharge	25	88%	88%	90%	100%
Fibrinolytic Medication Timing	0	-	21%	31%	100%
PCI Within 90 Minutes of Arrival	0	-	47%	54%	95%
Smoking Cessation Advice[1]	3	67%	84%	88%	100%
Heart Failure Care					
ACE Inhibitor or ARB for LVSD	59	86%	83%	82%	100%
Discharge Instructions	122	85%	67%	61%	93%
Evaluation of LVS Function	166	96%	88%	83%	99%
Smoking Cessation Advice[1]	21	90%	83%	82%	100%
Pneumonia Care					
Appropriate Initial Antibiotic	131	86%	83%	83%	94%
Blood Culture Timing	116	92%	91%	90%	100%
Influenza Vaccine	50	94%	63%	70%	100%
Initial Antibiotic Timing	164	89%	81%	80%	93%
Oxygenation Assessment	214	100%	99%	99%	100%
Pneumococcal Vaccine	134	98%	62%	69%	94%
Smoking Cessation Advice	51	98%	80%	80%	100%
Surgical Infection Prevention					
Prophylactic Antibiotic Given	374	97%	74%	77%	95%
Prophylactic Antibiotic Selection	100	95%	91%	90%	100%
Prophylactic Antibiotic Stopped	363	90%	67%	72%	95%
Pregnancy Care					
Inpatient Neonatal Mortality	-	-	-	-	-
Third or Fourth Degree Laceration	-	-	3.89%	3.63%	3.27%

Hammond-Henry Hospital

600 N College Avenue — Phone: 309-944-6431
Geneseo, IL 61254 — Fax: 309-944-5299
E-mail: hhh@hammondhenry.com
URL: www.hammondhenry.com
Ownership: Govt - Hospital District or Authority — Accredited: Yes
Emergency Services: Yes — Licensed Beds: 105

Key Personnel:
President/CEO. . . . . Bradley Solberg
Chief Medical Staff. . . . . L Gumidyala
ER Manager. . . . . Kurt Krueger
Emergency Room . . . . Lokanathum Gumadyala, MD
Surgery Manager. . . . . Robin Van Meenen
Infection Control Manager . . . . Geri Egert
Medical/Surgical/CCU Manager. . . . . Karen Crossman
Surgery Manager. . . . . Robin Van Meenen

Measure	Cases	This Hospital	State Average	U.S. Average	Top Hospital
Heart Attack Care					
ACE Inhibitor or ARB for LVSD[5]	-	-	79%	82%	100%
Aspirin at Arrival[5]	-	-	93%	92%	100%
Aspirin at Discharge[5]	-	-	90%	90%	100%
Beta Blocker at Arrival[5]	-	-	87%	87%	100%
Beta Blocker at Discharge[5]	-	-	88%	90%	100%
Fibrinolytic Medication Timing[5]	-	-	21%	31%	100%
PCI Within 90 Minutes of Arrival[5]	-	-	47%	54%	95%
Smoking Cessation Advice[5]	-	-	84%	88%	100%
Heart Failure Care					
ACE Inhibitor or ARB for LVSD[1]	5	100%	83%	82%	100%
Discharge Instructions[1]	13	92%	67%	61%	93%
Evaluation of LVS Function[1]	19	68%	88%	83%	99%
Smoking Cessation Advice[1]	2	100%	83%	82%	100%
Pneumonia Care					
Appropriate Initial Antibiotic	26	81%	83%	83%	94%
Blood Culture Timing[1]	12	83%	91%	90%	100%
Influenza Vaccine[1]	5	60%	63%	70%	100%
Initial Antibiotic Timing[1]	19	84%	81%	80%	93%
Oxygenation Assessment	32	100%	99%	99%	100%
Pneumococcal Vaccine[1]	20	85%	62%	69%	94%
Smoking Cessation Advice[1]	4	75%	80%	80%	100%
Surgical Infection Prevention					
Prophylactic Antibiotic Given	35	91%	74%	77%	95%
Prophylactic Antibiotic Selection[1]	11	91%	91%	90%	100%
Prophylactic Antibiotic Stopped	33	45%	67%	72%	95%
Pregnancy Care					
Inpatient Neonatal Mortality	-	-	-	-	-
Third or Fourth Degree Laceration	-	-	3.89%	3.63%	3.27%

Delnor Community Hospital

300 Randall Road — Phone: 630-208-3000
Geneva, IL 60134 — Fax: 630-208-3478
E-mail: info@delnor.com
URL: www.delnor.com
Ownership: Voluntary non-profit - Other — Accredited: Yes
Emergency Services: Yes — Licensed Beds: 118

Key Personnel:
President/CEO. . . . . Craig A Livermore
Medical/Surgical Nursing . . . . Katherine Barker
OB/GYN Womens Health. . . . . Judy O Smith
Respiratory/Cardiopulmonary. . . . . Rae Vicory

Measure	Cases	This Hospital	State Average	U.S. Average	Top Hospital
Heart Attack Care					
ACE Inhibitor or ARB for LVSD[1]	18	83%	79%	82%	100%
Aspirin at Arrival	98	99%	93%	92%	100%
Aspirin at Discharge	81	99%	90%	90%	100%
Beta Blocker at Arrival	91	99%	87%	87%	100%
Beta Blocker at Discharge	86	98%	88%	90%	100%
Fibrinolytic Medication Timing	0	-	21%	31%	100%
PCI Within 90 Minutes of Arrival[1]	6	33%	47%	54%	95%
Smoking Cessation Advice[1]	21	95%	84%	88%	100%
Heart Failure Care					
ACE Inhibitor or ARB for LVSD	62	87%	83%	82%	100%
Discharge Instructions	164	87%	67%	61%	93%
Evaluation of LVS Function	236	97%	88%	83%	99%
Smoking Cessation Advice	31	97%	83%	82%	100%
Pneumonia Care					
Appropriate Initial Antibiotic	128	92%	83%	83%	94%
Blood Culture Timing	114	89%	91%	90%	100%
Influenza Vaccine	44	100%	63%	70%	100%
Initial Antibiotic Timing	207	91%	81%	80%	93%
Oxygenation Assessment	243	100%	99%	99%	100%
Pneumococcal Vaccine	176	99%	62%	69%	94%
Smoking Cessation Advice[1]	23	78%	80%	80%	100%
Surgical Infection Prevention					
Prophylactic Antibiotic Given[2,3]	368	71%	74%	77%	95%
Prophylactic Antibiotic Selection[2]	89	79%	91%	90%	100%
Prophylactic Antibiotic Stopped[2,3]	353	65%	67%	72%	95%
Pregnancy Care					
Inpatient Neonatal Mortality	1,587	0.06%	-	-	-
Third or Fourth Degree Laceration	984	8.33%	3.89%	3.63%	3.27%

Gibson Community Hospital

1120 North Melvin Street — Phone: 217-784-4251
Gibson City, IL 60936 — Fax: 217-784-2610
URL: www.gibsonhospital.org
Ownership: Voluntary non-profit - Other — Accredited: Yes
Emergency Services: Yes — Licensed Beds: 82

Key Personnel:
CEO. . . . . Gary Peterson
Emergency Room . . . . Brenda Standerfer
Infection Control. . . . . Becki Garard
ICU . . . . Brenda Standerfer
Medical Surgical Nursing . . . . Denise Birky
Director OB Unit. . . . . Tina Frantz
Respiratory/Cardiopulmonary. . . . . Pat Harper

Measure	Cases	This Hospital	State Average	U.S. Average	Top Hospital
Heart Attack Care					
ACE Inhibitor or ARB for LVSD[3]	0	-	79%	82%	100%

NOTE: Hospital profiles are in alphabetical order by state, then city, then hospital within the city; Rankings are sorted by rate in descending order and exclude hospitals with less than 25 cases; (1) The number of cases is too small (n<25) for purposes of reliably predicting hospital performance; (2) Measure reflects the hospital's indication that its submission was based upon a sample of its relevant discharges; (3) Rate reflects fewer than the maximum possible quarters of data for the measure; (4) Inaccurate information submitted and suppressed for one or more quarters; (5) No data is available from the hospital for this measure; Please refer to the User's Guide for a full explanation of data

Measure	Cases	This Hospital	State Average	U.S. Average	Top Hospital
Aspirin at Arrival[1,3]	1	100%	93%	92%	100%
Aspirin at Discharge[3]	0	-	90%	90%	100%
Beta Blocker at Arrival[1,3]	1	100%	87%	87%	100%
Beta Blocker at Discharge[3]	0	-	88%	90%	100%
Fibrinolytic Medication Timing[3]	0	-	21%	31%	100%
PCI Within 90 Minutes of Arrival[5]	-	-	47%	54%	95%
Smoking Cessation Advice[3]	0	-	84%	88%	100%
Heart Failure Care					
ACE Inhibitor or ARB for LVSD[1]	8	62%	83%	82%	100%
Discharge Instructions[1]	8	38%	67%	61%	93%
Evaluation of LVS Function	25	88%	88%	83%	99%
Smoking Cessation Advice[1]	3	33%	83%	82%	100%
Pneumonia Care					
Appropriate Initial Antibiotic	32	94%	83%	83%	94%
Blood Culture Timing[1]	23	83%	91%	90%	100%
Influenza Vaccine[1]	11	73%	63%	70%	100%
Initial Antibiotic Timing	42	86%	81%	80%	93%
Oxygenation Assessment	57	100%	99%	99%	100%
Pneumococcal Vaccine	33	82%	62%	69%	94%
Smoking Cessation Advice[1]	10	90%	80%	80%	100%
Surgical Infection Prevention					
Prophylactic Antibiotic Given	31	84%	74%	77%	95%
Prophylactic Antibiotic Selection[1]	6	100%	91%	90%	100%
Prophylactic Antibiotic Stopped	31	29%	67%	72%	95%
Pregnancy Care					
Inpatient Neonatal Mortality	-	-	-	-	-
Third or Fourth Degree Laceration	-	-	3.89%	3.63%	3.27%

Adventist GlenOaks Hospital

701 Winthrop Avenue — Phone: 630-545-8000
Glendale Heights, IL 60139 — Fax: 630-545-3920
URL: www.keepingyouwell.com
Ownership: Voluntary non-profit - Other — Accredited: Yes
Emergency Services: Yes — Licensed Beds: 186

Key Personnel:

President/CEO . . . . Brinsley Lewis
Chief Medical Staff . . . . Lisa Wohl, MD
Cardiac Lab . . . . Richard Kenney
Catheterization Lab . . . . Tamara Dennis
Emergency Room . . . . Joseph Shanahan, MD
Emergency Room . . . . Mary Murphy
Infection Control . . . . Darlene Gallagher
ICU . . . . Josephine Baldo
OB/GYN Women's Health . . . . Pam Bamaung
Surgical Services . . . . Judy Papendorf
Director Respiratory Therapy . . . . Richard Kenney

Measure	Cases	This Hospital	State Average	U.S. Average	Top Hospital
Heart Attack Care					
ACE Inhibitor or ARB for LVSD[1,2]	4	75%	79%	82%	100%
Aspirin at Arrival[1,2]	22	100%	93%	92%	100%
Aspirin at Discharge[1,2]	3	67%	90%	90%	100%
Beta Blocker at Arrival[1,2]	15	87%	87%	87%	100%
Beta Blocker at Discharge[1,2]	9	78%	88%	90%	100%
Fibrinolytic Medication Timing[1,2]	2	50%	21%	31%	100%
PCI Within 90 Minutes of Arrival[2]	0	-	47%	54%	95%
Smoking Cessation Advice[1,2]	1	100%	84%	88%	100%
Heart Failure Care					
ACE Inhibitor or ARB for LVSD[1]	23	78%	83%	82%	100%
Discharge Instructions	43	70%	67%	61%	93%
Evaluation of LVS Function	73	88%	88%	83%	99%
Smoking Cessation Advice[1]	16	81%	83%	82%	100%
Pneumonia Care					
Appropriate Initial Antibiotic	35	89%	83%	83%	94%
Blood Culture Timing	63	98%	91%	90%	100%
Influenza Vaccine[1]	9	11%	63%	70%	100%
Initial Antibiotic Timing	76	95%	81%	80%	93%
Oxygenation Assessment	99	100%	99%	99%	100%
Pneumococcal Vaccine	57	77%	62%	69%	94%
Smoking Cessation Advice[1]	17	82%	80%	80%	100%
Surgical Infection Prevention					
Prophylactic Antibiotic Given[3]	37	86%	74%	77%	95%
Prophylactic Antibiotic Selection[1]	13	100%	91%	90%	100%
Prophylactic Antibiotic Stopped[3]	35	83%	67%	72%	95%
Pregnancy Care					
Inpatient Neonatal Mortality	-	-	-	-	-
Third or Fourth Degree Laceration	-	-	3.89%	3.63%	3.27%

Gateway Regional Medical Center

2100 Madison Avenue — Phone: 618-798-3000
Granite City, IL 62040 — Fax: 618-798-3853
URL: www.sehs.com
Ownership: Proprietary — Accredited: Yes
Emergency Services: Yes — Licensed Beds: 393

Key Personnel:

Administrator/President . . . . Ted Eilerman
Chief Medical Staff . . . . K Konzen, MD
Chief Catheterization Laboratory . . . . KM Patel, MD
Director Infection/Disease Control . . . . Ruth Ann Gabriel
CCU Spvg. Nurse . . . . Keith Werner
Director Medical/Surgical Nursing . . . . Carol Nesbit
OB/GYN Womens Health . . . . Y Shah, MD
Chief Radiology . . . . A Hammerman, MD
Director Respiratory Therapy . . . . Dan McDowell

Measure	Cases	This Hospital	State Average	U.S. Average	Top Hospital
Heart Attack Care					
ACE Inhibitor or ARB for LVSD[1]	18	94%	79%	82%	100%
Aspirin at Arrival	112	91%	93%	92%	100%
Aspirin at Discharge	91	96%	90%	90%	100%
Beta Blocker at Arrival	87	89%	87%	87%	100%
Beta Blocker at Discharge	87	98%	88%	90%	100%
Fibrinolytic Medication Timing[1]	2	0%	21%	31%	100%
PCI Within 90 Minutes of Arrival	0	-	47%	54%	95%
Smoking Cessation Advice	31	97%	84%	88%	100%
Heart Failure Care					
ACE Inhibitor or ARB for LVSD	81	91%	83%	82%	100%
Discharge Instructions	223	33%	67%	61%	93%
Evaluation of LVS Function	269	87%	88%	83%	99%
Smoking Cessation Advice	47	87%	83%	82%	100%
Pneumonia Care					
Appropriate Initial Antibiotic	142	80%	83%	83%	94%
Blood Culture Timing	103	93%	91%	90%	100%
Influenza Vaccine	28	54%	63%	70%	100%
Initial Antibiotic Timing	186	77%	81%	80%	93%
Oxygenation Assessment	198	99%	99%	99%	100%
Pneumococcal Vaccine	96	59%	62%	69%	94%
Smoking Cessation Advice	67	82%	80%	80%	100%
Surgical Infection Prevention					
Prophylactic Antibiotic Given[2,3]	177	30%	74%	77%	95%
Prophylactic Antibiotic Selection[2]	47	89%	91%	90%	100%
Prophylactic Antibiotic Stopped[2,3]	176	66%	67%	72%	95%
Pregnancy Care					
Inpatient Neonatal Mortality	-	-	-	-	-
Third or Fourth Degree Laceration	-	-	3.89%	3.63%	3.27%

Greenville Regional Hospital

200 Healthcare Drive — Phone: 618-664-1230
Greenville, IL 62246 — Fax: 618-664-9750
Ownership: Voluntary non-profit - Other — Accredited: Yes
Emergency Services: Yes — Licensed Beds: 50

Key Personnel:

CEO . . . . Morris Bond
Emergency Room . . . . Sara McPeak

Measure	Cases	This Hospital	State Average	U.S. Average	Top Hospital
Heart Attack Care					
ACE Inhibitor or ARB for LVSD	0	-	79%	82%	100%
Aspirin at Arrival[1]	9	78%	93%	92%	100%
Aspirin at Discharge[1]	6	100%	90%	90%	100%
Beta Blocker at Arrival[1]	6	67%	87%	87%	100%
Beta Blocker at Discharge[1]	6	100%	88%	90%	100%
Fibrinolytic Medication Timing	0	-	21%	31%	100%
PCI Within 90 Minutes of Arrival	0	-	47%	54%	95%
Smoking Cessation Advice	0	-	84%	88%	100%

NOTE: Hospital profiles are in alphabetical order by state, then city, then hospital within the city; Rankings are sorted by rate in descending order and exclude hospitals with less than 25 cases; (1) The number of cases is too small (n<25) for purposes of reliably predicting hospital performance; (2) Measure reflects the hospital's indication that its submission was based upon a sample of its relevant discharges; (3) Rate reflects fewer than the maximum possible quarters of data for the measure; (4) Inaccurate information submitted and suppressed for one or more quarters; (5) No data is available from the hospital for this measure; Please refer to the User's Guide for a full explanation of data

Measure	Cases	This Hospital	State Average	U.S. Average	Top Hospital
Heart Failure Care					
ACE Inhibitor or ARB for LVSD[1]	5	100%	83%	82%	100%
Discharge Instructions	29	52%	67%	61%	93%
Evaluation of LVS Function	47	83%	88%	83%	99%
Smoking Cessation Advice[1]	3	67%	83%	82%	100%
Pneumonia Care					
Appropriate Initial Antibiotic	63	73%	83%	83%	94%
Blood Culture Timing	60	93%	91%	90%	100%
Influenza Vaccine[1]	24	62%	63%	70%	100%
Initial Antibiotic Timing	98	77%	81%	80%	93%
Oxygenation Assessment	127	100%	99%	99%	100%
Pneumococcal Vaccine	85	35%	62%	69%	94%
Smoking Cessation Advice[1]	22	68%	80%	80%	100%
Surgical Infection Prevention					
Prophylactic Antibiotic Given[1]	22	55%	74%	77%	95%
Prophylactic Antibiotic Selection[1]	7	100%	91%	90%	100%
Prophylactic Antibiotic Stopped[1]	20	90%	67%	72%	95%
Pregnancy Care					
Inpatient Neonatal Mortality	130	0.00%	-	-	-
Third or Fourth Degree Laceration	76	10.53%	3.89%	3.63%	3.27%

Harrisburg Medical Center

100 Hospital Drive
PO Box 428
Harrisburg, IL 62946
E-mail: cchatterton@harrisburgmed.org
Phone: 618-253-7671
Fax: 618-252-7274
Ownership: Voluntary non-profit - Other
Emergency Services: Yes
Accredited: Yes
Licensed Beds: 86

Key Personnel:

Interim President/CEO . . . . Cindy Ford
Chief Medical Staff . . . . Vinai Mehta, MD
Emergency Room Medical Director . . . . Thomas J Bucinski, MD
Director Infection/Disease Control . . . . Brenda Duckworth, RN
CCU Spvg. Nurse . . . . Nancy Patton, RN
Director Medical/Surgical Nursing . . . . Rebecca Shaw
Cadiopulmonary/Rehab Nurse Manager . . . . . . Nancy Patton, RN
Director Respiratory Therapy . . . . Stan Harris

Measure	Cases	This Hospital	State Average	U.S. Average	Top Hospital
Heart Attack Care					
ACE Inhibitor or ARB for LVSD[1]	2	100%	79%	82%	100%
Aspirin at Arrival[1]	11	100%	93%	92%	100%
Aspirin at Discharge[1]	6	83%	90%	90%	100%
Beta Blocker at Arrival[1]	9	67%	87%	87%	100%
Beta Blocker at Discharge[1]	7	86%	88%	90%	100%
Fibrinolytic Medication Timing[1]	1	0%	21%	31%	100%
PCI Within 90 Minutes of Arrival	0	-	47%	54%	95%
Smoking Cessation Advice[1]	1	0%	84%	88%	100%
Heart Failure Care					
ACE Inhibitor or ARB for LVSD	29	86%	83%	82%	100%
Discharge Instructions	88	77%	67%	61%	93%
Evaluation of LVS Function	119	85%	88%	83%	99%
Smoking Cessation Advice[1]	18	67%	83%	82%	100%
Pneumonia Care					
Appropriate Initial Antibiotic	87	60%	83%	83%	94%
Blood Culture Timing	49	80%	91%	90%	100%
Influenza Vaccine[4,5]	-	-	63%	70%	100%
Initial Antibiotic Timing	143	83%	81%	80%	93%
Oxygenation Assessment	171	98%	99%	99%	100%
Pneumococcal Vaccine	108	55%	62%	69%	94%
Smoking Cessation Advice	28	79%	80%	80%	100%
Surgical Infection Prevention					
Prophylactic Antibiotic Given[1,3]	9	22%	74%	77%	95%
Prophylactic Antibiotic Selection[1]	4	25%	91%	90%	100%
Prophylactic Antibiotic Stopped[1,3]	9	67%	67%	72%	95%
Pregnancy Care					
Inpatient Neonatal Mortality	-	-	-	-	-
Third or Fourth Degree Laceration	-	-	3.89%	3.63%	3.27%

Mercy Harvard Hospital

901 Grant Street
Harvard, IL 60033
E-mail: custserv@mhsjvl.org
URL: www.mercyhealthsystem.org
Phone: 815-943-5431
Fax: 815-943-2493
Ownership: Voluntary non-profit - Private
Emergency Services: Yes
Accredited: Yes
Licensed Beds: 46

Key Personnel:

Administrator/CEO . . . . Dan Colby
Chief Medical Staff . . . . Joseph Levenstein, MD
Director Respiratory Therapy . . . . Susan Grindey

Measure	Cases	This Hospital	State Average	U.S. Average	Top Hospital
Heart Attack Care					
ACE Inhibitor or ARB for LVSD	0	-	79%	82%	100%
Aspirin at Arrival[1]	9	100%	93%	92%	100%
Aspirin at Discharge[1]	5	100%	90%	90%	100%
Beta Blocker at Arrival[1]	6	100%	87%	87%	100%
Beta Blocker at Discharge[1]	4	100%	88%	90%	100%
Fibrinolytic Medication Timing	0	-	21%	31%	100%
PCI Within 90 Minutes of Arrival	0	-	47%	54%	95%
Smoking Cessation Advice	0	-	84%	88%	100%
Heart Failure Care					
ACE Inhibitor or ARB for LVSD[1]	2	100%	83%	82%	100%
Discharge Instructions[1]	17	82%	67%	61%	93%
Evaluation of LVS Function	26	96%	88%	83%	99%
Smoking Cessation Advice[1]	1	100%	83%	82%	100%
Pneumonia Care					
Appropriate Initial Antibiotic[1]	16	94%	83%	83%	94%
Blood Culture Timing[1]	16	94%	91%	90%	100%
Influenza Vaccine[1]	6	83%	63%	70%	100%
Initial Antibiotic Timing	25	100%	81%	80%	93%
Oxygenation Assessment	28	100%	99%	99%	100%
Pneumococcal Vaccine[1]	20	90%	62%	69%	94%
Smoking Cessation Advice[1]	6	100%	80%	80%	100%
Surgical Infection Prevention					
Prophylactic Antibiotic Given	41	93%	74%	77%	95%
Prophylactic Antibiotic Selection[1]	6	100%	91%	90%	100%
Prophylactic Antibiotic Stopped	41	56%	67%	72%	95%
Pregnancy Care					
Inpatient Neonatal Mortality	-	-	-	-	-
Third or Fourth Degree Laceration	-	-	3.89%	3.63%	3.27%

Ingalls Memorial Hospital

One Ingalls Drive
Harvey, IL 60426
URL: www.ingalls.org
Phone: 708-333-2300
Fax: 708-915-2707
Ownership: Voluntary non-profit - Private
Emergency Services: Yes
Accredited: Yes
Licensed Beds: 563

Key Personnel:

President/CEO . . . . Kurt Johnson

Measure	Cases	This Hospital	State Average	U.S. Average	Top Hospital
Heart Attack Care					
ACE Inhibitor or ARB for LVSD[2]	46	76%	79%	82%	100%
Aspirin at Arrival[2]	175	94%	93%	92%	100%
Aspirin at Discharge[2]	177	85%	90%	90%	100%
Beta Blocker at Arrival[2]	157	85%	87%	87%	100%
Beta Blocker at Discharge[2]	189	87%	88%	90%	100%
Fibrinolytic Medication Timing[2]	0	-	21%	31%	100%
PCI Within 90 Minutes of Arrival[1,2]	2	50%	47%	54%	95%
Smoking Cessation Advice[2]	53	98%	84%	88%	100%
Heart Failure Care					
ACE Inhibitor or ARB for LVSD[2]	90	76%	83%	82%	100%
Discharge Instructions[2]	271	87%	67%	61%	93%
Evaluation of LVS Function[2]	303	83%	88%	83%	99%
Smoking Cessation Advice[2]	58	88%	83%	82%	100%
Pneumonia Care					
Appropriate Initial Antibiotic[2]	123	81%	83%	83%	94%
Blood Culture Timing[2]	99	73%	91%	90%	100%
Influenza Vaccine[1,2]	24	79%	63%	70%	100%
Initial Antibiotic Timing[2]	183	67%	81%	80%	93%
Oxygenation Assessment[2]	203	100%	99%	99%	100%

NOTE: Hospital profiles are in alphabetical order by state, then city, then hospital within the city; Rankings are sorted by rate in descending order and exclude hospitals with less than 25 cases; (1) The number of cases is too small (n<25) for purposes of reliably predicting hospital performance; (2) Measure reflects the hospital's indication that its submission was based upon a sample of its relevant discharges; (3) Rate reflects fewer than the maximum possible quarters of data for the measure; (4) Inaccurate information submitted and suppressed for one or more quarters; (5) No data is available from the hospital for this measure; Please refer to the User's Guide for a full explanation of data

Pneumococcal Vaccine[2]	98	68%	62%	69%	94%
Smoking Cessation Advice[2]	57	93%	80%	80%	100%
Surgical Infection Prevention					
Prophylactic Antibiotic Given[2,3]	407	88%	74%	77%	95%
Prophylactic Antibiotic Selection[2]	81	98%	91%	90%	100%
Prophylactic Antibiotic Stopped[2,3]	404	71%	67%	72%	95%
Pregnancy Care					
Inpatient Neonatal Mortality	1,461	0.55%	-	-	-
Third or Fourth Degree Laceration	1,067	2.06%	3.89%	3.63%	3.27%

Mason District Hospital

615 N Promenade St
Havana, IL 62644
E-mail: hwolin@fgi.net
URL: www.masondistricthospital.org
Ownership: Govt - Hospital District or Authority
Emergency Services: Yes
Phone: 309-543-8575
Fax: 309-543-8523
Accredited: Yes
Licensed Beds: 48

Key Personnel:
Administrator . . . . Harry Wolin
Chief Medical Staff. . . . . Tad A Yetter
Emergency Room . . . . Rhonda Hine, RN
Director Infection/Disease Control . . . . Lori Canada

Measure	Cases	This Hospital	State Average	U.S. Average	Top Hospital
Heart Attack Care					
ACE Inhibitor or ARB for LVSD[1,3]	1	100%	79%	82%	100%
Aspirin at Arrival[1,3]	3	100%	93%	92%	100%
Aspirin at Discharge[1,3]	3	100%	90%	90%	100%
Beta Blocker at Arrival[1,3]	3	100%	87%	87%	100%
Beta Blocker at Discharge[1,3]	4	100%	88%	90%	100%
Fibrinolytic Medication Timing[3]	0	-	21%	31%	100%
PCI Within 90 Minutes of Arrival[5]	-	-	47%	54%	95%
Smoking Cessation Advice[3]	0	-	84%	88%	100%
Heart Failure Care					
ACE Inhibitor or ARB for LVSD[1]	4	75%	83%	82%	100%
Discharge Instructions[1]	17	41%	67%	61%	93%
Evaluation of LVS Function	26	88%	88%	83%	99%
Smoking Cessation Advice[1]	2	50%	83%	82%	100%
Pneumonia Care					
Appropriate Initial Antibiotic	26	92%	83%	83%	94%
Blood Culture Timing[1]	22	100%	91%	90%	100%
Influenza Vaccine[1]	15	80%	63%	70%	100%
Initial Antibiotic Timing	44	82%	81%	80%	93%
Oxygenation Assessment	52	96%	99%	99%	100%
Pneumococcal Vaccine	42	74%	62%	69%	94%
Smoking Cessation Advice[1]	8	100%	80%	80%	100%
Surgical Infection Prevention					
Prophylactic Antibiotic Given[1]	13	46%	74%	77%	95%
Prophylactic Antibiotic Selection[1]	5	100%	91%	90%	100%
Prophylactic Antibiotic Stopped[1]	13	62%	67%	72%	95%
Pregnancy Care					
Inpatient Neonatal Mortality	-	-	-	-	-
Third or Fourth Degree Laceration	-	-	3.89%	3.63%	3.27%

Advocate South Suburban Hospital

17800 S Kedzie Avenue
Hazel Crest, IL 60429
E-mail: maureen.daugherty@advocatehealth.com
URL: www.advocatehealth.com
Ownership: Voluntary non-profit - Church
Emergency Services: Yes
Phone: 708-799-8000
Fax: 773-967-4217
Accredited: Yes
Licensed Beds: 291

Key Personnel:
CEO. . . . . Pat Martin
Chief Medical Staff. . . . . Asta Kelly, MD
Emergency Room . . . . Diane Warbuton
OB/GYN Women's Health . . . . Bridget McNitt, RN
Director Respiratory Therapy . . . . Scott Baker

Measure	Cases	This Hospital	State Average	U.S. Average	Top Hospital
Heart Attack Care					
ACE Inhibitor or ARB for LVSD	43	86%	79%	82%	100%
Aspirin at Arrival	188	94%	93%	92%	100%
Aspirin at Discharge	125	98%	90%	90%	100%
Beta Blocker at Arrival	149	93%	87%	87%	100%
Beta Blocker at Discharge	142	95%	88%	90%	100%
Fibrinolytic Medication Timing[1]	1	0%	21%	31%	100%
PCI Within 90 Minutes of Arrival[1]	9	33%	47%	54%	95%
Smoking Cessation Advice	51	100%	84%	88%	100%
Heart Failure Care					
ACE Inhibitor or ARB for LVSD[2]	146	86%	83%	82%	100%
Discharge Instructions[2]	296	75%	67%	61%	93%
Evaluation of LVS Function[2]	366	95%	88%	83%	99%
Smoking Cessation Advice[2]	65	100%	83%	82%	100%
Pneumonia Care					
Appropriate Initial Antibiotic[2]	105	90%	83%	83%	94%
Blood Culture Timing[2]	86	87%	91%	90%	100%
Influenza Vaccine[1]	21	90%	63%	70%	100%
Initial Antibiotic Timing[2]	164	68%	81%	80%	93%
Oxygenation Assessment[2]	187	98%	99%	99%	100%
Pneumococcal Vaccine[2]	118	75%	62%	69%	94%
Smoking Cessation Advice[2]	50	100%	80%	80%	100%
Surgical Infection Prevention					
Prophylactic Antibiotic Given[2]	236	85%	74%	77%	95%
Prophylactic Antibiotic Selection[2]	62	100%	91%	90%	100%
Prophylactic Antibiotic Stopped[2]	225	69%	67%	72%	95%
Pregnancy Care					
Inpatient Neonatal Mortality[2]	255	0.00%	-	-	-
Third or Fourth Degree Laceration[2]	343	1.75%	3.89%	3.63%	3.27%

Herrin Hospital

201 S 14th Street
Herrin, IL 62948
URL: www.sih.net
Ownership: Voluntary non-profit - Other
Emergency Services: Yes
Phone: 618-942-2171
Fax: 618-351-4929
Accredited: Yes
Licensed Beds: 92

Key Personnel:
CEO. . . . . Jack Buckley
Chief Medical Staff. . . . . Pramote Anantachai, MD
Emergency Room . . . . Daniel Bercu, MD
Director Infection/Disease Control . . . . Dottie Throgmorton, RN
CCU Spvg. Nurse . . . . Dottie Throgmorton
Medical Surgical Nursing Manager. . . . . Ann Coon, RN
Cardio-Pulmonary Services Manager. . . . . Joe Hutchcraft

Measure	Cases	This Hospital	State Average	U.S. Average	Top Hospital
Heart Attack Care					
ACE Inhibitor or ARB for LVSD[1]	7	86%	79%	82%	100%
Aspirin at Arrival[1]	16	100%	93%	92%	100%
Aspirin at Discharge[1]	11	91%	90%	90%	100%
Beta Blocker at Arrival[1]	18	100%	87%	87%	100%
Beta Blocker at Discharge[1]	15	93%	88%	90%	100%
Fibrinolytic Medication Timing	0	-	21%	31%	100%
PCI Within 90 Minutes of Arrival	0	-	47%	54%	95%
Smoking Cessation Advice[1]	2	50%	84%	88%	100%
Heart Failure Care					
ACE Inhibitor or ARB for LVSD	28	100%	83%	82%	100%
Discharge Instructions	141	79%	67%	61%	93%
Evaluation of LVS Function	173	89%	88%	83%	99%
Smoking Cessation Advice[1]	23	96%	83%	82%	100%
Pneumonia Care					
Appropriate Initial Antibiotic	116	76%	83%	83%	94%
Blood Culture Timing	107	93%	91%	90%	100%
Influenza Vaccine	29	86%	63%	70%	100%
Initial Antibiotic Timing	168	80%	81%	80%	93%
Oxygenation Assessment	210	100%	99%	99%	100%
Pneumococcal Vaccine	134	73%	62%	69%	94%
Smoking Cessation Advice	50	90%	80%	80%	100%
Surgical Infection Prevention					
Prophylactic Antibiotic Given	170	87%	74%	77%	95%
Prophylactic Antibiotic Selection	41	100%	91%	90%	100%
Prophylactic Antibiotic Stopped	151	79%	67%	72%	95%
Pregnancy Care					
Inpatient Neonatal Mortality	-	-	-	-	-
Third or Fourth Degree Laceration	-	-	3.89%	3.63%	3.27%

NOTE: Hospital profiles are in alphabetical order by state, then city, then hospital within the city; Rankings are sorted by rate in descending order and exclude hospitals with less than 25 cases; (1) The number of cases is too small (n<25) for purposes of reliably predicting hospital performance; (2) Measure reflects the hospital's indication that its submission was based upon a sample of its relevant discharges; (3) Rate reflects fewer than the maximum possible quarters of data for the measure; (4) Inaccurate information submitted and suppressed for one or more quarters; (5) No data is available from the hospital for this measure; Please refer to the User's Guide for a full explanation of data

Saint Joseph's Hospital

1515 Main Street
Highland, IL 62249
Ownership: Voluntary non-profit - Church
Emergency Services: Yes
Phone: 618-654-7421
Fax: 618-654-2012
Accredited: No
Licensed Beds: 106

Key Personnel:

CEO. . . . . Claudao Fort
Chief of Medical Staff. . . . . Greg Mirianda
Emergency Room . . . . Greg Mirianda, MD

Measure	Cases	This Hospital	State Average	U.S. Average	Top Hospital
Heart Attack Care					
ACE Inhibitor or ARB for LVSD[1]	1	100%	79%	82%	100%
Aspirin at Arrival[1]	8	62%	93%	92%	100%
Aspirin at Discharge[1]	6	67%	90%	90%	100%
Beta Blocker at Arrival[1]	6	67%	87%	87%	100%
Beta Blocker at Discharge[1]	5	80%	88%	90%	100%
Fibrinolytic Medication Timing	0	-	21%	31%	100%
PCI Within 90 Minutes of Arrival	0	-	47%	54%	95%
Smoking Cessation Advice	0	-	84%	88%	100%
Heart Failure Care					
ACE Inhibitor or ARB for LVSD[1]	8	88%	83%	82%	100%
Discharge Instructions	31	74%	67%	61%	93%
Evaluation of LVS Function	50	64%	88%	83%	99%
Smoking Cessation Advice[1]	4	100%	83%	82%	100%
Pneumonia Care					
Appropriate Initial Antibiotic	41	73%	83%	83%	94%
Blood Culture Timing	38	97%	91%	90%	100%
Influenza Vaccine[1]	13	69%	63%	70%	100%
Initial Antibiotic Timing	71	83%	81%	80%	93%
Oxygenation Assessment	81	100%	99%	99%	100%
Pneumococcal Vaccine	57	79%	62%	69%	94%
Smoking Cessation Advice[1]	13	100%	80%	80%	100%
Surgical Infection Prevention					
Prophylactic Antibiotic Given[5]	-	-	74%	77%	95%
Prophylactic Antibiotic Selection[5]	-	-	91%	90%	100%
Prophylactic Antibiotic Stopped[5]	-	-	67%	72%	95%
Pregnancy Care					
Inpatient Neonatal Mortality	-	-	-	-	-
Third or Fourth Degree Laceration	-	-	3.89%	3.63%	3.27%

Hinsdale Hospital

120 N Oak Street
Hinsdale, IL 60521
URL: www.keepingyouwell.com
Ownership: Voluntary non-profit - Church
Emergency Services: Yes
Phone: 630-856-9000
Fax: 630-856-7560
Accredited: Yes
Licensed Beds: 426

Key Personnel:

President . . . . Ernie Sadau
Chief Medical Officer . . . . Robert Zeck, MD
Director Emergency Services. . . . . Sue Smith
OB/GYN Womens Health. . . . . Betty Sue Netzel

Measure	Cases	This Hospital	State Average	U.S. Average	Top Hospital
Heart Attack Care					
ACE Inhibitor or ARB for LVSD	26	100%	79%	82%	100%
Aspirin at Arrival	132	98%	93%	92%	100%
Aspirin at Discharge	148	100%	90%	90%	100%
Beta Blocker at Arrival	120	97%	87%	87%	100%
Beta Blocker at Discharge	141	98%	88%	90%	100%
Fibrinolytic Medication Timing[1]	1	0%	21%	31%	100%
PCI Within 90 Minutes of Arrival[1]	4	75%	47%	54%	95%
Smoking Cessation Advice	37	100%	84%	88%	100%
Heart Failure Care					
ACE Inhibitor or ARB for LVSD	93	74%	83%	82%	100%
Discharge Instructions	200	80%	67%	61%	93%
Evaluation of LVS Function	273	96%	88%	83%	99%
Smoking Cessation Advice[1]	16	100%	83%	82%	100%
Pneumonia Care					
Appropriate Initial Antibiotic	156	87%	83%	83%	94%
Blood Culture Timing	252	96%	91%	90%	100%
Influenza Vaccine	62	90%	63%	70%	100%
Initial Antibiotic Timing	278	81%	81%	80%	93%
Oxygenation Assessment	375	100%	99%	99%	100%
Pneumococcal Vaccine	266	83%	62%	69%	94%
Smoking Cessation Advice	60	95%	80%	80%	100%
Surgical Infection Prevention					
Prophylactic Antibiotic Given[2,3]	175	79%	74%	77%	95%
Prophylactic Antibiotic Selection[2]	59	92%	91%	90%	100%
Prophylactic Antibiotic Stopped[2,3]	162	48%	67%	72%	95%
Pregnancy Care					
Inpatient Neonatal Mortality	-	-	-	-	-
Third or Fourth Degree Laceration	-	-	3.89%	3.63%	3.27%

Saint Alexius Medical Center

Alternate Name: Suburban Medical Center
1555 North Barrington Road
Hoffman Estates, IL 60194
E-mail: linda.baker@stalexius.net
Ownership: Voluntary non-profit - Church
Emergency Services: Yes
Phone: 847-843-2000
Fax: 847-755-7612
Accredited: Yes
Licensed Beds: 324

Key Personnel:

President/CEO. . . . . Edward M Goldberg
Cardiac Lab Supervisor . . . . Jeff Cook
Catheterization Lab . . . . Michelle Gallagher
Emergency Room . . . . Sue Emond, RN
Director Infection/Disease Control . . . . Darlene Gallagher, RN
ICU . . . . Cindy Carter, RN
Director Medical Surgical Nursing . . . . Robert Brown, RN
OB/GYN/Women's Health . . . . Jo Boros, RN
Director Respiratory Therapy . . . . Tonya Fuller

Measure	Cases	This Hospital	State Average	U.S. Average	Top Hospital
Heart Attack Care					
ACE Inhibitor or ARB for LVSD	44	84%	79%	82%	100%
Aspirin at Arrival	152	97%	93%	92%	100%
Aspirin at Discharge	123	93%	90%	90%	100%
Beta Blocker at Arrival	106	92%	87%	87%	100%
Beta Blocker at Discharge	129	100%	88%	90%	100%
Fibrinolytic Medication Timing	0	-	21%	31%	100%
PCI Within 90 Minutes of Arrival[1]	11	73%	47%	54%	95%
Smoking Cessation Advice	48	100%	84%	88%	100%
Heart Failure Care					
ACE Inhibitor or ARB for LVSD[2]	120	92%	83%	82%	100%
Discharge Instructions[2]	238	82%	67%	61%	93%
Evaluation of LVS Function[2]	315	97%	88%	83%	99%
Smoking Cessation Advice[2]	51	98%	83%	82%	100%
Pneumonia Care					
Appropriate Initial Antibiotic[2]	156	85%	83%	83%	94%
Blood Culture Timing[2]	205	99%	91%	90%	100%
Influenza Vaccine	47	64%	63%	70%	100%
Initial Antibiotic Timing[2]	274	89%	81%	80%	93%
Oxygenation Assessment[2]	315	100%	99%	99%	100%
Pneumococcal Vaccine[2]	193	75%	62%	69%	94%
Smoking Cessation Advice[2]	62	100%	80%	80%	100%
Surgical Infection Prevention					
Prophylactic Antibiotic Given[2]	287	92%	74%	77%	95%
Prophylactic Antibiotic Selection[2]	61	87%	91%	90%	100%
Prophylactic Antibiotic Stopped[2]	277	77%	67%	72%	95%
Pregnancy Care					
Inpatient Neonatal Mortality	-	-	-	-	-
Third or Fourth Degree Laceration	-	-	3.89%	3.63%	3.27%

Hoopeston Community Memorial Hospital

701 E Orange Street
Hoopeston, IL 60942
Ownership: Voluntary non-profit - Private
Emergency Services: Yes
Phone: 217-283-5531
Fax: 217-283-7991
Accredited: Yes
Licensed Beds: 25

Key Personnel:

President/CEO. . . . . Frank T Caruso
Chief Medical Staff. . . . . Daesun Oh, MD
Director Infection/Disease Control . . . . Carole Bond
Director Respiratory Therapy . . . . Jennifer Tweedy

Measure	Cases	This Hospital	State Average	U.S. Average	Top Hospital

NOTE: Hospital profiles are in alphabetical order by state, then city, then hospital within the city; Rankings are sorted by rate in descending order and exclude hospitals with less than 25 cases; (1) The number of cases is too small (n<25) for purposes of reliably predicting hospital performance; (2) Measure reflects the hospital's indication that its submission was based upon a sample of its relevant discharges; (3) Rate reflects fewer than the maximum possible quarters of data for the measure; (4) Inaccurate information submitted and suppressed for one or more quarters; (5) No data is available from the hospital for this measure; Please refer to the User's Guide for a full explanation of data

Measure	Cases	This Hospital	State Average	U.S. Average	Top Hospital
Heart Attack Care					
ACE Inhibitor or ARB for LVSD[3]	0	-	79%	82%	100%
Aspirin at Arrival[1,3]	4	100%	93%	92%	100%
Aspirin at Discharge[1,3]	2	50%	90%	90%	100%
Beta Blocker at Arrival[1,3]	2	100%	87%	87%	100%
Beta Blocker at Discharge[3]	0	-	88%	90%	100%
Fibrinolytic Medication Timing[3]	0	-	21%	31%	100%
PCI Within 90 Minutes of Arrival	0	-	47%	54%	95%
Smoking Cessation Advice[3]	0	-	84%	88%	100%
Heart Failure Care					
ACE Inhibitor or ARB for LVSD	0	-	83%	82%	100%
Discharge Instructions	28	4%	67%	61%	93%
Evaluation of LVS Function	27	4%	88%	83%	99%
Smoking Cessation Advice	0	-	83%	82%	100%
Pneumonia Care					
Appropriate Initial Antibiotic	52	85%	83%	83%	94%
Blood Culture Timing[1]	11	73%	91%	90%	100%
Influenza Vaccine[1]	10	30%	63%	70%	100%
Initial Antibiotic Timing	51	98%	81%	80%	93%
Oxygenation Assessment	60	100%	99%	99%	100%
Pneumococcal Vaccine	50	14%	62%	69%	94%
Smoking Cessation Advice[1]	13	23%	80%	80%	100%
Surgical Infection Prevention					
Prophylactic Antibiotic Given[5]	-	-	74%	77%	95%
Prophylactic Antibiotic Selection[5]	-	-	91%	90%	100%
Prophylactic Antibiotic Stopped[5]	-	-	67%	72%	95%
Pregnancy Care					
Inpatient Neonatal Mortality	-	-	-	-	-
Third or Fourth Degree Laceration	-	-	3.89%	3.63%	3.27%

Hopedale Medical Complex

107 Tremont Street
Hopedale, IL 61747
Phone: 309-449-3321
Ownership: Voluntary non-profit - Other
Accredited: No
Emergency Services: Yes

Measure	Cases	This Hospital	State Average	U.S. Average	Top Hospital
Heart Attack Care					
ACE Inhibitor or ARB for LVSD[5]	-	-	79%	82%	100%
Aspirin at Arrival[5]	-	-	93%	92%	100%
Aspirin at Discharge[5]	-	-	90%	90%	100%
Beta Blocker at Arrival[5]	-	-	87%	87%	100%
Beta Blocker at Discharge[5]	-	-	88%	90%	100%
Fibrinolytic Medication Timing[5]	-	-	21%	31%	100%
PCI Within 90 Minutes of Arrival[5]	-	-	47%	54%	95%
Smoking Cessation Advice[5]	-	-	84%	88%	100%
Heart Failure Care					
ACE Inhibitor or ARB for LVSD[5]	-	-	83%	82%	100%
Discharge Instructions[5]	-	-	67%	61%	93%
Evaluation of LVS Function[5]	-	-	88%	83%	99%
Smoking Cessation Advice[5]	-	-	83%	82%	100%
Pneumonia Care					
Appropriate Initial Antibiotic[5]	-	-	83%	83%	94%
Blood Culture Timing[5]	-	-	91%	90%	100%
Influenza Vaccine[5]	-	-	63%	70%	100%
Initial Antibiotic Timing[5]	-	-	81%	80%	93%
Oxygenation Assessment[5]	-	-	99%	99%	100%
Pneumococcal Vaccine[5]	-	-	62%	69%	94%
Smoking Cessation Advice[5]	-	-	80%	80%	100%
Surgical Infection Prevention					
Prophylactic Antibiotic Given[5]	-	-	74%	77%	95%
Prophylactic Antibiotic Selection[5]	-	-	91%	90%	100%
Prophylactic Antibiotic Stopped[5]	-	-	67%	72%	95%
Pregnancy Care					
Inpatient Neonatal Mortality	-	-	-	-	-
Third or Fourth Degree Laceration	-	-	3.89%	3.63%	3.27%

Passavant Memorial Area Hospital

Alternate Name: Passavant Area Hospital
1600 W Walnut Street
Jacksonville, IL 62650
Phone: 217-245-9541
Fax: 217-479-5637
E-mail: info@passavanthospital.com
URL: www.passavanthospital.com
Ownership: Voluntary non-profit - Other
Accredited: Yes
Emergency Services: Yes
Licensed Beds: 99

Key Personnel:

CEO. . . . . Chester A Wynn, CPA
Chief Medical Staff. . . . . Darr Leutz, MD
Emergency Room . . . . Phillip Malinosky, MD
Infection Control. . . . . Anne Beck
ICU . . . . Stephanie Meyer
Director Medical Surgical Nursing . . . . Karen Daum
Surgical Services . . . . Karen Daum
Respiratory/Cardiopulmonary. . . . . Janet Littig

Measure	Cases	This Hospital	State Average	U.S. Average	Top Hospital
Heart Attack Care					
ACE Inhibitor or ARB for LVSD[1]	3	100%	79%	82%	100%
Aspirin at Arrival[1]	19	63%	93%	92%	100%
Aspirin at Discharge[1]	11	82%	90%	90%	100%
Beta Blocker at Arrival[1]	18	72%	87%	87%	100%
Beta Blocker at Discharge[1]	12	83%	88%	90%	100%
Fibrinolytic Medication Timing	0	-	21%	31%	100%
PCI Within 90 Minutes of Arrival	0	-	47%	54%	95%
Smoking Cessation Advice[1]	3	100%	84%	88%	100%
Heart Failure Care					
ACE Inhibitor or ARB for LVSD	34	82%	83%	82%	100%
Discharge Instructions	96	76%	67%	61%	93%
Evaluation of LVS Function	153	95%	88%	83%	99%
Smoking Cessation Advice[1]	15	73%	83%	82%	100%
Pneumonia Care					
Appropriate Initial Antibiotic	117	91%	83%	83%	94%
Blood Culture Timing	134	80%	91%	90%	100%
Influenza Vaccine	41	90%	63%	70%	100%
Initial Antibiotic Timing	205	95%	81%	80%	93%
Oxygenation Assessment	252	100%	99%	99%	100%
Pneumococcal Vaccine	176	87%	62%	69%	94%
Smoking Cessation Advice	54	83%	80%	80%	100%
Surgical Infection Prevention					
Prophylactic Antibiotic Given	170	95%	74%	77%	95%
Prophylactic Antibiotic Selection	62	95%	91%	90%	100%
Prophylactic Antibiotic Stopped	161	93%	67%	72%	95%
Pregnancy Care					
Inpatient Neonatal Mortality	-	-	-	-	-
Third or Fourth Degree Laceration	-	-	3.89%	3.63%	3.27%

Jersey Community Hospital

400 Maple Summit Road
Jerseyville, IL 62052
Phone: 618-498-6402
Fax: 618-498-8492
Ownership: Govt - Hospital District or Authority
Accredited: Yes
Emergency Services: Yes
Licensed Beds: 67

Key Personnel:

CEO. . . . . Larry Bear
Chief of Medical Staff. Susan Vritweiser
Emergency Room . . . . Alvina Isringhausen
Director of Pulmonary/Respiratory Care. . . . . . . Beth Crane

Measure	Cases	This Hospital	State Average	U.S. Average	Top Hospital
Heart Attack Care					
ACE Inhibitor or ARB for LVSD[1]	8	62%	79%	82%	100%
Aspirin at Arrival	68	74%	93%	92%	100%
Aspirin at Discharge	51	84%	90%	90%	100%
Beta Blocker at Arrival	57	74%	87%	87%	100%
Beta Blocker at Discharge	52	73%	88%	90%	100%
Fibrinolytic Medication Timing	0	-	21%	31%	100%
PCI Within 90 Minutes of Arrival	0	-	47%	54%	95%
Smoking Cessation Advice[1]	7	86%	84%	88%	100%
Heart Failure Care					
ACE Inhibitor or ARB for LVSD	34	56%	83%	82%	100%
Discharge Instructions	76	42%	67%	61%	93%
Evaluation of LVS Function	114	69%	88%	83%	99%
Smoking Cessation Advice[1]	12	50%	83%	82%	100%

NOTE: Hospital profiles are in alphabetical order by state, then city, then hospital within the city; Rankings are sorted by rate in descending order and exclude hospitals with less than 25 cases; (1) The number of cases is too small (n<25) for purposes of reliably predicting hospital performance; (2) Measure reflects the hospital's indication that its submission was based upon a sample of its relevant discharges; (3) Rate reflects fewer than the maximum possible quarters of data for the measure; (4) Inaccurate information submitted and suppressed for one or more quarters; (5) No data is available from the hospital for this measure; Please refer to the User's Guide for a full explanation of data

Pneumonia Care					
Appropriate Initial Antibiotic	96	79%	83%	83%	94%
Blood Culture Timing	78	95%	91%	90%	100%
Influenza Vaccine	28	86%	63%	70%	100%
Initial Antibiotic Timing	113	88%	81%	80%	93%
Oxygenation Assessment	154	99%	99%	99%	100%
Pneumococcal Vaccine	112	62%	62%	69%	94%
Smoking Cessation Advice	25	56%	80%	80%	100%
Surgical Infection Prevention					
Prophylactic Antibiotic Given[1,3]	23	39%	74%	77%	95%
Prophylactic Antibiotic Selection[1]	3	100%	91%	90%	100%
Prophylactic Antibiotic Stopped[1,3]	21	57%	67%	72%	95%
Pregnancy Care					
Inpatient Neonatal Mortality	-	-	-	-	-
Third or Fourth Degree Laceration	-	-	3.89%	3.63%	3.27%

Saint Joseph Medical Center

333 N Madison Street
Joliet, IL 60435
URL: www.provenasaintjoe.org
Ownership: Voluntary non-profit - Church
Emergency Services: Yes

Phone: 815-725-7133
Fax: 815-741-7121
Accredited: Yes
Licensed Beds: 452

Key Personnel:

Emergency Room . . . . Dave Laurich
Emergency Room . . . . Rao Kilaru, MD
Chief Medical Officer . . . . Lon McPherson, MD
Director of Pulmonary/Respiratory Care. . . . . . . P Heidel

Measure	Cases	This Hospital	State Average	U.S. Average	Top Hospital
Heart Attack Care					
ACE Inhibitor or ARB for LVSD	73	77%	79%	82%	100%
Aspirin at Arrival	280	92%	93%	92%	100%
Aspirin at Discharge	290	95%	90%	90%	100%
Beta Blocker at Arrival	255	85%	87%	87%	100%
Beta Blocker at Discharge	292	91%	88%	90%	100%
Fibrinolytic Medication Timing[1]	1	0%	21%	31%	100%
PCI Within 90 Minutes of Arrival[1]	16	31%	47%	54%	95%
Smoking Cessation Advice	101	90%	84%	88%	100%
Heart Failure Care					
ACE Inhibitor or ARB for LVSD	287	78%	83%	82%	100%
Discharge Instructions	663	95%	67%	61%	93%
Evaluation of LVS Function	808	96%	88%	83%	99%
Smoking Cessation Advice	77	99%	83%	82%	100%
Pneumonia Care					
Appropriate Initial Antibiotic	420	79%	83%	83%	94%
Blood Culture Timing	74	95%	91%	90%	100%
Influenza Vaccine	117	41%	63%	70%	100%
Initial Antibiotic Timing	609	65%	81%	80%	93%
Oxygenation Assessment	673	100%	99%	99%	100%
Pneumococcal Vaccine	399	37%	62%	69%	94%
Smoking Cessation Advice	124	80%	80%	80%	100%
Surgical Infection Prevention					
Prophylactic Antibiotic Given[2]	989	75%	74%	77%	95%
Prophylactic Antibiotic Selection[2]	228	90%	91%	90%	100%
Prophylactic Antibiotic Stopped[2]	959	47%	67%	72%	95%
Pregnancy Care					
Inpatient Neonatal Mortality	1,926	0.21%	-	-	-
Third or Fourth Degree Laceration	1,202	4.16%	3.89%	3.63%	3.27%

Silver Cross Hospital

1200 Maple Road
Joliet, IL 60432
E-mail: tsimons@silvercross.org
URL: www.silvercross.org
Ownership: Voluntary non-profit - Private
Emergency Services: Yes

Phone: 815-740-1100
Fax: 815-740-3561
Accredited: Yes
Licensed Beds: 297

Key Personnel:

CEO. . . . . Paul Pawlak
Chief Medical Staff. . . . . Kishor Ajmere, MD
Manager Cardiac Services. . . . . Paula Simpson
Director Infection Control . . . . Margaret Rodegher
Director Maternal/Child Services . . . . Peggy Gricus
Manager Respiratory Therapy . . . . LuAnn Hubert

Measure	Cases	This Hospital	State Average	U.S. Average	Top Hospital
Heart Attack Care					
ACE Inhibitor or ARB for LVSD	41	95%	79%	82%	100%
Aspirin at Arrival	170	94%	93%	92%	100%
Aspirin at Discharge	143	93%	90%	90%	100%
Beta Blocker at Arrival	106	96%	87%	87%	100%
Beta Blocker at Discharge	151	95%	88%	90%	100%
Fibrinolytic Medication Timing	0	-	21%	31%	100%
PCI Within 90 Minutes of Arrival[1]	12	25%	47%	54%	95%
Smoking Cessation Advice	55	98%	84%	88%	100%
Heart Failure Care					
ACE Inhibitor or ARB for LVSD	179	93%	83%	82%	100%
Discharge Instructions	450	100%	67%	61%	93%
Evaluation of LVS Function	549	99%	88%	83%	99%
Smoking Cessation Advice	112	100%	83%	82%	100%
Pneumonia Care					
Appropriate Initial Antibiotic	250	91%	83%	83%	94%
Blood Culture Timing	257	88%	91%	90%	100%
Influenza Vaccine	77	39%	63%	70%	100%
Initial Antibiotic Timing	431	87%	81%	80%	93%
Oxygenation Assessment	468	100%	99%	99%	100%
Pneumococcal Vaccine	256	45%	62%	69%	94%
Smoking Cessation Advice	120	97%	80%	80%	100%
Surgical Infection Prevention					
Prophylactic Antibiotic Given	499	96%	74%	77%	95%
Prophylactic Antibiotic Selection	124	90%	91%	90%	100%
Prophylactic Antibiotic Stopped	463	75%	67%	72%	95%
Pregnancy Care					
Inpatient Neonatal Mortality	2,076	0.39%	-	-	-
Third or Fourth Degree Laceration	1,446	2.28%	3.89%	3.63%	3.27%

Riverside Medical Center

350 N Wall Street
Kankakee, IL 60901
URL: www.riversidehealthcare.org
Ownership: Voluntary non-profit - Other
Emergency Services: Yes

Phone: 815-933-1671
Fax: 815-935-7823
Accredited: Yes
Licensed Beds: 336

Key Personnel:

President/CEO. . . . . Phil Kambic
Emergency Room . . . . Crystal Allen
Director Medical/Surgical Nursing . . . . Jane Tarnow
Director Respiratory Therapy . . . . David Duda

Measure	Cases	This Hospital	State Average	U.S. Average	Top Hospital
Heart Attack Care					
ACE Inhibitor or ARB for LVSD[1]	23	100%	79%	82%	100%
Aspirin at Arrival	93	100%	93%	92%	100%
Aspirin at Discharge	100	100%	90%	90%	100%
Beta Blocker at Arrival	53	98%	87%	87%	100%
Beta Blocker at Discharge	97	98%	88%	90%	100%
Fibrinolytic Medication Timing[1]	2	100%	21%	31%	100%
PCI Within 90 Minutes of Arrival[1]	4	50%	47%	54%	95%
Smoking Cessation Advice	43	100%	84%	88%	100%
Heart Failure Care					
ACE Inhibitor or ARB for LVSD	145	94%	83%	82%	100%
Discharge Instructions	305	99%	67%	61%	93%
Evaluation of LVS Function	365	99%	88%	83%	99%
Smoking Cessation Advice	66	100%	83%	82%	100%
Pneumonia Care					
Appropriate Initial Antibiotic	124	85%	83%	83%	94%
Blood Culture Timing	177	97%	91%	90%	100%
Influenza Vaccine	52	44%	63%	70%	100%
Initial Antibiotic Timing	262	82%	81%	80%	93%
Oxygenation Assessment	304	100%	99%	99%	100%
Pneumococcal Vaccine	202	49%	62%	69%	94%
Smoking Cessation Advice	63	100%	80%	80%	100%
Surgical Infection Prevention					
Prophylactic Antibiotic Given[2,3]	402	79%	74%	77%	95%
Prophylactic Antibiotic Selection[2]	94	94%	91%	90%	100%
Prophylactic Antibiotic Stopped[2,3]	380	68%	67%	72%	95%
Pregnancy Care					

NOTE: Hospital profiles are in alphabetical order by state, then city, then hospital within the city; Rankings are sorted by rate in descending order and exclude hospitals with less than 25 cases; (1) The number of cases is too small (n<25) for purposes of reliably predicting hospital performance; (2) Measure reflects the hospital's indication that its submission was based upon a sample of its relevant discharges; (3) Rate reflects fewer than the maximum possible quarters of data for the measure; (4) Inaccurate information submitted and suppressed for one or more quarters; (5) No data is available from the hospital for this measure; Please refer to the User's Guide for a full explanation of data

Inpatient Neonatal Mortality	1,238	0.40%	-	-	-
Third or Fourth Degree Laceration	852	2.23%	3.89%	3.63%	3.27%

Saint Mary's Hospital of Kankakee

500 W Court Street
Kankakee, IL 60901
Phone: 815-937-2490
Fax: 815-937-8772
URL: www.provenastmarys.com
Ownership: Voluntary non-profit - Other
Accredited: Yes
Emergency Services: Yes
Licensed Beds: 210

Key Personnel:

CEO. . . . . George N Miller Jr
Chief Medical Staff. . . . . Hippen Hammer
Chief of Cardiology/Cardiac Lab. . . . . Michelle Hardesty
Emergency Room . . . . Tony Brunello
Infection Control. . . . . Julie Nehls
OB/GYN Womens Health. . . . . Linda Jones
Director Radiology . . . . Tony Hardesty
Respiratory/Cardiopulmonary. . . . . Linda Patnaude

Measure	Cases	This Hospital	State Average	U.S. Average	Top Hospital
Heart Attack Care					
ACE Inhibitor or ARB for LVSD[1]	16	81%	79%	82%	100%
Aspirin at Arrival	83	90%	93%	92%	100%
Aspirin at Discharge	61	90%	90%	90%	100%
Beta Blocker at Arrival	71	94%	87%	87%	100%
Beta Blocker at Discharge	60	95%	88%	90%	100%
Fibrinolytic Medication Timing	0	-	21%	31%	100%
PCI Within 90 Minutes of Arrival	0	-	47%	54%	95%
Smoking Cessation Advice	25	100%	84%	88%	100%
Heart Failure Care					
ACE Inhibitor or ARB for LVSD	96	85%	83%	82%	100%
Discharge Instructions	187	60%	67%	61%	93%
Evaluation of LVS Function	238	91%	88%	83%	99%
Smoking Cessation Advice	63	100%	83%	82%	100%
Pneumonia Care					
Appropriate Initial Antibiotic	210	76%	83%	83%	94%
Blood Culture Timing	217	86%	91%	90%	100%
Influenza Vaccine	51	71%	63%	70%	100%
Initial Antibiotic Timing	310	79%	81%	80%	93%
Oxygenation Assessment	362	100%	99%	99%	100%
Pneumococcal Vaccine	156	49%	62%	69%	94%
Smoking Cessation Advice	90	100%	80%	80%	100%
Surgical Infection Prevention					
Prophylactic Antibiotic Given[2]	336	86%	74%	77%	95%
Prophylactic Antibiotic Selection[2]	78	96%	91%	90%	100%
Prophylactic Antibiotic Stopped[2]	328	64%	67%	72%	95%
Pregnancy Care					
Inpatient Neonatal Mortality	553	0.00%	-	-	-
Third or Fourth Degree Laceration	387	3.88%	3.89%	3.63%	3.27%

Kewanee Hospital

719 Elliott Street
PO Box 747
Kewanee, IL 61443
Phone: 309-853-3361
Fax: 309-854-5209
E-mail: rlindner@kewaneehospital.com
URL: kewaneehospital.com
Ownership: Voluntary non-profit - Other
Accredited: No
Emergency Services: Yes
Licensed Beds: 82

Key Personnel:

Acting CEO . . . . Margaret Gustafson
Chief Medical Staff. . . . . Rick Cernovich, MD
Emergency Department Director . . . . Dianna Orr
Emergency Medical Services Director . . . . Adam Reading
Infection Control Coordinator . . . . Brenda Wager
Director Medical/Surgical/Pediatrics. . . . . Gayle Padilla
Surgical Services/Central Sterilization . . . . Karen Swan
Director Radiology . . . . Diannaine Orr
Director Respiratory Therapy . . . . Sue Van De Rostyne

Measure	Cases	This Hospital	State Average	U.S. Average	Top Hospital
Heart Attack Care					
ACE Inhibitor or ARB for LVSD[1,3]	2	0%	79%	82%	100%
Aspirin at Arrival[1,3]	6	33%	93%	92%	100%
Aspirin at Discharge[1,3]	4	50%	90%	90%	100%
Beta Blocker at Arrival[1,3]	5	60%	87%	87%	100%
Beta Blocker at Discharge[1,3]	5	80%	88%	90%	100%
Fibrinolytic Medication Timing[3]	0	-	21%	31%	100%
PCI Within 90 Minutes of Arrival	0	-	47%	54%	95%
Smoking Cessation Advice[3]	0	-	84%	88%	100%
Heart Failure Care					
ACE Inhibitor or ARB for LVSD[1]	11	91%	83%	82%	100%
Discharge Instructions	58	81%	67%	61%	93%
Evaluation of LVS Function	96	80%	88%	83%	99%
Smoking Cessation Advice[1]	9	78%	83%	82%	100%
Pneumonia Care					
Appropriate Initial Antibiotic	66	95%	83%	83%	94%
Blood Culture Timing	58	97%	91%	90%	100%
Influenza Vaccine[1]	15	60%	63%	70%	100%
Initial Antibiotic Timing	108	84%	81%	80%	93%
Oxygenation Assessment	123	100%	99%	99%	100%
Pneumococcal Vaccine	82	67%	62%	69%	94%
Smoking Cessation Advice[1]	23	74%	80%	80%	100%
Surgical Infection Prevention					
Prophylactic Antibiotic Given	34	74%	74%	77%	95%
Prophylactic Antibiotic Selection[1]	5	80%	91%	90%	100%
Prophylactic Antibiotic Stopped	33	70%	67%	72%	95%
Pregnancy Care					
Inpatient Neonatal Mortality	-	-	-	-	-
Third or Fourth Degree Laceration	-	-	3.89%	3.63%	3.27%

Adventist LaGrange Memorial Hospital

Alternate Name: LaGrange Memorial Hospital
5101 S Willow Springs Road
La Grange, IL 60525
Phone: 708-245-9000
Fax: 708-245-5627
E-mail: egervain@ahss.org
URL: www.keepingyouwell.com
Ownership: Voluntary non-profit - Other
Accredited: Yes
Emergency Services: Yes
Licensed Beds: 274

Key Personnel:

CEO. . . . . Tim Cook
Chief Medical Staff. . . . . Patrick Quirke, MD
Emergency Room . . . . Gail Weimer, RN
Director Medical/Surgical Nursing . . . . Karen Gonzalez
OB/GYN Womens Health. . . . . Michael Schied, MD
Chief Radiology . . . . Timothy N Merrill, MD
Manager Pulmonary Services . . . . Mary Ann Johnson, RN

Measure	Cases	This Hospital	State Average	U.S. Average	Top Hospital
Heart Attack Care					
ACE Inhibitor or ARB for LVSD	41	76%	79%	82%	100%
Aspirin at Arrival	134	94%	93%	92%	100%
Aspirin at Discharge	112	91%	90%	90%	100%
Beta Blocker at Arrival	104	90%	87%	87%	100%
Beta Blocker at Discharge	133	94%	88%	90%	100%
Fibrinolytic Medication Timing	0	-	21%	31%	100%
PCI Within 90 Minutes of Arrival[1]	4	75%	47%	54%	95%
Smoking Cessation Advice	39	90%	84%	88%	100%
Heart Failure Care					
ACE Inhibitor or ARB for LVSD	85	76%	83%	82%	100%
Discharge Instructions	293	61%	67%	61%	93%
Evaluation of LVS Function	385	85%	88%	83%	99%
Smoking Cessation Advice	33	91%	83%	82%	100%
Pneumonia Care					
Appropriate Initial Antibiotic	214	82%	83%	83%	94%
Blood Culture Timing	231	93%	91%	90%	100%
Influenza Vaccine	53	57%	63%	70%	100%
Initial Antibiotic Timing	307	78%	81%	80%	93%
Oxygenation Assessment	358	99%	99%	99%	100%
Pneumococcal Vaccine	228	52%	62%	69%	94%
Smoking Cessation Advice	55	89%	80%	80%	100%
Surgical Infection Prevention					
Prophylactic Antibiotic Given[2,3]	151	92%	74%	77%	95%
Prophylactic Antibiotic Selection[2]	56	98%	91%	90%	100%
Prophylactic Antibiotic Stopped[2,3]	146	81%	67%	72%	95%
Pregnancy Care					
Inpatient Neonatal Mortality	-	-	-	-	-

NOTE: Hospital profiles are in alphabetical order by state, then city, then hospital within the city; Rankings are sorted by rate in descending order and exclude hospitals with less than 25 cases; (1) The number of cases is too small (n<25) for purposes of reliably predicting hospital performance; (2) Measure reflects the hospital's indication that its submission was based upon a sample of its relevant discharges; (3) Rate reflects fewer than the maximum possible quarters of data for the measure; (4) Inaccurate information submitted and suppressed for one or more quarters; (5) No data is available from the hospital for this measure; Please refer to the User's Guide for a full explanation of data

Third or Fourth Degree Laceration	-	-	3.89%	3.63%	3.27%

Lake Forest Hospital

660 N Westmoreland Road
Lake Forest, IL 60045
URL: www.lakeforesthospital.com
Ownership: Voluntary non-profit - Other
Emergency Services: Yes
Phone: 847-234-5600
Fax: 847-535-7846
Accredited: Yes
Licensed Beds: 261

Key Personnel:
CEO. . . . . William Ries

Measure	Cases	This Hospital	State Average	U.S. Average	Top Hospital
Heart Attack Care					
ACE Inhibitor or ARB for LVSD[1]	3	67%	79%	82%	100%
Aspirin at Arrival	26	96%	93%	92%	100%
Aspirin at Discharge[1]	6	67%	90%	90%	100%
Beta Blocker at Arrival[1]	24	100%	87%	87%	100%
Beta Blocker at Discharge[1]	10	100%	88%	90%	100%
Fibrinolytic Medication Timing	0	-	21%	31%	100%
PCI Within 90 Minutes of Arrival	0	-	47%	54%	95%
Smoking Cessation Advice[1]	2	50%	84%	88%	100%
Heart Failure Care					
ACE Inhibitor or ARB for LVSD	45	87%	83%	82%	100%
Discharge Instructions	107	90%	67%	61%	93%
Evaluation of LVS Function	128	95%	88%	83%	99%
Smoking Cessation Advice[1]	13	100%	83%	82%	100%
Pneumonia Care					
Appropriate Initial Antibiotic	150	89%	83%	83%	94%
Blood Culture Timing	120	87%	91%	90%	100%
Influenza Vaccine	35	83%	63%	70%	100%
Initial Antibiotic Timing	159	85%	81%	80%	93%
Oxygenation Assessment	193	100%	99%	99%	100%
Pneumococcal Vaccine	135	78%	62%	69%	94%
Smoking Cessation Advice	26	88%	80%	80%	100%
Surgical Infection Prevention					
Prophylactic Antibiotic Given[3]	511	83%	74%	77%	95%
Prophylactic Antibiotic Selection	169	96%	91%	90%	100%
Prophylactic Antibiotic Stopped[3]	498	62%	67%	72%	95%
Pregnancy Care					
Inpatient Neonatal Mortality	-	-	-	-	-
Third or Fourth Degree Laceration	-	-	3.89%	3.63%	3.27%

Lawrence County Memorial Hospital

2200 W State Street
Lawrenceville, IL 62439
Ownership: Government - Local
Emergency Services: Yes
Phone: 618-943-1000
Fax: 618-943-7230
Accredited: No
Licensed Beds: 58

Key Personnel:
CEO. . . . . Silvia Pulleyblank
Chief Medical Staff. . . . . A Adekunle, MD
Emergency Room . . . . Rita Garvey
Respiratory Therapy. . . . . Maggie O'Haver

Measure	Cases	This Hospital	State Average	U.S. Average	Top Hospital
Heart Attack Care					
ACE Inhibitor or ARB for LVSD[1,3]	2	0%	79%	82%	100%
Aspirin at Arrival[1,3]	10	80%	93%	92%	100%
Aspirin at Discharge[1,3]	5	100%	90%	90%	100%
Beta Blocker at Arrival[1,3]	10	80%	87%	87%	100%
Beta Blocker at Discharge[1,3]	7	57%	88%	90%	100%
Fibrinolytic Medication Timing[3]	0	-	21%	31%	100%
PCI Within 90 Minutes of Arrival[5]	-	-	47%	54%	95%
Smoking Cessation Advice[1,3]	1	100%	84%	88%	100%
Heart Failure Care					
ACE Inhibitor or ARB for LVSD[1]	8	100%	83%	82%	100%
Discharge Instructions	34	97%	67%	61%	93%
Evaluation of LVS Function	53	94%	88%	83%	99%
Smoking Cessation Advice[1]	7	86%	83%	82%	100%
Pneumonia Care					
Appropriate Initial Antibiotic[1,3]	9	89%	83%	83%	94%
Blood Culture Timing[1]	23	83%	91%	90%	100%
Influenza Vaccine[1]	13	92%	63%	70%	100%
Initial Antibiotic Timing	42	90%	81%	80%	93%
Oxygenation Assessment	48	100%	99%	99%	100%
Pneumococcal Vaccine	39	64%	62%	69%	94%
Smoking Cessation Advice[1]	8	75%	80%	80%	100%
Surgical Infection Prevention					
Prophylactic Antibiotic Given[5]	-	-	74%	77%	95%
Prophylactic Antibiotic Selection[5]	-	-	91%	90%	100%
Prophylactic Antibiotic Stopped[5]	-	-	67%	72%	95%
Pregnancy Care					
Inpatient Neonatal Mortality	-	-	-	-	-
Third or Fourth Degree Laceration	-	-	3.89%	3.63%	3.27%

Condell Medical Center

801 S Milwaukee Avenue
Libertyville, IL 60048
URL: www.condell.org
Ownership: Voluntary non-profit - Other
Emergency Services: Yes
Phone: 847-362-2900
Fax: 847-362-1721
Accredited: Yes
Licensed Beds: 305

Key Personnel:
President/CEO. . . . . Eugene Pritchard
Emergency Room . . . . Tammy Koslenko
ICU Supervising Nurse. Sharon Reich
Director Radiology . . . . Ray Eiterman
Director Respiratory Therapy . . . . Robert Amodeo

Measure	Cases	This Hospital	State Average	U.S. Average	Top Hospital
Heart Attack Care					
ACE Inhibitor or ARB for LVSD	63	75%	79%	82%	100%
Aspirin at Arrival	216	93%	93%	92%	100%
Aspirin at Discharge	191	93%	90%	90%	100%
Beta Blocker at Arrival	182	82%	87%	87%	100%
Beta Blocker at Discharge	217	91%	88%	90%	100%
Fibrinolytic Medication Timing[1]	1	0%	21%	31%	100%
PCI Within 90 Minutes of Arrival[1]	15	27%	47%	54%	95%
Smoking Cessation Advice	70	96%	84%	88%	100%
Heart Failure Care					
ACE Inhibitor or ARB for LVSD[2]	129	70%	83%	82%	100%
Discharge Instructions[2]	314	37%	67%	61%	93%
Evaluation of LVS Function[2]	406	88%	88%	83%	99%
Smoking Cessation Advice[2]	60	80%	83%	82%	100%
Pneumonia Care					
Appropriate Initial Antibiotic[2]	161	72%	83%	83%	94%
Blood Culture Timing[2]	140	95%	91%	90%	100%
Influenza Vaccine[2]	34	74%	63%	70%	100%
Initial Antibiotic Timing[2]	200	73%	81%	80%	93%
Oxygenation Assessment[2]	264	100%	99%	99%	100%
Pneumococcal Vaccine[2]	151	67%	62%	69%	94%
Smoking Cessation Advice[2]	58	90%	80%	80%	100%
Surgical Infection Prevention					
Prophylactic Antibiotic Given[2,3]	503	78%	74%	77%	95%
Prophylactic Antibiotic Selection[2]	82	93%	91%	90%	100%
Prophylactic Antibiotic Stopped[2,3]	494	59%	67%	72%	95%
Pregnancy Care					
Inpatient Neonatal Mortality	-	-	-	-	-
Third or Fourth Degree Laceration	-	-	3.89%	3.63%	3.27%

Abraham Lincoln Memorial Hospital

315 8th Street
Lincoln, IL 62656
URL: www.almh.org
Ownership: Voluntary non-profit - Private
Emergency Services: Yes
Phone: 217-732-2161
Fax: 217-732-7481
Accredited: Yes
Licensed Beds: 66

Key Personnel:
Emergency Room . . . . Larry Pinter, MD
Director Infection/Disease Control . . . . Margaret Evers, RN
CCU Spvg. Nurse . . . . Judy Evans
Director Medical/Surgical Nursing . . . . Judy Evans
Director Respiratory Therapy . . . . Sharon Koester

Measure	Cases	This Hospital	State Average	U.S. Average	Top Hospital
Heart Attack Care					
ACE Inhibitor or ARB for LVSD	0	-	79%	82%	100%

NOTE: Hospital profiles are in alphabetical order by state, then city, then hospital within the city; Rankings are sorted by rate in descending order and exclude hospitals with less than 25 cases; (1) The number of cases is too small (n<25) for purposes of reliably predicting hospital performance; (2) Measure reflects the hospital's indication that its submission was based upon a sample of its relevant discharges; (3) Rate reflects fewer than the maximum possible quarters of data for the measure; (4) Inaccurate information submitted and suppressed for one or more quarters; (5) No data is available from the hospital for this measure; Please refer to the User's Guide for a full explanation of data

Aspirin at Arrival[1]	4	100%	93%	92%	100%
Aspirin at Discharge[1]	4	100%	90%	90%	100%
Beta Blocker at Arrival[1]	5	80%	87%	87%	100%
Beta Blocker at Discharge[1]	4	100%	88%	90%	100%
Fibrinolytic Medication Timing	0	-	21%	31%	100%
PCI Within 90 Minutes of Arrival	0	-	47%	54%	95%
Smoking Cessation Advice[1]	1	100%	84%	88%	100%
Heart Failure Care					
ACE Inhibitor or ARB for LVSD[1]	14	86%	83%	82%	100%
Discharge Instructions	26	88%	67%	61%	93%
Evaluation of LVS Function	54	96%	88%	83%	99%
Smoking Cessation Advice[1]	7	100%	83%	82%	100%
Pneumonia Care					
Appropriate Initial Antibiotic	67	87%	83%	83%	94%
Blood Culture Timing	55	93%	91%	90%	100%
Influenza Vaccine[1]	19	95%	63%	70%	100%
Initial Antibiotic Timing	77	94%	81%	80%	93%
Oxygenation Assessment	100	100%	99%	99%	100%
Pneumococcal Vaccine	69	87%	62%	69%	94%
Smoking Cessation Advice[1]	18	94%	80%	80%	100%
Surgical Infection Prevention					
Prophylactic Antibiotic Given	52	98%	74%	77%	95%
Prophylactic Antibiotic Selection[1]	12	100%	91%	90%	100%
Prophylactic Antibiotic Stopped	47	96%	67%	72%	95%
Pregnancy Care					
Inpatient Neonatal Mortality	-	-	-	-	-
Third or Fourth Degree Laceration	-	-	3.89%	3.63%	3.27%

Saint Francis Hospital

1215 Franciscan Drive
Litchfield, IL 62056
URL: www.stfrancis-litchfield.org
Ownership: Voluntary non-profit - Church
Emergency Services: Yes
Phone: 217-324-2191
Fax: 217-324-3081
Accredited: No
Licensed Beds: 138

Key Personnel:
Administrator . . . . Daniel Perryman
Chief Medical Staff . . . . Timothy Ishmael, MD
Emergency Room . . . . Vicky Fuller, RN
Infection Control . . . . Angie Tefteller, RN
ICU . . . . Pat Wernsing, RN
Director Medical Surgical Nursing . . . . Pat Wernsing, RN
OB/GYN Women's Health . . . . Elisa Feldmann, MD
Director Radiology . . . . Steve Sabo
Respiratory Therapy . . . . Karen Scheller

Measure	Cases	This Hospital	State Average	U.S. Average	Top Hospital
Heart Attack Care					
ACE Inhibitor or ARB for LVSD	0	-	79%	82%	100%
Aspirin at Arrival[1]	5	80%	93%	92%	100%
Aspirin at Discharge[1]	4	50%	90%	90%	100%
Beta Blocker at Arrival[1]	5	40%	87%	87%	100%
Beta Blocker at Discharge[1]	4	25%	88%	90%	100%
Fibrinolytic Medication Timing[1]	1	0%	21%	31%	100%
PCI Within 90 Minutes of Arrival	0	-	47%	54%	95%
Smoking Cessation Advice	0	-	84%	88%	100%
Heart Failure Care					
ACE Inhibitor or ARB for LVSD[1]	20	25%	83%	82%	100%
Discharge Instructions	61	54%	67%	61%	93%
Evaluation of LVS Function	91	64%	88%	83%	99%
Smoking Cessation Advice[1]	3	67%	83%	82%	100%
Pneumonia Care					
Appropriate Initial Antibiotic	98	53%	83%	83%	94%
Blood Culture Timing	48	92%	91%	90%	100%
Influenza Vaccine[1]	24	50%	63%	70%	100%
Initial Antibiotic Timing	159	82%	81%	80%	93%
Oxygenation Assessment	176	100%	99%	99%	100%
Pneumococcal Vaccine	121	45%	62%	69%	94%
Smoking Cessation Advice[1]	15	67%	80%	80%	100%
Surgical Infection Prevention					
Prophylactic Antibiotic Given[3]	40	42%	74%	77%	95%
Prophylactic Antibiotic Selection[1]	12	75%	91%	90%	100%
Prophylactic Antibiotic Stopped[3]	37	97%	67%	72%	95%
Pregnancy Care					

Inpatient Neonatal Mortality	-	-	-	-	-
Third or Fourth Degree Laceration	-	-	3.89%	3.63%	3.27%

McDonough District Hospital

525 E Grant Street
Macomb, IL 61455
URL: www.mdh.org
Ownership: Govt - Hospital District or Authority
Emergency Services: Yes
Phone: 309-833-4101
Fax: 309-836-1507
Accredited: Yes
Licensed Beds: 113

Key Personnel:
President/CEO . . . . Stephen R Hopper
President Medical Staff . . . . Dr David Miller, MD
Director Emergency Services . . . . Chris Dace
ER Medical Director . . . . George Roodhouse, DO
Infection Control . . . . Carol Rowland-Maguire, RN
Medical Surgical Nursing . . . . Betty Sherwood, RN
Director Surgical Services . . . . Christine Chase
Respiratory/Cardiopulmonary . . . . Debbie Jessen

Measure	Cases	This Hospital	State Average	U.S. Average	Top Hospital
Heart Attack Care					
ACE Inhibitor or ARB for LVSD[1]	8	75%	79%	82%	100%
Aspirin at Arrival[1]	16	69%	93%	92%	100%
Aspirin at Discharge[1]	6	33%	90%	90%	100%
Beta Blocker at Arrival[1]	9	67%	87%	87%	100%
Beta Blocker at Discharge[1]	10	60%	88%	90%	100%
Fibrinolytic Medication Timing	0	-	21%	31%	100%
PCI Within 90 Minutes of Arrival	0	-	47%	54%	95%
Smoking Cessation Advice[1]	2	100%	84%	88%	100%
Heart Failure Care					
ACE Inhibitor or ARB for LVSD	33	73%	83%	82%	100%
Discharge Instructions	58	72%	67%	61%	93%
Evaluation of LVS Function	95	76%	88%	83%	99%
Smoking Cessation Advice[1]	6	100%	83%	82%	100%
Pneumonia Care					
Appropriate Initial Antibiotic	110	93%	83%	83%	94%
Blood Culture Timing	59	97%	91%	90%	100%
Influenza Vaccine	31	94%	63%	70%	100%
Initial Antibiotic Timing	142	81%	81%	80%	93%
Oxygenation Assessment	191	100%	99%	99%	100%
Pneumococcal Vaccine	152	74%	62%	69%	94%
Smoking Cessation Advice	25	92%	80%	80%	100%
Surgical Infection Prevention					
Prophylactic Antibiotic Given	161	91%	74%	77%	95%
Prophylactic Antibiotic Selection	33	91%	91%	90%	100%
Prophylactic Antibiotic Stopped	154	82%	67%	72%	95%
Pregnancy Care					
Inpatient Neonatal Mortality	391	0.00%	-	-	-
Third or Fourth Degree Laceration	286	2.80%	3.89%	3.63%	3.27%

Heartland Regional Medical Center

3333 W De Young
Marion, IL 62959
Ownership: Proprietary
Emergency Services: Yes
Phone: 618-998-7000
Accredited: Yes

Measure	Cases	This Hospital	State Average	U.S. Average	Top Hospital
Heart Attack Care					
ACE Inhibitor or ARB for LVSD[1]	16	81%	79%	82%	100%
Aspirin at Arrival	63	97%	93%	92%	100%
Aspirin at Discharge	83	95%	90%	90%	100%
Beta Blocker at Arrival	65	95%	87%	87%	100%
Beta Blocker at Discharge	86	99%	88%	90%	100%
Fibrinolytic Medication Timing[1]	3	33%	21%	31%	100%
PCI Within 90 Minutes of Arrival[1]	3	0%	47%	54%	95%
Smoking Cessation Advice	34	97%	84%	88%	100%
Heart Failure Care					
ACE Inhibitor or ARB for LVSD	42	81%	83%	82%	100%
Discharge Instructions	125	77%	67%	61%	93%
Evaluation of LVS Function	167	90%	88%	83%	99%
Smoking Cessation Advice	25	88%	83%	82%	100%
Pneumonia Care					

NOTE: Hospital profiles are in alphabetical order by state, then city, then hospital within the city; Rankings are sorted by rate in descending order and exclude hospitals with less than 25 cases; (1) The number of cases is too small (n<25) for purposes of reliably predicting hospital performance; (2) Measure reflects the hospital's indication that its submission was based upon a sample of its relevant discharges; (3) Rate reflects fewer than the maximum possible quarters of data for the measure; (4) Inaccurate information submitted and suppressed for one or more quarters; (5) No data is available from the hospital for this measure; Please refer to the User's Guide for a full explanation of data

Appropriate Initial Antibiotic[2]	101	82%	83%	83%	94%
Blood Culture Timing[2]	98	94%	91%	90%	100%
Influenza Vaccine[2]	27	93%	63%	70%	100%
Initial Antibiotic Timing[2]	152	80%	81%	80%	93%
Oxygenation Assessment[2]	181	100%	99%	99%	100%
Pneumococcal Vaccine[2]	106	87%	62%	69%	94%
Smoking Cessation Advice[2]	44	98%	80%	80%	100%
Surgical Infection Prevention					
Prophylactic Antibiotic Given[2,3]	260	34%	74%	77%	95%
Prophylactic Antibiotic Selection[2]	75	89%	91%	90%	100%
Prophylactic Antibiotic Stopped[2,3]	239	44%	67%	72%	95%
Pregnancy Care					
Inpatient Neonatal Mortality	-	-	-	-	-
Third or Fourth Degree Laceration	-	-	3.89%	3.63%	3.27%

Anderson Hospital

6800 State Route #162
Maryville, IL 62062
URL: www.andersonhospital.org
Ownership: Voluntary non-profit - Private
Emergency Services: Yes
Phone: 618-288-5711
Fax: 618-288-4088
Accredited: Yes
Licensed Beds: 130

Key Personnel:

President/CEO . . . . R Coert Shepard
Administrator/COO . . . . Keith Page
Chief Medical Staff . . . . Rod Greeling, MD
Emergency Room . . . . Richard Nicol, MD
Director Infection/Disease Control . . . . Doris Driscoll, RN
CCU Spvg. Nurse . . . . Andrea Burns, RN
Director Medical/Surgical Nursing . . . . Sandy Riley, RN
OB/GYN Womens Health . . . . Gerard Malnar, MD
Chief Radiology . . . . Mohomed Megahy, MD
Director Respiratory Therapy . . . . Scott Ellner

Measure	Cases	This Hospital	State Average	U.S. Average	Top Hospital
Heart Attack Care					
ACE Inhibitor or ARB for LVSD[1]	15	80%	79%	82%	100%
Aspirin at Arrival	66	98%	93%	92%	100%
Aspirin at Discharge	35	91%	90%	90%	100%
Beta Blocker at Arrival	58	97%	87%	87%	100%
Beta Blocker at Discharge	33	97%	88%	90%	100%
Fibrinolytic Medication Timing[3]	0	-	21%	31%	100%
PCI Within 90 Minutes of Arrival	0	-	47%	54%	95%
Smoking Cessation Advice[1]	6	83%	84%	88%	100%
Heart Failure Care					
ACE Inhibitor or ARB for LVSD	53	100%	83%	82%	100%
Discharge Instructions	113	85%	67%	61%	93%
Evaluation of LVS Function	152	95%	88%	83%	99%
Smoking Cessation Advice[1]	18	89%	83%	82%	100%
Pneumonia Care					
Appropriate Initial Antibiotic	181	92%	83%	83%	94%
Blood Culture Timing	224	96%	91%	90%	100%
Influenza Vaccine[5]	-	-	63%	70%	100%
Initial Antibiotic Timing	249	79%	81%	80%	93%
Oxygenation Assessment	328	100%	99%	99%	100%
Pneumococcal Vaccine	221	78%	62%	69%	94%
Smoking Cessation Advice	69	91%	80%	80%	100%
Surgical Infection Prevention					
Prophylactic Antibiotic Given	568	93%	74%	77%	95%
Prophylactic Antibiotic Selection	118	95%	91%	90%	100%
Prophylactic Antibiotic Stopped	548	87%	67%	72%	95%
Pregnancy Care					
Inpatient Neonatal Mortality	-	-	-	-	-
Third or Fourth Degree Laceration	-	-	3.89%	3.63%	3.27%

Sarah Bush Lincoln Health Center

Alternate Name: Sarah Buch Lincoln Health Center
1000 Health Center Drive
Mattoon, IL 61938
E-mail: jpierce@sblhs.org
Ownership: Voluntary non-profit - Private
Emergency Services: Yes
Phone: 217-258-2525
Fax: 217-258-2111
Accredited: Yes
Licensed Beds: 202

Key Personnel:

CEO . . . . Gary Barnett
Chief Medical Staff . . . . William Houseworth
Emergency Room . . . . Joseph Burton, DO
Director Infection/Disease Control . . . . Ramona Tomshack
OB/GYN Womens Health . . . . Michelle Fenought, MD
Chief Radiology . . . . Jeffrey Lash, DO
Director Respiratory Therapy . . . . Joyce Cottingham

Measure	Cases	This Hospital	State Average	U.S. Average	Top Hospital
Heart Attack Care					
ACE Inhibitor or ARB for LVSD[1]	3	100%	79%	82%	100%
Aspirin at Arrival	36	100%	93%	92%	100%
Aspirin at Discharge[1]	13	100%	90%	90%	100%
Beta Blocker at Arrival	32	100%	87%	87%	100%
Beta Blocker at Discharge[1]	13	100%	88%	90%	100%
Fibrinolytic Medication Timing	0	-	21%	31%	100%
PCI Within 90 Minutes of Arrival	0	-	47%	54%	95%
Smoking Cessation Advice[1]	1	100%	84%	88%	100%
Heart Failure Care					
ACE Inhibitor or ARB for LVSD	74	100%	83%	82%	100%
Discharge Instructions	181	82%	67%	61%	93%
Evaluation of LVS Function	249	99%	88%	83%	99%
Smoking Cessation Advice	26	100%	83%	82%	100%
Pneumonia Care					
Appropriate Initial Antibiotic	168	88%	83%	83%	94%
Blood Culture Timing	124	80%	91%	90%	100%
Influenza Vaccine	45	82%	63%	70%	100%
Initial Antibiotic Timing	210	94%	81%	80%	93%
Oxygenation Assessment	272	100%	99%	99%	100%
Pneumococcal Vaccine	183	94%	62%	69%	94%
Smoking Cessation Advice	62	94%	80%	80%	100%
Surgical Infection Prevention					
Prophylactic Antibiotic Given	374	93%	74%	77%	95%
Prophylactic Antibiotic Selection	91	71%	91%	90%	100%
Prophylactic Antibiotic Stopped	365	63%	67%	72%	95%
Pregnancy Care					
Inpatient Neonatal Mortality	-	-	-	-	-
Third or Fourth Degree Laceration	-	-	3.89%	3.63%	3.27%

Loyola University Health System

2160 S First Avenue
Maywood, IL 60153
URL: www.luhs.org
Ownership: Voluntary non-profit - Other
Emergency Services: Yes
Phone: 708-216-9000
Fax: 708-216-5690
Accredited: Yes
Licensed Beds: 523

Key Personnel:

President/CEO . . . . Anthony L Barbato, MD
Chief Medical Staff . . . . Leonard L Vertuno, MD
Cardiac Lab . . . . David Wilber
Catheterization Lab . . . . Fred Leya, MD
Emergency Room . . . . Denise J Speed
Emergency Room . . . . Amber Spencer, BSN
Director Infection/Disease Control . . . . Paul O'Keefe, MD
ICU . . . . Martin Tobin, MD
Director Medical/Surgical Nursing . . . . Susan Flores
OB/GYN Womens Health . . . . John Gianopoulos, MD
Director Respiratory Therapy . . . . Dave Hauptman

Measure	Cases	This Hospital	State Average	U.S. Average	Top Hospital
Heart Attack Care					
ACE Inhibitor or ARB for LVSD	37	84%	79%	82%	100%
Aspirin at Arrival	169	100%	93%	92%	100%
Aspirin at Discharge	188	100%	90%	90%	100%
Beta Blocker at Arrival	160	98%	87%	87%	100%
Beta Blocker at Discharge	201	100%	88%	90%	100%
Fibrinolytic Medication Timing[1]	1	0%	21%	31%	100%
PCI Within 90 Minutes of Arrival[1]	7	43%	47%	54%	95%
Smoking Cessation Advice	60	100%	84%	88%	100%
Heart Failure Care					
ACE Inhibitor or ARB for LVSD	408	91%	83%	82%	100%
Discharge Instructions	693	66%	67%	61%	93%
Evaluation of LVS Function	754	99%	88%	83%	99%
Smoking Cessation Advice	155	90%	83%	82%	100%
Pneumonia Care					

NOTE: Hospital profiles are in alphabetical order by state, then city, then hospital within the city; Rankings are sorted by rate in descending order and exclude hospitals with less than 25 cases; (1) The number of cases is too small (n<25) for purposes of reliably predicting hospital performance; (2) Measure reflects the hospital's indication that its submission was based upon a sample of its relevant discharges; (3) Rate reflects fewer than the maximum possible quarters of data for the measure; (4) Inaccurate information submitted and suppressed for one or more quarters; (5) No data is available from the hospital for this measure; Please refer to the User's Guide for a full explanation of data

Appropriate Initial Antibiotic	120	85%	83%	83%	94%
Blood Culture Timing	145	94%	91%	90%	100%
Influenza Vaccine	35	80%	63%	70%	100%
Initial Antibiotic Timing	176	62%	81%	80%	93%
Oxygenation Assessment	254	100%	99%	99%	100%
Pneumococcal Vaccine	125	82%	62%	69%	94%
Smoking Cessation Advice	48	77%	80%	80%	100%
Surgical Infection Prevention					
Prophylactic Antibiotic Given[2,3]	283	95%	74%	77%	95%
Prophylactic Antibiotic Selection[2]	74	88%	91%	90%	100%
Prophylactic Antibiotic Stopped[2,3]	276	88%	67%	72%	95%
Pregnancy Care					
Inpatient Neonatal Mortality	1,895	2.27%	-	-	-
Third or Fourth Degree Laceration	997	2.41%	3.89%	3.63%	3.27%

Centegra Northern Illinois Medical Center

4201 Medical Center Drive | Phone: 815-344-5000
McHenry, IL 60050 | Fax: 815-759-8094
URL: www.centegra.org
Ownership: Voluntary non-profit - Other | Accredited: Yes
Emergency Services: Yes | Licensed Beds: 196

Key Personnel:
President/CEO . . . . Michael S Eesley
Chief Medical Staff . . . . Kanu Panchal, MD
Emergency Room . . . . Amy Moerschbaecher
Director Infection/Disease Control . . . . Pat Kinney
Director Medical/Surgical Nursing . . . . Suzan Buchaklian
OB/GYN Womens Health . . . . JoAnna White

Measure	Cases	This Hospital	State Average	U.S. Average	Top Hospital
Heart Attack Care					
ACE Inhibitor or ARB for LVSD[1]	17	88%	79%	82%	100%
Aspirin at Arrival	124	95%	93%	92%	100%
Aspirin at Discharge	123	96%	90%	90%	100%
Beta Blocker at Arrival	93	91%	87%	87%	100%
Beta Blocker at Discharge	137	97%	88%	90%	100%
Fibrinolytic Medication Timing[1]	1	100%	21%	31%	100%
PCI Within 90 Minutes of Arrival[1]	7	71%	47%	54%	95%
Smoking Cessation Advice	56	100%	84%	88%	100%
Heart Failure Care					
ACE Inhibitor or ARB for LVSD	116	84%	83%	82%	100%
Discharge Instructions	250	71%	67%	61%	93%
Evaluation of LVS Function	324	97%	88%	83%	99%
Smoking Cessation Advice	47	89%	83%	82%	100%
Pneumonia Care					
Appropriate Initial Antibiotic	146	85%	83%	83%	94%
Blood Culture Timing	186	94%	91%	90%	100%
Influenza Vaccine	35	51%	63%	70%	100%
Initial Antibiotic Timing	210	87%	81%	80%	93%
Oxygenation Assessment	261	100%	99%	99%	100%
Pneumococcal Vaccine	150	63%	62%	69%	94%
Smoking Cessation Advice	67	94%	80%	80%	100%
Surgical Infection Prevention					
Prophylactic Antibiotic Given[2]	544	81%	74%	77%	95%
Prophylactic Antibiotic Selection[2]	121	89%	91%	90%	100%
Prophylactic Antibiotic Stopped[2]	525	79%	67%	72%	95%
Pregnancy Care					
Inpatient Neonatal Mortality	-	-	-	-	-
Third or Fourth Degree Laceration	-	-	3.89%	3.63%	3.27%

Hamilton Memorial Hospital

611 South Marshall Avenue | Phone: 618-643-2361
McLeansboro, IL 62859 | Fax: 618-643-2875
URL: www.mcleansboro.com
Ownership: Govt - Hospital District or Authority | Accredited: Yes
Emergency Services: Yes | Licensed Beds: 85

Key Personnel:
CEO . . . . Randall W Dauby

Measure	Cases	This Hospital	State Average	U.S. Average	Top Hospital
Heart Attack Care					
ACE Inhibitor or ARB for LVSD[5]	-	-	79%	82%	100%
Aspirin at Arrival[5]	-	-	93%	92%	100%
Aspirin at Discharge[5]	-	-	90%	90%	100%
Beta Blocker at Arrival[5]	-	-	87%	87%	100%
Beta Blocker at Discharge[5]	-	-	88%	90%	100%
Fibrinolytic Medication Timing[5]	-	-	21%	31%	100%
PCI Within 90 Minutes of Arrival[5]	-	-	47%	54%	95%
Smoking Cessation Advice[5]	-	-	84%	88%	100%
Heart Failure Care					
ACE Inhibitor or ARB for LVSD[1]	9	89%	83%	82%	100%
Discharge Instructions	32	94%	67%	61%	93%
Evaluation of LVS Function	46	98%	88%	83%	99%
Smoking Cessation Advice[1]	4	100%	83%	82%	100%
Pneumonia Care					
Appropriate Initial Antibiotic	25	72%	83%	83%	94%
Blood Culture Timing[1]	5	80%	91%	90%	100%
Influenza Vaccine[1]	4	25%	63%	70%	100%
Initial Antibiotic Timing	38	92%	81%	80%	93%
Oxygenation Assessment	41	98%	99%	99%	100%
Pneumococcal Vaccine[1]	21	71%	62%	69%	94%
Smoking Cessation Advice[1]	11	100%	80%	80%	100%
Surgical Infection Prevention					
Prophylactic Antibiotic Given[5]	-	-	74%	77%	95%
Prophylactic Antibiotic Selection[5]	-	-	91%	90%	100%
Prophylactic Antibiotic Stopped[5]	-	-	67%	72%	95%
Pregnancy Care					
Inpatient Neonatal Mortality	-	-	-	-	-
Third or Fourth Degree Laceration	-	-	3.89%	3.63%	3.27%

Gottlieb Memorial Hospital

701 W North Avenue | Phone: 708-681-3200
Melrose Park, IL 60160 | Fax: 708-681-0078
URL: www.gottliebhospital.org
Ownership: Voluntary non-profit - Private | Accredited: Yes
Emergency Services: Yes | Licensed Beds: 247

Key Personnel:
President . . . . John Morgan
Chief Medical Staff . . . . Dr. Anand Lal
Emergency Room . . . . Laura Guerrieri, RN
Chairman Emergency Medicine . . . . Mark DeSilva, MD
Infection Control Coordinator . . . . Cathy Paulas
Chairman Cardiology . . . . Dragon Irkovic, MD
Chairman OB/GYN . . . . Jaafar Afshar, MD
Director Surgical Services . . . . Kathy Kozerski, RN
Respiratory Care Manager . . . . Gerry Arcaro

Measure	Cases	This Hospital	State Average	U.S. Average	Top Hospital
Heart Attack Care					
ACE Inhibitor or ARB for LVSD	29	97%	79%	82%	100%
Aspirin at Arrival	114	95%	93%	92%	100%
Aspirin at Discharge	103	95%	90%	90%	100%
Beta Blocker at Arrival	104	94%	87%	87%	100%
Beta Blocker at Discharge	101	97%	88%	90%	100%
Fibrinolytic Medication Timing	0	-	21%	31%	100%
PCI Within 90 Minutes of Arrival[1]	4	0%	47%	54%	95%
Smoking Cessation Advice	34	100%	84%	88%	100%
Heart Failure Care					
ACE Inhibitor or ARB for LVSD[2]	118	97%	83%	82%	100%
Discharge Instructions[2]	285	68%	67%	61%	93%
Evaluation of LVS Function[2]	348	96%	88%	83%	99%
Smoking Cessation Advice[2]	46	100%	83%	82%	100%
Pneumonia Care					
Appropriate Initial Antibiotic[2]	104	88%	83%	83%	94%
Blood Culture Timing[2]	128	99%	91%	90%	100%
Influenza Vaccine	26	88%	63%	70%	100%
Initial Antibiotic Timing[2]	153	86%	81%	80%	93%
Oxygenation Assessment[2]	186	100%	99%	99%	100%
Pneumococcal Vaccine[2]	110	92%	62%	69%	94%
Smoking Cessation Advice[2]	41	100%	80%	80%	100%
Surgical Infection Prevention					
Prophylactic Antibiotic Given[2,3]	167	89%	74%	77%	95%
Prophylactic Antibiotic Selection[2]	55	82%	91%	90%	100%
Prophylactic Antibiotic Stopped[2,3]	162	46%	67%	72%	95%
Pregnancy Care					

NOTE: Hospital profiles are in alphabetical order by state, then city, then hospital within the city; Rankings are sorted by rate in descending order and exclude hospitals with less than 25 cases; (1) The number of cases is too small (n<25) for purposes of reliably predicting hospital performance; (2) Measure reflects the hospital's indication that its submission was based upon a sample of its relevant discharges; (3) Rate reflects fewer than the maximum possible quarters of data for the measure; (4) Inaccurate information submitted and suppressed for one or more quarters; (5) No data is available from the hospital for this measure; Please refer to the User's Guide for a full explanation of data

Inpatient Neonatal Mortality	-	-	-	-	-
Third or Fourth Degree Laceration	-	-	3.89%	3.63%	3.27%

Westlake Community Hospital

1225 Lake Street
Melrose Park, IL 60160
URL: www.reshealth.org
Ownership: Voluntary non-profit - Church
Emergency Services: Yes
Phone: 708-681-3000
Fax: 708-938-7905
Accredited: Yes
Licensed Beds: 326

Key Personnel:
CEO. . . . . Pat Shehorn
Chief of Medical Staff. Nabil Saleh
Emergency Room . . . . Steve Meeks
OB/GYN Womens Health. . . . . Jean Alexandre', MD
Chief Radiology . . . . Robert Liebman, MD
Director Cardio-Pulmonary Services . . . . Romy Sison

Measure	Cases	This Hospital	State Average	U.S. Average	Top Hospital
Heart Attack Care					
ACE Inhibitor or ARB for LVSD[1]	18	78%	79%	82%	100%
Aspirin at Arrival	80	98%	93%	92%	100%
Aspirin at Discharge	68	99%	90%	90%	100%
Beta Blocker at Arrival	70	96%	87%	87%	100%
Beta Blocker at Discharge	65	94%	88%	90%	100%
Fibrinolytic Medication Timing	0	-	21%	31%	100%
PCI Within 90 Minutes of Arrival[1]	2	100%	47%	54%	95%
Smoking Cessation Advice[1]	21	86%	84%	88%	100%
Heart Failure Care					
ACE Inhibitor or ARB for LVSD	92	78%	83%	82%	100%
Discharge Instructions	221	54%	67%	61%	93%
Evaluation of LVS Function	288	92%	88%	83%	99%
Smoking Cessation Advice	57	88%	83%	82%	100%
Pneumonia Care					
Appropriate Initial Antibiotic	58	90%	83%	83%	94%
Blood Culture Timing	73	89%	91%	90%	100%
Influenza Vaccine[1]	23	43%	63%	70%	100%
Initial Antibiotic Timing	124	74%	81%	80%	93%
Oxygenation Assessment	153	100%	99%	99%	100%
Pneumococcal Vaccine	81	27%	62%	69%	94%
Smoking Cessation Advice	31	58%	80%	80%	100%
Surgical Infection Prevention					
Prophylactic Antibiotic Given[2]	197	89%	74%	77%	95%
Prophylactic Antibiotic Selection[2]	49	96%	91%	90%	100%
Prophylactic Antibiotic Stopped[2]	185	55%	67%	72%	95%
Pregnancy Care					
Inpatient Neonatal Mortality	-	-	-	-	-
Third or Fourth Degree Laceration	-	-	3.89%	3.63%	3.27%

Mendota Community Hospital

1315 Memorial Drive
Mendota, IL 61342
URL: www.mendotahospital.com
Ownership: Voluntary non-profit - Other
Emergency Services: Yes
Phone: 815-539-7461
Fax: 815-538-5516
Accredited: Yes
Licensed Beds: 68

Key Personnel:
Administrator . . . . Susan Urso
Chief Medical Staff. . . . . Mary Chin
OB/GYN Womens Health. . . . . Rebecca Salvanni, MD

Measure	Cases	This Hospital	State Average	U.S. Average	Top Hospital
Heart Attack Care					
ACE Inhibitor or ARB for LVSD[3]	0	-	79%	82%	100%
Aspirin at Arrival[1,3]	3	67%	93%	92%	100%
Aspirin at Discharge[3]	0	-	90%	90%	100%
Beta Blocker at Arrival[1,3]	3	100%	87%	87%	100%
Beta Blocker at Discharge[3]	0	-	88%	90%	100%
Fibrinolytic Medication Timing[3]	0	-	21%	31%	100%
PCI Within 90 Minutes of Arrival	0	-	47%	54%	95%
Smoking Cessation Advice[3]	0	-	84%	88%	100%
Heart Failure Care					
ACE Inhibitor or ARB for LVSD[1]	8	88%	83%	82%	100%
Discharge Instructions[1]	17	6%	67%	61%	93%
Evaluation of LVS Function	32	78%	88%	83%	99%
Smoking Cessation Advice[1]	4	50%	83%	82%	100%
Pneumonia Care					
Appropriate Initial Antibiotic[1]	18	78%	83%	83%	94%
Blood Culture Timing[1]	8	100%	91%	90%	100%
Influenza Vaccine[1]	6	83%	63%	70%	100%
Initial Antibiotic Timing	31	87%	81%	80%	93%
Oxygenation Assessment	44	98%	99%	99%	100%
Pneumococcal Vaccine	40	82%	62%	69%	94%
Smoking Cessation Advice[1]	4	100%	80%	80%	100%
Surgical Infection Prevention					
Prophylactic Antibiotic Given[1]	17	47%	74%	77%	95%
Prophylactic Antibiotic Selection[1]	2	100%	91%	90%	100%
Prophylactic Antibiotic Stopped[1]	16	12%	67%	72%	95%
Pregnancy Care					
Inpatient Neonatal Mortality	-	-	-	-	-
Third or Fourth Degree Laceration	-	-	3.89%	3.63%	3.27%

Community Medical Center

1000 W Harlem Avenue
Monmouth, IL 61462
URL: www.cmchospital.com
Ownership: Voluntary non-profit - Private
Emergency Services: No
Phone: 309-734-3141
Fax: 309-734-3029
Accredited: No
Licensed Beds: 68

Key Personnel:
President/CEO. . . . . Donald G Brown
Chief Medical Staff. . . . . Ruben Medrano
Emergency Room . . . . Beverly Vanriper
Director Radiology . . . . Mary Mowen
Director of Respiratory . . . . Kate Brislawn

Measure	Cases	This Hospital	State Average	U.S. Average	Top Hospital
Heart Attack Care					
ACE Inhibitor or ARB for LVSD[3]	0	-	79%	82%	100%
Aspirin at Arrival[1,3]	3	33%	93%	92%	100%
Aspirin at Discharge[1,3]	1	100%	90%	90%	100%
Beta Blocker at Arrival[1,3]	2	50%	87%	87%	100%
Beta Blocker at Discharge[1,3]	2	100%	88%	90%	100%
Fibrinolytic Medication Timing[3]	0	-	21%	31%	100%
PCI Within 90 Minutes of Arrival	0	-	47%	54%	95%
Smoking Cessation Advice[1,3]	2	100%	84%	88%	100%
Heart Failure Care					
ACE Inhibitor or ARB for LVSD[1]	6	83%	83%	82%	100%
Discharge Instructions[1]	21	100%	67%	61%	93%
Evaluation of LVS Function	39	72%	88%	83%	99%
Smoking Cessation Advice[1]	9	100%	83%	82%	100%
Pneumonia Care					
Appropriate Initial Antibiotic	43	84%	83%	83%	94%
Blood Culture Timing[1]	23	100%	91%	90%	100%
Influenza Vaccine[1]	12	67%	63%	70%	100%
Initial Antibiotic Timing	49	76%	81%	80%	93%
Oxygenation Assessment	65	100%	99%	99%	100%
Pneumococcal Vaccine	41	61%	62%	69%	94%
Smoking Cessation Advice[1]	14	100%	80%	80%	100%
Surgical Infection Prevention					
Prophylactic Antibiotic Given[1]	17	59%	74%	77%	95%
Prophylactic Antibiotic Selection[1]	2	100%	91%	90%	100%
Prophylactic Antibiotic Stopped[1]	15	20%	67%	72%	95%
Pregnancy Care					
Inpatient Neonatal Mortality	-	-	-	-	-
Third or Fourth Degree Laceration	-	-	3.89%	3.63%	3.27%

John & Mary Kirby Hospital

1111 N State Street
Monticello, IL 61856
Ownership: Voluntary non-profit - Other
Emergency Services: Yes
Phone: 217-762-2115
Fax: 217-762-6267
Accredited: Yes
Licensed Beds: 17

Key Personnel:
Administrator . . . . Thomas D Dixon

Measure	Cases	This Hospital	State Average	U.S. Average	Top Hospital
Heart Attack Care					

NOTE: Hospital profiles are in alphabetical order by state, then city, then hospital within the city; Rankings are sorted by rate in descending order and exclude hospitals with less than 25 cases; (1) The number of cases is too small (n<25) for purposes of reliably predicting hospital performance; (2) Measure reflects the hospital's indication that its submission was based upon a sample of its relevant discharges; (3) Rate reflects fewer than the maximum possible quarters of data for the measure; (4) Inaccurate information submitted and suppressed for one or more quarters; (5) No data is available from the hospital for this measure; Please refer to the User's Guide for a full explanation of data

ACE Inhibitor or ARB for LVSD[5]	-	-	79%	82%	100%
Aspirin at Arrival[5]	-	-	93%	92%	100%
Aspirin at Discharge[5]	-	-	90%	90%	100%
Beta Blocker at Arrival[5]	-	-	87%	87%	100%
Beta Blocker at Discharge[5]	-	-	88%	90%	100%
Fibrinolytic Medication Timing[5]	-	-	21%	31%	100%
PCI Within 90 Minutes of Arrival[5]	-	-	47%	54%	95%
Smoking Cessation Advice[5]	-	-	84%	88%	100%
Heart Failure Care					
ACE Inhibitor or ARB for LVSD[1]	6	100%	83%	82%	100%
Discharge Instructions[1]	14	64%	67%	61%	93%
Evaluation of LVS Function[1]	22	82%	88%	83%	99%
Smoking Cessation Advice[1]	1	0%	83%	82%	100%
Pneumonia Care					
Appropriate Initial Antibiotic	28	75%	83%	83%	94%
Blood Culture Timing[1]	21	90%	91%	90%	100%
Influenza Vaccine[1]	13	31%	63%	70%	100%
Initial Antibiotic Timing	50	64%	81%	80%	93%
Oxygenation Assessment	60	98%	99%	99%	100%
Pneumococcal Vaccine	50	52%	62%	69%	94%
Smoking Cessation Advice[1]	6	17%	80%	80%	100%
Surgical Infection Prevention					
Prophylactic Antibiotic Given[5]	-	-	74%	77%	95%
Prophylactic Antibiotic Selection[5]	-	-	91%	90%	100%
Prophylactic Antibiotic Stopped[5]	-	-	67%	72%	95%
Pregnancy Care					
Inpatient Neonatal Mortality	-	-	-	-	-
Third or Fourth Degree Laceration	-	-	3.89%	3.63%	3.27%

Morris Hospital

150 W High Street
Morris, IL 60450
Phone: 815-942-2932
Fax: 815-942-3154
E-mail: info@morrishospital.org
URL: www.morrishospital.org
Ownership: Voluntary non-profit - Private
Accredited: Yes
Emergency Services: Yes
Licensed Beds: 82

Key Personnel:

CEO. . . . . Coissord Corbett

Measure	Cases	This Hospital	State Average	U.S. Average	Top Hospital
Heart Attack Care					
ACE Inhibitor or ARB for LVSD[1]	9	89%	79%	82%	100%
Aspirin at Arrival	40	98%	93%	92%	100%
Aspirin at Discharge[1]	24	100%	90%	90%	100%
Beta Blocker at Arrival[1]	22	82%	87%	87%	100%
Beta Blocker at Discharge	32	91%	88%	90%	100%
Fibrinolytic Medication Timing	0	-	21%	31%	100%
PCI Within 90 Minutes of Arrival[1]	2	100%	47%	54%	95%
Smoking Cessation Advice[1]	10	100%	84%	88%	100%
Heart Failure Care					
ACE Inhibitor or ARB for LVSD	50	90%	83%	82%	100%
Discharge Instructions	130	90%	67%	61%	93%
Evaluation of LVS Function	168	99%	88%	83%	99%
Smoking Cessation Advice	25	100%	83%	82%	100%
Pneumonia Care					
Appropriate Initial Antibiotic	118	89%	83%	83%	94%
Blood Culture Timing	118	89%	91%	90%	100%
Influenza Vaccine	44	52%	63%	70%	100%
Initial Antibiotic Timing	212	90%	81%	80%	93%
Oxygenation Assessment	228	100%	99%	99%	100%
Pneumococcal Vaccine	163	57%	62%	69%	94%
Smoking Cessation Advice	43	100%	80%	80%	100%
Surgical Infection Prevention					
Prophylactic Antibiotic Given[2]	216	79%	74%	77%	95%
Prophylactic Antibiotic Selection[2]	42	95%	91%	90%	100%
Prophylactic Antibiotic Stopped[2]	207	61%	67%	72%	95%
Pregnancy Care					
Inpatient Neonatal Mortality	-	-	-	-	-
Third or Fourth Degree Laceration	-	-	3.89%	3.63%	3.27%

Wabash General Hospital

1418 College Drive
Mount Carmel, IL 62863
Phone: 618-262-8621
Fax: 618-263-6461
URL: www.wabashgeneral.com
Ownership: Govt - Hospital District or Authority
Accredited: Yes
Emergency Services: Yes
Licensed Beds: 56

Key Personnel:

CEO. . . . . Jay Turvis
Head of Radiology . . . . Debbie Dilbeck
Respiratory Care . . . . Marie Caddell

Measure	Cases	This Hospital	State Average	U.S. Average	Top Hospital
Heart Attack Care					
ACE Inhibitor or ARB for LVSD[1,3]	3	100%	79%	82%	100%
Aspirin at Arrival[1,3]	6	67%	93%	92%	100%
Aspirin at Discharge[1,3]	5	80%	90%	90%	100%
Beta Blocker at Arrival[1,3]	4	75%	87%	87%	100%
Beta Blocker at Discharge[1,3]	4	75%	88%	90%	100%
Fibrinolytic Medication Timing[3]	0	-	21%	31%	100%
PCI Within 90 Minutes of Arrival[5]	-	-	47%	54%	95%
Smoking Cessation Advice[3]	0	-	84%	88%	100%
Heart Failure Care					
ACE Inhibitor or ARB for LVSD[1]	8	88%	83%	82%	100%
Discharge Instructions	34	71%	67%	61%	93%
Evaluation of LVS Function	49	88%	88%	83%	99%
Smoking Cessation Advice[1]	4	100%	83%	82%	100%
Pneumonia Care					
Appropriate Initial Antibiotic	42	83%	83%	83%	94%
Blood Culture Timing	35	97%	91%	90%	100%
Influenza Vaccine[1]	15	67%	63%	70%	100%
Initial Antibiotic Timing	67	88%	81%	80%	93%
Oxygenation Assessment	90	100%	99%	99%	100%
Pneumococcal Vaccine	67	70%	62%	69%	94%
Smoking Cessation Advice[1]	12	42%	80%	80%	100%
Surgical Infection Prevention					
Prophylactic Antibiotic Given[1]	7	14%	74%	77%	95%
Prophylactic Antibiotic Selection	0	-	91%	90%	100%
Prophylactic Antibiotic Stopped[1]	5	100%	67%	72%	95%
Pregnancy Care					
Inpatient Neonatal Mortality	-	-	-	-	-
Third or Fourth Degree Laceration	-	-	3.89%	3.63%	3.27%

Crossroads Community Hospital

8 Doctor Parks Road
Mount Vernon, IL 62864
Phone: 618-244-5500
Fax: 618-244-5566
URL: www.crossroadscommnityhospital.com
Ownership: Proprietary
Accredited: Yes
Emergency Services: Yes
Licensed Beds: 55

Key Personnel:

President/CEO. . . . . Gregory F Simsniel, RN
Chief of Medical Staff. Alan Sroehling
Emergency Room/Medical Director . . . . Thurman Phemister, MD
Infection Control. . . . . Mike Beirman, RN
ICU . . . . Brandi Hill, RN
Medical Surgical Nursing . . . . Carla Wood, RN
Registered Surgical Nurse/CNO. . . . . Stacey Mavey, RN
Respiratory/Cardiopulmonary. . . . . Karen Harbin
Director Radiology . . . . Kerri Carr, BS
Director of Respiratory . . . . Jennifer Ice

Measure	Cases	This Hospital	State Average	U.S. Average	Top Hospital
Heart Attack Care					
ACE Inhibitor or ARB for LVSD[1]	3	100%	79%	82%	100%
Aspirin at Arrival[1]	7	100%	93%	92%	100%
Aspirin at Discharge[1]	5	100%	90%	90%	100%
Beta Blocker at Arrival[1]	6	83%	87%	87%	100%
Beta Blocker at Discharge[1]	3	67%	88%	90%	100%
Fibrinolytic Medication Timing[1]	2	0%	21%	31%	100%
PCI Within 90 Minutes of Arrival	0	-	47%	54%	95%
Smoking Cessation Advice[1]	1	0%	84%	88%	100%
Heart Failure Care					
ACE Inhibitor or ARB for LVSD[1]	16	88%	83%	82%	100%
Discharge Instructions	26	62%	67%	61%	93%

NOTE: Hospital profiles are in alphabetical order by state, then city, then hospital within the city; Rankings are sorted by rate in descending order and exclude hospitals with less than 25 cases; (1) The number of cases is too small (n<25) for purposes of reliably predicting hospital performance; (2) Measure reflects the hospital's indication that its submission was based upon a sample of its relevant discharges; (3) Rate reflects fewer than the maximum possible quarters of data for the measure; (4) Inaccurate information submitted and suppressed for one or more quarters; (5) No data is available from the hospital for this measure; Please refer to the User's Guide for a full explanation of data

Measure	Cases	This Hospital	State Average	U.S. Average	Top Hospital
Evaluation of LVS Function	45	78%	88%	83%	99%
Smoking Cessation Advice[1]	3	100%	83%	82%	100%
Pneumonia Care					
Appropriate Initial Antibiotic	106	75%	83%	83%	94%
Blood Culture Timing	56	96%	91%	90%	100%
Influenza Vaccine	27	96%	63%	70%	100%
Initial Antibiotic Timing	136	76%	81%	80%	93%
Oxygenation Assessment	161	100%	99%	99%	100%
Pneumococcal Vaccine	83	88%	62%	69%	94%
Smoking Cessation Advice	50	88%	80%	80%	100%
Surgical Infection Prevention					
Prophylactic Antibiotic Given[2,3]	113	25%	74%	77%	95%
Prophylactic Antibiotic Selection[2]	30	97%	91%	90%	100%
Prophylactic Antibiotic Stopped[2,3]	112	90%	67%	72%	95%
Pregnancy Care					
Inpatient Neonatal Mortality	-	-	-	-	-
Third or Fourth Degree Laceration	-	-	3.89%	3.63%	3.27%

Good Samaritan Regional Health Center

Alternate Name: Saint Mary's Good Samaritan
605 N 12th Street
Mount Vernon, IL 62864
Phone: 618-241-2000
Fax: 618-242-3196
Ownership: Voluntary non-profit - Church
Accredited: Yes
Emergency Services: Yes
Licensed Beds: 175

Key Personnel:

President/CEO . . . . Leo F Childers, Jr
Chief Medical Staff . . . . Jitendra Trivedi, MD
Chief Catheterization Laboratory . . . . M Haseeb, MD
Emergency Room . . . . Scott Roustio, MD
Director Infection/Disease Control . . . . Jeralee Sargent, RN
CCU Spvg. Nurse . . . . Darren Bock
Director Medical/Surgical Nursing . . . . Lynn Lenker, RN
Chief Radiology . . . . Jerrold Willis, MD
Director Respiratory Therapy . . . . Trisha Barczweski

Measure	Cases	This Hospital	State Average	U.S. Average	Top Hospital
Heart Attack Care					
ACE Inhibitor or ARB for LVSD	42	100%	79%	82%	100%
Aspirin at Arrival	98	98%	93%	92%	100%
Aspirin at Discharge	202	100%	90%	90%	100%
Beta Blocker at Arrival	77	95%	87%	87%	100%
Beta Blocker at Discharge	221	100%	88%	90%	100%
Fibrinolytic Medication Timing[1]	1	0%	21%	31%	100%
PCI Within 90 Minutes of Arrival[1]	5	20%	47%	54%	95%
Smoking Cessation Advice	92	96%	84%	88%	100%
Heart Failure Care					
ACE Inhibitor or ARB for LVSD	94	88%	83%	82%	100%
Discharge Instructions	238	63%	67%	61%	93%
Evaluation of LVS Function	273	97%	88%	83%	99%
Smoking Cessation Advice	46	91%	83%	82%	100%
Pneumonia Care					
Appropriate Initial Antibiotic	150	90%	83%	83%	94%
Blood Culture Timing	151	92%	91%	90%	100%
Influenza Vaccine	60	72%	63%	70%	100%
Initial Antibiotic Timing	238	88%	81%	80%	93%
Oxygenation Assessment	272	99%	99%	99%	100%
Pneumococcal Vaccine	188	69%	62%	69%	94%
Smoking Cessation Advice	57	84%	80%	80%	100%
Surgical Infection Prevention					
Prophylactic Antibiotic Given	442	86%	74%	77%	95%
Prophylactic Antibiotic Selection	102	92%	91%	90%	100%
Prophylactic Antibiotic Stopped	426	73%	67%	72%	95%
Pregnancy Care					
Inpatient Neonatal Mortality	739	0.00%	-	-	-
Third or Fourth Degree Laceration	476	3.36%	3.89%	3.63%	3.27%

Saint Joseph Memorial Hospital

2 S Hospital Drive
Murphysboro, IL 62966
Phone: 618-684-3156
Fax: 618-529-0535
E-mail: info@sih.net
URL: www.sih.net
Ownership: Voluntary non-profit - Private
Accredited: No
Emergency Services: Yes
Licensed Beds: 59

Key Personnel:

Administrator . . . . Elizabeth Gaffney
Chief Medical Staff . . . . Dale Blaise, MD
Emergency Room . . . . Karen Robert
Director Infection/Disease Control . . . . Tammy Jurgens
CCU Spvg. Nurse . . . . Ann Smith, RN
Director Medical/Surgical Nursing . . . . Ann Smith, RN
OB/GYN Womens Health . . . . Ann Smith
Director Respiratory Therapy . . . . Dana Troutman

Measure	Cases	This Hospital	State Average	U.S. Average	Top Hospital
Heart Attack Care					
ACE Inhibitor or ARB for LVSD[1]	3	67%	79%	82%	100%
Aspirin at Arrival[1]	10	80%	93%	92%	100%
Aspirin at Discharge[1]	6	83%	90%	90%	100%
Beta Blocker at Arrival[1]	10	60%	87%	87%	100%
Beta Blocker at Discharge[1]	6	67%	88%	90%	100%
Fibrinolytic Medication Timing	0	-	21%	31%	100%
PCI Within 90 Minutes of Arrival	0	-	47%	54%	95%
Smoking Cessation Advice	0	-	84%	88%	100%
Heart Failure Care					
ACE Inhibitor or ARB for LVSD[1]	10	80%	83%	82%	100%
Discharge Instructions	50	74%	67%	61%	93%
Evaluation of LVS Function	57	74%	88%	83%	99%
Smoking Cessation Advice[1]	13	85%	83%	82%	100%
Pneumonia Care					
Appropriate Initial Antibiotic	41	83%	83%	83%	94%
Blood Culture Timing	29	90%	91%	90%	100%
Influenza Vaccine[1]	6	67%	63%	70%	100%
Initial Antibiotic Timing	50	88%	81%	80%	93%
Oxygenation Assessment	59	100%	99%	99%	100%
Pneumococcal Vaccine	40	50%	62%	69%	94%
Smoking Cessation Advice[1]	13	100%	80%	80%	100%
Surgical Infection Prevention					
Prophylactic Antibiotic Given[5]	-	-	74%	77%	95%
Prophylactic Antibiotic Selection[5]	-	-	91%	90%	100%
Prophylactic Antibiotic Stopped[5]	-	-	67%	72%	95%
Pregnancy Care					
Inpatient Neonatal Mortality	-	-	-	-	-
Third or Fourth Degree Laceration	-	-	3.89%	3.63%	3.27%

Edward Hospital

801 S Washington Street
Naperville, IL 60540
Phone: 630-527-3000
Fax: 630-961-4910
URL: www.edward.org
Ownership: Voluntary non-profit - Private
Accredited: Yes
Emergency Services: Yes
Licensed Beds: 179

Key Personnel:

President/CEO . . . . Pamela Meyer-Davis
Chief Medical Staff . . . . Glenn Grobe
Chief Catheterization Laboratory . . . . Mark Goodwin, MD
Emergency Room . . . . Alan Kaplan
Director Infection/Disease Control . . . . Robert Chase, MD
OB/GYN Womens Health . . . . Karen Druzak
Chief Radiology . . . . Steven Papagiannopoulo, MD
Director Respiratory Therapy . . . . Lynn Wagner

Measure	Cases	This Hospital	State Average	U.S. Average	Top Hospital
Heart Attack Care					
ACE Inhibitor or ARB for LVSD	58	100%	79%	82%	100%
Aspirin at Arrival	263	100%	93%	92%	100%
Aspirin at Discharge	268	100%	90%	90%	100%
Beta Blocker at Arrival	229	100%	87%	87%	100%
Beta Blocker at Discharge	264	100%	88%	90%	100%
Fibrinolytic Medication Timing	0	-	21%	31%	100%

NOTE: Hospital profiles are in alphabetical order by state, then city, then hospital within the city; Rankings are sorted by rate in descending order and exclude hospitals with less than 25 cases; (1) The number of cases is too small (n<25) for purposes of reliably predicting hospital performance; (2) Measure reflects the hospital's indication that its submission was based upon a sample of its relevant discharges; (3) Rate reflects fewer than the maximum possible quarters of data for the measure; (4) Inaccurate information submitted and suppressed for one or more quarters; (5) No data is available from the hospital for this measure; Please refer to the User's Guide for a full explanation of data

PCI Within 90 Minutes of Arrival[1]	15	80%	47%	54%	95%
Smoking Cessation Advice	71	100%	84%	88%	100%
Heart Failure Care					
ACE Inhibitor or ARB for LVSD	215	93%	83%	82%	100%
Discharge Instructions	402	91%	67%	61%	93%
Evaluation of LVS Function	517	98%	88%	83%	99%
Smoking Cessation Advice	68	99%	83%	82%	100%
Pneumonia Care					
Appropriate Initial Antibiotic	271	91%	83%	83%	94%
Blood Culture Timing	370	96%	91%	90%	100%
Influenza Vaccine[4,5]	-	-	63%	70%	100%
Initial Antibiotic Timing	439	81%	81%	80%	93%
Oxygenation Assessment	577	100%	99%	99%	100%
Pneumococcal Vaccine	395	70%	62%	69%	94%
Smoking Cessation Advice	80	91%	80%	80%	100%
Surgical Infection Prevention					
Prophylactic Antibiotic Given[3]	983	83%	74%	77%	95%
Prophylactic Antibiotic Selection	335	99%	91%	90%	100%
Prophylactic Antibiotic Stopped[3]	954	42%	67%	72%	95%
Pregnancy Care					
Inpatient Neonatal Mortality	3,972	0.55%	-	-	-
Third or Fourth Degree Laceration	2,506	6.58%	3.89%	3.63%	3.27%

Bromenn Healthcare

1304 Franklin Avenue
Normal, IL 61761
Phone: 309-454-1400
Ownership: Voluntary non-profit - Church
Accredited: Yes
Emergency Services: Yes

Measure	Cases	This Hospital	State Average	U.S. Average	Top Hospital
Heart Attack Care					
ACE Inhibitor or ARB for LVSD[1]	23	100%	79%	82%	100%
Aspirin at Arrival	132	98%	93%	92%	100%
Aspirin at Discharge	143	99%	90%	90%	100%
Beta Blocker at Arrival	99	90%	87%	87%	100%
Beta Blocker at Discharge	141	99%	88%	90%	100%
Fibrinolytic Medication Timing	0	-	21%	31%	100%
PCI Within 90 Minutes of Arrival[1]	9	56%	47%	54%	95%
Smoking Cessation Advice	49	100%	84%	88%	100%
Heart Failure Care					
ACE Inhibitor or ARB for LVSD	93	95%	83%	82%	100%
Discharge Instructions	151	79%	67%	61%	93%
Evaluation of LVS Function	202	96%	88%	83%	99%
Smoking Cessation Advice	25	100%	83%	82%	100%
Pneumonia Care					
Appropriate Initial Antibiotic	106	89%	83%	83%	94%
Blood Culture Timing	145	83%	91%	90%	100%
Influenza Vaccine	51	92%	63%	70%	100%
Initial Antibiotic Timing	182	80%	81%	80%	93%
Oxygenation Assessment	236	100%	99%	99%	100%
Pneumococcal Vaccine	167	87%	62%	69%	94%
Smoking Cessation Advice	53	98%	80%	80%	100%
Surgical Infection Prevention					
Prophylactic Antibiotic Given	1,056	86%	74%	77%	95%
Prophylactic Antibiotic Selection	241	97%	91%	90%	100%
Prophylactic Antibiotic Stopped	1,022	67%	67%	72%	95%
Pregnancy Care					
Inpatient Neonatal Mortality	-	-	-	-	-
Third or Fourth Degree Laceration	-	-	3.89%	3.63%	3.27%

Oak Forest Hospital of Cook County

15900 South Cicero Avenue
Oak Forest, IL 60452
Phone: 708-687-7200
Fax: 708-687-7979
URL: www.cchil.org/cch/oak.htm
Ownership: Government - Local
Accredited: Yes
Emergency Services: Yes
Licensed Beds: 550

Key Personnel:
Emergency Room . . . . Shams Shafiei, MD
Director Infection/Disease Control . . . . Patricia DeMarais, MD
Director Radiology . . . . Tunisia Pinkley
Director Respiratory Therapy . . . . John Karnaus

Measure	Cases	This Hospital	State Average	U.S. Average	Top Hospital
Heart Attack Care					
ACE Inhibitor or ARB for LVSD	0	-	79%	82%	100%
Aspirin at Arrival[1]	11	100%	93%	92%	100%
Aspirin at Discharge[1]	3	100%	90%	90%	100%
Beta Blocker at Arrival[1]	9	100%	87%	87%	100%
Beta Blocker at Discharge[1]	5	100%	88%	90%	100%
Fibrinolytic Medication Timing	0	-	21%	31%	100%
PCI Within 90 Minutes of Arrival	0	-	47%	54%	95%
Smoking Cessation Advice	0	-	84%	88%	100%
Heart Failure Care					
ACE Inhibitor or ARB for LVSD	73	93%	83%	82%	100%
Discharge Instructions	137	80%	67%	61%	93%
Evaluation of LVS Function	145	97%	88%	83%	99%
Smoking Cessation Advice	68	99%	83%	82%	100%
Pneumonia Care					
Appropriate Initial Antibiotic	54	87%	83%	83%	94%
Blood Culture Timing	49	96%	91%	90%	100%
Influenza Vaccine[1]	4	100%	63%	70%	100%
Initial Antibiotic Timing	63	71%	81%	80%	93%
Oxygenation Assessment	72	100%	99%	99%	100%
Pneumococcal Vaccine[1]	6	100%	62%	69%	94%
Smoking Cessation Advice	43	95%	80%	80%	100%
Surgical Infection Prevention					
Prophylactic Antibiotic Given[3]	28	82%	74%	77%	95%
Prophylactic Antibiotic Selection[1]	6	100%	91%	90%	100%
Prophylactic Antibiotic Stopped[3]	25	36%	67%	72%	95%
Pregnancy Care					
Inpatient Neonatal Mortality	-	-	-	-	-
Third or Fourth Degree Laceration	-	-	3.89%	3.63%	3.27%

Advocate Christ Med Ctr/Hope Children's

4440 W 95th Street
Oak Lawn, IL 60453
Phone: 708-684-8000
Fax: 708-864-4440
URL: www.advocatehealth.com
Ownership: Voluntary non-profit - Church
Accredited: Yes
Emergency Services: Yes
Licensed Beds: 64

Measure	Cases	This Hospital	State Average	U.S. Average	Top Hospital
Heart Attack Care					
ACE Inhibitor or ARB for LVSD[2]	83	90%	79%	82%	100%
Aspirin at Arrival[2]	190	99%	93%	92%	100%
Aspirin at Discharge[2]	214	100%	90%	90%	100%
Beta Blocker at Arrival[2]	147	98%	87%	87%	100%
Beta Blocker at Discharge[2]	239	99%	88%	90%	100%
Fibrinolytic Medication Timing[2]	0	-	21%	31%	100%
PCI Within 90 Minutes of Arrival[1,2]	6	67%	47%	54%	95%
Smoking Cessation Advice[2]	86	94%	84%	88%	100%
Heart Failure Care					
ACE Inhibitor or ARB for LVSD[2]	154	88%	83%	82%	100%
Discharge Instructions[2]	263	69%	67%	61%	93%
Evaluation of LVS Function[2]	340	96%	88%	83%	99%
Smoking Cessation Advice[2]	50	94%	83%	82%	100%
Pneumonia Care					
Appropriate Initial Antibiotic[2]	85	85%	83%	83%	94%
Blood Culture Timing[2]	93	90%	91%	90%	100%
Influenza Vaccine[1]	23	61%	63%	70%	100%
Initial Antibiotic Timing[2]	161	78%	81%	80%	93%
Oxygenation Assessment[2]	171	100%	99%	99%	100%
Pneumococcal Vaccine[2]	106	65%	62%	69%	94%
Smoking Cessation Advice[1,2]	24	96%	80%	80%	100%
Surgical Infection Prevention					
Prophylactic Antibiotic Given[2]	345	92%	74%	77%	95%
Prophylactic Antibiotic Selection[2]	88	72%	91%	90%	100%
Prophylactic Antibiotic Stopped[2]	337	89%	67%	72%	95%
Pregnancy Care					
Inpatient Neonatal Mortality[2]	871	1.03%	-	-	-
Third or Fourth Degree Laceration[2]	642	4.05%	3.89%	3.63%	3.27%

NOTE: Hospital profiles are in alphabetical order by state, then city, then hospital within the city; Rankings are sorted by rate in descending order and exclude hospitals with less than 25 cases; (1) The number of cases is too small (n<25) for purposes of reliably predicting hospital performance; (2) Measure reflects the hospital's indication that its submission was based upon a sample of its relevant discharges; (3) Rate reflects fewer than the maximum possible quarters of data for the measure; (4) Inaccurate information submitted and suppressed for one or more quarters; (5) No data is available from the hospital for this measure; Please refer to the User's Guide for a full explanation of data

Rush Oak Park Hospital

520 South Maple Avenue
Oak Park, IL 60304
E-mail: ROPH_HR@rush.edu
URL: www.oakparkhospital.org
Ownership: Voluntary non-profit - Church
Emergency Services: Yes
Phone: 708-383-9300
Fax: 708-660-6658
Accredited: Yes
Licensed Beds: 296

Key Personnel:

President/CEO . . . . Bruce M Elegant
President Medical Staff . . . . Judy Carter, MD
VP . . . . Jim Kaese
Catheterization Lab . . . . LuAnn Smith
Emergency Room . . . . Daniel Noonan, MD
Emergency Room . . . . Sonia Winanay
VP Medical/Surgical Nursing . . . . Mickie Opalecky
Chief Radiology . . . . William Mollihan, MD
Director Respiratory Therapy . . . . Lori Majewski

Measure	Cases	This Hospital	State Average	U.S. Average	Top Hospital
Heart Attack Care					
ACE Inhibitor or ARB for LVSD[1,2]	9	67%	79%	82%	100%
Aspirin at Arrival[2]	53	96%	93%	92%	100%
Aspirin at Discharge[2]	38	89%	90%	90%	100%
Beta Blocker at Arrival[2]	40	95%	87%	87%	100%
Beta Blocker at Discharge[2]	39	92%	88%	90%	100%
Fibrinolytic Medication Timing[1,2]	8	62%	21%	31%	100%
PCI Within 90 Minutes of Arrival[2]	0	-	47%	54%	95%
Smoking Cessation Advice[1,2]	6	100%	84%	88%	100%
Heart Failure Care					
ACE Inhibitor or ARB for LVSD	62	76%	83%	82%	100%
Discharge Instructions	203	65%	67%	61%	93%
Evaluation of LVS Function	255	87%	88%	83%	99%
Smoking Cessation Advice	52	90%	83%	82%	100%
Pneumonia Care					
Appropriate Initial Antibiotic	96	86%	83%	83%	94%
Blood Culture Timing	129	94%	91%	90%	100%
Influenza Vaccine	35	71%	63%	70%	100%
Initial Antibiotic Timing	155	81%	81%	80%	93%
Oxygenation Assessment	193	100%	99%	99%	100%
Pneumococcal Vaccine	108	70%	62%	69%	94%
Smoking Cessation Advice	40	98%	80%	80%	100%
Surgical Infection Prevention					
Prophylactic Antibiotic Given[2,3]	80	80%	74%	77%	95%
Prophylactic Antibiotic Selection[2]	26	100%	91%	90%	100%
Prophylactic Antibiotic Stopped[2,3]	77	36%	67%	72%	95%
Pregnancy Care					
Inpatient Neonatal Mortality	-	-	-	-	-
Third or Fourth Degree Laceration	-	-	3.89%	3.63%	3.27%

West Suburban Medical Center

3 Erie Court
Oak Park, IL 60302
URL: www.wshmc.org
Ownership: Voluntary non-profit - Other
Emergency Services: Yes
Toll-Free: 877-931-8782
Phone: 708-383-6200
Fax: 708-386-9246
Accredited: Yes
Licensed Beds: 245

Key Personnel:

CEO . . . . Jay Kreuzer
Chief Medical Staff . . . . Roy Horras, MD
Director of Pulmonary/Respiratory Care . . . . Carol Glab

Measure	Cases	This Hospital	State Average	U.S. Average	Top Hospital
Heart Attack Care					
ACE Inhibitor or ARB for LVSD	25	72%	79%	82%	100%
Aspirin at Arrival	120	97%	93%	92%	100%
Aspirin at Discharge	98	83%	90%	90%	100%
Beta Blocker at Arrival	127	96%	87%	87%	100%
Beta Blocker at Discharge	113	81%	88%	90%	100%
Fibrinolytic Medication Timing[1]	11	36%	21%	31%	100%
PCI Within 90 Minutes of Arrival[1]	1	100%	47%	54%	95%
Smoking Cessation Advice	54	98%	84%	88%	100%
Heart Failure Care					
ACE Inhibitor or ARB for LVSD	195	78%	83%	82%	100%
Discharge Instructions	522	80%	67%	61%	93%
Evaluation of LVS Function	568	98%	88%	83%	99%
Smoking Cessation Advice	131	98%	83%	82%	100%
Pneumonia Care					
Appropriate Initial Antibiotic	178	82%	83%	83%	94%
Blood Culture Timing	169	94%	91%	90%	100%
Influenza Vaccine[4,5]	-	-	63%	70%	100%
Initial Antibiotic Timing	250	75%	81%	80%	93%
Oxygenation Assessment	285	100%	99%	99%	100%
Pneumococcal Vaccine	122	48%	62%	69%	94%
Smoking Cessation Advice	93	94%	80%	80%	100%
Surgical Infection Prevention					
Prophylactic Antibiotic Given	468	83%	74%	77%	95%
Prophylactic Antibiotic Selection	105	94%	91%	90%	100%
Prophylactic Antibiotic Stopped	448	50%	67%	72%	95%
Pregnancy Care					
Inpatient Neonatal Mortality	-	-	-	-	-
Third or Fourth Degree Laceration	-	-	3.89%	3.63%	3.27%

Richland Memorial Hospital

800 E Locust Street
Olney, IL 62450
URL: www.richlandmemorial.com
Ownership: Voluntary non-profit - Private
Emergency Services: Yes
Phone: 618-395-2131
Fax: 618-392-3228
Accredited: Yes
Licensed Beds: 135

Key Personnel:

CEO . . . . Harvey Pettry
Chief of Medical Staff . . . . Michael Joseph
Emergency Room . . . . Antonio Rodrigeuez
Infection Control . . . . Penni Kuenstler
ICU . . . . Jane Bailey
Respiratory Therapy . . . . Joni Cox

Measure	Cases	This Hospital	State Average	U.S. Average	Top Hospital
Heart Attack Care					
ACE Inhibitor or ARB for LVSD[1]	2	50%	79%	82%	100%
Aspirin at Arrival[1]	11	91%	93%	92%	100%
Aspirin at Discharge[1]	8	62%	90%	90%	100%
Beta Blocker at Arrival[1]	7	71%	87%	87%	100%
Beta Blocker at Discharge[1]	7	100%	88%	90%	100%
Fibrinolytic Medication Timing[1]	1	0%	21%	31%	100%
PCI Within 90 Minutes of Arrival	0	-	47%	54%	95%
Smoking Cessation Advice[1]	1	0%	84%	88%	100%
Heart Failure Care					
ACE Inhibitor or ARB for LVSD	25	76%	83%	82%	100%
Discharge Instructions	48	54%	67%	61%	93%
Evaluation of LVS Function	73	89%	88%	83%	99%
Smoking Cessation Advice[1]	6	33%	83%	82%	100%
Pneumonia Care					
Appropriate Initial Antibiotic	58	81%	83%	83%	94%
Blood Culture Timing	46	98%	91%	90%	100%
Influenza Vaccine[1]	19	74%	63%	70%	100%
Initial Antibiotic Timing	83	88%	81%	80%	93%
Oxygenation Assessment	108	100%	99%	99%	100%
Pneumococcal Vaccine	72	51%	62%	69%	94%
Smoking Cessation Advice	28	61%	80%	80%	100%
Surgical Infection Prevention					
Prophylactic Antibiotic Given[2,3]	85	86%	74%	77%	95%
Prophylactic Antibiotic Selection[2]	27	81%	91%	90%	100%
Prophylactic Antibiotic Stopped[2,3]	82	57%	67%	72%	95%
Pregnancy Care					
Inpatient Neonatal Mortality	-	-	-	-	-
Third or Fourth Degree Laceration	-	-	3.89%	3.63%	3.27%

Saint James Hospital and Health Center

20201 S Crawford Avenue
Olympia Fields, IL 60461
Ownership: Proprietary
Emergency Services: Yes
Phone: 708-747-4000
Fax: 708-756-6763
Accredited: Yes
Licensed Beds: 201

Key Personnel:

CEO . . . . Peter J Murphy
Chief Medical Staff . . . . Aswatch Subram, MD

NOTE: Hospital profiles are in alphabetical order by state, then city, then hospital within the city; Rankings are sorted by rate in descending order and exclude hospitals with less than 25 cases; (1) The number of cases is too small (n<25) for purposes of reliably predicting hospital performance; (2) Measure reflects the hospital's indication that its submission was based upon a sample of its relevant discharges; (3) Rate reflects fewer than the maximum possible quarters of data for the measure; (4) Inaccurate information submitted and suppressed for one or more quarters; (5) No data is available from the hospital for this measure; Please refer to the User's Guide for a full explanation of data

Measure	Cases	This Hospital	State Average	U.S. Average	Top Hospital
Heart Attack Care					
ACE Inhibitor or ARB for LVSD	56	84%	79%	82%	100%
Aspirin at Arrival	246	91%	93%	92%	100%
Aspirin at Discharge	197	95%	90%	90%	100%
Beta Blocker at Arrival	160	85%	87%	87%	100%
Beta Blocker at Discharge	198	93%	88%	90%	100%
Fibrinolytic Medication Timing	0	-	21%	31%	100%
PCI Within 90 Minutes of Arrival[1]	12	17%	47%	54%	95%
Smoking Cessation Advice	79	97%	84%	88%	100%
Heart Failure Care					
ACE Inhibitor or ARB for LVSD[2]	106	85%	83%	82%	100%
Discharge Instructions[2]	292	40%	67%	61%	93%
Evaluation of LVS Function[2]	353	94%	88%	83%	99%
Smoking Cessation Advice[2]	59	100%	83%	82%	100%
Pneumonia Care					
Appropriate Initial Antibiotic[2]	131	82%	83%	83%	94%
Blood Culture Timing[2]	131	94%	91%	90%	100%
Influenza Vaccine[2]	33	70%	63%	70%	100%
Initial Antibiotic Timing[2]	221	68%	81%	80%	93%
Oxygenation Assessment[2]	280	99%	99%	99%	100%
Pneumococcal Vaccine[2]	146	60%	62%	69%	94%
Smoking Cessation Advice[2]	66	95%	80%	80%	100%
Surgical Infection Prevention					
Prophylactic Antibiotic Given[2]	379	84%	74%	77%	95%
Prophylactic Antibiotic Selection[2]	93	89%	91%	90%	100%
Prophylactic Antibiotic Stopped[2]	365	55%	67%	72%	95%
Pregnancy Care					
Inpatient Neonatal Mortality	-	-	-	-	-
Third or Fourth Degree Laceration	-	-	3.89%	3.63%	3.27%

Community Hospital of Ottawa

1100 E Norris Drive
Ottawa, IL 61350
Phone: 815-433-3100
Fax: 815-431-5500
URL: www.community-hospital.org
Ownership: Voluntary non-profit - Private
Accredited: Yes
Emergency Services: Yes
Licensed Beds: 124

Key Personnel:

President/CEO. . . . . Robert I Schmelter
Chief Medical Staff. . . . . Joseph S Kokoszka, MD
Emergency Room . . . . Linda Grey, RN
Director Infection/Disease Control . . . . Kerry Gerding
CCU Spvg. Nurse . . . . Kathy Jakubek, RN
Director Medical/Surgical Nursing . . . . Barbara Beer
Chief Radiology . . . . N Lobo, MD
Director Respiratory Therapy . . . . Helen Kelly

Measure	Cases	This Hospital	State Average	U.S. Average	Top Hospital
Heart Attack Care					
ACE Inhibitor or ARB for LVSD[1]	2	100%	79%	82%	100%
Aspirin at Arrival[1]	15	93%	93%	92%	100%
Aspirin at Discharge[1]	9	100%	90%	90%	100%
Beta Blocker at Arrival[1]	13	92%	87%	87%	100%
Beta Blocker at Discharge[1]	10	90%	88%	90%	100%
Fibrinolytic Medication Timing	0	-	21%	31%	100%
PCI Within 90 Minutes of Arrival	0	-	47%	54%	95%
Smoking Cessation Advice[1]	2	100%	84%	88%	100%
Heart Failure Care					
ACE Inhibitor or ARB for LVSD[1]	16	81%	83%	82%	100%
Discharge Instructions	74	89%	67%	61%	93%
Evaluation of LVS Function	98	91%	88%	83%	99%
Smoking Cessation Advice[1]	8	100%	83%	82%	100%
Pneumonia Care					
Appropriate Initial Antibiotic	93	88%	83%	83%	94%
Blood Culture Timing	74	92%	91%	90%	100%
Influenza Vaccine	25	76%	63%	70%	100%
Initial Antibiotic Timing	138	93%	81%	80%	93%
Oxygenation Assessment	173	99%	99%	99%	100%
Pneumococcal Vaccine	127	84%	62%	69%	94%
Smoking Cessation Advice[1]	22	86%	80%	80%	100%
Surgical Infection Prevention					
Prophylactic Antibiotic Given[1,3]	23	65%	74%	77%	95%
Prophylactic Antibiotic Selection[5]	-	-	91%	90%	100%
Prophylactic Antibiotic Stopped[1,3]	19	21%	67%	72%	95%
Pregnancy Care					
Inpatient Neonatal Mortality	288	1.04%	-	-	-
Third or Fourth Degree Laceration	220	2.27%	3.89%	3.63%	3.27%

Palos Community Hospital

12251 S 80th Avenue
Palos Heights, IL 60463
Phone: 708-923-4000
Fax: 708-923-4620
URL: www.paloscommunityhospital.org
Ownership: Voluntary non-profit - Private
Accredited: Yes
Emergency Services: Yes
Licensed Beds: 369

Key Personnel:

President/CEO. . . . . Sr Margaret Wright
Chief Medical Staff. . . . . Thomas Lavery
Manager Cardiology. . . . . Julie Callahan
Director Emergency Room. . . . . Lori Stott
Manager Respiratory Therapy . . . . Tim Tkach

Measure	Cases	This Hospital	State Average	U.S. Average	Top Hospital
Heart Attack Care					
ACE Inhibitor or ARB for LVSD[2]	32	81%	79%	82%	100%
Aspirin at Arrival[2]	264	100%	93%	92%	100%
Aspirin at Discharge[2]	213	97%	90%	90%	100%
Beta Blocker at Arrival[2]	217	98%	87%	87%	100%
Beta Blocker at Discharge[2]	211	93%	88%	90%	100%
Fibrinolytic Medication Timing[2]	0	-	21%	31%	100%
PCI Within 90 Minutes of Arrival[1,2]	13	46%	47%	54%	95%
Smoking Cessation Advice[2]	68	96%	84%	88%	100%
Heart Failure Care					
ACE Inhibitor or ARB for LVSD[2]	64	58%	83%	82%	100%
Discharge Instructions[2]	211	61%	67%	61%	93%
Evaluation of LVS Function[2]	290	93%	88%	83%	99%
Smoking Cessation Advice[2]	29	86%	83%	82%	100%
Pneumonia Care					
Appropriate Initial Antibiotic[2]	120	93%	83%	83%	94%
Blood Culture Timing[2]	127	98%	91%	90%	100%
Influenza Vaccine[2]	31	61%	63%	70%	100%
Initial Antibiotic Timing[2]	153	65%	81%	80%	93%
Oxygenation Assessment[2]	203	100%	99%	99%	100%
Pneumococcal Vaccine[2]	142	61%	62%	69%	94%
Smoking Cessation Advice[2]	40	85%	80%	80%	100%
Surgical Infection Prevention					
Prophylactic Antibiotic Given[2,3]	221	81%	74%	77%	95%
Prophylactic Antibiotic Selection[2]	73	78%	91%	90%	100%
Prophylactic Antibiotic Stopped[2,3]	213	56%	67%	72%	95%
Pregnancy Care					
Inpatient Neonatal Mortality	-	-	-	-	-
Third or Fourth Degree Laceration	-	-	3.89%	3.63%	3.27%

Pana Community Hospital

101 E 9th Street
Pana, IL 62557
Phone: 217-562-2131
Fax: 217-562-6270
Ownership: Voluntary non-profit - Private
Accredited: No
Emergency Services: Yes
Licensed Beds: 44

Key Personnel:

CEO. . . . . Roland Carlson
Chief Medical Staff. . . . . Allen Frigy, MD
Director Infection/Disease Control . . . . Sheri Trexler
Director Medical/Surgical Nursing . . . . Joyce Schmits

Measure	Cases	This Hospital	State Average	U.S. Average	Top Hospital
Heart Attack Care					
ACE Inhibitor or ARB for LVSD[1]	2	100%	79%	82%	100%
Aspirin at Arrival[1]	4	100%	93%	92%	100%
Aspirin at Discharge[1]	4	100%	90%	90%	100%
Beta Blocker at Arrival[1]	4	75%	87%	87%	100%
Beta Blocker at Discharge[1]	4	75%	88%	90%	100%
Fibrinolytic Medication Timing[3]	0	-	21%	31%	100%
PCI Within 90 Minutes of Arrival[5]	-	-	47%	54%	95%
Smoking Cessation Advice[1]	1	0%	84%	88%	100%
Heart Failure Care					

NOTE: Hospital profiles are in alphabetical order by state, then city, then hospital within the city; Rankings are sorted by rate in descending order and exclude hospitals with less than 25 cases; (1) The number of cases is too small (n<25) for purposes of reliably predicting hospital performance; (2) Measure reflects the hospital's indication that its submission was based upon a sample of its relevant discharges; (3) Rate reflects fewer than the maximum possible quarters of data for the measure; (4) Inaccurate information submitted and suppressed for one or more quarters; (5) No data is available from the hospital for this measure; Please refer to the User's Guide for a full explanation of data

ACE Inhibitor or ARB for LVSD[1]	9	78%	83%	82%	100%
Discharge Instructions	27	56%	67%	61%	93%
Evaluation of LVS Function	41	56%	88%	83%	99%
Smoking Cessation Advice[1]	8	75%	83%	82%	100%
Pneumonia Care					
Appropriate Initial Antibiotic[1]	20	75%	83%	83%	94%
Blood Culture Timing[1]	20	85%	91%	90%	100%
Influenza Vaccine[1]	5	20%	63%	70%	100%
Initial Antibiotic Timing	30	80%	81%	80%	93%
Oxygenation Assessment	37	100%	99%	99%	100%
Pneumococcal Vaccine[1]	22	68%	62%	69%	94%
Smoking Cessation Advice[1]	3	100%	80%	80%	100%
Surgical Infection Prevention					
Prophylactic Antibiotic Given[5]	-	-	74%	77%	95%
Prophylactic Antibiotic Selection[5]	-	-	91%	90%	100%
Prophylactic Antibiotic Stopped[5]	-	-	67%	72%	95%
Pregnancy Care					
Inpatient Neonatal Mortality	-	-	-	-	-
Third or Fourth Degree Laceration	-	-	3.89%	3.63%	3.27%

Paris Community Hospital

721 E Court Street
Paris, IL 61944
Phone: 217-465-4141
Fax: 217-463-2096
URL: www.pariscommunityhospital.com
Ownership: Voluntary non-profit - Other
Accredited: Yes
Emergency Services: Yes
Licensed Beds: 49

Key Personnel:

CEO. . . . . John Fajt
Chief Medical Staff. . . . . Daniel R Gilbert, DO
Emergency Room . . . . Jeffrey Hatcher, DO
VP . . . . Ollie Smith
Infection Control. . . . . Tammy Hewitt, RN
ICU . . . . Rachel Young, RN
Medical Surgical Nursing . . . . Chris Bloodworth, RN
Surgical Services . . . . Katrina Conine, RN
Respiratory/Cardiopulmonary. . . . . David Wilson, CRT/RCP

Measure	Cases	This Hospital	State Average	U.S. Average	Top Hospital
Heart Attack Care					
ACE Inhibitor or ARB for LVSD[5]	-	-	79%	82%	100%
Aspirin at Arrival[5]	-	-	93%	92%	100%
Aspirin at Discharge[5]	-	-	90%	90%	100%
Beta Blocker at Arrival[5]	-	-	87%	87%	100%
Beta Blocker at Discharge[5]	-	-	88%	90%	100%
Fibrinolytic Medication Timing[5]	-	-	21%	31%	100%
PCI Within 90 Minutes of Arrival[5]	-	-	47%	54%	95%
Smoking Cessation Advice[5]	-	-	84%	88%	100%
Heart Failure Care					
ACE Inhibitor or ARB for LVSD[5]	-	-	83%	82%	100%
Discharge Instructions[5]	-	-	67%	61%	93%
Evaluation of LVS Function[5]	-	-	88%	83%	99%
Smoking Cessation Advice[5]	-	-	83%	82%	100%
Pneumonia Care					
Appropriate Initial Antibiotic[5]	-	-	83%	83%	94%
Blood Culture Timing[5]	-	-	91%	90%	100%
Influenza Vaccine[5]	-	-	63%	70%	100%
Initial Antibiotic Timing[5]	-	-	81%	80%	93%
Oxygenation Assessment[5]	-	-	99%	99%	100%
Pneumococcal Vaccine[5]	-	-	62%	69%	94%
Smoking Cessation Advice[5]	-	-	80%	80%	100%
Surgical Infection Prevention					
Prophylactic Antibiotic Given[5]	-	-	74%	77%	95%
Prophylactic Antibiotic Selection[5]	-	-	91%	90%	100%
Prophylactic Antibiotic Stopped[5]	-	-	67%	72%	95%
Pregnancy Care					
Inpatient Neonatal Mortality	-	-	-	-	-
Third or Fourth Degree Laceration	-	-	3.89%	3.63%	3.27%

Advocate Lutheran General Children's Hospital

1775 Dempster Street
Park Ridge, IL 60068
Phone: 847-723-2210
Fax: 847-696-2612
URL: www.advocatehealth.com
Ownership: Voluntary non-profit - Church
Accredited: Yes
Emergency Services: Yes

Measure	Cases	This Hospital	State Average	U.S. Average	Top Hospital
Heart Attack Care					
ACE Inhibitor or ARB for LVSD	77	92%	79%	82%	100%
Aspirin at Arrival	268	100%	93%	92%	100%
Aspirin at Discharge	244	99%	90%	90%	100%
Beta Blocker at Arrival	225	99%	87%	87%	100%
Beta Blocker at Discharge	259	98%	88%	90%	100%
Fibrinolytic Medication Timing	0	-	21%	31%	100%
PCI Within 90 Minutes of Arrival[1]	8	88%	47%	54%	95%
Smoking Cessation Advice	66	98%	84%	88%	100%
Heart Failure Care					
ACE Inhibitor or ARB for LVSD	228	93%	83%	82%	100%
Discharge Instructions	455	79%	67%	61%	93%
Evaluation of LVS Function	624	97%	88%	83%	99%
Smoking Cessation Advice	47	87%	83%	82%	100%
Pneumonia Care					
Appropriate Initial Antibiotic	206	85%	83%	83%	94%
Blood Culture Timing	242	95%	91%	90%	100%
Influenza Vaccine	66	74%	63%	70%	100%
Initial Antibiotic Timing	328	86%	81%	80%	93%
Oxygenation Assessment	436	100%	99%	99%	100%
Pneumococcal Vaccine	321	81%	62%	69%	94%
Smoking Cessation Advice	68	82%	80%	80%	100%
Surgical Infection Prevention					
Prophylactic Antibiotic Given[2]	559	94%	74%	77%	95%
Prophylactic Antibiotic Selection[2]	81	98%	91%	90%	100%
Prophylactic Antibiotic Stopped[2]	528	65%	67%	72%	95%
Pregnancy Care					
Inpatient Neonatal Mortality[2]	822	1.09%	-	-	-
Third or Fourth Degree Laceration[2]	630	4.76%	3.89%	3.63%	3.27%

Pekin Hospital

600 S 13th Street
Pekin, IL 61554
Phone: 309-347-1151
Fax: 309-347-5453
URL: www.pekinhospital.org
Ownership: Voluntary non-profit - Private
Accredited: Yes
Emergency Services: Yes
Licensed Beds: 125

Key Personnel:

CEO. . . . . Robert Moore
Director Cardio-Pulmonary Services . . . . Kerry Howard

Measure	Cases	This Hospital	State Average	U.S. Average	Top Hospital
Heart Attack Care					
ACE Inhibitor or ARB for LVSD[1]	6	100%	79%	82%	100%
Aspirin at Arrival	29	97%	93%	92%	100%
Aspirin at Discharge[1]	14	93%	90%	90%	100%
Beta Blocker at Arrival	31	100%	87%	87%	100%
Beta Blocker at Discharge[1]	21	90%	88%	90%	100%
Fibrinolytic Medication Timing[1]	1	0%	21%	31%	100%
PCI Within 90 Minutes of Arrival	0	-	47%	54%	95%
Smoking Cessation Advice[1]	7	71%	84%	88%	100%
Heart Failure Care					
ACE Inhibitor or ARB for LVSD	50	90%	83%	82%	100%
Discharge Instructions	86	71%	67%	61%	93%
Evaluation of LVS Function	128	93%	88%	83%	99%
Smoking Cessation Advice[1]	19	95%	83%	82%	100%
Pneumonia Care					
Appropriate Initial Antibiotic	99	88%	83%	83%	94%
Blood Culture Timing	106	94%	91%	90%	100%
Influenza Vaccine	33	12%	63%	70%	100%
Initial Antibiotic Timing	187	86%	81%	80%	93%
Oxygenation Assessment	224	99%	99%	99%	100%
Pneumococcal Vaccine	157	41%	62%	69%	94%
Smoking Cessation Advice	50	72%	80%	80%	100%

NOTE: Hospital profiles are in alphabetical order by state, then city, then hospital within the city; Rankings are sorted by rate in descending order and exclude hospitals with less than 25 cases; (1) The number of cases is too small (n<25) for purposes of reliably predicting hospital performance; (2) Measure reflects the hospital's indication that its submission was based upon a sample of its relevant discharges; (3) Rate reflects fewer than the maximum possible quarters of data for the measure; (4) Inaccurate information submitted and suppressed for one or more quarters; (5) No data is available from the hospital for this measure; Please refer to the User's Guide for a full explanation of data

Surgical Infection Prevention					
Prophylactic Antibiotic Given	299	78%	74%	77%	95%
Prophylactic Antibiotic Selection	77	92%	91%	90%	100%
Prophylactic Antibiotic Stopped	287	56%	67%	72%	95%
Pregnancy Care					
Inpatient Neonatal Mortality	-	-	-	-	-
Third or Fourth Degree Laceration	-	-	3.89%	3.63%	3.27%

Methodist Medical Center of Illinois

221 NE Glen Oak Avenue
Peoria, IL 61636
URL: www.mmci.org
Ownership: Voluntary non-profit - Other
Emergency Services: Yes
Phone: 309-672-5522
Fax: 309-671-8303
Accredited: Yes
Licensed Beds: 342

Key Personnel:
CEO. . . . . W Michael Bryant
Chief Medical Staff. . . . . Fred Holser, MD
Cardiac Lab . . . . Jeanine Spain, RN
Director Emergency Room. . . . . Margie Cobb
Infection Control. . . . . Tammy Durenback
Director Radiology . . . . Tony Howard

Measure	Cases	This Hospital	State Average	U.S. Average	Top Hospital
Heart Attack Care					
ACE Inhibitor or ARB for LVSD	49	96%	79%	82%	100%
Aspirin at Arrival	114	97%	93%	92%	100%
Aspirin at Discharge	183	99%	90%	90%	100%
Beta Blocker at Arrival	96	94%	87%	87%	100%
Beta Blocker at Discharge	213	98%	88%	90%	100%
Fibrinolytic Medication Timing	0	-	21%	31%	100%
PCI Within 90 Minutes of Arrival[1]	2	50%	47%	54%	95%
Smoking Cessation Advice	92	99%	84%	88%	100%
Heart Failure Care					
ACE Inhibitor or ARB for LVSD	156	96%	83%	82%	100%
Discharge Instructions	294	75%	67%	61%	93%
Evaluation of LVS Function	370	97%	88%	83%	99%
Smoking Cessation Advice	93	94%	83%	82%	100%
Pneumonia Care					
Appropriate Initial Antibiotic	159	93%	83%	83%	94%
Blood Culture Timing	147	96%	91%	90%	100%
Influenza Vaccine	51	96%	63%	70%	100%
Initial Antibiotic Timing	237	81%	81%	80%	93%
Oxygenation Assessment	327	100%	99%	99%	100%
Pneumococcal Vaccine	204	98%	62%	69%	94%
Smoking Cessation Advice	96	96%	80%	80%	100%
Surgical Infection Prevention					
Prophylactic Antibiotic Given[3]	681	91%	74%	77%	95%
Prophylactic Antibiotic Selection	243	91%	91%	90%	100%
Prophylactic Antibiotic Stopped[3]	650	89%	67%	72%	95%
Pregnancy Care					
Inpatient Neonatal Mortality	-	-	-	-	-
Third or Fourth Degree Laceration	-	-	3.89%	3.63%	3.27%

Proctor Hospital

5409 N Knoxville
Peoria, IL 61614
E-mail: information@proctor.org
URL: www.proctor.org
Ownership: Voluntary non-profit - Private
Emergency Services: Yes
Phone: 309-691-1000
Fax: 309-689-6062
Accredited: Yes
Licensed Beds: 163

Key Personnel:
President/CEO. . . . . Norman H LaConte

Measure	Cases	This Hospital	State Average	U.S. Average	Top Hospital
Heart Attack Care					
ACE Inhibitor or ARB for LVSD	27	100%	79%	82%	100%
Aspirin at Arrival	88	98%	93%	92%	100%
Aspirin at Discharge	93	99%	90%	90%	100%
Beta Blocker at Arrival	90	99%	87%	87%	100%
Beta Blocker at Discharge	111	100%	88%	90%	100%
Fibrinolytic Medication Timing	0	-	21%	31%	100%
PCI Within 90 Minutes of Arrival[1]	5	80%	47%	54%	95%
Smoking Cessation Advice	29	100%	84%	88%	100%
Heart Failure Care					
ACE Inhibitor or ARB for LVSD	71	99%	83%	82%	100%
Discharge Instructions	145	97%	67%	61%	93%
Evaluation of LVS Function	201	100%	88%	83%	99%
Smoking Cessation Advice[1]	24	92%	83%	82%	100%
Pneumonia Care					
Appropriate Initial Antibiotic	147	88%	83%	83%	94%
Blood Culture Timing	181	95%	91%	90%	100%
Influenza Vaccine	38	97%	63%	70%	100%
Initial Antibiotic Timing	214	95%	81%	80%	93%
Oxygenation Assessment	267	100%	99%	99%	100%
Pneumococcal Vaccine	205	98%	62%	69%	94%
Smoking Cessation Advice	50	90%	80%	80%	100%
Surgical Infection Prevention					
Prophylactic Antibiotic Given	634	85%	74%	77%	95%
Prophylactic Antibiotic Selection	164	96%	91%	90%	100%
Prophylactic Antibiotic Stopped	623	86%	67%	72%	95%
Pregnancy Care					
Inpatient Neonatal Mortality	-	-	-	-	-
Third or Fourth Degree Laceration	-	-	3.89%	3.63%	3.27%

Saint Francis Medical Center

530 NE Glen Oak Avenue
Peoria, IL 61637
URL: www.osfsaintfrancis.org
Ownership: Voluntary non-profit - Church
Emergency Services: Yes
Phone: 309-655-2000
Fax: 309-671-8996
Accredited: Yes
Licensed Beds: 731

Key Personnel:
Administrator . . . . Keith Steffen
Chief Medical Staff. . . . . Tim Miller, MD
Director Cardiology Services . . . . Delmar Smith
Chief Catheterization Laboratory . . . . Robert Crawford, MD
Emergency Room . . . . George Hevesy, MD
Coordinator Infection Control . . . . Patricia Ham
ICU . . . . Cathy Bingham
CCU Spvg. Nurse . . . . Judy Ritchie, RN
Director Medical/Surgical Nursing . . . . Susan Ehlers
OB/GYN Womens Health. . . . . Yolanda Renfroe, MD
Manager Respiratory Therapy . . . . Brenda Arians
Chief Surgery. . . . . Judy Winkler, MD

Measure	Cases	This Hospital	State Average	U.S. Average	Top Hospital
Heart Attack Care					
ACE Inhibitor or ARB for LVSD	155	90%	79%	82%	100%
Aspirin at Arrival	246	98%	93%	92%	100%
Aspirin at Discharge	511	98%	90%	90%	100%
Beta Blocker at Arrival	228	95%	87%	87%	100%
Beta Blocker at Discharge	595	99%	88%	90%	100%
Fibrinolytic Medication Timing	0	-	21%	31%	100%
PCI Within 90 Minutes of Arrival[1]	16	38%	47%	54%	95%
Smoking Cessation Advice	212	100%	84%	88%	100%
Heart Failure Care					
ACE Inhibitor or ARB for LVSD	272	88%	83%	82%	100%
Discharge Instructions	455	56%	67%	61%	93%
Evaluation of LVS Function	574	91%	88%	83%	99%
Smoking Cessation Advice	146	94%	83%	82%	100%
Pneumonia Care					
Appropriate Initial Antibiotic	273	92%	83%	83%	94%
Blood Culture Timing	199	94%	91%	90%	100%
Influenza Vaccine	80	85%	63%	70%	100%
Initial Antibiotic Timing	409	82%	81%	80%	93%
Oxygenation Assessment	460	100%	99%	99%	100%
Pneumococcal Vaccine	282	79%	62%	69%	94%
Smoking Cessation Advice	136	97%	80%	80%	100%
Surgical Infection Prevention					
Prophylactic Antibiotic Given[2]	1,730	90%	74%	77%	95%
Prophylactic Antibiotic Selection[2]	406	87%	91%	90%	100%
Prophylactic Antibiotic Stopped[2]	1,707	87%	67%	72%	95%
Pregnancy Care					
Inpatient Neonatal Mortality	-	-	-	-	-
Third or Fourth Degree Laceration	-	-	3.89%	3.63%	3.27%

NOTE: Hospital profiles are in alphabetical order by state, then city, then hospital within the city; Rankings are sorted by rate in descending order and exclude hospitals with less than 25 cases; (1) The number of cases is too small (n<25) for purposes of reliably predicting hospital performance; (2) Measure reflects the hospital's indication that its submission was based upon a sample of its relevant discharges; (3) Rate reflects fewer than the maximum possible quarters of data for the measure; (4) Inaccurate information submitted and suppressed for one or more quarters; (5) No data is available from the hospital for this measure; Please refer to the User's Guide for a full explanation of data

Illinois Valley Community Hospital

925 W Street
Peru, IL 61354
E-mail: prelate@ivch.org
URL: www.ivch.org
Ownership: Voluntary non-profit - Other
Emergency Services: Yes
Phone: 815-223-3300
Fax: 815-223-3394
Accredited: Yes

Key Personnel:

Administrator . . . . Willis F Fry
Chief Medical Staff . . . . Mario Cote, MD
Emergency Room . . . . Greg Guard, MD
Director Infection/Disease Control . . . . Deb Patyk
Chief Radiology . . . . Merle Piacenti, MD

Measure	Cases	This Hospital	State Average	U.S. Average	Top Hospital
Heart Attack Care					
ACE Inhibitor or ARB for LVSD[1]	3	67%	79%	82%	100%
Aspirin at Arrival[1]	9	89%	93%	92%	100%
Aspirin at Discharge[1]	7	86%	90%	90%	100%
Beta Blocker at Arrival[1]	11	91%	87%	87%	100%
Beta Blocker at Discharge[1]	8	88%	88%	90%	100%
Fibrinolytic Medication Timing	0	-	21%	31%	100%
PCI Within 90 Minutes of Arrival	0	-	47%	54%	95%
Smoking Cessation Advice[1]	1	100%	84%	88%	100%
Heart Failure Care					
ACE Inhibitor or ARB for LVSD	28	82%	83%	82%	100%
Discharge Instructions	74	68%	67%	61%	93%
Evaluation of LVS Function	113	80%	88%	83%	99%
Smoking Cessation Advice[1]	16	88%	83%	82%	100%
Pneumonia Care					
Appropriate Initial Antibiotic	101	79%	83%	83%	94%
Blood Culture Timing	98	82%	91%	90%	100%
Influenza Vaccine	35	34%	63%	70%	100%
Initial Antibiotic Timing	160	91%	81%	80%	93%
Oxygenation Assessment	178	99%	99%	99%	100%
Pneumococcal Vaccine	131	54%	62%	69%	94%
Smoking Cessation Advice	25	76%	80%	80%	100%
Surgical Infection Prevention					
Prophylactic Antibiotic Given	184	48%	74%	77%	95%
Prophylactic Antibiotic Selection	46	96%	91%	90%	100%
Prophylactic Antibiotic Stopped	181	57%	67%	72%	95%
Pregnancy Care					
Inpatient Neonatal Mortality	-	-	-	-	-
Third or Fourth Degree Laceration	-	-	3.89%	3.63%	3.27%

Pinckneyville Community Hospital

101 N Walnut Street
Pinckneyville, IL 62274
Ownership: Govt - Hospital District or Authority
Emergency Services: No
Phone: 618-357-2187
Fax: 618-357-6740
Accredited: No
Licensed Beds: 85

Key Personnel:

Chief Medical Staff . . . . Craig Fovard

Measure	Cases	This Hospital	State Average	U.S. Average	Top Hospital
Heart Attack Care					
ACE Inhibitor or ARB for LVSD[1,3]	1	0%	79%	82%	100%
Aspirin at Arrival[1,3]	5	100%	93%	92%	100%
Aspirin at Discharge[1,3]	4	75%	90%	90%	100%
Beta Blocker at Arrival[1,3]	5	80%	87%	87%	100%
Beta Blocker at Discharge[1,3]	4	75%	88%	90%	100%
Fibrinolytic Medication Timing[3]	0	-	21%	31%	100%
PCI Within 90 Minutes of Arrival[5]	-	-	47%	54%	95%
Smoking Cessation Advice[3]	0	-	84%	88%	100%
Heart Failure Care					
ACE Inhibitor or ARB for LVSD[1]	8	62%	83%	82%	100%
Discharge Instructions[1]	20	55%	67%	61%	93%
Evaluation of LVS Function	28	79%	88%	83%	99%
Smoking Cessation Advice[1]	1	0%	83%	82%	100%
Pneumonia Care					
Appropriate Initial Antibiotic[3]	41	78%	83%	83%	94%
Blood Culture Timing[3]	0	-	91%	90%	100%
Influenza Vaccine[1]	10	70%	63%	70%	100%
Initial Antibiotic Timing[3]	33	94%	81%	80%	93%
Oxygenation Assessment[3]	46	96%	99%	99%	100%
Pneumococcal Vaccine[3]	40	70%	62%	69%	94%
Smoking Cessation Advice[1,3]	9	56%	80%	80%	100%
Surgical Infection Prevention					
Prophylactic Antibiotic Given[1,3]	4	0%	74%	77%	95%
Prophylactic Antibiotic Selection[1]	2	100%	91%	90%	100%
Prophylactic Antibiotic Stopped[1,3]	4	25%	67%	72%	95%
Pregnancy Care					
Inpatient Neonatal Mortality	-	-	-	-	-
Third or Fourth Degree Laceration	-	-	3.89%	3.63%	3.27%

Illini Community Hospital

640 W Washington Street
Pittsfield, IL 62363
URL: www.illinihospital.org
Ownership: Voluntary non-profit - Private
Emergency Services: Yes
Phone: 217-285-2113
Fax: 217-285-5090
Accredited: Yes
Licensed Beds: 37

Key Personnel:

President/CEO . . . . Connie Schroeder
President Medical Staff . . . . James Grete, MD
Manager Emergency Room . . . . Kathy Willman
Infection Control/Operating Room Manager . . . . RoseAnn Hamilton
Manager Medical Surgery Nursing . . . . Rachel Griselman
Manager Radiology . . . . Jeanne Krutmeier

Measure	Cases	This Hospital	State Average	U.S. Average	Top Hospital
Heart Attack Care					
ACE Inhibitor or ARB for LVSD[1]	1	0%	79%	82%	100%
Aspirin at Arrival[1]	10	70%	93%	92%	100%
Aspirin at Discharge[1]	6	50%	90%	90%	100%
Beta Blocker at Arrival[1]	8	75%	87%	87%	100%
Beta Blocker at Discharge[1]	6	83%	88%	90%	100%
Fibrinolytic Medication Timing	0	-	21%	31%	100%
PCI Within 90 Minutes of Arrival	0	-	47%	54%	95%
Smoking Cessation Advice	0	-	84%	88%	100%
Heart Failure Care					
ACE Inhibitor or ARB for LVSD[1]	7	71%	83%	82%	100%
Discharge Instructions[1]	16	88%	67%	61%	93%
Evaluation of LVS Function	25	92%	88%	83%	99%
Smoking Cessation Advice[1]	3	100%	83%	82%	100%
Pneumonia Care					
Appropriate Initial Antibiotic	33	100%	83%	83%	94%
Blood Culture Timing[1]	5	100%	91%	90%	100%
Influenza Vaccine[1]	11	100%	63%	70%	100%
Initial Antibiotic Timing	45	80%	81%	80%	93%
Oxygenation Assessment	60	98%	99%	99%	100%
Pneumococcal Vaccine	49	82%	62%	69%	94%
Smoking Cessation Advice[1]	9	100%	80%	80%	100%
Surgical Infection Prevention					
Prophylactic Antibiotic Given[1,3]	5	40%	74%	77%	95%
Prophylactic Antibiotic Selection[1]	3	33%	91%	90%	100%
Prophylactic Antibiotic Stopped[1,3]	2	0%	67%	72%	95%
Pregnancy Care					
Inpatient Neonatal Mortality	-	-	-	-	-
Third or Fourth Degree Laceration	-	-	3.89%	3.63%	3.27%

Saint James OSF

Alternate Name: Saint James Hospital
610 E Water Street
Pontiac, IL 61764
Ownership: Voluntary non-profit - Church
Emergency Services: Yes
Phone: 815-842-2828
Fax: 815-842-4912
Accredited: Yes
Licensed Beds: 89

Key Personnel:

Administrator . . . . David Ochs
Emergency Room . . . . Nan Marx

Measure	Cases	This Hospital	State Average	U.S. Average	Top Hospital
Heart Attack Care					
ACE Inhibitor or ARB for LVSD[1]	1	100%	79%	82%	100%
Aspirin at Arrival[1]	14	100%	93%	92%	100%
Aspirin at Discharge[1]	9	89%	90%	90%	100%
Beta Blocker at Arrival[1]	13	92%	87%	87%	100%

NOTE: Hospital profiles are in alphabetical order by state, then city, then hospital within the city; Rankings are sorted by rate in descending order and exclude hospitals with less than 25 cases; (1) The number of cases is too small (n<25) for purposes of reliably predicting hospital performance; (2) Measure reflects the hospital's indication that its submission was based upon a sample of its relevant discharges; (3) Rate reflects fewer than the maximum possible quarters of data for the measure; (4) Inaccurate information submitted and suppressed for one or more quarters; (5) No data is available from the hospital for this measure; Please refer to the User's Guide for a full explanation of data

Measure	Cases	This Hospital	State Average	U.S. Average	Top Hospital
Beta Blocker at Discharge[1]	9	100%	88%	90%	100%
Fibrinolytic Medication Timing	0	-	21%	31%	100%
PCI Within 90 Minutes of Arrival	0	-	47%	54%	95%
Smoking Cessation Advice	0	-	84%	88%	100%
Heart Failure Care					
ACE Inhibitor or ARB for LVSD	25	76%	83%	82%	100%
Discharge Instructions	35	77%	67%	61%	93%
Evaluation of LVS Function	63	97%	88%	83%	99%
Smoking Cessation Advice[1]	6	100%	83%	82%	100%
Pneumonia Care					
Appropriate Initial Antibiotic	50	84%	83%	83%	94%
Blood Culture Timing	34	94%	91%	90%	100%
Influenza Vaccine[1]	11	100%	63%	70%	100%
Initial Antibiotic Timing	49	92%	81%	80%	93%
Oxygenation Assessment	65	100%	99%	99%	100%
Pneumococcal Vaccine	42	88%	62%	69%	94%
Smoking Cessation Advice[1]	14	64%	80%	80%	100%
Surgical Infection Prevention					
Prophylactic Antibiotic Given	116	93%	74%	77%	95%
Prophylactic Antibiotic Selection	31	100%	91%	90%	100%
Prophylactic Antibiotic Stopped	112	46%	67%	72%	95%
Pregnancy Care					
Inpatient Neonatal Mortality	226	0.44%	-	-	-
Third or Fourth Degree Laceration	140	3.57%	3.89%	3.63%	3.27%

Perry Memorial Hospital

530 Park Avenue E
Princeton, IL 61356
Phone: 815-875-2811
Fax: 815-872-6006
URL: www.perry-memorial.org
Ownership: Government - State
Accredited: No
Emergency Services: Yes
Licensed Beds: 98

Key Personnel:

President/CEO. . . . . Robert Senneff
Chief Medical Staff. . . . . E Doran, MD
Emergency Room . . . . Dr. Earel Belford
Director Radiology . . . . Scott Hartman

Measure	Cases	This Hospital	State Average	U.S. Average	Top Hospital
Heart Attack Care					
ACE Inhibitor or ARB for LVSD[1]	3	100%	79%	82%	100%
Aspirin at Arrival[1]	16	75%	93%	92%	100%
Aspirin at Discharge[1]	11	55%	90%	90%	100%
Beta Blocker at Arrival[1]	16	62%	87%	87%	100%
Beta Blocker at Discharge[1]	11	82%	88%	90%	100%
Fibrinolytic Medication Timing	0	-	21%	31%	100%
PCI Within 90 Minutes of Arrival	0	-	47%	54%	95%
Smoking Cessation Advice	0	-	84%	88%	100%
Heart Failure Care					
ACE Inhibitor or ARB for LVSD[1]	9	67%	83%	82%	100%
Discharge Instructions	55	85%	67%	61%	93%
Evaluation of LVS Function	88	85%	88%	83%	99%
Smoking Cessation Advice[1]	4	100%	83%	82%	100%
Pneumonia Care					
Appropriate Initial Antibiotic	46	85%	83%	83%	94%
Blood Culture Timing[1]	22	95%	91%	90%	100%
Influenza Vaccine[1]	13	15%	63%	70%	100%
Initial Antibiotic Timing	59	97%	81%	80%	93%
Oxygenation Assessment	81	100%	99%	99%	100%
Pneumococcal Vaccine	58	24%	62%	69%	94%
Smoking Cessation Advice[1]	9	89%	80%	80%	100%
Surgical Infection Prevention					
Prophylactic Antibiotic Given[5]	-	-	74%	77%	95%
Prophylactic Antibiotic Selection[5]	-	-	91%	90%	100%
Prophylactic Antibiotic Stopped[5]	-	-	67%	72%	95%
Pregnancy Care					
Inpatient Neonatal Mortality	-	-	-	-	-
Third or Fourth Degree Laceration	-	-	3.89%	3.63%	3.27%

Blessing Hospital

Broadway at 11th Street
Quincy, IL 62305
Phone: 217-223-1200
Fax: 217-223-1200
E-mail: sfelde@blessinghospital.com
URL: www.blessinghealthsystem.org
Ownership: Voluntary non-profit - Other
Accredited: Yes
Emergency Services: Yes
Licensed Beds: 426

Key Personnel:

CEO. . . . . Maureen A Kahn
Surgery Director. . . . . Barb Hagmeier, RN
Supervisor Catheterization Laboratory . . . . Debbie Heinecke, RN
Infection Control Coordinator . . . . Carleen Orton, RN
Director Maternal-Child Services . . . . Joan Hynek, RN
Director Surgical Services . . . . Barb Hagmeier, RN
Director Respiratory SVS . . . . Jolene Beaber

Measure	Cases	This Hospital	State Average	U.S. Average	Top Hospital
Heart Attack Care					
ACE Inhibitor or ARB for LVSD	54	85%	79%	82%	100%
Aspirin at Arrival	206	98%	93%	92%	100%
Aspirin at Discharge	211	97%	90%	90%	100%
Beta Blocker at Arrival	152	95%	87%	87%	100%
Beta Blocker at Discharge	234	98%	88%	90%	100%
Fibrinolytic Medication Timing[1]	6	67%	21%	31%	100%
PCI Within 90 Minutes of Arrival[1]	8	88%	47%	54%	95%
Smoking Cessation Advice	90	96%	84%	88%	100%
Heart Failure Care					
ACE Inhibitor or ARB for LVSD	88	88%	83%	82%	100%
Discharge Instructions	226	64%	67%	61%	93%
Evaluation of LVS Function	325	84%	88%	83%	99%
Smoking Cessation Advice	54	91%	83%	82%	100%
Pneumonia Care					
Appropriate Initial Antibiotic	290	94%	83%	83%	94%
Blood Culture Timing	449	92%	91%	90%	100%
Influenza Vaccine	117	87%	63%	70%	100%
Initial Antibiotic Timing	519	87%	81%	80%	93%
Oxygenation Assessment	688	100%	99%	99%	100%
Pneumococcal Vaccine	479	87%	62%	69%	94%
Smoking Cessation Advice	149	87%	80%	80%	100%
Surgical Infection Prevention					
Prophylactic Antibiotic Given[3]	226	85%	74%	77%	95%
Prophylactic Antibiotic Selection	112	77%	91%	90%	100%
Prophylactic Antibiotic Stopped[3]	214	63%	67%	72%	95%
Pregnancy Care					
Inpatient Neonatal Mortality	-	-	-	-	-
Third or Fourth Degree Laceration	-	-	3.89%	3.63%	3.27%

Red Bud Regional Hospital

Alternate Name: Saint Clement Hospital
1 Saint Clement Boulevard
Red Bud, IL 62278
Phone: 618-282-3831
Fax: 618-282-6101
Ownership: Proprietary
Accredited: No
Emergency Services: Yes
Licensed Beds: 202

Key Personnel:

CEO/President. . . . . Bob Moore
Chief Medical Staff. . . . . Chung Khan
Emergency Room . . . . Bob Wagner
OB/GYN Womens Health. . . . . Susan Sviantek
Director of Pulmonary . . . . Linda Harbison

Measure	Cases	This Hospital	State Average	U.S. Average	Top Hospital
Heart Attack Care					
ACE Inhibitor or ARB for LVSD[3]	0	-	79%	82%	100%
Aspirin at Arrival[1,3]	1	100%	93%	92%	100%
Aspirin at Discharge[3]	0	-	90%	90%	100%
Beta Blocker at Arrival[1,3]	1	0%	87%	87%	100%
Beta Blocker at Discharge[3]	0	-	88%	90%	100%
Fibrinolytic Medication Timing[3]	0	-	21%	31%	100%
PCI Within 90 Minutes of Arrival	0	-	47%	54%	95%
Smoking Cessation Advice[3]	0	-	84%	88%	100%
Heart Failure Care					
ACE Inhibitor or ARB for LVSD[1]	8	75%	83%	82%	100%
Discharge Instructions	30	87%	67%	61%	93%

NOTE: Hospital profiles are in alphabetical order by state, then city, then hospital within the city; Rankings are sorted by rate in descending order and exclude hospitals with less than 25 cases; (1) The number of cases is too small (n<25) for purposes of reliably predicting hospital performance; (2) Measure reflects the hospital's indication that its submission was based upon a sample of its relevant discharges; (3) Rate reflects fewer than the maximum possible quarters of data for the measure; (4) Inaccurate information submitted and suppressed for one or more quarters; (5) No data is available from the hospital for this measure; Please refer to the User's Guide for a full explanation of data

Evaluation of LVS Function	61	87%	88%	83%	99%
Smoking Cessation Advice[1]	9	100%	83%	82%	100%
Pneumonia Care					
Appropriate Initial Antibiotic	42	98%	83%	83%	94%
Blood Culture Timing	52	98%	91%	90%	100%
Influenza Vaccine[1]	17	94%	63%	70%	100%
Initial Antibiotic Timing	63	89%	81%	80%	93%
Oxygenation Assessment	88	100%	99%	99%	100%
Pneumococcal Vaccine	51	78%	62%	69%	94%
Smoking Cessation Advice[1]	14	100%	80%	80%	100%
Surgical Infection Prevention					
Prophylactic Antibiotic Given[2,3]	29	62%	74%	77%	95%
Prophylactic Antibiotic Selection[1,2]	4	100%	91%	90%	100%
Prophylactic Antibiotic Stopped[2,3]	27	81%	67%	72%	95%
Pregnancy Care					
Inpatient Neonatal Mortality	-	-	-	-	-
Third or Fourth Degree Laceration	-	-	3.89%	3.63%	3.27%

Crawford Memorial Hospital

1000 N Allen Street
Robinson, IL 62454
E-mail: debbie.robinson@crawfordmh.org
URL: www.crawfordmh.com
Phone: 618-544-3131
Fax: 618-546-2600
Ownership: Govt - Hospital District or Authority
Accredited: Yes
Emergency Services: Yes
Licensed Beds: 93

Key Personnel:

CEO. . . . . Randy Simmons, MHA
Chief Medical Staff. . . . . Michael Elliott, MD

Measure	Cases	This Hospital	State Average	U.S. Average	Top Hospital
Heart Attack Care					
ACE Inhibitor or ARB for LVSD[1]	2	50%	79%	82%	100%
Aspirin at Arrival[1]	17	88%	93%	92%	100%
Aspirin at Discharge[1]	13	85%	90%	90%	100%
Beta Blocker at Arrival[1]	15	47%	87%	87%	100%
Beta Blocker at Discharge[1]	12	58%	88%	90%	100%
Fibrinolytic Medication Timing[3]	0	-	21%	31%	100%
PCI Within 90 Minutes of Arrival[5]	-	-	47%	54%	95%
Smoking Cessation Advice[1]	4	0%	84%	88%	100%
Heart Failure Care					
ACE Inhibitor or ARB for LVSD[1]	4	75%	83%	82%	100%
Discharge Instructions[1]	21	38%	67%	61%	93%
Evaluation of LVS Function	30	73%	88%	83%	99%
Smoking Cessation Advice[1]	5	0%	83%	82%	100%
Pneumonia Care					
Appropriate Initial Antibiotic[1,3]	8	62%	83%	83%	94%
Blood Culture Timing[1]	15	93%	91%	90%	100%
Influenza Vaccine[1]	8	62%	63%	70%	100%
Initial Antibiotic Timing	30	57%	81%	80%	93%
Oxygenation Assessment	35	94%	99%	99%	100%
Pneumococcal Vaccine	25	52%	62%	69%	94%
Smoking Cessation Advice[1]	7	43%	80%	80%	100%
Surgical Infection Prevention					
Prophylactic Antibiotic Given	67	72%	74%	77%	95%
Prophylactic Antibiotic Selection[1]	12	75%	91%	90%	100%
Prophylactic Antibiotic Stopped	63	51%	67%	72%	95%
Pregnancy Care					
Inpatient Neonatal Mortality	-	-	-	-	-
Third or Fourth Degree Laceration	-	-	3.89%	3.63%	3.27%

Rochelle Community Hospital

900 N 2nd Street
Rochelle, IL 61068
URL: www.rcha.net
Phone: 815-562-2181
Fax: 815-562-5474
Ownership: Voluntary non-profit - Private
Accredited: Yes
Emergency Services: Yes
Licensed Beds: 42

Key Personnel:

CEO. . . . . Greggory Olson
Chief Medical Staff. . . . . John Prabbaker, MD
Emergency Room . . . . Janet Lodico, RN
Infection Control. . . . . Dorrie Kasman

Measure	Cases	This Hospital	State Average	U.S. Average	Top Hospital
Heart Attack Care					
ACE Inhibitor or ARB for LVSD[3]	0	-	79%	82%	100%
Aspirin at Arrival[1,3]	3	67%	93%	92%	100%
Aspirin at Discharge[1,3]	2	100%	90%	90%	100%
Beta Blocker at Arrival[1,3]	3	100%	87%	87%	100%
Beta Blocker at Discharge[1,3]	2	100%	88%	90%	100%
Fibrinolytic Medication Timing[3]	0	-	21%	31%	100%
PCI Within 90 Minutes of Arrival	0	-	47%	54%	95%
Smoking Cessation Advice[3]	0	-	84%	88%	100%
Heart Failure Care					
ACE Inhibitor or ARB for LVSD[1,3]	4	50%	83%	82%	100%
Discharge Instructions[1,3]	17	47%	67%	61%	93%
Evaluation of LVS Function[1,3]	23	78%	88%	83%	99%
Smoking Cessation Advice[1,3]	1	0%	83%	82%	100%
Pneumonia Care					
Appropriate Initial Antibiotic[1,3]	22	82%	83%	83%	94%
Blood Culture Timing[1,3]	7	100%	91%	90%	100%
Influenza Vaccine[5]	-	-	63%	70%	100%
Initial Antibiotic Timing[3]	33	79%	81%	80%	93%
Oxygenation Assessment[3]	38	100%	99%	99%	100%
Pneumococcal Vaccine[1,3]	19	37%	62%	69%	94%
Smoking Cessation Advice[1,3]	10	30%	80%	80%	100%
Surgical Infection Prevention					
Prophylactic Antibiotic Given[1,3]	7	100%	74%	77%	95%
Prophylactic Antibiotic Selection[1]	7	100%	91%	90%	100%
Prophylactic Antibiotic Stopped[1,3]	7	100%	67%	72%	95%
Pregnancy Care					
Inpatient Neonatal Mortality	-	-	-	-	-
Third or Fourth Degree Laceration	-	-	3.89%	3.63%	3.27%

Trinity Medical Center

West Campus
2701 17th Street
Rock Island, IL 61201
URL: www.trinityqc.com
Phone: 309-779-5000
Fax: 309-779-2695
Ownership: Voluntary non-profit - Private
Accredited: No
Emergency Services: Yes
Licensed Beds: 349

Key Personnel:

Administrator . . . . Eric Crowell
Chief Medical Staff. . . . . Harry Wallner, MD
Emergency Room . . . . Jack Buzek, MD
Director Infection/Disease Control . . . . Marilynn Van Vliete, RN
CCU Spvg. Nurse . . . . Laurie Schultz, RN
OB/GYN Womens Health. . . . . Shashi Upadhya, MD
Chief Radiology . . . . Craig Tillman, MD

Measure	Cases	This Hospital	State Average	U.S. Average	Top Hospital
Heart Attack Care					
ACE Inhibitor or ARB for LVSD	82	87%	79%	82%	100%
Aspirin at Arrival	291	96%	93%	92%	100%
Aspirin at Discharge	394	94%	90%	90%	100%
Beta Blocker at Arrival	260	95%	87%	87%	100%
Beta Blocker at Discharge	371	95%	88%	90%	100%
Fibrinolytic Medication Timing	0	-	21%	31%	100%
PCI Within 90 Minutes of Arrival[1]	12	75%	47%	54%	95%
Smoking Cessation Advice	117	100%	84%	88%	100%
Heart Failure Care					
ACE Inhibitor or ARB for LVSD	173	81%	83%	82%	100%
Discharge Instructions	429	89%	67%	61%	93%
Evaluation of LVS Function	559	96%	88%	83%	99%
Smoking Cessation Advice	113	99%	83%	82%	100%
Pneumonia Care					
Appropriate Initial Antibiotic[2]	96	83%	83%	83%	94%
Blood Culture Timing[2]	91	95%	91%	90%	100%
Influenza Vaccine[2]	28	93%	63%	70%	100%
Initial Antibiotic Timing[2]	123	91%	81%	80%	93%
Oxygenation Assessment[2]	156	99%	99%	99%	100%
Pneumococcal Vaccine[2]	112	83%	62%	69%	94%
Smoking Cessation Advice[2]	47	96%	80%	80%	100%
Surgical Infection Prevention					
Prophylactic Antibiotic Given[2]	281	93%	74%	77%	95%

NOTE: Hospital profiles are in alphabetical order by state, then city, then hospital within the city; Rankings are sorted by rate in descending order and exclude hospitals with less than 25 cases; (1) The number of cases is too small (n<25) for purposes of reliably predicting hospital performance; (2) Measure reflects the hospital's indication that its submission was based upon a sample of its relevant discharges; (3) Rate reflects fewer than the maximum possible quarters of data for the measure; (4) Inaccurate information submitted and suppressed for one or more quarters; (5) No data is available from the hospital for this measure; Please refer to the User's Guide for a full explanation of data

Prophylactic Antibiotic Selection[2]	66	95%	91%	90%	100%
Prophylactic Antibiotic Stopped[2]	269	74%	67%	72%	95%
Pregnancy Care					
Inpatient Neonatal Mortality	-	-	-	-	-
Third or Fourth Degree Laceration	-	-	3.89%	3.63%	3.27%

Rockford Memorial Hospital

2400 N Rockton Avenue
Rockford, IL 61103
URL: www.rhsnet.org
Ownership: Voluntary non-profit - Private
Emergency Services: Yes

Phone: 815-971-5000
Fax: 815-971-6167
Accredited: Yes
Licensed Beds: 396

Key Personnel:
President/CEO . . . . Gary Kaatz
Emergency Room . . . . Dennis Veharra, MD
Chief Medical Officer . . . . Milton Schmitt, MD

Measure	Cases	This Hospital	State Average	U.S. Average	Top Hospital
Heart Attack Care					
ACE Inhibitor or ARB for LVSD	54	85%	79%	82%	100%
Aspirin at Arrival	196	98%	93%	92%	100%
Aspirin at Discharge	272	97%	90%	90%	100%
Beta Blocker at Arrival	189	95%	87%	87%	100%
Beta Blocker at Discharge	284	100%	88%	90%	100%
Fibrinolytic Medication Timing	0	-	21%	31%	100%
PCI Within 90 Minutes of Arrival[1]	8	100%	47%	54%	95%
Smoking Cessation Advice	98	93%	84%	88%	100%
Heart Failure Care					
ACE Inhibitor or ARB for LVSD[2]	108	91%	83%	82%	100%
Discharge Instructions[2]	239	90%	67%	61%	93%
Evaluation of LVS Function[2]	320	98%	88%	83%	99%
Smoking Cessation Advice[2]	62	98%	83%	82%	100%
Pneumonia Care					
Appropriate Initial Antibiotic[2]	103	92%	83%	83%	94%
Blood Culture Timing[2]	158	97%	91%	90%	100%
Influenza Vaccine[2]	31	77%	63%	70%	100%
Initial Antibiotic Timing[2]	192	80%	81%	80%	93%
Oxygenation Assessment[2]	238	100%	99%	99%	100%
Pneumococcal Vaccine[2]	159	67%	62%	69%	94%
Smoking Cessation Advice[2]	51	88%	80%	80%	100%
Surgical Infection Prevention					
Prophylactic Antibiotic Given[2,3]	506	89%	74%	77%	95%
Prophylactic Antibiotic Selection[2]	106	97%	91%	90%	100%
Prophylactic Antibiotic Stopped[2,3]	498	85%	67%	72%	95%
Pregnancy Care					
Inpatient Neonatal Mortality	-	-	-	-	-
Third or Fourth Degree Laceration	-	-	3.89%	3.63%	3.27%

Saint Anthony Medical Center

5666 E State Street
Rockford, IL 61108

URL: www.osfhealth.com
Ownership: Voluntary non-profit - Church
Emergency Services: Yes

Toll-Free: 800-343-3185
Phone: 815-226-2000
Fax: 815-395-5449
Accredited: Yes
Licensed Beds: 254

Key Personnel:
President/CEO . . . . David A Schertz
Chief Medical Staff . . . . Robert White, MD
Cardiac Lab . . . . Anne Hammes
Catheterization Lab . . . . Darcie Chamberlain
Emergency Room . . . . Lisa Marie Johnson
Infection Control . . . . Larry Brown, RN
ICU . . . . Laura Nie, RN
Intensive Coronary Care . . . . Brenda Schroeder, RN
Medical/Surgical Nursing . . . . Carol King, RN
OB/GYN Women's Health . . . . RE Field, MD
Respiratory/Cardiopulmonary . . . . Ken Templeton

Measure	Cases	This Hospital	State Average	U.S. Average	Top Hospital
Heart Attack Care					
ACE Inhibitor or ARB for LVSD	69	94%	79%	82%	100%
Aspirin at Arrival	228	99%	93%	92%	100%
Aspirin at Discharge	321	99%	90%	90%	100%
Beta Blocker at Arrival	205	97%	87%	87%	100%
Beta Blocker at Discharge	306	97%	88%	90%	100%
Fibrinolytic Medication Timing	0	-	21%	31%	100%
PCI Within 90 Minutes of Arrival[1]	11	45%	47%	54%	95%
Smoking Cessation Advice	104	98%	84%	88%	100%
Heart Failure Care					
ACE Inhibitor or ARB for LVSD	146	90%	83%	82%	100%
Discharge Instructions	302	88%	67%	61%	93%
Evaluation of LVS Function	406	99%	88%	83%	99%
Smoking Cessation Advice	56	96%	83%	82%	100%
Pneumonia Care					
Appropriate Initial Antibiotic	195	84%	83%	83%	94%
Blood Culture Timing	193	94%	91%	90%	100%
Influenza Vaccine	47	89%	63%	70%	100%
Initial Antibiotic Timing	290	79%	81%	80%	93%
Oxygenation Assessment	347	99%	99%	99%	100%
Pneumococcal Vaccine	239	80%	62%	69%	94%
Smoking Cessation Advice	53	92%	80%	80%	100%
Surgical Infection Prevention					
Prophylactic Antibiotic Given	1,107	92%	74%	77%	95%
Prophylactic Antibiotic Selection	280	99%	91%	90%	100%
Prophylactic Antibiotic Stopped	1,077	85%	67%	72%	95%
Pregnancy Care					
Inpatient Neonatal Mortality	-	-	-	-	-
Third or Fourth Degree Laceration	-	-	3.89%	3.63%	3.27%

Swedish American Hospital

1401 E State Street
Rockford, IL 61104
E-mail: webmaster@swedishamerican.org
URL: www.swedishamerican.org
Ownership: Voluntary non-profit - Other
Emergency Services: Yes

Phone: 815-968-4400
Fax: 815-961-2445
Accredited: Yes
Licensed Beds: 357

Key Personnel:
Administrator/President . . . . Robert B Klint, MD
Chief Medical Staff . . . . Lee Bach, MD
Chief Catheterization Laboratory . . . . Ashoha Nautujal, MD
Emergency Room . . . . Robert Porter, MD
Director Infection/Disease Control . . . . Gary Rifkin, MD
CCU Spvg. Nurse . . . . Kathy Arnold
OB/GYN Womens Health . . . . Richard Ragsdale, MD
Chief Radiology . . . . Steven Rodman, MD
Director Respiratory Therapy . . . . Ken Scrivano

Measure	Cases	This Hospital	State Average	U.S. Average	Top Hospital
Heart Attack Care					
ACE Inhibitor or ARB for LVSD	80	94%	79%	82%	100%
Aspirin at Arrival	234	99%	93%	92%	100%
Aspirin at Discharge	290	100%	90%	90%	100%
Beta Blocker at Arrival	135	95%	87%	87%	100%
Beta Blocker at Discharge	327	99%	88%	90%	100%
Fibrinolytic Medication Timing[1]	1	0%	21%	31%	100%
PCI Within 90 Minutes of Arrival[1]	13	54%	47%	54%	95%
Smoking Cessation Advice	146	97%	84%	88%	100%
Heart Failure Care					
ACE Inhibitor or ARB for LVSD	209	94%	83%	82%	100%
Discharge Instructions	367	97%	67%	61%	93%
Evaluation of LVS Function	470	98%	88%	83%	99%
Smoking Cessation Advice	88	93%	83%	82%	100%
Pneumonia Care					
Appropriate Initial Antibiotic	174	91%	83%	83%	94%
Blood Culture Timing	142	93%	91%	90%	100%
Influenza Vaccine	35	69%	63%	70%	100%
Initial Antibiotic Timing	226	84%	81%	80%	93%
Oxygenation Assessment	275	100%	99%	99%	100%
Pneumococcal Vaccine	169	76%	62%	69%	94%
Smoking Cessation Advice	75	97%	80%	80%	100%
Surgical Infection Prevention					
Prophylactic Antibiotic Given	1,114	94%	74%	77%	95%
Prophylactic Antibiotic Selection	247	96%	91%	90%	100%
Prophylactic Antibiotic Stopped	1,100	68%	67%	72%	95%
Pregnancy Care					
Inpatient Neonatal Mortality	2,300	0.17%	-	-	-

NOTE: Hospital profiles are in alphabetical order by state, then city, then hospital within the city; Rankings are sorted by rate in descending order and exclude hospitals with less than 25 cases; (1) The number of cases is too small (n<25) for purposes of reliably predicting hospital performance; (2) Measure reflects the hospital's indication that its submission was based upon a sample of its relevant discharges; (3) Rate reflects fewer than the maximum possible quarters of data for the measure; (4) Inaccurate information submitted and suppressed for one or more quarters; (5) No data is available from the hospital for this measure; Please refer to the User's Guide for a full explanation of data

Third or Fourth Degree Laceration	1,572	3.82%	3.89%	3.63%	3.27%

Hardin County General Hospital

Ferrell Road
Rosiclare, IL 62982
Ownership: Voluntary non-profit - Private
Emergency Services: No

Phone: 618-285-6634
Fax: 618-285-6651
Accredited: No
Licensed Beds: 48

Key Personnel:
CEO. . . . . Roby Williams
Chief Medical Staff. . . . . Marcos Sunga, MD
Emergency Room . . . . Donna Oxford

Measure	Cases	This Hospital	State Average	U.S. Average	Top Hospital
Heart Attack Care					
ACE Inhibitor or ARB for LVSD[5]	-	-	79%	82%	100%
Aspirin at Arrival[5]	-	-	93%	92%	100%
Aspirin at Discharge[5]	-	-	90%	90%	100%
Beta Blocker at Arrival[5]	-	-	87%	87%	100%
Beta Blocker at Discharge[5]	-	-	88%	90%	100%
Fibrinolytic Medication Timing[5]	-	-	21%	31%	100%
PCI Within 90 Minutes of Arrival[5]	-	-	47%	54%	95%
Smoking Cessation Advice[5]	-	-	84%	88%	100%
Heart Failure Care					
ACE Inhibitor or ARB for LVSD[1]	7	100%	83%	82%	100%
Discharge Instructions	38	100%	67%	61%	93%
Evaluation of LVS Function	51	100%	88%	83%	99%
Smoking Cessation Advice[1]	8	100%	83%	82%	100%
Pneumonia Care					
Appropriate Initial Antibiotic	26	81%	83%	83%	94%
Blood Culture Timing	34	100%	91%	90%	100%
Influenza Vaccine[1]	8	100%	63%	70%	100%
Initial Antibiotic Timing	46	93%	81%	80%	93%
Oxygenation Assessment	55	96%	99%	99%	100%
Pneumococcal Vaccine	34	100%	62%	69%	94%
Smoking Cessation Advice[1]	13	100%	80%	80%	100%
Surgical Infection Prevention					
Prophylactic Antibiotic Given[5]	-	-	74%	77%	95%
Prophylactic Antibiotic Selection[5]	-	-	91%	90%	100%
Prophylactic Antibiotic Stopped[5]	-	-	67%	72%	95%
Pregnancy Care					
Inpatient Neonatal Mortality	-	-	-	-	-
Third or Fourth Degree Laceration	-	-	3.89%	3.63%	3.27%

Culbertson Memorial Hospital

Alternate Name: Sarah D Culbertson Memorial Hospital
238 S Congress
Rushville, IL 62681
E-mail: CMH@CMHospital.com
URL: www.cmhospital.com
Ownership: Govt - Hospital District or Authority
Emergency Services: Yes

Phone: 217-322-4321
Fax: 217-322-6425
Accredited: No
Licensed Beds: 64

Key Personnel:
CEO. . . . . David Sniff
Chief Medical Staff. . . . . Lisa Downs, RN
Emergency Room . . . . Lisa Downs, RN

Measure	Cases	This Hospital	State Average	U.S. Average	Top Hospital
Heart Attack Care					
ACE Inhibitor or ARB for LVSD[5]	-	-	79%	82%	100%
Aspirin at Arrival[5]	-	-	93%	92%	100%
Aspirin at Discharge[5]	-	-	90%	90%	100%
Beta Blocker at Arrival[5]	-	-	87%	87%	100%
Beta Blocker at Discharge[5]	-	-	88%	90%	100%
Fibrinolytic Medication Timing[5]	-	-	21%	31%	100%
PCI Within 90 Minutes of Arrival[5]	-	-	47%	54%	95%
Smoking Cessation Advice[5]	-	-	84%	88%	100%
Heart Failure Care					
ACE Inhibitor or ARB for LVSD[1]	7	71%	83%	82%	100%
Discharge Instructions[1]	19	63%	67%	61%	93%
Evaluation of LVS Function	34	94%	88%	83%	99%
Smoking Cessation Advice[1]	4	75%	83%	82%	100%
Pneumonia Care					
Appropriate Initial Antibiotic[1]	24	92%	83%	83%	94%
Blood Culture Timing[1]	13	92%	91%	90%	100%
Influenza Vaccine[1]	10	100%	63%	70%	100%
Initial Antibiotic Timing	38	84%	81%	80%	93%
Oxygenation Assessment	51	100%	99%	99%	100%
Pneumococcal Vaccine	35	97%	62%	69%	94%
Smoking Cessation Advice[1]	7	100%	80%	80%	100%
Surgical Infection Prevention					
Prophylactic Antibiotic Given[5]	-	-	74%	77%	95%
Prophylactic Antibiotic Selection[5]	-	-	91%	90%	100%
Prophylactic Antibiotic Stopped[5]	-	-	67%	72%	95%
Pregnancy Care					
Inpatient Neonatal Mortality	-	-	-	-	-
Third or Fourth Degree Laceration	-	-	3.89%	3.63%	3.27%

Salem Township Hospital

Alternate Name: Public Hospital of the Town of Salem
1201 Ricker Drive
Salem, IL 62881
Ownership: Voluntary non-profit - Other
Emergency Services: Yes

Phone: 618-548-3194
Fax: 618-548-6831
Accredited: Yes
Licensed Beds: 46

Key Personnel:
President/CEO . . . . Rithilll Rennegarve
Chief Medical Staff. . . . . A T Aguilar
Emergency Room Director. . . . . Roberto Parcias
Director Infection/Disease Control . . . . Wilma Gott, RN, B
Chief Radiology . . . . Preecha Tawjareon, MD
Director Respiratory Therapy . . . . Chris Jahn, RT

Measure	Cases	This Hospital	State Average	U.S. Average	Top Hospital
Heart Attack Care					
ACE Inhibitor or ARB for LVSD	0	-	79%	82%	100%
Aspirin at Arrival[1]	8	88%	93%	92%	100%
Aspirin at Discharge[1]	8	88%	90%	90%	100%
Beta Blocker at Arrival[1]	7	86%	87%	87%	100%
Beta Blocker at Discharge[1]	8	75%	88%	90%	100%
Fibrinolytic Medication Timing	0	-	21%	31%	100%
PCI Within 90 Minutes of Arrival	0	-	47%	54%	95%
Smoking Cessation Advice	0	-	84%	88%	100%
Heart Failure Care					
ACE Inhibitor or ARB for LVSD[1]	6	67%	83%	82%	100%
Discharge Instructions	30	80%	67%	61%	93%
Evaluation of LVS Function	47	34%	88%	83%	99%
Smoking Cessation Advice[1]	6	83%	83%	82%	100%
Pneumonia Care					
Appropriate Initial Antibiotic	60	77%	83%	83%	94%
Blood Culture Timing[1]	20	85%	91%	90%	100%
Influenza Vaccine[1]	17	0%	63%	70%	100%
Initial Antibiotic Timing	87	77%	81%	80%	93%
Oxygenation Assessment	90	90%	99%	99%	100%
Pneumococcal Vaccine	71	3%	62%	69%	94%
Smoking Cessation Advice[1]	10	80%	80%	80%	100%
Surgical Infection Prevention					
Prophylactic Antibiotic Given[1,3]	4	25%	74%	77%	95%
Prophylactic Antibiotic Selection[1]	2	100%	91%	90%	100%
Prophylactic Antibiotic Stopped[1,3]	4	100%	67%	72%	95%
Pregnancy Care					
Inpatient Neonatal Mortality	-	-	-	-	-
Third or Fourth Degree Laceration	-	-	3.89%	3.63%	3.27%

Valley West Community Hospital

Alternate Name: Sandwich Community Hospital
11 E Pleasant Avenue
Sandwich, IL 60548
E-mail: sandhosp@snd.softfarm.com/sandhosp
URL: www.snd.softfarm.com/sandhosp
Ownership: Voluntary non-profit - Other
Emergency Services: Yes

Phone: 815-786-8484
Fax: 815-786-3705
Accredited: No
Licensed Beds: 84

Key Personnel:
CEO. . . . . Brad Topple
Chief Medical Staff. . . . . Martin Brauweiler
Emergency Room . . . . Richard Arribiello
Emergency Room . . . . Victor Garber, MD

NOTE: Hospital profiles are in alphabetical order by state, then city, then hospital within the city; Rankings are sorted by rate in descending order and exclude hospitals with less than 25 cases; (1) The number of cases is too small (n<25) for purposes of reliably predicting hospital performance; (2) Measure reflects the hospital's indication that its submission was based upon a sample of its relevant discharges; (3) Rate reflects fewer than the maximum possible quarters of data for the measure; (4) Inaccurate information submitted and suppressed for one or more quarters; (5) No data is available from the hospital for this measure; Please refer to the User's Guide for a full explanation of data

Director Infection/Disease Control . . . . Carol Vignali
Director Medical/Surgical Nursing . . . . Pam Michel
Chief Radiology . . . . Burji Singh, MD
Director Respiratory Therapy . . . . Paul Rothenbach

Measure	Cases	This Hospital	State Average	U.S. Average	Top Hospital
Heart Attack Care					
ACE Inhibitor or ARB for LVSD[1]	1	0%	79%	82%	100%
Aspirin at Arrival[1]	5	100%	93%	92%	100%
Aspirin at Discharge[1]	5	100%	90%	90%	100%
Beta Blocker at Arrival[1]	3	67%	87%	87%	100%
Beta Blocker at Discharge[1]	2	0%	88%	90%	100%
Fibrinolytic Medication Timing[1]	1	0%	21%	31%	100%
PCI Within 90 Minutes of Arrival	0	-	47%	54%	95%
Smoking Cessation Advice[1]	2	100%	84%	88%	100%
Heart Failure Care					
ACE Inhibitor or ARB for LVSD[1]	3	67%	83%	82%	100%
Discharge Instructions[1]	22	68%	67%	61%	93%
Evaluation of LVS Function	27	89%	88%	83%	99%
Smoking Cessation Advice[1]	4	100%	83%	82%	100%
Pneumonia Care					
Appropriate Initial Antibiotic[2]	46	80%	83%	83%	94%
Blood Culture Timing[2]	28	93%	91%	90%	100%
Influenza Vaccine[1]	12	75%	63%	70%	100%
Initial Antibiotic Timing[1,2]	20	85%	81%	80%	93%
Oxygenation Assessment[2]	63	100%	99%	99%	100%
Pneumococcal Vaccine[2]	35	83%	62%	69%	94%
Smoking Cessation Advice[1,2]	11	91%	80%	80%	100%
Surgical Infection Prevention					
Prophylactic Antibiotic Given[3]	35	83%	74%	77%	95%
Prophylactic Antibiotic Selection[1]	10	70%	91%	90%	100%
Prophylactic Antibiotic Stopped[3]	34	26%	67%	72%	95%
Pregnancy Care					
Inpatient Neonatal Mortality	-	-	-	-	-
Third or Fourth Degree Laceration	-	-	3.89%	3.63%	3.27%

Shelby Memorial Hospital

200 S Cedar
Shelbyville, IL 62565
Ownership: Voluntary non-profit - Private
Emergency Services: No
Phone: 217-774-3961
Fax: 217-774-5100
Accredited: Yes
Licensed Beds: 54

Key Personnel:

Administrator . . . . John Bennett
Emergency Room . . . . U Dauz, MD
Director Infection/Disease Control . . . . Meredith Barnes
Director Medical/Surgical Nursing . . . . Kelle Endris, RN
Chief Radiology . . . . Lynn Turner, MD
Director Respiratory Therapy . . . . Gary Blurton

Measure	Cases	This Hospital	State Average	U.S. Average	Top Hospital
Heart Attack Care					
ACE Inhibitor or ARB for LVSD[1,3]	1	100%	79%	82%	100%
Aspirin at Arrival[1,3]	1	100%	93%	92%	100%
Aspirin at Discharge[1,3]	1	100%	90%	90%	100%
Beta Blocker at Arrival[1,3]	1	100%	87%	87%	100%
Beta Blocker at Discharge[1,3]	1	100%	88%	90%	100%
Fibrinolytic Medication Timing[3]	0	-	21%	31%	100%
PCI Within 90 Minutes of Arrival[5]	-	-	47%	54%	95%
Smoking Cessation Advice[3]	0	-	84%	88%	100%
Heart Failure Care					
ACE Inhibitor or ARB for LVSD[1]	15	100%	83%	82%	100%
Discharge Instructions	25	56%	67%	61%	93%
Evaluation of LVS Function	104	91%	88%	83%	99%
Smoking Cessation Advice[1]	3	67%	83%	82%	100%
Pneumonia Care					
Appropriate Initial Antibiotic	36	72%	83%	83%	94%
Blood Culture Timing[1]	17	100%	91%	90%	100%
Influenza Vaccine[4,5]	-	-	63%	70%	100%
Initial Antibiotic Timing	42	88%	81%	80%	93%
Oxygenation Assessment	72	100%	99%	99%	100%
Pneumococcal Vaccine	52	65%	62%	69%	94%
Smoking Cessation Advice[1]	11	82%	80%	80%	100%

Measure	Cases	This Hospital	State Average	U.S. Average	Top Hospital
Surgical Infection Prevention					
Prophylactic Antibiotic Given[1,3]	3	33%	74%	77%	95%
Prophylactic Antibiotic Selection[1]	3	100%	91%	90%	100%
Prophylactic Antibiotic Stopped[1,3]	3	100%	67%	72%	95%
Pregnancy Care					
Inpatient Neonatal Mortality	-	-	-	-	-
Third or Fourth Degree Laceration	-	-	3.89%	3.63%	3.27%

Genesis Medical Center-Illini Campus

801 Illini Road
Silvis, IL 61282
Ownership: Voluntary non-profit - Private
Emergency Services: Yes
Phone: 309-792-9363
Fax: 309-792-4274
Accredited: Yes
Licensed Beds: 150

Key Personnel:

CEO. . . . . Charles Bruhn
Chief of Medical Staff. Thomas VonGilliern, MD
Cardiology Director . . . . Andy Nelson
Emergency Room . . . . Kathy Christofferson
Emergency Room . . . . Janet Eckhart, RN
Infection Control. . . . . Anne Lewis
Director of Respiratory . . . . Andy Nelson

Measure	Cases	This Hospital	State Average	U.S. Average	Top Hospital
Heart Attack Care					
ACE Inhibitor or ARB for LVSD	66	79%	79%	82%	100%
Aspirin at Arrival	99	94%	93%	92%	100%
Aspirin at Discharge	103	86%	90%	90%	100%
Beta Blocker at Arrival	90	91%	87%	87%	100%
Beta Blocker at Discharge	101	89%	88%	90%	100%
Fibrinolytic Medication Timing	0	-	21%	31%	100%
PCI Within 90 Minutes of Arrival[1]	5	40%	47%	54%	95%
Smoking Cessation Advice	43	81%	84%	88%	100%
Heart Failure Care					
ACE Inhibitor or ARB for LVSD	59	80%	83%	82%	100%
Discharge Instructions	150	88%	67%	61%	93%
Evaluation of LVS Function	207	88%	88%	83%	99%
Smoking Cessation Advice	39	90%	83%	82%	100%
Pneumonia Care					
Appropriate Initial Antibiotic	90	72%	83%	83%	94%
Blood Culture Timing	69	84%	91%	90%	100%
Influenza Vaccine	26	62%	63%	70%	100%
Initial Antibiotic Timing	127	71%	81%	80%	93%
Oxygenation Assessment	149	100%	99%	99%	100%
Pneumococcal Vaccine	100	72%	62%	69%	94%
Smoking Cessation Advice	37	70%	80%	80%	100%
Surgical Infection Prevention					
Prophylactic Antibiotic Given[3]	92	96%	74%	77%	95%
Prophylactic Antibiotic Selection	92	99%	91%	90%	100%
Prophylactic Antibiotic Stopped[3]	91	73%	67%	72%	95%
Pregnancy Care					
Inpatient Neonatal Mortality	780	0.00%	-	-	-
Third or Fourth Degree Laceration	545	3.49%	3.89%	3.63%	3.27%

Rush North Shore Medical Center

9600 Gross Point Road
Skokie, IL 60076
Ownership: Voluntary non-profit - Other
Emergency Services: Yes
Phone: 847-677-9600
Fax: 847-933-6439
Accredited: Yes
Licensed Beds: 268

Key Personnel:

CEO. . . . . James Frankenbach
Director Respiratory Therapy . . . . Sue Victor

Measure	Cases	This Hospital	State Average	U.S. Average	Top Hospital
Heart Attack Care					
ACE Inhibitor or ARB for LVSD[1]	22	82%	79%	82%	100%
Aspirin at Arrival	106	96%	93%	92%	100%
Aspirin at Discharge	95	97%	90%	90%	100%
Beta Blocker at Arrival	86	92%	87%	87%	100%
Beta Blocker at Discharge	99	92%	88%	90%	100%
Fibrinolytic Medication Timing	0	-	21%	31%	100%
PCI Within 90 Minutes of Arrival[1]	3	33%	47%	54%	95%
Smoking Cessation Advice[1]	12	92%	84%	88%	100%

NOTE: Hospital profiles are in alphabetical order by state, then city, then hospital within the city; Rankings are sorted by rate in descending order and exclude hospitals with less than 25 cases; (1) The number of cases is too small (n<25) for purposes of reliably predicting hospital performance; (2) Measure reflects the hospital's indication that its submission was based upon a sample of its relevant discharges; (3) Rate reflects fewer than the maximum possible quarters of data for the measure; (4) Inaccurate information submitted and suppressed for one or more quarters; (5) No data is available from the hospital for this measure; Please refer to the User's Guide for a full explanation of data

Measure	Cases	This Hospital	State Average	U.S. Average	Top Hospital
Heart Failure Care					
ACE Inhibitor or ARB for LVSD	146	79%	83%	82%	100%
Discharge Instructions	285	45%	67%	61%	93%
Evaluation of LVS Function	418	96%	88%	83%	99%
Smoking Cessation Advice[1]	21	81%	83%	82%	100%
Pneumonia Care					
Appropriate Initial Antibiotic	138	80%	83%	83%	94%
Blood Culture Timing	156	96%	91%	90%	100%
Influenza Vaccine	47	60%	63%	70%	100%
Initial Antibiotic Timing	233	85%	81%	80%	93%
Oxygenation Assessment	278	100%	99%	99%	100%
Pneumococcal Vaccine	213	58%	62%	69%	94%
Smoking Cessation Advice	25	60%	80%	80%	100%
Surgical Infection Prevention					
Prophylactic Antibiotic Given[2,3]	194	96%	74%	77%	95%
Prophylactic Antibiotic Selection[2]	68	100%	91%	90%	100%
Prophylactic Antibiotic Stopped[2,3]	192	88%	67%	72%	95%
Pregnancy Care					
Inpatient Neonatal Mortality	-	-	-	-	-
Third or Fourth Degree Laceration	-	-	3.89%	3.63%	3.27%

Sparta Community Hospital

818 E Broadway
Sparta, IL 62286
E-mail: hertzingp@spartahospital.com
URL: www.spartahospital.com
Ownership: Govt - Hospital District or Authority
Emergency Services: Yes

Phone: 618-443-2177
Fax: 618-443-1383
Accredited: Yes
Licensed Beds: 39

Key Personnel:

Administrator . . . . Joann Emge
Chief Medical Staff. . . . . Wim Sippo, MD
Emergency Room . . . . Sharon Hall, MD
Director Infection/Disease Control . . . . Donna Chappell, RN
Director Medical/Surgical Nursing . . . . Ruth Holloway, RN
OB/GYN Womens Health. . . . . MD George Lukats, MD
Chief Radiology . . . . Josh Greten
Director Respiratory Therapy . . . . Betty Birchler

Measure	Cases	This Hospital	State Average	U.S. Average	Top Hospital
Heart Attack Care					
ACE Inhibitor or ARB for LVSD[3]	0	-	79%	82%	100%
Aspirin at Arrival[1,3]	3	100%	93%	92%	100%
Aspirin at Discharge[1,3]	2	50%	90%	90%	100%
Beta Blocker at Arrival[1,3]	4	50%	87%	87%	100%
Beta Blocker at Discharge[1,3]	2	50%	88%	90%	100%
Fibrinolytic Medication Timing[3]	0	-	21%	31%	100%
PCI Within 90 Minutes of Arrival	0	-	47%	54%	95%
Smoking Cessation Advice[3]	0	-	84%	88%	100%
Heart Failure Care					
ACE Inhibitor or ARB for LVSD[1]	13	77%	83%	82%	100%
Discharge Instructions	26	73%	67%	61%	93%
Evaluation of LVS Function	39	82%	88%	83%	99%
Smoking Cessation Advice[1]	2	100%	83%	82%	100%
Pneumonia Care					
Appropriate Initial Antibiotic	28	75%	83%	83%	94%
Blood Culture Timing	25	84%	91%	90%	100%
Influenza Vaccine[1]	11	73%	63%	70%	100%
Initial Antibiotic Timing	45	73%	81%	80%	93%
Oxygenation Assessment	52	100%	99%	99%	100%
Pneumococcal Vaccine	32	81%	62%	69%	94%
Smoking Cessation Advice[1]	8	100%	80%	80%	100%
Surgical Infection Prevention					
Prophylactic Antibiotic Given[5]	-	-	74%	77%	95%
Prophylactic Antibiotic Selection[5]	-	-	91%	90%	100%
Prophylactic Antibiotic Stopped[5]	-	-	67%	72%	95%
Pregnancy Care					
Inpatient Neonatal Mortality	-	-	-	-	-
Third or Fourth Degree Laceration	-	-	3.89%	3.63%	3.27%

Saint Margaret's Hospital

600 E 1st Street
Spring Valley, IL 61362
E-mail: hrdir@st-margarets.com
Ownership: Voluntary non-profit - Church
Emergency Services: Yes

Phone: 815-664-5311
Fax: 815-664-1608
Accredited: Yes
Licensed Beds: 155

Key Personnel:

President/CEO. . . . . Tim Muntz
Chief of Medical Staff. . . . . Marshal Cummings

Measure	Cases	This Hospital	State Average	U.S. Average	Top Hospital
Heart Attack Care					
ACE Inhibitor or ARB for LVSD[1]	1	0%	79%	82%	100%
Aspirin at Arrival[1]	4	100%	93%	92%	100%
Aspirin at Discharge[1]	3	100%	90%	90%	100%
Beta Blocker at Arrival[1]	7	86%	87%	87%	100%
Beta Blocker at Discharge[1]	6	83%	88%	90%	100%
Fibrinolytic Medication Timing[1]	3	33%	21%	31%	100%
PCI Within 90 Minutes of Arrival	0	-	47%	54%	95%
Smoking Cessation Advice	0	-	84%	88%	100%
Heart Failure Care					
ACE Inhibitor or ARB for LVSD[1]	22	91%	83%	82%	100%
Discharge Instructions	74	68%	67%	61%	93%
Evaluation of LVS Function	98	93%	88%	83%	99%
Smoking Cessation Advice[1]	11	82%	83%	82%	100%
Pneumonia Care					
Appropriate Initial Antibiotic	70	77%	83%	83%	94%
Blood Culture Timing	81	94%	91%	90%	100%
Influenza Vaccine[1]	21	71%	63%	70%	100%
Initial Antibiotic Timing	128	91%	81%	80%	93%
Oxygenation Assessment	168	100%	99%	99%	100%
Pneumococcal Vaccine	108	32%	62%	69%	94%
Smoking Cessation Advice	25	68%	80%	80%	100%
Surgical Infection Prevention					
Prophylactic Antibiotic Given	244	89%	74%	77%	95%
Prophylactic Antibiotic Selection	53	98%	91%	90%	100%
Prophylactic Antibiotic Stopped	239	31%	67%	72%	95%
Pregnancy Care					
Inpatient Neonatal Mortality	-	-	-	-	-
Third or Fourth Degree Laceration	-	-	3.89%	3.63%	3.27%

Memorial Medical Center

701 N 1st Street
Springfield, IL 62781
URL: www.memorialmedical.com
Ownership: Voluntary non-profit - Private
Emergency Services: Yes

Phone: 217-788-3000
Fax: 217-788-5594
Accredited: Yes
Licensed Beds: 562

Key Personnel:

President/CEO. . . . . Robert T Clarke
Chief Medical Staff. . . . . Robert Vautrain, MD
Administrator . . . . Charles D Callahan, PhD
Executive Director . . . . Barb Sullivan
Director Infection/Disease Control . . . . Margaret Roth, RN
Supervising Nurse Coronary Care Unit . . . . Donna Crompton, RN
Respiratory/Cardiopulmonary. . . . . Karen Baur
VP . . . . Jim Brote

Measure	Cases	This Hospital	State Average	U.S. Average	Top Hospital
Heart Attack Care					
ACE Inhibitor or ARB for LVSD	128	95%	79%	82%	100%
Aspirin at Arrival	295	98%	93%	92%	100%
Aspirin at Discharge	507	99%	90%	90%	100%
Beta Blocker at Arrival	255	94%	87%	87%	100%
Beta Blocker at Discharge	539	99%	88%	90%	100%
Fibrinolytic Medication Timing	0	-	21%	31%	100%
PCI Within 90 Minutes of Arrival[1]	16	81%	47%	54%	95%
Smoking Cessation Advice	201	100%	84%	88%	100%
Heart Failure Care					
ACE Inhibitor or ARB for LVSD	207	95%	83%	82%	100%
Discharge Instructions	400	90%	67%	61%	93%
Evaluation of LVS Function	504	100%	88%	83%	99%
Smoking Cessation Advice	84	100%	83%	82%	100%
Pneumonia Care					

NOTE: Hospital profiles are in alphabetical order by state, then city, then hospital within the city; Rankings are sorted by rate in descending order and exclude hospitals with less than 25 cases; (1) The number of cases is too small (n<25) for purposes of reliably predicting hospital performance; (2) Measure reflects the hospital's indication that its submission was based upon a sample of its relevant discharges; (3) Rate reflects fewer than the maximum possible quarters of data for the measure; (4) Inaccurate information submitted and suppressed for one or more quarters; (5) No data is available from the hospital for this measure; Please refer to the User's Guide for a full explanation of data

Appropriate Initial Antibiotic	261	91%	83%	83%	94%
Blood Culture Timing	331	84%	91%	90%	100%
Influenza Vaccine	81	78%	63%	70%	100%
Initial Antibiotic Timing	433	83%	81%	80%	93%
Oxygenation Assessment	561	100%	99%	99%	100%
Pneumococcal Vaccine	358	77%	62%	69%	94%
Smoking Cessation Advice	144	100%	80%	80%	100%
Surgical Infection Prevention					
Prophylactic Antibiotic Given[2]	1,496	94%	74%	77%	95%
Prophylactic Antibiotic Selection[2]	84	88%	91%	90%	100%
Prophylactic Antibiotic Stopped[2]	1,456	93%	67%	72%	95%
Pregnancy Care					
Inpatient Neonatal Mortality	-	-	-	-	-
Third or Fourth Degree Laceration	-	-	3.89%	3.63%	3.27%

Saint John's Hospital

800 E Carpenter Street
Springfield, IL 62769
URL: www.st-johns.org
Ownership: Voluntary non-profit - Church
Emergency Services: Yes
Phone: 217-544-6464
Fax: 217-535-3989
Accredited: Yes
Licensed Beds: 742

Key Personnel:

CEO/EVP. . . . . Allison Laabs
Chief Medical Staff. . . . . Ron Deering, MD
Chief Catheterization Laboratory . . . . Pete Garvey
Emergency Room . . . . Marilyn Rigney
Director Infection/Disease Control . . . . Carol Coleman, RN
CCU Spvg. Nurse . . . . Diane Lueders, RN
Director Medical/Surgical Nursing . . . . Jo Ellen Bretz
Director Radiology . . . . John Loscher
Director Respiratory Therapy . . . . Debbie Brooks

Measure	Cases	This Hospital	State Average	U.S. Average	Top Hospital
Heart Attack Care					
ACE Inhibitor or ARB for LVSD	237	87%	79%	82%	100%
Aspirin at Arrival	180	99%	93%	92%	100%
Aspirin at Discharge	553	99%	90%	90%	100%
Beta Blocker at Arrival	138	98%	87%	87%	100%
Beta Blocker at Discharge	639	98%	88%	90%	100%
Fibrinolytic Medication Timing	0	-	21%	31%	100%
PCI Within 90 Minutes of Arrival[1]	14	79%	47%	54%	95%
Smoking Cessation Advice	275	99%	84%	88%	100%
Heart Failure Care					
ACE Inhibitor or ARB for LVSD	274	78%	83%	82%	100%
Discharge Instructions	437	54%	67%	61%	93%
Evaluation of LVS Function	528	98%	88%	83%	99%
Smoking Cessation Advice	110	96%	83%	82%	100%
Pneumonia Care					
Appropriate Initial Antibiotic	151	90%	83%	83%	94%
Blood Culture Timing	157	96%	91%	90%	100%
Influenza Vaccine	49	43%	63%	70%	100%
Initial Antibiotic Timing	262	88%	81%	80%	93%
Oxygenation Assessment	302	100%	99%	99%	100%
Pneumococcal Vaccine	190	93%	62%	69%	94%
Smoking Cessation Advice	98	85%	80%	80%	100%
Surgical Infection Prevention					
Prophylactic Antibiotic Given[2]	359	88%	74%	77%	95%
Prophylactic Antibiotic Selection[2]	86	90%	91%	90%	100%
Prophylactic Antibiotic Stopped[2]	354	92%	67%	72%	95%
Pregnancy Care					
Inpatient Neonatal Mortality	-	-	-	-	-
Third or Fourth Degree Laceration	-	-	3.89%	3.63%	3.27%

Community Memorial Hospital

400 Caldwell Street
Staunton, IL 62088
E-mail: mbellovich@stauntonhospital.org
URL: www.stauntonhospital.org
Ownership: Voluntary non-profit - Other
Emergency Services: Yes
Phone: 618-635-2200
Fax: 618-635-3400
Accredited: No
Licensed Beds: 49

Key Personnel:

CEO. . . . . Patrick B Heise
Chief Medical Staff. . . . . Manish Mathur
Emergency Room . . . . Sue Laughoin
Emergency Room . . . . Roberta Monsholt, RN
Director Infection/Disease Control . . . . Judy Matteson, RN
Director Medical/Surgical Nursing . . . . Bernice Henke
Chief Radiology . . . . Dennis Toon, RT
Director Respiratory Therapy . . . . JoAnn Baum

Measure	Cases	This Hospital	State Average	U.S. Average	Top Hospital
Heart Attack Care					
ACE Inhibitor or ARB for LVSD[1]	1	100%	79%	82%	100%
Aspirin at Arrival[1]	13	77%	93%	92%	100%
Aspirin at Discharge[1]	8	62%	90%	90%	100%
Beta Blocker at Arrival[1]	12	67%	87%	87%	100%
Beta Blocker at Discharge[1]	7	71%	88%	90%	100%
Fibrinolytic Medication Timing	0	-	21%	31%	100%
PCI Within 90 Minutes of Arrival	0	-	47%	54%	95%
Smoking Cessation Advice	0	-	84%	88%	100%
Heart Failure Care					
ACE Inhibitor or ARB for LVSD[1]	10	70%	83%	82%	100%
Discharge Instructions[1]	13	31%	67%	61%	93%
Evaluation of LVS Function	27	63%	88%	83%	99%
Smoking Cessation Advice[1]	4	75%	83%	82%	100%
Pneumonia Care					
Appropriate Initial Antibiotic[1]	21	57%	83%	83%	94%
Blood Culture Timing	0	-	91%	90%	100%
Influenza Vaccine[1]	10	0%	63%	70%	100%
Initial Antibiotic Timing[1]	23	87%	81%	80%	93%
Oxygenation Assessment	32	100%	99%	99%	100%
Pneumococcal Vaccine[1]	23	0%	62%	69%	94%
Smoking Cessation Advice[1]	8	38%	80%	80%	100%
Surgical Infection Prevention					
Prophylactic Antibiotic Given[1,3]	2	0%	74%	77%	95%
Prophylactic Antibiotic Selection	0	-	91%	90%	100%
Prophylactic Antibiotic Stopped[1,3]	2	100%	67%	72%	95%
Pregnancy Care					
Inpatient Neonatal Mortality	-	-	-	-	-
Third or Fourth Degree Laceration	-	-	3.89%	3.63%	3.27%

CGH Medical Center

100 E LeFevre Road
Sterling, IL 61081
URL: www.cghmc.com
Ownership: Government - Local
Emergency Services: Yes
Phone: 815-625-0400
Fax: 815-625-4825
Accredited: Yes
Licensed Beds: 139

Key Personnel:

President/CEO. . . . . Ed Andersen
Chief Medical Staff. . . . . Angel Biazquez, MD
Emergency Room . . . . Val Menis, MD
Director Infection/Disease Control . . . . Sandra Westbo, RN
CCU Spvg. Nurse . . . . Alice Vetter, RN
Director Medical/Surgical Nursing . . . . Linda Olds-Steinert
OB/GYN Womens Health. . . . . Frank Tugwell, MD
Chief Radiology . . . . Surjit Herman, MD
Director Respiratory Therapy . . . . Alice Vetter

Measure	Cases	This Hospital	State Average	U.S. Average	Top Hospital
Heart Attack Care					
ACE Inhibitor or ARB for LVSD[1]	16	69%	79%	82%	100%
Aspirin at Arrival	72	96%	93%	92%	100%
Aspirin at Discharge	55	80%	90%	90%	100%
Beta Blocker at Arrival	71	93%	87%	87%	100%
Beta Blocker at Discharge	55	93%	88%	90%	100%
Fibrinolytic Medication Timing	0	-	21%	31%	100%
PCI Within 90 Minutes of Arrival[1]	3	33%	47%	54%	95%
Smoking Cessation Advice[1]	18	100%	84%	88%	100%
Heart Failure Care					
ACE Inhibitor or ARB for LVSD	55	89%	83%	82%	100%
Discharge Instructions	154	97%	67%	61%	93%
Evaluation of LVS Function	197	81%	88%	83%	99%
Smoking Cessation Advice[1]	17	100%	83%	82%	100%
Pneumonia Care					
Appropriate Initial Antibiotic	146	82%	83%	83%	94%
Blood Culture Timing	87	93%	91%	90%	100%

NOTE: Hospital profiles are in alphabetical order by state, then city, then hospital within the city; Rankings are sorted by rate in descending order and exclude hospitals with less than 25 cases; (1) The number of cases is too small (n<25) for purposes of reliably predicting hospital performance; (2) Measure reflects the hospital's indication that its submission was based upon a sample of its relevant discharges; (3) Rate reflects fewer than the maximum possible quarters of data for the measure; (4) Inaccurate information submitted and suppressed for one or more quarters; (5) No data is available from the hospital for this measure; Please refer to the User's Guide for a full explanation of data

Measure	Cases	This Hospital	State Average	U.S. Average	Top Hospital
Influenza Vaccine	26	54%	63%	70%	100%
Initial Antibiotic Timing	159	84%	81%	80%	93%
Oxygenation Assessment	191	96%	99%	99%	100%
Pneumococcal Vaccine	121	56%	62%	69%	94%
Smoking Cessation Advice	34	100%	80%	80%	100%
Surgical Infection Prevention					
Prophylactic Antibiotic Given[2]	311	93%	74%	77%	95%
Prophylactic Antibiotic Selection[2]	73	100%	91%	90%	100%
Prophylactic Antibiotic Stopped[2]	298	70%	67%	72%	95%
Pregnancy Care					
Inpatient Neonatal Mortality	-	-	-	-	-
Third or Fourth Degree Laceration	-	-	3.89%	3.63%	3.27%

Saint Mary's Hospital

111 Spring Street
Streator, IL 61364
URL: www.stmaryshospital.org
Ownership: Voluntary non-profit - Church
Emergency Services: Yes
Phone: 815-673-2311
Fax: 815-673-4592
Accredited: Yes
Licensed Beds: 251

Key Personnel:
CEO. . . . . Marker Heller
Chief of Medical Staff. . . . . Glen Ricca
Emergency Room Director. . . . . Sandy Knight
Emergency Room . . . . . Susan Taylor, RN
OB/GYN Womens Health. . . . . Chaoming Chen, MD
Chief Radiology . . . . . Mark Hilborn, MD
Director Respiratory Therapy . . . . . Jackie Yackl

Measure	Cases	This Hospital	State Average	U.S. Average	Top Hospital
Heart Attack Care					
ACE Inhibitor or ARB for LVSD[1]	4	100%	79%	82%	100%
Aspirin at Arrival[1]	12	92%	93%	92%	100%
Aspirin at Discharge[1]	7	86%	90%	90%	100%
Beta Blocker at Arrival[1]	9	100%	87%	87%	100%
Beta Blocker at Discharge[1]	11	100%	88%	90%	100%
Fibrinolytic Medication Timing	0	-	21%	31%	100%
PCI Within 90 Minutes of Arrival	0	-	47%	54%	95%
Smoking Cessation Advice[1]	2	100%	84%	88%	100%
Heart Failure Care					
ACE Inhibitor or ARB for LVSD	42	93%	83%	82%	100%
Discharge Instructions	79	80%	67%	61%	93%
Evaluation of LVS Function	124	94%	88%	83%	99%
Smoking Cessation Advice[1]	16	94%	83%	82%	100%
Pneumonia Care					
Appropriate Initial Antibiotic	94	91%	83%	83%	94%
Blood Culture Timing	111	91%	91%	90%	100%
Influenza Vaccine	31	87%	63%	70%	100%
Initial Antibiotic Timing	182	92%	81%	80%	93%
Oxygenation Assessment	217	100%	99%	99%	100%
Pneumococcal Vaccine	170	83%	62%	69%	94%
Smoking Cessation Advice	31	100%	80%	80%	100%
Surgical Infection Prevention					
Prophylactic Antibiotic Given[2]	154	75%	74%	77%	95%
Prophylactic Antibiotic Selection[2]	34	100%	91%	90%	100%
Prophylactic Antibiotic Stopped[2]	134	73%	67%	72%	95%
Pregnancy Care					
Inpatient Neonatal Mortality	215	0.00%	-	-	-
Third or Fourth Degree Laceration	162	2.47%	3.89%	3.63%	3.27%

Taylorville Memorial Hospital

Alternate Name: Saint Vincent Memorial Hospital
201 East Pleasant Street
Taylorville, IL 62568
URL: www.svmh.org
Ownership: Voluntary non-profit - Church
Emergency Services: No
Phone: 217-824-3331
Fax: 217-824-1638
Accredited: No
Licensed Beds: 40

Key Personnel:
President/CEO. . . . . Dan Raab
Emergency Room . . . . . Jeri Frye

Measure	Cases	This Hospital	State Average	U.S. Average	Top Hospital
Heart Attack Care					
ACE Inhibitor or ARB for LVSD[1]	4	75%	79%	82%	100%
Aspirin at Arrival[1]	9	78%	93%	92%	100%
Aspirin at Discharge[1]	8	100%	90%	90%	100%
Beta Blocker at Arrival[1]	7	100%	87%	87%	100%
Beta Blocker at Discharge[1]	9	67%	88%	90%	100%
Fibrinolytic Medication Timing	0	-	21%	31%	100%
PCI Within 90 Minutes of Arrival	0	-	47%	54%	95%
Smoking Cessation Advice[1]	3	67%	84%	88%	100%
Heart Failure Care					
ACE Inhibitor or ARB for LVSD	35	91%	83%	82%	100%
Discharge Instructions	81	98%	67%	61%	93%
Evaluation of LVS Function	110	91%	88%	83%	99%
Smoking Cessation Advice[1]	10	70%	83%	82%	100%
Pneumonia Care					
Appropriate Initial Antibiotic	44	82%	83%	83%	94%
Blood Culture Timing	66	95%	91%	90%	100%
Influenza Vaccine	26	88%	63%	70%	100%
Initial Antibiotic Timing	98	93%	81%	80%	93%
Oxygenation Assessment	136	100%	99%	99%	100%
Pneumococcal Vaccine	103	95%	62%	69%	94%
Smoking Cessation Advice	26	96%	80%	80%	100%
Surgical Infection Prevention					
Prophylactic Antibiotic Given[3]	44	66%	74%	77%	95%
Prophylactic Antibiotic Selection[1]	11	82%	91%	90%	100%
Prophylactic Antibiotic Stopped[3]	41	80%	67%	72%	95%
Pregnancy Care					
Inpatient Neonatal Mortality	-	-	-	-	-
Third or Fourth Degree Laceration	-	-	3.89%	3.63%	3.27%

Carle Foundation Hospital

611 W Park Street
Urbana, IL 61801
URL: www.carle.com
Ownership: Voluntary non-profit - Other
Emergency Services: Yes
Phone: 217-383-3311
Fax: 217-383-3373
Accredited: Yes
Licensed Beds: 300

Key Personnel:
CEO. . . . . John Snyber
Chief Medical Staff. . . . . David Graham, MD
Emergency Room . . . . . Jay Yambert
OB/GYN Womens Health. . . . . TW Frank, MD
Chief Radiology . . . . . Jon Hendrickson, MD
Director of Pulmonary . . . . . Donald Greele

Measure	Cases	This Hospital	State Average	U.S. Average	Top Hospital
Heart Attack Care					
ACE Inhibitor or ARB for LVSD[2]	49	69%	79%	82%	100%
Aspirin at Arrival[2]	158	99%	93%	92%	100%
Aspirin at Discharge[2]	249	99%	90%	90%	100%
Beta Blocker at Arrival[2]	140	94%	87%	87%	100%
Beta Blocker at Discharge[2]	256	94%	88%	90%	100%
Fibrinolytic Medication Timing[2]	0	-	21%	31%	100%
PCI Within 90 Minutes of Arrival[1,2]	5	20%	47%	54%	95%
Smoking Cessation Advice[2]	93	89%	84%	88%	100%
Heart Failure Care					
ACE Inhibitor or ARB for LVSD[2]	96	88%	83%	82%	100%
Discharge Instructions[2]	205	56%	67%	61%	93%
Evaluation of LVS Function[2]	283	87%	88%	83%	99%
Smoking Cessation Advice[2]	33	76%	83%	82%	100%
Pneumonia Care					
Appropriate Initial Antibiotic[2]	91	87%	83%	83%	94%
Blood Culture Timing[2]	95	85%	91%	90%	100%
Influenza Vaccine[1,2]	20	90%	63%	70%	100%
Initial Antibiotic Timing[2]	116	76%	81%	80%	93%
Oxygenation Assessment[2]	142	100%	99%	99%	100%
Pneumococcal Vaccine[2]	108	73%	62%	69%	94%
Smoking Cessation Advice[2]	37	84%	80%	80%	100%
Surgical Infection Prevention					
Prophylactic Antibiotic Given[2,3]	215	66%	74%	77%	95%
Prophylactic Antibiotic Selection[2]	71	82%	91%	90%	100%
Prophylactic Antibiotic Stopped[2,3]	205	78%	67%	72%	95%
Pregnancy Care					
Inpatient Neonatal Mortality	-	-	-	-	-

NOTE: Hospital profiles are in alphabetical order by state, then city, then hospital within the city; Rankings are sorted by rate in descending order and exclude hospitals with less than 25 cases; (1) The number of cases is too small (n<25) for purposes of reliably predicting hospital performance; (2) Measure reflects the hospital's indication that its submission was based upon a sample of its relevant discharges; (3) Rate reflects fewer than the maximum possible quarters of data for the measure; (4) Inaccurate information submitted and suppressed for one or more quarters; (5) No data is available from the hospital for this measure; Please refer to the User's Guide for a full explanation of data

Third or Fourth Degree Laceration	-	-	3.89%	3.63%	3.27%

Provena Covenant Medical Center

1400 W Park Avenue
Urbana, IL 61801
Phone: 217-337-2000
Fax: 217-337-2619
URL: www.provena.org/covenant
Ownership: Voluntary non-profit - Church
Accredited: Yes
Emergency Services: Yes
Licensed Beds: 268

Key Personnel:

CEO. . . . . Diane Friedman
OB/GYN Womens Health. . . . . Barbara Michell, MD
Director Radiology . . . . Ed Mabry
Director Respiratory Therapy . . . . Kathy Johnson

Measure	Cases	This Hospital	State Average	U.S. Average	Top Hospital
Heart Attack Care					
ACE Inhibitor or ARB for LVSD	45	96%	79%	82%	100%
Aspirin at Arrival	107	97%	93%	92%	100%
Aspirin at Discharge	249	99%	90%	90%	100%
Beta Blocker at Arrival	56	89%	87%	87%	100%
Beta Blocker at Discharge	227	99%	88%	90%	100%
Fibrinolytic Medication Timing[1]	4	50%	21%	31%	100%
PCI Within 90 Minutes of Arrival[1]	4	75%	47%	54%	95%
Smoking Cessation Advice	100	97%	84%	88%	100%
Heart Failure Care					
ACE Inhibitor or ARB for LVSD	120	98%	83%	82%	100%
Discharge Instructions	292	83%	67%	61%	93%
Evaluation of LVS Function	373	99%	88%	83%	99%
Smoking Cessation Advice	59	85%	83%	82%	100%
Pneumonia Care					
Appropriate Initial Antibiotic	119	91%	83%	83%	94%
Blood Culture Timing	155	97%	91%	90%	100%
Influenza Vaccine	46	48%	63%	70%	100%
Initial Antibiotic Timing	230	70%	81%	80%	93%
Oxygenation Assessment	283	100%	99%	99%	100%
Pneumococcal Vaccine	183	56%	62%	69%	94%
Smoking Cessation Advice	64	95%	80%	80%	100%
Surgical Infection Prevention					
Prophylactic Antibiotic Given[2]	603	82%	74%	77%	95%
Prophylactic Antibiotic Selection[2]	153	86%	91%	90%	100%
Prophylactic Antibiotic Stopped[2]	585	66%	67%	72%	95%
Pregnancy Care					
Inpatient Neonatal Mortality	1,236	0.32%	-	-	-
Third or Fourth Degree Laceration	890	3.15%	3.89%	3.63%	3.27%

Iroquois Memorial Hospital & Resident Home

200 Fairman Avenue
Watseka, IL 60970
Toll-Free: 800-242-2731
Phone: 815-432-5841
Fax: 815-432-7821
E-mail: info@iroquoimemorial.com
URL: www.iroquoismemorial.com
Ownership: Voluntary non-profit - Private
Accredited: Yes
Emergency Services: Yes
Licensed Beds: 94

Key Personnel:

Administrator/CEO . . . . Rex Conger
VP . . . . Chuck Bohlmann
Emergency Room . . . . Abby Purvis, RN
Emergency Room Medical Director . . . . John Timmons, MD
Director Infection/Disease Control . . . . Lou Wonna Bell
ICU . . . . Peggy Jaskula, RN
Intensive Coronary Care . . . . Peggy Jaskula
Medical Surgical Nursing . . . . Nancy Dickenson, RN
OB/GYN/Women's Health . . . . Sharon Hilgendorf, RN
Respiratory/Cardiopulmonary. . . . . Peggy Jaskula, RN

Measure	Cases	This Hospital	State Average	U.S. Average	Top Hospital
Heart Attack Care					
ACE Inhibitor or ARB for LVSD[1]	2	100%	79%	82%	100%
Aspirin at Arrival	40	98%	93%	92%	100%
Aspirin at Discharge[1]	14	100%	90%	90%	100%
Beta Blocker at Arrival	30	83%	87%	87%	100%
Beta Blocker at Discharge[1]	15	93%	88%	90%	100%
Fibrinolytic Medication Timing[1]	8	12%	21%	31%	100%
PCI Within 90 Minutes of Arrival	0	-	47%	54%	95%
Smoking Cessation Advice[1]	2	100%	84%	88%	100%
Heart Failure Care					
ACE Inhibitor or ARB for LVSD[1]	17	88%	83%	82%	100%
Discharge Instructions	80	56%	67%	61%	93%
Evaluation of LVS Function	125	84%	88%	83%	99%
Smoking Cessation Advice	25	92%	83%	82%	100%
Pneumonia Care					
Appropriate Initial Antibiotic	122	81%	83%	83%	94%
Blood Culture Timing	146	92%	91%	90%	100%
Influenza Vaccine[4,5]	-	-	63%	70%	100%
Initial Antibiotic Timing	217	89%	81%	80%	93%
Oxygenation Assessment	275	100%	99%	99%	100%
Pneumococcal Vaccine	198	73%	62%	69%	94%
Smoking Cessation Advice	50	86%	80%	80%	100%
Surgical Infection Prevention					
Prophylactic Antibiotic Given[1,3]	14	50%	74%	77%	95%
Prophylactic Antibiotic Selection[1]	1	100%	91%	90%	100%
Prophylactic Antibiotic Stopped[1,3]	14	57%	67%	72%	95%
Pregnancy Care					
Inpatient Neonatal Mortality	-	-	-	-	-
Third or Fourth Degree Laceration	-	-	3.89%	3.63%	3.27%

Vista Medical Center East

1324 N Sheridan Road
Waukegan, IL 60085
Phone: 847-360-3000
Fax: 847-360-4230
URL: www.vistahealth.com
Ownership: Voluntary non-profit - Other
Accredited: Yes
Emergency Services: Yes
Licensed Beds: 299

Key Personnel:

CEO. . . . . Timothy Harrington
Director Respiratory Therapy . . . . Kim Needham

Measure	Cases	This Hospital	State Average	U.S. Average	Top Hospital
Heart Attack Care					
ACE Inhibitor or ARB for LVSD[1]	24	79%	79%	82%	100%
Aspirin at Arrival	137	92%	93%	92%	100%
Aspirin at Discharge	112	89%	90%	90%	100%
Beta Blocker at Arrival	123	83%	87%	87%	100%
Beta Blocker at Discharge	115	91%	88%	90%	100%
Fibrinolytic Medication Timing	0	-	21%	31%	100%
PCI Within 90 Minutes of Arrival[1]	5	40%	47%	54%	95%
Smoking Cessation Advice	43	100%	84%	88%	100%
Heart Failure Care					
ACE Inhibitor or ARB for LVSD	123	78%	83%	82%	100%
Discharge Instructions	269	28%	67%	61%	93%
Evaluation of LVS Function	347	91%	88%	83%	99%
Smoking Cessation Advice	82	99%	83%	82%	100%
Pneumonia Care					
Appropriate Initial Antibiotic	156	76%	83%	83%	94%
Blood Culture Timing	235	90%	91%	90%	100%
Influenza Vaccine	64	38%	63%	70%	100%
Initial Antibiotic Timing	398	66%	81%	80%	93%
Oxygenation Assessment	428	99%	99%	99%	100%
Pneumococcal Vaccine	225	39%	62%	69%	94%
Smoking Cessation Advice	89	98%	80%	80%	100%
Surgical Infection Prevention					
Prophylactic Antibiotic Given[3]	263	74%	74%	77%	95%
Prophylactic Antibiotic Selection	72	65%	91%	90%	100%
Prophylactic Antibiotic Stopped[3]	259	64%	67%	72%	95%
Pregnancy Care					
Inpatient Neonatal Mortality	-	-	-	-	-
Third or Fourth Degree Laceration	-	-	3.89%	3.63%	3.27%

Vista Medical Center West

2615 Washington Street
Waukegan, IL 60085
Phone: 847-249-3900
Fax: 847-360-4230
URL: www.vistahealth.com
Ownership: Voluntary non-profit - Church
Accredited: Yes
Emergency Services: Yes
Licensed Beds: 388

Key Personnel:

President/CEO. . . . . Timothy J Harrington
Manager Emergency Room . . . . Denise Tucker, RN

NOTE: Hospital profiles are in alphabetical order by state, then city, then hospital within the city; Rankings are sorted by rate in descending order and exclude hospitals with less than 25 cases; (1) The number of cases is too small (n<25) for purposes of reliably predicting hospital performance; (2) Measure reflects the hospital's indication that its submission was based upon a sample of its relevant discharges; (3) Rate reflects fewer than the maximum possible quarters of data for the measure; (4) Inaccurate information submitted and suppressed for one or more quarters; (5) No data is available from the hospital for this measure; Please refer to the User's Guide for a full explanation of data

Infection Control. . . . . Karen VanBuren
Director Surgical Services . . . . Marianne Finlay
Director Respiratory Services. . . . . Kimberly Needham

Measure	Cases	This Hospital	State Average	U.S. Average	Top Hospital
Heart Attack Care					
ACE Inhibitor or ARB for LVSD[5]	-	-	79%	82%	100%
Aspirin at Arrival[5]	-	-	93%	92%	100%
Aspirin at Discharge[5]	-	-	90%	90%	100%
Beta Blocker at Arrival[5]	-	-	87%	87%	100%
Beta Blocker at Discharge[5]	-	-	88%	90%	100%
Fibrinolytic Medication Timing[5]	-	-	21%	31%	100%
PCI Within 90 Minutes of Arrival[5]	-	-	47%	54%	95%
Smoking Cessation Advice[5]	-	-	84%	88%	100%
Heart Failure Care					
ACE Inhibitor or ARB for LVSD[5]	-	-	83%	82%	100%
Discharge Instructions[5]	-	-	67%	61%	93%
Evaluation of LVS Function[5]	-	-	88%	83%	99%
Smoking Cessation Advice[5]	-	-	83%	82%	100%
Pneumonia Care					
Appropriate Initial Antibiotic[5]	-	-	83%	83%	94%
Blood Culture Timing[5]	-	-	91%	90%	100%
Influenza Vaccine[5]	-	-	63%	70%	100%
Initial Antibiotic Timing[5]	-	-	81%	80%	93%
Oxygenation Assessment[5]	-	-	99%	99%	100%
Pneumococcal Vaccine[5]	-	-	62%	69%	94%
Smoking Cessation Advice[5]	-	-	80%	80%	100%
Surgical Infection Prevention					
Prophylactic Antibiotic Given[5]	-	-	74%	77%	95%
Prophylactic Antibiotic Selection[5]	-	-	91%	90%	100%
Prophylactic Antibiotic Stopped[5]	-	-	67%	72%	95%
Pregnancy Care					
Inpatient Neonatal Mortality	-	-	-	-	-
Third or Fourth Degree Laceration	-	-	3.89%	3.63%	3.27%

Central DuPage Hospital

25 N Winfield Road — Phone: 630-933-1600
Winfield, IL 60190 — Fax: 630-933-1300
E-mail: cdh_information@cdh.org
URL: www.cdh.org
Ownership: Voluntary non-profit - Private — Accredited: Yes
Emergency Services: Yes — Licensed Beds: 361
Key Personnel:
President/CEO. . . . . Luke McGuinness

Measure	Cases	This Hospital	State Average	U.S. Average	Top Hospital
Heart Attack Care					
ACE Inhibitor or ARB for LVSD	34	76%	79%	82%	100%
Aspirin at Arrival	180	97%	93%	92%	100%
Aspirin at Discharge	167	96%	90%	90%	100%
Beta Blocker at Arrival	146	93%	87%	87%	100%
Beta Blocker at Discharge	168	96%	88%	90%	100%
Fibrinolytic Medication Timing	0	-	21%	31%	100%
PCI Within 90 Minutes of Arrival[1]	10	80%	47%	54%	95%
Smoking Cessation Advice	53	100%	84%	88%	100%
Heart Failure Care					
ACE Inhibitor or ARB for LVSD	152	73%	83%	82%	100%
Discharge Instructions	309	62%	67%	61%	93%
Evaluation of LVS Function	421	96%	88%	83%	99%
Smoking Cessation Advice	55	98%	83%	82%	100%
Pneumonia Care					
Appropriate Initial Antibiotic	192	90%	83%	83%	94%
Blood Culture Timing	226	93%	91%	90%	100%
Influenza Vaccine	45	62%	63%	70%	100%
Initial Antibiotic Timing	277	82%	81%	80%	93%
Oxygenation Assessment	348	100%	99%	99%	100%
Pneumococcal Vaccine	225	63%	62%	69%	94%
Smoking Cessation Advice	64	97%	80%	80%	100%
Surgical Infection Prevention					
Prophylactic Antibiotic Given[2]	297	71%	74%	77%	95%
Prophylactic Antibiotic Selection[2]	77	100%	91%	90%	100%
Prophylactic Antibiotic Stopped[2]	289	68%	67%	72%	95%
Pregnancy Care					
Inpatient Neonatal Mortality	-	-	-	-	-
Third or Fourth Degree Laceration	-	-	3.89%	3.63%	3.27%

Memorial Medical Center

Alternate Name: Centegra Memorial Medical Center
3701 Doty Road — Phone: 815-338-2500
Woodstock, IL 60098 — Fax: 815-334-3948
URL: www.centegra.prg
Ownership: Voluntary non-profit - Other — Accredited: Yes
Emergency Services: Yes — Licensed Beds: 154
Key Personnel:
CEO. . . . . Paul Laubick

Measure	Cases	This Hospital	State Average	U.S. Average	Top Hospital
Heart Attack Care					
ACE Inhibitor or ARB for LVSD[1]	5	60%	79%	82%	100%
Aspirin at Arrival	35	94%	93%	92%	100%
Aspirin at Discharge[1]	12	92%	90%	90%	100%
Beta Blocker at Arrival	27	89%	87%	87%	100%
Beta Blocker at Discharge[1]	23	96%	88%	90%	100%
Fibrinolytic Medication Timing[1]	1	0%	21%	31%	100%
PCI Within 90 Minutes of Arrival	0	-	47%	54%	95%
Smoking Cessation Advice[1]	5	80%	84%	88%	100%
Heart Failure Care					
ACE Inhibitor or ARB for LVSD	64	73%	83%	82%	100%
Discharge Instructions	171	78%	67%	61%	93%
Evaluation of LVS Function	230	99%	88%	83%	99%
Smoking Cessation Advice	41	80%	83%	82%	100%
Pneumonia Care					
Appropriate Initial Antibiotic	139	87%	83%	83%	94%
Blood Culture Timing	164	96%	91%	90%	100%
Influenza Vaccine	43	60%	63%	70%	100%
Initial Antibiotic Timing	205	90%	81%	80%	93%
Oxygenation Assessment	251	100%	99%	99%	100%
Pneumococcal Vaccine	157	68%	62%	69%	94%
Smoking Cessation Advice	39	87%	80%	80%	100%
Surgical Infection Prevention					
Prophylactic Antibiotic Given[2]	326	90%	74%	77%	95%
Prophylactic Antibiotic Selection[2]	74	85%	91%	90%	100%
Prophylactic Antibiotic Stopped[2]	311	77%	67%	72%	95%
Pregnancy Care					
Inpatient Neonatal Mortality	-	-	-	-	-
Third or Fourth Degree Laceration	-	-	3.89%	3.63%	3.27%

Midwestern Regional Medical Center

Alternate Name: American International Hospital
2520 Elisha Avenue — Toll-Free: 800-322-9183
Zion, IL 60099 — Phone: 847-872-4561
Fax: 847-872-6222
E-mail: susan.thomas@mrmc-ctca.com
URL: www.cancercare.com
Ownership: Proprietary — Accredited: Yes
Emergency Services: Yes — Licensed Beds: 95
Key Personnel:
President/CEO. . . . . Roger Cary
Chief Medical Staff. . . . . Joel Granitk
Emergency Room . . . . Peter Senatore, DO
Director Infection/Disease Control . . . . Debra Horton
Director Medical/Surgical Nursing . . . . Carmelita Mangubat
Chief Radiology . . . . Pakorn Sirijintakarn, MD
Director Respiratory Therapy . . . . Jerry Butts

Measure	Cases	This Hospital	State Average	U.S. Average	Top Hospital
Heart Attack Care					
ACE Inhibitor or ARB for LVSD[3]	0	-	79%	82%	100%
Aspirin at Arrival[1,3]	1	100%	93%	92%	100%
Aspirin at Discharge[1,3]	1	100%	90%	90%	100%
Beta Blocker at Arrival[1,3]	1	100%	87%	87%	100%
Beta Blocker at Discharge[1,3]	1	100%	88%	90%	100%
Fibrinolytic Medication Timing[3]	0	-	21%	31%	100%
PCI Within 90 Minutes of Arrival	0	-	47%	54%	95%
Smoking Cessation Advice[3]	0	-	84%	88%	100%

NOTE: Hospital profiles are in alphabetical order by state, then city, then hospital within the city; Rankings are sorted by rate in descending order and exclude hospitals with less than 25 cases; (1) The number of cases is too small (n<25) for purposes of reliably predicting hospital performance; (2) Measure reflects the hospital's indication that its submission was based upon a sample of its relevant discharges; (3) Rate reflects fewer than the maximum possible quarters of data for the measure; (4) Inaccurate information submitted and suppressed for one or more quarters; (5) No data is available from the hospital for this measure; Please refer to the User's Guide for a full explanation of data

Heart Failure Care					
ACE Inhibitor or ARB for LVSD[1]	4	75%	83%	82%	100%
Discharge Instructions[1,3]	1	100%	67%	61%	93%
Evaluation of LVS Function[1]	23	96%	88%	83%	99%
Smoking Cessation Advice[1,3]	1	100%	83%	82%	100%
Pneumonia Care					
Appropriate Initial Antibiotic[1,3]	4	100%	83%	83%	94%
Blood Culture Timing[1,3]	10	100%	91%	90%	100%
Influenza Vaccine[5]	-	-	63%	70%	100%
Initial Antibiotic Timing	50	60%	81%	80%	93%
Oxygenation Assessment	62	100%	99%	99%	100%
Pneumococcal Vaccine[1]	18	22%	62%	69%	94%
Smoking Cessation Advice[1,3]	3	100%	80%	80%	100%
Surgical Infection Prevention					
Prophylactic Antibiotic Given[1,3]	15	73%	74%	77%	95%
Prophylactic Antibiotic Selection[5]	-	-	91%	90%	100%
Prophylactic Antibiotic Stopped[1,3]	14	21%	67%	72%	95%
Pregnancy Care					
Inpatient Neonatal Mortality	-	-	-	-	-
Third or Fourth Degree Laceration	-	-	3.89%	3.63%	3.27%

NOTE: Hospital profiles are in alphabetical order by state, then city, then hospital within the city; Rankings are sorted by rate in descending order and exclude hospitals with less than 25 cases; (1) The number of cases is too small (n<25) for purposes of reliably predicting hospital performance; (2) Measure reflects the hospital's indication that its submission was based upon a sample of its relevant discharges; (3) Rate reflects fewer than the maximum possible quarters of data for the measure; (4) Inaccurate information submitted and suppressed for one or more quarters; (5) No data is available from the hospital for this measure; Please refer to the User's Guide for a full explanation of data

Heart Attack Care

1. ACE Inhibitor or ARB for LVSD

Hospital Name	City	Rate	Cases
Elkhart General Hospital	Elkhart	98%	55
Indiana Heart Hospital	Indianapolis	98%	125
Reid Hospital and Health Care Services	Richmond	98%	60
Wishard Memorial Hospital	Indianapolis	98%	42
Good Samaritan Hospital	Vincennes	96%	50
Columbus Regional Hospital	Columbus	95%	42
Bloomington Hospital	Bloomington	94%	83
Parkview Memorial Hospital	Fort Wayne	92%	39
Saint Vincent Heart Center of Indiana	Indianapolis	91%	307
Union Hospital	Terre Haute	91%	86
Community Hospital South	Indianapolis	90%	40
Floyd Memorial Hospital and Health Services	New Albany	87%	60
Ball Memorial Hospital	Muncie	86%	114
Lutheran Hospital of Indiana	Fort Wayne	86%	144
Memorial Hospital and Health Care Center	Jasper	86%	35
Methodist Hospital of Indiana	Indianapolis	86%	146
Saint Vincent Indianapolis Hospital	Indianapolis	84%	167
Porter Memorial Health System	Valparaiso	83%	46
Community Health Network	Indianapolis	82%	38
Deaconess Hospital	Evansville	82%	182
Saint Margaret Mercy Healthcare Centers	Dyer	81%	27
Terre Haute Regional Hospital	Terre Haute	81%	54
Saint Francis Beech Grove	Beech Grove	80%	45
Clark Memorial Hospital	Jeffersonville	79%	43
Methodist Hospitals-North Lake Campus	Gary	79%	47
Saint Mary's Medical Center	Evansville	79%	118
Saint Anthony Medical Center	Crown Point	78%	32
Community Hospital	Hammond	76%	33
Saint Elizabeth Medical Center	Lafayette	74%	65
Memorial Hospital of South Bend	South Bend	70%	54
Saint Francis at Indianapolis	Indianapolis	70%	27
Saint Margaret Mercy Healthcare Centers	Hammond	60%	55

2. Aspirin at Arrival

Hospital Name	City	Rate	Cases
Community Hosp of Anderson & Madison Co	Anderson	100%	33
Dearborn County Hospital	Lawrenceburg	100%	35
Floyd Memorial Hospital and Health Services	New Albany	100%	208
Reid Hospital and Health Care Services	Richmond	100%	296
Riverview Hospital	Noblesville	100%	95
Saint Joseph's Reg Med Ctr-Plymouth Campus	Plymouth	100%	39
Saint Margaret Mercy Healthcare Centers	Dyer	100%	94
Ball Memorial Hospital	Muncie	99%	297
Clark Memorial Hospital	Jeffersonville	99%	148
Columbus Regional Hospital	Columbus	99%	159
Community Hospital South	Indianapolis	99%	110
Parkview Memorial Hospital	Fort Wayne	99%	130
Saint Elizabeth Medical Center	Lafayette	99%	243
Saint Vincent Heart Center of Indiana	Indianapolis	99%	113
Wishard Memorial Hospital	Indianapolis	99%	181
Bloomington Hospital	Bloomington	98%	246
Community Hospital	Hammond	98%	171
Elkhart General Hospital	Elkhart	98%	289
Hendricks Regional Health	Danville	98%	88
Saint Anthony Memorial Health Centers	Michigan City	98%	109
Saint Francis at Indianapolis	Indianapolis	98%	113
Saint Joseph Hospital	Fort Wayne	98%	85
Saint Mary's Medical Center	Evansville	98%	260
Saint Vincent Indianapolis Hospital	Indianapolis	98%	308
Howard Regional Health System	Kokomo	97%	30
Kosciusko Community Hospital	Warsaw	97%	38
Memorial Hospital of South Bend	South Bend	97%	234
Methodist Hospital of Indiana	Indianapolis	97%	361
Saint Joseph's Regional Medical Center	South Bend	97%	164
Terre Haute Regional Hospital	Terre Haute	97%	96
Union Hospital	Terre Haute	97%	228
Community Health Network	Indianapolis	96%	127
Deaconess Hospital	Evansville	96%	394
Indiana Heart Hospital	Indianapolis	96%	149
Lutheran Hospital of Indiana	Fort Wayne	96%	285
Porter Memorial Health System	Valparaiso	96%	173
Saint Joseph Regional Med Ctr-Mishawaka	Mishawaka	96%	53
Saint Mary's Medical Center	Hobart	96%	83
Goshen General Hospital	Goshen	95%	44
Saint Catherine Hospital of East Chicago	East Chicago	95%	57
Saint Margaret Mercy Healthcare Centers	Hammond	95%	207
Bluffton Regional Medical Center	Bluffton	94%	31
LaPorte Hospital	La Porte	94%	90
Memorial Hospital and Health Care Center	Jasper	94%	90
Saint Anthony Medical Center	Crown Point	94%	155
Saint John's Health System	Anderson	94%	72
Clarian West Medical Center	Avon	93%	29
Dunn Memorial Hospital	Bedford	93%	75
Good Samaritan Hospital	Vincennes	93%	127
King's Daughters Hospital	Madison	91%	35
Methodist Hospitals-North Lake Campus	Gary	90%	194
Saint Francis Beech Grove	Beech Grove	88%	207
Marion General Hospital	Marion	87%	31
Fayette Memorial Hospital	Connersville	86%	37

3. Aspirin at Discharge

Hospital Name	City	Rate	Cases
Indiana Heart Hospital	Indianapolis	100%	402
Parkview Memorial Hospital	Fort Wayne	100%	215
Riverview Hospital	Noblesville	100%	120
Saint Joseph Regional Med Ctr-Mishawaka	Mishawaka	100%	48
Saint Vincent Heart Center of Indiana	Indianapolis	100%	1036
Bloomington Hospital	Bloomington	99%	349
Columbus Regional Hospital	Columbus	99%	201
Community Health Network	Indianapolis	99%	111
Community Hospital South	Indianapolis	99%	137
Floyd Memorial Hospital and Health Services	New Albany	99%	226
Good Samaritan Hospital	Vincennes	99%	152
Reid Hospital and Health Care Services	Richmond	99%	287
Saint Anthony Memorial Health Centers	Michigan City	99%	88
Saint Joseph Hospital	Fort Wayne	99%	103
Saint Joseph's Regional Medical Center	South Bend	99%	221
Saint Margaret Mercy Healthcare Centers	Dyer	99%	88
Wishard Memorial Hospital	Indianapolis	99%	155
Elkhart General Hospital	Elkhart	98%	319
Lutheran Hospital of Indiana	Fort Wayne	98%	667
Saint Elizabeth Medical Center	Lafayette	98%	346
Saint Francis Beech Grove	Beech Grove	98%	268
Saint Vincent Indianapolis Hospital	Indianapolis	98%	493
Ball Memorial Hospital	Muncie	97%	386
Bluffton Regional Medical Center	Bluffton	97%	30
Clark Memorial Hospital	Jeffersonville	97%	190
Deaconess Hospital	Evansville	97%	653
Porter Memorial Health System	Valparaiso	97%	179
Saint Francis at Indianapolis	Indianapolis	97%	172
Saint Mary's Medical Center	Evansville	97%	336
Terre Haute Regional Hospital	Terre Haute	97%	181
Goshen General Hospital	Goshen	96%	27
Howard Regional Health System	Kokomo	96%	27
Memorial Hospital of South Bend	South Bend	96%	245
Methodist Hospital of Indiana	Indianapolis	96%	437
Saint Catherine Hospital of East Chicago	East Chicago	96%	55
Community Hospital	Hammond	95%	147
Dunn Memorial Hospital	Bedford	95%	77
Memorial Hospital and Health Care Center	Jasper	95%	129
Hendricks Regional Health	Danville	94%	33
LaPorte Hospital	La Porte	94%	93
Saint Anthony Medical Center	Crown Point	94%	126
Saint Margaret Mercy Healthcare Centers	Hammond	94%	212
Union Hospital	Terre Haute	94%	259
Saint John's Health System	Anderson	90%	48
Saint Mary's Medical Center	Hobart	90%	92
Methodist Hospitals-North Lake Campus	Gary	82%	165
Fayette Memorial Hospital	Connersville	58%	26

4. Beta Blocker at Arrival

Hospital Name	City	Rate	Cases
Community Hosp of Anderson & Madison Co	Anderson	100%	29
Goshen General Hospital	Goshen	100%	27
Riverview Hospital	Noblesville	100%	74
Clark Memorial Hospital	Jeffersonville	99%	122
Reid Hospital and Health Care Services	Richmond	99%	217
Saint Anthony Memorial Health Centers	Michigan City	99%	98
Columbus Regional Hospital	Columbus	98%	141
Community Hospital South	Indianapolis	98%	49
Saint Joseph's Regional Medical Center	South Bend	98%	85
Saint Vincent Indianapolis Hospital	Indianapolis	98%	281
Ball Memorial Hospital	Muncie	97%	254
King's Daughters Hospital	Madison	97%	30
Saint Francis at Indianapolis	Indianapolis	97%	115
Saint Joseph's Reg Med Ctr-Plymouth Campus	Plymouth	97%	37
Saint Margaret Mercy Healthcare Centers	Dyer	97%	69
Saint Vincent Heart Center of Indiana	Indianapolis	97%	102
Wishard Memorial Hospital	Indianapolis	97%	161
Bluffton Regional Medical Center	Bluffton	96%	27
Elkhart General Hospital	Elkhart	96%	233
Indiana Heart Hospital	Indianapolis	96%	84
Floyd Memorial Hospital and Health Services	New Albany	95%	176
Hendricks Regional Health	Danville	95%	87

NOTE: Hospital profiles are in alphabetical order by state, then city, then hospital within the city; Rankings are sorted by rate in descending order and exclude hospitals with less than 25 cases; (1) The number of cases is too small (n<25) for purposes of reliably predicting hospital performance; (2) Measure reflects the hospital's indication that its submission was based upon a sample of its relevant discharges; (3) Rate reflects fewer than the maximum possible quarters of data for the measure; (4) Inaccurate information submitted and suppressed for one or more quarters; (5) No data is available from the hospital for this measure; Please refer to the User's Guide for a full explanation of data

Hospital Name	City	Rate	Cases
Saint Joseph Regional Med Ctr-Mishawaka	Mishawaka	95%	39
Saint Mary's Medical Center	Evansville	95%	198
Bloomington Hospital	Bloomington	94%	199
Methodist Hospital of Indiana	Indianapolis	94%	270
Saint Elizabeth Medical Center	Lafayette	94%	185
Union Hospital	Terre Haute	94%	177
Memorial Hospital and Health Care Center	Jasper	93%	90
Parkview Memorial Hospital	Fort Wayne	93%	55
Saint Joseph Hospital	Fort Wayne	93%	81
Saint Margaret Mercy Healthcare Centers	Hammond	93%	151
Community Health Network	Indianapolis	92%	75
Community Hospital	Hammond	91%	110
Dunn Memorial Hospital	Bedford	91%	65
Lutheran Hospital of Indiana	Fort Wayne	91%	239
Memorial Hospital of South Bend	South Bend	91%	152
Saint John's Health System	Anderson	90%	73
Saint Mary's Medical Center	Hobart	90%	81
LaPorte Hospital	La Porte	89%	64
Deaconess Hospital	Evansville	88%	332
Good Samaritan Hospital	Vincennes	88%	98
Porter Memorial Health System	Valparaiso	88%	114
Saint Anthony Medical Center	Crown Point	87%	127
Saint Francis Beech Grove	Beech Grove	87%	197
Saint Catherine Hospital of East Chicago	East Chicago	86%	44
Terre Haute Regional Hospital	Terre Haute	86%	72
Marion General Hospital	Marion	82%	33
Methodist Hospitals-North Lake Campus	Gary	81%	166
Howard Regional Health System	Kokomo	77%	26
Clarian West Medical Center	Avon	76%	29
Fayette Memorial Hospital	Connersville	50%	34

5. Beta Blocker at Discharge

Hospital Name	City	Rate	Cases
Bluffton Regional Medical Center	Bluffton	100%	30
Community Hospital South	Indianapolis	100%	109
Goshen General Hospital	Goshen	100%	26
Saint Anthony Memorial Health Centers	Michigan City	100%	86
Saint Margaret Mercy Healthcare Centers	Dyer	100%	87
Saint Vincent Heart Center of Indiana	Indianapolis	100%	1027
Ball Memorial Hospital	Muncie	99%	352
Columbus Regional Hospital	Columbus	99%	190
Community Health Network	Indianapolis	99%	102
Dunn Memorial Hospital	Bedford	99%	83
Elkhart General Hospital	Elkhart	99%	296
Indiana Heart Hospital	Indianapolis	99%	386
Parkview Memorial Hospital	Fort Wayne	99%	224
Reid Hospital and Health Care Services	Richmond	99%	321
Riverview Hospital	Noblesville	99%	112
Saint Mary's Medical Center	Evansville	99%	335
Saint Vincent Indianapolis Hospital	Indianapolis	99%	485
Wishard Memorial Hospital	Indianapolis	99%	151
Bloomington Hospital	Bloomington	98%	339
Memorial Hospital and Health Care Center	Jasper	98%	127
Saint John's Health System	Anderson	98%	53
Terre Haute Regional Hospital	Terre Haute	98%	182
Clark Memorial Hospital	Jeffersonville	97%	188
Good Samaritan Hospital	Vincennes	97%	152
Hendricks Regional Health	Danville	97%	38
Methodist Hospital of Indiana	Indianapolis	97%	445
Porter Memorial Health System	Valparaiso	97%	176
Saint Francis Beech Grove	Beech Grove	97%	271
Howard Regional Health System	Kokomo	96%	26
Lutheran Hospital of Indiana	Fort Wayne	96%	657
Saint Francis at Indianapolis	Indianapolis	96%	176
Saint Joseph Regional Med Ctr-Mishawaka	Mishawaka	96%	51
Saint Joseph's Regional Medical Center	South Bend	96%	194
Union Hospital	Terre Haute	96%	293
Floyd Memorial Hospital and Health Services	New Albany	95%	211
Saint Elizabeth Medical Center	Lafayette	95%	391
Saint Joseph Hospital	Fort Wayne	95%	98
Deaconess Hospital	Evansville	94%	640
LaPorte Hospital	La Porte	94%	94
Memorial Hospital of South Bend	South Bend	94%	265
Community Hospital	Hammond	93%	164
Saint Margaret Mercy Healthcare Centers	Hammond	92%	237
Saint Catherine Hospital of East Chicago	East Chicago	90%	50
Saint Mary's Medical Center	Hobart	90%	97
Methodist Hospitals-North Lake Campus	Gary	86%	179
Saint Anthony Medical Center	Crown Point	86%	134
Fayette Memorial Hospital	Connersville	66%	29

6. Fibrinolytic Medication Timing

Hospital Name	City	Rate	Cases
Reid Hospital and Health Care Services	Richmond	88%	33

8. Smoking Cessation Advice

Hospital Name	City	Rate	Cases
Bloomington Hospital	Bloomington	100%	156
Columbus Regional Hospital	Columbus	100%	89
Community Health Network	Indianapolis	100%	54
Community Hospital South	Indianapolis	100%	62
Dunn Memorial Hospital	Bedford	100%	27
Good Samaritan Hospital	Vincennes	100%	62
Indiana Heart Hospital	Indianapolis	100%	229
LaPorte Hospital	La Porte	100%	32
Memorial Hospital and Health Care Center	Jasper	100%	51
Methodist Hospitals-North Lake Campus	Gary	100%	86
Reid Hospital and Health Care Services	Richmond	100%	114
Riverview Hospital	Noblesville	100%	31
Saint Anthony Memorial Health Centers	Michigan City	100%	36
Saint Joseph Hospital	Fort Wayne	100%	44
Saint Mary's Medical Center	Hobart	100%	43
Terre Haute Regional Hospital	Terre Haute	100%	80
Clark Memorial Hospital	Jeffersonville	99%	78
Deaconess Hospital	Evansville	99%	273
Lutheran Hospital of Indiana	Fort Wayne	99%	268
Saint Mary's Medical Center	Evansville	99%	145
Union Hospital	Terre Haute	98%	103
Ball Memorial Hospital	Muncie	97%	132
Methodist Hospital of Indiana	Indianapolis	96%	233
Saint Joseph's Regional Medical Center	South Bend	96%	97
Floyd Memorial Hospital and Health Services	New Albany	95%	109
Saint Francis at Indianapolis	Indianapolis	95%	96
Saint Vincent Indianapolis Hospital	Indianapolis	95%	166
Saint Anthony Medical Center	Crown Point	94%	48
Saint Vincent Heart Center of Indiana	Indianapolis	94%	400
Parkview Memorial Hospital	Fort Wayne	92%	113
Saint Francis Beech Grove	Beech Grove	91%	102
Wishard Memorial Hospital	Indianapolis	91%	98
Saint Elizabeth Medical Center	Lafayette	90%	145
Elkhart General Hospital	Elkhart	89%	120
Memorial Hospital of South Bend	South Bend	82%	111
Saint Margaret Mercy Healthcare Centers	Hammond	82%	79
Saint Margaret Mercy Healthcare Centers	Dyer	78%	32

Heart Failure Care

9. ACE Inhibitor or ARB for LVSD

Hospital Name	City	Rate	Cases
Bedford Regional Medical Center	Bedford	100%	34
Goshen General Hospital	Goshen	100%	45
Indiana Heart Hospital	Indianapolis	100%	122
Reid Hospital and Health Care Services	Richmond	100%	78
Riverview Hospital	Noblesville	100%	49
Saint Joseph Hospital	Kokomo	100%	60
Bluffton Regional Medical Center	Bluffton	98%	42
Columbus Regional Hospital	Columbus	98%	90
Porter Memorial Health System	Valparaiso	98%	172
Morgan Hospital Medical Centre	Martinsville	97%	63
Wishard Memorial Hospital	Indianapolis	97%	250
Saint Anthony Memorial Health Centers	Michigan City	96%	68
Saint Catherine Hospital of East Chicago	East Chicago	96%	164
King's Daughters Hospital	Madison	94%	36
Kosciusko Community Hospital	Warsaw	94%	32
Major Hospital	Shelbyville	94%	31
Saint John's Health System	Anderson	94%	84
Schneck Medical Center	Seymour	94%	31
Community Hosp of Anderson & Madison Co	Anderson	92%	50
Marion General Hospital	Marion	92%	62
Henry County Memorial Hospital	New Castle	91%	34
Good Samaritan Hospital	Vincennes	90%	109
Parkview Memorial Hospital	Fort Wayne	89%	85
Saint Vincent Heart Center of Indiana	Indianapolis	89%	258
Saint Mary's Medical Center	Hobart	88%	127
Saint Vincent Indianapolis Hospital	Indianapolis	88%	226
Union Hospital	Terre Haute	88%	145
Bloomington Hospital	Bloomington	87%	127
Saint Joseph's Regional Medical Center	South Bend	87%	121
Saint Mary's Medical Center	Evansville	87%	129
Adams Memorial Hospital	Decatur	86%	28
Memorial Hospital of South Bend	South Bend	86%	169
Memorial Hospital and Health Care Center	Jasper	84%	77
Ball Memorial Hospital	Muncie	83%	201
Dunn Memorial Hospital	Bedford	83%	30
Saint Francis at Indianapolis	Indianapolis	83%	48
Saint Joseph Hospital	Fort Wayne	83%	70
Saint Margaret Mercy Healthcare Centers	Dyer	83%	87
Floyd Memorial Hospital and Health Services	New Albany	82%	118
Deaconess Hospital	Evansville	80%	317

NOTE: Hospital profiles are in alphabetical order by state, then city, then hospital within the city; Rankings are sorted by rate in descending order and exclude hospitals with less than 25 cases; (1) The number of cases is too small (n<25) for purposes of reliably predicting hospital performance; (2) Measure reflects the hospital's indication that its submission was based upon a sample of its relevant discharges; (3) Rate reflects fewer than the maximum possible quarters of data for the measure; (4) Inaccurate information submitted and suppressed for one or more quarters; (5) No data is available from the hospital for this measure; Please refer to the User's Guide for a full explanation of data

Howard Regional Health System	Kokomo	80%	71
Methodist Hospital of Indiana	Indianapolis	80%	556
Hancock Memorial Hospital and Health Services	Greenfield	79%	33
Saint Joseph Regional Med Ctr-Mishawaka	Mishawaka	79%	33
Elkhart General Hospital	Elkhart	78%	211
Lutheran Hospital of Indiana	Fort Wayne	78%	255
Methodist Hospitals-North Lake Campus	Gary	78%	392
Saint Anthony Medical Center	Crown Point	78%	116
Saint Francis Beech Grove	Beech Grove	78%	127
Hendricks Regional Health	Danville	77%	70
LaPorte Hospital	La Porte	77%	102
Community Hospital South	Indianapolis	76%	51
Saint Margaret Mercy Healthcare Centers	Hammond	76%	107
Community Hospital	Hammond	75%	310
Community Health Network	Indianapolis	74%	136
Clarian West Medical Center	Avon	73%	41
Harrison County Hospital	Corydon	73%	26
Terre Haute Regional Hospital	Terre Haute	72%	141
Clark Memorial Hospital	Jeffersonville	69%	94
Dearborn County Hospital	Lawrenceburg	68%	44
Saint Elizabeth Medical Center	Lafayette	68%	117
Fayette Memorial Hospital	Connersville	62%	29
Daviess Community Hospital	Washington	53%	34
Saint Clare Medical Center	Crawfordsville	53%	30

10. Discharge Instructions

Hospital Name	City	Rate	Cases
Bluffton Regional Medical Center	Bluffton	100%	73
Morgan Hospital Medical Centre	Martinsville	100%	28
Saint Mary's Warrick Hospital	Boonville	100%	25
Saint Vincent Williamsport	Williamsport	100%	35
Reid Hospital and Health Care Services	Richmond	99%	299
Saint Catherine Hospital of East Chicago	East Chicago	99%	91
Saint Joseph Hospital	Kokomo	99%	113
Indiana Heart Hospital	Indianapolis	98%	234
Henry County Memorial Hospital	New Castle	97%	59
Saint Mary's Medical Center	Evansville	97%	235
Riverview Hospital	Noblesville	96%	99
Saint Joseph Hospital	Fort Wayne	96%	162
Union Hospital	Terre Haute	95%	332
Witham Memorial Hospital	Lebanon	95%	42
Porter Memorial Health System	Valparaiso	94%	79
Bedford Regional Medical Center	Bedford	93%	57
Community Hosp of Anderson & Madison Co	Anderson	91%	138
Saint Mary's Medical Center	Hobart	91%	314
Schneck Medical Center	Seymour	91%	74
King's Daughters Hospital	Madison	90%	103
Kosciusko Community Hospital	Warsaw	90%	68
Dekalb Memorial Hospital	Auburn	88%	40
Columbus Regional Hospital	Columbus	87%	255
Goshen General Hospital	Goshen	86%	117
Saint Vincent Heart Center of Indiana	Indianapolis	86%	339
Saint Joseph's Regional Medical Center	South Bend	85%	293
Saint Vincent Indianapolis Hospital	Indianapolis	85%	502
Major Hospital	Shelbyville	84%	67
Scott Memorial Hospital	Scottsburg	84%	68
Bloomington Hospital	Bloomington	83%	229
Marion General Hospital	Marion	83%	145
Parkview Huntington Hospital	Huntington	82%	33
Saint John's Health System	Anderson	81%	157
Decatur County Memorial Hospital	Greensburg	80%	40
Greene County General Hospital	Linton	80%	35
Saint Anthony Memorial Health Centers	Michigan City	80%	167
Ball Memorial Hospital	Muncie	79%	372
Floyd Memorial Hospital and Health Services	New Albany	79%	233
Good Samaritan Hospital	Vincennes	79%	235
Hendricks Regional Health	Danville	79%	126
LaPorte Hospital	La Porte	78%	179
Memorial Hospital of South Bend	South Bend	78%	384
Saint Margaret Mercy Healthcare Centers	Dyer	78%	194
Tipton Hospital	Tipton	78%	37
Dukes Memorial Hospital	Peru	77%	43
Gibson General Hospital	Princeton	77%	35
Saint Elizabeth Medical Center	Lafayette	76%	250
West Central Community Hospital	Clinton	74%	35
Logansport Memorial Hospital	Logansport	73%	44
Methodist Hospital of Indiana	Indianapolis	73%	847
Saint Joseph's Reg Med Ctr-Plymouth Campus	Plymouth	73%	56
Adams Memorial Hospital	Decatur	72%	54
Community Hospital	Hammond	72%	139
Saint Margaret Mercy Healthcare Centers	Hammond	72%	253
Johnson Memorial Hospital	Franklin	70%	64
Terre Haute Regional Hospital	Terre Haute	68%	320
Parkview Noble Hospital	Kendallville	67%	67
Saint Francis at Indianapolis	Indianapolis	67%	90
Howard Regional Health System	Kokomo	65%	139
Deaconess Hospital	Evansville	63%	631
Saint Joseph Regional Med Ctr-Mishawaka	Mishawaka	62%	72
Dunn Memorial Hospital	Bedford	61%	57
Saint Anthony Medical Center	Crown Point	59%	272
Clark Memorial Hospital	Jeffersonville	58%	250
Dupont Hospital	Fort Wayne	58%	26
Lutheran Hospital of Indiana	Fort Wayne	58%	477
Parkview Whitley Hospital	Columbia City	58%	33
Parkview Memorial Hospital	Fort Wayne	56%	209
Memorial Hospital and Health Care Center	Jasper	55%	113
Community Hospital South	Indianapolis	54%	108
Saint Vincent Frankfort Hospital	Frankfort	52%	27
Westview Hospital	Indianapolis	52%	62
Jasper County Hospital	Rensselaer	51%	37
Lafayette Home Hospital	Lafayette	50%	54
Margaret Mary Community Hospital	Batesville	50%	34
Saint Francis Beech Grove	Beech Grove	50%	253
Sullivan County Community Hospital	Sullivan	45%	33
Community Health Network	Indianapolis	43%	213
Elkhart General Hospital	Elkhart	43%	417
Saint Clare Medical Center	Crawfordsville	42%	64
Dearborn County Hospital	Lawrenceburg	39%	82
Starke Memorial Hospital	Knox	39%	38
Wishard Memorial Hospital	Indianapolis	39%	333
Fayette Memorial Hospital	Connersville	30%	102
Methodist Hospitals-North Lake Campus	Gary	29%	852
Hancock Memorial Hospital and Health Services	Greenfield	25%	55
Cameron Memorial Community Hospital	Angola	21%	29
Harrison County Hospital	Corydon	20%	46
Daviess Community Hospital	Washington	11%	44
Saint Vincent Carmel Hospital	Carmel	4%	26

11. Evaluation of LVS Function

Hospital Name	City	Rate	Cases
Bedford Regional Medical Center	Bedford	100%	77
Dekalb Memorial Hospital	Auburn	100%	60
Dupont Hospital	Fort Wayne	100%	33
Harrison County Hospital	Corydon	100%	59
Major Hospital	Shelbyville	100%	87
Porter Memorial Health System	Valparaiso	100%	426
Bluffton Regional Medical Center	Bluffton	99%	105
Henry County Memorial Hospital	New Castle	99%	85
Indiana Heart Hospital	Indianapolis	99%	298
King's Daughters Hospital	Madison	99%	147
Kosciusko Community Hospital	Warsaw	99%	99
Reid Hospital and Health Care Services	Richmond	99%	398
Riverview Hospital	Noblesville	99%	134
Saint Anthony Memorial Health Centers	Michigan City	99%	205
Saint Catherine Hospital of East Chicago	East Chicago	99%	494
Saint John's Health System	Anderson	99%	205
Saint Joseph Regional Med Ctr-Mishawaka	Mishawaka	99%	97
Saint Vincent Heart Center of Indiana	Indianapolis	99%	373
Methodist Hospital of Indiana	Indianapolis	98%	1026
Saint Mary's Warrick Hospital	Boonville	98%	48
Wishard Memorial Hospital	Indianapolis	98%	377
Clarian West Medical Center	Avon	97%	98
Community Hosp of Anderson & Madison Co	Anderson	97%	185
Goshen General Hospital	Goshen	97%	158
Marion General Hospital	Marion	97%	196
Saint Francis at Indianapolis	Indianapolis	97%	108
Saint Joseph's Regional Medical Center	South Bend	97%	378
Saint Mary's Medical Center	Hobart	97%	386
Union Hospital	Terre Haute	97%	405
Ball Memorial Hospital	Muncie	96%	515
Columbus Regional Hospital	Columbus	96%	314
Floyd Memorial Hospital and Health Services	New Albany	96%	312
Memorial Hospital of South Bend	South Bend	96%	459
Saint Joseph Hospital	Fort Wayne	96%	218
Saint Margaret Mercy Healthcare Centers	Dyer	96%	225
Saint Vincent Indianapolis Hospital	Indianapolis	96%	643
Johnson Memorial Hospital	Franklin	95%	98
Saint Vincent Williamsport	Williamsport	95%	55
Dunn Memorial Hospital	Bedford	94%	66
Hendricks Regional Health	Danville	94%	180
Saint Mary's Medical Center	Evansville	93%	305
Schneck Medical Center	Seymour	93%	98
Parkview Memorial Hospital	Fort Wayne	92%	285
Bloomington Hospital	Bloomington	91%	293
Community Hospital South	Indianapolis	91%	153
Howard Regional Health System	Kokomo	91%	193
Lutheran Hospital of Indiana	Fort Wayne	91%	590
Tipton Hospital	Tipton	91%	46

NOTE: Hospital profiles are in alphabetical order by state, then city, then hospital within the city; Rankings are sorted by rate in descending order and exclude hospitals with less than 25 cases; (1) The number of cases is too small (n<25) for purposes of reliably predicting hospital performance; (2) Measure reflects the hospital's indication that its submission was based upon a sample of its relevant discharges; (3) Rate reflects fewer than the maximum possible quarters of data for the measure; (4) Inaccurate information submitted and suppressed for one or more quarters; (5) No data is available from the hospital for this measure; Please refer to the User's Guide for a full explanation of data

Westview Hospital	Indianapolis	91%	82
Community Health Network	Indianapolis	90%	306
Community Hospital	Hammond	90%	800
Deaconess Hospital	Evansville	90%	801
Dearborn County Hospital	Lawrenceburg	90%	82
Dukes Memorial Hospital	Peru	90%	63
Gibson General Hospital	Princeton	90%	61
Saint Joseph's Reg Med Ctr-Plymouth Campus	Plymouth	89%	79
Good Samaritan Hospital	Vincennes	88%	307
LaPorte Hospital	La Porte	88%	243
Lafayette Home Hospital	Lafayette	88%	80
Saint Francis Beech Grove	Beech Grove	88%	395
Morgan Hospital Medical Centre	Martinsville	87%	159
Parkview Noble Hospital	Kendallville	87%	95
Decatur County Memorial Hospital	Greensburg	86%	63
Terre Haute Regional Hospital	Terre Haute	86%	377
Community Hospital of Bremen	Bremen	85%	26
Daviess Community Hospital	Washington	84%	62
Greene County General Hospital	Linton	84%	58
Hancock Memorial Hospital and Health Services	Greenfield	84%	90
Memorial Hospital and Health Care Center	Jasper	84%	160
Parkview Whitley Hospital	Columbia City	84%	45
Saint Joseph Hospital	Kokomo	84%	143
Logansport Memorial Hospital	Logansport	83%	77
Starke Memorial Hospital	Knox	83%	48
Wabash County Hospital	Wabash	83%	30
West Central Community Hospital	Clinton	83%	58
Elkhart General Hospital	Elkhart	82%	488
Clark Memorial Hospital	Jeffersonville	81%	343
Saint Elizabeth Medical Center	Lafayette	81%	348
Medical Center of Southern Indiana	Charlestown	79%	29
Methodist Hospitals-North Lake Campus	Gary	79%	1070
Parkview Huntington Hospital	Huntington	79%	47
Margaret Mary Community Hospital	Batesville	78%	50
Saint Vincent Clay Hospital	Brazil	78%	40
White County Memorial Hospital	Monticello	78%	40
Jasper County Hospital	Rensselaer	77%	56
Saint Anthony Medical Center	Crown Point	77%	355
Saint Margaret Mercy Healthcare Centers	Hammond	74%	289
Saint Vincent Carmel Hospital	Carmel	74%	43
Witham Memorial Hospital	Lebanon	74%	50
Heartland Memorial Hospital	Munster	73%	81
Adams Memorial Hospital	Decatur	72%	83
Saint Vincent Frankfort Hospital	Frankfort	69%	26
Saint Clare Medical Center	Crawfordsville	64%	104
Scott Memorial Hospital	Scottsburg	61%	80
Fayette Memorial Hospital	Connersville	55%	143
Sullivan County Community Hospital	Sullivan	50%	48
Cameron Memorial Community Hospital	Angola	38%	39

12. Smoking Cessation Advice

Hospital Name	City	Rate	Cases
Bloomington Hospital	Bloomington	100%	60
Columbus Regional Hospital	Columbus	100%	82
Community Health Network	Indianapolis	100%	75
Indiana Heart Hospital	Indianapolis	100%	57
Reid Hospital and Health Care Services	Richmond	100%	55
Saint Anthony Memorial Health Centers	Michigan City	100%	35
Saint Joseph Hospital	Fort Wayne	100%	46
Saint Mary's Medical Center	Evansville	100%	52
Terre Haute Regional Hospital	Terre Haute	100%	85
Deaconess Hospital	Evansville	99%	182
Lutheran Hospital of Indiana	Fort Wayne	99%	125
Saint Mary's Medical Center	Hobart	98%	49
Marion General Hospital	Marion	97%	33
Union Hospital	Terre Haute	96%	47
Methodist Hospitals-North Lake Campus	Gary	95%	260
Saint Joseph's Regional Medical Center	South Bend	95%	60
Ball Memorial Hospital	Muncie	93%	76
Methodist Hospital of Indiana	Indianapolis	93%	230
Saint John's Health System	Anderson	93%	42
Saint Vincent Indianapolis Hospital	Indianapolis	93%	71
Wishard Memorial Hospital	Indianapolis	93%	135
Parkview Memorial Hospital	Fort Wayne	88%	49
Saint Francis at Indianapolis	Indianapolis	88%	26
LaPorte Hospital	La Porte	87%	39
Memorial Hospital of South Bend	South Bend	86%	113
Floyd Memorial Hospital and Health Services	New Albany	84%	64
Saint Vincent Heart Center of Indiana	Indianapolis	82%	45
Clark Memorial Hospital	Jeffersonville	81%	70
Saint Margaret Mercy Healthcare Centers	Hammond	81%	68
Good Samaritan Hospital	Vincennes	73%	37
Saint Elizabeth Medical Center	Lafayette	70%	64
Saint Margaret Mercy Healthcare Centers	Dyer	69%	32
Saint Anthony Medical Center	Crown Point	68%	37
Elkhart General Hospital	Elkhart	62%	72
Saint Francis Beech Grove	Beech Grove	62%	73
Adams Memorial Hospital	Decatur	40%	25
Fayette Memorial Hospital	Connersville	37%	27

Pneumonia Care

13. Appropriate Initial Antibiotic

Hospital Name	City	Rate	Cases
Dekalb Memorial Hospital	Auburn	98%	106
Community Hosp of Anderson & Madison Co	Anderson	96%	165
Parkview Whitley Hospital	Columbia City	96%	57
Marion General Hospital	Marion	95%	111
Major Hospital	Shelbyville	94%	117
Reid Hospital and Health Care Services	Richmond	94%	318
Cameron Memorial Community Hospital	Angola	93%	59
Columbus Regional Hospital	Columbus	93%	133
Floyd Memorial Hospital and Health Services	New Albany	93%	199
Logansport Memorial Hospital	Logansport	93%	44
Parkview Noble Hospital	Kendallville	93%	68
Saint Joseph Regional Med Ctr-Mishawaka	Mishawaka	93%	59
Deaconess Hospital	Evansville	92%	320
Kosciusko Community Hospital	Warsaw	92%	121
LaGrange Community Hospital	LaGrange	92%	64
LaPorte Hospital	La Porte	92%	108
Parkview Memorial Hospital	Fort Wayne	92%	102
Bluffton Regional Medical Center	Bluffton	91%	110
Johnson Memorial Hospital	Franklin	91%	107
Lutheran Hospital of Indiana	Fort Wayne	91%	144
Saint Anthony Memorial Health Centers	Michigan City	91%	180
Ball Memorial Hospital	Muncie	90%	283
Saint John's Health System	Anderson	90%	139
Saint Joseph's Regional Medical Center	South Bend	90%	143
Dearborn County Hospital	Lawrenceburg	89%	119
Elkhart General Hospital	Elkhart	89%	183
Memorial Hospital of South Bend	South Bend	89%	230
Porter Memorial Health System	Valparaiso	89%	38
Saint Francis Beech Grove	Beech Grove	89%	115
Westview Hospital	Indianapolis	89%	65
Bloomington Hospital	Bloomington	88%	200
Community Hospital South	Indianapolis	88%	125
Henry County Memorial Hospital	New Castle	88%	125
King's Daughters Hospital	Madison	88%	180
Saint Francis at Indianapolis	Indianapolis	88%	41
Saint Margaret Mercy Healthcare Centers	Dyer	88%	98
Saint Mary's Medical Center	Hobart	88%	182
Riverview Hospital	Noblesville	87%	76
Saint Mary's Medical Center	Evansville	87%	180
Wishard Memorial Hospital	Indianapolis	87%	93
Daviess Community Hospital	Washington	86%	142
Hendricks Regional Health	Danville	86%	170
Howard Regional Health System	Kokomo	86%	177
Saint Mary's Warrick Hospital	Boonville	86%	64
Saint Vincent Carmel Hospital	Carmel	86%	73
Schneck Medical Center	Seymour	86%	128
West Central Community Hospital	Clinton	86%	65
Adams Memorial Hospital	Decatur	85%	60
Community Health Network	Indianapolis	85%	191
Goshen General Hospital	Goshen	85%	109
Methodist Hospital of Indiana	Indianapolis	85%	106
Saint Joseph Hospital	Fort Wayne	85%	33
Dupont Hospital	Fort Wayne	84%	44
Margaret Mary Community Hospital	Batesville	84%	91
Parkview Huntington Hospital	Huntington	84%	49
Saint Margaret Mercy Healthcare Centers	Hammond	84%	133
Starke Memorial Hospital	Knox	84%	99
Dukes Memorial Hospital	Peru	83%	47
Saint Anthony Medical Center	Crown Point	83%	224
Union Hospital	Terre Haute	83%	199
Clark Memorial Hospital	Jeffersonville	81%	188
Greene County General Hospital	Linton	81%	31
Saint Joseph's Reg Med Ctr-Plymouth Campus	Plymouth	81%	79
Scott Memorial Hospital	Scottsburg	81%	118
Wabash County Hospital	Wabash	81%	52
Saint Vincent Indianapolis Hospital	Indianapolis	80%	228
Saint Vincent Williamsport	Williamsport	80%	40
Sullivan County Community Hospital	Sullivan	80%	59
Bedford Regional Medical Center	Bedford	79%	57
Hancock Memorial Hospital and Health Services	Greenfield	79%	190
Terre Haute Regional Hospital	Terre Haute	79%	97
Saint Vincent Mercy Hospital	Elwood	78%	77
Saint Vincent Clay Hospital	Brazil	77%	39
Community Hospital	Hammond	76%	46

NOTE: Hospital profiles are in alphabetical order by state, then city, then hospital within the city; Rankings are sorted by rate in descending order and exclude hospitals with less than 25 cases; (1) The number of cases is too small (n<25) for purposes of reliably predicting hospital performance; (2) Measure reflects the hospital's indication that its submission was based upon a sample of its relevant discharges; (3) Rate reflects fewer than the maximum possible quarters of data for the measure; (4) Inaccurate information submitted and suppressed for one or more quarters; (5) No data is available from the hospital for this measure; Please refer to the User's Guide for a full explanation of data

Hospital Name	City	Rate	Cases
Methodist Hospitals-North Lake Campus	Gary	76%	202
White County Memorial Hospital	Monticello	76%	46
Decatur County Memorial Hospital	Greensburg	75%	55
Fayette Memorial Hospital	Connersville	74%	62
Memorial Hospital and Health Care Center	Jasper	71%	182
Saint Elizabeth Medical Center	Lafayette	71%	143
Saint Joseph Hospital	Kokomo	69%	149
Good Samaritan Hospital	Vincennes	67%	99
Lafayette Home Hospital	Lafayette	67%	113
Saint Vincent Frankfort Hospital	Frankfort	67%	48
Witham Memorial Hospital	Lebanon	66%	77
Harrison County Hospital	Corydon	64%	102
Saint Clare Medical Center	Crawfordsville	63%	102
Dunn Memorial Hospital	Bedford	60%	63
Tipton Hospital	Tipton	54%	48
Jasper County Hospital	Rensselaer	44%	63

14. Blood Culture Timing

Hospital Name	City	Rate	Cases
Dupont Hospital	Fort Wayne	100%	36
Fayette Memorial Hospital	Connersville	100%	30
Greene County General Hospital	Linton	100%	26
Dekalb Memorial Hospital	Auburn	99%	78
Saint Mary's Medical Center	Hobart	99%	177
Bluffton Regional Medical Center	Bluffton	98%	92
Columbus Regional Hospital	Columbus	98%	64
Community Hospital	Hammond	98%	52
Reid Hospital and Health Care Services	Richmond	98%	392
Memorial Hospital and Health Care Center	Jasper	97%	91
Saint Elizabeth Medical Center	Lafayette	97%	212
Saint Joseph's Regional Medical Center	South Bend	97%	141
Terre Haute Regional Hospital	Terre Haute	97%	94
Westview Hospital	Indianapolis	97%	78
Community Hosp of Anderson & Madison Co	Anderson	96%	109
Dunn Memorial Hospital	Bedford	96%	45
Riverview Hospital	Noblesville	96%	47
Saint Vincent Mercy Hospital	Elwood	96%	51
Schneck Medical Center	Seymour	96%	100
Union Hospital	Terre Haute	96%	148
Floyd Memorial Hospital and Health Services	New Albany	95%	276
Howard Regional Health System	Kokomo	95%	101
Parkview Noble Hospital	Kendallville	95%	62
Community Health Network	Indianapolis	94%	172
Kosciusko Community Hospital	Warsaw	94%	121
Lafayette Home Hospital	Lafayette	94%	98
Lutheran Hospital of Indiana	Fort Wayne	94%	207
Bedford Regional Medical Center	Bedford	93%	58
Goshen General Hospital	Goshen	93%	69
Logansport Memorial Hospital	Logansport	93%	45
Major Hospital	Shelbyville	93%	106
Saint Francis at Indianapolis	Indianapolis	93%	30
Saint Joseph's Reg Med Ctr-Plymouth Campus	Plymouth	93%	57
Saint Margaret Mercy Healthcare Centers	Hammond	93%	131
Saint Mary's Warrick Hospital	Boonville	93%	58
Saint Vincent Indianapolis Hospital	Indianapolis	93%	208
Parkview Huntington Hospital	Huntington	92%	52
Parkview Memorial Hospital	Fort Wayne	92%	97
Parkview Whitley Hospital	Columbia City	92%	49
Porter Memorial Health System	Valparaiso	92%	49
Saint Joseph Hospital	Kokomo	92%	93
Saint Margaret Mercy Healthcare Centers	Dyer	92%	106
Bloomington Hospital	Bloomington	91%	171
Saint Anthony Medical Center	Crown Point	91%	143
Saint Joseph Hospital	Fort Wayne	91%	33
Sullivan County Community Hospital	Sullivan	91%	44
Deaconess Hospital	Evansville	90%	318
King's Daughters Hospital	Madison	90%	127
LaPorte Hospital	La Porte	90%	89
Margaret Mary Community Hospital	Batesville	90%	68
Saint John's Health System	Anderson	90%	121
West Central Community Hospital	Clinton	90%	61
White County Memorial Hospital	Monticello	90%	39
Community Hospital South	Indianapolis	89%	76
Good Samaritan Hospital	Vincennes	89%	74
Saint Anthony Memorial Health Centers	Michigan City	89%	95
Saint Francis Beech Grove	Beech Grove	89%	80
Saint Joseph Regional Med Ctr-Mishawaka	Mishawaka	89%	37
Saint Mary's Medical Center	Evansville	89%	151
Saint Vincent Frankfort Hospital	Frankfort	89%	35
Cameron Memorial Community Hospital	Angola	88%	49
Memorial Hospital of South Bend	South Bend	88%	212
Ball Memorial Hospital	Muncie	87%	248
Dearborn County Hospital	Lawrenceburg	87%	126
Dukes Memorial Hospital	Peru	87%	38

Hospital Name	City	Rate	Cases
Daviess Community Hospital	Washington	86%	125
Methodist Hospitals-North Lake Campus	Gary	86%	106
Johnson Memorial Hospital	Franklin	85%	88
Saint Clare Medical Center	Crawfordsville	85%	27
Starke Memorial Hospital	Knox	84%	55
Wabash County Hospital	Wabash	84%	31
Clark Memorial Hospital	Jeffersonville	83%	116
Hendricks Regional Health	Danville	83%	99
Wishard Memorial Hospital	Indianapolis	83%	54
Scott Memorial Hospital	Scottsburg	82%	61
Methodist Hospital of Indiana	Indianapolis	80%	69
Witham Memorial Hospital	Lebanon	80%	54
Harrison County Hospital	Corydon	79%	29
Marion General Hospital	Marion	79%	110
Hancock Memorial Hospital and Health Services	Greenfield	74%	160
Henry County Memorial Hospital	New Castle	68%	76

15. Influenza Vaccine

Hospital Name	City	Rate	Cases
Dekalb Memorial Hospital	Auburn	100%	28
Reid Hospital and Health Care Services	Richmond	98%	88
Floyd Memorial Hospital and Health Services	New Albany	97%	74
Saint Margaret Mercy Healthcare Centers	Hammond	97%	31
Riverview Hospital	Noblesville	96%	25
Columbus Regional Hospital	Columbus	95%	39
Lutheran Hospital of Indiana	Fort Wayne	94%	66
Saint Joseph Hospital	Kokomo	93%	30
Ball Memorial Hospital	Muncie	92%	61
Hendricks Regional Health	Danville	92%	36
Johnson Memorial Hospital	Franklin	92%	26
Kosciusko Community Hospital	Warsaw	90%	31
Saint Joseph's Regional Medical Center	South Bend	89%	44
Union Hospital	Terre Haute	88%	48
Deaconess Hospital	Evansville	87%	104
Saint Francis Beech Grove	Beech Grove	87%	31
Saint Mary's Medical Center	Hobart	83%	58
Bloomington Hospital	Bloomington	82%	50
Howard Regional Health System	Kokomo	81%	48
Major Hospital	Shelbyville	81%	37
Memorial Hospital of South Bend	South Bend	77%	65
Saint Mary's Medical Center	Evansville	77%	61
Terre Haute Regional Hospital	Terre Haute	77%	30
LaPorte Hospital	La Porte	76%	25
Lafayette Home Hospital	Lafayette	74%	34
Saint Elizabeth Medical Center	Lafayette	71%	55
Good Samaritan Hospital	Vincennes	70%	33
Parkview Memorial Hospital	Fort Wayne	68%	25
Saint Anthony Memorial Health Centers	Michigan City	65%	26
Harrison County Hospital	Corydon	64%	28
Community Health Network	Indianapolis	59%	39
Daviess Community Hospital	Washington	53%	32
Saint John's Health System	Anderson	53%	58
Methodist Hospitals-North Lake Campus	Gary	51%	63
Elkhart General Hospital	Elkhart	50%	36
Saint Anthony Medical Center	Crown Point	45%	33
Saint Vincent Indianapolis Hospital	Indianapolis	39%	72
Hancock Memorial Hospital and Health Services	Greenfield	35%	46
Dearborn County Hospital	Lawrenceburg	24%	34
Clark Memorial Hospital	Jeffersonville	6%	33
Memorial Hospital and Health Care Center	Jasper	3%	38

16. Initial Antibiotic Timing

Hospital Name	City	Rate	Cases
Dekalb Memorial Hospital	Auburn	98%	118
Bluffton Regional Medical Center	Bluffton	97%	140
Gibson General Hospital	Princeton	97%	32
Medical Center of Southern Indiana	Charlestown	97%	31
Dukes Memorial Hospital	Peru	96%	55
Columbus Regional Hospital	Columbus	95%	176
Morgan Hospital Medical Centre	Martinsville	95%	126
Wabash County Hospital	Wabash	95%	57
West Central Community Hospital	Clinton	95%	120
Greene County General Hospital	Linton	94%	52
Reid Hospital and Health Care Services	Richmond	94%	459
Saint Joseph's Reg Med Ctr-Plymouth Campus	Plymouth	94%	107
Saint Vincent Clay Hospital	Brazil	94%	34
Community Hosp of Anderson & Madison Co	Anderson	93%	256
King's Daughters Hospital	Madison	93%	194
Kosciusko Community Hospital	Warsaw	93%	141
Daviess Community Hospital	Washington	92%	155
Henry County Memorial Hospital	New Castle	92%	168
Riverview Hospital	Noblesville	92%	92
Bedford Regional Medical Center	Bedford	91%	78
LaGrange Community Hospital	LaGrange	91%	57

NOTE: Hospital profiles are in alphabetical order by state, then city, then hospital within the city; Rankings are sorted by rate in descending order and exclude hospitals with less than 25 cases; (1) The number of cases is too small (n<25) for purposes of reliably predicting hospital performance; (2) Measure reflects the hospital's indication that its submission was based upon a sample of its relevant discharges; (3) Rate reflects fewer than the maximum possible quarters of data for the measure; (4) Inaccurate information submitted and suppressed for one or more quarters; (5) No data is available from the hospital for this measure; Please refer to the User's Guide for a full explanation of data

Hospital Name	City	Rate	Cases
Saint Joseph Regional Med Ctr-Mishawaka	Mishawaka	91%	75
Decatur County Memorial Hospital	Greensburg	90%	63
Saint Mary's Warrick Hospital	Boonville	90%	69
Hendricks Regional Health	Danville	89%	272
Major Hospital	Shelbyville	89%	183
Parkview Noble Hospital	Kendallville	89%	85
Saint Vincent Carmel Hospital	Carmel	89%	73
Schneck Medical Center	Seymour	89%	156
Union Hospital	Terre Haute	89%	284
Witham Memorial Hospital	Lebanon	89%	104
Dupont Hospital	Fort Wayne	88%	42
Johnson Memorial Hospital	Franklin	88%	112
Saint Mary's Medical Center	Hobart	88%	274
Sullivan County Community Hospital	Sullivan	88%	78
Bloomington Hospital	Bloomington	87%	250
Cameron Memorial Community Hospital	Angola	87%	70
Marion General Hospital	Marion	87%	166
Saint Elizabeth Medical Center	Lafayette	87%	262
Saint Vincent Frankfort Hospital	Frankfort	87%	53
White County Memorial Hospital	Monticello	87%	47
Adams Memorial Hospital	Decatur	86%	84
Good Samaritan Hospital	Vincennes	86%	136
Goshen General Hospital	Goshen	86%	116
Hancock Memorial Hospital and Health Services	Greenfield	86%	257
Howard Regional Health System	Kokomo	86%	220
Lutheran Hospital of Indiana	Fort Wayne	86%	260
Saint John's Health System	Anderson	86%	274
Starke Memorial Hospital	Knox	86%	125
LaPorte Hospital	La Porte	85%	138
Saint Anthony Memorial Health Centers	Michigan City	85%	187
Clarian West Medical Center	Avon	84%	122
Elkhart General Hospital	Elkhart	84%	290
Saint Vincent Mercy Hospital	Elwood	84%	90
Ball Memorial Hospital	Muncie	83%	339
Community Hospital South	Indianapolis	83%	141
Parkview Huntington Hospital	Huntington	83%	88
Saint Francis Beech Grove	Beech Grove	83%	126
Saint Joseph Hospital	Fort Wayne	83%	59
Saint Joseph's Regional Medical Center	South Bend	83%	222
Margaret Mary Community Hospital	Batesville	82%	131
Parkview Memorial Hospital	Fort Wayne	82%	132
Parkview Whitley Hospital	Columbia City	82%	65
Community Health Network	Indianapolis	81%	271
Saint Joseph Hospital	Kokomo	81%	149
Saint Margaret Mercy Healthcare Centers	Dyer	81%	134
Scott Memorial Hospital	Scottsburg	81%	112
Wishard Memorial Hospital	Indianapolis	81%	120
Lafayette Home Hospital	Lafayette	80%	149
Saint Vincent Williamsport	Williamsport	80%	50
Terre Haute Regional Hospital	Terre Haute	80%	174
Dearborn County Hospital	Lawrenceburg	79%	183
Floyd Memorial Hospital and Health Services	New Albany	79%	366
Porter Memorial Health System	Valparaiso	79%	324
Deaconess Hospital	Evansville	78%	479
Logansport Memorial Hospital	Logansport	78%	69
Saint Catherine Hospital of East Chicago	East Chicago	78%	148
Westview Hospital	Indianapolis	78%	106
Clark Memorial Hospital	Jeffersonville	77%	210
Saint Clare Medical Center	Crawfordsville	77%	108
Dunn Memorial Hospital	Bedford	76%	71
Saint Vincent Indianapolis Hospital	Indianapolis	75%	321
Tipton Hospital	Tipton	75%	57
Community Hospital	Hammond	74%	325
Memorial Hospital and Health Care Center	Jasper	74%	154
Methodist Hospital of Indiana	Indianapolis	74%	187
Saint Margaret Mercy Healthcare Centers	Hammond	74%	174
Jasper County Hospital	Rensselaer	73%	71
Memorial Hospital of South Bend	South Bend	73%	313
Saint Anthony Medical Center	Crown Point	73%	209
Harrison County Hospital	Corydon	72%	130
Saint Francis at Indianapolis	Indianapolis	68%	37
Saint Mary's Medical Center	Evansville	68%	257
Fayette Memorial Hospital	Connersville	66%	88
Methodist Hospitals-North Lake Campus	Gary	57%	357

17. Oxygenation Assessment

Hospital Name	City	Rate	Cases
Ball Memorial Hospital	Muncie	100%	429
Bedford Regional Medical Center	Bedford	100%	102
Bloomington Hospital	Bloomington	100%	322
Bluffton Regional Medical Center	Bluffton	100%	165
Cameron Memorial Community Hospital	Angola	100%	85
Clarian North Medical Center	Carmel	100%	26
Clarian West Medical Center	Avon	100%	133
Clark Memorial Hospital	Jeffersonville	100%	259
Columbus Regional Hospital	Columbus	100%	232
Community Health Network	Indianapolis	100%	317
Community Hospital	Hammond	100%	370
Community Hospital South	Indianapolis	100%	171
Community Hosp of Anderson & Madison Co	Anderson	100%	292
Community Hospital of Bremen	Bremen	100%	25
Daviess Community Hospital	Washington	100%	206
Deaconess Hospital	Evansville	100%	615
Dearborn County Hospital	Lawrenceburg	100%	229
Dekalb Memorial Hospital	Auburn	100%	157
Dukes Memorial Hospital	Peru	100%	65
Dupont Hospital	Fort Wayne	100%	55
Fayette Memorial Hospital	Connersville	100%	104
Gibson General Hospital	Princeton	100%	45
Goshen General Hospital	Goshen	100%	146
Greene County General Hospital	Linton	100%	62
Harrison County Hospital	Corydon	100%	140
Hendricks Regional Health	Danville	100%	274
Henry County Memorial Hospital	New Castle	100%	212
Johnson Memorial Hospital	Franklin	100%	148
King's Daughters Hospital	Madison	100%	236
Kosciusko Community Hospital	Warsaw	100%	177
LaGrange Community Hospital	LaGrange	100%	70
Logansport Memorial Hospital	Logansport	100%	91
Lutheran Hospital of Indiana	Fort Wayne	100%	337
Margaret Mary Community Hospital	Batesville	100%	155
Marion General Hospital	Marion	100%	198
Memorial Hospital of South Bend	South Bend	100%	407
Methodist Hospital of Indiana	Indianapolis	100%	248
Methodist Hospitals-North Lake Campus	Gary	100%	432
Morgan Hospital Medical Centre	Martinsville	100%	144
Parkview Huntington Hospital	Huntington	100%	108
Parkview Memorial Hospital	Fort Wayne	100%	177
Parkview Noble Hospital	Kendallville	100%	115
Parkview Whitley Hospital	Columbia City	100%	86
Porter Memorial Health System	Valparaiso	100%	379
Reid Hospital and Health Care Services	Richmond	100%	596
Riverview Hospital	Noblesville	100%	118
Saint Anthony Medical Center	Crown Point	100%	268
Saint Francis Beech Grove	Beech Grove	100%	180
Saint Francis at Indianapolis	Indianapolis	100%	49
Saint John's Health System	Anderson	100%	342
Saint Joseph Hospital	Fort Wayne	100%	67
Saint Joseph Hospital	Kokomo	100%	168
Saint Joseph Regional Med Ctr-Mishawaka	Mishawaka	100%	87
Saint Joseph's Regional Medical Center	South Bend	100%	269
Saint Joseph's Reg Med Ctr-Plymouth Campus	Plymouth	100%	143
Saint Margaret Mercy Healthcare Centers	Dyer	100%	168
Saint Margaret Mercy Healthcare Centers	Hammond	100%	205
Saint Mary's Medical Center	Hobart	100%	313
Saint Vincent Indianapolis Hospital	Indianapolis	100%	422
Saint Vincent Williamsport	Williamsport	100%	66
Scott Memorial Hospital	Scottsburg	100%	139
Starke Memorial Hospital	Knox	100%	133
Sullivan County Community Hospital	Sullivan	100%	84
Terre Haute Regional Hospital	Terre Haute	100%	200
Tipton Hospital	Tipton	100%	65
Union Hospital	Terre Haute	100%	339
Wabash County Hospital	Wabash	100%	66
Westview Hospital	Indianapolis	100%	113
Wishard Memorial Hospital	Indianapolis	100%	127
Decatur County Memorial Hospital	Greensburg	99%	77
Floyd Memorial Hospital and Health Services	New Albany	99%	471
Good Samaritan Hospital	Vincennes	99%	187
Hancock Memorial Hospital and Health Services	Greenfield	99%	286
Howard Regional Health System	Kokomo	99%	282
Lafayette Home Hospital	Lafayette	99%	187
Major Hospital	Shelbyville	99%	204
Saint Elizabeth Medical Center	Lafayette	99%	326
Saint Mary's Medical Center	Evansville	99%	332
Saint Vincent Carmel Hospital	Carmel	99%	108
Saint Vincent Frankfort Hospital	Frankfort	99%	67
Saint Vincent Mercy Hospital	Elwood	99%	102
West Central Community Hospital	Clinton	99%	148
Witham Memorial Hospital	Lebanon	99%	113
Dunn Memorial Hospital	Bedford	98%	104
Elkhart General Hospital	Elkhart	98%	308
Jasper County Hospital	Rensselaer	98%	84
LaPorte Hospital	La Porte	98%	164
Saint Clare Medical Center	Crawfordsville	98%	121
Saint Vincent Clay Hospital	Brazil	98%	56
Schneck Medical Center	Seymour	98%	199
Adams Memorial Hospital	Decatur	97%	94
Medical Center of Southern Indiana	Charlestown	97%	32

NOTE: Hospital profiles are in alphabetical order by state, then city, then hospital within the city; Rankings are sorted by rate in descending order and exclude hospitals with less than 25 cases; (1) The number of cases is too small (n<25) for purposes of reliably predicting hospital performance; (2) Measure reflects the hospital's indication that its submission was based upon a sample of its relevant discharges; (3) Rate reflects fewer than the maximum possible quarters of data for the measure; (4) Inaccurate information submitted and suppressed for one or more quarters; (5) No data is available from the hospital for this measure; Please refer to the User's Guide for a full explanation of data

Hospital Name	City	Rate	Cases
Saint Catherine Hospital of East Chicago	East Chicago	97%	162
Saint Mary's Warrick Hospital	Boonville	97%	91
Memorial Hospital and Health Care Center	Jasper	96%	194
Saint Anthony Memorial Health Centers	Michigan City	95%	220
White County Memorial Hospital	Monticello	94%	68

18. Pneumococcal Vaccine

Hospital Name	City	Rate	Cases
Bedford Regional Medical Center	Bedford	100%	68
Community Hosp of Anderson & Madison Co	Anderson	100%	191
Dekalb Memorial Hospital	Auburn	100%	100
Bluffton Regional Medical Center	Bluffton	99%	101
King's Daughters Hospital	Madison	99%	148
Schneck Medical Center	Seymour	99%	125
Dupont Hospital	Fort Wayne	97%	29
Marion General Hospital	Marion	97%	117
Floyd Memorial Hospital and Health Services	New Albany	96%	271
Kosciusko Community Hospital	Warsaw	96%	108
Saint Francis at Indianapolis	Indianapolis	96%	28
Reid Hospital and Health Care Services	Richmond	95%	332
Riverview Hospital	Noblesville	95%	81
Saint Joseph Regional Med Ctr-Mishawaka	Mishawaka	95%	56
Columbus Regional Hospital	Columbus	94%	136
Parkview Noble Hospital	Kendallville	94%	65
Lutheran Hospital of Indiana	Fort Wayne	93%	241
West Central Community Hospital	Clinton	93%	92
Goshen General Hospital	Goshen	92%	91
Saint Joseph Hospital	Fort Wayne	92%	39
Union Hospital	Terre Haute	92%	203
Decatur County Memorial Hospital	Greensburg	91%	44
Ball Memorial Hospital	Muncie	90%	242
LaPorte Hospital	La Porte	89%	119
Memorial Hospital of South Bend	South Bend	89%	256
Dukes Memorial Hospital	Peru	88%	33
Major Hospital	Shelbyville	88%	137
Wabash County Hospital	Wabash	88%	40
Cameron Memorial Community Hospital	Angola	86%	56
Deaconess Hospital	Evansville	86%	404
Johnson Memorial Hospital	Franklin	85%	78
Sullivan County Community Hospital	Sullivan	85%	53
Community Hospital South	Indianapolis	84%	100
Greene County General Hospital	Linton	84%	45
Parkview Huntington Hospital	Huntington	84%	68
Bloomington Hospital	Bloomington	83%	217
Gibson General Hospital	Princeton	83%	30
Saint Francis Beech Grove	Beech Grove	83%	136
Saint Joseph's Regional Medical Center	South Bend	83%	168
Community Hospital	Hammond	82%	213
Logansport Memorial Hospital	Logansport	82%	51
Saint Vincent Clay Hospital	Brazil	82%	34
Howard Regional Health System	Kokomo	81%	182
Memorial Hospital and Health Care Center	Jasper	81%	129
Margaret Mary Community Hospital	Batesville	80%	111
Saint John's Health System	Anderson	80%	231
Saint Joseph Hospital	Kokomo	79%	113
Saint Margaret Mercy Healthcare Centers	Hammond	79%	124
Wishard Memorial Hospital	Indianapolis	79%	34
Saint Catherine Hospital of East Chicago	East Chicago	78%	74
Adams Memorial Hospital	Decatur	77%	66
Clarian West Medical Center	Avon	77%	88
Saint Mary's Medical Center	Hobart	77%	220
Witham Memorial Hospital	Lebanon	77%	77
Community Health Network	Indianapolis	75%	186
Good Samaritan Hospital	Vincennes	75%	129
Parkview Whitley Hospital	Columbia City	75%	53
Hendricks Regional Health	Danville	73%	162
Clark Memorial Hospital	Jeffersonville	72%	155
Harrison County Hospital	Corydon	72%	78
Henry County Memorial Hospital	New Castle	72%	123
Methodist Hospital of Indiana	Indianapolis	72%	116
Saint Margaret Mercy Healthcare Centers	Dyer	72%	95
Saint Mary's Medical Center	Evansville	72%	192
Terre Haute Regional Hospital	Terre Haute	72%	130
Saint Mary's Warrick Hospital	Boonville	70%	64
White County Memorial Hospital	Monticello	70%	47
Morgan Hospital Medical Centre	Martinsville	68%	95
Daviess Community Hospital	Washington	67%	123
Dearborn County Hospital	Lawrenceburg	67%	139
Saint Anthony Memorial Health Centers	Michigan City	67%	126
Saint Vincent Mercy Hospital	Elwood	67%	66
Hancock Memorial Hospital and Health Services	Greenfield	66%	193
Dunn Memorial Hospital	Bedford	64%	72
Saint Elizabeth Medical Center	Lafayette	64%	227
Saint Vincent Williamsport	Williamsport	64%	36
LaGrange Community Hospital	LaGrange	63%	43
Parkview Memorial Hospital	Fort Wayne	63%	109
Saint Joseph's Reg Med Ctr-Plymouth Campus	Plymouth	63%	97
Scott Memorial Hospital	Scottsburg	63%	65
Jasper County Hospital	Rensselaer	62%	68
Lafayette Home Hospital	Lafayette	61%	117
Porter Memorial Health System	Valparaiso	60%	277
Tipton Hospital	Tipton	58%	43
Starke Memorial Hospital	Knox	57%	69
Westview Hospital	Indianapolis	57%	69
Methodist Hospitals-North Lake Campus	Gary	52%	214
Saint Anthony Medical Center	Crown Point	51%	171
Saint Vincent Indianapolis Hospital	Indianapolis	51%	274
Saint Vincent Frankfort Hospital	Frankfort	49%	37
Elkhart General Hospital	Elkhart	42%	184
Saint Clare Medical Center	Crawfordsville	38%	80
Fayette Memorial Hospital	Connersville	35%	66
Saint Vincent Carmel Hospital	Carmel	23%	62

19. Smoking Cessation Advice

Hospital Name	City	Rate	Cases
Bluffton Regional Medical Center	Bluffton	100%	34
Columbus Regional Hospital	Columbus	100%	75
Community Health Network	Indianapolis	100%	64
Community Hospital South	Indianapolis	100%	37
Kosciusko Community Hospital	Warsaw	100%	50
Memorial Hospital and Health Care Center	Jasper	100%	33
Reid Hospital and Health Care Services	Richmond	100%	131
Saint Anthony Memorial Health Centers	Michigan City	100%	49
Saint Joseph Hospital	Kokomo	100%	54
Saint Joseph's Reg Med Ctr-Plymouth Campus	Plymouth	100%	31
Terre Haute Regional Hospital	Terre Haute	100%	73
Wishard Memorial Hospital	Indianapolis	100%	39
Community Hosp of Anderson & Madison Co	Anderson	99%	78
Union Hospital	Terre Haute	99%	98
Deaconess Hospital	Evansville	98%	183
Lutheran Hospital of Indiana	Fort Wayne	97%	93
West Central Community Hospital	Clinton	97%	37
Marion General Hospital	Marion	96%	51
Bloomington Hospital	Bloomington	95%	95
Saint Mary's Medical Center	Hobart	95%	81
Schneck Medical Center	Seymour	95%	40
Dekalb Memorial Hospital	Auburn	94%	36
King's Daughters Hospital	Madison	94%	54
Saint John's Health System	Anderson	94%	68
Howard Regional Health System	Kokomo	93%	70
Floyd Memorial Hospital and Health Services	New Albany	92%	130
Methodist Hospitals-North Lake Campus	Gary	92%	111
Johnson Memorial Hospital	Franklin	91%	35
Henry County Memorial Hospital	New Castle	90%	50
Saint Mary's Medical Center	Evansville	90%	100
LaPorte Hospital	La Porte	88%	40
Goshen General Hospital	Goshen	86%	28
Saint Margaret Mercy Healthcare Centers	Dyer	86%	42
Dearborn County Hospital	Lawrenceburg	85%	68
Hendricks Regional Health	Danville	85%	54
Major Hospital	Shelbyville	84%	55
Parkview Noble Hospital	Kendallville	84%	37
Methodist Hospital of Indiana	Indianapolis	81%	73
Parkview Memorial Hospital	Fort Wayne	81%	42
Saint Joseph Regional Med Ctr-Mishawaka	Mishawaka	80%	30
Margaret Mary Community Hospital	Batesville	78%	36
Westview Hospital	Indianapolis	78%	32
Dunn Memorial Hospital	Bedford	76%	25
Saint Clare Medical Center	Crawfordsville	76%	25
Saint Vincent Mercy Hospital	Elwood	76%	29
Ball Memorial Hospital	Muncie	75%	118
Daviess Community Hospital	Washington	75%	40
Lafayette Home Hospital	Lafayette	75%	44
Saint Joseph's Regional Medical Center	South Bend	75%	52
Saint Margaret Mercy Healthcare Centers	Hammond	75%	57
Clark Memorial Hospital	Jeffersonville	74%	76
Saint Francis Beech Grove	Beech Grove	72%	50
Saint Elizabeth Medical Center	Lafayette	70%	81
Good Samaritan Hospital	Vincennes	69%	42
Scott Memorial Hospital	Scottsburg	68%	47
Elkhart General Hospital	Elkhart	62%	81
Memorial Hospital of South Bend	South Bend	62%	78
Hancock Memorial Hospital and Health Services	Greenfield	57%	63
Saint Vincent Indianapolis Hospital	Indianapolis	49%	80
Harrison County Hospital	Corydon	45%	33
Starke Memorial Hospital	Knox	44%	39
Saint Anthony Medical Center	Crown Point	27%	41

NOTE: Hospital profiles are in alphabetical order by state, then city, then hospital within the city; Rankings are sorted by rate in descending order and exclude hospitals with less than 25 cases; (1) The number of cases is too small (n<25) for purposes of reliably predicting hospital performance; (2) Measure reflects the hospital's indication that its submission was based upon a sample of its relevant discharges; (3) Rate reflects fewer than the maximum possible quarters of data for the measure; (4) Inaccurate information submitted and suppressed for one or more quarters; (5) No data is available from the hospital for this measure; Please refer to the User's Guide for a full explanation of data

Surgical Infection Prevention

20. Prophylactic Antibiotic Given

Hospital Name	City	Rate	Cases
Saint Vincent Heart Center of Indiana	Indianapolis	99%	143
Bluffton Regional Medical Center	Bluffton	98%	161
King's Daughters Hospital	Madison	98%	133
Community Hosp of Anderson & Madison Co	Anderson	96%	400
Dekalb Memorial Hospital	Auburn	96%	46
Reid Hospital and Health Care Services	Richmond	96%	357
Women's Hospital	Newburgh	96%	449
Dearborn County Hospital	Lawrenceburg	95%	234
Indiana Heart Hospital	Indianapolis	95%	444
LaPorte Hospital	La Porte	95%	377
Saint Vincent Carmel Hospital	Carmel	95%	134
Floyd Memorial Hospital and Health Services	New Albany	94%	364
Riverview Hospital	Noblesville	94%	391
Community Hospital South	Indianapolis	93%	59
Saint Margaret Mercy Healthcare Centers	Dyer	93%	198
Schneck Medical Center	Seymour	93%	202
Clarian West Medical Center	Avon	92%	36
Goshen General Hospital	Goshen	92%	356
Henry County Memorial Hospital	New Castle	92%	176
Kosciusko Community Hospital	Warsaw	92%	239
Methodist Hospital of Indiana	Indianapolis	92%	360
Saint Anthony Medical Center	Crown Point	92%	583
Bloomington Hospital	Bloomington	91%	895
Saint Anthony Memorial Health Centers	Michigan City	91%	284
Saint Joseph's Regional Medical Center	South Bend	91%	925
Saint Margaret Mercy Healthcare Centers	Hammond	91%	294
West Central Community Hospital	Clinton	91%	33
Clarian North Medical Center	Carmel	90%	39
Clark Memorial Hospital	Jeffersonville	90%	126
Bedford Regional Medical Center	Bedford	89%	65
Parkview Huntington Hospital	Huntington	89%	111
Community Hospital	Hammond	88%	88
Indiana Orthopaedic Hospital	Indianapolis	88%	26
Johnson Memorial Hospital	Franklin	88%	121
Columbus Regional Hospital	Columbus	87%	631
Lafayette Home Hospital	Lafayette	87%	766
Major Hospital	Shelbyville	87%	92
Saint Francis at Mooresville	Mooresville	87%	353
Saint Joseph's Reg Med Ctr-Plymouth Campus	Plymouth	87%	171
Terre Haute Regional Hospital	Terre Haute	87%	188
Union Hospital	Terre Haute	87%	854
Saint Elizabeth Medical Center	Lafayette	86%	523
Ball Memorial Hospital	Muncie	85%	1006
Hancock Memorial Hospital and Health Services	Greenfield	85%	186
Saint Francis at Indianapolis	Indianapolis	85%	163
Daviess Community Hospital	Washington	83%	30
Logansport Memorial Hospital	Logansport	82%	165
Marion General Hospital	Marion	82%	271
Memorial Hospital of South Bend	South Bend	82%	519
Parkview Noble Hospital	Kendallville	82%	78
Saint John's Health System	Anderson	82%	502
Saint Joseph Regional Med Ctr-Mishawaka	Mishawaka	81%	109
Cameron Memorial Community Hospital	Angola	79%	39
Dupont Hospital	Fort Wayne	79%	623
Hendricks Regional Health	Danville	79%	315
Saint Francis Beech Grove	Beech Grove	79%	351
Saint Clare Medical Center	Crawfordsville	78%	138
Wishard Memorial Hospital	Indianapolis	78%	158
Deaconess Hospital	Evansville	77%	1072
Saint Vincent Indianapolis Hospital	Indianapolis	75%	227
Elkhart General Hospital	Elkhart	72%	1152
Lutheran Hospital of Indiana	Fort Wayne	72%	1709
Saint Joseph Hospital	Fort Wayne	72%	163
Harrison County Hospital	Corydon	71%	56
Howard Regional Health System	Kokomo	70%	147
Parkview Whitley Hospital	Columbia City	70%	61
Westview Hospital	Indianapolis	70%	82
Porter Memorial Health System	Valparaiso	67%	66
Parkview Memorial Hospital	Fort Wayne	66%	314
Saint Mary's Medical Center	Evansville	66%	335
Dunn Memorial Hospital	Bedford	65%	31
Decatur County Memorial Hospital	Greensburg	64%	66
Good Samaritan Hospital	Vincennes	63%	514
Methodist Hospitals-North Lake Campus	Gary	63%	383
Witham Memorial Hospital	Lebanon	62%	34
Fayette Memorial Hospital	Connersville	56%	100
Memorial Hospital and Health Care Center	Jasper	56%	345
Saint Mary's Medical Center	Hobart	54%	209
Community Health Network	Indianapolis	52%	79
Saint Vincent Frankfort Hospital	Frankfort	52%	31
Saint Joseph Hospital	Kokomo	46%	139
Dukes Memorial Hospital	Peru	44%	36
Margaret Mary Community Hospital	Batesville	44%	126
Adams Memorial Hospital	Decatur	43%	35
Saint Catherine Hospital of East Chicago	East Chicago	29%	63

21. Prophylactic Antibiotic Selection

Hospital Name	City	Rate	Cases
Community Hosp of Anderson & Madison Co	Anderson	100%	96
Daviess Community Hospital	Washington	100%	30
Henry County Memorial Hospital	New Castle	100%	44
Indiana Heart Hospital	Indianapolis	100%	169
King's Daughters Hospital	Madison	100%	41
Saint Clare Medical Center	Crawfordsville	100%	33
Saint Joseph Hospital	Fort Wayne	100%	42
Saint Joseph Regional Med Ctr-Mishawaka	Mishawaka	100%	32
Saint Vincent Carmel Hospital	Carmel	100%	44
Saint Vincent Heart Center of Indiana	Indianapolis	100%	64
Methodist Hospital of Indiana	Indianapolis	99%	67
Saint Joseph's Regional Medical Center	South Bend	99%	309
Goshen General Hospital	Goshen	98%	82
Hancock Memorial Hospital and Health Services	Greenfield	98%	41
LaPorte Hospital	La Porte	98%	92
Memorial Hospital of South Bend	South Bend	98%	172
Saint Margaret Mercy Healthcare Centers	Hammond	98%	59
Schneck Medical Center	Seymour	98%	41
Bloomington Hospital	Bloomington	97%	209
Floyd Memorial Hospital and Health Services	New Albany	97%	109
Logansport Memorial Hospital	Logansport	97%	37
Margaret Mary Community Hospital	Batesville	97%	35
Parkview Memorial Hospital	Fort Wayne	97%	79
Saint Francis at Indianapolis	Indianapolis	97%	92
Saint Francis at Mooresville	Mooresville	97%	75
Saint Joseph's Reg Med Ctr-Plymouth Campus	Plymouth	97%	64
Ball Memorial Hospital	Muncie	96%	214
Bluffton Regional Medical Center	Bluffton	96%	51
Dearborn County Hospital	Lawrenceburg	96%	50
Lutheran Hospital of Indiana	Fort Wayne	96%	437
Reid Hospital and Health Care Services	Richmond	96%	102
Saint John's Health System	Anderson	96%	122
Saint Mary's Medical Center	Evansville	96%	121
Women's Hospital	Newburgh	96%	78
Columbus Regional Hospital	Columbus	95%	149
Deaconess Hospital	Evansville	95%	297
Dupont Hospital	Fort Wayne	95%	173
Elkhart General Hospital	Elkhart	95%	277
Saint Anthony Memorial Health Centers	Michigan City	95%	91
Saint Vincent Indianapolis Hospital	Indianapolis	95%	104
Union Hospital	Terre Haute	95%	212
Wishard Memorial Hospital	Indianapolis	95%	43
Kosciusko Community Hospital	Warsaw	94%	70
Howard Regional Health System	Kokomo	93%	46
Memorial Hospital and Health Care Center	Jasper	93%	111
Saint Anthony Medical Center	Crown Point	93%	131
Saint Margaret Mercy Healthcare Centers	Dyer	93%	60
Hendricks Regional Health	Danville	92%	71
Saint Francis Beech Grove	Beech Grove	91%	46
Clark Memorial Hospital	Jeffersonville	89%	122
Lafayette Home Hospital	Lafayette	88%	185
Good Samaritan Hospital	Vincennes	87%	164
Terre Haute Regional Hospital	Terre Haute	85%	80
Methodist Hospitals-North Lake Campus	Gary	80%	127
Saint Elizabeth Medical Center	Lafayette	80%	120
Saint Mary's Medical Center	Hobart	80%	65
Riverview Hospital	Noblesville	79%	99
Marion General Hospital	Marion	78%	88

22. Prophylactic Antibiotic Stopped

Hospital Name	City	Rate	Cases
Bluffton Regional Medical Center	Bluffton	99%	156
Saint Joseph Hospital	Kokomo	99%	129
Clark Memorial Hospital	Jeffersonville	96%	117
Johnson Memorial Hospital	Franklin	96%	114
Reid Hospital and Health Care Services	Richmond	96%	315
Saint Vincent Heart Center of Indiana	Indianapolis	96%	137
Dekalb Memorial Hospital	Auburn	95%	43
Indiana Heart Hospital	Indianapolis	95%	422
Saint Vincent Carmel Hospital	Carmel	94%	133
Saint Vincent Frankfort Hospital	Frankfort	93%	29
Saint Joseph's Regional Medical Center	South Bend	92%	897
Schneck Medical Center	Seymour	92%	186
King's Daughters Hospital	Madison	91%	130
Parkview Huntington Hospital	Huntington	91%	108
Bloomington Hospital	Bloomington	89%	853

NOTE: Hospital profiles are in alphabetical order by state, then city, then hospital within the city; Rankings are sorted by rate in descending order and exclude hospitals with less than 25 cases; (1) The number of cases is too small (n<25) for purposes of reliably predicting hospital performance; (2) Measure reflects the hospital's indication that its submission was based upon a sample of its relevant discharges; (3) Rate reflects fewer than the maximum possible quarters of data for the measure; (4) Inaccurate information submitted and suppressed for one or more quarters; (5) No data is available from the hospital for this measure; Please refer to the User's Guide for a full explanation of data

Hospital Name	City	Rate	Cases
Riverview Hospital	Noblesville	89%	384
Marion General Hospital	Marion	88%	260
Witham Memorial Hospital	Lebanon	88%	34
Women's Hospital	Newburgh	88%	438
LaPorte Hospital	La Porte	87%	363
Logansport Memorial Hospital	Logansport	87%	167
Memorial Hospital of South Bend	South Bend	86%	487
Saint Francis at Mooresville	Mooresville	86%	348
Ball Memorial Hospital	Muncie	84%	976
Floyd Memorial Hospital and Health Services	New Albany	84%	351
Saint Francis at Indianapolis	Indianapolis	84%	154
Saint Vincent Indianapolis Hospital	Indianapolis	84%	226
Wishard Memorial Hospital	Indianapolis	84%	150
Community Hosp of Anderson & Madison Co	Anderson	83%	380
Dukes Memorial Hospital	Peru	83%	36
Saint John's Health System	Anderson	83%	501
Goshen General Hospital	Goshen	81%	345
Harrison County Hospital	Corydon	80%	54
Saint Francis Beech Grove	Beech Grove	79%	335
Community Hospital South	Indianapolis	78%	59
Fayette Memorial Hospital	Connersville	78%	87
Good Samaritan Hospital	Vincennes	76%	502
Saint Joseph's Reg Med Ctr-Plymouth Campus	Plymouth	76%	168
Clarian North Medical Center	Carmel	74%	39
Dearborn County Hospital	Lawrenceburg	74%	212
Dupont Hospital	Fort Wayne	74%	600
Kosciusko Community Hospital	Warsaw	74%	238
Memorial Hospital and Health Care Center	Jasper	74%	337
Parkview Noble Hospital	Kendallville	73%	75
Clarian West Medical Center	Avon	72%	32
Howard Regional Health System	Kokomo	72%	137
Lutheran Hospital of Indiana	Fort Wayne	71%	1624
Methodist Hospital of Indiana	Indianapolis	71%	341
Saint Joseph Hospital	Fort Wayne	71%	162
Saint Joseph Regional Med Ctr-Mishawaka	Mishawaka	71%	99
Saint Mary's Medical Center	Evansville	71%	327
Saint Margaret Mercy Healthcare Centers	Hammond	70%	290
Columbus Regional Hospital	Columbus	69%	593
Indiana Orthopaedic Hospital	Indianapolis	69%	26
West Central Community Hospital	Clinton	69%	32
Cameron Memorial Community Hospital	Angola	67%	39
Daviess Community Hospital	Washington	67%	30
Saint Anthony Memorial Health Centers	Michigan City	67%	278
Union Hospital	Terre Haute	67%	809
Porter Memorial Health System	Valparaiso	66%	61
Community Health Network	Indianapolis	65%	72
Hendricks Regional Health	Danville	61%	309
Lafayette Home Hospital	Lafayette	60%	752
Saint Mary's Medical Center	Hobart	60%	205
Dunn Memorial Hospital	Bedford	58%	31
Elkhart General Hospital	Elkhart	58%	1120
Saint Elizabeth Medical Center	Lafayette	58%	513
Saint Margaret Mercy Healthcare Centers	Dyer	58%	195
Westview Hospital	Indianapolis	58%	78
Parkview Memorial Hospital	Fort Wayne	57%	306
Methodist Hospitals-North Lake Campus	Gary	56%	363
Deaconess Hospital	Evansville	53%	1037
Saint Anthony Medical Center	Crown Point	51%	573
Hancock Memorial Hospital and Health Services	Greenfield	49%	182
Major Hospital	Shelbyville	49%	89
Parkview Whitley Hospital	Columbia City	48%	58
Community Hospital	Hammond	47%	86
Terre Haute Regional Hospital	Terre Haute	43%	185
Bedford Regional Medical Center	Bedford	39%	61
Adams Memorial Hospital	Decatur	32%	34
Margaret Mary Community Hospital	Batesville	32%	124
Decatur County Memorial Hospital	Greensburg	30%	64
Saint Catherine Hospital of East Chicago	East Chicago	29%	63
Saint Clare Medical Center	Crawfordsville	25%	137
Henry County Memorial Hospital	New Castle	21%	169

Pregnancy Care

23. Inpatient Neonatal Mortality

Hospital Name	City	Rate	Cases
Bluffton Regional Medical Center	Bluffton	0.00%	274
Community Hosp of Anderson & Madison Co	Anderson	0.00%	1008
Daviess Community Hospital	Washington	0.00%	402
LaPorte Hospital	La Porte	0.00%	693
Morgan Hospital Medical Centre	Martinsville	0.00%	213
Saint Joseph's Reg Med Ctr-Plymouth Campus	Plymouth	0.00%	411
Dupont Hospital	Fort Wayne	0.09%	2296
Clarian West Medical Center	Avon	0.11%	933
Goshen General Hospital	Goshen	0.12%	1637
Porter Memorial Health System	Valparaiso	0.14%	1390
Community Hospital South	Indianapolis	0.15%	657
Saint Joseph Regional Med Ctr-Mishawaka	Mishawaka	0.30%	659
Community Health Network	Indianapolis	0.35%	1713
Women's Hospital	Newburgh	0.44%	3217
Clarian North Medical Center	Carmel	0.45%	1553
Community Hospital	Hammond	0.56%	2308
Lutheran Hospital of Indiana	Fort Wayne	0.59%	1849
Saint Joseph's Regional Medical Center	South Bend	1.08%	1206

24. Third or Fourth Degree Laceration

Hospital Name	City	Rate	Cases
Saint Joseph Regional Med Ctr-Mishawaka	Mishawaka	1.15%	521
LaPorte Hospital	La Porte	1.41%	498
Community Hospital	Hammond	2.43%	1441
Saint Joseph's Regional Medical Center	South Bend	2.60%	845
Community Hosp of Anderson & Madison Co	Anderson	2.65%	717
Morgan Hospital Medical Centre	Martinsville	2.72%	147
Saint Joseph's Reg Med Ctr-Plymouth Campus	Plymouth	2.72%	294
Goshen General Hospital	Goshen	2.81%	1316
Lutheran Hospital of Indiana	Fort Wayne	2.82%	1133
Bluffton Regional Medical Center	Bluffton	2.96%	203
Daviess Community Hospital	Washington	3.63%	303
Porter Memorial Health System	Valparaiso	3.63%	936
Clarian West Medical Center	Avon	4.51%	621
Dupont Hospital	Fort Wayne	4.76%	1640
Clarian North Medical Center	Carmel	5.67%	970
Community Health Network	Indianapolis	6.24%	2019
Women's Hospital	Newburgh	6.35%	2001
Community Hospital South	Indianapolis	8.07%	471

NOTE: Hospital profiles are in alphabetical order by state, then city, then hospital within the city; Rankings are sorted by rate in descending order and exclude hospitals with less than 25 cases; (1) The number of cases is too small (n<25) for purposes of reliably predicting hospital performance; (2) Measure reflects the hospital's indication that its submission was based upon a sample of its relevant discharges; (3) Rate reflects fewer than the maximum possible quarters of data for the measure; (4) Inaccurate information submitted and suppressed for one or more quarters; (5) No data is available from the hospital for this measure; Please refer to the User's Guide for a full explanation of data

Community Hosp of Anderson & Madison Co

Alternate Name: Community Hospital
1515 N Madison Avenue
Anderson, IN 46011
Phone: 765-298-4242
Fax: 765-298-5819
Ownership: Voluntary non-profit - Private
Accredited: Yes
Emergency Services: Yes
Licensed Beds: 207

Key Personnel:

CEO . . . . Williams Vanneff
Chief Medical Staff . . . . Ronald Harmening, MD
Director Infection/Disease Control . . . . Linda Robinson
ICU Supervising Nurse . . . . Evelyn Bertram
Cardiology . . . . Michael Ball
Director Medical/Surgical Nursing . . . . Lois Meeker
Director Medical/Surgical Nursing . . . . Pat Gorman
Chief OB/GYN . . . . William Gist, MD
Chief Radiology . . . . Bob Reed
Pulmonary . . . . Saiful Kabir

Measure	Cases	This Hospital	State Average	U.S. Average	Top Hospital
Heart Attack Care					
ACE Inhibitor or ARB for LVSD[1]	2	100%	83%	82%	100%
Aspirin at Arrival	33	100%	91%	92%	100%
Aspirin at Discharge[1]	21	100%	91%	90%	100%
Beta Blocker at Arrival	29	100%	84%	87%	100%
Beta Blocker at Discharge[1]	21	100%	91%	90%	100%
Fibrinolytic Medication Timing[1]	6	83%	44%	31%	100%
PCI Within 90 Minutes of Arrival	0	-	56%	54%	95%
Smoking Cessation Advice[1]	6	100%	90%	88%	100%
Heart Failure Care					
ACE Inhibitor or ARB for LVSD	50	92%	81%	82%	100%
Discharge Instructions	138	91%	69%	61%	93%
Evaluation of LVS Function	185	97%	87%	83%	99%
Smoking Cessation Advice[1]	21	100%	84%	82%	100%
Pneumonia Care					
Appropriate Initial Antibiotic[2]	165	96%	83%	83%	94%
Blood Culture Timing[2]	109	96%	90%	90%	100%
Influenza Vaccine[4,5]	-	-	74%	70%	100%
Initial Antibiotic Timing[2]	256	93%	84%	80%	93%
Oxygenation Assessment[2]	292	100%	99%	99%	100%
Pneumococcal Vaccine[2]	191	100%	77%	69%	94%
Smoking Cessation Advice[2]	78	99%	81%	80%	100%
Surgical Infection Prevention					
Prophylactic Antibiotic Given	400	96%	76%	77%	95%
Prophylactic Antibiotic Selection	96	100%	92%	90%	100%
Prophylactic Antibiotic Stopped	380	83%	70%	72%	95%
Pregnancy Care					
Inpatient Neonatal Mortality	1,008	0.00%	-	-	-
Third or Fourth Degree Laceration	717	2.65%	4.02%	3.63%	3.27%

Saint John's Health System

2015 Jackson Street
Anderson, IN 46016
Phone: 765-649-2511
Fax: 765-646-8504
URL: www.stjohnshealthsystem.org
Ownership: Voluntary non-profit - Private
Accredited: Yes
Emergency Services: No
Licensed Beds: 332

Key Personnel:

President . . . . Kyle De Fur
Director of Cardiopulmonary . . . . Ross Brodhead
Head of Emergency Room . . . . Robert Steele
VP/Chief Medical Officer . . . . Gary Brazel, MD
Chief OB/GYN . . . . Jeffrey Blake, MD
Chief Radiology . . . . Henry Jones, MD
Director Respiratory Therapy . . . . Tim Thompson

Measure	Cases	This Hospital	State Average	U.S. Average	Top Hospital
Heart Attack Care					
ACE Inhibitor or ARB for LVSD[1]	19	89%	83%	82%	100%
Aspirin at Arrival	72	94%	91%	92%	100%
Aspirin at Discharge	48	90%	91%	90%	100%
Beta Blocker at Arrival	73	90%	84%	87%	100%
Beta Blocker at Discharge	53	98%	91%	90%	100%
Fibrinolytic Medication Timing	0	-	44%	31%	100%
PCI Within 90 Minutes of Arrival	0	-	56%	54%	95%
Smoking Cessation Advice[1]	9	78%	90%	88%	100%
Heart Failure Care					
ACE Inhibitor or ARB for LVSD	84	94%	81%	82%	100%
Discharge Instructions	157	81%	69%	61%	93%
Evaluation of LVS Function	205	99%	87%	83%	99%
Smoking Cessation Advice	42	93%	84%	82%	100%
Pneumonia Care					
Appropriate Initial Antibiotic	139	90%	83%	83%	94%
Blood Culture Timing	121	90%	90%	90%	100%
Influenza Vaccine	58	53%	74%	70%	100%
Initial Antibiotic Timing	274	86%	84%	80%	93%
Oxygenation Assessment	342	100%	99%	99%	100%
Pneumococcal Vaccine	231	80%	77%	69%	94%
Smoking Cessation Advice	68	94%	81%	80%	100%
Surgical Infection Prevention					
Prophylactic Antibiotic Given	502	82%	76%	77%	95%
Prophylactic Antibiotic Selection	122	96%	92%	90%	100%
Prophylactic Antibiotic Stopped	501	83%	70%	72%	95%
Pregnancy Care					
Inpatient Neonatal Mortality	-	-	-	-	-
Third or Fourth Degree Laceration	-	-	4.02%	3.63%	3.27%

Cameron Memorial Community Hospital

416 E Maumee Street
Angola, IN 46703
Toll-Free: 800-942-9583
Phone: 260-665-2141
Fax: 260-665-2879
URL: www.cameronmch.com
Ownership: Government - Local
Accredited: No
Emergency Services: Yes
Licensed Beds: 25

Key Personnel:

CEO/Administrator . . . . Dennis L Knapp

Measure	Cases	This Hospital	State Average	U.S. Average	Top Hospital
Heart Attack Care					
ACE Inhibitor or ARB for LVSD[5]	-	-	83%	82%	100%
Aspirin at Arrival[5]	-	-	91%	92%	100%
Aspirin at Discharge[5]	-	-	91%	90%	100%
Beta Blocker at Arrival[5]	-	-	84%	87%	100%
Beta Blocker at Discharge[5]	-	-	91%	90%	100%
Fibrinolytic Medication Timing[5]	-	-	44%	31%	100%
PCI Within 90 Minutes of Arrival[5]	-	-	56%	54%	95%
Smoking Cessation Advice[5]	-	-	90%	88%	100%
Heart Failure Care					
ACE Inhibitor or ARB for LVSD[1]	3	33%	81%	82%	100%
Discharge Instructions	29	21%	69%	61%	93%
Evaluation of LVS Function	39	38%	87%	83%	99%
Smoking Cessation Advice[1]	1	100%	84%	82%	100%
Pneumonia Care					
Appropriate Initial Antibiotic	59	93%	83%	83%	94%
Blood Culture Timing	49	88%	90%	90%	100%
Influenza Vaccine[1]	12	58%	74%	70%	100%
Initial Antibiotic Timing	70	87%	84%	80%	93%
Oxygenation Assessment	85	100%	99%	99%	100%
Pneumococcal Vaccine	56	86%	77%	69%	94%
Smoking Cessation Advice[1]	20	80%	81%	80%	100%
Surgical Infection Prevention					
Prophylactic Antibiotic Given	39	79%	76%	77%	95%
Prophylactic Antibiotic Selection[1]	7	57%	92%	90%	100%
Prophylactic Antibiotic Stopped	39	67%	70%	72%	95%
Pregnancy Care					
Inpatient Neonatal Mortality	-	-	-	-	-
Third or Fourth Degree Laceration	-	-	4.02%	3.63%	3.27%

Dekalb Memorial Hospital

1316 E Seventh Street
Auburn, IN 46706
Phone: 260-925-4600
Fax: 260-925-4733
E-mail: info@dekalbmemorial.com
URL: www.dekalbmemorial.com
Ownership: Voluntary non-profit - Other
Accredited: No
Emergency Services: Yes
Licensed Beds: 47

Key Personnel:

President/CEO . . . . JM Corey
Chief Medical Staff . . . . Khin Mar Oo, MD

NOTE: Hospital profiles are in alphabetical order by state, then city, then hospital within the city; Rankings are sorted by rate in descending order and exclude hospitals with less than 25 cases; (1) The number of cases is too small (n<25) for purposes of reliably predicting hospital performance; (2) Measure reflects the hospital's indication that its submission was based upon a sample of its relevant discharges; (3) Rate reflects fewer than the maximum possible quarters of data for the measure; (4) Inaccurate information submitted and suppressed for one or more quarters; (5) No data is available from the hospital for this measure; Please refer to the User's Guide for a full explanation of data

Emergency Room . . . . Mark Souder, MD
Director Infection/Disease Control . . . . Mary Bigelow, RN
CCU Spvg. Nurse . . . . Jackie Myers, RN
OB/GYN Womens Health. . . . . Michael Webb, MD
Chief Radiology . . . . Mitchell Travis, MD
Director Respiratory Therapy . . . . Rob Miller

Measure	Cases	This Hospital	State Average	U.S. Average	Top Hospital
Heart Attack Care					
ACE Inhibitor or ARB for LVSD	0	-	83%	82%	100%
Aspirin at Arrival[1]	9	100%	91%	92%	100%
Aspirin at Discharge[1]	4	100%	91%	90%	100%
Beta Blocker at Arrival[1]	11	91%	84%	87%	100%
Beta Blocker at Discharge[1]	4	100%	91%	90%	100%
Fibrinolytic Medication Timing	0	-	44%	31%	100%
PCI Within 90 Minutes of Arrival	0	-	56%	54%	95%
Smoking Cessation Advice[1]	1	100%	90%	88%	100%
Heart Failure Care					
ACE Inhibitor or ARB for LVSD[1]	14	93%	81%	82%	100%
Discharge Instructions	40	88%	69%	61%	93%
Evaluation of LVS Function	60	100%	87%	83%	99%
Smoking Cessation Advice[1]	7	100%	84%	82%	100%
Pneumonia Care					
Appropriate Initial Antibiotic	106	98%	83%	83%	94%
Blood Culture Timing	78	99%	90%	90%	100%
Influenza Vaccine	28	100%	74%	70%	100%
Initial Antibiotic Timing	118	98%	84%	80%	93%
Oxygenation Assessment	157	100%	99%	99%	100%
Pneumococcal Vaccine	100	100%	77%	69%	94%
Smoking Cessation Advice	36	94%	81%	80%	100%
Surgical Infection Prevention					
Prophylactic Antibiotic Given	46	96%	76%	77%	95%
Prophylactic Antibiotic Selection[1]	11	100%	92%	90%	100%
Prophylactic Antibiotic Stopped	43	95%	70%	72%	95%
Pregnancy Care					
Inpatient Neonatal Mortality	-	-	-	-	-
Third or Fourth Degree Laceration	-	-	4.02%	3.63%	3.27%

Clarian West Medical Center

1111 North Ronald Reagan Pky
Avon, IN 46123
Phone: 317-217-3000
Ownership: Voluntary non-profit - Private
Accredited: Yes
Emergency Services: Yes

Measure	Cases	This Hospital	State Average	U.S. Average	Top Hospital
Heart Attack Care					
ACE Inhibitor or ARB for LVSD[1]	3	33%	83%	82%	100%
Aspirin at Arrival	29	93%	91%	92%	100%
Aspirin at Discharge[1]	13	85%	91%	90%	100%
Beta Blocker at Arrival	29	76%	84%	87%	100%
Beta Blocker at Discharge[1]	14	64%	91%	90%	100%
Fibrinolytic Medication Timing[3]	0	-	44%	31%	100%
PCI Within 90 Minutes of Arrival	0	-	56%	54%	95%
Smoking Cessation Advice[1,3]	1	100%	90%	88%	100%
Heart Failure Care					
ACE Inhibitor or ARB for LVSD	41	73%	81%	82%	100%
Discharge Instructions[1,3]	24	88%	69%	61%	93%
Evaluation of LVS Function	98	97%	87%	83%	99%
Smoking Cessation Advice[1,3]	2	100%	84%	82%	100%
Pneumonia Care					
Appropriate Initial Antibiotic[1,3]	15	67%	83%	83%	94%
Blood Culture Timing[1,3]	16	75%	90%	90%	100%
Influenza Vaccine[5]	-	-	74%	70%	100%
Initial Antibiotic Timing	122	84%	84%	80%	93%
Oxygenation Assessment	133	100%	99%	99%	100%
Pneumococcal Vaccine	88	77%	77%	69%	94%
Smoking Cessation Advice[1,3]	4	100%	81%	80%	100%
Surgical Infection Prevention					
Prophylactic Antibiotic Given[2,3]	36	92%	76%	77%	95%
Prophylactic Antibiotic Selection[5]	-	-	92%	90%	100%
Prophylactic Antibiotic Stopped[2,3]	32	72%	70%	72%	95%
Pregnancy Care					
Inpatient Neonatal Mortality	933	0.11%	-	-	-
Third or Fourth Degree Laceration	621	4.51%	4.02%	3.63%	3.27%

Margaret Mary Community Hospital

321 Mitchell Avenue
Batesville, IN 47006
Phone: 812-934-6624
Fax: 812-934-5373
E-mail: mmch@venus.net
URL: www.mmch.org
Ownership: Government - Local
Accredited: Yes
Emergency Services: No
Licensed Beds: 79

Key Personnel:
President . . . . James L Amos
Chief of Medical Staff . . . . Kim Kick, MD
Emergency Room Manager . . . . Sharon Kreuzman
Infection Control . . . . Lisa Banks
ICU . . . . Bonnie Weber
Medical Surgical Nursing . . . . Bonnie Weber
Obstetrics Manager . . . . Cathy Bauer
Cardiopulmonary Manager . . . . Kathy Newell

Measure	Cases	This Hospital	State Average	U.S. Average	Top Hospital
Heart Attack Care					
ACE Inhibitor or ARB for LVSD[1]	1	100%	83%	82%	100%
Aspirin at Arrival[1]	10	80%	91%	92%	100%
Aspirin at Discharge[1]	4	75%	91%	90%	100%
Beta Blocker at Arrival[1]	7	86%	84%	87%	100%
Beta Blocker at Discharge[1]	5	80%	91%	90%	100%
Fibrinolytic Medication Timing	0	-	44%	31%	100%
PCI Within 90 Minutes of Arrival	0	-	56%	54%	95%
Smoking Cessation Advice	0	-	90%	88%	100%
Heart Failure Care					
ACE Inhibitor or ARB for LVSD[1]	16	69%	81%	82%	100%
Discharge Instructions	34	50%	69%	61%	93%
Evaluation of LVS Function	50	78%	87%	83%	99%
Smoking Cessation Advice[1]	5	80%	84%	82%	100%
Pneumonia Care					
Appropriate Initial Antibiotic	91	84%	83%	83%	94%
Blood Culture Timing	68	90%	90%	90%	100%
Influenza Vaccine[1]	15	87%	74%	70%	100%
Initial Antibiotic Timing	131	82%	84%	80%	93%
Oxygenation Assessment	155	100%	99%	99%	100%
Pneumococcal Vaccine	111	80%	77%	69%	94%
Smoking Cessation Advice	36	78%	81%	80%	100%
Surgical Infection Prevention					
Prophylactic Antibiotic Given	126	44%	76%	77%	95%
Prophylactic Antibiotic Selection	35	97%	92%	90%	100%
Prophylactic Antibiotic Stopped	124	32%	70%	72%	95%
Pregnancy Care					
Inpatient Neonatal Mortality	-	-	-	-	-
Third or Fourth Degree Laceration	-	-	4.02%	3.63%	3.27%

Bedford Regional Medical Center

Alternate Name: Bedford Medical Center
2900 West 16th Street
Bedford, IN 47421
Toll-Free: 800-755-3734
Phone: 812-275-1200
Fax: 812-275-1450
E-mail: kellis@kiva.net
URL: www.brmchealthcare.com
Ownership: Government - Local
Accredited: Yes
Emergency Services: Yes
Licensed Beds: 49

Key Personnel:
President/CEO . . . . Bradford W Dykes

Measure	Cases	This Hospital	State Average	U.S. Average	Top Hospital
Heart Attack Care					
ACE Inhibitor or ARB for LVSD[1]	4	100%	83%	82%	100%
Aspirin at Arrival[1]	20	90%	91%	92%	100%
Aspirin at Discharge[1]	11	100%	91%	90%	100%
Beta Blocker at Arrival[1]	14	100%	84%	87%	100%
Beta Blocker at Discharge[1]	13	100%	91%	90%	100%
Fibrinolytic Medication Timing	0	-	44%	31%	100%
PCI Within 90 Minutes of Arrival	0	-	56%	54%	95%
Smoking Cessation Advice	0	-	90%	88%	100%

NOTE: Hospital profiles are in alphabetical order by state, then city, then hospital within the city; Rankings are sorted by rate in descending order and exclude hospitals with less than 25 cases; (1) The number of cases is too small (n<25) for purposes of reliably predicting hospital performance; (2) Measure reflects the hospital's indication that its submission was based upon a sample of its relevant discharges; (3) Rate reflects fewer than the maximum possible quarters of data for the measure; (4) Inaccurate information submitted and suppressed for one or more quarters; (5) No data is available from the hospital for this measure; Please refer to the User's Guide for a full explanation of data

Heart Failure Care					
ACE Inhibitor or ARB for LVSD	34	100%	81%	82%	100%
Discharge Instructions	57	93%	69%	61%	93%
Evaluation of LVS Function	77	100%	87%	83%	99%
Smoking Cessation Advice[1]	6	100%	84%	82%	100%
Pneumonia Care					
Appropriate Initial Antibiotic	57	79%	83%	83%	94%
Blood Culture Timing	58	93%	90%	90%	100%
Influenza Vaccine[1]	20	85%	74%	70%	100%
Initial Antibiotic Timing	78	91%	84%	80%	93%
Oxygenation Assessment	102	100%	99%	99%	100%
Pneumococcal Vaccine	68	100%	77%	69%	94%
Smoking Cessation Advice[1]	24	92%	81%	80%	100%
Surgical Infection Prevention					
Prophylactic Antibiotic Given[3]	65	89%	76%	77%	95%
Prophylactic Antibiotic Selection[1]	20	100%	92%	90%	100%
Prophylactic Antibiotic Stopped[3]	61	39%	70%	72%	95%
Pregnancy Care					
Inpatient Neonatal Mortality	-	-	-	-	-
Third or Fourth Degree Laceration	-	-	4.02%	3.63%	3.27%

Dunn Memorial Hospital

1600 23rd Street
Bedford, IN 47421
Ownership: Government - Local
Emergency Services: Yes

Phone: 812-275-3331
Fax: 812-276-1211
Accredited: Yes
Licensed Beds: 137

Key Personnel:
CEO/President. . . . . D Bruner
Chief Medical Staff. . . . . RB Kalari
Emergency Room Director. . . . . M McCool
Director of Pulmonary/Respiratory Care. . . . . . . Connie Salm

Measure	Cases	This Hospital	State Average	U.S. Average	Top Hospital
Heart Attack Care					
ACE Inhibitor or ARB for LVSD[1]	17	94%	83%	82%	100%
Aspirin at Arrival	75	93%	91%	92%	100%
Aspirin at Discharge	77	95%	91%	90%	100%
Beta Blocker at Arrival	65	91%	84%	87%	100%
Beta Blocker at Discharge	83	99%	91%	90%	100%
Fibrinolytic Medication Timing	0	-	44%	31%	100%
PCI Within 90 Minutes of Arrival[1]	3	33%	56%	54%	95%
Smoking Cessation Advice	27	100%	90%	88%	100%
Heart Failure Care					
ACE Inhibitor or ARB for LVSD	30	83%	81%	82%	100%
Discharge Instructions	57	61%	69%	61%	93%
Evaluation of LVS Function	66	94%	87%	83%	99%
Smoking Cessation Advice[1]	10	70%	84%	82%	100%
Pneumonia Care					
Appropriate Initial Antibiotic	63	60%	83%	83%	94%
Blood Culture Timing	45	96%	90%	90%	100%
Influenza Vaccine[1]	20	85%	74%	70%	100%
Initial Antibiotic Timing	71	76%	84%	80%	93%
Oxygenation Assessment	104	98%	99%	99%	100%
Pneumococcal Vaccine	72	64%	77%	69%	94%
Smoking Cessation Advice	25	76%	81%	80%	100%
Surgical Infection Prevention					
Prophylactic Antibiotic Given	31	65%	76%	77%	95%
Prophylactic Antibiotic Selection[1]	3	33%	92%	90%	100%
Prophylactic Antibiotic Stopped	31	58%	70%	72%	95%
Pregnancy Care					
Inpatient Neonatal Mortality	-	-	-	-	-
Third or Fourth Degree Laceration	-	-	4.02%	3.63%	3.27%

Saint Francis Beech Grove

1600 Albany Street
Beech Grove, IN 46107
URL: www.stfrancis-indy.org
Ownership: Voluntary non-profit - Church
Emergency Services: Yes

Phone: 317-787-3311
Fax: 317-784-4675
Accredited: Yes
Licensed Beds: 500

Key Personnel:
Administrator/President . . . . Bob Brody
Chief Medical Staff. . . . . Donald Kerner
Manager of Cardiology. . . . . Paula Phillips
Emergency Room . . . . Claire Roembke, RN
Director Infection/Disease Control . . . . Cindy Eagan
OB/GYN Womens Health. . . . . Katrina Seltz, MD
Manager of Radiology . . . . Charisse Mershon

Measure	Cases	This Hospital	State Average	U.S. Average	Top Hospital
Heart Attack Care					
ACE Inhibitor or ARB for LVSD	45	80%	83%	82%	100%
Aspirin at Arrival	207	88%	91%	92%	100%
Aspirin at Discharge	268	98%	91%	90%	100%
Beta Blocker at Arrival	197	87%	84%	87%	100%
Beta Blocker at Discharge	271	97%	91%	90%	100%
Fibrinolytic Medication Timing	0	-	44%	31%	100%
PCI Within 90 Minutes of Arrival	0	-	56%	54%	95%
Smoking Cessation Advice	102	91%	90%	88%	100%
Heart Failure Care					
ACE Inhibitor or ARB for LVSD	127	78%	81%	82%	100%
Discharge Instructions	253	50%	69%	61%	93%
Evaluation of LVS Function	395	88%	87%	83%	99%
Smoking Cessation Advice	73	62%	84%	82%	100%
Pneumonia Care					
Appropriate Initial Antibiotic[2]	115	89%	83%	83%	94%
Blood Culture Timing[2]	80	89%	90%	90%	100%
Influenza Vaccine[2]	31	87%	74%	70%	100%
Initial Antibiotic Timing[2]	126	83%	84%	80%	93%
Oxygenation Assessment[2]	180	100%	99%	99%	100%
Pneumococcal Vaccine[2]	136	83%	77%	69%	94%
Smoking Cessation Advice[2]	50	72%	81%	80%	100%
Surgical Infection Prevention					
Prophylactic Antibiotic Given[2]	351	79%	76%	77%	95%
Prophylactic Antibiotic Selection[2]	46	91%	92%	90%	100%
Prophylactic Antibiotic Stopped[2]	335	79%	70%	72%	95%
Pregnancy Care					
Inpatient Neonatal Mortality	-	-	-	-	-
Third or Fourth Degree Laceration	-	-	4.02%	3.63%	3.27%

Bloomington Hospital

601 West Second Street
PO Box 1149
Bloomington, IN 47402
E-mail: BHHSWebMaster@bloomhealth.org
URL: www.bhhs.org
Ownership: Voluntary non-profit - Private
Emergency Services: Yes

Phone: 812-336-6821
Fax: 812-336-9519
Accredited: Yes
Licensed Beds: 355

Key Personnel:
President/CEO. . . . . Mark Moore
Director Medical/Surgical Nurses . . . . Dawn Jacquard, RN
OB/GYN Womens Health. . . . . Lillette Wood, MD
Director Radiology . . . . Phil Lewis
Director Respiratory Therapy . . . . Ed Getts

Measure	Cases	This Hospital	State Average	U.S. Average	Top Hospital
Heart Attack Care					
ACE Inhibitor or ARB for LVSD	83	94%	83%	82%	100%
Aspirin at Arrival	246	98%	91%	92%	100%
Aspirin at Discharge	349	99%	91%	90%	100%
Beta Blocker at Arrival	199	94%	84%	87%	100%
Beta Blocker at Discharge	339	98%	91%	90%	100%
Fibrinolytic Medication Timing	0	-	44%	31%	100%
PCI Within 90 Minutes of Arrival[1]	23	74%	56%	54%	95%
Smoking Cessation Advice	156	100%	90%	88%	100%
Heart Failure Care					
ACE Inhibitor or ARB for LVSD	127	87%	81%	82%	100%
Discharge Instructions	229	83%	69%	61%	93%
Evaluation of LVS Function	293	91%	87%	83%	99%
Smoking Cessation Advice	60	100%	84%	82%	100%
Pneumonia Care					
Appropriate Initial Antibiotic	200	88%	83%	83%	94%
Blood Culture Timing	171	91%	90%	90%	100%
Influenza Vaccine	50	82%	74%	70%	100%
Initial Antibiotic Timing	250	87%	84%	80%	93%
Oxygenation Assessment	322	100%	99%	99%	100%

NOTE: Hospital profiles are in alphabetical order by state, then city, then hospital within the city; Rankings are sorted by rate in descending order and exclude hospitals with less than 25 cases; (1) The number of cases is too small (n<25) for purposes of reliably predicting hospital performance; (2) Measure reflects the hospital's indication that its submission was based upon a sample of its relevant discharges; (3) Rate reflects fewer than the maximum possible quarters of data for the measure; (4) Inaccurate information submitted and suppressed for one or more quarters; (5) No data is available from the hospital for this measure; Please refer to the User's Guide for a full explanation of data

Pneumococcal Vaccine	217	83%	77%	69%	94%
Smoking Cessation Advice	95	95%	81%	80%	100%
Surgical Infection Prevention					
Prophylactic Antibiotic Given	895	91%	76%	77%	95%
Prophylactic Antibiotic Selection	209	97%	92%	90%	100%
Prophylactic Antibiotic Stopped	853	89%	70%	72%	95%
Pregnancy Care					
Inpatient Neonatal Mortality	-	-	-	-	-
Third or Fourth Degree Laceration	-	-	4.02%	3.63%	3.27%

Bluffton Regional Medical Center

303 South Main Street
Bluffton, IN 46714

Toll-Free: 888-919-3557
Phone: 260-824-3210
Fax: 260-919-3851

URL: www.blufftonregional.com
Ownership: Proprietary
Emergency Services: Yes

Accredited: Yes
Licensed Beds: 79

Key Personnel:
President/CEO. . . . . Thomas Clark
Emergency Room . . . . Derrick Williams
Respiratory Care . . . . Linda Sliger

Measure	Cases	This Hospital	State Average	U.S. Average	Top Hospital
Heart Attack Care					
ACE Inhibitor or ARB for LVSD[1]	10	100%	83%	82%	100%
Aspirin at Arrival	31	94%	91%	92%	100%
Aspirin at Discharge	30	97%	91%	90%	100%
Beta Blocker at Arrival	27	96%	84%	87%	100%
Beta Blocker at Discharge	30	100%	91%	90%	100%
Fibrinolytic Medication Timing	0	-	44%	31%	100%
PCI Within 90 Minutes of Arrival	0	-	56%	54%	95%
Smoking Cessation Advice[1]	5	100%	90%	88%	100%
Heart Failure Care					
ACE Inhibitor or ARB for LVSD	42	98%	81%	82%	100%
Discharge Instructions	73	100%	69%	61%	93%
Evaluation of LVS Function	105	99%	87%	83%	99%
Smoking Cessation Advice[1]	11	100%	84%	82%	100%
Pneumonia Care					
Appropriate Initial Antibiotic	110	91%	83%	83%	94%
Blood Culture Timing	92	98%	90%	90%	100%
Influenza Vaccine[1]	18	100%	74%	70%	100%
Initial Antibiotic Timing	140	97%	84%	80%	93%
Oxygenation Assessment	165	100%	99%	99%	100%
Pneumococcal Vaccine	101	99%	77%	69%	94%
Smoking Cessation Advice	34	100%	81%	80%	100%
Surgical Infection Prevention					
Prophylactic Antibiotic Given	161	98%	76%	77%	95%
Prophylactic Antibiotic Selection	51	96%	92%	90%	100%
Prophylactic Antibiotic Stopped	156	99%	70%	72%	95%
Pregnancy Care					
Inpatient Neonatal Mortality	274	0.00%	-	-	-
Third or Fourth Degree Laceration	203	2.96%	4.02%	3.63%	3.27%

Saint Mary's Warrick Hospital

1116 Millis Avenue
Boonville, IN 47601

Toll-Free: 800-897-3831
Phone: 812-897-4800
Fax: 812-897-7375

URL: www.stmarys.org
Ownership: Voluntary non-profit - Private
Emergency Services: Yes

Accredited: Yes
Licensed Beds: 25

Key Personnel:
President/CEO. . . . . Marc Dooley
Chief Medical Staff. . . . . Syed Ali
Chief Medical Staff. . . . . David Vaughn
Emergency Room . . . . David Baughn
Director of Pulmonary/Respiratory Care. . . . . . . James Mooney

Measure	Cases	This Hospital	State Average	U.S. Average	Top Hospital
Heart Attack Care					
ACE Inhibitor or ARB for LVSD[1]	5	80%	83%	82%	100%
Aspirin at Arrival[1]	16	100%	91%	92%	100%
Aspirin at Discharge[1]	12	92%	91%	90%	100%
Beta Blocker at Arrival[1]	17	88%	84%	87%	100%
Beta Blocker at Discharge[1]	15	80%	91%	90%	100%
Fibrinolytic Medication Timing	0	-	44%	31%	100%
PCI Within 90 Minutes of Arrival	0	-	56%	54%	95%
Smoking Cessation Advice[1]	1	100%	90%	88%	100%
Heart Failure Care					
ACE Inhibitor or ARB for LVSD[1]	8	100%	81%	82%	100%
Discharge Instructions	25	100%	69%	61%	93%
Evaluation of LVS Function	48	98%	87%	83%	99%
Smoking Cessation Advice[1]	4	100%	84%	82%	100%
Pneumonia Care					
Appropriate Initial Antibiotic	64	86%	83%	83%	94%
Blood Culture Timing	58	93%	90%	90%	100%
Influenza Vaccine[1]	10	60%	74%	70%	100%
Initial Antibiotic Timing	69	90%	84%	80%	93%
Oxygenation Assessment	91	97%	99%	99%	100%
Pneumococcal Vaccine	64	70%	77%	69%	94%
Smoking Cessation Advice[1]	22	100%	81%	80%	100%
Surgical Infection Prevention					
Prophylactic Antibiotic Given[5]	-	-	76%	77%	95%
Prophylactic Antibiotic Selection[5]	-	-	92%	90%	100%
Prophylactic Antibiotic Stopped[5]	-	-	70%	72%	95%
Pregnancy Care					
Inpatient Neonatal Mortality	-	-	-	-	-
Third or Fourth Degree Laceration	-	-	4.02%	3.63%	3.27%

Saint Vincent Clay Hospital

1206 E National Avenue
Brazil, IN 47834
URL: www.stvincent.org/faccen/clay
Ownership: Voluntary non-profit - Private
Emergency Services: Yes

Phone: 812-442-2500
Fax: 812-442-2605

Accredited: Yes
Licensed Beds: 58

Key Personnel:
President/CEO. . . . . Jerry Laue
Chief Medical Staff. . . . . Catherine Brush
Emergency Room . . . . R Curtis Oehler, MD
Chief Radiology . . . . Jessie Lund, DDS
Director Respiratory Therapy . . . . Lisa Mathis

Measure	Cases	This Hospital	State Average	U.S. Average	Top Hospital
Heart Attack Care					
ACE Inhibitor or ARB for LVSD[1,3]	2	100%	83%	82%	100%
Aspirin at Arrival[1,3]	3	100%	91%	92%	100%
Aspirin at Discharge[1,3]	3	67%	91%	90%	100%
Beta Blocker at Arrival[1,3]	3	100%	84%	87%	100%
Beta Blocker at Discharge[1,3]	3	100%	91%	90%	100%
Fibrinolytic Medication Timing[3]	0	-	44%	31%	100%
PCI Within 90 Minutes of Arrival[5]	-	-	56%	54%	95%
Smoking Cessation Advice[3]	0	-	90%	88%	100%
Heart Failure Care					
ACE Inhibitor or ARB for LVSD[1]	13	69%	81%	82%	100%
Discharge Instructions[1]	17	41%	69%	61%	93%
Evaluation of LVS Function	40	78%	87%	83%	99%
Smoking Cessation Advice[1]	4	50%	84%	82%	100%
Pneumonia Care					
Appropriate Initial Antibiotic	39	77%	83%	83%	94%
Blood Culture Timing[1]	23	91%	90%	90%	100%
Influenza Vaccine[1]	14	57%	74%	70%	100%
Initial Antibiotic Timing	34	94%	84%	80%	93%
Oxygenation Assessment	56	98%	99%	99%	100%
Pneumococcal Vaccine	34	82%	77%	69%	94%
Smoking Cessation Advice[1]	10	70%	81%	80%	100%
Surgical Infection Prevention					
Prophylactic Antibiotic Given[5]	-	-	76%	77%	95%
Prophylactic Antibiotic Selection[5]	-	-	92%	90%	100%
Prophylactic Antibiotic Stopped[5]	-	-	70%	72%	95%
Pregnancy Care					
Inpatient Neonatal Mortality	-	-	-	-	-
Third or Fourth Degree Laceration	-	-	4.02%	3.63%	3.27%

NOTE: Hospital profiles are in alphabetical order by state, then city, then hospital within the city; Rankings are sorted by rate in descending order and exclude hospitals with less than 25 cases; (1) The number of cases is too small (n<25) for purposes of reliably predicting hospital performance; (2) Measure reflects the hospital's indication that its submission was based upon a sample of its relevant discharges; (3) Rate reflects fewer than the maximum possible quarters of data for the measure; (4) Inaccurate information submitted and suppressed for one or more quarters; (5) No data is available from the hospital for this measure; Please refer to the User's Guide for a full explanation of data

Community Hospital of Bremen

411 South Whitlock Street
PO Box 8
Bremen, IN 46506
E-mail: pboard@bremenhospital.com
URL: www.bremenhospital.com
Ownership: Voluntary non-profit - Private
Emergency Services: Yes

Phone: 574-546-2211
Fax: 574-546-4312

Accredited: No
Licensed Beds: 24

Key Personnel:
President/CEO . . . . Scott Graybill
Chief Medical Staff . . . . Carey Gear, MD
Emergency Room . . . . Carey Gear, MD
Director Infection/Disease Control . . . . Teresa Brown, RN

Measure	Cases	This Hospital	State Average	U.S. Average	Top Hospital
Heart Attack Care					
ACE Inhibitor or ARB for LVSD[3]	0	-	83%	82%	100%
Aspirin at Arrival[1,3]	2	100%	91%	92%	100%
Aspirin at Discharge[1,3]	3	100%	91%	90%	100%
Beta Blocker at Arrival[1,3]	1	100%	84%	87%	100%
Beta Blocker at Discharge[1,3]	3	100%	91%	90%	100%
Fibrinolytic Medication Timing[3]	0	-	44%	31%	100%
PCI Within 90 Minutes of Arrival[5]	-	-	56%	54%	95%
Smoking Cessation Advice[3]	0	-	90%	88%	100%
Heart Failure Care					
ACE Inhibitor or ARB for LVSD[1]	2	100%	81%	82%	100%
Discharge Instructions[1]	13	62%	69%	61%	93%
Evaluation of LVS Function	26	85%	87%	83%	99%
Smoking Cessation Advice[1]	2	100%	84%	82%	100%
Pneumonia Care					
Appropriate Initial Antibiotic[1]	20	80%	83%	83%	94%
Blood Culture Timing[1]	12	100%	90%	90%	100%
Influenza Vaccine[1]	4	100%	74%	70%	100%
Initial Antibiotic Timing[1]	19	95%	84%	80%	93%
Oxygenation Assessment	25	100%	99%	99%	100%
Pneumococcal Vaccine[1]	16	94%	77%	69%	94%
Smoking Cessation Advice[1]	6	67%	81%	80%	100%
Surgical Infection Prevention					
Prophylactic Antibiotic Given[5]	-	-	76%	77%	95%
Prophylactic Antibiotic Selection[5]	-	-	92%	90%	100%
Prophylactic Antibiotic Stopped[5]	-	-	70%	72%	95%
Pregnancy Care					
Inpatient Neonatal Mortality	-	-	-	-	-
Third or Fourth Degree Laceration	-	-	4.02%	3.63%	3.27%

Clarian North Medical Center

11700 N Meridian St
Carmel, IN 46032
Ownership: Proprietary
Emergency Services: Yes

Phone: 317-688-2000

Accredited: Yes

Measure	Cases	This Hospital	State Average	U.S. Average	Top Hospital
Heart Attack Care					
ACE Inhibitor or ARB for LVSD[1,3]	1	100%	83%	82%	100%
Aspirin at Arrival[1,3]	4	75%	91%	92%	100%
Aspirin at Discharge[1,3]	4	100%	91%	90%	100%
Beta Blocker at Arrival[1,3]	6	33%	84%	87%	100%
Beta Blocker at Discharge[1,3]	6	50%	91%	90%	100%
Fibrinolytic Medication Timing[3]	0	-	44%	31%	100%
PCI Within 90 Minutes of Arrival	0	-	56%	54%	95%
Smoking Cessation Advice[3]	0	-	90%	88%	100%
Heart Failure Care					
ACE Inhibitor or ARB for LVSD[1]	8	88%	81%	82%	100%
Discharge Instructions[1,3]	2	50%	69%	61%	93%
Evaluation of LVS Function[1]	15	93%	87%	83%	99%
Smoking Cessation Advice[1,3]	1	0%	84%	82%	100%
Pneumonia Care					
Appropriate Initial Antibiotic[1,3]	9	56%	83%	83%	94%
Blood Culture Timing[1,3]	3	100%	90%	90%	100%
Influenza Vaccine[5]	-	-	74%	70%	100%
Initial Antibiotic Timing[1]	17	65%	84%	80%	93%
Oxygenation Assessment	26	100%	99%	99%	100%
Pneumococcal Vaccine[1]	17	76%	77%	69%	94%
Smoking Cessation Advice[1,3]	2	100%	81%	80%	100%
Surgical Infection Prevention					
Prophylactic Antibiotic Given[2,3]	39	90%	76%	77%	95%
Prophylactic Antibiotic Selection[5]	-	-	92%	90%	100%
Prophylactic Antibiotic Stopped[2,3]	39	74%	70%	72%	95%
Pregnancy Care					
Inpatient Neonatal Mortality	1,553	0.45%	-	-	-
Third or Fourth Degree Laceration	970	5.67%	4.02%	3.63%	3.27%

Saint Vincent Carmel Hospital

13500 N Meridian
Carmel, IN 46032
URL: www.stvincent.org/faccen/carmel
Ownership: Voluntary non-profit - Church
Emergency Services: Yes

Phone: 317-582-7171
Fax: 317-582-7492

Accredited: Yes
Licensed Beds: 100

Key Personnel:
Administrator . . . . Michael D Chittenden
Chief Medical Staff . . . . Steve Priddy, MD

Measure	Cases	This Hospital	State Average	U.S. Average	Top Hospital
Heart Attack Care					
ACE Inhibitor or ARB for LVSD[1]	4	50%	83%	82%	100%
Aspirin at Arrival[1]	7	100%	91%	92%	100%
Aspirin at Discharge[1]	5	100%	91%	90%	100%
Beta Blocker at Arrival[1]	7	57%	84%	87%	100%
Beta Blocker at Discharge[1]	6	83%	91%	90%	100%
Fibrinolytic Medication Timing	0	-	44%	31%	100%
PCI Within 90 Minutes of Arrival	0	-	56%	54%	95%
Smoking Cessation Advice	0	-	90%	88%	100%
Heart Failure Care					
ACE Inhibitor or ARB for LVSD[1]	10	80%	81%	82%	100%
Discharge Instructions	26	4%	69%	61%	93%
Evaluation of LVS Function	43	74%	87%	83%	99%
Smoking Cessation Advice[1]	6	0%	84%	82%	100%
Pneumonia Care					
Appropriate Initial Antibiotic	73	86%	83%	83%	94%
Blood Culture Timing[1]	17	82%	90%	90%	100%
Influenza Vaccine[1]	13	31%	74%	70%	100%
Initial Antibiotic Timing	73	89%	84%	80%	93%
Oxygenation Assessment	108	99%	99%	99%	100%
Pneumococcal Vaccine	62	23%	77%	69%	94%
Smoking Cessation Advice[1]	11	18%	81%	80%	100%
Surgical Infection Prevention					
Prophylactic Antibiotic Given[2,3]	134	95%	76%	77%	95%
Prophylactic Antibiotic Selection[2]	44	100%	92%	90%	100%
Prophylactic Antibiotic Stopped[2,3]	133	94%	70%	72%	95%
Pregnancy Care					
Inpatient Neonatal Mortality	-	-	-	-	-
Third or Fourth Degree Laceration	-	-	4.02%	3.63%	3.27%

Medical Center of Southern Indiana

2200 Market Street
Charlestown, IN 47111
E-mail: wobertate@altavista.net
Ownership: Voluntary non-profit - Private
Emergency Services: Yes

Phone: 812-256-1070
Fax: 812-256-0201

Accredited: No
Licensed Beds: 96

Measure	Cases	This Hospital	State Average	U.S. Average	Top Hospital
Heart Attack Care					
ACE Inhibitor or ARB for LVSD[1,3]	2	100%	83%	82%	100%
Aspirin at Arrival[1,3]	3	67%	91%	92%	100%
Aspirin at Discharge[1,3]	3	100%	91%	90%	100%
Beta Blocker at Arrival[1,3]	3	67%	84%	87%	100%
Beta Blocker at Discharge[1,3]	3	100%	91%	90%	100%
Fibrinolytic Medication Timing[3]	0	-	44%	31%	100%
PCI Within 90 Minutes of Arrival	0	-	56%	54%	95%
Smoking Cessation Advice[1,3]	1	100%	90%	88%	100%
Heart Failure Care					
ACE Inhibitor or ARB for LVSD[1,3]	7	86%	81%	82%	100%
Discharge Instructions[1,3]	15	87%	69%	61%	93%
Evaluation of LVS Function[3]	29	79%	87%	83%	99%

NOTE: Hospital profiles are in alphabetical order by state, then city, then hospital within the city; Rankings are sorted by rate in descending order and exclude hospitals with less than 25 cases; (1) The number of cases is too small (n<25) for purposes of reliably predicting hospital performance; (2) Measure reflects the hospital's indication that its submission was based upon a sample of its relevant discharges; (3) Rate reflects fewer than the maximum possible quarters of data for the measure; (4) Inaccurate information submitted and suppressed for one or more quarters; (5) No data is available from the hospital for this measure; Please refer to the User's Guide for a full explanation of data

Smoking Cessation Advice[1,3]	4	100%	84%	82%	100%
Pneumonia Care					
Appropriate Initial Antibiotic[1,3]	18	94%	83%	83%	94%
Blood Culture Timing[1,3]	4	25%	90%	90%	100%
Influenza Vaccine[5]	-	-	74%	70%	100%
Initial Antibiotic Timing[3]	31	97%	84%	80%	93%
Oxygenation Assessment[3]	32	97%	99%	99%	100%
Pneumococcal Vaccine[1,3]	15	100%	77%	69%	94%
Smoking Cessation Advice[1,3]	6	100%	81%	80%	100%
Surgical Infection Prevention					
Prophylactic Antibiotic Given[1,3]	2	0%	76%	77%	95%
Prophylactic Antibiotic Selection[5]	-	-	92%	90%	100%
Prophylactic Antibiotic Stopped[1,3]	2	50%	70%	72%	95%
Pregnancy Care					
Inpatient Neonatal Mortality	-	-	-	-	-
Third or Fourth Degree Laceration	-	-	4.02%	3.63%	3.27%

West Central Community Hospital

801 S Main Street
Clinton, IN 47842
Phone: 765-832-1203
Ownership: Voluntary non-profit - Private
Accredited: No
Emergency Services: No

Measure	Cases	This Hospital	State Average	U.S. Average	Top Hospital
Heart Attack Care					
ACE Inhibitor or ARB for LVSD[1]	1	0%	83%	82%	100%
Aspirin at Arrival[1]	15	93%	91%	92%	100%
Aspirin at Discharge[1]	10	50%	91%	90%	100%
Beta Blocker at Arrival[1]	14	64%	84%	87%	100%
Beta Blocker at Discharge[1]	9	67%	91%	90%	100%
Fibrinolytic Medication Timing[3]	0	-	44%	31%	100%
PCI Within 90 Minutes of Arrival[5]	-	-	56%	54%	95%
Smoking Cessation Advice[1]	1	100%	90%	88%	100%
Heart Failure Care					
ACE Inhibitor or ARB for LVSD[1]	19	74%	81%	82%	100%
Discharge Instructions	35	74%	69%	61%	93%
Evaluation of LVS Function	58	83%	87%	83%	99%
Smoking Cessation Advice[1]	10	100%	84%	82%	100%
Pneumonia Care					
Appropriate Initial Antibiotic	65	86%	83%	83%	94%
Blood Culture Timing	61	90%	90%	90%	100%
Influenza Vaccine[1]	15	100%	74%	70%	100%
Initial Antibiotic Timing	120	95%	84%	80%	93%
Oxygenation Assessment	148	99%	99%	99%	100%
Pneumococcal Vaccine	92	93%	77%	69%	94%
Smoking Cessation Advice	37	97%	81%	80%	100%
Surgical Infection Prevention					
Prophylactic Antibiotic Given	33	91%	76%	77%	95%
Prophylactic Antibiotic Selection[1]	6	67%	92%	90%	100%
Prophylactic Antibiotic Stopped	32	69%	70%	72%	95%
Pregnancy Care					
Inpatient Neonatal Mortality	-	-	-	-	-
Third or Fourth Degree Laceration	-	-	4.02%	3.63%	3.27%

Parkview Whitley Hospital

Alternate Name: Whitley County Memorial Hospital
353 N Oak Street
Columbia City, IN 46725
Toll-Free: 800-325-1338
Phone: 260-248-9000
Fax: 260-248-9107
URL: www.parkview.com
Ownership: Voluntary non-profit - Private
Accredited: Yes
Emergency Services: Yes
Licensed Beds: 45
Key Personnel:
Chief of Medical Staff. Dr Jeff Brookes

Measure	Cases	This Hospital	State Average	U.S. Average	Top Hospital
Heart Attack Care					
ACE Inhibitor or ARB for LVSD[1]	1	100%	83%	82%	100%
Aspirin at Arrival[1]	6	67%	91%	92%	100%
Aspirin at Discharge[1]	5	100%	91%	90%	100%
Beta Blocker at Arrival[1]	5	80%	84%	87%	100%
Beta Blocker at Discharge[1]	7	86%	91%	90%	100%
Fibrinolytic Medication Timing	0	-	44%	31%	100%
PCI Within 90 Minutes of Arrival	0	-	56%	54%	95%
Smoking Cessation Advice	0	-	90%	88%	100%
Heart Failure Care					
ACE Inhibitor or ARB for LVSD[1]	21	67%	81%	82%	100%
Discharge Instructions	33	58%	69%	61%	93%
Evaluation of LVS Function	45	84%	87%	83%	99%
Smoking Cessation Advice[1]	8	75%	84%	82%	100%
Pneumonia Care					
Appropriate Initial Antibiotic	57	96%	83%	83%	94%
Blood Culture Timing	49	92%	90%	90%	100%
Influenza Vaccine[1]	14	93%	74%	70%	100%
Initial Antibiotic Timing	65	82%	84%	80%	93%
Oxygenation Assessment	86	100%	99%	99%	100%
Pneumococcal Vaccine	53	75%	77%	69%	94%
Smoking Cessation Advice[1]	24	58%	81%	80%	100%
Surgical Infection Prevention					
Prophylactic Antibiotic Given	61	70%	76%	77%	95%
Prophylactic Antibiotic Selection[1]	20	90%	92%	90%	100%
Prophylactic Antibiotic Stopped	58	48%	70%	72%	95%
Pregnancy Care					
Inpatient Neonatal Mortality	-	-	-	-	-
Third or Fourth Degree Laceration	-	-	4.02%	3.63%	3.27%

Columbus Regional Hospital

Alternate Name: Bartholomew County Hospital
2400 E 17th Street
Columbus, IN 47201
Phone: 812-379-4441
Fax: 812-376-5001
Ownership: Government - Local
Accredited: Yes
Emergency Services: Yes
Licensed Beds: 325
Key Personnel:
CEO. . . . . Douglas Lenord
Chief Medical Staff. . . . . D Sauderman
Director Infection/Disease Control . . . . Cindy Fields
Director of Pulmonary . . . . David Wilson

Measure	Cases	This Hospital	State Average	U.S. Average	Top Hospital
Heart Attack Care					
ACE Inhibitor or ARB for LVSD	42	95%	83%	82%	100%
Aspirin at Arrival	159	99%	91%	92%	100%
Aspirin at Discharge	201	99%	91%	90%	100%
Beta Blocker at Arrival	141	98%	84%	87%	100%
Beta Blocker at Discharge	190	99%	91%	90%	100%
Fibrinolytic Medication Timing[1]	9	78%	44%	31%	100%
PCI Within 90 Minutes of Arrival[1]	5	100%	56%	54%	95%
Smoking Cessation Advice	89	100%	90%	88%	100%
Heart Failure Care					
ACE Inhibitor or ARB for LVSD	90	98%	81%	82%	100%
Discharge Instructions	255	87%	69%	61%	93%
Evaluation of LVS Function	314	96%	87%	83%	99%
Smoking Cessation Advice	82	100%	84%	82%	100%
Pneumonia Care					
Appropriate Initial Antibiotic	133	93%	83%	83%	94%
Blood Culture Timing	64	98%	90%	90%	100%
Influenza Vaccine	39	95%	74%	70%	100%
Initial Antibiotic Timing	176	95%	84%	80%	93%
Oxygenation Assessment	232	100%	99%	99%	100%
Pneumococcal Vaccine	136	94%	77%	69%	94%
Smoking Cessation Advice	75	100%	81%	80%	100%
Surgical Infection Prevention					
Prophylactic Antibiotic Given	631	87%	76%	77%	95%
Prophylactic Antibiotic Selection	149	95%	92%	90%	100%
Prophylactic Antibiotic Stopped	593	69%	70%	72%	95%
Pregnancy Care					
Inpatient Neonatal Mortality	-	-	-	-	-
Third or Fourth Degree Laceration	-	-	4.02%	3.63%	3.27%

NOTE: Hospital profiles are in alphabetical order by state, then city, then hospital within the city; Rankings are sorted by rate in descending order and exclude hospitals with less than 25 cases; (1) The number of cases is too small (n<25) for purposes of reliably predicting hospital performance; (2) Measure reflects the hospital's indication that its submission was based upon a sample of its relevant discharges; (3) Rate reflects fewer than the maximum possible quarters of data for the measure; (4) Inaccurate information submitted and suppressed for one or more quarters; (5) No data is available from the hospital for this measure; Please refer to the User's Guide for a full explanation of data

Fayette Memorial Hospital

1941 Virginia Avenue
Connersville, IN 47331
Phone: 765-825-5131
Fax: 765-827-7775
URL: www.fayettememorial.org
Ownership: Voluntary non-profit - Private
Accredited: Yes
Emergency Services: Yes
Licensed Beds: 140

Key Personnel:

President/CEO . . . . David R Brandon
Chief Medical Staff . . . . Wayne White
Cardiology . . . . Joan Baum, DO
Emergency Room . . . . Shelley Millor
OB/GYN Womens Health . . . . Wayne B White, MD
Chief Radiology . . . . John E DePersio, MD
Director of Pulmonary . . . . Mark Schafer

Measure	Cases	This Hospital	State Average	U.S. Average	Top Hospital
Heart Attack Care					
ACE Inhibitor or ARB for LVSD[1]	3	33%	83%	82%	100%
Aspirin at Arrival	37	86%	91%	92%	100%
Aspirin at Discharge	26	58%	91%	90%	100%
Beta Blocker at Arrival	34	50%	84%	87%	100%
Beta Blocker at Discharge	29	66%	91%	90%	100%
Fibrinolytic Medication Timing	0	-	44%	31%	100%
PCI Within 90 Minutes of Arrival	0	-	56%	54%	95%
Smoking Cessation Advice[1]	7	57%	90%	88%	100%
Heart Failure Care					
ACE Inhibitor or ARB for LVSD	29	62%	81%	82%	100%
Discharge Instructions	102	30%	69%	61%	93%
Evaluation of LVS Function	143	55%	87%	83%	99%
Smoking Cessation Advice	27	37%	84%	82%	100%
Pneumonia Care					
Appropriate Initial Antibiotic	62	74%	83%	83%	94%
Blood Culture Timing	30	100%	90%	90%	100%
Influenza Vaccine[1]	14	71%	74%	70%	100%
Initial Antibiotic Timing	88	66%	84%	80%	93%
Oxygenation Assessment	104	100%	99%	99%	100%
Pneumococcal Vaccine	66	35%	77%	69%	94%
Smoking Cessation Advice[1]	18	11%	81%	80%	100%
Surgical Infection Prevention					
Prophylactic Antibiotic Given	100	56%	76%	77%	95%
Prophylactic Antibiotic Selection[1]	14	100%	92%	90%	100%
Prophylactic Antibiotic Stopped	87	78%	70%	72%	95%
Pregnancy Care					
Inpatient Neonatal Mortality	-	-	-	-	-
Third or Fourth Degree Laceration	-	-	4.02%	3.63%	3.27%

Harrison County Hospital

245 Atwood Street
Corydon, IN 47112
Phone: 812-738-4251
Fax: 812-738-7829
URL: www.hchin.org
Ownership: Government - Local
Accredited: No
Emergency Services: Yes
Licensed Beds: 68

Key Personnel:

CEO . . . . Steve Taylor
Chief Medical Staff . . . . Reggie Lyell, MD
Emergency Room . . . . Ruth Donahue, RN
Director Infection/Disease Control . . . . Debra Gibson
Director Medical/Surgical Nursing . . . . Diane Clark, RN
OB/GYN Womens Health . . . . Richard Brown, RN
Director Respiratory Therapy . . . . Karen Keigher

Measure	Cases	This Hospital	State Average	U.S. Average	Top Hospital
Heart Attack Care					
ACE Inhibitor or ARB for LVSD[1]	4	75%	83%	82%	100%
Aspirin at Arrival[1]	11	91%	91%	92%	100%
Aspirin at Discharge[1]	6	83%	91%	90%	100%
Beta Blocker at Arrival[1]	10	70%	84%	87%	100%
Beta Blocker at Discharge[1]	6	83%	91%	90%	100%
Fibrinolytic Medication Timing[3]	0	-	44%	31%	100%
PCI Within 90 Minutes of Arrival[5]	-	-	56%	54%	95%
Smoking Cessation Advice	0	-	90%	88%	100%
Heart Failure Care					
ACE Inhibitor or ARB for LVSD	26	73%	81%	82%	100%
Discharge Instructions	46	20%	69%	61%	93%
Evaluation of LVS Function	59	100%	87%	83%	99%
Smoking Cessation Advice[1]	10	70%	84%	82%	100%
Pneumonia Care					
Appropriate Initial Antibiotic	102	64%	83%	83%	94%
Blood Culture Timing	29	79%	90%	90%	100%
Influenza Vaccine	28	64%	74%	70%	100%
Initial Antibiotic Timing	130	72%	84%	80%	93%
Oxygenation Assessment	140	100%	99%	99%	100%
Pneumococcal Vaccine	78	72%	77%	69%	94%
Smoking Cessation Advice	33	45%	81%	80%	100%
Surgical Infection Prevention					
Prophylactic Antibiotic Given	56	71%	76%	77%	95%
Prophylactic Antibiotic Selection[1]	12	83%	92%	90%	100%
Prophylactic Antibiotic Stopped	54	80%	70%	72%	95%
Pregnancy Care					
Inpatient Neonatal Mortality	-	-	-	-	-
Third or Fourth Degree Laceration	-	-	4.02%	3.63%	3.27%

Saint Clare Medical Center

1710 Lafayette Road
Crawfordsville, IN 47933
Phone: 765-362-2800
Fax: 765-364-9010
URL: www.stclaremedical.org
Ownership: Voluntary non-profit - Church
Accredited: Yes
Emergency Services: Yes
Licensed Beds: 120

Key Personnel:

Executive Director . . . . Jeffrey C Zeh

Measure	Cases	This Hospital	State Average	U.S. Average	Top Hospital
Heart Attack Care					
ACE Inhibitor or ARB for LVSD[1]	5	60%	83%	82%	100%
Aspirin at Arrival[1]	13	77%	91%	92%	100%
Aspirin at Discharge[1]	8	50%	91%	90%	100%
Beta Blocker at Arrival[1]	14	14%	84%	87%	100%
Beta Blocker at Discharge[1]	7	71%	91%	90%	100%
Fibrinolytic Medication Timing[1]	1	100%	44%	31%	100%
PCI Within 90 Minutes of Arrival	0	-	56%	54%	95%
Smoking Cessation Advice[1]	2	50%	90%	88%	100%
Heart Failure Care					
ACE Inhibitor or ARB for LVSD	30	53%	81%	82%	100%
Discharge Instructions	64	42%	69%	61%	93%
Evaluation of LVS Function	104	64%	87%	83%	99%
Smoking Cessation Advice[1]	12	92%	84%	82%	100%
Pneumonia Care					
Appropriate Initial Antibiotic	102	63%	83%	83%	94%
Blood Culture Timing	27	85%	90%	90%	100%
Influenza Vaccine[1]	20	40%	74%	70%	100%
Initial Antibiotic Timing	108	77%	84%	80%	93%
Oxygenation Assessment	121	98%	99%	99%	100%
Pneumococcal Vaccine	80	38%	77%	69%	94%
Smoking Cessation Advice	25	76%	81%	80%	100%
Surgical Infection Prevention					
Prophylactic Antibiotic Given	138	78%	76%	77%	95%
Prophylactic Antibiotic Selection	33	100%	92%	90%	100%
Prophylactic Antibiotic Stopped	137	25%	70%	72%	95%
Pregnancy Care					
Inpatient Neonatal Mortality	-	-	-	-	-
Third or Fourth Degree Laceration	-	-	4.02%	3.63%	3.27%

Saint Anthony Medical Center

1201 South Main Street
Crown Point, IN 46307
Phone: 219-738-2100
Fax: 219-757-6242
URL: www.stanthonymedicalcenter.com
Ownership: Voluntary non-profit - Church
Accredited: Yes
Emergency Services: Yes
Licensed Beds: 411

Key Personnel:

President . . . . Seth Warren
Chief Medical Staff . . . . John King, MD
Director of Emergency . . . . Daniel Netluch
Emergency Room . . . . Crystal Allen
Director Infection/Disease Control . . . . Chris Shakula
Director Medical/Surgical Nursing . . . . Carla McArdle

NOTE: Hospital profiles are in alphabetical order by state, then city, then hospital within the city; Rankings are sorted by rate in descending order and exclude hospitals with less than 25 cases; (1) The number of cases is too small (n<25) for purposes of reliably predicting hospital performance; (2) Measure reflects the hospital's indication that its submission was based upon a sample of its relevant discharges; (3) Rate reflects fewer than the maximum possible quarters of data for the measure; (4) Inaccurate information submitted and suppressed for one or more quarters; (5) No data is available from the hospital for this measure; Please refer to the User's Guide for a full explanation of data

Measure	Cases	This Hospital	State Average	U.S. Average	Top Hospital
Heart Attack Care					
ACE Inhibitor or ARB for LVSD	32	78%	83%	82%	100%
Aspirin at Arrival	155	94%	91%	92%	100%
Aspirin at Discharge	126	94%	91%	90%	100%
Beta Blocker at Arrival	127	87%	84%	87%	100%
Beta Blocker at Discharge	134	86%	91%	90%	100%
Fibrinolytic Medication Timing	0	-	44%	31%	100%
PCI Within 90 Minutes of Arrival[1]	5	60%	56%	54%	95%
Smoking Cessation Advice	48	94%	90%	88%	100%
Heart Failure Care					
ACE Inhibitor or ARB for LVSD	116	78%	81%	82%	100%
Discharge Instructions	272	59%	69%	61%	93%
Evaluation of LVS Function	355	77%	87%	83%	99%
Smoking Cessation Advice	37	68%	84%	82%	100%
Pneumonia Care					
Appropriate Initial Antibiotic	224	83%	83%	83%	94%
Blood Culture Timing	143	91%	90%	90%	100%
Influenza Vaccine	33	45%	74%	70%	100%
Initial Antibiotic Timing	209	73%	84%	80%	93%
Oxygenation Assessment	268	100%	99%	99%	100%
Pneumococcal Vaccine	171	51%	77%	69%	94%
Smoking Cessation Advice	41	27%	81%	80%	100%
Surgical Infection Prevention					
Prophylactic Antibiotic Given	583	92%	76%	77%	95%
Prophylactic Antibiotic Selection	131	93%	92%	90%	100%
Prophylactic Antibiotic Stopped	573	51%	70%	72%	95%
Pregnancy Care					
Inpatient Neonatal Mortality	-	-	-	-	-
Third or Fourth Degree Laceration	-	-	4.02%	3.63%	3.27%

Hendricks Regional Health

1000 East Main Street
Danville, IN 46122
URL: www.hendricksregional.org
Ownership: Government - Local
Emergency Services: No

Phone: 317-745-4451
Fax: 317-745-8325

Accredited: Yes
Licensed Beds: 141

Key Personnel:

President/CEO . . . . Dennis W Dawes
Director Emergency Room . . . . Anne Miller
Director Intensive Coronary . . . . Jo Morton
Director Medical Surgical Nursing . . . . Marcia Tracey
Director OB/GYN/Women's Health . . . . Deb Case
Director Radiology . . . . Stan Metzger

Measure	Cases	This Hospital	State Average	U.S. Average	Top Hospital
Heart Attack Care					
ACE Inhibitor or ARB for LVSD[1]	18	78%	83%	82%	100%
Aspirin at Arrival	88	98%	91%	92%	100%
Aspirin at Discharge	33	94%	91%	90%	100%
Beta Blocker at Arrival	87	95%	84%	87%	100%
Beta Blocker at Discharge	38	97%	91%	90%	100%
Fibrinolytic Medication Timing[1]	3	67%	44%	31%	100%
PCI Within 90 Minutes of Arrival	0	-	56%	54%	95%
Smoking Cessation Advice[1]	3	100%	90%	88%	100%
Heart Failure Care					
ACE Inhibitor or ARB for LVSD	70	77%	81%	82%	100%
Discharge Instructions	126	79%	69%	61%	93%
Evaluation of LVS Function	180	94%	87%	83%	99%
Smoking Cessation Advice[1]	16	94%	84%	82%	100%
Pneumonia Care					
Appropriate Initial Antibiotic	170	86%	83%	83%	94%
Blood Culture Timing	99	83%	90%	90%	100%
Influenza Vaccine	36	92%	74%	70%	100%
Initial Antibiotic Timing	272	89%	84%	80%	93%
Oxygenation Assessment	274	100%	99%	99%	100%
Pneumococcal Vaccine	162	73%	77%	69%	94%
Smoking Cessation Advice	54	85%	81%	80%	100%
Surgical Infection Prevention					
Prophylactic Antibiotic Given	315	79%	76%	77%	95%
Prophylactic Antibiotic Selection	71	92%	92%	90%	100%
Prophylactic Antibiotic Stopped	309	61%	70%	72%	95%

Pregnancy Care					
Inpatient Neonatal Mortality	-	-	-	-	-
Third or Fourth Degree Laceration	-	-	4.02%	3.63%	3.27%

Adams Memorial Hospital

1100 Mercer Street
PO Box 151
Decatur, IN 46733
URL: www.adamshospital.com
Ownership: Government - Local
Emergency Services: Yes

Phone: 260-724-2145
Fax: 260-728-3865

Accredited: Yes
Licensed Beds: 87

Key Personnel:

Chief Medical Staff . . . . Brian Zurcher, MD
Director of Cardiology/Cardiac Lab . . . . Ronda Brune
Emergency Room . . . . Scott Smith, MD
Emergency Room . . . . Lesley Scholl, MD
Director Infection/Disease Control . . . . Peggy LaFountaine
Director Medical/Surgical Nursing . . . . Jo McIntire
Respiratory Care . . . . Lousina Thatcher

Measure	Cases	This Hospital	State Average	U.S. Average	Top Hospital
Heart Attack Care					
ACE Inhibitor or ARB for LVSD[1]	4	100%	83%	82%	100%
Aspirin at Arrival[1]	21	86%	91%	92%	100%
Aspirin at Discharge[1]	14	86%	91%	90%	100%
Beta Blocker at Arrival[1]	18	67%	84%	87%	100%
Beta Blocker at Discharge[1]	14	100%	91%	90%	100%
Fibrinolytic Medication Timing	0	-	44%	31%	100%
PCI Within 90 Minutes of Arrival	0	-	56%	54%	95%
Smoking Cessation Advice[1]	1	0%	90%	88%	100%
Heart Failure Care					
ACE Inhibitor or ARB for LVSD	28	86%	81%	82%	100%
Discharge Instructions	54	72%	69%	61%	93%
Evaluation of LVS Function	83	72%	87%	83%	99%
Smoking Cessation Advice	25	40%	84%	82%	100%
Pneumonia Care					
Appropriate Initial Antibiotic	60	85%	83%	83%	94%
Blood Culture Timing[1,3]	14	100%	90%	90%	100%
Influenza Vaccine[1]	22	82%	74%	70%	100%
Initial Antibiotic Timing	84	86%	84%	80%	93%
Oxygenation Assessment	94	97%	99%	99%	100%
Pneumococcal Vaccine	66	77%	77%	69%	94%
Smoking Cessation Advice[1]	13	62%	81%	80%	100%
Surgical Infection Prevention					
Prophylactic Antibiotic Given	35	43%	76%	77%	95%
Prophylactic Antibiotic Selection[1]	11	91%	92%	90%	100%
Prophylactic Antibiotic Stopped	34	32%	70%	72%	95%
Pregnancy Care					
Inpatient Neonatal Mortality	-	-	-	-	-
Third or Fourth Degree Laceration	-	-	4.02%	3.63%	3.27%

Saint Margaret Mercy Healthcare Centers

Alternate Name: South Campus
24 Joliet Street
Dyer, IN 46311
URL: www.smmhc.com
Ownership: Voluntary non-profit - Church
Emergency Services: Yes

Phone: 219-865-2141
Fax: 219-864-2585

Accredited: Yes
Licensed Beds: 794

Key Personnel:

President/CEO . . . . Gene Diamond
Chief Medical Staff . . . . R Kanuru, MD
Cardiac Lab . . . . Dora Slupsizi
Emergency Room . . . . Bryan Staffin
ICU . . . . Linda Ray
Medical Surgical Nursing . . . . Deb Kolosh
OB/GYN Womens Health . . . . Linda Krairo
Respiratory/Cardiopulmonary . . . . George Buozik

Measure	Cases	This Hospital	State Average	U.S. Average	Top Hospital
Heart Attack Care					
ACE Inhibitor or ARB for LVSD	27	81%	83%	82%	100%
Aspirin at Arrival	94	100%	91%	92%	100%
Aspirin at Discharge	88	99%	91%	90%	100%

NOTE: Hospital profiles are in alphabetical order by state, then city, then hospital within the city; Rankings are sorted by rate in descending order and exclude hospitals with less than 25 cases; (1) The number of cases is too small (n<25) for purposes of reliably predicting hospital performance; (2) Measure reflects the hospital's indication that its submission was based upon a sample of its relevant discharges; (3) Rate reflects fewer than the maximum possible quarters of data for the measure; (4) Inaccurate information submitted and suppressed for one or more quarters; (5) No data is available from the hospital for this measure; Please refer to the User's Guide for a full explanation of data

Measure	Cases	This Hospital	State Average	U.S. Average	Top Hospital
Beta Blocker at Arrival	69	97%	84%	87%	100%
Beta Blocker at Discharge	87	100%	91%	90%	100%
Fibrinolytic Medication Timing	0	-	44%	31%	100%
PCI Within 90 Minutes of Arrival[1]	3	33%	56%	54%	95%
Smoking Cessation Advice	32	78%	90%	88%	100%
Heart Failure Care					
ACE Inhibitor or ARB for LVSD	87	83%	81%	82%	100%
Discharge Instructions	194	78%	69%	61%	93%
Evaluation of LVS Function	225	96%	87%	83%	99%
Smoking Cessation Advice	32	69%	84%	82%	100%
Pneumonia Care					
Appropriate Initial Antibiotic	98	88%	83%	83%	94%
Blood Culture Timing	106	92%	90%	90%	100%
Influenza Vaccine[4,5]	-	-	74%	70%	100%
Initial Antibiotic Timing	134	81%	84%	80%	93%
Oxygenation Assessment	168	100%	99%	99%	100%
Pneumococcal Vaccine	95	72%	77%	69%	94%
Smoking Cessation Advice	42	86%	81%	80%	100%
Surgical Infection Prevention					
Prophylactic Antibiotic Given	198	93%	76%	77%	95%
Prophylactic Antibiotic Selection	60	93%	92%	90%	100%
Prophylactic Antibiotic Stopped	195	58%	70%	72%	95%
Pregnancy Care					
Inpatient Neonatal Mortality	-	-	-	-	-
Third or Fourth Degree Laceration	-	-	4.02%	3.63%	3.27%

Saint Catherine Hospital of East Chicago

4321 Fir Street
East Chicago, IN 46312
URL: www.comhs.org/stcatherine
Ownership: Voluntary non-profit - Private
Emergency Services: No
Phone: 219-392-1700
Fax: 219-392-7622
Accredited: Yes
Licensed Beds: 290

Key Personnel:
Administrator . . . . JoAnn Birdzell
Chief Medical Staff. . . . . John Griep
Emergency Room . . . . Jeffery Dubnow
OB/GYN Womens Health. . . . . Michael Linton, MD
Respiratory Care . . . . Elliot Stoker

Measure	Cases	This Hospital	State Average	U.S. Average	Top Hospital
Heart Attack Care					
ACE Inhibitor or ARB for LVSD[1]	12	75%	83%	82%	100%
Aspirin at Arrival	57	95%	91%	92%	100%
Aspirin at Discharge	55	96%	91%	90%	100%
Beta Blocker at Arrival	44	86%	84%	87%	100%
Beta Blocker at Discharge	50	90%	91%	90%	100%
Fibrinolytic Medication Timing[3]	0	-	44%	31%	100%
PCI Within 90 Minutes of Arrival[1]	4	25%	56%	54%	95%
Smoking Cessation Advice[1,3]	5	100%	90%	88%	100%
Heart Failure Care					
ACE Inhibitor or ARB for LVSD	164	96%	81%	82%	100%
Discharge Instructions[3]	91	99%	69%	61%	93%
Evaluation of LVS Function	494	99%	87%	83%	99%
Smoking Cessation Advice[1,3]	24	100%	84%	82%	100%
Pneumonia Care					
Appropriate Initial Antibiotic[1,3]	17	94%	83%	83%	94%
Blood Culture Timing[1,3]	19	95%	90%	90%	100%
Influenza Vaccine[5]	-	-	74%	70%	100%
Initial Antibiotic Timing	148	78%	84%	80%	93%
Oxygenation Assessment	162	97%	99%	99%	100%
Pneumococcal Vaccine	74	78%	77%	69%	94%
Smoking Cessation Advice[1,3]	10	60%	81%	80%	100%
Surgical Infection Prevention					
Prophylactic Antibiotic Given[3]	63	29%	76%	77%	95%
Prophylactic Antibiotic Selection[5]	-	-	92%	90%	100%
Prophylactic Antibiotic Stopped[3]	63	29%	70%	72%	95%
Pregnancy Care					
Inpatient Neonatal Mortality	-	-	-	-	-
Third or Fourth Degree Laceration	-	-	4.02%	3.63%	3.27%

Elkhart General Hospital

600 East Boulevard
Elkhart, IN 46514
URL: www.egh.org
Ownership: Voluntary non-profit - Other
Emergency Services: Yes
Phone: 574-294-2621
Fax: 574-523-3495
Accredited: Yes
Licensed Beds: 365

Key Personnel:
CEO. . . . . Gregory W Lintjer
Emergency Room . . . . Colleen Nowlin
Director Cardio-Pulmonary Services . . . . Cindie McPhie

Measure	Cases	This Hospital	State Average	U.S. Average	Top Hospital
Heart Attack Care					
ACE Inhibitor or ARB for LVSD	55	98%	83%	82%	100%
Aspirin at Arrival	289	98%	91%	92%	100%
Aspirin at Discharge	319	98%	91%	90%	100%
Beta Blocker at Arrival	233	96%	84%	87%	100%
Beta Blocker at Discharge	296	99%	91%	90%	100%
Fibrinolytic Medication Timing	0	-	44%	31%	100%
PCI Within 90 Minutes of Arrival[1]	12	75%	56%	54%	95%
Smoking Cessation Advice	120	89%	90%	88%	100%
Heart Failure Care					
ACE Inhibitor or ARB for LVSD	211	78%	81%	82%	100%
Discharge Instructions	417	43%	69%	61%	93%
Evaluation of LVS Function	488	82%	87%	83%	99%
Smoking Cessation Advice	72	62%	84%	82%	100%
Pneumonia Care					
Appropriate Initial Antibiotic	183	89%	83%	83%	94%
Blood Culture Timing[1]	2	100%	90%	90%	100%
Influenza Vaccine	36	50%	74%	70%	100%
Initial Antibiotic Timing	290	84%	84%	80%	93%
Oxygenation Assessment	308	98%	99%	99%	100%
Pneumococcal Vaccine	184	42%	77%	69%	94%
Smoking Cessation Advice	81	62%	81%	80%	100%
Surgical Infection Prevention					
Prophylactic Antibiotic Given	1,152	72%	76%	77%	95%
Prophylactic Antibiotic Selection	277	95%	92%	90%	100%
Prophylactic Antibiotic Stopped	1,120	58%	70%	72%	95%
Pregnancy Care					
Inpatient Neonatal Mortality	-	-	-	-	-
Third or Fourth Degree Laceration	-	-	4.02%	3.63%	3.27%

Saint Vincent Mercy Hospital

Alternate Name: Mercy Hospital
1331 South A Street
Elwood, IN 46036
URL: www.stvincent.org
Ownership: Voluntary non-profit - Church
Emergency Services: No
Phone: 765-552-4600
Fax: 765-552-4700
Accredited: Yes
Licensed Beds: 25

Key Personnel:
Chief of Medical Staff. . . . . Robert Helm, MD
Emergency Room . . . . Brad Hayes
Director Infection/Disease Control . . . . Candy Robinson
OB/GYN Womens Health. . . . . Dean Paulsen, MD
Director of Pulmonary/Respiratory Care. . . . . . . Caren Myer

Measure	Cases	This Hospital	State Average	U.S. Average	Top Hospital
Heart Attack Care					
ACE Inhibitor or ARB for LVSD[3]	0	-	83%	82%	100%
Aspirin at Arrival[1,3]	1	100%	91%	92%	100%
Aspirin at Discharge[3]	0	-	91%	90%	100%
Beta Blocker at Arrival[1,3]	1	100%	84%	87%	100%
Beta Blocker at Discharge[3]	0	-	91%	90%	100%
Fibrinolytic Medication Timing[3]	0	-	44%	31%	100%
PCI Within 90 Minutes of Arrival[5]	-	-	56%	54%	95%
Smoking Cessation Advice[3]	0	-	90%	88%	100%
Heart Failure Care					
ACE Inhibitor or ARB for LVSD[1]	5	80%	81%	82%	100%
Discharge Instructions[1]	10	60%	69%	61%	93%
Evaluation of LVS Function[1]	14	57%	87%	83%	99%
Smoking Cessation Advice[1]	1	0%	84%	82%	100%
Pneumonia Care					
Appropriate Initial Antibiotic	77	78%	83%	83%	94%

NOTE: Hospital profiles are in alphabetical order by state, then city, then hospital within the city; Rankings are sorted by rate in descending order and exclude hospitals with less than 25 cases; (1) The number of cases is too small (n<25) for purposes of reliably predicting hospital performance; (2) Measure reflects the hospital's indication that its submission was based upon a sample of its relevant discharges; (3) Rate reflects fewer than the maximum possible quarters of data for the measure; (4) Inaccurate information submitted and suppressed for one or more quarters; (5) No data is available from the hospital for this measure; Please refer to the User's Guide for a full explanation of data

Blood Culture Timing	51	96%	90%	90%	100%
Influenza Vaccine[1]	15	93%	74%	70%	100%
Initial Antibiotic Timing	90	84%	84%	80%	93%
Oxygenation Assessment	102	99%	99%	99%	100%
Pneumococcal Vaccine	66	67%	77%	69%	94%
Smoking Cessation Advice	29	76%	81%	80%	100%
Surgical Infection Prevention					
Prophylactic Antibiotic Given[3]	0	-	76%	77%	95%
Prophylactic Antibiotic Selection	0	-	92%	90%	100%
Prophylactic Antibiotic Stopped[3]	0	-	70%	72%	95%
Pregnancy Care					
Inpatient Neonatal Mortality	-	-	-	-	-
Third or Fourth Degree Laceration	-	-	4.02%	3.63%	3.27%

Deaconess Hospital

600 Mary Street
Evansville, IN 47747
URL: www.deaconess.com
Ownership: Voluntary non-profit - Private
Emergency Services: Yes

Phone: 812-450-5000
Fax: 812-450-6051
Accredited: Yes
Licensed Beds: 400

Key Personnel:

President/CEO . . . . Harry L Smith Jr
CEO . . . . Wallace Simmons
Infection Control . . . . Mellodee Montgomery

Measure	Cases	This Hospital	State Average	U.S. Average	Top Hospital
Heart Attack Care					
ACE Inhibitor or ARB for LVSD	182	82%	83%	82%	100%
Aspirin at Arrival	394	96%	91%	92%	100%
Aspirin at Discharge	653	97%	91%	90%	100%
Beta Blocker at Arrival	332	88%	84%	87%	100%
Beta Blocker at Discharge	640	94%	91%	90%	100%
Fibrinolytic Medication Timing	0	-	44%	31%	100%
PCI Within 90 Minutes of Arrival[1]	16	75%	56%	54%	95%
Smoking Cessation Advice	273	99%	90%	88%	100%
Heart Failure Care					
ACE Inhibitor or ARB for LVSD	317	80%	81%	82%	100%
Discharge Instructions	631	63%	69%	61%	93%
Evaluation of LVS Function	801	90%	87%	83%	99%
Smoking Cessation Advice	182	99%	84%	82%	100%
Pneumonia Care					
Appropriate Initial Antibiotic	320	92%	83%	83%	94%
Blood Culture Timing	318	90%	90%	90%	100%
Influenza Vaccine	104	87%	74%	70%	100%
Initial Antibiotic Timing	479	78%	84%	80%	93%
Oxygenation Assessment	615	100%	99%	99%	100%
Pneumococcal Vaccine	404	86%	77%	69%	94%
Smoking Cessation Advice	183	98%	81%	80%	100%
Surgical Infection Prevention					
Prophylactic Antibiotic Given[2,3]	1,072	77%	76%	77%	95%
Prophylactic Antibiotic Selection[2]	297	95%	92%	90%	100%
Prophylactic Antibiotic Stopped[2,3]	1,037	53%	70%	72%	95%
Pregnancy Care					
Inpatient Neonatal Mortality	-	-	-	-	-
Third or Fourth Degree Laceration	-	-	4.02%	3.63%	3.27%

Saint Mary's Medical Center

3700 Washington Avenue
Evansville, IN 47734
URL: www.stmarys.org
Ownership: Voluntary non-profit - Church
Emergency Services: Yes

Phone: 812-485-4000
Fax: 812-485-7800
Accredited: Yes
Licensed Beds: 564

Key Personnel:

President/CEO . . . . Timothy Flesch
Emergency Room . . . . Amy Stamman
Emergency Room . . . . Connie Brandes
Director Infection/Disease Control . . . . Donna Bratt
Chief Medical Officer . . . . John Gallagher, MD
OB/GYN Womens Health . . . . Nelson Graham, MD
Chief Radiology . . . . Paul Hargan, MD
Director Cardio-Pulmonary Services . . . . Becky Dicus

Measure	Cases	This Hospital	State Average	U.S. Average	Top Hospital
Heart Attack Care					
ACE Inhibitor or ARB for LVSD	118	79%	83%	82%	100%
Aspirin at Arrival	260	98%	91%	92%	100%
Aspirin at Discharge	336	97%	91%	90%	100%
Beta Blocker at Arrival	198	95%	84%	87%	100%
Beta Blocker at Discharge	335	99%	91%	90%	100%
Fibrinolytic Medication Timing[1]	2	0%	44%	31%	100%
PCI Within 90 Minutes of Arrival[1]	8	38%	56%	54%	95%
Smoking Cessation Advice	145	99%	90%	88%	100%
Heart Failure Care					
ACE Inhibitor or ARB for LVSD	129	87%	81%	82%	100%
Discharge Instructions	235	97%	69%	61%	93%
Evaluation of LVS Function	305	93%	87%	83%	99%
Smoking Cessation Advice	52	100%	84%	82%	100%
Pneumonia Care					
Appropriate Initial Antibiotic[2]	180	87%	83%	83%	94%
Blood Culture Timing[2]	151	89%	90%	90%	100%
Influenza Vaccine	61	77%	74%	70%	100%
Initial Antibiotic Timing[2]	257	68%	84%	80%	93%
Oxygenation Assessment[2]	332	99%	99%	99%	100%
Pneumococcal Vaccine[2]	192	72%	77%	69%	94%
Smoking Cessation Advice[2]	100	90%	81%	80%	100%
Surgical Infection Prevention					
Prophylactic Antibiotic Given[2,3]	335	66%	76%	77%	95%
Prophylactic Antibiotic Selection[2]	121	96%	92%	90%	100%
Prophylactic Antibiotic Stopped[2,3]	327	71%	70%	72%	95%
Pregnancy Care					
Inpatient Neonatal Mortality	-	-	-	-	-
Third or Fourth Degree Laceration	-	-	4.02%	3.63%	3.27%

Dupont Hospital

2520 E Dupont Rd
Fort Wayne, IN 46825
Ownership: Proprietary
Emergency Services: Yes

Phone: 260-416-3000
Accredited: Yes

Measure	Cases	This Hospital	State Average	U.S. Average	Top Hospital
Heart Attack Care					
ACE Inhibitor or ARB for LVSD[1,3]	1	100%	83%	82%	100%
Aspirin at Arrival[1,3]	7	71%	91%	92%	100%
Aspirin at Discharge[1,3]	4	100%	91%	90%	100%
Beta Blocker at Arrival[1,3]	9	78%	84%	87%	100%
Beta Blocker at Discharge[1,3]	5	100%	91%	90%	100%
Fibrinolytic Medication Timing[3]	0	-	44%	31%	100%
PCI Within 90 Minutes of Arrival	0	-	56%	54%	95%
Smoking Cessation Advice[1,3]	1	100%	90%	88%	100%
Heart Failure Care					
ACE Inhibitor or ARB for LVSD[1]	11	55%	81%	82%	100%
Discharge Instructions	26	58%	69%	61%	93%
Evaluation of LVS Function	33	100%	87%	83%	99%
Smoking Cessation Advice[1]	4	100%	84%	82%	100%
Pneumonia Care					
Appropriate Initial Antibiotic	44	84%	83%	83%	94%
Blood Culture Timing	36	100%	90%	90%	100%
Influenza Vaccine[1]	8	75%	74%	70%	100%
Initial Antibiotic Timing	42	88%	84%	80%	93%
Oxygenation Assessment	55	100%	99%	99%	100%
Pneumococcal Vaccine	29	97%	77%	69%	94%
Smoking Cessation Advice[1]	11	91%	81%	80%	100%
Surgical Infection Prevention					
Prophylactic Antibiotic Given[2]	623	79%	76%	77%	95%
Prophylactic Antibiotic Selection[2]	173	95%	92%	90%	100%
Prophylactic Antibiotic Stopped[2]	600	74%	70%	72%	95%
Pregnancy Care					
Inpatient Neonatal Mortality	2,296	0.09%	-	-	-
Third or Fourth Degree Laceration	1,640	4.76%	4.02%	3.63%	3.27%

NOTE: Hospital profiles are in alphabetical order by state, then city, then hospital within the city; Rankings are sorted by rate in descending order and exclude hospitals with less than 25 cases; (1) The number of cases is too small (n<25) for purposes of reliably predicting hospital performance; (2) Measure reflects the hospital's indication that its submission was based upon a sample of its relevant discharges; (3) Rate reflects fewer than the maximum possible quarters of data for the measure; (4) Inaccurate information submitted and suppressed for one or more quarters; (5) No data is available from the hospital for this measure; Please refer to the User's Guide for a full explanation of data

Lutheran Hospital of Indiana

7950 W Jefferson Boulevard
Fort Wayne, IN 46804
URL: www.lutheranhospital.com
Ownership: Voluntary non-profit - Private
Emergency Services: Yes
Phone: 260-435-7001
Fax: 260-435-7640
Accredited: Yes
Licensed Beds: 366

Key Personnel:
CEO. . . . . Thomas D Miller
Chief Medical Staff. . . . . B.V. House, MD

Measure	Cases	This Hospital	State Average	U.S. Average	Top Hospital
Heart Attack Care					
ACE Inhibitor or ARB for LVSD	144	86%	83%	82%	100%
Aspirin at Arrival	285	96%	91%	92%	100%
Aspirin at Discharge	667	98%	91%	90%	100%
Beta Blocker at Arrival	239	91%	84%	87%	100%
Beta Blocker at Discharge	657	96%	91%	90%	100%
Fibrinolytic Medication Timing	0	-	44%	31%	100%
PCI Within 90 Minutes of Arrival[1]	24	58%	56%	54%	95%
Smoking Cessation Advice	268	99%	90%	88%	100%
Heart Failure Care					
ACE Inhibitor or ARB for LVSD	255	78%	81%	82%	100%
Discharge Instructions	477	58%	69%	61%	93%
Evaluation of LVS Function	590	91%	87%	83%	99%
Smoking Cessation Advice	125	99%	84%	82%	100%
Pneumonia Care					
Appropriate Initial Antibiotic	144	91%	83%	83%	94%
Blood Culture Timing	207	94%	90%	90%	100%
Influenza Vaccine	66	94%	74%	70%	100%
Initial Antibiotic Timing	260	86%	84%	80%	93%
Oxygenation Assessment	337	100%	99%	99%	100%
Pneumococcal Vaccine	241	93%	77%	69%	94%
Smoking Cessation Advice	93	97%	81%	80%	100%
Surgical Infection Prevention					
Prophylactic Antibiotic Given	1,709	72%	76%	77%	95%
Prophylactic Antibiotic Selection	437	96%	92%	90%	100%
Prophylactic Antibiotic Stopped	1,624	71%	70%	72%	95%
Pregnancy Care					
Inpatient Neonatal Mortality	1,849	0.59%	-	-	-
Third or Fourth Degree Laceration	1,133	2.82%	4.02%	3.63%	3.27%

Parkview Memorial Hospital

2200 Ranhallin Drive
Fort Wayne, IN 46805
Toll-Free: 888-856-2522
Phone: 260-484-6636
Fax: 260-483-1373
E-mail: fdb@parkview.com
URL: www.parkview.com
Ownership: Voluntary non-profit - Private
Emergency Services: Yes
Accredited: Yes
Licensed Beds: 656

Key Personnel:
President/CEO. . . . . Frank D Byrne, MD
Chief Medical Staff. . . . . Richard Neilsen, MD
Chief Catheterization Laboratory . . . . Dennis Warner
Emergency Room . . . . Dan Garman
Director Infection/Disease Control . . . . Joan Kennedy, RN
CCU Spvg. Nurse . . . . Cheri Shaw, RN
OB/GYN Womens Health. . . . . Bev Mills, RN
Chief Radiology . . . . Tom Sarosi, MD
Director Respiratory Therapy . . . . Eileen Brackett

Measure	Cases	This Hospital	State Average	U.S. Average	Top Hospital
Heart Attack Care					
ACE Inhibitor or ARB for LVSD	39	92%	83%	82%	100%
Aspirin at Arrival	130	99%	91%	92%	100%
Aspirin at Discharge	215	100%	91%	90%	100%
Beta Blocker at Arrival	55	93%	84%	87%	100%
Beta Blocker at Discharge	224	99%	91%	90%	100%
Fibrinolytic Medication Timing[1]	9	67%	44%	31%	100%
PCI Within 90 Minutes of Arrival[1]	11	73%	56%	54%	95%
Smoking Cessation Advice	113	92%	90%	88%	100%
Heart Failure Care					
ACE Inhibitor or ARB for LVSD	85	89%	81%	82%	100%
Discharge Instructions	209	56%	69%	61%	93%
Evaluation of LVS Function	285	92%	87%	83%	99%
Smoking Cessation Advice	49	88%	84%	82%	100%
Pneumonia Care					
Appropriate Initial Antibiotic	102	92%	83%	83%	94%
Blood Culture Timing	97	92%	90%	90%	100%
Influenza Vaccine	25	68%	74%	70%	100%
Initial Antibiotic Timing	132	82%	84%	80%	93%
Oxygenation Assessment	177	100%	99%	99%	100%
Pneumococcal Vaccine	109	63%	77%	69%	94%
Smoking Cessation Advice	42	81%	81%	80%	100%
Surgical Infection Prevention					
Prophylactic Antibiotic Given	314	66%	76%	77%	95%
Prophylactic Antibiotic Selection	79	97%	92%	90%	100%
Prophylactic Antibiotic Stopped	306	57%	70%	72%	95%
Pregnancy Care					
Inpatient Neonatal Mortality	-	-	-	-	-
Third or Fourth Degree Laceration	-	-	4.02%	3.63%	3.27%

Saint Joseph Hospital

700 Broadway
Fort Wayne, IN 46802
URL: www.stjoehospital.com
Ownership: Proprietary
Emergency Services: Yes
Phone: 260-425-3000
Fax: 260-425-3013
Accredited: Yes
Licensed Beds: 191

Key Personnel:
CEO. . . . . Kirk Bay
Emergency Room . . . . Jernice Watson, RN
OB/GYN Womens Health. . . . . Joan Landin, RN
Director Radiology . . . . Rob Snyder
Director Cardio-Pulmonary Services . . . . Randy Batt
Director Surgery. . . . . Bernice Ewing

Measure	Cases	This Hospital	State Average	U.S. Average	Top Hospital
Heart Attack Care					
ACE Inhibitor or ARB for LVSD[1]	20	100%	83%	82%	100%
Aspirin at Arrival	85	98%	91%	92%	100%
Aspirin at Discharge	103	99%	91%	90%	100%
Beta Blocker at Arrival	81	93%	84%	87%	100%
Beta Blocker at Discharge	98	95%	91%	90%	100%
Fibrinolytic Medication Timing[1]	1	0%	44%	31%	100%
PCI Within 90 Minutes of Arrival[1]	8	38%	56%	54%	95%
Smoking Cessation Advice	44	100%	90%	88%	100%
Heart Failure Care					
ACE Inhibitor or ARB for LVSD	70	83%	81%	82%	100%
Discharge Instructions	162	96%	69%	61%	93%
Evaluation of LVS Function	218	96%	87%	83%	99%
Smoking Cessation Advice	46	100%	84%	82%	100%
Pneumonia Care					
Appropriate Initial Antibiotic	33	85%	83%	83%	94%
Blood Culture Timing	33	91%	90%	90%	100%
Influenza Vaccine[1]	12	83%	74%	70%	100%
Initial Antibiotic Timing	59	83%	84%	80%	93%
Oxygenation Assessment	67	100%	99%	99%	100%
Pneumococcal Vaccine	39	92%	77%	69%	94%
Smoking Cessation Advice[1]	17	94%	81%	80%	100%
Surgical Infection Prevention					
Prophylactic Antibiotic Given	163	72%	76%	77%	95%
Prophylactic Antibiotic Selection	42	100%	92%	90%	100%
Prophylactic Antibiotic Stopped	162	71%	70%	72%	95%
Pregnancy Care					
Inpatient Neonatal Mortality	-	-	-	-	-
Third or Fourth Degree Laceration	-	-	4.02%	3.63%	3.27%

Saint Vincent Frankfort Hospital

1300 S Jackson Street
Frankfort, IN 46041
URL: www.stvincent.org
Ownership: Voluntary non-profit - Church
Emergency Services: No
Phone: 765-656-3000
Fax: 765-654-6881
Accredited: Yes
Licensed Beds: 25

Key Personnel:
Chief Medical Staff. . . . . Stephen D Thorp, MD
Emergency Room . . . . James Rudolph, MD
CCU Spvg. Nurse . . . . Debbie Lineback, RN

NOTE: Hospital profiles are in alphabetical order by state, then city, then hospital within the city; Rankings are sorted by rate in descending order and exclude hospitals with less than 25 cases; (1) The number of cases is too small (n<25) for purposes of reliably predicting hospital performance; (2) Measure reflects the hospital's indication that its submission was based upon a sample of its relevant discharges; (3) Rate reflects fewer than the maximum possible quarters of data for the measure; (4) Inaccurate information submitted and suppressed for one or more quarters; (5) No data is available from the hospital for this measure; Please refer to the User's Guide for a full explanation of data

Director Medical/Surgical Nursing . . . . Debbie Lineback, RN
OB/GYN Womens Health. . . . . Alan Wagoner, MD
Chief Radiology . . . . Richard T Beeler, MD
Director Respiratory Therapy . . . . Joanne Miller

Measure	Cases	This Hospital	State Average	U.S. Average	Top Hospital
Heart Attack Care					
ACE Inhibitor or ARB for LVSD[1]	2	100%	83%	82%	100%
Aspirin at Arrival[1]	4	100%	91%	92%	100%
Aspirin at Discharge[1]	4	100%	91%	90%	100%
Beta Blocker at Arrival[1]	5	60%	84%	87%	100%
Beta Blocker at Discharge[1]	5	100%	91%	90%	100%
Fibrinolytic Medication Timing	0	-	44%	31%	100%
PCI Within 90 Minutes of Arrival[5]	-	-	56%	54%	95%
Smoking Cessation Advice	0	-	90%	88%	100%
Heart Failure Care					
ACE Inhibitor or ARB for LVSD[1]	12	92%	81%	82%	100%
Discharge Instructions	27	52%	69%	61%	93%
Evaluation of LVS Function	26	69%	87%	83%	99%
Smoking Cessation Advice	0	-	84%	82%	100%
Pneumonia Care					
Appropriate Initial Antibiotic	48	67%	83%	83%	94%
Blood Culture Timing	35	89%	90%	90%	100%
Influenza Vaccine[1]	8	75%	74%	70%	100%
Initial Antibiotic Timing	53	87%	84%	80%	93%
Oxygenation Assessment	67	99%	99%	99%	100%
Pneumococcal Vaccine	37	49%	77%	69%	94%
Smoking Cessation Advice[1]	17	59%	81%	80%	100%
Surgical Infection Prevention					
Prophylactic Antibiotic Given	31	52%	76%	77%	95%
Prophylactic Antibiotic Selection[1]	8	100%	92%	90%	100%
Prophylactic Antibiotic Stopped	29	93%	70%	72%	95%
Pregnancy Care					
Inpatient Neonatal Mortality	-	-	-	-	-
Third or Fourth Degree Laceration	-	-	4.02%	3.63%	3.27%

Johnson Memorial Hospital

1125 W Jefferson
Franklin, IN 46131
Phone: 317-736-3300
Fax: 317-738-7894
URL: www.johnsonmemorial.org
Ownership: Government - Local
Emergency Services: No
Accredited: Yes
Licensed Beds: 161

Key Personnel:
President . . . . Gregg Bechtold
Chief Medical Staff. . . . . Paul Vessely, MD
Director Emergency Department . . . . Carla M Taylor
Director Medical/Surgical . . . . Pamela Ribelin
Director Surgical Services . . . . Vickie McCullough
Director Radiology . . . . Randy Collins

Measure	Cases	This Hospital	State Average	U.S. Average	Top Hospital
Heart Attack Care					
ACE Inhibitor or ARB for LVSD[1]	1	100%	83%	82%	100%
Aspirin at Arrival[1]	23	100%	91%	92%	100%
Aspirin at Discharge[1]	5	100%	91%	90%	100%
Beta Blocker at Arrival[1]	19	95%	84%	87%	100%
Beta Blocker at Discharge[1]	4	100%	91%	90%	100%
Fibrinolytic Medication Timing[1]	4	50%	44%	31%	100%
PCI Within 90 Minutes of Arrival	0	-	56%	54%	95%
Smoking Cessation Advice[1]	1	0%	90%	88%	100%
Heart Failure Care					
ACE Inhibitor or ARB for LVSD[1]	19	79%	81%	82%	100%
Discharge Instructions	64	70%	69%	61%	93%
Evaluation of LVS Function	98	95%	87%	83%	99%
Smoking Cessation Advice[1]	19	68%	84%	82%	100%
Pneumonia Care					
Appropriate Initial Antibiotic	107	91%	83%	83%	94%
Blood Culture Timing	88	85%	90%	90%	100%
Influenza Vaccine	26	92%	74%	70%	100%
Initial Antibiotic Timing	112	88%	84%	80%	93%
Oxygenation Assessment	148	100%	99%	99%	100%
Pneumococcal Vaccine	78	85%	77%	69%	94%
Smoking Cessation Advice	35	91%	81%	80%	100%
Surgical Infection Prevention					
Prophylactic Antibiotic Given	121	88%	76%	77%	95%
Prophylactic Antibiotic Selection[1]	23	100%	92%	90%	100%
Prophylactic Antibiotic Stopped	114	96%	70%	72%	95%
Pregnancy Care					
Inpatient Neonatal Mortality	-	-	-	-	-
Third or Fourth Degree Laceration	-	-	4.02%	3.63%	3.27%

Methodist Hospitals-North Lake Campus

600 Grant Street
Gary, IN 46402
Phone: 219-886-4000
Fax: 219-886-4592
URL: www.methodisthospital.org
Ownership: Voluntary non-profit - Private
Emergency Services: No
Accredited: Yes
Licensed Beds: 469

Key Personnel:
President . . . . Andre Artis, MD
Chief Cardiology Subspecialty Director . . . . Nazzal Obaid, MD
Chief Obstetrics/Gynecology . . . . Anthony Iwuagwu, MD
Chief Radiology . . . . Tulsi Sawlani, MD

Measure	Cases	This Hospital	State Average	U.S. Average	Top Hospital
Heart Attack Care					
ACE Inhibitor or ARB for LVSD	47	79%	83%	82%	100%
Aspirin at Arrival	194	90%	91%	92%	100%
Aspirin at Discharge	165	82%	91%	90%	100%
Beta Blocker at Arrival	166	81%	84%	87%	100%
Beta Blocker at Discharge	179	86%	91%	90%	100%
Fibrinolytic Medication Timing[1]	3	0%	44%	31%	100%
PCI Within 90 Minutes of Arrival[1]	9	11%	56%	54%	95%
Smoking Cessation Advice	86	100%	90%	88%	100%
Heart Failure Care					
ACE Inhibitor or ARB for LVSD	392	78%	81%	82%	100%
Discharge Instructions	852	29%	69%	61%	93%
Evaluation of LVS Function	1,070	79%	87%	83%	99%
Smoking Cessation Advice	260	95%	84%	82%	100%
Pneumonia Care					
Appropriate Initial Antibiotic	202	76%	83%	83%	94%
Blood Culture Timing	106	86%	90%	90%	100%
Influenza Vaccine	63	51%	74%	70%	100%
Initial Antibiotic Timing	357	57%	84%	80%	93%
Oxygenation Assessment	432	100%	99%	99%	100%
Pneumococcal Vaccine	214	52%	77%	69%	94%
Smoking Cessation Advice	111	92%	81%	80%	100%
Surgical Infection Prevention					
Prophylactic Antibiotic Given[3]	383	63%	76%	77%	95%
Prophylactic Antibiotic Selection	127	80%	92%	90%	100%
Prophylactic Antibiotic Stopped[3]	363	56%	70%	72%	95%
Pregnancy Care					
Inpatient Neonatal Mortality	-	-	-	-	-
Third or Fourth Degree Laceration	-	-	4.02%	3.63%	3.27%

Goshen General Hospital

200 High Park Avenue
Goshen, IN 46526
Phone: 574-535-2666
Fax: 574-535-2859
E-mail: ksearcy@goshenhealth.com
URL: www.goshenhalth.com
Ownership: Voluntary non-profit - Private
Emergency Services: Yes
Accredited: Yes
Licensed Beds: 160

Key Personnel:
President/CEO. . . . . James Dague
Chief of Medical Staff. . . . . Randy Cammengade
Director of Cardiology/Cardiac Lab. . . . . Scott Ereksen
Emergency Room Director. . . . . Candes Andersen
Director Surgery. . . . . Wil Beachy
Respiratory Care . . . . Laura Graber

Measure	Cases	This Hospital	State Average	U.S. Average	Top Hospital
Heart Attack Care					
ACE Inhibitor or ARB for LVSD[1]	7	100%	83%	82%	100%
Aspirin at Arrival	44	95%	91%	92%	100%
Aspirin at Discharge	27	96%	91%	90%	100%
Beta Blocker at Arrival	27	100%	84%	87%	100%

NOTE: Hospital profiles are in alphabetical order by state, then city, then hospital within the city; Rankings are sorted by rate in descending order and exclude hospitals with less than 25 cases; (1) The number of cases is too small (n<25) for purposes of reliably predicting hospital performance; (2) Measure reflects the hospital's indication that its submission was based upon a sample of its relevant discharges; (3) Rate reflects fewer than the maximum possible quarters of data for the measure; (4) Inaccurate information submitted and suppressed for one or more quarters; (5) No data is available from the hospital for this measure; Please refer to the User's Guide for a full explanation of data

Measure	Cases	This Hospital	State Average	U.S. Average	Top Hospital
Beta Blocker at Discharge	26	100%	91%	90%	100%
Fibrinolytic Medication Timing	0	-	44%	31%	100%
PCI Within 90 Minutes of Arrival	0	-	56%	54%	95%
Smoking Cessation Advice[1]	5	100%	90%	88%	100%
Heart Failure Care					
ACE Inhibitor or ARB for LVSD	45	100%	81%	82%	100%
Discharge Instructions	117	86%	69%	61%	93%
Evaluation of LVS Function	158	97%	87%	83%	99%
Smoking Cessation Advice[1]	18	89%	84%	82%	100%
Pneumonia Care					
Appropriate Initial Antibiotic	109	85%	83%	83%	94%
Blood Culture Timing	69	93%	90%	90%	100%
Influenza Vaccine[1]	24	88%	74%	70%	100%
Initial Antibiotic Timing	116	86%	84%	80%	93%
Oxygenation Assessment	146	100%	99%	99%	100%
Pneumococcal Vaccine	91	92%	77%	69%	94%
Smoking Cessation Advice	28	86%	81%	80%	100%
Surgical Infection Prevention					
Prophylactic Antibiotic Given[2]	356	92%	76%	77%	95%
Prophylactic Antibiotic Selection[2]	82	98%	92%	90%	100%
Prophylactic Antibiotic Stopped[2]	345	81%	70%	72%	95%
Pregnancy Care					
Inpatient Neonatal Mortality	1,637	0.12%	-	-	-
Third or Fourth Degree Laceration	1,316	2.81%	4.02%	3.63%	3.27%

Hancock Memorial Hospital and Health Services

Alternate Name: Hancock Memorial Hospital
801 N State Street — Phone: 317-462-5544
Greenfield, IN 46140
URL: www.hmhhs.org
Ownership: Government - Local — Accredited: Yes
Emergency Services: Yes — Licensed Beds: 120

Key Personnel:
President/CEO. . . . . Robert C Keen, MD
Chief of Medical Staff. . . . . D Fletcher, MD
Emergency Room . . . . Wayne O'Conner
Medical/Surgical Nursing . . . . Jane Garin, RN
OB/GYN Womens Health. . . . . Cindy Pendlum
Respiratory/Cardiopulmonary. . . . . Bobbie Dunne

Measure	Cases	This Hospital	State Average	U.S. Average	Top Hospital
Heart Attack Care					
ACE Inhibitor or ARB for LVSD[1]	3	100%	83%	82%	100%
Aspirin at Arrival[1]	15	100%	91%	92%	100%
Aspirin at Discharge[1]	7	71%	91%	90%	100%
Beta Blocker at Arrival[1]	12	92%	84%	87%	100%
Beta Blocker at Discharge[1]	8	62%	91%	90%	100%
Fibrinolytic Medication Timing	0	-	44%	31%	100%
PCI Within 90 Minutes of Arrival	0	-	56%	54%	95%
Smoking Cessation Advice[1]	3	67%	90%	88%	100%
Heart Failure Care					
ACE Inhibitor or ARB for LVSD	33	79%	81%	82%	100%
Discharge Instructions	55	25%	69%	61%	93%
Evaluation of LVS Function	90	84%	87%	83%	99%
Smoking Cessation Advice[1]	14	57%	84%	82%	100%
Pneumonia Care					
Appropriate Initial Antibiotic	190	79%	83%	83%	94%
Blood Culture Timing	160	74%	90%	90%	100%
Influenza Vaccine	46	35%	74%	70%	100%
Initial Antibiotic Timing	257	86%	84%	80%	93%
Oxygenation Assessment	286	99%	99%	99%	100%
Pneumococcal Vaccine	193	66%	77%	69%	94%
Smoking Cessation Advice	63	57%	81%	80%	100%
Surgical Infection Prevention					
Prophylactic Antibiotic Given[2]	186	85%	76%	77%	95%
Prophylactic Antibiotic Selection[2]	41	98%	92%	90%	100%
Prophylactic Antibiotic Stopped[2]	182	49%	70%	72%	95%
Pregnancy Care					
Inpatient Neonatal Mortality	-	-	-	-	-
Third or Fourth Degree Laceration	-	-	4.02%	3.63%	3.27%

Decatur County Memorial Hospital

720 N Lincoln Street — Phone: 812-663-4331
Greensburg, IN 47240 — Fax: 812-663-9738
URL: www.dcmh.net
Ownership: Government - Local — Accredited: Yes
Emergency Services: Yes — Licensed Beds: 115

Key Personnel:
CEO. . . . . David Trexler
Infection Control. . . . . Pat Barnes, RN
ICU . . . . Cindy Grote, RN
Respiratory/Cardiopulmonary. . . . . James Heaney

Measure	Cases	This Hospital	State Average	U.S. Average	Top Hospital
Heart Attack Care					
ACE Inhibitor or ARB for LVSD[1]	3	67%	83%	82%	100%
Aspirin at Arrival[1]	11	91%	91%	92%	100%
Aspirin at Discharge[1]	6	83%	91%	90%	100%
Beta Blocker at Arrival[1]	9	78%	84%	87%	100%
Beta Blocker at Discharge[1]	9	44%	91%	90%	100%
Fibrinolytic Medication Timing[3]	0	-	44%	31%	100%
PCI Within 90 Minutes of Arrival	0	-	56%	54%	95%
Smoking Cessation Advice[1]	1	100%	90%	88%	100%
Heart Failure Care					
ACE Inhibitor or ARB for LVSD[1]	15	80%	81%	82%	100%
Discharge Instructions	40	80%	69%	61%	93%
Evaluation of LVS Function	63	86%	87%	83%	99%
Smoking Cessation Advice[1]	10	80%	84%	82%	100%
Pneumonia Care					
Appropriate Initial Antibiotic	55	75%	83%	83%	94%
Blood Culture Timing[1]	23	87%	90%	90%	100%
Influenza Vaccine[1]	7	86%	74%	70%	100%
Initial Antibiotic Timing	63	90%	84%	80%	93%
Oxygenation Assessment	77	99%	99%	99%	100%
Pneumococcal Vaccine	44	91%	77%	69%	94%
Smoking Cessation Advice[1]	16	88%	81%	80%	100%
Surgical Infection Prevention					
Prophylactic Antibiotic Given[3]	66	64%	76%	77%	95%
Prophylactic Antibiotic Selection[1]	20	100%	92%	90%	100%
Prophylactic Antibiotic Stopped[3]	64	30%	70%	72%	95%
Pregnancy Care					
Inpatient Neonatal Mortality	-	-	-	-	-
Third or Fourth Degree Laceration	-	-	4.02%	3.63%	3.27%

Saint Margaret Mercy Healthcare Centers

5454 Hohman Avenue — Phone: 219-932-2300
Hammond, IN 46320 — Fax: 219-933-2585
URL: www.smmhc.com
Ownership: Voluntary non-profit - Church — Accredited: Yes
Emergency Services: Yes — Licensed Beds: 475

Key Personnel:
CEO. . . . . Jean Diamond
Chief Medical Staff. . . . . J Patel
Emergency Room . . . . Brian Staffin, DO
Director Infection/Disease Control . . . . Sally Bola
OB/GYN Womens Health. . . . . S Zabaneh
Director Radiology . . . . Richard Peterson
Director Pulmonary Therapy . . . . Bird Piper

Measure	Cases	This Hospital	State Average	U.S. Average	Top Hospital
Heart Attack Care					
ACE Inhibitor or ARB for LVSD[2]	55	60%	83%	82%	100%
Aspirin at Arrival[2]	207	95%	91%	92%	100%
Aspirin at Discharge[2]	212	94%	91%	90%	100%
Beta Blocker at Arrival[2]	151	93%	84%	87%	100%
Beta Blocker at Discharge[2]	237	92%	91%	90%	100%
Fibrinolytic Medication Timing[2]	0	-	44%	31%	100%
PCI Within 90 Minutes of Arrival[1,2]	10	30%	56%	54%	95%
Smoking Cessation Advice[2]	79	82%	90%	88%	100%
Heart Failure Care					
ACE Inhibitor or ARB for LVSD[2]	107	76%	81%	82%	100%
Discharge Instructions[2]	253	72%	69%	61%	93%
Evaluation of LVS Function[2]	289	74%	87%	83%	99%
Smoking Cessation Advice[2]	68	81%	84%	82%	100%

NOTE: Hospital profiles are in alphabetical order by state, then city, then hospital within the city; Rankings are sorted by rate in descending order and exclude hospitals with less than 25 cases; (1) The number of cases is too small (n<25) for purposes of reliably predicting hospital performance; (2) Measure reflects the hospital's indication that its submission was based upon a sample of its relevant discharges; (3) Rate reflects fewer than the maximum possible quarters of data for the measure; (4) Inaccurate information submitted and suppressed for one or more quarters; (5) No data is available from the hospital for this measure; Please refer to the User's Guide for a full explanation of data

Measure	Cases	This Hospital	State Average	U.S. Average	Top Hospital
Pneumonia Care					
Appropriate Initial Antibiotic[2]	133	84%	83%	83%	94%
Blood Culture Timing[2]	131	93%	90%	90%	100%
Influenza Vaccine[2]	31	97%	74%	70%	100%
Initial Antibiotic Timing[2]	174	74%	84%	80%	93%
Oxygenation Assessment[2]	205	100%	99%	99%	100%
Pneumococcal Vaccine[2]	124	79%	77%	69%	94%
Smoking Cessation Advice[2]	57	75%	81%	80%	100%
Surgical Infection Prevention					
Prophylactic Antibiotic Given[2]	294	91%	76%	77%	95%
Prophylactic Antibiotic Selection[2]	59	98%	92%	90%	100%
Prophylactic Antibiotic Stopped[2]	290	70%	70%	72%	95%
Pregnancy Care					
Inpatient Neonatal Mortality	-	-	-	-	-
Third or Fourth Degree Laceration	-	-	4.02%	3.63%	3.27%

Saint Mary's Medical Center

1500 S Lake Park Ave
Hobart, IN 46342
Phone: 219-942-0551
Ownership: Voluntary non-profit - Private
Accredited: Yes
Emergency Services: Yes

Measure	Cases	This Hospital	State Average	U.S. Average	Top Hospital
Heart Attack Care					
ACE Inhibitor or ARB for LVSD[1]	13	69%	83%	82%	100%
Aspirin at Arrival	83	96%	91%	92%	100%
Aspirin at Discharge	92	90%	91%	90%	100%
Beta Blocker at Arrival	81	90%	84%	87%	100%
Beta Blocker at Discharge	97	90%	91%	90%	100%
Fibrinolytic Medication Timing	0	-	44%	31%	100%
PCI Within 90 Minutes of Arrival[1]	13	0%	56%	54%	95%
Smoking Cessation Advice	43	100%	90%	88%	100%
Heart Failure Care					
ACE Inhibitor or ARB for LVSD[2]	127	88%	81%	82%	100%
Discharge Instructions[2]	314	91%	69%	61%	93%
Evaluation of LVS Function[2]	386	97%	87%	83%	99%
Smoking Cessation Advice[2]	49	98%	84%	82%	100%
Pneumonia Care					
Appropriate Initial Antibiotic	182	88%	83%	83%	94%
Blood Culture Timing	177	99%	90%	90%	100%
Influenza Vaccine	58	83%	74%	70%	100%
Initial Antibiotic Timing	274	88%	84%	80%	93%
Oxygenation Assessment	313	100%	99%	99%	100%
Pneumococcal Vaccine	220	77%	77%	69%	94%
Smoking Cessation Advice	81	95%	81%	80%	100%
Surgical Infection Prevention					
Prophylactic Antibiotic Given[2,3]	209	54%	76%	77%	95%
Prophylactic Antibiotic Selection[2]	65	80%	92%	90%	100%
Prophylactic Antibiotic Stopped[2,3]	205	60%	70%	72%	95%
Pregnancy Care					
Inpatient Neonatal Mortality	-	-	-	-	-
Third or Fourth Degree Laceration	-	-	4.02%	3.63%	3.27%

Parkview Huntington Hospital

2001 Stults Road
Huntington, IN 46750
Toll-Free: 800-533-2252
Phone: 260-356-3000
Fax: 260-355-3346
URL: www.parkview.com
Ownership: Voluntary non-profit - Private
Accredited: Yes
Emergency Services: Yes
Licensed Beds: 36

Key Personnel:

Chief Medical Staff . . . . James Edlund, MD
Chief Medical Staff . . . . Jeffrey Brookes
Manager Emergency Room . . . . Mary Johnson, RN
Director Pulmonary . . . . John Mathew

Measure	Cases	This Hospital	State Average	U.S. Average	Top Hospital
Heart Attack Care					
ACE Inhibitor or ARB for LVSD[1]	3	67%	83%	82%	100%
Aspirin at Arrival[1]	8	75%	91%	92%	100%
Aspirin at Discharge[1]	2	100%	91%	90%	100%
Beta Blocker at Arrival[1]	8	75%	84%	87%	100%
Beta Blocker at Discharge[1]	6	100%	91%	90%	100%
Fibrinolytic Medication Timing	0	-	44%	31%	100%
PCI Within 90 Minutes of Arrival	0	-	56%	54%	95%
Smoking Cessation Advice[1]	1	0%	90%	88%	100%
Heart Failure Care					
ACE Inhibitor or ARB for LVSD[1]	14	64%	81%	82%	100%
Discharge Instructions	33	82%	69%	61%	93%
Evaluation of LVS Function	47	79%	87%	83%	99%
Smoking Cessation Advice[1]	8	100%	84%	82%	100%
Pneumonia Care					
Appropriate Initial Antibiotic	49	84%	83%	83%	94%
Blood Culture Timing	52	92%	90%	90%	100%
Influenza Vaccine[1]	10	90%	74%	70%	100%
Initial Antibiotic Timing	88	83%	84%	80%	93%
Oxygenation Assessment	108	100%	99%	99%	100%
Pneumococcal Vaccine	68	84%	77%	69%	94%
Smoking Cessation Advice[1]	22	82%	81%	80%	100%
Surgical Infection Prevention					
Prophylactic Antibiotic Given	111	89%	76%	77%	95%
Prophylactic Antibiotic Selection[1]	23	100%	92%	90%	100%
Prophylactic Antibiotic Stopped	108	91%	70%	72%	95%
Pregnancy Care					
Inpatient Neonatal Mortality	-	-	-	-	-
Third or Fourth Degree Laceration	-	-	4.02%	3.63%	3.27%

Community Health Network

1500 N Ritter Avenue
Indianapolis, IN 46219
Phone: 317-355-1411
Fax: 317-351-7726
URL: www.ecommunity.com
Ownership: Voluntary non-profit - Private
Accredited: Yes
Emergency Services: Yes
Licensed Beds: 1,025

Key Personnel:

Chief Medical Staff . . . . James Ehlich
Emergency Room . . . . Chris Burke
Director Infection/Disease Control . . . . . . Robert Baker, MD
CCU Spvg. Nurse . . . . Susan Holbrook-Presto
OB/GYN Womens Health . . . . Mary Miser
Chief Radiology . . . . Michael Mullinix, MD
Director Respiratory Therapy . . . . Curlie Morrow

Measure	Cases	This Hospital	State Average	U.S. Average	Top Hospital
Heart Attack Care					
ACE Inhibitor or ARB for LVSD	38	82%	83%	82%	100%
Aspirin at Arrival	127	96%	91%	92%	100%
Aspirin at Discharge	111	99%	91%	90%	100%
Beta Blocker at Arrival	75	92%	84%	87%	100%
Beta Blocker at Discharge	102	99%	91%	90%	100%
Fibrinolytic Medication Timing[1]	4	0%	44%	31%	100%
PCI Within 90 Minutes of Arrival[1]	11	73%	56%	54%	95%
Smoking Cessation Advice	54	100%	90%	88%	100%
Heart Failure Care					
ACE Inhibitor or ARB for LVSD	136	74%	81%	82%	100%
Discharge Instructions	213	43%	69%	61%	93%
Evaluation of LVS Function	306	90%	87%	83%	99%
Smoking Cessation Advice	75	100%	84%	82%	100%
Pneumonia Care					
Appropriate Initial Antibiotic[2]	191	85%	83%	83%	94%
Blood Culture Timing[2]	172	94%	90%	90%	100%
Influenza Vaccine[2]	39	59%	74%	70%	100%
Initial Antibiotic Timing[2]	271	81%	84%	80%	93%
Oxygenation Assessment[2]	317	100%	99%	99%	100%
Pneumococcal Vaccine[2]	186	75%	77%	69%	94%
Smoking Cessation Advice[2]	64	100%	81%	80%	100%
Surgical Infection Prevention					
Prophylactic Antibiotic Given[2,3]	79	52%	76%	77%	95%
Prophylactic Antibiotic Selection[5]	-	-	92%	90%	100%
Prophylactic Antibiotic Stopped[2,3]	72	65%	70%	72%	95%
Pregnancy Care					
Inpatient Neonatal Mortality	1,713	0.35%	-	-	-
Third or Fourth Degree Laceration	2,019	6.24%	4.02%	3.63%	3.27%

NOTE: Hospital profiles are in alphabetical order by state, then city, then hospital within the city; Rankings are sorted by rate in descending order and exclude hospitals with less than 25 cases; (1) The number of cases is too small (n<25) for purposes of reliably predicting hospital performance; (2) Measure reflects the hospital's indication that its submission was based upon a sample of its relevant discharges; (3) Rate reflects fewer than the maximum possible quarters of data for the measure; (4) Inaccurate information submitted and suppressed for one or more quarters; (5) No data is available from the hospital for this measure; Please refer to the User's Guide for a full explanation of data

Community Hospital South

1402 E County Line Road S
Indianapolis, IN 46227
URL: www.ecommunity.com/south
Ownership: Voluntary non-profit - Private
Emergency Services: Yes
Phone: 317-887-7000
Fax: 317-887-4670
Accredited: Yes

Key Personnel:
Administrator . . . . Mike Blanchet
Chief Medical Staff . . . . Carolyn Waymire
Catheterization Lab . . . . Cathy Cook
Emergency Room . . . . Kandy Alspach
Infection Control . . . . Gayle Walsh
ICU . . . . Kerry Sawin
Intensive Coronary . . . . Kerry Sawin
Medical/Surgical Nursing . . . . Kerry Sawin
OB/GYN/Womens Health . . . . Dana Matthews
Respiratory/Cardiopulmonary . . . . Jose Lougaria

Measure	Cases	This Hospital	State Average	U.S. Average	Top Hospital
Heart Attack Care					
ACE Inhibitor or ARB for LVSD	40	90%	83%	82%	100%
Aspirin at Arrival	110	99%	91%	92%	100%
Aspirin at Discharge	137	99%	91%	90%	100%
Beta Blocker at Arrival	49	98%	84%	87%	100%
Beta Blocker at Discharge	109	100%	91%	90%	100%
Fibrinolytic Medication Timing	0	-	44%	31%	100%
PCI Within 90 Minutes of Arrival[1]	11	82%	56%	54%	95%
Smoking Cessation Advice	62	100%	90%	88%	100%
Heart Failure Care					
ACE Inhibitor or ARB for LVSD	51	76%	81%	82%	100%
Discharge Instructions	108	54%	69%	61%	93%
Evaluation of LVS Function	153	91%	87%	83%	99%
Smoking Cessation Advice[1]	19	100%	84%	82%	100%
Pneumonia Care					
Appropriate Initial Antibiotic[2]	125	88%	83%	83%	94%
Blood Culture Timing[2]	76	89%	90%	90%	100%
Influenza Vaccine[1,2]	24	54%	74%	70%	100%
Initial Antibiotic Timing[2]	141	83%	84%	80%	93%
Oxygenation Assessment[2]	171	100%	99%	99%	100%
Pneumococcal Vaccine[2]	100	84%	77%	69%	94%
Smoking Cessation Advice[2]	37	100%	81%	80%	100%
Surgical Infection Prevention					
Prophylactic Antibiotic Given[2,3]	59	93%	76%	77%	95%
Prophylactic Antibiotic Selection[5]	-	-	92%	90%	100%
Prophylactic Antibiotic Stopped[2,3]	59	78%	70%	72%	95%
Pregnancy Care					
Inpatient Neonatal Mortality	657	0.15%	-	-	-
Third or Fourth Degree Laceration	471	8.07%	4.02%	3.63%	3.27%

Indiana Heart Hospital

8075 N Shadeland Avenue
Indianapolis, IN 46250
URL: www.hearthospital.com
Ownership: Government - Local
Emergency Services: No
Phone: 317-621-8000
Fax: 317-621-8111
Accredited: Yes
Licensed Beds: 72

Key Personnel:
Interim CEO . . . . Mark Dixon
Chief Medical Officer . . . . Michael Venturini, MD/FACC

Measure	Cases	This Hospital	State Average	U.S. Average	Top Hospital
Heart Attack Care					
ACE Inhibitor or ARB for LVSD	125	98%	83%	82%	100%
Aspirin at Arrival	149	96%	91%	92%	100%
Aspirin at Discharge	402	100%	91%	90%	100%
Beta Blocker at Arrival	84	96%	84%	87%	100%
Beta Blocker at Discharge	386	99%	91%	90%	100%
Fibrinolytic Medication Timing[1]	3	100%	44%	31%	100%
PCI Within 90 Minutes of Arrival[1]	13	77%	56%	54%	95%
Smoking Cessation Advice	229	100%	90%	88%	100%
Heart Failure Care					
ACE Inhibitor or ARB for LVSD	122	100%	81%	82%	100%
Discharge Instructions	234	98%	69%	61%	93%
Evaluation of LVS Function	298	99%	87%	83%	99%
Smoking Cessation Advice	57	100%	84%	82%	100%
Pneumonia Care					
Appropriate Initial Antibiotic[1]	6	67%	83%	83%	94%
Blood Culture Timing[1]	6	83%	90%	90%	100%
Influenza Vaccine	0	-	74%	70%	100%
Initial Antibiotic Timing[1]	6	83%	84%	80%	93%
Oxygenation Assessment[1]	8	100%	99%	99%	100%
Pneumococcal Vaccine[1]	3	100%	77%	69%	94%
Smoking Cessation Advice[1]	2	100%	81%	80%	100%
Surgical Infection Prevention					
Prophylactic Antibiotic Given[3]	444	95%	76%	77%	95%
Prophylactic Antibiotic Selection	169	100%	92%	90%	100%
Prophylactic Antibiotic Stopped[3]	422	95%	70%	72%	95%
Pregnancy Care					
Inpatient Neonatal Mortality	-	-	-	-	-
Third or Fourth Degree Laceration	-	-	4.02%	3.63%	3.27%

Indiana Orthopaedic Hospital

8400 Northwest Boulevard
Indianapolis, IN 46278
Ownership: Proprietary
Emergency Services: No
Phone: 317-956-1000
Accredited: No

Measure	Cases	This Hospital	State Average	U.S. Average	Top Hospital
Heart Attack Care					
ACE Inhibitor or ARB for LVSD[5]	-	-	83%	82%	100%
Aspirin at Arrival[5]	-	-	91%	92%	100%
Aspirin at Discharge[5]	-	-	91%	90%	100%
Beta Blocker at Arrival[5]	-	-	84%	87%	100%
Beta Blocker at Discharge[5]	-	-	91%	90%	100%
Fibrinolytic Medication Timing[5]	-	-	44%	31%	100%
PCI Within 90 Minutes of Arrival[5]	-	-	56%	54%	95%
Smoking Cessation Advice[5]	-	-	90%	88%	100%
Heart Failure Care					
ACE Inhibitor or ARB for LVSD[5]	-	-	81%	82%	100%
Discharge Instructions[5]	-	-	69%	61%	93%
Evaluation of LVS Function[5]	-	-	87%	83%	99%
Smoking Cessation Advice[5]	-	-	84%	82%	100%
Pneumonia Care					
Appropriate Initial Antibiotic[5]	-	-	83%	83%	94%
Blood Culture Timing[5]	-	-	90%	90%	100%
Influenza Vaccine[5]	-	-	74%	70%	100%
Initial Antibiotic Timing[5]	-	-	84%	80%	93%
Oxygenation Assessment[5]	-	-	99%	99%	100%
Pneumococcal Vaccine[5]	-	-	77%	69%	94%
Smoking Cessation Advice[5]	-	-	81%	80%	100%
Surgical Infection Prevention					
Prophylactic Antibiotic Given[2,3]	26	88%	76%	77%	95%
Prophylactic Antibiotic Selection[5]	-	-	92%	90%	100%
Prophylactic Antibiotic Stopped[2,3]	26	69%	70%	72%	95%
Pregnancy Care					
Inpatient Neonatal Mortality	-	-	-	-	-
Third or Fourth Degree Laceration	-	-	4.02%	3.63%	3.27%

Methodist Hospital of Indiana

Alternate Name: Clarian Health Partners
1701 N Senate Boulevard
Indianapolis, IN 46206
Ownership: Voluntary non-profit - Private
Emergency Services: Yes
Phone: 317-929-2000
Fax: 317-962-1867
Accredited: Yes
Licensed Beds: 1,120

Key Personnel:
President/CEO . . . . William J Loveday
Chief Medical Staff . . . . Richard F Graffis, MD
Chief Catheterization Laboratory . . . . Kirk Parr, MD
Emergency Room . . . . Joseph D Phillips, MD
Director Infection/Disease Control . . . . Diana Korpal, RN
OB/GYN Womens Health . . . . J Thomas Benson, MD
Director Respiratory Therapy . . . . David B Cook, MD

Measure	Cases	This Hospital	State Average	U.S. Average	Top Hospital
Heart Attack Care					
ACE Inhibitor or ARB for LVSD	146	86%	83%	82%	100%

NOTE: Hospital profiles are in alphabetical order by state, then city, then hospital within the city; Rankings are sorted by rate in descending order and exclude hospitals with less than 25 cases; (1) The number of cases is too small (n<25) for purposes of reliably predicting hospital performance; (2) Measure reflects the hospital's indication that its submission was based upon a sample of its relevant discharges; (3) Rate reflects fewer than the maximum possible quarters of data for the measure; (4) Inaccurate information submitted and suppressed for one or more quarters; (5) No data is available from the hospital for this measure; Please refer to the User's Guide for a full explanation of data

Aspirin at Arrival	361	97%	91%	92%	100%
Aspirin at Discharge	437	96%	91%	90%	100%
Beta Blocker at Arrival	270	94%	84%	87%	100%
Beta Blocker at Discharge	445	97%	91%	90%	100%
Fibrinolytic Medication Timing[1]	3	0%	44%	31%	100%
PCI Within 90 Minutes of Arrival[1]	19	68%	56%	54%	95%
Smoking Cessation Advice	233	96%	90%	88%	100%
Heart Failure Care					
ACE Inhibitor or ARB for LVSD	556	80%	81%	82%	100%
Discharge Instructions	847	73%	69%	61%	93%
Evaluation of LVS Function	1,026	98%	87%	83%	99%
Smoking Cessation Advice	230	93%	84%	82%	100%
Pneumonia Care					
Appropriate Initial Antibiotic[2]	106	85%	83%	83%	94%
Blood Culture Timing[2]	69	80%	90%	90%	100%
Influenza Vaccine[1,2]	15	87%	74%	70%	100%
Initial Antibiotic Timing[2]	187	74%	84%	80%	93%
Oxygenation Assessment[2]	248	100%	99%	99%	100%
Pneumococcal Vaccine[2]	116	72%	77%	69%	94%
Smoking Cessation Advice[2]	73	81%	81%	80%	100%
Surgical Infection Prevention					
Prophylactic Antibiotic Given[2,3]	360	92%	76%	77%	95%
Prophylactic Antibiotic Selection[2]	67	99%	92%	90%	100%
Prophylactic Antibiotic Stopped[2,3]	341	71%	70%	72%	95%
Pregnancy Care					
Inpatient Neonatal Mortality	-	-	-	-	-
Third or Fourth Degree Laceration	-	-	4.02%	3.63%	3.27%

Saint Francis at Indianapolis

8111 S Emerson Avenue
Indianapolis, IN 46237
Phone: 317-865-5000
Fax: 317-783-8152
URL: www.stfrancishospitals.org
Ownership: Voluntary non-profit - Church
Accredited: Yes
Emergency Services: Yes

Key Personnel:
President/CEO. . . . . Robert Brody
Chief Medical Staff. . . . . Allen Gillespie, MD

Measure	Cases	This Hospital	State Average	U.S. Average	Top Hospital
Heart Attack Care					
ACE Inhibitor or ARB for LVSD[3]	27	70%	83%	82%	100%
Aspirin at Arrival[3]	113	98%	91%	92%	100%
Aspirin at Discharge[3]	172	97%	91%	90%	100%
Beta Blocker at Arrival[3]	115	97%	84%	87%	100%
Beta Blocker at Discharge[3]	176	96%	91%	90%	100%
Fibrinolytic Medication Timing[3]	0	-	44%	31%	100%
PCI Within 90 Minutes of Arrival[1]	15	100%	56%	54%	95%
Smoking Cessation Advice[3]	96	95%	90%	88%	100%
Heart Failure Care					
ACE Inhibitor or ARB for LVSD[3]	48	83%	81%	82%	100%
Discharge Instructions[3]	90	67%	69%	61%	93%
Evaluation of LVS Function[3]	108	97%	87%	83%	99%
Smoking Cessation Advice[3]	26	88%	84%	82%	100%
Pneumonia Care					
Appropriate Initial Antibiotic[3]	41	88%	83%	83%	94%
Blood Culture Timing[3]	30	93%	90%	90%	100%
Influenza Vaccine[5]	-	-	74%	70%	100%
Initial Antibiotic Timing[3]	37	68%	84%	80%	93%
Oxygenation Assessment[3]	49	100%	99%	99%	100%
Pneumococcal Vaccine[3]	28	96%	77%	69%	94%
Smoking Cessation Advice[1,3]	13	85%	81%	80%	100%
Surgical Infection Prevention					
Prophylactic Antibiotic Given[3]	163	85%	76%	77%	95%
Prophylactic Antibiotic Selection	92	97%	92%	90%	100%
Prophylactic Antibiotic Stopped[3]	154	84%	70%	72%	95%
Pregnancy Care					
Inpatient Neonatal Mortality	-	-	-	-	-
Third or Fourth Degree Laceration	-	-	4.02%	3.63%	3.27%

Saint Vincent Heart Center of Indiana

10580 N Meridian Street
Indianapolis, IN 46290
Toll-Free: 866-432-7830
Phone: 317-583-5000
Fax: 317-583-5002
E-mail: marketing@theheartcenter.com
URL: www.theheartcenter.com
Ownership: Proprietary
Accredited: Yes
Emergency Services: Yes
Licensed Beds: 60

Key Personnel:
President/CEO. . . . . John Stewart
Chief Medical Staff. . . . . William Store
Director Cardiology . . . . Gregg Elsener

Measure	Cases	This Hospital	State Average	U.S. Average	Top Hospital
Heart Attack Care					
ACE Inhibitor or ARB for LVSD	307	91%	83%	82%	100%
Aspirin at Arrival	113	99%	91%	92%	100%
Aspirin at Discharge	1,036	100%	91%	90%	100%
Beta Blocker at Arrival	102	97%	84%	87%	100%
Beta Blocker at Discharge	1,027	100%	91%	90%	100%
Fibrinolytic Medication Timing	0	-	44%	31%	100%
PCI Within 90 Minutes of Arrival[1]	6	100%	56%	54%	95%
Smoking Cessation Advice	400	94%	90%	88%	100%
Heart Failure Care					
ACE Inhibitor or ARB for LVSD	258	89%	81%	82%	100%
Discharge Instructions	339	86%	69%	61%	93%
Evaluation of LVS Function	373	99%	87%	83%	99%
Smoking Cessation Advice	45	82%	84%	82%	100%
Pneumonia Care					
Appropriate Initial Antibiotic[1]	6	100%	83%	83%	94%
Blood Culture Timing[1]	1	100%	90%	90%	100%
Influenza Vaccine[1]	2	0%	74%	70%	100%
Initial Antibiotic Timing[1]	7	86%	84%	80%	93%
Oxygenation Assessment[1]	8	88%	99%	99%	100%
Pneumococcal Vaccine[1]	7	57%	77%	69%	94%
Smoking Cessation Advice	0	-	81%	80%	100%
Surgical Infection Prevention					
Prophylactic Antibiotic Given[2,3]	143	99%	76%	77%	95%
Prophylactic Antibiotic Selection[2]	64	100%	92%	90%	100%
Prophylactic Antibiotic Stopped[2,3]	137	96%	70%	72%	95%
Pregnancy Care					
Inpatient Neonatal Mortality	-	-	-	-	-
Third or Fourth Degree Laceration	-	-	4.02%	3.63%	3.27%

Saint Vincent Indianapolis Hospital

2001 W 86th Street
Indianapolis, IN 46240
Phone: 317-338-2345
Fax: 317-338-7005
URL: www.indianapolis.stvincent.org
Ownership: Voluntary non-profit - Church
Accredited: Yes
Emergency Services: Yes
Licensed Beds: 650

Key Personnel:
President/CEO. . . . . Anthony R Tersigni, EdD
Manager Infection/Disease Control . . . . Carolyn Davee
OB/GYN Womens Health. . . . . David Kenley, MD
Chief Radiology . . . . Homer Beltz, MD

Measure	Cases	This Hospital	State Average	U.S. Average	Top Hospital
Heart Attack Care					
ACE Inhibitor or ARB for LVSD	167	84%	83%	82%	100%
Aspirin at Arrival	308	98%	91%	92%	100%
Aspirin at Discharge	493	98%	91%	90%	100%
Beta Blocker at Arrival	281	98%	84%	87%	100%
Beta Blocker at Discharge	485	99%	91%	90%	100%
Fibrinolytic Medication Timing	0	-	44%	31%	100%
PCI Within 90 Minutes of Arrival[1]	15	47%	56%	54%	95%
Smoking Cessation Advice	166	95%	90%	88%	100%
Heart Failure Care					
ACE Inhibitor or ARB for LVSD	226	88%	81%	82%	100%
Discharge Instructions	502	85%	69%	61%	93%
Evaluation of LVS Function	643	96%	87%	83%	99%
Smoking Cessation Advice	71	93%	84%	82%	100%
Pneumonia Care					
Appropriate Initial Antibiotic	228	80%	83%	83%	94%

NOTE: Hospital profiles are in alphabetical order by state, then city, then hospital within the city; Rankings are sorted by rate in descending order and exclude hospitals with less than 25 cases; (1) The number of cases is too small (n<25) for purposes of reliably predicting hospital performance; (2) Measure reflects the hospital's indication that its submission was based upon a sample of its relevant discharges; (3) Rate reflects fewer than the maximum possible quarters of data for the measure; (4) Inaccurate information submitted and suppressed for one or more quarters; (5) No data is available from the hospital for this measure; Please refer to the User's Guide for a full explanation of data

Blood Culture Timing	208	93%	90%	90%	100%
Influenza Vaccine	72	39%	74%	70%	100%
Initial Antibiotic Timing	321	75%	84%	80%	93%
Oxygenation Assessment	422	100%	99%	99%	100%
Pneumococcal Vaccine	274	51%	77%	69%	94%
Smoking Cessation Advice	80	49%	81%	80%	100%
Surgical Infection Prevention					
Prophylactic Antibiotic Given[2,3]	227	75%	76%	77%	95%
Prophylactic Antibiotic Selection[2]	104	95%	92%	90%	100%
Prophylactic Antibiotic Stopped[2,3]	226	84%	70%	72%	95%
Pregnancy Care					
Inpatient Neonatal Mortality	-	-	-	-	-
Third or Fourth Degree Laceration	-	-	4.02%	3.63%	3.27%

Westview Hospital

3630 Guion Road
Indianapolis, IN 46222
E-mail: info@westviewhospital.org
URL: www.westviewhospital.org
Ownership: Voluntary non-profit - Private
Emergency Services: Yes
Phone: 317-920-8439
Fax: 317-920-7551
Accredited: Yes
Licensed Beds: 116

Key Personnel:
CEO. . . . . Jerry Porter

Measure	Cases	This Hospital	State Average	U.S. Average	Top Hospital
Heart Attack Care					
ACE Inhibitor or ARB for LVSD[1]	1	100%	83%	82%	100%
Aspirin at Arrival[1]	7	100%	91%	92%	100%
Aspirin at Discharge[1]	5	100%	91%	90%	100%
Beta Blocker at Arrival[1]	10	90%	84%	87%	100%
Beta Blocker at Discharge[1]	7	86%	91%	90%	100%
Fibrinolytic Medication Timing[1]	1	0%	44%	31%	100%
PCI Within 90 Minutes of Arrival	0	-	56%	54%	95%
Smoking Cessation Advice[1]	1	100%	90%	88%	100%
Heart Failure Care					
ACE Inhibitor or ARB for LVSD[1]	18	94%	81%	82%	100%
Discharge Instructions	62	52%	69%	61%	93%
Evaluation of LVS Function	82	91%	87%	83%	99%
Smoking Cessation Advice[1]	18	78%	84%	82%	100%
Pneumonia Care					
Appropriate Initial Antibiotic	65	89%	83%	83%	94%
Blood Culture Timing	78	97%	90%	90%	100%
Influenza Vaccine[1]	19	63%	74%	70%	100%
Initial Antibiotic Timing	106	78%	84%	80%	93%
Oxygenation Assessment	113	100%	99%	99%	100%
Pneumococcal Vaccine	69	57%	77%	69%	94%
Smoking Cessation Advice	32	78%	81%	80%	100%
Surgical Infection Prevention					
Prophylactic Antibiotic Given	82	70%	76%	77%	95%
Prophylactic Antibiotic Selection[1]	20	90%	92%	90%	100%
Prophylactic Antibiotic Stopped	78	58%	70%	72%	95%
Pregnancy Care					
Inpatient Neonatal Mortality	-	-	-	-	-
Third or Fourth Degree Laceration	-	-	4.02%	3.63%	3.27%

Wishard Memorial Hospital

1001 W Tenth Street
Indianapolis, IN 46202
URL: www.wishard.edu
Ownership: Govt - Hospital District or Authority
Emergency Services: Yes
Phone: 317-639-6671
Fax: 317-630-7678
Accredited: Yes
Licensed Beds: 354

Key Personnel:
CEO/Medical Director . . . . Lisa E Harris, MD
Executive VP/CFO . . . . Gordon King

Measure	Cases	This Hospital	State Average	U.S. Average	Top Hospital
Heart Attack Care					
ACE Inhibitor or ARB for LVSD[2]	42	98%	83%	82%	100%
Aspirin at Arrival[2]	181	99%	91%	92%	100%
Aspirin at Discharge[2]	155	99%	91%	90%	100%
Beta Blocker at Arrival[2]	161	97%	84%	87%	100%
Beta Blocker at Discharge[2]	151	99%	91%	90%	100%
Fibrinolytic Medication Timing[1,2]	14	57%	44%	31%	100%
PCI Within 90 Minutes of Arrival[1,2]	2	0%	56%	54%	95%
Smoking Cessation Advice[2]	98	91%	90%	88%	100%
Heart Failure Care					
ACE Inhibitor or ARB for LVSD[2]	250	97%	81%	82%	100%
Discharge Instructions[2]	333	39%	69%	61%	93%
Evaluation of LVS Function[2]	377	98%	87%	83%	99%
Smoking Cessation Advice[2]	135	93%	84%	82%	100%
Pneumonia Care					
Appropriate Initial Antibiotic[2]	93	87%	83%	83%	94%
Blood Culture Timing[2]	54	83%	90%	90%	100%
Influenza Vaccine[1,2]	8	62%	74%	70%	100%
Initial Antibiotic Timing[2]	120	81%	84%	80%	93%
Oxygenation Assessment[2]	127	100%	99%	99%	100%
Pneumococcal Vaccine[2]	34	79%	77%	69%	94%
Smoking Cessation Advice[2]	39	100%	81%	80%	100%
Surgical Infection Prevention					
Prophylactic Antibiotic Given[2,3]	158	78%	76%	77%	95%
Prophylactic Antibiotic Selection[2]	43	95%	92%	90%	100%
Prophylactic Antibiotic Stopped[2,3]	150	84%	70%	72%	95%
Pregnancy Care					
Inpatient Neonatal Mortality	-	-	-	-	-
Third or Fourth Degree Laceration	-	-	4.02%	3.63%	3.27%

Memorial Hospital and Health Care Center

800 W 9th Street
Jasper, IN 47546
URL: www.mhhcc.org
Ownership: Voluntary non-profit - Church
Emergency Services: Yes
Toll-Free: 800-852-7279
Phone: 812-482-2345
Fax: 812-482-0302
Accredited: Yes
Licensed Beds: 131

Key Personnel:
President/CEO. . . . . Ray Snowden
Chief Medical Staff. . . . . Cindy Caser, DO
Emergency Room . . . . Stephen O'Connor, MD
Director Infection/Disease Control . . . . Susan Roberts, RN
CCU Spvg. Nurse . . . . Kathy Howell
Director Medical/Surgical Nursing . . . . Jan Wallhauser, RN
OB/GYN Womens Health. . . . . Terry Brown, MD
Chief Radiology . . . . Timothy M McClure, MD
Director Respiratory Therapy . . . . Ron Gehlhausen

Measure	Cases	This Hospital	State Average	U.S. Average	Top Hospital
Heart Attack Care					
ACE Inhibitor or ARB for LVSD	35	86%	83%	82%	100%
Aspirin at Arrival	90	94%	91%	92%	100%
Aspirin at Discharge	129	95%	91%	90%	100%
Beta Blocker at Arrival	90	93%	84%	87%	100%
Beta Blocker at Discharge	127	98%	91%	90%	100%
Fibrinolytic Medication Timing[1]	1	100%	44%	31%	100%
PCI Within 90 Minutes of Arrival[1]	5	40%	56%	54%	95%
Smoking Cessation Advice	51	100%	90%	88%	100%
Heart Failure Care					
ACE Inhibitor or ARB for LVSD	77	84%	81%	82%	100%
Discharge Instructions	113	55%	69%	61%	93%
Evaluation of LVS Function	160	84%	87%	83%	99%
Smoking Cessation Advice[1]	22	100%	84%	82%	100%
Pneumonia Care					
Appropriate Initial Antibiotic	182	71%	83%	83%	94%
Blood Culture Timing	91	97%	90%	90%	100%
Influenza Vaccine	38	3%	74%	70%	100%
Initial Antibiotic Timing	154	74%	84%	80%	93%
Oxygenation Assessment	194	96%	99%	99%	100%
Pneumococcal Vaccine	129	81%	77%	69%	94%
Smoking Cessation Advice	33	100%	81%	80%	100%
Surgical Infection Prevention					
Prophylactic Antibiotic Given[3]	345	56%	76%	77%	95%
Prophylactic Antibiotic Selection	111	93%	92%	90%	100%
Prophylactic Antibiotic Stopped[3]	337	74%	70%	72%	95%
Pregnancy Care					
Inpatient Neonatal Mortality	-	-	-	-	-
Third or Fourth Degree Laceration	-	-	4.02%	3.63%	3.27%

NOTE: Hospital profiles are in alphabetical order by state, then city, then hospital within the city; Rankings are sorted by rate in descending order and exclude hospitals with less than 25 cases; (1) The number of cases is too small (n<25) for purposes of reliably predicting hospital performance; (2) Measure reflects the hospital's indication that its submission was based upon a sample of its relevant discharges; (3) Rate reflects fewer than the maximum possible quarters of data for the measure; (4) Inaccurate information submitted and suppressed for one or more quarters; (5) No data is available from the hospital for this measure; Please refer to the User's Guide for a full explanation of data

Clark Memorial Hospital

1220 Missouri Avenue
Jeffersonville, IN 47130
Phone: 812-282-6631
Fax: 812-283-2688
E-mail: paula.lamb@clarkmemorial.org
URL: www.clarkmemorial.org
Ownership: Government - Local
Accredited: Yes
Emergency Services: Yes
Licensed Beds: 241

Key Personnel:

CEO. . . . . Merle E Stepp
Emergency Room . . . . Maiken Himmel
Emergency Room . . . . Lynn Meuer
Director Medical/Surgical Nursing . . . . Kathy Neuner
Chief Radiology . . . . Steve Matthews, MD
Director of Pulmonary/Respiratory Care. . . . . . . Christi Norris

Measure	Cases	This Hospital	State Average	U.S. Average	Top Hospital
Heart Attack Care					
ACE Inhibitor or ARB for LVSD	43	79%	83%	82%	100%
Aspirin at Arrival	148	99%	91%	92%	100%
Aspirin at Discharge	190	97%	91%	90%	100%
Beta Blocker at Arrival	122	99%	84%	87%	100%
Beta Blocker at Discharge	188	97%	91%	90%	100%
Fibrinolytic Medication Timing[1]	11	82%	44%	31%	100%
PCI Within 90 Minutes of Arrival[1]	4	50%	56%	54%	95%
Smoking Cessation Advice	78	99%	90%	88%	100%
Heart Failure Care					
ACE Inhibitor or ARB for LVSD	94	69%	81%	82%	100%
Discharge Instructions	250	58%	69%	61%	93%
Evaluation of LVS Function	343	81%	87%	83%	99%
Smoking Cessation Advice	70	81%	84%	82%	100%
Pneumonia Care					
Appropriate Initial Antibiotic	188	81%	83%	83%	94%
Blood Culture Timing	116	83%	90%	90%	100%
Influenza Vaccine	33	6%	74%	70%	100%
Initial Antibiotic Timing	210	77%	84%	80%	93%
Oxygenation Assessment	259	100%	99%	99%	100%
Pneumococcal Vaccine	155	72%	77%	69%	94%
Smoking Cessation Advice	76	74%	81%	80%	100%
Surgical Infection Prevention					
Prophylactic Antibiotic Given[3]	126	90%	76%	77%	95%
Prophylactic Antibiotic Selection	122	89%	92%	90%	100%
Prophylactic Antibiotic Stopped[3]	117	96%	70%	72%	95%
Pregnancy Care					
Inpatient Neonatal Mortality	-	-	-	-	-
Third or Fourth Degree Laceration	-	-	4.02%	3.63%	3.27%

Parkview Noble Hospital

401 Sawyer Road
Kendallville, IN 46755
Phone: 260-347-8700
E-mail: mashek4126@aol.com
URL: www.parkview.com
Ownership: Government - Local
Accredited: Yes
Emergency Services: No
Licensed Beds: 66

Key Personnel:

President/CEO. . . . . John Berhow
Chief Medical Staff. . . . . Abdali Jan, MD
Emergency Room . . . . Mindy Kurtz
Emergency Room . . . . Kim Horan
Director Infection/Disease Control . . . . Karen Denny
ICU . . . . Mindy Kurtz
Medical Surgical Nursing . . . . Kris Graft
Chief Radiology . . . . Ted Wallace
Respiratory/Cardiopulmonary. . . . . Greg Hein

Measure	Cases	This Hospital	State Average	U.S. Average	Top Hospital
Heart Attack Care					
ACE Inhibitor or ARB for LVSD[1]	1	100%	83%	82%	100%
Aspirin at Arrival[1]	6	100%	91%	92%	100%
Aspirin at Discharge[1]	5	80%	91%	90%	100%
Beta Blocker at Arrival[1]	3	100%	84%	87%	100%
Beta Blocker at Discharge[1]	3	100%	91%	90%	100%
Fibrinolytic Medication Timing	0	-	44%	31%	100%
PCI Within 90 Minutes of Arrival	0	-	56%	54%	95%
Smoking Cessation Advice	0	-	90%	88%	100%
Heart Failure Care					
ACE Inhibitor or ARB for LVSD[1]	20	75%	81%	82%	100%
Discharge Instructions	67	67%	69%	61%	93%
Evaluation of LVS Function	95	87%	87%	83%	99%
Smoking Cessation Advice[1]	17	100%	84%	82%	100%
Pneumonia Care					
Appropriate Initial Antibiotic	68	93%	83%	83%	94%
Blood Culture Timing	62	95%	90%	90%	100%
Influenza Vaccine[1]	20	90%	74%	70%	100%
Initial Antibiotic Timing	85	89%	84%	80%	93%
Oxygenation Assessment	115	100%	99%	99%	100%
Pneumococcal Vaccine	65	94%	77%	69%	94%
Smoking Cessation Advice	37	84%	81%	80%	100%
Surgical Infection Prevention					
Prophylactic Antibiotic Given	78	82%	76%	77%	95%
Prophylactic Antibiotic Selection[1]	24	92%	92%	90%	100%
Prophylactic Antibiotic Stopped	75	73%	70%	72%	95%
Pregnancy Care					
Inpatient Neonatal Mortality	-	-	-	-	-
Third or Fourth Degree Laceration	-	-	4.02%	3.63%	3.27%

Starke Memorial Hospital

102 E Culver Road
PO Box 339
Knox, IN 46534
Phone: 574-772-6231
Fax: 574-772-1144
E-mail: info@starkememorial.com
URL: www.starkememorial.com
Ownership: Proprietary
Accredited: Yes
Emergency Services: Yes
Licensed Beds: 53

Key Personnel:

CEO. . . . . Michael Meadows
Chief Medical Staff. . . . . Walter Fritz, MD
Chief Medical Staff. . . . . Patricia Alexander
Emergency Room . . . . Kathie Jones, RN

Measure	Cases	This Hospital	State Average	U.S. Average	Top Hospital
Heart Attack Care					
ACE Inhibitor or ARB for LVSD	0	-	83%	82%	100%
Aspirin at Arrival[1]	9	67%	91%	92%	100%
Aspirin at Discharge[1]	3	67%	91%	90%	100%
Beta Blocker at Arrival[1]	6	67%	84%	87%	100%
Beta Blocker at Discharge[1]	3	67%	91%	90%	100%
Fibrinolytic Medication Timing	0	-	44%	31%	100%
PCI Within 90 Minutes of Arrival	0	-	56%	54%	95%
Smoking Cessation Advice	0	-	90%	88%	100%
Heart Failure Care					
ACE Inhibitor or ARB for LVSD[1]	10	50%	81%	82%	100%
Discharge Instructions	38	39%	69%	61%	93%
Evaluation of LVS Function	48	83%	87%	83%	99%
Smoking Cessation Advice[1]	11	45%	84%	82%	100%
Pneumonia Care					
Appropriate Initial Antibiotic	99	84%	83%	83%	94%
Blood Culture Timing	55	84%	90%	90%	100%
Influenza Vaccine[1]	21	86%	74%	70%	100%
Initial Antibiotic Timing	125	86%	84%	80%	93%
Oxygenation Assessment	133	100%	99%	99%	100%
Pneumococcal Vaccine	69	57%	77%	69%	94%
Smoking Cessation Advice	39	44%	81%	80%	100%
Surgical Infection Prevention					
Prophylactic Antibiotic Given[1,3]	7	14%	76%	77%	95%
Prophylactic Antibiotic Selection[1]	1	100%	92%	90%	100%
Prophylactic Antibiotic Stopped[1,3]	7	0%	70%	72%	95%
Pregnancy Care					
Inpatient Neonatal Mortality	-	-	-	-	-
Third or Fourth Degree Laceration	-	-	4.02%	3.63%	3.27%

NOTE: Hospital profiles are in alphabetical order by state, then city, then hospital within the city; Rankings are sorted by rate in descending order and exclude hospitals with less than 25 cases; (1) The number of cases is too small (n<25) for purposes of reliably predicting hospital performance; (2) Measure reflects the hospital's indication that its submission was based upon a sample of its relevant discharges; (3) Rate reflects fewer than the maximum possible quarters of data for the measure; (4) Inaccurate information submitted and suppressed for one or more quarters; (5) No data is available from the hospital for this measure; Please refer to the User's Guide for a full explanation of data

Howard Regional Health System

3500 South Lafountain Street
Kokomo, IN 46902
URL: www.howardcommunity.org
Ownership: Government - Local
Emergency Services: Yes
Phone: 765-453-0702
Fax: 765-453-8087
Accredited: Yes
Licensed Beds: 150

Key Personnel:
President/CEO. . . . . James P Alender
Chief Medical Staff. . . . . Bruce Hughes, MD
Director Infection/Disease Control . . . . Danel Peterson
Director Respiratory Therapy . . . . Jeff Plough

Measure	Cases	This Hospital	State Average	U.S. Average	Top Hospital
Heart Attack Care					
ACE Inhibitor or ARB for LVSD[1]	5	80%	83%	82%	100%
Aspirin at Arrival	30	97%	91%	92%	100%
Aspirin at Discharge	27	96%	91%	90%	100%
Beta Blocker at Arrival	26	77%	84%	87%	100%
Beta Blocker at Discharge	26	96%	91%	90%	100%
Fibrinolytic Medication Timing	0	-	44%	31%	100%
PCI Within 90 Minutes of Arrival[1]	2	50%	56%	54%	95%
Smoking Cessation Advice[1]	8	100%	90%	88%	100%
Heart Failure Care					
ACE Inhibitor or ARB for LVSD	71	80%	81%	82%	100%
Discharge Instructions	139	65%	69%	61%	93%
Evaluation of LVS Function	193	91%	87%	83%	99%
Smoking Cessation Advice[1]	21	86%	84%	82%	100%
Pneumonia Care					
Appropriate Initial Antibiotic	177	86%	83%	83%	94%
Blood Culture Timing	101	95%	90%	90%	100%
Influenza Vaccine	48	81%	74%	70%	100%
Initial Antibiotic Timing	220	86%	84%	80%	93%
Oxygenation Assessment	282	99%	99%	99%	100%
Pneumococcal Vaccine	182	81%	77%	69%	94%
Smoking Cessation Advice	70	93%	81%	80%	100%
Surgical Infection Prevention					
Prophylactic Antibiotic Given[3]	147	70%	76%	77%	95%
Prophylactic Antibiotic Selection	46	93%	92%	90%	100%
Prophylactic Antibiotic Stopped[3]	137	72%	70%	72%	95%
Pregnancy Care					
Inpatient Neonatal Mortality	-	-	-	-	-
Third or Fourth Degree Laceration	-	-	4.02%	3.63%	3.27%

Saint Joseph Hospital

1907 W Sycamore Street
Kokomo, IN 46901
URL: www.stvincent.org
Ownership: Voluntary non-profit - Church
Emergency Services: Yes
Phone: 765-456-5433
Fax: 765-456-5779
Accredited: Yes
Licensed Beds: 156

Key Personnel:
CEO. . . . . Darcy Burghay
Chief Medical Staff. . . . . RJ Steele, MD
Emergency Room . . . . Monette Allen
OB/GYN Womens Health. . . . . RJ Kinsey, MD
Director Radiology . . . . J Green, MD
Director Respiratory Therapy . . . . Karen Hughes

Measure	Cases	This Hospital	State Average	U.S. Average	Top Hospital
Heart Attack Care					
ACE Inhibitor or ARB for LVSD[1]	3	100%	83%	82%	100%
Aspirin at Arrival[1]	14	100%	91%	92%	100%
Aspirin at Discharge[1]	7	100%	91%	90%	100%
Beta Blocker at Arrival[1]	16	100%	84%	87%	100%
Beta Blocker at Discharge[1]	8	100%	91%	90%	100%
Fibrinolytic Medication Timing[1]	2	0%	44%	31%	100%
PCI Within 90 Minutes of Arrival	0	-	56%	54%	95%
Smoking Cessation Advice[1]	2	100%	90%	88%	100%
Heart Failure Care					
ACE Inhibitor or ARB for LVSD	60	100%	81%	82%	100%
Discharge Instructions	113	99%	69%	61%	93%
Evaluation of LVS Function	143	84%	87%	83%	99%
Smoking Cessation Advice[1]	23	100%	84%	82%	100%
Pneumonia Care					
Appropriate Initial Antibiotic	149	69%	83%	83%	94%
Blood Culture Timing	93	92%	90%	90%	100%
Influenza Vaccine	30	93%	74%	70%	100%
Initial Antibiotic Timing	149	81%	84%	80%	93%
Oxygenation Assessment	168	100%	99%	99%	100%
Pneumococcal Vaccine	113	79%	77%	69%	94%
Smoking Cessation Advice	54	100%	81%	80%	100%
Surgical Infection Prevention					
Prophylactic Antibiotic Given[3]	139	46%	76%	77%	95%
Prophylactic Antibiotic Selection[1]	5	0%	92%	90%	100%
Prophylactic Antibiotic Stopped[3]	129	99%	70%	72%	95%
Pregnancy Care					
Inpatient Neonatal Mortality	-	-	-	-	-
Third or Fourth Degree Laceration	-	-	4.02%	3.63%	3.27%

LaPorte Hospital

1007 Lincoln Way
La Porte, IN 46350
Toll-Free: 800-235-6204
Phone: 219-326-1234
Fax: 219-326-2509
URL: www.laportehealth.org
Ownership: Voluntary non-profit - Private
Emergency Services: Yes
Accredited: Yes
Licensed Beds: 227

Key Personnel:
President/CEO. . . . . Michael Haley
Chief of Medical Staff. Dabi Baughman
Director Medical/Surgical Nursing . . . . Linda Satkoski
Coordinator Surgical Services . . . . Jan Thode, RN
Manager Radiology . . . . Nancy Bowers

Measure	Cases	This Hospital	State Average	U.S. Average	Top Hospital
Heart Attack Care					
ACE Inhibitor or ARB for LVSD[1]	20	70%	83%	82%	100%
Aspirin at Arrival	90	94%	91%	92%	100%
Aspirin at Discharge	93	94%	91%	90%	100%
Beta Blocker at Arrival	64	89%	84%	87%	100%
Beta Blocker at Discharge	94	94%	91%	90%	100%
Fibrinolytic Medication Timing	0	-	44%	31%	100%
PCI Within 90 Minutes of Arrival[1]	6	83%	56%	54%	95%
Smoking Cessation Advice	32	100%	90%	88%	100%
Heart Failure Care					
ACE Inhibitor or ARB for LVSD	102	77%	81%	82%	100%
Discharge Instructions	179	78%	69%	61%	93%
Evaluation of LVS Function	243	88%	87%	83%	99%
Smoking Cessation Advice	39	87%	84%	82%	100%
Pneumonia Care					
Appropriate Initial Antibiotic	108	92%	83%	83%	94%
Blood Culture Timing	89	90%	90%	90%	100%
Influenza Vaccine	25	76%	74%	70%	100%
Initial Antibiotic Timing	138	85%	84%	80%	93%
Oxygenation Assessment	164	98%	99%	99%	100%
Pneumococcal Vaccine	119	89%	77%	69%	94%
Smoking Cessation Advice	40	88%	81%	80%	100%
Surgical Infection Prevention					
Prophylactic Antibiotic Given	377	95%	76%	77%	95%
Prophylactic Antibiotic Selection	92	98%	92%	90%	100%
Prophylactic Antibiotic Stopped	363	87%	70%	72%	95%
Pregnancy Care					
Inpatient Neonatal Mortality	693	0.00%	-	-	-
Third or Fourth Degree Laceration	498	1.41%	4.02%	3.63%	3.27%

Lafayette Home Hospital

2400 South Street
Lafayette, IN 47904
URL: www.glhsi.org
Ownership: Voluntary non-profit - Church
Emergency Services: Yes
Phone: 765-447-6811
Fax: 765-423-6475
Accredited: Yes
Licensed Beds: 365

Key Personnel:
President/CEO. . . . . Terrance E Wilson
Director Infection/Disease Control . . . . Patricia Boardman
Director Respiratory Therapy . . . . Brad Richards

Measure	Cases	This Hospital	State Average	U.S. Average	Top Hospital

NOTE: Hospital profiles are in alphabetical order by state, then city, then hospital within the city; Rankings are sorted by rate in descending order and exclude hospitals with less than 25 cases; (1) The number of cases is too small (n<25) for purposes of reliably predicting hospital performance; (2) Measure reflects the hospital's indication that its submission was based upon a sample of its relevant discharges; (3) Rate reflects fewer than the maximum possible quarters of data for the measure; (4) Inaccurate information submitted and suppressed for one or more quarters; (5) No data is available from the hospital for this measure; Please refer to the User's Guide for a full explanation of data

Measure	Cases	This Hospital	State Average	U.S. Average	Top Hospital
Heart Attack Care					
ACE Inhibitor or ARB for LVSD[1]	4	50%	83%	82%	100%
Aspirin at Arrival[1]	22	100%	91%	92%	100%
Aspirin at Discharge[1]	11	73%	91%	90%	100%
Beta Blocker at Arrival[1]	11	73%	84%	87%	100%
Beta Blocker at Discharge[1]	13	92%	91%	90%	100%
Fibrinolytic Medication Timing	0	-	44%	31%	100%
PCI Within 90 Minutes of Arrival	0	-	56%	54%	95%
Smoking Cessation Advice[1]	3	100%	90%	88%	100%
Heart Failure Care					
ACE Inhibitor or ARB for LVSD[1]	19	89%	81%	82%	100%
Discharge Instructions	54	50%	69%	61%	93%
Evaluation of LVS Function	80	88%	87%	83%	99%
Smoking Cessation Advice[1]	17	88%	84%	82%	100%
Pneumonia Care					
Appropriate Initial Antibiotic	113	67%	83%	83%	94%
Blood Culture Timing	98	94%	90%	90%	100%
Influenza Vaccine	34	74%	74%	70%	100%
Initial Antibiotic Timing	149	80%	84%	80%	93%
Oxygenation Assessment	187	99%	99%	99%	100%
Pneumococcal Vaccine	117	61%	77%	69%	94%
Smoking Cessation Advice	44	75%	81%	80%	100%
Surgical Infection Prevention					
Prophylactic Antibiotic Given	766	87%	76%	77%	95%
Prophylactic Antibiotic Selection	185	88%	92%	90%	100%
Prophylactic Antibiotic Stopped	752	60%	70%	72%	95%
Pregnancy Care					
Inpatient Neonatal Mortality	-	-	-	-	-
Third or Fourth Degree Laceration	-	-	4.02%	3.63%	3.27%

Saint Elizabeth Medical Center

Alternate Name: Greater LaFayette Health Services
1501 Hartford Street
PO Box 7501
Lafayette, IN 47903
URL: www.glhsi.org
Toll-Free: 800-371-6011
Phone: 765-423-6011
Fax: 765-423-6925
Ownership: Voluntary non-profit - Church
Emergency Services: Yes
Accredited: Yes
Licensed Beds: 375

Key Personnel:
President/CEO . . . . Terrence Wilson
Chief Medical Staff . . . . Donald Edelen, MD
Cardio Laboratory . . . . Larry Drummond
Chief Catheterization Laboratory . . . . G Brodell, MD
Emergency Room . . . . TN Petry, MD
Director Infection/Disease Control . . . . Patricia Boardman, RN
Division Director Respiratory Therapy . . . . Brad Richards

Measure	Cases	This Hospital	State Average	U.S. Average	Top Hospital
Heart Attack Care					
ACE Inhibitor or ARB for LVSD[2]	65	74%	83%	82%	100%
Aspirin at Arrival[2]	243	99%	91%	92%	100%
Aspirin at Discharge[2]	346	98%	91%	90%	100%
Beta Blocker at Arrival[2]	185	94%	84%	87%	100%
Beta Blocker at Discharge[2]	391	95%	91%	90%	100%
Fibrinolytic Medication Timing[1,2]	1	100%	44%	31%	100%
PCI Within 90 Minutes of Arrival[1,2]	8	62%	56%	54%	95%
Smoking Cessation Advice[2]	145	90%	90%	88%	100%
Heart Failure Care					
ACE Inhibitor or ARB for LVSD[2]	117	68%	81%	82%	100%
Discharge Instructions[2]	250	76%	69%	61%	93%
Evaluation of LVS Function[2]	348	81%	87%	83%	99%
Smoking Cessation Advice[2]	64	70%	84%	82%	100%
Pneumonia Care					
Appropriate Initial Antibiotic[2]	143	71%	83%	83%	94%
Blood Culture Timing[2]	212	97%	90%	90%	100%
Influenza Vaccine	55	71%	74%	70%	100%
Initial Antibiotic Timing[2]	262	87%	84%	80%	93%
Oxygenation Assessment[2]	326	99%	99%	99%	100%
Pneumococcal Vaccine[2]	227	64%	77%	69%	94%
Smoking Cessation Advice[2]	81	70%	81%	80%	100%
Surgical Infection Prevention					
Prophylactic Antibiotic Given[2]	523	86%	76%	77%	95%
Prophylactic Antibiotic Selection[2]	120	80%	92%	90%	100%
Prophylactic Antibiotic Stopped[2]	513	58%	70%	72%	95%
Pregnancy Care					
Inpatient Neonatal Mortality	-	-	-	-	-
Third or Fourth Degree Laceration	-	-	4.02%	3.63%	3.27%

LaGrange Community Hospital

Alternate Name: LaGrange Hospital
207 N Townline Road
LaGrange, IN 46761
Phone: 260-463-2143
Fax: 260-463-3190
Ownership: Voluntary non-profit - Private
Emergency Services: Yes
Accredited: Yes
Licensed Beds: 62

Key Personnel:
Administrator . . . . Shelleye Hicks
Chief Medical Staff . . . . Shashank Kashyap, MD
Emergency Room . . . . Scott Smith, MD
Infection Control . . . . Jane Case
Chief Radiology . . . . James Wehrenberg, MD
Director Respiratory Therapy . . . . Jim Cleveland

Measure	Cases	This Hospital	State Average	U.S. Average	Top Hospital
Heart Attack Care					
ACE Inhibitor or ARB for LVSD[3]	0	-	83%	82%	100%
Aspirin at Arrival[1,3]	3	100%	91%	92%	100%
Aspirin at Discharge[1,3]	3	100%	91%	90%	100%
Beta Blocker at Arrival[1,3]	2	100%	84%	87%	100%
Beta Blocker at Discharge[1,3]	2	100%	91%	90%	100%
Fibrinolytic Medication Timing[3]	0	-	44%	31%	100%
PCI Within 90 Minutes of Arrival	0	-	56%	54%	95%
Smoking Cessation Advice[3]	0	-	90%	88%	100%
Heart Failure Care					
ACE Inhibitor or ARB for LVSD[1]	2	50%	81%	82%	100%
Discharge Instructions[1]	19	16%	69%	61%	93%
Evaluation of LVS Function[1]	22	55%	87%	83%	99%
Smoking Cessation Advice[1]	4	100%	84%	82%	100%
Pneumonia Care					
Appropriate Initial Antibiotic	64	92%	83%	83%	94%
Blood Culture Timing[1]	24	96%	90%	90%	100%
Influenza Vaccine[1]	18	83%	74%	70%	100%
Initial Antibiotic Timing	57	91%	84%	80%	93%
Oxygenation Assessment	70	100%	99%	99%	100%
Pneumococcal Vaccine	43	63%	77%	69%	94%
Smoking Cessation Advice[1]	19	100%	81%	80%	100%
Surgical Infection Prevention					
Prophylactic Antibiotic Given[1]	21	67%	76%	77%	95%
Prophylactic Antibiotic Selection[1]	3	100%	92%	90%	100%
Prophylactic Antibiotic Stopped[1]	20	10%	70%	72%	95%
Pregnancy Care					
Inpatient Neonatal Mortality	-	-	-	-	-
Third or Fourth Degree Laceration	-	-	4.02%	3.63%	3.27%

Dearborn County Hospital

600 Wilson Creek Road
Lawrenceburg, IN 47025
Toll-Free: 800-676-5572
Phone: 812-537-1010
Fax: 812-537-2897
E-mail: hhinds@dch.org
URL: www.dhc.org
Ownership: Government - Local
Emergency Services: Yes
Accredited: Yes
Licensed Beds: 144

Key Personnel:
Executive Director . . . . Peter V Resnick
Chief Medical Staff . . . . Richard Cardosi, MD
Director Cath Lab . . . . Ashok Penmetsa, MD
Emergency Room . . . . Steven Gunderson, MO
Director Medical Surgical . . . . Ann Beckett, RN
Chief of OB . . . . Reshma Khan, MD

Measure	Cases	This Hospital	State Average	U.S. Average	Top Hospital
Heart Attack Care					
ACE Inhibitor or ARB for LVSD[1]	6	67%	83%	82%	100%
Aspirin at Arrival	35	100%	91%	92%	100%
Aspirin at Discharge[1]	16	88%	91%	90%	100%
Beta Blocker at Arrival[1]	24	100%	84%	87%	100%
Beta Blocker at Discharge[1]	20	100%	91%	90%	100%

NOTE: Hospital profiles are in alphabetical order by state, then city, then hospital within the city; Rankings are sorted by rate in descending order and exclude hospitals with less than 25 cases; (1) The number of cases is too small (n<25) for purposes of reliably predicting hospital performance; (2) Measure reflects the hospital's indication that its submission was based upon a sample of its relevant discharges; (3) Rate reflects fewer than the maximum possible quarters of data for the measure; (4) Inaccurate information submitted and suppressed for one or more quarters; (5) No data is available from the hospital for this measure; Please refer to the User's Guide for a full explanation of data

Fibrinolytic Medication Timing[1]	6	33%	44%	31%	100%
PCI Within 90 Minutes of Arrival	0	-	56%	54%	95%
Smoking Cessation Advice[1]	4	100%	90%	88%	100%
Heart Failure Care					
ACE Inhibitor or ARB for LVSD	44	68%	81%	82%	100%
Discharge Instructions	82	39%	69%	61%	93%
Evaluation of LVS Function	82	90%	87%	83%	99%
Smoking Cessation Advice[1]	20	90%	84%	82%	100%
Pneumonia Care					
Appropriate Initial Antibiotic	119	89%	83%	83%	94%
Blood Culture Timing	126	87%	90%	90%	100%
Influenza Vaccine	34	24%	74%	70%	100%
Initial Antibiotic Timing	183	79%	84%	80%	93%
Oxygenation Assessment	229	100%	99%	99%	100%
Pneumococcal Vaccine	139	67%	77%	69%	94%
Smoking Cessation Advice	68	85%	81%	80%	100%
Surgical Infection Prevention					
Prophylactic Antibiotic Given	234	95%	76%	77%	95%
Prophylactic Antibiotic Selection	50	96%	92%	90%	100%
Prophylactic Antibiotic Stopped	212	74%	70%	72%	95%
Pregnancy Care					
Inpatient Neonatal Mortality	-	-	-	-	-
Third or Fourth Degree Laceration	-	-	4.02%	3.63%	3.27%

Witham Memorial Hospital

2605 N Lebanon Street
Lebanon, IN 46052

Toll-Free: 877-494-8426
Phone: 765-485-8000
Fax: 765-482-8688

URL: www.witham.org
Ownership: Government - Local
Emergency Services: No

Accredited: Yes
Licensed Beds: 80

Key Personnel:
President/CEO. . . . . Raymond Ingham
Clinical Coordinator Intensive Coronary . . . . Cindy Line
Manager Cardiopulmonary. . . . . Linda Smith

Measure	Cases	This Hospital	State Average	U.S. Average	Top Hospital
Heart Attack Care					
ACE Inhibitor or ARB for LVSD[1]	2	100%	83%	82%	100%
Aspirin at Arrival[1]	19	95%	91%	92%	100%
Aspirin at Discharge[1]	14	100%	91%	90%	100%
Beta Blocker at Arrival[1]	17	76%	84%	87%	100%
Beta Blocker at Discharge[1]	12	92%	91%	90%	100%
Fibrinolytic Medication Timing[3]	0	-	44%	31%	100%
PCI Within 90 Minutes of Arrival	0	-	56%	54%	95%
Smoking Cessation Advice[1]	1	100%	90%	88%	100%
Heart Failure Care					
ACE Inhibitor or ARB for LVSD[1]	24	83%	81%	82%	100%
Discharge Instructions	42	95%	69%	61%	93%
Evaluation of LVS Function	50	74%	87%	83%	99%
Smoking Cessation Advice[1]	7	100%	84%	82%	100%
Pneumonia Care					
Appropriate Initial Antibiotic	77	66%	83%	83%	94%
Blood Culture Timing	54	80%	90%	90%	100%
Influenza Vaccine[1]	18	44%	74%	70%	100%
Initial Antibiotic Timing	104	89%	84%	80%	93%
Oxygenation Assessment	113	99%	99%	99%	100%
Pneumococcal Vaccine	77	77%	77%	69%	94%
Smoking Cessation Advice[1]	17	100%	81%	80%	100%
Surgical Infection Prevention					
Prophylactic Antibiotic Given	34	62%	76%	77%	95%
Prophylactic Antibiotic Selection[1]	7	100%	92%	90%	100%
Prophylactic Antibiotic Stopped	34	88%	70%	72%	95%
Pregnancy Care					
Inpatient Neonatal Mortality	-	-	-	-	-
Third or Fourth Degree Laceration	-	-	4.02%	3.63%	3.27%

Greene County General Hospital

RR 1
Box 1000
Linton, IN 47441
URL: www.greenecountyhospital.com
Ownership: Government - Local
Emergency Services: Yes

Phone: 812-847-2281
Fax: 812-847-6166
Accredited: Yes
Licensed Beds: 76

Key Personnel:
Chief Medical Staff. . . . . Fred Ridge
Emergency Room . . . . Tim Hale
Infection Control. . . . . Cheryl Corbin
ICU . . . . Amy Miller
Director Radiology . . . . Benjamin Wendell, MD

Measure	Cases	This Hospital	State Average	U.S. Average	Top Hospital
Heart Attack Care					
ACE Inhibitor or ARB for LVSD	0	-	83%	82%	100%
Aspirin at Arrival[1]	8	100%	91%	92%	100%
Aspirin at Discharge[1]	3	67%	91%	90%	100%
Beta Blocker at Arrival[1]	4	50%	84%	87%	100%
Beta Blocker at Discharge[1]	3	67%	91%	90%	100%
Fibrinolytic Medication Timing[1]	1	0%	44%	31%	100%
PCI Within 90 Minutes of Arrival[5]	-	-	56%	54%	95%
Smoking Cessation Advice	0	-	90%	88%	100%
Heart Failure Care					
ACE Inhibitor or ARB for LVSD[1]	20	75%	81%	82%	100%
Discharge Instructions	35	80%	69%	61%	93%
Evaluation of LVS Function	58	84%	87%	83%	99%
Smoking Cessation Advice[1]	4	50%	84%	82%	100%
Pneumonia Care					
Appropriate Initial Antibiotic	31	81%	83%	83%	94%
Blood Culture Timing	26	100%	90%	90%	100%
Influenza Vaccine[1]	12	75%	74%	70%	100%
Initial Antibiotic Timing	52	94%	84%	80%	93%
Oxygenation Assessment	62	100%	99%	99%	100%
Pneumococcal Vaccine	45	84%	77%	69%	94%
Smoking Cessation Advice[1]	13	69%	81%	80%	100%
Surgical Infection Prevention					
Prophylactic Antibiotic Given[5]	-	-	76%	77%	95%
Prophylactic Antibiotic Selection[5]	-	-	92%	90%	100%
Prophylactic Antibiotic Stopped[5]	-	-	70%	72%	95%
Pregnancy Care					
Inpatient Neonatal Mortality	-	-	-	-	-
Third or Fourth Degree Laceration	-	-	4.02%	3.63%	3.27%

Logansport Memorial Hospital

1101 Michigan Avenue
PO Box 7013
Logansport, IN 46947
E-mail: info@mhlogan.org
URL: www.mhlogan.org
Ownership: Government - Local
Emergency Services: Yes

Toll-Free: 800-243-4512
Phone: 574-753-7541
Accredited: Yes
Licensed Beds: 104

Key Personnel:
CEO. . . . . Brian Shockney
Emergency Room . . . . Zahid Hussan
Emergency Room . . . . Lazo Krysteyski, MD
Director Infection/Disease Control . . . . Sebrena Ide, RN
ICU . . . . Angela Cleland, RN
CCU Spvg. Nurse . . . . Angela Cleland, RN
Manager Medical/Surgical Nursing. . . . . Jennifer Albright, RN
Chief of Pulmonary/Respiratory Care. . . . . Suzane Vin-Podel

Measure	Cases	This Hospital	State Average	U.S. Average	Top Hospital
Heart Attack Care					
ACE Inhibitor or ARB for LVSD[1]	1	100%	83%	82%	100%
Aspirin at Arrival[1]	17	94%	91%	92%	100%
Aspirin at Discharge[1]	5	100%	91%	90%	100%
Beta Blocker at Arrival[1]	16	81%	84%	87%	100%
Beta Blocker at Discharge[1]	4	75%	91%	90%	100%
Fibrinolytic Medication Timing	0	-	44%	31%	100%
PCI Within 90 Minutes of Arrival	0	-	56%	54%	95%
Smoking Cessation Advice	0	-	90%	88%	100%

NOTE: Hospital profiles are in alphabetical order by state, then city, then hospital within the city; Rankings are sorted by rate in descending order and exclude hospitals with less than 25 cases; (1) The number of cases is too small (n<25) for purposes of reliably predicting hospital performance; (2) Measure reflects the hospital's indication that its submission was based upon a sample of its relevant discharges; (3) Rate reflects fewer than the maximum possible quarters of data for the measure; (4) Inaccurate information submitted and suppressed for one or more quarters; (5) No data is available from the hospital for this measure; Please refer to the User's Guide for a full explanation of data

Measure	Cases	This Hospital	State Average	U.S. Average	Top Hospital
Heart Failure Care					
ACE Inhibitor or ARB for LVSD[1]	22	77%	81%	82%	100%
Discharge Instructions	44	73%	69%	61%	93%
Evaluation of LVS Function	77	83%	87%	83%	99%
Smoking Cessation Advice[1]	13	46%	84%	82%	100%
Pneumonia Care					
Appropriate Initial Antibiotic	44	93%	83%	83%	94%
Blood Culture Timing	45	93%	90%	90%	100%
Influenza Vaccine[1]	11	91%	74%	70%	100%
Initial Antibiotic Timing	69	78%	84%	80%	93%
Oxygenation Assessment	91	100%	99%	99%	100%
Pneumococcal Vaccine	51	82%	77%	69%	94%
Smoking Cessation Advice[1]	24	29%	81%	80%	100%
Surgical Infection Prevention					
Prophylactic Antibiotic Given	165	82%	76%	77%	95%
Prophylactic Antibiotic Selection	37	97%	92%	90%	100%
Prophylactic Antibiotic Stopped	167	87%	70%	72%	95%
Pregnancy Care					
Inpatient Neonatal Mortality	-	-	-	-	-
Third or Fourth Degree Laceration	-	-	4.02%	3.63%	3.27%

King's Daughters Hospital

One King's Daughters' Drive
Madison, IN 47250
E-mail: kdh@seida.com
URL: www.kdhhs.org
Phone: 812-265-5211
Fax: 812-265-0680
Ownership: Voluntary non-profit - Private
Emergency Services: Yes
Accredited: Yes
Licensed Beds: 142

Key Personnel:

Administrator/President . . . . Roger Allman
Chief Medical Staff. . . . . William Estes, MD
Emergency Room . . . . Tim Deckert
Director Infection/Disease Control . . . . Vikki Conners, RN
CCU Spvg. Nurse . . . . Nick James, RN
Director Medical/Surgical Nursing . . . . Kathy Brown
Chief Radiology . . . . Melvin Skiles, MD
Director Cardio-Pulmonary Services . . . . Connie Wolf

Measure	Cases	This Hospital	State Average	U.S. Average	Top Hospital
Heart Attack Care					
ACE Inhibitor or ARB for LVSD[1]	3	100%	83%	82%	100%
Aspirin at Arrival	35	91%	91%	92%	100%
Aspirin at Discharge[1]	20	90%	91%	90%	100%
Beta Blocker at Arrival	30	97%	84%	87%	100%
Beta Blocker at Discharge[1]	17	88%	91%	90%	100%
Fibrinolytic Medication Timing	0	-	44%	31%	100%
PCI Within 90 Minutes of Arrival	0	-	56%	54%	95%
Smoking Cessation Advice[1]	2	100%	90%	88%	100%
Heart Failure Care					
ACE Inhibitor or ARB for LVSD	36	94%	81%	82%	100%
Discharge Instructions	103	90%	69%	61%	93%
Evaluation of LVS Function	147	99%	87%	83%	99%
Smoking Cessation Advice[1]	17	94%	84%	82%	100%
Pneumonia Care					
Appropriate Initial Antibiotic	180	88%	83%	83%	94%
Blood Culture Timing	127	90%	90%	90%	100%
Influenza Vaccine[4,5]	-	-	74%	70%	100%
Initial Antibiotic Timing	194	93%	84%	80%	93%
Oxygenation Assessment	236	100%	99%	99%	100%
Pneumococcal Vaccine	148	99%	77%	69%	94%
Smoking Cessation Advice	54	94%	81%	80%	100%
Surgical Infection Prevention					
Prophylactic Antibiotic Given	133	98%	76%	77%	95%
Prophylactic Antibiotic Selection	41	100%	92%	90%	100%
Prophylactic Antibiotic Stopped	130	91%	70%	72%	95%
Pregnancy Care					
Inpatient Neonatal Mortality	-	-	-	-	-
Third or Fourth Degree Laceration	-	-	4.02%	3.63%	3.27%

Marion General Hospital

441 N Wabash Avenue
Marion, IN 46952
Phone: 765-662-4684
Fax: 765-662-4842
Ownership: Voluntary non-profit - Other
Emergency Services: Yes
Accredited: Yes
Licensed Beds: 191

Key Personnel:

Chief Medical Staff. . . . . James Camarata
Director Medical/Surgical Nursing . . . . Sherry Howell
Director Respiratory Therapy . . . . Debbie Briscoe

Measure	Cases	This Hospital	State Average	U.S. Average	Top Hospital
Heart Attack Care					
ACE Inhibitor or ARB for LVSD[1]	8	100%	83%	82%	100%
Aspirin at Arrival	31	87%	91%	92%	100%
Aspirin at Discharge[1]	17	76%	91%	90%	100%
Beta Blocker at Arrival	33	82%	84%	87%	100%
Beta Blocker at Discharge[1]	19	100%	91%	90%	100%
Fibrinolytic Medication Timing	0	-	44%	31%	100%
PCI Within 90 Minutes of Arrival	0	-	56%	54%	95%
Smoking Cessation Advice[1]	3	100%	90%	88%	100%
Heart Failure Care					
ACE Inhibitor or ARB for LVSD	62	92%	81%	82%	100%
Discharge Instructions	145	83%	69%	61%	93%
Evaluation of LVS Function	196	97%	87%	83%	99%
Smoking Cessation Advice	33	97%	84%	82%	100%
Pneumonia Care					
Appropriate Initial Antibiotic	111	95%	83%	83%	94%
Blood Culture Timing	110	79%	90%	90%	100%
Influenza Vaccine[1]	22	95%	74%	70%	100%
Initial Antibiotic Timing	166	87%	84%	80%	93%
Oxygenation Assessment	198	100%	99%	99%	100%
Pneumococcal Vaccine	117	97%	77%	69%	94%
Smoking Cessation Advice	51	96%	81%	80%	100%
Surgical Infection Prevention					
Prophylactic Antibiotic Given[3]	271	82%	76%	77%	95%
Prophylactic Antibiotic Selection	88	78%	92%	90%	100%
Prophylactic Antibiotic Stopped[3]	260	88%	70%	72%	95%
Pregnancy Care					
Inpatient Neonatal Mortality	-	-	-	-	-
Third or Fourth Degree Laceration	-	-	4.02%	3.63%	3.27%

Morgan Hospital Medical Centre

2209 John R Wooden Drive
Martinsville, IN 46151
Phone: 765-349-6500
Fax: 765-349-5411
Ownership: Government - Local
Emergency Services: No
Accredited: Yes
Licensed Beds: 106

Key Personnel:

President/CEO. . . . . Thomas W Laux
Chief Medical Staff. . . . . Dr Worren Gray
Director of Cardiology/Cardiac Lab. . . . . Terri Ridenour
Emergency Room Director. . . . . Debbie Aderf
Infection Control. . . . . Deanna Skaggs
Director Medical Surgery . . . . Shirley East
Director OB/Women's Care/Children . . . . Laurie Helms
Director Radiology . . . . Linda Sheets

Measure	Cases	This Hospital	State Average	U.S. Average	Top Hospital
Heart Attack Care					
ACE Inhibitor or ARB for LVSD[1]	3	100%	83%	82%	100%
Aspirin at Arrival[1]	15	100%	91%	92%	100%
Aspirin at Discharge[1]	5	100%	91%	90%	100%
Beta Blocker at Arrival[1]	13	92%	84%	87%	100%
Beta Blocker at Discharge[1]	6	100%	91%	90%	100%
Fibrinolytic Medication Timing[3]	0	-	44%	31%	100%
PCI Within 90 Minutes of Arrival	0	-	56%	54%	95%
Smoking Cessation Advice[3]	0	-	90%	88%	100%
Heart Failure Care					
ACE Inhibitor or ARB for LVSD	63	97%	81%	82%	100%
Discharge Instructions[3]	28	100%	69%	61%	93%
Evaluation of LVS Function	159	87%	87%	83%	99%
Smoking Cessation Advice[1,3]	8	100%	84%	82%	100%
Pneumonia Care					
Appropriate Initial Antibiotic[1,3]	9	89%	83%	83%	94%

NOTE: Hospital profiles are in alphabetical order by state, then city, then hospital within the city; Rankings are sorted by rate in descending order and exclude hospitals with less than 25 cases; (1) The number of cases is too small (n<25) for purposes of reliably predicting hospital performance; (2) Measure reflects the hospital's indication that its submission was based upon a sample of its relevant discharges; (3) Rate reflects fewer than the maximum possible quarters of data for the measure; (4) Inaccurate information submitted and suppressed for one or more quarters; (5) No data is available from the hospital for this measure; Please refer to the User's Guide for a full explanation of data

Blood Culture Timing[1,3]	20	85%	90%	90%	100%
Influenza Vaccine[5]	-	-	74%	70%	100%
Initial Antibiotic Timing	126	95%	84%	80%	93%
Oxygenation Assessment	144	100%	99%	99%	100%
Pneumococcal Vaccine	95	68%	77%	69%	94%
Smoking Cessation Advice[1,3]	6	100%	81%	80%	100%
Surgical Infection Prevention					
Prophylactic Antibiotic Given[1,3]	14	50%	76%	77%	95%
Prophylactic Antibiotic Selection[5]	-	-	92%	90%	100%
Prophylactic Antibiotic Stopped[1,3]	14	93%	70%	72%	95%
Pregnancy Care					
Inpatient Neonatal Mortality	213	0.00%	-	-	-
Third or Fourth Degree Laceration	147	2.72%	4.02%	3.63%	3.27%

Saint Anthony Memorial Health Centers

301 West Homer Street — Phone: 219-879-8511
Michigan City, IN 46360 — Fax: 219-877-1684
URL: www.samhc.org
Ownership: Voluntary non-profit - Church — Accredited: Yes
Emergency Services: Yes — Licensed Beds: 310

Key Personnel:

President/CEO. . . . . Bruce Rampage
Chief Medical Staff. . . . . James Callaghan, MD
Cardiac Lab . . . . Linda Rempala
Catheterization Lab . . . . Linda Rempala
Emergency Room . . . . Alice Ulm, RN
Infection Control. . . . . Janene Gumz-Pulaski
ICU . . . . Dorothy Tomlin
OB/GYN/Women's Health . . . . Lynn Stevens, NP
Respiratory/Cardiopulmonary. . . . . Kathy Mosley

Measure	Cases	This Hospital	State Average	U.S. Average	Top Hospital
Heart Attack Care					
ACE Inhibitor or ARB for LVSD[1]	22	91%	83%	82%	100%
Aspirin at Arrival	109	98%	91%	92%	100%
Aspirin at Discharge	88	99%	91%	90%	100%
Beta Blocker at Arrival	98	99%	84%	87%	100%
Beta Blocker at Discharge	86	100%	91%	90%	100%
Fibrinolytic Medication Timing	0	-	44%	31%	100%
PCI Within 90 Minutes of Arrival[1]	9	44%	56%	54%	95%
Smoking Cessation Advice	36	100%	90%	88%	100%
Heart Failure Care					
ACE Inhibitor or ARB for LVSD	68	96%	81%	82%	100%
Discharge Instructions	167	80%	69%	61%	93%
Evaluation of LVS Function	205	99%	87%	83%	99%
Smoking Cessation Advice	35	100%	84%	82%	100%
Pneumonia Care					
Appropriate Initial Antibiotic	180	91%	83%	83%	94%
Blood Culture Timing	95	89%	90%	90%	100%
Influenza Vaccine	26	65%	74%	70%	100%
Initial Antibiotic Timing	187	85%	84%	80%	93%
Oxygenation Assessment	220	95%	99%	99%	100%
Pneumococcal Vaccine	126	67%	77%	69%	94%
Smoking Cessation Advice	49	100%	81%	80%	100%
Surgical Infection Prevention					
Prophylactic Antibiotic Given	284	91%	76%	77%	95%
Prophylactic Antibiotic Selection	91	95%	92%	90%	100%
Prophylactic Antibiotic Stopped	278	67%	70%	72%	95%
Pregnancy Care					
Inpatient Neonatal Mortality	-	-	-	-	-
Third or Fourth Degree Laceration	-	-	4.02%	3.63%	3.27%

Saint Joseph Regional Med Ctr-Mishawaka

215 W 4th Street — Phone: 574-259-2431
Mishawaka, IN 46544 — Fax: 574-247-5401
URL: www.sjmed.com
Ownership: Voluntary non-profit - Church — Accredited: Yes
Emergency Services: Yes — Licensed Beds: 125

Key Personnel:

CEO. . . . . Lori Terce
Chief of Medical Staff. . . . . Norbet Sphear
Emergency Room . . . . Iceses Seltenight
Respiratory Care . . . . Brett Broviak

Measure	Cases	This Hospital	State Average	U.S. Average	Top Hospital
Heart Attack Care					
ACE Inhibitor or ARB for LVSD[1]	6	67%	83%	82%	100%
Aspirin at Arrival	53	96%	91%	92%	100%
Aspirin at Discharge	48	100%	91%	90%	100%
Beta Blocker at Arrival	39	95%	84%	87%	100%
Beta Blocker at Discharge	51	96%	91%	90%	100%
Fibrinolytic Medication Timing	0	-	44%	31%	100%
PCI Within 90 Minutes of Arrival[1]	6	100%	56%	54%	95%
Smoking Cessation Advice[1]	15	87%	90%	88%	100%
Heart Failure Care					
ACE Inhibitor or ARB for LVSD	33	79%	81%	82%	100%
Discharge Instructions	72	62%	69%	61%	93%
Evaluation of LVS Function	97	99%	87%	83%	99%
Smoking Cessation Advice[1]	24	71%	84%	82%	100%
Pneumonia Care					
Appropriate Initial Antibiotic	59	93%	83%	83%	94%
Blood Culture Timing	37	89%	90%	90%	100%
Influenza Vaccine[1]	15	73%	74%	70%	100%
Initial Antibiotic Timing	75	91%	84%	80%	93%
Oxygenation Assessment	87	100%	99%	99%	100%
Pneumococcal Vaccine	56	95%	77%	69%	94%
Smoking Cessation Advice	30	80%	81%	80%	100%
Surgical Infection Prevention					
Prophylactic Antibiotic Given[3]	109	81%	76%	77%	95%
Prophylactic Antibiotic Selection	32	100%	92%	90%	100%
Prophylactic Antibiotic Stopped[3]	99	71%	70%	72%	95%
Pregnancy Care					
Inpatient Neonatal Mortality	659	0.30%	-	-	-
Third or Fourth Degree Laceration	521	1.15%	4.02%	3.63%	3.27%

White County Memorial Hospital

1101 O'Connor Boulevard — Phone: 574-583-7111
Monticello, IN 47960 — Fax: 574-583-1703
URL: www.whitecmh.org
Ownership: Government - Local — Accredited: Yes
Emergency Services: Yes — Licensed Beds: 25

Key Personnel:

CEO. . . . . Paul Pardwell
Chief Medical Staff. . . . . David Bailey
Emergency Room . . . . Denise Voetz
Infection Control. . . . . Robin Smith
Medical/Surgical Nursing . . . . Connie Jordan
OB/GYN Womens Health. . . . . Joanie Kahl

Measure	Cases	This Hospital	State Average	U.S. Average	Top Hospital
Heart Attack Care					
ACE Inhibitor or ARB for LVSD[1,3]	1	100%	83%	82%	100%
Aspirin at Arrival[1,3]	4	0%	91%	92%	100%
Aspirin at Discharge[1,3]	2	50%	91%	90%	100%
Beta Blocker at Arrival[1,3]	4	25%	84%	87%	100%
Beta Blocker at Discharge[1,3]	2	100%	91%	90%	100%
Fibrinolytic Medication Timing[5]	-	-	44%	31%	100%
PCI Within 90 Minutes of Arrival[5]	-	-	56%	54%	95%
Smoking Cessation Advice[1,3]	1	0%	90%	88%	100%
Heart Failure Care					
ACE Inhibitor or ARB for LVSD[1,3]	11	73%	81%	82%	100%
Discharge Instructions[1,3]	18	78%	69%	61%	93%
Evaluation of LVS Function[3]	40	78%	87%	83%	99%
Smoking Cessation Advice[1,3]	8	62%	84%	82%	100%
Pneumonia Care					
Appropriate Initial Antibiotic[3]	46	76%	83%	83%	94%
Blood Culture Timing	39	90%	90%	90%	100%
Influenza Vaccine[1]	13	62%	74%	70%	100%
Initial Antibiotic Timing[3]	47	87%	84%	80%	93%
Oxygenation Assessment[3]	68	94%	99%	99%	100%
Pneumococcal Vaccine[3]	47	70%	77%	69%	94%
Smoking Cessation Advice[1,3]	14	79%	81%	80%	100%
Surgical Infection Prevention					
Prophylactic Antibiotic Given[1,3]	21	81%	76%	77%	95%
Prophylactic Antibiotic Selection[1]	5	100%	92%	90%	100%
Prophylactic Antibiotic Stopped[1,3]	20	80%	70%	72%	95%

NOTE: Hospital profiles are in alphabetical order by state, then city, then hospital within the city; Rankings are sorted by rate in descending order and exclude hospitals with less than 25 cases; (1) The number of cases is too small (n<25) for purposes of reliably predicting hospital performance; (2) Measure reflects the hospital's indication that its submission was based upon a sample of its relevant discharges; (3) Rate reflects fewer than the maximum possible quarters of data for the measure; (4) Inaccurate information submitted and suppressed for one or more quarters; (5) No data is available from the hospital for this measure; Please refer to the User's Guide for a full explanation of data

Pregnancy Care					
Inpatient Neonatal Mortality	-	-	-	-	-
Third or Fourth Degree Laceration	-	-	4.02%	3.63%	3.27%

Saint Francis at Mooresville

1201 Hadley Road
Mooresville, IN 46158
Ownership: Voluntary non-profit - Church
Emergency Services: No
Phone: 317-831-1160
Fax: 317-831-9315
Accredited: Yes

Measure	Cases	This Hospital	State Average	U.S. Average	Top Hospital
Heart Attack Care					
ACE Inhibitor or ARB for LVSD[5]	-	-	83%	82%	100%
Aspirin at Arrival[5]	-	-	91%	92%	100%
Aspirin at Discharge[5]	-	-	91%	90%	100%
Beta Blocker at Arrival[5]	-	-	84%	87%	100%
Beta Blocker at Discharge[5]	-	-	91%	90%	100%
Fibrinolytic Medication Timing[5]	-	-	44%	31%	100%
PCI Within 90 Minutes of Arrival[5]	-	-	56%	54%	95%
Smoking Cessation Advice[5]	-	-	90%	88%	100%
Heart Failure Care					
ACE Inhibitor or ARB for LVSD	0	-	81%	82%	100%
Discharge Instructions[1]	4	25%	69%	61%	93%
Evaluation of LVS Function[1]	4	25%	87%	83%	99%
Smoking Cessation Advice	0	-	84%	82%	100%
Pneumonia Care					
Appropriate Initial Antibiotic[1,3]	1	100%	83%	83%	94%
Blood Culture Timing[5]	-	-	90%	90%	100%
Influenza Vaccine[5]	-	-	74%	70%	100%
Initial Antibiotic Timing[1,3]	1	100%	84%	80%	93%
Oxygenation Assessment[1,3]	1	100%	99%	99%	100%
Pneumococcal Vaccine[3]	0	-	77%	69%	94%
Smoking Cessation Advice[3]	0	-	81%	80%	100%
Surgical Infection Prevention					
Prophylactic Antibiotic Given[2]	353	87%	76%	77%	95%
Prophylactic Antibiotic Selection[2]	75	97%	92%	90%	100%
Prophylactic Antibiotic Stopped[2]	348	86%	70%	72%	95%
Pregnancy Care					
Inpatient Neonatal Mortality	-	-	-	-	-
Third or Fourth Degree Laceration	-	-	4.02%	3.63%	3.27%

Ball Memorial Hospital

2401 W University Avenue
Muncie, IN 47303
URL: www.ballhospital.org
Ownership: Voluntary non-profit - Private
Emergency Services: Yes
Phone: 765-747-3111
Fax: 765-747-3404
Accredited: Yes
Licensed Beds: 436

Key Personnel:
President . . . . Brent L Batman
VP of Medical Staff. . . . . Charles Sanders
Head of Emergency Room. . . . . Karla Kirby
Emergency Room . . . . John Nahre, MD
Director Infection/Disease Control . . . . Michael Langona
CCU Spvg. Nurse . . . . Alexis Neal
Director Medical/Surgical Nursing . . . . Judy Bernhardt
Chief Radiology . . . . Charles Leiphart, MD
Director Respiratory Therapy . . . . Mike Owens

Measure	Cases	This Hospital	State Average	U.S. Average	Top Hospital
Heart Attack Care					
ACE Inhibitor or ARB for LVSD	114	86%	83%	82%	100%
Aspirin at Arrival	297	99%	91%	92%	100%
Aspirin at Discharge	386	97%	91%	90%	100%
Beta Blocker at Arrival	254	97%	84%	87%	100%
Beta Blocker at Discharge	352	99%	91%	90%	100%
Fibrinolytic Medication Timing	0	-	44%	31%	100%
PCI Within 90 Minutes of Arrival[1]	12	75%	56%	54%	95%
Smoking Cessation Advice	132	97%	90%	88%	100%
Heart Failure Care					
ACE Inhibitor or ARB for LVSD	201	83%	81%	82%	100%
Discharge Instructions	372	79%	69%	61%	93%
Evaluation of LVS Function	515	96%	87%	83%	99%
Smoking Cessation Advice	76	93%	84%	82%	100%
Pneumonia Care					
Appropriate Initial Antibiotic	283	90%	83%	83%	94%
Blood Culture Timing	248	87%	90%	90%	100%
Influenza Vaccine	61	92%	74%	70%	100%
Initial Antibiotic Timing	339	83%	84%	80%	93%
Oxygenation Assessment	429	100%	99%	99%	100%
Pneumococcal Vaccine	242	90%	77%	69%	94%
Smoking Cessation Advice	118	75%	81%	80%	100%
Surgical Infection Prevention					
Prophylactic Antibiotic Given[2]	1,006	85%	76%	77%	95%
Prophylactic Antibiotic Selection[2]	214	96%	92%	90%	100%
Prophylactic Antibiotic Stopped[2]	976	84%	70%	72%	95%
Pregnancy Care					
Inpatient Neonatal Mortality	-	-	-	-	-
Third or Fourth Degree Laceration	-	-	4.02%	3.63%	3.27%

Community Hospital

901 MacArthur Boulevard
Hammond, IN 46321
URL: www.comhs.org/community
Ownership: Voluntary non-profit - Private
Emergency Services: Yes
Phone: 219-836-1600
Fax: 219-836-6380
Accredited: Yes
Licensed Beds: 350

Key Personnel:
Administrator . . . . Edward P Robinson
Emergency Room . . . . Robert L Cavens, MD
Director Medical/Surgical Nursing . . . . Sharon Desancic

Measure	Cases	This Hospital	State Average	U.S. Average	Top Hospital
Heart Attack Care					
ACE Inhibitor or ARB for LVSD	33	76%	83%	82%	100%
Aspirin at Arrival	171	98%	91%	92%	100%
Aspirin at Discharge	147	95%	91%	90%	100%
Beta Blocker at Arrival	110	91%	84%	87%	100%
Beta Blocker at Discharge	164	93%	91%	90%	100%
Fibrinolytic Medication Timing[3]	0	-	44%	31%	100%
PCI Within 90 Minutes of Arrival[1]	15	13%	56%	54%	95%
Smoking Cessation Advice[1,3]	19	95%	90%	88%	100%
Heart Failure Care					
ACE Inhibitor or ARB for LVSD	310	75%	81%	82%	100%
Discharge Instructions[3]	139	72%	69%	61%	93%
Evaluation of LVS Function	800	90%	87%	83%	99%
Smoking Cessation Advice[1,3]	21	90%	84%	82%	100%
Pneumonia Care					
Appropriate Initial Antibiotic[3]	46	76%	83%	83%	94%
Blood Culture Timing[3]	52	98%	90%	90%	100%
Influenza Vaccine[5]	-	-	74%	70%	100%
Initial Antibiotic Timing	325	74%	84%	80%	93%
Oxygenation Assessment	370	100%	99%	99%	100%
Pneumococcal Vaccine	213	82%	77%	69%	94%
Smoking Cessation Advice[1,3]	21	90%	81%	80%	100%
Surgical Infection Prevention					
Prophylactic Antibiotic Given[2,3]	88	88%	76%	77%	95%
Prophylactic Antibiotic Selection[5]	-	-	92%	90%	100%
Prophylactic Antibiotic Stopped[2,3]	86	47%	70%	72%	95%
Pregnancy Care					
Inpatient Neonatal Mortality	2,308	0.56%	-	-	-
Third or Fourth Degree Laceration	1,441	2.43%	4.02%	3.63%	3.27%

Heartland Memorial Hospital

701 Superior Ave
Munster, IN 46321
Ownership: Proprietary
Emergency Services: No
Phone: 219-924-1300
Accredited: Yes

Measure	Cases	This Hospital	State Average	U.S. Average	Top Hospital
Heart Attack Care					
ACE Inhibitor or ARB for LVSD[1,3]	1	0%	83%	82%	100%
Aspirin at Arrival[1,3]	7	86%	91%	92%	100%
Aspirin at Discharge[1,3]	9	67%	91%	90%	100%
Beta Blocker at Arrival[1,3]	7	14%	84%	87%	100%
Beta Blocker at Discharge[1,3]	8	25%	91%	90%	100%

NOTE: Hospital profiles are in alphabetical order by state, then city, then hospital within the city; Rankings are sorted by rate in descending order and exclude hospitals with less than 25 cases; (1) The number of cases is too small (n<25) for purposes of reliably predicting hospital performance; (2) Measure reflects the hospital's indication that its submission was based upon a sample of its relevant discharges; (3) Rate reflects fewer than the maximum possible quarters of data for the measure; (4) Inaccurate information submitted and suppressed for one or more quarters; (5) No data is available from the hospital for this measure; Please refer to the User's Guide for a full explanation of data

Measure	Cases	This Hospital	State Average	U.S. Average	Top Hospital
Fibrinolytic Medication Timing[3]	0	-	44%	31%	100%
PCI Within 90 Minutes of Arrival	0	-	56%	54%	95%
Smoking Cessation Advice[3]	0	-	90%	88%	100%
Heart Failure Care					
ACE Inhibitor or ARB for LVSD[1]	22	41%	81%	82%	100%
Discharge Instructions[1,3]	18	22%	69%	61%	93%
Evaluation of LVS Function	81	73%	87%	83%	99%
Smoking Cessation Advice[1,3]	3	0%	84%	82%	100%
Pneumonia Care					
Appropriate Initial Antibiotic[1,3]	1	0%	83%	83%	94%
Blood Culture Timing[3]	0	-	90%	90%	100%
Influenza Vaccine[5]	-	-	74%	70%	100%
Initial Antibiotic Timing[1,3]	8	62%	84%	80%	93%
Oxygenation Assessment[1,3]	12	100%	99%	99%	100%
Pneumococcal Vaccine[1,3]	8	50%	77%	69%	94%
Smoking Cessation Advice[3]	0	-	81%	80%	100%
Surgical Infection Prevention					
Prophylactic Antibiotic Given[1,3]	20	30%	76%	77%	95%
Prophylactic Antibiotic Selection[5]	-	-	92%	90%	100%
Prophylactic Antibiotic Stopped[1,3]	20	50%	70%	72%	95%
Pregnancy Care					
Inpatient Neonatal Mortality	-	-	-	-	-
Third or Fourth Degree Laceration	-	-	4.02%	3.63%	3.27%

Floyd Memorial Hospital and Health Services

1850 State Street Phone: 812-944-7701
New Albany, IN 47150 Fax: 812-949-5607
URL: www.floydmedical.org
Ownership: Government - Local Accredited: Yes
Emergency Services: Yes Licensed Beds: 245

Key Personnel:
CEO. . . . . Bryant R Hanson
Emergency Room . . . . Ruth Heideman
Director Medical/Surgical Nursing . . . . Ginny Ehrlich, RN
OB/GYN Womens Health. . . . . Steve Baldwin, MD
Director Respiratory Therapy . . . . Janice Fessel

Measure	Cases	This Hospital	State Average	U.S. Average	Top Hospital
Heart Attack Care					
ACE Inhibitor or ARB for LVSD	60	87%	83%	82%	100%
Aspirin at Arrival	208	100%	91%	92%	100%
Aspirin at Discharge	226	99%	91%	90%	100%
Beta Blocker at Arrival	176	95%	84%	87%	100%
Beta Blocker at Discharge	211	95%	91%	90%	100%
Fibrinolytic Medication Timing[1,3]	1	0%	44%	31%	100%
PCI Within 90 Minutes of Arrival[1]	11	36%	56%	54%	95%
Smoking Cessation Advice	109	95%	90%	88%	100%
Heart Failure Care					
ACE Inhibitor or ARB for LVSD	118	82%	81%	82%	100%
Discharge Instructions	233	79%	69%	61%	93%
Evaluation of LVS Function	312	96%	87%	83%	99%
Smoking Cessation Advice	64	84%	84%	82%	100%
Pneumonia Care					
Appropriate Initial Antibiotic	199	93%	83%	83%	94%
Blood Culture Timing	276	95%	90%	90%	100%
Influenza Vaccine	74	97%	74%	70%	100%
Initial Antibiotic Timing	366	79%	84%	80%	93%
Oxygenation Assessment	471	99%	99%	99%	100%
Pneumococcal Vaccine	271	96%	77%	69%	94%
Smoking Cessation Advice	130	92%	81%	80%	100%
Surgical Infection Prevention					
Prophylactic Antibiotic Given[3]	364	94%	76%	77%	95%
Prophylactic Antibiotic Selection	109	97%	92%	90%	100%
Prophylactic Antibiotic Stopped[3]	351	84%	70%	72%	95%
Pregnancy Care					
Inpatient Neonatal Mortality	-	-	-	-	-
Third or Fourth Degree Laceration	-	-	4.02%	3.63%	3.27%

Henry County Memorial Hospital

1000 N 16th Street Phone: 765-521-0890
New Castle, IN 47362 Fax: 765-521-1555
URL: www.hcmhcares.org
Ownership: Government - Local Accredited: Yes
Emergency Services: No Licensed Beds: 107

Key Personnel:
President/CEO . . . . Blake Dye
Emergency Room . . . . Louann Glesser
Emergency Room . . . . Mark Doyle
Director Medical/Surgical Nursing . . . . Sue Chew, RN
Director of Respiratory . . . . Chlquica Keith

Measure	Cases	This Hospital	State Average	U.S. Average	Top Hospital
Heart Attack Care					
ACE Inhibitor or ARB for LVSD[1]	3	67%	83%	82%	100%
Aspirin at Arrival[1]	10	90%	91%	92%	100%
Aspirin at Discharge[1]	4	75%	91%	90%	100%
Beta Blocker at Arrival[1]	5	80%	84%	87%	100%
Beta Blocker at Discharge[1]	4	100%	91%	90%	100%
Fibrinolytic Medication Timing	0	-	44%	31%	100%
PCI Within 90 Minutes of Arrival	0	-	56%	54%	95%
Smoking Cessation Advice	0	-	90%	88%	100%
Heart Failure Care					
ACE Inhibitor or ARB for LVSD	34	91%	81%	82%	100%
Discharge Instructions	59	97%	69%	61%	93%
Evaluation of LVS Function	85	99%	87%	83%	99%
Smoking Cessation Advice[1]	6	100%	84%	82%	100%
Pneumonia Care					
Appropriate Initial Antibiotic	125	88%	83%	83%	94%
Blood Culture Timing	76	68%	90%	90%	100%
Influenza Vaccine[1]	21	90%	74%	70%	100%
Initial Antibiotic Timing	168	92%	84%	80%	93%
Oxygenation Assessment	212	100%	99%	99%	100%
Pneumococcal Vaccine	123	72%	77%	69%	94%
Smoking Cessation Advice	50	90%	81%	80%	100%
Surgical Infection Prevention					
Prophylactic Antibiotic Given	176	92%	76%	77%	95%
Prophylactic Antibiotic Selection	44	100%	92%	90%	100%
Prophylactic Antibiotic Stopped	169	21%	70%	72%	95%
Pregnancy Care					
Inpatient Neonatal Mortality	-	-	-	-	-
Third or Fourth Degree Laceration	-	-	4.02%	3.63%	3.27%

Women's Hospital

4199 Gateway Blvd Phone: 812-842-4222
Newburgh, IN 47630
Ownership: Proprietary Accredited: Yes
Emergency Services: No

Measure	Cases	This Hospital	State Average	U.S. Average	Top Hospital
Heart Attack Care					
ACE Inhibitor or ARB for LVSD[5]	-	-	83%	82%	100%
Aspirin at Arrival[5]	-	-	91%	92%	100%
Aspirin at Discharge[5]	-	-	91%	90%	100%
Beta Blocker at Arrival[5]	-	-	84%	87%	100%
Beta Blocker at Discharge[5]	-	-	91%	90%	100%
Fibrinolytic Medication Timing[5]	-	-	44%	31%	100%
PCI Within 90 Minutes of Arrival[5]	-	-	56%	54%	95%
Smoking Cessation Advice[5]	-	-	90%	88%	100%
Heart Failure Care					
ACE Inhibitor or ARB for LVSD[5]	-	-	81%	82%	100%
Discharge Instructions[5]	-	-	69%	61%	93%
Evaluation of LVS Function[5]	-	-	87%	83%	99%
Smoking Cessation Advice[5]	-	-	84%	82%	100%
Pneumonia Care					
Appropriate Initial Antibiotic[5]	-	-	83%	83%	94%
Blood Culture Timing[5]	-	-	90%	90%	100%
Influenza Vaccine[5]	-	-	74%	70%	100%
Initial Antibiotic Timing[5]	-	-	84%	80%	93%
Oxygenation Assessment[5]	-	-	99%	99%	100%
Pneumococcal Vaccine[5]	-	-	77%	69%	94%

NOTE: Hospital profiles are in alphabetical order by state, then city, then hospital within the city; Rankings are sorted by rate in descending order and exclude hospitals with less than 25 cases; (1) The number of cases is too small (n<25) for purposes of reliably predicting hospital performance; (2) Measure reflects the hospital's indication that its submission was based upon a sample of its relevant discharges; (3) Rate reflects fewer than the maximum possible quarters of data for the measure; (4) Inaccurate information submitted and suppressed for one or more quarters; (5) No data is available from the hospital for this measure; Please refer to the User's Guide for a full explanation of data

Smoking Cessation Advice[5]	-	-	81%	80%	100%
Surgical Infection Prevention					
Prophylactic Antibiotic Given[2]	449	96%	76%	77%	95%
Prophylactic Antibiotic Selection[2]	78	96%	92%	90%	100%
Prophylactic Antibiotic Stopped[2]	438	88%	70%	72%	95%
Pregnancy Care					
Inpatient Neonatal Mortality	3,217	0.44%	-	-	-
Third or Fourth Degree Laceration	2,001	6.35%	4.02%	3.63%	3.27%

Riverview Hospital

395 Westfield Road
Noblesville, IN 46060

Toll-Free: 800-523-6001
Phone: 317-773-0760
Fax: 317-776-7134

URL: www.riverviewhospital.org
Ownership: Government - Local
Emergency Services: Yes

Accredited: Yes
Licensed Beds: 161

Key Personnel:
President/CEO. . . . . Patricia K Fox

Measure	Cases	This Hospital	State Average	U.S. Average	Top Hospital
Heart Attack Care					
ACE Inhibitor or ARB for LVSD[1]	23	96%	83%	82%	100%
Aspirin at Arrival	95	100%	91%	92%	100%
Aspirin at Discharge	120	100%	91%	90%	100%
Beta Blocker at Arrival	74	100%	84%	87%	100%
Beta Blocker at Discharge	112	99%	91%	90%	100%
Fibrinolytic Medication Timing	0	-	44%	31%	100%
PCI Within 90 Minutes of Arrival[1]	5	100%	56%	54%	95%
Smoking Cessation Advice	31	100%	90%	88%	100%
Heart Failure Care					
ACE Inhibitor or ARB for LVSD	49	100%	81%	82%	100%
Discharge Instructions	99	96%	69%	61%	93%
Evaluation of LVS Function	134	99%	87%	83%	99%
Smoking Cessation Advice[1]	16	100%	84%	82%	100%
Pneumonia Care					
Appropriate Initial Antibiotic	76	87%	83%	83%	94%
Blood Culture Timing	47	96%	90%	90%	100%
Influenza Vaccine	25	96%	74%	70%	100%
Initial Antibiotic Timing	92	92%	84%	80%	93%
Oxygenation Assessment	118	100%	99%	99%	100%
Pneumococcal Vaccine	81	95%	77%	69%	94%
Smoking Cessation Advice[1]	19	100%	81%	80%	100%
Surgical Infection Prevention					
Prophylactic Antibiotic Given	391	94%	76%	77%	95%
Prophylactic Antibiotic Selection	99	79%	92%	90%	100%
Prophylactic Antibiotic Stopped	384	89%	70%	72%	95%
Pregnancy Care					
Inpatient Neonatal Mortality	-	-	-	-	-
Third or Fourth Degree Laceration	-	-	4.02%	3.63%	3.27%

Dukes Memorial Hospital

Alternate Name: Dukes
275 W 12th Street
Peru, IN 46970
URL: www.dukesmemorialhosp.com
Ownership: Proprietary
Emergency Services: Yes

Phone: 765-472-8000
Fax: 765-473-8244

Accredited: Yes
Licensed Beds: 158

Key Personnel:
CEO. . . . . Mike Funk
Chief Medical Staff. . . . . Neo Stalker
Infection Control Nurse. Gail Berkheiser
ICU . . . . Sally Piper
Pulmonary Manager. . . . . Sharon Anderson

Measure	Cases	This Hospital	State Average	U.S. Average	Top Hospital
Heart Attack Care					
ACE Inhibitor or ARB for LVSD[1]	1	100%	83%	82%	100%
Aspirin at Arrival[1]	9	67%	91%	92%	100%
Aspirin at Discharge[1]	7	100%	91%	90%	100%
Beta Blocker at Arrival[1]	9	44%	84%	87%	100%
Beta Blocker at Discharge[1]	7	100%	91%	90%	100%
Fibrinolytic Medication Timing	0	-	44%	31%	100%
PCI Within 90 Minutes of Arrival	0	-	56%	54%	95%
Smoking Cessation Advice[1]	1	100%	90%	88%	100%
Heart Failure Care					
ACE Inhibitor or ARB for LVSD[1]	8	88%	81%	82%	100%
Discharge Instructions	43	77%	69%	61%	93%
Evaluation of LVS Function	63	90%	87%	83%	99%
Smoking Cessation Advice[1]	5	100%	84%	82%	100%
Pneumonia Care					
Appropriate Initial Antibiotic	47	83%	83%	83%	94%
Blood Culture Timing	38	87%	90%	90%	100%
Influenza Vaccine[1]	13	92%	74%	70%	100%
Initial Antibiotic Timing	55	96%	84%	80%	93%
Oxygenation Assessment	65	100%	99%	99%	100%
Pneumococcal Vaccine	33	88%	77%	69%	94%
Smoking Cessation Advice[1]	21	100%	81%	80%	100%
Surgical Infection Prevention					
Prophylactic Antibiotic Given	36	44%	76%	77%	95%
Prophylactic Antibiotic Selection[1]	3	100%	92%	90%	100%
Prophylactic Antibiotic Stopped	36	83%	70%	72%	95%
Pregnancy Care					
Inpatient Neonatal Mortality	-	-	-	-	-
Third or Fourth Degree Laceration	-	-	4.02%	3.63%	3.27%

Saint Joseph's Reg Med Ctr-Plymouth Campus

Alternate Name: Saint Joseph's Hospital of Marshall County
1915 Lake Avenue
Plymouth, IN 46563
URL: www.sjmed.com
Ownership: Voluntary non-profit - Church
Emergency Services: No

Phone: 574-936-3181
Fax: 574-935-2250

Accredited: Yes
Licensed Beds: 58

Key Personnel:
CEO. . . . . Lori Price
Chief Medical Staff. . . . . Todd Stillson, MD
Emergency Room . . . . Joan Hum

Measure	Cases	This Hospital	State Average	U.S. Average	Top Hospital
Heart Attack Care					
ACE Inhibitor or ARB for LVSD[1]	5	100%	83%	82%	100%
Aspirin at Arrival	39	100%	91%	92%	100%
Aspirin at Discharge[1]	23	96%	91%	90%	100%
Beta Blocker at Arrival	37	97%	84%	87%	100%
Beta Blocker at Discharge[1]	23	96%	91%	90%	100%
Fibrinolytic Medication Timing[1]	2	0%	44%	31%	100%
PCI Within 90 Minutes of Arrival	0	-	56%	54%	95%
Smoking Cessation Advice[1]	3	100%	90%	88%	100%
Heart Failure Care					
ACE Inhibitor or ARB for LVSD[1]	16	88%	81%	82%	100%
Discharge Instructions	56	73%	69%	61%	93%
Evaluation of LVS Function	79	89%	87%	83%	99%
Smoking Cessation Advice[1]	11	100%	84%	82%	100%
Pneumonia Care					
Appropriate Initial Antibiotic	79	81%	83%	83%	94%
Blood Culture Timing	57	93%	90%	90%	100%
Influenza Vaccine[1]	18	56%	74%	70%	100%
Initial Antibiotic Timing	107	94%	84%	80%	93%
Oxygenation Assessment	143	100%	99%	99%	100%
Pneumococcal Vaccine	97	63%	77%	69%	94%
Smoking Cessation Advice	31	100%	81%	80%	100%
Surgical Infection Prevention					
Prophylactic Antibiotic Given[3]	171	87%	76%	77%	95%
Prophylactic Antibiotic Selection	64	97%	92%	90%	100%
Prophylactic Antibiotic Stopped[3]	168	76%	70%	72%	95%
Pregnancy Care					
Inpatient Neonatal Mortality	411	0.00%	-	-	-
Third or Fourth Degree Laceration	294	2.72%	4.02%	3.63%	3.27%

Gibson General Hospital

1808 Sherman Drive
Princeton, IN 47670
Ownership: Voluntary non-profit - Private
Emergency Services: Yes

Phone: 812-385-3401
Fax: 812-385-9323
Accredited: Yes
Licensed Beds: 109

Key Personnel:
Interim CEO. . . . . Tonya Heim

NOTE: Hospital profiles are in alphabetical order by state, then city, then hospital within the city; Rankings are sorted by rate in descending order and exclude hospitals with less than 25 cases; (1) The number of cases is too small (n<25) for purposes of reliably predicting hospital performance; (2) Measure reflects the hospital's indication that its submission was based upon a sample of its relevant discharges; (3) Rate reflects fewer than the maximum possible quarters of data for the measure; (4) Inaccurate information submitted and suppressed for one or more quarters; (5) No data is available from the hospital for this measure; Please refer to the User's Guide for a full explanation of data

Chief of Medical Staff . . . . Krishna Murthy, MD
Emergency Room . . . . Richard Griffin, Dir

Measure	Cases	This Hospital	State Average	U.S. Average	Top Hospital
Heart Attack Care					
ACE Inhibitor or ARB for LVSD[5]	-	-	83%	82%	100%
Aspirin at Arrival[5]	-	-	91%	92%	100%
Aspirin at Discharge[5]	-	-	91%	90%	100%
Beta Blocker at Arrival[5]	-	-	84%	87%	100%
Beta Blocker at Discharge[5]	-	-	91%	90%	100%
Fibrinolytic Medication Timing[5]	-	-	44%	31%	100%
PCI Within 90 Minutes of Arrival[5]	-	-	56%	54%	95%
Smoking Cessation Advice[5]	-	-	90%	88%	100%
Heart Failure Care					
ACE Inhibitor or ARB for LVSD[1]	13	92%	81%	82%	100%
Discharge Instructions	35	77%	69%	61%	93%
Evaluation of LVS Function	61	90%	87%	83%	99%
Smoking Cessation Advice[1]	5	80%	84%	82%	100%
Pneumonia Care					
Appropriate Initial Antibiotic[1]	24	100%	83%	83%	94%
Blood Culture Timing[1]	23	78%	90%	90%	100%
Influenza Vaccine[1]	10	90%	74%	70%	100%
Initial Antibiotic Timing	32	97%	84%	80%	93%
Oxygenation Assessment	45	100%	99%	99%	100%
Pneumococcal Vaccine	30	83%	77%	69%	94%
Smoking Cessation Advice[1]	14	71%	81%	80%	100%
Surgical Infection Prevention					
Prophylactic Antibiotic Given[5]	-	-	76%	77%	95%
Prophylactic Antibiotic Selection[5]	-	-	92%	90%	100%
Prophylactic Antibiotic Stopped[5]	-	-	70%	72%	95%
Pregnancy Care					
Inpatient Neonatal Mortality	-	-	-	-	-
Third or Fourth Degree Laceration	-	-	4.02%	3.63%	3.27%

Jasper County Hospital

1104 E Grace Street
Rensselaer, IN 47978
URL: www.jchh.com
Ownership: Government - Local
Emergency Services: Yes

Phone: 219-866-5141
Fax: 219-866-3234

Accredited: No
Licensed Beds: 86

Key Personnel:
President/CEO . . . . Tim Schreeg
Chief of Medical Staff . . . . Robert Darnady
Emergency Room . . . . Ramish Daud

Measure	Cases	This Hospital	State Average	U.S. Average	Top Hospital
Heart Attack Care					
ACE Inhibitor or ARB for LVSD[1]	1	100%	83%	82%	100%
Aspirin at Arrival[1]	6	33%	91%	92%	100%
Aspirin at Discharge[1]	2	50%	91%	90%	100%
Beta Blocker at Arrival[1]	8	75%	84%	87%	100%
Beta Blocker at Discharge[1]	2	50%	91%	90%	100%
Fibrinolytic Medication Timing	0	-	44%	31%	100%
PCI Within 90 Minutes of Arrival[5]	-	-	56%	54%	95%
Smoking Cessation Advice	0	-	90%	88%	100%
Heart Failure Care					
ACE Inhibitor or ARB for LVSD[1]	20	30%	81%	82%	100%
Discharge Instructions	37	51%	69%	61%	93%
Evaluation of LVS Function	56	77%	87%	83%	99%
Smoking Cessation Advice[1]	9	78%	84%	82%	100%
Pneumonia Care					
Appropriate Initial Antibiotic	63	44%	83%	83%	94%
Blood Culture Timing[1]	24	96%	90%	90%	100%
Influenza Vaccine[1]	10	70%	74%	70%	100%
Initial Antibiotic Timing	71	73%	84%	80%	93%
Oxygenation Assessment	84	98%	99%	99%	100%
Pneumococcal Vaccine	68	62%	77%	69%	94%
Smoking Cessation Advice[1]	12	8%	81%	80%	100%
Surgical Infection Prevention					
Prophylactic Antibiotic Given[1,3]	2	50%	76%	77%	95%
Prophylactic Antibiotic Selection[1]	2	100%	92%	90%	100%
Prophylactic Antibiotic Stopped[1,3]	2	100%	70%	72%	95%

Measure	Cases	This Hospital	State Average	U.S. Average	Top Hospital
Pregnancy Care					
Inpatient Neonatal Mortality	-	-	-	-	-
Third or Fourth Degree Laceration	-	-	4.02%	3.63%	3.27%

Reid Hospital and Health Care Services

1401 Chester Boulevard
Richmond, IN 47374

Toll-Free: 800-382-7343
Phone: 765-983-3000
Fax: 765-983-3219

URL: www.reidhosp.com
Ownership: Voluntary non-profit - Other
Emergency Services: Yes

Accredited: Yes
Licensed Beds: 233

Key Personnel:
President . . . . Barry S MacDowell
Cardiac Services . . . . Jeanette Sullivan
Cardiac Cath . . . . Brenda McClure
Emergency Room . . . . Michael Baldwin, MD
Emergency Room . . . . Nancy Newman, RN
OB/GYN Womens Health. . . . . M Scott Haswell, MD
Surgical Services . . . . Jackie Stucky
Director Respiratory Therapy . . . . LuAnne Christofaro

Measure	Cases	This Hospital	State Average	U.S. Average	Top Hospital
Heart Attack Care					
ACE Inhibitor or ARB for LVSD	60	98%	83%	82%	100%
Aspirin at Arrival	296	100%	91%	92%	100%
Aspirin at Discharge	287	99%	91%	90%	100%
Beta Blocker at Arrival	217	99%	84%	87%	100%
Beta Blocker at Discharge	321	99%	91%	90%	100%
Fibrinolytic Medication Timing	33	88%	44%	31%	100%
PCI Within 90 Minutes of Arrival[1]	1	100%	56%	54%	95%
Smoking Cessation Advice	114	100%	90%	88%	100%
Heart Failure Care					
ACE Inhibitor or ARB for LVSD	78	100%	81%	82%	100%
Discharge Instructions	299	99%	69%	61%	93%
Evaluation of LVS Function	398	99%	87%	83%	99%
Smoking Cessation Advice	55	100%	84%	82%	100%
Pneumonia Care					
Appropriate Initial Antibiotic	318	94%	83%	83%	94%
Blood Culture Timing	392	98%	90%	90%	100%
Influenza Vaccine	88	98%	74%	70%	100%
Initial Antibiotic Timing	459	94%	84%	80%	93%
Oxygenation Assessment	596	100%	99%	99%	100%
Pneumococcal Vaccine	332	95%	77%	69%	94%
Smoking Cessation Advice	131	100%	81%	80%	100%
Surgical Infection Prevention					
Prophylactic Antibiotic Given[3]	357	96%	76%	77%	95%
Prophylactic Antibiotic Selection	102	96%	92%	90%	100%
Prophylactic Antibiotic Stopped[3]	315	96%	70%	72%	95%
Pregnancy Care					
Inpatient Neonatal Mortality	-	-	-	-	-
Third or Fourth Degree Laceration	-	-	4.02%	3.63%	3.27%

Scott Memorial Hospital

1451 N Gardener
Scottsburg, IN 47170
E-mail: jwells@hsonline.net
Ownership: Government - Local
Emergency Services: Yes

Phone: 812-752-8552
Fax: 812-752-5884

Accredited: Yes
Licensed Beds: 107

Key Personnel:
CEO. . . . . Cariff Nay
Chief Medical Staff . . . . Meera Ummat, MD
Chief Medical Staff . . . . Shane Avery
Emergency Room . . . . John Croasdell, MD
Respiratory Care . . . . Neva Randolph

Measure	Cases	This Hospital	State Average	U.S. Average	Top Hospital
Heart Attack Care					
ACE Inhibitor or ARB for LVSD[1]	5	40%	83%	82%	100%
Aspirin at Arrival[1]	15	73%	91%	92%	100%
Aspirin at Discharge[1]	6	50%	91%	90%	100%
Beta Blocker at Arrival[1]	16	62%	84%	87%	100%
Beta Blocker at Discharge[1]	7	71%	91%	90%	100%
Fibrinolytic Medication Timing[1]	1	100%	44%	31%	100%

NOTE: Hospital profiles are in alphabetical order by state, then city, then hospital within the city; Rankings are sorted by rate in descending order and exclude hospitals with less than 25 cases; (1) The number of cases is too small (n<25) for purposes of reliably predicting hospital performance; (2) Measure reflects the hospital's indication that its submission was based upon a sample of its relevant discharges; (3) Rate reflects fewer than the maximum possible quarters of data for the measure; (4) Inaccurate information submitted and suppressed for one or more quarters; (5) No data is available from the hospital for this measure; Please refer to the User's Guide for a full explanation of data

Measure	Cases	This Hospital	State Average	U.S. Average	Top Hospital
PCI Within 90 Minutes of Arrival[5]	-	-	56%	54%	95%
Smoking Cessation Advice[1]	1	100%	90%	88%	100%
Heart Failure Care					
ACE Inhibitor or ARB for LVSD[1]	21	71%	81%	82%	100%
Discharge Instructions	68	84%	69%	61%	93%
Evaluation of LVS Function	80	61%	87%	83%	99%
Smoking Cessation Advice[1]	20	40%	84%	82%	100%
Pneumonia Care					
Appropriate Initial Antibiotic	118	81%	83%	83%	94%
Blood Culture Timing	61	82%	90%	90%	100%
Influenza Vaccine[1]	20	55%	74%	70%	100%
Initial Antibiotic Timing	112	81%	84%	80%	93%
Oxygenation Assessment	139	100%	99%	99%	100%
Pneumococcal Vaccine	65	63%	77%	69%	94%
Smoking Cessation Advice	47	68%	81%	80%	100%
Surgical Infection Prevention					
Prophylactic Antibiotic Given[5]	-	-	76%	77%	95%
Prophylactic Antibiotic Selection[5]	-	-	92%	90%	100%
Prophylactic Antibiotic Stopped[5]	-	-	70%	72%	95%
Pregnancy Care					
Inpatient Neonatal Mortality	-	-	-	-	-
Third or Fourth Degree Laceration	-	-	4.02%	3.63%	3.27%

Schneck Medical Center

411 W Tipton Street
Seymour, IN 47274
Phone: 812-522-2349
Fax: 812-522-0544
E-mail: info@schneckmed.org
URL: www.schneckmed.org
Ownership: Government - Local
Emergency Services: Yes
Accredited: Yes
Licensed Beds: 166

Key Personnel:

President/CEO. . . . . Gary A Meyer, MHA
Director Infection/Disease Control . . . . Judy Tape

Measure	Cases	This Hospital	State Average	U.S. Average	Top Hospital
Heart Attack Care					
ACE Inhibitor or ARB for LVSD[1]	4	100%	83%	82%	100%
Aspirin at Arrival[1]	17	100%	91%	92%	100%
Aspirin at Discharge[1]	9	100%	91%	90%	100%
Beta Blocker at Arrival[1]	17	100%	84%	87%	100%
Beta Blocker at Discharge[1]	9	100%	91%	90%	100%
Fibrinolytic Medication Timing	0	-	44%	31%	100%
PCI Within 90 Minutes of Arrival	0	-	56%	54%	95%
Smoking Cessation Advice[1]	1	100%	90%	88%	100%
Heart Failure Care					
ACE Inhibitor or ARB for LVSD	31	94%	81%	82%	100%
Discharge Instructions	74	91%	69%	61%	93%
Evaluation of LVS Function	98	93%	87%	83%	99%
Smoking Cessation Advice[1]	15	100%	84%	82%	100%
Pneumonia Care					
Appropriate Initial Antibiotic	128	86%	83%	83%	94%
Blood Culture Timing	100	96%	90%	90%	100%
Influenza Vaccine[4,5]	-	-	74%	70%	100%
Initial Antibiotic Timing	156	89%	84%	80%	93%
Oxygenation Assessment	199	98%	99%	99%	100%
Pneumococcal Vaccine	125	99%	77%	69%	94%
Smoking Cessation Advice	40	95%	81%	80%	100%
Surgical Infection Prevention					
Prophylactic Antibiotic Given	202	93%	76%	77%	95%
Prophylactic Antibiotic Selection	41	98%	92%	90%	100%
Prophylactic Antibiotic Stopped	186	92%	70%	72%	95%
Pregnancy Care					
Inpatient Neonatal Mortality	-	-	-	-	-
Third or Fourth Degree Laceration	-	-	4.02%	3.63%	3.27%

Major Hospital

150 W Washington Street
Shelbyville, IN 46176
Phone: 317-392-3211
Fax: 317-398-5253
E-mail: info@majorhospital.com
URL: www.majorhospital.com
Ownership: Government - Local
Emergency Services: Yes
Accredited: Yes
Licensed Beds: 89

Key Personnel:

President/CEO. . . . . Anthony B Lennen
Chief Medical Staff. . . . . Ed Stone, MD
Emergency Room . . . . David Moser, MD
Director Infection/Disease Control . . . . Candy Oliger
OB/GYN Womens Health. . . . . Lloyd Lewis, Jr, MD
Director Respiratory Therapy . . . . Linda Burke

Measure	Cases	This Hospital	State Average	U.S. Average	Top Hospital
Heart Attack Care					
ACE Inhibitor or ARB for LVSD[1]	2	100%	83%	82%	100%
Aspirin at Arrival[1]	13	100%	91%	92%	100%
Aspirin at Discharge[1]	9	100%	91%	90%	100%
Beta Blocker at Arrival[1]	11	100%	84%	87%	100%
Beta Blocker at Discharge[1]	6	100%	91%	90%	100%
Fibrinolytic Medication Timing[3]	0	-	44%	31%	100%
PCI Within 90 Minutes of Arrival	0	-	56%	54%	95%
Smoking Cessation Advice	0	-	90%	88%	100%
Heart Failure Care					
ACE Inhibitor or ARB for LVSD	31	94%	81%	82%	100%
Discharge Instructions	67	84%	69%	61%	93%
Evaluation of LVS Function	87	100%	87%	83%	99%
Smoking Cessation Advice[1]	10	100%	84%	82%	100%
Pneumonia Care					
Appropriate Initial Antibiotic	117	94%	83%	83%	94%
Blood Culture Timing	106	93%	90%	90%	100%
Influenza Vaccine	37	81%	74%	70%	100%
Initial Antibiotic Timing	183	89%	84%	80%	93%
Oxygenation Assessment	204	99%	99%	99%	100%
Pneumococcal Vaccine	137	88%	77%	69%	94%
Smoking Cessation Advice	55	84%	81%	80%	100%
Surgical Infection Prevention					
Prophylactic Antibiotic Given	92	87%	76%	77%	95%
Prophylactic Antibiotic Selection[1]	17	100%	92%	90%	100%
Prophylactic Antibiotic Stopped	89	49%	70%	72%	95%
Pregnancy Care					
Inpatient Neonatal Mortality	-	-	-	-	-
Third or Fourth Degree Laceration	-	-	4.02%	3.63%	3.27%

Memorial Hospital of South Bend

615 N Michigan Street
South Bend, IN 46601
Phone: 574-647-1000
Fax: 574-647-3670
E-mail: ltatum@memorialsb.org
URL: www.qualityoflife.org
Ownership: Voluntary non-profit - Other
Emergency Services: Yes
Accredited: Yes
Licensed Beds: 526

Key Personnel:

Administrator/President . . . . Philip A Newbold
Chief Medical Staff. . . . . John Mathis, MD
Emergency Room . . . . Bev Teegarden
Director Infection/Disease Control . . . . Susan Kraska
CCU Spvg. Nurse . . . . Connie McCahill
VP Medical & Surgical Nursing. . . . . Connie McCahill
OB/GYN Womens Health. . . . . Carlton Lyons, MD
Chief Radiology . . . . Gerard DuPrat, MD
Director Respiratory Therapy . . . . Patricia Wise

Measure	Cases	This Hospital	State Average	U.S. Average	Top Hospital
Heart Attack Care					
ACE Inhibitor or ARB for LVSD	54	70%	83%	82%	100%
Aspirin at Arrival	234	97%	91%	92%	100%
Aspirin at Discharge	245	96%	91%	90%	100%
Beta Blocker at Arrival	152	91%	84%	87%	100%
Beta Blocker at Discharge	265	94%	91%	90%	100%
Fibrinolytic Medication Timing	0	-	44%	31%	100%
PCI Within 90 Minutes of Arrival[1]	12	75%	56%	54%	95%

NOTE: Hospital profiles are in alphabetical order by state, then city, then hospital within the city; Rankings are sorted by rate in descending order and exclude hospitals with less than 25 cases; (1) The number of cases is too small (n<25) for purposes of reliably predicting hospital performance; (2) Measure reflects the hospital's indication that its submission was based upon a sample of its relevant discharges; (3) Rate reflects fewer than the maximum possible quarters of data for the measure; (4) Inaccurate information submitted and suppressed for one or more quarters; (5) No data is available from the hospital for this measure; Please refer to the User's Guide for a full explanation of data

Smoking Cessation Advice	111	82%	90%	88%	100%
Heart Failure Care					
ACE Inhibitor or ARB for LVSD	169	86%	81%	82%	100%
Discharge Instructions	384	78%	69%	61%	93%
Evaluation of LVS Function	459	96%	87%	83%	99%
Smoking Cessation Advice	113	86%	84%	82%	100%
Pneumonia Care					
Appropriate Initial Antibiotic	230	89%	83%	83%	94%
Blood Culture Timing	212	88%	90%	90%	100%
Influenza Vaccine	65	77%	74%	70%	100%
Initial Antibiotic Timing	313	73%	84%	80%	93%
Oxygenation Assessment	407	100%	99%	99%	100%
Pneumococcal Vaccine	256	89%	77%	69%	94%
Smoking Cessation Advice	78	62%	81%	80%	100%
Surgical Infection Prevention					
Prophylactic Antibiotic Given[3]	519	82%	76%	77%	95%
Prophylactic Antibiotic Selection	172	98%	92%	90%	100%
Prophylactic Antibiotic Stopped[3]	487	86%	70%	72%	95%
Pregnancy Care					
Inpatient Neonatal Mortality	-	-	-	-	-
Third or Fourth Degree Laceration	-	-	4.02%	3.63%	3.27%

Saint Joseph's Regional Medical Center

801 E LaSalle Avenue
South Bend, IN 46617
URL: www.sjmed.com
Phone: 574-237-7111
Fax: 574-237-7077
Ownership: Voluntary non-profit - Other
Accredited: Yes
Emergency Services: Yes
Licensed Beds: 339

Key Personnel:

President/CEO . . . . Robert Beyer
Administrator/COO. . . . . J Thomas Hardy, DO
Chief Medical Staff. . . . . Daniel Scherb, MD
Chief Catheterization Laboratory . . . . Donald Westerhausen, MD
Emergency Room . . . . Jennifer Lackman, MD
Director Infection/Disease Control . . . . Chris Costello
CCU Spvg. Nurse . . . . Monica Cates
Director Medical/Surgical Nursing . . . . Carol Norris
OB/GYN Womens Health. . . . . Mark Lewis, DO
Chief Radiology . . . . Michael McCrea

Measure	Cases	This Hospital	State Average	U.S. Average	Top Hospital
Heart Attack Care					
ACE Inhibitor or ARB for LVSD[1]	21	86%	83%	82%	100%
Aspirin at Arrival	164	97%	91%	92%	100%
Aspirin at Discharge	221	99%	91%	90%	100%
Beta Blocker at Arrival	85	98%	84%	87%	100%
Beta Blocker at Discharge	194	96%	91%	90%	100%
Fibrinolytic Medication Timing	0	-	44%	31%	100%
PCI Within 90 Minutes of Arrival[1]	11	73%	56%	54%	95%
Smoking Cessation Advice	97	96%	90%	88%	100%
Heart Failure Care					
ACE Inhibitor or ARB for LVSD	121	87%	81%	82%	100%
Discharge Instructions	293	85%	69%	61%	93%
Evaluation of LVS Function	378	97%	87%	83%	99%
Smoking Cessation Advice	60	95%	84%	82%	100%
Pneumonia Care					
Appropriate Initial Antibiotic	143	90%	83%	83%	94%
Blood Culture Timing	141	97%	90%	90%	100%
Influenza Vaccine	44	89%	74%	70%	100%
Initial Antibiotic Timing	222	83%	84%	80%	93%
Oxygenation Assessment	269	100%	99%	99%	100%
Pneumococcal Vaccine	168	83%	77%	69%	94%
Smoking Cessation Advice	52	75%	81%	80%	100%
Surgical Infection Prevention					
Prophylactic Antibiotic Given[3]	925	91%	76%	77%	95%
Prophylactic Antibiotic Selection	309	99%	92%	90%	100%
Prophylactic Antibiotic Stopped[3]	897	92%	70%	72%	95%
Pregnancy Care					
Inpatient Neonatal Mortality	1,206	1.08%	-	-	-
Third or Fourth Degree Laceration	845	2.60%	4.02%	3.63%	3.27%

Sullivan County Community Hospital

Alternate Name: Mary Sherman Hospital
2200 N Section Street
PO Box 10
Sullivan, IN 47882
Phone: 812-268-4311
Fax: 812-268-2570
E-mail: denisebrashear@schosp.com
URL: www.schosp.com
Ownership: Voluntary non-profit - Other
Accredited: Yes
Emergency Services: Yes

Key Personnel:

President/CEO . . . . Michelle Sly-Smith
Chief Medical Staff. . . . . Gene Bourgasser, MD
Emergency Room . . . . Jeanna Lusman, RN
Infection Control. . . . . Marti Bradbury, RN
ICU . . . . Marian Bynum, RN
OB/GYN/Women's Health . . . . Rebecca Norris, RN
Respiratory/Cardiopulmonary. . . . . Susan Mikiskia

Measure	Cases	This Hospital	State Average	U.S. Average	Top Hospital
Heart Attack Care					
ACE Inhibitor or ARB for LVSD[1]	2	100%	83%	82%	100%
Aspirin at Arrival[1]	15	73%	91%	92%	100%
Aspirin at Discharge[1]	9	89%	91%	90%	100%
Beta Blocker at Arrival[1]	16	75%	84%	87%	100%
Beta Blocker at Discharge[1]	8	88%	91%	90%	100%
Fibrinolytic Medication Timing	0	-	44%	31%	100%
PCI Within 90 Minutes of Arrival	0	-	56%	54%	95%
Smoking Cessation Advice[1]	2	100%	90%	88%	100%
Heart Failure Care					
ACE Inhibitor or ARB for LVSD[1]	13	62%	81%	82%	100%
Discharge Instructions	33	45%	69%	61%	93%
Evaluation of LVS Function	48	50%	87%	83%	99%
Smoking Cessation Advice[1]	14	79%	84%	82%	100%
Pneumonia Care					
Appropriate Initial Antibiotic	59	80%	83%	83%	94%
Blood Culture Timing	44	91%	90%	90%	100%
Influenza Vaccine[1]	18	72%	74%	70%	100%
Initial Antibiotic Timing	78	88%	84%	80%	93%
Oxygenation Assessment	84	100%	99%	99%	100%
Pneumococcal Vaccine	53	85%	77%	69%	94%
Smoking Cessation Advice[1]	20	70%	81%	80%	100%
Surgical Infection Prevention					
Prophylactic Antibiotic Given[1]	24	92%	76%	77%	95%
Prophylactic Antibiotic Selection[1]	9	100%	92%	90%	100%
Prophylactic Antibiotic Stopped[1]	24	67%	70%	72%	95%
Pregnancy Care					
Inpatient Neonatal Mortality	-	-	-	-	-
Third or Fourth Degree Laceration	-	-	4.02%	3.63%	3.27%

Terre Haute Regional Hospital

3901 S 7th Street
Terre Haute, IN 47802
Toll-Free: 800-678-8474
Phone: 812-232-0021
Fax: 812-237-9514
Ownership: Proprietary
Accredited: Yes
Emergency Services: No
Licensed Beds: 278

Key Personnel:

CEO. . . . . Ken Hutchenrider
Catheterization Lab . . . . Joe Hansel
Emergency Room . . . . Julie VanOven
Infection Control. . . . . Kathy Hand
Intensive Coronary Care . . . . Deb Girton
Medical Surgical Nursing . . . . John Williams
OB/GYN Womens Health. . . . . Michelle Farris

Measure	Cases	This Hospital	State Average	U.S. Average	Top Hospital
Heart Attack Care					
ACE Inhibitor or ARB for LVSD	54	81%	83%	82%	100%
Aspirin at Arrival	96	97%	91%	92%	100%
Aspirin at Discharge	181	97%	91%	90%	100%
Beta Blocker at Arrival	72	86%	84%	87%	100%
Beta Blocker at Discharge	182	98%	91%	90%	100%
Fibrinolytic Medication Timing	0	-	44%	31%	100%
PCI Within 90 Minutes of Arrival[1]	4	0%	56%	54%	95%

NOTE: Hospital profiles are in alphabetical order by state, then city, then hospital within the city; Rankings are sorted by rate in descending order and exclude hospitals with less than 25 cases; (1) The number of cases is too small (n<25) for purposes of reliably predicting hospital performance; (2) Measure reflects the hospital's indication that its submission was based upon a sample of its relevant discharges; (3) Rate reflects fewer than the maximum possible quarters of data for the measure; (4) Inaccurate information submitted and suppressed for one or more quarters; (5) No data is available from the hospital for this measure; Please refer to the User's Guide for a full explanation of data

Smoking Cessation Advice	80	100%	90%	88%	100%
Heart Failure Care					
ACE Inhibitor or ARB for LVSD	141	72%	81%	82%	100%
Discharge Instructions	320	68%	69%	61%	93%
Evaluation of LVS Function	377	86%	87%	83%	99%
Smoking Cessation Advice	85	100%	84%	82%	100%
Pneumonia Care					
Appropriate Initial Antibiotic	97	79%	83%	83%	94%
Blood Culture Timing	94	97%	90%	90%	100%
Influenza Vaccine	30	77%	74%	70%	100%
Initial Antibiotic Timing	174	80%	84%	80%	93%
Oxygenation Assessment	200	100%	99%	99%	100%
Pneumococcal Vaccine	130	72%	77%	69%	94%
Smoking Cessation Advice	73	100%	81%	80%	100%
Surgical Infection Prevention					
Prophylactic Antibiotic Given[2,3]	188	87%	76%	77%	95%
Prophylactic Antibiotic Selection[2]	80	85%	92%	90%	100%
Prophylactic Antibiotic Stopped[2,3]	185	43%	70%	72%	95%
Pregnancy Care					
Inpatient Neonatal Mortality	-	-	-	-	-
Third or Fourth Degree Laceration	-	-	4.02%	3.63%	3.27%

Union Hospital

1606 North 7th Street
Terre Haute, IN 47804
Phone: 812-238-7000
Ownership: Voluntary non-profit - Other
Accredited: Yes
Emergency Services: Yes

Measure	Cases	This Hospital	State Average	U.S. Average	Top Hospital
Heart Attack Care					
ACE Inhibitor or ARB for LVSD[2]	86	91%	83%	82%	100%
Aspirin at Arrival[2]	228	97%	91%	92%	100%
Aspirin at Discharge[2]	259	94%	91%	90%	100%
Beta Blocker at Arrival[2]	177	94%	84%	87%	100%
Beta Blocker at Discharge[2]	293	96%	91%	90%	100%
Fibrinolytic Medication Timing[1,2]	2	0%	44%	31%	100%
PCI Within 90 Minutes of Arrival[1,2]	5	20%	56%	54%	95%
Smoking Cessation Advice[2]	103	98%	90%	88%	100%
Heart Failure Care					
ACE Inhibitor or ARB for LVSD[2]	145	88%	81%	82%	100%
Discharge Instructions[2]	332	95%	69%	61%	93%
Evaluation of LVS Function[2]	405	97%	87%	83%	99%
Smoking Cessation Advice[2]	47	96%	84%	82%	100%
Pneumonia Care					
Appropriate Initial Antibiotic[2]	199	83%	83%	83%	94%
Blood Culture Timing[2]	148	96%	90%	90%	100%
Influenza Vaccine	48	88%	74%	70%	100%
Initial Antibiotic Timing[2]	284	89%	84%	80%	93%
Oxygenation Assessment[2]	339	100%	99%	99%	100%
Pneumococcal Vaccine[2]	203	92%	77%	69%	94%
Smoking Cessation Advice[2]	98	99%	81%	80%	100%
Surgical Infection Prevention					
Prophylactic Antibiotic Given	854	87%	76%	77%	95%
Prophylactic Antibiotic Selection	212	95%	92%	90%	100%
Prophylactic Antibiotic Stopped	809	67%	70%	72%	95%
Pregnancy Care					
Inpatient Neonatal Mortality	-	-	-	-	-
Third or Fourth Degree Laceration	-	-	4.02%	3.63%	3.27%

Tipton Hospital

1000 S Main Street
Tipton, IN 46072
Phone: 765-675-8500
Fax: 765-675-8222
URL: www.tiptonhospital.org
Ownership: Government - Local
Accredited: Yes
Emergency Services: Yes
Licensed Beds: 102

Key Personnel:

President/CEO . . . . Michael L Harlowe, CHE
Emergency Room . . . . Jo Ellen Scott
Director Infection/Disease Control . . . . Trina Delph
CCU Spvg. Nurse . . . . JoEllen Scott
Director Medical/Surgical Nursing . . . . Teresa Burns
Director Respiratory Therapy . . . . Pamela Melander

Measure	Cases	This Hospital	State Average	U.S. Average	Top Hospital
Heart Attack Care					
ACE Inhibitor or ARB for LVSD[1]	1	100%	83%	82%	100%
Aspirin at Arrival[1]	3	100%	91%	92%	100%
Aspirin at Discharge[1]	1	100%	91%	90%	100%
Beta Blocker at Arrival[1]	4	75%	84%	87%	100%
Beta Blocker at Discharge[1]	2	100%	91%	90%	100%
Fibrinolytic Medication Timing	0	-	44%	31%	100%
PCI Within 90 Minutes of Arrival	0	-	56%	54%	95%
Smoking Cessation Advice	0	-	90%	88%	100%
Heart Failure Care					
ACE Inhibitor or ARB for LVSD[1]	15	87%	81%	82%	100%
Discharge Instructions	37	78%	69%	61%	93%
Evaluation of LVS Function	46	91%	87%	83%	99%
Smoking Cessation Advice[1]	8	88%	84%	82%	100%
Pneumonia Care					
Appropriate Initial Antibiotic	48	54%	83%	83%	94%
Blood Culture Timing[1]	19	89%	90%	90%	100%
Influenza Vaccine[1]	8	75%	74%	70%	100%
Initial Antibiotic Timing	57	75%	84%	80%	93%
Oxygenation Assessment	65	100%	99%	99%	100%
Pneumococcal Vaccine	43	58%	77%	69%	94%
Smoking Cessation Advice[1]	15	80%	81%	80%	100%
Surgical Infection Prevention					
Prophylactic Antibiotic Given[1,3]	18	28%	76%	77%	95%
Prophylactic Antibiotic Selection[1]	18	56%	92%	90%	100%
Prophylactic Antibiotic Stopped[1,3]	18	78%	70%	72%	95%
Pregnancy Care					
Inpatient Neonatal Mortality	-	-	-	-	-
Third or Fourth Degree Laceration	-	-	4.02%	3.63%	3.27%

Porter Memorial Health System

814 La Porte Avenue
Valparaiso, IN 46383
Phone: 219-463-4600
Fax: 219-463-4882
URL: www.portermemorial.org
Ownership: Voluntary non-profit - Private
Accredited: Yes
Emergency Services: Yes
Licensed Beds: 402

Key Personnel:

President/CEO . . . . Ronald C Winger
Emergency Room . . . . John Johnson, MD
Director Infection/Disease Control . . . . Julie Downey, RN
CCU Spvg. Nurse . . . . Kaaren Erdelles, RN
Chief Medical Officer . . . . Ramireddy Tummuru, MD
OB/GYN Womens Health. . . . . Frank Sturdevant
Chief Radiology . . . . Anil Kothari, MD
Director Respiratory Therapy . . . . Dennis Kniat

Measure	Cases	This Hospital	State Average	U.S. Average	Top Hospital
Heart Attack Care					
ACE Inhibitor or ARB for LVSD	46	83%	83%	82%	100%
Aspirin at Arrival	173	96%	91%	92%	100%
Aspirin at Discharge	179	97%	91%	90%	100%
Beta Blocker at Arrival	114	88%	84%	87%	100%
Beta Blocker at Discharge	176	97%	91%	90%	100%
Fibrinolytic Medication Timing[3]	0	-	44%	31%	100%
PCI Within 90 Minutes of Arrival[1]	10	70%	56%	54%	95%
Smoking Cessation Advice[1,3]	24	100%	90%	88%	100%
Heart Failure Care					
ACE Inhibitor or ARB for LVSD	172	98%	81%	82%	100%
Discharge Instructions[3]	79	94%	69%	61%	93%
Evaluation of LVS Function	426	100%	87%	83%	99%
Smoking Cessation Advice[1,3]	22	100%	84%	82%	100%
Pneumonia Care					
Appropriate Initial Antibiotic[3]	38	89%	83%	83%	94%
Blood Culture Timing[3]	49	92%	90%	90%	100%
Influenza Vaccine[5]	-	-	74%	70%	100%
Initial Antibiotic Timing	324	79%	84%	80%	93%
Oxygenation Assessment	379	100%	99%	99%	100%
Pneumococcal Vaccine	277	60%	77%	69%	94%
Smoking Cessation Advice[1,3]	23	61%	81%	80%	100%
Surgical Infection Prevention					
Prophylactic Antibiotic Given[3]	66	67%	76%	77%	95%

NOTE: Hospital profiles are in alphabetical order by state, then city, then hospital within the city; Rankings are sorted by rate in descending order and exclude hospitals with less than 25 cases; (1) The number of cases is too small (n<25) for purposes of reliably predicting hospital performance; (2) Measure reflects the hospital's indication that its submission was based upon a sample of its relevant discharges; (3) Rate reflects fewer than the maximum possible quarters of data for the measure; (4) Inaccurate information submitted and suppressed for one or more quarters; (5) No data is available from the hospital for this measure; Please refer to the User's Guide for a full explanation of data

Prophylactic Antibiotic Selection[5]	-	-	92%	90%	100%
Prophylactic Antibiotic Stopped[3]	61	66%	70%	72%	95%
Pregnancy Care					
Inpatient Neonatal Mortality	1,390	0.14%	-	-	-
Third or Fourth Degree Laceration	936	3.63%	4.02%	3.63%	3.27%

Good Samaritan Hospital

520 S 7th Street
Vincennes, IN 47591
URL: www,gshvin.org
Ownership: Government - Local
Emergency Services: Yes

Phone: 812-882-5220
Fax: 812-885-3961

Accredited: Yes
Licensed Beds: 271

Key Personnel:

President/CEO . . . . . Matthew D. Bailey
Chief Medical Staff . . . . . Charles Hedde, MD
Emergency Room . . . . . Thomas Dagney
Infection Control . . . . . Robin Riley
Director Medical/Surgical Nursing . . . . . Sandra Haggart
OB/GYN Womens Health . . . . . Joseph Mohammed, MD
Surgical Services . . . . . Debra Brand
Director of Respiratory Therapy . . . . . Janet Sievers

Measure	Cases	This Hospital	State Average	U.S. Average	Top Hospital
Heart Attack Care					
ACE Inhibitor or ARB for LVSD	50	96%	83%	82%	100%
Aspirin at Arrival	127	93%	91%	92%	100%
Aspirin at Discharge	152	99%	91%	90%	100%
Beta Blocker at Arrival	98	88%	84%	87%	100%
Beta Blocker at Discharge	152	97%	91%	90%	100%
Fibrinolytic Medication Timing	0	-	44%	31%	100%
PCI Within 90 Minutes of Arrival[1]	7	29%	56%	54%	95%
Smoking Cessation Advice	62	100%	90%	88%	100%
Heart Failure Care					
ACE Inhibitor or ARB for LVSD	109	90%	81%	82%	100%
Discharge Instructions	235	79%	69%	61%	93%
Evaluation of LVS Function	307	88%	87%	83%	99%
Smoking Cessation Advice	37	73%	84%	82%	100%
Pneumonia Care					
Appropriate Initial Antibiotic	99	67%	83%	83%	94%
Blood Culture Timing	74	89%	90%	90%	100%
Influenza Vaccine	33	70%	74%	70%	100%
Initial Antibiotic Timing	136	86%	84%	80%	93%
Oxygenation Assessment	187	99%	99%	99%	100%
Pneumococcal Vaccine	129	75%	77%	69%	94%
Smoking Cessation Advice	42	69%	81%	80%	100%
Surgical Infection Prevention					
Prophylactic Antibiotic Given[3]	514	63%	76%	77%	95%
Prophylactic Antibiotic Selection	164	87%	92%	90%	100%
Prophylactic Antibiotic Stopped[3]	502	76%	70%	72%	95%
Pregnancy Care					
Inpatient Neonatal Mortality	-	-	-	-	-
Third or Fourth Degree Laceration	-	-	4.02%	3.63%	3.27%

Wabash County Hospital

710 N E Street
Wabash, IN 46992

Toll-Free: 800-346-2110
Phone: 260-563-3131
Fax: 260-569-2410

URL: www.wchospital.com
Ownership: Government - Local
Emergency Services: Yes

Accredited: Yes
Licensed Beds: 25

Key Personnel:

Administrator/CEO . . . . . David C Hunter
Emergency Room . . . . . Jonathan Grandstaff-Dunp
Director Infection/Disease Control . . . . . Mike Vogel, RN
CCU Spvg. Nurse . . . . . Sandy Wright, RN
Director Medical/Surgical Nursing . . . . . Sandy Wright, RN
Chief Radiology . . . . . Mike Saint, RT
Director Respiratory Therapy . . . . . Pam Smith, RN

Measure	Cases	This Hospital	State Average	U.S. Average	Top Hospital
Heart Attack Care					
ACE Inhibitor or ARB for LVSD[3]	0	-	83%	82%	100%
Aspirin at Arrival[1,3]	2	50%	91%	92%	100%
Aspirin at Discharge[1,3]	2	100%	91%	90%	100%
Beta Blocker at Arrival[1,3]	2	50%	84%	87%	100%
Beta Blocker at Discharge[1,3]	2	100%	91%	90%	100%
Fibrinolytic Medication Timing[3]	0	-	44%	31%	100%
PCI Within 90 Minutes of Arrival[5]	-	-	56%	54%	95%
Smoking Cessation Advice[3]	0	-	90%	88%	100%
Heart Failure Care					
ACE Inhibitor or ARB for LVSD[1]	8	75%	81%	82%	100%
Discharge Instructions[1]	16	88%	69%	61%	93%
Evaluation of LVS Function	30	83%	87%	83%	99%
Smoking Cessation Advice[1]	1	100%	84%	82%	100%
Pneumonia Care					
Appropriate Initial Antibiotic	52	81%	83%	83%	94%
Blood Culture Timing	31	84%	90%	90%	100%
Influenza Vaccine[1]	7	100%	74%	70%	100%
Initial Antibiotic Timing	57	95%	84%	80%	93%
Oxygenation Assessment	66	100%	99%	99%	100%
Pneumococcal Vaccine	40	88%	77%	69%	94%
Smoking Cessation Advice[1]	19	100%	81%	80%	100%
Surgical Infection Prevention					
Prophylactic Antibiotic Given[5]	-	-	76%	77%	95%
Prophylactic Antibiotic Selection[5]	-	-	92%	90%	100%
Prophylactic Antibiotic Stopped[5]	-	-	70%	72%	95%
Pregnancy Care					
Inpatient Neonatal Mortality	-	-	-	-	-
Third or Fourth Degree Laceration	-	-	4.02%	3.63%	3.27%

Kosciusko Community Hospital

2101 E Dubois Drive
Warsaw, IN 46580

Toll-Free: 800-828-5628
Phone: 574-267-3200
Fax: 574-372-7816

URL: www.kch.com
Ownership: Proprietary
Emergency Services: Yes

Accredited: Yes
Licensed Beds: 72

Key Personnel:

CEO . . . . . Jerry Beasley
Chief Medical Staff . . . . . Gregory Haase, DO
Emergency Room . . . . . Linda Law, MD
Director Infection/Disease Control . . . . . Thomas Kocoshis, MD
Director Medical/Surgical Nursing . . . . . Sandy Rader, RN
Director Radiology . . . . . Steph Damon

Measure	Cases	This Hospital	State Average	U.S. Average	Top Hospital
Heart Attack Care					
ACE Inhibitor or ARB for LVSD[1]	3	100%	83%	82%	100%
Aspirin at Arrival	38	97%	91%	92%	100%
Aspirin at Discharge[1]	21	100%	91%	90%	100%
Beta Blocker at Arrival[1]	24	100%	84%	87%	100%
Beta Blocker at Discharge[1]	17	100%	91%	90%	100%
Fibrinolytic Medication Timing	0	-	44%	31%	100%
PCI Within 90 Minutes of Arrival	0	-	56%	54%	95%
Smoking Cessation Advice[1]	2	100%	90%	88%	100%
Heart Failure Care					
ACE Inhibitor or ARB for LVSD	32	94%	81%	82%	100%
Discharge Instructions	68	90%	69%	61%	93%
Evaluation of LVS Function	99	99%	87%	83%	99%
Smoking Cessation Advice[1]	7	100%	84%	82%	100%
Pneumonia Care					
Appropriate Initial Antibiotic	121	92%	83%	83%	94%
Blood Culture Timing	121	94%	90%	90%	100%
Influenza Vaccine	31	90%	74%	70%	100%
Initial Antibiotic Timing	141	93%	84%	80%	93%
Oxygenation Assessment	177	100%	99%	99%	100%
Pneumococcal Vaccine	108	96%	77%	69%	94%
Smoking Cessation Advice	50	100%	81%	80%	100%
Surgical Infection Prevention					
Prophylactic Antibiotic Given	239	92%	76%	77%	95%
Prophylactic Antibiotic Selection	70	94%	92%	90%	100%
Prophylactic Antibiotic Stopped	238	74%	70%	72%	95%
Pregnancy Care					
Inpatient Neonatal Mortality	-	-	-	-	-
Third or Fourth Degree Laceration	-	-	4.02%	3.63%	3.27%

NOTE: Hospital profiles are in alphabetical order by state, then city, then hospital within the city; Rankings are sorted by rate in descending order and exclude hospitals with less than 25 cases; (1) The number of cases is too small (n<25) for purposes of reliably predicting hospital performance; (2) Measure reflects the hospital's indication that its submission was based upon a sample of its relevant discharges; (3) Rate reflects fewer than the maximum possible quarters of data for the measure; (4) Inaccurate information submitted and suppressed for one or more quarters; (5) No data is available from the hospital for this measure; Please refer to the User's Guide for a full explanation of data

Daviess Community Hospital

1314 E Walnut St
Washington, IN 47501
E-mail: msmith@dchosp.org
URL: www.dchosp.org
Ownership: Government - Local
Emergency Services: Yes

Phone: 812-254-2760
Fax: 812-254-8897

Accredited: Yes
Licensed Beds: 120

Key Personnel:

CEO. . . . . Robert J Heckert
Chief Medical Staff. . . . . James Filler
Director Cardiology . . . . Phillip Dawkins, MD
Emergency Room . . . . Tina Dumil
Director Infection/Disease Control . . . . Carol Matteson
Director Medical/Surgical Nursing . . . . Konnie Ball
Director Radiology . . . . E M Cha, MD
Director Respiratory Therapy . . . . Val Roark

Measure	Cases	This Hospital	State Average	U.S. Average	Top Hospital
Heart Attack Care					
ACE Inhibitor or ARB for LVSD[1]	9	67%	83%	82%	100%
Aspirin at Arrival[1]	23	96%	91%	92%	100%
Aspirin at Discharge[1]	15	93%	91%	90%	100%
Beta Blocker at Arrival[1]	22	91%	84%	87%	100%
Beta Blocker at Discharge[1]	14	93%	91%	90%	100%
Fibrinolytic Medication Timing	0	-	44%	31%	100%
PCI Within 90 Minutes of Arrival	0	-	56%	54%	95%
Smoking Cessation Advice[1]	1	100%	90%	88%	100%
Heart Failure Care					
ACE Inhibitor or ARB for LVSD	34	53%	81%	82%	100%
Discharge Instructions	44	11%	69%	61%	93%
Evaluation of LVS Function	62	84%	87%	83%	99%
Smoking Cessation Advice[1]	7	86%	84%	82%	100%
Pneumonia Care					
Appropriate Initial Antibiotic	142	86%	83%	83%	94%
Blood Culture Timing	125	86%	90%	90%	100%
Influenza Vaccine	32	53%	74%	70%	100%
Initial Antibiotic Timing	155	92%	84%	80%	93%
Oxygenation Assessment	206	100%	99%	99%	100%
Pneumococcal Vaccine	123	67%	77%	69%	94%
Smoking Cessation Advice	40	75%	81%	80%	100%
Surgical Infection Prevention					
Prophylactic Antibiotic Given[3]	30	83%	76%	77%	95%
Prophylactic Antibiotic Selection	30	100%	92%	90%	100%
Prophylactic Antibiotic Stopped[3]	30	67%	70%	72%	95%
Pregnancy Care					
Inpatient Neonatal Mortality	402	0.00%	-	-	-
Third or Fourth Degree Laceration	303	3.63%	4.02%	3.63%	3.27%

Saint Vincent Williamsport

Alternate Name: Community Hospital
412 N Monroe Street
Williamsport, IN 47993
URL: www.stvincent.org
Ownership: Voluntary non-profit - Church
Emergency Services: Yes

Phone: 765-762-4000
Fax: 765-762-4126

Accredited: Yes
Licensed Beds: 16

Key Personnel:

Chief Medical Staff. . . . . Dr. Tahir Hafeez
Emergency Room . . . . H Brenner, MD

Measure	Cases	This Hospital	State Average	U.S. Average	Top Hospital
Heart Attack Care					
ACE Inhibitor or ARB for LVSD[1,3]	4	25%	83%	82%	100%
Aspirin at Arrival[1,3]	10	60%	91%	92%	100%
Aspirin at Discharge[1,3]	7	71%	91%	90%	100%
Beta Blocker at Arrival[1,3]	11	55%	84%	87%	100%
Beta Blocker at Discharge[1,3]	8	75%	91%	90%	100%
Fibrinolytic Medication Timing[5]	-	-	44%	31%	100%
PCI Within 90 Minutes of Arrival[5]	-	-	56%	54%	95%
Smoking Cessation Advice[3]	0	-	90%	88%	100%
Heart Failure Care					
ACE Inhibitor or ARB for LVSD[1]	15	93%	81%	82%	100%
Discharge Instructions	35	100%	69%	61%	93%
Evaluation of LVS Function	55	95%	87%	83%	99%
Smoking Cessation Advice[1]	8	88%	84%	82%	100%
Pneumonia Care					
Appropriate Initial Antibiotic	40	80%	83%	83%	94%
Blood Culture Timing[1]	13	77%	90%	90%	100%
Influenza Vaccine[1]	7	86%	74%	70%	100%
Initial Antibiotic Timing	50	80%	84%	80%	93%
Oxygenation Assessment	66	100%	99%	99%	100%
Pneumococcal Vaccine	36	64%	77%	69%	94%
Smoking Cessation Advice[1]	22	91%	81%	80%	100%
Surgical Infection Prevention					
Prophylactic Antibiotic Given[1,3]	1	0%	76%	77%	95%
Prophylactic Antibiotic Selection[1]	1	100%	92%	90%	100%
Prophylactic Antibiotic Stopped[1,3]	1	0%	70%	72%	95%
Pregnancy Care					
Inpatient Neonatal Mortality	-	-	-	-	-
Third or Fourth Degree Laceration	-	-	4.02%	3.63%	3.27%

NOTE: Hospital profiles are in alphabetical order by state, then city, then hospital within the city; Rankings are sorted by rate in descending order and exclude hospitals with less than 25 cases; (1) The number of cases is too small (n<25) for purposes of reliably predicting hospital performance; (2) Measure reflects the hospital's indication that its submission was based upon a sample of its relevant discharges; (3) Rate reflects fewer than the maximum possible quarters of data for the measure; (4) Inaccurate information submitted and suppressed for one or more quarters; (5) No data is available from the hospital for this measure; Please refer to the User's Guide for a full explanation of data

Heart Attack Care

1. ACE Inhibitor or ARB for LVSD

Hospital Name	City	Rate	Cases
Trinity Regional Medical Center	Fort Dodge	100%	46
Mercy Medical Center-Des Moines	Des Moines	99%	178
Mercy Medical Center-North Iowa	Mason City	97%	61
Iowa Lutheran Hospital	Des Moines	95%	42
Mercy Medical Center	Cedar Rapids	95%	37
Mercy Medical Center-Dubuque	Dubuque	95%	59
Mercy Medical Center	Sioux City	91%	57
Saint Luke's Hospital	Cedar Rapids	88%	41
Mercy Hospital	Iowa City	86%	50
Mary Greeley Medical Center	Ames	85%	39
Allen Memorial Hospital	Waterloo	83%	78
University of Iowa Hospitals and Clinics	Iowa City	82%	60
Genesis Medical Center-Davenport	Davenport	81%	119
Iowa Methodist Medical Center	Des Moines	79%	124

2. Aspirin at Arrival

Hospital Name	City	Rate	Cases
Genesis Medical Center-Davenport	Davenport	100%	267
Great River Medical Center	West Burlington	100%	97
Mercy Hospital	Council Bluffs	100%	46
Mercy Medical Center	Cedar Rapids	100%	175
Mercy Medical Center-Des Moines	Des Moines	100%	331
University of Iowa Hospitals and Clinics	Iowa City	100%	79
Iowa Lutheran Hospital	Des Moines	99%	85
Mercy Medical Center	Sioux City	99%	190
Saint Luke's Hospital	Cedar Rapids	99%	191
Allen Memorial Hospital	Waterloo	98%	153
Mercy Hospital	Iowa City	98%	131
Mercy Medical Center-Dubuque	Dubuque	98%	190
Trinity Regional Medical Center	Fort Dodge	98%	121
Mercy Medical Center-North Iowa	Mason City	97%	172
Ottumwa Regional Health Center	Ottumwa	97%	71
Trinity-Terrace Park Campus	Bettendorf	97%	32
Iowa Methodist Medical Center	Des Moines	96%	149
Jennie Edmundson Memorial Hospital	Council Bluffs	96%	76
Saint Luke's Regional Medical Center	Sioux City	96%	53
Mary Greeley Medical Center	Ames	95%	113
Samaritan Health System	Clinton	94%	144
Finley Hospital	Dubuque	91%	47

3. Aspirin at Discharge

Hospital Name	City	Rate	Cases
Jennie Edmundson Memorial Hospital	Council Bluffs	100%	63
Mercy Hospital	Council Bluffs	100%	30
Mercy Medical Center	Cedar Rapids	100%	160
Mercy Medical Center-Des Moines	Des Moines	100%	586
Mercy Medical Center-North Iowa	Mason City	100%	270
Trinity Regional Medical Center	Fort Dodge	100%	206
Allen Memorial Hospital	Waterloo	99%	235
Iowa Lutheran Hospital	Des Moines	99%	77
Mary Greeley Medical Center	Ames	99%	142
Mercy Hospital	Iowa City	99%	219
Mercy Medical Center	Sioux City	99%	343
Saint Luke's Hospital	Cedar Rapids	99%	213
University of Iowa Hospitals and Clinics	Iowa City	99%	240
Genesis Medical Center-Davenport	Davenport	98%	500
Mercy Medical Center-Dubuque	Dubuque	98%	289
Saint Luke's Regional Medical Center	Sioux City	98%	43
Finley Hospital	Dubuque	97%	30
Iowa Methodist Medical Center	Des Moines	97%	273
Great River Medical Center	West Burlington	95%	42
Ottumwa Regional Health Center	Ottumwa	95%	40
Samaritan Health System	Clinton	92%	119
Trinity-Terrace Park Campus	Bettendorf	92%	36

4. Beta Blocker at Arrival

Hospital Name	City	Rate	Cases
Mercy Hospital	Council Bluffs	100%	36
Trinity-Terrace Park Campus	Bettendorf	100%	27
Jennie Edmundson Memorial Hospital	Council Bluffs	99%	74
Mercy Medical Center	Cedar Rapids	99%	114
University of Iowa Hospitals and Clinics	Iowa City	99%	67
Great River Medical Center	West Burlington	98%	94
Mercy Medical Center	Sioux City	98%	186
Mercy Medical Center-Des Moines	Des Moines	98%	262
Saint Luke's Regional Medical Center	Sioux City	98%	42
Saint Luke's Hospital	Cedar Rapids	97%	157
Genesis Medical Center-Davenport	Davenport	96%	239
Iowa Methodist Medical Center	Des Moines	96%	110
Mary Greeley Medical Center	Ames	96%	101
Trinity Regional Medical Center	Fort Dodge	96%	105
Mercy Medical Center-Dubuque	Dubuque	95%	172
Mercy Medical Center-North Iowa	Mason City	95%	148
Ottumwa Regional Health Center	Ottumwa	95%	81
Allen Memorial Hospital	Waterloo	94%	133
Samaritan Health System	Clinton	93%	85
Mercy Hospital	Iowa City	92%	117
Finley Hospital	Dubuque	89%	35
Iowa Lutheran Hospital	Des Moines	87%	68

5. Beta Blocker at Discharge

Hospital Name	City	Rate	Cases
Mercy Hospital	Council Bluffs	100%	38
Mercy Medical Center-Des Moines	Des Moines	100%	554
Saint Luke's Regional Medical Center	Sioux City	100%	38
University of Iowa Hospitals and Clinics	Iowa City	100%	263
Mercy Medical Center	Cedar Rapids	99%	182
Mercy Medical Center-North Iowa	Mason City	99%	268
Iowa Lutheran Hospital	Des Moines	98%	95
Mary Greeley Medical Center	Ames	98%	140
Mercy Medical Center	Sioux City	98%	343
Trinity Regional Medical Center	Fort Dodge	98%	190
Allen Memorial Hospital	Waterloo	97%	270
Iowa Methodist Medical Center	Des Moines	97%	286
Jennie Edmundson Memorial Hospital	Council Bluffs	97%	65
Mercy Medical Center-Dubuque	Dubuque	97%	267
Saint Luke's Hospital	Cedar Rapids	97%	239
Genesis Medical Center-Davenport	Davenport	96%	482
Great River Medical Center	West Burlington	96%	46
Ottumwa Regional Health Center	Ottumwa	96%	51
Mercy Hospital	Iowa City	95%	235
Trinity-Terrace Park Campus	Bettendorf	94%	35
Finley Hospital	Dubuque	91%	35
Samaritan Health System	Clinton	91%	117

8. Smoking Cessation Advice

Hospital Name	City	Rate	Cases
Mary Greeley Medical Center	Ames	100%	33
Mercy Medical Center	Sioux City	100%	122
Mercy Medical Center-Des Moines	Des Moines	100%	280
Genesis Medical Center-Davenport	Davenport	99%	191
Mercy Medical Center	Cedar Rapids	99%	76
Mercy Medical Center-North Iowa	Mason City	99%	86
Trinity Regional Medical Center	Fort Dodge	99%	69
Allen Memorial Hospital	Waterloo	98%	107
Saint Luke's Hospital	Cedar Rapids	98%	94
Iowa Lutheran Hospital	Des Moines	97%	33
Jennie Edmundson Memorial Hospital	Council Bluffs	97%	30
Mercy Hospital	Iowa City	97%	59
Iowa Methodist Medical Center	Des Moines	96%	91
University of Iowa Hospitals and Clinics	Iowa City	96%	113
Mercy Medical Center-Dubuque	Dubuque	95%	85
Samaritan Health System	Clinton	94%	36

Heart Failure Care

9. ACE Inhibitor or ARB for LVSD

Hospital Name	City	Rate	Cases
Broadlawns Medical Center	Des Moines	100%	47
Mercy Hospital	Council Bluffs	100%	39
Saint Luke's Regional Medical Center	Sioux City	100%	38
Mercy Medical Center-Des Moines	Des Moines	99%	285
Jennie Edmundson Memorial Hospital	Council Bluffs	98%	65
Fort Madison Community Hospital	Fort Madison	97%	30
Great River Medical Center	West Burlington	97%	37
Mary Greeley Medical Center	Ames	97%	95
Mercy Medical Center-North Iowa	Mason City	94%	139
Samaritan Health System	Clinton	93%	41
Trinity Regional Medical Center	Fort Dodge	93%	107
Trinity-Terrace Park Campus	Bettendorf	93%	27
Mercy Medical Center	Sioux City	92%	100
Iowa Lutheran Hospital	Des Moines	91%	104
Iowa Methodist Medical Center	Des Moines	89%	148
Mercy Medical Center	Cedar Rapids	87%	53
Mercy Medical Center-Dubuque	Dubuque	85%	75
University of Iowa Hospitals and Clinics	Iowa City	84%	188
Mercy Hospital	Iowa City	83%	81
Ottumwa Regional Health Center	Ottumwa	83%	30
Genesis Medical Center-Davenport	Davenport	81%	127
Saint Luke's Hospital	Cedar Rapids	80%	96
Allen Memorial Hospital	Waterloo	79%	139

NOTE: Hospital profiles are in alphabetical order by state, then city, then hospital within the city; Rankings are sorted by rate in descending order and exclude hospitals with less than 25 cases; (1) The number of cases is too small (n<25) for purposes of reliably predicting hospital performance; (2) Measure reflects the hospital's indication that its submission was based upon a sample of its relevant discharges; (3) Rate reflects fewer than the maximum possible quarters of data for the measure; (4) Inaccurate information submitted and suppressed for one or more quarters; (5) No data is available from the hospital for this measure; Please refer to the User's Guide for a full explanation of data

Hospital Name	City	Rate	Cases
Covenant Medical Center	Waterloo	74%	34

10. Discharge Instructions

Hospital Name	City	Rate	Cases
Fort Madison Community Hospital	Fort Madison	98%	54
Mercy Hospital	Council Bluffs	98%	83
Mercy Medical Center-Des Moines	Des Moines	98%	734
Floyd Valley Hospital	Le Mars	96%	27
Marshalltown Medical & Surgical Center	Marshalltown	95%	59
Saint Luke's Regional Medical Center	Sioux City	95%	81
Finley Hospital	Dubuque	94%	69
Great River Medical Center	West Burlington	93%	135
Mercy Medical Center	Cedar Rapids	91%	159
Trinity Regional Medical Center	Fort Dodge	90%	174
Mercy Medical Center-North Iowa	Mason City	89%	249
Covenant Medical Center	Waterloo	88%	82
Saint Luke's Hospital	Cedar Rapids	88%	191
Mercy Hospital	Iowa City	86%	187
Spencer Hospital	Spencer	86%	37
Mary Greeley Medical Center	Ames	85%	170
Northwest Iowa Health Center	Sheldon	85%	34
Jennie Edmundson Memorial Hospital	Council Bluffs	84%	113
Grinnell Regional Medical Center	Grinnell	83%	52
Samaritan Health System	Clinton	83%	177
Trinity-Terrace Park Campus	Bettendorf	79%	47
University of Iowa Hospitals and Clinics	Iowa City	79%	253
Keokuk Area Hospital	Keokuk	78%	60
Mercy Medical Center	Sioux City	77%	197
Allen Memorial Hospital	Waterloo	67%	252
Broadlawns Medical Center	Des Moines	67%	75
Iowa Lutheran Hospital	Des Moines	65%	193
Iowa Methodist Medical Center	Des Moines	65%	235
Boone County Hospital	Boone	60%	30
Hamilton County Public Hospital	Webster City	60%	52
Genesis Medical Center-Davenport	Davenport	59%	273
Mercy Medical Center-Dubuque	Dubuque	56%	162
Ottumwa Regional Health Center	Ottumwa	56%	86
Skiff Medical Center	Newton	56%	48
Unity Hospital	Muscatine	48%	25
Davis County Hospital	Bloomfield	37%	27
Lakes Regional Healthcare	Spirit Lake	0%	25

11. Evaluation of LVS Function

Hospital Name	City	Rate	Cases
Broadlawns Medical Center	Des Moines	100%	81
Fort Madison Community Hospital	Fort Madison	100%	88
Mercy Hospital	Council Bluffs	100%	105
Mercy Medical Center-Des Moines	Des Moines	100%	888
Montgomery County Memorial Hospital	Red Oak	100%	42
Sartori Memorial Hospital	Cedar Falls	100%	27
Shelby County Myrtue Memorial Hospital	Harlan	100%	64
Great River Medical Center	West Burlington	99%	192
Saint Luke's Regional Medical Center	Sioux City	99%	118
Covenant Medical Center	Waterloo	98%	121
Iowa Methodist Medical Center	Des Moines	98%	284
Mary Greeley Medical Center	Ames	98%	224
Mercy Medical Center-North Iowa	Mason City	98%	332
University of Iowa Hospitals and Clinics	Iowa City	98%	280
Cass County Memorial Hospital	Atlantic	97%	31
Hamilton County Public Hospital	Webster City	97%	72
Trinity-Terrace Park Campus	Bettendorf	97%	58
Knoxville Hospital & Clinics	Knoxville	96%	25
Iowa Lutheran Hospital	Des Moines	95%	228
Jennie Edmundson Memorial Hospital	Council Bluffs	95%	143
Keokuk Area Hospital	Keokuk	95%	101
Mercy Medical Center	Sioux City	95%	242
Mercy Medical Center-Centerville	Centerville	95%	40
Trinity Regional Medical Center	Fort Dodge	95%	240
Genesis Medical Center-Davenport	Davenport	94%	310
Saint Luke's Hospital	Cedar Rapids	94%	254
Samaritan Health System	Clinton	94%	218
Winneshiek County Memorial Hospital	Decorah	94%	35
Marshalltown Medical & Surgical Center	Marshalltown	93%	97
Mercy Hospital	Iowa City	93%	230
Mercy Medical Center-Dubuque	Dubuque	93%	189
Ottumwa Regional Health Center	Ottumwa	93%	99
Allen Memorial Hospital	Waterloo	92%	323
Mercy Medical Center	Cedar Rapids	92%	201
Pella Regional Health Center	Pella	92%	26
Grinnell Regional Medical Center	Grinnell	89%	93
Jefferson County Hospital	Fairfield	89%	27
Finley Hospital	Dubuque	87%	95
Saint Anthony Regional Hospital	Carroll	86%	59
Spencer Hospital	Spencer	86%	71
Mercy Hospital of Franciscan Sisters	Oelwein	85%	34
Floyd Valley Hospital	Le Mars	82%	49
Unity Hospital	Muscatine	80%	46
Regional Medical Center of Northeast Iowa	Manchester	79%	28
Van Buren County Hospital	Keosauqua	71%	41
Northwest Iowa Health Center	Sheldon	70%	46
Buena Vista Regional Medical Center	Storm Lake	67%	46
Crawford County Memorial Hospital	Denison	61%	41
Lakes Regional Healthcare	Spirit Lake	61%	38
Skiff Medical Center	Newton	61%	72
Henry County Health Center	Mount Pleasant	52%	42
Greene County Medical Center	Jefferson	46%	28
Boone County Hospital	Boone	42%	48
Ellsworth Municipal Hospital	Iowa Falls	41%	29
Greater Regional Medical Center	Creston	28%	32
Davis County Hospital	Bloomfield	21%	33

12. Smoking Cessation Advice

Hospital Name	City	Rate	Cases
Iowa Lutheran Hospital	Des Moines	100%	57
Jennie Edmundson Memorial Hospital	Council Bluffs	100%	27
Mercy Medical Center-Des Moines	Des Moines	100%	145
Iowa Methodist Medical Center	Des Moines	98%	41
Mercy Medical Center	Sioux City	98%	42
Mercy Medical Center-North Iowa	Mason City	97%	36
Mercy Hospital	Iowa City	94%	32
Samaritan Health System	Clinton	94%	36
Allen Memorial Hospital	Waterloo	92%	60
Saint Luke's Hospital	Cedar Rapids	88%	26
Trinity Regional Medical Center	Fort Dodge	85%	47
University of Iowa Hospitals and Clinics	Iowa City	85%	81
Genesis Medical Center-Davenport	Davenport	81%	48
Broadlawns Medical Center	Des Moines	49%	41

Pneumonia Care

13. Appropriate Initial Antibiotic

Hospital Name	City	Rate	Cases
Alegent Health Community Memorial Hospital	Missouri Valley	100%	28
Northwest Iowa Health Center	Sheldon	98%	48
Cherokee Regional Medical Center	Cherokee	97%	29
Mercy Hospital	Council Bluffs	97%	108
Mercy Medical Center-Des Moines	Des Moines	97%	352
Mercy Hospital of Franciscan Sisters	Oelwein	96%	45
Pella Regional Health Center	Pella	96%	46
Allen Memorial Hospital	Waterloo	95%	149
Saint Luke's Regional Medical Center	Sioux City	95%	175
Saint Luke's Hospital	Cedar Rapids	94%	85
Shelby County Myrtue Memorial Hospital	Harlan	94%	49
Shenandoah Medical Center	Shenandoah	94%	32
Sioux Center Community Hospital	Sioux Center	94%	33
Unity Hospital	Muscatine	94%	80
Covenant Medical Center	Waterloo	92%	108
Regional Medical Center of Northeast Iowa	Manchester	92%	26
Trinity Regional Medical Center	Fort Dodge	92%	160
Genesis Medical Center-Davenport	Davenport	91%	100
Iowa Lutheran Hospital	Des Moines	91%	102
Jones Regional Medical Center	Anamosa	91%	35
Mary Greeley Medical Center	Ames	91%	133
Spencer Hospital	Spencer	91%	44
Madison County Memorial Hospital	Winterset	89%	55
Marshalltown Medical & Surgical Center	Marshalltown	89%	89
Trinity-Terrace Park Campus	Bettendorf	89%	53
Mercy Medical Center	Sioux City	88%	132
Montgomery County Memorial Hospital	Red Oak	88%	32
Samaritan Health System	Clinton	88%	165
Broadlawns Medical Center	Des Moines	87%	55
Mercy Medical Center	Cedar Rapids	87%	173
Mercy Medical Center-Dubuque	Dubuque	87%	108
Mercy Medical Center-North Iowa	Mason City	87%	142
Ellsworth Municipal Hospital	Iowa Falls	86%	29
Stewart Memorial Community Hospital	Lake City	86%	43
Cass County Memorial Hospital	Atlantic	85%	27
Finley Hospital	Dubuque	85%	61
Grinnell Regional Medical Center	Grinnell	85%	75
Ottumwa Regional Health Center	Ottumwa	85%	127
Fort Madison Community Hospital	Fort Madison	83%	58
Jennie Edmundson Memorial Hospital	Council Bluffs	83%	113
Skiff Medical Center	Newton	83%	47
Winneshiek County Memorial Hospital	Decorah	82%	57
Great River Medical Center	West Burlington	81%	134
Mercy Hospital	Iowa City	81%	108
Clarinda Regional Health Center	Clarinda	80%	30
Hamilton County Public Hospital	Webster City	80%	41

NOTE: Hospital profiles are in alphabetical order by state, then city, then hospital within the city; Rankings are sorted by rate in descending order and exclude hospitals with less than 25 cases; (1) The number of cases is too small (n<25) for purposes of reliably predicting hospital performance; (2) Measure reflects the hospital's indication that its submission was based upon a sample of its relevant discharges; (3) Rate reflects fewer than the maximum possible quarters of data for the measure; (4) Inaccurate information submitted and suppressed for one or more quarters; (5) No data is available from the hospital for this measure; Please refer to the User's Guide for a full explanation of data

Hospital Name	City	Rate	Cases
Henry County Health Center	Mount Pleasant	80%	35
Sartori Memorial Hospital	Cedar Falls	80%	46
University of Iowa Hospitals and Clinics	Iowa City	80%	50
Davis County Hospital	Bloomfield	78%	51
Iowa Methodist Medical Center	Des Moines	78%	88
Boone County Hospital	Boone	77%	48
Washington County Hospital	Washington	76%	25
Lakes Regional Healthcare	Spirit Lake	71%	45
Keokuk Area Hospital	Keokuk	70%	103
Crawford County Memorial Hospital	Denison	65%	31
Greater Regional Medical Center	Creston	62%	40

14. Blood Culture Timing

Hospital Name	City	Rate	Cases
Alegent Health Community Memorial Hospital	Missouri Valley	100%	25
Finley Hospital	Dubuque	100%	72
Fort Madison Community Hospital	Fort Madison	100%	58
Northwest Iowa Health Center	Sheldon	100%	25
Shelby County Myrtue Memorial Hospital	Harlan	100%	54
Mercy Hospital	Council Bluffs	99%	137
Mercy Medical Center	Sioux City	99%	138
Grinnell Regional Medical Center	Grinnell	98%	54
Mercy Hospital of Franciscan Sisters	Oelwein	98%	43
Saint Luke's Regional Medical Center	Sioux City	98%	131
Trinity Regional Medical Center	Fort Dodge	98%	209
Boone County Hospital	Boone	97%	31
Iowa Lutheran Hospital	Des Moines	97%	67
Keokuk Area Hospital	Keokuk	97%	75
Lakes Regional Healthcare	Spirit Lake	97%	29
Mercy Medical Center	Cedar Rapids	97%	193
Spencer Hospital	Spencer	97%	36
Cass County Memorial Hospital	Atlantic	96%	27
Hamilton County Public Hospital	Webster City	96%	27
Iowa Methodist Medical Center	Des Moines	96%	52
Marshalltown Medical & Surgical Center	Marshalltown	96%	77
Mercy Hospital	Iowa City	96%	93
Saint Luke's Hospital	Cedar Rapids	96%	107
Mercy Medical Center-Des Moines	Des Moines	95%	348
Ottumwa Regional Health Center	Ottumwa	95%	115
Sartori Memorial Hospital	Cedar Falls	95%	58
Great River Medical Center	West Burlington	94%	158
Jennie Edmundson Memorial Hospital	Council Bluffs	94%	115
Trinity-Terrace Park Campus	Bettendorf	94%	48
Unity Hospital	Muscatine	94%	54
Genesis Medical Center-Davenport	Davenport	91%	86
Pella Regional Health Center	Pella	91%	46
Winneshiek County Memorial Hospital	Decorah	91%	58
Allen Memorial Hospital	Waterloo	89%	137
Covenant Medical Center	Waterloo	89%	81
Mary Greeley Medical Center	Ames	89%	110
Broadlawns Medical Center	Des Moines	88%	43
Mercy Medical Center-Dubuque	Dubuque	88%	97
Skiff Medical Center	Newton	85%	27
University of Iowa Hospitals and Clinics	Iowa City	85%	52
Mercy Medical Center-North Iowa	Mason City	84%	140
Samaritan Health System	Clinton	77%	106

15. Influenza Vaccine

Hospital Name	City	Rate	Cases
Mercy Hospital	Council Bluffs	100%	39
Saint Luke's Regional Medical Center	Sioux City	100%	52
Mercy Medical Center-Des Moines	Des Moines	97%	110
Mercy Medical Center-North Iowa	Mason City	97%	39
Great River Medical Center	West Burlington	96%	50
Marshalltown Medical & Surgical Center	Marshalltown	96%	28
Mary Greeley Medical Center	Ames	96%	68
Saint Luke's Hospital	Cedar Rapids	96%	25
Mercy Medical Center	Cedar Rapids	93%	58
Keokuk Area Hospital	Keokuk	92%	38
Mercy Medical Center-Dubuque	Dubuque	92%	26
Trinity Regional Medical Center	Fort Dodge	91%	65
Allen Memorial Hospital	Waterloo	89%	55
Covenant Medical Center	Waterloo	84%	25
Mercy Medical Center	Sioux City	84%	43
Jennie Edmundson Memorial Hospital	Council Bluffs	79%	43
Mercy Hospital	Iowa City	79%	28
Iowa Lutheran Hospital	Des Moines	76%	29
Genesis Medical Center-Davenport	Davenport	73%	26
Samaritan Health System	Clinton	67%	58
Ottumwa Regional Health Center	Ottumwa	16%	31

16. Initial Antibiotic Timing

Hospital Name	City	Rate	Cases
Northwest Iowa Health Center	Sheldon	100%	56
Alegent Health Community Memorial Hospital	Missouri Valley	98%	40
Mercy Hospital	Council Bluffs	98%	169
Cass County Memorial Hospital	Atlantic	97%	39
Mercy Medical Center-Centerville	Centerville	97%	31
Trinity Regional Medical Center	Fort Dodge	96%	249
Winneshiek County Memorial Hospital	Decorah	96%	73
Fort Madison Community Hospital	Fort Madison	95%	85
Saint Anthony Regional Hospital	Carroll	94%	54
Finley Hospital	Dubuque	93%	95
Jennie Edmundson Memorial Hospital	Council Bluffs	93%	161
Shelby County Myrtue Memorial Hospital	Harlan	93%	84
Spencer Hospital	Spencer	93%	67
Jackson County Public Hospital	Maquoketa	92%	26
Keokuk Area Hospital	Keokuk	92%	160
Madison County Memorial Hospital	Winterset	92%	61
Mercy Medical Center-North Iowa	Mason City	92%	168
Saint Luke's Regional Medical Center	Sioux City	92%	220
Sartori Memorial Hospital	Cedar Falls	92%	80
Cherokee Regional Medical Center	Cherokee	91%	34
Hamilton County Public Hospital	Webster City	91%	65
Montgomery County Memorial Hospital	Red Oak	91%	44
Unity Hospital	Muscatine	91%	80
Van Buren County Hospital	Keosauqua	91%	32
Crawford County Memorial Hospital	Denison	90%	39
Ellsworth Municipal Hospital	Iowa Falls	90%	49
Pella Regional Health Center	Pella	90%	68
Ringgold County Hospital	Mount Ayr	90%	29
Marshalltown Medical & Surgical Center	Marshalltown	89%	131
Trinity-Terrace Park Campus	Bettendorf	89%	66
Allen Memorial Hospital	Waterloo	88%	233
Grinnell Regional Medical Center	Grinnell	88%	107
Mercy Medical Center	Cedar Rapids	88%	243
Samaritan Health System	Clinton	88%	280
Sioux Center Community Hospital	Sioux Center	88%	25
Broadlawns Medical Center	Des Moines	87%	60
Iowa Lutheran Hospital	Des Moines	87%	143
Lakes Regional Healthcare	Spirit Lake	87%	53
Saint Luke's Hospital	Cedar Rapids	87%	127
Boone County Hospital	Boone	86%	79
Genesis Medical Center-Davenport	Davenport	86%	169
Jefferson County Hospital	Fairfield	86%	28
Knoxville Hospital & Clinics	Knoxville	86%	36
Mercy Hospital of Franciscan Sisters	Oelwein	86%	49
Regional Medical Center of Northeast Iowa	Manchester	86%	35
Mercy Medical Center	Sioux City	85%	206
Mercy Medical Center-Des Moines	Des Moines	85%	517
Great River Medical Center	West Burlington	84%	209
Shenandoah Medical Center	Shenandoah	84%	49
Floyd Valley Hospital	Le Mars	83%	35
Stewart Memorial Community Hospital	Lake City	83%	59
Iowa Methodist Medical Center	Des Moines	82%	114
Mary Greeley Medical Center	Ames	82%	220
Genesis Medical Center-Dewitt	Dewitt	81%	26
Covenant Medical Center	Waterloo	80%	141
Davis County Hospital	Bloomfield	80%	41
Mercy Hospital	Iowa City	79%	137
Jones Regional Medical Center	Anamosa	78%	41
Greater Regional Medical Center	Creston	77%	44
Buena Vista Regional Medical Center	Storm Lake	76%	51
Mercy Medical Center-Dubuque	Dubuque	73%	175
Henry County Health Center	Mount Pleasant	71%	31
Skiff Medical Center	Newton	71%	65
Washington County Hospital	Washington	70%	50
Ottumwa Regional Health Center	Ottumwa	69%	162
Clarinda Regional Health Center	Clarinda	68%	37
University of Iowa Hospitals and Clinics	Iowa City	67%	101

17. Oxygenation Assessment

Hospital Name	City	Rate	Cases
Alegent Health Community Memorial Hospital	Missouri Valley	100%	53
Allen Memorial Hospital	Waterloo	100%	268
Boone County Hospital	Boone	100%	96
Broadlawns Medical Center	Des Moines	100%	67
Buchanan County Health Center	Independence	100%	34
Buena Vista Regional Medical Center	Storm Lake	100%	79
Cass County Memorial Hospital	Atlantic	100%	51
Cherokee Regional Medical Center	Cherokee	100%	46
Clarinda Regional Health Center	Clarinda	100%	58
Covenant Medical Center	Waterloo	100%	189
Crawford County Memorial Hospital	Denison	100%	51
Davis County Hospital	Bloomfield	100%	54

NOTE: Hospital profiles are in alphabetical order by state, then city, then hospital within the city; Rankings are sorted by rate in descending order and exclude hospitals with less than 25 cases; (1) The number of cases is too small (n<25) for purposes of reliably predicting hospital performance; (2) Measure reflects the hospital's indication that its submission was based upon a sample of its relevant discharges; (3) Rate reflects fewer than the maximum possible quarters of data for the measure; (4) Inaccurate information submitted and suppressed for one or more quarters; (5) No data is available from the hospital for this measure; Please refer to the User's Guide for a full explanation of data

Ellsworth Municipal Hospital	Iowa Falls	100%	62
Finley Hospital	Dubuque	100%	144
Floyd Valley Hospital	Le Mars	100%	41
Fort Madison Community Hospital	Fort Madison	100%	101
Genesis Medical Center-Davenport	Davenport	100%	190
Genesis Medical Center-Dewitt	Dewitt	100%	35
Great River Medical Center	West Burlington	100%	261
Greater Regional Medical Center	Creston	100%	65
Grinnell Regional Medical Center	Grinnell	100%	126
Hamilton County Public Hospital	Webster City	100%	77
Henry County Health Center	Mount Pleasant	100%	38
Iowa Lutheran Hospital	Des Moines	100%	167
Iowa Methodist Medical Center	Des Moines	100%	140
Jackson County Public Hospital	Maquoketa	100%	31
Jones Regional Medical Center	Anamosa	100%	44
Keokuk Area Hospital	Keokuk	100%	200
Knoxville Hospital & Clinics	Knoxville	100%	43
Lakes Regional Healthcare	Spirit Lake	100%	69
Madison County Memorial Hospital	Winterset	100%	78
Marshalltown Medical & Surgical Center	Marshalltown	100%	160
Mercy Hospital	Council Bluffs	100%	204
Mercy Hospital of Franciscan Sisters	Oelwein	100%	70
Mercy Medical Center	Cedar Rapids	100%	348
Mercy Medical Center	Sioux City	100%	258
Mercy Medical Center-Centerville	Centerville	100%	36
Mercy Medical Center-Des Moines	Des Moines	100%	659
Mercy Medical Center-North Iowa	Mason City	100%	216
Montgomery County Memorial Hospital	Red Oak	100%	60
Northwest Iowa Health Center	Sheldon	100%	70
Ottumwa Regional Health Center	Ottumwa	100%	217
Pella Regional Health Center	Pella	100%	80
Regional Medical Center of Northeast Iowa	Manchester	100%	42
Ringgold County Hospital	Mount Ayr	100%	33
Saint Anthony Regional Hospital	Carroll	100%	96
Saint Luke's Hospital	Cedar Rapids	100%	165
Saint Luke's Regional Medical Center	Sioux City	100%	280
Sartori Memorial Hospital	Cedar Falls	100%	97
Shelby County Myrtue Memorial Hospital	Harlan	100%	98
Shenandoah Medical Center	Shenandoah	100%	60
Skiff Medical Center	Newton	100%	74
Spencer Hospital	Spencer	100%	76
Stewart Memorial Community Hospital	Lake City	100%	71
Trinity Regional Medical Center	Fort Dodge	100%	297
Trinity-Terrace Park Campus	Bettendorf	100%	90
Unity Hospital	Muscatine	100%	107
University of Iowa Hospitals and Clinics	Iowa City	100%	124
Van Buren County Hospital	Keosauqua	100%	36
Washington County Hospital	Washington	100%	61
Wayne County Hospital	Corydon	100%	25
Winneshiek County Memorial Hospital	Decorah	100%	89
Mercy Hospital	Iowa City	99%	168
Mercy Medical Center-Dubuque	Dubuque	99%	214
Jennie Edmundson Memorial Hospital	Council Bluffs	98%	201
Mary Greeley Medical Center	Ames	98%	261
Jefferson County Hospital	Fairfield	97%	35
Samaritan Health System	Clinton	97%	346
Sioux Center Community Hospital	Sioux Center	97%	36
Veterans Memorial Hospital	Waukon	97%	31

18. Pneumococcal Vaccine

Hospital Name	City	Rate	Cases
Cass County Memorial Hospital	Atlantic	100%	38
Mercy Hospital	Council Bluffs	100%	128
Buena Vista Regional Medical Center	Storm Lake	98%	63
Montgomery County Memorial Hospital	Red Oak	98%	48
Pella Regional Health Center	Pella	98%	64
Spencer Hospital	Spencer	98%	53
Fort Madison Community Hospital	Fort Madison	96%	78
Mercy Hospital of Franciscan Sisters	Oelwein	96%	49
Mercy Medical Center-Des Moines	Des Moines	95%	435
Allen Memorial Hospital	Waterloo	94%	188
Great River Medical Center	West Burlington	94%	195
Marshalltown Medical & Surgical Center	Marshalltown	94%	110
Mary Greeley Medical Center	Ames	94%	193
Regional Medical Center of Northeast Iowa	Manchester	94%	32
Ringgold County Hospital	Mount Ayr	94%	31
Sartori Memorial Hospital	Cedar Falls	94%	80
Shelby County Myrtue Memorial Hospital	Harlan	94%	79
Trinity Regional Medical Center	Fort Dodge	94%	218
Winneshiek County Memorial Hospital	Decorah	94%	66
Alegent Health Community Memorial Hospital	Missouri Valley	93%	43
Mercy Medical Center-North Iowa	Mason City	93%	162
Stewart Memorial Community Hospital	Lake City	93%	56
Trinity-Terrace Park Campus	Bettendorf	93%	59
Ellsworth Municipal Hospital	Iowa Falls	92%	48
Grinnell Regional Medical Center	Grinnell	92%	90
Saint Luke's Hospital	Cedar Rapids	92%	118
Saint Luke's Regional Medical Center	Sioux City	92%	183
Unity Hospital	Muscatine	92%	75
Cherokee Regional Medical Center	Cherokee	91%	34
Clarinda Regional Health Center	Clarinda	91%	45
Finley Hospital	Dubuque	90%	115
Hamilton County Public Hospital	Webster City	88%	49
Saint Anthony Regional Hospital	Carroll	88%	78
Jennie Edmundson Memorial Hospital	Council Bluffs	87%	141
Genesis Medical Center-Davenport	Davenport	86%	126
Keokuk Area Hospital	Keokuk	86%	140
Mercy Medical Center-Dubuque	Dubuque	86%	166
Covenant Medical Center	Waterloo	85%	123
Floyd Valley Hospital	Le Mars	85%	33
Sioux Center Community Hospital	Sioux Center	85%	27
Boone County Hospital	Boone	84%	69
Mercy Medical Center	Cedar Rapids	84%	241
Crawford County Memorial Hospital	Denison	80%	45
Ottumwa Regional Health Center	Ottumwa	79%	140
Samaritan Health System	Clinton	79%	236
Mercy Hospital	Iowa City	78%	123
Iowa Methodist Medical Center	Des Moines	76%	108
Jones Regional Medical Center	Anamosa	75%	36
Iowa Lutheran Hospital	Des Moines	74%	109
Mercy Medical Center	Sioux City	74%	176
Mercy Medical Center-Centerville	Centerville	73%	26
Skiff Medical Center	Newton	73%	37
Knoxville Hospital & Clinics	Knoxville	68%	31
Lakes Regional Healthcare	Spirit Lake	68%	50
Northwest Iowa Health Center	Sheldon	68%	41
Shenandoah Medical Center	Shenandoah	67%	45
Veterans Memorial Hospital	Waukon	64%	25
University of Iowa Hospitals and Clinics	Iowa City	56%	59
Davis County Hospital	Bloomfield	55%	33
Greater Regional Medical Center	Creston	53%	38
Madison County Memorial Hospital	Winterset	53%	55
Washington County Hospital	Washington	53%	47

19. Smoking Cessation Advice

Hospital Name	City	Rate	Cases
Jennie Edmundson Memorial Hospital	Council Bluffs	100%	33
Mercy Hospital	Council Bluffs	100%	65
Covenant Medical Center	Waterloo	98%	45
Mercy Medical Center-North Iowa	Mason City	98%	43
Saint Luke's Regional Medical Center	Sioux City	98%	66
Mercy Medical Center	Sioux City	97%	66
Saint Luke's Hospital	Cedar Rapids	96%	27
Allen Memorial Hospital	Waterloo	95%	61
Great River Medical Center	West Burlington	95%	60
Mercy Medical Center-Des Moines	Des Moines	95%	184
Trinity Regional Medical Center	Fort Dodge	95%	42
Marshalltown Medical & Surgical Center	Marshalltown	92%	26
Mercy Medical Center-Dubuque	Dubuque	92%	26
Iowa Lutheran Hospital	Des Moines	89%	37
Mary Greeley Medical Center	Ames	87%	39
Ottumwa Regional Health Center	Ottumwa	86%	44
Mercy Hospital	Iowa City	85%	33
Samaritan Health System	Clinton	85%	81
Keokuk Area Hospital	Keokuk	84%	43
Genesis Medical Center-Davenport	Davenport	77%	60
Broadlawns Medical Center	Des Moines	76%	45
Mercy Medical Center	Cedar Rapids	73%	74
Iowa Methodist Medical Center	Des Moines	65%	31
University of Iowa Hospitals and Clinics	Iowa City	35%	48

Surgical Infection Prevention

20. Prophylactic Antibiotic Given

Hospital Name	City	Rate	Cases
Finley Hospital	Dubuque	97%	158
Allen Memorial Hospital	Waterloo	96%	653
Marshalltown Medical & Surgical Center	Marshalltown	96%	284
Jennie Edmundson Memorial Hospital	Council Bluffs	95%	399
Mercy Hospital	Council Bluffs	95%	327
Spencer Hospital	Spencer	95%	291
Iowa Lutheran Hospital	Des Moines	94%	234
Iowa Methodist Medical Center	Des Moines	94%	332
Mercy Hospital	Iowa City	94%	379
Saint Anthony Regional Hospital	Carroll	94%	53
Covenant Medical Center	Waterloo	93%	237
Mercy Medical Center-Dubuque	Dubuque	92%	455
Pella Regional Health Center	Pella	92%	103

NOTE: Hospital profiles are in alphabetical order by state, then city, then hospital within the city; Rankings are sorted by rate in descending order and exclude hospitals with less than 25 cases; (1) The number of cases is too small (n<25) for purposes of reliably predicting hospital performance; (2) Measure reflects the hospital's indication that its submission was based upon a sample of its relevant discharges; (3) Rate reflects fewer than the maximum possible quarters of data for the measure; (4) Inaccurate information submitted and suppressed for one or more quarters; (5) No data is available from the hospital for this measure; Please refer to the User's Guide for a full explanation of data

Hospital Name	City	Rate	Cases
Grinnell Regional Medical Center	Grinnell	91%	111
Mercy Medical Center	Cedar Rapids	91%	152
Fort Madison Community Hospital	Fort Madison	90%	105
Mercy Medical Center-North Iowa	Mason City	90%	703
Trinity-Terrace Park Campus	Bettendorf	90%	157
Mercy Medical Center	Sioux City	89%	536
Mercy Medical Center-Des Moines	Des Moines	89%	479
Saint Luke's Hospital	Cedar Rapids	89%	281
Saint Luke's Regional Medical Center	Sioux City	89%	670
Sartori Memorial Hospital	Cedar Falls	88%	52
Genesis Medical Center-Davenport	Davenport	87%	91
Skiff Medical Center	Newton	86%	181
Keokuk Area Hospital	Keokuk	84%	31
Trinity Regional Medical Center	Fort Dodge	84%	234
Great River Medical Center	West Burlington	83%	300
Jefferson County Hospital	Fairfield	83%	52
Mary Greeley Medical Center	Ames	82%	208
Samaritan Health System	Clinton	81%	100
University of Iowa Hospitals and Clinics	Iowa City	80%	499
Broadlawns Medical Center	Des Moines	79%	52
Greater Regional Medical Center	Creston	78%	36
Mercy Medical Center-Centerville	Centerville	73%	41
Lakes Regional Healthcare	Spirit Lake	72%	116
Ottumwa Regional Health Center	Ottumwa	72%	196
Unity Hospital	Muscatine	72%	99
Hamilton County Public Hospital	Webster City	71%	28

21. Prophylactic Antibiotic Selection

Hospital Name	City	Rate	Cases
Allen Memorial Hospital	Waterloo	100%	61
Fort Madison Community Hospital	Fort Madison	100%	42
Trinity Regional Medical Center	Fort Dodge	100%	57
Great River Medical Center	West Burlington	99%	67
Mary Greeley Medical Center	Ames	99%	126
Mercy Hospital	Iowa City	99%	217
Mercy Medical Center	Sioux City	99%	70
Mercy Medical Center-North Iowa	Mason City	98%	235
Grinnell Regional Medical Center	Grinnell	97%	31
Iowa Lutheran Hospital	Des Moines	97%	59
Mercy Medical Center-Dubuque	Dubuque	97%	94
Trinity-Terrace Park Campus	Bettendorf	97%	34
Saint Anthony Regional Hospital	Carroll	96%	54
Saint Luke's Regional Medical Center	Sioux City	96%	151
Genesis Medical Center-Davenport	Davenport	95%	93
Marshalltown Medical & Surgical Center	Marshalltown	95%	58
Mercy Medical Center-Des Moines	Des Moines	95%	136
Saint Luke's Hospital	Cedar Rapids	95%	73
Finley Hospital	Dubuque	94%	36
Jennie Edmundson Memorial Hospital	Council Bluffs	93%	98
Lakes Regional Healthcare	Spirit Lake	93%	28
Mercy Medical Center	Cedar Rapids	93%	57
Pella Regional Health Center	Pella	93%	29
Unity Hospital	Muscatine	92%	36
Covenant Medical Center	Waterloo	91%	66
Iowa Methodist Medical Center	Des Moines	91%	85
Mercy Hospital	Council Bluffs	89%	38
Ottumwa Regional Health Center	Ottumwa	89%	46
Samaritan Health System	Clinton	87%	45
Skiff Medical Center	Newton	84%	44
Spencer Hospital	Spencer	78%	46
University of Iowa Hospitals and Clinics	Iowa City	71%	70

22. Prophylactic Antibiotic Stopped

Hospital Name	City	Rate	Cases
Allen Memorial Hospital	Waterloo	96%	625
Greater Regional Medical Center	Creston	94%	36
Lakes Regional Healthcare	Spirit Lake	94%	114
Mercy Hospital	Council Bluffs	94%	319
Pella Regional Health Center	Pella	93%	102
Mercy Medical Center-Des Moines	Des Moines	92%	449
Jennie Edmundson Memorial Hospital	Council Bluffs	91%	399
Saint Anthony Regional Hospital	Carroll	91%	53
Trinity-Terrace Park Campus	Bettendorf	90%	154
Genesis Medical Center-Davenport	Davenport	88%	85
Spencer Hospital	Spencer	88%	286
Mercy Medical Center-North Iowa	Mason City	87%	694
Keokuk Area Hospital	Keokuk	86%	29
Saint Luke's Regional Medical Center	Sioux City	85%	651
Finley Hospital	Dubuque	84%	154
Saint Luke's Hospital	Cedar Rapids	83%	232
Fort Madison Community Hospital	Fort Madison	82%	100
Great River Medical Center	West Burlington	82%	289
Ottumwa Regional Health Center	Ottumwa	82%	180
Jefferson County Hospital	Fairfield	80%	45
Mercy Medical Center-Dubuque	Dubuque	80%	447
Mercy Medical Center	Sioux City	79%	530
Trinity Regional Medical Center	Fort Dodge	78%	226
Iowa Lutheran Hospital	Des Moines	73%	226
Iowa Methodist Medical Center	Des Moines	73%	324
Broadlawns Medical Center	Des Moines	69%	49
Grinnell Regional Medical Center	Grinnell	68%	101
Mercy Medical Center-Centerville	Centerville	67%	39
Mercy Hospital	Iowa City	65%	376
Unity Hospital	Muscatine	64%	92
University of Iowa Hospitals and Clinics	Iowa City	64%	481
Mercy Medical Center	Cedar Rapids	63%	142
Skiff Medical Center	Newton	60%	178
Mary Greeley Medical Center	Ames	59%	194
Covenant Medical Center	Waterloo	49%	230
Marshalltown Medical & Surgical Center	Marshalltown	48%	278
Samaritan Health System	Clinton	44%	101
Hamilton County Public Hospital	Webster City	35%	26
Sartori Memorial Hospital	Cedar Falls	35%	51

Pregnancy Care

23. Inpatient Neonatal Mortality

Hospital Name	City	Rate	Cases
Genesis Medical Center-Davenport	Davenport	0.08%	2372
Mercy Medical Center-Dubuque	Dubuque	0.11%	937
Saint Luke's Regional Medical Center	Sioux City	0.14%	2137
Allen Memorial Hospital	Waterloo	0.16%	619
Samaritan Health System	Clinton	0.17%	572
University of Iowa Hospitals and Clinics	Iowa City	2.08%	2022

24. Third or Fourth Degree Laceration

Hospital Name	City	Rate	Cases
Samaritan Health System	Clinton	1.80%	388
Mercy Medical Center-Dubuque	Dubuque	2.51%	677
Genesis Medical Center-Davenport	Davenport	3.65%	1646
Saint Luke's Regional Medical Center	Sioux City	3.78%	1454
Allen Memorial Hospital	Waterloo	4.73%	465
University of Iowa Hospitals and Clinics	Iowa City	5.72%	1084

NOTE: Hospital profiles are in alphabetical order by state, then city, then hospital within the city; Rankings are sorted by rate in descending order and exclude hospitals with less than 25 cases; (1) The number of cases is too small (n<25) for purposes of reliably predicting hospital performance; (2) Measure reflects the hospital's indication that its submission was based upon a sample of its relevant discharges; (3) Rate reflects fewer than the maximum possible quarters of data for the measure; (4) Inaccurate information submitted and suppressed for one or more quarters; (5) No data is available from the hospital for this measure; Please refer to the User's Guide for a full explanation of data

Mary Greeley Medical Center

1111 Duff Avenue
Ames, IA 50010
Phone: 515-239-2011
Fax: 515-239-2007
E-mail: yourhealth.mgmc@mgmc.com
URL: www.mgmc.org
Ownership: Government - Local
Accredited: Yes
Emergency Services: Yes
Licensed Beds: 220

Key Personnel:

President/CEO . . . . Kimberly Russel
Director Emergency Department . . . . Marylin Polito
Emergency Room . . . . Richard Watts
Infection Control Specialist . . . . Betty Fosse
OB/GYN Women's Health . . . . Linda Torres
Director Surgical Services . . . . Bonnie Herrin
Director Radiology . . . . Brian Smith
Director Respiratory Therapy . . . . Tammy Jarnagin

Measure	Cases	This Hospital	State Average	U.S. Average	Top Hospital
Heart Attack Care					
ACE Inhibitor or ARB for LVSD	39	85%	86%	82%	100%
Aspirin at Arrival	113	95%	89%	92%	100%
Aspirin at Discharge	142	99%	90%	90%	100%
Beta Blocker at Arrival	101	96%	91%	87%	100%
Beta Blocker at Discharge	140	98%	91%	90%	100%
Fibrinolytic Medication Timing	0	-	33%	31%	100%
PCI Within 90 Minutes of Arrival[1]	5	80%	73%	54%	95%
Smoking Cessation Advice	33	100%	92%	88%	100%
Heart Failure Care					
ACE Inhibitor or ARB for LVSD	95	97%	84%	82%	100%
Discharge Instructions	170	85%	62%	61%	93%
Evaluation of LVS Function	224	98%	75%	83%	99%
Smoking Cessation Advice[1]	19	95%	78%	82%	100%
Pneumonia Care					
Appropriate Initial Antibiotic	133	91%	85%	83%	94%
Blood Culture Timing	110	89%	95%	90%	100%
Influenza Vaccine	68	96%	85%	70%	100%
Initial Antibiotic Timing	220	82%	87%	80%	93%
Oxygenation Assessment	261	98%	99%	99%	100%
Pneumococcal Vaccine	193	94%	83%	69%	94%
Smoking Cessation Advice	39	87%	75%	80%	100%
Surgical Infection Prevention					
Prophylactic Antibiotic Given[2,3]	208	82%	79%	77%	95%
Prophylactic Antibiotic Selection[2]	126	99%	89%	90%	100%
Prophylactic Antibiotic Stopped[2,3]	194	59%	76%	72%	95%
Pregnancy Care					
Inpatient Neonatal Mortality	-	-	-	-	-
Third or Fourth Degree Laceration	-	-	-	3.63%	3.27%

Jones Regional Medical Center

Alternate Name: Anamosa Community Hospital
104 Broadway Place
Anamosa, IA 52205
Phone: 319-462-6135
Fax: 319-462-4689
E-mail: secrisdr@castlukes.com
URL: www.jonesregional.org
Ownership: Voluntary non-profit - Private
Accredited: No
Emergency Services: Yes
Licensed Beds: 38

Key Personnel:

CEO . . . . Sean Williams
Emergency Room . . . . M Weston

Measure	Cases	This Hospital	State Average	U.S. Average	Top Hospital
Heart Attack Care					
ACE Inhibitor or ARB for LVSD[5]	-	-	86%	82%	100%
Aspirin at Arrival[5]	-	-	89%	92%	100%
Aspirin at Discharge[5]	-	-	90%	90%	100%
Beta Blocker at Arrival[5]	-	-	91%	87%	100%
Beta Blocker at Discharge[5]	-	-	91%	90%	100%
Fibrinolytic Medication Timing[5]	-	-	33%	31%	100%
PCI Within 90 Minutes of Arrival[5]	-	-	73%	54%	95%
Smoking Cessation Advice[5]	-	-	92%	88%	100%
Heart Failure Care					
ACE Inhibitor or ARB for LVSD[1,2]	2	0%	84%	82%	100%
Discharge Instructions[1,2]	9	11%	62%	61%	93%
Evaluation of LVS Function[1,2]	16	81%	75%	83%	99%
Smoking Cessation Advice[2]	0	-	78%	82%	100%
Pneumonia Care					
Appropriate Initial Antibiotic[2]	35	91%	85%	83%	94%
Blood Culture Timing[1,2]	20	95%	95%	90%	100%
Influenza Vaccine[1]	7	57%	85%	70%	100%
Initial Antibiotic Timing[2]	41	78%	87%	80%	93%
Oxygenation Assessment[2]	44	100%	99%	99%	100%
Pneumococcal Vaccine[2]	36	75%	83%	69%	94%
Smoking Cessation Advice[1,2]	12	75%	75%	80%	100%
Surgical Infection Prevention					
Prophylactic Antibiotic Given[5]	-	-	79%	77%	95%
Prophylactic Antibiotic Selection[5]	-	-	89%	90%	100%
Prophylactic Antibiotic Stopped[5]	-	-	76%	72%	95%
Pregnancy Care					
Inpatient Neonatal Mortality	-	-	-	-	-
Third or Fourth Degree Laceration	-	-	-	3.63%	3.27%

Cass County Memorial Hospital

1501 East Tenth Street
Atlantic, IA 50022
Phone: 712-243-3250
Ownership: Government - Local
Accredited: No
Emergency Services: No

Measure	Cases	This Hospital	State Average	U.S. Average	Top Hospital
Heart Attack Care					
ACE Inhibitor or ARB for LVSD	0	-	86%	82%	100%
Aspirin at Arrival[1]	7	57%	89%	92%	100%
Aspirin at Discharge[1]	4	100%	90%	90%	100%
Beta Blocker at Arrival[1]	6	67%	91%	87%	100%
Beta Blocker at Discharge[1]	4	100%	91%	90%	100%
Fibrinolytic Medication Timing	0	-	33%	31%	100%
PCI Within 90 Minutes of Arrival[5]	-	-	73%	54%	95%
Smoking Cessation Advice	0	-	92%	88%	100%
Heart Failure Care					
ACE Inhibitor or ARB for LVSD[1]	12	67%	84%	82%	100%
Discharge Instructions[1]	13	85%	62%	61%	93%
Evaluation of LVS Function	31	97%	75%	83%	99%
Smoking Cessation Advice[1]	5	100%	78%	82%	100%
Pneumonia Care					
Appropriate Initial Antibiotic	27	85%	85%	83%	94%
Blood Culture Timing	27	96%	95%	90%	100%
Influenza Vaccine[1]	9	100%	85%	70%	100%
Initial Antibiotic Timing	39	97%	87%	80%	93%
Oxygenation Assessment	51	100%	99%	99%	100%
Pneumococcal Vaccine	38	100%	83%	69%	94%
Smoking Cessation Advice[1]	9	78%	75%	80%	100%
Surgical Infection Prevention					
Prophylactic Antibiotic Given[1]	14	71%	79%	77%	95%
Prophylactic Antibiotic Selection[1]	4	100%	89%	90%	100%
Prophylactic Antibiotic Stopped[1]	13	77%	76%	72%	95%
Pregnancy Care					
Inpatient Neonatal Mortality	-	-	-	-	-
Third or Fourth Degree Laceration	-	-	-	3.63%	3.27%

Audubon County Memorial Hospital

515 Pacific Street
Audubon, IA 50025
Phone: 712-563-2611
Fax: 712-563-5277
E-mail: acmhhosp@netins.net
URL: www.acmhhosp.org
Ownership: Voluntary non-profit - Other
Accredited: No
Emergency Services: Yes
Licensed Beds: 25

Key Personnel:

CEO . . . . Thomas Smith
Chief Medical Staff . . . . James M Cunningham, DO
Emergency Room . . . . Bonnie Tigges, RN
Medical/Surgical Nursing . . . . Bonnie Tigges, RN
Director Respiratory Therapy . . . . Cindy Benson

Measure	Cases	This Hospital	State Average	U.S. Average	Top Hospital
Heart Attack Care					
ACE Inhibitor or ARB for LVSD[3]	0	-	86%	82%	100%

NOTE: Hospital profiles are in alphabetical order by state, then city, then hospital within the city; Rankings are sorted by rate in descending order and exclude hospitals with less than 25 cases; (1) The number of cases is too small (n<25) for purposes of reliably predicting hospital performance; (2) Measure reflects the hospital's indication that its submission was based upon a sample of its relevant discharges; (3) Rate reflects fewer than the maximum possible quarters of data for the measure; (4) Inaccurate information submitted and suppressed for one or more quarters; (5) No data is available from the hospital for this measure; Please refer to the User's Guide for a full explanation of data

Measure	Cases	This Hospital	State Average	U.S. Average	Top Hospital
Aspirin at Arrival[1,3]	4	100%	89%	92%	100%
Aspirin at Discharge[1,3]	4	100%	90%	90%	100%
Beta Blocker at Arrival[1,3]	3	67%	91%	87%	100%
Beta Blocker at Discharge[1,3]	3	100%	91%	90%	100%
Fibrinolytic Medication Timing[3]	0	-	33%	31%	100%
PCI Within 90 Minutes of Arrival[5]	-	-	73%	54%	95%
Smoking Cessation Advice[3]	0	-	92%	88%	100%
Heart Failure Care					
ACE Inhibitor or ARB for LVSD[1]	2	100%	84%	82%	100%
Discharge Instructions[1]	5	40%	62%	61%	93%
Evaluation of LVS Function[1]	9	100%	75%	83%	99%
Smoking Cessation Advice	0	-	78%	82%	100%
Pneumonia Care					
Appropriate Initial Antibiotic[1]	10	80%	85%	83%	94%
Blood Culture Timing[1]	4	100%	95%	90%	100%
Influenza Vaccine[1]	5	80%	85%	70%	100%
Initial Antibiotic Timing[1]	12	92%	87%	80%	93%
Oxygenation Assessment[1]	15	100%	99%	99%	100%
Pneumococcal Vaccine[1]	10	90%	83%	69%	94%
Smoking Cessation Advice[1]	1	0%	75%	80%	100%
Surgical Infection Prevention					
Prophylactic Antibiotic Given[1,3]	2	50%	79%	77%	95%
Prophylactic Antibiotic Selection[5]	-	-	89%	90%	100%
Prophylactic Antibiotic Stopped[1,3]	2	50%	76%	72%	95%
Pregnancy Care					
Inpatient Neonatal Mortality	-	-	-	-	-
Third or Fourth Degree Laceration	-	-	-	3.63%	3.27%

Trinity-Terrace Park Campus

4500 Utica Ridge Road
Bettendorf, IA 52722
URL: www.trinityqc.com
Ownership: Voluntary non-profit - Private
Emergency Services: Yes

Phone: 563-742-5000
Fax: 563-779-2260
Accredited: Yes
Licensed Beds: 150

Measure	Cases	This Hospital	State Average	U.S. Average	Top Hospital
Heart Attack Care					
ACE Inhibitor or ARB for LVSD[1]	5	80%	86%	82%	100%
Aspirin at Arrival	32	97%	89%	92%	100%
Aspirin at Discharge	36	92%	90%	90%	100%
Beta Blocker at Arrival	27	100%	91%	87%	100%
Beta Blocker at Discharge	35	94%	91%	90%	100%
Fibrinolytic Medication Timing[3]	0	-	33%	31%	100%
PCI Within 90 Minutes of Arrival[1]	1	100%	73%	54%	95%
Smoking Cessation Advice[1]	10	100%	92%	88%	100%
Heart Failure Care					
ACE Inhibitor or ARB for LVSD	27	93%	84%	82%	100%
Discharge Instructions	47	79%	62%	61%	93%
Evaluation of LVS Function	58	97%	75%	83%	99%
Smoking Cessation Advice[1]	14	100%	78%	82%	100%
Pneumonia Care					
Appropriate Initial Antibiotic[2]	53	89%	85%	83%	94%
Blood Culture Timing[2]	48	94%	95%	90%	100%
Influenza Vaccine[1,2]	15	100%	85%	70%	100%
Initial Antibiotic Timing[2]	66	89%	87%	80%	93%
Oxygenation Assessment[2]	90	100%	99%	99%	100%
Pneumococcal Vaccine[2]	59	93%	83%	69%	94%
Smoking Cessation Advice[1,2]	17	100%	75%	80%	100%
Surgical Infection Prevention					
Prophylactic Antibiotic Given[2]	157	90%	79%	77%	95%
Prophylactic Antibiotic Selection[2]	34	97%	89%	90%	100%
Prophylactic Antibiotic Stopped[2]	154	90%	76%	72%	95%
Pregnancy Care					
Inpatient Neonatal Mortality	-	-	-	-	-
Third or Fourth Degree Laceration	-	-	-	3.63%	3.27%

Davis County Hospital

509 North Madison Street
Bloomfield, IA 52537
E-mail: webmaster@daviscountyhospital.org
URL: www.daviscountyhospital.org
Ownership: Govt - Hospital District or Authority
Emergency Services: Yes

Phone: 641-664-2145
Fax: 641-664-1669
Accredited: No
Licensed Beds: 57

Key Personnel:

President/CEO. . . . . Deb Herzberg
Chief Medical Staff. . . . . Donald Wirtanen, DO
Emergency Room . . . . Pam Cyrene
Emergency Room . . . . Theresa Tuvera
Director Infection/Disease Control . . . . Joan Morris
Medical/Surgical Nursing . . . . Connie Roberts
Lead Respiratory Therapy . . . . Renee Wirtanen

Measure	Cases	This Hospital	State Average	U.S. Average	Top Hospital
Heart Attack Care					
ACE Inhibitor or ARB for LVSD[3]	0	-	86%	82%	100%
Aspirin at Arrival[3]	0	-	89%	92%	100%
Aspirin at Discharge[3]	0	-	90%	90%	100%
Beta Blocker at Arrival[1,3]	1	100%	91%	87%	100%
Beta Blocker at Discharge[3]	0	-	91%	90%	100%
Fibrinolytic Medication Timing[3]	0	-	33%	31%	100%
PCI Within 90 Minutes of Arrival[5]	-	-	73%	54%	95%
Smoking Cessation Advice[3]	0	-	92%	88%	100%
Heart Failure Care					
ACE Inhibitor or ARB for LVSD[1]	3	0%	84%	82%	100%
Discharge Instructions	27	37%	62%	61%	93%
Evaluation of LVS Function	33	21%	75%	83%	99%
Smoking Cessation Advice[1]	3	67%	78%	82%	100%
Pneumonia Care					
Appropriate Initial Antibiotic	51	78%	85%	83%	94%
Blood Culture Timing[1]	4	100%	95%	90%	100%
Influenza Vaccine[4,5]	-	-	85%	70%	100%
Initial Antibiotic Timing	41	80%	87%	80%	93%
Oxygenation Assessment	54	100%	99%	99%	100%
Pneumococcal Vaccine	33	55%	83%	69%	94%
Smoking Cessation Advice[1]	10	80%	75%	80%	100%
Surgical Infection Prevention					
Prophylactic Antibiotic Given[3]	0	-	79%	77%	95%
Prophylactic Antibiotic Selection	0	-	89%	90%	100%
Prophylactic Antibiotic Stopped[3]	0	-	76%	72%	95%
Pregnancy Care					
Inpatient Neonatal Mortality	-	-	-	-	-
Third or Fourth Degree Laceration	-	-	-	3.63%	3.27%

Boone County Hospital

1015 Union Street
Boone, IA 50036

Toll-Free: 888-324-4849
Phone: 515-432-3140
Fax: 515-433-8926

E-mail: dibaltimore@boonecountyhospital.com.
URL: www.boonehospital.com
Ownership: Voluntary non-profit - Other
Emergency Services: Yes

Accredited: No
Licensed Beds: 48

Key Personnel:

President/CEO. . . . . Joseph S Smith
Chief Medical Staff. . . . . Scott L Thiel, MD
Emergency Room . . . . Matthew Byrnes, DO
Director Emergency Room. . . . . Deana Purdy
Infection Control. . . . . Karlene Millang

Measure	Cases	This Hospital	State Average	U.S. Average	Top Hospital
Heart Attack Care					
ACE Inhibitor or ARB for LVSD	0	-	86%	82%	100%
Aspirin at Arrival[1]	7	100%	89%	92%	100%
Aspirin at Discharge[1]	3	67%	90%	90%	100%
Beta Blocker at Arrival[1]	5	100%	91%	87%	100%
Beta Blocker at Discharge[1]	3	67%	91%	90%	100%
Fibrinolytic Medication Timing	0	-	33%	31%	100%
PCI Within 90 Minutes of Arrival	0	-	73%	54%	95%
Smoking Cessation Advice	0	-	92%	88%	100%
Heart Failure Care					

NOTE: Hospital profiles are in alphabetical order by state, then city, then hospital within the city; Rankings are sorted by rate in descending order and exclude hospitals with less than 25 cases; (1) The number of cases is too small (n<25) for purposes of reliably predicting hospital performance; (2) Measure reflects the hospital's indication that its submission was based upon a sample of its relevant discharges; (3) Rate reflects fewer than the maximum possible quarters of data for the measure; (4) Inaccurate information submitted and suppressed for one or more quarters; (5) No data is available from the hospital for this measure; Please refer to the User's Guide for a full explanation of data

Measure	Cases	This Hospital	State Average	U.S. Average	Top Hospital
ACE Inhibitor or ARB for LVSD[1]	7	86%	84%	82%	100%
Discharge Instructions	30	60%	62%	61%	93%
Evaluation of LVS Function	48	42%	75%	83%	99%
Smoking Cessation Advice[1]	8	62%	78%	82%	100%
Pneumonia Care					
Appropriate Initial Antibiotic	48	77%	85%	83%	94%
Blood Culture Timing	31	97%	95%	90%	100%
Influenza Vaccine[1]	17	88%	85%	70%	100%
Initial Antibiotic Timing	79	86%	87%	80%	93%
Oxygenation Assessment	96	100%	99%	99%	100%
Pneumococcal Vaccine	69	84%	83%	69%	94%
Smoking Cessation Advice[1]	18	50%	75%	80%	100%
Surgical Infection Prevention					
Prophylactic Antibiotic Given[5]	-	-	79%	77%	95%
Prophylactic Antibiotic Selection[5]	-	-	89%	90%	100%
Prophylactic Antibiotic Stopped[5]	-	-	76%	72%	95%
Pregnancy Care					
Inpatient Neonatal Mortality	-	-	-	-	-
Third or Fourth Degree Laceration	-	-	-	3.63%	3.27%

Saint Anthony Regional Hospital

311 S Clark Street
Carroll, IA 51401
Phone: 712-792-3581
Fax: 712-792-2124
URL: www.stanthonyhospital.org
Ownership: Voluntary non-profit - Church
Accredited: No
Emergency Services: Yes
Licensed Beds: 178

Key Personnel:

CEO. . . . . Gary P Riedmann
Chief Medical Staff. . . . . John Evin, MD
Chief Medical Staff. . . . . LouAnn Lease
Director Emergency Room. . . . . Sheryll Stolman
Director Medical/Surgical Nursing . . . . Joyce Ryberg
Director Respiratory Therapy . . . . Cindy Klocke

Measure	Cases	This Hospital	State Average	U.S. Average	Top Hospital
Heart Attack Care					
ACE Inhibitor or ARB for LVSD	0	-	86%	82%	100%
Aspirin at Arrival[1]	11	91%	89%	92%	100%
Aspirin at Discharge[1]	5	100%	90%	90%	100%
Beta Blocker at Arrival[1]	6	83%	91%	87%	100%
Beta Blocker at Discharge[1]	5	80%	91%	90%	100%
Fibrinolytic Medication Timing[3]	0	-	33%	31%	100%
PCI Within 90 Minutes of Arrival	0	-	73%	54%	95%
Smoking Cessation Advice[3]	0	-	92%	88%	100%
Heart Failure Care					
ACE Inhibitor or ARB for LVSD[1]	9	89%	84%	82%	100%
Discharge Instructions[1,3]	12	8%	62%	61%	93%
Evaluation of LVS Function	59	86%	75%	83%	99%
Smoking Cessation Advice[1,3]	1	100%	78%	82%	100%
Pneumonia Care					
Appropriate Initial Antibiotic[1,3]	9	78%	85%	83%	94%
Blood Culture Timing[1,3]	6	100%	95%	90%	100%
Influenza Vaccine[5]	-	-	85%	70%	100%
Initial Antibiotic Timing	54	94%	87%	80%	93%
Oxygenation Assessment	96	100%	99%	99%	100%
Pneumococcal Vaccine	78	88%	83%	69%	94%
Smoking Cessation Advice[1,3]	2	100%	75%	80%	100%
Surgical Infection Prevention					
Prophylactic Antibiotic Given[2,3]	53	94%	79%	77%	95%
Prophylactic Antibiotic Selection[2]	54	96%	89%	90%	100%
Prophylactic Antibiotic Stopped[2,3]	53	91%	76%	72%	95%
Pregnancy Care					
Inpatient Neonatal Mortality	-	-	-	-	-
Third or Fourth Degree Laceration	-	-	-	3.63%	3.27%

Sartori Memorial Hospital

515 College Street
Cedar Falls, IA 50613
Phone: 319-268-3000
Fax: 319-268-3270
E-mail: schaeferk@covhealth.com
URL: www.covhealth.com/sartori.asp
Ownership: Voluntary non-profit - Church
Accredited: Yes
Emergency Services: Yes
Licensed Beds: 100

Key Personnel:

President/CEO. . . . . Richard A Schrupp
Administrator . . . . Sherri Greenwood
Chief Medical Staff. . . . . Carl Vanderkooi
Emergency Room . . . . Maureen Beckman, RN
Infection Control. . . . . Nancy Kiehne, RN
ICU . . . . Denise Lampman, RN
Medical Surgical Nursing . . . . Denise Lampman, RN
Respiratory/Cardiopulmonary. . . . . Donna Camarata

Measure	Cases	This Hospital	State Average	U.S. Average	Top Hospital
Heart Attack Care					
ACE Inhibitor or ARB for LVSD[1]	3	100%	86%	82%	100%
Aspirin at Arrival[1]	12	92%	89%	92%	100%
Aspirin at Discharge[1]	9	100%	90%	90%	100%
Beta Blocker at Arrival[1]	12	100%	91%	87%	100%
Beta Blocker at Discharge[1]	11	100%	91%	90%	100%
Fibrinolytic Medication Timing	0	-	33%	31%	100%
PCI Within 90 Minutes of Arrival	0	-	73%	54%	95%
Smoking Cessation Advice[1]	2	100%	92%	88%	100%
Heart Failure Care					
ACE Inhibitor or ARB for LVSD[1]	10	100%	84%	82%	100%
Discharge Instructions[1]	14	86%	62%	61%	93%
Evaluation of LVS Function	27	100%	75%	83%	99%
Smoking Cessation Advice[1]	2	100%	78%	82%	100%
Pneumonia Care					
Appropriate Initial Antibiotic	46	80%	85%	83%	94%
Blood Culture Timing	58	95%	95%	90%	100%
Influenza Vaccine[1]	20	95%	85%	70%	100%
Initial Antibiotic Timing	80	92%	87%	80%	93%
Oxygenation Assessment	97	100%	99%	99%	100%
Pneumococcal Vaccine	80	94%	83%	69%	94%
Smoking Cessation Advice[1]	12	92%	75%	80%	100%
Surgical Infection Prevention					
Prophylactic Antibiotic Given[3]	52	88%	79%	77%	95%
Prophylactic Antibiotic Selection[1]	21	90%	89%	90%	100%
Prophylactic Antibiotic Stopped[3]	51	35%	76%	72%	95%
Pregnancy Care					
Inpatient Neonatal Mortality	-	-	-	-	-
Third or Fourth Degree Laceration	-	-	-	3.63%	3.27%

Mercy Medical Center

701 10th Street SE
Cedar Rapids, IA 52403
Phone: 319-398-6011
Fax: 319-398-6912
URL: www.mercycare.org
Ownership: Voluntary non-profit - Church
Accredited: Yes
Emergency Services: Yes
Licensed Beds: 365

Key Personnel:

President/CEO. . . . . A James Tinker
Chief Medical Staff. . . . . Margie Ebel
Director Infection/Disease Control . . . . Jolene Utt
CCU Spvg. Nurse . . . . Rose Hutchcroft
Director Respiratory Therapy . . . . George Zeman

Measure	Cases	This Hospital	State Average	U.S. Average	Top Hospital
Heart Attack Care					
ACE Inhibitor or ARB for LVSD	37	95%	86%	82%	100%
Aspirin at Arrival	175	100%	89%	92%	100%
Aspirin at Discharge	160	100%	90%	90%	100%
Beta Blocker at Arrival	114	99%	91%	87%	100%
Beta Blocker at Discharge	182	99%	91%	90%	100%
Fibrinolytic Medication Timing[1]	2	0%	33%	31%	100%
PCI Within 90 Minutes of Arrival[1]	8	75%	73%	54%	95%
Smoking Cessation Advice	76	99%	92%	88%	100%
Heart Failure Care					
ACE Inhibitor or ARB for LVSD	53	87%	84%	82%	100%

NOTE: Hospital profiles are in alphabetical order by state, then city, then hospital within the city; Rankings are sorted by rate in descending order and exclude hospitals with less than 25 cases; (1) The number of cases is too small (n<25) for purposes of reliably predicting hospital performance; (2) Measure reflects the hospital's indication that its submission was based upon a sample of its relevant discharges; (3) Rate reflects fewer than the maximum possible quarters of data for the measure; (4) Inaccurate information submitted and suppressed for one or more quarters; (5) No data is available from the hospital for this measure; Please refer to the User's Guide for a full explanation of data

Discharge Instructions	159	91%	62%	61%	93%
Evaluation of LVS Function	201	92%	75%	83%	99%
Smoking Cessation Advice[1]	19	95%	78%	82%	100%
Pneumonia Care					
Appropriate Initial Antibiotic	173	87%	85%	83%	94%
Blood Culture Timing	193	97%	95%	90%	100%
Influenza Vaccine	58	93%	85%	70%	100%
Initial Antibiotic Timing	243	88%	87%	80%	93%
Oxygenation Assessment	348	100%	99%	99%	100%
Pneumococcal Vaccine	241	84%	83%	69%	94%
Smoking Cessation Advice	74	73%	75%	80%	100%
Surgical Infection Prevention					
Prophylactic Antibiotic Given[3]	152	91%	79%	77%	95%
Prophylactic Antibiotic Selection	57	93%	89%	90%	100%
Prophylactic Antibiotic Stopped[3]	142	63%	76%	72%	95%
Pregnancy Care					
Inpatient Neonatal Mortality	-	-	-	-	-
Third or Fourth Degree Laceration	-	-	-	3.63%	3.27%

Saint Luke's Hospital

1026 A Avenue NE
Cedar Rapids, IA 52402
URL: www.crstlukes.com
Ownership: Voluntary non-profit - Private
Emergency Services: Yes
Phone: 319-369-7211
Fax: 319-369-8036
Accredited: Yes
Licensed Beds: 560

Key Personnel:
President/CEO. . . . . Theodore Townsend
Chief Medical Staff. . . . . James R. LaMorgese, MD
Cardiology . . . . Peg Bradke
Emergency Room . . . . Craig Hovda, MD
Director Infection/Disease Control . . . . Brenda Depue
CCU Spvg. Nurse . . . . Mary Ann Osborne
Director Medical/Surgical Nursing . . . . Gail Stork, RN
Surgical Services . . . . Janna Petersen
Chief Radiology . . . . Michael Harleman
Director Respiratory Therapy . . . . Dean Bleadorn

Measure	Cases	This Hospital	State Average	U.S. Average	Top Hospital
Heart Attack Care					
ACE Inhibitor or ARB for LVSD[2]	41	88%	86%	82%	100%
Aspirin at Arrival[2]	191	99%	89%	92%	100%
Aspirin at Discharge[2]	213	99%	90%	90%	100%
Beta Blocker at Arrival[2]	157	97%	91%	87%	100%
Beta Blocker at Discharge[2]	239	97%	91%	90%	100%
Fibrinolytic Medication Timing[1,2]	1	0%	33%	31%	100%
PCI Within 90 Minutes of Arrival[1,2]	20	65%	73%	54%	95%
Smoking Cessation Advice[2]	94	98%	92%	88%	100%
Heart Failure Care					
ACE Inhibitor or ARB for LVSD[2]	96	80%	84%	82%	100%
Discharge Instructions[2]	191	88%	62%	61%	93%
Evaluation of LVS Function[2]	254	94%	75%	83%	99%
Smoking Cessation Advice[2]	26	88%	78%	82%	100%
Pneumonia Care					
Appropriate Initial Antibiotic[2]	85	94%	85%	83%	94%
Blood Culture Timing[2]	107	96%	95%	90%	100%
Influenza Vaccine[2]	25	96%	85%	70%	100%
Initial Antibiotic Timing[2]	127	87%	87%	80%	93%
Oxygenation Assessment[2]	165	100%	99%	99%	100%
Pneumococcal Vaccine[2]	118	92%	83%	69%	94%
Smoking Cessation Advice[2]	27	96%	75%	80%	100%
Surgical Infection Prevention					
Prophylactic Antibiotic Given[2]	281	89%	79%	77%	95%
Prophylactic Antibiotic Selection[2]	73	95%	89%	90%	100%
Prophylactic Antibiotic Stopped[2]	232	83%	76%	72%	95%
Pregnancy Care					
Inpatient Neonatal Mortality	-	-	-	-	-
Third or Fourth Degree Laceration	-	-	-	3.63%	3.27%

Mercy Medical Center-Centerville

Alternate Name: Saint Joseph's Mercy Hospital
1 Saint Joseph's Drive
Centerville, IA 52544
URL: www.mercycenterville.org
Ownership: Voluntary non-profit - Church
Emergency Services: Yes
Phone: 641-437-4111
Fax: 641-437-3422
Accredited: No
Licensed Beds: 58

Key Personnel:
CEO/President. . . . . Clint Christensen
Chief Medical Staff. . . . . LG Heikes, MD
Emergency Room . . . . Mary Lou Sales, RN
Director Medical/Surgical Nursing . . . . Cindy Keene, RN
OB/GYN Womens Health. . . . . DB Fraser, MD
Chief Radiology . . . . Tim Schroeder
Director Respiratory Therapy . . . . Susan Henderson

Measure	Cases	This Hospital	State Average	U.S. Average	Top Hospital
Heart Attack Care					
ACE Inhibitor or ARB for LVSD[1,3]	2	100%	86%	82%	100%
Aspirin at Arrival[1,3]	7	100%	89%	92%	100%
Aspirin at Discharge[1,3]	6	100%	90%	90%	100%
Beta Blocker at Arrival[1,3]	8	100%	91%	87%	100%
Beta Blocker at Discharge[1,3]	8	100%	91%	90%	100%
Fibrinolytic Medication Timing[3]	0	-	33%	31%	100%
PCI Within 90 Minutes of Arrival	0	-	73%	54%	95%
Smoking Cessation Advice[3]	0	-	92%	88%	100%
Heart Failure Care					
ACE Inhibitor or ARB for LVSD[1]	17	88%	84%	82%	100%
Discharge Instructions[1]	20	70%	62%	61%	93%
Evaluation of LVS Function	40	95%	75%	83%	99%
Smoking Cessation Advice[1]	3	67%	78%	82%	100%
Pneumonia Care					
Appropriate Initial Antibiotic[1]	19	58%	85%	83%	94%
Blood Culture Timing[1]	17	88%	95%	90%	100%
Influenza Vaccine[1]	2	100%	85%	70%	100%
Initial Antibiotic Timing	31	97%	87%	80%	93%
Oxygenation Assessment	36	100%	99%	99%	100%
Pneumococcal Vaccine	26	73%	83%	69%	94%
Smoking Cessation Advice[1]	4	75%	75%	80%	100%
Surgical Infection Prevention					
Prophylactic Antibiotic Given	41	73%	79%	77%	95%
Prophylactic Antibiotic Selection[1]	14	86%	89%	90%	100%
Prophylactic Antibiotic Stopped	39	67%	76%	72%	95%
Pregnancy Care					
Inpatient Neonatal Mortality	-	-	-	-	-
Third or Fourth Degree Laceration	-	-	-	3.63%	3.27%

Lucas County Health Center

1200 N 7th Street
Chariton, IA 50049
Ownership: Voluntary non-profit - Other
Emergency Services: Yes
Phone: 641-774-3000
Fax: 641-774-3233
Accredited: No
Licensed Beds: 56

Key Personnel:
CEO. . . . . Daniel Minkoff
Director Medical/Surgical Nursing . . . . Sonya Newsom

Measure	Cases	This Hospital	State Average	U.S. Average	Top Hospital
Heart Attack Care					
ACE Inhibitor or ARB for LVSD[5]	-	-	86%	82%	100%
Aspirin at Arrival[5]	-	-	89%	92%	100%
Aspirin at Discharge[5]	-	-	90%	90%	100%
Beta Blocker at Arrival[5]	-	-	91%	87%	100%
Beta Blocker at Discharge[5]	-	-	91%	90%	100%
Fibrinolytic Medication Timing[5]	-	-	33%	31%	100%
PCI Within 90 Minutes of Arrival[5]	-	-	73%	54%	95%
Smoking Cessation Advice[5]	-	-	92%	88%	100%
Heart Failure Care					
ACE Inhibitor or ARB for LVSD[5]	-	-	84%	82%	100%
Discharge Instructions[5]	-	-	62%	61%	93%
Evaluation of LVS Function[5]	-	-	75%	83%	99%
Smoking Cessation Advice[5]	-	-	78%	82%	100%
Pneumonia Care					
Appropriate Initial Antibiotic[5]	-	-	85%	83%	94%
Blood Culture Timing[5]	-	-	95%	90%	100%
Influenza Vaccine[5]	-	-	85%	70%	100%

NOTE: Hospital profiles are in alphabetical order by state, then city, then hospital within the city; Rankings are sorted by rate in descending order and exclude hospitals with less than 25 cases; (1) The number of cases is too small (n<25) for purposes of reliably predicting hospital performance; (2) Measure reflects the hospital's indication that its submission was based upon a sample of its relevant discharges; (3) Rate reflects fewer than the maximum possible quarters of data for the measure; (4) Inaccurate information submitted and suppressed for one or more quarters; (5) No data is available from the hospital for this measure; Please refer to the User's Guide for a full explanation of data

Measure	Cases	This Hospital	State Average	U.S. Average	Top Hospital
Initial Antibiotic Timing[5]	-	-	87%	80%	93%
Oxygenation Assessment[5]	-	-	99%	99%	100%
Pneumococcal Vaccine[5]	-	-	83%	69%	94%
Smoking Cessation Advice[5]	-	-	75%	80%	100%
Surgical Infection Prevention					
Prophylactic Antibiotic Given[5]	-	-	79%	77%	95%
Prophylactic Antibiotic Selection[5]	-	-	89%	90%	100%
Prophylactic Antibiotic Stopped[5]	-	-	76%	72%	95%
Pregnancy Care					
Inpatient Neonatal Mortality	-	-	-	-	-
Third or Fourth Degree Laceration	-	-	-	3.63%	3.27%

Cherokee Regional Medical Center

300 Sioux Valley Drive
Cherokee, IA 51012
Toll-Free: 800-942-3859
Phone: 712-225-5101
Fax: 712-225-6870
URL: www.cherokeermc.org
Ownership: Voluntary non-profit - Other
Accredited: No
Emergency Services: Yes
Licensed Beds: 25

Key Personnel:

CEO. . . . . John Comstock
Senior Vice President. . . . . Barry Goettsch
President Medical Staff . . . . Timothy Rice, DO
Emergency Room . . . . Doyle Kruger, RN
Coordinator Infection Control/QI. . . . . Susie Haselhoff
Intensive Coronary. . . . . Wesley Parker, MD
President . . . . Stephen Veit, MD
OB/GYN Womens Health. . . . . Patricia Harrison, MD
Manager Radiology . . . . Mary Groher
Manager Respiratory Therapy . . . . Chris Rausch

Measure	Cases	This Hospital	State Average	U.S. Average	Top Hospital
Heart Attack Care					
ACE Inhibitor or ARB for LVSD[5]	-	-	86%	82%	100%
Aspirin at Arrival[5]	-	-	89%	92%	100%
Aspirin at Discharge[5]	-	-	90%	90%	100%
Beta Blocker at Arrival[5]	-	-	91%	87%	100%
Beta Blocker at Discharge[5]	-	-	91%	90%	100%
Fibrinolytic Medication Timing[5]	-	-	33%	31%	100%
PCI Within 90 Minutes of Arrival[5]	-	-	73%	54%	95%
Smoking Cessation Advice[5]	-	-	92%	88%	100%
Heart Failure Care					
ACE Inhibitor or ARB for LVSD[1,2]	3	100%	84%	82%	100%
Discharge Instructions[1,2]	13	77%	62%	61%	93%
Evaluation of LVS Function[5]	-	-	75%	83%	99%
Smoking Cessation Advice[5]	-	-	78%	82%	100%
Pneumonia Care					
Appropriate Initial Antibiotic[2]	29	97%	85%	83%	94%
Blood Culture Timing[1,2]	11	91%	95%	90%	100%
Influenza Vaccine[1,2]	14	100%	85%	70%	100%
Initial Antibiotic Timing[2]	34	91%	87%	80%	93%
Oxygenation Assessment[2]	46	100%	99%	99%	100%
Pneumococcal Vaccine[2]	34	91%	83%	69%	94%
Smoking Cessation Advice[1,2]	7	86%	75%	80%	100%
Surgical Infection Prevention					
Prophylactic Antibiotic Given[1,2,3]	12	100%	79%	77%	95%
Prophylactic Antibiotic Selection[1,2]	5	100%	89%	90%	100%
Prophylactic Antibiotic Stopped[1,2,3]	12	92%	76%	72%	95%
Pregnancy Care					
Inpatient Neonatal Mortality	-	-	-	-	-
Third or Fourth Degree Laceration	-	-	-	3.63%	3.27%

Clarinda Regional Health Center

823 South 17th Street
PO Box 217
Clarinda, IA 51632
Phone: 712-542-2176
Fax: 712-542-3380
E-mail: rudys@clarinda.heartland.net
URL: www.clarindahealth.com
Ownership: Government - Local
Accredited: No
Emergency Services: Yes
Licensed Beds: 47

Key Personnel:

CEO. . . . . Keith Heuser
Chief Medical Staff. . . . . Jim Schlichtmann, MD
Emergency Room . . . . Kathy Burweril
OB/GYN Womens Health. . . . . Maggie Brown
Director Respiratory Therapy . . . . Ryan Barr

Measure	Cases	This Hospital	State Average	U.S. Average	Top Hospital
Heart Attack Care					
ACE Inhibitor or ARB for LVSD[3]	0	-	86%	82%	100%
Aspirin at Arrival[1,3]	6	100%	89%	92%	100%
Aspirin at Discharge[1,3]	3	100%	90%	90%	100%
Beta Blocker at Arrival[1,3]	5	100%	91%	87%	100%
Beta Blocker at Discharge[1,3]	3	100%	91%	90%	100%
Fibrinolytic Medication Timing[3]	0	-	33%	31%	100%
PCI Within 90 Minutes of Arrival[5]	-	-	73%	54%	95%
Smoking Cessation Advice[3]	0	-	92%	88%	100%
Heart Failure Care					
ACE Inhibitor or ARB for LVSD[3]	0	-	84%	82%	100%
Discharge Instructions[1,3]	1	0%	62%	61%	93%
Evaluation of LVS Function[1,3]	7	71%	75%	83%	99%
Smoking Cessation Advice[1,3]	1	100%	78%	82%	100%
Pneumonia Care					
Appropriate Initial Antibiotic	30	80%	85%	83%	94%
Blood Culture Timing[1]	15	93%	95%	90%	100%
Influenza Vaccine[1]	11	82%	85%	70%	100%
Initial Antibiotic Timing	37	68%	87%	80%	93%
Oxygenation Assessment	58	100%	99%	99%	100%
Pneumococcal Vaccine	45	91%	83%	69%	94%
Smoking Cessation Advice[1]	9	78%	75%	80%	100%
Surgical Infection Prevention					
Prophylactic Antibiotic Given[5]	-	-	79%	77%	95%
Prophylactic Antibiotic Selection[5]	-	-	89%	90%	100%
Prophylactic Antibiotic Stopped[5]	-	-	76%	72%	95%
Pregnancy Care					
Inpatient Neonatal Mortality	-	-	-	-	-
Third or Fourth Degree Laceration	-	-	-	3.63%	3.27%

Wright Medical Center

1316 S Main Street
Clarion, IA 50525
Toll-Free: 866-426-4188
Phone: 515-532-2811
Fax: 515-532-3443
E-mail: wmc@wrightmed.com
URL: www.wrightmed.com
Ownership: Government - Local
Accredited: No
Emergency Services: Yes
Licensed Beds: 25

Key Personnel:

CEO. . . . . Steve Simonin
Chief Medical Staff. . . . . Dustin Smith, MD
Emergency Room . . . . Vinny Frank, PA-C
Infection Control. . . . . Tara Wagner, RN
Medical Surgery. . . . . Colleen Parks
Staff Respiratory Therapist. . . . . Deb Akers

Measure	Cases	This Hospital	State Average	U.S. Average	Top Hospital
Heart Attack Care					
ACE Inhibitor or ARB for LVSD[5]	-	-	86%	82%	100%
Aspirin at Arrival[5]	-	-	89%	92%	100%
Aspirin at Discharge[5]	-	-	90%	90%	100%
Beta Blocker at Arrival[5]	-	-	91%	87%	100%
Beta Blocker at Discharge[5]	-	-	91%	90%	100%
Fibrinolytic Medication Timing[5]	-	-	33%	31%	100%
PCI Within 90 Minutes of Arrival[5]	-	-	73%	54%	95%
Smoking Cessation Advice[5]	-	-	92%	88%	100%
Heart Failure Care					
ACE Inhibitor or ARB for LVSD[5]	-	-	84%	82%	100%
Discharge Instructions[5]	-	-	62%	61%	93%
Evaluation of LVS Function[5]	-	-	75%	83%	99%
Smoking Cessation Advice[5]	-	-	78%	82%	100%
Pneumonia Care					
Appropriate Initial Antibiotic[5]	-	-	85%	83%	94%
Blood Culture Timing[5]	-	-	95%	90%	100%
Influenza Vaccine[5]	-	-	85%	70%	100%
Initial Antibiotic Timing[5]	-	-	87%	80%	93%
Oxygenation Assessment[5]	-	-	99%	99%	100%

NOTE: Hospital profiles are in alphabetical order by state, then city, then hospital within the city; Rankings are sorted by rate in descending order and exclude hospitals with less than 25 cases; (1) The number of cases is too small (n<25) for purposes of reliably predicting hospital performance; (2) Measure reflects the hospital's indication that its submission was based upon a sample of its relevant discharges; (3) Rate reflects fewer than the maximum possible quarters of data for the measure; (4) Inaccurate information submitted and suppressed for one or more quarters; (5) No data is available from the hospital for this measure; Please refer to the User's Guide for a full explanation of data

Pneumococcal Vaccine[5]	-	-	83%	69%	94%
Smoking Cessation Advice[5]	-	-	75%	80%	100%
Surgical Infection Prevention					
Prophylactic Antibiotic Given[5]	-	-	79%	77%	95%
Prophylactic Antibiotic Selection[5]	-	-	89%	90%	100%
Prophylactic Antibiotic Stopped[5]	-	-	76%	72%	95%
Pregnancy Care					
Inpatient Neonatal Mortality	-	-	-	-	-
Third or Fourth Degree Laceration	-	-	-	3.63%	3.27%

Samaritan Health System

Alternate Name: Mercy Medical Center-Clinton
1410 N 4th Street
Clinton, IA 52732
Ownership: Voluntary non-profit - Church
Emergency Services: Yes
Phone: 563-244-3535
Fax: 563-244-5592
Accredited: Yes
Licensed Beds: 171

Key Personnel:
CEO. . . . . Donna Oliver
Director Medical/Surgical Nursing . . . . Roseanne Peska
Chief Radiology . . . . Juergen Holl, MD
Director Respiratory Therapy . . . . Bill Vogel

Measure	Cases	This Hospital	State Average	U.S. Average	Top Hospital
Heart Attack Care					
ACE Inhibitor or ARB for LVSD[1]	18	83%	86%	82%	100%
Aspirin at Arrival	144	94%	89%	92%	100%
Aspirin at Discharge	119	92%	90%	90%	100%
Beta Blocker at Arrival	85	93%	91%	87%	100%
Beta Blocker at Discharge	117	91%	91%	90%	100%
Fibrinolytic Medication Timing[1]	15	80%	33%	31%	100%
PCI Within 90 Minutes of Arrival	0	-	73%	54%	95%
Smoking Cessation Advice	36	94%	92%	88%	100%
Heart Failure Care					
ACE Inhibitor or ARB for LVSD	41	93%	84%	82%	100%
Discharge Instructions	177	83%	62%	61%	93%
Evaluation of LVS Function	218	94%	75%	83%	99%
Smoking Cessation Advice	36	94%	78%	82%	100%
Pneumonia Care					
Appropriate Initial Antibiotic	165	88%	85%	83%	94%
Blood Culture Timing	106	77%	95%	90%	100%
Influenza Vaccine	58	67%	85%	70%	100%
Initial Antibiotic Timing	280	88%	87%	80%	93%
Oxygenation Assessment	346	97%	99%	99%	100%
Pneumococcal Vaccine	236	79%	83%	69%	94%
Smoking Cessation Advice	81	85%	75%	80%	100%
Surgical Infection Prevention					
Prophylactic Antibiotic Given[3]	100	81%	79%	77%	95%
Prophylactic Antibiotic Selection	45	87%	89%	90%	100%
Prophylactic Antibiotic Stopped[3]	101	44%	76%	72%	95%
Pregnancy Care					
Inpatient Neonatal Mortality	572	0.17%	-	-	-
Third or Fourth Degree Laceration	388	1.80%	-	3.63%	3.27%

Alegent Health Mercy Hospital

603 Rosary Drive
PO Box 368
Corning, IA 50841
URL: www.alegent.com
Ownership: Voluntary non-profit - Church
Emergency Services: Yes
Phone: 641-322-3121
Fax: 641-322-3616
Accredited: No
Licensed Beds: 25

Key Personnel:
Director Cardiology . . . . Rosy Bissell
Emergency Room . . . . Jo Beldeing
Respiratory Care . . . . Sherry Johnson

Measure	Cases	This Hospital	State Average	U.S. Average	Top Hospital
Heart Attack Care					
ACE Inhibitor or ARB for LVSD[3]	0	-	86%	82%	100%
Aspirin at Arrival[1,3]	1	0%	89%	92%	100%
Aspirin at Discharge[1,3]	2	0%	90%	90%	100%
Beta Blocker at Arrival[3]	0	-	91%	87%	100%
Beta Blocker at Discharge[1,3]	1	0%	91%	90%	100%
Fibrinolytic Medication Timing[1,3]	1	0%	33%	31%	100%
PCI Within 90 Minutes of Arrival[5]	-	-	73%	54%	95%
Smoking Cessation Advice[3]	0	-	92%	88%	100%
Heart Failure Care					
ACE Inhibitor or ARB for LVSD[1]	2	100%	84%	82%	100%
Discharge Instructions[1]	18	78%	62%	61%	93%
Evaluation of LVS Function[1]	21	95%	75%	83%	99%
Smoking Cessation Advice[1]	3	100%	78%	82%	100%
Pneumonia Care					
Appropriate Initial Antibiotic[1,3]	12	67%	85%	83%	94%
Blood Culture Timing[1,3]	4	100%	95%	90%	100%
Influenza Vaccine[1]	3	67%	85%	70%	100%
Initial Antibiotic Timing[1,3]	12	58%	87%	80%	93%
Oxygenation Assessment[1,3]	18	100%	99%	99%	100%
Pneumococcal Vaccine[1,3]	13	77%	83%	69%	94%
Smoking Cessation Advice[1,3]	1	0%	75%	80%	100%
Surgical Infection Prevention					
Prophylactic Antibiotic Given[1,3]	8	50%	79%	77%	95%
Prophylactic Antibiotic Selection[1]	1	100%	89%	90%	100%
Prophylactic Antibiotic Stopped[1,3]	8	100%	76%	72%	95%
Pregnancy Care					
Inpatient Neonatal Mortality	-	-	-	-	-
Third or Fourth Degree Laceration	-	-	-	3.63%	3.27%

Wayne County Hospital

417 S E Street
Corydon, IA 50060
Ownership: Government - Local
Emergency Services: Yes
Phone: 641-872-2260
Fax: 641-872-3116
Accredited: No
Licensed Beds: 28

Key Personnel:
Administrator . . . . Brian Burnside
CEO. . . . . Brian Burnside
Chief of Medical Staff. . . . . Joel Baker
Emergency Room . . . . Patrick Frankl
Cardiologist . . . . Martin Aronow
Director of Pulmonary/Respiratory Care. . . . . . Keith Garber

Measure	Cases	This Hospital	State Average	U.S. Average	Top Hospital
Heart Attack Care					
ACE Inhibitor or ARB for LVSD[1,3]	2	100%	86%	82%	100%
Aspirin at Arrival[1,3]	3	100%	89%	92%	100%
Aspirin at Discharge[1,3]	4	100%	90%	90%	100%
Beta Blocker at Arrival[1,3]	4	100%	91%	87%	100%
Beta Blocker at Discharge[1,3]	4	100%	91%	90%	100%
Fibrinolytic Medication Timing[3]	0	-	33%	31%	100%
PCI Within 90 Minutes of Arrival[5]	-	-	73%	54%	95%
Smoking Cessation Advice[3]	0	-	92%	88%	100%
Heart Failure Care					
ACE Inhibitor or ARB for LVSD[1]	3	100%	84%	82%	100%
Discharge Instructions[1]	10	20%	62%	61%	93%
Evaluation of LVS Function[1]	14	64%	75%	83%	99%
Smoking Cessation Advice[1]	1	0%	78%	82%	100%
Pneumonia Care					
Appropriate Initial Antibiotic[1]	12	67%	85%	83%	94%
Blood Culture Timing[1]	2	100%	95%	90%	100%
Influenza Vaccine[1]	4	75%	85%	70%	100%
Initial Antibiotic Timing[1]	19	95%	87%	80%	93%
Oxygenation Assessment	25	100%	99%	99%	100%
Pneumococcal Vaccine[1]	19	79%	83%	69%	94%
Smoking Cessation Advice[1]	5	60%	75%	80%	100%
Surgical Infection Prevention					
Prophylactic Antibiotic Given[3]	0	-	79%	77%	95%
Prophylactic Antibiotic Selection[1]	2	100%	89%	90%	100%
Prophylactic Antibiotic Stopped[3]	0	-	76%	72%	95%
Pregnancy Care					
Inpatient Neonatal Mortality	-	-	-	-	-
Third or Fourth Degree Laceration	-	-	-	3.63%	3.27%

NOTE: Hospital profiles are in alphabetical order by state, then city, then hospital within the city; Rankings are sorted by rate in descending order and exclude hospitals with less than 25 cases; (1) The number of cases is too small (n<25) for purposes of reliably predicting hospital performance; (2) Measure reflects the hospital's indication that its submission was based upon a sample of its relevant discharges; (3) Rate reflects fewer than the maximum possible quarters of data for the measure; (4) Inaccurate information submitted and suppressed for one or more quarters; (5) No data is available from the hospital for this measure; Please refer to the User's Guide for a full explanation of data

Jennie Edmundson Memorial Hospital

933 E Pierce Street
Council Bluffs, IA 51503
URL: www.bestcare.org
Phone: 712-396-6000
Fax: 712-396-7617
Ownership: Voluntary non-profit - Private
Emergency Services: Yes
Accredited: Yes
Licensed Beds: 118

Key Personnel:

CEO/President. . . . . David M Holcomb
Chief Medical Staff. . . . . John A Okerbloom, MD

Measure	Cases	This Hospital	State Average	U.S. Average	Top Hospital
Heart Attack Care					
ACE Inhibitor or ARB for LVSD[1]	13	92%	86%	82%	100%
Aspirin at Arrival	76	96%	89%	92%	100%
Aspirin at Discharge	63	100%	90%	90%	100%
Beta Blocker at Arrival	74	99%	91%	87%	100%
Beta Blocker at Discharge	65	97%	91%	90%	100%
Fibrinolytic Medication Timing[1]	5	80%	33%	31%	100%
PCI Within 90 Minutes of Arrival	0	-	73%	54%	95%
Smoking Cessation Advice	30	97%	92%	88%	100%
Heart Failure Care					
ACE Inhibitor or ARB for LVSD	65	98%	84%	82%	100%
Discharge Instructions	113	84%	62%	61%	93%
Evaluation of LVS Function	143	95%	75%	83%	99%
Smoking Cessation Advice	27	100%	78%	82%	100%
Pneumonia Care					
Appropriate Initial Antibiotic	113	83%	85%	83%	94%
Blood Culture Timing	115	94%	95%	90%	100%
Influenza Vaccine	43	79%	85%	70%	100%
Initial Antibiotic Timing	161	93%	87%	80%	93%
Oxygenation Assessment	201	98%	99%	99%	100%
Pneumococcal Vaccine	141	87%	83%	69%	94%
Smoking Cessation Advice	33	100%	75%	80%	100%
Surgical Infection Prevention					
Prophylactic Antibiotic Given	399	95%	79%	77%	95%
Prophylactic Antibiotic Selection	98	93%	89%	90%	100%
Prophylactic Antibiotic Stopped	399	91%	76%	72%	95%
Pregnancy Care					
Inpatient Neonatal Mortality	-	-	-	-	-
Third or Fourth Degree Laceration	-	-	-	3.63%	3.27%

Mercy Hospital

800 Mercy Drive
Council Bluffs, IA 51503
URL: www.alegent.com/mercy
Phone: 712-328-5000
Fax: 712-328-5088
Ownership: Voluntary non-profit - Church
Emergency Services: Yes
Accredited: Yes
Licensed Beds: 324

Key Personnel:

CEO/President. . . . . Wayne Sensor
Chief Medical Staff. . . . . David Hanks, MD
Emergency Room . . . . Barb Roenfeld
Emergency Room . . . . Joe Hoagbin, Dr
Director Medical/Surgical Nursing . . . . Cindy Kallsen
OB/GYN Womens Health. . . . . Jorge Sotolongo, MD
Chief Radiology . . . . Donald Van De Water
Chief Respiratory Care. Chris Wolf

Measure	Cases	This Hospital	State Average	U.S. Average	Top Hospital
Heart Attack Care					
ACE Inhibitor or ARB for LVSD[1]	9	100%	86%	82%	100%
Aspirin at Arrival	46	100%	89%	92%	100%
Aspirin at Discharge	30	100%	90%	90%	100%
Beta Blocker at Arrival	36	100%	91%	87%	100%
Beta Blocker at Discharge	38	100%	91%	90%	100%
Fibrinolytic Medication Timing[1]	6	67%	33%	31%	100%
PCI Within 90 Minutes of Arrival[1]	4	75%	73%	54%	95%
Smoking Cessation Advice[1]	16	100%	92%	88%	100%
Heart Failure Care					
ACE Inhibitor or ARB for LVSD	39	100%	84%	82%	100%
Discharge Instructions	83	98%	62%	61%	93%
Evaluation of LVS Function	105	100%	75%	83%	99%
Smoking Cessation Advice[1]	23	100%	78%	82%	100%
Pneumonia Care					
Appropriate Initial Antibiotic	108	97%	85%	83%	94%
Blood Culture Timing	137	99%	95%	90%	100%
Influenza Vaccine	39	100%	85%	70%	100%
Initial Antibiotic Timing	169	98%	87%	80%	93%
Oxygenation Assessment	204	100%	99%	99%	100%
Pneumococcal Vaccine	128	100%	83%	69%	94%
Smoking Cessation Advice	65	100%	75%	80%	100%
Surgical Infection Prevention					
Prophylactic Antibiotic Given[2,3]	327	95%	79%	77%	95%
Prophylactic Antibiotic Selection[2]	38	89%	89%	90%	100%
Prophylactic Antibiotic Stopped[2,3]	319	94%	76%	72%	95%
Pregnancy Care					
Inpatient Neonatal Mortality	-	-	-	-	-
Third or Fourth Degree Laceration	-	-	-	3.63%	3.27%

Greater Regional Medical Center

1700 W Townline Rd
Creston, IA 50801
URL: www.greaterch.com
Phone: 641-782-7091
Fax: 641-782-3801
Ownership: Voluntary non-profit - Other
Emergency Services: Yes
Accredited: No
Licensed Beds: 80

Key Personnel:

Administrator/CEO . . . . Monte Neitzel
Chief Medical Staff. . . . . Tom Young, DO
Medical Surgical Nursing . . . . Deb Risser
OB/GYN/Women's Health . . . . Diana Huntington
Chief Radiology . . . . Todd Kucera, MD
Director Respiratory Therapy . . . . Larry Wagner

Measure	Cases	This Hospital	State Average	U.S. Average	Top Hospital
Heart Attack Care					
ACE Inhibitor or ARB for LVSD	0	-	86%	82%	100%
Aspirin at Arrival[1]	15	93%	89%	92%	100%
Aspirin at Discharge[1]	9	100%	90%	90%	100%
Beta Blocker at Arrival[1]	16	94%	91%	87%	100%
Beta Blocker at Discharge[1]	9	89%	91%	90%	100%
Fibrinolytic Medication Timing	0	-	33%	31%	100%
PCI Within 90 Minutes of Arrival	0	-	73%	54%	95%
Smoking Cessation Advice[1]	2	100%	92%	88%	100%
Heart Failure Care					
ACE Inhibitor or ARB for LVSD[1]	4	75%	84%	82%	100%
Discharge Instructions[1]	22	91%	62%	61%	93%
Evaluation of LVS Function	32	28%	75%	83%	99%
Smoking Cessation Advice[1]	3	67%	78%	82%	100%
Pneumonia Care					
Appropriate Initial Antibiotic	40	62%	85%	83%	94%
Blood Culture Timing[1]	7	100%	95%	90%	100%
Influenza Vaccine[1]	12	67%	85%	70%	100%
Initial Antibiotic Timing	44	77%	87%	80%	93%
Oxygenation Assessment	65	100%	99%	99%	100%
Pneumococcal Vaccine	38	53%	83%	69%	94%
Smoking Cessation Advice[1]	11	55%	75%	80%	100%
Surgical Infection Prevention					
Prophylactic Antibiotic Given	36	78%	79%	77%	95%
Prophylactic Antibiotic Selection[1]	5	80%	89%	90%	100%
Prophylactic Antibiotic Stopped	36	94%	76%	72%	95%
Pregnancy Care					
Inpatient Neonatal Mortality	-	-	-	-	-
Third or Fourth Degree Laceration	-	-	-	3.63%	3.27%

Genesis Medical Center-Davenport

Alternate Name: Saint Luke's Hospital & Mercy Hospital
1227 E Rusholme Street
Davenport, IA 52803
URL: www.genesishealth.com
Phone: 563-421-1000
Fax: 563-421-6279
Ownership: Voluntary non-profit - Other
Emergency Services: Yes
Accredited: Yes
Licensed Beds: 502

Key Personnel:

President/CEO. . . . . Leo Bressanelli
Chief Medical Staff. . . . . Frank Claudy, MD
Catheterization Lab . . . . Cindy McGee
Emergency Room . . . . Colleen Mulholland
Emergency Room . . . . Patty Garrols

NOTE: Hospital profiles are in alphabetical order by state, then city, then hospital within the city; Rankings are sorted by rate in descending order and exclude hospitals with less than 25 cases; (1) The number of cases is too small (n<25) for purposes of reliably predicting hospital performance; (2) Measure reflects the hospital's indication that its submission was based upon a sample of its relevant discharges; (3) Rate reflects fewer than the maximum possible quarters of data for the measure; (4) Inaccurate information submitted and suppressed for one or more quarters; (5) No data is available from the hospital for this measure; Please refer to the User's Guide for a full explanation of data

Infection Control. . . . . Lisa Caffery
Medical/Surgical Nursing . . . . Dianna Paustiah
Respiratory/Cardiopulmonary. . . . . Dennis Harker

Measure	Cases	This Hospital	State Average	U.S. Average	Top Hospital
Heart Attack Care					
ACE Inhibitor or ARB for LVSD[2]	119	81%	86%	82%	100%
Aspirin at Arrival[2]	267	100%	89%	92%	100%
Aspirin at Discharge[2]	500	98%	90%	90%	100%
Beta Blocker at Arrival[2]	239	96%	91%	87%	100%
Beta Blocker at Discharge[2]	482	96%	91%	90%	100%
Fibrinolytic Medication Timing[2]	0	-	33%	31%	100%
PCI Within 90 Minutes of Arrival[1,2]	9	89%	73%	54%	95%
Smoking Cessation Advice[2]	191	99%	92%	88%	100%
Heart Failure Care					
ACE Inhibitor or ARB for LVSD[2]	127	81%	84%	82%	100%
Discharge Instructions[2]	273	59%	62%	61%	93%
Evaluation of LVS Function[2]	310	94%	75%	83%	99%
Smoking Cessation Advice[2]	48	81%	78%	82%	100%
Pneumonia Care					
Appropriate Initial Antibiotic[2]	100	91%	85%	83%	94%
Blood Culture Timing[2]	86	91%	95%	90%	100%
Influenza Vaccine[2]	26	73%	85%	70%	100%
Initial Antibiotic Timing[2]	169	86%	87%	80%	93%
Oxygenation Assessment[2]	190	100%	99%	99%	100%
Pneumococcal Vaccine[2]	126	86%	83%	69%	94%
Smoking Cessation Advice[2]	60	77%	75%	80%	100%
Surgical Infection Prevention					
Prophylactic Antibiotic Given[2,3]	91	87%	79%	77%	95%
Prophylactic Antibiotic Selection[2]	93	95%	89%	90%	100%
Prophylactic Antibiotic Stopped[2,3]	85	88%	76%	72%	95%
Pregnancy Care					
Inpatient Neonatal Mortality	2,372	0.08%	-	-	-
Third or Fourth Degree Laceration	1,646	3.65%	-	3.63%	3.27%

Winneshiek County Memorial Hospital

901 Montgomery Street
Decorah, IA 52101
Phone: 563-382-2911
Fax: 563-387-3102
URL: www.winmedical.org
Ownership: Voluntary non-profit - Other
Accredited: No
Emergency Services: Yes
Licensed Beds: 83

Key Personnel:

Medical Staff President . . . . Kurt Swanson, MD
Emergency Room . . . . Tudy Belay
Infection Control. . . . . Brenda Schwan, RN
Director Medical/Surgical Nursing . . . . Cindy Clausen
Head of Radiology . . . . Julie Katzer

Measure	Cases	This Hospital	State Average	U.S. Average	Top Hospital
Heart Attack Care					
ACE Inhibitor or ARB for LVSD[1]	1	100%	86%	82%	100%
Aspirin at Arrival[1]	4	100%	89%	92%	100%
Aspirin at Discharge[1]	4	100%	90%	90%	100%
Beta Blocker at Arrival[1]	4	100%	91%	87%	100%
Beta Blocker at Discharge[1]	4	100%	91%	90%	100%
Fibrinolytic Medication Timing	0	-	33%	31%	100%
PCI Within 90 Minutes of Arrival	0	-	73%	54%	95%
Smoking Cessation Advice	0	-	92%	88%	100%
Heart Failure Care					
ACE Inhibitor or ARB for LVSD[1]	16	94%	84%	82%	100%
Discharge Instructions[1]	22	77%	62%	61%	93%
Evaluation of LVS Function	35	94%	75%	83%	99%
Smoking Cessation Advice[1]	5	100%	78%	82%	100%
Pneumonia Care					
Appropriate Initial Antibiotic	57	82%	85%	83%	94%
Blood Culture Timing	58	91%	95%	90%	100%
Influenza Vaccine[1]	17	100%	85%	70%	100%
Initial Antibiotic Timing	73	96%	87%	80%	93%
Oxygenation Assessment	89	100%	99%	99%	100%
Pneumococcal Vaccine	66	94%	83%	69%	94%
Smoking Cessation Advice[1]	12	67%	75%	80%	100%
Surgical Infection Prevention					
Prophylactic Antibiotic Given[5]	-	-	79%	77%	95%
Prophylactic Antibiotic Selection[5]	-	-	89%	90%	100%
Prophylactic Antibiotic Stopped[5]	-	-	76%	72%	95%
Pregnancy Care					
Inpatient Neonatal Mortality	-	-	-	-	-
Third or Fourth Degree Laceration	-	-	-	3.63%	3.27%

Crawford County Memorial Hospital

2020 1st Avenue S
Denison, IA 51442
Toll-Free: 888-747-0852
Phone: 712-263-5021
Fax: 712-263-1711
E-mail: edgast@ccmhia.com
URL: www.ccmhia.com
Ownership: Government - Local
Accredited: No
Emergency Services: Yes
Licensed Beds: 72

Key Personnel:

CEO. . . . . Edwin A Gast
Emergency Room . . . . Laurie Powres
Director Medical/Surgical Nursing . . . . Corrine Reitz
Director Radiology . . . . Kari Boyens
Director Respiratory Therapy . . . . Susan Schmedke

Measure	Cases	This Hospital	State Average	U.S. Average	Top Hospital
Heart Attack Care					
ACE Inhibitor or ARB for LVSD	0	-	86%	82%	100%
Aspirin at Arrival[1]	6	100%	89%	92%	100%
Aspirin at Discharge[1]	2	50%	90%	90%	100%
Beta Blocker at Arrival[1]	6	50%	91%	87%	100%
Beta Blocker at Discharge[1]	4	75%	91%	90%	100%
Fibrinolytic Medication Timing	0	-	33%	31%	100%
PCI Within 90 Minutes of Arrival	0	-	73%	54%	95%
Smoking Cessation Advice	0	-	92%	88%	100%
Heart Failure Care					
ACE Inhibitor or ARB for LVSD[1]	10	70%	84%	82%	100%
Discharge Instructions[1]	20	5%	62%	61%	93%
Evaluation of LVS Function	41	61%	75%	83%	99%
Smoking Cessation Advice[1]	3	0%	78%	82%	100%
Pneumonia Care					
Appropriate Initial Antibiotic	31	65%	85%	83%	94%
Blood Culture Timing[1]	15	93%	95%	90%	100%
Influenza Vaccine[1]	16	50%	85%	70%	100%
Initial Antibiotic Timing	39	90%	87%	80%	93%
Oxygenation Assessment	51	100%	99%	99%	100%
Pneumococcal Vaccine	45	80%	83%	69%	94%
Smoking Cessation Advice[1]	5	40%	75%	80%	100%
Surgical Infection Prevention					
Prophylactic Antibiotic Given[5]	-	-	79%	77%	95%
Prophylactic Antibiotic Selection[5]	-	-	89%	90%	100%
Prophylactic Antibiotic Stopped[5]	-	-	76%	72%	95%
Pregnancy Care					
Inpatient Neonatal Mortality	-	-	-	-	-
Third or Fourth Degree Laceration	-	-	-	3.63%	3.27%

Broadlawns Medical Center

1801 Hickman Road
Des Moines, IA 50314
Phone: 515-282-2200
Fax: 515-282-5785
E-mail: externalrelations@broadlawns.org
URL: www.broadlawns.org
Ownership: Government - Local
Accredited: Yes
Emergency Services: Yes
Licensed Beds: 200

Key Personnel:

President/CEO. . . . . Robert J Lundin, II
Chief Medical Officer . . . . Donald Jensen, MD
Director Medical/Surgical Nursing . . . . Carolyn Ruggles
OB/GYN Department Chief . . . . Larry Lindell, MD
Chief Radiology . . . . Steve Cooper, MD
Director Respiratory Therapy . . . . Robert Lambuth

Measure	Cases	This Hospital	State Average	U.S. Average	Top Hospital
Heart Attack Care					
ACE Inhibitor or ARB for LVSD[1]	3	67%	86%	82%	100%
Aspirin at Arrival[1]	12	83%	89%	92%	100%
Aspirin at Discharge[1]	8	88%	90%	90%	100%

NOTE: Hospital profiles are in alphabetical order by state, then city, then hospital within the city; Rankings are sorted by rate in descending order and exclude hospitals with less than 25 cases; (1) The number of cases is too small (n<25) for purposes of reliably predicting hospital performance; (2) Measure reflects the hospital's indication that its submission was based upon a sample of its relevant discharges; (3) Rate reflects fewer than the maximum possible quarters of data for the measure; (4) Inaccurate information submitted and suppressed for one or more quarters; (5) No data is available from the hospital for this measure; Please refer to the User's Guide for a full explanation of data

Beta Blocker at Arrival[1]	9	89%	91%	87%	100%
Beta Blocker at Discharge[1]	7	86%	91%	90%	100%
Fibrinolytic Medication Timing	0	-	33%	31%	100%
PCI Within 90 Minutes of Arrival	0	-	73%	54%	95%
Smoking Cessation Advice[1]	3	67%	92%	88%	100%
Heart Failure Care					
ACE Inhibitor or ARB for LVSD	47	100%	84%	82%	100%
Discharge Instructions	75	67%	62%	61%	93%
Evaluation of LVS Function	81	100%	75%	83%	99%
Smoking Cessation Advice	41	49%	78%	82%	100%
Pneumonia Care					
Appropriate Initial Antibiotic	55	87%	85%	83%	94%
Blood Culture Timing	43	88%	95%	90%	100%
Influenza Vaccine[1]	4	50%	85%	70%	100%
Initial Antibiotic Timing	60	87%	87%	80%	93%
Oxygenation Assessment	67	100%	99%	99%	100%
Pneumococcal Vaccine[1]	9	89%	83%	69%	94%
Smoking Cessation Advice	45	76%	75%	80%	100%
Surgical Infection Prevention					
Prophylactic Antibiotic Given	52	79%	79%	77%	95%
Prophylactic Antibiotic Selection[1]	16	100%	89%	90%	100%
Prophylactic Antibiotic Stopped	49	69%	76%	72%	95%
Pregnancy Care					
Inpatient Neonatal Mortality	-	-	-	-	-
Third or Fourth Degree Laceration	-	-	-	3.63%	3.27%

Iowa Lutheran Hospital

700 E University
Des Moines, IA 50316
URL: ihsdesmoines.org
Ownership: Voluntary non-profit - Church
Emergency Services: Yes

Phone: 515-241-6212
Fax: 515-241-5994
Accredited: Yes
Licensed Beds: 465

Key Personnel:
President/CEO. . . . . Eric Crowell
Chief Medical Staff. . . . . Kent Croskey, DO
Emergency Room . . . . Larry Baker, DO
Emergency Room . . . . Pam Ballard
Respiratory/Cardiopulmonary. . . . . Mike Wheeler

Measure	Cases	This Hospital	State Average	U.S. Average	Top Hospital
Heart Attack Care					
ACE Inhibitor or ARB for LVSD[2]	42	95%	86%	82%	100%
Aspirin at Arrival[2]	85	99%	89%	92%	100%
Aspirin at Discharge[2]	77	99%	90%	90%	100%
Beta Blocker at Arrival[2]	68	87%	91%	87%	100%
Beta Blocker at Discharge[2]	95	98%	91%	90%	100%
Fibrinolytic Medication Timing[2]	0	-	33%	31%	100%
PCI Within 90 Minutes of Arrival[1,2]	4	75%	73%	54%	95%
Smoking Cessation Advice[2]	33	97%	92%	88%	100%
Heart Failure Care					
ACE Inhibitor or ARB for LVSD[2]	104	91%	84%	82%	100%
Discharge Instructions[2]	193	65%	62%	61%	93%
Evaluation of LVS Function[2]	228	95%	75%	83%	99%
Smoking Cessation Advice[2]	57	100%	78%	82%	100%
Pneumonia Care					
Appropriate Initial Antibiotic[2]	102	91%	85%	83%	94%
Blood Culture Timing[2]	67	97%	95%	90%	100%
Influenza Vaccine[2]	29	76%	85%	70%	100%
Initial Antibiotic Timing[2]	143	87%	87%	80%	93%
Oxygenation Assessment[2]	167	100%	99%	99%	100%
Pneumococcal Vaccine[2]	109	74%	83%	69%	94%
Smoking Cessation Advice[2]	37	89%	75%	80%	100%
Surgical Infection Prevention					
Prophylactic Antibiotic Given[2]	234	94%	79%	77%	95%
Prophylactic Antibiotic Selection[2]	59	97%	89%	90%	100%
Prophylactic Antibiotic Stopped[2]	226	73%	76%	72%	95%
Pregnancy Care					
Inpatient Neonatal Mortality	-	-	-	-	-
Third or Fourth Degree Laceration	-	-	-	3.63%	3.27%

Iowa Methodist Medical Center

Alternate Name: Iowa Health Des Moines
1200 Pleasant Street
Des Moines, IA 50309
URL: www.ihsdesmoines.com
Ownership: Voluntary non-profit - Private
Emergency Services: Yes

Phone: 515-241-6212
Fax: 515-241-8580
Accredited: Yes
Licensed Beds: 373

Key Personnel:
President/CEO. . . . . Eric Crowell
Chief Medical Staff. . . . . Dr Josephson
Director Cardiology . . . . Steve House
Director Emergency Room. . . . . Lynda Schumaker

Measure	Cases	This Hospital	State Average	U.S. Average	Top Hospital
Heart Attack Care					
ACE Inhibitor or ARB for LVSD[2]	124	79%	86%	82%	100%
Aspirin at Arrival[2]	149	96%	89%	92%	100%
Aspirin at Discharge[2]	273	97%	90%	90%	100%
Beta Blocker at Arrival[2]	110	96%	91%	87%	100%
Beta Blocker at Discharge[2]	286	97%	91%	90%	100%
Fibrinolytic Medication Timing[2]	0	-	33%	31%	100%
PCI Within 90 Minutes of Arrival[1,2]	16	62%	73%	54%	95%
Smoking Cessation Advice[2]	91	96%	92%	88%	100%
Heart Failure Care					
ACE Inhibitor or ARB for LVSD[2]	148	89%	84%	82%	100%
Discharge Instructions[2]	235	65%	62%	61%	93%
Evaluation of LVS Function[2]	284	98%	75%	83%	99%
Smoking Cessation Advice[2]	41	98%	78%	82%	100%
Pneumonia Care					
Appropriate Initial Antibiotic[2]	88	78%	85%	83%	94%
Blood Culture Timing[2]	52	96%	95%	90%	100%
Influenza Vaccine[1,2]	19	74%	85%	70%	100%
Initial Antibiotic Timing[2]	114	82%	87%	80%	93%
Oxygenation Assessment[2]	140	100%	99%	99%	100%
Pneumococcal Vaccine[2]	108	76%	83%	69%	94%
Smoking Cessation Advice[2]	31	65%	75%	80%	100%
Surgical Infection Prevention					
Prophylactic Antibiotic Given[2]	332	94%	79%	77%	95%
Prophylactic Antibiotic Selection[2]	85	91%	89%	90%	100%
Prophylactic Antibiotic Stopped[2]	324	73%	76%	72%	95%
Pregnancy Care					
Inpatient Neonatal Mortality	-	-	-	-	-
Third or Fourth Degree Laceration	-	-	-	3.63%	3.27%

Mercy Medical Center-Des Moines

1111 6th Avenue
Des Moines, IA 50314
URL: www.mercydesmoines.org
Ownership: Voluntary non-profit - Church
Emergency Services: Yes

Phone: 515-247-3121
Fax: 515-643-8498
Accredited: Yes
Licensed Beds: 673

Key Personnel:
President/CEO. . . . . David Vellinga
Chief Medical Staff. . . . . RoseMary Mullin
Chief Catheterization Laboratory . . . . Liberto Iannone, MD
Emergency Room . . . . David Stilley, MD
Director Infection/Disease Control . . . . Connie Grout
CCU Spvg. Nurse . . . . Sharon Meadowcroft
OB/GYN Womens Health. . . . . Frederic Sager, DO
Chief Radiology . . . . Ruben Koehler, MD

Measure	Cases	This Hospital	State Average	U.S. Average	Top Hospital
Heart Attack Care					
ACE Inhibitor or ARB for LVSD	178	99%	86%	82%	100%
Aspirin at Arrival	331	100%	89%	92%	100%
Aspirin at Discharge	586	100%	90%	90%	100%
Beta Blocker at Arrival	262	98%	91%	87%	100%
Beta Blocker at Discharge	554	100%	91%	90%	100%
Fibrinolytic Medication Timing[1]	1	0%	33%	31%	100%
PCI Within 90 Minutes of Arrival[1]	20	95%	73%	54%	95%
Smoking Cessation Advice	280	100%	92%	88%	100%
Heart Failure Care					
ACE Inhibitor or ARB for LVSD	285	99%	84%	82%	100%
Discharge Instructions	734	98%	62%	61%	93%
Evaluation of LVS Function	888	100%	75%	83%	99%
Smoking Cessation Advice	145	100%	78%	82%	100%

NOTE: Hospital profiles are in alphabetical order by state, then city, then hospital within the city; Rankings are sorted by rate in descending order and exclude hospitals with less than 25 cases; (1) The number of cases is too small (n<25) for purposes of reliably predicting hospital performance; (2) Measure reflects the hospital's indication that its submission was based upon a sample of its relevant discharges; (3) Rate reflects fewer than the maximum possible quarters of data for the measure; (4) Inaccurate information submitted and suppressed for one or more quarters; (5) No data is available from the hospital for this measure; Please refer to the User's Guide for a full explanation of data

Pneumonia Care					
Appropriate Initial Antibiotic	352	97%	85%	83%	94%
Blood Culture Timing	348	95%	95%	90%	100%
Influenza Vaccine	110	97%	85%	70%	100%
Initial Antibiotic Timing	517	85%	87%	80%	93%
Oxygenation Assessment	659	100%	99%	99%	100%
Pneumococcal Vaccine	435	95%	83%	69%	94%
Smoking Cessation Advice	184	95%	75%	80%	100%
Surgical Infection Prevention					
Prophylactic Antibiotic Given	479	89%	79%	77%	95%
Prophylactic Antibiotic Selection	136	95%	89%	90%	100%
Prophylactic Antibiotic Stopped	449	92%	76%	72%	95%
Pregnancy Care					
Inpatient Neonatal Mortality	-	-	-	-	-
Third or Fourth Degree Laceration	-	-	-	3.63%	3.27%

Genesis Medical Center-Dewitt

1118 11th Street
Dewitt, IA 52742
Phone: 563-659-4200
URL: www.genesishealth.com
Ownership: Voluntary non-profit - Private
Accredited: Yes
Emergency Services: Yes
Licensed Beds: 90

Key Personnel:
President/CEO . . . . Jeffrey Cooper
Director Medical/Surgical Nursing . . . . Theresa Brock
Director Respiratory Therapy . . . . Peg Naughton

Measure	Cases	This Hospital	State Average	U.S. Average	Top Hospital
Heart Attack Care					
ACE Inhibitor or ARB for LVSD[5]	-	-	86%	82%	100%
Aspirin at Arrival[5]	-	-	89%	92%	100%
Aspirin at Discharge[5]	-	-	90%	90%	100%
Beta Blocker at Arrival[5]	-	-	91%	87%	100%
Beta Blocker at Discharge[5]	-	-	91%	90%	100%
Fibrinolytic Medication Timing[5]	-	-	33%	31%	100%
PCI Within 90 Minutes of Arrival[5]	-	-	73%	54%	95%
Smoking Cessation Advice[5]	-	-	92%	88%	100%
Heart Failure Care					
ACE Inhibitor or ARB for LVSD[1]	1	100%	84%	82%	100%
Discharge Instructions[1]	3	0%	62%	61%	93%
Evaluation of LVS Function[1]	4	50%	75%	83%	99%
Smoking Cessation Advice	0	-	78%	82%	100%
Pneumonia Care					
Appropriate Initial Antibiotic[1]	9	78%	85%	83%	94%
Blood Culture Timing[1]	15	80%	95%	90%	100%
Influenza Vaccine[1]	11	91%	85%	70%	100%
Initial Antibiotic Timing	26	81%	87%	80%	93%
Oxygenation Assessment	35	100%	99%	99%	100%
Pneumococcal Vaccine[1]	24	88%	83%	69%	94%
Smoking Cessation Advice[1]	4	100%	75%	80%	100%
Surgical Infection Prevention					
Prophylactic Antibiotic Given[5]	-	-	79%	77%	95%
Prophylactic Antibiotic Selection[5]	-	-	89%	90%	100%
Prophylactic Antibiotic Stopped[5]	-	-	76%	72%	95%
Pregnancy Care					
Inpatient Neonatal Mortality	-	-	-	-	-
Third or Fourth Degree Laceration	-	-	-	3.63%	3.27%

Finley Hospital

350 N Grandview Avenue
Dubuque, IA 52001
Toll-Free: 800-528-1891
Phone: 563-582-1881
Fax: 563-589-2620

E-mail: cr@finleyhospital.org
URL: www.finleyhospital.org
Ownership: Voluntary non-profit - Private
Accredited: Yes
Emergency Services: Yes
Licensed Beds: 158

Key Personnel:
CEO . . . . John E Knox
President Medical Staff . . . . Thomas J Bende Jr, MD
Director Womens/Childrens Services . . . . Jan Pacholke, MD
Director Surgical Services . . . . Lavern Bird
Director Respiratory Therapy . . . . Doug Becker

Measure	Cases	This Hospital	State Average	U.S. Average	Top Hospital
Heart Attack Care					
ACE Inhibitor or ARB for LVSD[1]	12	83%	86%	82%	100%
Aspirin at Arrival	47	91%	89%	92%	100%
Aspirin at Discharge	30	97%	90%	90%	100%
Beta Blocker at Arrival	35	89%	91%	87%	100%
Beta Blocker at Discharge	35	91%	91%	90%	100%
Fibrinolytic Medication Timing	0	-	33%	31%	100%
PCI Within 90 Minutes of Arrival	0	-	73%	54%	95%
Smoking Cessation Advice[1]	5	100%	92%	88%	100%
Heart Failure Care					
ACE Inhibitor or ARB for LVSD[1]	24	79%	84%	82%	100%
Discharge Instructions	69	94%	62%	61%	93%
Evaluation of LVS Function	95	87%	75%	83%	99%
Smoking Cessation Advice[1]	14	86%	78%	82%	100%
Pneumonia Care					
Appropriate Initial Antibiotic[2]	61	85%	85%	83%	94%
Blood Culture Timing[2]	72	100%	95%	90%	100%
Influenza Vaccine[1,2]	21	90%	85%	70%	100%
Initial Antibiotic Timing[2]	95	93%	87%	80%	93%
Oxygenation Assessment[2]	144	100%	99%	99%	100%
Pneumococcal Vaccine[2]	115	90%	83%	69%	94%
Smoking Cessation Advice[1,2]	20	90%	75%	80%	100%
Surgical Infection Prevention					
Prophylactic Antibiotic Given[2]	158	97%	79%	77%	95%
Prophylactic Antibiotic Selection[2]	36	94%	89%	90%	100%
Prophylactic Antibiotic Stopped[2]	154	84%	76%	72%	95%
Pregnancy Care					
Inpatient Neonatal Mortality	-	-	-	-	-
Third or Fourth Degree Laceration	-	-	-	3.63%	3.27%

Mercy Medical Center-Dubuque

250 Mercy Drive
Dubuque, IA 52001
Phone: 563-589-8000
Ownership: Voluntary non-profit - Church
Accredited: Yes
Emergency Services: Yes

Measure	Cases	This Hospital	State Average	U.S. Average	Top Hospital
Heart Attack Care					
ACE Inhibitor or ARB for LVSD	59	95%	86%	82%	100%
Aspirin at Arrival	190	98%	89%	92%	100%
Aspirin at Discharge	289	98%	90%	90%	100%
Beta Blocker at Arrival	172	95%	91%	87%	100%
Beta Blocker at Discharge	267	97%	91%	90%	100%
Fibrinolytic Medication Timing	0	-	33%	31%	100%
PCI Within 90 Minutes of Arrival[1]	10	50%	73%	54%	95%
Smoking Cessation Advice	85	95%	92%	88%	100%
Heart Failure Care					
ACE Inhibitor or ARB for LVSD	75	85%	84%	82%	100%
Discharge Instructions	162	56%	62%	61%	93%
Evaluation of LVS Function	189	93%	75%	83%	99%
Smoking Cessation Advice[1]	19	89%	78%	82%	100%
Pneumonia Care					
Appropriate Initial Antibiotic	108	87%	85%	83%	94%
Blood Culture Timing	97	88%	95%	90%	100%
Influenza Vaccine	26	92%	85%	70%	100%
Initial Antibiotic Timing	175	73%	87%	80%	93%
Oxygenation Assessment	214	99%	99%	99%	100%
Pneumococcal Vaccine	166	86%	83%	69%	94%
Smoking Cessation Advice	26	92%	75%	80%	100%
Surgical Infection Prevention					
Prophylactic Antibiotic Given[2,3]	455	92%	79%	77%	95%
Prophylactic Antibiotic Selection[2]	94	97%	89%	90%	100%
Prophylactic Antibiotic Stopped[2,3]	447	80%	76%	72%	95%
Pregnancy Care					
Inpatient Neonatal Mortality	937	0.11%	-	-	-
Third or Fourth Degree Laceration	677	2.51%	-	3.63%	3.27%

Mercy Medical Center-Dyersville

Alternate Name: Mercy Health Center-Saint Marys

NOTE: Hospital profiles are in alphabetical order by state, then city, then hospital within the city; Rankings are sorted by rate in descending order and exclude hospitals with less than 25 cases; (1) The number of cases is too small (n<25) for purposes of reliably predicting hospital performance; (2) Measure reflects the hospital's indication that its submission was based upon a sample of its relevant discharges; (3) Rate reflects fewer than the maximum possible quarters of data for the measure; (4) Inaccurate information submitted and suppressed for one or more quarters; (5) No data is available from the hospital for this measure; Please refer to the User's Guide for a full explanation of data

1111 3rd Street SW
Dyersville, IA 52040
Ownership: Voluntary non-profit - Other
Emergency Services: Yes
Phone: 563-875-7101
Fax: 563-875-2904
Accredited: No
Licensed Beds: 95

Key Personnel:
CEO. . . . . Rusty Knight

Measure	Cases	This Hospital	State Average	U.S. Average	Top Hospital
Heart Attack Care					
ACE Inhibitor or ARB for LVSD[5]	-	-	86%	82%	100%
Aspirin at Arrival[5]	-	-	89%	92%	100%
Aspirin at Discharge[5]	-	-	90%	90%	100%
Beta Blocker at Arrival[5]	-	-	91%	87%	100%
Beta Blocker at Discharge[5]	-	-	91%	90%	100%
Fibrinolytic Medication Timing[5]	-	-	33%	31%	100%
PCI Within 90 Minutes of Arrival[5]	-	-	73%	54%	95%
Smoking Cessation Advice[5]	-	-	92%	88%	100%
Heart Failure Care					
ACE Inhibitor or ARB for LVSD[3]	0	-	84%	82%	100%
Discharge Instructions[3]	0	-	62%	61%	93%
Evaluation of LVS Function[1,3]	1	0%	75%	83%	99%
Smoking Cessation Advice[3]	0	-	78%	82%	100%
Pneumonia Care					
Appropriate Initial Antibiotic[1,3]	3	100%	85%	83%	94%
Blood Culture Timing[1,3]	2	100%	95%	90%	100%
Influenza Vaccine[1]	2	100%	85%	70%	100%
Initial Antibiotic Timing[1,3]	5	60%	87%	80%	93%
Oxygenation Assessment[1,3]	5	100%	99%	99%	100%
Pneumococcal Vaccine[1,3]	3	67%	83%	69%	94%
Smoking Cessation Advice[3]	0	-	75%	80%	100%
Surgical Infection Prevention					
Prophylactic Antibiotic Given[5]	-	-	79%	77%	95%
Prophylactic Antibiotic Selection[5]	-	-	89%	90%	100%
Prophylactic Antibiotic Stopped[5]	-	-	76%	72%	95%
Pregnancy Care					
Inpatient Neonatal Mortality	-	-	-	-	-
Third or Fourth Degree Laceration	-	-	-	3.63%	3.27%

Jefferson County Hospital

400 Highland
Fairfield, IA 52556
URL: www.jchospital.org
Ownership: Government - State
Emergency Services: Yes
Phone: 641-472-4111
Fax: 641-469-4375
Accredited: No
Licensed Beds: 67

Key Personnel:
CEO/President. . . . . Ralph Paulding
Chief of Medical Staff. . . . . Deb Cardin
Emergency Room . . . . Curt Smith
Manager Radiology . . . . Linda Marlay
Director Respiratory Therapy . . . . Ross De Boer, RT

Measure	Cases	This Hospital	State Average	U.S. Average	Top Hospital
Heart Attack Care					
ACE Inhibitor or ARB for LVSD	0	-	86%	82%	100%
Aspirin at Arrival[1]	4	50%	89%	92%	100%
Aspirin at Discharge[1]	3	100%	90%	90%	100%
Beta Blocker at Arrival[1]	2	50%	91%	87%	100%
Beta Blocker at Discharge[1]	2	100%	91%	90%	100%
Fibrinolytic Medication Timing	0	-	33%	31%	100%
PCI Within 90 Minutes of Arrival	0	-	73%	54%	95%
Smoking Cessation Advice	0	-	92%	88%	100%
Heart Failure Care					
ACE Inhibitor or ARB for LVSD[1]	6	100%	84%	82%	100%
Discharge Instructions[1]	9	56%	62%	61%	93%
Evaluation of LVS Function	27	89%	75%	83%	99%
Smoking Cessation Advice[1]	2	0%	78%	82%	100%
Pneumonia Care					
Appropriate Initial Antibiotic[1]	22	82%	85%	83%	94%
Blood Culture Timing[1]	15	93%	95%	90%	100%
Influenza Vaccine[1]	2	100%	85%	70%	100%
Initial Antibiotic Timing	28	86%	87%	80%	93%
Oxygenation Assessment	35	97%	99%	99%	100%
Pneumococcal Vaccine[1]	21	52%	83%	69%	94%
Smoking Cessation Advice[1]	4	25%	75%	80%	100%
Surgical Infection Prevention					
Prophylactic Antibiotic Given	52	83%	79%	77%	95%
Prophylactic Antibiotic Selection[1]	10	100%	89%	90%	100%
Prophylactic Antibiotic Stopped	45	80%	76%	72%	95%
Pregnancy Care					
Inpatient Neonatal Mortality	-	-	-	-	-
Third or Fourth Degree Laceration	-	-	-	3.63%	3.27%

Trinity Regional Medical Center

802 Kenyon Road
Fort Dodge, IA 50501
URL: www.trmc.org
Ownership: Voluntary non-profit - Private
Emergency Services: Yes
Phone: 515-573-3101
Fax: 515-573-8710
Accredited: Yes
Licensed Beds: 200

Key Personnel:
CEO. . . . . Thomas F Tibbits
Chief Medical Staff. . . . . Kenneth Adams, DO
Cardiac/Laboratory. . . . . Eric Anderson
Catheterization Laboratory . . . . Eric Anderson
Emergency Room . . . . Paylane Wilweath
Infection Control. . . . . Linda Opheim
ICU . . . . Sheryl Rogers
Medical/Surgical Nursing . . . . Deb Schriver
OB/GYN. . . . . Joan Hisler
Respiratory Therapy. . . . . Paul Goldman

Measure	Cases	This Hospital	State Average	U.S. Average	Top Hospital
Heart Attack Care					
ACE Inhibitor or ARB for LVSD	46	100%	86%	82%	100%
Aspirin at Arrival	121	98%	89%	92%	100%
Aspirin at Discharge	206	100%	90%	90%	100%
Beta Blocker at Arrival	105	96%	91%	87%	100%
Beta Blocker at Discharge	190	98%	91%	90%	100%
Fibrinolytic Medication Timing[3]	0	-	33%	31%	100%
PCI Within 90 Minutes of Arrival[1]	3	100%	73%	54%	95%
Smoking Cessation Advice	69	99%	92%	88%	100%
Heart Failure Care					
ACE Inhibitor or ARB for LVSD	107	93%	84%	82%	100%
Discharge Instructions	174	90%	62%	61%	93%
Evaluation of LVS Function	240	95%	75%	83%	99%
Smoking Cessation Advice	47	85%	78%	82%	100%
Pneumonia Care					
Appropriate Initial Antibiotic	160	92%	85%	83%	94%
Blood Culture Timing	209	98%	95%	90%	100%
Influenza Vaccine	65	91%	85%	70%	100%
Initial Antibiotic Timing	249	96%	87%	80%	93%
Oxygenation Assessment	297	100%	99%	99%	100%
Pneumococcal Vaccine	218	94%	83%	69%	94%
Smoking Cessation Advice	42	95%	75%	80%	100%
Surgical Infection Prevention					
Prophylactic Antibiotic Given[2]	234	84%	79%	77%	95%
Prophylactic Antibiotic Selection[2]	57	100%	89%	90%	100%
Prophylactic Antibiotic Stopped[2]	226	78%	76%	72%	95%
Pregnancy Care					
Inpatient Neonatal Mortality	-	-	-	-	-
Third or Fourth Degree Laceration	-	-	-	3.63%	3.27%

Fort Madison Community Hospital

5545 Avenue O
Fort Madison, IA 52627
E-mail: jplatt@fmchosp.com
URL: www.fmchosp.com
Ownership: Proprietary
Emergency Services: Yes
Phone: 319-372-6530
Fax: 319-372-9119
Accredited: Yes
Licensed Beds: 50

Key Personnel:
CEO. . . . . C James Platt
Chief Medical Staff. . . . . David Wenger Keller, MD
Emergency Room . . . . Debbie Magel
Chief Radiology . . . . Tim Reiners, MD
Director Respiratory Therapy . . . . Mona Meyers

NOTE: Hospital profiles are in alphabetical order by state, then city, then hospital within the city; Rankings are sorted by rate in descending order and exclude hospitals with less than 25 cases; (1) The number of cases is too small (n<25) for purposes of reliably predicting hospital performance; (2) Measure reflects the hospital's indication that its submission was based upon a sample of its relevant discharges; (3) Rate reflects fewer than the maximum possible quarters of data for the measure; (4) Inaccurate information submitted and suppressed for one or more quarters; (5) No data is available from the hospital for this measure; Please refer to the User's Guide for a full explanation of data

Measure	Cases	This Hospital	State Average	U.S. Average	Top Hospital
Heart Attack Care					
ACE Inhibitor or ARB for LVSD[1]	5	100%	86%	82%	100%
Aspirin at Arrival[1]	9	100%	89%	92%	100%
Aspirin at Discharge[1]	5	100%	90%	90%	100%
Beta Blocker at Arrival[1]	10	100%	91%	87%	100%
Beta Blocker at Discharge[1]	5	100%	91%	90%	100%
Fibrinolytic Medication Timing	0	-	33%	31%	100%
PCI Within 90 Minutes of Arrival	0	-	73%	54%	95%
Smoking Cessation Advice	0	-	92%	88%	100%
Heart Failure Care					
ACE Inhibitor or ARB for LVSD	30	97%	84%	82%	100%
Discharge Instructions	54	98%	62%	61%	93%
Evaluation of LVS Function	88	100%	75%	83%	99%
Smoking Cessation Advice[1]	8	100%	78%	82%	100%
Pneumonia Care					
Appropriate Initial Antibiotic	58	83%	85%	83%	94%
Blood Culture Timing	58	100%	95%	90%	100%
Influenza Vaccine[1]	13	100%	85%	70%	100%
Initial Antibiotic Timing	85	95%	87%	80%	93%
Oxygenation Assessment	101	100%	99%	99%	100%
Pneumococcal Vaccine	78	96%	83%	69%	94%
Smoking Cessation Advice[1]	16	100%	75%	80%	100%
Surgical Infection Prevention					
Prophylactic Antibiotic Given[3]	105	90%	79%	77%	95%
Prophylactic Antibiotic Selection	42	100%	89%	90%	100%
Prophylactic Antibiotic Stopped[3]	100	82%	76%	72%	95%
Pregnancy Care					
Inpatient Neonatal Mortality	-	-	-	-	-
Third or Fourth Degree Laceration	-	-	-	3.63%	3.27%

Adair County Memorial Hospital

609 SE Kent
Greenfield, IA 50849
Phone: 641-743-2123
Fax: 641-743-2610
URL: www.adaircountyhealthsystem.org
Ownership: Government - Local
Accredited: No
Emergency Services: Yes
Licensed Beds: 31

Key Personnel:

CEO. . . . . M Gandal
Administrator . . . . Myrna Erb-Gondel
Chief Medical Staff. . . . . Troy Renaud
Director Infection/Disease Control . . . . Deb Tindle, RN

Measure	Cases	This Hospital	State Average	U.S. Average	Top Hospital
Heart Attack Care					
ACE Inhibitor or ARB for LVSD[5]	-	-	86%	82%	100%
Aspirin at Arrival[5]	-	-	89%	92%	100%
Aspirin at Discharge[5]	-	-	90%	90%	100%
Beta Blocker at Arrival[5]	-	-	91%	87%	100%
Beta Blocker at Discharge[5]	-	-	91%	90%	100%
Fibrinolytic Medication Timing[5]	-	-	33%	31%	100%
PCI Within 90 Minutes of Arrival[5]	-	-	73%	54%	95%
Smoking Cessation Advice[5]	-	-	92%	88%	100%
Heart Failure Care					
ACE Inhibitor or ARB for LVSD[3]	0	-	84%	82%	100%
Discharge Instructions[1,3]	10	80%	62%	61%	93%
Evaluation of LVS Function[1,3]	12	17%	75%	83%	99%
Smoking Cessation Advice[1,3]	1	0%	78%	82%	100%
Pneumonia Care					
Appropriate Initial Antibiotic[1]	12	67%	85%	83%	94%
Blood Culture Timing[1]	4	100%	95%	90%	100%
Influenza Vaccine[4,5]	-	-	85%	70%	100%
Initial Antibiotic Timing[1]	12	92%	87%	80%	93%
Oxygenation Assessment[1]	18	100%	99%	99%	100%
Pneumococcal Vaccine[1]	15	100%	83%	69%	94%
Smoking Cessation Advice[1]	3	100%	75%	80%	100%
Surgical Infection Prevention					
Prophylactic Antibiotic Given[5]	-	-	79%	77%	95%
Prophylactic Antibiotic Selection[5]	-	-	89%	90%	100%
Prophylactic Antibiotic Stopped[5]	-	-	76%	72%	95%
Pregnancy Care					
Inpatient Neonatal Mortality	-	-	-	-	-
Third or Fourth Degree Laceration	-	-	-	3.63%	3.27%

Grinnell Regional Medical Center

Alternate Name: Grinnell General Hospital
210 4th Avenue
Grinnell, IA 50112
Phone: 641-236-7511
Fax: 641-236-2995
URL: www.grmc.us
Ownership: Voluntary non-profit - Private
Accredited: No
Emergency Services: Yes
Licensed Beds: 81

Key Personnel:

President/CEO. . . . . Todd C Linden
Medical Staff President . . . . Roy Doorebos, MD
Director Surgical Services . . . . Deb Reding

Measure	Cases	This Hospital	State Average	U.S. Average	Top Hospital
Heart Attack Care					
ACE Inhibitor or ARB for LVSD[1]	1	100%	86%	82%	100%
Aspirin at Arrival[1]	7	100%	89%	92%	100%
Aspirin at Discharge[1]	7	100%	90%	90%	100%
Beta Blocker at Arrival[1]	5	100%	91%	87%	100%
Beta Blocker at Discharge[1]	6	100%	91%	90%	100%
Fibrinolytic Medication Timing[1]	1	100%	33%	31%	100%
PCI Within 90 Minutes of Arrival	0	-	73%	54%	95%
Smoking Cessation Advice[1]	1	100%	92%	88%	100%
Heart Failure Care					
ACE Inhibitor or ARB for LVSD[1]	8	75%	84%	82%	100%
Discharge Instructions	52	83%	62%	61%	93%
Evaluation of LVS Function	93	89%	75%	83%	99%
Smoking Cessation Advice[1]	11	91%	78%	82%	100%
Pneumonia Care					
Appropriate Initial Antibiotic	75	85%	85%	83%	94%
Blood Culture Timing	54	98%	95%	90%	100%
Influenza Vaccine[1]	18	100%	85%	70%	100%
Initial Antibiotic Timing	107	88%	87%	80%	93%
Oxygenation Assessment	126	100%	99%	99%	100%
Pneumococcal Vaccine	90	92%	83%	69%	94%
Smoking Cessation Advice[1]	16	62%	75%	80%	100%
Surgical Infection Prevention					
Prophylactic Antibiotic Given[2]	111	91%	79%	77%	95%
Prophylactic Antibiotic Selection[2]	31	97%	89%	90%	100%
Prophylactic Antibiotic Stopped[2]	101	68%	76%	72%	95%
Pregnancy Care					
Inpatient Neonatal Mortality	-	-	-	-	-
Third or Fourth Degree Laceration	-	-	-	3.63%	3.27%

Grundy County Memorial Hospital

201 E J Avenue
Grundy Center, IA 50638
Phone: 319-824-5421
Fax: 319-824-3337
E-mail: janicem@gcmuni.net
URL: www.grundyhospital.com
Ownership: Voluntary non-profit - Other
Accredited: No
Emergency Services: Yes
Licensed Beds: 25

Key Personnel:

CEO. . . . . Pamela Delagardelle
Chief Medical Staff. . . . . Robert Thompson, MD
Emergency Room/Operating Room Director . . . Elizabeth Ash, RN

Measure	Cases	This Hospital	State Average	U.S. Average	Top Hospital
Heart Attack Care					
ACE Inhibitor or ARB for LVSD[5]	-	-	86%	82%	100%
Aspirin at Arrival[5]	-	-	89%	92%	100%
Aspirin at Discharge[5]	-	-	90%	90%	100%
Beta Blocker at Arrival[5]	-	-	91%	87%	100%
Beta Blocker at Discharge[5]	-	-	91%	90%	100%
Fibrinolytic Medication Timing[5]	-	-	33%	31%	100%
PCI Within 90 Minutes of Arrival[5]	-	-	73%	54%	95%
Smoking Cessation Advice[5]	-	-	92%	88%	100%
Heart Failure Care					
ACE Inhibitor or ARB for LVSD[3]	0	-	84%	82%	100%
Discharge Instructions[1,3]	2	0%	62%	61%	93%
Evaluation of LVS Function[1,3]	5	40%	75%	83%	99%

NOTE: Hospital profiles are in alphabetical order by state, then city, then hospital within the city; Rankings are sorted by rate in descending order and exclude hospitals with less than 25 cases; (1) The number of cases is too small (n<25) for purposes of reliably predicting hospital performance; (2) Measure reflects the hospital's indication that its submission was based upon a sample of its relevant discharges; (3) Rate reflects fewer than the maximum possible quarters of data for the measure; (4) Inaccurate information submitted and suppressed for one or more quarters; (5) No data is available from the hospital for this measure; Please refer to the User's Guide for a full explanation of data

Measure	Cases	This Hospital	State Average	U.S. Average	Top Hospital
Smoking Cessation Advice[3]	0	-	78%	82%	100%
Pneumonia Care					
Appropriate Initial Antibiotic[1,3]	4	100%	85%	83%	94%
Blood Culture Timing[3]	0	-	95%	90%	100%
Influenza Vaccine[5]	-	-	85%	70%	100%
Initial Antibiotic Timing[1,3]	2	100%	87%	80%	93%
Oxygenation Assessment[1,3]	4	100%	99%	99%	100%
Pneumococcal Vaccine[1,3]	4	100%	83%	69%	94%
Smoking Cessation Advice[3]	0	-	75%	80%	100%
Surgical Infection Prevention					
Prophylactic Antibiotic Given[1,3]	2	100%	79%	77%	95%
Prophylactic Antibiotic Selection[1]	2	100%	89%	90%	100%
Prophylactic Antibiotic Stopped[1,3]	2	100%	76%	72%	95%
Pregnancy Care					
Inpatient Neonatal Mortality	-	-	-	-	-
Third or Fourth Degree Laceration	-	-	-	3.63%	3.27%

Guttenberg Municipal Hospital

2nd & Main Streets
PO Box 550
Guttenberg, IA 52052
Phone: 563-252-1121
Fax: 563-252-3120
URL: www.guttenberghospital.org
Ownership: Government - Local
Accredited: No
Emergency Services: Yes
Licensed Beds: 25

Key Personnel:

CEO . . . . Kimberly A Gau
Chief Staff . . . . Robert Merrick, MD
Cardiac Lab . . . . Doreen Roberts
Emergency Room . . . . Andrew Smith-Liason, MD
Infection Control . . . . Robin Scott, RN
CEO & Chief Nurse Executive . . . . Kim Gau, RN
Respiratory/Cardiopulmonary . . . . Doreen Roberts

Measure	Cases	This Hospital	State Average	U.S. Average	Top Hospital
Heart Attack Care					
ACE Inhibitor or ARB for LVSD[1]	1	100%	86%	82%	100%
Aspirin at Arrival[1]	9	78%	89%	92%	100%
Aspirin at Discharge[1]	9	89%	90%	90%	100%
Beta Blocker at Arrival[1]	11	73%	91%	87%	100%
Beta Blocker at Discharge[1]	12	92%	91%	90%	100%
Fibrinolytic Medication Timing[1]	2	0%	33%	31%	100%
PCI Within 90 Minutes of Arrival	0	-	73%	54%	95%
Smoking Cessation Advice[1]	1	100%	92%	88%	100%
Heart Failure Care					
ACE Inhibitor or ARB for LVSD[1]	2	100%	84%	82%	100%
Discharge Instructions[1]	12	33%	62%	61%	93%
Evaluation of LVS Function[1]	20	60%	75%	83%	99%
Smoking Cessation Advice[1]	1	0%	78%	82%	100%
Pneumonia Care					
Appropriate Initial Antibiotic[1]	7	86%	85%	83%	94%
Blood Culture Timing[1]	5	80%	95%	90%	100%
Influenza Vaccine[1]	3	100%	85%	70%	100%
Initial Antibiotic Timing[1]	5	80%	87%	80%	93%
Oxygenation Assessment[1]	13	69%	99%	99%	100%
Pneumococcal Vaccine[1]	9	100%	83%	69%	94%
Smoking Cessation Advice	0	-	75%	80%	100%
Surgical Infection Prevention					
Prophylactic Antibiotic Given[1,3]	1	0%	79%	77%	95%
Prophylactic Antibiotic Selection[5]	-	-	89%	90%	100%
Prophylactic Antibiotic Stopped[1,3]	1	100%	76%	72%	95%
Pregnancy Care					
Inpatient Neonatal Mortality	-	-	-	-	-
Third or Fourth Degree Laceration	-	-	-	3.63%	3.27%

Shelby County Myrtue Memorial Hospital

1213 Garfield Avenue
Harlan, IA 51537
Phone: 712-755-5161
Fax: 712-755-2640
URL: www.shelbycohealth.com
Ownership: Government - State
Accredited: No
Emergency Services: Yes
Licensed Beds: 52

Key Personnel:

CEO . . . . Mark Woodring
Chief Medical Staff . . . . Timothy Brelje
Chief Medical Staff . . . . Don Klilgaard
Emergency Room . . . . Scott Markham
Director Respiratory Therapy . . . . John Bolton

Measure	Cases	This Hospital	State Average	U.S. Average	Top Hospital
Heart Attack Care					
ACE Inhibitor or ARB for LVSD[1,3]	1	100%	86%	82%	100%
Aspirin at Arrival[1,3]	1	100%	89%	92%	100%
Aspirin at Discharge[1,3]	2	100%	90%	90%	100%
Beta Blocker at Arrival[1,3]	1	100%	91%	87%	100%
Beta Blocker at Discharge[1,3]	2	100%	91%	90%	100%
Fibrinolytic Medication Timing[3]	0	-	33%	31%	100%
PCI Within 90 Minutes of Arrival	0	-	73%	54%	95%
Smoking Cessation Advice[3]	0	-	92%	88%	100%
Heart Failure Care					
ACE Inhibitor or ARB for LVSD[1]	17	100%	84%	82%	100%
Discharge Instructions[1]	20	95%	62%	61%	93%
Evaluation of LVS Function	64	100%	75%	83%	99%
Smoking Cessation Advice[1]	4	100%	78%	82%	100%
Pneumonia Care					
Appropriate Initial Antibiotic	49	94%	85%	83%	94%
Blood Culture Timing	54	100%	95%	90%	100%
Influenza Vaccine[1]	24	100%	85%	70%	100%
Initial Antibiotic Timing	84	93%	87%	80%	93%
Oxygenation Assessment	98	100%	99%	99%	100%
Pneumococcal Vaccine	79	94%	83%	69%	94%
Smoking Cessation Advice[1]	7	86%	75%	80%	100%
Surgical Infection Prevention					
Prophylactic Antibiotic Given[1,2]	10	100%	79%	77%	95%
Prophylactic Antibiotic Selection[1,2]	2	100%	89%	90%	100%
Prophylactic Antibiotic Stopped[1,2]	10	80%	76%	72%	95%
Pregnancy Care					
Inpatient Neonatal Mortality	-	-	-	-	-
Third or Fourth Degree Laceration	-	-	-	3.63%	3.27%

Hawarden Community Hospital

1111 11th Street
Hawarden, IA 51023
Phone: 712-551-3100
Fax: 712-551-3106
E-mail: commhosp@acsnet.com
URL: www.acsnet.com
Ownership: Government - Local
Accredited: No
Emergency Services: Yes
Licensed Beds: 18

Key Personnel:

CEO . . . . Chad Markham
Emergency Room . . . . Lorna Westra
Chief of Respiratory/Pulmonary Therapy . . . . . . Glenda VanYhe

Measure	Cases	This Hospital	State Average	U.S. Average	Top Hospital
Heart Attack Care					
ACE Inhibitor or ARB for LVSD[5]	-	-	86%	82%	100%
Aspirin at Arrival[5]	-	-	89%	92%	100%
Aspirin at Discharge[5]	-	-	90%	90%	100%
Beta Blocker at Arrival[5]	-	-	91%	87%	100%
Beta Blocker at Discharge[5]	-	-	91%	90%	100%
Fibrinolytic Medication Timing[5]	-	-	33%	31%	100%
PCI Within 90 Minutes of Arrival[5]	-	-	73%	54%	95%
Smoking Cessation Advice[5]	-	-	92%	88%	100%
Heart Failure Care					
ACE Inhibitor or ARB for LVSD[1,2,3]	1	100%	84%	82%	100%
Discharge Instructions[1,2,3]	5	20%	62%	61%	93%
Evaluation of LVS Function[1,2,3]	4	25%	75%	83%	99%
Smoking Cessation Advice[2,3]	0	-	78%	82%	100%
Pneumonia Care					
Appropriate Initial Antibiotic[1,2,3]	6	100%	85%	83%	94%
Blood Culture Timing[1,2,3]	3	100%	95%	90%	100%
Influenza Vaccine[1,2]	3	100%	85%	70%	100%
Initial Antibiotic Timing[1,2,3]	7	86%	87%	80%	93%
Oxygenation Assessment[1,2,3]	8	100%	99%	99%	100%
Pneumococcal Vaccine[1,2,3]	8	100%	83%	69%	94%
Smoking Cessation Advice[1,2,3]	2	100%	75%	80%	100%
Surgical Infection Prevention					
Prophylactic Antibiotic Given[5]	-	-	79%	77%	95%

NOTE: Hospital profiles are in alphabetical order by state, then city, then hospital within the city; Rankings are sorted by rate in descending order and exclude hospitals with less than 25 cases; (1) The number of cases is too small (n<25) for purposes of reliably predicting hospital performance; (2) Measure reflects the hospital's indication that its submission was based upon a sample of its relevant discharges; (3) Rate reflects fewer than the maximum possible quarters of data for the measure; (4) Inaccurate information submitted and suppressed for one or more quarters; (5) No data is available from the hospital for this measure; Please refer to the User's Guide for a full explanation of data

Prophylactic Antibiotic Selection[5]	-	-	89%	90%	100%
Prophylactic Antibiotic Stopped[5]	-	-	76%	72%	95%
Pregnancy Care					
Inpatient Neonatal Mortality	-	-	-	-	-
Third or Fourth Degree Laceration	-	-	-	3.63%	3.27%

Horn Memorial Hospital

701 E 2nd Street
Ida Grove, IA 51445
Phone: 712-364-3311
Fax: 712-364-4341
E-mail: dellis@hornmemorialhospital.org
URL: www.hornmemorialhospital.org
Ownership: Voluntary non-profit - Private
Accredited: No
Emergency Services: Yes
Licensed Beds: 25

Key Personnel:

CEO. . . . . Dan Ellis
Chief Medical Staff. . . . . Albert Veltri, MD
Manager Emergency Room . . . . Betsy Dettman, RN
Infection Control. . . . . Kay Zediker, RN
Director Radiology . . . . Jerri Down

Measure	Cases	This Hospital	State Average	U.S. Average	Top Hospital
Heart Attack Care					
ACE Inhibitor or ARB for LVSD[5]	-	-	86%	82%	100%
Aspirin at Arrival[5]	-	-	89%	92%	100%
Aspirin at Discharge[5]	-	-	90%	90%	100%
Beta Blocker at Arrival[5]	-	-	91%	87%	100%
Beta Blocker at Discharge[5]	-	-	91%	90%	100%
Fibrinolytic Medication Timing[5]	-	-	33%	31%	100%
PCI Within 90 Minutes of Arrival[5]	-	-	73%	54%	95%
Smoking Cessation Advice[5]	-	-	92%	88%	100%
Heart Failure Care					
ACE Inhibitor or ARB for LVSD[1]	2	50%	84%	82%	100%
Discharge Instructions[1]	11	36%	62%	61%	93%
Evaluation of LVS Function[1]	21	38%	75%	83%	99%
Smoking Cessation Advice[1]	3	0%	78%	82%	100%
Pneumonia Care					
Appropriate Initial Antibiotic[5]	-	-	85%	83%	94%
Blood Culture Timing[5]	-	-	95%	90%	100%
Influenza Vaccine[5]	-	-	85%	70%	100%
Initial Antibiotic Timing[5]	-	-	87%	80%	93%
Oxygenation Assessment[5]	-	-	99%	99%	100%
Pneumococcal Vaccine[5]	-	-	83%	69%	94%
Smoking Cessation Advice[5]	-	-	75%	80%	100%
Surgical Infection Prevention					
Prophylactic Antibiotic Given[5]	-	-	79%	77%	95%
Prophylactic Antibiotic Selection[5]	-	-	89%	90%	100%
Prophylactic Antibiotic Stopped[5]	-	-	76%	72%	95%
Pregnancy Care					
Inpatient Neonatal Mortality	-	-	-	-	-
Third or Fourth Degree Laceration	-	-	-	3.63%	3.27%

Buchanan County Health Center

1600 1st Street E
Independence, IA 50644
Phone: 319-334-6071
Fax: 319-334-6149
URL: www.bchealth.info
Ownership: Voluntary non-profit - Other
Accredited: No
Emergency Services: Yes
Licensed Beds: 84

Key Personnel:

CEO. . . . . Robert J Richard
Chief Medical Staff. . . . . Julia Sprusall
Chief Medical Staff. . . . . Dr Julie Sandell
Director Cardiology . . . . Deb Recker
Emergency Room . . . . Roslind Gibbs
Infection Control. . . . . Mary Schmitt
Director Medical/Surgical Nursing . . . . Julie Sproull
Chief Radiology . . . . Inez Kremer
Director Respiratory Therapy . . . . Linda Faust

Measure	Cases	This Hospital	State Average	U.S. Average	Top Hospital
Heart Attack Care					
ACE Inhibitor or ARB for LVSD[5]	-	-	86%	82%	100%
Aspirin at Arrival[5]	-	-	89%	92%	100%
Aspirin at Discharge[5]	-	-	90%	90%	100%
Beta Blocker at Arrival[5]	-	-	91%	87%	100%
Beta Blocker at Discharge[5]	-	-	91%	90%	100%
Fibrinolytic Medication Timing[5]	-	-	33%	31%	100%
PCI Within 90 Minutes of Arrival[5]	-	-	73%	54%	95%
Smoking Cessation Advice[5]	-	-	92%	88%	100%
Heart Failure Care					
ACE Inhibitor or ARB for LVSD[1]	2	50%	84%	82%	100%
Discharge Instructions[1]	13	54%	62%	61%	93%
Evaluation of LVS Function[1]	16	38%	75%	83%	99%
Smoking Cessation Advice	0	-	78%	82%	100%
Pneumonia Care					
Appropriate Initial Antibiotic[1]	24	79%	85%	83%	94%
Blood Culture Timing[1]	4	100%	95%	90%	100%
Influenza Vaccine[1]	5	80%	85%	70%	100%
Initial Antibiotic Timing[1]	22	77%	87%	80%	93%
Oxygenation Assessment	34	100%	99%	99%	100%
Pneumococcal Vaccine[1]	24	79%	83%	69%	94%
Smoking Cessation Advice[1]	9	44%	75%	80%	100%
Surgical Infection Prevention					
Prophylactic Antibiotic Given[5]	-	-	79%	77%	95%
Prophylactic Antibiotic Selection[5]	-	-	89%	90%	100%
Prophylactic Antibiotic Stopped[5]	-	-	76%	72%	95%
Pregnancy Care					
Inpatient Neonatal Mortality	-	-	-	-	-
Third or Fourth Degree Laceration	-	-	-	3.63%	3.27%

Mercy Hospital

Alternate Name: Mercy Iowa City
500 E Market Street
Iowa City, IA 52245
Phone: 319-339-0300
Fax: 319-339-3788
URL: www.mercyiowacity.org
Ownership: Voluntary non-profit - Church
Accredited: Yes
Emergency Services: Yes
Licensed Beds: 240

Key Personnel:

President/CEO. . . . . Ronald R Reed

Measure	Cases	This Hospital	State Average	U.S. Average	Top Hospital
Heart Attack Care					
ACE Inhibitor or ARB for LVSD	50	86%	86%	82%	100%
Aspirin at Arrival	131	98%	89%	92%	100%
Aspirin at Discharge	219	99%	90%	90%	100%
Beta Blocker at Arrival	117	92%	91%	87%	100%
Beta Blocker at Discharge	235	95%	91%	90%	100%
Fibrinolytic Medication Timing	0	-	33%	31%	100%
PCI Within 90 Minutes of Arrival[1]	9	22%	73%	54%	95%
Smoking Cessation Advice	59	97%	92%	88%	100%
Heart Failure Care					
ACE Inhibitor or ARB for LVSD	81	83%	84%	82%	100%
Discharge Instructions	187	86%	62%	61%	93%
Evaluation of LVS Function	230	93%	75%	83%	99%
Smoking Cessation Advice	32	94%	78%	82%	100%
Pneumonia Care					
Appropriate Initial Antibiotic	108	81%	85%	83%	94%
Blood Culture Timing	93	96%	95%	90%	100%
Influenza Vaccine	28	79%	85%	70%	100%
Initial Antibiotic Timing	137	79%	87%	80%	93%
Oxygenation Assessment	168	99%	99%	99%	100%
Pneumococcal Vaccine	123	78%	83%	69%	94%
Smoking Cessation Advice	33	85%	75%	80%	100%
Surgical Infection Prevention					
Prophylactic Antibiotic Given[3]	379	94%	79%	77%	95%
Prophylactic Antibiotic Selection	217	99%	89%	90%	100%
Prophylactic Antibiotic Stopped[3]	376	65%	76%	72%	95%
Pregnancy Care					
Inpatient Neonatal Mortality	-	-	-	-	-
Third or Fourth Degree Laceration	-	-	-	3.63%	3.27%

NOTE: Hospital profiles are in alphabetical order by state, then city, then hospital within the city; Rankings are sorted by rate in descending order and exclude hospitals with less than 25 cases; (1) The number of cases is too small (n<25) for purposes of reliably predicting hospital performance; (2) Measure reflects the hospital's indication that its submission was based upon a sample of its relevant discharges; (3) Rate reflects fewer than the maximum possible quarters of data for the measure; (4) Inaccurate information submitted and suppressed for one or more quarters; (5) No data is available from the hospital for this measure; Please refer to the User's Guide for a full explanation of data

University of Iowa Hospitals and Clinics

200 Hawkins Drive
Iowa City, IA 52242
URL: www.uihealthcare.com
Ownership: Government - State
Emergency Services: Yes

Phone: 319-356-1616
Fax: 319-356-3862

Accredited: Yes
Licensed Beds: 762

Key Personnel:

President/CEO. . . . . Donna Katen-Bahensky
Chief Medical Staff. . . . . Eva Tsalikian
Emergency Room . . . . Eric Dickson, MD
Associate Medical/Surgical Nursing . . . . Joelle Jensen, RN
Chief Medical Officer . . . . Craig Syrop, MD
OB/GYN Womens Health. . . . . Jennifer R Niebyl, MD
Director Respiratory . . . . Twila J Martin

Measure	Cases	This Hospital	State Average	U.S. Average	Top Hospital
Heart Attack Care					
ACE Inhibitor or ARB for LVSD[2]	60	82%	86%	82%	100%
Aspirin at Arrival[2]	79	100%	89%	92%	100%
Aspirin at Discharge[2]	240	99%	90%	90%	100%
Beta Blocker at Arrival[2]	67	99%	91%	87%	100%
Beta Blocker at Discharge[2]	263	100%	91%	90%	100%
Fibrinolytic Medication Timing[2]	0	-	33%	31%	100%
PCI Within 90 Minutes of Arrival[1,2]	5	40%	73%	54%	95%
Smoking Cessation Advice[2]	113	96%	92%	88%	100%
Heart Failure Care					
ACE Inhibitor or ARB for LVSD[2]	188	84%	84%	82%	100%
Discharge Instructions[2]	253	79%	62%	61%	93%
Evaluation of LVS Function[2]	280	98%	75%	83%	99%
Smoking Cessation Advice[2]	81	85%	78%	82%	100%
Pneumonia Care					
Appropriate Initial Antibiotic[2]	50	80%	85%	83%	94%
Blood Culture Timing[2]	52	85%	95%	90%	100%
Influenza Vaccine[1,2]	21	62%	85%	70%	100%
Initial Antibiotic Timing[2]	101	67%	87%	80%	93%
Oxygenation Assessment[2]	124	100%	99%	99%	100%
Pneumococcal Vaccine[2]	59	56%	83%	69%	94%
Smoking Cessation Advice[2]	48	35%	75%	80%	100%
Surgical Infection Prevention					
Prophylactic Antibiotic Given[2]	499	80%	79%	77%	95%
Prophylactic Antibiotic Selection[2]	70	71%	89%	90%	100%
Prophylactic Antibiotic Stopped[2]	481	64%	76%	72%	95%
Pregnancy Care					
Inpatient Neonatal Mortality	2,022	2.08%	-	-	-
Third or Fourth Degree Laceration	1,084	5.72%	-	3.63%	3.27%

Ellsworth Municipal Hospital

110 Rocksylvania Avenue
Iowa Falls, IA 50126
URL: www.emhia.com
Ownership: Government - Local
Emergency Services: Yes

Phone: 641-648-4631
Fax: 641-648-2850

Accredited: No
Licensed Beds: 42

Key Personnel:

CEO. . . . . John O'Brien
Administrator . . . . John O'Brien
Chief Medical Staff. . . . . David VanGord
Director Infection/Disease Control . . . . Ann Holmguard
Director Medical/Surgical Nursing . . . . Mary Brooks
Chief OB/GYN . . . . Zane Craig
Chief Radiology . . . . David Dennis
Director Cardio-Pulmonary Services . . . . Katie Rieks

Measure	Cases	This Hospital	State Average	U.S. Average	Top Hospital
Heart Attack Care					
ACE Inhibitor or ARB for LVSD	0	-	86%	82%	100%
Aspirin at Arrival[1]	2	0%	89%	92%	100%
Aspirin at Discharge[1]	2	0%	90%	90%	100%
Beta Blocker at Arrival[1]	2	100%	91%	87%	100%
Beta Blocker at Discharge[1]	2	100%	91%	90%	100%
Fibrinolytic Medication Timing[1]	1	0%	33%	31%	100%
PCI Within 90 Minutes of Arrival	0	-	73%	54%	95%
Smoking Cessation Advice	0	-	92%	88%	100%
Heart Failure Care					
ACE Inhibitor or ARB for LVSD[1]	1	100%	84%	82%	100%
Discharge Instructions[1]	16	88%	62%	61%	93%
Evaluation of LVS Function	29	41%	75%	83%	99%
Smoking Cessation Advice[1]	2	50%	78%	82%	100%
Pneumonia Care					
Appropriate Initial Antibiotic	29	86%	85%	83%	94%
Blood Culture Timing[1]	13	100%	95%	90%	100%
Influenza Vaccine[1]	9	67%	85%	70%	100%
Initial Antibiotic Timing	49	90%	87%	80%	93%
Oxygenation Assessment	62	100%	99%	99%	100%
Pneumococcal Vaccine	48	92%	83%	69%	94%
Smoking Cessation Advice[1]	7	71%	75%	80%	100%
Surgical Infection Prevention					
Prophylactic Antibiotic Given[5]	-	-	79%	77%	95%
Prophylactic Antibiotic Selection[5]	-	-	89%	90%	100%
Prophylactic Antibiotic Stopped[5]	-	-	76%	72%	95%
Pregnancy Care					
Inpatient Neonatal Mortality	-	-	-	-	-
Third or Fourth Degree Laceration	-	-	-	3.63%	3.27%

Greene County Medical Center

1000 West Lincolnway
Jefferson, IA 50129
URL: www.gcmchealth.com
Ownership: Government - Local
Emergency Services: Yes

Phone: 515-386-2114
Fax: 515-386-3695

Accredited: No
Licensed Beds: 127

Key Personnel:

President/CEO. . . . . Karen Bossard
Emergency Room . . . . Jeri Reese, RN
Infection Control. . . . . Amy Love
Respiratory/Cardiopulmonary. . . . . Phyllis Drake

Measure	Cases	This Hospital	State Average	U.S. Average	Top Hospital
Heart Attack Care					
ACE Inhibitor or ARB for LVSD[3]	0	-	86%	82%	100%
Aspirin at Arrival[1]	3	100%	89%	92%	100%
Aspirin at Discharge[1,3]	3	100%	90%	90%	100%
Beta Blocker at Arrival[1]	3	100%	91%	87%	100%
Beta Blocker at Discharge[1,3]	3	100%	91%	90%	100%
Fibrinolytic Medication Timing[3]	0	-	33%	31%	100%
PCI Within 90 Minutes of Arrival	0	-	73%	54%	95%
Smoking Cessation Advice[3]	0	-	92%	88%	100%
Heart Failure Care					
ACE Inhibitor or ARB for LVSD[1]	4	0%	84%	82%	100%
Discharge Instructions[1]	14	93%	62%	61%	93%
Evaluation of LVS Function	28	46%	75%	83%	99%
Smoking Cessation Advice[1]	6	67%	78%	82%	100%
Pneumonia Care					
Appropriate Initial Antibiotic[1]	12	83%	85%	83%	94%
Blood Culture Timing[1]	9	100%	95%	90%	100%
Influenza Vaccine[1]	5	60%	85%	70%	100%
Initial Antibiotic Timing[1]	14	100%	87%	80%	93%
Oxygenation Assessment[1]	21	100%	99%	99%	100%
Pneumococcal Vaccine[1]	14	93%	83%	69%	94%
Smoking Cessation Advice[1]	3	100%	75%	80%	100%
Surgical Infection Prevention					
Prophylactic Antibiotic Given[1,3]	2	50%	79%	77%	95%
Prophylactic Antibiotic Selection[1]	1	0%	89%	90%	100%
Prophylactic Antibiotic Stopped[1,3]	2	50%	76%	72%	95%
Pregnancy Care					
Inpatient Neonatal Mortality	-	-	-	-	-
Third or Fourth Degree Laceration	-	-	-	3.63%	3.27%

Keokuk Area Hospital

1600 Morgan Street
Keokuk, IA 52632

Toll-Free: 800-383-9087
Phone: 319-524-7150
Fax: 319-524-5317

URL: www.keokukhealthsystems.org
Ownership: Voluntary non-profit - Other
Emergency Services: Yes

Accredited: Yes
Licensed Beds: 120

Key Personnel:

CEO. . . . . Allan W Zastrow
Chief Medical Staff. . . . . Satyan Kantamneni, MD

NOTE: Hospital profiles are in alphabetical order by state, then city, then hospital within the city; Rankings are sorted by rate in descending order and exclude hospitals with less than 25 cases; (1) The number of cases is too small (n<25) for purposes of reliably predicting hospital performance; (2) Measure reflects the hospital's indication that its submission was based upon a sample of its relevant discharges; (3) Rate reflects fewer than the maximum possible quarters of data for the measure; (4) Inaccurate information submitted and suppressed for one or more quarters; (5) No data is available from the hospital for this measure; Please refer to the User's Guide for a full explanation of data

Emergency Room . . . . Linda Cockrell
Director Infection/Disease Control . . . . Ardath Tweedy, RN
Director Medical/Surgical Nursing . . . . Linda Daughters
Director Radiology . . . . Cathy Beelman
Director Respiratory Therapy . . . . Donna Myers

Measure	Cases	This Hospital	State Average	U.S. Average	Top Hospital
Heart Attack Care					
ACE Inhibitor or ARB for LVSD[1]	3	100%	86%	82%	100%
Aspirin at Arrival[1]	10	90%	89%	92%	100%
Aspirin at Discharge[1]	2	100%	90%	90%	100%
Beta Blocker at Arrival[1]	7	100%	91%	87%	100%
Beta Blocker at Discharge[1]	3	100%	91%	90%	100%
Fibrinolytic Medication Timing[1]	8	38%	33%	31%	100%
PCI Within 90 Minutes of Arrival	0	-	73%	54%	95%
Smoking Cessation Advice	0	-	92%	88%	100%
Heart Failure Care					
ACE Inhibitor or ARB for LVSD[1]	24	92%	84%	82%	100%
Discharge Instructions	60	78%	62%	61%	93%
Evaluation of LVS Function	101	95%	75%	83%	99%
Smoking Cessation Advice[1]	17	100%	78%	82%	100%
Pneumonia Care					
Appropriate Initial Antibiotic	103	70%	85%	83%	94%
Blood Culture Timing	75	97%	95%	90%	100%
Influenza Vaccine	38	92%	85%	70%	100%
Initial Antibiotic Timing	160	92%	87%	80%	93%
Oxygenation Assessment	200	100%	99%	99%	100%
Pneumococcal Vaccine	140	86%	83%	69%	94%
Smoking Cessation Advice	43	84%	75%	80%	100%
Surgical Infection Prevention					
Prophylactic Antibiotic Given[3]	31	84%	79%	77%	95%
Prophylactic Antibiotic Selection[1]	12	92%	89%	90%	100%
Prophylactic Antibiotic Stopped[3]	29	86%	76%	72%	95%
Pregnancy Care					
Inpatient Neonatal Mortality	-	-	-	-	-
Third or Fourth Degree Laceration	-	-	-	3.63%	3.27%

Van Buren County Hospital

340 Frankin Highway 1N
Keosauqua, IA 52565

Toll-Free: 800-225-8244
Phone: 319-293-3171
Fax: 319-293-3142

URL: www.netins.net/showcase/forhealth
Ownership: Government - Local
Accredited: No
Emergency Services: Yes

Key Personnel:
CEO. . . . . Lisa Schnedler
Director Nursing/Emergency Room . . . . Vicki L Robertson, RN, DON
Director Respiratory Therapy . . . . Dixie Daugherty

Measure	Cases	This Hospital	State Average	U.S. Average	Top Hospital
Heart Attack Care					
ACE Inhibitor or ARB for LVSD[3]	0	-	86%	82%	100%
Aspirin at Arrival[1,3]	2	100%	89%	92%	100%
Aspirin at Discharge[1,3]	2	100%	90%	90%	100%
Beta Blocker at Arrival[1,3]	2	100%	91%	87%	100%
Beta Blocker at Discharge[1,3]	2	100%	91%	90%	100%
Fibrinolytic Medication Timing[3]	0	-	33%	31%	100%
PCI Within 90 Minutes of Arrival	0	-	73%	54%	95%
Smoking Cessation Advice[1,3]	1	100%	92%	88%	100%
Heart Failure Care					
ACE Inhibitor or ARB for LVSD[1]	9	89%	84%	82%	100%
Discharge Instructions[1]	15	60%	62%	61%	93%
Evaluation of LVS Function	41	71%	75%	83%	99%
Smoking Cessation Advice[1]	6	100%	78%	82%	100%
Pneumonia Care					
Appropriate Initial Antibiotic[1]	19	89%	85%	83%	94%
Blood Culture Timing[1]	15	87%	95%	90%	100%
Influenza Vaccine[1]	6	100%	85%	70%	100%
Initial Antibiotic Timing	32	91%	87%	80%	93%
Oxygenation Assessment	36	100%	99%	99%	100%
Pneumococcal Vaccine[1]	24	83%	83%	69%	94%
Smoking Cessation Advice[1]	7	86%	75%	80%	100%
Surgical Infection Prevention					
Prophylactic Antibiotic Given[5]	-	-	79%	77%	95%
Prophylactic Antibiotic Selection[5]	-	-	89%	90%	100%
Prophylactic Antibiotic Stopped[5]	-	-	76%	72%	95%
Pregnancy Care					
Inpatient Neonatal Mortality	-	-	-	-	-
Third or Fourth Degree Laceration	-	-	-	3.63%	3.27%

Knoxville Hospital & Clinics

1002 South Lincoln
Knoxville, IA 50138
Phone: 641-842-2151
Ownership: Voluntary non-profit - Private
Accredited: No
Emergency Services: Yes

Measure	Cases	This Hospital	State Average	U.S. Average	Top Hospital
Heart Attack Care					
ACE Inhibitor or ARB for LVSD[3]	0	-	86%	82%	100%
Aspirin at Arrival[1,3]	4	100%	89%	92%	100%
Aspirin at Discharge[1,3]	3	100%	90%	90%	100%
Beta Blocker at Arrival[1,3]	2	100%	91%	87%	100%
Beta Blocker at Discharge[1,3]	2	100%	91%	90%	100%
Fibrinolytic Medication Timing[3]	0	-	33%	31%	100%
PCI Within 90 Minutes of Arrival[5]	-	-	73%	54%	95%
Smoking Cessation Advice[3]	0	-	92%	88%	100%
Heart Failure Care					
ACE Inhibitor or ARB for LVSD[1]	5	60%	84%	82%	100%
Discharge Instructions[1]	13	69%	62%	61%	93%
Evaluation of LVS Function	25	96%	75%	83%	99%
Smoking Cessation Advice[1]	1	100%	78%	82%	100%
Pneumonia Care					
Appropriate Initial Antibiotic[1]	17	94%	85%	83%	94%
Blood Culture Timing[1]	17	100%	95%	90%	100%
Influenza Vaccine[1]	7	86%	85%	70%	100%
Initial Antibiotic Timing	36	86%	87%	80%	93%
Oxygenation Assessment	43	100%	99%	99%	100%
Pneumococcal Vaccine	31	68%	83%	69%	94%
Smoking Cessation Advice[1]	5	80%	75%	80%	100%
Surgical Infection Prevention					
Prophylactic Antibiotic Given[1,3]	1	100%	79%	77%	95%
Prophylactic Antibiotic Selection[1]	2	100%	89%	90%	100%
Prophylactic Antibiotic Stopped[1,3]	1	100%	76%	72%	95%
Pregnancy Care					
Inpatient Neonatal Mortality	-	-	-	-	-
Third or Fourth Degree Laceration	-	-	-	3.63%	3.27%

Stewart Memorial Community Hospital

1301 W Main
Lake City, IA 51449

Toll-Free: 800-262-2614
Phone: 712-464-3171
Fax: 712-464-3269

URL: www.stewartmemorial.org
Ownership: Voluntary non-profit - Private
Accredited: No
Emergency Services: Yes
Licensed Beds: 25

Key Personnel:
CEO. . . . . Kris Baumgart
Chief Medical Staff. . . . . Linda Iler, MD
Emergency Room . . . . Vikki Roby
Director Respiratory Therapy . . . . Lorra Brown

Measure	Cases	This Hospital	State Average	U.S. Average	Top Hospital
Heart Attack Care					
ACE Inhibitor or ARB for LVSD[1,3]	1	100%	86%	82%	100%
Aspirin at Arrival[1,3]	2	100%	89%	92%	100%
Aspirin at Discharge[1,3]	2	100%	90%	90%	100%
Beta Blocker at Arrival[1,3]	2	50%	91%	87%	100%
Beta Blocker at Discharge[1,3]	2	50%	91%	90%	100%
Fibrinolytic Medication Timing[3]	0	-	33%	31%	100%
PCI Within 90 Minutes of Arrival	0	-	73%	54%	95%
Smoking Cessation Advice[3]	0	-	92%	88%	100%
Heart Failure Care					
ACE Inhibitor or ARB for LVSD	0	-	84%	82%	100%
Discharge Instructions[1]	9	78%	62%	61%	93%
Evaluation of LVS Function[1]	18	33%	75%	83%	99%

NOTE: Hospital profiles are in alphabetical order by state, then city, then hospital within the city; Rankings are sorted by rate in descending order and exclude hospitals with less than 25 cases; (1) The number of cases is too small (n<25) for purposes of reliably predicting hospital performance; (2) Measure reflects the hospital's indication that its submission was based upon a sample of its relevant discharges; (3) Rate reflects fewer than the maximum possible quarters of data for the measure; (4) Inaccurate information submitted and suppressed for one or more quarters; (5) No data is available from the hospital for this measure; Please refer to the User's Guide for a full explanation of data

Measure	Cases	This Hospital	State Average	U.S. Average	Top Hospital
Smoking Cessation Advice[1]	1	100%	78%	82%	100%
Pneumonia Care					
Appropriate Initial Antibiotic	43	86%	85%	83%	94%
Blood Culture Timing[1]	9	100%	95%	90%	100%
Influenza Vaccine[1]	7	100%	85%	70%	100%
Initial Antibiotic Timing	59	83%	87%	80%	93%
Oxygenation Assessment	71	100%	99%	99%	100%
Pneumococcal Vaccine	56	93%	83%	69%	94%
Smoking Cessation Advice[1]	9	89%	75%	80%	100%
Surgical Infection Prevention					
Prophylactic Antibiotic Given[1,3]	4	100%	79%	77%	95%
Prophylactic Antibiotic Selection[1]	2	50%	89%	90%	100%
Prophylactic Antibiotic Stopped[1,3]	3	100%	76%	72%	95%
Pregnancy Care					
Inpatient Neonatal Mortality	-	-	-	-	-
Third or Fourth Degree Laceration	-	-	-	3.63%	3.27%

Floyd Valley Hospital

714 Lincoln Street NE
PO Box 10
Le Mars, IA 51031
Phone: 712-546-7871
Fax: 712-546-3352
URL: www.floydvalleyhospital.org
Ownership: Government - Local
Accredited: No
Emergency Services: Yes
Licensed Beds: 44

Key Personnel:

Administrator . . . . Michael Donlin
Chief Medical Staff. . . . . Paul Parmelee, DO
Cardiac Rehab Coordinator . . . . Lavonne Galles
Surgery Supervisor . . . . Janet Haack, RN
Infection Control Coordinator . . . . Robert Norfolk
Director Medical/Surgical Nursing . . . . Loretta Myers, RN
Surgery Surevisor . . . . Gina Vacuna
Director Respiratory Therapy . . . . Wanda MaComb

Measure	Cases	This Hospital	State Average	U.S. Average	Top Hospital
Heart Attack Care					
ACE Inhibitor or ARB for LVSD[1]	4	100%	86%	82%	100%
Aspirin at Arrival[1]	11	100%	89%	92%	100%
Aspirin at Discharge[1]	8	100%	90%	90%	100%
Beta Blocker at Arrival[1]	11	82%	91%	87%	100%
Beta Blocker at Discharge[1]	6	83%	91%	90%	100%
Fibrinolytic Medication Timing	0	-	33%	31%	100%
PCI Within 90 Minutes of Arrival	0	-	73%	54%	95%
Smoking Cessation Advice	0	-	92%	88%	100%
Heart Failure Care					
ACE Inhibitor or ARB for LVSD[1]	9	78%	84%	82%	100%
Discharge Instructions	27	96%	62%	61%	93%
Evaluation of LVS Function	49	82%	75%	83%	99%
Smoking Cessation Advice[1]	1	100%	78%	82%	100%
Pneumonia Care					
Appropriate Initial Antibiotic[1]	15	87%	85%	83%	94%
Blood Culture Timing[1]	10	90%	95%	90%	100%
Influenza Vaccine[1]	7	100%	85%	70%	100%
Initial Antibiotic Timing	35	83%	87%	80%	93%
Oxygenation Assessment	41	100%	99%	99%	100%
Pneumococcal Vaccine	33	85%	83%	69%	94%
Smoking Cessation Advice[1]	6	83%	75%	80%	100%
Surgical Infection Prevention					
Prophylactic Antibiotic Given[5]	-	-	79%	77%	95%
Prophylactic Antibiotic Selection[5]	-	-	89%	90%	100%
Prophylactic Antibiotic Stopped[5]	-	-	76%	72%	95%
Pregnancy Care					
Inpatient Neonatal Mortality	-	-	-	-	-
Third or Fourth Degree Laceration	-	-	-	3.63%	3.27%

Decatur County Hospital

1405 NW Church Street
Leon, IA 50144
Phone: 641-446-4871
Fax: 641-446-2201
URL: www.decaturcountyhospital.org
Ownership: Voluntary non-profit - Other
Accredited: No
Emergency Services: Yes
Licensed Beds: 25

Key Personnel:

President/CEO . . . . Darrell Vondrak
Chief of Medical Staff. . . . . Larry Richard
Emergency Room . . . . Alison Reynolds
Surgery Director. . . . . Mary Jane Applegate

Measure	Cases	This Hospital	State Average	U.S. Average	Top Hospital
Heart Attack Care					
ACE Inhibitor or ARB for LVSD[5]	-	-	86%	82%	100%
Aspirin at Arrival[5]	-	-	89%	92%	100%
Aspirin at Discharge[5]	-	-	90%	90%	100%
Beta Blocker at Arrival[5]	-	-	91%	87%	100%
Beta Blocker at Discharge[5]	-	-	91%	90%	100%
Fibrinolytic Medication Timing[5]	-	-	33%	31%	100%
PCI Within 90 Minutes of Arrival[5]	-	-	73%	54%	95%
Smoking Cessation Advice[5]	-	-	92%	88%	100%
Heart Failure Care					
ACE Inhibitor or ARB for LVSD[3]	0	-	84%	82%	100%
Discharge Instructions[1,3]	1	100%	62%	61%	93%
Evaluation of LVS Function[1,3]	1	0%	75%	83%	99%
Smoking Cessation Advice[3]	0	-	78%	82%	100%
Pneumonia Care					
Appropriate Initial Antibiotic[1,3]	2	50%	85%	83%	94%
Blood Culture Timing[3]	0	-	95%	90%	100%
Influenza Vaccine[5]	-	-	85%	70%	100%
Initial Antibiotic Timing[1,3]	2	100%	87%	80%	93%
Oxygenation Assessment[1,3]	2	100%	99%	99%	100%
Pneumococcal Vaccine[1,3]	2	50%	83%	69%	94%
Smoking Cessation Advice[3]	0	-	75%	80%	100%
Surgical Infection Prevention					
Prophylactic Antibiotic Given[5]	-	-	79%	77%	95%
Prophylactic Antibiotic Selection[5]	-	-	89%	90%	100%
Prophylactic Antibiotic Stopped[5]	-	-	76%	72%	95%
Pregnancy Care					
Inpatient Neonatal Mortality	-	-	-	-	-
Third or Fourth Degree Laceration	-	-	-	3.63%	3.27%

Regional Medical Center of Northeast Iowa

Alternate Name: Delaware County Memorial Hospital
709 W Main Street
Box 359
Manchester, IA 52057
Phone: 563-927-3232
Fax: 563-927-7444
URL: www.regmedctr.org
Ownership: Government - Local
Accredited: No
Emergency Services: Yes
Licensed Beds: 25

Key Personnel:

CEO. . . . . Lon Butikofer, RN
Director Medical/Surgical Nursing . . . . Rose Downs, RN, B
Director Respiratory Therapy . . . . Ann Wilson

Measure	Cases	This Hospital	State Average	U.S. Average	Top Hospital
Heart Attack Care					
ACE Inhibitor or ARB for LVSD[3]	0	-	86%	82%	100%
Aspirin at Arrival[1,3]	2	100%	89%	92%	100%
Aspirin at Discharge[1,3]	3	100%	90%	90%	100%
Beta Blocker at Arrival[1,3]	3	100%	91%	87%	100%
Beta Blocker at Discharge[1,3]	3	67%	91%	90%	100%
Fibrinolytic Medication Timing[3]	0	-	33%	31%	100%
PCI Within 90 Minutes of Arrival[5]	-	-	73%	54%	95%
Smoking Cessation Advice[1,3]	1	100%	92%	88%	100%
Heart Failure Care					
ACE Inhibitor or ARB for LVSD[1]	3	100%	84%	82%	100%
Discharge Instructions[1]	19	84%	62%	61%	93%
Evaluation of LVS Function	28	79%	75%	83%	99%
Smoking Cessation Advice	0	-	78%	82%	100%
Pneumonia Care					
Appropriate Initial Antibiotic	26	92%	85%	83%	94%
Blood Culture Timing[1]	21	95%	95%	90%	100%
Influenza Vaccine[1]	8	75%	85%	70%	100%
Initial Antibiotic Timing	35	86%	87%	80%	93%
Oxygenation Assessment	42	100%	99%	99%	100%
Pneumococcal Vaccine	32	94%	83%	69%	94%
Smoking Cessation Advice[1]	5	60%	75%	80%	100%
Surgical Infection Prevention					

NOTE: Hospital profiles are in alphabetical order by state, then city, then hospital within the city; Rankings are sorted by rate in descending order and exclude hospitals with less than 25 cases; (1) The number of cases is too small (n<25) for purposes of reliably predicting hospital performance; (2) Measure reflects the hospital's indication that its submission was based upon a sample of its relevant discharges; (3) Rate reflects fewer than the maximum possible quarters of data for the measure; (4) Inaccurate information submitted and suppressed for one or more quarters; (5) No data is available from the hospital for this measure; Please refer to the User's Guide for a full explanation of data

Prophylactic Antibiotic Given[5]	-	-	79%	77%	95%
Prophylactic Antibiotic Selection[5]	-	-	89%	90%	100%
Prophylactic Antibiotic Stopped[5]	-	-	76%	72%	95%
Pregnancy Care					
Inpatient Neonatal Mortality	-	-	-	-	-
Third or Fourth Degree Laceration	-	-	-	3.63%	3.27%

Manning Regional Healthcare Center

410 Main Street
Manning, IA 51455
URL: www.mrhcia.com
Ownership: Voluntary non-profit - Other
Emergency Services: Yes

Phone: 712-655-2072
Fax: 712-655-2216

Accredited: No
Licensed Beds: 41

Key Personnel:
CEO. . . . . Jenne Goche
Chief Medical Staff. . . . . Daphney Gonsalzes, MD
Emergency Room . . . . Cynthia Genzen
OB/GYN Womens Health. . . . . Barbara Hodne, DO
Director Respiratory Therapy . . . . Linda Vinke

Measure	Cases	This Hospital	State Average	U.S. Average	Top Hospital
Heart Attack Care					
ACE Inhibitor or ARB for LVSD[5]	-	-	86%	82%	100%
Aspirin at Arrival[5]	-	-	89%	92%	100%
Aspirin at Discharge[5]	-	-	90%	90%	100%
Beta Blocker at Arrival[5]	-	-	91%	87%	100%
Beta Blocker at Discharge[5]	-	-	91%	90%	100%
Fibrinolytic Medication Timing[5]	-	-	33%	31%	100%
PCI Within 90 Minutes of Arrival[5]	-	-	73%	54%	95%
Smoking Cessation Advice[5]	-	-	92%	88%	100%
Heart Failure Care					
ACE Inhibitor or ARB for LVSD[5]	-	-	84%	82%	100%
Discharge Instructions[5]	-	-	62%	61%	93%
Evaluation of LVS Function[5]	-	-	75%	83%	99%
Smoking Cessation Advice[5]	-	-	78%	82%	100%
Pneumonia Care					
Appropriate Initial Antibiotic[1]	3	100%	85%	83%	94%
Blood Culture Timing	0	-	95%	90%	100%
Influenza Vaccine[1]	5	100%	85%	70%	100%
Initial Antibiotic Timing[1]	10	100%	87%	80%	93%
Oxygenation Assessment[1]	11	100%	99%	99%	100%
Pneumococcal Vaccine[1]	11	100%	83%	69%	94%
Smoking Cessation Advice	0	-	75%	80%	100%
Surgical Infection Prevention					
Prophylactic Antibiotic Given[5]	-	-	79%	77%	95%
Prophylactic Antibiotic Selection[5]	-	-	89%	90%	100%
Prophylactic Antibiotic Stopped[5]	-	-	76%	72%	95%
Pregnancy Care					
Inpatient Neonatal Mortality	-	-	-	-	-
Third or Fourth Degree Laceration	-	-	-	3.63%	3.27%

Jackson County Public Hospital

700 W Grove Street
Maquoketa, IA 52060
Ownership: Government - Local
Emergency Services: Yes

Phone: 563-652-2474
Fax: 563-652-4018
Accredited: Yes
Licensed Beds: 43

Key Personnel:
President/CEO. . . . . Curt Coleman
Chief Medical Staff. . . . . Curt Giswein, MD
Emergency Room . . . . Cheryl Wagner
Director Infection/Disease Control . . . . Sandra Rockwell

Measure	Cases	This Hospital	State Average	U.S. Average	Top Hospital
Heart Attack Care					
ACE Inhibitor or ARB for LVSD[5]	-	-	86%	82%	100%
Aspirin at Arrival[5]	-	-	89%	92%	100%
Aspirin at Discharge[5]	-	-	90%	90%	100%
Beta Blocker at Arrival[5]	-	-	91%	87%	100%
Beta Blocker at Discharge[5]	-	-	91%	90%	100%
Fibrinolytic Medication Timing[5]	-	-	33%	31%	100%
PCI Within 90 Minutes of Arrival[5]	-	-	73%	54%	95%
Smoking Cessation Advice[5]	-	-	92%	88%	100%
Heart Failure Care					
ACE Inhibitor or ARB for LVSD[1]	4	100%	84%	82%	100%
Discharge Instructions[1]	11	55%	62%	61%	93%
Evaluation of LVS Function[1]	14	71%	75%	83%	99%
Smoking Cessation Advice[1]	3	67%	78%	82%	100%
Pneumonia Care					
Appropriate Initial Antibiotic[1]	24	67%	85%	83%	94%
Blood Culture Timing[1]	10	90%	95%	90%	100%
Influenza Vaccine[1]	7	86%	85%	70%	100%
Initial Antibiotic Timing	26	92%	87%	80%	93%
Oxygenation Assessment	31	100%	99%	99%	100%
Pneumococcal Vaccine[1]	24	79%	83%	69%	94%
Smoking Cessation Advice[1]	3	67%	75%	80%	100%
Surgical Infection Prevention					
Prophylactic Antibiotic Given[5]	-	-	79%	77%	95%
Prophylactic Antibiotic Selection[5]	-	-	89%	90%	100%
Prophylactic Antibiotic Stopped[5]	-	-	76%	72%	95%
Pregnancy Care					
Inpatient Neonatal Mortality	-	-	-	-	-
Third or Fourth Degree Laceration	-	-	-	3.63%	3.27%

Marengo Memorial Hospital

300 W May Street
PO Box 228
Marengo, IA 52301
URL: www.marengohospital.org
Ownership: Government - Local
Emergency Services: Yes

Phone: 319-642-5543
Fax: 319-642-8007

Accredited: No
Licensed Beds: 25

Key Personnel:
CEO. . . . . Genny Morac
Chief Medical Staff. . . . . Sylvia Chang
Head of Emergency Room. . . . . Teresa Sauerai
Emergency Room . . . . Malcom Findlater, MD
Infection Control. . . . . Sharon Schulte, RN
Head of Respiratory . . . . Lorie Christy

Measure	Cases	This Hospital	State Average	U.S. Average	Top Hospital
Heart Attack Care					
ACE Inhibitor or ARB for LVSD[5]	-	-	86%	82%	100%
Aspirin at Arrival[5]	-	-	89%	92%	100%
Aspirin at Discharge[5]	-	-	90%	90%	100%
Beta Blocker at Arrival[5]	-	-	91%	87%	100%
Beta Blocker at Discharge[5]	-	-	91%	90%	100%
Fibrinolytic Medication Timing[5]	-	-	33%	31%	100%
PCI Within 90 Minutes of Arrival[5]	-	-	73%	54%	95%
Smoking Cessation Advice[5]	-	-	92%	88%	100%
Heart Failure Care					
ACE Inhibitor or ARB for LVSD[5]	-	-	84%	82%	100%
Discharge Instructions[5]	-	-	62%	61%	93%
Evaluation of LVS Function[5]	-	-	75%	83%	99%
Smoking Cessation Advice[5]	-	-	78%	82%	100%
Pneumonia Care					
Appropriate Initial Antibiotic[5]	-	-	85%	83%	94%
Blood Culture Timing[5]	-	-	95%	90%	100%
Influenza Vaccine[5]	-	-	85%	70%	100%
Initial Antibiotic Timing[5]	-	-	87%	80%	93%
Oxygenation Assessment[5]	-	-	99%	99%	100%
Pneumococcal Vaccine[5]	-	-	83%	69%	94%
Smoking Cessation Advice[5]	-	-	75%	80%	100%
Surgical Infection Prevention					
Prophylactic Antibiotic Given[5]	-	-	79%	77%	95%
Prophylactic Antibiotic Selection[5]	-	-	89%	90%	100%
Prophylactic Antibiotic Stopped[5]	-	-	76%	72%	95%
Pregnancy Care					
Inpatient Neonatal Mortality	-	-	-	-	-
Third or Fourth Degree Laceration	-	-	-	3.63%	3.27%

NOTE: Hospital profiles are in alphabetical order by state, then city, then hospital within the city; Rankings are sorted by rate in descending order and exclude hospitals with less than 25 cases; (1) The number of cases is too small (n<25) for purposes of reliably predicting hospital performance; (2) Measure reflects the hospital's indication that its submission was based upon a sample of its relevant discharges; (3) Rate reflects fewer than the maximum possible quarters of data for the measure; (4) Inaccurate information submitted and suppressed for one or more quarters; (5) No data is available from the hospital for this measure; Please refer to the User's Guide for a full explanation of data

Marshalltown Medical & Surgical Center

3 S 4th Avenue
Marshalltown, IA 50158
Phone: 641-754-5151
Fax: 641-753-2570
URL: www.everydaychampions.org
Ownership: Voluntary non-profit - Private
Accredited: Yes
Emergency Services: Yes
Licensed Beds: 105

Key Personnel:

CEO. . . . . Rob Cooper
Chief of Medical Staff. . . . . Gary Peasley
Emergency Room . . . . Pat Whitmord
Emergency Room . . . . Donna Schuster
Director Medical/Surgical Nursing . . . . Chris Schill
Chief Radiology . . . . Roy Struve
Director Respiratory Therapy . . . . Marsh Deaker

Measure	Cases	This Hospital	State Average	U.S. Average	Top Hospital
Heart Attack Care					
ACE Inhibitor or ARB for LVSD[1]	3	100%	86%	82%	100%
Aspirin at Arrival[1]	24	96%	89%	92%	100%
Aspirin at Discharge[1]	16	81%	90%	90%	100%
Beta Blocker at Arrival[1]	21	100%	91%	87%	100%
Beta Blocker at Discharge[1]	16	100%	91%	90%	100%
Fibrinolytic Medication Timing	0	-	33%	31%	100%
PCI Within 90 Minutes of Arrival	0	-	73%	54%	95%
Smoking Cessation Advice	0	-	92%	88%	100%
Heart Failure Care					
ACE Inhibitor or ARB for LVSD[1]	16	100%	84%	82%	100%
Discharge Instructions	59	95%	62%	61%	93%
Evaluation of LVS Function	97	93%	75%	83%	99%
Smoking Cessation Advice[1]	13	100%	78%	82%	100%
Pneumonia Care					
Appropriate Initial Antibiotic	89	89%	85%	83%	94%
Blood Culture Timing	77	96%	95%	90%	100%
Influenza Vaccine	28	96%	85%	70%	100%
Initial Antibiotic Timing	131	89%	87%	80%	93%
Oxygenation Assessment	160	100%	99%	99%	100%
Pneumococcal Vaccine	110	94%	83%	69%	94%
Smoking Cessation Advice	26	92%	75%	80%	100%
Surgical Infection Prevention					
Prophylactic Antibiotic Given[2]	284	96%	79%	77%	95%
Prophylactic Antibiotic Selection[2]	58	95%	89%	90%	100%
Prophylactic Antibiotic Stopped[2]	278	48%	76%	72%	95%
Pregnancy Care					
Inpatient Neonatal Mortality	-	-	-	-	-
Third or Fourth Degree Laceration	-	-	-	3.63%	3.27%

Mercy Medical Center-North Iowa

Alternate Name: North Iowa Mercy Health Center
1000 4th Street SW
Mason City, IA 50401
Toll-Free: 800-433-3883
Phone: 641-422-7000
Fax: 641-422-7827
URL: www.mercynorthiowa.com
Ownership: Voluntary non-profit - Church
Accredited: Yes
Emergency Services: Yes
Licensed Beds: 346

Key Personnel:

President/CEO. . . . . James G Fitzpatrick
Chief Medical Staff. . . . . Ron Moeller, MD
Director Emergency Services. . . . . Paul Leavens

Measure	Cases	This Hospital	State Average	U.S. Average	Top Hospital
Heart Attack Care					
ACE Inhibitor or ARB for LVSD	61	97%	86%	82%	100%
Aspirin at Arrival	172	97%	89%	92%	100%
Aspirin at Discharge	270	100%	90%	90%	100%
Beta Blocker at Arrival	148	95%	91%	87%	100%
Beta Blocker at Discharge	268	99%	91%	90%	100%
Fibrinolytic Medication Timing	0	-	33%	31%	100%
PCI Within 90 Minutes of Arrival[1]	16	62%	73%	54%	95%
Smoking Cessation Advice	86	99%	92%	88%	100%
Heart Failure Care					
ACE Inhibitor or ARB for LVSD	139	94%	84%	82%	100%
Discharge Instructions	249	89%	62%	61%	93%
Evaluation of LVS Function	332	98%	75%	83%	99%
Smoking Cessation Advice	36	97%	78%	82%	100%
Pneumonia Care					
Appropriate Initial Antibiotic	142	87%	85%	83%	94%
Blood Culture Timing	140	84%	95%	90%	100%
Influenza Vaccine	39	97%	85%	70%	100%
Initial Antibiotic Timing	168	92%	87%	80%	93%
Oxygenation Assessment	216	100%	99%	99%	100%
Pneumococcal Vaccine	162	93%	83%	69%	94%
Smoking Cessation Advice	43	98%	75%	80%	100%
Surgical Infection Prevention					
Prophylactic Antibiotic Given[3]	703	90%	79%	77%	95%
Prophylactic Antibiotic Selection	235	98%	89%	90%	100%
Prophylactic Antibiotic Stopped[3]	694	87%	76%	72%	95%
Pregnancy Care					
Inpatient Neonatal Mortality	-	-	-	-	-
Third or Fourth Degree Laceration	-	-	-	3.63%	3.27%

Alegent Health Community Memorial Hospital

Alternate Name: Community Memorial Hospital
631 N 8th Street
Missouri Valley, IA 51555
Phone: 712-642-2784
Fax: 712-642-2760
URL: www.alegent.org
Ownership: Voluntary non-profit - Other
Accredited: No
Emergency Services: Yes
Licensed Beds: 25

Key Personnel:

President/CEO. . . . . Robert Sellers
Chief Medical Staff. . . . . Charles B Johnson, MD
Lead Cardio-Pulmonary . . . . Shelley LeValley
Emergency Room . . . . Kathy Lovell, RN
Coordinator Outpatient Surgical Services. . . . . . Sheri Spark

Measure	Cases	This Hospital	State Average	U.S. Average	Top Hospital
Heart Attack Care					
ACE Inhibitor or ARB for LVSD[1]	1	100%	86%	82%	100%
Aspirin at Arrival[1]	3	67%	89%	92%	100%
Aspirin at Discharge[1]	2	100%	90%	90%	100%
Beta Blocker at Arrival[1]	4	100%	91%	87%	100%
Beta Blocker at Discharge[1]	2	100%	91%	90%	100%
Fibrinolytic Medication Timing[3]	0	-	33%	31%	100%
PCI Within 90 Minutes of Arrival	0	-	73%	54%	95%
Smoking Cessation Advice	0	-	92%	88%	100%
Heart Failure Care					
ACE Inhibitor or ARB for LVSD[1]	6	33%	84%	82%	100%
Discharge Instructions[1]	10	60%	62%	61%	93%
Evaluation of LVS Function[1]	22	100%	75%	83%	99%
Smoking Cessation Advice[1]	3	33%	78%	82%	100%
Pneumonia Care					
Appropriate Initial Antibiotic	28	100%	85%	83%	94%
Blood Culture Timing	25	100%	95%	90%	100%
Influenza Vaccine[1]	8	100%	85%	70%	100%
Initial Antibiotic Timing	40	98%	87%	80%	93%
Oxygenation Assessment	53	100%	99%	99%	100%
Pneumococcal Vaccine	43	93%	83%	69%	94%
Smoking Cessation Advice[1]	6	83%	75%	80%	100%
Surgical Infection Prevention					
Prophylactic Antibiotic Given[5]	-	-	79%	77%	95%
Prophylactic Antibiotic Selection[5]	-	-	89%	90%	100%
Prophylactic Antibiotic Stopped[5]	-	-	76%	72%	95%
Pregnancy Care					
Inpatient Neonatal Mortality	-	-	-	-	-
Third or Fourth Degree Laceration	-	-	-	3.63%	3.27%

Ringgold County Hospital

211 Shellway Drive
Mount Ayr, IA 50854
Phone: 641-464-3226
Fax: 641-464-4420
Ownership: Government - Federal
Accredited: No
Emergency Services: Yes
Licensed Beds: 23

Key Personnel:

President/CEO. . . . . Gordon Winkler
Chief Medical Staff. . . . . Dane Johnson, DO
Respiratory/Cardiopulmonary. . . . . John Schafer

NOTE: Hospital profiles are in alphabetical order by state, then city, then hospital within the city; Rankings are sorted by rate in descending order and exclude hospitals with less than 25 cases; (1) The number of cases is too small (n<25) for purposes of reliably predicting hospital performance; (2) Measure reflects the hospital's indication that its submission was based upon a sample of its relevant discharges; (3) Rate reflects fewer than the maximum possible quarters of data for the measure; (4) Inaccurate information submitted and suppressed for one or more quarters; (5) No data is available from the hospital for this measure; Please refer to the User's Guide for a full explanation of data

Measure	Cases	This Hospital	State Average	U.S. Average	Top Hospital
Heart Attack Care					
ACE Inhibitor or ARB for LVSD[1,3]	1	0%	86%	82%	100%
Aspirin at Arrival[3]	0	-	89%	92%	100%
Aspirin at Discharge[3]	0	-	90%	90%	100%
Beta Blocker at Arrival[1,3]	1	100%	91%	87%	100%
Beta Blocker at Discharge[3]	0	-	91%	90%	100%
Fibrinolytic Medication Timing[3]	0	-	33%	31%	100%
PCI Within 90 Minutes of Arrival[5]	-	-	73%	54%	95%
Smoking Cessation Advice[3]	0	-	92%	88%	100%
Heart Failure Care					
ACE Inhibitor or ARB for LVSD	0	-	84%	82%	100%
Discharge Instructions[1]	7	14%	62%	61%	93%
Evaluation of LVS Function[1]	8	50%	75%	83%	99%
Smoking Cessation Advice[1]	1	100%	78%	82%	100%
Pneumonia Care					
Appropriate Initial Antibiotic[1]	16	100%	85%	83%	94%
Blood Culture Timing[1]	10	80%	95%	90%	100%
Influenza Vaccine[1]	10	100%	85%	70%	100%
Initial Antibiotic Timing	29	90%	87%	80%	93%
Oxygenation Assessment	33	100%	99%	99%	100%
Pneumococcal Vaccine	31	94%	83%	69%	94%
Smoking Cessation Advice[1]	3	67%	75%	80%	100%
Surgical Infection Prevention					
Prophylactic Antibiotic Given[5]	-	-	79%	77%	95%
Prophylactic Antibiotic Selection[5]	-	-	89%	90%	100%
Prophylactic Antibiotic Stopped[5]	-	-	76%	72%	95%
Pregnancy Care					
Inpatient Neonatal Mortality	-	-	-	-	-
Third or Fourth Degree Laceration	-	-	-	3.63%	3.27%

Henry County Health Center

407 S White
Mount Pleasant, IA 52641
E-mail: miller@hchc.org
URL: www.hchc.org
Ownership: Government - Local
Emergency Services: Yes

Phone: 319-385-3141
Fax: 319-385-6731
Accredited: No
Licensed Beds: 74

Key Personnel:
CEO. . . . . Dan Sheehan
Chief Medical Staff. . . . . Steven Davis, MD
Chief Medical Staff. . . . . Dave Wess
Emergency Room . . . . Vicky Oge, RN
Chief Radiology . . . . Steven Davis, MD
Director Respiratory Therapy . . . . Darin Shull, RT

Measure	Cases	This Hospital	State Average	U.S. Average	Top Hospital
Heart Attack Care					
ACE Inhibitor or ARB for LVSD[1]	1	100%	86%	82%	100%
Aspirin at Arrival[1]	15	60%	89%	92%	100%
Aspirin at Discharge[1]	11	82%	90%	90%	100%
Beta Blocker at Arrival[1]	16	75%	91%	87%	100%
Beta Blocker at Discharge[1]	10	80%	91%	90%	100%
Fibrinolytic Medication Timing	0	-	33%	31%	100%
PCI Within 90 Minutes of Arrival	0	-	73%	54%	95%
Smoking Cessation Advice[1]	1	0%	92%	88%	100%
Heart Failure Care					
ACE Inhibitor or ARB for LVSD[1]	8	88%	84%	82%	100%
Discharge Instructions[1]	19	5%	62%	61%	93%
Evaluation of LVS Function	42	52%	75%	83%	99%
Smoking Cessation Advice[1]	3	67%	78%	82%	100%
Pneumonia Care					
Appropriate Initial Antibiotic	35	80%	85%	83%	94%
Blood Culture Timing[1]	4	100%	95%	90%	100%
Influenza Vaccine[1]	4	0%	85%	70%	100%
Initial Antibiotic Timing	31	71%	87%	80%	93%
Oxygenation Assessment	38	100%	99%	99%	100%
Pneumococcal Vaccine[1]	22	9%	83%	69%	94%
Smoking Cessation Advice[1]	10	50%	75%	80%	100%
Surgical Infection Prevention					
Prophylactic Antibiotic Given[1,3]	8	62%	79%	77%	95%
Prophylactic Antibiotic Selection[1]	8	88%	89%	90%	100%
Prophylactic Antibiotic Stopped[1,3]	7	86%	76%	72%	95%
Pregnancy Care					
Inpatient Neonatal Mortality	-	-	-	-	-
Third or Fourth Degree Laceration	-	-	-	3.63%	3.27%

Unity Hospital

1518 Mulberry Avenue
Muscatine, IA 52761
E-mail: tvanwey@unityiowa.org
URL: www.unityiowa.org
Ownership: Voluntary non-profit - Private
Emergency Services: Yes

Phone: 563-264-9100
Fax: 563-264-9463
Accredited: Yes
Licensed Beds: 80

Key Personnel:
President/CEO. . . . . Karmon Bjella
Chief Medical Staff. . . . . Steven Paulsrud, DO
Surgical Care Director . . . . Judy Maxwell
Emergency Room . . . . Reineer Van Tonder, MD
Infection Control Coordinator . . . . Teresa Coder, RN
Surgical Services Director . . . . Lynn Volkyl
Director Radiology . . . . Jeri Bailey
Cardiopulmonary Services Director . . . . Connie Cooling

Measure	Cases	This Hospital	State Average	U.S. Average	Top Hospital
Heart Attack Care					
ACE Inhibitor or ARB for LVSD[1]	3	67%	86%	82%	100%
Aspirin at Arrival[1]	10	100%	89%	92%	100%
Aspirin at Discharge[1]	8	75%	90%	90%	100%
Beta Blocker at Arrival[1]	14	93%	91%	87%	100%
Beta Blocker at Discharge[1]	11	73%	91%	90%	100%
Fibrinolytic Medication Timing	0	-	33%	31%	100%
PCI Within 90 Minutes of Arrival	0	-	73%	54%	95%
Smoking Cessation Advice	0	-	92%	88%	100%
Heart Failure Care					
ACE Inhibitor or ARB for LVSD[1]	20	70%	84%	82%	100%
Discharge Instructions	25	48%	62%	61%	93%
Evaluation of LVS Function	46	80%	75%	83%	99%
Smoking Cessation Advice[1]	5	80%	78%	82%	100%
Pneumonia Care					
Appropriate Initial Antibiotic	80	94%	85%	83%	94%
Blood Culture Timing	54	94%	95%	90%	100%
Influenza Vaccine[1]	12	92%	85%	70%	100%
Initial Antibiotic Timing	80	91%	87%	80%	93%
Oxygenation Assessment	107	100%	99%	99%	100%
Pneumococcal Vaccine	75	92%	83%	69%	94%
Smoking Cessation Advice[1]	18	94%	75%	80%	100%
Surgical Infection Prevention					
Prophylactic Antibiotic Given[2,3]	99	72%	79%	77%	95%
Prophylactic Antibiotic Selection[2]	36	92%	89%	90%	100%
Prophylactic Antibiotic Stopped[2,3]	92	64%	76%	72%	95%
Pregnancy Care					
Inpatient Neonatal Mortality	-	-	-	-	-
Third or Fourth Degree Laceration	-	-	-	3.63%	3.27%

Skiff Medical Center

204 N 4th Avenue E
Newton, IA 50208
E-mail: info@skiffmed.com
URL: www.skiffmed.com
Ownership: Government - Local
Emergency Services: Yes

Phone: 641-792-1273
Fax: 641-792-4603
Accredited: Yes
Licensed Beds: 68

Key Personnel:
President/CEO. . . . . Eric Lothe
Chief Medical Staff. . . . . P L Clevenger, DO
ER/SCU Director . . . . Susan Carzoli, RN
Infection Control. . . . . Lisa Guldberg, RN BSN
Director Medical Surgical Nursing . . . . Kris Hoyt
OR/OP Surgery Director . . . . Glenda Palmer, RN
Director Radiology . . . . Jane Maury
Director Respiratory Therapy . . . . William Lahart

Measure	Cases	This Hospital	State Average	U.S. Average	Top Hospital
Heart Attack Care					
ACE Inhibitor or ARB for LVSD[1]	2	100%	86%	82%	100%

NOTE: Hospital profiles are in alphabetical order by state, then city, then hospital within the city; Rankings are sorted by rate in descending order and exclude hospitals with less than 25 cases; (1) The number of cases is too small (n<25) for purposes of reliably predicting hospital performance; (2) Measure reflects the hospital's indication that its submission was based upon a sample of its relevant discharges; (3) Rate reflects fewer than the maximum possible quarters of data for the measure; (4) Inaccurate information submitted and suppressed for one or more quarters; (5) No data is available from the hospital for this measure; Please refer to the User's Guide for a full explanation of data

Measure	Cases	This Hospital	State Average	U.S. Average	Top Hospital
Aspirin at Arrival[1]	10	50%	89%	92%	100%
Aspirin at Discharge[1]	5	60%	90%	90%	100%
Beta Blocker at Arrival[1]	12	50%	91%	87%	100%
Beta Blocker at Discharge[1]	7	86%	91%	90%	100%
Fibrinolytic Medication Timing	0	-	33%	31%	100%
PCI Within 90 Minutes of Arrival	0	-	73%	54%	95%
Smoking Cessation Advice	0	-	92%	88%	100%
Heart Failure Care					
ACE Inhibitor or ARB for LVSD[1]	13	54%	84%	82%	100%
Discharge Instructions	48	56%	62%	61%	93%
Evaluation of LVS Function	72	61%	75%	83%	99%
Smoking Cessation Advice[1]	9	67%	78%	82%	100%
Pneumonia Care					
Appropriate Initial Antibiotic	47	83%	85%	83%	94%
Blood Culture Timing	27	85%	95%	90%	100%
Influenza Vaccine[1]	10	70%	85%	70%	100%
Initial Antibiotic Timing	65	71%	87%	80%	93%
Oxygenation Assessment	74	100%	99%	99%	100%
Pneumococcal Vaccine	37	73%	83%	69%	94%
Smoking Cessation Advice[1]	15	73%	75%	80%	100%
Surgical Infection Prevention					
Prophylactic Antibiotic Given[2]	181	86%	79%	77%	95%
Prophylactic Antibiotic Selection[2]	44	84%	89%	90%	100%
Prophylactic Antibiotic Stopped[2]	178	60%	76%	72%	95%
Pregnancy Care					
Inpatient Neonatal Mortality	-	-	-	-	-
Third or Fourth Degree Laceration	-	-	-	3.63%	3.27%

Mercy Hospital of Franciscan Sisters

201 8th Avenue SE
Oelwein, IA 50662
Phone: 319-283-6000
Fax: 319-283-6004
URL: www.covhealth.com
Ownership: Voluntary non-profit - Private
Accredited: No
Emergency Services: Yes
Licensed Beds: 64

Key Personnel:

CEO . . . . Katherine Hintz
Emergency Room . . . . Judy Malget, RN
Director Medical/Surgical Nursing . . . . John Fox, RN, B
Director Respiratory Therapy . . . . Bridget Frank

Measure	Cases	This Hospital	State Average	U.S. Average	Top Hospital
Heart Attack Care					
ACE Inhibitor or ARB for LVSD[5]	-	-	86%	82%	100%
Aspirin at Arrival[5]	-	-	89%	92%	100%
Aspirin at Discharge[5]	-	-	90%	90%	100%
Beta Blocker at Arrival[5]	-	-	91%	87%	100%
Beta Blocker at Discharge[5]	-	-	91%	90%	100%
Fibrinolytic Medication Timing[5]	-	-	33%	31%	100%
PCI Within 90 Minutes of Arrival[5]	-	-	73%	54%	95%
Smoking Cessation Advice[5]	-	-	92%	88%	100%
Heart Failure Care					
ACE Inhibitor or ARB for LVSD[1]	13	77%	84%	82%	100%
Discharge Instructions[1]	15	93%	62%	61%	93%
Evaluation of LVS Function	34	85%	75%	83%	99%
Smoking Cessation Advice[1]	5	80%	78%	82%	100%
Pneumonia Care					
Appropriate Initial Antibiotic	45	96%	85%	83%	94%
Blood Culture Timing	43	98%	95%	90%	100%
Influenza Vaccine[1]	11	82%	85%	70%	100%
Initial Antibiotic Timing	49	86%	87%	80%	93%
Oxygenation Assessment	70	100%	99%	99%	100%
Pneumococcal Vaccine	49	96%	83%	69%	94%
Smoking Cessation Advice[1]	11	91%	75%	80%	100%
Surgical Infection Prevention					
Prophylactic Antibiotic Given[1,3]	5	80%	79%	77%	95%
Prophylactic Antibiotic Selection[1]	2	50%	89%	90%	100%
Prophylactic Antibiotic Stopped[1,3]	5	20%	76%	72%	95%
Pregnancy Care					
Inpatient Neonatal Mortality	-	-	-	-	-
Third or Fourth Degree Laceration	-	-	-	3.63%	3.27%

Orange City Area Health System

400 Central Avenue NW
Orange City, IA 51041
Toll-Free: 800-808-6264
Phone: 712-737-4984
Fax: 712-737-5252
URL: www.ochealthsystem.org
Ownership: Government - Local
Accredited: No
Emergency Services: Yes
Licensed Beds: 63

Key Personnel:

CEO . . . . Martin W Guthmiller
Chief Medical Staff . . . . John Weber, MD
Emergency Room . . . . Amy Van Beck
Infection Control . . . . Val Droog
Medical/Surgical Nursing . . . . Karie Stamer
Chief Radiology . . . . Darin Blankespoor
Respiratory/Cardiopulmonary . . . . Patty DeKock

Measure	Cases	This Hospital	State Average	U.S. Average	Top Hospital
Heart Attack Care					
ACE Inhibitor or ARB for LVSD[1,3]	2	100%	86%	82%	100%
Aspirin at Arrival[1,3]	7	86%	89%	92%	100%
Aspirin at Discharge[1,3]	5	80%	90%	90%	100%
Beta Blocker at Arrival[1,3]	7	100%	91%	87%	100%
Beta Blocker at Discharge[1,3]	5	100%	91%	90%	100%
Fibrinolytic Medication Timing[1,3]	1	0%	33%	31%	100%
PCI Within 90 Minutes of Arrival[5]	-	-	73%	54%	95%
Smoking Cessation Advice[3]	0	-	92%	88%	100%
Heart Failure Care					
ACE Inhibitor or ARB for LVSD[1]	5	100%	84%	82%	100%
Discharge Instructions[1]	10	40%	62%	61%	93%
Evaluation of LVS Function[1]	18	72%	75%	83%	99%
Smoking Cessation Advice	0	-	78%	82%	100%
Pneumonia Care					
Appropriate Initial Antibiotic[1,2,3]	20	65%	85%	83%	94%
Blood Culture Timing[1,2,3]	3	100%	95%	90%	100%
Influenza Vaccine[1]	4	100%	85%	70%	100%
Initial Antibiotic Timing[1,2,3]	22	77%	87%	80%	93%
Oxygenation Assessment[1,2,3]	24	100%	99%	99%	100%
Pneumococcal Vaccine[1,2,3]	21	95%	83%	69%	94%
Smoking Cessation Advice[1,2,3]	3	67%	75%	80%	100%
Surgical Infection Prevention					
Prophylactic Antibiotic Given[1,3]	4	0%	79%	77%	95%
Prophylactic Antibiotic Selection[5]	-	-	89%	90%	100%
Prophylactic Antibiotic Stopped[1,3]	4	100%	76%	72%	95%
Pregnancy Care					
Inpatient Neonatal Mortality	-	-	-	-	-
Third or Fourth Degree Laceration	-	-	-	3.63%	3.27%

Clarke County Hospital

800 S Fillmore Street
Osceola, IA 50213
Phone: 641-342-2184
Fax: 641-342-5378
URL: www.clarkehosp.org
Ownership: Government - Local
Accredited: No
Emergency Services: Yes
Licensed Beds: 25

Key Personnel:

CEO . . . . Brian Evans
Chief of Medical Staff . . . . Wilson Raglor
Emergency Room . . . . Neline Halls
Director Infection/Disease Control . . . . Cindy Johnson
Manager Radiology . . . . Janelle Baker
Respiratory Care . . . . Luann Hennstra

Measure	Cases	This Hospital	State Average	U.S. Average	Top Hospital
Heart Attack Care					
ACE Inhibitor or ARB for LVSD[3]	0	-	86%	82%	100%
Aspirin at Arrival[1,3]	2	100%	89%	92%	100%
Aspirin at Discharge[1,3]	1	100%	90%	90%	100%
Beta Blocker at Arrival[1,3]	2	50%	91%	87%	100%
Beta Blocker at Discharge[1,3]	1	100%	91%	90%	100%
Fibrinolytic Medication Timing[3]	0	-	33%	31%	100%
PCI Within 90 Minutes of Arrival	0	-	73%	54%	95%
Smoking Cessation Advice[3]	0	-	92%	88%	100%
Heart Failure Care					
ACE Inhibitor or ARB for LVSD[1]	5	100%	84%	82%	100%

NOTE: Hospital profiles are in alphabetical order by state, then city, then hospital within the city; Rankings are sorted by rate in descending order and exclude hospitals with less than 25 cases; (1) The number of cases is too small (n<25) for purposes of reliably predicting hospital performance; (2) Measure reflects the hospital's indication that its submission was based upon a sample of its relevant discharges; (3) Rate reflects fewer than the maximum possible quarters of data for the measure; (4) Inaccurate information submitted and suppressed for one or more quarters; (5) No data is available from the hospital for this measure; Please refer to the User's Guide for a full explanation of data

Measure	Cases	This Hospital	State Average	U.S. Average	Top Hospital
Discharge Instructions[1]	13	0%	62%	61%	93%
Evaluation of LVS Function[1]	15	67%	75%	83%	99%
Smoking Cessation Advice[1]	1	100%	78%	82%	100%
Pneumonia Care					
Appropriate Initial Antibiotic[1]	11	100%	85%	83%	94%
Blood Culture Timing[1]	6	100%	95%	90%	100%
Influenza Vaccine[1]	4	75%	85%	70%	100%
Initial Antibiotic Timing[1]	17	82%	87%	80%	93%
Oxygenation Assessment[1]	19	100%	99%	99%	100%
Pneumococcal Vaccine[1]	11	91%	83%	69%	94%
Smoking Cessation Advice[1]	6	83%	75%	80%	100%
Surgical Infection Prevention					
Prophylactic Antibiotic Given[5]	-	-	79%	77%	95%
Prophylactic Antibiotic Selection[5]	-	-	89%	90%	100%
Prophylactic Antibiotic Stopped[5]	-	-	76%	72%	95%
Pregnancy Care					
Inpatient Neonatal Mortality	-	-	-	-	-
Third or Fourth Degree Laceration	-	-	-	3.63%	3.27%

Ottumwa Regional Health Center

1001 Pennsylvania Avenue
Ottumwa, IA 52501

Toll-Free: 800-933-6742
Phone: 641-682-2300
Fax: 641-684-3154

E-mail: webmaster@orhc.com
URL: www.orhc.com
Ownership: Voluntary non-profit - Private
Emergency Services: Yes
Accredited: Yes
Licensed Beds: 94

Key Personnel:

President/CEO . . . . . Tom Siemers
Chief Medical Staff . . . . . Kenneth Wayne
Emergency Room . . . . . Fred Neujahr
Infection Control . . . . . Paula Simplot
Diretor Medical Surgical Nursing . . . . . Barbara Gardner
Director Womens/Family Care . . . . . Johnni Burns
Director Surgical Services . . . . . Brenda Jeffers
Manager Radiology . . . . . Lynn Manning
Director Cardiopulmonary . . . . . Deb McLeland

Measure	Cases	This Hospital	State Average	U.S. Average	Top Hospital
Heart Attack Care					
ACE Inhibitor or ARB for LVSD[1]	10	70%	86%	82%	100%
Aspirin at Arrival	71	97%	89%	92%	100%
Aspirin at Discharge	40	95%	90%	90%	100%
Beta Blocker at Arrival	81	95%	91%	87%	100%
Beta Blocker at Discharge	51	96%	91%	90%	100%
Fibrinolytic Medication Timing	0	-	33%	31%	100%
PCI Within 90 Minutes of Arrival	0	-	73%	54%	95%
Smoking Cessation Advice[1]	3	100%	92%	88%	100%
Heart Failure Care					
ACE Inhibitor or ARB for LVSD	30	83%	84%	82%	100%
Discharge Instructions	86	56%	62%	61%	93%
Evaluation of LVS Function	99	93%	75%	83%	99%
Smoking Cessation Advice[1]	7	100%	78%	82%	100%
Pneumonia Care					
Appropriate Initial Antibiotic	127	85%	85%	83%	94%
Blood Culture Timing	115	95%	95%	90%	100%
Influenza Vaccine	31	16%	85%	70%	100%
Initial Antibiotic Timing	162	69%	87%	80%	93%
Oxygenation Assessment	217	100%	99%	99%	100%
Pneumococcal Vaccine	140	79%	83%	69%	94%
Smoking Cessation Advice	44	86%	75%	80%	100%
Surgical Infection Prevention					
Prophylactic Antibiotic Given	196	72%	79%	77%	95%
Prophylactic Antibiotic Selection	46	89%	89%	90%	100%
Prophylactic Antibiotic Stopped	180	82%	76%	72%	95%
Pregnancy Care					
Inpatient Neonatal Mortality	-	-	-	-	-
Third or Fourth Degree Laceration	-	-	-	3.63%	3.27%

Pella Regional Health Center

Alternate Name: Pella Community Hospital

404 Jefferson Street
Pella, IA 50219

Toll-Free: 800-628-3150
Phone: 641-628-3150
Fax: 641-628-8901

E-mail: info@pellahealth.org
URL: www.pellahealth.org
Ownership: Voluntary non-profit - Other
Emergency Services: Yes
Accredited: Yes
Licensed Beds: 25

Key Personnel:

President/CEO . . . . . Bob Kroese
Chief Medical Staff . . . . . Jeff Hartung, MD
Cardiac Lab . . . . . Sherilyn Nickel
Emergency Room . . . . . Jan Chapman, RN
Urgent Care . . . . . Marilou Houk, RN
Director Infection/Disease Control . . . . . Cheryl Thomson, RN
ICU . . . . . Joan Vandekrol, RN
OB/GYN/Women's Health . . . . . Karen Westercamp, RN
Chief Radiology . . . . . Lee Henry, DO
Director Respiratory Therapy . . . . . David Cornelder

Measure	Cases	This Hospital	State Average	U.S. Average	Top Hospital
Heart Attack Care					
ACE Inhibitor or ARB for LVSD[1]	3	67%	86%	82%	100%
Aspirin at Arrival[1]	7	86%	89%	92%	100%
Aspirin at Discharge[1]	4	75%	90%	90%	100%
Beta Blocker at Arrival[1]	7	100%	91%	87%	100%
Beta Blocker at Discharge[1]	5	100%	91%	90%	100%
Fibrinolytic Medication Timing	0	-	33%	31%	100%
PCI Within 90 Minutes of Arrival	0	-	73%	54%	95%
Smoking Cessation Advice	0	-	92%	88%	100%
Heart Failure Care					
ACE Inhibitor or ARB for LVSD[1]	11	91%	84%	82%	100%
Discharge Instructions[1]	17	71%	62%	61%	93%
Evaluation of LVS Function	26	92%	75%	83%	99%
Smoking Cessation Advice[1]	2	100%	78%	82%	100%
Pneumonia Care					
Appropriate Initial Antibiotic	46	96%	85%	83%	94%
Blood Culture Timing	46	91%	95%	90%	100%
Influenza Vaccine[1]	21	100%	85%	70%	100%
Initial Antibiotic Timing	68	90%	87%	80%	93%
Oxygenation Assessment	80	100%	99%	99%	100%
Pneumococcal Vaccine	64	98%	83%	69%	94%
Smoking Cessation Advice[1]	10	50%	75%	80%	100%
Surgical Infection Prevention					
Prophylactic Antibiotic Given[2]	103	92%	79%	77%	95%
Prophylactic Antibiotic Selection[2]	29	93%	89%	90%	100%
Prophylactic Antibiotic Stopped[2]	102	93%	76%	72%	95%
Pregnancy Care					
Inpatient Neonatal Mortality	-	-	-	-	-
Third or Fourth Degree Laceration	-	-	-	3.63%	3.27%

Baum Harmon Mercy Hospital

255 N Welch Avenue
Primghar, IA 51245

Phone: 712-757-2300
Fax: 712-757-0300

URL: www.baumharmon.org
Ownership: Voluntary non-profit - Church
Emergency Services: Yes
Accredited: No
Licensed Beds: 13

Key Personnel:

President/CEO . . . . . Robert Monical
Chief Medical Staff . . . . . Danniel Rithcer, MD
Emergency Room . . . . . Linda Bindner
Infection Control . . . . . Tracy Lenz
Medical/Surgical Nursing . . . . . Linda Bindner

Measure	Cases	This Hospital	State Average	U.S. Average	Top Hospital
Heart Attack Care					
ACE Inhibitor or ARB for LVSD[5]	-	-	86%	82%	100%
Aspirin at Arrival[5]	-	-	89%	92%	100%
Aspirin at Discharge[5]	-	-	90%	90%	100%
Beta Blocker at Arrival[5]	-	-	91%	87%	100%
Beta Blocker at Discharge[5]	-	-	91%	90%	100%
Fibrinolytic Medication Timing[5]	-	-	33%	31%	100%
PCI Within 90 Minutes of Arrival[5]	-	-	73%	54%	95%
Smoking Cessation Advice[5]	-	-	92%	88%	100%

NOTE: Hospital profiles are in alphabetical order by state, then city, then hospital within the city; Rankings are sorted by rate in descending order and exclude hospitals with less than 25 cases; (1) The number of cases is too small (n<25) for purposes of reliably predicting hospital performance; (2) Measure reflects the hospital's indication that its submission was based upon a sample of its relevant discharges; (3) Rate reflects fewer than the maximum possible quarters of data for the measure; (4) Inaccurate information submitted and suppressed for one or more quarters; (5) No data is available from the hospital for this measure; Please refer to the User's Guide for a full explanation of data

Measure	Cases	This Hospital	State Average	U.S. Average	Top Hospital
Heart Failure Care					
ACE Inhibitor or ARB for LVSD[3]	0	-	84%	82%	100%
Discharge Instructions[1,3]	5	20%	62%	61%	93%
Evaluation of LVS Function[1,3]	8	50%	75%	83%	99%
Smoking Cessation Advice[1,3]	2	100%	78%	82%	100%
Pneumonia Care					
Appropriate Initial Antibiotic[1,3]	3	67%	85%	83%	94%
Blood Culture Timing[1,3]	1	100%	95%	90%	100%
Influenza Vaccine[5]	-	-	85%	70%	100%
Initial Antibiotic Timing[1,3]	2	100%	87%	80%	93%
Oxygenation Assessment[1,3]	3	100%	99%	99%	100%
Pneumococcal Vaccine[1,3]	2	100%	83%	69%	94%
Smoking Cessation Advice[3]	0	-	75%	80%	100%
Surgical Infection Prevention					
Prophylactic Antibiotic Given[5]	-	-	79%	77%	95%
Prophylactic Antibiotic Selection[5]	-	-	89%	90%	100%
Prophylactic Antibiotic Stopped[5]	-	-	76%	72%	95%
Pregnancy Care					
Inpatient Neonatal Mortality	-	-	-	-	-
Third or Fourth Degree Laceration	-	-	-	3.63%	3.27%

Montgomery County Memorial Hospital

2301 Eastern Avenue
PO Box 498
Red Oak, IA 51566
Phone: 712-623-7000
Fax: 712-623-7180
URL: www.mcmh.org
Ownership: Government - Local
Accredited: No
Emergency Services: Yes
Licensed Beds: 40

Key Personnel:

CEO. . . . . Allen E Pohren
Director Medical/Surgical Nursing . . . . Sue Allen
OB/GYN Womens Health. . . . . Cyril Newman
Chief Radiology . . . . Joyce Siebels
Director Respiratory Therapy . . . . Cindy Arett

Measure	Cases	This Hospital	State Average	U.S. Average	Top Hospital
Heart Attack Care					
ACE Inhibitor or ARB for LVSD	0	-	86%	82%	100%
Aspirin at Arrival[1]	10	60%	89%	92%	100%
Aspirin at Discharge[1]	5	80%	90%	90%	100%
Beta Blocker at Arrival[1]	11	82%	91%	87%	100%
Beta Blocker at Discharge[1]	6	83%	91%	90%	100%
Fibrinolytic Medication Timing	0	-	33%	31%	100%
PCI Within 90 Minutes of Arrival	0	-	73%	54%	95%
Smoking Cessation Advice[1]	1	100%	92%	88%	100%
Heart Failure Care					
ACE Inhibitor or ARB for LVSD[1]	12	92%	84%	82%	100%
Discharge Instructions[1]	23	74%	62%	61%	93%
Evaluation of LVS Function	42	100%	75%	83%	99%
Smoking Cessation Advice[1]	1	100%	78%	82%	100%
Pneumonia Care					
Appropriate Initial Antibiotic	32	88%	85%	83%	94%
Blood Culture Timing[1]	13	100%	95%	90%	100%
Influenza Vaccine[1]	14	100%	85%	70%	100%
Initial Antibiotic Timing	44	91%	87%	80%	93%
Oxygenation Assessment	60	100%	99%	99%	100%
Pneumococcal Vaccine	48	98%	83%	69%	94%
Smoking Cessation Advice[1]	9	89%	75%	80%	100%
Surgical Infection Prevention					
Prophylactic Antibiotic Given[1]	16	88%	79%	77%	95%
Prophylactic Antibiotic Selection[1]	1	100%	89%	90%	100%
Prophylactic Antibiotic Stopped[1]	16	100%	76%	72%	95%
Pregnancy Care					
Inpatient Neonatal Mortality	-	-	-	-	-
Third or Fourth Degree Laceration	-	-	-	3.63%	3.27%

Merrill Pioneer Community Hospital

801 S Greene Street
Rock Rapids, IA 51246
Phone: 712-472-2591
Fax: 712-472-2552
URL: www.merrillpioneer.org
Ownership: Voluntary non-profit - Private
Accredited: No
Emergency Services: No
Licensed Beds: 25

Key Personnel:

CEO. . . . . Gordy Smith
Medical Staff President . . . . David Springer, MD
Emergency Room . . . . Cathy Huff
Infection Control. . . . . Linda Brinkhous

Measure	Cases	This Hospital	State Average	U.S. Average	Top Hospital
Heart Attack Care					
ACE Inhibitor or ARB for LVSD[5]	-	-	86%	82%	100%
Aspirin at Arrival[5]	-	-	89%	92%	100%
Aspirin at Discharge[5]	-	-	90%	90%	100%
Beta Blocker at Arrival[5]	-	-	91%	87%	100%
Beta Blocker at Discharge[5]	-	-	91%	90%	100%
Fibrinolytic Medication Timing[5]	-	-	33%	31%	100%
PCI Within 90 Minutes of Arrival[5]	-	-	73%	54%	95%
Smoking Cessation Advice[5]	-	-	92%	88%	100%
Heart Failure Care					
ACE Inhibitor or ARB for LVSD[1]	2	50%	84%	82%	100%
Discharge Instructions[1]	3	100%	62%	61%	93%
Evaluation of LVS Function[1]	14	43%	75%	83%	99%
Smoking Cessation Advice	0	-	78%	82%	100%
Pneumonia Care					
Appropriate Initial Antibiotic[1]	5	100%	85%	83%	94%
Blood Culture Timing[1]	2	100%	95%	90%	100%
Influenza Vaccine[1]	2	100%	85%	70%	100%
Initial Antibiotic Timing[1]	7	100%	87%	80%	93%
Oxygenation Assessment[1]	8	100%	99%	99%	100%
Pneumococcal Vaccine[1]	6	83%	83%	69%	94%
Smoking Cessation Advice	0	-	75%	80%	100%
Surgical Infection Prevention					
Prophylactic Antibiotic Given[1]	7	57%	79%	77%	95%
Prophylactic Antibiotic Selection[1]	1	0%	89%	90%	100%
Prophylactic Antibiotic Stopped[1]	7	43%	76%	72%	95%
Pregnancy Care					
Inpatient Neonatal Mortality	-	-	-	-	-
Third or Fourth Degree Laceration	-	-	-	3.63%	3.27%

Hegg Memorial Hospital

1202 21st Avenue
Rock Valley, IA 51247
Phone: 712-476-8000
Fax: 712-476-8090
URL: www.heggmemorialhealthcenter.org
Ownership: Voluntary non-profit - Private
Accredited: No
Emergency Services: Yes
Licensed Beds: 120

Key Personnel:

President/CEO. . . . . Glenn Zevenbergen

Measure	Cases	This Hospital	State Average	U.S. Average	Top Hospital
Heart Attack Care					
ACE Inhibitor or ARB for LVSD[5]	-	-	86%	82%	100%
Aspirin at Arrival[5]	-	-	89%	92%	100%
Aspirin at Discharge[5]	-	-	90%	90%	100%
Beta Blocker at Arrival[5]	-	-	91%	87%	100%
Beta Blocker at Discharge[5]	-	-	91%	90%	100%
Fibrinolytic Medication Timing[5]	-	-	33%	31%	100%
PCI Within 90 Minutes of Arrival[5]	-	-	73%	54%	95%
Smoking Cessation Advice[5]	-	-	92%	88%	100%
Heart Failure Care					
ACE Inhibitor or ARB for LVSD[1]	1	100%	84%	82%	100%
Discharge Instructions[1]	2	0%	62%	61%	93%
Evaluation of LVS Function[1]	8	88%	75%	83%	99%
Smoking Cessation Advice	0	-	78%	82%	100%
Pneumonia Care					
Appropriate Initial Antibiotic[1,3]	4	75%	85%	83%	94%
Blood Culture Timing[3]	0	-	95%	90%	100%
Influenza Vaccine[1]	1	100%	85%	70%	100%
Initial Antibiotic Timing[1,3]	8	100%	87%	80%	93%

NOTE: Hospital profiles are in alphabetical order by state, then city, then hospital within the city; Rankings are sorted by rate in descending order and exclude hospitals with less than 25 cases; (1) The number of cases is too small (n<25) for purposes of reliably predicting hospital performance; (2) Measure reflects the hospital's indication that its submission was based upon a sample of its relevant discharges; (3) Rate reflects fewer than the maximum possible quarters of data for the measure; (4) Inaccurate information submitted and suppressed for one or more quarters; (5) No data is available from the hospital for this measure; Please refer to the User's Guide for a full explanation of data

Measure	Cases	This Hospital	State Average	U.S. Average	Top Hospital
Oxygenation Assessment[1,3]	9	100%	99%	99%	100%
Pneumococcal Vaccine[1,3]	9	67%	83%	69%	94%
Smoking Cessation Advice[1,3]	1	100%	75%	80%	100%
Surgical Infection Prevention					
Prophylactic Antibiotic Given[5]	-	-	79%	77%	95%
Prophylactic Antibiotic Selection[5]	-	-	89%	90%	100%
Prophylactic Antibiotic Stopped[5]	-	-	76%	72%	95%
Pregnancy Care					
Inpatient Neonatal Mortality	-	-	-	-	-
Third or Fourth Degree Laceration	-	-	-	3.63%	3.27%

Northwest Iowa Health Center

118 N 7th Avenue
Sheldon, IA 51201

Toll-Free: 800-568-4320
Phone: 712-324-5041
Fax: 712-324-6015

URL: www.nwiowahealthcenter.org
Ownership: Voluntary non-profit - Private
Emergency Services: Yes

Accredited: No
Licensed Beds: 28

Key Personnel:
CEO. . . . . Charles R Miller
Chief Medical Staff. . . . . Scott Lichby, MD
Emergency Room . . . . Kathy Altena, RN
Director Medical/Surgical Nursing . . . . Kathy Altena, RN
Chief Radiology . . . . Harold Elchmann
Director Respiratory Therapy . . . . Marcus Buresh

Measure	Cases	This Hospital	State Average	U.S. Average	Top Hospital
Heart Attack Care					
ACE Inhibitor or ARB for LVSD[3]	0	-	86%	82%	100%
Aspirin at Arrival[1,3]	6	100%	89%	92%	100%
Aspirin at Discharge[1,3]	4	75%	90%	90%	100%
Beta Blocker at Arrival[1,3]	5	80%	91%	87%	100%
Beta Blocker at Discharge[1,3]	5	100%	91%	90%	100%
Fibrinolytic Medication Timing[3]	0	-	33%	31%	100%
PCI Within 90 Minutes of Arrival[5]	-	-	73%	54%	95%
Smoking Cessation Advice[3]	0	-	92%	88%	100%
Heart Failure Care					
ACE Inhibitor or ARB for LVSD[1]	11	82%	84%	82%	100%
Discharge Instructions	34	85%	62%	61%	93%
Evaluation of LVS Function	46	70%	75%	83%	99%
Smoking Cessation Advice[1]	7	100%	78%	82%	100%
Pneumonia Care					
Appropriate Initial Antibiotic	48	98%	85%	83%	94%
Blood Culture Timing	25	100%	95%	90%	100%
Influenza Vaccine[1]	14	79%	85%	70%	100%
Initial Antibiotic Timing	56	100%	87%	80%	93%
Oxygenation Assessment	70	100%	99%	99%	100%
Pneumococcal Vaccine	41	68%	83%	69%	94%
Smoking Cessation Advice[1]	13	85%	75%	80%	100%
Surgical Infection Prevention					
Prophylactic Antibiotic Given[5]	-	-	79%	77%	95%
Prophylactic Antibiotic Selection[5]	-	-	89%	90%	100%
Prophylactic Antibiotic Stopped[5]	-	-	76%	72%	95%
Pregnancy Care					
Inpatient Neonatal Mortality	-	-	-	-	-
Third or Fourth Degree Laceration	-	-	-	3.63%	3.27%

Shenandoah Medical Center

300 Pershing Avenue
Shenandoah, IA 51601

Phone: 712-246-1230
Fax: 712-246-4737

URL: www.shenandoahmedcenter.com
Ownership: Voluntary non-profit - Other
Emergency Services: Yes

Accredited: No
Licensed Beds: 44

Key Personnel:
CEO. . . . . Charles Millburg
Emergency Room . . . . Tammy Franks
Director Medical/Surgical Nursing . . . . Melodee Picray
Chief Radiology . . . . David Halsey
Director Respiratory Therapy . . . . Neal Petersen

Measure	Cases	This Hospital	State Average	U.S. Average	Top Hospital
Heart Attack Care					
ACE Inhibitor or ARB for LVSD[1,3]	1	100%	86%	82%	100%
Aspirin at Arrival[1,3]	5	100%	89%	92%	100%
Aspirin at Discharge[1,3]	3	100%	90%	90%	100%
Beta Blocker at Arrival[1,3]	4	100%	91%	87%	100%
Beta Blocker at Discharge[1,3]	3	100%	91%	90%	100%
Fibrinolytic Medication Timing[3]	0	-	33%	31%	100%
PCI Within 90 Minutes of Arrival[5]	-	-	73%	54%	95%
Smoking Cessation Advice[1,3]	1	0%	92%	88%	100%
Heart Failure Care					
ACE Inhibitor or ARB for LVSD[1]	1	100%	84%	82%	100%
Discharge Instructions[1]	6	83%	62%	61%	93%
Evaluation of LVS Function[1]	9	89%	75%	83%	99%
Smoking Cessation Advice[1]	1	100%	78%	82%	100%
Pneumonia Care					
Appropriate Initial Antibiotic	32	94%	85%	83%	94%
Blood Culture Timing[1]	23	100%	95%	90%	100%
Influenza Vaccine[1]	7	86%	85%	70%	100%
Initial Antibiotic Timing	49	84%	87%	80%	93%
Oxygenation Assessment	60	100%	99%	99%	100%
Pneumococcal Vaccine	45	67%	83%	69%	94%
Smoking Cessation Advice[1]	15	67%	75%	80%	100%
Surgical Infection Prevention					
Prophylactic Antibiotic Given[1]	16	25%	79%	77%	95%
Prophylactic Antibiotic Selection[1]	3	67%	89%	90%	100%
Prophylactic Antibiotic Stopped[1]	16	69%	76%	72%	95%
Pregnancy Care					
Inpatient Neonatal Mortality	-	-	-	-	-
Third or Fourth Degree Laceration	-	-	-	3.63%	3.27%

Osceola Community Hospital

9th Avenue N
Sibley, IA 51249

Toll-Free: 800-859-1419
Phone: 712-754-2574
Fax: 712-754-3782

URL: www.osceolacommunityhospital.org
Ownership: Voluntary non-profit - Private
Emergency Services: Yes

Accredited: No
Licensed Beds: 25

Key Personnel:
CEO. . . . . Janet Dykstra
Chief Medical Staff. . . . . SR Helmers, MD
Chief Medical Staff. . . . . W Hicks
Chief Radiology . . . . Brenda Thole
Director Respiratory Therapy . . . . Martha Rolfes

Measure	Cases	This Hospital	State Average	U.S. Average	Top Hospital
Heart Attack Care					
ACE Inhibitor or ARB for LVSD[3]	0	-	86%	82%	100%
Aspirin at Arrival[1,3]	1	100%	89%	92%	100%
Aspirin at Discharge[1,3]	1	0%	90%	90%	100%
Beta Blocker at Arrival[1,3]	1	100%	91%	87%	100%
Beta Blocker at Discharge[1,3]	1	100%	91%	90%	100%
Fibrinolytic Medication Timing[3]	0	-	33%	31%	100%
PCI Within 90 Minutes of Arrival[5]	-	-	73%	54%	95%
Smoking Cessation Advice[3]	0	-	92%	88%	100%
Heart Failure Care					
ACE Inhibitor or ARB for LVSD[1]	1	100%	84%	82%	100%
Discharge Instructions[1]	7	29%	62%	61%	93%
Evaluation of LVS Function[1]	8	38%	75%	83%	99%
Smoking Cessation Advice	0	-	78%	82%	100%
Pneumonia Care					
Appropriate Initial Antibiotic[1,3]	15	93%	85%	83%	94%
Blood Culture Timing[1,3]	3	100%	95%	90%	100%
Influenza Vaccine[1]	1	100%	85%	70%	100%
Initial Antibiotic Timing[1,3]	12	92%	87%	80%	93%
Oxygenation Assessment[1,3]	17	100%	99%	99%	100%
Pneumococcal Vaccine[1,3]	12	25%	83%	69%	94%
Smoking Cessation Advice[3]	0	-	75%	80%	100%
Surgical Infection Prevention					
Prophylactic Antibiotic Given[1,3]	8	38%	79%	77%	95%
Prophylactic Antibiotic Selection[1]	1	100%	89%	90%	100%
Prophylactic Antibiotic Stopped[1,3]	8	88%	76%	72%	95%
Pregnancy Care					
Inpatient Neonatal Mortality	-	-	-	-	-
Third or Fourth Degree Laceration	-	-	-	3.63%	3.27%

NOTE: Hospital profiles are in alphabetical order by state, then city, then hospital within the city; Rankings are sorted by rate in descending order and exclude hospitals with less than 25 cases; (1) The number of cases is too small (n<25) for purposes of reliably predicting hospital performance; (2) Measure reflects the hospital's indication that its submission was based upon a sample of its relevant discharges; (3) Rate reflects fewer than the maximum possible quarters of data for the measure; (4) Inaccurate information submitted and suppressed for one or more quarters; (5) No data is available from the hospital for this measure; Please refer to the User's Guide for a full explanation of data

Sioux Center Community Hospital

605 S Main Avenue
Sioux Center, IA 51250
Phone: 712-722-1271
Fax: 712-722-0787
URL: www.schospital.org
Ownership: Voluntary non-profit - Private
Accredited: No
Emergency Services: Yes
Licensed Beds: 90

Key Personnel:

CEO. . . . . Mike Seda
Chief of Medical Staff. . . . . Robert Clemens
Director Medical/Surgical Nursing . . . . Marilyn Ver Meer

Measure	Cases	This Hospital	State Average	U.S. Average	Top Hospital
Heart Attack Care					
ACE Inhibitor or ARB for LVSD[5]	-	-	86%	82%	100%
Aspirin at Arrival[5]	-	-	89%	92%	100%
Aspirin at Discharge[5]	-	-	90%	90%	100%
Beta Blocker at Arrival[5]	-	-	91%	87%	100%
Beta Blocker at Discharge[5]	-	-	91%	90%	100%
Fibrinolytic Medication Timing[5]	-	-	33%	31%	100%
PCI Within 90 Minutes of Arrival[5]	-	-	73%	54%	95%
Smoking Cessation Advice[5]	-	-	92%	88%	100%
Heart Failure Care					
ACE Inhibitor or ARB for LVSD[1]	1	100%	84%	82%	100%
Discharge Instructions[1]	7	86%	62%	61%	93%
Evaluation of LVS Function[1]	16	19%	75%	83%	99%
Smoking Cessation Advice	0	-	78%	82%	100%
Pneumonia Care					
Appropriate Initial Antibiotic	33	94%	85%	83%	94%
Blood Culture Timing[1]	7	100%	95%	90%	100%
Influenza Vaccine[1]	5	80%	85%	70%	100%
Initial Antibiotic Timing	25	88%	87%	80%	93%
Oxygenation Assessment	36	97%	99%	99%	100%
Pneumococcal Vaccine	27	85%	83%	69%	94%
Smoking Cessation Advice[1]	4	25%	75%	80%	100%
Surgical Infection Prevention					
Prophylactic Antibiotic Given[1]	13	62%	79%	77%	95%
Prophylactic Antibiotic Selection[1]	4	100%	89%	90%	100%
Prophylactic Antibiotic Stopped[1]	12	92%	76%	72%	95%
Pregnancy Care					
Inpatient Neonatal Mortality	-	-	-	-	-
Third or Fourth Degree Laceration	-	-	-	3.63%	3.27%

Mercy Medical Center

801 Fifth Street
Sioux City, IA 51102
Phone: 712-279-2010
Fax: 712-279-5624
URL: www.mercysiouxcity.com
Ownership: Voluntary non-profit - Church
Accredited: Yes
Emergency Services: Yes
Licensed Beds: 483

Key Personnel:

President/CEO. . . . . Mari Kaptain-Dahlen
Chief Medical Staff. . . . . Bruce Miller, MD
Emergency Room . . . . Tom Benzoni, DO
Director Infection/Disease Control . . . . Diane Priekfat
Intensive/Coronary Care . . . . Mitchell Horowitz, MD
OB/GYN Womens Health. . . . . Kevin Hamburger, MD
Chief Radiology . . . . Jonathan C Beeler, MD

Measure	Cases	This Hospital	State Average	U.S. Average	Top Hospital
Heart Attack Care					
ACE Inhibitor or ARB for LVSD	57	91%	86%	82%	100%
Aspirin at Arrival	190	99%	89%	92%	100%
Aspirin at Discharge	343	99%	90%	90%	100%
Beta Blocker at Arrival	186	98%	91%	87%	100%
Beta Blocker at Discharge	343	98%	91%	90%	100%
Fibrinolytic Medication Timing	0	-	33%	31%	100%
PCI Within 90 Minutes of Arrival[1]	13	77%	73%	54%	95%
Smoking Cessation Advice	122	100%	92%	88%	100%
Heart Failure Care					
ACE Inhibitor or ARB for LVSD	100	92%	84%	82%	100%
Discharge Instructions	197	77%	62%	61%	93%
Evaluation of LVS Function	242	95%	75%	83%	99%
Smoking Cessation Advice	42	98%	78%	82%	100%
Pneumonia Care					
Appropriate Initial Antibiotic	132	88%	85%	83%	94%
Blood Culture Timing	138	99%	95%	90%	100%
Influenza Vaccine	43	84%	85%	70%	100%
Initial Antibiotic Timing	206	85%	87%	80%	93%
Oxygenation Assessment	258	100%	99%	99%	100%
Pneumococcal Vaccine	176	74%	83%	69%	94%
Smoking Cessation Advice	66	97%	75%	80%	100%
Surgical Infection Prevention					
Prophylactic Antibiotic Given[2,3]	536	89%	79%	77%	95%
Prophylactic Antibiotic Selection[2]	70	99%	89%	90%	100%
Prophylactic Antibiotic Stopped[2,3]	530	79%	76%	72%	95%
Pregnancy Care					
Inpatient Neonatal Mortality	-	-	-	-	-
Third or Fourth Degree Laceration	-	-	-	3.63%	3.27%

Saint Luke's Regional Medical Center

2720 Stone Park Boulevard
Sioux City, IA 51104
Toll-Free: 800-541-2304
Phone: 712-279-3500
Fax: 712-279-7958
URL: www.stlukes.org
Ownership: Voluntary non-profit - Private
Accredited: Yes
Emergency Services: Yes
Licensed Beds: 353

Key Personnel:

Administrator/President . . . . Peter Thoreen
Chief Medical Staff. . . . . John Redwine, DO
Chief Catheterization Laboratory . . . . Michael Chandra, MD
Emergency Room . . . . Paul Berger, MD
Director Infection/Disease Control . . . . Dee Pedersen, RN
Director Medical/Surgical Nursing . . . . Ronda Keenan, RN
OB/GYN Womens Health. . . . . WN Vereen, DO
Chief Radiology . . . . Gregory R Jackson, MD
Director Cardio-Pulmonary Services . . . . Mark Scott

Measure	Cases	This Hospital	State Average	U.S. Average	Top Hospital
Heart Attack Care					
ACE Inhibitor or ARB for LVSD[1]	15	87%	86%	82%	100%
Aspirin at Arrival	53	96%	89%	92%	100%
Aspirin at Discharge	43	98%	90%	90%	100%
Beta Blocker at Arrival	42	98%	91%	87%	100%
Beta Blocker at Discharge	38	100%	91%	90%	100%
Fibrinolytic Medication Timing	0	-	33%	31%	100%
PCI Within 90 Minutes of Arrival	0	-	73%	54%	95%
Smoking Cessation Advice[1]	12	100%	92%	88%	100%
Heart Failure Care					
ACE Inhibitor or ARB for LVSD	38	100%	84%	82%	100%
Discharge Instructions	81	95%	62%	61%	93%
Evaluation of LVS Function	118	99%	75%	83%	99%
Smoking Cessation Advice[1]	17	100%	78%	82%	100%
Pneumonia Care					
Appropriate Initial Antibiotic	175	95%	85%	83%	94%
Blood Culture Timing	131	98%	95%	90%	100%
Influenza Vaccine	52	100%	85%	70%	100%
Initial Antibiotic Timing	220	92%	87%	80%	93%
Oxygenation Assessment	280	100%	99%	99%	100%
Pneumococcal Vaccine	183	92%	83%	69%	94%
Smoking Cessation Advice	66	98%	75%	80%	100%
Surgical Infection Prevention					
Prophylactic Antibiotic Given	670	89%	79%	77%	95%
Prophylactic Antibiotic Selection	151	96%	89%	90%	100%
Prophylactic Antibiotic Stopped	651	85%	76%	72%	95%
Pregnancy Care					
Inpatient Neonatal Mortality	2,137	0.14%	-	-	-
Third or Fourth Degree Laceration	1,454	3.78%	-	3.63%	3.27%

Spencer Hospital

1200 First Avenue E
Spencer, IA 51301
Phone: 712-264-6111
Fax: 712-264-6404
E-mail: ddoorn@spencerhospital.org
URL: www.spencerhospital.org
Ownership: Government - Local
Accredited: No
Emergency Services: Yes
Licensed Beds: 85

Key Personnel:

CEO. . . . . Doug Doorn

NOTE: Hospital profiles are in alphabetical order by state, then city, then hospital within the city; Rankings are sorted by rate in descending order and exclude hospitals with less than 25 cases; (1) The number of cases is too small (n<25) for purposes of reliably predicting hospital performance; (2) Measure reflects the hospital's indication that its submission was based upon a sample of its relevant discharges; (3) Rate reflects fewer than the maximum possible quarters of data for the measure; (4) Inaccurate information submitted and suppressed for one or more quarters; (5) No data is available from the hospital for this measure; Please refer to the User's Guide for a full explanation of data

Cardio-Pulmonary Services . . . . Jason Trierweiler
Emergency Room . . . . Deb Brodersen
OB/GYN Womens Health. . . . . Daryll Forsland
Surgical Services . . . . Dee Hoger

Measure	Cases	This Hospital	State Average	U.S. Average	Top Hospital
Heart Attack Care					
ACE Inhibitor or ARB for LVSD[1]	3	100%	86%	82%	100%
Aspirin at Arrival[1]	10	100%	89%	92%	100%
Aspirin at Discharge[1]	6	100%	90%	90%	100%
Beta Blocker at Arrival[1]	12	100%	91%	87%	100%
Beta Blocker at Discharge[1]	8	100%	91%	90%	100%
Fibrinolytic Medication Timing[3]	0	-	33%	31%	100%
PCI Within 90 Minutes of Arrival	0	-	73%	54%	95%
Smoking Cessation Advice[1]	1	100%	92%	88%	100%
Heart Failure Care					
ACE Inhibitor or ARB for LVSD[1]	14	86%	84%	82%	100%
Discharge Instructions	37	86%	62%	61%	93%
Evaluation of LVS Function	71	86%	75%	83%	99%
Smoking Cessation Advice[1]	6	67%	78%	82%	100%
Pneumonia Care					
Appropriate Initial Antibiotic	44	91%	85%	83%	94%
Blood Culture Timing	36	97%	95%	90%	100%
Influenza Vaccine[1]	13	85%	85%	70%	100%
Initial Antibiotic Timing	67	93%	87%	80%	93%
Oxygenation Assessment	76	100%	99%	99%	100%
Pneumococcal Vaccine	53	98%	83%	69%	94%
Smoking Cessation Advice[1]	10	90%	75%	80%	100%
Surgical Infection Prevention					
Prophylactic Antibiotic Given[2]	291	95%	79%	77%	95%
Prophylactic Antibiotic Selection[2]	46	78%	89%	90%	100%
Prophylactic Antibiotic Stopped[2]	286	88%	76%	72%	95%
Pregnancy Care					
Inpatient Neonatal Mortality	-	-	-	-	-
Third or Fourth Degree Laceration	-	-	-	3.63%	3.27%

Lakes Regional Healthcare

Highway 71 South
Spirit Lake, IA 51360
Phone: 712-336-1230
Fax: 712-336-8626
URL: www.lakeshealth.org
Ownership: Government - Local
Accredited: No
Emergency Services: No
Licensed Beds: 49

Key Personnel:

CEO. . . . . Richard Kielman
Chief Medical Staff. . . . . Timothy Taylor
Emergency Room . . . . Geoff Messerole
Director Respiratory Therapy . . . . W Hutchinson

Measure	Cases	This Hospital	State Average	U.S. Average	Top Hospital
Heart Attack Care					
ACE Inhibitor or ARB for LVSD	0	-	86%	82%	100%
Aspirin at Arrival[1]	11	91%	89%	92%	100%
Aspirin at Discharge[1]	8	100%	90%	90%	100%
Beta Blocker at Arrival[1]	10	90%	91%	87%	100%
Beta Blocker at Discharge[1]	7	86%	91%	90%	100%
Fibrinolytic Medication Timing[1]	1	100%	33%	31%	100%
PCI Within 90 Minutes of Arrival	0	-	73%	54%	95%
Smoking Cessation Advice	0	-	92%	88%	100%
Heart Failure Care					
ACE Inhibitor or ARB for LVSD[1]	8	62%	84%	82%	100%
Discharge Instructions	25	0%	62%	61%	93%
Evaluation of LVS Function	38	61%	75%	83%	99%
Smoking Cessation Advice[1]	5	40%	78%	82%	100%
Pneumonia Care					
Appropriate Initial Antibiotic	45	71%	85%	83%	94%
Blood Culture Timing	29	97%	95%	90%	100%
Influenza Vaccine[1]	8	75%	85%	70%	100%
Initial Antibiotic Timing	53	87%	87%	80%	93%
Oxygenation Assessment	69	100%	99%	99%	100%
Pneumococcal Vaccine	50	68%	83%	69%	94%
Smoking Cessation Advice[1]	10	60%	75%	80%	100%
Surgical Infection Prevention					
Prophylactic Antibiotic Given	116	72%	79%	77%	95%
Prophylactic Antibiotic Selection	28	93%	89%	90%	100%
Prophylactic Antibiotic Stopped	114	94%	76%	72%	95%
Pregnancy Care					
Inpatient Neonatal Mortality	-	-	-	-	-
Third or Fourth Degree Laceration	-	-	-	3.63%	3.27%

Buena Vista Regional Medical Center

1525 West 5th Street
PO Box 309
Storm Lake, IA 50588
Toll-Free: 888-712-5433
Phone: 712-732-4030
Fax: 712-213-1233
E-mail: marketing-info@bvrmc.org
URL: www.bvrmc.org
Ownership: Government - Local
Accredited: Yes
Emergency Services: Yes
Licensed Beds: 42

Key Personnel:

CEO. . . . . Todd Hudspeth
Emergency Room . . . . Denise Haisch
Infection Control. . . . . Judy Kropf
Medical Surgical Nursing . . . . Barb Jorgensen
Director Respiratory Therapy . . . . Larry Schubert

Measure	Cases	This Hospital	State Average	U.S. Average	Top Hospital
Heart Attack Care					
ACE Inhibitor or ARB for LVSD[1]	2	50%	86%	82%	100%
Aspirin at Arrival[1]	13	92%	89%	92%	100%
Aspirin at Discharge[1]	7	100%	90%	90%	100%
Beta Blocker at Arrival[1]	6	100%	91%	87%	100%
Beta Blocker at Discharge[1]	6	100%	91%	90%	100%
Fibrinolytic Medication Timing	0	-	33%	31%	100%
PCI Within 90 Minutes of Arrival	0	-	73%	54%	95%
Smoking Cessation Advice	0	-	92%	88%	100%
Heart Failure Care					
ACE Inhibitor or ARB for LVSD[1]	6	83%	84%	82%	100%
Discharge Instructions[1]	22	50%	62%	61%	93%
Evaluation of LVS Function	46	67%	75%	83%	99%
Smoking Cessation Advice[1]	5	80%	78%	82%	100%
Pneumonia Care					
Appropriate Initial Antibiotic[1]	24	92%	85%	83%	94%
Blood Culture Timing[1]	18	94%	95%	90%	100%
Influenza Vaccine[1]	11	100%	85%	70%	100%
Initial Antibiotic Timing	51	76%	87%	80%	93%
Oxygenation Assessment	79	100%	99%	99%	100%
Pneumococcal Vaccine	63	98%	83%	69%	94%
Smoking Cessation Advice[1]	10	50%	75%	80%	100%
Surgical Infection Prevention					
Prophylactic Antibiotic Given[5]	-	-	79%	77%	95%
Prophylactic Antibiotic Selection[5]	-	-	89%	90%	100%
Prophylactic Antibiotic Stopped[5]	-	-	76%	72%	95%
Pregnancy Care					
Inpatient Neonatal Mortality	-	-	-	-	-
Third or Fourth Degree Laceration	-	-	-	3.63%	3.27%

Washington County Hospital

400 E Polk Street
Washington, IA 52353
Phone: 319-653-5481
Fax: 319-653-3401
URL: www.wchc.org
Ownership: Voluntary non-profit - Other
Accredited: No
Emergency Services: Yes
Licensed Beds: 68

Key Personnel:

CEO. . . . . Donald Patterson
Emergency Room . . . . Cathy Buffington
Chief Radiology . . . . Letha Sylvester

Measure	Cases	This Hospital	State Average	U.S. Average	Top Hospital
Heart Attack Care					
ACE Inhibitor or ARB for LVSD[5]	-	-	86%	82%	100%
Aspirin at Arrival[5]	-	-	89%	92%	100%
Aspirin at Discharge[5]	-	-	90%	90%	100%
Beta Blocker at Arrival[5]	-	-	91%	87%	100%
Beta Blocker at Discharge[5]	-	-	91%	90%	100%
Fibrinolytic Medication Timing[5]	-	-	33%	31%	100%
PCI Within 90 Minutes of Arrival[5]	-	-	73%	54%	95%

NOTE: Hospital profiles are in alphabetical order by state, then city, then hospital within the city; Rankings are sorted by rate in descending order and exclude hospitals with less than 25 cases; (1) The number of cases is too small (n<25) for purposes of reliably predicting hospital performance; (2) Measure reflects the hospital's indication that its submission was based upon a sample of its relevant discharges; (3) Rate reflects fewer than the maximum possible quarters of data for the measure; (4) Inaccurate information submitted and suppressed for one or more quarters; (5) No data is available from the hospital for this measure; Please refer to the User's Guide for a full explanation of data

Smoking Cessation Advice[5]	-	-	92%	88%	100%
Heart Failure Care					
ACE Inhibitor or ARB for LVSD[1,3]	7	71%	84%	82%	100%
Discharge Instructions[1,3]	10	30%	62%	61%	93%
Evaluation of LVS Function[1,3]	24	62%	75%	83%	99%
Smoking Cessation Advice[1,3]	2	0%	78%	82%	100%
Pneumonia Care					
Appropriate Initial Antibiotic	25	76%	85%	83%	94%
Blood Culture Timing[1]	11	100%	95%	90%	100%
Influenza Vaccine[1]	16	62%	85%	70%	100%
Initial Antibiotic Timing	50	70%	87%	80%	93%
Oxygenation Assessment	61	100%	99%	99%	100%
Pneumococcal Vaccine	47	53%	83%	69%	94%
Smoking Cessation Advice[1]	9	67%	75%	80%	100%
Surgical Infection Prevention					
Prophylactic Antibiotic Given[5]	-	-	79%	77%	95%
Prophylactic Antibiotic Selection[5]	-	-	89%	90%	100%
Prophylactic Antibiotic Stopped[5]	-	-	76%	72%	95%
Pregnancy Care					
Inpatient Neonatal Mortality	-	-	-	-	-
Third or Fourth Degree Laceration	-	-	-	3.63%	3.27%

Allen Memorial Hospital

1825 Logan Avenue — Phone: 319-235-3941
Waterloo, IA 50703 — Fax: 319-235-3461
URL: www.allenhospital.org
Ownership: Voluntary non-profit - Private — Accredited: Yes
Emergency Services: Yes — Licensed Beds: 234

Key Personnel:

President/CEO . . . . Richard A Seidler
Chief Medical Staff . . . . Thomas Gorsche, MD
Cardiac Lab . . . . Lois Benefas
Catheterization Lab . . . . Lois Bonefas
Emergency Room . . . . Deb Gingrich
Emergency Room . . . . Roberta Southworth
Infection Control . . . . Bill Farmer
ICU . . . . Deb Gingrish
Intensive/Coronary Care . . . . Deb Gingrich
Medical/Surgical Nursing . . . . Deb Gingrich
OB/GYN Womens Health . . . . Marilee Tarkett
Respiratory/Cardiopulmonary . . . . Lois Bonefas

Measure	Cases	This Hospital	State Average	U.S. Average	Top Hospital
Heart Attack Care					
ACE Inhibitor or ARB for LVSD	78	83%	86%	82%	100%
Aspirin at Arrival	153	98%	89%	92%	100%
Aspirin at Discharge	235	99%	90%	90%	100%
Beta Blocker at Arrival	133	94%	91%	87%	100%
Beta Blocker at Discharge	270	97%	91%	90%	100%
Fibrinolytic Medication Timing[1]	1	0%	33%	31%	100%
PCI Within 90 Minutes of Arrival[1]	9	67%	73%	54%	95%
Smoking Cessation Advice	107	98%	92%	88%	100%
Heart Failure Care					
ACE Inhibitor or ARB for LVSD	139	79%	84%	82%	100%
Discharge Instructions	252	67%	62%	61%	93%
Evaluation of LVS Function	323	92%	75%	83%	99%
Smoking Cessation Advice	60	92%	78%	82%	100%
Pneumonia Care					
Appropriate Initial Antibiotic	149	95%	85%	83%	94%
Blood Culture Timing	137	89%	95%	90%	100%
Influenza Vaccine	55	89%	85%	70%	100%
Initial Antibiotic Timing	233	88%	87%	80%	93%
Oxygenation Assessment	268	100%	99%	99%	100%
Pneumococcal Vaccine	188	94%	83%	69%	94%
Smoking Cessation Advice	61	95%	75%	80%	100%
Surgical Infection Prevention					
Prophylactic Antibiotic Given	653	96%	79%	77%	95%
Prophylactic Antibiotic Selection	61	100%	89%	90%	100%
Prophylactic Antibiotic Stopped	625	96%	76%	72%	95%
Pregnancy Care					
Inpatient Neonatal Mortality[2]	619	0.16%	-	-	-
Third or Fourth Degree Laceration[2]	465	4.73%	-	3.63%	3.27%

Covenant Medical Center

3421 W 9th Street — Phone: 319-272-8000
Waterloo, IA 50702 — Fax: 319-272-7313
URL: www.covhealth.com
Ownership: Voluntary non-profit - Church — Accredited: Yes
Emergency Services: Yes — Licensed Beds: 281

Key Personnel:

Administrator/President . . . . Jack Dusenbery
Chief Medical Staff . . . . Cassandra Foensr, MD
Chief ER Services . . . . Geoffrey Miller, MD
Emergency Room . . . . Niki Maas
Director Infection/Disease Control . . . . Nancy Schuler
Coordinator CCU . . . . Denise Lampman
Medical/Surgical Nursing . . . . Marcia Dlouhy
OB/GYN Womens Health . . . . Edward Sandy, MD
Chief Radiology . . . . Lawrence Furlong, MD
Director Respiratory Therapy . . . . Donna Camaratta

Measure	Cases	This Hospital	State Average	U.S. Average	Top Hospital
Heart Attack Care					
ACE Inhibitor or ARB for LVSD[1]	1	0%	86%	82%	100%
Aspirin at Arrival[1]	20	100%	89%	92%	100%
Aspirin at Discharge[1]	11	100%	90%	90%	100%
Beta Blocker at Arrival[1]	17	94%	91%	87%	100%
Beta Blocker at Discharge[1]	11	100%	91%	90%	100%
Fibrinolytic Medication Timing[1]	1	0%	33%	31%	100%
PCI Within 90 Minutes of Arrival	0	-	73%	54%	95%
Smoking Cessation Advice	0	-	92%	88%	100%
Heart Failure Care					
ACE Inhibitor or ARB for LVSD	34	74%	84%	82%	100%
Discharge Instructions	82	88%	62%	61%	93%
Evaluation of LVS Function	121	98%	75%	83%	99%
Smoking Cessation Advice[1]	20	95%	78%	82%	100%
Pneumonia Care					
Appropriate Initial Antibiotic	108	92%	85%	83%	94%
Blood Culture Timing	81	89%	95%	90%	100%
Influenza Vaccine	25	84%	85%	70%	100%
Initial Antibiotic Timing	141	80%	87%	80%	93%
Oxygenation Assessment	189	100%	99%	99%	100%
Pneumococcal Vaccine	123	85%	83%	69%	94%
Smoking Cessation Advice	45	98%	75%	80%	100%
Surgical Infection Prevention					
Prophylactic Antibiotic Given[3]	237	93%	79%	77%	95%
Prophylactic Antibiotic Selection	66	91%	89%	90%	100%
Prophylactic Antibiotic Stopped[3]	230	49%	76%	72%	95%
Pregnancy Care					
Inpatient Neonatal Mortality	-	-	-	-	-
Third or Fourth Degree Laceration	-	-	-	3.63%	3.27%

Veterans Memorial Hospital

40 1st Street SE — Phone: 563-568-3411
Waukon, IA 52172 — Fax: 563-568-5550
URL: www.vmhospital.com
Ownership: Government - Local — Accredited: No
Emergency Services: Yes — Licensed Beds: 25

Key Personnel:

CEO . . . . Michael D Myers
Chief Medical Staff . . . . David Schwartz
Chief of Medical Staff . . . . Larry Bartel
Emergency Room . . . . Diane Butikofer

Measure	Cases	This Hospital	State Average	U.S. Average	Top Hospital
Heart Attack Care					
ACE Inhibitor or ARB for LVSD[3]	0	-	86%	82%	100%
Aspirin at Arrival[1,3]	5	100%	89%	92%	100%
Aspirin at Discharge[1,3]	3	100%	90%	90%	100%
Beta Blocker at Arrival[1,3]	3	100%	91%	87%	100%
Beta Blocker at Discharge[1,3]	3	67%	91%	90%	100%
Fibrinolytic Medication Timing[3]	0	-	33%	31%	100%
PCI Within 90 Minutes of Arrival[5]	-	-	73%	54%	95%
Smoking Cessation Advice[3]	0	-	92%	88%	100%
Heart Failure Care					
ACE Inhibitor or ARB for LVSD[1]	6	67%	84%	82%	100%

NOTE: Hospital profiles are in alphabetical order by state, then city, then hospital within the city; Rankings are sorted by rate in descending order and exclude hospitals with less than 25 cases; (1) The number of cases is too small (n<25) for purposes of reliably predicting hospital performance; (2) Measure reflects the hospital's indication that its submission was based upon a sample of its relevant discharges; (3) Rate reflects fewer than the maximum possible quarters of data for the measure; (4) Inaccurate information submitted and suppressed for one or more quarters; (5) No data is available from the hospital for this measure; Please refer to the User's Guide for a full explanation of data

Discharge Instructions[1]	13	54%	62%	61%	93%
Evaluation of LVS Function[1]	24	71%	75%	83%	99%
Smoking Cessation Advice[1]	3	67%	78%	82%	100%
Pneumonia Care					
Appropriate Initial Antibiotic[1]	15	100%	85%	83%	94%
Blood Culture Timing[1]	10	90%	95%	90%	100%
Influenza Vaccine[1]	4	75%	85%	70%	100%
Initial Antibiotic Timing[1]	22	91%	87%	80%	93%
Oxygenation Assessment	31	97%	99%	99%	100%
Pneumococcal Vaccine	25	64%	83%	69%	94%
Smoking Cessation Advice[1]	4	50%	75%	80%	100%
Surgical Infection Prevention					
Prophylactic Antibiotic Given[1]	19	42%	79%	77%	95%
Prophylactic Antibiotic Selection[1]	7	86%	89%	90%	100%
Prophylactic Antibiotic Stopped[1]	18	11%	76%	72%	95%
Pregnancy Care					
Inpatient Neonatal Mortality	-	-	-	-	-
Third or Fourth Degree Laceration	-	-	-	3.63%	3.27%

Waverly Health Center

312 9th Street SW
Waverly, IA 50677
Phone: 319-352-4120
Fax: 319-352-3992
E-mail: aflessner@wavhosp.org
URL: www.waverlyhealthcenter.org
Ownership: Government - Local
Accredited: Yes
Emergency Services: Yes
Licensed Beds: 25

Key Personnel:

CEO. . . . . Michael Trachta
Director Medical/Surgical Nursing . . . . Mary Conway
OB/GYN Womens Health. . . . . Lee Fagre, MD
Chief Radiology . . . . Leah Briggs
Director Respiratory Therapy . . . . Ethel Manross

Measure	Cases	This Hospital	State Average	U.S. Average	Top Hospital
Heart Attack Care					
ACE Inhibitor or ARB for LVSD[1,3]	1	100%	86%	82%	100%
Aspirin at Arrival[1,3]	2	50%	89%	92%	100%
Aspirin at Discharge[1,3]	2	100%	90%	90%	100%
Beta Blocker at Arrival[1,3]	2	50%	91%	87%	100%
Beta Blocker at Discharge[1,3]	2	100%	91%	90%	100%
Fibrinolytic Medication Timing[3]	0	-	33%	31%	100%
PCI Within 90 Minutes of Arrival[5]	-	-	73%	54%	95%
Smoking Cessation Advice[3]	0	-	92%	88%	100%
Heart Failure Care					
ACE Inhibitor or ARB for LVSD[1,3]	4	100%	84%	82%	100%
Discharge Instructions[1,3]	8	38%	62%	61%	93%
Evaluation of LVS Function[1,3]	9	67%	75%	83%	99%
Smoking Cessation Advice[1,3]	1	100%	78%	82%	100%
Pneumonia Care					
Appropriate Initial Antibiotic[1,3]	4	75%	85%	83%	94%
Blood Culture Timing[1,3]	6	67%	95%	90%	100%
Influenza Vaccine[5]	-	-	85%	70%	100%
Initial Antibiotic Timing[1,3]	8	75%	87%	80%	93%
Oxygenation Assessment[1,3]	9	100%	99%	99%	100%
Pneumococcal Vaccine[1,3]	8	50%	83%	69%	94%
Smoking Cessation Advice[1,3]	1	100%	75%	80%	100%
Surgical Infection Prevention					
Prophylactic Antibiotic Given[1,3]	23	87%	79%	77%	95%
Prophylactic Antibiotic Selection[1]	16	88%	89%	90%	100%
Prophylactic Antibiotic Stopped[1,3]	23	87%	76%	72%	95%
Pregnancy Care					
Inpatient Neonatal Mortality	-	-	-	-	-
Third or Fourth Degree Laceration	-	-	-	3.63%	3.27%

Hamilton County Public Hospital

800 Ohio Street
Webster City, IA 50595
Phone: 515-832-9400
Fax: 515-832-9420
URL: www.hamiltonhospital.com
Ownership: Government - Local
Accredited: No
Emergency Services: Yes
Licensed Beds: 25

Key Personnel:

CEO. . . . . Palmer Schneider
Chief Medical Staff. . . . . Stephen Sundberg, MD
Emergency Room . . . . Kendra Cook
Emergency Room . . . . Claudia Boff
Director Medical/Surgical Nursing . . . . Joan Hisler
Chief Radiology . . . . Tom Fink, DO
Director Respiratory Therapy . . . . Jay Bell

Measure	Cases	This Hospital	State Average	U.S. Average	Top Hospital
Heart Attack Care					
ACE Inhibitor or ARB for LVSD[1]	2	50%	86%	82%	100%
Aspirin at Arrival[1]	5	60%	89%	92%	100%
Aspirin at Discharge[1]	4	50%	90%	90%	100%
Beta Blocker at Arrival[1]	7	71%	91%	87%	100%
Beta Blocker at Discharge[1]	7	86%	91%	90%	100%
Fibrinolytic Medication Timing	0	-	33%	31%	100%
PCI Within 90 Minutes of Arrival[5]	-	-	73%	54%	95%
Smoking Cessation Advice	0	-	92%	88%	100%
Heart Failure Care					
ACE Inhibitor or ARB for LVSD[1]	5	100%	84%	82%	100%
Discharge Instructions	52	60%	62%	61%	93%
Evaluation of LVS Function	72	97%	75%	83%	99%
Smoking Cessation Advice[1]	5	60%	78%	82%	100%
Pneumonia Care					
Appropriate Initial Antibiotic	41	80%	85%	83%	94%
Blood Culture Timing	27	96%	95%	90%	100%
Influenza Vaccine[1]	10	90%	85%	70%	100%
Initial Antibiotic Timing	65	91%	87%	80%	93%
Oxygenation Assessment	77	100%	99%	99%	100%
Pneumococcal Vaccine	49	88%	83%	69%	94%
Smoking Cessation Advice[1]	9	78%	75%	80%	100%
Surgical Infection Prevention					
Prophylactic Antibiotic Given	28	71%	79%	77%	95%
Prophylactic Antibiotic Selection[1]	6	100%	89%	90%	100%
Prophylactic Antibiotic Stopped	26	35%	76%	72%	95%
Pregnancy Care					
Inpatient Neonatal Mortality	-	-	-	-	-
Third or Fourth Degree Laceration	-	-	-	3.63%	3.27%

Great River Medical Center

1221 S Gear Avenue
West Burlington, IA 52655
Phone: 319-768-1000
Fax: 319-768-3306
URL: www.greatrivermedical.org
Ownership: Voluntary non-profit - Other
Accredited: Yes
Emergency Services: Yes
Licensed Beds: 378

Key Personnel:

President/CEO. . . . . Mark Richardson
Chief Medical Staff. . . . . Sherman Williams, MD
Chief Radiology . . . . Donald Gale, MD
Director Respiratory Therapy . . . . Kermit Dieterich, RRT

Measure	Cases	This Hospital	State Average	U.S. Average	Top Hospital
Heart Attack Care					
ACE Inhibitor or ARB for LVSD[1]	10	100%	86%	82%	100%
Aspirin at Arrival	97	100%	89%	92%	100%
Aspirin at Discharge	42	95%	90%	90%	100%
Beta Blocker at Arrival	94	98%	91%	87%	100%
Beta Blocker at Discharge	46	96%	91%	90%	100%
Fibrinolytic Medication Timing[1]	19	58%	33%	31%	100%
PCI Within 90 Minutes of Arrival[1]	1	100%	73%	54%	95%
Smoking Cessation Advice[1]	12	100%	92%	88%	100%
Heart Failure Care					
ACE Inhibitor or ARB for LVSD	37	97%	84%	82%	100%
Discharge Instructions	135	93%	62%	61%	93%
Evaluation of LVS Function	192	99%	75%	83%	99%
Smoking Cessation Advice[1]	22	100%	78%	82%	100%
Pneumonia Care					
Appropriate Initial Antibiotic	134	81%	85%	83%	94%
Blood Culture Timing	158	94%	95%	90%	100%
Influenza Vaccine	50	96%	85%	70%	100%
Initial Antibiotic Timing	209	84%	87%	80%	93%
Oxygenation Assessment	261	100%	99%	99%	100%
Pneumococcal Vaccine	195	94%	83%	69%	94%
Smoking Cessation Advice	60	95%	75%	80%	100%

NOTE: Hospital profiles are in alphabetical order by state, then city, then hospital within the city; Rankings are sorted by rate in descending order and exclude hospitals with less than 25 cases; (1) The number of cases is too small (n<25) for purposes of reliably predicting hospital performance; (2) Measure reflects the hospital's indication that its submission was based upon a sample of its relevant discharges; (3) Rate reflects fewer than the maximum possible quarters of data for the measure; (4) Inaccurate information submitted and suppressed for one or more quarters; (5) No data is available from the hospital for this measure; Please refer to the User's Guide for a full explanation of data

Measure	Cases	This Hospital	State Average	U.S. Average	Top Hospital
Surgical Infection Prevention					
Prophylactic Antibiotic Given[2,3]	300	83%	79%	77%	95%
Prophylactic Antibiotic Selection[2]	67	99%	89%	90%	100%
Prophylactic Antibiotic Stopped[2,3]	289	82%	76%	72%	95%
Pregnancy Care					
Inpatient Neonatal Mortality	-	-	-	-	-
Third or Fourth Degree Laceration	-	-	-	3.63%	3.27%

Palmer Lutheran Health Center

112 Jefferson
West Union, IA 52175
Ownership: Voluntary non-profit - Private
Emergency Services: Yes
Phone: 563-422-3811
Fax: 563-422-3664
Accredited: No
Licensed Beds: 25

Key Personnel:

CEO . . . . Debrah Chensvold
Chief of Medical Staff . . . . Chaudri Rasool
Supervisor ER . . . . Jani Rothlisberger, RN
Director of Surgery . . . . Sue Schnieder
Respiratory/Cardiopulmonary . . . . Deb Schmidt

Measure	Cases	This Hospital	State Average	U.S. Average	Top Hospital
Heart Attack Care					
ACE Inhibitor or ARB for LVSD[5]	-	-	86%	82%	100%
Aspirin at Arrival[5]	-	-	89%	92%	100%
Aspirin at Discharge[5]	-	-	90%	90%	100%
Beta Blocker at Arrival[5]	-	-	91%	87%	100%
Beta Blocker at Discharge[5]	-	-	91%	90%	100%
Fibrinolytic Medication Timing[5]	-	-	33%	31%	100%
PCI Within 90 Minutes of Arrival[5]	-	-	73%	54%	95%
Smoking Cessation Advice[5]	-	-	92%	88%	100%
Heart Failure Care					
ACE Inhibitor or ARB for LVSD[1,3]	1	100%	84%	82%	100%
Discharge Instructions[1,3]	1	100%	62%	61%	93%
Evaluation of LVS Function[1,3]	1	100%	75%	83%	99%
Smoking Cessation Advice[3]	0	-	78%	82%	100%
Pneumonia Care					
Appropriate Initial Antibiotic[1,3]	5	100%	85%	83%	94%
Blood Culture Timing[1]	7	86%	95%	90%	100%
Influenza Vaccine[1]	4	100%	85%	70%	100%
Initial Antibiotic Timing[1]	17	94%	87%	80%	93%
Oxygenation Assessment[1]	19	100%	99%	99%	100%
Pneumococcal Vaccine[1]	17	100%	83%	69%	94%
Smoking Cessation Advice[1]	1	0%	75%	80%	100%
Surgical Infection Prevention					
Prophylactic Antibiotic Given[5]	-	-	79%	77%	95%
Prophylactic Antibiotic Selection[5]	-	-	89%	90%	100%
Prophylactic Antibiotic Stopped[5]	-	-	76%	72%	95%
Pregnancy Care					
Inpatient Neonatal Mortality	-	-	-	-	-
Third or Fourth Degree Laceration	-	-	-	3.63%	3.27%

Madison County Memorial Hospital

300 Hutchings Street
Winterset, IA 50273
URL: www.madisonhealth.com
Ownership: Government - Local
Emergency Services: Yes
Phone: 515-462-2373
Fax: 515-462-5008
Accredited: No
Licensed Beds: 25

Key Personnel:

CEO . . . . Marcia Harris
Chief of Medical Staff . . . . Sherrie Broadbent
Emergency Room . . . . Cindy Frank
Director Medical/Surgical Nursing . . . . Trish Hubbard
Chief Radiology . . . . Stephan Cooper, MD
Director Respiratory Therapy . . . . Trish Hubbard

Measure	Cases	This Hospital	State Average	U.S. Average	Top Hospital
Heart Attack Care					
ACE Inhibitor or ARB for LVSD[3]	0	-	86%	82%	100%
Aspirin at Arrival[1,3]	2	100%	89%	92%	100%
Aspirin at Discharge[1,3]	1	100%	90%	90%	100%
Beta Blocker at Arrival[1,3]	3	100%	91%	87%	100%
Beta Blocker at Discharge[1,3]	1	0%	91%	90%	100%
Fibrinolytic Medication Timing[3]	0	-	33%	31%	100%
PCI Within 90 Minutes of Arrival[5]	-	-	73%	54%	95%
Smoking Cessation Advice[3]	0	-	92%	88%	100%
Heart Failure Care					
ACE Inhibitor or ARB for LVSD[1]	2	100%	84%	82%	100%
Discharge Instructions[1]	10	0%	62%	61%	93%
Evaluation of LVS Function[1]	19	32%	75%	83%	99%
Smoking Cessation Advice[1]	1	0%	78%	82%	100%
Pneumonia Care					
Appropriate Initial Antibiotic	55	89%	85%	83%	94%
Blood Culture Timing[1]	2	100%	95%	90%	100%
Influenza Vaccine[1]	11	27%	85%	70%	100%
Initial Antibiotic Timing	61	92%	87%	80%	93%
Oxygenation Assessment	78	100%	99%	99%	100%
Pneumococcal Vaccine	55	53%	83%	69%	94%
Smoking Cessation Advice[1]	15	33%	75%	80%	100%
Surgical Infection Prevention					
Prophylactic Antibiotic Given[1,3]	1	100%	79%	77%	95%
Prophylactic Antibiotic Selection[5]	-	-	89%	90%	100%
Prophylactic Antibiotic Stopped[1,3]	1	100%	76%	72%	95%
Pregnancy Care					
Inpatient Neonatal Mortality	-	-	-	-	-
Third or Fourth Degree Laceration	-	-	-	3.63%	3.27%

NOTE: Hospital profiles are in alphabetical order by state, then city, then hospital within the city; Rankings are sorted by rate in descending order and exclude hospitals with less than 25 cases; (1) The number of cases is too small (n<25) for purposes of reliably predicting hospital performance; (2) Measure reflects the hospital's indication that its submission was based upon a sample of its relevant discharges; (3) Rate reflects fewer than the maximum possible quarters of data for the measure; (4) Inaccurate information submitted and suppressed for one or more quarters; (5) No data is available from the hospital for this measure; Please refer to the User's Guide for a full explanation of data

Heart Attack Care

1. ACE Inhibitor or ARB for LVSD

Hospital Name	City	Rate	Cases
Shawnee Mission Medical Center	Shawnee Mission	96%	55
Providence Medical Center	Kansas City	94%	66
University of Kansas Medical Center	Kansas City	92%	61
Salina Regional Health Center	Salina	91%	35
Wesley Medical Center	Wichita	90%	69
Kansas Heart Hospital	Wichita	89%	27
Stormont-Vail Healthcare	Topeka	89%	37
Hays Medical Center	Hays	87%	39
Saint Francis Health Center	Topeka	86%	77
Hutchinson Hospital	Hutchinson	85%	55
Via Christi Regional Medical Center	Wichita	85%	153
Overland Park Regional Medical Center	Overland Park	84%	25
Olathe Medical Center	Olathe	82%	40

2. Aspirin at Arrival

Hospital Name	City	Rate	Cases
Lawrence Memorial Hospital	Lawrence	100%	53
Mount Carmel Regional Medical Center	Pittsburg	100%	67
Saint Luke's South	Overland Park	100%	43
Shawnee Mission Medical Center	Shawnee Mission	100%	209
University of Kansas Medical Center	Kansas City	100%	110
Saint Francis Health Center	Topeka	99%	136
Hutchinson Hospital	Hutchinson	98%	178
Olathe Medical Center	Olathe	98%	129
Overland Park Regional Medical Center	Overland Park	98%	84
Menorah Medical Center	Shawnee Mission	97%	62
Wesley Medical Center	Wichita	97%	258
Providence Medical Center	Kansas City	96%	153
Stormont-Vail Healthcare	Topeka	96%	184
Western Plains Medical Company	Dodge City	96%	28
Salina Regional Health Center	Salina	95%	120
Via Christi Regional Medical Center	Wichita	95%	581
Hays Medical Center	Hays	94%	64
Coffeyville Regional Medical Center	Coffeyville	89%	28
Galichia Heart Hospital	Wichita	82%	28

3. Aspirin at Discharge

Hospital Name	City	Rate	Cases
Lawrence Memorial Hospital	Lawrence	100%	37
Shawnee Mission Medical Center	Shawnee Mission	99%	211
Kansas Heart Hospital	Wichita	98%	172
Olathe Medical Center	Olathe	98%	157
University of Kansas Medical Center	Kansas City	98%	245
Menorah Medical Center	Shawnee Mission	97%	75
Stormont-Vail Healthcare	Topeka	97%	233
Wesley Medical Center	Wichita	97%	291
Hays Medical Center	Hays	96%	156
Providence Medical Center	Kansas City	96%	172
Salina Regional Health Center	Salina	96%	194
Mount Carmel Regional Medical Center	Pittsburg	95%	55
Overland Park Regional Medical Center	Overland Park	95%	81
Saint Francis Health Center	Topeka	95%	247
Saint Luke's South	Overland Park	95%	42
Hutchinson Hospital	Hutchinson	94%	214
Via Christi Regional Medical Center	Wichita	93%	715
Galichia Heart Hospital	Wichita	89%	62

4. Beta Blocker at Arrival

Hospital Name	City	Rate	Cases
Lawrence Memorial Hospital	Lawrence	100%	47
Shawnee Mission Medical Center	Shawnee Mission	99%	189
University of Kansas Medical Center	Kansas City	99%	106
Stormont-Vail Healthcare	Topeka	98%	171
Wesley Medical Center	Wichita	98%	187
Providence Medical Center	Kansas City	97%	118
Mount Carmel Regional Medical Center	Pittsburg	95%	58
Saint Francis Health Center	Topeka	95%	101
Olathe Medical Center	Olathe	93%	113
Via Christi Regional Medical Center	Wichita	93%	531
Hutchinson Hospital	Hutchinson	92%	149
Overland Park Regional Medical Center	Overland Park	92%	76
Saint Luke's South	Overland Park	92%	40
Menorah Medical Center	Shawnee Mission	91%	46
Hays Medical Center	Hays	89%	54
Salina Regional Health Center	Salina	88%	115
Galichia Heart Hospital	Wichita	83%	29
Coffeyville Regional Medical Center	Coffeyville	61%	28

5. Beta Blocker at Discharge

Hospital Name	City	Rate	Cases
Lawrence Memorial Hospital	Lawrence	100%	37
Stormont-Vail Healthcare	Topeka	100%	229
Overland Park Regional Medical Center	Overland Park	99%	79
Shawnee Mission Medical Center	Shawnee Mission	99%	203
University of Kansas Medical Center	Kansas City	99%	242
Kansas Heart Hospital	Wichita	98%	162
Providence Medical Center	Kansas City	98%	180
Saint Luke's South	Overland Park	98%	41
Menorah Medical Center	Shawnee Mission	97%	66
Olathe Medical Center	Olathe	97%	187
Wesley Medical Center	Wichita	97%	321
Saint Francis Health Center	Topeka	96%	270
Hays Medical Center	Hays	94%	158
Mount Carmel Regional Medical Center	Pittsburg	94%	53
Via Christi Regional Medical Center	Wichita	93%	691
Salina Regional Health Center	Salina	87%	192
Hutchinson Hospital	Hutchinson	86%	198
Galichia Heart Hospital	Wichita	85%	65

8. Smoking Cessation Advice

Hospital Name	City	Rate	Cases
Menorah Medical Center	Shawnee Mission	100%	27
Olathe Medical Center	Olathe	100%	94
Overland Park Regional Medical Center	Overland Park	100%	25
Providence Medical Center	Kansas City	100%	71
Stormont-Vail Healthcare	Topeka	100%	74
University of Kansas Medical Center	Kansas City	100%	111
Saint Francis Health Center	Topeka	99%	91
Hays Medical Center	Hays	98%	42
Salina Regional Health Center	Salina	97%	73
Wesley Medical Center	Wichita	97%	170
Kansas Heart Hospital	Wichita	96%	67
Shawnee Mission Medical Center	Shawnee Mission	96%	77
Via Christi Regional Medical Center	Wichita	95%	301
Galichia Heart Hospital	Wichita	86%	29
Hutchinson Hospital	Hutchinson	84%	70

Heart Failure Care

9. ACE Inhibitor or ARB for LVSD

Hospital Name	City	Rate	Cases
Lawrence Memorial Hospital	Lawrence	100%	68
Shawnee Mission Medical Center	Shawnee Mission	99%	136
Kansas Heart Hospital	Wichita	95%	59
Salina Regional Health Center	Salina	95%	60
University of Kansas Medical Center	Kansas City	93%	165
Hays Medical Center	Hays	92%	48
Mount Carmel Regional Medical Center	Pittsburg	91%	45
Olathe Medical Center	Olathe	91%	105
Saint Francis Health Center	Topeka	91%	90
Hutchinson Hospital	Hutchinson	89%	64
Stormont-Vail Healthcare	Topeka	89%	118
Overland Park Regional Medical Center	Overland Park	88%	67
Mercy Health Center	Fort Scott	84%	32
Mercy Regional Health Center	Manhattan	84%	37
Providence Medical Center	Kansas City	83%	209
Saint Luke's South	Overland Park	83%	41
Menorah Medical Center	Shawnee Mission	81%	42
Via Christi Regional Medical Center	Wichita	78%	360
Wesley Medical Center	Wichita	78%	136
Galichia Heart Hospital	Wichita	67%	102
Coffeyville Regional Medical Center	Coffeyville	55%	47
Labette County Medical Center	Parsons	44%	34

10. Discharge Instructions

Hospital Name	City	Rate	Cases
Geary Community Hospital	Junction City	98%	52
Galichia Heart Hospital	Wichita	94%	239
Mercy Hospital-Independence	Independence	93%	46
Susan B Allen Memorial Hospital	El Dorado	92%	26
University of Kansas Medical Center	Kansas City	89%	261
Saint John Hospital	Leavenworth	88%	43
Lawrence Memorial Hospital	Lawrence	87%	82
Mercy Health Center	Fort Scott	85%	81
Kansas Heart Hospital	Wichita	82%	103
Ransom Memorial Hospital	Ottawa	79%	33
Southwest Medical Center	Liberal	79%	28
Saint Francis Health Center	Topeka	78%	180
Menorah Medical Center	Shawnee Mission	76%	98
Olathe Medical Center	Olathe	74%	243

NOTE: Hospital profiles are in alphabetical order by state, then city, then hospital within the city; Rankings are sorted by rate in descending order and exclude hospitals with less than 25 cases; (1) The number of cases is too small (n<25) for purposes of reliably predicting hospital performance; (2) Measure reflects the hospital's indication that its submission was based upon a sample of its relevant discharges; (3) Rate reflects fewer than the maximum possible quarters of data for the measure; (4) Inaccurate information submitted and suppressed for one or more quarters; (5) No data is available from the hospital for this measure; Please refer to the User's Guide for a full explanation of data

Hays Medical Center	Hays	73%	106
Overland Park Regional Medical Center	Overland Park	72%	119
Stormont-Vail Healthcare	Topeka	71%	216
Allen County Hospital	Iola	69%	26
Newton Medical Center	Newton	69%	62
Coffeyville Regional Medical Center	Coffeyville	68%	98
Newman Regional Health	Emporia	68%	69
Providence Medical Center	Kansas City	65%	394
Saint Catherine's Hospital	Garden City	65%	31
Saint Luke's South	Overland Park	60%	70
Mount Carmel Regional Medical Center	Pittsburg	58%	105
Via Christi Regional Medical Center	Wichita	57%	707
Hutchinson Hospital	Hutchinson	56%	156
Wesley Medical Center	Wichita	56%	331
Western Plains Medical Company	Dodge City	56%	48
Salina Regional Health Center	Salina	50%	137
Pratt Regional Medical Center	Pratt	42%	26
Shawnee Mission Medical Center	Shawnee Mission	40%	284
Cushing Memorial Hospital	Leavenworth	37%	38
Neosho Memorial Regional Medical Center	Chanute	37%	41
Labette County Medical Center	Parsons	28%	68
Mercy Regional Health Center	Manhattan	27%	83
Coffey County Hospital	Burlington	26%	34
Atchison Hospital	Atchison	18%	34
Central Kansas Medical Center	Great Bend	18%	28
Memorial Hospital	McPherson	18%	34
Mitchell County Hospital	Beloit	6%	31
South Central Kansas Regional Medical Center	Arkansas City	4%	26

11. Evaluation of LVS Function

Hospital Name	City	Rate	Cases
Kansas Heart Hospital	Wichita	100%	115
Olathe Medical Center	Olathe	100%	308
Saint Francis Health Center	Topeka	99%	230
University of Kansas Medical Center	Kansas City	99%	295
Cushing Memorial Hospital	Leavenworth	98%	52
Lawrence Memorial Hospital	Lawrence	98%	125
Menorah Medical Center	Shawnee Mission	98%	132
Saint Luke's South	Overland Park	98%	89
Shawnee Mission Medical Center	Shawnee Mission	98%	372
Stormont-Vail Healthcare	Topeka	98%	298
Mount Carmel Regional Medical Center	Pittsburg	97%	151
Providence Medical Center	Kansas City	97%	476
Wesley Medical Center	Wichita	95%	430
Overland Park Regional Medical Center	Overland Park	94%	174
Galichia Heart Hospital	Wichita	92%	263
Mercy Hospital-Independence	Independence	92%	71
Mercy Health Center	Fort Scott	91%	111
Ransom Memorial Hospital	Ottawa	91%	44
Mercy Regional Health Center	Manhattan	89%	125
Via Christi Regional Medical Center	Wichita	89%	842
Hays Medical Center	Hays	86%	145
William Newton Memorial Hospital	Winfield	85%	26
Southwest Medical Center	Liberal	81%	37
Saint John Hospital	Leavenworth	80%	50
Mitchell County Hospital	Beloit	78%	54
Newton Medical Center	Newton	77%	101
Salina Regional Health Center	Salina	76%	186
Neosho Memorial Regional Medical Center	Chanute	75%	68
Western Plains Medical Company	Dodge City	74%	65
Labette County Medical Center	Parsons	73%	81
Susan B Allen Memorial Hospital	El Dorado	73%	64
Coffeyville Regional Medical Center	Coffeyville	72%	146
Hutchinson Hospital	Hutchinson	72%	206
Hiawatha Community Hospital	Hiawatha	71%	42
Newman Regional Health	Emporia	65%	104
Geary Community Hospital	Junction City	64%	66
Central Kansas Medical Center	Great Bend	62%	45
Memorial Hospital	McPherson	59%	54
Atchison Hospital	Atchison	58%	55
Saint Catherine's Hospital	Garden City	57%	42
Allen County Hospital	Iola	53%	30
Ellsworth County Medical Center	Ellsworth	51%	43
Pratt Regional Medical Center	Pratt	50%	30
Morton County Hospital	Elkhart	49%	37
Memorial Health System	Abilene	44%	32
Girard Medical Center	Girard	41%	34
Saint Luke Hospital & Living Center	Marion	41%	27
South Central Kansas Regional Medical Center	Arkansas City	41%	44
Community Hospital-Onaga	Onaga	38%	37
Coffey County Hospital	Burlington	37%	52
Greenwood County Hospital	Eureka	28%	32
Fredonia Regional Hospital	Fredonia	26%	27

12. Smoking Cessation Advice

Hospital Name	City	Rate	Cases
Hays Medical Center	Hays	100%	26
Olathe Medical Center	Olathe	100%	50
Stormont-Vail Healthcare	Topeka	100%	48
Providence Medical Center	Kansas City	98%	131
Via Christi Regional Medical Center	Wichita	97%	159
Wesley Medical Center	Wichita	97%	89
University of Kansas Medical Center	Kansas City	96%	81
Hutchinson Hospital	Hutchinson	93%	28
Saint Francis Health Center	Topeka	91%	47
Salina Regional Health Center	Salina	86%	28
Galichia Heart Hospital	Wichita	68%	34
Shawnee Mission Medical Center	Shawnee Mission	65%	51

Pneumonia Care

13. Appropriate Initial Antibiotic

Hospital Name	City	Rate	Cases
Stormont-Vail Healthcare	Topeka	98%	166
Allen County Hospital	Iola	97%	32
Ransom Memorial Hospital	Ottawa	96%	69
Central Kansas Medical Center	Great Bend	94%	35
Mercy Regional Health Center	Manhattan	93%	68
Saint Francis Health Center	Topeka	91%	157
University of Kansas Medical Center	Kansas City	91%	134
Mercy Health Center	Fort Scott	90%	71
Mercy Hospital-Independence	Independence	90%	48
Lawrence Memorial Hospital	Lawrence	89%	75
Coffey County Hospital	Burlington	88%	43
Miami County Medical Center	Paola	88%	33
Newton Medical Center	Newton	88%	96
Overland Park Regional Medical Center	Overland Park	88%	93
Neosho Memorial Regional Medical Center	Chanute	87%	61
Menorah Medical Center	Shawnee Mission	86%	86
Saint Luke's South	Overland Park	86%	66
Salina Regional Health Center	Salina	86%	120
Geary Community Hospital	Junction City	85%	65
Susan B Allen Memorial Hospital	El Dorado	85%	53
William Newton Memorial Hospital	Winfield	85%	26
Memorial Hospital	McPherson	84%	50
Newman Regional Health	Emporia	84%	68
Olathe Medical Center	Olathe	84%	113
Saint Catherine's Hospital	Garden City	84%	74
Saint John Hospital	Leavenworth	83%	35
Shawnee Mission Medical Center	Shawnee Mission	83%	215
Providence Medical Center	Kansas City	82%	148
Memorial Health System	Abilene	81%	31
Mount Carmel Regional Medical Center	Pittsburg	80%	75
Kingman Community Hospital	Kingman	79%	38
South Central Kansas Regional Medical Center	Arkansas City	78%	58
Wesley Medical Center	Wichita	78%	223
Cushing Memorial Hospital	Leavenworth	76%	63
Hutchinson Hospital	Hutchinson	74%	148
Mitchell County Hospital	Beloit	74%	38
Cloud County Health Center	Concordia	73%	59
Coffeyville Regional Medical Center	Coffeyville	73%	105
Pratt Regional Medical Center	Pratt	72%	36
Via Christi Regional Medical Center	Wichita	72%	197
Hays Medical Center	Hays	70%	80
Labette County Medical Center	Parsons	70%	70
Western Plains Medical Company	Dodge City	70%	57
Clay County Medical Center	Clay Center	68%	63
Southwest Medical Center	Liberal	68%	28
Greenwood County Hospital	Eureka	62%	69
Fredonia Regional Hospital	Fredonia	53%	51
Meade District Hospital	Meade	51%	41
Republic County Hospital	Belleville	49%	69

14. Blood Culture Timing

Hospital Name	City	Rate	Cases
Cushing Memorial Hospital	Leavenworth	100%	34
Labette County Medical Center	Parsons	100%	43
Mercy Regional Health Center	Manhattan	100%	49
Mitchell County Hospital	Beloit	100%	30
Menorah Medical Center	Shawnee Mission	99%	74
Mount Carmel Regional Medical Center	Pittsburg	99%	92
Western Plains Medical Company	Dodge City	98%	42
Miami County Medical Center	Paola	96%	25
Neosho Memorial Regional Medical Center	Chanute	96%	49
Stormont-Vail Healthcare	Topeka	96%	204
Hutchinson Hospital	Hutchinson	95%	74
Mercy Health Center	Fort Scott	95%	39

NOTE: Hospital profiles are in alphabetical order by state, then city, then hospital within the city; Rankings are sorted by rate in descending order and exclude hospitals with less than 25 cases; (1) The number of cases is too small (n<25) for purposes of reliably predicting hospital performance; (2) Measure reflects the hospital's indication that its submission was based upon a sample of its relevant discharges; (3) Rate reflects fewer than the maximum possible quarters of data for the measure; (4) Inaccurate information submitted and suppressed for one or more quarters; (5) No data is available from the hospital for this measure; Please refer to the User's Guide for a full explanation of data

Mercy Hospital-Independence	Independence	95%	39
Providence Medical Center	Kansas City	95%	152
Ransom Memorial Hospital	Ottawa	95%	55
Saint Luke's South	Overland Park	95%	43
Salina Regional Health Center	Salina	95%	110
Shawnee Mission Medical Center	Shawnee Mission	95%	187
Coffeyville Regional Medical Center	Coffeyville	94%	54
Saint Catherine's Hospital	Garden City	94%	48
University of Kansas Medical Center	Kansas City	94%	142
Wesley Medical Center	Wichita	94%	218
Memorial Hospital	McPherson	93%	30
Olathe Medical Center	Olathe	93%	75
Saint Francis Health Center	Topeka	92%	65
Hays Medical Center	Hays	90%	42
Newton Medical Center	Newton	89%	44
Overland Park Regional Medical Center	Overland Park	89%	89
Via Christi Regional Medical Center	Wichita	89%	81
Newman Regional Health	Emporia	88%	40
Lawrence Memorial Hospital	Lawrence	87%	60

15. Influenza Vaccine

Hospital Name	City	Rate	Cases
Ransom Memorial Hospital	Ottawa	97%	34
Providence Medical Center	Kansas City	95%	39
Saint Francis Health Center	Topeka	94%	54
Olathe Medical Center	Olathe	91%	32
Stormont-Vail Healthcare	Topeka	90%	72
University of Kansas Medical Center	Kansas City	89%	35
Via Christi Regional Medical Center	Wichita	86%	28
Mount Carmel Regional Medical Center	Pittsburg	83%	46
Hutchinson Hospital	Hutchinson	77%	44
Newton Medical Center	Newton	76%	38
Shawnee Mission Medical Center	Shawnee Mission	74%	69
Wesley Medical Center	Wichita	74%	74
Neosho Memorial Regional Medical Center	Chanute	73%	26
South Central Kansas Regional Medical Center	Arkansas City	64%	25
Coffeyville Regional Medical Center	Coffeyville	53%	49
Salina Regional Health Center	Salina	53%	53
Overland Park Regional Medical Center	Overland Park	52%	25
Coffey County Hospital	Burlington	4%	26
Greenwood County Hospital	Eureka	0%	30

16. Initial Antibiotic Timing

Hospital Name	City	Rate	Cases
Morris County Hospital	Council Grove	94%	34
Menorah Medical Center	Shawnee Mission	93%	111
Miami County Medical Center	Paola	93%	41
Ransom Memorial Hospital	Ottawa	93%	97
Southwest Medical Center	Liberal	93%	46
Lawrence Memorial Hospital	Lawrence	92%	93
Lindsborg Community Hospital	Lindsborg	92%	37
Neosho Memorial Regional Medical Center	Chanute	92%	75
Central Kansas Medical Center	Great Bend	91%	45
Coffey County Hospital	Burlington	91%	67
Mount Carmel Regional Medical Center	Pittsburg	91%	119
Cloud County Health Center	Concordia	90%	51
Providence Medical Center	Kansas City	90%	191
Saint Luke's South	Overland Park	90%	78
Geary Community Hospital	Junction City	89%	85
Fredonia Regional Hospital	Fredonia	88%	59
Hays Medical Center	Hays	88%	98
Memorial Health System	Abilene	88%	32
Mercy Health Center	Fort Scott	88%	92
Morton County Hospital	Elkhart	88%	50
Susan B Allen Memorial Hospital	El Dorado	88%	73
Kingman Community Hospital	Kingman	87%	47
Republic County Hospital	Belleville	87%	54
William Newton Memorial Hospital	Winfield	86%	35
Clay County Medical Center	Clay Center	85%	65
Newman Regional Health	Emporia	85%	93
Overland Park Regional Medical Center	Overland Park	85%	128
Saint John Hospital	Leavenworth	85%	55
Allen County Hospital	Iola	84%	49
Mitchell County Hospital	Beloit	84%	62
Pratt Regional Medical Center	Pratt	84%	58
Cushing Memorial Hospital	Leavenworth	83%	71
Via Christi Regional Medical Center	Wichita	83%	184
Saint Catherine's Hospital	Garden City	82%	79
Saint Francis Health Center	Topeka	82%	224
University of Kansas Medical Center	Kansas City	82%	202
Goodland Regional Medical Center	Goodland	81%	31
Memorial Hospital	McPherson	81%	70
Mercy Regional Health Center	Manhattan	81%	97
Ellsworth County Medical Center	Ellsworth	80%	40
Coffeyville Regional Medical Center	Coffeyville	79%	219
Shawnee Mission Medical Center	Shawnee Mission	79%	297
Meade District Hospital	Meade	78%	51
Newton Medical Center	Newton	78%	111
Western Plains Medical Company	Dodge City	77%	90
Atchison Hospital	Atchison	76%	33
Salina Regional Health Center	Salina	76%	173
Stormont-Vail Healthcare	Topeka	76%	250
Wesley Medical Center	Wichita	76%	317
Girard Medical Center	Girard	73%	30
Mercy Hospital-Independence	Independence	73%	71
Olathe Medical Center	Olathe	72%	156
South Central Kansas Regional Medical Center	Arkansas City	71%	58
Labette County Medical Center	Parsons	68%	76
Hutchinson Hospital	Hutchinson	65%	211

17. Oxygenation Assessment

Hospital Name	City	Rate	Cases
Allen County Hospital	Iola	100%	57
Anderson County Hospital	Garnett	100%	26
Atchison Hospital	Atchison	100%	43
Bob Wilson Memorial Grant Hospital	Ulysses	100%	27
Central Kansas Medical Center	Great Bend	100%	59
Cloud County Health Center	Concordia	100%	64
Coffey County Hospital	Burlington	100%	75
Coffeyville Regional Medical Center	Coffeyville	100%	226
Cushing Memorial Hospital	Leavenworth	100%	75
Ellsworth County Medical Center	Ellsworth	100%	52
Fredonia Regional Hospital	Fredonia	100%	68
Geary Community Hospital	Junction City	100%	91
Girard Medical Center	Girard	100%	39
Goodland Regional Medical Center	Goodland	100%	37
Greenwood County Hospital	Eureka	100%	93
Hays Medical Center	Hays	100%	131
Hutchinson Hospital	Hutchinson	100%	277
Labette County Medical Center	Parsons	100%	125
Lawrence Memorial Hospital	Lawrence	100%	135
Lindsborg Community Hospital	Lindsborg	100%	45
Meade District Hospital	Meade	100%	75
Memorial Health System	Abilene	100%	38
Mercy Health Center	Fort Scott	100%	107
Mercy Hospital-Independence	Independence	100%	81
Mercy Regional Health Center	Manhattan	100%	130
Miami County Medical Center	Paola	100%	58
Mitchell County Hospital	Beloit	100%	88
Morris County Hospital	Council Grove	100%	47
Morton County Hospital	Elkhart	100%	66
Mount Carmel Regional Medical Center	Pittsburg	100%	155
Neosho Memorial Regional Medical Center	Chanute	100%	102
Newman Regional Health	Emporia	100%	106
Newton Medical Center	Newton	100%	138
Olathe Medical Center	Olathe	100%	213
Overland Park Regional Medical Center	Overland Park	100%	170
Pratt Regional Medical Center	Pratt	100%	61
Providence Medical Center	Kansas City	100%	246
Ransom Memorial Hospital	Ottawa	100%	116
Sabetha Community Hospital	Sabetha	100%	33
Saint Catherine's Hospital	Garden City	100%	94
Saint Francis Health Center	Topeka	100%	264
Saint Luke Hospital & Living Center	Marion	100%	28
Saint Luke's South	Overland Park	100%	94
Salina Regional Health Center	Salina	100%	211
Shawnee Mission Medical Center	Shawnee Mission	100%	340
South Central Kansas Regional Medical Center	Arkansas City	100%	71
Southwest Medical Center	Liberal	100%	68
Stormont-Vail Healthcare	Topeka	100%	331
Susan B Allen Memorial Hospital	El Dorado	100%	89
University of Kansas Medical Center	Kansas City	100%	265
Via Christi Regional Medical Center	Wichita	100%	262
Wesley Medical Center	Wichita	100%	387
Western Plains Medical Company	Dodge City	100%	107
Clay County Medical Center	Clay Center	99%	75
Memorial Hospital	McPherson	99%	90
Kingman Community Hospital	Kingman	98%	57
Saint John Hospital	Leavenworth	98%	66
William Newton Memorial Hospital	Winfield	98%	46
Menorah Medical Center	Shawnee Mission	97%	140
Republic County Hospital	Belleville	97%	79
Sumner Regional Medical Center	Wellington	96%	25
Community Hospital-Onaga	Onaga	93%	27

18. Pneumococcal Vaccine

Hospital Name	City	Rate	Cases
Lindsborg Community Hospital	Lindsborg	97%	35

NOTE: Hospital profiles are in alphabetical order by state, then city, then hospital within the city; Rankings are sorted by rate in descending order and exclude hospitals with less than 25 cases; (1) The number of cases is too small (n<25) for purposes of reliably predicting hospital performance; (2) Measure reflects the hospital's indication that its submission was based upon a sample of its relevant discharges; (3) Rate reflects fewer than the maximum possible quarters of data for the measure; (4) Inaccurate information submitted and suppressed for one or more quarters; (5) No data is available from the hospital for this measure; Please refer to the User's Guide for a full explanation of data

Hospital Name	City	Rate	Cases
Clay County Medical Center	Clay Center	96%	56
Lawrence Memorial Hospital	Lawrence	96%	98
Cushing Memorial Hospital	Leavenworth	92%	38
Saint Francis Health Center	Topeka	92%	173
Saint Luke's South	Overland Park	92%	64
Menorah Medical Center	Shawnee Mission	91%	109
Meade District Hospital	Meade	90%	58
Olathe Medical Center	Olathe	90%	133
Ransom Memorial Hospital	Ottawa	89%	83
University of Kansas Medical Center	Kansas City	89%	90
Newman Regional Health	Emporia	88%	74
Stormont-Vail Healthcare	Topeka	88%	221
Susan B Allen Memorial Hospital	El Dorado	88%	51
William Newton Memorial Hospital	Winfield	88%	40
Hays Medical Center	Hays	86%	99
Providence Medical Center	Kansas City	86%	134
Cloud County Health Center	Concordia	85%	47
Mercy Health Center	Fort Scott	84%	64
Miami County Medical Center	Paola	84%	32
Mount Carmel Regional Medical Center	Pittsburg	83%	101
Western Plains Medical Company	Dodge City	82%	68
Saint John Hospital	Leavenworth	81%	36
Newton Medical Center	Newton	78%	91
Mercy Hospital-Independence	Independence	77%	56
Mercy Regional Health Center	Manhattan	76%	83
Wesley Medical Center	Wichita	76%	240
Atchison Hospital	Atchison	74%	31
Republic County Hospital	Belleville	71%	62
Via Christi Regional Medical Center	Wichita	70%	161
Pratt Regional Medical Center	Pratt	69%	49
Shawnee Mission Medical Center	Shawnee Mission	69%	228
Sabetha Community Hospital	Sabetha	68%	25
Saint Catherine's Hospital	Garden City	67%	48
Memorial Hospital	McPherson	62%	66
Neosho Memorial Regional Medical Center	Chanute	62%	65
Overland Park Regional Medical Center	Overland Park	62%	104
Southwest Medical Center	Liberal	59%	34
Kingman Community Hospital	Kingman	58%	40
Coffey County Hospital	Burlington	56%	54
Ellsworth County Medical Center	Ellsworth	55%	44
Hutchinson Hospital	Hutchinson	55%	178
Morton County Hospital	Elkhart	53%	47
Salina Regional Health Center	Salina	53%	147
Labette County Medical Center	Parsons	50%	80
Coffeyville Regional Medical Center	Coffeyville	47%	159
Allen County Hospital	Iola	46%	37
Geary Community Hospital	Junction City	46%	59
Central Kansas Medical Center	Great Bend	43%	47
Goodland Regional Medical Center	Goodland	41%	29
Girard Medical Center	Girard	36%	28
Mitchell County Hospital	Beloit	30%	69
South Central Kansas Regional Medical Center	Arkansas City	22%	49
Morris County Hospital	Council Grove	15%	41
Saint Luke Hospital & Living Center	Marion	8%	25
Community Hospital-Onaga	Onaga	4%	26
Memorial Health System	Abilene	3%	29
Fredonia Regional Hospital	Fredonia	2%	40
Greenwood County Hospital	Eureka	0%	56

19. Smoking Cessation Advice

Hospital Name	City	Rate	Cases
Lawrence Memorial Hospital	Lawrence	100%	27
Ransom Memorial Hospital	Ottawa	100%	32
Stormont-Vail Healthcare	Topeka	100%	102
Providence Medical Center	Kansas City	99%	93
Olathe Medical Center	Olathe	97%	61
University of Kansas Medical Center	Kansas City	95%	99
Saint Francis Health Center	Topeka	91%	85
Hutchinson Hospital	Hutchinson	87%	61
Overland Park Regional Medical Center	Overland Park	87%	30
Via Christi Regional Medical Center	Wichita	82%	77
Wesley Medical Center	Wichita	82%	110
Mercy Health Center	Fort Scott	77%	35
Neosho Memorial Regional Medical Center	Chanute	76%	29
Salina Regional Health Center	Salina	76%	55
Shawnee Mission Medical Center	Shawnee Mission	70%	54
Western Plains Medical Company	Dodge City	68%	28
Coffeyville Regional Medical Center	Coffeyville	67%	45
Mount Carmel Regional Medical Center	Pittsburg	60%	35
Mercy Regional Health Center	Manhattan	58%	31

Surgical Infection Prevention

20. Prophylactic Antibiotic Given

Hospital Name	City	Rate	Cases
Kansas City Orthopaedic Institute	Leawood	97%	96
William Newton Memorial Hospital	Winfield	97%	62
Kansas Heart Hospital	Wichita	95%	205
Olathe Medical Center	Olathe	95%	624
Mercy Health Center	Fort Scott	94%	93
Saint Luke's South	Overland Park	94%	211
Via Christi Regional Medical Center	Wichita	94%	790
Mitchell County Hospital	Beloit	93%	29
Pratt Regional Medical Center	Pratt	93%	112
Salina Surgical Hospital	Salina	93%	374
Kansas Surgery & Recovery Center	Wichita	92%	198
Salina Regional Health Center	Salina	92%	623
Providence Medical Center	Kansas City	91%	478
Hutchinson Hospital	Hutchinson	90%	803
Overland Park Regional Medical Center	Overland Park	89%	240
Stormont-Vail Healthcare	Topeka	89%	431
University of Kansas Medical Center	Kansas City	85%	342
Hays Medical Center	Hays	84%	322
Newton Medical Center	Newton	84%	333
Heartland Surgical Specialty Hospital	Overland Park	83%	58
Mercy Hospital-Independence	Independence	83%	103
Mount Carmel Regional Medical Center	Pittsburg	83%	169
Saint Francis Health Center	Topeka	83%	218
Lawrence Memorial Hospital	Lawrence	82%	378
Susan B Allen Memorial Hospital	El Dorado	81%	79
Wesley Medical Center	Wichita	79%	325
Coffeyville Regional Medical Center	Coffeyville	78%	49
Saint John Hospital	Leavenworth	78%	37
Newman Regional Health	Emporia	77%	99
Neosho Memorial Regional Medical Center	Chanute	76%	76
Geary Community Hospital	Junction City	75%	65
Mercy Regional Health Center	Manhattan	74%	92
Shawnee Mission Medical Center	Shawnee Mission	74%	627
Labette County Medical Center	Parsons	73%	390
Atchison Hospital	Atchison	72%	39
Menorah Medical Center	Shawnee Mission	71%	246
Southwest Medical Center	Liberal	68%	98
Saint Catherine's Hospital	Garden City	67%	371
Republic County Hospital	Belleville	63%	43
Western Plains Medical Company	Dodge City	63%	90
Hiawatha Community Hospital	Hiawatha	61%	36
Manhattan Surgical Hospital	Manhattan	61%	219
Memorial Hospital	McPherson	61%	31
Miami County Medical Center	Paola	60%	52
Girard Medical Center	Girard	47%	36
Galichia Heart Hospital	Wichita	46%	37
South Central Kansas Regional Medical Center	Arkansas City	43%	49
Ransom Memorial Hospital	Ottawa	41%	27
Central Kansas Medical Center	Great Bend	22%	146

21. Prophylactic Antibiotic Selection

Hospital Name	City	Rate	Cases
Salina Surgical Hospital	Salina	99%	103
Kansas Heart Hospital	Wichita	98%	45
Lawrence Memorial Hospital	Lawrence	98%	105
Manhattan Surgical Hospital	Manhattan	98%	56
Labette County Medical Center	Parsons	97%	88
Saint Francis Health Center	Topeka	97%	73
Hutchinson Hospital	Hutchinson	96%	182
Kansas Surgery & Recovery Center	Wichita	96%	51
Mercy Hospital-Independence	Independence	96%	25
Salina Regional Health Center	Salina	96%	143
Stormont-Vail Healthcare	Topeka	96%	67
Susan B Allen Memorial Hospital	El Dorado	96%	27
Via Christi Regional Medical Center	Wichita	96%	136
Mercy Regional Health Center	Manhattan	95%	92
Olathe Medical Center	Olathe	95%	197
Overland Park Regional Medical Center	Overland Park	95%	111
University of Kansas Medical Center	Kansas City	95%	74
Central Kansas Medical Center	Great Bend	94%	49
Saint Luke's South	Overland Park	94%	81
Shawnee Mission Medical Center	Shawnee Mission	93%	59
Hays Medical Center	Hays	91%	80
Newman Regional Health	Emporia	90%	29
Galichia Heart Hospital	Wichita	89%	38
Newton Medical Center	Newton	89%	80
Pratt Regional Medical Center	Pratt	89%	35
Providence Medical Center	Kansas City	87%	143
Western Plains Medical Company	Dodge City	87%	31
Menorah Medical Center	Shawnee Mission	84%	116

NOTE: Hospital profiles are in alphabetical order by state, then city, then hospital within the city; Rankings are sorted by rate in descending order and exclude hospitals with less than 25 cases; (1) The number of cases is too small (n<25) for purposes of reliably predicting hospital performance; (2) Measure reflects the hospital's indication that its submission was based upon a sample of its relevant discharges; (3) Rate reflects fewer than the maximum possible quarters of data for the measure; (4) Inaccurate information submitted and suppressed for one or more quarters; (5) No data is available from the hospital for this measure; Please refer to the User's Guide for a full explanation of data

Mount Carmel Regional Medical Center	Pittsburg	81%	52
Wesley Medical Center	Wichita	60%	154
Saint Catherine's Hospital	Garden City	44%	108

22. Prophylactic Antibiotic Stopped

Hospital Name	City	Rate	Cases
Memorial Hospital	McPherson	97%	29
Pratt Regional Medical Center	Pratt	97%	110
South Central Kansas Regional Medical Center	Arkansas City	97%	36
Manhattan Surgical Hospital	Manhattan	96%	215
Mitchell County Hospital	Beloit	93%	28
William Newton Memorial Hospital	Winfield	92%	62
Hiawatha Community Hospital	Hiawatha	91%	34
Stormont-Vail Healthcare	Topeka	91%	411
Coffeyville Regional Medical Center	Coffeyville	88%	48
Newton Medical Center	Newton	87%	315
Saint Francis Health Center	Topeka	87%	213
Heartland Surgical Specialty Hospital	Overland Park	85%	54
Providence Medical Center	Kansas City	85%	428
Hutchinson Hospital	Hutchinson	84%	787
Kansas City Orthopaedic Institute	Leawood	81%	96
Mercy Hospital-Independence	Independence	81%	97
Saint Luke's South	Overland Park	80%	206
Labette County Medical Center	Parsons	78%	361
Mercy Regional Health Center	Manhattan	78%	86
Lawrence Memorial Hospital	Lawrence	77%	360
Wesley Medical Center	Wichita	77%	312
Salina Surgical Hospital	Salina	76%	372
Olathe Medical Center	Olathe	75%	602
Saint John Hospital	Leavenworth	74%	31
Overland Park Regional Medical Center	Overland Park	73%	221
Geary Community Hospital	Junction City	70%	61
Newman Regional Health	Emporia	70%	81
Mercy Health Center	Fort Scott	69%	84
Mount Carmel Regional Medical Center	Pittsburg	66%	166
Shawnee Mission Medical Center	Shawnee Mission	66%	620
Susan B Allen Memorial Hospital	El Dorado	63%	76
Neosho Memorial Regional Medical Center	Chanute	61%	64
Saint Catherine's Hospital	Garden City	61%	375
Salina Regional Health Center	Salina	61%	604
University of Kansas Medical Center	Kansas City	61%	330
Kansas Heart Hospital	Wichita	59%	203
Atchison Hospital	Atchison	54%	35
Menorah Medical Center	Shawnee Mission	53%	235
Hays Medical Center	Hays	48%	308
Western Plains Medical Company	Dodge City	48%	83
Galichia Heart Hospital	Wichita	42%	36
Southwest Medical Center	Liberal	42%	97
Republic County Hospital	Belleville	41%	44
Kansas Surgery & Recovery Center	Wichita	39%	198
Via Christi Regional Medical Center	Wichita	38%	763
Ransom Memorial Hospital	Ottawa	35%	26
Girard Medical Center	Girard	31%	32
Central Kansas Medical Center	Great Bend	11%	145
Miami County Medical Center	Paola	2%	50

Pregnancy Care

23. Inpatient Neonatal Mortality

Hospital Name	City	Rate	Cases
Hays Medical Center	Hays	0.00%	244
Saint Catherine's Hospital	Garden City	0.00%	925
Saint Francis Health Center	Topeka	0.00%	925
Saint John Hospital	Leavenworth	0.00%	258
Susan B Allen Memorial Hospital	El Dorado	0.00%	292
Shawnee Mission Medical Center	Shawnee Mission	0.06%	3593
Providence Medical Center	Kansas City	0.13%	1559
Via Christi Regional Medical Center	Wichita	0.34%	2940
Overland Park Regional Medical Center	Overland Park	0.91%	2737
Central Kansas Medical Center	Great Bend	0.92%	433

24. Third or Fourth Degree Laceration

Hospital Name	City	Rate	Cases
Saint John Hospital	Leavenworth	1.57%	191
Providence Medical Center	Kansas City	2.67%	1161
Via Christi Regional Medical Center	Wichita	3.20%	2091
Central Kansas Medical Center	Great Bend	3.62%	276
Susan B Allen Memorial Hospital	El Dorado	3.68%	190
Saint Catherine's Hospital	Garden City	3.91%	665
Shawnee Mission Medical Center	Shawnee Mission	4.21%	2447
Overland Park Regional Medical Center	Overland Park	4.41%	1657
Saint Francis Health Center	Topeka	4.76%	715
Hays Medical Center	Hays	9.68%	155

NOTE: Hospital profiles are in alphabetical order by state, then city, then hospital within the city; Rankings are sorted by rate in descending order and exclude hospitals with less than 25 cases; (1) The number of cases is too small (n<25) for purposes of reliably predicting hospital performance; (2) Measure reflects the hospital's indication that its submission was based upon a sample of its relevant discharges; (3) Rate reflects fewer than the maximum possible quarters of data for the measure; (4) Inaccurate information submitted and suppressed for one or more quarters; (5) No data is available from the hospital for this measure; Please refer to the User's Guide for a full explanation of data

Memorial Health System

511 NE 10th Street
PO Box 69
Abilene, KS 67410
URL: www.mhsks.org
Phone: 785-263-2100
Fax: 785-263-6622
Ownership: Govt - Hospital District or Authority
Accredited: No
Emergency Services: No
Licensed Beds: 49

Key Personnel:

CEO. . . . . Mark A Miller
Chief Medical Staff. . . . . Brian Holmes, MD
CNO. . . . . Trish Berns
Infection Control. . . . . Carol Landis, RN
Director Radiology . . . . Jim Barten

Measure	Cases	This Hospital	State Average	U.S. Average	Top Hospital
Heart Attack Care					
ACE Inhibitor or ARB for LVSD[1,3]	1	100%	78%	82%	100%
Aspirin at Arrival[1,3]	7	86%	90%	92%	100%
Aspirin at Discharge[1,3]	5	80%	88%	90%	100%
Beta Blocker at Arrival[1,3]	7	100%	82%	87%	100%
Beta Blocker at Discharge[1,3]	5	100%	82%	90%	100%
Fibrinolytic Medication Timing[3]	0	-	24%	31%	100%
PCI Within 90 Minutes of Arrival	0	-	55%	54%	95%
Smoking Cessation Advice[3]	0	-	86%	88%	100%
Heart Failure Care					
ACE Inhibitor or ARB for LVSD[1,3]	6	67%	72%	82%	100%
Discharge Instructions[1,3]	11	18%	41%	61%	93%
Evaluation of LVS Function[3]	32	44%	65%	83%	99%
Smoking Cessation Advice[1,3]	1	100%	67%	82%	100%
Pneumonia Care					
Appropriate Initial Antibiotic[3]	31	81%	78%	83%	94%
Blood Culture Timing[1,3]	7	86%	93%	90%	100%
Influenza Vaccine[5]	-	-	63%	70%	100%
Initial Antibiotic Timing[3]	32	88%	85%	80%	93%
Oxygenation Assessment[3]	38	100%	99%	99%	100%
Pneumococcal Vaccine[3]	29	3%	59%	69%	94%
Smoking Cessation Advice[1,3]	4	50%	60%	80%	100%
Surgical Infection Prevention					
Prophylactic Antibiotic Given[5]	-	-	74%	77%	95%
Prophylactic Antibiotic Selection[5]	-	-	91%	90%	100%
Prophylactic Antibiotic Stopped[5]	-	-	72%	72%	95%
Pregnancy Care					
Inpatient Neonatal Mortality	-	-	-	-	-
Third or Fourth Degree Laceration	-	-	3.82%	3.63%	3.27%

Kansas Medical Center

1124 West 21st Street
Andover, KS 67002
Phone: 316-300-4000
Ownership: Voluntary non-profit - Private
Accredited: No
Emergency Services: No

Measure	Cases	This Hospital	State Average	U.S. Average	Top Hospital
Heart Attack Care					
ACE Inhibitor or ARB for LVSD[5]	-	-	78%	82%	100%
Aspirin at Arrival[5]	-	-	90%	92%	100%
Aspirin at Discharge[5]	-	-	88%	90%	100%
Beta Blocker at Arrival[5]	-	-	82%	87%	100%
Beta Blocker at Discharge[5]	-	-	82%	90%	100%
Fibrinolytic Medication Timing[5]	-	-	24%	31%	100%
PCI Within 90 Minutes of Arrival[5]	-	-	55%	54%	95%
Smoking Cessation Advice[5]	-	-	86%	88%	100%
Heart Failure Care					
ACE Inhibitor or ARB for LVSD[5]	-	-	72%	82%	100%
Discharge Instructions[5]	-	-	41%	61%	93%
Evaluation of LVS Function[5]	-	-	65%	83%	99%
Smoking Cessation Advice[5]	-	-	67%	82%	100%
Pneumonia Care					
Appropriate Initial Antibiotic[5]	-	-	78%	83%	94%
Blood Culture Timing[5]	-	-	93%	90%	100%
Influenza Vaccine[5]	-	-	63%	70%	100%
Initial Antibiotic Timing[5]	-	-	85%	80%	93%
Oxygenation Assessment[5]	-	-	99%	99%	100%
Pneumococcal Vaccine[5]	-	-	59%	69%	94%
Smoking Cessation Advice[5]	-	-	60%	80%	100%
Surgical Infection Prevention					
Prophylactic Antibiotic Given[5]	-	-	74%	77%	95%
Prophylactic Antibiotic Selection[5]	-	-	91%	90%	100%
Prophylactic Antibiotic Stopped[5]	-	-	72%	72%	95%
Pregnancy Care					
Inpatient Neonatal Mortality	-	-	-	-	-
Third or Fourth Degree Laceration	-	-	3.82%	3.63%	3.27%

South Central Kansas Regional Medical Center

Alternate Name: Arkansas City Memorial Hospital
216 W Birch Avenue
PO Box 1107
Arkansas City, KS 67005
E-mail: ceo@sckrmc.com
URL: www.sckrmc.com
Phone: 620-442-2500
Fax: 620-441-5966
Ownership: Voluntary non-profit - Other
Accredited: No
Emergency Services: Yes
Licensed Beds: 85

Key Personnel:

CEO. . . . . Joe Jirinec
Chief Medical Staff. . . . . Kamran Shahzada, MD

Measure	Cases	This Hospital	State Average	U.S. Average	Top Hospital
Heart Attack Care					
ACE Inhibitor or ARB for LVSD[1]	3	33%	78%	82%	100%
Aspirin at Arrival[1]	12	75%	90%	92%	100%
Aspirin at Discharge[1]	9	44%	88%	90%	100%
Beta Blocker at Arrival[1]	11	45%	82%	87%	100%
Beta Blocker at Discharge[1]	8	50%	82%	90%	100%
Fibrinolytic Medication Timing	0	-	24%	31%	100%
PCI Within 90 Minutes of Arrival	0	-	55%	54%	95%
Smoking Cessation Advice[1]	1	0%	86%	88%	100%
Heart Failure Care					
ACE Inhibitor or ARB for LVSD[1]	5	60%	72%	82%	100%
Discharge Instructions	26	4%	41%	61%	93%
Evaluation of LVS Function	44	41%	65%	83%	99%
Smoking Cessation Advice[1]	8	38%	67%	82%	100%
Pneumonia Care					
Appropriate Initial Antibiotic	58	78%	78%	83%	94%
Blood Culture Timing[1]	3	67%	93%	90%	100%
Influenza Vaccine	25	64%	63%	70%	100%
Initial Antibiotic Timing	58	71%	85%	80%	93%
Oxygenation Assessment	71	100%	99%	99%	100%
Pneumococcal Vaccine	49	22%	59%	69%	94%
Smoking Cessation Advice[1]	18	50%	60%	80%	100%
Surgical Infection Prevention					
Prophylactic Antibiotic Given[3]	49	43%	74%	77%	95%
Prophylactic Antibiotic Selection[1]	16	94%	91%	90%	100%
Prophylactic Antibiotic Stopped[3]	36	97%	72%	72%	95%
Pregnancy Care					
Inpatient Neonatal Mortality	-	-	-	-	-
Third or Fourth Degree Laceration	-	-	3.82%	3.63%	3.27%

Ashland District Hospital

709 Oak Street
Ashland, KS 67831
Phone: 620-635-2241
Fax: 620-635-2229
Ownership: Voluntary non-profit - Other
Accredited: No
Emergency Services: Yes
Licensed Beds: 12

Key Personnel:

CEO. . . . . Daryl Marshall
Chief Medical Staff. . . . . Neal Suthers
Chief Medical Staff. . . . . Samuel Todd Stephens
Director of Cardiology/Cardiac . . . . Samuel Todd Stephens, MD
Emergency Room . . . . Michelle Moore
Pulmonary/Respiratory Care . . . . Joe Glave

Measure	Cases	This Hospital	State Average	U.S. Average	Top Hospital
Heart Attack Care					
ACE Inhibitor or ARB for LVSD[5]	-	-	78%	82%	100%
Aspirin at Arrival[5]	-	-	90%	92%	100%
Aspirin at Discharge[5]	-	-	88%	90%	100%
Beta Blocker at Arrival[5]	-	-	82%	87%	100%

NOTE: Hospital profiles are in alphabetical order by state, then city, then hospital within the city; Rankings are sorted by rate in descending order and exclude hospitals with less than 25 cases; (1) The number of cases is too small (n<25) for purposes of reliably predicting hospital performance; (2) Measure reflects the hospital's indication that its submission was based upon a sample of its relevant discharges; (3) Rate reflects fewer than the maximum possible quarters of data for the measure; (4) Inaccurate information submitted and suppressed for one or more quarters; (5) No data is available from the hospital for this measure; Please refer to the User's Guide for a full explanation of data

Measure	Cases	This Hospital	State Average	U.S. Average	Top Hospital
Beta Blocker at Discharge[5]	-	-	82%	90%	100%
Fibrinolytic Medication Timing[5]	-	-	24%	31%	100%
PCI Within 90 Minutes of Arrival[5]	-	-	55%	54%	95%
Smoking Cessation Advice[5]	-	-	86%	88%	100%
Heart Failure Care					
ACE Inhibitor or ARB for LVSD[3]	0	-	72%	82%	100%
Discharge Instructions[1,3]	1	0%	41%	61%	93%
Evaluation of LVS Function[1,3]	5	0%	65%	83%	99%
Smoking Cessation Advice[3]	0	-	67%	82%	100%
Pneumonia Care					
Appropriate Initial Antibiotic[1,3]	7	71%	78%	83%	94%
Blood Culture Timing[1,3]	1	100%	93%	90%	100%
Influenza Vaccine[5]	-	-	63%	70%	100%
Initial Antibiotic Timing[1,3]	5	80%	85%	80%	93%
Oxygenation Assessment[1,3]	7	100%	99%	99%	100%
Pneumococcal Vaccine[1,3]	6	67%	59%	69%	94%
Smoking Cessation Advice[3]	0	-	60%	80%	100%
Surgical Infection Prevention					
Prophylactic Antibiotic Given[5]	-	-	74%	77%	95%
Prophylactic Antibiotic Selection[5]	-	-	91%	90%	100%
Prophylactic Antibiotic Stopped[5]	-	-	72%	72%	95%
Pregnancy Care					
Inpatient Neonatal Mortality	-	-	-	-	-
Third or Fourth Degree Laceration	-	-	3.82%	3.63%	3.27%

Atchison Hospital

1301 N 2nd
Atchison, KS 66002

Toll-Free: 800-559-2135
Phone: 913-367-2131
Fax: 913-367-2913

Ownership: Voluntary non-profit - Private
Emergency Services: Yes
Accredited: No
Licensed Beds: 67

Key Personnel:

President/CEO . . . . John Jacobson
Chief Medical Staff . . . . Ryan Thomas, MD
Emergency Room . . . . Wayne O Wallace Jr, MD
Manager Emergency Room . . . . Theresa Miller
Infection Control Clinician . . . . Jim Brown
Manager Surgery . . . . Jean Ober
Manager Radiology . . . . Mary Ann Turpin
Manager Respiratory/Cardiopulmonary . . . . JoAnn Rajca

Measure	Cases	This Hospital	State Average	U.S. Average	Top Hospital
Heart Attack Care					
ACE Inhibitor or ARB for LVSD	0	-	78%	82%	100%
Aspirin at Arrival[1]	5	80%	90%	92%	100%
Aspirin at Discharge[1]	2	100%	88%	90%	100%
Beta Blocker at Arrival[1]	3	100%	82%	87%	100%
Beta Blocker at Discharge[1]	1	0%	82%	90%	100%
Fibrinolytic Medication Timing	0	-	24%	31%	100%
PCI Within 90 Minutes of Arrival	0	-	55%	54%	95%
Smoking Cessation Advice	0	-	86%	88%	100%
Heart Failure Care					
ACE Inhibitor or ARB for LVSD[1]	13	54%	72%	82%	100%
Discharge Instructions	34	18%	41%	61%	93%
Evaluation of LVS Function	55	58%	65%	83%	99%
Smoking Cessation Advice[1]	3	33%	67%	82%	100%
Pneumonia Care					
Appropriate Initial Antibiotic[1]	23	83%	78%	83%	94%
Blood Culture Timing[1]	16	100%	93%	90%	100%
Influenza Vaccine[1]	5	100%	63%	70%	100%
Initial Antibiotic Timing	33	76%	85%	80%	93%
Oxygenation Assessment	43	100%	99%	99%	100%
Pneumococcal Vaccine	31	74%	59%	69%	94%
Smoking Cessation Advice[1]	10	50%	60%	80%	100%
Surgical Infection Prevention					
Prophylactic Antibiotic Given	39	72%	74%	77%	95%
Prophylactic Antibiotic Selection[1]	7	86%	91%	90%	100%
Prophylactic Antibiotic Stopped	35	54%	72%	72%	95%
Pregnancy Care					
Inpatient Neonatal Mortality	-	-	-	-	-
Third or Fourth Degree Laceration	-	-	3.82%	3.63%	3.27%

Republic County Hospital

2420 G Street
Belleville, KS 66935
E-mail: rchospital1@nckcn.com
URL: www.republiccountyhospital.org

Phone: 785-527-2254
Fax: 785-527-2324

Ownership: Voluntary non-profit - Other
Emergency Services: No
Accredited: No
Licensed Beds: 48

Key Personnel:

Administrator . . . . Blaine Miller

Measure	Cases	This Hospital	State Average	U.S. Average	Top Hospital
Heart Attack Care					
ACE Inhibitor or ARB for LVSD	0	-	78%	82%	100%
Aspirin at Arrival[1]	7	100%	90%	92%	100%
Aspirin at Discharge[1]	6	67%	88%	90%	100%
Beta Blocker at Arrival[1]	8	75%	82%	87%	100%
Beta Blocker at Discharge[1]	7	71%	82%	90%	100%
Fibrinolytic Medication Timing[1]	2	0%	24%	31%	100%
PCI Within 90 Minutes of Arrival	0	-	55%	54%	95%
Smoking Cessation Advice[1]	1	100%	86%	88%	100%
Heart Failure Care					
ACE Inhibitor or ARB for LVSD[5]	-	-	72%	82%	100%
Discharge Instructions[5]	-	-	41%	61%	93%
Evaluation of LVS Function[5]	-	-	65%	83%	99%
Smoking Cessation Advice[5]	-	-	67%	82%	100%
Pneumonia Care					
Appropriate Initial Antibiotic	69	49%	78%	83%	94%
Blood Culture Timing[1]	4	100%	93%	90%	100%
Influenza Vaccine[1]	20	65%	63%	70%	100%
Initial Antibiotic Timing	54	87%	85%	80%	93%
Oxygenation Assessment	79	97%	99%	99%	100%
Pneumococcal Vaccine	62	71%	59%	69%	94%
Smoking Cessation Advice[1]	13	69%	60%	80%	100%
Surgical Infection Prevention					
Prophylactic Antibiotic Given	43	63%	74%	77%	95%
Prophylactic Antibiotic Selection[1]	10	90%	91%	90%	100%
Prophylactic Antibiotic Stopped	44	41%	72%	72%	95%
Pregnancy Care					
Inpatient Neonatal Mortality	-	-	-	-	-
Third or Fourth Degree Laceration	-	-	3.82%	3.63%	3.27%

Mitchell County Hospital

400 W 8th Street
Beloit, KS 67420
URL: www.gpha.com

Phone: 785-738-2266
Fax: 785-738-9503

Ownership: Voluntary non-profit - Private
Emergency Services: Yes
Accredited: No
Licensed Beds: 89

Key Personnel:

President/CEO . . . . David Dick
Chief of Medical Staff . . . . Cristine Marozes
Emergency Room . . . . Mary Grey
Director of Pulmonary/Respiratory . . . . Con Cammon

Measure	Cases	This Hospital	State Average	U.S. Average	Top Hospital
Heart Attack Care					
ACE Inhibitor or ARB for LVSD[1,3]	1	100%	78%	82%	100%
Aspirin at Arrival[1,3]	6	100%	90%	92%	100%
Aspirin at Discharge[1,3]	2	100%	88%	90%	100%
Beta Blocker at Arrival[1,3]	6	83%	82%	87%	100%
Beta Blocker at Discharge[1,3]	3	100%	82%	90%	100%
Fibrinolytic Medication Timing[1,3]	2	100%	24%	31%	100%
PCI Within 90 Minutes of Arrival[5]	-	-	55%	54%	95%
Smoking Cessation Advice[3]	0	-	86%	88%	100%
Heart Failure Care					
ACE Inhibitor or ARB for LVSD[1]	7	86%	72%	82%	100%
Discharge Instructions	31	6%	41%	61%	93%
Evaluation of LVS Function	54	78%	65%	83%	99%
Smoking Cessation Advice[1]	1	0%	67%	82%	100%
Pneumonia Care					
Appropriate Initial Antibiotic	38	74%	78%	83%	94%
Blood Culture Timing	30	100%	93%	90%	100%
Influenza Vaccine[1]	14	36%	63%	70%	100%
Initial Antibiotic Timing	62	84%	85%	80%	93%

NOTE: Hospital profiles are in alphabetical order by state, then city, then hospital within the city; Rankings are sorted by rate in descending order and exclude hospitals with less than 25 cases; (1) The number of cases is too small (n<25) for purposes of reliably predicting hospital performance; (2) Measure reflects the hospital's indication that its submission was based upon a sample of its relevant discharges; (3) Rate reflects fewer than the maximum possible quarters of data for the measure; (4) Inaccurate information submitted and suppressed for one or more quarters; (5) No data is available from the hospital for this measure; Please refer to the User's Guide for a full explanation of data

Oxygenation Assessment	88	100%	99%	99%	100%
Pneumococcal Vaccine	69	30%	59%	69%	94%
Smoking Cessation Advice[1]	7	43%	60%	80%	100%
Surgical Infection Prevention					
Prophylactic Antibiotic Given	29	93%	74%	77%	95%
Prophylactic Antibiotic Selection[1]	5	80%	91%	90%	100%
Prophylactic Antibiotic Stopped	28	93%	72%	72%	95%
Pregnancy Care					
Inpatient Neonatal Mortality	-	-	-	-	-
Third or Fourth Degree Laceration	-	-	3.82%	3.63%	3.27%

Coffey County Hospital

801 N 4th Street
Burlington, KS 66839
URL: www.coffeyhealth.org
Ownership: Government - Local
Emergency Services: Yes

Phone: 620-364-2121
Fax: 620-364-2605
Accredited: No
Licensed Beds: 36

Key Personnel:

President/CEO . . . . Dennis George
Chief Medical Staff . . . . John Shell, MD
Emergency Room . . . . John Shell
Infection Control . . . . Elaine Weston, RN
Medical Surgical Nursing . . . . Shirley Ulrich, RN
Respiratory/Cardiopulmonary . . . . Melinda Pattinson

Measure	Cases	This Hospital	State Average	U.S. Average	Top Hospital
Heart Attack Care					
ACE Inhibitor or ARB for LVSD[3]	0	-	78%	82%	100%
Aspirin at Arrival[1,3]	2	50%	90%	92%	100%
Aspirin at Discharge[1,3]	1	100%	88%	90%	100%
Beta Blocker at Arrival[1,3]	2	50%	82%	87%	100%
Beta Blocker at Discharge[1,3]	1	0%	82%	90%	100%
Fibrinolytic Medication Timing[1,3]	3	100%	24%	31%	100%
PCI Within 90 Minutes of Arrival	0	-	55%	54%	95%
Smoking Cessation Advice[3]	0	-	86%	88%	100%
Heart Failure Care					
ACE Inhibitor or ARB for LVSD[1]	6	50%	72%	82%	100%
Discharge Instructions	34	26%	41%	61%	93%
Evaluation of LVS Function	52	37%	65%	83%	99%
Smoking Cessation Advice[1]	4	75%	67%	82%	100%
Pneumonia Care					
Appropriate Initial Antibiotic	43	88%	78%	83%	94%
Blood Culture Timing[1]	1	100%	93%	90%	100%
Influenza Vaccine	26	4%	63%	70%	100%
Initial Antibiotic Timing	67	91%	85%	80%	93%
Oxygenation Assessment	75	100%	99%	99%	100%
Pneumococcal Vaccine	54	56%	59%	69%	94%
Smoking Cessation Advice[1]	16	88%	60%	80%	100%
Surgical Infection Prevention					
Prophylactic Antibiotic Given[1]	22	23%	74%	77%	95%
Prophylactic Antibiotic Selection[1]	3	100%	91%	90%	100%
Prophylactic Antibiotic Stopped[1]	17	71%	72%	72%	95%
Pregnancy Care					
Inpatient Neonatal Mortality	-	-	-	-	-
Third or Fourth Degree Laceration	-	-	3.82%	3.63%	3.27%

Neosho Memorial Regional Medical Center

629 S Plummer
PO Box 426
Chanute, KS 66720
URL: www.nmrmc.com
Ownership: Proprietary
Emergency Services: Yes

Phone: 620-431-4000
Fax: 620-431-7556
Accredited: No
Licensed Beds: 97

Key Personnel:

President/CEO . . . . Murray L Brown
Chief Medical Staff . . . . DeAnna Vaugh, MD
Emergency Room . . . . Todd Morrison, MD
Emergency Room . . . . Pat Lucke, RN
Infection Control . . . . Kathy Wicker, RN
ICU . . . . Sandy Froemming, RN
Respiratory/Cardiopulmonary . . . . Jeff Scobee

Measure	Cases	This Hospital	State Average	U.S. Average	Top Hospital
Heart Attack Care					
ACE Inhibitor or ARB for LVSD[1]	1	100%	78%	82%	100%
Aspirin at Arrival[1]	8	75%	90%	92%	100%
Aspirin at Discharge[1]	6	100%	88%	90%	100%
Beta Blocker at Arrival[1]	8	100%	82%	87%	100%
Beta Blocker at Discharge[1]	7	86%	82%	90%	100%
Fibrinolytic Medication Timing	0	-	24%	31%	100%
PCI Within 90 Minutes of Arrival	0	-	55%	54%	95%
Smoking Cessation Advice	0	-	86%	88%	100%
Heart Failure Care					
ACE Inhibitor or ARB for LVSD[1]	18	44%	72%	82%	100%
Discharge Instructions	41	37%	41%	61%	93%
Evaluation of LVS Function	68	75%	65%	83%	99%
Smoking Cessation Advice[1]	15	53%	67%	82%	100%
Pneumonia Care					
Appropriate Initial Antibiotic	61	87%	78%	83%	94%
Blood Culture Timing	49	96%	93%	90%	100%
Influenza Vaccine	26	73%	63%	70%	100%
Initial Antibiotic Timing	75	92%	85%	80%	93%
Oxygenation Assessment	102	100%	99%	99%	100%
Pneumococcal Vaccine	65	62%	59%	69%	94%
Smoking Cessation Advice	29	76%	60%	80%	100%
Surgical Infection Prevention					
Prophylactic Antibiotic Given	76	76%	74%	77%	95%
Prophylactic Antibiotic Selection[1]	13	100%	91%	90%	100%
Prophylactic Antibiotic Stopped	64	61%	72%	72%	95%
Pregnancy Care					
Inpatient Neonatal Mortality	-	-	-	-	-
Third or Fourth Degree Laceration	-	-	3.82%	3.63%	3.27%

Clay County Medical Center

617 Liberty
Clay Center, KS 67432
Ownership: Government - Local
Emergency Services: Yes

Phone: 785-632-2144
Accredited: No

Measure	Cases	This Hospital	State Average	U.S. Average	Top Hospital
Heart Attack Care					
ACE Inhibitor or ARB for LVSD	0	-	78%	82%	100%
Aspirin at Arrival[1]	4	75%	90%	92%	100%
Aspirin at Discharge	0	-	88%	90%	100%
Beta Blocker at Arrival[1]	3	67%	82%	87%	100%
Beta Blocker at Discharge	0	-	82%	90%	100%
Fibrinolytic Medication Timing[1]	2	0%	24%	31%	100%
PCI Within 90 Minutes of Arrival[5]	-	-	55%	54%	95%
Smoking Cessation Advice	0	-	86%	88%	100%
Heart Failure Care					
ACE Inhibitor or ARB for LVSD[1]	3	67%	72%	82%	100%
Discharge Instructions[1]	6	17%	41%	61%	93%
Evaluation of LVS Function[1]	15	80%	65%	83%	99%
Smoking Cessation Advice[1]	2	0%	67%	82%	100%
Pneumonia Care					
Appropriate Initial Antibiotic	63	68%	78%	83%	94%
Blood Culture Timing[1]	10	100%	93%	90%	100%
Influenza Vaccine[1]	12	92%	63%	70%	100%
Initial Antibiotic Timing	65	85%	85%	80%	93%
Oxygenation Assessment	75	99%	99%	99%	100%
Pneumococcal Vaccine	56	96%	59%	69%	94%
Smoking Cessation Advice[1]	8	50%	60%	80%	100%
Surgical Infection Prevention					
Prophylactic Antibiotic Given[1,3]	3	67%	74%	77%	95%
Prophylactic Antibiotic Selection[1]	1	100%	91%	90%	100%
Prophylactic Antibiotic Stopped[1,3]	3	100%	72%	72%	95%
Pregnancy Care					
Inpatient Neonatal Mortality	-	-	-	-	-
Third or Fourth Degree Laceration	-	-	3.82%	3.63%	3.27%

NOTE: Hospital profiles are in alphabetical order by state, then city, then hospital within the city; Rankings are sorted by rate in descending order and exclude hospitals with less than 25 cases; (1) The number of cases is too small (n<25) for purposes of reliably predicting hospital performance; (2) Measure reflects the hospital's indication that its submission was based upon a sample of its relevant discharges; (3) Rate reflects fewer than the maximum possible quarters of data for the measure; (4) Inaccurate information submitted and suppressed for one or more quarters; (5) No data is available from the hospital for this measure; Please refer to the User's Guide for a full explanation of data

Coffeyville Regional Medical Center

1400 W 4th Street
Coffeyville, KS 67337

Toll-Free: 800-914-8732
Phone: 620-252-1500
Fax: 620-252-1562

E-mail: humanresources@crmcinc.com
URL: www.crmcinc.com
Ownership: Government - Local
Emergency Services: Yes

Accredited: Yes
Licensed Beds: 105

Key Personnel:
CEO. . . . . Jerry Marquette

Measure	Cases	This Hospital	State Average	U.S. Average	Top Hospital
Heart Attack Care					
ACE Inhibitor or ARB for LVSD[1]	7	57%	78%	82%	100%
Aspirin at Arrival	28	89%	90%	92%	100%
Aspirin at Discharge[1]	12	83%	88%	90%	100%
Beta Blocker at Arrival	28	61%	82%	87%	100%
Beta Blocker at Discharge[1]	13	54%	82%	90%	100%
Fibrinolytic Medication Timing[1]	1	0%	24%	31%	100%
PCI Within 90 Minutes of Arrival	0	-	55%	54%	95%
Smoking Cessation Advice[1]	2	50%	86%	88%	100%
Heart Failure Care					
ACE Inhibitor or ARB for LVSD	47	55%	72%	82%	100%
Discharge Instructions	98	68%	41%	61%	93%
Evaluation of LVS Function	146	72%	65%	83%	99%
Smoking Cessation Advice[1]	14	50%	67%	82%	100%
Pneumonia Care					
Appropriate Initial Antibiotic	105	73%	78%	83%	94%
Blood Culture Timing	54	94%	93%	90%	100%
Influenza Vaccine	49	53%	63%	70%	100%
Initial Antibiotic Timing	219	79%	85%	80%	93%
Oxygenation Assessment	226	100%	99%	99%	100%
Pneumococcal Vaccine	159	47%	59%	69%	94%
Smoking Cessation Advice	45	67%	60%	80%	100%
Surgical Infection Prevention					
Prophylactic Antibiotic Given[3]	49	78%	74%	77%	95%
Prophylactic Antibiotic Selection[1]	17	35%	91%	90%	100%
Prophylactic Antibiotic Stopped[3]	48	88%	72%	72%	95%
Pregnancy Care					
Inpatient Neonatal Mortality	-	-	-	-	-
Third or Fourth Degree Laceration	-	-	3.82%	3.63%	3.27%

Comanche County Hospital

202 Frisco Street
HC 65 Box 8A
Coldwater, KS 67029
URL: www.gpha.com
Ownership: Government - Local
Emergency Services: Yes

Phone: 620-582-2144
Fax: 620-582-2572

Accredited: No
Licensed Beds: 14

Key Personnel:
Administrator . . . . Nancy Zimmerman

Measure	Cases	This Hospital	State Average	U.S. Average	Top Hospital
Heart Attack Care					
ACE Inhibitor or ARB for LVSD[5]	-	-	78%	82%	100%
Aspirin at Arrival[5]	-	-	90%	92%	100%
Aspirin at Discharge[5]	-	-	88%	90%	100%
Beta Blocker at Arrival[5]	-	-	82%	87%	100%
Beta Blocker at Discharge[5]	-	-	82%	90%	100%
Fibrinolytic Medication Timing[5]	-	-	24%	31%	100%
PCI Within 90 Minutes of Arrival[5]	-	-	55%	54%	95%
Smoking Cessation Advice[5]	-	-	86%	88%	100%
Heart Failure Care					
ACE Inhibitor or ARB for LVSD[5]	-	-	72%	82%	100%
Discharge Instructions[5]	-	-	41%	61%	93%
Evaluation of LVS Function[5]	-	-	65%	83%	99%
Smoking Cessation Advice[5]	-	-	67%	82%	100%
Pneumonia Care					
Appropriate Initial Antibiotic[1,3]	12	50%	78%	83%	94%
Blood Culture Timing[1,3]	1	100%	93%	90%	100%
Influenza Vaccine[5]	-	-	63%	70%	100%
Initial Antibiotic Timing[1,3]	11	91%	85%	80%	93%
Oxygenation Assessment[1,3]	15	100%	99%	99%	100%
Pneumococcal Vaccine[1,3]	12	17%	59%	69%	94%
Smoking Cessation Advice[1,3]	1	100%	60%	80%	100%
Surgical Infection Prevention					
Prophylactic Antibiotic Given[5]	-	-	74%	77%	95%
Prophylactic Antibiotic Selection[5]	-	-	91%	90%	100%
Prophylactic Antibiotic Stopped[5]	-	-	72%	72%	95%
Pregnancy Care					
Inpatient Neonatal Mortality	-	-	-	-	-
Third or Fourth Degree Laceration	-	-	3.82%	3.63%	3.27%

Cloud County Health Center

Alternate Name: Saint Joseph Hospital
1100 Highland Drive
Concordia, KS 66901
URL: www.cchc.com
Ownership: Voluntary non-profit - Private
Emergency Services: Yes

Phone: 785-243-1234
Fax: 785-243-8411

Accredited: No
Licensed Beds: 25

Key Personnel:
CEO. . . . . James E Wahlmeier
Chief Medical Staff. . . . . Justin Poore, MD
Emergency Room . . . . Justin Poore
CCU Supervisor. . . . . Laura Ottert
Director Cardiopulmonary . . . . Kris Copple

Measure	Cases	This Hospital	State Average	U.S. Average	Top Hospital
Heart Attack Care					
ACE Inhibitor or ARB for LVSD[3]	0	-	78%	82%	100%
Aspirin at Arrival[1,3]	3	100%	90%	92%	100%
Aspirin at Discharge[1,3]	3	67%	88%	90%	100%
Beta Blocker at Arrival[1,3]	3	100%	82%	87%	100%
Beta Blocker at Discharge[1,3]	3	100%	82%	90%	100%
Fibrinolytic Medication Timing[3]	0	-	24%	31%	100%
PCI Within 90 Minutes of Arrival[5]	-	-	55%	54%	95%
Smoking Cessation Advice[1,3]	1	0%	86%	88%	100%
Heart Failure Care					
ACE Inhibitor or ARB for LVSD[1]	3	67%	72%	82%	100%
Discharge Instructions[1]	16	56%	41%	61%	93%
Evaluation of LVS Function[1]	21	76%	65%	83%	99%
Smoking Cessation Advice	0	-	67%	82%	100%
Pneumonia Care					
Appropriate Initial Antibiotic	59	73%	78%	83%	94%
Blood Culture Timing[1]	5	80%	93%	90%	100%
Influenza Vaccine[1]	17	82%	63%	70%	100%
Initial Antibiotic Timing	51	90%	85%	80%	93%
Oxygenation Assessment	64	100%	99%	99%	100%
Pneumococcal Vaccine	47	85%	59%	69%	94%
Smoking Cessation Advice[1]	10	40%	60%	80%	100%
Surgical Infection Prevention					
Prophylactic Antibiotic Given[5]	-	-	74%	77%	95%
Prophylactic Antibiotic Selection[5]	-	-	91%	90%	100%
Prophylactic Antibiotic Stopped[5]	-	-	72%	72%	95%
Pregnancy Care					
Inpatient Neonatal Mortality	-	-	-	-	-
Third or Fourth Degree Laceration	-	-	3.82%	3.63%	3.27%

Morris County Hospital

600 N Washington Street
Council Grove, KS 66846
URL: www.mrchosp.com
Ownership: Government - Local
Emergency Services: Yes

Phone: 620-767-6811
Fax: 620-767-5611

Accredited: No
Licensed Beds: 28

Key Personnel:
President/CEO. . . . . James H Reagan Jr, MD
Chief of Medical Staff. Daniel Frese
Emergency Room . . . . Joel Hornung

Measure	Cases	This Hospital	State Average	U.S. Average	Top Hospital
Heart Attack Care					
ACE Inhibitor or ARB for LVSD	0	-	78%	82%	100%
Aspirin at Arrival[1]	1	100%	90%	92%	100%
Aspirin at Discharge[1]	1	100%	88%	90%	100%
Beta Blocker at Arrival[1]	1	0%	82%	87%	100%

NOTE: Hospital profiles are in alphabetical order by state, then city, then hospital within the city; Rankings are sorted by rate in descending order and exclude hospitals with less than 25 cases; (1) The number of cases is too small (n<25) for purposes of reliably predicting hospital performance; (2) Measure reflects the hospital's indication that its submission was based upon a sample of its relevant discharges; (3) Rate reflects fewer than the maximum possible quarters of data for the measure; (4) Inaccurate information submitted and suppressed for one or more quarters; (5) No data is available from the hospital for this measure; Please refer to the User's Guide for a full explanation of data

Beta Blocker at Discharge[1]	1	0%	82%	90%	100%
Fibrinolytic Medication Timing	0	-	24%	31%	100%
PCI Within 90 Minutes of Arrival	0	-	55%	54%	95%
Smoking Cessation Advice	0	-	86%	88%	100%
Heart Failure Care					
ACE Inhibitor or ARB for LVSD[1]	3	100%	72%	82%	100%
Discharge Instructions[1]	14	36%	41%	61%	93%
Evaluation of LVS Function[1]	23	35%	65%	83%	99%
Smoking Cessation Advice[1]	2	0%	67%	82%	100%
Pneumonia Care					
Appropriate Initial Antibiotic[1]	20	75%	78%	83%	94%
Blood Culture Timing[1]	1	100%	93%	90%	100%
Influenza Vaccine[1]	9	22%	63%	70%	100%
Initial Antibiotic Timing	34	94%	85%	80%	93%
Oxygenation Assessment	47	100%	99%	99%	100%
Pneumococcal Vaccine	41	15%	59%	69%	94%
Smoking Cessation Advice[1]	4	75%	60%	80%	100%
Surgical Infection Prevention					
Prophylactic Antibiotic Given[5]	-	-	74%	77%	95%
Prophylactic Antibiotic Selection[5]	-	-	91%	90%	100%
Prophylactic Antibiotic Stopped[5]	-	-	72%	72%	95%
Pregnancy Care					
Inpatient Neonatal Mortality	-	-	-	-	-
Third or Fourth Degree Laceration	-	-	3.82%	3.63%	3.27%

Western Plains Medical Company

Alternate Name: Humana Hospital Dodge City
3001 Avenue A
Dodge City, KS 67801
Phone: 620-225-8400
Fax: 620-225-8403
URL: www.westernplainsmc.com
Ownership: Proprietary
Accredited: No
Emergency Services: No
Licensed Beds: 99

Key Personnel:
CEO. . . . . Steven Daniel
Chief Medical Staff. . . . . D Trotter, MD
Emergency Room . . . . Phillis Williams
Director of Respiratory . . . . Debra Bauer

Measure	Cases	This Hospital	State Average	U.S. Average	Top Hospital
Heart Attack Care					
ACE Inhibitor or ARB for LVSD[1]	3	67%	78%	82%	100%
Aspirin at Arrival	28	96%	90%	92%	100%
Aspirin at Discharge[1]	23	100%	88%	90%	100%
Beta Blocker at Arrival[1]	20	80%	82%	87%	100%
Beta Blocker at Discharge[1]	22	77%	82%	90%	100%
Fibrinolytic Medication Timing	0	-	24%	31%	100%
PCI Within 90 Minutes of Arrival[1]	4	25%	55%	54%	95%
Smoking Cessation Advice[1]	11	82%	86%	88%	100%
Heart Failure Care					
ACE Inhibitor or ARB for LVSD[1]	20	75%	72%	82%	100%
Discharge Instructions	48	56%	41%	61%	93%
Evaluation of LVS Function	65	74%	65%	83%	99%
Smoking Cessation Advice[1]	6	83%	67%	82%	100%
Pneumonia Care					
Appropriate Initial Antibiotic	57	70%	78%	83%	94%
Blood Culture Timing	42	98%	93%	90%	100%
Influenza Vaccine[1]	22	55%	63%	70%	100%
Initial Antibiotic Timing	90	77%	85%	80%	93%
Oxygenation Assessment	107	100%	99%	99%	100%
Pneumococcal Vaccine	68	82%	59%	69%	94%
Smoking Cessation Advice	28	68%	60%	80%	100%
Surgical Infection Prevention					
Prophylactic Antibiotic Given[2,3]	90	63%	74%	77%	95%
Prophylactic Antibiotic Selection[2]	31	87%	91%	90%	100%
Prophylactic Antibiotic Stopped[2,3]	83	48%	72%	72%	95%
Pregnancy Care					
Inpatient Neonatal Mortality	-	-	-	-	-
Third or Fourth Degree Laceration	-	-	3.82%	3.63%	3.27%

Susan B Allen Memorial Hospital

720 West Central
El Dorado, KS 67042
Phone: 316-321-3300
Fax: 316-321-2916
URL: www.sbamh.com
Ownership: Voluntary non-profit - Private
Accredited: Yes
Emergency Services: Yes
Licensed Beds: 103

Key Personnel:
President/CEO. . . . . Jim Wilson

Measure	Cases	This Hospital	State Average	U.S. Average	Top Hospital
Heart Attack Care					
ACE Inhibitor or ARB for LVSD	0	-	78%	82%	100%
Aspirin at Arrival[1]	7	100%	90%	92%	100%
Aspirin at Discharge[1]	4	100%	88%	90%	100%
Beta Blocker at Arrival[1]	4	100%	82%	87%	100%
Beta Blocker at Discharge[1]	3	100%	82%	90%	100%
Fibrinolytic Medication Timing	0	-	24%	31%	100%
PCI Within 90 Minutes of Arrival	0	-	55%	54%	95%
Smoking Cessation Advice[1]	1	100%	86%	88%	100%
Heart Failure Care					
ACE Inhibitor or ARB for LVSD[1]	6	100%	72%	82%	100%
Discharge Instructions	26	92%	41%	61%	93%
Evaluation of LVS Function	64	73%	65%	83%	99%
Smoking Cessation Advice[1]	9	100%	67%	82%	100%
Pneumonia Care					
Appropriate Initial Antibiotic	53	85%	78%	83%	94%
Blood Culture Timing[1]	3	100%	93%	90%	100%
Influenza Vaccine[1]	17	88%	63%	70%	100%
Initial Antibiotic Timing	73	88%	85%	80%	93%
Oxygenation Assessment	89	100%	99%	99%	100%
Pneumococcal Vaccine	51	88%	59%	69%	94%
Smoking Cessation Advice[1]	24	88%	60%	80%	100%
Surgical Infection Prevention					
Prophylactic Antibiotic Given	79	81%	74%	77%	95%
Prophylactic Antibiotic Selection	27	96%	91%	90%	100%
Prophylactic Antibiotic Stopped	76	63%	72%	72%	95%
Pregnancy Care					
Inpatient Neonatal Mortality	292	0.00%	-	-	-
Third or Fourth Degree Laceration	190	3.68%	3.82%	3.63%	3.27%

Morton County Hospital

445 Hilltop Street
Elkhart, KS 67950
Phone: 620-697-2141
Fax: 620-697-4766
URL: www.mchswecare.com
Ownership: Government - Local
Accredited: No
Emergency Services: Yes
Licensed Beds: 40

Key Personnel:
President/CEO. . . . . Leonard Hernandez
Chief Medical Staff. . . . . D Perido, MD
Director of Pulmonary/Respiratory Care. . . . . . . S Jones

Measure	Cases	This Hospital	State Average	U.S. Average	Top Hospital
Heart Attack Care					
ACE Inhibitor or ARB for LVSD	0	-	78%	82%	100%
Aspirin at Arrival[1]	3	33%	90%	92%	100%
Aspirin at Discharge[1]	2	50%	88%	90%	100%
Beta Blocker at Arrival[1]	3	67%	82%	87%	100%
Beta Blocker at Discharge[1]	2	50%	82%	90%	100%
Fibrinolytic Medication Timing[1,3]	1	0%	24%	31%	100%
PCI Within 90 Minutes of Arrival	0	-	55%	54%	95%
Smoking Cessation Advice[3]	0	-	86%	88%	100%
Heart Failure Care					
ACE Inhibitor or ARB for LVSD[1]	4	50%	72%	82%	100%
Discharge Instructions[1,3]	5	0%	41%	61%	93%
Evaluation of LVS Function	37	49%	65%	83%	99%
Smoking Cessation Advice[1,3]	1	100%	67%	82%	100%
Pneumonia Care					
Appropriate Initial Antibiotic[1,3]	3	100%	78%	83%	94%
Blood Culture Timing[3]	0	-	93%	90%	100%
Influenza Vaccine[5]	-	-	63%	70%	100%
Initial Antibiotic Timing	50	88%	85%	80%	93%
Oxygenation Assessment	66	100%	99%	99%	100%

NOTE: Hospital profiles are in alphabetical order by state, then city, then hospital within the city; Rankings are sorted by rate in descending order and exclude hospitals with less than 25 cases; (1) The number of cases is too small (n<25) for purposes of reliably predicting hospital performance; (2) Measure reflects the hospital's indication that its submission was based upon a sample of its relevant discharges; (3) Rate reflects fewer than the maximum possible quarters of data for the measure; (4) Inaccurate information submitted and suppressed for one or more quarters; (5) No data is available from the hospital for this measure; Please refer to the User's Guide for a full explanation of data

Measure	Cases	This Hospital	State Average	U.S. Average	Top Hospital
Pneumococcal Vaccine	47	53%	59%	69%	94%
Smoking Cessation Advice[1,3]	1	100%	60%	80%	100%
Surgical Infection Prevention					
Prophylactic Antibiotic Given[1,2,3]	7	29%	74%	77%	95%
Prophylactic Antibiotic Selection[5]	-	-	91%	90%	100%
Prophylactic Antibiotic Stopped[1,2,3]	7	100%	72%	72%	95%
Pregnancy Care					
Inpatient Neonatal Mortality	-	-	-	-	-
Third or Fourth Degree Laceration	-	-	3.82%	3.63%	3.27%

Ellinwood District Hospital

605 N Main Street
Ellinwood, KS 67526
URL: www.gpha.com
Ownership: Govt - Hospital District or Authority
Emergency Services: Yes
Phone: 620-564-2549
Fax: 620-564-3117
Accredited: No
Licensed Beds: 12

Key Personnel:
CEO. . . . . David Haneke

Measure	Cases	This Hospital	State Average	U.S. Average	Top Hospital
Heart Attack Care					
ACE Inhibitor or ARB for LVSD[5]	-	-	78%	82%	100%
Aspirin at Arrival[5]	-	-	90%	92%	100%
Aspirin at Discharge[5]	-	-	88%	90%	100%
Beta Blocker at Arrival[5]	-	-	82%	87%	100%
Beta Blocker at Discharge[5]	-	-	82%	90%	100%
Fibrinolytic Medication Timing[5]	-	-	24%	31%	100%
PCI Within 90 Minutes of Arrival[5]	-	-	55%	54%	95%
Smoking Cessation Advice[5]	-	-	86%	88%	100%
Heart Failure Care					
ACE Inhibitor or ARB for LVSD[5]	-	-	72%	82%	100%
Discharge Instructions[5]	-	-	41%	61%	93%
Evaluation of LVS Function[5]	-	-	65%	83%	99%
Smoking Cessation Advice[5]	-	-	67%	82%	100%
Pneumonia Care					
Appropriate Initial Antibiotic[5]	-	-	78%	83%	94%
Blood Culture Timing[5]	-	-	93%	90%	100%
Influenza Vaccine[5]	-	-	63%	70%	100%
Initial Antibiotic Timing[5]	-	-	85%	80%	93%
Oxygenation Assessment[5]	-	-	99%	99%	100%
Pneumococcal Vaccine[5]	-	-	59%	69%	94%
Smoking Cessation Advice[5]	-	-	60%	80%	100%
Surgical Infection Prevention					
Prophylactic Antibiotic Given[5]	-	-	74%	77%	95%
Prophylactic Antibiotic Selection[5]	-	-	91%	90%	100%
Prophylactic Antibiotic Stopped[5]	-	-	72%	72%	95%
Pregnancy Care					
Inpatient Neonatal Mortality	-	-	-	-	-
Third or Fourth Degree Laceration	-	-	3.82%	3.63%	3.27%

Ellsworth County Medical Center

Alternate Name: Ellsworth County Veterans Memorial Hospital
1604 Aylward Street
PO Box 87
Ellsworth, KS 67439
URL: www.ewmed.com
Ownership: Government - Local
Emergency Services: Yes
Phone: 785-472-3111
Fax: 785-472-5760
Accredited: No
Licensed Beds: 20

Key Personnel:
CEO. . . . . Roger Pearson
Chief Medical Staff. . . . . Ronald Whitmer, DO
Emergency Room . . . . Betsy Prisco
Director Radiology . . . . Randy Packard
Director Respiratory/Cardiopulmonary . . . . Mona Wermen

Measure	Cases	This Hospital	State Average	U.S. Average	Top Hospital
Heart Attack Care					
ACE Inhibitor or ARB for LVSD[1]	1	0%	78%	82%	100%
Aspirin at Arrival[1]	5	80%	90%	92%	100%
Aspirin at Discharge[1]	4	25%	88%	90%	100%
Beta Blocker at Arrival[1]	7	86%	82%	87%	100%
Beta Blocker at Discharge[1]	5	20%	82%	90%	100%
Fibrinolytic Medication Timing	0	-	24%	31%	100%
PCI Within 90 Minutes of Arrival	0	-	55%	54%	95%
Smoking Cessation Advice	0	-	86%	88%	100%
Heart Failure Care					
ACE Inhibitor or ARB for LVSD[1]	5	20%	72%	82%	100%
Discharge Instructions[1]	20	5%	41%	61%	93%
Evaluation of LVS Function	43	51%	65%	83%	99%
Smoking Cessation Advice	0	-	67%	82%	100%
Pneumonia Care					
Appropriate Initial Antibiotic[1]	24	79%	78%	83%	94%
Blood Culture Timing[1]	10	100%	93%	90%	100%
Influenza Vaccine[1]	21	62%	63%	70%	100%
Initial Antibiotic Timing	40	80%	85%	80%	93%
Oxygenation Assessment	52	100%	99%	99%	100%
Pneumococcal Vaccine	44	55%	59%	69%	94%
Smoking Cessation Advice[1]	6	100%	60%	80%	100%
Surgical Infection Prevention					
Prophylactic Antibiotic Given[5]	-	-	74%	77%	95%
Prophylactic Antibiotic Selection[5]	-	-	91%	90%	100%
Prophylactic Antibiotic Stopped[5]	-	-	72%	72%	95%
Pregnancy Care					
Inpatient Neonatal Mortality	-	-	-	-	-
Third or Fourth Degree Laceration	-	-	3.82%	3.63%	3.27%

Emporia Surgical Hospital

1602 West 15th Street
Emporia, KS 66801
Ownership: Voluntary non-profit - Other
Emergency Services: No
Phone: 620-342-8822
Accredited: No

Measure	Cases	This Hospital	State Average	U.S. Average	Top Hospital
Heart Attack Care					
ACE Inhibitor or ARB for LVSD[5]	-	-	78%	82%	100%
Aspirin at Arrival[5]	-	-	90%	92%	100%
Aspirin at Discharge[5]	-	-	88%	90%	100%
Beta Blocker at Arrival[5]	-	-	82%	87%	100%
Beta Blocker at Discharge[5]	-	-	82%	90%	100%
Fibrinolytic Medication Timing[5]	-	-	24%	31%	100%
PCI Within 90 Minutes of Arrival[5]	-	-	55%	54%	95%
Smoking Cessation Advice[5]	-	-	86%	88%	100%
Heart Failure Care					
ACE Inhibitor or ARB for LVSD[5]	-	-	72%	82%	100%
Discharge Instructions[5]	-	-	41%	61%	93%
Evaluation of LVS Function[5]	-	-	65%	83%	99%
Smoking Cessation Advice[5]	-	-	67%	82%	100%
Pneumonia Care					
Appropriate Initial Antibiotic[5]	-	-	78%	83%	94%
Blood Culture Timing[5]	-	-	93%	90%	100%
Influenza Vaccine[5]	-	-	63%	70%	100%
Initial Antibiotic Timing[5]	-	-	85%	80%	93%
Oxygenation Assessment[5]	-	-	99%	99%	100%
Pneumococcal Vaccine[5]	-	-	59%	69%	94%
Smoking Cessation Advice[5]	-	-	60%	80%	100%
Surgical Infection Prevention					
Prophylactic Antibiotic Given[1,3]	2	100%	74%	77%	95%
Prophylactic Antibiotic Selection	0	-	91%	90%	100%
Prophylactic Antibiotic Stopped[1,3]	2	100%	72%	72%	95%
Pregnancy Care					
Inpatient Neonatal Mortality	-	-	-	-	-
Third or Fourth Degree Laceration	-	-	3.82%	3.63%	3.27%

Newman Regional Health

1201 W 12th Avenue
Emporia, KS 66801
URL: www.newmanrh.org
Ownership: Government - Local
Emergency Services: Yes
Phone: 620-343-6800
Fax: 620-341-7801
Accredited: Yes
Licensed Beds: 122

Key Personnel:
President/CEO. . . . . Terry R Lambert
Chief Medical Staff. . . . . Cy Anderson, MD
Cardiac Lab . . . . Jim Pelch
Catheterization Lab . . . . Jim Pelch

NOTE: Hospital profiles are in alphabetical order by state, then city, then hospital within the city; Rankings are sorted by rate in descending order and exclude hospitals with less than 25 cases; (1) The number of cases is too small (n<25) for purposes of reliably predicting hospital performance; (2) Measure reflects the hospital's indication that its submission was based upon a sample of its relevant discharges; (3) Rate reflects fewer than the maximum possible quarters of data for the measure; (4) Inaccurate information submitted and suppressed for one or more quarters; (5) No data is available from the hospital for this measure; Please refer to the User's Guide for a full explanation of data

Emergency Room . . . . Pam Kvas
Infection Control. . . . . Jami White
ICU . . . . Amy Jarvis
Medical Surgical Nursing . . . . Amy Jarvis
OB/GYN/Women's Health . . . . Cathy McCurdy
Respiratory/Cardiopulmonary. . . . . Jim Pelch

Measure	Cases	This Hospital	State Average	U.S. Average	Top Hospital
Heart Attack Care					
ACE Inhibitor or ARB for LVSD[1]	2	100%	78%	82%	100%
Aspirin at Arrival[1]	15	93%	90%	92%	100%
Aspirin at Discharge[1]	7	100%	88%	90%	100%
Beta Blocker at Arrival[1]	14	93%	82%	87%	100%
Beta Blocker at Discharge[1]	6	100%	82%	90%	100%
Fibrinolytic Medication Timing	0	-	24%	31%	100%
PCI Within 90 Minutes of Arrival	0	-	55%	54%	95%
Smoking Cessation Advice	0	-	86%	88%	100%
Heart Failure Care					
ACE Inhibitor or ARB for LVSD[1]	19	74%	72%	82%	100%
Discharge Instructions	69	68%	41%	61%	93%
Evaluation of LVS Function	104	65%	65%	83%	99%
Smoking Cessation Advice[1]	14	100%	67%	82%	100%
Pneumonia Care					
Appropriate Initial Antibiotic	68	84%	78%	83%	94%
Blood Culture Timing	40	88%	93%	90%	100%
Influenza Vaccine[1]	17	76%	63%	70%	100%
Initial Antibiotic Timing	93	85%	85%	80%	93%
Oxygenation Assessment	106	100%	99%	99%	100%
Pneumococcal Vaccine	74	88%	59%	69%	94%
Smoking Cessation Advice[1]	23	100%	60%	80%	100%
Surgical Infection Prevention					
Prophylactic Antibiotic Given[3]	99	77%	74%	77%	95%
Prophylactic Antibiotic Selection	29	90%	91%	90%	100%
Prophylactic Antibiotic Stopped[3]	81	70%	72%	72%	95%
Pregnancy Care					
Inpatient Neonatal Mortality	-	-	-	-	-
Third or Fourth Degree Laceration	-	-	3.82%	3.63%	3.27%

Greenwood County Hospital

100 W 16th Street
Eureka, KS 67045
Phone: 620-583-7451
Fax: 620-583-6884
Ownership: Government - Local
Accredited: No
Emergency Services: Yes
Licensed Beds: 25

Key Personnel:

CEO. . . . . Bruce Birchell

Measure	Cases	This Hospital	State Average	U.S. Average	Top Hospital
Heart Attack Care					
ACE Inhibitor or ARB for LVSD[5]	-	-	78%	82%	100%
Aspirin at Arrival[5]	-	-	90%	92%	100%
Aspirin at Discharge[5]	-	-	88%	90%	100%
Beta Blocker at Arrival[5]	-	-	82%	87%	100%
Beta Blocker at Discharge[5]	-	-	82%	90%	100%
Fibrinolytic Medication Timing[5]	-	-	24%	31%	100%
PCI Within 90 Minutes of Arrival[5]	-	-	55%	54%	95%
Smoking Cessation Advice[5]	-	-	86%	88%	100%
Heart Failure Care					
ACE Inhibitor or ARB for LVSD[1]	5	20%	72%	82%	100%
Discharge Instructions[1]	9	0%	41%	61%	93%
Evaluation of LVS Function	32	28%	65%	83%	99%
Smoking Cessation Advice[1]	3	33%	67%	82%	100%
Pneumonia Care					
Appropriate Initial Antibiotic[3]	69	62%	78%	83%	94%
Blood Culture Timing[1,3]	19	89%	93%	90%	100%
Influenza Vaccine	30	0%	63%	70%	100%
Initial Antibiotic Timing[1,3]	22	73%	85%	80%	93%
Oxygenation Assessment[3]	93	100%	99%	99%	100%
Pneumococcal Vaccine[3]	56	0%	59%	69%	94%
Smoking Cessation Advice[1,3]	20	15%	60%	80%	100%
Surgical Infection Prevention					
Prophylactic Antibiotic Given[5]	-	-	74%	77%	95%
Prophylactic Antibiotic Selection[5]	-	-	91%	90%	100%
Prophylactic Antibiotic Stopped[5]	-	-	72%	72%	95%
Pregnancy Care					
Inpatient Neonatal Mortality	-	-	-	-	-
Third or Fourth Degree Laceration	-	-	3.82%	3.63%	3.27%

Mercy Health Center

401 Woodland Hills Blvd
Fort Scott, KS 66701
Phone: 316-223-7057
Ownership: Voluntary non-profit - Church
Accredited: Yes
Emergency Services: Yes

Measure	Cases	This Hospital	State Average	U.S. Average	Top Hospital
Heart Attack Care					
ACE Inhibitor or ARB for LVSD[1]	2	100%	78%	82%	100%
Aspirin at Arrival[1]	15	93%	90%	92%	100%
Aspirin at Discharge[1]	10	100%	88%	90%	100%
Beta Blocker at Arrival[1]	13	85%	82%	87%	100%
Beta Blocker at Discharge[1]	11	82%	82%	90%	100%
Fibrinolytic Medication Timing	0	-	24%	31%	100%
PCI Within 90 Minutes of Arrival	0	-	55%	54%	95%
Smoking Cessation Advice[1]	1	100%	86%	88%	100%
Heart Failure Care					
ACE Inhibitor or ARB for LVSD	32	84%	72%	82%	100%
Discharge Instructions	81	85%	41%	61%	93%
Evaluation of LVS Function	111	91%	65%	83%	99%
Smoking Cessation Advice[1]	11	100%	67%	82%	100%
Pneumonia Care					
Appropriate Initial Antibiotic	71	90%	78%	83%	94%
Blood Culture Timing	39	95%	93%	90%	100%
Influenza Vaccine[1]	18	39%	63%	70%	100%
Initial Antibiotic Timing	92	88%	85%	80%	93%
Oxygenation Assessment	107	100%	99%	99%	100%
Pneumococcal Vaccine	64	84%	59%	69%	94%
Smoking Cessation Advice	35	77%	60%	80%	100%
Surgical Infection Prevention					
Prophylactic Antibiotic Given	93	94%	74%	77%	95%
Prophylactic Antibiotic Selection[1]	17	100%	91%	90%	100%
Prophylactic Antibiotic Stopped	84	69%	72%	72%	95%
Pregnancy Care					
Inpatient Neonatal Mortality	-	-	-	-	-
Third or Fourth Degree Laceration	-	-	3.82%	3.63%	3.27%

Fredonia Regional Hospital

1527 Madison Street
Fredonia, KS 66736
Phone: 620-378-2121
Fax: 620-378-3169
URL: www.gpha.com
Ownership: Voluntary non-profit - Other
Accredited: No
Emergency Services: Yes
Licensed Beds: 51

Key Personnel:

President/CEO. . . . . Terry Deschaine
Chief Medical Staff. . . . . Oswaldo Bacami
Emergency Room . . . . Kim Buttler
Infection Control. . . . . Peggy Dole
Respiratory/Cardiopulmonary. . . . . Heather McKenna

Measure	Cases	This Hospital	State Average	U.S. Average	Top Hospital
Heart Attack Care					
ACE Inhibitor or ARB for LVSD[3]	0	-	78%	82%	100%
Aspirin at Arrival[1,3]	1	100%	90%	92%	100%
Aspirin at Discharge[1,3]	2	100%	88%	90%	100%
Beta Blocker at Arrival[1,3]	2	50%	82%	87%	100%
Beta Blocker at Discharge[1,3]	2	50%	82%	90%	100%
Fibrinolytic Medication Timing[3]	0	-	24%	31%	100%
PCI Within 90 Minutes of Arrival[5]	-	-	55%	54%	95%
Smoking Cessation Advice[1,3]	1	0%	86%	88%	100%
Heart Failure Care					
ACE Inhibitor or ARB for LVSD[1]	1	0%	72%	82%	100%
Discharge Instructions[1]	17	0%	41%	61%	93%
Evaluation of LVS Function	27	26%	65%	83%	99%
Smoking Cessation Advice[1]	6	0%	67%	82%	100%
Pneumonia Care					
Appropriate Initial Antibiotic	51	53%	78%	83%	94%

NOTE: Hospital profiles are in alphabetical order by state, then city, then hospital within the city; Rankings are sorted by rate in descending order and exclude hospitals with less than 25 cases; (1) The number of cases is too small (n<25) for purposes of reliably predicting hospital performance; (2) Measure reflects the hospital's indication that its submission was based upon a sample of its relevant discharges; (3) Rate reflects fewer than the maximum possible quarters of data for the measure; (4) Inaccurate information submitted and suppressed for one or more quarters; (5) No data is available from the hospital for this measure; Please refer to the User's Guide for a full explanation of data

Blood Culture Timing[1]	1	0%	93%	90%	100%
Influenza Vaccine[1]	24	4%	63%	70%	100%
Initial Antibiotic Timing	59	88%	85%	80%	93%
Oxygenation Assessment	68	100%	99%	99%	100%
Pneumococcal Vaccine	40	2%	59%	69%	94%
Smoking Cessation Advice[1]	19	5%	60%	80%	100%
Surgical Infection Prevention					
Prophylactic Antibiotic Given[5]	-	-	74%	77%	95%
Prophylactic Antibiotic Selection[5]	-	-	91%	90%	100%
Prophylactic Antibiotic Stopped[5]	-	-	72%	72%	95%
Pregnancy Care					
Inpatient Neonatal Mortality	-	-	-	-	-
Third or Fourth Degree Laceration	-	-	3.82%	3.63%	3.27%

Saint Catherine's Hospital

401 E Spruce
Garden City, KS 67846
URL: www.stcath-hosp.org
Ownership: Voluntary non-profit - Church
Emergency Services: Yes
Phone: 620-272-2222
Fax: 620-272-2528
Accredited: Yes

Key Personnel:
CEO. . . . . Scott Taylor

Measure	Cases	This Hospital	State Average	U.S. Average	Top Hospital
Heart Attack Care					
ACE Inhibitor or ARB for LVSD	0	-	78%	82%	100%
Aspirin at Arrival[1]	9	89%	90%	92%	100%
Aspirin at Discharge[1]	3	100%	88%	90%	100%
Beta Blocker at Arrival[1]	9	67%	82%	87%	100%
Beta Blocker at Discharge[1]	3	67%	82%	90%	100%
Fibrinolytic Medication Timing	0	-	24%	31%	100%
PCI Within 90 Minutes of Arrival	0	-	55%	54%	95%
Smoking Cessation Advice[1]	1	100%	86%	88%	100%
Heart Failure Care					
ACE Inhibitor or ARB for LVSD[1]	10	60%	72%	82%	100%
Discharge Instructions	31	65%	41%	61%	93%
Evaluation of LVS Function	42	57%	65%	83%	99%
Smoking Cessation Advice[1]	6	83%	67%	82%	100%
Pneumonia Care					
Appropriate Initial Antibiotic	74	84%	78%	83%	94%
Blood Culture Timing	48	94%	93%	90%	100%
Influenza Vaccine[4,5]	-	-	63%	70%	100%
Initial Antibiotic Timing	79	82%	85%	80%	93%
Oxygenation Assessment	94	100%	99%	99%	100%
Pneumococcal Vaccine	48	67%	59%	69%	94%
Smoking Cessation Advice[1]	16	50%	60%	80%	100%
Surgical Infection Prevention					
Prophylactic Antibiotic Given	371	67%	74%	77%	95%
Prophylactic Antibiotic Selection	108	44%	91%	90%	100%
Prophylactic Antibiotic Stopped	375	61%	72%	72%	95%
Pregnancy Care					
Inpatient Neonatal Mortality	925	0.00%	-	-	-
Third or Fourth Degree Laceration	665	3.91%	3.82%	3.63%	3.27%

Meadowbrook Rehabilitation Hospital

Alternate Name: Meadowbrook Hospital
427 W Main Street
Gardner, KS 66030
E-mail: meadowbrookadm@clcofltc.org
URL: www.meadowbrookrh.org
Ownership: Voluntary non-profit - Private
Emergency Services: No
Phone: 913-856-8748
Fax: 913-856-8339
Accredited: No
Licensed Beds: 74

Key Personnel:
Administrator . . . . Sharon Bingham
Chief Medical Staff. . . . . Alan Berman
Infection Control. . . . . Carrie Moore
Respiratory/Cardiopulmonary. . . . . David Guardino

Measure	Cases	This Hospital	State Average	U.S. Average	Top Hospital
Heart Attack Care					
ACE Inhibitor or ARB for LVSD[5]	-	-	78%	82%	100%
Aspirin at Arrival[5]	-	-	90%	92%	100%
Aspirin at Discharge[5]	-	-	88%	90%	100%
Beta Blocker at Arrival[5]	-	-	82%	87%	100%
Beta Blocker at Discharge[5]	-	-	82%	90%	100%
Fibrinolytic Medication Timing[5]	-	-	24%	31%	100%
PCI Within 90 Minutes of Arrival[5]	-	-	55%	54%	95%
Smoking Cessation Advice[5]	-	-	86%	88%	100%
Heart Failure Care					
ACE Inhibitor or ARB for LVSD[5]	-	-	72%	82%	100%
Discharge Instructions[5]	-	-	41%	61%	93%
Evaluation of LVS Function[5]	-	-	65%	83%	99%
Smoking Cessation Advice[5]	-	-	67%	82%	100%
Pneumonia Care					
Appropriate Initial Antibiotic[5]	-	-	78%	83%	94%
Blood Culture Timing[5]	-	-	93%	90%	100%
Influenza Vaccine[5]	-	-	63%	70%	100%
Initial Antibiotic Timing[5]	-	-	85%	80%	93%
Oxygenation Assessment[5]	-	-	99%	99%	100%
Pneumococcal Vaccine[5]	-	-	59%	69%	94%
Smoking Cessation Advice[5]	-	-	60%	80%	100%
Surgical Infection Prevention					
Prophylactic Antibiotic Given[5]	-	-	74%	77%	95%
Prophylactic Antibiotic Selection[5]	-	-	91%	90%	100%
Prophylactic Antibiotic Stopped[5]	-	-	72%	72%	95%
Pregnancy Care					
Inpatient Neonatal Mortality	-	-	-	-	-
Third or Fourth Degree Laceration	-	-	3.82%	3.63%	3.27%

Anderson County Hospital

421 South Maple
Garnett, KS 66032
URL: www.saint-lukes.org
Ownership: Voluntary non-profit - Private
Emergency Services: Yes
Phone: 785-448-3131
Fax: 785-448-3118
Accredited: No
Licensed Beds: 47

Key Personnel:
CEO. . . . . Dennis A Hachenberg

Measure	Cases	This Hospital	State Average	U.S. Average	Top Hospital
Heart Attack Care					
ACE Inhibitor or ARB for LVSD[3]	0	-	78%	82%	100%
Aspirin at Arrival[1,3]	1	100%	90%	92%	100%
Aspirin at Discharge[1,3]	1	100%	88%	90%	100%
Beta Blocker at Arrival[3]	0	-	82%	87%	100%
Beta Blocker at Discharge[3]	0	-	82%	90%	100%
Fibrinolytic Medication Timing[3]	0	-	24%	31%	100%
PCI Within 90 Minutes of Arrival[5]	-	-	55%	54%	95%
Smoking Cessation Advice[3]	0	-	86%	88%	100%
Heart Failure Care					
ACE Inhibitor or ARB for LVSD[1]	5	60%	72%	82%	100%
Discharge Instructions[1]	8	50%	41%	61%	93%
Evaluation of LVS Function[1]	16	100%	65%	83%	99%
Smoking Cessation Advice[1]	2	50%	67%	82%	100%
Pneumonia Care					
Appropriate Initial Antibiotic[1]	17	94%	78%	83%	94%
Blood Culture Timing[1]	6	100%	93%	90%	100%
Influenza Vaccine[1]	10	30%	63%	70%	100%
Initial Antibiotic Timing[1]	22	77%	85%	80%	93%
Oxygenation Assessment	26	100%	99%	99%	100%
Pneumococcal Vaccine[1]	15	40%	59%	69%	94%
Smoking Cessation Advice[1]	8	62%	60%	80%	100%
Surgical Infection Prevention					
Prophylactic Antibiotic Given[1,3]	4	75%	74%	77%	95%
Prophylactic Antibiotic Selection[5]	-	-	91%	90%	100%
Prophylactic Antibiotic Stopped[1,3]	4	100%	72%	72%	95%
Pregnancy Care					
Inpatient Neonatal Mortality	-	-	-	-	-
Third or Fourth Degree Laceration	-	-	3.82%	3.63%	3.27%

NOTE: Hospital profiles are in alphabetical order by state, then city, then hospital within the city; Rankings are sorted by rate in descending order and exclude hospitals with less than 25 cases; (1) The number of cases is too small (n<25) for purposes of reliably predicting hospital performance; (2) Measure reflects the hospital's indication that its submission was based upon a sample of its relevant discharges; (3) Rate reflects fewer than the maximum possible quarters of data for the measure; (4) Inaccurate information submitted and suppressed for one or more quarters; (5) No data is available from the hospital for this measure; Please refer to the User's Guide for a full explanation of data

Girard Medical Center

302 N Hospital Drive
Girard, KS 66743
URL: www.hd1cc.com
Ownership: Govt - Hospital District or Authority
Emergency Services: Yes
Phone: 620-724-8291
Fax: 620-724-6332
Accredited: No
Licensed Beds: 38

Key Personnel:

President /CEO . . . . Kenneth Boyd Jr
Chief Medical Staff . . . . Ronald Edwards, MD
Emergency Room . . . . Simon Howayek
ICU . . . . Tammy Simon
Intensive/Coronary . . . . Tammy Simon
Medical Surgical Director . . . . Elaine Weber
Obstetrics Manager . . . . Karen Tompkins-Dobbs
Surgical Services . . . . Carol Diskin, RN
Respiratory/Cardiology . . . . Mark Laforte

Measure	Cases	This Hospital	State Average	U.S. Average	Top Hospital
Heart Attack Care					
ACE Inhibitor or ARB for LVSD[3]	0	-	78%	82%	100%
Aspirin at Arrival[1,3]	2	100%	90%	92%	100%
Aspirin at Discharge[1,3]	1	0%	88%	90%	100%
Beta Blocker at Arrival[1,3]	2	0%	82%	87%	100%
Beta Blocker at Discharge[1,3]	1	0%	82%	90%	100%
Fibrinolytic Medication Timing[1,3]	1	0%	24%	31%	100%
PCI Within 90 Minutes of Arrival[5]	-	-	55%	54%	95%
Smoking Cessation Advice[3]	0	-	86%	88%	100%
Heart Failure Care					
ACE Inhibitor or ARB for LVSD[1]	4	25%	72%	82%	100%
Discharge Instructions[1]	13	69%	41%	61%	93%
Evaluation of LVS Function	34	41%	65%	83%	99%
Smoking Cessation Advice[1]	1	100%	67%	82%	100%
Pneumonia Care					
Appropriate Initial Antibiotic[1]	23	83%	78%	83%	94%
Blood Culture Timing[1,3]	6	100%	93%	90%	100%
Influenza Vaccine[1]	7	57%	63%	70%	100%
Initial Antibiotic Timing	30	73%	85%	80%	93%
Oxygenation Assessment	39	100%	99%	99%	100%
Pneumococcal Vaccine	28	36%	59%	69%	94%
Smoking Cessation Advice[1]	8	62%	60%	80%	100%
Surgical Infection Prevention					
Prophylactic Antibiotic Given	36	47%	74%	77%	95%
Prophylactic Antibiotic Selection[1]	2	100%	91%	90%	100%
Prophylactic Antibiotic Stopped	32	31%	72%	72%	95%
Pregnancy Care					
Inpatient Neonatal Mortality	-	-	-	-	-
Third or Fourth Degree Laceration	-	-	3.82%	3.63%	3.27%

Goodland Regional Medical Center

Alternate Name: Northwest Regional Medical Center
220 W 2nd Street
Goodland, KS 67735
Ownership: Government - Local
Emergency Services: Yes
Phone: 785-890-3625
Fax: 785-890-7209
Accredited: No
Licensed Beds: 25

Key Personnel:

CEO . . . . Jay Jolly
Chief of Medical Staff . . . . Travis Daise, MD
Emergency Room . . . . Kathy Erickson, RN
Infection Control . . . . Karen Hooker, RRT
Medical Surgical Nursing . . . . Candi Douthit, RN
Respiratory/Cardiopulmonary . . . . Karen Hooker, RRT

Measure	Cases	This Hospital	State Average	U.S. Average	Top Hospital
Heart Attack Care					
ACE Inhibitor or ARB for LVSD[2,3]	0	-	78%	82%	100%
Aspirin at Arrival[1,2,3]	1	100%	90%	92%	100%
Aspirin at Discharge[1,2,3]	1	100%	88%	90%	100%
Beta Blocker at Arrival[1,2,3]	1	100%	82%	87%	100%
Beta Blocker at Discharge[1,2,3]	1	100%	82%	90%	100%
Fibrinolytic Medication Timing[2,3]	0	-	24%	31%	100%
PCI Within 90 Minutes of Arrival[2]	0	-	55%	54%	95%
Smoking Cessation Advice[2,3]	0	-	86%	88%	100%
Heart Failure Care					
ACE Inhibitor or ARB for LVSD[1,2]	4	50%	72%	82%	100%
Discharge Instructions[1,2]	9	33%	41%	61%	93%
Evaluation of LVS Function[1,2]	18	56%	65%	83%	99%
Smoking Cessation Advice[1,2]	1	100%	67%	82%	100%
Pneumonia Care					
Appropriate Initial Antibiotic[1,2]	18	89%	78%	83%	94%
Blood Culture Timing[1,2]	5	100%	93%	90%	100%
Influenza Vaccine[1,2]	13	8%	63%	70%	100%
Initial Antibiotic Timing[2]	31	81%	85%	80%	93%
Oxygenation Assessment[2]	37	100%	99%	99%	100%
Pneumococcal Vaccine[2]	29	41%	59%	69%	94%
Smoking Cessation Advice[1,2]	4	25%	60%	80%	100%
Surgical Infection Prevention					
Prophylactic Antibiotic Given[5]	-	-	74%	77%	95%
Prophylactic Antibiotic Selection[5]	-	-	91%	90%	100%
Prophylactic Antibiotic Stopped[5]	-	-	72%	72%	95%
Pregnancy Care					
Inpatient Neonatal Mortality	-	-	-	-	-
Third or Fourth Degree Laceration	-	-	3.82%	3.63%	3.27%

Central Kansas Medical Center

Alternate Name: Saint Rose Hospital Campus
3515 Broadway Street
Great Bend, KS 67530
URL: www.ckmc.org
Ownership: Voluntary non-profit - Church
Emergency Services: Yes
Phone: 620-792-2511
Fax: 620-786-6298
Accredited: Yes
Licensed Beds: 367

Key Personnel:

President/CEO . . . . Chris Thomas
Chief Medical Staff . . . . William Slater, MD
Manager OB/GYN Womens Health . . . . Jennifer Johnson
Manager Radiology . . . . Elaine Felke

Measure	Cases	This Hospital	State Average	U.S. Average	Top Hospital
Heart Attack Care					
ACE Inhibitor or ARB for LVSD	0	-	78%	82%	100%
Aspirin at Arrival[1]	14	93%	90%	92%	100%
Aspirin at Discharge[1]	6	100%	88%	90%	100%
Beta Blocker at Arrival[1]	13	62%	82%	87%	100%
Beta Blocker at Discharge[1]	10	70%	82%	90%	100%
Fibrinolytic Medication Timing	0	-	24%	31%	100%
PCI Within 90 Minutes of Arrival	0	-	55%	54%	95%
Smoking Cessation Advice	0	-	86%	88%	100%
Heart Failure Care					
ACE Inhibitor or ARB for LVSD[1]	7	57%	72%	82%	100%
Discharge Instructions	28	18%	41%	61%	93%
Evaluation of LVS Function	45	62%	65%	83%	99%
Smoking Cessation Advice[1]	4	75%	67%	82%	100%
Pneumonia Care					
Appropriate Initial Antibiotic	35	94%	78%	83%	94%
Blood Culture Timing[1]	12	100%	93%	90%	100%
Influenza Vaccine[1]	10	50%	63%	70%	100%
Initial Antibiotic Timing	45	91%	85%	80%	93%
Oxygenation Assessment	59	100%	99%	99%	100%
Pneumococcal Vaccine	47	43%	59%	69%	94%
Smoking Cessation Advice[1]	8	75%	60%	80%	100%
Surgical Infection Prevention					
Prophylactic Antibiotic Given[3]	146	22%	74%	77%	95%
Prophylactic Antibiotic Selection	49	94%	91%	90%	100%
Prophylactic Antibiotic Stopped[3]	145	11%	72%	72%	95%
Pregnancy Care					
Inpatient Neonatal Mortality	433	0.92%	-	-	-
Third or Fourth Degree Laceration	276	3.62%	3.82%	3.63%	3.27%

Surgical and Diagnostic Center of Great Bend

514 Cleveland Street
Great Bend, KS 67530
Ownership: Proprietary
Emergency Services: No
Phone: 620-792-8833
Accredited: No

Measure	Cases	This Hospital	State Average	U.S. Average	Top Hospital
Heart Attack Care					

NOTE: Hospital profiles are in alphabetical order by state, then city, then hospital within the city; Rankings are sorted by rate in descending order and exclude hospitals with less than 25 cases; (1) The number of cases is too small (n<25) for purposes of reliably predicting hospital performance; (2) Measure reflects the hospital's indication that its submission was based upon a sample of its relevant discharges; (3) Rate reflects fewer than the maximum possible quarters of data for the measure; (4) Inaccurate information submitted and suppressed for one or more quarters; (5) No data is available from the hospital for this measure; Please refer to the User's Guide for a full explanation of data

Measure	Cases	This Hospital	State Average	U.S. Average	Top Hospital
ACE Inhibitor or ARB for LVSD[5]	-	-	78%	82%	100%
Aspirin at Arrival[5]	-	-	90%	92%	100%
Aspirin at Discharge[5]	-	-	88%	90%	100%
Beta Blocker at Arrival[5]	-	-	82%	87%	100%
Beta Blocker at Discharge[5]	-	-	82%	90%	100%
Fibrinolytic Medication Timing[5]	-	-	24%	31%	100%
PCI Within 90 Minutes of Arrival[5]	-	-	55%	54%	95%
Smoking Cessation Advice[5]	-	-	86%	88%	100%
Heart Failure Care					
ACE Inhibitor or ARB for LVSD[5]	-	-	72%	82%	100%
Discharge Instructions[5]	-	-	41%	61%	93%
Evaluation of LVS Function[5]	-	-	65%	83%	99%
Smoking Cessation Advice[5]	-	-	67%	82%	100%
Pneumonia Care					
Appropriate Initial Antibiotic[5]	-	-	78%	83%	94%
Blood Culture Timing[5]	-	-	93%	90%	100%
Influenza Vaccine[5]	-	-	63%	70%	100%
Initial Antibiotic Timing[5]	-	-	85%	80%	93%
Oxygenation Assessment[5]	-	-	99%	99%	100%
Pneumococcal Vaccine[5]	-	-	59%	69%	94%
Smoking Cessation Advice[5]	-	-	60%	80%	100%
Surgical Infection Prevention					
Prophylactic Antibiotic Given[1,2,3]	23	91%	74%	77%	95%
Prophylactic Antibiotic Selection[5]	-	-	91%	90%	100%
Prophylactic Antibiotic Stopped[1,2,3]	23	30%	72%	72%	95%
Pregnancy Care					
Inpatient Neonatal Mortality	-	-	-	-	-
Third or Fourth Degree Laceration	-	-	3.82%	3.63%	3.27%

Harper Hospital/District #5

Alternate Name: Harper Hospital
1204 Maple Street
Harper, KS 67058
URL: www.harperhosp.com
Ownership: Govt - Hospital District or Authority
Emergency Services: Yes

Phone: 620-896-7324
Fax: 620-896-7127
Accredited: No
Licensed Beds: 25

Key Personnel:
CEO. . . . . Kim Cinelli
Chief Medical Staff. . . . . Dr R E Bellar
Emergency Room . . . . Martha Ediger
Infection Control. . . . . Nearaj Vasishtha
Surgical Services . . . . Donald Ransom, DO

Measure	Cases	This Hospital	State Average	U.S. Average	Top Hospital
Heart Attack Care					
ACE Inhibitor or ARB for LVSD[3]	0	-	78%	82%	100%
Aspirin at Arrival[1,3]	1	100%	90%	92%	100%
Aspirin at Discharge[3]	0	-	88%	90%	100%
Beta Blocker at Arrival[1,3]	1	100%	82%	87%	100%
Beta Blocker at Discharge[3]	0	-	82%	90%	100%
Fibrinolytic Medication Timing[3]	0	-	24%	31%	100%
PCI Within 90 Minutes of Arrival[5]	-	-	55%	54%	95%
Smoking Cessation Advice[3]	0	-	86%	88%	100%
Heart Failure Care					
ACE Inhibitor or ARB for LVSD[1]	3	33%	72%	82%	100%
Discharge Instructions[1]	5	0%	41%	61%	93%
Evaluation of LVS Function[1]	17	29%	65%	83%	99%
Smoking Cessation Advice[1]	1	0%	67%	82%	100%
Pneumonia Care					
Appropriate Initial Antibiotic[1,3]	22	86%	78%	83%	94%
Blood Culture Timing[1,3]	2	100%	93%	90%	100%
Influenza Vaccine[1]	10	0%	63%	70%	100%
Initial Antibiotic Timing[1,3]	22	100%	85%	80%	93%
Oxygenation Assessment[1,3]	24	100%	99%	99%	100%
Pneumococcal Vaccine[1,3]	20	5%	59%	69%	94%
Smoking Cessation Advice[1,3]	4	0%	60%	80%	100%
Surgical Infection Prevention					
Prophylactic Antibiotic Given[1,3]	1	0%	74%	77%	95%
Prophylactic Antibiotic Selection[5]	-	-	91%	90%	100%
Prophylactic Antibiotic Stopped[1,3]	1	100%	72%	72%	95%
Pregnancy Care					
Inpatient Neonatal Mortality	-	-	-	-	-
Third or Fourth Degree Laceration	-	-	3.82%	3.63%	3.27%

Hays Medical Center

2220 Canterbury Drive
Hays, KS 67601
URL: www.haysmed.com
Ownership: Voluntary non-profit - Private
Emergency Services: Yes

Phone: 785-623-5000
Fax: 785-623-5627
Accredited: Yes
Licensed Beds: 158

Key Personnel:
CEO. . . . . John Jeter

Measure	Cases	This Hospital	State Average	U.S. Average	Top Hospital
Heart Attack Care					
ACE Inhibitor or ARB for LVSD	39	87%	78%	82%	100%
Aspirin at Arrival	64	94%	90%	92%	100%
Aspirin at Discharge	156	96%	88%	90%	100%
Beta Blocker at Arrival	54	89%	82%	87%	100%
Beta Blocker at Discharge	158	94%	82%	90%	100%
Fibrinolytic Medication Timing	0	-	24%	31%	100%
PCI Within 90 Minutes of Arrival[1]	8	75%	55%	54%	95%
Smoking Cessation Advice	42	98%	86%	88%	100%
Heart Failure Care					
ACE Inhibitor or ARB for LVSD	48	92%	72%	82%	100%
Discharge Instructions	106	73%	41%	61%	93%
Evaluation of LVS Function	145	86%	65%	83%	99%
Smoking Cessation Advice	26	100%	67%	82%	100%
Pneumonia Care					
Appropriate Initial Antibiotic[2]	80	70%	78%	83%	94%
Blood Culture Timing[2]	42	90%	93%	90%	100%
Influenza Vaccine[1,2]	21	86%	63%	70%	100%
Initial Antibiotic Timing[2]	98	88%	85%	80%	93%
Oxygenation Assessment[2]	131	100%	99%	99%	100%
Pneumococcal Vaccine[2]	99	86%	59%	69%	94%
Smoking Cessation Advice[1,2]	20	95%	60%	80%	100%
Surgical Infection Prevention					
Prophylactic Antibiotic Given[2]	322	84%	74%	77%	95%
Prophylactic Antibiotic Selection[2]	80	91%	91%	90%	100%
Prophylactic Antibiotic Stopped[2]	308	48%	72%	72%	95%
Pregnancy Care					
Inpatient Neonatal Mortality[2]	244	0.00%	-	-	-
Third or Fourth Degree Laceration[2]	155	9.68%	3.82%	3.63%	3.27%

Herington Municipal Hospital

100 E Helen
Herington, KS 67449
Ownership: Government - Local
Emergency Services: Yes

Phone: 785-258-2207
Fax: 785-258-5127
Accredited: No
Licensed Beds: 20

Key Personnel:
Administrator . . . . Mary Steiner
Chief Medical Staff. . . . . John Mosier
Director Infection/Disease Control . . . . Marge Bergstrom, RN
OB/GYN Womens Health. . . . . John R Whitehead, DO
Chief Radiology . . . . Gary Copeland, MD
Director Respiratory Therapy . . . . Colleen Greenemeyer

Measure	Cases	This Hospital	State Average	U.S. Average	Top Hospital
Heart Attack Care					
ACE Inhibitor or ARB for LVSD[3]	0	-	78%	82%	100%
Aspirin at Arrival[1,3]	1	100%	90%	92%	100%
Aspirin at Discharge[3]	0	-	88%	90%	100%
Beta Blocker at Arrival[3]	0	-	82%	87%	100%
Beta Blocker at Discharge[3]	0	-	82%	90%	100%
Fibrinolytic Medication Timing[3]	0	-	24%	31%	100%
PCI Within 90 Minutes of Arrival[5]	-	-	55%	54%	95%
Smoking Cessation Advice[3]	0	-	86%	88%	100%
Heart Failure Care					
ACE Inhibitor or ARB for LVSD[3]	0	-	72%	82%	100%
Discharge Instructions[3]	0	-	41%	61%	93%
Evaluation of LVS Function[3]	0	-	65%	83%	99%
Smoking Cessation Advice[3]	0	-	67%	82%	100%
Pneumonia Care					

NOTE: Hospital profiles are in alphabetical order by state, then city, then hospital within the city; Rankings are sorted by rate in descending order and exclude hospitals with less than 25 cases; (1) The number of cases is too small (n<25) for purposes of reliably predicting hospital performance; (2) Measure reflects the hospital's indication that its submission was based upon a sample of its relevant discharges; (3) Rate reflects fewer than the maximum possible quarters of data for the measure; (4) Inaccurate information submitted and suppressed for one or more quarters; (5) No data is available from the hospital for this measure; Please refer to the User's Guide for a full explanation of data

Measure	Cases	This Hospital	State Average	U.S. Average	Top Hospital
Appropriate Initial Antibiotic[1,3]	12	92%	78%	83%	94%
Blood Culture Timing[3]	0	-	93%	90%	100%
Influenza Vaccine[1]	8	88%	63%	70%	100%
Initial Antibiotic Timing[1,3]	15	87%	85%	80%	93%
Oxygenation Assessment[1,3]	16	100%	99%	99%	100%
Pneumococcal Vaccine[1,3]	11	64%	59%	69%	94%
Smoking Cessation Advice[1,3]	2	50%	60%	80%	100%
Surgical Infection Prevention					
Prophylactic Antibiotic Given[5]	-	-	74%	77%	95%
Prophylactic Antibiotic Selection[5]	-	-	91%	90%	100%
Prophylactic Antibiotic Stopped[5]	-	-	72%	72%	95%
Pregnancy Care					
Inpatient Neonatal Mortality	-	-	-	-	-
Third or Fourth Degree Laceration	-	-	3.82%	3.63%	3.27%

Hiawatha Community Hospital

300 Utah Street
Hiawatha, KS 66434
Phone: 785-742-2131
Ownership: Voluntary non-profit - Private
Accredited: No
Emergency Services: Yes

Measure	Cases	This Hospital	State Average	U.S. Average	Top Hospital
Heart Attack Care					
ACE Inhibitor or ARB for LVSD[1,3]	1	0%	78%	82%	100%
Aspirin at Arrival[1,3]	2	100%	90%	92%	100%
Aspirin at Discharge[1,3]	2	100%	88%	90%	100%
Beta Blocker at Arrival[1,3]	1	100%	82%	87%	100%
Beta Blocker at Discharge[1,3]	2	100%	82%	90%	100%
Fibrinolytic Medication Timing[3]	0	-	24%	31%	100%
PCI Within 90 Minutes of Arrival	0	-	55%	54%	95%
Smoking Cessation Advice[3]	0	-	86%	88%	100%
Heart Failure Care					
ACE Inhibitor or ARB for LVSD[1]	10	90%	72%	82%	100%
Discharge Instructions[1]	21	5%	41%	61%	93%
Evaluation of LVS Function	42	71%	65%	83%	99%
Smoking Cessation Advice[1]	7	14%	67%	82%	100%
Pneumonia Care					
Appropriate Initial Antibiotic[1]	13	85%	78%	83%	94%
Blood Culture Timing[1]	3	100%	93%	90%	100%
Influenza Vaccine[1]	5	80%	63%	70%	100%
Initial Antibiotic Timing[1]	20	90%	85%	80%	93%
Oxygenation Assessment[1]	23	100%	99%	99%	100%
Pneumococcal Vaccine[1]	17	71%	59%	69%	94%
Smoking Cessation Advice[1]	5	0%	60%	80%	100%
Surgical Infection Prevention					
Prophylactic Antibiotic Given	36	61%	74%	77%	95%
Prophylactic Antibiotic Selection[1]	11	100%	91%	90%	100%
Prophylactic Antibiotic Stopped	34	91%	72%	72%	95%
Pregnancy Care					
Inpatient Neonatal Mortality	-	-	-	-	-
Third or Fourth Degree Laceration	-	-	3.82%	3.63%	3.27%

Hillsboro Community Medical Center

Alternate Name: Salem Hospital
701 S Main Street
Hillsboro, KS 67063
Phone: 620-947-3114
Fax: 620-947-5690
E-mail: comf@southwind.net
URL: www.hillsboromedicalcenter.org
Ownership: Voluntary non-profit - Private
Accredited: No
Emergency Services: Yes
Licensed Beds: 79

Key Personnel:

Administrator/CEO . . . . Michael Ryan
Chief Medical Staff . . . . A Randal Claassen
Director Infection/Disease Control . . . . Cayle Goertzen, MT
Director Medical/Surgical Nursing . . . . Jan Fenske, RN
OB/GYN Womens Health . . . . Jan Fenske, RN
Director Radiology . . . . Billie Kueser
Director Respiratory Therapy . . . . Ken Johnson, RT

Measure	Cases	This Hospital	State Average	U.S. Average	Top Hospital
Heart Attack Care					
ACE Inhibitor or ARB for LVSD[1,3]	1	100%	78%	82%	100%
Aspirin at Arrival[1,3]	1	100%	90%	92%	100%
Aspirin at Discharge[3]	0	-	88%	90%	100%
Beta Blocker at Arrival[1,3]	2	100%	82%	87%	100%
Beta Blocker at Discharge[1,3]	2	100%	82%	90%	100%
Fibrinolytic Medication Timing[3]	0	-	24%	31%	100%
PCI Within 90 Minutes of Arrival	0	-	55%	54%	95%
Smoking Cessation Advice[3]	0	-	86%	88%	100%
Heart Failure Care					
ACE Inhibitor or ARB for LVSD[1]	1	100%	72%	82%	100%
Discharge Instructions[1]	2	0%	41%	61%	93%
Evaluation of LVS Function[1]	15	53%	65%	83%	99%
Smoking Cessation Advice[1]	1	0%	67%	82%	100%
Pneumonia Care					
Appropriate Initial Antibiotic[1,3]	5	60%	78%	83%	94%
Blood Culture Timing[3]	0	-	93%	90%	100%
Influenza Vaccine[1]	2	0%	63%	70%	100%
Initial Antibiotic Timing[1,3]	5	100%	85%	80%	93%
Oxygenation Assessment[1,3]	9	100%	99%	99%	100%
Pneumococcal Vaccine[1,3]	5	0%	59%	69%	94%
Smoking Cessation Advice[3]	0	-	60%	80%	100%
Surgical Infection Prevention					
Prophylactic Antibiotic Given[5]	-	-	74%	77%	95%
Prophylactic Antibiotic Selection[5]	-	-	91%	90%	100%
Prophylactic Antibiotic Stopped[5]	-	-	72%	72%	95%
Pregnancy Care					
Inpatient Neonatal Mortality	-	-	-	-	-
Third or Fourth Degree Laceration	-	-	3.82%	3.63%	3.27%

Holton Community Hospital

1110 Columbine Dr
Holton, KS 66436
Phone: 785-364-9645
Ownership: Voluntary non-profit - Private
Accredited: No
Emergency Services: Yes

Measure	Cases	This Hospital	State Average	U.S. Average	Top Hospital
Heart Attack Care					
ACE Inhibitor or ARB for LVSD[5]	-	-	78%	82%	100%
Aspirin at Arrival[5]	-	-	90%	92%	100%
Aspirin at Discharge[5]	-	-	88%	90%	100%
Beta Blocker at Arrival[5]	-	-	82%	87%	100%
Beta Blocker at Discharge[5]	-	-	82%	90%	100%
Fibrinolytic Medication Timing[5]	-	-	24%	31%	100%
PCI Within 90 Minutes of Arrival[5]	-	-	55%	54%	95%
Smoking Cessation Advice[5]	-	-	86%	88%	100%
Heart Failure Care					
ACE Inhibitor or ARB for LVSD[1]	5	80%	72%	82%	100%
Discharge Instructions[1]	14	7%	41%	61%	93%
Evaluation of LVS Function[1]	17	47%	65%	83%	99%
Smoking Cessation Advice[1]	1	100%	67%	82%	100%
Pneumonia Care					
Appropriate Initial Antibiotic[1]	11	36%	78%	83%	94%
Blood Culture Timing[1]	1	100%	93%	90%	100%
Influenza Vaccine	0	-	63%	70%	100%
Initial Antibiotic Timing[1]	9	89%	85%	80%	93%
Oxygenation Assessment[1]	13	92%	99%	99%	100%
Pneumococcal Vaccine[1]	5	80%	59%	69%	94%
Smoking Cessation Advice[1]	2	100%	60%	80%	100%
Surgical Infection Prevention					
Prophylactic Antibiotic Given[5]	-	-	74%	77%	95%
Prophylactic Antibiotic Selection[5]	-	-	91%	90%	100%
Prophylactic Antibiotic Stopped[5]	-	-	72%	72%	95%
Pregnancy Care					
Inpatient Neonatal Mortality	-	-	-	-	-
Third or Fourth Degree Laceration	-	-	3.82%	3.63%	3.27%

NOTE: Hospital profiles are in alphabetical order by state, then city, then hospital within the city; Rankings are sorted by rate in descending order and exclude hospitals with less than 25 cases; (1) The number of cases is too small (n<25) for purposes of reliably predicting hospital performance; (2) Measure reflects the hospital's indication that its submission was based upon a sample of its relevant discharges; (3) Rate reflects fewer than the maximum possible quarters of data for the measure; (4) Inaccurate information submitted and suppressed for one or more quarters; (5) No data is available from the hospital for this measure; Please refer to the User's Guide for a full explanation of data

Hutchinson Hospital

1701 E 23rd Street
Hutchinson, KS 67502
E-mail: info@hhosp.com
URL: hutchinsonhospital.com
Ownership: Government - Federal
Emergency Services: Yes
Phone: 620-665-2000
Fax: 620-513-3811
Accredited: No
Licensed Beds: 200

Key Personnel:
President/CEO. . . . . Gene E Schmidt

Measure	Cases	This Hospital	State Average	U.S. Average	Top Hospital
Heart Attack Care					
ACE Inhibitor or ARB for LVSD	55	85%	78%	82%	100%
Aspirin at Arrival	178	98%	90%	92%	100%
Aspirin at Discharge	214	94%	88%	90%	100%
Beta Blocker at Arrival	149	92%	82%	87%	100%
Beta Blocker at Discharge	198	86%	82%	90%	100%
Fibrinolytic Medication Timing	0	-	24%	31%	100%
PCI Within 90 Minutes of Arrival[1]	10	100%	55%	54%	95%
Smoking Cessation Advice	70	84%	86%	88%	100%
Heart Failure Care					
ACE Inhibitor or ARB for LVSD	64	89%	72%	82%	100%
Discharge Instructions	156	56%	41%	61%	93%
Evaluation of LVS Function	206	72%	65%	83%	99%
Smoking Cessation Advice	28	93%	67%	82%	100%
Pneumonia Care					
Appropriate Initial Antibiotic	148	74%	78%	83%	94%
Blood Culture Timing	74	95%	93%	90%	100%
Influenza Vaccine	44	77%	63%	70%	100%
Initial Antibiotic Timing	211	65%	85%	80%	93%
Oxygenation Assessment	277	100%	99%	99%	100%
Pneumococcal Vaccine	178	55%	59%	69%	94%
Smoking Cessation Advice	61	87%	60%	80%	100%
Surgical Infection Prevention					
Prophylactic Antibiotic Given[2]	803	90%	74%	77%	95%
Prophylactic Antibiotic Selection[2]	182	96%	91%	90%	100%
Prophylactic Antibiotic Stopped[2]	787	84%	72%	72%	95%
Pregnancy Care					
Inpatient Neonatal Mortality	-	-	-	-	-
Third or Fourth Degree Laceration	-	-	3.82%	3.63%	3.27%

Summit Surgical

1818 East 23rd Avenue
Hutchinson, KS 67502
Ownership: Proprietary
Emergency Services: No
Phone: 620-663-4800
Accredited: No

Measure	Cases	This Hospital	State Average	U.S. Average	Top Hospital
Heart Attack Care					
ACE Inhibitor or ARB for LVSD[5]	-	-	78%	82%	100%
Aspirin at Arrival[5]	-	-	90%	92%	100%
Aspirin at Discharge[5]	-	-	88%	90%	100%
Beta Blocker at Arrival[5]	-	-	82%	87%	100%
Beta Blocker at Discharge[5]	-	-	82%	90%	100%
Fibrinolytic Medication Timing[5]	-	-	24%	31%	100%
PCI Within 90 Minutes of Arrival[5]	-	-	55%	54%	95%
Smoking Cessation Advice[5]	-	-	86%	88%	100%
Heart Failure Care					
ACE Inhibitor or ARB for LVSD[5]	-	-	72%	82%	100%
Discharge Instructions[5]	-	-	41%	61%	93%
Evaluation of LVS Function[5]	-	-	65%	83%	99%
Smoking Cessation Advice[5]	-	-	67%	82%	100%
Pneumonia Care					
Appropriate Initial Antibiotic[5]	-	-	78%	83%	94%
Blood Culture Timing[5]	-	-	93%	90%	100%
Influenza Vaccine[5]	-	-	63%	70%	100%
Initial Antibiotic Timing[5]	-	-	85%	80%	93%
Oxygenation Assessment[5]	-	-	99%	99%	100%
Pneumococcal Vaccine[5]	-	-	59%	69%	94%
Smoking Cessation Advice[5]	-	-	60%	80%	100%
Surgical Infection Prevention					
Prophylactic Antibiotic Given[5]	-	-	74%	77%	95%
Prophylactic Antibiotic Selection[5]	-	-	91%	90%	100%
Prophylactic Antibiotic Stopped[5]	-	-	72%	72%	95%
Pregnancy Care					
Inpatient Neonatal Mortality	-	-	-	-	-
Third or Fourth Degree Laceration	-	-	3.82%	3.63%	3.27%

Mercy Hospital-Independence

800 W Myrtle
Independence, KS 67301
URL: www.mercykansas.com
Ownership: Voluntary non-profit - Church
Emergency Services: Yes
Phone: 620-331-2200
Fax: 620-332-3270
Accredited: Yes
Licensed Beds: 93

Key Personnel:
CEO. . . . . John Woodrich
Chief Medical Staff. . . . . Cathey Henisey
Emergency Room . . . . Charles Empson, MD
Director Infection/Disease Control . . . . Michelle Foreman
CCU Spvg. Nurse . . . . Michelle Foreman
Chief Radiology . . . . Kevin Hamm, MD
Director Respiratory Therapy . . . . Todd Kahler

Measure	Cases	This Hospital	State Average	U.S. Average	Top Hospital
Heart Attack Care					
ACE Inhibitor or ARB for LVSD[1,3]	1	100%	78%	82%	100%
Aspirin at Arrival[1,3]	5	80%	90%	92%	100%
Aspirin at Discharge[1,3]	2	100%	88%	90%	100%
Beta Blocker at Arrival[1,3]	5	100%	82%	87%	100%
Beta Blocker at Discharge[1,3]	3	100%	82%	90%	100%
Fibrinolytic Medication Timing[3]	0	-	24%	31%	100%
PCI Within 90 Minutes of Arrival	0	-	55%	54%	95%
Smoking Cessation Advice[3]	0	-	86%	88%	100%
Heart Failure Care					
ACE Inhibitor or ARB for LVSD[1]	16	100%	72%	82%	100%
Discharge Instructions	46	93%	41%	61%	93%
Evaluation of LVS Function	71	92%	65%	83%	99%
Smoking Cessation Advice[1]	11	100%	67%	82%	100%
Pneumonia Care					
Appropriate Initial Antibiotic	48	90%	78%	83%	94%
Blood Culture Timing	39	95%	93%	90%	100%
Influenza Vaccine[1]	16	50%	63%	70%	100%
Initial Antibiotic Timing	71	73%	85%	80%	93%
Oxygenation Assessment	81	100%	99%	99%	100%
Pneumococcal Vaccine	56	77%	59%	69%	94%
Smoking Cessation Advice[1]	17	100%	60%	80%	100%
Surgical Infection Prevention					
Prophylactic Antibiotic Given	103	83%	74%	77%	95%
Prophylactic Antibiotic Selection	25	96%	91%	90%	100%
Prophylactic Antibiotic Stopped	97	81%	72%	72%	95%
Pregnancy Care					
Inpatient Neonatal Mortality	-	-	-	-	-
Third or Fourth Degree Laceration	-	-	3.82%	3.63%	3.27%

Allen County Hospital

101 S First Street
Iola, KS 66749
URL: www.allencountyhospital.com
Ownership: Proprietary
Emergency Services: Yes
Toll-Free: 888-922-3131
Phone: 620-365-1000
Fax: 620-365-1140
Accredited: No
Licensed Beds: 25

Key Personnel:
CEO. . . . . Jennifer Jackman

Measure	Cases	This Hospital	State Average	U.S. Average	Top Hospital
Heart Attack Care					
ACE Inhibitor or ARB for LVSD[3]	0	-	78%	82%	100%
Aspirin at Arrival[1,3]	1	100%	90%	92%	100%
Aspirin at Discharge[1,3]	1	100%	88%	90%	100%
Beta Blocker at Arrival[1,3]	1	100%	82%	87%	100%
Beta Blocker at Discharge[1,3]	1	100%	82%	90%	100%
Fibrinolytic Medication Timing[3]	0	-	24%	31%	100%
PCI Within 90 Minutes of Arrival[5]	-	-	55%	54%	95%
Smoking Cessation Advice[3]	0	-	86%	88%	100%

NOTE: Hospital profiles are in alphabetical order by state, then city, then hospital within the city; Rankings are sorted by rate in descending order and exclude hospitals with less than 25 cases; (1) The number of cases is too small (n<25) for purposes of reliably predicting hospital performance; (2) Measure reflects the hospital's indication that its submission was based upon a sample of its relevant discharges; (3) Rate reflects fewer than the maximum possible quarters of data for the measure; (4) Inaccurate information submitted and suppressed for one or more quarters; (5) No data is available from the hospital for this measure; Please refer to the User's Guide for a full explanation of data

Measure	Cases	This Hospital	State Average	U.S. Average	Top Hospital
Heart Failure Care					
ACE Inhibitor or ARB for LVSD[1]	3	100%	72%	82%	100%
Discharge Instructions	26	69%	41%	61%	93%
Evaluation of LVS Function	30	53%	65%	83%	99%
Smoking Cessation Advice	0	-	67%	82%	100%
Pneumonia Care					
Appropriate Initial Antibiotic	32	97%	78%	83%	94%
Blood Culture Timing[1]	19	95%	93%	90%	100%
Influenza Vaccine[1]	10	40%	63%	70%	100%
Initial Antibiotic Timing	49	84%	85%	80%	93%
Oxygenation Assessment	57	100%	99%	99%	100%
Pneumococcal Vaccine	37	46%	59%	69%	94%
Smoking Cessation Advice[1]	15	100%	60%	80%	100%
Surgical Infection Prevention					
Prophylactic Antibiotic Given[1,2,3]	24	92%	74%	77%	95%
Prophylactic Antibiotic Selection[1,2]	9	100%	91%	90%	100%
Prophylactic Antibiotic Stopped[1,2,3]	23	100%	72%	72%	95%
Pregnancy Care					
Inpatient Neonatal Mortality	-	-	-	-	-
Third or Fourth Degree Laceration	-	-	3.82%	3.63%	3.27%

Geary Community Hospital

1102 St Marys Road
PO Box 490
Junction City, KS 66441
E-mail: ceo@gchks.org
URL: www.gchks.org
Ownership: Government - Local
Emergency Services: Yes

Phone: 785-238-4131
Fax: 785-238-5278
Accredited: Yes
Licensed Beds: 92

Key Personnel:
President/CEO. . . . . David K Bradley, CHE
Chief Medical Staff. . . . . Charles Bollman, MD
Emergency Room . . . . Louise Buxman, RN
Infection Control. . . . . Sandy Grant, RN
ICU . . . . Jolene Stackhouse, RN
Medical/Surgical Nursing . . . . Laurel Peterson, RN
OB/GYN Womens Health. . . . . Dawn Engel
Respiratory/Cardiopulmonary. . . . . Bob Kimbrell

Measure	Cases	This Hospital	State Average	U.S. Average	Top Hospital
Heart Attack Care					
ACE Inhibitor or ARB for LVSD	0	-	78%	82%	100%
Aspirin at Arrival[1]	8	75%	90%	92%	100%
Aspirin at Discharge[1]	2	50%	88%	90%	100%
Beta Blocker at Arrival[1]	5	60%	82%	87%	100%
Beta Blocker at Discharge[1]	3	67%	82%	90%	100%
Fibrinolytic Medication Timing[1]	1	0%	24%	31%	100%
PCI Within 90 Minutes of Arrival	0	-	55%	54%	95%
Smoking Cessation Advice	0	-	86%	88%	100%
Heart Failure Care					
ACE Inhibitor or ARB for LVSD[1]	22	82%	72%	82%	100%
Discharge Instructions	52	98%	41%	61%	93%
Evaluation of LVS Function	66	64%	65%	83%	99%
Smoking Cessation Advice[1]	19	95%	67%	82%	100%
Pneumonia Care					
Appropriate Initial Antibiotic	65	85%	78%	83%	94%
Blood Culture Timing[1]	18	89%	93%	90%	100%
Influenza Vaccine[1]	17	41%	63%	70%	100%
Initial Antibiotic Timing	85	89%	85%	80%	93%
Oxygenation Assessment	91	100%	99%	99%	100%
Pneumococcal Vaccine	59	46%	59%	69%	94%
Smoking Cessation Advice[1]	19	95%	60%	80%	100%
Surgical Infection Prevention					
Prophylactic Antibiotic Given[3]	65	75%	74%	77%	95%
Prophylactic Antibiotic Selection[1]	16	88%	91%	90%	100%
Prophylactic Antibiotic Stopped[3]	61	70%	72%	72%	95%
Pregnancy Care					
Inpatient Neonatal Mortality	-	-	-	-	-
Third or Fourth Degree Laceration	-	-	3.82%	3.63%	3.27%

Providence Medical Center

Alternate Name: Providence Health
8929 Parallel Parkway
Kansas City, KS 66112
URL: www.providence-health.org
Ownership: Voluntary non-profit - Church
Emergency Services: Yes

Phone: 913-596-4000
Fax: 913-596-4324
Accredited: Yes
Licensed Beds: 400

Key Personnel:
President/CEO. . . . . James P Paquette
CEO/Executive Director . . . . Juanita Roy
Emergency Room . . . . Richard Rosenthal, MD
ICU . . . . Patty Geiger
Medical/Surgical Nursing . . . . Anne Healy
Respiratory/Cardiopulmonary. . . . . Ben Wano

Measure	Cases	This Hospital	State Average	U.S. Average	Top Hospital
Heart Attack Care					
ACE Inhibitor or ARB for LVSD	66	94%	78%	82%	100%
Aspirin at Arrival	153	96%	90%	92%	100%
Aspirin at Discharge	172	96%	88%	90%	100%
Beta Blocker at Arrival	118	97%	82%	87%	100%
Beta Blocker at Discharge	180	98%	82%	90%	100%
Fibrinolytic Medication Timing	0	-	24%	31%	100%
PCI Within 90 Minutes of Arrival[1]	9	44%	55%	54%	95%
Smoking Cessation Advice	71	100%	86%	88%	100%
Heart Failure Care					
ACE Inhibitor or ARB for LVSD	209	83%	72%	82%	100%
Discharge Instructions	394	65%	41%	61%	93%
Evaluation of LVS Function	476	97%	65%	83%	99%
Smoking Cessation Advice	131	98%	67%	82%	100%
Pneumonia Care					
Appropriate Initial Antibiotic	148	82%	78%	83%	94%
Blood Culture Timing	152	95%	93%	90%	100%
Influenza Vaccine	39	95%	63%	70%	100%
Initial Antibiotic Timing	191	90%	85%	80%	93%
Oxygenation Assessment	246	100%	99%	99%	100%
Pneumococcal Vaccine	134	86%	59%	69%	94%
Smoking Cessation Advice	93	99%	60%	80%	100%
Surgical Infection Prevention					
Prophylactic Antibiotic Given[3]	478	91%	74%	77%	95%
Prophylactic Antibiotic Selection	143	87%	91%	90%	100%
Prophylactic Antibiotic Stopped[3]	428	85%	72%	72%	95%
Pregnancy Care					
Inpatient Neonatal Mortality	1,559	0.13%	-	-	-
Third or Fourth Degree Laceration	1,161	2.67%	3.82%	3.63%	3.27%

University of Kansas Medical Center

3901 Rainbow Boulevard
Kansas City, KS 66160
URL: www.kumc.edu
Ownership: Government - State
Emergency Services: Yes

Phone: 913-588-5000
Fax: 913-588-5863
Accredited: Yes
Licensed Beds: 620

Key Personnel:
President/CEO. . . . . Irene Cumming
Cardiovascular Services. . . . . Patricia Kinsman
Infection Control. . . . . Daivd Woods
Obstetrics and Gynecology . . . . Norma Turner
Operating Room Surgery . . . . Laurie Wood
Respiratory Therapy. . . . . Lynn Lewman

Measure	Cases	This Hospital	State Average	U.S. Average	Top Hospital
Heart Attack Care					
ACE Inhibitor or ARB for LVSD	61	92%	78%	82%	100%
Aspirin at Arrival	110	100%	90%	92%	100%
Aspirin at Discharge	245	98%	88%	90%	100%
Beta Blocker at Arrival	106	99%	82%	87%	100%
Beta Blocker at Discharge	242	99%	82%	90%	100%
Fibrinolytic Medication Timing	0	-	24%	31%	100%
PCI Within 90 Minutes of Arrival[1]	8	75%	55%	54%	95%
Smoking Cessation Advice	111	100%	86%	88%	100%
Heart Failure Care					
ACE Inhibitor or ARB for LVSD	165	93%	72%	82%	100%
Discharge Instructions	261	89%	41%	61%	93%
Evaluation of LVS Function	295	99%	65%	83%	99%
Smoking Cessation Advice	81	96%	67%	82%	100%

NOTE: Hospital profiles are in alphabetical order by state, then city, then hospital within the city; Rankings are sorted by rate in descending order and exclude hospitals with less than 25 cases; (1) The number of cases is too small (n<25) for purposes of reliably predicting hospital performance; (2) Measure reflects the hospital's indication that its submission was based upon a sample of its relevant discharges; (3) Rate reflects fewer than the maximum possible quarters of data for the measure; (4) Inaccurate information submitted and suppressed for one or more quarters; (5) No data is available from the hospital for this measure; Please refer to the User's Guide for a full explanation of data

Measure	Cases	This Hospital	State Average	U.S. Average	Top Hospital
Pneumonia Care					
Appropriate Initial Antibiotic	134	91%	78%	83%	94%
Blood Culture Timing	142	94%	93%	90%	100%
Influenza Vaccine	35	89%	63%	70%	100%
Initial Antibiotic Timing	202	82%	85%	80%	93%
Oxygenation Assessment	265	100%	99%	99%	100%
Pneumococcal Vaccine	90	89%	59%	69%	94%
Smoking Cessation Advice	99	95%	60%	80%	100%
Surgical Infection Prevention					
Prophylactic Antibiotic Given[2,3]	342	85%	74%	77%	95%
Prophylactic Antibiotic Selection[2]	74	95%	91%	90%	100%
Prophylactic Antibiotic Stopped[2,3]	330	61%	72%	72%	95%
Pregnancy Care					
Inpatient Neonatal Mortality	-	-	-	-	-
Third or Fourth Degree Laceration	-	-	3.82%	3.63%	3.27%

Kingman Community Hospital

750 West D Avenue
Kingman, KS 67068

Toll-Free: 800-530-5853
Phone: 620-532-3147
Fax: 620-532-5221

E-mail: nvhs@ink.org
URL: www.nvhsinc.com
Ownership: Voluntary non-profit - Private
Emergency Services: No
Accredited: No
Licensed Beds: 50

Key Personnel:
Administrator/CEO . . . . Gary Tiller
Chief Medical Staff . . . . Victoria Moots, DO
Emergency Room . . . . Nita McFarland
Director Medical/Surgical Nursing . . . . Rogene Jarmer, RN
Director Radiology . . . . Connie Johnson
Respiratory Care . . . . Sheila Elpers

Measure	Cases	This Hospital	State Average	U.S. Average	Top Hospital
Heart Attack Care					
ACE Inhibitor or ARB for LVSD[1]	1	100%	78%	82%	100%
Aspirin at Arrival[1]	4	75%	90%	92%	100%
Aspirin at Discharge[1]	4	100%	88%	90%	100%
Beta Blocker at Arrival[1]	6	83%	82%	87%	100%
Beta Blocker at Discharge[1]	4	100%	82%	90%	100%
Fibrinolytic Medication Timing	0	-	24%	31%	100%
PCI Within 90 Minutes of Arrival	0	-	55%	54%	95%
Smoking Cessation Advice	0	-	86%	88%	100%
Heart Failure Care					
ACE Inhibitor or ARB for LVSD[1]	7	71%	72%	82%	100%
Discharge Instructions[1]	10	20%	41%	61%	93%
Evaluation of LVS Function[1]	23	52%	65%	83%	99%
Smoking Cessation Advice[1]	3	33%	67%	82%	100%
Pneumonia Care					
Appropriate Initial Antibiotic	38	79%	78%	83%	94%
Blood Culture Timing[1]	6	100%	93%	90%	100%
Influenza Vaccine[4,5]	-	-	63%	70%	100%
Initial Antibiotic Timing	47	87%	85%	80%	93%
Oxygenation Assessment	57	98%	99%	99%	100%
Pneumococcal Vaccine	40	58%	59%	69%	94%
Smoking Cessation Advice[1]	15	27%	60%	80%	100%
Surgical Infection Prevention					
Prophylactic Antibiotic Given[1]	10	100%	74%	77%	95%
Prophylactic Antibiotic Selection[1]	1	100%	91%	90%	100%
Prophylactic Antibiotic Stopped[1]	10	100%	72%	72%	95%
Pregnancy Care					
Inpatient Neonatal Mortality	-	-	-	-	-
Third or Fourth Degree Laceration	-	-	3.82%	3.63%	3.27%

Kearny County Hospital

500 Thorpe Street
Lakin, KS 67860
URL: www.kearnycountyhospital.com
Ownership: Government - Local
Emergency Services: Yes

Phone: 620-355-7111
Fax: 620-355-1527
Accredited: No
Licensed Beds: 90

Key Personnel:
Administrator . . . . John Loebl
Infection Control . . . . Ken Barnett, RN
Respiratory Care . . . . Kem Barnett

Measure	Cases	This Hospital	State Average	U.S. Average	Top Hospital
Heart Attack Care					
ACE Inhibitor or ARB for LVSD[5]	-	-	78%	82%	100%
Aspirin at Arrival[5]	-	-	90%	92%	100%
Aspirin at Discharge[5]	-	-	88%	90%	100%
Beta Blocker at Arrival[5]	-	-	82%	87%	100%
Beta Blocker at Discharge[5]	-	-	82%	90%	100%
Fibrinolytic Medication Timing[5]	-	-	24%	31%	100%
PCI Within 90 Minutes of Arrival[5]	-	-	55%	54%	95%
Smoking Cessation Advice[5]	-	-	86%	88%	100%
Heart Failure Care					
ACE Inhibitor or ARB for LVSD[3]	0	-	72%	82%	100%
Discharge Instructions[1,3]	8	25%	41%	61%	93%
Evaluation of LVS Function[1,3]	11	0%	65%	83%	99%
Smoking Cessation Advice[3]	0	-	67%	82%	100%
Pneumonia Care					
Appropriate Initial Antibiotic[1]	5	100%	78%	83%	94%
Blood Culture Timing	0	-	93%	90%	100%
Influenza Vaccine	0	-	63%	70%	100%
Initial Antibiotic Timing[1]	6	100%	85%	80%	93%
Oxygenation Assessment[1]	6	100%	99%	99%	100%
Pneumococcal Vaccine[1]	3	100%	59%	69%	94%
Smoking Cessation Advice[1]	1	0%	60%	80%	100%
Surgical Infection Prevention					
Prophylactic Antibiotic Given[5]	-	-	74%	77%	95%
Prophylactic Antibiotic Selection[5]	-	-	91%	90%	100%
Prophylactic Antibiotic Stopped[5]	-	-	72%	72%	95%
Pregnancy Care					
Inpatient Neonatal Mortality	-	-	-	-	-
Third or Fourth Degree Laceration	-	-	3.82%	3.63%	3.27%

Lawrence Memorial Hospital

325 Maine Street
Lawrence, KS 66044
URL: www.lmh.org
Ownership: Government - Local
Emergency Services: Yes

Phone: 785-749-6100
Fax: 785-749-6126
Accredited: Yes
Licensed Beds: 173

Key Personnel:
President/CEO . . . . Gene Meyer
Chief Medical Staff . . . . Mike Zabel, MD
Emergency Room . . . . Joan Arenas
Infection Control . . . . Janet Wehrle
ICU . . . . Carol Cockrett
Medical/Surgical Nursing . . . . Dana Hale
Director Respiratory Therapy . . . . David Dempsey

Measure	Cases	This Hospital	State Average	U.S. Average	Top Hospital
Heart Attack Care					
ACE Inhibitor or ARB for LVSD[1]	7	100%	78%	82%	100%
Aspirin at Arrival	53	100%	90%	92%	100%
Aspirin at Discharge	37	100%	88%	90%	100%
Beta Blocker at Arrival	47	100%	82%	87%	100%
Beta Blocker at Discharge	37	100%	82%	90%	100%
Fibrinolytic Medication Timing[1]	2	0%	24%	31%	100%
PCI Within 90 Minutes of Arrival[1]	2	0%	55%	54%	95%
Smoking Cessation Advice[1]	16	94%	86%	88%	100%
Heart Failure Care					
ACE Inhibitor or ARB for LVSD	68	100%	72%	82%	100%
Discharge Instructions	82	87%	41%	61%	93%
Evaluation of LVS Function	125	98%	65%	83%	99%
Smoking Cessation Advice[1]	24	100%	67%	82%	100%
Pneumonia Care					
Appropriate Initial Antibiotic	75	89%	78%	83%	94%
Blood Culture Timing	60	87%	93%	90%	100%
Influenza Vaccine[1]	22	77%	63%	70%	100%
Initial Antibiotic Timing	93	92%	85%	80%	93%
Oxygenation Assessment	135	100%	99%	99%	100%
Pneumococcal Vaccine	98	96%	59%	69%	94%
Smoking Cessation Advice	27	100%	60%	80%	100%
Surgical Infection Prevention					
Prophylactic Antibiotic Given	378	82%	74%	77%	95%
Prophylactic Antibiotic Selection	105	98%	91%	90%	100%

NOTE: Hospital profiles are in alphabetical order by state, then city, then hospital within the city; Rankings are sorted by rate in descending order and exclude hospitals with less than 25 cases; (1) The number of cases is too small (n<25) for purposes of reliably predicting hospital performance; (2) Measure reflects the hospital's indication that its submission was based upon a sample of its relevant discharges; (3) Rate reflects fewer than the maximum possible quarters of data for the measure; (4) Inaccurate information submitted and suppressed for one or more quarters; (5) No data is available from the hospital for this measure; Please refer to the User's Guide for a full explanation of data

Prophylactic Antibiotic Stopped	360	77%	72%	72%	95%
Pregnancy Care					
Inpatient Neonatal Mortality	-	-	-	-	-
Third or Fourth Degree Laceration	-	-	3.82%	3.63%	3.27%

Cushing Memorial Hospital

711 Marshall Street
Leavenworth, KS 66048
URL: www.cushinghospital.org
Ownership: Voluntary non-profit - Private
Emergency Services: Yes

Phone: 913-684-1100
Fax: 913-684-1390

Accredited: Yes
Licensed Beds: 74

Key Personnel:

CEO. . . . . Bob S Edward Jr
Chief Medical Staff. . . . . Dr Habib
Head Emergency Room. . . . . Fondra Fausalt
Director Respiratory . . . . Paul Rumends

Measure	Cases	This Hospital	State Average	U.S. Average	Top Hospital
Heart Attack Care					
ACE Inhibitor or ARB for LVSD[1]	1	0%	78%	82%	100%
Aspirin at Arrival[1]	7	100%	90%	92%	100%
Aspirin at Discharge[1]	2	100%	88%	90%	100%
Beta Blocker at Arrival[1]	5	100%	82%	87%	100%
Beta Blocker at Discharge[1]	2	100%	82%	90%	100%
Fibrinolytic Medication Timing	0	-	24%	31%	100%
PCI Within 90 Minutes of Arrival	0	-	55%	54%	95%
Smoking Cessation Advice[1]	1	100%	86%	88%	100%
Heart Failure Care					
ACE Inhibitor or ARB for LVSD[1]	15	80%	72%	82%	100%
Discharge Instructions	38	37%	41%	61%	93%
Evaluation of LVS Function	52	98%	65%	83%	99%
Smoking Cessation Advice[1]	11	100%	67%	82%	100%
Pneumonia Care					
Appropriate Initial Antibiotic	63	76%	78%	83%	94%
Blood Culture Timing	34	100%	93%	90%	100%
Influenza Vaccine[1]	11	100%	63%	70%	100%
Initial Antibiotic Timing	71	83%	85%	80%	93%
Oxygenation Assessment	75	100%	99%	99%	100%
Pneumococcal Vaccine	38	92%	59%	69%	94%
Smoking Cessation Advice[1]	21	95%	60%	80%	100%
Surgical Infection Prevention					
Prophylactic Antibiotic Given[1]	17	88%	74%	77%	95%
Prophylactic Antibiotic Selection[1]	7	57%	91%	90%	100%
Prophylactic Antibiotic Stopped[1]	14	93%	72%	72%	95%
Pregnancy Care					
Inpatient Neonatal Mortality	-	-	-	-	-
Third or Fourth Degree Laceration	-	-	3.82%	3.63%	3.27%

Saint John Hospital

3500 S Fourth Street Trafficway
Leavenworth, KS 66048
URL: www.providence-health.org
Ownership: Voluntary non-profit - Other
Emergency Services: Yes

Phone: 913-680-6000
Fax: 913-680-6013

Accredited: Yes
Licensed Beds: 76

Key Personnel:

Chief Medical Staff. . . . . Greg Madsen
Emergency Room . . . . Jodi Fincher
Emergency Room . . . . Mark Scarborough, MD
Director Infection/Disease Control . . . . Barbara McNett, RN
Director Medical/Surgical Nursing . . . . Peg Williams
Chief Radiology . . . . Caprice Olomon, MD
Director Respiratory Therapy . . . . Denice Brown

Measure	Cases	This Hospital	State Average	U.S. Average	Top Hospital
Heart Attack Care					
ACE Inhibitor or ARB for LVSD[1]	4	25%	78%	82%	100%
Aspirin at Arrival[1]	10	80%	90%	92%	100%
Aspirin at Discharge[1]	9	67%	88%	90%	100%
Beta Blocker at Arrival[1]	9	67%	82%	87%	100%
Beta Blocker at Discharge[1]	8	50%	82%	90%	100%
Fibrinolytic Medication Timing	0	-	24%	31%	100%
PCI Within 90 Minutes of Arrival	0	-	55%	54%	95%
Smoking Cessation Advice	0	-	86%	88%	100%
Heart Failure Care					
ACE Inhibitor or ARB for LVSD[1]	15	73%	72%	82%	100%
Discharge Instructions	43	88%	41%	61%	93%
Evaluation of LVS Function	50	80%	65%	83%	99%
Smoking Cessation Advice[1]	15	100%	67%	82%	100%
Pneumonia Care					
Appropriate Initial Antibiotic	35	83%	78%	83%	94%
Blood Culture Timing[1]	23	96%	93%	90%	100%
Influenza Vaccine[1]	7	71%	63%	70%	100%
Initial Antibiotic Timing	55	85%	85%	80%	93%
Oxygenation Assessment	66	98%	99%	99%	100%
Pneumococcal Vaccine	36	81%	59%	69%	94%
Smoking Cessation Advice[1]	13	100%	60%	80%	100%
Surgical Infection Prevention					
Prophylactic Antibiotic Given[3]	37	78%	74%	77%	95%
Prophylactic Antibiotic Selection[1]	10	90%	91%	90%	100%
Prophylactic Antibiotic Stopped[3]	31	74%	72%	72%	95%
Pregnancy Care					
Inpatient Neonatal Mortality	258	0.00%	-	-	-
Third or Fourth Degree Laceration	191	1.57%	3.82%	3.63%	3.27%

Doctors Hospital

4901 College Blvd
Leawood, KS 66211
Ownership: Proprietary
Emergency Services: No

Phone: 913-529-1801

Accredited: Yes

Measure	Cases	This Hospital	State Average	U.S. Average	Top Hospital
Heart Attack Care					
ACE Inhibitor or ARB for LVSD[5]	-	-	78%	82%	100%
Aspirin at Arrival[5]	-	-	90%	92%	100%
Aspirin at Discharge[5]	-	-	88%	90%	100%
Beta Blocker at Arrival[5]	-	-	82%	87%	100%
Beta Blocker at Discharge[5]	-	-	82%	90%	100%
Fibrinolytic Medication Timing[5]	-	-	24%	31%	100%
PCI Within 90 Minutes of Arrival[5]	-	-	55%	54%	95%
Smoking Cessation Advice[5]	-	-	86%	88%	100%
Heart Failure Care					
ACE Inhibitor or ARB for LVSD[5]	-	-	72%	82%	100%
Discharge Instructions[5]	-	-	41%	61%	93%
Evaluation of LVS Function[5]	-	-	65%	83%	99%
Smoking Cessation Advice[5]	-	-	67%	82%	100%
Pneumonia Care					
Appropriate Initial Antibiotic[1,3]	1	0%	78%	83%	94%
Blood Culture Timing[3]	0	-	93%	90%	100%
Influenza Vaccine	0	-	63%	70%	100%
Initial Antibiotic Timing[3]	0	-	85%	80%	93%
Oxygenation Assessment[1,3]	1	100%	99%	99%	100%
Pneumococcal Vaccine[3]	0	-	59%	69%	94%
Smoking Cessation Advice[1,3]	1	0%	60%	80%	100%
Surgical Infection Prevention					
Prophylactic Antibiotic Given[1]	17	94%	74%	77%	95%
Prophylactic Antibiotic Selection[1]	3	100%	91%	90%	100%
Prophylactic Antibiotic Stopped[1]	16	94%	72%	72%	95%
Pregnancy Care					
Inpatient Neonatal Mortality	-	-	-	-	-
Third or Fourth Degree Laceration	-	-	3.82%	3.63%	3.27%

Kansas City Orthopaedic Institute

3651 College Blvd
Leawood, KS 66211
Ownership: Proprietary
Emergency Services: No

Phone: 913-319-7633

Accredited: No

Measure	Cases	This Hospital	State Average	U.S. Average	Top Hospital
Heart Attack Care					
ACE Inhibitor or ARB for LVSD[5]	-	-	78%	82%	100%
Aspirin at Arrival[5]	-	-	90%	92%	100%
Aspirin at Discharge[5]	-	-	88%	90%	100%
Beta Blocker at Arrival[5]	-	-	82%	87%	100%
Beta Blocker at Discharge[5]	-	-	82%	90%	100%
Fibrinolytic Medication Timing[5]	-	-	24%	31%	100%

NOTE: Hospital profiles are in alphabetical order by state, then city, then hospital within the city; Rankings are sorted by rate in descending order and exclude hospitals with less than 25 cases; (1) The number of cases is too small (n<25) for purposes of reliably predicting hospital performance; (2) Measure reflects the hospital's indication that its submission was based upon a sample of its relevant discharges; (3) Rate reflects fewer than the maximum possible quarters of data for the measure; (4) Inaccurate information submitted and suppressed for one or more quarters; (5) No data is available from the hospital for this measure; Please refer to the User's Guide for a full explanation of data

Measure	Cases	This Hospital	State Average	U.S. Average	Top Hospital
PCI Within 90 Minutes of Arrival[5]	-	-	55%	54%	95%
Smoking Cessation Advice[5]	-	-	86%	88%	100%
Heart Failure Care					
ACE Inhibitor or ARB for LVSD[5]	-	-	72%	82%	100%
Discharge Instructions[5]	-	-	41%	61%	93%
Evaluation of LVS Function[5]	-	-	65%	83%	99%
Smoking Cessation Advice[5]	-	-	67%	82%	100%
Pneumonia Care					
Appropriate Initial Antibiotic[5]	-	-	78%	83%	94%
Blood Culture Timing[5]	-	-	93%	90%	100%
Influenza Vaccine[5]	-	-	63%	70%	100%
Initial Antibiotic Timing[5]	-	-	85%	80%	93%
Oxygenation Assessment[5]	-	-	99%	99%	100%
Pneumococcal Vaccine[5]	-	-	59%	69%	94%
Smoking Cessation Advice[5]	-	-	60%	80%	100%
Surgical Infection Prevention					
Prophylactic Antibiotic Given[2]	96	97%	74%	77%	95%
Prophylactic Antibiotic Selection[1,2]	22	100%	91%	90%	100%
Prophylactic Antibiotic Stopped[2]	96	81%	72%	72%	95%
Pregnancy Care					
Inpatient Neonatal Mortality	-	-	-	-	-
Third or Fourth Degree Laceration	-	-	3.82%	3.63%	3.27%

Southwest Medical Center

315 W 15th St
Liberal, KS 67905
Phone: 620-624-1651
Fax: 620-629-2442
Ownership: Government - Local
Accredited: Yes
Emergency Services: Yes
Licensed Beds: 101

Key Personnel:
Administrator . . . . Anthony Daigle
Chief of Medical Staff . . . . David Fitzgerald, MD
Infection Control . . . . Sandra Wiswell
ICU Supervising Nurse . . . . Diane Miller
Nurse Manager Surgical Floor . . . . Sandy Meade
OB/GYN Women's Health . . . . Dennis Knudsen, MD

Measure	Cases	This Hospital	State Average	U.S. Average	Top Hospital
Heart Attack Care					
ACE Inhibitor or ARB for LVSD[1]	1	100%	78%	82%	100%
Aspirin at Arrival[1]	11	100%	90%	92%	100%
Aspirin at Discharge[1]	7	86%	88%	90%	100%
Beta Blocker at Arrival[1]	8	100%	82%	87%	100%
Beta Blocker at Discharge[1]	5	80%	82%	90%	100%
Fibrinolytic Medication Timing[1]	1	0%	24%	31%	100%
PCI Within 90 Minutes of Arrival	0	-	55%	54%	95%
Smoking Cessation Advice	0	-	86%	88%	100%
Heart Failure Care					
ACE Inhibitor or ARB for LVSD[1]	8	75%	72%	82%	100%
Discharge Instructions	28	79%	41%	61%	93%
Evaluation of LVS Function	37	81%	65%	83%	99%
Smoking Cessation Advice[1]	3	33%	67%	82%	100%
Pneumonia Care					
Appropriate Initial Antibiotic	28	68%	78%	83%	94%
Blood Culture Timing[1]	14	100%	93%	90%	100%
Influenza Vaccine[1]	13	62%	63%	70%	100%
Initial Antibiotic Timing	46	93%	85%	80%	93%
Oxygenation Assessment	68	100%	99%	99%	100%
Pneumococcal Vaccine	34	59%	59%	69%	94%
Smoking Cessation Advice[1]	14	36%	60%	80%	100%
Surgical Infection Prevention					
Prophylactic Antibiotic Given[3]	98	68%	74%	77%	95%
Prophylactic Antibiotic Selection[1]	23	39%	91%	90%	100%
Prophylactic Antibiotic Stopped[3]	97	42%	72%	72%	95%
Pregnancy Care					
Inpatient Neonatal Mortality	-	-	-	-	-
Third or Fourth Degree Laceration	-	-	3.82%	3.63%	3.27%

Lindsborg Community Hospital

605 W Lincoln Street
Lindsborg, KS 67456
Phone: 785-227-3308
Fax: 785-227-4130
E-mail: lch@lindsborghospital.org
URL: www.lindsborghospital.org
Ownership: Voluntary non-profit - Other
Accredited: No
Emergency Services: Yes
Licensed Beds: 25

Key Personnel:
CEO/Administrator . . . . Greg Lundstrom
Chief of Medical Staff . . . . Susan Chrislip
Director Infection/Disease Control . . . . Beth Hedberg, RN
Director Medical/Surgical Nursing . . . . Joanie Worthen, RN

Measure	Cases	This Hospital	State Average	U.S. Average	Top Hospital
Heart Attack Care					
ACE Inhibitor or ARB for LVSD[3]	0	-	78%	82%	100%
Aspirin at Arrival[1,3]	1	100%	90%	92%	100%
Aspirin at Discharge[3]	0	-	88%	90%	100%
Beta Blocker at Arrival[1,3]	1	100%	82%	87%	100%
Beta Blocker at Discharge[3]	0	-	82%	90%	100%
Fibrinolytic Medication Timing[3]	0	-	24%	31%	100%
PCI Within 90 Minutes of Arrival	0	-	55%	54%	95%
Smoking Cessation Advice[3]	0	-	86%	88%	100%
Heart Failure Care					
ACE Inhibitor or ARB for LVSD[1,3]	2	50%	72%	82%	100%
Discharge Instructions[1,3]	2	0%	41%	61%	93%
Evaluation of LVS Function[1,3]	7	86%	65%	83%	99%
Smoking Cessation Advice[1,3]	1	100%	67%	82%	100%
Pneumonia Care					
Appropriate Initial Antibiotic[1]	23	87%	78%	83%	94%
Blood Culture Timing[1]	4	100%	93%	90%	100%
Influenza Vaccine[1]	12	92%	63%	70%	100%
Initial Antibiotic Timing	37	92%	85%	80%	93%
Oxygenation Assessment	45	100%	99%	99%	100%
Pneumococcal Vaccine	35	97%	59%	69%	94%
Smoking Cessation Advice[1]	6	83%	60%	80%	100%
Surgical Infection Prevention					
Prophylactic Antibiotic Given[5]	-	-	74%	77%	95%
Prophylactic Antibiotic Selection[5]	-	-	91%	90%	100%
Prophylactic Antibiotic Stopped[5]	-	-	72%	72%	95%
Pregnancy Care					
Inpatient Neonatal Mortality	-	-	-	-	-
Third or Fourth Degree Laceration	-	-	3.82%	3.63%	3.27%

Manhattan Surgical Hospital

1829 College Avenue
Manhattan, KS 66502
Phone: 785-776-5100
Ownership: Proprietary
Accredited: No
Emergency Services: No

Measure	Cases	This Hospital	State Average	U.S. Average	Top Hospital
Heart Attack Care					
ACE Inhibitor or ARB for LVSD[5]	-	-	78%	82%	100%
Aspirin at Arrival[5]	-	-	90%	92%	100%
Aspirin at Discharge[5]	-	-	88%	90%	100%
Beta Blocker at Arrival[5]	-	-	82%	87%	100%
Beta Blocker at Discharge[5]	-	-	82%	90%	100%
Fibrinolytic Medication Timing[5]	-	-	24%	31%	100%
PCI Within 90 Minutes of Arrival[5]	-	-	55%	54%	95%
Smoking Cessation Advice[5]	-	-	86%	88%	100%
Heart Failure Care					
ACE Inhibitor or ARB for LVSD[5]	-	-	72%	82%	100%
Discharge Instructions[5]	-	-	41%	61%	93%
Evaluation of LVS Function[5]	-	-	65%	83%	99%
Smoking Cessation Advice[5]	-	-	67%	82%	100%
Pneumonia Care					
Appropriate Initial Antibiotic[5]	-	-	78%	83%	94%
Blood Culture Timing[5]	-	-	93%	90%	100%
Influenza Vaccine[5]	-	-	63%	70%	100%
Initial Antibiotic Timing[5]	-	-	85%	80%	93%
Oxygenation Assessment[5]	-	-	99%	99%	100%
Pneumococcal Vaccine[5]	-	-	59%	69%	94%

NOTE: Hospital profiles are in alphabetical order by state, then city, then hospital within the city; Rankings are sorted by rate in descending order and exclude hospitals with less than 25 cases; (1) The number of cases is too small (n<25) for purposes of reliably predicting hospital performance; (2) Measure reflects the hospital's indication that its submission was based upon a sample of its relevant discharges; (3) Rate reflects fewer than the maximum possible quarters of data for the measure; (4) Inaccurate information submitted and suppressed for one or more quarters; (5) No data is available from the hospital for this measure; Please refer to the User's Guide for a full explanation of data

Smoking Cessation Advice[5]	-	-	60%	80%	100%
Surgical Infection Prevention					
Prophylactic Antibiotic Given	219	61%	74%	77%	95%
Prophylactic Antibiotic Selection	56	98%	91%	90%	100%
Prophylactic Antibiotic Stopped	215	96%	72%	72%	95%
Pregnancy Care					
Inpatient Neonatal Mortality	-	-	-	-	-
Third or Fourth Degree Laceration	-	-	3.82%	3.63%	3.27%

Mercy Regional Health Center

1823 College Avenue
Manhattan, KS 66502
URL: www.mercyregional.org
Ownership: Voluntary non-profit - Church
Emergency Services: Yes
Phone: 785-776-3322
Fax: 785-776-2804
Accredited: Yes
Licensed Beds: 150

Key Personnel:
President/CEO . . . . Richard L Allen
Chief Medical Staff . . . . Joe Philipp
Director Cardiac Laboratory . . . . Don Hedden
Infection Control . . . . Vivian Nutsch
Supervising Nurse CCU . . . . Cynthia Whitaker
Medical/Surgical Nursing . . . . Chris Holden
CEO . . . . Richard Allen
Director Women's Health . . . . Angie Elliot
Cardiopulmonary . . . . Don Hedden

Measure	Cases	This Hospital	State Average	U.S. Average	Top Hospital
Heart Attack Care					
ACE Inhibitor or ARB for LVSD[1,2]	2	50%	78%	82%	100%
Aspirin at Arrival[1,2]	21	100%	90%	92%	100%
Aspirin at Discharge[1,2]	11	91%	88%	90%	100%
Beta Blocker at Arrival[1,2]	15	93%	82%	87%	100%
Beta Blocker at Discharge[1,2]	11	91%	82%	90%	100%
Fibrinolytic Medication Timing[2]	0	-	24%	31%	100%
PCI Within 90 Minutes of Arrival[2]	0	-	55%	54%	95%
Smoking Cessation Advice[1,2]	3	100%	86%	88%	100%
Heart Failure Care					
ACE Inhibitor or ARB for LVSD	37	84%	72%	82%	100%
Discharge Instructions	83	27%	41%	61%	93%
Evaluation of LVS Function	125	89%	65%	83%	99%
Smoking Cessation Advice[1]	19	53%	67%	82%	100%
Pneumonia Care					
Appropriate Initial Antibiotic[2]	68	93%	78%	83%	94%
Blood Culture Timing[2]	49	100%	93%	90%	100%
Influenza Vaccine[1]	14	86%	63%	70%	100%
Initial Antibiotic Timing[2]	97	81%	85%	80%	93%
Oxygenation Assessment[2]	130	100%	99%	99%	100%
Pneumococcal Vaccine[2]	83	76%	59%	69%	94%
Smoking Cessation Advice[2]	31	58%	60%	80%	100%
Surgical Infection Prevention					
Prophylactic Antibiotic Given[2,3]	92	74%	74%	77%	95%
Prophylactic Antibiotic Selection[2]	92	95%	91%	90%	100%
Prophylactic Antibiotic Stopped[2,3]	86	78%	72%	72%	95%
Pregnancy Care					
Inpatient Neonatal Mortality	-	-	-	-	-
Third or Fourth Degree Laceration	-	-	3.82%	3.63%	3.27%

Saint Luke Hospital & Living Center

535 South Freeborn
Marion, KS 66861
URL: www.slhmarion.org
Ownership: Voluntary non-profit - Private
Emergency Services: Yes
Phone: 620-382-2177
Fax: 620-382-9104
Accredited: No
Licensed Beds: 54

Key Personnel:
CEO/Administrator . . . . Jeremy Armstrong
Chief Medical Staff . . . . Don Hudson, MD
Emergency Room . . . . Linda Kennedy
Director Medical/Surgical Nursing . . . . Patti Thomas
Chief Radiology . . . . Jerry Berg, MD

Measure	Cases	This Hospital	State Average	U.S. Average	Top Hospital
Heart Attack Care					
ACE Inhibitor or ARB for LVSD[5]	-	-	78%	82%	100%
Aspirin at Arrival[5]	-	-	90%	92%	100%
Aspirin at Discharge[5]	-	-	88%	90%	100%
Beta Blocker at Arrival[5]	-	-	82%	87%	100%
Beta Blocker at Discharge[5]	-	-	82%	90%	100%
Fibrinolytic Medication Timing[5]	-	-	24%	31%	100%
PCI Within 90 Minutes of Arrival[5]	-	-	55%	54%	95%
Smoking Cessation Advice[5]	-	-	86%	88%	100%
Heart Failure Care					
ACE Inhibitor or ARB for LVSD[1]	4	75%	72%	82%	100%
Discharge Instructions[1]	13	8%	41%	61%	93%
Evaluation of LVS Function	27	41%	65%	83%	99%
Smoking Cessation Advice[1]	2	0%	67%	82%	100%
Pneumonia Care					
Appropriate Initial Antibiotic[1]	14	86%	78%	83%	94%
Blood Culture Timing[1]	1	100%	93%	90%	100%
Influenza Vaccine[1]	8	25%	63%	70%	100%
Initial Antibiotic Timing[1]	16	94%	85%	80%	93%
Oxygenation Assessment	28	100%	99%	99%	100%
Pneumococcal Vaccine	25	8%	59%	69%	94%
Smoking Cessation Advice[1]	4	25%	60%	80%	100%
Surgical Infection Prevention					
Prophylactic Antibiotic Given[1,3]	1	100%	74%	77%	95%
Prophylactic Antibiotic Selection[1]	1	100%	91%	90%	100%
Prophylactic Antibiotic Stopped[1,3]	1	100%	72%	72%	95%
Pregnancy Care					
Inpatient Neonatal Mortality	-	-	-	-	-
Third or Fourth Degree Laceration	-	-	3.82%	3.63%	3.27%

Community Memorial Hospital

708 N 18th Street
Marysville, KS 66508
Ownership: Voluntary non-profit - Private
Emergency Services: Yes
Phone: 785-562-2311
Fax: 785-562-2348
Accredited: No
Licensed Beds: 109

Key Personnel:
Administrator . . . . J Canter
Chief Medical Staff . . . . Randy Brown, MD
Director Infection/Disease Control . . . . Mayme Easton

Measure	Cases	This Hospital	State Average	U.S. Average	Top Hospital
Heart Attack Care					
ACE Inhibitor or ARB for LVSD[5]	-	-	78%	82%	100%
Aspirin at Arrival[5]	-	-	90%	92%	100%
Aspirin at Discharge[5]	-	-	88%	90%	100%
Beta Blocker at Arrival[5]	-	-	82%	87%	100%
Beta Blocker at Discharge[5]	-	-	82%	90%	100%
Fibrinolytic Medication Timing[5]	-	-	24%	31%	100%
PCI Within 90 Minutes of Arrival[5]	-	-	55%	54%	95%
Smoking Cessation Advice[5]	-	-	86%	88%	100%
Heart Failure Care					
ACE Inhibitor or ARB for LVSD[5]	-	-	72%	82%	100%
Discharge Instructions[5]	-	-	41%	61%	93%
Evaluation of LVS Function[5]	-	-	65%	83%	99%
Smoking Cessation Advice[5]	-	-	67%	82%	100%
Pneumonia Care					
Appropriate Initial Antibiotic[1,3]	4	25%	78%	83%	94%
Blood Culture Timing[3]	0	-	93%	90%	100%
Influenza Vaccine[5]	-	-	63%	70%	100%
Initial Antibiotic Timing[1,3]	10	80%	85%	80%	93%
Oxygenation Assessment[1,3]	10	100%	99%	99%	100%
Pneumococcal Vaccine[1,3]	5	20%	59%	69%	94%
Smoking Cessation Advice[1,3]	4	25%	60%	80%	100%
Surgical Infection Prevention					
Prophylactic Antibiotic Given[5]	-	-	74%	77%	95%
Prophylactic Antibiotic Selection[5]	-	-	91%	90%	100%
Prophylactic Antibiotic Stopped[5]	-	-	72%	72%	95%
Pregnancy Care					
Inpatient Neonatal Mortality	-	-	-	-	-
Third or Fourth Degree Laceration	-	-	3.82%	3.63%	3.27%

NOTE: Hospital profiles are in alphabetical order by state, then city, then hospital within the city; Rankings are sorted by rate in descending order and exclude hospitals with less than 25 cases; (1) The number of cases is too small (n<25) for purposes of reliably predicting hospital performance; (2) Measure reflects the hospital's indication that its submission was based upon a sample of its relevant discharges; (3) Rate reflects fewer than the maximum possible quarters of data for the measure; (4) Inaccurate information submitted and suppressed for one or more quarters; (5) No data is available from the hospital for this measure; Please refer to the User's Guide for a full explanation of data

Memorial Hospital

1000 Hospital Drive
McPherson, KS 67460
Ownership: Voluntary non-profit - Private
Emergency Services: Yes
Phone: 620-241-2250
Fax: 620-245-9153
Accredited: No
Licensed Beds: 70

Key Personnel:
President/CEO . . . . . Rex Walk
Chief Medical Staff . . . . . Trish Goad
Emergency Room . . . . . Daryel Patrick
Director Infection/Disease Control . . . . . Kathy Rishel
Director Medical/Surgical Nursing . . . . . Sue Unruh, RN
Director Respiratory Therapy . . . . . Glenn Tammen

Measure	Cases	This Hospital	State Average	U.S. Average	Top Hospital
Heart Attack Care					
ACE Inhibitor or ARB for LVSD[1,3]	1	100%	78%	82%	100%
Aspirin at Arrival[3]	0	-	90%	92%	100%
Aspirin at Discharge[3]	0	-	88%	90%	100%
Beta Blocker at Arrival[1,3]	1	100%	82%	87%	100%
Beta Blocker at Discharge[1,3]	1	100%	82%	90%	100%
Fibrinolytic Medication Timing[3]	0	-	24%	31%	100%
PCI Within 90 Minutes of Arrival[5]	-	-	55%	54%	95%
Smoking Cessation Advice[3]	0	-	86%	88%	100%
Heart Failure Care					
ACE Inhibitor or ARB for LVSD[1]	11	55%	72%	82%	100%
Discharge Instructions	34	18%	41%	61%	93%
Evaluation of LVS Function	54	59%	65%	83%	99%
Smoking Cessation Advice[1]	4	0%	67%	82%	100%
Pneumonia Care					
Appropriate Initial Antibiotic	50	84%	78%	83%	94%
Blood Culture Timing	30	93%	93%	90%	100%
Influenza Vaccine[1]	16	69%	63%	70%	100%
Initial Antibiotic Timing	70	81%	85%	80%	93%
Oxygenation Assessment	90	99%	99%	99%	100%
Pneumococcal Vaccine	66	62%	59%	69%	94%
Smoking Cessation Advice[1]	9	11%	60%	80%	100%
Surgical Infection Prevention					
Prophylactic Antibiotic Given[2]	31	61%	74%	77%	95%
Prophylactic Antibiotic Selection[1,2]	6	100%	91%	90%	100%
Prophylactic Antibiotic Stopped[2]	29	97%	72%	72%	95%
Pregnancy Care					
Inpatient Neonatal Mortality	-	-	-	-	-
Third or Fourth Degree Laceration	-	-	3.82%	3.63%	3.27%

Meade District Hospital

510 E Carthage PO Box 820
Meade, KS 67864
Ownership: Govt - Hospital District or Authority
Emergency Services: No
Phone: 620-873-5500
Accredited: No

Measure	Cases	This Hospital	State Average	U.S. Average	Top Hospital
Heart Attack Care					
ACE Inhibitor or ARB for LVSD[5]	-	-	78%	82%	100%
Aspirin at Arrival[5]	-	-	90%	92%	100%
Aspirin at Discharge[5]	-	-	88%	90%	100%
Beta Blocker at Arrival[5]	-	-	82%	87%	100%
Beta Blocker at Discharge[5]	-	-	82%	90%	100%
Fibrinolytic Medication Timing[5]	-	-	24%	31%	100%
PCI Within 90 Minutes of Arrival[5]	-	-	55%	54%	95%
Smoking Cessation Advice[5]	-	-	86%	88%	100%
Heart Failure Care					
ACE Inhibitor or ARB for LVSD[1,3]	1	0%	72%	82%	100%
Discharge Instructions[1,3]	7	0%	41%	61%	93%
Evaluation of LVS Function[1,3]	10	30%	65%	83%	99%
Smoking Cessation Advice[3]	0	-	67%	82%	100%
Pneumonia Care					
Appropriate Initial Antibiotic	41	51%	78%	83%	94%
Blood Culture Timing[1]	1	100%	93%	90%	100%
Influenza Vaccine[1]	17	100%	63%	70%	100%
Initial Antibiotic Timing	51	78%	85%	80%	93%
Oxygenation Assessment	75	100%	99%	99%	100%
Pneumococcal Vaccine	58	90%	59%	69%	94%
Smoking Cessation Advice[1]	11	0%	60%	80%	100%
Surgical Infection Prevention					
Prophylactic Antibiotic Given[5]	-	-	74%	77%	95%
Prophylactic Antibiotic Selection[5]	-	-	91%	90%	100%
Prophylactic Antibiotic Stopped[5]	-	-	72%	72%	95%
Pregnancy Care					
Inpatient Neonatal Mortality	-	-	-	-	-
Third or Fourth Degree Laceration	-	-	3.82%	3.63%	3.27%

Mercy Hospital

218 E Pack Street
Moundridge, KS 67107
Ownership: Voluntary non-profit - Church
Emergency Services: No
Phone: 620-345-6391
Fax: 620-345-6344
Accredited: No
Licensed Beds: 21

Key Personnel:
Administrator . . . . . Doyle K Johnson
Emergency Room . . . . . Donnella Unruh, RN
Director Medical Surgical Nursing . . . . . Donnella Unruh, RN
Respiratory/Cardiopulmonary . . . . . Donella Unruh

Measure	Cases	This Hospital	State Average	U.S. Average	Top Hospital
Heart Attack Care					
ACE Inhibitor or ARB for LVSD[3]	0	-	78%	82%	100%
Aspirin at Arrival[1,3]	3	100%	90%	92%	100%
Aspirin at Discharge[1,3]	3	100%	88%	90%	100%
Beta Blocker at Arrival[1,3]	3	67%	82%	87%	100%
Beta Blocker at Discharge[1,3]	3	67%	82%	90%	100%
Fibrinolytic Medication Timing[3]	0	-	24%	31%	100%
PCI Within 90 Minutes of Arrival	0	-	55%	54%	95%
Smoking Cessation Advice[3]	0	-	86%	88%	100%
Heart Failure Care					
ACE Inhibitor or ARB for LVSD[1]	5	80%	72%	82%	100%
Discharge Instructions[1,3]	1	0%	41%	61%	93%
Evaluation of LVS Function[1]	20	70%	65%	83%	99%
Smoking Cessation Advice[3]	0	-	67%	82%	100%
Pneumonia Care					
Appropriate Initial Antibiotic[1,3]	4	75%	78%	83%	94%
Blood Culture Timing[1,3]	1	100%	93%	90%	100%
Influenza Vaccine[5]	-	-	63%	70%	100%
Initial Antibiotic Timing[1]	17	88%	85%	80%	93%
Oxygenation Assessment[1]	23	100%	99%	99%	100%
Pneumococcal Vaccine[1]	22	68%	59%	69%	94%
Smoking Cessation Advice[3]	0	-	60%	80%	100%
Surgical Infection Prevention					
Prophylactic Antibiotic Given[5]	-	-	74%	77%	95%
Prophylactic Antibiotic Selection[5]	-	-	91%	90%	100%
Prophylactic Antibiotic Stopped[5]	-	-	72%	72%	95%
Pregnancy Care					
Inpatient Neonatal Mortality	-	-	-	-	-
Third or Fourth Degree Laceration	-	-	3.82%	3.63%	3.27%

Wilson County Hospital

205 Mill Street
Neodesha, KS 66757
URL: www.wilsoncountyhospital.org
Ownership: Government - Local
Emergency Services: Yes
Phone: 620-325-2611
Fax: 620-325-2907
Accredited: No
Licensed Beds: 38

Key Personnel:
CEO/Administrator . . . . . Deanna Pittman

Measure	Cases	This Hospital	State Average	U.S. Average	Top Hospital
Heart Attack Care					
ACE Inhibitor or ARB for LVSD[5]	-	-	78%	82%	100%
Aspirin at Arrival[5]	-	-	90%	92%	100%
Aspirin at Discharge[5]	-	-	88%	90%	100%
Beta Blocker at Arrival[5]	-	-	82%	87%	100%
Beta Blocker at Discharge[5]	-	-	82%	90%	100%
Fibrinolytic Medication Timing[5]	-	-	24%	31%	100%
PCI Within 90 Minutes of Arrival[5]	-	-	55%	54%	95%
Smoking Cessation Advice[5]	-	-	86%	88%	100%
Heart Failure Care					
ACE Inhibitor or ARB for LVSD[5]	-	-	72%	82%	100%

NOTE: Hospital profiles are in alphabetical order by state, then city, then hospital within the city; Rankings are sorted by rate in descending order and exclude hospitals with less than 25 cases; (1) The number of cases is too small (n<25) for purposes of reliably predicting hospital performance; (2) Measure reflects the hospital's indication that its submission was based upon a sample of its relevant discharges; (3) Rate reflects fewer than the maximum possible quarters of data for the measure; (4) Inaccurate information submitted and suppressed for one or more quarters; (5) No data is available from the hospital for this measure; Please refer to the User's Guide for a full explanation of data

Measure	Cases	This Hospital	State Average	U.S. Average	Top Hospital
Discharge Instructions[5]	-	-	41%	61%	93%
Evaluation of LVS Function[5]	-	-	65%	83%	99%
Smoking Cessation Advice[5]	-	-	67%	82%	100%
Pneumonia Care					
Appropriate Initial Antibiotic[5]	-	-	78%	83%	94%
Blood Culture Timing[5]	-	-	93%	90%	100%
Influenza Vaccine[5]	-	-	63%	70%	100%
Initial Antibiotic Timing[5]	-	-	85%	80%	93%
Oxygenation Assessment[5]	-	-	99%	99%	100%
Pneumococcal Vaccine[5]	-	-	59%	69%	94%
Smoking Cessation Advice[5]	-	-	60%	80%	100%
Surgical Infection Prevention					
Prophylactic Antibiotic Given[5]	-	-	74%	77%	95%
Prophylactic Antibiotic Selection[5]	-	-	91%	90%	100%
Prophylactic Antibiotic Stopped[5]	-	-	72%	72%	95%
Pregnancy Care					
Inpatient Neonatal Mortality	-	-	-	-	-
Third or Fourth Degree Laceration	-	-	3.82%	3.63%	3.27%

Ness County Hospital District #2

312 Custer Street — Phone: 785-798-2291
Ness City, KS 67560 — Fax: 785-798-3435
E-mail: nesshosp@gbta.net
Ownership: Govt - Hospital District or Authority — Accredited: No
Emergency Services: Yes — Licensed Beds: 25

Key Personnel:
Administrator . . . . CT McCracken
Emergency Room . . . . Jaci Dumler, RN
Director Infection/Disease Control . . . . Jackie Foos, RN
Chief Radiology . . . . Lomon Reile

Measure	Cases	This Hospital	State Average	U.S. Average	Top Hospital
Heart Attack Care					
ACE Inhibitor or ARB for LVSD[5]	-	-	78%	82%	100%
Aspirin at Arrival[5]	-	-	90%	92%	100%
Aspirin at Discharge[5]	-	-	88%	90%	100%
Beta Blocker at Arrival[5]	-	-	82%	87%	100%
Beta Blocker at Discharge[5]	-	-	82%	90%	100%
Fibrinolytic Medication Timing[5]	-	-	24%	31%	100%
PCI Within 90 Minutes of Arrival[5]	-	-	55%	54%	95%
Smoking Cessation Advice[5]	-	-	86%	88%	100%
Heart Failure Care					
ACE Inhibitor or ARB for LVSD[5]	-	-	72%	82%	100%
Discharge Instructions[5]	-	-	41%	61%	93%
Evaluation of LVS Function[5]	-	-	65%	83%	99%
Smoking Cessation Advice[5]	-	-	67%	82%	100%
Pneumonia Care					
Appropriate Initial Antibiotic[3]	0	-	78%	83%	94%
Blood Culture Timing[3]	0	-	93%	90%	100%
Influenza Vaccine[5]	-	-	63%	70%	100%
Initial Antibiotic Timing[1,3]	1	100%	85%	80%	93%
Oxygenation Assessment[1,3]	1	100%	99%	99%	100%
Pneumococcal Vaccine[1,3]	1	0%	59%	69%	94%
Smoking Cessation Advice[3]	0	-	60%	80%	100%
Surgical Infection Prevention					
Prophylactic Antibiotic Given[5]	-	-	74%	77%	95%
Prophylactic Antibiotic Selection[5]	-	-	91%	90%	100%
Prophylactic Antibiotic Stopped[5]	-	-	72%	72%	95%
Pregnancy Care					
Inpatient Neonatal Mortality	-	-	-	-	-
Third or Fourth Degree Laceration	-	-	3.82%	3.63%	3.27%

Newton Medical Center

600 Medical Center Drive — Phone: 316-283-2700
PO Box 308 — Fax: 316-804-6260
Newton, KS 67114
E-mail: nmcinfor@newmedCenterorg
URL: www.newtonmedicalcenter.com
Ownership: Voluntary non-profit - Private — Accredited: Yes
Emergency Services: Yes — Licensed Beds: 83

Key Personnel:
President/CEO . . . . Steven G Kelly, FACHE

Measure	Cases	This Hospital	State Average	U.S. Average	Top Hospital
Heart Attack Care					
ACE Inhibitor or ARB for LVSD[1]	2	100%	78%	82%	100%
Aspirin at Arrival[1]	16	100%	90%	92%	100%
Aspirin at Discharge[1]	12	100%	88%	90%	100%
Beta Blocker at Arrival[1]	16	81%	82%	87%	100%
Beta Blocker at Discharge[1]	12	92%	82%	90%	100%
Fibrinolytic Medication Timing[1]	7	57%	24%	31%	100%
PCI Within 90 Minutes of Arrival	0	-	55%	54%	95%
Smoking Cessation Advice	0	-	86%	88%	100%
Heart Failure Care					
ACE Inhibitor or ARB for LVSD[1]	18	78%	72%	82%	100%
Discharge Instructions	62	69%	41%	61%	93%
Evaluation of LVS Function	101	77%	65%	83%	99%
Smoking Cessation Advice[1]	12	58%	67%	82%	100%
Pneumonia Care					
Appropriate Initial Antibiotic	96	88%	78%	83%	94%
Blood Culture Timing	44	89%	93%	90%	100%
Influenza Vaccine	38	76%	63%	70%	100%
Initial Antibiotic Timing	111	78%	85%	80%	93%
Oxygenation Assessment	138	100%	99%	99%	100%
Pneumococcal Vaccine	91	78%	59%	69%	94%
Smoking Cessation Advice[1]	19	47%	60%	80%	100%
Surgical Infection Prevention					
Prophylactic Antibiotic Given	333	84%	74%	77%	95%
Prophylactic Antibiotic Selection	80	89%	91%	90%	100%
Prophylactic Antibiotic Stopped	315	87%	72%	72%	95%
Pregnancy Care					
Inpatient Neonatal Mortality	-	-	-	-	-
Third or Fourth Degree Laceration	-	-	3.82%	3.63%	3.27%

Olathe Medical Center

Alternate Name: Olathe Community Hospital
20333 W 151st Street — Phone: 913-791-4200
Olathe, KS 66061 — Fax: 913-791-4393
URL: www.ohsi.com
Ownership: Voluntary non-profit - Other — Accredited: Yes
Emergency Services: Yes — Licensed Beds: 200

Key Personnel:
Administrator/President . . . . Frank H Devocelle
Chief of Medical Staff. . . . . Bruce Snider, MD
Director Emergency Room Department . . . . Cindy Kolich
Director Infection Control . . . . Elaine Fitzmaurice
Director Surgical Services . . . . Dave Wayatt
Director of Pulmonary . . . . Eric Shroeder, MD

Measure	Cases	This Hospital	State Average	U.S. Average	Top Hospital
Heart Attack Care					
ACE Inhibitor or ARB for LVSD	40	82%	78%	82%	100%
Aspirin at Arrival	129	98%	90%	92%	100%
Aspirin at Discharge	157	98%	88%	90%	100%
Beta Blocker at Arrival	113	93%	82%	87%	100%
Beta Blocker at Discharge	187	97%	82%	90%	100%
Fibrinolytic Medication Timing	0	-	24%	31%	100%
PCI Within 90 Minutes of Arrival[1]	10	70%	55%	54%	95%
Smoking Cessation Advice	94	100%	86%	88%	100%
Heart Failure Care					
ACE Inhibitor or ARB for LVSD	105	91%	72%	82%	100%
Discharge Instructions	243	74%	41%	61%	93%
Evaluation of LVS Function	308	100%	65%	83%	99%
Smoking Cessation Advice	50	100%	67%	82%	100%
Pneumonia Care					
Appropriate Initial Antibiotic	113	84%	78%	83%	94%
Blood Culture Timing	75	93%	93%	90%	100%
Influenza Vaccine	32	91%	63%	70%	100%
Initial Antibiotic Timing	156	72%	85%	80%	93%
Oxygenation Assessment	213	100%	99%	99%	100%
Pneumococcal Vaccine	133	90%	59%	69%	94%
Smoking Cessation Advice	61	97%	60%	80%	100%
Surgical Infection Prevention					
Prophylactic Antibiotic Given[3]	624	95%	74%	77%	95%
Prophylactic Antibiotic Selection	197	95%	91%	90%	100%

NOTE: Hospital profiles are in alphabetical order by state, then city, then hospital within the city; Rankings are sorted by rate in descending order and exclude hospitals with less than 25 cases; (1) The number of cases is too small (n<25) for purposes of reliably predicting hospital performance; (2) Measure reflects the hospital's indication that its submission was based upon a sample of its relevant discharges; (3) Rate reflects fewer than the maximum possible quarters of data for the measure; (4) Inaccurate information submitted and suppressed for one or more quarters; (5) No data is available from the hospital for this measure; Please refer to the User's Guide for a full explanation of data

Prophylactic Antibiotic Stopped[3]	602	75%	72%	72%	95%
Pregnancy Care					
Inpatient Neonatal Mortality	-	-	-	-	-
Third or Fourth Degree Laceration	-	-	3.82%	3.63%	3.27%

Community Hospital-Onaga

120 W 8th
Onaga, KS 66521
URL: www.chcs-ks.org
Ownership: Voluntary non-profit - Private
Emergency Services: Yes
Phone: 785-889-4272
Fax: 785-889-7163
Accredited: No
Licensed Beds: 30

Key Personnel:
CEO. . . . . Greg Unruh
Chief of Medical Staff. . . . . Nancy J Zidek
Director Infection/Disease Control . . . . Cathy VanDonge
Chief Radiology . . . . Kari Bowhay
Supervisor Respiratory Care . . . . Missi McCormick

Measure	Cases	This Hospital	State Average	U.S. Average	Top Hospital
Heart Attack Care					
ACE Inhibitor or ARB for LVSD	0	-	78%	82%	100%
Aspirin at Arrival[1]	4	75%	90%	92%	100%
Aspirin at Discharge[1]	4	75%	88%	90%	100%
Beta Blocker at Arrival[1]	4	75%	82%	87%	100%
Beta Blocker at Discharge[1]	4	75%	82%	90%	100%
Fibrinolytic Medication Timing[1]	1	0%	24%	31%	100%
PCI Within 90 Minutes of Arrival	0	-	55%	54%	95%
Smoking Cessation Advice	0	-	86%	88%	100%
Heart Failure Care					
ACE Inhibitor or ARB for LVSD[1]	6	67%	72%	82%	100%
Discharge Instructions[1]	14	7%	41%	61%	93%
Evaluation of LVS Function	37	38%	65%	83%	99%
Smoking Cessation Advice[1]	1	100%	67%	82%	100%
Pneumonia Care					
Appropriate Initial Antibiotic[1]	18	56%	78%	83%	94%
Blood Culture Timing[1]	2	100%	93%	90%	100%
Influenza Vaccine[1]	8	0%	63%	70%	100%
Initial Antibiotic Timing[1]	17	82%	85%	80%	93%
Oxygenation Assessment	27	93%	99%	99%	100%
Pneumococcal Vaccine	26	4%	59%	69%	94%
Smoking Cessation Advice[1]	6	33%	60%	80%	100%
Surgical Infection Prevention					
Prophylactic Antibiotic Given[5]	-	-	74%	77%	95%
Prophylactic Antibiotic Selection[5]	-	-	91%	90%	100%
Prophylactic Antibiotic Stopped[5]	-	-	72%	72%	95%
Pregnancy Care					
Inpatient Neonatal Mortality	-	-	-	-	-
Third or Fourth Degree Laceration	-	-	3.82%	3.63%	3.27%

Osborne County Memorial Hospital

424 New Hampshire
PO Box 70
Osborne, KS 67473
URL: www.ocmh.org
Ownership: Government - Local
Emergency Services: No
Phone: 785-346-2121
Fax: 785-346-5498
Accredited: No
Licensed Beds: 25

Key Personnel:
Chief of Medical Staff. . . . . Barbara Brown

Measure	Cases	This Hospital	State Average	U.S. Average	Top Hospital
Heart Attack Care					
ACE Inhibitor or ARB for LVSD[5]	-	-	78%	82%	100%
Aspirin at Arrival[5]	-	-	90%	92%	100%
Aspirin at Discharge[5]	-	-	88%	90%	100%
Beta Blocker at Arrival[5]	-	-	82%	87%	100%
Beta Blocker at Discharge[5]	-	-	82%	90%	100%
Fibrinolytic Medication Timing[5]	-	-	24%	31%	100%
PCI Within 90 Minutes of Arrival[5]	-	-	55%	54%	95%
Smoking Cessation Advice[5]	-	-	86%	88%	100%
Heart Failure Care					
ACE Inhibitor or ARB for LVSD[5]	-	-	72%	82%	100%
Discharge Instructions[5]	-	-	41%	61%	93%
Evaluation of LVS Function[5]	-	-	65%	83%	99%
Smoking Cessation Advice[5]	-	-	67%	82%	100%
Pneumonia Care					
Appropriate Initial Antibiotic[5]	-	-	78%	83%	94%
Blood Culture Timing[5]	-	-	93%	90%	100%
Influenza Vaccine[5]	-	-	63%	70%	100%
Initial Antibiotic Timing[5]	-	-	85%	80%	93%
Oxygenation Assessment[5]	-	-	99%	99%	100%
Pneumococcal Vaccine[5]	-	-	59%	69%	94%
Smoking Cessation Advice[5]	-	-	60%	80%	100%
Surgical Infection Prevention					
Prophylactic Antibiotic Given[5]	-	-	74%	77%	95%
Prophylactic Antibiotic Selection[5]	-	-	91%	90%	100%
Prophylactic Antibiotic Stopped[5]	-	-	72%	72%	95%
Pregnancy Care					
Inpatient Neonatal Mortality	-	-	-	-	-
Third or Fourth Degree Laceration	-	-	3.82%	3.63%	3.27%

Ransom Memorial Hospital

1301 S Main Street
Ottawa, KS 66067
URL: www.ransom.org
Ownership: Government - Local
Emergency Services: Yes
Phone: 785-229-8200
Fax: 785-242-8339
Accredited: Yes
Licensed Beds: 55

Key Personnel:
CEO. . . . . Larry Felix
Director Cardiopulmonary Services . . . . Brian Marsh
Director Infection Control . . . . Linda Reed
Director Surgery. . . . . Rick Coffman

Measure	Cases	This Hospital	State Average	U.S. Average	Top Hospital
Heart Attack Care					
ACE Inhibitor or ARB for LVSD[1]	1	100%	78%	82%	100%
Aspirin at Arrival[1]	5	100%	90%	92%	100%
Aspirin at Discharge[1]	4	100%	88%	90%	100%
Beta Blocker at Arrival[1]	3	100%	82%	87%	100%
Beta Blocker at Discharge[1]	4	75%	82%	90%	100%
Fibrinolytic Medication Timing	0	-	24%	31%	100%
PCI Within 90 Minutes of Arrival	0	-	55%	54%	95%
Smoking Cessation Advice[1]	1	100%	86%	88%	100%
Heart Failure Care					
ACE Inhibitor or ARB for LVSD[1]	15	73%	72%	82%	100%
Discharge Instructions	33	79%	41%	61%	93%
Evaluation of LVS Function	44	91%	65%	83%	99%
Smoking Cessation Advice[1]	3	100%	67%	82%	100%
Pneumonia Care					
Appropriate Initial Antibiotic	69	96%	78%	83%	94%
Blood Culture Timing	55	95%	93%	90%	100%
Influenza Vaccine	34	97%	63%	70%	100%
Initial Antibiotic Timing	97	93%	85%	80%	93%
Oxygenation Assessment	116	100%	99%	99%	100%
Pneumococcal Vaccine	83	89%	59%	69%	94%
Smoking Cessation Advice	32	100%	60%	80%	100%
Surgical Infection Prevention					
Prophylactic Antibiotic Given[3]	27	41%	74%	77%	95%
Prophylactic Antibiotic Selection[1]	7	100%	91%	90%	100%
Prophylactic Antibiotic Stopped[3]	26	35%	72%	72%	95%
Pregnancy Care					
Inpatient Neonatal Mortality	-	-	-	-	-
Third or Fourth Degree Laceration	-	-	3.82%	3.63%	3.27%

Heartland Surgical Specialty Hospital

10720 Nall
Overland Park, KS 66211
Ownership: Proprietary
Emergency Services: No
Phone: 913-754-4505
Accredited: Yes

Measure	Cases	This Hospital	State Average	U.S. Average	Top Hospital
Heart Attack Care					
ACE Inhibitor or ARB for LVSD[5]	-	-	78%	82%	100%
Aspirin at Arrival[5]	-	-	90%	92%	100%
Aspirin at Discharge[5]	-	-	88%	90%	100%

NOTE: Hospital profiles are in alphabetical order by state, then city, then hospital within the city; Rankings are sorted by rate in descending order and exclude hospitals with less than 25 cases; (1) The number of cases is too small (n<25) for purposes of reliably predicting hospital performance; (2) Measure reflects the hospital's indication that its submission was based upon a sample of its relevant discharges; (3) Rate reflects fewer than the maximum possible quarters of data for the measure; (4) Inaccurate information submitted and suppressed for one or more quarters; (5) No data is available from the hospital for this measure; Please refer to the User's Guide for a full explanation of data

Measure	Cases	This Hospital	State Average	U.S. Average	Top Hospital
Beta Blocker at Arrival[5]	-	-	82%	87%	100%
Beta Blocker at Discharge[5]	-	-	82%	90%	100%
Fibrinolytic Medication Timing[5]	-	-	24%	31%	100%
PCI Within 90 Minutes of Arrival[5]	-	-	55%	54%	95%
Smoking Cessation Advice[5]	-	-	86%	88%	100%
Heart Failure Care					
ACE Inhibitor or ARB for LVSD[5]	-	-	72%	82%	100%
Discharge Instructions[5]	-	-	41%	61%	93%
Evaluation of LVS Function[5]	-	-	65%	83%	99%
Smoking Cessation Advice[5]	-	-	67%	82%	100%
Pneumonia Care					
Appropriate Initial Antibiotic[5]	-	-	78%	83%	94%
Blood Culture Timing[5]	-	-	93%	90%	100%
Influenza Vaccine[5]	-	-	63%	70%	100%
Initial Antibiotic Timing[5]	-	-	85%	80%	93%
Oxygenation Assessment[5]	-	-	99%	99%	100%
Pneumococcal Vaccine[5]	-	-	59%	69%	94%
Smoking Cessation Advice[5]	-	-	60%	80%	100%
Surgical Infection Prevention					
Prophylactic Antibiotic Given	58	83%	74%	77%	95%
Prophylactic Antibiotic Selection[1]	20	95%	91%	90%	100%
Prophylactic Antibiotic Stopped	54	85%	72%	72%	95%
Pregnancy Care					
Inpatient Neonatal Mortality	-	-	-	-	-
Third or Fourth Degree Laceration	-	-	3.82%	3.63%	3.27%

Menorah Medical Center

5721 W 119th Street
Shawnee Mission, KS 66209
URL: www.menorahmedicalcenter.com
Ownership: Voluntary non-profit - Other
Emergency Services: Yes
Phone: 913-498-6000
Fax: 913-498-7106
Accredited: Yes
Licensed Beds: 158

Key Personnel:
CEO. . . . . Steven Wilkinson

Measure	Cases	This Hospital	State Average	U.S. Average	Top Hospital
Heart Attack Care					
ACE Inhibitor or ARB for LVSD[1]	13	77%	78%	82%	100%
Aspirin at Arrival	62	97%	90%	92%	100%
Aspirin at Discharge	75	97%	88%	90%	100%
Beta Blocker at Arrival	46	91%	82%	87%	100%
Beta Blocker at Discharge	66	97%	82%	90%	100%
Fibrinolytic Medication Timing	0	-	24%	31%	100%
PCI Within 90 Minutes of Arrival[1]	5	20%	55%	54%	95%
Smoking Cessation Advice	27	100%	86%	88%	100%
Heart Failure Care					
ACE Inhibitor or ARB for LVSD	42	81%	72%	82%	100%
Discharge Instructions	98	76%	41%	61%	93%
Evaluation of LVS Function	132	98%	65%	83%	99%
Smoking Cessation Advice[1]	20	100%	67%	82%	100%
Pneumonia Care					
Appropriate Initial Antibiotic	86	86%	78%	83%	94%
Blood Culture Timing	74	99%	93%	90%	100%
Influenza Vaccine[1]	23	83%	63%	70%	100%
Initial Antibiotic Timing	111	93%	85%	80%	93%
Oxygenation Assessment	140	97%	99%	99%	100%
Pneumococcal Vaccine	109	91%	59%	69%	94%
Smoking Cessation Advice[1]	22	100%	60%	80%	100%
Surgical Infection Prevention					
Prophylactic Antibiotic Given[2,3]	246	71%	74%	77%	95%
Prophylactic Antibiotic Selection[2]	116	84%	91%	90%	100%
Prophylactic Antibiotic Stopped[2,3]	235	53%	72%	72%	95%
Pregnancy Care					
Inpatient Neonatal Mortality	-	-	-	-	-
Third or Fourth Degree Laceration	-	-	3.82%	3.63%	3.27%

Overland Park Regional Medical Center

10500 Quivira Road
Overland Park, KS 66215
URL: www.oprmc.com
Ownership: Proprietary
Emergency Services: Yes
Phone: 913-541-5000
Fax: 913-541-5790
Accredited: No
Licensed Beds: 256

Key Personnel:
CEO. . . . . Kevin J Hicks

Measure	Cases	This Hospital	State Average	U.S. Average	Top Hospital
Heart Attack Care					
ACE Inhibitor or ARB for LVSD	25	84%	78%	82%	100%
Aspirin at Arrival	84	98%	90%	92%	100%
Aspirin at Discharge	81	95%	88%	90%	100%
Beta Blocker at Arrival	76	92%	82%	87%	100%
Beta Blocker at Discharge	79	99%	82%	90%	100%
Fibrinolytic Medication Timing	0	-	24%	31%	100%
PCI Within 90 Minutes of Arrival[1]	5	80%	55%	54%	95%
Smoking Cessation Advice	25	100%	86%	88%	100%
Heart Failure Care					
ACE Inhibitor or ARB for LVSD	67	88%	72%	82%	100%
Discharge Instructions	119	72%	41%	61%	93%
Evaluation of LVS Function	174	94%	65%	83%	99%
Smoking Cessation Advice[1]	19	74%	67%	82%	100%
Pneumonia Care					
Appropriate Initial Antibiotic	93	88%	78%	83%	94%
Blood Culture Timing	89	89%	93%	90%	100%
Influenza Vaccine	25	52%	63%	70%	100%
Initial Antibiotic Timing	128	85%	85%	80%	93%
Oxygenation Assessment	170	100%	99%	99%	100%
Pneumococcal Vaccine	104	62%	59%	69%	94%
Smoking Cessation Advice	30	87%	60%	80%	100%
Surgical Infection Prevention					
Prophylactic Antibiotic Given[2,3]	240	89%	74%	77%	95%
Prophylactic Antibiotic Selection[2]	111	95%	91%	90%	100%
Prophylactic Antibiotic Stopped[2,3]	221	73%	72%	72%	95%
Pregnancy Care					
Inpatient Neonatal Mortality	2,737	0.91%	-	-	-
Third or Fourth Degree Laceration	1,657	4.41%	3.82%	3.63%	3.27%

Saint Luke's South

12300 Metcalf Avenue
Overland Park, KS 66213
URL: www.saintlukeshealthsystem.org
Ownership: Voluntary non-profit - Other
Emergency Services: Yes
Phone: 913-317-7000
Fax: 913-317-7672
Accredited: Yes
Licensed Beds: 75

Key Personnel:
CEO. . . . . Julie L Quirin

Measure	Cases	This Hospital	State Average	U.S. Average	Top Hospital
Heart Attack Care					
ACE Inhibitor or ARB for LVSD[1]	4	100%	78%	82%	100%
Aspirin at Arrival	43	100%	90%	92%	100%
Aspirin at Discharge	42	95%	88%	90%	100%
Beta Blocker at Arrival	40	92%	82%	87%	100%
Beta Blocker at Discharge	41	98%	82%	90%	100%
Fibrinolytic Medication Timing	0	-	24%	31%	100%
PCI Within 90 Minutes of Arrival[1]	3	100%	55%	54%	95%
Smoking Cessation Advice[1]	17	100%	86%	88%	100%
Heart Failure Care					
ACE Inhibitor or ARB for LVSD	41	83%	72%	82%	100%
Discharge Instructions	70	60%	41%	61%	93%
Evaluation of LVS Function	89	98%	65%	83%	99%
Smoking Cessation Advice[1]	7	100%	67%	82%	100%
Pneumonia Care					
Appropriate Initial Antibiotic	66	86%	78%	83%	94%
Blood Culture Timing	43	95%	93%	90%	100%
Influenza Vaccine[1]	23	87%	63%	70%	100%
Initial Antibiotic Timing	78	90%	85%	80%	93%
Oxygenation Assessment	94	100%	99%	99%	100%
Pneumococcal Vaccine	64	92%	59%	69%	94%
Smoking Cessation Advice[1]	10	100%	60%	80%	100%

NOTE: Hospital profiles are in alphabetical order by state, then city, then hospital within the city; Rankings are sorted by rate in descending order and exclude hospitals with less than 25 cases; (1) The number of cases is too small (n<25) for purposes of reliably predicting hospital performance; (2) Measure reflects the hospital's indication that its submission was based upon a sample of its relevant discharges; (3) Rate reflects fewer than the maximum possible quarters of data for the measure; (4) Inaccurate information submitted and suppressed for one or more quarters; (5) No data is available from the hospital for this measure; Please refer to the User's Guide for a full explanation of data

Measure	Cases	This Hospital	State Average	U.S. Average	Top Hospital
Surgical Infection Prevention					
Prophylactic Antibiotic Given[3]	211	94%	74%	77%	95%
Prophylactic Antibiotic Selection	81	94%	91%	90%	100%
Prophylactic Antibiotic Stopped[3]	206	80%	72%	72%	95%
Pregnancy Care					
Inpatient Neonatal Mortality	-	-	-	-	-
Third or Fourth Degree Laceration	-	-	3.82%	3.63%	3.27%

Miami County Medical Center

2100 Baptiste Drive
Paola, KS 66071
Phone: 913-294-2327
Fax: 913-294-5919
Ownership: Govt - Hospital District or Authority
Accredited: Yes
Emergency Services: Yes
Licensed Beds: 39

Key Personnel:
Chief Medical Staff. . . . . Jack Campbell
Emergency Room Manager. . . . . Stacy Steiner
Director Infection/Disease Control . . . . Kathy Auten
Manager Medical/Surgical Nursing. . . . . Wendy Richardson
Manager Respiratory Therapy . . . . Stacy Steiner

Measure	Cases	This Hospital	State Average	U.S. Average	Top Hospital
Heart Attack Care					
ACE Inhibitor or ARB for LVSD[1,3]	1	100%	78%	82%	100%
Aspirin at Arrival[1,3]	2	100%	90%	92%	100%
Aspirin at Discharge[1,3]	2	100%	88%	90%	100%
Beta Blocker at Arrival[1,3]	1	100%	82%	87%	100%
Beta Blocker at Discharge[1,3]	2	100%	82%	90%	100%
Fibrinolytic Medication Timing[3]	0	-	24%	31%	100%
PCI Within 90 Minutes of Arrival[5]	-	-	55%	54%	95%
Smoking Cessation Advice[3]	0	-	86%	88%	100%
Heart Failure Care					
ACE Inhibitor or ARB for LVSD[1]	3	100%	72%	82%	100%
Discharge Instructions[1]	8	50%	41%	61%	93%
Evaluation of LVS Function[1]	13	92%	65%	83%	99%
Smoking Cessation Advice	0	-	67%	82%	100%
Pneumonia Care					
Appropriate Initial Antibiotic	33	88%	78%	83%	94%
Blood Culture Timing	25	96%	93%	90%	100%
Influenza Vaccine[1]	12	100%	63%	70%	100%
Initial Antibiotic Timing	41	93%	85%	80%	93%
Oxygenation Assessment	58	100%	99%	99%	100%
Pneumococcal Vaccine	32	84%	59%	69%	94%
Smoking Cessation Advice[1]	20	100%	60%	80%	100%
Surgical Infection Prevention					
Prophylactic Antibiotic Given[3]	52	60%	74%	77%	95%
Prophylactic Antibiotic Selection[1]	17	100%	91%	90%	100%
Prophylactic Antibiotic Stopped[3]	50	2%	72%	72%	95%
Pregnancy Care					
Inpatient Neonatal Mortality	-	-	-	-	-
Third or Fourth Degree Laceration	-	-	3.82%	3.63%	3.27%

Labette County Medical Center

1902 S US Highway 59
Parsons, KS 67357
Toll-Free: 800-843-5262
Phone: 620-421-4880
Fax: 620-421-5042
URL: www.lcmc.com
Ownership: Govt - Hospital District or Authority
Accredited: Yes
Emergency Services: Yes
Licensed Beds: 109

Key Personnel:
CEO. . . . . William Mahoney
Chief of Medical Staff. . . . . Dr Rothstein
Emergency Room . . . . Linda West
Infection Control. . . . . Carol Hale
ICU . . . . Kathy McKinney
Medical/Surgical Nursing . . . . Kathy McKinney
OB/GYN Womens Health. . . . . Donna Vitt

Measure	Cases	This Hospital	State Average	U.S. Average	Top Hospital
Heart Attack Care					
ACE Inhibitor or ARB for LVSD	0	-	78%	82%	100%
Aspirin at Arrival[1]	7	71%	90%	92%	100%
Aspirin at Discharge[1]	2	100%	88%	90%	100%
Beta Blocker at Arrival[1]	7	29%	82%	87%	100%
Beta Blocker at Discharge[1]	3	67%	82%	90%	100%
Fibrinolytic Medication Timing	0	-	24%	31%	100%
PCI Within 90 Minutes of Arrival	0	-	55%	54%	95%
Smoking Cessation Advice	0	-	86%	88%	100%
Heart Failure Care					
ACE Inhibitor or ARB for LVSD	34	44%	72%	82%	100%
Discharge Instructions	68	28%	41%	61%	93%
Evaluation of LVS Function	81	73%	65%	83%	99%
Smoking Cessation Advice[1]	14	57%	67%	82%	100%
Pneumonia Care					
Appropriate Initial Antibiotic	70	70%	78%	83%	94%
Blood Culture Timing	43	100%	93%	90%	100%
Influenza Vaccine[1]	20	55%	63%	70%	100%
Initial Antibiotic Timing[3]	76	68%	85%	80%	93%
Oxygenation Assessment	125	100%	99%	99%	100%
Pneumococcal Vaccine	80	50%	59%	69%	94%
Smoking Cessation Advice[1]	24	50%	60%	80%	100%
Surgical Infection Prevention					
Prophylactic Antibiotic Given	390	73%	74%	77%	95%
Prophylactic Antibiotic Selection	88	97%	91%	90%	100%
Prophylactic Antibiotic Stopped	361	78%	72%	72%	95%
Pregnancy Care					
Inpatient Neonatal Mortality	-	-	-	-	-
Third or Fourth Degree Laceration	-	-	3.82%	3.63%	3.27%

Phillips County Hospital

1150 State Street
Phillipsburg, KS 67661
Phone: 785-543-5226
Fax: 785-543-6272
Ownership: Government - Local
Accredited: No
Emergency Services: Yes
Licensed Beds: 62

Key Personnel:
President/CEO. . . . . Heather Harper

Measure	Cases	This Hospital	State Average	U.S. Average	Top Hospital
Heart Attack Care					
ACE Inhibitor or ARB for LVSD[3]	0	-	78%	82%	100%
Aspirin at Arrival[3]	0	-	90%	92%	100%
Aspirin at Discharge[3]	0	-	88%	90%	100%
Beta Blocker at Arrival[1,3]	1	100%	82%	87%	100%
Beta Blocker at Discharge[1,3]	1	100%	82%	90%	100%
Fibrinolytic Medication Timing[3]	0	-	24%	31%	100%
PCI Within 90 Minutes of Arrival[5]	-	-	55%	54%	95%
Smoking Cessation Advice[3]	0	-	86%	88%	100%
Heart Failure Care					
ACE Inhibitor or ARB for LVSD[1]	6	100%	72%	82%	100%
Discharge Instructions[1]	5	0%	41%	61%	93%
Evaluation of LVS Function[1]	15	40%	65%	83%	99%
Smoking Cessation Advice[1]	1	0%	67%	82%	100%
Pneumonia Care					
Appropriate Initial Antibiotic[1]	10	70%	78%	83%	94%
Blood Culture Timing[1]	3	67%	93%	90%	100%
Influenza Vaccine[1]	8	88%	63%	70%	100%
Initial Antibiotic Timing[1]	10	80%	85%	80%	93%
Oxygenation Assessment[1]	18	100%	99%	99%	100%
Pneumococcal Vaccine[1]	15	60%	59%	69%	94%
Smoking Cessation Advice[1]	2	50%	60%	80%	100%
Surgical Infection Prevention					
Prophylactic Antibiotic Given[5]	-	-	74%	77%	95%
Prophylactic Antibiotic Selection[5]	-	-	91%	90%	100%
Prophylactic Antibiotic Stopped[5]	-	-	72%	72%	95%
Pregnancy Care					
Inpatient Neonatal Mortality	-	-	-	-	-
Third or Fourth Degree Laceration	-	-	3.82%	3.63%	3.27%

Mount Carmel Regional Medical Center

1102 E Centennial
Pittsburg, KS 66762
Phone: 620-231-6100
Fax: 620-232-0493
URL: www.mtcarmel.org
Ownership: Voluntary non-profit - Church
Accredited: Yes
Emergency Services: Yes
Licensed Beds: 188

Key Personnel:
President/CEO. . . . . Jonathan Davis

NOTE: Hospital profiles are in alphabetical order by state, then city, then hospital within the city; Rankings are sorted by rate in descending order and exclude hospitals with less than 25 cases; (1) The number of cases is too small (n<25) for purposes of reliably predicting hospital performance; (2) Measure reflects the hospital's indication that its submission was based upon a sample of its relevant discharges; (3) Rate reflects fewer than the maximum possible quarters of data for the measure; (4) Inaccurate information submitted and suppressed for one or more quarters; (5) No data is available from the hospital for this measure; Please refer to the User's Guide for a full explanation of data

Chief Medical Staff. . . . . Renee Bartlett, MD
Director Surgery/PAR/Day Surgery . . . . Brenda Lemmons
Director Heart Center. . . . . Bill Kellogg
Director Cardiopulmonary/Emergency Svcs. . . . Tom Pryor
Infection Control Nurse. Wayne MeDown
Intensive Coronary. . . . . Lois Scofield
Director Women's Services . . . . SanDee McChristy
Director Surgery. . . . . Brenda Lemmons
Director Cardiopulmonary Services . . . . Tom Pryor

Measure	Cases	This Hospital	State Average	U.S. Average	Top Hospital
Heart Attack Care					
ACE Inhibitor or ARB for LVSD[1]	11	91%	78%	82%	100%
Aspirin at Arrival	67	100%	90%	92%	100%
Aspirin at Discharge	55	95%	88%	90%	100%
Beta Blocker at Arrival	58	95%	82%	87%	100%
Beta Blocker at Discharge	53	94%	82%	90%	100%
Fibrinolytic Medication Timing[1]	4	50%	24%	31%	100%
PCI Within 90 Minutes of Arrival[1]	1	100%	55%	54%	95%
Smoking Cessation Advice[1]	18	100%	86%	88%	100%
Heart Failure Care					
ACE Inhibitor or ARB for LVSD	45	91%	72%	82%	100%
Discharge Instructions	105	58%	41%	61%	93%
Evaluation of LVS Function	151	97%	65%	83%	99%
Smoking Cessation Advice[1]	18	89%	67%	82%	100%
Pneumonia Care					
Appropriate Initial Antibiotic	75	80%	78%	83%	94%
Blood Culture Timing	92	99%	93%	90%	100%
Influenza Vaccine	46	83%	63%	70%	100%
Initial Antibiotic Timing	119	91%	85%	80%	93%
Oxygenation Assessment	155	100%	99%	99%	100%
Pneumococcal Vaccine	101	83%	59%	69%	94%
Smoking Cessation Advice	35	60%	60%	80%	100%
Surgical Infection Prevention					
Prophylactic Antibiotic Given[3]	169	83%	74%	77%	95%
Prophylactic Antibiotic Selection	52	81%	91%	90%	100%
Prophylactic Antibiotic Stopped[3]	166	66%	72%	72%	95%
Pregnancy Care					
Inpatient Neonatal Mortality	-	-	-	-	-
Third or Fourth Degree Laceration	-	-	3.82%	3.63%	3.27%

Pratt Regional Medical Center

200 Commodore
Pratt, KS 67124

Toll-Free: 888-900-7762
Phone: 620-672-6476
Fax: 620-672-2113

E-mail: spage@prmc.org
URL: www.prmc.org
Ownership: Voluntary non-profit - Private
Emergency Services: Yes
Accredited: No
Licensed Beds: 84

Key Personnel:
President/CEO. . . . . Susan Page
Chief Medical Staff. . . . . Wakon Fowler, MD
Infection Control Nurse. . . . . Cecile Pearce, RN
CEO. . . . . Susan Page
Cardiopulmonary Services . . . . Bill Rea

Measure	Cases	This Hospital	State Average	U.S. Average	Top Hospital
Heart Attack Care					
ACE Inhibitor or ARB for LVSD[3]	0	-	78%	82%	100%
Aspirin at Arrival[1,3]	2	100%	90%	92%	100%
Aspirin at Discharge[3]	0	-	88%	90%	100%
Beta Blocker at Arrival[1,3]	2	100%	82%	87%	100%
Beta Blocker at Discharge[3]	0	-	82%	90%	100%
Fibrinolytic Medication Timing[3]	0	-	24%	31%	100%
PCI Within 90 Minutes of Arrival	0	-	55%	54%	95%
Smoking Cessation Advice[3]	0	-	86%	88%	100%
Heart Failure Care					
ACE Inhibitor or ARB for LVSD[1]	3	67%	72%	82%	100%
Discharge Instructions	26	42%	41%	61%	93%
Evaluation of LVS Function	30	50%	65%	83%	99%
Smoking Cessation Advice[1]	8	50%	67%	82%	100%
Pneumonia Care					
Appropriate Initial Antibiotic	36	72%	78%	83%	94%
Blood Culture Timing[1]	19	95%	93%	90%	100%
Influenza Vaccine[1]	12	67%	63%	70%	100%
Initial Antibiotic Timing	58	84%	85%	80%	93%
Oxygenation Assessment	61	100%	99%	99%	100%
Pneumococcal Vaccine	49	69%	59%	69%	94%
Smoking Cessation Advice[1]	7	57%	60%	80%	100%
Surgical Infection Prevention					
Prophylactic Antibiotic Given[2]	112	93%	74%	77%	95%
Prophylactic Antibiotic Selection[2]	35	89%	91%	90%	100%
Prophylactic Antibiotic Stopped[2]	110	97%	72%	72%	95%
Pregnancy Care					
Inpatient Neonatal Mortality	-	-	-	-	-
Third or Fourth Degree Laceration	-	-	3.82%	3.63%	3.27%

Grisell Memorial Hospital

210 S Vermont Avenue
PO Box 268
Ransom, KS 67572
Ownership: Govt - Hospital District or Authority
Emergency Services: No

Phone: 785-731-2231
Fax: 785-731-2895
Accredited: No
Licensed Beds: 46

Key Personnel:
CEO. . . . . Kris Ochs
Chief Medical Staff. . . . . Allen McLean, MD
Emergency Room . . . . Allen McLean, MD

Measure	Cases	This Hospital	State Average	U.S. Average	Top Hospital
Heart Attack Care					
ACE Inhibitor or ARB for LVSD[5]	-	-	78%	82%	100%
Aspirin at Arrival[5]	-	-	90%	92%	100%
Aspirin at Discharge[5]	-	-	88%	90%	100%
Beta Blocker at Arrival[5]	-	-	82%	87%	100%
Beta Blocker at Discharge[5]	-	-	82%	90%	100%
Fibrinolytic Medication Timing[5]	-	-	24%	31%	100%
PCI Within 90 Minutes of Arrival[5]	-	-	55%	54%	95%
Smoking Cessation Advice[5]	-	-	86%	88%	100%
Heart Failure Care					
ACE Inhibitor or ARB for LVSD[5]	-	-	72%	82%	100%
Discharge Instructions[5]	-	-	41%	61%	93%
Evaluation of LVS Function[5]	-	-	65%	83%	99%
Smoking Cessation Advice[5]	-	-	67%	82%	100%
Pneumonia Care					
Appropriate Initial Antibiotic[5]	-	-	78%	83%	94%
Blood Culture Timing[5]	-	-	93%	90%	100%
Influenza Vaccine[5]	-	-	63%	70%	100%
Initial Antibiotic Timing[5]	-	-	85%	80%	93%
Oxygenation Assessment[5]	-	-	99%	99%	100%
Pneumococcal Vaccine[5]	-	-	59%	69%	94%
Smoking Cessation Advice[5]	-	-	60%	80%	100%
Surgical Infection Prevention					
Prophylactic Antibiotic Given[5]	-	-	74%	77%	95%
Prophylactic Antibiotic Selection[5]	-	-	91%	90%	100%
Prophylactic Antibiotic Stopped[5]	-	-	72%	72%	95%
Pregnancy Care					
Inpatient Neonatal Mortality	-	-	-	-	-
Third or Fourth Degree Laceration	-	-	3.82%	3.63%	3.27%

Sabetha Community Hospital

14th & Oregon Streets
Sabetha, KS 66534
Ownership: Voluntary non-profit - Other
Emergency Services: No

Phone: 785-284-2121
Fax: 785-284-2516
Accredited: No
Licensed Beds: 27

Key Personnel:
President/CEO. . . . . Rita Buurman

Measure	Cases	This Hospital	State Average	U.S. Average	Top Hospital
Heart Attack Care					
ACE Inhibitor or ARB for LVSD	0	-	78%	82%	100%
Aspirin at Arrival[1]	2	100%	90%	92%	100%
Aspirin at Discharge[1]	2	100%	88%	90%	100%
Beta Blocker at Arrival[1]	1	0%	82%	87%	100%
Beta Blocker at Discharge[1]	2	100%	82%	90%	100%
Fibrinolytic Medication Timing	0	-	24%	31%	100%

NOTE: Hospital profiles are in alphabetical order by state, then city, then hospital within the city; Rankings are sorted by rate in descending order and exclude hospitals with less than 25 cases; (1) The number of cases is too small (n<25) for purposes of reliably predicting hospital performance; (2) Measure reflects the hospital's indication that its submission was based upon a sample of its relevant discharges; (3) Rate reflects fewer than the maximum possible quarters of data for the measure; (4) Inaccurate information submitted and suppressed for one or more quarters; (5) No data is available from the hospital for this measure; Please refer to the User's Guide for a full explanation of data

PCI Within 90 Minutes of Arrival	0	-	55%	54%	95%
Smoking Cessation Advice	0	-	86%	88%	100%
Heart Failure Care					
ACE Inhibitor or ARB for LVSD[1]	4	75%	72%	82%	100%
Discharge Instructions[1]	3	0%	41%	61%	93%
Evaluation of LVS Function[1]	11	73%	65%	83%	99%
Smoking Cessation Advice	0	-	67%	82%	100%
Pneumonia Care					
Appropriate Initial Antibiotic[1]	17	100%	78%	83%	94%
Blood Culture Timing[1]	1	100%	93%	90%	100%
Influenza Vaccine[1]	3	67%	63%	70%	100%
Initial Antibiotic Timing[1]	22	95%	85%	80%	93%
Oxygenation Assessment	33	100%	99%	99%	100%
Pneumococcal Vaccine	25	68%	59%	69%	94%
Smoking Cessation Advice[1]	4	50%	60%	80%	100%
Surgical Infection Prevention					
Prophylactic Antibiotic Given[1,3]	4	75%	74%	77%	95%
Prophylactic Antibiotic Selection[5]	-	-	91%	90%	100%
Prophylactic Antibiotic Stopped[1,3]	4	75%	72%	72%	95%
Pregnancy Care					
Inpatient Neonatal Mortality	-	-	-	-	-
Third or Fourth Degree Laceration	-	-	3.82%	3.63%	3.27%

Cheyenne County Hospital

210 W 1st Street
PO Box 547
Saint Francis, KS 67756
Phone: 785-332-2104
Fax: 785-332-2106
E-mail: llacy@cheyennecountyhospital.com
URL: cheyennecountyhospital.com
Ownership: Government - Local
Accredited: No
Emergency Services: Yes
Licensed Beds: 16

Key Personnel:
Administrator . . . . Leslie Lacy, RN
CEO. . . . . Leslie Lacey
Emergency Room . . . . Craig Button

Measure	Cases	This Hospital	State Average	U.S. Average	Top Hospital
Heart Attack Care					
ACE Inhibitor or ARB for LVSD[3]	0	-	78%	82%	100%
Aspirin at Arrival[1,3]	4	100%	90%	92%	100%
Aspirin at Discharge[1,3]	4	100%	88%	90%	100%
Beta Blocker at Arrival[1,3]	3	33%	82%	87%	100%
Beta Blocker at Discharge[1,3]	3	100%	82%	90%	100%
Fibrinolytic Medication Timing[1,3]	1	0%	24%	31%	100%
PCI Within 90 Minutes of Arrival[5]	-	-	55%	54%	95%
Smoking Cessation Advice[3]	0	-	86%	88%	100%
Heart Failure Care					
ACE Inhibitor or ARB for LVSD[3]	0	-	72%	82%	100%
Discharge Instructions[1,3]	3	0%	41%	61%	93%
Evaluation of LVS Function[1,3]	3	0%	65%	83%	99%
Smoking Cessation Advice[3]	0	-	67%	82%	100%
Pneumonia Care					
Appropriate Initial Antibiotic[1,3]	15	100%	78%	83%	94%
Blood Culture Timing[1,3]	1	100%	93%	90%	100%
Influenza Vaccine[1]	5	60%	63%	70%	100%
Initial Antibiotic Timing[1,3]	15	67%	85%	80%	93%
Oxygenation Assessment[1,3]	21	100%	99%	99%	100%
Pneumococcal Vaccine[1,3]	16	44%	59%	69%	94%
Smoking Cessation Advice[1,3]	4	25%	60%	80%	100%
Surgical Infection Prevention					
Prophylactic Antibiotic Given[5]	-	-	74%	77%	95%
Prophylactic Antibiotic Selection[5]	-	-	91%	90%	100%
Prophylactic Antibiotic Stopped[5]	-	-	72%	72%	95%
Pregnancy Care					
Inpatient Neonatal Mortality	-	-	-	-	-
Third or Fourth Degree Laceration	-	-	3.82%	3.63%	3.27%

Salina Regional Health Center

400 S Santa Fe
Salina, KS 67401
Phone: 785-452-7000
Fax: 785-452-6963
E-mail: srhc@midusa.net
URL: www.srhc.com
Ownership: Voluntary non-profit - Private
Accredited: Yes
Emergency Services: Yes
Licensed Beds: 385

Key Personnel:
President/CEO. . . . . Randy Peterson
Chief Medical Staff. . . . . Mark Mikinski, MD
Director Surgical Services . . . . Craig Koppen
Manager Non-Invasive Cardiac Lab. . . . . Janice Hanson
Supervisor Cardiac Catheterization Lab. . . . . . . Ann Alexandres
Director Emergency Department . . . . Emma Doherty
Infection Control Coordinator . . . . Kelli Olson
Director Medical/Surgical Nursing . . . . Joyce Roegge
Director Women/Children Services . . . . Deb Hyman
Director Women & Children Services. . . . . Deb Hyman
Director Radiology . . . . Terry Hauschel
Director Respiratory Therapy . . . . Troy Gooch

Measure	Cases	This Hospital	State Average	U.S. Average	Top Hospital
Heart Attack Care					
ACE Inhibitor or ARB for LVSD	35	91%	78%	82%	100%
Aspirin at Arrival	120	95%	90%	92%	100%
Aspirin at Discharge	194	96%	88%	90%	100%
Beta Blocker at Arrival	115	88%	82%	87%	100%
Beta Blocker at Discharge	192	87%	82%	90%	100%
Fibrinolytic Medication Timing[1]	13	62%	24%	31%	100%
PCI Within 90 Minutes of Arrival[1]	3	0%	55%	54%	95%
Smoking Cessation Advice	73	97%	86%	88%	100%
Heart Failure Care					
ACE Inhibitor or ARB for LVSD	60	95%	72%	82%	100%
Discharge Instructions	137	50%	41%	61%	93%
Evaluation of LVS Function	186	76%	65%	83%	99%
Smoking Cessation Advice	28	86%	67%	82%	100%
Pneumonia Care					
Appropriate Initial Antibiotic	120	86%	78%	83%	94%
Blood Culture Timing	110	95%	93%	90%	100%
Influenza Vaccine	53	53%	63%	70%	100%
Initial Antibiotic Timing	173	76%	85%	80%	93%
Oxygenation Assessment	211	100%	99%	99%	100%
Pneumococcal Vaccine	147	53%	59%	69%	94%
Smoking Cessation Advice	55	76%	60%	80%	100%
Surgical Infection Prevention					
Prophylactic Antibiotic Given[2]	623	92%	74%	77%	95%
Prophylactic Antibiotic Selection[2]	143	96%	91%	90%	100%
Prophylactic Antibiotic Stopped[2]	604	61%	72%	72%	95%
Pregnancy Care					
Inpatient Neonatal Mortality	-	-	-	-	-
Third or Fourth Degree Laceration	-	-	3.82%	3.63%	3.27%

Salina Surgical Hospital

401 South Santa Fe
Salina, KS 67401
Phone: 785-827-0610
Ownership: Proprietary
Accredited: No
Emergency Services: No

Measure	Cases	This Hospital	State Average	U.S. Average	Top Hospital
Heart Attack Care					
ACE Inhibitor or ARB for LVSD[5]	-	-	78%	82%	100%
Aspirin at Arrival[5]	-	-	90%	92%	100%
Aspirin at Discharge[5]	-	-	88%	90%	100%
Beta Blocker at Arrival[5]	-	-	82%	87%	100%
Beta Blocker at Discharge[5]	-	-	82%	90%	100%
Fibrinolytic Medication Timing[5]	-	-	24%	31%	100%
PCI Within 90 Minutes of Arrival[5]	-	-	55%	54%	95%
Smoking Cessation Advice[5]	-	-	86%	88%	100%
Heart Failure Care					
ACE Inhibitor or ARB for LVSD[5]	-	-	72%	82%	100%
Discharge Instructions[5]	-	-	41%	61%	93%
Evaluation of LVS Function[5]	-	-	65%	83%	99%
Smoking Cessation Advice[5]	-	-	67%	82%	100%

NOTE: Hospital profiles are in alphabetical order by state, then city, then hospital within the city; Rankings are sorted by rate in descending order and exclude hospitals with less than 25 cases; (1) The number of cases is too small (n<25) for purposes of reliably predicting hospital performance; (2) Measure reflects the hospital's indication that its submission was based upon a sample of its relevant discharges; (3) Rate reflects fewer than the maximum possible quarters of data for the measure; (4) Inaccurate information submitted and suppressed for one or more quarters; (5) No data is available from the hospital for this measure; Please refer to the User's Guide for a full explanation of data

Measure	Cases	This Hospital	State Average	U.S. Average	Top Hospital
Pneumonia Care					
Appropriate Initial Antibiotic[5]	-	-	78%	83%	94%
Blood Culture Timing[5]	-	-	93%	90%	100%
Influenza Vaccine[5]	-	-	63%	70%	100%
Initial Antibiotic Timing[5]	-	-	85%	80%	93%
Oxygenation Assessment[5]	-	-	99%	99%	100%
Pneumococcal Vaccine[5]	-	-	59%	69%	94%
Smoking Cessation Advice[5]	-	-	60%	80%	100%
Surgical Infection Prevention					
Prophylactic Antibiotic Given	374	93%	74%	77%	95%
Prophylactic Antibiotic Selection	103	99%	91%	90%	100%
Prophylactic Antibiotic Stopped	372	76%	72%	72%	95%
Pregnancy Care					
Inpatient Neonatal Mortality	-	-	-	-	-
Third or Fourth Degree Laceration	-	-	3.82%	3.63%	3.27%

Scott County Hospital

310 E 3rd Street
Scott City, KS 67871
URL: www.scotthospital.net
Ownership: Government - Local
Emergency Services: Yes

Phone: 620-872-5811
Fax: 620-872-7193
Accredited: No
Licensed Beds: 27

Key Personnel:

President/CEO . . . . Mark Burnett
Chief of Medical Staff . . . . Christian Cupp
Director Infection/Disease Control . . . . Thea Beckman
Surgical Services . . . . Deanna Kennedy
Respiratory Care . . . . Isidro Morales

Measure	Cases	This Hospital	State Average	U.S. Average	Top Hospital
Heart Attack Care					
ACE Inhibitor or ARB for LVSD[5]	-	-	78%	82%	100%
Aspirin at Arrival[5]	-	-	90%	92%	100%
Aspirin at Discharge[5]	-	-	88%	90%	100%
Beta Blocker at Arrival[5]	-	-	82%	87%	100%
Beta Blocker at Discharge[5]	-	-	82%	90%	100%
Fibrinolytic Medication Timing[5]	-	-	24%	31%	100%
PCI Within 90 Minutes of Arrival[5]	-	-	55%	54%	95%
Smoking Cessation Advice[5]	-	-	86%	88%	100%
Heart Failure Care					
ACE Inhibitor or ARB for LVSD[5]	-	-	72%	82%	100%
Discharge Instructions[5]	-	-	41%	61%	93%
Evaluation of LVS Function[5]	-	-	65%	83%	99%
Smoking Cessation Advice[5]	-	-	67%	82%	100%
Pneumonia Care					
Appropriate Initial Antibiotic[5]	-	-	78%	83%	94%
Blood Culture Timing[5]	-	-	93%	90%	100%
Influenza Vaccine[5]	-	-	63%	70%	100%
Initial Antibiotic Timing[5]	-	-	85%	80%	93%
Oxygenation Assessment[5]	-	-	99%	99%	100%
Pneumococcal Vaccine[5]	-	-	59%	69%	94%
Smoking Cessation Advice[5]	-	-	60%	80%	100%
Surgical Infection Prevention					
Prophylactic Antibiotic Given[5]	-	-	74%	77%	95%
Prophylactic Antibiotic Selection[5]	-	-	91%	90%	100%
Prophylactic Antibiotic Stopped[5]	-	-	72%	72%	95%
Pregnancy Care					
Inpatient Neonatal Mortality	-	-	-	-	-
Third or Fourth Degree Laceration	-	-	3.82%	3.63%	3.27%

Nemaha Valley Community Hospital

1600 Community Drive
Seneca, KS 66538

Ownership: Voluntary non-profit - Other
Emergency Services: Yes

Toll-Free: 888-697-6181
Phone: 785-336-6181
Fax: 785-336-3052
Accredited: No
Licensed Beds: 24

Key Personnel:

Administrator/CEO . . . . Stan Regehr
Director Infection/Disease Control . . . . Donna Stallbuam
OB/GYN Womens Health . . . . James Lueger, MD

Measure	Cases	This Hospital	State Average	U.S. Average	Top Hospital
Heart Attack Care					
ACE Inhibitor or ARB for LVSD[5]	-	-	78%	82%	100%
Aspirin at Arrival[5]	-	-	90%	92%	100%
Aspirin at Discharge[5]	-	-	88%	90%	100%
Beta Blocker at Arrival[5]	-	-	82%	87%	100%
Beta Blocker at Discharge[5]	-	-	82%	90%	100%
Fibrinolytic Medication Timing[5]	-	-	24%	31%	100%
PCI Within 90 Minutes of Arrival[5]	-	-	55%	54%	95%
Smoking Cessation Advice[5]	-	-	86%	88%	100%
Heart Failure Care					
ACE Inhibitor or ARB for LVSD[5]	-	-	72%	82%	100%
Discharge Instructions[5]	-	-	41%	61%	93%
Evaluation of LVS Function[5]	-	-	65%	83%	99%
Smoking Cessation Advice[5]	-	-	67%	82%	100%
Pneumonia Care					
Appropriate Initial Antibiotic[5]	-	-	78%	83%	94%
Blood Culture Timing[5]	-	-	93%	90%	100%
Influenza Vaccine[5]	-	-	63%	70%	100%
Initial Antibiotic Timing[5]	-	-	85%	80%	93%
Oxygenation Assessment[5]	-	-	99%	99%	100%
Pneumococcal Vaccine[5]	-	-	59%	69%	94%
Smoking Cessation Advice[5]	-	-	60%	80%	100%
Surgical Infection Prevention					
Prophylactic Antibiotic Given[5]	-	-	74%	77%	95%
Prophylactic Antibiotic Selection[5]	-	-	91%	90%	100%
Prophylactic Antibiotic Stopped[5]	-	-	72%	72%	95%
Pregnancy Care					
Inpatient Neonatal Mortality	-	-	-	-	-
Third or Fourth Degree Laceration	-	-	3.82%	3.63%	3.27%

Shawnee Mission Medical Center

9100 W 74th Street
Shawnee Mission, KS 66204
E-mail: webmaster@shawneemission.org
URL: www.shawneemission.org
Ownership: Voluntary non-profit - Church
Emergency Services: Yes

Phone: 913-676-2000
Fax: 913-676-7724
Accredited: Yes
Licensed Beds: 383

Key Personnel:

President/CEO . . . . Samuel H Turner, Sr
Director of Pulmonary . . . . Janie Hoffman

Measure	Cases	This Hospital	State Average	U.S. Average	Top Hospital
Heart Attack Care					
ACE Inhibitor or ARB for LVSD	55	96%	78%	82%	100%
Aspirin at Arrival	209	100%	90%	92%	100%
Aspirin at Discharge	211	99%	88%	90%	100%
Beta Blocker at Arrival	189	99%	82%	87%	100%
Beta Blocker at Discharge	203	99%	82%	90%	100%
Fibrinolytic Medication Timing	0	-	24%	31%	100%
PCI Within 90 Minutes of Arrival[1]	14	57%	55%	54%	95%
Smoking Cessation Advice	77	96%	86%	88%	100%
Heart Failure Care					
ACE Inhibitor or ARB for LVSD	136	99%	72%	82%	100%
Discharge Instructions	284	40%	41%	61%	93%
Evaluation of LVS Function	372	98%	65%	83%	99%
Smoking Cessation Advice	51	65%	67%	82%	100%
Pneumonia Care					
Appropriate Initial Antibiotic	215	83%	78%	83%	94%
Blood Culture Timing	187	95%	93%	90%	100%
Influenza Vaccine	69	74%	63%	70%	100%
Initial Antibiotic Timing	297	79%	85%	80%	93%
Oxygenation Assessment	340	100%	99%	99%	100%
Pneumococcal Vaccine	228	69%	59%	69%	94%
Smoking Cessation Advice	54	70%	60%	80%	100%
Surgical Infection Prevention					
Prophylactic Antibiotic Given[3]	627	74%	74%	77%	95%
Prophylactic Antibiotic Selection	59	93%	91%	90%	100%
Prophylactic Antibiotic Stopped[3]	620	66%	72%	72%	95%
Pregnancy Care					
Inpatient Neonatal Mortality	3,593	0.06%	-	-	-
Third or Fourth Degree Laceration	2,447	4.21%	3.82%	3.63%	3.27%

NOTE: Hospital profiles are in alphabetical order by state, then city, then hospital within the city; Rankings are sorted by rate in descending order and exclude hospitals with less than 25 cases; (1) The number of cases is too small (n<25) for purposes of reliably predicting hospital performance; (2) Measure reflects the hospital's indication that its submission was based upon a sample of its relevant discharges; (3) Rate reflects fewer than the maximum possible quarters of data for the measure; (4) Inaccurate information submitted and suppressed for one or more quarters; (5) No data is available from the hospital for this measure; Please refer to the User's Guide for a full explanation of data

Smith County Memorial Hospital

Alternate Name: Great Plains of Smith County
614 S Main Street
Smith Center, KS 66967
Ownership: Government - Local
Emergency Services: Yes

Phone: 785-282-6845
Fax: 785-282-6331
Accredited: No
Licensed Beds: 54

Key Personnel:
Administrator . . . . Carolyn K Hess
Chief Medical Staff. . . . . Joe Barnes, MD
Emergency Room . . . . Jodie Frydendall
Director Infection/Disease Control . . . . Karen Herndon
OB/GYN Womens Health. . . . . Paula Hayes, RN
Chief Radiology . . . . Penny McKenzie

Measure	Cases	This Hospital	State Average	U.S. Average	Top Hospital
Heart Attack Care					
ACE Inhibitor or ARB for LVSD[3]	0	-	78%	82%	100%
Aspirin at Arrival[1,3]	4	100%	90%	92%	100%
Aspirin at Discharge[1,3]	3	67%	88%	90%	100%
Beta Blocker at Arrival[1,3]	4	50%	82%	87%	100%
Beta Blocker at Discharge[1,3]	3	100%	82%	90%	100%
Fibrinolytic Medication Timing[1,3]	2	50%	24%	31%	100%
PCI Within 90 Minutes of Arrival	0	-	55%	54%	95%
Smoking Cessation Advice[3]	0	-	86%	88%	100%
Heart Failure Care					
ACE Inhibitor or ARB for LVSD[1,3]	1	100%	72%	82%	100%
Discharge Instructions[1,3]	17	35%	41%	61%	93%
Evaluation of LVS Function[1,3]	24	58%	65%	83%	99%
Smoking Cessation Advice[3]	0	-	67%	82%	100%
Pneumonia Care					
Appropriate Initial Antibiotic[1]	16	88%	78%	83%	94%
Blood Culture Timing[1]	3	100%	93%	90%	100%
Influenza Vaccine[1]	5	60%	63%	70%	100%
Initial Antibiotic Timing[1]	15	93%	85%	80%	93%
Oxygenation Assessment[1]	21	100%	99%	99%	100%
Pneumococcal Vaccine[1]	14	93%	59%	69%	94%
Smoking Cessation Advice[1]	2	50%	60%	80%	100%
Surgical Infection Prevention					
Prophylactic Antibiotic Given[5]	-	-	74%	77%	95%
Prophylactic Antibiotic Selection[5]	-	-	91%	90%	100%
Prophylactic Antibiotic Stopped[5]	-	-	72%	72%	95%
Pregnancy Care					
Inpatient Neonatal Mortality	-	-	-	-	-
Third or Fourth Degree Laceration	-	-	3.82%	3.63%	3.27%

Hamilton County Hospital

700 N Huser Street
PO Box 948
Syracuse, KS 67878
URL: www.hamiltoncountyhospital.net
Ownership: Government - Local
Emergency Services: No

Phone: 620-384-7461
Fax: 620-384-5500
Accredited: No
Licensed Beds: 29

Key Personnel:
CEO. . . . . Edwin E Hurysz
Emergency Room . . . . Joseph Rehal, MD
Director Medical/Surgical Nursing . . . . Cynthia Akers, RN

Measure	Cases	This Hospital	State Average	U.S. Average	Top Hospital
Heart Attack Care					
ACE Inhibitor or ARB for LVSD[3]	0	-	78%	82%	100%
Aspirin at Arrival[1,3]	1	100%	90%	92%	100%
Aspirin at Discharge[1,3]	1	100%	88%	90%	100%
Beta Blocker at Arrival[1,3]	1	100%	82%	87%	100%
Beta Blocker at Discharge[1,3]	1	100%	82%	90%	100%
Fibrinolytic Medication Timing[3]	0	-	24%	31%	100%
PCI Within 90 Minutes of Arrival[5]	-	-	55%	54%	95%
Smoking Cessation Advice[3]	0	-	86%	88%	100%
Heart Failure Care					
ACE Inhibitor or ARB for LVSD[3]	0	-	72%	82%	100%
Discharge Instructions[1,3]	1	0%	41%	61%	93%
Evaluation of LVS Function[1,3]	2	0%	65%	83%	99%
Smoking Cessation Advice[3]	0	-	67%	82%	100%
Pneumonia Care					
Appropriate Initial Antibiotic[1]	7	71%	78%	83%	94%
Blood Culture Timing	0	-	93%	90%	100%
Influenza Vaccine[1]	4	50%	63%	70%	100%
Initial Antibiotic Timing[1]	5	100%	85%	80%	93%
Oxygenation Assessment[1]	8	100%	99%	99%	100%
Pneumococcal Vaccine[1]	7	29%	59%	69%	94%
Smoking Cessation Advice[1]	1	0%	60%	80%	100%
Surgical Infection Prevention					
Prophylactic Antibiotic Given[5]	-	-	74%	77%	95%
Prophylactic Antibiotic Selection[5]	-	-	91%	90%	100%
Prophylactic Antibiotic Stopped[5]	-	-	72%	72%	95%
Pregnancy Care					
Inpatient Neonatal Mortality	-	-	-	-	-
Third or Fourth Degree Laceration	-	-	3.82%	3.63%	3.27%

Saint Francis Health Center

1700 SW 7th Street
Topeka, KS 66606
E-mail: cr@stfrancistopeka.org
URL: www.stfrancistopeka.org
Ownership: Voluntary non-profit - Church
Emergency Services: Yes

Phone: 785-295-8000
Fax: 785-295-7854
Accredited: Yes
Licensed Beds: 378

Key Personnel:
President/CEO. . . . . Loretto Marie Colwell
Chief Medical Staff. . . . . John Kleinholz, MD
Infection Control Nurse. Nancy Krohe
Cardiology . . . . Moussa Elbayoumy
Respiratory . . . . David Niller

Measure	Cases	This Hospital	State Average	U.S. Average	Top Hospital
Heart Attack Care					
ACE Inhibitor or ARB for LVSD	77	86%	78%	82%	100%
Aspirin at Arrival	136	99%	90%	92%	100%
Aspirin at Discharge	247	95%	88%	90%	100%
Beta Blocker at Arrival	101	95%	82%	87%	100%
Beta Blocker at Discharge	270	96%	82%	90%	100%
Fibrinolytic Medication Timing[1]	1	0%	24%	31%	100%
PCI Within 90 Minutes of Arrival[1]	6	33%	55%	54%	95%
Smoking Cessation Advice	91	99%	86%	88%	100%
Heart Failure Care					
ACE Inhibitor or ARB for LVSD	90	91%	72%	82%	100%
Discharge Instructions	180	78%	41%	61%	93%
Evaluation of LVS Function	230	99%	65%	83%	99%
Smoking Cessation Advice	47	91%	67%	82%	100%
Pneumonia Care					
Appropriate Initial Antibiotic	157	91%	78%	83%	94%
Blood Culture Timing	65	92%	93%	90%	100%
Influenza Vaccine	54	94%	63%	70%	100%
Initial Antibiotic Timing	224	82%	85%	80%	93%
Oxygenation Assessment	264	100%	99%	99%	100%
Pneumococcal Vaccine	173	92%	59%	69%	94%
Smoking Cessation Advice	85	91%	60%	80%	100%
Surgical Infection Prevention					
Prophylactic Antibiotic Given[2,3]	218	83%	74%	77%	95%
Prophylactic Antibiotic Selection[2]	73	97%	91%	90%	100%
Prophylactic Antibiotic Stopped[2,3]	213	87%	72%	72%	95%
Pregnancy Care					
Inpatient Neonatal Mortality	925	0.00%	-	-	-
Third or Fourth Degree Laceration	715	4.76%	3.82%	3.63%	3.27%

Stormont-Vail Healthcare

Alternate Name: Stormont-Vail Regional Health Center
1500 SW 10th Avenue
Topeka, KS 66604
URL: www.stormontvail.org
Ownership: Voluntary non-profit - Private
Emergency Services: Yes

Phone: 785-354-6121
Fax: 785-354-5123
Accredited: Yes
Licensed Beds: 586

Key Personnel:
President/CEO. . . . . Maynard Ohverius
Chief Medical Staff. . . . . Kent Palmberg, MD
Director Surgical Services . . . . Jane Asher, RN
Director Surgery Services . . . . Jane Asher

NOTE: Hospital profiles are in alphabetical order by state, then city, then hospital within the city; Rankings are sorted by rate in descending order and exclude hospitals with less than 25 cases; (1) The number of cases is too small (n<25) for purposes of reliably predicting hospital performance; (2) Measure reflects the hospital's indication that its submission was based upon a sample of its relevant discharges; (3) Rate reflects fewer than the maximum possible quarters of data for the measure; (4) Inaccurate information submitted and suppressed for one or more quarters; (5) No data is available from the hospital for this measure; Please refer to the User's Guide for a full explanation of data

Measure	Cases	This Hospital	State Average	U.S. Average	Top Hospital
Heart Attack Care					
ACE Inhibitor or ARB for LVSD	37	89%	78%	82%	100%
Aspirin at Arrival	184	96%	90%	92%	100%
Aspirin at Discharge	233	97%	88%	90%	100%
Beta Blocker at Arrival	171	98%	82%	87%	100%
Beta Blocker at Discharge	229	100%	82%	90%	100%
Fibrinolytic Medication Timing[1]	3	33%	24%	31%	100%
PCI Within 90 Minutes of Arrival[1]	14	100%	55%	54%	95%
Smoking Cessation Advice	74	100%	86%	88%	100%
Heart Failure Care					
ACE Inhibitor or ARB for LVSD	118	89%	72%	82%	100%
Discharge Instructions	216	71%	41%	61%	93%
Evaluation of LVS Function	298	98%	65%	83%	99%
Smoking Cessation Advice	48	100%	67%	82%	100%
Pneumonia Care					
Appropriate Initial Antibiotic	166	98%	78%	83%	94%
Blood Culture Timing	204	96%	93%	90%	100%
Influenza Vaccine	72	90%	63%	70%	100%
Initial Antibiotic Timing	250	76%	85%	80%	93%
Oxygenation Assessment	331	100%	99%	99%	100%
Pneumococcal Vaccine	221	88%	59%	69%	94%
Smoking Cessation Advice	102	100%	60%	80%	100%
Surgical Infection Prevention					
Prophylactic Antibiotic Given	431	89%	74%	77%	95%
Prophylactic Antibiotic Selection	67	96%	91%	90%	100%
Prophylactic Antibiotic Stopped	411	91%	72%	72%	95%
Pregnancy Care					
Inpatient Neonatal Mortality	-	-	-	-	-
Third or Fourth Degree Laceration	-	-	3.82%	3.63%	3.27%

Greeley County Hospital & LTCU

506 3rd Street
PO Box 338
Tribune, KS 67879
Phone: 620-376-4221
Fax: 620-376-2406
Ownership: Voluntary non-profit - Other
Emergency Services: Yes
Accredited: No
Licensed Beds: 18

Key Personnel:

Administrator . . . . Todd Burch
Chief Medical Staff. . . . . Robert P Moser, MD
Emergency Room . . . . Robert P Moser, MD
Director Infection/Disease Control . . . . Linda Peterson, RN
Director Respiratory Therapy . . . . Dalene Moser

Measure	Cases	This Hospital	State Average	U.S. Average	Top Hospital
Heart Attack Care					
ACE Inhibitor or ARB for LVSD[2,3]	0	-	78%	82%	100%
Aspirin at Arrival[1,2,3]	1	100%	90%	92%	100%
Aspirin at Discharge[1,2,3]	1	100%	88%	90%	100%
Beta Blocker at Arrival[1,2,3]	1	100%	82%	87%	100%
Beta Blocker at Discharge[1,2,3]	1	100%	82%	90%	100%
Fibrinolytic Medication Timing[1,2,3]	1	0%	24%	31%	100%
PCI Within 90 Minutes of Arrival[5]	-	-	55%	54%	95%
Smoking Cessation Advice[2,3]	0	-	86%	88%	100%
Heart Failure Care					
ACE Inhibitor or ARB for LVSD[1,3]	2	50%	72%	82%	100%
Discharge Instructions[1,3]	3	0%	41%	61%	93%
Evaluation of LVS Function[1,3]	11	36%	65%	83%	99%
Smoking Cessation Advice[1,3]	3	0%	67%	82%	100%
Pneumonia Care					
Appropriate Initial Antibiotic[1,3]	10	60%	78%	83%	94%
Blood Culture Timing[1,3]	3	100%	93%	90%	100%
Influenza Vaccine[1]	4	50%	63%	70%	100%
Initial Antibiotic Timing[3]	0	-	85%	80%	93%
Oxygenation Assessment[1,3]	13	100%	99%	99%	100%
Pneumococcal Vaccine[1,3]	9	44%	59%	69%	94%
Smoking Cessation Advice[1,3]	5	0%	60%	80%	100%
Surgical Infection Prevention					
Prophylactic Antibiotic Given[5]	-	-	74%	77%	95%
Prophylactic Antibiotic Selection[5]	-	-	91%	90%	100%
Prophylactic Antibiotic Stopped[5]	-	-	72%	72%	95%
Pregnancy Care					
Inpatient Neonatal Mortality	-	-	-	-	-
Third or Fourth Degree Laceration	-	-	3.82%	3.63%	3.27%

Bob Wilson Memorial Grant Hospital

415 N Main Street
Ulysses, KS 67880
URL: bwmgch.com
Phone: 620-356-1266
Fax: 620-356-2302
Ownership: Voluntary non-profit - Church
Emergency Services: Yes
Accredited: No
Licensed Beds: 46

Key Personnel:

President/CEO . . . . Steve Daniel

Measure	Cases	This Hospital	State Average	U.S. Average	Top Hospital
Heart Attack Care					
ACE Inhibitor or ARB for LVSD[1,3]	2	0%	78%	82%	100%
Aspirin at Arrival[1,3]	3	100%	90%	92%	100%
Aspirin at Discharge[1,3]	2	50%	88%	90%	100%
Beta Blocker at Arrival[1,3]	4	100%	82%	87%	100%
Beta Blocker at Discharge[1,3]	2	100%	82%	90%	100%
Fibrinolytic Medication Timing[3]	0	-	24%	31%	100%
PCI Within 90 Minutes of Arrival[5]	-	-	55%	54%	95%
Smoking Cessation Advice[3]	0	-	86%	88%	100%
Heart Failure Care					
ACE Inhibitor or ARB for LVSD[1,3]	9	67%	72%	82%	100%
Discharge Instructions[1,3]	9	44%	41%	61%	93%
Evaluation of LVS Function[1,3]	14	71%	65%	83%	99%
Smoking Cessation Advice[3]	0	-	67%	82%	100%
Pneumonia Care					
Appropriate Initial Antibiotic[1]	19	79%	78%	83%	94%
Blood Culture Timing[1]	3	100%	93%	90%	100%
Influenza Vaccine[1]	7	71%	63%	70%	100%
Initial Antibiotic Timing[1]	23	100%	85%	80%	93%
Oxygenation Assessment	27	100%	99%	99%	100%
Pneumococcal Vaccine[1]	17	53%	59%	69%	94%
Smoking Cessation Advice[1]	4	100%	60%	80%	100%
Surgical Infection Prevention					
Prophylactic Antibiotic Given[1,3]	2	0%	74%	77%	95%
Prophylactic Antibiotic Selection[1]	2	100%	91%	90%	100%
Prophylactic Antibiotic Stopped[1,3]	2	50%	72%	72%	95%
Pregnancy Care					
Inpatient Neonatal Mortality	-	-	-	-	-
Third or Fourth Degree Laceration	-	-	3.82%	3.63%	3.27%

Trego County-Lemke Memorial Hospital

320 13th Street
WaKeeney, KS 67672
Phone: 785-743-2182
Fax: 785-743-6317
Ownership: Government - Local
Emergency Services: Yes
Accredited: No
Licensed Beds: 25

Key Personnel:

CEO. . . . . Stacey Malson
Emergency Room . . . . Judy Hearting
Director Infection/Disease Control . . . . Mary Jo McClannahan
Chief Radiology . . . . Lisa Kuhn

Measure	Cases	This Hospital	State Average	U.S. Average	Top Hospital
Heart Attack Care					
ACE Inhibitor or ARB for LVSD[2,3]	0	-	78%	82%	100%
Aspirin at Arrival[1,2,3]	1	100%	90%	92%	100%
Aspirin at Discharge[1,2,3]	1	100%	88%	90%	100%
Beta Blocker at Arrival[1,2,3]	1	100%	82%	87%	100%
Beta Blocker at Discharge[1,2,3]	1	100%	82%	90%	100%
Fibrinolytic Medication Timing[2,3]	0	-	24%	31%	100%
PCI Within 90 Minutes of Arrival[5]	-	-	55%	54%	95%
Smoking Cessation Advice[2,3]	0	-	86%	88%	100%
Heart Failure Care					
ACE Inhibitor or ARB for LVSD[1,2,3]	2	0%	72%	82%	100%
Discharge Instructions[1,2,3]	6	100%	41%	61%	93%
Evaluation of LVS Function[1,2,3]	10	40%	65%	83%	99%
Smoking Cessation Advice[2,3]	0	-	67%	82%	100%
Pneumonia Care					
Appropriate Initial Antibiotic[1,2,3]	22	55%	78%	83%	94%
Blood Culture Timing[1,2,3]	2	100%	93%	90%	100%

NOTE: Hospital profiles are in alphabetical order by state, then city, then hospital within the city; Rankings are sorted by rate in descending order and exclude hospitals with less than 25 cases; (1) The number of cases is too small (n<25) for purposes of reliably predicting hospital performance; (2) Measure reflects the hospital's indication that its submission was based upon a sample of its relevant discharges; (3) Rate reflects fewer than the maximum possible quarters of data for the measure; (4) Inaccurate information submitted and suppressed for one or more quarters; (5) No data is available from the hospital for this measure; Please refer to the User's Guide for a full explanation of data

Measure	Cases	This Hospital	State Average	U.S. Average	Top Hospital
Influenza Vaccine[5]	-	-	63%	70%	100%
Initial Antibiotic Timing[1,2,3]	23	78%	85%	80%	93%
Oxygenation Assessment[1,2,3]	24	100%	99%	99%	100%
Pneumococcal Vaccine[1,2,3]	21	67%	59%	69%	94%
Smoking Cessation Advice[1,2,3]	3	0%	60%	80%	100%
Surgical Infection Prevention					
Prophylactic Antibiotic Given[5]	-	-	74%	77%	95%
Prophylactic Antibiotic Selection[5]	-	-	91%	90%	100%
Prophylactic Antibiotic Stopped[5]	-	-	72%	72%	95%
Pregnancy Care					
Inpatient Neonatal Mortality	-	-	-	-	-
Third or Fourth Degree Laceration	-	-	3.82%	3.63%	3.27%

Wamego City Hospital

711 Genn Drive
Wamego, KS 66547
URL: www.wamegocityhospital.com
Ownership: Voluntary non-profit - Other
Emergency Services: Yes

Phone: 785-456-2295
Fax: 785-456-6916

Accredited: No
Licensed Beds: 26

Measure	Cases	This Hospital	State Average	U.S. Average	Top Hospital
Heart Attack Care					
ACE Inhibitor or ARB for LVSD[3]	0	-	78%	82%	100%
Aspirin at Arrival[1,3]	1	0%	90%	92%	100%
Aspirin at Discharge[1,3]	1	100%	88%	90%	100%
Beta Blocker at Arrival[3]	0	-	82%	87%	100%
Beta Blocker at Discharge[1,3]	1	100%	82%	90%	100%
Fibrinolytic Medication Timing[3]	0	-	24%	31%	100%
PCI Within 90 Minutes of Arrival	0	-	55%	54%	95%
Smoking Cessation Advice[3]	0	-	86%	88%	100%
Heart Failure Care					
ACE Inhibitor or ARB for LVSD[1,3]	2	100%	72%	82%	100%
Discharge Instructions[1,3]	10	0%	41%	61%	93%
Evaluation of LVS Function[1,3]	13	23%	65%	83%	99%
Smoking Cessation Advice[3]	0	-	67%	82%	100%
Pneumonia Care					
Appropriate Initial Antibiotic[1,3]	4	100%	78%	83%	94%
Blood Culture Timing[1,3]	1	0%	93%	90%	100%
Influenza Vaccine[5]	-	-	63%	70%	100%
Initial Antibiotic Timing[1,3]	7	100%	85%	80%	93%
Oxygenation Assessment[1,3]	12	100%	99%	99%	100%
Pneumococcal Vaccine[1,3]	10	10%	59%	69%	94%
Smoking Cessation Advice[3]	0	-	60%	80%	100%
Surgical Infection Prevention					
Prophylactic Antibiotic Given[5]	-	-	74%	77%	95%
Prophylactic Antibiotic Selection[5]	-	-	91%	90%	100%
Prophylactic Antibiotic Stopped[5]	-	-	72%	72%	95%
Pregnancy Care					
Inpatient Neonatal Mortality	-	-	-	-	-
Third or Fourth Degree Laceration	-	-	3.82%	3.63%	3.27%

Washington County Hospital

304 E 3rd Street
Washington, KS 66968
Ownership: Government - Local
Emergency Services: Yes

Phone: 785-325-2211
Fax: 785-325-3224
Accredited: No
Licensed Beds: 27

Key Personnel:
CEO. . . . . Everett Lutjemeier
Chief Medical Staff. . . . . David Hodgson
Emergency Room . . . . Marry Walter

Measure	Cases	This Hospital	State Average	U.S. Average	Top Hospital
Heart Attack Care					
ACE Inhibitor or ARB for LVSD[5]	-	-	78%	82%	100%
Aspirin at Arrival[5]	-	-	90%	92%	100%
Aspirin at Discharge[5]	-	-	88%	90%	100%
Beta Blocker at Arrival[5]	-	-	82%	87%	100%
Beta Blocker at Discharge[5]	-	-	82%	90%	100%
Fibrinolytic Medication Timing[5]	-	-	24%	31%	100%
PCI Within 90 Minutes of Arrival[5]	-	-	55%	54%	95%
Smoking Cessation Advice[5]	-	-	86%	88%	100%
Heart Failure Care					
ACE Inhibitor or ARB for LVSD[3]	0	-	72%	82%	100%
Discharge Instructions[1,3]	5	20%	41%	61%	93%
Evaluation of LVS Function[1,3]	4	50%	65%	83%	99%
Smoking Cessation Advice[3]	0	-	67%	82%	100%
Pneumonia Care					
Appropriate Initial Antibiotic[1,3]	9	78%	78%	83%	94%
Blood Culture Timing[3]	0	-	93%	90%	100%
Influenza Vaccine[1]	4	100%	63%	70%	100%
Initial Antibiotic Timing[1,3]	7	100%	85%	80%	93%
Oxygenation Assessment[1,3]	10	100%	99%	99%	100%
Pneumococcal Vaccine[1,3]	10	100%	59%	69%	94%
Smoking Cessation Advice[1,3]	1	0%	60%	80%	100%
Surgical Infection Prevention					
Prophylactic Antibiotic Given[5]	-	-	74%	77%	95%
Prophylactic Antibiotic Selection[5]	-	-	91%	90%	100%
Prophylactic Antibiotic Stopped[5]	-	-	72%	72%	95%
Pregnancy Care					
Inpatient Neonatal Mortality	-	-	-	-	-
Third or Fourth Degree Laceration	-	-	3.82%	3.63%	3.27%

Sumner Regional Medical Center

Alternate Name: Saint Lukes Hospital
1323 North A Street
Wellington, KS 67152

Toll-Free: 866-326-7451
Phone: 620-326-7451
Fax: 620-326-2225

URL: www.srmcks.org
Ownership: Government - Local
Emergency Services: Yes

Accredited: No
Licensed Beds: 80

Key Personnel:
President/CEO. . . . . Robert H Bean, PhD
Chief of Medical Staff. Larry Anderson
Respiratory Therapy Manager . . . . Wendy Herron

Measure	Cases	This Hospital	State Average	U.S. Average	Top Hospital
Heart Attack Care					
ACE Inhibitor or ARB for LVSD[3]	0	-	78%	82%	100%
Aspirin at Arrival[1,3]	3	33%	90%	92%	100%
Aspirin at Discharge[1,3]	3	0%	88%	90%	100%
Beta Blocker at Arrival[1,3]	3	67%	82%	87%	100%
Beta Blocker at Discharge[1,3]	3	33%	82%	90%	100%
Fibrinolytic Medication Timing[3]	0	-	24%	31%	100%
PCI Within 90 Minutes of Arrival	0	-	55%	54%	95%
Smoking Cessation Advice[3]	0	-	86%	88%	100%
Heart Failure Care					
ACE Inhibitor or ARB for LVSD[1,3]	1	100%	72%	82%	100%
Discharge Instructions[1,3]	16	0%	41%	61%	93%
Evaluation of LVS Function[1,3]	22	9%	65%	83%	99%
Smoking Cessation Advice[1,3]	3	33%	67%	82%	100%
Pneumonia Care					
Appropriate Initial Antibiotic[1,3]	15	60%	78%	83%	94%
Blood Culture Timing[1,3]	2	100%	93%	90%	100%
Influenza Vaccine[5]	-	-	63%	70%	100%
Initial Antibiotic Timing[1,3]	21	76%	85%	80%	93%
Oxygenation Assessment[3]	25	96%	99%	99%	100%
Pneumococcal Vaccine[1,3]	19	0%	59%	69%	94%
Smoking Cessation Advice[1,3]	4	0%	60%	80%	100%
Surgical Infection Prevention					
Prophylactic Antibiotic Given[1,3]	7	43%	74%	77%	95%
Prophylactic Antibiotic Selection[1]	3	100%	91%	90%	100%
Prophylactic Antibiotic Stopped[1,3]	7	100%	72%	72%	95%
Pregnancy Care					
Inpatient Neonatal Mortality	-	-	-	-	-
Third or Fourth Degree Laceration	-	-	3.82%	3.63%	3.27%

Galichia Heart Hospital

2610 N Woodlawn
Wichita, KS 67220
URL: www.ghhospital.com
Ownership: Proprietary
Emergency Services: No

Phone: 316-858-2610
Fax: 316-858-2790

Accredited: No
Licensed Beds: 80

Key Personnel:
CEO. . . . . Tom Nester

NOTE: Hospital profiles are in alphabetical order by state, then city, then hospital within the city; Rankings are sorted by rate in descending order and exclude hospitals with less than 25 cases; (1) The number of cases is too small (n<25) for purposes of reliably predicting hospital performance; (2) Measure reflects the hospital's indication that its submission was based upon a sample of its relevant discharges; (3) Rate reflects fewer than the maximum possible quarters of data for the measure; (4) Inaccurate information submitted and suppressed for one or more quarters; (5) No data is available from the hospital for this measure; Please refer to the User's Guide for a full explanation of data

Measure	Cases	This Hospital	State Average	U.S. Average	Top Hospital
Heart Attack Care					
ACE Inhibitor or ARB for LVSD[1]	14	57%	78%	82%	100%
Aspirin at Arrival	28	82%	90%	92%	100%
Aspirin at Discharge	62	89%	88%	90%	100%
Beta Blocker at Arrival	29	83%	82%	87%	100%
Beta Blocker at Discharge	65	85%	82%	90%	100%
Fibrinolytic Medication Timing[1]	3	33%	24%	31%	100%
PCI Within 90 Minutes of Arrival[1]	2	0%	55%	54%	95%
Smoking Cessation Advice	29	86%	86%	88%	100%
Heart Failure Care					
ACE Inhibitor or ARB for LVSD[2]	102	67%	72%	82%	100%
Discharge Instructions[2]	239	94%	41%	61%	93%
Evaluation of LVS Function[2]	263	92%	65%	83%	99%
Smoking Cessation Advice[2]	34	68%	67%	82%	100%
Pneumonia Care					
Appropriate Initial Antibiotic[1,2]	15	67%	78%	83%	94%
Blood Culture Timing[1,2]	5	100%	93%	90%	100%
Influenza Vaccine[1]	4	25%	63%	70%	100%
Initial Antibiotic Timing[1,2]	16	50%	85%	80%	93%
Oxygenation Assessment[1,2]	23	91%	99%	99%	100%
Pneumococcal Vaccine[1,2]	18	39%	59%	69%	94%
Smoking Cessation Advice[1,2]	5	60%	60%	80%	100%
Surgical Infection Prevention					
Prophylactic Antibiotic Given[3]	37	46%	74%	77%	95%
Prophylactic Antibiotic Selection	38	89%	91%	90%	100%
Prophylactic Antibiotic Stopped[3]	36	42%	72%	72%	95%
Pregnancy Care					
Inpatient Neonatal Mortality	-	-	-	-	-
Third or Fourth Degree Laceration	-	-	3.82%	3.63%	3.27%

Kansas Heart Hospital

3601 N Webb Road
Wichita, KS 67226
URL: www.kansasheart.com
Ownership: Proprietary
Emergency Services: No

Phone: 316-630-5000
Fax: 316-630-5050
Accredited: No
Licensed Beds: 54

Key Personnel:
CEO. . . . . Thomas L Aschom, MD

Measure	Cases	This Hospital	State Average	U.S. Average	Top Hospital
Heart Attack Care					
ACE Inhibitor or ARB for LVSD	27	89%	78%	82%	100%
Aspirin at Arrival[1]	17	100%	90%	92%	100%
Aspirin at Discharge	172	98%	88%	90%	100%
Beta Blocker at Arrival[1]	11	91%	82%	87%	100%
Beta Blocker at Discharge	162	98%	82%	90%	100%
Fibrinolytic Medication Timing	0	-	24%	31%	100%
PCI Within 90 Minutes of Arrival	0	-	55%	54%	95%
Smoking Cessation Advice	67	96%	86%	88%	100%
Heart Failure Care					
ACE Inhibitor or ARB for LVSD	59	95%	72%	82%	100%
Discharge Instructions	103	82%	41%	61%	93%
Evaluation of LVS Function	115	100%	65%	83%	99%
Smoking Cessation Advice[1]	24	83%	67%	82%	100%
Pneumonia Care					
Appropriate Initial Antibiotic	0	-	78%	83%	94%
Blood Culture Timing	0	-	93%	90%	100%
Influenza Vaccine	0	-	63%	70%	100%
Initial Antibiotic Timing	0	-	85%	80%	93%
Oxygenation Assessment	0	-	99%	99%	100%
Pneumococcal Vaccine[1]	2	0%	59%	69%	94%
Smoking Cessation Advice	0	-	60%	80%	100%
Surgical Infection Prevention					
Prophylactic Antibiotic Given[2]	205	95%	74%	77%	95%
Prophylactic Antibiotic Selection[2]	45	98%	91%	90%	100%
Prophylactic Antibiotic Stopped[2]	203	59%	72%	72%	95%
Pregnancy Care					
Inpatient Neonatal Mortality	-	-	-	-	-
Third or Fourth Degree Laceration	-	-	3.82%	3.63%	3.27%

Kansas Spine Hospital

3333 N Webb Road
Wichita, KS 67226
Ownership: Proprietary
Emergency Services: No

Phone: 316-462-5338
Accredited: No

Measure	Cases	This Hospital	State Average	U.S. Average	Top Hospital
Heart Attack Care					
ACE Inhibitor or ARB for LVSD[5]	-	-	78%	82%	100%
Aspirin at Arrival[5]	-	-	90%	92%	100%
Aspirin at Discharge[5]	-	-	88%	90%	100%
Beta Blocker at Arrival[5]	-	-	82%	87%	100%
Beta Blocker at Discharge[5]	-	-	82%	90%	100%
Fibrinolytic Medication Timing[5]	-	-	24%	31%	100%
PCI Within 90 Minutes of Arrival[5]	-	-	55%	54%	95%
Smoking Cessation Advice[5]	-	-	86%	88%	100%
Heart Failure Care					
ACE Inhibitor or ARB for LVSD[5]	-	-	72%	82%	100%
Discharge Instructions[5]	-	-	41%	61%	93%
Evaluation of LVS Function[5]	-	-	65%	83%	99%
Smoking Cessation Advice[5]	-	-	67%	82%	100%
Pneumonia Care					
Appropriate Initial Antibiotic[5]	-	-	78%	83%	94%
Blood Culture Timing[5]	-	-	93%	90%	100%
Influenza Vaccine[5]	-	-	63%	70%	100%
Initial Antibiotic Timing[5]	-	-	85%	80%	93%
Oxygenation Assessment[5]	-	-	99%	99%	100%
Pneumococcal Vaccine[5]	-	-	59%	69%	94%
Smoking Cessation Advice[5]	-	-	60%	80%	100%
Surgical Infection Prevention					
Prophylactic Antibiotic Given[2,3]	0	-	74%	77%	95%
Prophylactic Antibiotic Selection[2]	0	-	91%	90%	100%
Prophylactic Antibiotic Stopped[2,3]	0	-	72%	72%	95%
Pregnancy Care					
Inpatient Neonatal Mortality	-	-	-	-	-
Third or Fourth Degree Laceration	-	-	3.82%	3.63%	3.27%

Kansas Surgery & Recovery Center

2770 N Webb Road
Wichita, KS 67226
Ownership: Voluntary non-profit - Private
Emergency Services: No

Phone: 316-634-0090
Accredited: No

Measure	Cases	This Hospital	State Average	U.S. Average	Top Hospital
Heart Attack Care					
ACE Inhibitor or ARB for LVSD[5]	-	-	78%	82%	100%
Aspirin at Arrival[5]	-	-	90%	92%	100%
Aspirin at Discharge[5]	-	-	88%	90%	100%
Beta Blocker at Arrival[5]	-	-	82%	87%	100%
Beta Blocker at Discharge[5]	-	-	82%	90%	100%
Fibrinolytic Medication Timing[5]	-	-	24%	31%	100%
PCI Within 90 Minutes of Arrival[5]	-	-	55%	54%	95%
Smoking Cessation Advice[5]	-	-	86%	88%	100%
Heart Failure Care					
ACE Inhibitor or ARB for LVSD[5]	-	-	72%	82%	100%
Discharge Instructions[5]	-	-	41%	61%	93%
Evaluation of LVS Function[5]	-	-	65%	83%	99%
Smoking Cessation Advice[5]	-	-	67%	82%	100%
Pneumonia Care					
Appropriate Initial Antibiotic[5]	-	-	78%	83%	94%
Blood Culture Timing[5]	-	-	93%	90%	100%
Influenza Vaccine[5]	-	-	63%	70%	100%
Initial Antibiotic Timing[5]	-	-	85%	80%	93%
Oxygenation Assessment[5]	-	-	99%	99%	100%
Pneumococcal Vaccine[5]	-	-	59%	69%	94%
Smoking Cessation Advice[5]	-	-	60%	80%	100%
Surgical Infection Prevention					
Prophylactic Antibiotic Given[2]	198	92%	74%	77%	95%
Prophylactic Antibiotic Selection[2]	51	96%	91%	90%	100%
Prophylactic Antibiotic Stopped[2]	198	39%	72%	72%	95%
Pregnancy Care					
Inpatient Neonatal Mortality	-	-	-	-	-

NOTE: Hospital profiles are in alphabetical order by state, then city, then hospital within the city; Rankings are sorted by rate in descending order and exclude hospitals with less than 25 cases; (1) The number of cases is too small (n<25) for purposes of reliably predicting hospital performance; (2) Measure reflects the hospital's indication that its submission was based upon a sample of its relevant discharges; (3) Rate reflects fewer than the maximum possible quarters of data for the measure; (4) Inaccurate information submitted and suppressed for one or more quarters; (5) No data is available from the hospital for this measure; Please refer to the User's Guide for a full explanation of data

Third or Fourth Degree Laceration	-	-	3.82%	3.63%	3.27%

Via Christi Regional Medical Center

Alternate Name: Saint Joseph Medical Center
929 N Saint Francis
Wichita, KS 67214
URL: www.via-christi.org
Ownership: Voluntary non-profit - Church
Emergency Services: Yes
Phone: 316-268-5000
Fax: 316-291-4570
Accredited: Yes
Licensed Beds: 1,532

Key Personnel:
President/CEO. . . . . Larry Schumacher
Director Infection/Disease Control . . . . Susan Hendrickson

Measure	Cases	This Hospital	State Average	U.S. Average	Top Hospital
Heart Attack Care					
ACE Inhibitor or ARB for LVSD	153	85%	78%	82%	100%
Aspirin at Arrival	581	95%	90%	92%	100%
Aspirin at Discharge	715	93%	88%	90%	100%
Beta Blocker at Arrival	531	93%	82%	87%	100%
Beta Blocker at Discharge	691	93%	82%	90%	100%
Fibrinolytic Medication Timing[1]	4	25%	24%	31%	100%
PCI Within 90 Minutes of Arrival[1]	15	47%	55%	54%	95%
Smoking Cessation Advice	301	95%	86%	88%	100%
Heart Failure Care					
ACE Inhibitor or ARB for LVSD	360	78%	72%	82%	100%
Discharge Instructions	707	57%	41%	61%	93%
Evaluation of LVS Function	842	89%	65%	83%	99%
Smoking Cessation Advice	159	97%	67%	82%	100%
Pneumonia Care					
Appropriate Initial Antibiotic[2]	197	72%	78%	83%	94%
Blood Culture Timing[2]	81	89%	93%	90%	100%
Influenza Vaccine[2]	28	86%	63%	70%	100%
Initial Antibiotic Timing[2]	184	83%	85%	80%	93%
Oxygenation Assessment[2]	262	100%	99%	99%	100%
Pneumococcal Vaccine[2]	161	70%	59%	69%	94%
Smoking Cessation Advice[2]	77	82%	60%	80%	100%
Surgical Infection Prevention					
Prophylactic Antibiotic Given[2]	790	94%	74%	77%	95%
Prophylactic Antibiotic Selection[2]	136	96%	91%	90%	100%
Prophylactic Antibiotic Stopped[2]	763	38%	72%	72%	95%
Pregnancy Care					
Inpatient Neonatal Mortality	2,940	0.34%	-	-	-
Third or Fourth Degree Laceration	2,091	3.20%	3.82%	3.63%	3.27%

Wesley Medical Center

Alternate Name: HCA Wesley Medical Center
550 N Hillside Avenue
Wichita, KS 67214
URL: www.wesleymc.com
Ownership: Proprietary
Emergency Services: Yes
Phone: 316-962-2000
Fax: 316-962-7076
Accredited: Yes
Licensed Beds: 670

Key Personnel:
CEO/Executive Director . . . . David Nevill
Chief Medical Staff. . . . . Francie Ekengren
Emergency Room . . . . Diane Lippolt
OB/GYN Womens Health. . . . . Douglas Horbelt, MD
Chief Radiology . . . . Richard Ahlstrand, MD
Director Respiratory Therapy . . . . Jerry Regehr

Measure	Cases	This Hospital	State Average	U.S. Average	Top Hospital
Heart Attack Care					
ACE Inhibitor or ARB for LVSD[2]	69	90%	78%	82%	100%
Aspirin at Arrival[2]	258	97%	90%	92%	100%
Aspirin at Discharge[2]	291	97%	88%	90%	100%
Beta Blocker at Arrival[2]	187	98%	82%	87%	100%
Beta Blocker at Discharge[2]	321	97%	82%	90%	100%
Fibrinolytic Medication Timing[2]	0	-	24%	31%	100%
PCI Within 90 Minutes of Arrival[1,2]	12	58%	55%	54%	95%
Smoking Cessation Advice[2]	170	97%	86%	88%	100%
Heart Failure Care					
ACE Inhibitor or ARB for LVSD[2]	136	78%	72%	82%	100%
Discharge Instructions[2]	331	56%	41%	61%	93%
Evaluation of LVS Function[2]	430	95%	65%	83%	99%
Smoking Cessation Advice[2]	89	97%	67%	82%	100%
Pneumonia Care					
Appropriate Initial Antibiotic[2]	223	78%	78%	83%	94%
Blood Culture Timing[2]	218	94%	93%	90%	100%
Influenza Vaccine	74	74%	63%	70%	100%
Initial Antibiotic Timing[2]	317	76%	85%	80%	93%
Oxygenation Assessment[2]	387	100%	99%	99%	100%
Pneumococcal Vaccine[2]	240	76%	59%	69%	94%
Smoking Cessation Advice[2]	110	82%	60%	80%	100%
Surgical Infection Prevention					
Prophylactic Antibiotic Given[2,3]	325	79%	74%	77%	95%
Prophylactic Antibiotic Selection[2]	154	60%	91%	90%	100%
Prophylactic Antibiotic Stopped[2,3]	312	77%	72%	72%	95%
Pregnancy Care					
Inpatient Neonatal Mortality	-	-	-	-	-
Third or Fourth Degree Laceration	-	-	3.82%	3.63%	3.27%

William Newton Memorial Hospital

1300 E 5th Street
Winfield, KS 67156
URL: www.wnmh.org
Ownership: Voluntary non-profit - Other
Emergency Services: Yes
Phone: 620-221-2300
Fax: 620-221-3594
Accredited: No
Licensed Beds: 99

Key Personnel:
Administrator . . . . Richard Vaught
Chief Medical Staff. . . . . Tom Embers
Emergency Room . . . . Greg Faimon, MD
Director Infection/Disease Control . . . . Linda King, RN
ICU . . . . Barbara Humpert, RN
Director Medical/Surgical Nursing . . . . Kristi Ball, RN
Chief Radiology . . . . Melissa Rosenquist, MD
Director Respiratory Therapy . . . . Ray German, RRT

Measure	Cases	This Hospital	State Average	U.S. Average	Top Hospital
Heart Attack Care					
ACE Inhibitor or ARB for LVSD[3]	0	-	78%	82%	100%
Aspirin at Arrival[1,3]	3	67%	90%	92%	100%
Aspirin at Discharge[1,3]	1	100%	88%	90%	100%
Beta Blocker at Arrival[1,3]	3	100%	82%	87%	100%
Beta Blocker at Discharge[1,3]	2	100%	82%	90%	100%
Fibrinolytic Medication Timing[3]	0	-	24%	31%	100%
PCI Within 90 Minutes of Arrival	0	-	55%	54%	95%
Smoking Cessation Advice[1,3]	1	100%	86%	88%	100%
Heart Failure Care					
ACE Inhibitor or ARB for LVSD[1,3]	6	83%	72%	82%	100%
Discharge Instructions[1,3]	20	70%	41%	61%	93%
Evaluation of LVS Function[3]	26	85%	65%	83%	99%
Smoking Cessation Advice[1,3]	1	100%	67%	82%	100%
Pneumonia Care					
Appropriate Initial Antibiotic[3]	26	85%	78%	83%	94%
Blood Culture Timing[1]	19	89%	93%	90%	100%
Influenza Vaccine[1]	18	89%	63%	70%	100%
Initial Antibiotic Timing[3]	35	86%	85%	80%	93%
Oxygenation Assessment[3]	46	98%	99%	99%	100%
Pneumococcal Vaccine[3]	40	88%	59%	69%	94%
Smoking Cessation Advice[1,3]	4	75%	60%	80%	100%
Surgical Infection Prevention					
Prophylactic Antibiotic Given[3]	62	97%	74%	77%	95%
Prophylactic Antibiotic Selection[1]	22	86%	91%	90%	100%
Prophylactic Antibiotic Stopped[3]	62	92%	72%	72%	95%
Pregnancy Care					
Inpatient Neonatal Mortality	-	-	-	-	-
Third or Fourth Degree Laceration	-	-	3.82%	3.63%	3.27%

NOTE: Hospital profiles are in alphabetical order by state, then city, then hospital within the city; Rankings are sorted by rate in descending order and exclude hospitals with less than 25 cases; (1) The number of cases is too small (n<25) for purposes of reliably predicting hospital performance; (2) Measure reflects the hospital's indication that its submission was based upon a sample of its relevant discharges; (3) Rate reflects fewer than the maximum possible quarters of data for the measure; (4) Inaccurate information submitted and suppressed for one or more quarters; (5) No data is available from the hospital for this measure; Please refer to the User's Guide for a full explanation of data

Heart Attack Care

1. ACE Inhibitor or ARB for LVSD

Hospital Name	City	Rate	Cases
Saint Joseph Mercy Oakland	Pontiac	100%	97
Saint Joseph's Healthcare	Clinton Township	100%	54
Saint Joseph Mercy Hospital	Ann Arbor	98%	163
Providence Hospital	Southfield	97%	112
Saint John Macomb Hospital	Warren	97%	105
Saint Mary Mercy Hospital	Livonia	97%	32
University of Michigan Medical Center	Ann Arbor	97%	70
Garden City Hospital	Garden City	96%	27
Henry Ford Hospital	Detroit	96%	68
Ingham Regional Medical Center	Lansing	95%	111
Saint John's Hospital and Medical Center	Detroit	95%	147
Mercy General Health Partners	Muskegon	94%	126
Spectrum Health	Grand Rapids	93%	202
William Beaumont Hospital	Troy	93%	90
Botsford General Hospital	Farmington	92%	48
Oakwood Hospital & Medical Center	Dearborn	92%	339
William Beaumont Hospital	Royal Oak	91%	128
Detroit Receiving Hosp & Univ Health Ctr	Detroit	90%	42
Munson Medical Center	Traverse City	90%	220
Hurley Medical Center	Flint	88%	26
Oakwood Annapolis Hospital	Wayne	88%	33
Foote Health System	Jackson	87%	38
Marquette General Hospital	Marquette	86%	58
Northern Michigan Hospital	Petoskey	85%	61
Port Huron Hospital	Port Huron	85%	52
Bay Regional Medical Center	Bay City	82%	77
Sinai-Grace Hospital	Detroit	81%	85
Bronson Methodist Hospital	Kalamazoo	80%	124
Covenant Medical Center	Saginaw	80%	145
Sparrow Hospital	Lansing	80%	112
Genesys Regional Medical Center	Grand Blanc	79%	103
Harper University Hospital	Detroit	79%	56
Lakeland Hospital-Saint Joseph	Saint Joseph	79%	72
Borgess Medical Center	Kalamazoo	78%	59
Henry Ford Wyandotte Hospital	Wyandotte	72%	54
Mount Clemens Regional Medical Center	Mount Clemens	69%	65
Saint Mary's of Michigan	Saginaw	68%	71
McLaren Regional Medical Center	Flint	63%	86

2. Aspirin at Arrival

Hospital Name	City	Rate	Cases
Botsford General Hospital	Farmington	100%	249
Hackley Hospital	Muskegon	100%	62
Hillsdale Community Health Center	Hillsdale	100%	29
Mecosta County Medical Center	Big Rapids	100%	26
Mercy General Health Partners	Muskegon	100%	229
Mercy Hospital-Grayling	Grayling	100%	29
Metro Health Hospital	Grand Rapids	100%	103
North Oakland Medical Center	Pontiac	100%	31
Saint John Detroit Riverview Hospital	Detroit	100%	38
Saint Joseph Mercy Oakland	Pontiac	100%	280
Spectrum Health	Grand Rapids	100%	508
University of Michigan Medical Center	Ann Arbor	100%	273
Alpena Regional Medical Center	Alpena	99%	69
Garden City Hospital	Garden City	99%	148
Henry Ford Hospital	Detroit	99%	236
Holland Community Hospital	Holland	99%	128
Ingham Regional Medical Center	Lansing	99%	290
Marquette General Hospital	Marquette	99%	92
Saint Joseph Mercy Hospital	Ann Arbor	99%	415
Saint Joseph's Healthcare	Clinton Township	99%	323
Saint Mary Mercy Hospital	Livonia	99%	230
Bronson Methodist Hospital	Kalamazoo	98%	280
Crittenton Hospital Medical Center	Rochester	98%	90
Detroit Receiving Hosp & Univ Health Ctr	Detroit	98%	196
Genesys Regional Medical Center	Grand Blanc	98%	651
Harper University Hospital	Detroit	98%	83
Mercy Hospital	Cadillac	98%	66
Mount Clemens Regional Medical Center	Mount Clemens	98%	173
Northern Michigan Hospital	Petoskey	98%	95
Oakwood Heritage Hospital	Taylor	98%	56
Providence Hospital	Southfield	98%	319
Saint John Macomb Hospital	Warren	98%	310
Saint John Oakland Hospital	Madison Heights	98%	47
Sparrow Hospital	Lansing	98%	245
Bon Secours Cottage Health Services	Grosse Point	97%	68
Borgess Medical Center	Kalamazoo	97%	89
Central Michigan Community Hospital	Mount Pleasant	97%	35
Hurley Medical Center	Flint	97%	163
McLaren Regional Medical Center	Flint	97%	299
MidMichigan Medical Center	Midland	97%	132
Munson Medical Center	Traverse City	97%	348
Oakwood Annapolis Hospital	Wayne	97%	118
Oakwood Southshore Medical Center	Trenton	97%	115
Saint John's Hospital and Medical Center	Detroit	97%	342
William Beaumont Hospital	Royal Oak	97%	356
Covenant Medical Center	Saginaw	96%	296
Lakeland Hospital-Saint Joseph	Saint Joseph	96%	303
Saint Mary's Health Care	Grand Rapids	96%	145
Saint Mary's of Michigan	Saginaw	96%	94
Dickinson County Healthcare System	Iron Mountain	95%	38
Foote Health System	Jackson	95%	259
Henry Ford Bi-County Hospital	Warren	95%	88
Mercy Hospital	Port Huron	95%	37
Mercy Memorial Hospital System	Monroe	95%	126
Oakwood Hospital & Medical Center	Dearborn	95%	535
Port Huron Hospital	Port Huron	95%	206
Sinai-Grace Hospital	Detroit	95%	391
West Branch Regional Medical Center	West Branch	95%	57
William Beaumont Hospital	Troy	95%	296
Huron Valley-Sinai Hospital	Commerce Twp	94%	100
Lapeer Regional Medical Center	Lapeer	94%	85
POH Medical Center	Pontiac	94%	71
Saint Francis Hospital	Escanaba	94%	32
Battle Creek Health System	Battle Creek	93%	105
Bay Regional Medical Center	Bay City	93%	213
Henry Ford Wyandotte Hospital	Wyandotte	93%	273
Bixby Medical Center	Adrian	92%	39
Gratiot Medical Center	Alma	92%	51
Pennock Hospital	Hastings	89%	28
Memorial Healthcare Center	Owosso	88%	34
Chippewa County War Memorial Hospital	Sault Ste Marie	85%	27

3. Aspirin at Discharge

Hospital Name	City	Rate	Cases
Bon Secours Cottage Health Services	Grosse Point	100%	48
Holland Community Hospital	Holland	100%	85
Lapeer Regional Medical Center	Lapeer	100%	40
Mercy General Health Partners	Muskegon	100%	406
Metro Health Hospital	Grand Rapids	100%	64
Northern Michigan Hospital	Petoskey	100%	253
Oakwood Heritage Hospital	Taylor	100%	26
Saint Joseph Mercy Oakland	Pontiac	100%	409
University of Michigan Medical Center	Ann Arbor	100%	396
William Beaumont Hospital	Troy	100%	252
Crittenton Hospital Medical Center	Rochester	99%	81
Henry Ford Hospital	Detroit	99%	316
Ingham Regional Medical Center	Lansing	99%	420
Munson Medical Center	Traverse City	99%	713
Saint Joseph Mercy Hospital	Ann Arbor	99%	642
Saint Joseph's Healthcare	Clinton Township	99%	308
Saint Mary Mercy Hospital	Livonia	99%	154
Sparrow Hospital	Lansing	99%	408
Spectrum Health	Grand Rapids	99%	1025
William Beaumont Hospital	Royal Oak	99%	409
Borgess Medical Center	Kalamazoo	98%	275
Bronson Methodist Hospital	Kalamazoo	98%	388
Hurley Medical Center	Flint	98%	99
Marquette General Hospital	Marquette	98%	297
MidMichigan Medical Center	Midland	98%	92
Oakwood Hospital & Medical Center	Dearborn	98%	861
Providence Hospital	Southfield	98%	471
Saint John's Hospital and Medical Center	Detroit	98%	508
Bay Regional Medical Center	Bay City	97%	332
Detroit Receiving Hosp & Univ Health Ctr	Detroit	97%	169
Lakeland Hospital-Saint Joseph	Saint Joseph	97%	298
Mount Clemens Regional Medical Center	Mount Clemens	97%	143
Oakwood Annapolis Hospital	Wayne	97%	65
Port Huron Hospital	Port Huron	97%	289
Saint John Macomb Hospital	Warren	97%	341
Saint Mary's Health Care	Grand Rapids	97%	100
Saint Mary's of Michigan	Saginaw	97%	235
Foote Health System	Jackson	96%	137
Genesys Regional Medical Center	Grand Blanc	96%	592
Hackley Hospital	Muskegon	96%	28
Harper University Hospital	Detroit	96%	117
Sinai-Grace Hospital	Detroit	96%	359
Garden City Hospital	Garden City	95%	104
Huron Valley-Sinai Hospital	Commerce Twp	95%	56
Covenant Medical Center	Saginaw	94%	338
McLaren Regional Medical Center	Flint	93%	386
Oakwood Southshore Medical Center	Trenton	93%	58
Botsford General Hospital	Farmington	92%	168
Dickinson County Healthcare System	Iron Mountain	92%	26

NOTE: Hospital profiles are in alphabetical order by state, then city, then hospital within the city; Rankings are sorted by rate in descending order and exclude hospitals with less than 25 cases; (1) The number of cases is too small (n<25) for purposes of reliably predicting hospital performance; (2) Measure reflects the hospital's indication that its submission was based upon a sample of its relevant discharges; (3) Rate reflects fewer than the maximum possible quarters of data for the measure; (4) Inaccurate information submitted and suppressed for one or more quarters; (5) No data is available from the hospital for this measure; Please refer to the User's Guide for a full explanation of data

Battle Creek Health System	Battle Creek	90%	63
Mercy Memorial Hospital System	Monroe	89%	47
Mercy Hospital	Cadillac	88%	26
Henry Ford Bi-County Hospital	Warren	87%	46
Henry Ford Wyandotte Hospital	Wyandotte	87%	180
Alpena Regional Medical Center	Alpena	86%	36
POH Medical Center	Pontiac	69%	35

4. Beta Blocker at Arrival

Hospital Name	City	Rate	Cases
Garden City Hospital	Garden City	100%	94
Hillsdale Community Health Center	Hillsdale	100%	27
North Oakland Medical Center	Pontiac	100%	25
Oakwood Heritage Hospital	Taylor	100%	31
Oakwood Southshore Medical Center	Trenton	100%	82
Saint John Detroit Riverview Hospital	Detroit	100%	34
Botsford General Hospital	Farmington	99%	231
Henry Ford Hospital	Detroit	99%	197
Mercy General Health Partners	Muskegon	99%	187
Metro Health Hospital	Grand Rapids	99%	91
Saint Joseph Mercy Oakland	Pontiac	99%	248
Saint Joseph's Healthcare	Clinton Township	99%	278
Saint Mary Mercy Hospital	Livonia	99%	216
Spectrum Health	Grand Rapids	99%	414
University of Michigan Medical Center	Ann Arbor	99%	240
Hackley Hospital	Muskegon	98%	61
Hurley Medical Center	Flint	98%	132
Oakwood Annapolis Hospital	Wayne	98%	87
Saint Mary's Health Care	Grand Rapids	98%	110
West Branch Regional Medical Center	West Branch	98%	60
Detroit Receiving Hosp & Univ Health Ctr	Detroit	97%	186
Henry Ford Bi-County Hospital	Warren	97%	58
Mercy Hospital	Cadillac	97%	62
Mercy Hospital	Port Huron	97%	34
MidMichigan Medical Center	Midland	97%	122
Oakwood Hospital & Medical Center	Dearborn	97%	350
Saint John Oakland Hospital	Madison Heights	97%	38
Alpena Regional Medical Center	Alpena	96%	52
Bixby Medical Center	Adrian	96%	28
Huron Valley-Sinai Hospital	Commerce Twp	96%	76
Lakeland Hospital-Saint Joseph	Saint Joseph	96%	266
Mount Clemens Regional Medical Center	Mount Clemens	96%	122
Northern Michigan Hospital	Petoskey	96%	76
Pennock Hospital	Hastings	96%	25
Providence Hospital	Southfield	96%	280
Saint John's Hospital and Medical Center	Detroit	96%	259
Bronson Methodist Hospital	Kalamazoo	95%	257
Genesys Regional Medical Center	Grand Blanc	95%	508
Holland Community Hospital	Holland	95%	96
Ingham Regional Medical Center	Lansing	95%	211
Saint Joseph Mercy Hospital	Ann Arbor	95%	314
William Beaumont Hospital	Royal Oak	95%	298
Saint John Macomb Hospital	Warren	94%	244
William Beaumont Hospital	Troy	94%	216
Battle Creek Health System	Battle Creek	93%	57
McLaren Regional Medical Center	Flint	93%	190
Mercy Memorial Hospital System	Monroe	93%	88
Munson Medical Center	Traverse City	93%	272
Saint Francis Hospital	Escanaba	93%	30
Sinai-Grace Hospital	Detroit	93%	311
Sparrow Hospital	Lansing	93%	211
Borgess Medical Center	Kalamazoo	92%	73
Foote Health System	Jackson	92%	222
Harper University Hospital	Detroit	92%	72
Lapeer Regional Medical Center	Lapeer	92%	80
Bon Secours Cottage Health Services	Grosse Point	91%	64
Crittenton Hospital Medical Center	Rochester	91%	68
POH Medical Center	Pontiac	91%	69
Port Huron Hospital	Port Huron	91%	187
Saint Mary's of Michigan	Saginaw	91%	79
Henry Ford Wyandotte Hospital	Wyandotte	90%	290
Gratiot Medical Center	Alma	89%	36
Bay Regional Medical Center	Bay City	88%	208
Covenant Medical Center	Saginaw	88%	224
Marquette General Hospital	Marquette	88%	65
Chippewa County War Memorial Hospital	Sault Ste Marie	87%	30
Central Michigan Community Hospital	Mount Pleasant	86%	36
Dickinson County Healthcare System	Iron Mountain	83%	29
Mercy Hospital-Grayling	Grayling	83%	29

5. Beta Blocker at Discharge

Hospital Name	City	Rate	Cases
Alpena Regional Medical Center	Alpena	100%	48
Holland Community Hospital	Holland	100%	88
Mercy Hospital	Cadillac	100%	27
Metro Health Hospital	Grand Rapids	100%	66
MidMichigan Medical Center	Midland	100%	94
Oakwood Annapolis Hospital	Wayne	100%	77
Saint Joseph's Healthcare	Clinton Township	100%	305
Spectrum Health	Grand Rapids	100%	998
University of Michigan Medical Center	Ann Arbor	100%	386
West Branch Regional Medical Center	West Branch	100%	28
Henry Ford Hospital	Detroit	99%	315
Ingham Regional Medical Center	Lansing	99%	444
Mercy General Health Partners	Muskegon	99%	406
Northern Michigan Hospital	Petoskey	99%	304
Oakwood Southshore Medical Center	Trenton	99%	74
Saint Joseph Mercy Hospital	Ann Arbor	99%	640
Saint Joseph Mercy Oakland	Pontiac	99%	398
Saint Mary Mercy Hospital	Livonia	99%	155
William Beaumont Hospital	Royal Oak	99%	478
William Beaumont Hospital	Troy	99%	273
Bon Secours Cottage Health Services	Grosse Point	98%	57
Bronson Methodist Hospital	Kalamazoo	98%	428
Detroit Receiving Hosp & Univ Health Ctr	Detroit	98%	161
Foote Health System	Jackson	98%	168
Garden City Hospital	Garden City	98%	109
Munson Medical Center	Traverse City	98%	779
Oakwood Hospital & Medical Center	Dearborn	98%	995
Port Huron Hospital	Port Huron	98%	291
Providence Hospital	Southfield	98%	477
Saint John Macomb Hospital	Warren	98%	330
Saint John's Hospital and Medical Center	Detroit	98%	570
Saint Mary's Health Care	Grand Rapids	98%	106
Sparrow Hospital	Lansing	98%	410
Botsford General Hospital	Farmington	97%	174
Mount Clemens Regional Medical Center	Mount Clemens	97%	168
Oakwood Heritage Hospital	Taylor	97%	37
Borgess Medical Center	Kalamazoo	96%	273
Hackley Hospital	Muskegon	96%	26
Harper University Hospital	Detroit	96%	152
Marquette General Hospital	Marquette	96%	301
Saint John Oakland Hospital	Madison Heights	96%	25
Saint Mary's of Michigan	Saginaw	96%	255
Covenant Medical Center	Saginaw	95%	454
Crittenton Hospital Medical Center	Rochester	95%	81
Genesys Regional Medical Center	Grand Blanc	95%	640
Hurley Medical Center	Flint	95%	107
Lakeland Hospital-Saint Joseph	Saint Joseph	95%	302
Lapeer Regional Medical Center	Lapeer	95%	42
Mercy Memorial Hospital System	Monroe	95%	55
Sinai-Grace Hospital	Detroit	95%	353
Huron Valley-Sinai Hospital	Commerce Twp	94%	64
Battle Creek Health System	Battle Creek	93%	72
Bay Regional Medical Center	Bay City	93%	322
Henry Ford Bi-County Hospital	Warren	93%	46
McLaren Regional Medical Center	Flint	92%	396
Mercy Hospital	Port Huron	88%	25
Saint Francis Hospital	Escanaba	88%	25
Dickinson County Healthcare System	Iron Mountain	87%	30
Henry Ford Wyandotte Hospital	Wyandotte	86%	205
POH Medical Center	Pontiac	84%	37

7. PCI Within 90 Minutes of Arrival

Hospital Name	City	Rate	Cases
Spectrum Health	Grand Rapids	92%	37
Genesys Regional Medical Center	Grand Blanc	36%	25

8. Smoking Cessation Advice

Hospital Name	City	Rate	Cases
Covenant Medical Center	Saginaw	100%	199
Crittenton Hospital Medical Center	Rochester	100%	26
Henry Ford Wyandotte Hospital	Wyandotte	100%	53
Holland Community Hospital	Holland	100%	27
Ingham Regional Medical Center	Lansing	100%	157
McLaren Regional Medical Center	Flint	100%	146
Mercy General Health Partners	Muskegon	100%	36
Northern Michigan Hospital	Petoskey	100%	112
Oakwood Annapolis Hospital	Wayne	100%	26
Saint Joseph Mercy Oakland	Pontiac	100%	136
Saint Joseph's Healthcare	Clinton Township	100%	95
Saint Mary Mercy Hospital	Livonia	100%	36
William Beaumont Hospital	Troy	100%	85
Bay Regional Medical Center	Bay City	99%	122
Borgess Medical Center	Kalamazoo	99%	99
Bronson Methodist Hospital	Kalamazoo	99%	141
Genesys Regional Medical Center	Grand Blanc	99%	226
Marquette General Hospital	Marquette	99%	112

NOTE: Hospital profiles are in alphabetical order by state, then city, then hospital within the city; Rankings are sorted by rate in descending order and exclude hospitals with less than 25 cases; (1) The number of cases is too small (n<25) for purposes of reliably predicting hospital performance; (2) Measure reflects the hospital's indication that its submission was based upon a sample of its relevant discharges; (3) Rate reflects fewer than the maximum possible quarters of data for the measure; (4) Inaccurate information submitted and suppressed for one or more quarters; (5) No data is available from the hospital for this measure; Please refer to the User's Guide for a full explanation of data

Hospital Name	City	Rate	Cases
Munson Medical Center	Traverse City	99%	280
Oakwood Hospital & Medical Center	Dearborn	99%	399
Spectrum Health	Grand Rapids	99%	380
William Beaumont Hospital	Royal Oak	99%	163
Hurley Medical Center	Flint	98%	49
Lakeland Hospital-Saint Joseph	Saint Joseph	98%	109
Saint John Macomb Hospital	Warren	98%	122
Saint Joseph Mercy Hospital	Ann Arbor	98%	263
University of Michigan Medical Center	Ann Arbor	98%	125
Battle Creek Health System	Battle Creek	97%	29
Foote Health System	Jackson	97%	61
Henry Ford Hospital	Detroit	97%	108
Saint Mary's Health Care	Grand Rapids	97%	29
Port Huron Hospital	Port Huron	96%	89
Providence Hospital	Southfield	96%	135
Saint John's Hospital and Medical Center	Detroit	96%	217
Mount Clemens Regional Medical Center	Mount Clemens	95%	77
Detroit Receiving Hosp & Univ Health Ctr	Detroit	94%	86
Garden City Hospital	Garden City	94%	48
Sinai-Grace Hospital	Detroit	93%	147
Sparrow Hospital	Lansing	93%	145
Harper University Hospital	Detroit	92%	63
Saint Mary's of Michigan	Saginaw	89%	110
Botsford General Hospital	Farmington	84%	32

Hospital Name	City	Rate	Cases
Sinai-Grace Hospital	Detroit	84%	485
Hurley Medical Center	Flint	83%	209
Oakwood Southshore Medical Center	Trenton	83%	121
Borgess Medical Center	Kalamazoo	82%	137
Mercy Memorial Hospital System	Monroe	82%	114
Oakwood Annapolis Hospital	Wayne	82%	173
MidMichigan Medical Center	Midland	81%	81
Saint Mary's of Michigan	Saginaw	81%	131
Bon Secours Cottage Health Services	Grosse Point	80%	190
Genesys Regional Medical Center	Grand Blanc	80%	206
McLaren Regional Medical Center	Flint	80%	145
Saint Joseph Health System	Tawas City	80%	35
William Beaumont Hospital	Troy	80%	260
Mount Clemens Regional Medical Center	Mount Clemens	79%	251
Alpena Regional Medical Center	Alpena	78%	81
Dickinson County Healthcare System	Iron Mountain	76%	25
Gratiot Medical Center	Alma	76%	51
Sturgis Hospital	Sturgis	76%	25
Bay Regional Medical Center	Bay City	74%	310
Memorial Healthcare Center	Owosso	74%	39
Covenant Medical Center	Saginaw	73%	360
Mercy Hospital	Port Huron	73%	55
POH Medical Center	Pontiac	73%	131
Henry Ford Bi-County Hospital	Warren	67%	94
Saint Francis Hospital	Escanaba	62%	34
Chippewa County War Memorial Hospital	Sault Ste Marie	43%	30

Heart Failure Care

9. ACE Inhibitor or ARB for LVSD

Hospital Name	City	Rate	Cases
Metro Health Hospital	Grand Rapids	100%	57
Saint Joseph Mercy Oakland	Pontiac	100%	261
Oakwood Heritage Hospital	Taylor	99%	80
Saint Joseph's Healthcare	Clinton Township	99%	158
Hillsdale Community Health Center	Hillsdale	98%	40
Mercy Hospital	Cadillac	98%	40
Providence Hospital	Southfield	98%	403
Saint John Oakland Hospital	Madison Heights	98%	127
Saint John River District Hospital-East China	East China Twp	98%	47
Saint John Detroit Riverview Hospital	Detroit	97%	211
Saint John's Hospital and Medical Center	Detroit	97%	294
Hackley Hospital	Muskegon	96%	48
University of Michigan Medical Center	Ann Arbor	96%	279
Saint John Macomb Hospital	Warren	95%	227
Garden City Hospital	Garden City	94%	113
Ingham Regional Medical Center	Lansing	94%	152
Oaklawn Hospital	Marshall	94%	33
Pennock Hospital	Hastings	94%	64
Spectrum Health	Grand Rapids	94%	335
West Branch Regional Medical Center	West Branch	94%	52
Saint Joseph Mercy Hospital	Ann Arbor	93%	330
William Beaumont Hospital	Royal Oak	93%	225
Botsford General Hospital	Farmington	92%	200
Mecosta County Medical Center	Big Rapids	92%	25
Saint Mary's Health Care	Grand Rapids	92%	103
Zeeland Community Hospital	Zeeland	92%	26
Detroit Receiving Hosp & Univ Health Ctr	Detroit	91%	386
Henry Ford Hospital	Detroit	91%	184
Mercy General Health Partners	Muskegon	91%	100
Northern Michigan Hospital	Petoskey	91%	105
Saint Mary Mercy Hospital	Livonia	91%	141
Oakwood Hospital & Medical Center	Dearborn	90%	563
Otsego Memorial Hospital	Gaylord	90%	31
Foote Health System	Jackson	89%	138
Gerber Memorial Health Services	Fremont	89%	28
Holland Community Hospital	Holland	89%	70
Port Huron Hospital	Port Huron	89%	127
Sparrow Hospital	Lansing	89%	244
Spectrum Health-Reed City Campus	Reed City	89%	28
Borgess-Lee Memorial Hospital	Dowagiac	88%	33
Bronson Methodist Hospital	Kalamazoo	88%	190
Central Michigan Community Hospital	Mount Pleasant	88%	34
Crittenton Hospital Medical Center	Rochester	88%	113
Lakeland Hospital-Saint Joseph	Saint Joseph	88%	199
Saint Joseph Mercy Livingston Hospital	Howell	88%	41
Harper University Hospital	Detroit	87%	388
Lapeer Regional Medical Center	Lapeer	87%	70
Memorial Medical Center West Michigan	Ludington	87%	45
Munson Medical Center	Traverse City	87%	170
Henry Ford Wyandotte Hospital	Wyandotte	86%	101
North Oakland Medical Center	Pontiac	86%	63
Huron Valley-Sinai Hospital	Commerce Twp	85%	68
Mercy Hospital-Grayling	Grayling	85%	26
Battle Creek Health System	Battle Creek	84%	181
Marquette General Hospital	Marquette	84%	68

10. Discharge Instructions

Hospital Name	City	Rate	Cases
Cheboygan Memorial Hospital	Cheboygan	100%	65
Ingham Regional Medical Center	Lansing	98%	454
Kelsey Memorial Hospital	Lakeview	97%	30
Oakwood Heritage Hospital	Taylor	97%	132
Mercy Hospital	Cadillac	96%	79
Metro Health Hospital	Grand Rapids	96%	122
University of Michigan Medical Center	Ann Arbor	96%	569
Saint Joseph Health System	Tawas City	95%	94
Spectrum Health-Reed City Campus	Reed City	95%	59
Bay Regional Medical Center	Bay City	94%	686
Bronson Methodist Hospital	Kalamazoo	94%	539
Holland Community Hospital	Holland	94%	137
Zeeland Community Hospital	Zeeland	94%	54
Mercy Hospital	Port Huron	93%	162
Saint John River District Hospital-East China	East China Twp	93%	112
Sinai-Grace Hospital	Detroit	92%	931
Central Michigan Community Hospital	Mount Pleasant	90%	103
Otsego Memorial Hospital	Gaylord	89%	65
United Memorial Health Center	Greenville	89%	87
MidMichigan Medical Center-Gladwin	Gladwin	88%	56
Spectrum Health	Grand Rapids	88%	826
Chelsea Community Hospital	Chelsea	87%	45
MidMichigan Medical Center	Midland	87%	224
Munson Medical Center	Traverse City	87%	357
Oaklawn Hospital	Marshall	87%	78
Saint Joseph Mercy Oakland	Pontiac	87%	585
Saint Joseph's Healthcare	Clinton Township	87%	530
Eaton Rapids Medical Center	Eaton Rapids	84%	32
Saint John Oakland Hospital	Madison Heights	84%	276
Carson City Hospital	Carson City	83%	30
Detroit Receiving Hosp & Univ Health Ctr	Detroit	83%	672
Hackley Hospital	Muskegon	83%	121
Lapeer Regional Medical Center	Lapeer	83%	178
Lakeland Hospital-Saint Joseph	Saint Joseph	82%	416
Memorial Healthcare Center	Owosso	82%	88
Saint John Macomb Hospital	Warren	82%	579
Saint Joseph Mercy Livingston Hospital	Howell	82%	103
Saint Joseph Mercy Saline Hospital	Saline	82%	40
Hurley Medical Center	Flint	81%	499
Port Huron Hospital	Port Huron	81%	302
Saint John Detroit Riverview Hospital	Detroit	81%	447
Sturgis Hospital	Sturgis	81%	94
Alpena Regional Medical Center	Alpena	80%	176
North Oakland Medical Center	Pontiac	80%	40
Saint John's Hospital and Medical Center	Detroit	80%	642
Saint Mary's of Michigan	Saginaw	80%	268
Garden City Hospital	Garden City	79%	346
Northern Michigan Hospital	Petoskey	79%	217
Saint Francis Hospital	Escanaba	78%	86
Gratiot Medical Center	Alma	77%	168
Mercy General Health Partners	Muskegon	77%	75
Providence Hospital	Southfield	77%	893
Borgess Medical Center	Kalamazoo	76%	240
Mecosta County Medical Center	Big Rapids	76%	67
Oakwood Southshore Medical Center	Trenton	75%	244

NOTE: Hospital profiles are in alphabetical order by state, then city, then hospital within the city; Rankings are sorted by rate in descending order and exclude hospitals with less than 25 cases; (1) The number of cases is too small (n<25) for purposes of reliably predicting hospital performance; (2) Measure reflects the hospital's indication that its submission was based upon a sample of its relevant discharges; (3) Rate reflects fewer than the maximum possible quarters of data for the measure; (4) Inaccurate information submitted and suppressed for one or more quarters; (5) No data is available from the hospital for this measure; Please refer to the User's Guide for a full explanation of data

West Shore Medical Center	Manistee	75%	32
Bixby Medical Center	Adrian	74%	54
Covenant Medical Center	Saginaw	74%	691
Hillsdale Community Health Center	Hillsdale	74%	70
Ionia County Memorial Hospital	Ionia	74%	38
Community Health Center of Branch County	Coldwater	73%	83
Marquette General Hospital	Marquette	73%	145
MidMichigan Medical Center-Clare	Clare	73%	116
Saint Joseph Mercy Hospital	Ann Arbor	72%	745
Dickinson County Healthcare System	Iron Mountain	71%	83
North Ottawa Community Hospital	Grand Haven	71%	42
Oakwood Hospital & Medical Center	Dearborn	71%	1037
Foote Health System	Jackson	70%	327
Gerber Memorial Health Services	Fremont	70%	80
Pennock Hospital	Hastings	70%	109
Harper University Hospital	Detroit	69%	813
Mount Clemens Regional Medical Center	Mount Clemens	69%	420
West Branch Regional Medical Center	West Branch	69%	159
Iron County Community Hospitals	Iron River	68%	44
Marlette Community Hospital	Marlette	68%	25
Crittenton Hospital Medical Center	Rochester	67%	281
Botsford General Hospital	Farmington	66%	481
Mercy Memorial Hospital System	Monroe	66%	338
Oakwood Annapolis Hospital	Wayne	66%	381
Three Rivers Area Hospital	Three Rivers	65%	46
McLaren Regional Medical Center	Flint	64%	284
William Beaumont Hospital	Royal Oak	64%	476
Borgess-Lee Memorial Hospital	Dowagiac	63%	65
Genesys Regional Medical Center	Grand Blanc	63%	589
Bon Secours Cottage Health Services	Grosse Point	61%	474
South Haven Community Hospital	South Haven	61%	33
Sparrow Hospital	Lansing	61%	493
Hayes Green Beach Memorial Hospital	Charlotte	60%	45
Mercy Hospital-Grayling	Grayling	58%	83
Battle Creek Health System	Battle Creek	55%	350
Saint Mary's Health Care	Grand Rapids	54%	267
Allegan General Hospital	Allegan	49%	55
Huron Valley-Sinai Hospital	Commerce Twp	49%	225
Henry Ford Hospital	Detroit	48%	414
Henry Ford Wyandotte Hospital	Wyandotte	48%	227
Herrick Memorial Hospital	Tecumseh	48%	25
Saint Mary Mercy Hospital	Livonia	47%	343
William Beaumont Hospital	Troy	45%	543
Clinton Memorial Hospital	Saint Johns	43%	30
Memorial Medical Center West Michigan	Ludington	42%	79
Hills & Dales General Hospital	Cass City	40%	30
Henry Ford Bi-County Hospital	Warren	37%	268
POH Medical Center	Pontiac	26%	198
Chippewa County War Memorial Hospital	Sault Ste Marie	13%	85
Huron Medical Center	Bad Axe	7%	58

11. Evaluation of LVS Function

Hospital Name	City	Rate	Cases
Gratiot Medical Center	Alma	100%	232
Kelsey Memorial Hospital	Lakeview	100%	41
Oakwood Heritage Hospital	Taylor	100%	216
Saint John Oakland Hospital	Madison Heights	100%	306
Saint Joseph Mercy Oakland	Pontiac	100%	685
Saint Joseph's Healthcare	Clinton Township	100%	693
Spectrum Health-Reed City Campus	Reed City	100%	69
University of Michigan Medical Center	Ann Arbor	100%	634
William Beaumont Hospital	Royal Oak	100%	592
Bronson Methodist Hospital	Kalamazoo	99%	664
Cheboygan Memorial Hospital	Cheboygan	99%	79
Harper University Hospital	Detroit	99%	872
Holland Community Hospital	Holland	99%	180
Saint John Detroit Riverview Hospital	Detroit	99%	531
Saint Joseph Mercy Hospital	Ann Arbor	99%	917
Saint Joseph Mercy Livingston Hospital	Howell	99%	150
Sinai-Grace Hospital	Detroit	99%	1083
Spectrum Health	Grand Rapids	99%	1009
United Memorial Health Center	Greenville	99%	115
William Beaumont Hospital	Troy	99%	666
Borgess Medical Center	Kalamazoo	98%	280
Chelsea Community Hospital	Chelsea	98%	61
Covenant Medical Center	Saginaw	98%	808
Crittenton Hospital Medical Center	Rochester	98%	343
Detroit Receiving Hosp & Univ Health Ctr	Detroit	98%	720
Gerber Memorial Health Services	Fremont	98%	92
Henry Ford Hospital	Detroit	98%	466
Huron Valley-Sinai Hospital	Commerce Twp	98%	272
Mercy General Health Partners	Muskegon	98%	306
Mount Clemens Regional Medical Center	Mount Clemens	98%	488
Oakwood Hospital & Medical Center	Dearborn	98%	1236
POH Medical Center	Pontiac	98%	251
Pennock Hospital	Hastings	98%	146
Saint John's Hospital and Medical Center	Detroit	98%	729
Saint Mary's of Michigan	Saginaw	98%	314
Battle Creek Health System	Battle Creek	97%	437
Bay Regional Medical Center	Bay City	97%	803
Carson City Hospital	Carson City	97%	39
Hackley Hospital	Muskegon	97%	153
Henry Ford Bi-County Hospital	Warren	97%	319
Ingham Regional Medical Center	Lansing	97%	515
Metro Health Hospital	Grand Rapids	97%	157
MidMichigan Medical Center	Midland	97%	266
MidMichigan Medical Center-Gladwin	Gladwin	97%	76
Munson Medical Center	Traverse City	97%	403
Oaklawn Hospital	Marshall	97%	92
Providence Hospital	Southfield	97%	1046
Saint Mary Mercy Hospital	Livonia	97%	533
Saint Mary's Health Care	Grand Rapids	97%	338
Garden City Hospital	Garden City	96%	438
Lapeer Regional Medical Center	Lapeer	96%	212
North Oakland Medical Center	Pontiac	96%	221
Oakwood Annapolis Hospital	Wayne	96%	475
Botsford General Hospital	Farmington	95%	622
Foote Health System	Jackson	95%	401
Marquette General Hospital	Marquette	95%	168
Mercy Hospital	Cadillac	95%	99
Mercy Hospital	Port Huron	95%	193
Port Huron Hospital	Port Huron	95%	370
Saint Francis Hospital	Escanaba	95%	102
Saint John Macomb Hospital	Warren	95%	714
Saint Joseph Mercy Saline Hospital	Saline	95%	60
Central Michigan Community Hospital	Mount Pleasant	94%	141
Hurley Medical Center	Flint	94%	562
Lakeland Hospital-Saint Joseph	Saint Joseph	94%	469
Saint John River District Hospital-East China	East China Twp	94%	140
Bixby Medical Center	Adrian	93%	68
Northern Michigan Hospital	Petoskey	93%	236
Oakwood Southshore Medical Center	Trenton	93%	324
Portage Health System	Hancock	93%	30
Sturgis Hospital	Sturgis	93%	119
Alpena Regional Medical Center	Alpena	92%	223
Bon Secours Cottage Health Services	Grosse Point	92%	549
Memorial Medical Center West Michigan	Ludington	92%	98
Saint Joseph Health System	Tawas City	92%	106
Zeeland Community Hospital	Zeeland	92%	78
Eaton Rapids Medical Center	Eaton Rapids	91%	34
Genesys Regional Medical Center	Grand Blanc	91%	662
Otsego Memorial Hospital	Gaylord	91%	76
Sparrow Hospital	Lansing	91%	588
West Branch Regional Medical Center	West Branch	91%	184
Ionia County Memorial Hospital	Ionia	90%	49
Henry Ford Wyandotte Hospital	Wyandotte	89%	285
Memorial Healthcare Center	Owosso	88%	113
Dickinson County Healthcare System	Iron Mountain	87%	123
Herrick Memorial Hospital	Tecumseh	87%	31
Hillsdale Community Health Center	Hillsdale	87%	90
McLaren Regional Medical Center	Flint	86%	338
Clinton Memorial Hospital	Saint Johns	85%	33
North Ottawa Community Hospital	Grand Haven	85%	59
Chippewa County War Memorial Hospital	Sault Ste Marie	84%	108
Mercy Hospital-Grayling	Grayling	84%	99
Mercy Memorial Hospital System	Monroe	84%	438
MidMichigan Medical Center-Clare	Clare	84%	126
Hayes Green Beach Memorial Hospital	Charlotte	82%	57
Three Rivers Area Hospital	Three Rivers	82%	60
Mecosta County Medical Center	Big Rapids	79%	80
Allegan General Hospital	Allegan	76%	71
Borgess-Lee Memorial Hospital	Dowagiac	76%	71
South Haven Community Hospital	South Haven	76%	38
West Shore Medical Center	Manistee	72%	46
Community Health Center of Branch County	Coldwater	65%	105
Community Hospital Watervliet	Watervliet	64%	84
Marlette Community Hospital	Marlette	62%	26
Huron Medical Center	Bad Axe	57%	77
Iron County Community Hospitals	Iron River	56%	61
Hills & Dales General Hospital	Cass City	24%	42

12. Smoking Cessation Advice

Hospital Name	City	Rate	Cases
Gratiot Medical Center	Alma	100%	29
Holland Community Hospital	Holland	100%	26
Ingham Regional Medical Center	Lansing	100%	90
Lapeer Regional Medical Center	Lapeer	100%	33
McLaren Regional Medical Center	Flint	100%	59

NOTE: Hospital profiles are in alphabetical order by state, then city, then hospital within the city; Rankings are sorted by rate in descending order and exclude hospitals with less than 25 cases; (1) The number of cases is too small (n<25) for purposes of reliably predicting hospital performance; (2) Measure reflects the hospital's indication that its submission was based upon a sample of its relevant discharges; (3) Rate reflects fewer than the maximum possible quarters of data for the measure; (4) Inaccurate information submitted and suppressed for one or more quarters; (5) No data is available from the hospital for this measure; Please refer to the User's Guide for a full explanation of data

Mercy Hospital	Port Huron	100%	36
Metro Health Hospital	Grand Rapids	100%	25
Mount Clemens Regional Medical Center	Mount Clemens	100%	79
Oakwood Annapolis Hospital	Wayne	100%	127
Oakwood Heritage Hospital	Taylor	100%	44
Oakwood Hospital & Medical Center	Dearborn	100%	270
Saint Joseph Mercy Oakland	Pontiac	100%	105
Saint Joseph's Healthcare	Clinton Township	100%	75
William Beaumont Hospital	Troy	100%	62
Bay Regional Medical Center	Bay City	99%	116
Lakeland Hospital-Saint Joseph	Saint Joseph	99%	74
Spectrum Health	Grand Rapids	99%	155
Crittenton Hospital Medical Center	Rochester	98%	42
Genesys Regional Medical Center	Grand Blanc	98%	109
Henry Ford Wyandotte Hospital	Wyandotte	98%	40
Saint Mary Mercy Hospital	Livonia	98%	44
Battle Creek Health System	Battle Creek	97%	114
Covenant Medical Center	Saginaw	97%	180
Foote Health System	Jackson	97%	70
Harper University Hospital	Detroit	97%	185
Huron Valley-Sinai Hospital	Commerce Twp	97%	32
Northern Michigan Hospital	Petoskey	97%	37
Oakwood Southshore Medical Center	Trenton	97%	65
Port Huron Hospital	Port Huron	97%	64
Botsford General Hospital	Farmington	96%	113
Saint Mary's Health Care	Grand Rapids	96%	71
University of Michigan Medical Center	Ann Arbor	96%	120
Saint John Detroit Riverview Hospital	Detroit	95%	183
William Beaumont Hospital	Royal Oak	95%	78
Borgess Medical Center	Kalamazoo	94%	53
Saint John's Hospital and Medical Center	Detroit	94%	203
Central Michigan Community Hospital	Mount Pleasant	93%	27
Detroit Receiving Hosp & Univ Health Ctr	Detroit	93%	323
Munson Medical Center	Traverse City	93%	55
Saint John Oakland Hospital	Madison Heights	93%	70
Sinai-Grace Hospital	Detroit	93%	406
Bronson Methodist Hospital	Kalamazoo	90%	130
Garden City Hospital	Garden City	90%	72
Henry Ford Hospital	Detroit	90%	123
Mercy Memorial Hospital System	Monroe	90%	69
Saint Joseph Mercy Hospital	Ann Arbor	89%	142
Hurley Medical Center	Flint	87%	202
Providence Hospital	Southfield	87%	188
MidMichigan Medical Center	Midland	83%	30
Saint John Macomb Hospital	Warren	83%	102
Sparrow Hospital	Lansing	83%	87
Saint Mary's of Michigan	Saginaw	80%	70
Henry Ford Bi-County Hospital	Warren	73%	45
MidMichigan Medical Center-Clare	Clare	73%	26
POH Medical Center	Pontiac	72%	76
Bon Secours Cottage Health Services	Grosse Point	65%	62

Pneumonia Care

13. Appropriate Initial Antibiotic

Hospital Name	City	Rate	Cases
Chelsea Community Hospital	Chelsea	100%	86
Munson Medical Center	Traverse City	98%	184
Bronson Methodist Hospital	Kalamazoo	97%	222
Metro Health Hospital	Grand Rapids	97%	117
Spectrum Health	Grand Rapids	97%	593
MidMichigan Medical Center-Clare	Clare	96%	112
Oaklawn Hospital	Marshall	96%	96
Oakwood Southshore Medical Center	Trenton	96%	179
Bixby Medical Center	Adrian	95%	74
Oakwood Annapolis Hospital	Wayne	95%	215
Oakwood Heritage Hospital	Taylor	95%	131
POH Medical Center	Pontiac	95%	122
Saint Joseph Mercy Livingston Hospital	Howell	95%	110
Saint Joseph Mercy Oakland	Pontiac	95%	186
West Shore Medical Center	Manistee	95%	76
William Beaumont Hospital	Troy	95%	262
Zeeland Community Hospital	Zeeland	95%	64
Borgess-Lee Memorial Hospital	Dowagiac	94%	66
Lapeer Regional Medical Center	Lapeer	94%	159
Providence Hospital	Southfield	94%	374
Garden City Hospital	Garden City	93%	281
Genesys Regional Medical Center	Grand Blanc	93%	294
Henry Ford Hospital	Detroit	93%	114
McLaren Regional Medical Center	Flint	93%	166
Oakwood Hospital & Medical Center	Dearborn	93%	432
Otsego Memorial Hospital	Gaylord	93%	59
Port Huron Hospital	Port Huron	93%	215
Saint John Oakland Hospital	Madison Heights	93%	75
William Beaumont Hospital	Royal Oak	93%	242
Alpena Regional Medical Center	Alpena	92%	165
Carson City Hospital	Carson City	92%	53
Cheboygan Memorial Hospital	Cheboygan	92%	64
Dickinson County Healthcare System	Iron Mountain	92%	76
Saint John's Hospital and Medical Center	Detroit	92%	394
Saint Joseph Health System	Tawas City	92%	73
Saint Mary's of Michigan	Saginaw	92%	103
Bay Regional Medical Center	Bay City	91%	233
Gerber Memorial Health Services	Fremont	91%	75
Ionia County Memorial Hospital	Ionia	91%	67
Mercy Hospital	Cadillac	91%	116
Mercy Hospital-Grayling	Grayling	91%	193
MidMichigan Medical Center	Midland	91%	141
MidMichigan Medical Center-Gladwin	Gladwin	91%	46
Mount Clemens Regional Medical Center	Mount Clemens	91%	154
Saint Joseph's Healthcare	Clinton Township	91%	292
Borgess Medical Center	Kalamazoo	90%	81
Covenant Medical Center	Saginaw	90%	290
Foote Health System	Jackson	90%	128
Herrick Memorial Hospital	Tecumseh	90%	50
Kelsey Memorial Hospital	Lakeview	90%	41
Marquette General Hospital	Marquette	90%	83
Mecosta County Medical Center	Big Rapids	90%	88
Saint John Detroit Riverview Hospital	Detroit	90%	115
Saint Joseph Mercy Hospital	Ann Arbor	90%	301
Saint Joseph Mercy Saline Hospital	Saline	90%	41
Mercy Hospital	Port Huron	89%	122
Spectrum Health-Reed City Campus	Reed City	89%	63
United Memorial Health Center	Greenville	89%	147
Crittenton Hospital Medical Center	Rochester	88%	167
Gratiot Medical Center	Alma	88%	109
Hayes Green Beach Memorial Hospital	Charlotte	88%	56
Portage Health System	Hancock	88%	59
Three Rivers Area Hospital	Three Rivers	88%	77
Battle Creek Health System	Battle Creek	87%	221
Central Michigan Community Hospital	Mount Pleasant	87%	101
Hackley Hospital	Muskegon	87%	119
Hillsdale Community Health Center	Hillsdale	87%	118
Hurley Medical Center	Flint	87%	239
Ingham Regional Medical Center	Lansing	87%	211
Marlette Community Hospital	Marlette	87%	30
North Ottawa Community Hospital	Grand Haven	87%	38
Saint John Macomb Hospital	Warren	87%	317
Sinai-Grace Hospital	Detroit	87%	206
Botsford General Hospital	Farmington	86%	243
Henry Ford Bi-County Hospital	Warren	86%	140
Huron Valley-Sinai Hospital	Commerce Twp	86%	107
Pennock Hospital	Hastings	86%	105
Saint John River District Hospital-East China	East China Twp	86%	79
Community Health Center of Branch County	Coldwater	85%	121
Mercy Memorial Hospital System	Monroe	85%	192
Northern Michigan Hospital	Petoskey	85%	67
University of Michigan Medical Center	Ann Arbor	85%	240
Lakeland Hospital-Saint Joseph	Saint Joseph	84%	223
Saint Mary's Health Care	Grand Rapids	84%	205
Allegan General Hospital	Allegan	83%	60
Henry Ford Wyandotte Hospital	Wyandotte	83%	113
Memorial Medical Center West Michigan	Ludington	83%	60
Sparrow Hospital	Lansing	83%	221
Harper University Hospital	Detroit	82%	90
Saint Mary Mercy Hospital	Livonia	81%	378
Bon Secours Cottage Health Services	Grosse Point	80%	247
Detroit Receiving Hosp & Univ Health Ctr	Detroit	80%	266
Holland Community Hospital	Holland	80%	178
West Branch Regional Medical Center	West Branch	80%	108
Clinton Memorial Hospital	Saint Johns	79%	34
Memorial Healthcare Center	Owosso	79%	121
Saint Francis Hospital	Escanaba	79%	104
Hills & Dales General Hospital	Cass City	78%	36
Sturgis Hospital	Sturgis	76%	67
Huron Medical Center	Bad Axe	70%	67
South Haven Community Hospital	South Haven	70%	71
Iron County Community Hospitals	Iron River	67%	27
Chippewa County War Memorial Hospital	Sault Ste Marie	64%	119

14. Blood Culture Timing

Hospital Name	City	Rate	Cases
Kelsey Memorial Hospital	Lakeview	100%	28
Marquette General Hospital	Marquette	100%	92
Mercy General Health Partners	Muskegon	100%	29
Pennock Hospital	Hastings	99%	93
Saint Joseph Mercy Livingston Hospital	Howell	99%	150
Garden City Hospital	Garden City	98%	342

NOTE: Hospital profiles are in alphabetical order by state, then city, then hospital within the city; Rankings are sorted by rate in descending order and exclude hospitals with less than 25 cases; (1) The number of cases is too small (n<25) for purposes of reliably predicting hospital performance; (2) Measure reflects the hospital's indication that its submission was based upon a sample of its relevant discharges; (3) Rate reflects fewer than the maximum possible quarters of data for the measure; (4) Inaccurate information submitted and suppressed for one or more quarters; (5) No data is available from the hospital for this measure; Please refer to the User's Guide for a full explanation of data

Oakwood Annapolis Hospital	Wayne	98%	307
Oakwood Southshore Medical Center	Trenton	98%	234
Spectrum Health-Reed City Campus	Reed City	98%	66
Sturgis Hospital	Sturgis	98%	46
Cheboygan Memorial Hospital	Cheboygan	97%	64
Oakwood Heritage Hospital	Taylor	97%	239
Portage Health System	Hancock	97%	37
Saint John Oakland Hospital	Madison Heights	97%	124
Saint Joseph Mercy Hospital	Ann Arbor	97%	370
Zeeland Community Hospital	Zeeland	97%	76
Alpena Regional Medical Center	Alpena	96%	149
Gratiot Medical Center	Alma	96%	134
Henry Ford Bi-County Hospital	Warren	96%	157
Mecosta County Medical Center	Big Rapids	96%	95
Mercy Memorial Hospital System	Monroe	96%	186
Metro Health Hospital	Grand Rapids	96%	142
MidMichigan Medical Center	Midland	96%	188
Northern Michigan Hospital	Petoskey	96%	73
Oaklawn Hospital	Marshall	96%	109
Saint Joseph Mercy Saline Hospital	Saline	96%	50
Central Michigan Community Hospital	Mount Pleasant	95%	87
Chippewa County War Memorial Hospital	Sault Ste Marie	95%	78
Dickinson County Healthcare System	Iron Mountain	95%	74
Gerber Memorial Health Services	Fremont	95%	80
Herrick Memorial Hospital	Tecumseh	95%	39
Memorial Medical Center West Michigan	Ludington	95%	79
Oakwood Hospital & Medical Center	Dearborn	95%	515
Saint Francis Hospital	Escanaba	95%	113
West Shore Medical Center	Manistee	95%	62
Chelsea Community Hospital	Chelsea	94%	98
Foote Health System	Jackson	94%	89
Harper University Hospital	Detroit	94%	117
Ionia County Memorial Hospital	Ionia	94%	36
Lakeland Hospital-Saint Joseph	Saint Joseph	94%	200
Lapeer Regional Medical Center	Lapeer	94%	198
Mount Clemens Regional Medical Center	Mount Clemens	94%	184
Munson Medical Center	Traverse City	94%	215
United Memorial Health Center	Greenville	94%	157
West Branch Regional Medical Center	West Branch	94%	102
William Beaumont Hospital	Troy	94%	295
Borgess Medical Center	Kalamazoo	93%	87
Crittenton Hospital Medical Center	Rochester	93%	179
Port Huron Hospital	Port Huron	93%	162
South Haven Community Hospital	South Haven	93%	46
William Beaumont Hospital	Royal Oak	93%	271
Carson City Hospital	Carson City	92%	26
Huron Valley-Sinai Hospital	Commerce Twp	92%	107
McLaren Regional Medical Center	Flint	92%	186
MidMichigan Medical Center-Clare	Clare	92%	124
MidMichigan Medical Center-Gladwin	Gladwin	92%	76
Otsego Memorial Hospital	Gaylord	92%	61
Saint Mary Mercy Hospital	Livonia	92%	378
University of Michigan Medical Center	Ann Arbor	92%	357
Bay Regional Medical Center	Bay City	91%	211
Bronson Methodist Hospital	Kalamazoo	91%	280
Community Health Center of Branch County	Coldwater	91%	92
Holland Community Hospital	Holland	91%	182
Covenant Medical Center	Saginaw	90%	351
Hayes Green Beach Memorial Hospital	Charlotte	90%	30
Hurley Medical Center	Flint	90%	230
North Ottawa Community Hospital	Grand Haven	90%	40
Saint John Macomb Hospital	Warren	90%	382
Saint Joseph Mercy Oakland	Pontiac	90%	303
Bixby Medical Center	Adrian	89%	76
Iron County Community Hospitals	Iron River	89%	44
Saint Mary's Health Care	Grand Rapids	89%	177
Borgess-Lee Memorial Hospital	Dowagiac	88%	57
Mercy Hospital-Grayling	Grayling	88%	152
North Oakland Medical Center	Pontiac	88%	25
Saint Joseph Health System	Tawas City	88%	67
Bon Secours Cottage Health Services	Grosse Point	87%	146
Botsford General Hospital	Farmington	87%	306
Henry Ford Hospital	Detroit	87%	134
Saint Mary's of Michigan	Saginaw	87%	139
Battle Creek Health System	Battle Creek	86%	231
Hackley Hospital	Muskegon	86%	94
Mercy Hospital	Cadillac	86%	102
Saint John's Hospital and Medical Center	Detroit	86%	419
Sinai-Grace Hospital	Detroit	86%	301
Spectrum Health	Grand Rapids	86%	728
Three Rivers Area Hospital	Three Rivers	86%	73
Genesys Regional Medical Center	Grand Blanc	85%	376
Henry Ford Wyandotte Hospital	Wyandotte	85%	124
Providence Hospital	Southfield	85%	358
Detroit Receiving Hosp & Univ Health Ctr	Detroit	84%	210
Mercy Hospital	Port Huron	84%	88
Allegan General Hospital	Allegan	83%	54
Hills & Dales General Hospital	Cass City	83%	29
Hillsdale Community Health Center	Hillsdale	83%	63
Sparrow Hospital	Lansing	83%	221
Memorial Healthcare Center	Owosso	82%	76
Saint John River District Hospital-East China	East China Twp	81%	93
Saint John Detroit Riverview Hospital	Detroit	70%	141
Ingham Regional Medical Center	Lansing	69%	218
Saint Joseph's Healthcare	Clinton Township	60%	301
Huron Medical Center	Bad Axe	58%	50
POH Medical Center	Pontiac	47%	112

15. Influenza Vaccine

Hospital Name	City	Rate	Cases
Oakwood Heritage Hospital	Taylor	100%	58
United Memorial Health Center	Greenville	100%	25
Holland Community Hospital	Holland	98%	50
Lapeer Regional Medical Center	Lapeer	96%	49
Saint Joseph Mercy Livingston Hospital	Howell	96%	28
Gratiot Medical Center	Alma	94%	32
Oaklawn Hospital	Marshall	93%	27
Saint Mary's Health Care	Grand Rapids	93%	60
Oakwood Annapolis Hospital	Wayne	92%	74
Bon Secours Cottage Health Services	Grosse Point	91%	44
Spectrum Health	Grand Rapids	91%	150
Foote Health System	Jackson	90%	30
Mount Clemens Regional Medical Center	Mount Clemens	89%	46
Sinai-Grace Hospital	Detroit	89%	57
MidMichigan Medical Center	Midland	88%	43
Munson Medical Center	Traverse City	88%	48
Covenant Medical Center	Saginaw	87%	68
Saint Joseph's Healthcare	Clinton Township	87%	68
Alpena Regional Medical Center	Alpena	86%	36
Lakeland Hospital-Saint Joseph	Saint Joseph	86%	43
Oakwood Hospital & Medical Center	Dearborn	85%	94
Oakwood Southshore Medical Center	Trenton	85%	60
Saint Joseph Mercy Oakland	Pontiac	85%	72
William Beaumont Hospital	Troy	82%	71
University of Michigan Medical Center	Ann Arbor	80%	70
Mercy Hospital	Port Huron	79%	29
MidMichigan Medical Center-Clare	Clare	79%	33
Hurley Medical Center	Flint	78%	36
Bronson Methodist Hospital	Kalamazoo	77%	71
Detroit Receiving Hosp & Univ Health Ctr	Detroit	76%	34
McLaren Regional Medical Center	Flint	76%	34
Port Huron Hospital	Port Huron	76%	49
Garden City Hospital	Garden City	74%	76
Providence Hospital	Southfield	74%	80
Saint John's Hospital and Medical Center	Detroit	74%	85
Mercy Memorial Hospital System	Monroe	73%	45
Hillsdale Community Health Center	Hillsdale	71%	35
Saint John Macomb Hospital	Warren	70%	90
Huron Valley-Sinai Hospital	Commerce Twp	69%	26
Harper University Hospital	Detroit	68%	38
Ingham Regional Medical Center	Lansing	67%	67
Saint Joseph Mercy Hospital	Ann Arbor	67%	104
West Branch Regional Medical Center	West Branch	63%	27
Community Health Center of Branch County	Coldwater	62%	26
Bay Regional Medical Center	Bay City	60%	63
Sparrow Hospital	Lansing	60%	60
Saint Mary's of Michigan	Saginaw	58%	26
Mercy Hospital-Grayling	Grayling	54%	48
Henry Ford Bi-County Hospital	Warren	52%	33
Crittenton Hospital Medical Center	Rochester	50%	48
Genesys Regional Medical Center	Grand Blanc	38%	130
Saint John Detroit Riverview Hospital	Detroit	27%	45
Saint John Oakland Hospital	Madison Heights	24%	25
William Beaumont Hospital	Royal Oak	13%	61

16. Initial Antibiotic Timing

Hospital Name	City	Rate	Cases
Kelsey Memorial Hospital	Lakeview	97%	35
Hackley Hospital	Muskegon	96%	127
Herrick Memorial Hospital	Tecumseh	96%	45
Mecosta County Medical Center	Big Rapids	95%	110
Zeeland Community Hospital	Zeeland	95%	88
Oaklawn Hospital	Marshall	94%	146
Saint Joseph Mercy Saline Hospital	Saline	94%	68
Spectrum Health-Reed City Campus	Reed City	94%	94
United Memorial Health Center	Greenville	94%	195
Hills & Dales General Hospital	Cass City	93%	44
West Shore Medical Center	Manistee	93%	90
Chelsea Community Hospital	Chelsea	92%	100

NOTE: Hospital profiles are in alphabetical order by state, then city, then hospital within the city; Rankings are sorted by rate in descending order and exclude hospitals with less than 25 cases; (1) The number of cases is too small (n<25) for purposes of reliably predicting hospital performance; (2) Measure reflects the hospital's indication that its submission was based upon a sample of its relevant discharges; (3) Rate reflects fewer than the maximum possible quarters of data for the measure; (4) Inaccurate information submitted and suppressed for one or more quarters; (5) No data is available from the hospital for this measure; Please refer to the User's Guide for a full explanation of data

Huron Medical Center	Bad Axe	92%	79
Metro Health Hospital	Grand Rapids	92%	174
Saint John Oakland Hospital	Madison Heights	92%	137
Saint Joseph Health System	Tawas City	92%	78
Borgess-Lee Memorial Hospital	Dowagiac	91%	79
Mercy Hospital	Cadillac	90%	125
Oakwood Southshore Medical Center	Trenton	90%	287
Portage Health System	Hancock	90%	69
Providence Hospital	Southfield	90%	507
Saint Francis Hospital	Escanaba	90%	156
Community Hospital Watervliet	Watervliet	89%	74
Huron Valley-Sinai Hospital	Commerce Twp	89%	148
Memorial Medical Center West Michigan	Ludington	89%	89
MidMichigan Medical Center-Clare	Clare	89%	159
POH Medical Center	Pontiac	89%	150
Saint Joseph Mercy Livingston Hospital	Howell	89%	166
Dickinson County Healthcare System	Iron Mountain	88%	103
Mercy Hospital-Grayling	Grayling	88%	211
Northern Michigan Hospital	Petoskey	88%	96
Otsego Memorial Hospital	Gaylord	88%	73
Saint John Macomb Hospital	Warren	88%	481
Spectrum Health	Grand Rapids	88%	860
Alpena Regional Medical Center	Alpena	87%	205
Borgess Medical Center	Kalamazoo	87%	110
Garden City Hospital	Garden City	87%	385
Gerber Memorial Health Services	Fremont	87%	95
Pennock Hospital	Hastings	87%	152
Allegan General Hospital	Allegan	86%	84
Bay Regional Medical Center	Bay City	86%	354
Gratiot Medical Center	Alma	86%	170
Henry Ford Wyandotte Hospital	Wyandotte	86%	172
Munson Medical Center	Traverse City	86%	266
Oakwood Heritage Hospital	Taylor	86%	262
Saint Joseph Mercy Oakland	Pontiac	86%	380
Carson City Hospital	Carson City	85%	54
Eaton Rapids Medical Center	Eaton Rapids	85%	27
Oakwood Annapolis Hospital	Wayne	85%	403
Clinton Memorial Hospital	Saint Johns	84%	31
Community Health Center of Branch County	Coldwater	84%	115
Crittenton Hospital Medical Center	Rochester	84%	225
Mercy General Health Partners	Muskegon	84%	150
MidMichigan Medical Center	Midland	84%	262
North Ottawa Community Hospital	Grand Haven	84%	51
Three Rivers Area Hospital	Three Rivers	84%	91
Covenant Medical Center	Saginaw	83%	427
Genesys Regional Medical Center	Grand Blanc	83%	652
Ingham Regional Medical Center	Lansing	83%	296
Ionia County Memorial Hospital	Ionia	83%	59
Port Huron Hospital	Port Huron	83%	266
Saint John River District Hospital-East China	East China Twp	83%	93
Holland Community Hospital	Holland	82%	245
MidMichigan Medical Center-Gladwin	Gladwin	82%	103
Saint Joseph Mercy Hospital	Ann Arbor	82%	512
Botsford General Hospital	Farmington	81%	393
Bronson Methodist Hospital	Kalamazoo	81%	300
Central Michigan Community Hospital	Mount Pleasant	81%	139
Cheboygan Memorial Hospital	Cheboygan	81%	96
Lakeland Hospital-Saint Joseph	Saint Joseph	81%	280
Mercy Hospital	Port Huron	81%	151
Saint Mary Mercy Hospital	Livonia	81%	550
Saint Mary's of Michigan	Saginaw	81%	161
Battle Creek Health System	Battle Creek	80%	326
Saint John Detroit Riverview Hospital	Detroit	80%	199
Chippewa County War Memorial Hospital	Sault Ste Marie	79%	132
Iron County Community Hospitals	Iron River	79%	53
Lapeer Regional Medical Center	Lapeer	79%	220
Marquette General Hospital	Marquette	79%	133
McLaren Regional Medical Center	Flint	79%	243
Mercy Memorial Hospital System	Monroe	79%	231
Saint John's Hospital and Medical Center	Detroit	79%	575
Saint Joseph's Healthcare	Clinton Township	79%	386
Bixby Medical Center	Adrian	78%	112
Foote Health System	Jackson	78%	169
Hayes Green Beach Memorial Hospital	Charlotte	78%	58
Henry Ford Hospital	Detroit	77%	173
Saint Mary's Health Care	Grand Rapids	77%	328
Sinai-Grace Hospital	Detroit	77%	434
Henry Ford Bi-County Hospital	Warren	75%	207
Memorial Healthcare Center	Owosso	75%	136
Mount Clemens Regional Medical Center	Mount Clemens	75%	187
Sturgis Hospital	Sturgis	75%	65
Hillsdale Community Health Center	Hillsdale	74%	124
Bon Secours Cottage Health Services	Grosse Point	73%	246
Sparrow Hospital	Lansing	73%	328
University of Michigan Medical Center	Ann Arbor	73%	397
Hurley Medical Center	Flint	72%	319
South Haven Community Hospital	South Haven	72%	75
West Branch Regional Medical Center	West Branch	70%	132
William Beaumont Hospital	Troy	69%	381
North Oakland Medical Center	Pontiac	68%	162
William Beaumont Hospital	Royal Oak	68%	379
Oakwood Hospital & Medical Center	Dearborn	67%	642
Detroit Receiving Hosp & Univ Health Ctr	Detroit	65%	322
Karmanos Cancer Center	Detroit	65%	43
Harper University Hospital	Detroit	63%	196

17. Oxygenation Assessment

Hospital Name	City	Rate	Cases
Alpena Regional Medical Center	Alpena	100%	255
Battle Creek Health System	Battle Creek	100%	390
Bay Regional Medical Center	Bay City	100%	414
Borgess Medical Center	Kalamazoo	100%	139
Borgess-Lee Memorial Hospital	Dowagiac	100%	101
Botsford General Hospital	Farmington	100%	475
Bronson Methodist Hospital	Kalamazoo	100%	426
Carson City Hospital	Carson City	100%	72
Central Michigan Community Hospital	Mount Pleasant	100%	172
Cheboygan Memorial Hospital	Cheboygan	100%	114
Chelsea Community Hospital	Chelsea	100%	127
Clinton Memorial Hospital	Saint Johns	100%	40
Community Health Center of Branch County	Coldwater	100%	149
Covenant Medical Center	Saginaw	100%	541
Crittenton Hospital Medical Center	Rochester	100%	287
Detroit Receiving Hosp & Univ Health Ctr	Detroit	100%	349
Dickinson County Healthcare System	Iron Mountain	100%	147
Eaton Rapids Medical Center	Eaton Rapids	100%	31
Foote Health System	Jackson	100%	202
Garden City Hospital	Garden City	100%	489
Genesys Regional Medical Center	Grand Blanc	100%	784
Gerber Memorial Health Services	Fremont	100%	122
Gratiot Medical Center	Alma	100%	219
Hackley Hospital	Muskegon	100%	175
Harper University Hospital	Detroit	100%	222
Hayes Green Beach Memorial Hospital	Charlotte	100%	75
Henry Ford Hospital	Detroit	100%	204
Henry Ford Wyandotte Hospital	Wyandotte	100%	180
Hillsdale Community Health Center	Hillsdale	100%	172
Holland Community Hospital	Holland	100%	287
Huron Valley-Sinai Hospital	Commerce Twp	100%	190
Ingham Regional Medical Center	Lansing	100%	359
Ionia County Memorial Hospital	Ionia	100%	72
Iron County Community Hospitals	Iron River	100%	79
Karmanos Cancer Center	Detroit	100%	49
Kelsey Memorial Hospital	Lakeview	100%	52
Lakeland Hospital-Saint Joseph	Saint Joseph	100%	329
Lapeer Regional Medical Center	Lapeer	100%	254
Marlette Community Hospital	Marlette	100%	33
McLaren Regional Medical Center	Flint	100%	281
Mecosta County Medical Center	Big Rapids	100%	137
Memorial Healthcare Center	Owosso	100%	166
Memorial Medical Center West Michigan	Ludington	100%	110
Mercy General Health Partners	Muskegon	100%	195
Mercy Hospital	Port Huron	100%	195
Mercy Hospital-Grayling	Grayling	100%	272
Mercy Memorial Hospital System	Monroe	100%	326
Metro Health Hospital	Grand Rapids	100%	210
MidMichigan Medical Center	Midland	100%	304
MidMichigan Medical Center-Clare	Clare	100%	182
MidMichigan Medical Center-Gladwin	Gladwin	100%	118
Mount Clemens Regional Medical Center	Mount Clemens	100%	260
North Ottawa Community Hospital	Grand Haven	100%	63
Northern Michigan Hospital	Petoskey	100%	122
Oakwood Annapolis Hospital	Wayne	100%	475
Oakwood Heritage Hospital	Taylor	100%	327
Oakwood Hospital & Medical Center	Dearborn	100%	803
Oakwood Southshore Medical Center	Trenton	100%	353
Otsego Memorial Hospital	Gaylord	100%	98
POH Medical Center	Pontiac	100%	186
Pennock Hospital	Hastings	100%	172
Port Huron Hospital	Port Huron	100%	318
Portage Health System	Hancock	100%	76
Providence Hospital	Southfield	100%	591
Saint Francis Hospital	Escanaba	100%	194
Saint John Detroit Riverview Hospital	Detroit	100%	240
Saint John North Shores Hospital	Harrison Township	100%	26
Saint John Oakland Hospital	Madison Heights	100%	175
Saint John's Hospital and Medical Center	Detroit	100%	666
Saint Joseph Health System	Tawas City	100%	115
Saint Joseph Mercy Hospital	Ann Arbor	100%	655

NOTE: Hospital profiles are in alphabetical order by state, then city, then hospital within the city; Rankings are sorted by rate in descending order and exclude hospitals with less than 25 cases; (1) The number of cases is too small (n<25) for purposes of reliably predicting hospital performance; (2) Measure reflects the hospital's indication that its submission was based upon a sample of its relevant discharges; (3) Rate reflects fewer than the maximum possible quarters of data for the measure; (4) Inaccurate information submitted and suppressed for one or more quarters; (5) No data is available from the hospital for this measure; Please refer to the User's Guide for a full explanation of data

Saint Joseph Mercy Livingston Hospital	Howell	100%	220
Saint Joseph Mercy Oakland	Pontiac	100%	469
Saint Joseph Mercy Saline Hospital	Saline	100%	78
Saint Joseph's Healthcare	Clinton Township	100%	447
Saint Mary Mercy Hospital	Livonia	100%	687
Saint Mary's Health Care	Grand Rapids	100%	404
Saint Mary's of Michigan	Saginaw	100%	208
Sinai-Grace Hospital	Detroit	100%	519
South Haven Community Hospital	South Haven	100%	87
Sparrow Hospital	Lansing	100%	399
Spectrum Health	Grand Rapids	100%	1061
Spectrum Health-Reed City Campus	Reed City	100%	99
Sturgis Hospital	Sturgis	100%	81
Three Rivers Area Hospital	Three Rivers	100%	102
United Memorial Health Center	Greenville	100%	228
University of Michigan Medical Center	Ann Arbor	100%	561
West Branch Regional Medical Center	West Branch	100%	161
West Shore Medical Center	Manistee	100%	125
William Beaumont Hospital	Royal Oak	100%	501
William Beaumont Hospital	Troy	100%	496
Zeeland Community Hospital	Zeeland	100%	108
Bixby Medical Center	Adrian	99%	139
Community Hospital Watervliet	Watervliet	99%	94
Henry Ford Bi-County Hospital	Warren	99%	244
Hurley Medical Center	Flint	99%	374
Huron Medical Center	Bad Axe	99%	89
Marquette General Hospital	Marquette	99%	168
Mercy Hospital	Cadillac	99%	160
Munson Medical Center	Traverse City	99%	341
North Oakland Medical Center	Pontiac	99%	193
Oaklawn Hospital	Marshall	99%	173
Saint John Macomb Hospital	Warren	99%	551
Bon Secours Cottage Health Services	Grosse Point	98%	300
Herrick Memorial Hospital	Tecumseh	98%	64
Allegan General Hospital	Allegan	97%	89
Hills & Dales General Hospital	Cass City	97%	61
Saint John River District Hospital-East China	East China Twp	97%	124
Chippewa County War Memorial Hospital	Sault Ste Marie	93%	149

18. Pneumococcal Vaccine

Hospital Name	City	Rate	Cases
Kelsey Memorial Hospital	Lakeview	100%	33
MidMichigan Medical Center-Gladwin	Gladwin	100%	79
Chelsea Community Hospital	Chelsea	99%	96
Oakwood Heritage Hospital	Taylor	99%	192
Spectrum Health-Reed City Campus	Reed City	98%	62
Zeeland Community Hospital	Zeeland	97%	77
Metro Health Hospital	Grand Rapids	95%	116
Cheboygan Memorial Hospital	Cheboygan	94%	72
Hackley Hospital	Muskegon	94%	109
Lapeer Regional Medical Center	Lapeer	94%	152
Pennock Hospital	Hastings	94%	102
Saint John River District Hospital-East China	East China Twp	94%	78
Saint Joseph Mercy Livingston Hospital	Howell	94%	145
Spectrum Health	Grand Rapids	94%	661
Central Michigan Community Hospital	Mount Pleasant	93%	94
Memorial Healthcare Center	Owosso	93%	92
Munson Medical Center	Traverse City	93%	246
Oaklawn Hospital	Marshall	93%	116
Oakwood Annapolis Hospital	Wayne	93%	260
United Memorial Health Center	Greenville	93%	133
Holland Community Hospital	Holland	92%	182
Alpena Regional Medical Center	Alpena	91%	181
Bixby Medical Center	Adrian	91%	96
MidMichigan Medical Center	Midland	91%	218
Otsego Memorial Hospital	Gaylord	90%	60
Saint Joseph Health System	Tawas City	90%	80
Mecosta County Medical Center	Big Rapids	89%	80
Oakwood Southshore Medical Center	Trenton	89%	230
Saint Francis Hospital	Escanaba	89%	125
Covenant Medical Center	Saginaw	88%	320
Gratiot Medical Center	Alma	88%	151
Saint Joseph's Healthcare	Clinton Township	88%	298
Foote Health System	Jackson	87%	117
Battle Creek Health System	Battle Creek	86%	238
Borgess Medical Center	Kalamazoo	86%	95
Saint Joseph Mercy Saline Hospital	Saline	85%	61
Herrick Memorial Hospital	Tecumseh	84%	45
Mercy Hospital	Cadillac	84%	103
Saint Joseph Mercy Oakland	Pontiac	84%	293
Oakwood Hospital & Medical Center	Dearborn	83%	472
University of Michigan Medical Center	Ann Arbor	83%	293
William Beaumont Hospital	Troy	83%	320
Memorial Medical Center West Michigan	Ludington	81%	81
Mercy General Health Partners	Muskegon	81%	111
Bronson Methodist Hospital	Kalamazoo	80%	285
Dickinson County Healthcare System	Iron Mountain	80%	103
Mercy Memorial Hospital System	Monroe	80%	166
Mount Clemens Regional Medical Center	Mount Clemens	80%	156
Northern Michigan Hospital	Petoskey	80%	84
Carson City Hospital	Carson City	79%	43
Port Huron Hospital	Port Huron	79%	196
North Ottawa Community Hospital	Grand Haven	78%	41
Bon Secours Cottage Health Services	Grosse Point	77%	178
Bay Regional Medical Center	Bay City	76%	291
Gerber Memorial Health Services	Fremont	76%	87
Saint John Detroit Riverview Hospital	Detroit	76%	90
Lakeland Hospital-Saint Joseph	Saint Joseph	74%	192
North Oakland Medical Center	Pontiac	74%	93
Saint Mary's Health Care	Grand Rapids	74%	225
Allegan General Hospital	Allegan	73%	59
Hurley Medical Center	Flint	73%	136
Clinton Memorial Hospital	Saint Johns	72%	25
Hillsdale Community Health Center	Hillsdale	72%	112
Huron Valley-Sinai Hospital	Commerce Twp	72%	100
MidMichigan Medical Center-Clare	Clare	72%	122
Saint John Macomb Hospital	Warren	72%	393
Saint John's Hospital and Medical Center	Detroit	72%	327
Saint Mary's of Michigan	Saginaw	72%	128
Three Rivers Area Hospital	Three Rivers	72%	60
Community Hospital Watervliet	Watervliet	70%	63
Garden City Hospital	Garden City	70%	312
Harper University Hospital	Detroit	69%	90
Mercy Hospital	Port Huron	69%	118
Portage Health System	Hancock	69%	54
Sinai-Grace Hospital	Detroit	69%	203
Providence Hospital	Southfield	65%	340
Iron County Community Hospitals	Iron River	64%	56
Sparrow Hospital	Lansing	64%	249
Botsford General Hospital	Farmington	59%	289
Detroit Receiving Hosp & Univ Health Ctr	Detroit	59%	76
Henry Ford Hospital	Detroit	59%	91
McLaren Regional Medical Center	Flint	59%	177
Saint Joseph Mercy Hospital	Ann Arbor	59%	466
Mercy Hospital-Grayling	Grayling	57%	160
Henry Ford Wyandotte Hospital	Wyandotte	54%	123
Ingham Regional Medical Center	Lansing	54%	217
Marquette General Hospital	Marquette	54%	111
Saint John Oakland Hospital	Madison Heights	54%	89
West Branch Regional Medical Center	West Branch	51%	85
Saint Mary Mercy Hospital	Livonia	49%	500
South Haven Community Hospital	South Haven	49%	45
Community Health Center of Branch County	Coldwater	47%	90
Genesys Regional Medical Center	Grand Blanc	47%	496
William Beaumont Hospital	Royal Oak	46%	333
Ionia County Memorial Hospital	Ionia	45%	47
Borgess-Lee Memorial Hospital	Dowagiac	44%	52
Crittenton Hospital Medical Center	Rochester	42%	212
Henry Ford Bi-County Hospital	Warren	42%	128
POH Medical Center	Pontiac	42%	69
Hayes Green Beach Memorial Hospital	Charlotte	37%	46
Chippewa County War Memorial Hospital	Sault Ste Marie	36%	90
West Shore Medical Center	Manistee	20%	80
Hills & Dales General Hospital	Cass City	13%	38
Sturgis Hospital	Sturgis	6%	53
Huron Medical Center	Bad Axe	3%	61

19. Smoking Cessation Advice

Hospital Name	City	Rate	Cases
Chelsea Community Hospital	Chelsea	100%	26
Gratiot Medical Center	Alma	100%	35
Lapeer Regional Medical Center	Lapeer	100%	73
Marquette General Hospital	Marquette	100%	54
Mercy Hospital	Cadillac	100%	33
Metro Health Hospital	Grand Rapids	100%	56
Oakwood Heritage Hospital	Taylor	100%	92
Port Huron Hospital	Port Huron	100%	83
Saint Joseph's Healthcare	Clinton Township	100%	104
Spectrum Health-Reed City Campus	Reed City	100%	30
William Beaumont Hospital	Troy	99%	100
Bay Regional Medical Center	Bay City	98%	84
Covenant Medical Center	Saginaw	98%	148
Henry Ford Wyandotte Hospital	Wyandotte	98%	47
Huron Valley-Sinai Hospital	Commerce Twp	98%	50
Mercy Hospital	Port Huron	98%	55
Oakwood Annapolis Hospital	Wayne	98%	160
Gerber Memorial Health Services	Fremont	97%	29
Ingham Regional Medical Center	Lansing	97%	78

NOTE: Hospital profiles are in alphabetical order by state, then city, then hospital within the city; Rankings are sorted by rate in descending order and exclude hospitals with less than 25 cases; (1) The number of cases is too small (n<25) for purposes of reliably predicting hospital performance; (2) Measure reflects the hospital's indication that its submission was based upon a sample of its relevant discharges; (3) Rate reflects fewer than the maximum possible quarters of data for the measure; (4) Inaccurate information submitted and suppressed for one or more quarters; (5) No data is available from the hospital for this measure; Please refer to the User's Guide for a full explanation of data

Oakwood Southshore Medical Center	Trenton	97%	87
Otsego Memorial Hospital	Gaylord	97%	30
Central Michigan Community Hospital	Mount Pleasant	96%	51
Munson Medical Center	Traverse City	96%	82
Battle Creek Health System	Battle Creek	95%	120
Crittenton Hospital Medical Center	Rochester	95%	43
Genesys Regional Medical Center	Grand Blanc	95%	187
Hackley Hospital	Muskegon	95%	39
Lakeland Hospital-Saint Joseph	Saint Joseph	95%	65
Mount Clemens Regional Medical Center	Mount Clemens	95%	76
United Memorial Health Center	Greenville	95%	59
Bronson Methodist Hospital	Kalamazoo	94%	104
Foote Health System	Jackson	94%	54
Oakwood Hospital & Medical Center	Dearborn	94%	231
Holland Community Hospital	Holland	93%	69
Oaklawn Hospital	Marshall	93%	44
Saint Francis Hospital	Escanaba	93%	29
Harper University Hospital	Detroit	92%	53
McLaren Regional Medical Center	Flint	92%	53
Saint John Oakland Hospital	Madison Heights	92%	53
Saint Mary Mercy Hospital	Livonia	92%	83
Saint Mary's Health Care	Grand Rapids	92%	110
Saint Joseph Mercy Oakland	Pontiac	90%	124
University of Michigan Medical Center	Ann Arbor	90%	110
William Beaumont Hospital	Royal Oak	90%	93
Mecosta County Medical Center	Big Rapids	89%	45
MidMichigan Medical Center	Midland	89%	56
Providence Hospital	Southfield	89%	118
Three Rivers Area Hospital	Three Rivers	89%	28
Alpena Regional Medical Center	Alpena	88%	51
Pennock Hospital	Hastings	88%	34
Saint John Detroit Riverview Hospital	Detroit	87%	79
Spectrum Health	Grand Rapids	87%	271
Borgess Medical Center	Kalamazoo	86%	50
Botsford General Hospital	Farmington	86%	97
Henry Ford Hospital	Detroit	86%	49
Memorial Healthcare Center	Owosso	86%	37
West Shore Medical Center	Manistee	86%	35
Mercy Memorial Hospital System	Monroe	85%	97
Bon Secours Cottage Health Services	Grosse Point	84%	74
Detroit Receiving Hosp & Univ Health Ctr	Detroit	83%	183
Dickinson County Healthcare System	Iron Mountain	83%	29
Hillsdale Community Health Center	Hillsdale	83%	48
Bixby Medical Center	Adrian	82%	28
Henry Ford Bi-County Hospital	Warren	82%	71
MidMichigan Medical Center-Clare	Clare	82%	44
Saint John's Hospital and Medical Center	Detroit	82%	192
Saint Joseph Mercy Livingston Hospital	Howell	82%	38
Sinai-Grace Hospital	Detroit	82%	146
Hurley Medical Center	Flint	78%	133
POH Medical Center	Pontiac	77%	82
Sparrow Hospital	Lansing	76%	106
West Branch Regional Medical Center	West Branch	75%	40
Garden City Hospital	Garden City	73%	96
Saint Joseph Mercy Hospital	Ann Arbor	73%	152
Community Health Center of Branch County	Coldwater	71%	38
Mercy Hospital-Grayling	Grayling	70%	70
Saint Mary's of Michigan	Saginaw	70%	50
Borgess-Lee Memorial Hospital	Dowagiac	69%	26
Saint John Macomb Hospital	Warren	68%	108
Chippewa County War Memorial Hospital	Sault Ste Marie	31%	26

Surgical Infection Prevention

20. Prophylactic Antibiotic Given

Hospital Name	City	Rate	Cases
Spectrum Health-Reed City Campus	Reed City	100%	38
Chelsea Community Hospital	Chelsea	99%	640
Henry Ford Bi-County Hospital	Warren	99%	253
Saint Joseph Mercy Oakland	Pontiac	99%	1264
Karmanos Cancer Center	Detroit	98%	44
Saint John's Hospital and Medical Center	Detroit	97%	1006
United Memorial Health Center	Greenville	97%	146
Bronson Methodist Hospital	Kalamazoo	96%	1653
Carson City Hospital	Carson City	96%	176
Garden City Hospital	Garden City	96%	411
Cheboygan Memorial Hospital	Cheboygan	95%	154
Huron Valley-Sinai Hospital	Commerce Twp	95%	625
Otsego Memorial Hospital	Gaylord	95%	110
Pennock Hospital	Hastings	95%	253
Providence Hospital	Southfield	95%	624
Oakwood Annapolis Hospital	Wayne	94%	344
Oakwood Heritage Hospital	Taylor	94%	156
Saint Joseph's Healthcare	Clinton Township	94%	1270
University of Michigan Medical Center	Ann Arbor	94%	1437
Community Hospital Watervliet	Watervliet	93%	152
Dickinson County Healthcare System	Iron Mountain	93%	255
Henry Ford Hospital	Detroit	93%	431
Oaklawn Hospital	Marshall	93%	371
Oakwood Hospital & Medical Center	Dearborn	93%	1503
Saint John Oakland Hospital	Madison Heights	93%	107
Saint Joseph Health System	Tawas City	93%	188
Ingham Regional Medical Center	Lansing	92%	1642
Lapeer Regional Medical Center	Lapeer	92%	404
Mercy Hospital	Port Huron	92%	499
Saint John River District Hospital-East China	East China Twp	92%	112
William Beaumont Hospital	Royal Oak	92%	478
Zeeland Community Hospital	Zeeland	92%	221
Bay Regional Medical Center	Bay City	91%	1106
Central Michigan Community Hospital	Mount Pleasant	91%	278
Hackley Hospital	Muskegon	91%	466
Holland Community Hospital	Holland	91%	543
Munson Medical Center	Traverse City	91%	612
Oakwood Southshore Medical Center	Trenton	91%	270
Saint Joseph Mercy Hospital	Ann Arbor	91%	374
Saint Joseph Mercy Livingston Hospital	Howell	91%	174
Saint Joseph Mercy Saline Hospital	Saline	91%	35
William Beaumont Hospital	Troy	91%	712
Allegan General Hospital	Allegan	90%	60
Foote Health System	Jackson	90%	190
Mercy Hospital	Cadillac	90%	213
Alpena Regional Medical Center	Alpena	89%	419
Botsford General Hospital	Farmington	89%	396
Genesys Regional Medical Center	Grand Blanc	89%	517
Harper University Hospital	Detroit	89%	952
Marquette General Hospital	Marquette	89%	211
Memorial Healthcare Center	Owosso	89%	238
MidMichigan Medical Center	Midland	89%	722
Sinai-Grace Hospital	Detroit	89%	784
Community Health Center of Branch County	Coldwater	88%	285
Gerber Memorial Health Services	Fremont	88%	228
Crittenton Hospital Medical Center	Rochester	87%	456
Saint Mary's Health Care	Grand Rapids	87%	313
Bon Secours Cottage Health Services	Grosse Point	86%	659
Spectrum Health	Grand Rapids	86%	372
West Shore Medical Center	Manistee	86%	106
Detroit Receiving Hosp & Univ Health Ctr	Detroit	85%	96
Saint Mary Mercy Hospital	Livonia	85%	504
Hurley Medical Center	Flint	84%	495
North Oakland Medical Center	Pontiac	84%	67
Covenant Medical Center	Saginaw	83%	583
Mercy General Health Partners	Muskegon	83%	199
POH Medical Center	Pontiac	83%	179
Port Huron Hospital	Port Huron	83%	640
Borgess Medical Center	Kalamazoo	82%	347
Gratiot Medical Center	Alma	82%	143
Mecosta County Medical Center	Big Rapids	82%	147
Memorial Medical Center West Michigan	Ludington	82%	160
Saint Mary's of Michigan	Saginaw	82%	258
Battle Creek Health System	Battle Creek	81%	715
North Ottawa Community Hospital	Grand Haven	81%	119
Saint John Detroit Riverview Hospital	Detroit	81%	183
Mercy Memorial Hospital System	Monroe	80%	551
Mount Clemens Regional Medical Center	Mount Clemens	80%	723
Metro Health Hospital	Grand Rapids	79%	253
Henry Ford Wyandotte Hospital	Wyandotte	78%	213
Saint John Macomb Hospital	Warren	78%	429
Portage Health System	Hancock	75%	77
Sparrow Hospital	Lansing	75%	1523
South Haven Community Hospital	South Haven	74%	73
Saint Francis Hospital	Escanaba	73%	138
Northern Michigan Hospital	Petoskey	71%	192
Lakeland Hospital-Saint Joseph	Saint Joseph	70%	272
West Branch Regional Medical Center	West Branch	65%	223
Bixby Medical Center	Adrian	64%	216
McLaren Regional Medical Center	Flint	64%	410
Sturgis Hospital	Sturgis	63%	99
Hayes Green Beach Memorial Hospital	Charlotte	62%	68
Mercy Hospital-Grayling	Grayling	60%	136
Marlette Community Hospital	Marlette	54%	41
Hillsdale Community Health Center	Hillsdale	49%	199
Huron Medical Center	Bad Axe	45%	110
Three Rivers Area Hospital	Three Rivers	24%	41
MidMichigan Medical Center-Clare	Clare	22%	64
Chippewa County War Memorial Hospital	Sault Ste Marie	21%	107

NOTE: Hospital profiles are in alphabetical order by state, then city, then hospital within the city; Rankings are sorted by rate in descending order and exclude hospitals with less than 25 cases; (1) The number of cases is too small (n<25) for purposes of reliably predicting hospital performance; (2) Measure reflects the hospital's indication that its submission was based upon a sample of its relevant discharges; (3) Rate reflects fewer than the maximum possible quarters of data for the measure; (4) Inaccurate information submitted and suppressed for one or more quarters; (5) No data is available from the hospital for this measure; Please refer to the User's Guide for a full explanation of data

21. Prophylactic Antibiotic Selection

Hospital Name	City	Rate	Cases
Battle Creek Health System	Battle Creek	100%	164
Cheboygan Memorial Hospital	Cheboygan	100%	40
Dickinson County Healthcare System	Iron Mountain	100%	58
Henry Ford Bi-County Hospital	Warren	100%	54
Huron Medical Center	Bad Axe	100%	41
Lapeer Regional Medical Center	Lapeer	100%	107
Memorial Medical Center West Michigan	Ludington	100%	60
Oakwood Heritage Hospital	Taylor	100%	30
Saint John River District Hospital-East China	East China Twp	100%	36
United Memorial Health Center	Greenville	100%	43
Garden City Hospital	Garden City	99%	96
Munson Medical Center	Traverse City	99%	154
Oaklawn Hospital	Marshall	99%	110
Oakwood Southshore Medical Center	Trenton	99%	71
Saint John's Hospital and Medical Center	Detroit	99%	317
Saint Joseph Mercy Oakland	Pontiac	99%	312
Alpena Regional Medical Center	Alpena	98%	110
Bronson Methodist Hospital	Kalamazoo	98%	408
Chelsea Community Hospital	Chelsea	98%	153
Community Hospital Watervliet	Watervliet	98%	41
Mercy Hospital	Cadillac	98%	60
North Ottawa Community Hospital	Grand Haven	98%	42
Oakwood Hospital & Medical Center	Dearborn	98%	390
Providence Hospital	Southfield	98%	279
Saint Joseph Health System	Tawas City	98%	45
Saint Joseph Mercy Livingston Hospital	Howell	98%	44
Sinai-Grace Hospital	Detroit	98%	198
William Beaumont Hospital	Troy	98%	187
Central Michigan Community Hospital	Mount Pleasant	97%	72
Crittenton Hospital Medical Center	Rochester	97%	148
Genesys Regional Medical Center	Grand Blanc	97%	180
Hackley Hospital	Muskegon	97%	161
Huron Valley-Sinai Hospital	Commerce Twp	97%	163
Mercy Hospital	Port Huron	97%	178
Northern Michigan Hospital	Petoskey	97%	67
Otsego Memorial Hospital	Gaylord	97%	37
Port Huron Hospital	Port Huron	97%	142
Saint John Oakland Hospital	Madison Heights	97%	36
Saint Mary's of Michigan	Saginaw	97%	91
University of Michigan Medical Center	Ann Arbor	97%	473
West Branch Regional Medical Center	West Branch	97%	68
West Shore Medical Center	Manistee	97%	31
Bay Regional Medical Center	Bay City	96%	244
Covenant Medical Center	Saginaw	96%	143
Henry Ford Hospital	Detroit	96%	111
Karmanos Cancer Center	Detroit	96%	46
Marquette General Hospital	Marquette	96%	67
Pennock Hospital	Hastings	96%	54
Saint John Detroit Riverview Hospital	Detroit	96%	69
Saint Joseph Mercy Hospital	Ann Arbor	96%	91
Saint Joseph's Healthcare	Clinton Township	96%	336
Bon Secours Cottage Health Services	Grosse Point	95%	233
Foote Health System	Jackson	95%	60
Botsford General Hospital	Farmington	94%	154
Carson City Hospital	Carson City	94%	35
Mercy Hospital-Grayling	Grayling	94%	31
Metro Health Hospital	Grand Rapids	94%	65
Oakwood Annapolis Hospital	Wayne	94%	99
Saint Mary's Health Care	Grand Rapids	94%	97
Sturgis Hospital	Sturgis	94%	36
Memorial Healthcare Center	Owosso	93%	72
Portage Health System	Hancock	93%	27
Saint Mary Mercy Hospital	Livonia	93%	176
Hurley Medical Center	Flint	92%	131
Ingham Regional Medical Center	Lansing	92%	519
Mercy Memorial Hospital System	Monroe	92%	146
POH Medical Center	Pontiac	92%	39
William Beaumont Hospital	Royal Oak	92%	119
Holland Community Hospital	Holland	91%	139
McLaren Regional Medical Center	Flint	91%	123
Chippewa County War Memorial Hospital	Sault Ste Marie	90%	31
Gerber Memorial Health Services	Fremont	90%	58
Borgess Medical Center	Kalamazoo	89%	84
Mecosta County Medical Center	Big Rapids	89%	56
Saint Francis Hospital	Escanaba	89%	36
Saint John Macomb Hospital	Warren	89%	257
Spectrum Health	Grand Rapids	89%	119
Bixby Medical Center	Adrian	88%	73
Community Health Center of Branch County	Coldwater	88%	65
Mount Clemens Regional Medical Center	Mount Clemens	88%	175
Sparrow Hospital	Lansing	88%	354
Zeeland Community Hospital	Zeeland	88%	59
Gratiot Medical Center	Alma	86%	49
Henry Ford Wyandotte Hospital	Wyandotte	86%	72
Lakeland Hospital-Saint Joseph	Saint Joseph	86%	88
Detroit Receiving Hosp & Univ Health Ctr	Detroit	85%	26
Harper University Hospital	Detroit	84%	203
South Haven Community Hospital	South Haven	83%	30
Three Rivers Area Hospital	Three Rivers	81%	27
Allegan General Hospital	Allegan	80%	30
Hillsdale Community Health Center	Hillsdale	79%	67
MidMichigan Medical Center	Midland	74%	214

22. Prophylactic Antibiotic Stopped

Hospital Name	City	Rate	Cases
Mercy Hospital	Cadillac	100%	213
Spectrum Health-Reed City Campus	Reed City	100%	38
Three Rivers Area Hospital	Three Rivers	100%	40
Saint Joseph Health System	Tawas City	99%	173
Cheboygan Memorial Hospital	Cheboygan	98%	148
Henry Ford Wyandotte Hospital	Wyandotte	97%	157
Chelsea Community Hospital	Chelsea	96%	628
Marlette Community Hospital	Marlette	95%	40
Oaklawn Hospital	Marshall	95%	362
Saint Joseph Mercy Oakland	Pontiac	95%	1175
Carson City Hospital	Carson City	94%	172
Gerber Memorial Health Services	Fremont	94%	218
Pennock Hospital	Hastings	94%	244
United Memorial Health Center	Greenville	94%	134
Allegan General Hospital	Allegan	93%	59
Alpena Regional Medical Center	Alpena	93%	406
Garden City Hospital	Garden City	93%	387
Karmanos Cancer Center	Detroit	93%	44
North Ottawa Community Hospital	Grand Haven	93%	118
Oakwood Heritage Hospital	Taylor	93%	150
MidMichigan Medical Center	Midland	92%	701
North Oakland Medical Center	Pontiac	92%	63
Saint John Oakland Hospital	Madison Heights	92%	100
Sinai-Grace Hospital	Detroit	92%	718
Hackley Hospital	Muskegon	91%	457
Huron Valley-Sinai Hospital	Commerce Twp	91%	607
Otsego Memorial Hospital	Gaylord	91%	110
Saint John's Hospital and Medical Center	Detroit	91%	962
Zeeland Community Hospital	Zeeland	91%	218
Bay Regional Medical Center	Bay City	90%	1065
Bronson Methodist Hospital	Kalamazoo	90%	1605
Henry Ford Bi-County Hospital	Warren	90%	241
Saint Joseph Mercy Hospital	Ann Arbor	90%	357
Spectrum Health	Grand Rapids	90%	363
William Beaumont Hospital	Royal Oak	90%	465
Central Michigan Community Hospital	Mount Pleasant	89%	275
Community Hospital Watervliet	Watervliet	89%	151
Dickinson County Healthcare System	Iron Mountain	89%	247
Henry Ford Hospital	Detroit	89%	417
Holland Community Hospital	Holland	89%	519
Lapeer Regional Medical Center	Lapeer	89%	381
Memorial Medical Center West Michigan	Ludington	89%	148
Providence Hospital	Southfield	89%	577
Saint Joseph Mercy Saline Hospital	Saline	89%	35
South Haven Community Hospital	South Haven	89%	72
William Beaumont Hospital	Troy	89%	662
Battle Creek Health System	Battle Creek	87%	666
Community Health Center of Branch County	Coldwater	87%	267
Ingham Regional Medical Center	Lansing	87%	1539
Munson Medical Center	Traverse City	87%	591
Saint Joseph's Healthcare	Clinton Township	87%	1212
Oakwood Southshore Medical Center	Trenton	86%	248
Port Huron Hospital	Port Huron	86%	624
Saint Mary's Health Care	Grand Rapids	86%	300
Sturgis Hospital	Sturgis	86%	97
Foote Health System	Jackson	85%	178
Saint Joseph Mercy Livingston Hospital	Howell	85%	168
Borgess Medical Center	Kalamazoo	84%	330
Botsford General Hospital	Farmington	84%	370
Mercy Hospital-Grayling	Grayling	84%	122
Saint John River District Hospital-East China	East China Twp	84%	102
Bixby Medical Center	Adrian	83%	209
Metro Health Hospital	Grand Rapids	83%	244
Oakwood Hospital & Medical Center	Dearborn	83%	1425
Hurley Medical Center	Flint	82%	464
Northern Michigan Hospital	Petoskey	82%	196
Bon Secours Cottage Health Services	Grosse Point	81%	641
Genesys Regional Medical Center	Grand Blanc	81%	459
Saint John Macomb Hospital	Warren	81%	401
Mercy General Health Partners	Muskegon	80%	193
Huron Medical Center	Bad Axe	79%	107

NOTE: Hospital profiles are in alphabetical order by state, then city, then hospital within the city; Rankings are sorted by rate in descending order and exclude hospitals with less than 25 cases; (1) The number of cases is too small (n<25) for purposes of reliably predicting hospital performance; (2) Measure reflects the hospital's indication that its submission was based upon a sample of its relevant discharges; (3) Rate reflects fewer than the maximum possible quarters of data for the measure; (4) Inaccurate information submitted and suppressed for one or more quarters; (5) No data is available from the hospital for this measure; Please refer to the User's Guide for a full explanation of data

Crittenton Hospital Medical Center	Rochester	78%	447
Oakwood Annapolis Hospital	Wayne	78%	325
Saint Mary Mercy Hospital	Livonia	78%	481
Memorial Healthcare Center	Owosso	77%	222
Mercy Memorial Hospital System	Monroe	77%	533
Saint Mary's of Michigan	Saginaw	77%	252
University of Michigan Medical Center	Ann Arbor	76%	1341
Mecosta County Medical Center	Big Rapids	75%	142
Saint Francis Hospital	Escanaba	75%	120
West Shore Medical Center	Manistee	73%	101
Harper University Hospital	Detroit	70%	908
Mount Clemens Regional Medical Center	Mount Clemens	70%	698
POH Medical Center	Pontiac	70%	166
Sparrow Hospital	Lansing	70%	1483
Gratiot Medical Center	Alma	69%	131
Hayes Green Beach Memorial Hospital	Charlotte	69%	67
Covenant Medical Center	Saginaw	66%	559
Mercy Hospital	Port Huron	65%	425
Detroit Receiving Hosp & Univ Health Ctr	Detroit	63%	81
Chippewa County War Memorial Hospital	Sault Ste Marie	61%	99
McLaren Regional Medical Center	Flint	61%	389
Lakeland Hospital-Saint Joseph	Saint Joseph	60%	267
Portage Health System	Hancock	57%	65
Marquette General Hospital	Marquette	54%	206
MidMichigan Medical Center-Clare	Clare	54%	63
Saint John Detroit Riverview Hospital	Detroit	53%	175
West Branch Regional Medical Center	West Branch	45%	217
Hillsdale Community Health Center	Hillsdale	11%	195

Pregnancy Care

23. Inpatient Neonatal Mortality

Hospital Name	City	Rate	Cases
Saint Francis Hospital	Escanaba	0.00%	250
South Haven Community Hospital	South Haven	0.00%	430
Three Rivers Area Hospital	Three Rivers	0.00%	347
Holland Community Hospital	Holland	0.11%	1788
Saint Mary Mercy Hospital	Livonia	0.14%	711
Sturgis Hospital	Sturgis	0.24%	424
Battle Creek Health System	Battle Creek	0.28%	1067
Chippewa County War Memorial Hospital	Sault Ste Marie	0.30%	333
Gratiot Medical Center	Alma	0.30%	656
Cheboygan Memorial Hospital	Cheboygan	0.41%	244
Marquette General Hospital	Marquette	0.45%	888
Spectrum Health	Grand Rapids	0.49%	8861
North Oakland Medical Center	Pontiac	0.59%	511
Harper University Hospital	Detroit	1.15%	5568

24. Third or Fourth Degree Laceration

Hospital Name	City	Rate	Cases
Three Rivers Area Hospital	Three Rivers	0.00%	278
South Haven Community Hospital	South Haven	0.29%	342
Harper University Hospital	Detroit	1.18%	3893
Spectrum Health	Grand Rapids	2.15%	5726
Saint Mary Mercy Hospital	Livonia	2.22%	992
Battle Creek Health System	Battle Creek	2.80%	857
Cheboygan Memorial Hospital	Cheboygan	3.05%	164
Gratiot Medical Center	Alma	3.36%	446
North Oakland Medical Center	Pontiac	3.97%	982
Sturgis Hospital	Sturgis	4.78%	293
Saint Francis Hospital	Escanaba	5.44%	147
Chippewa County War Memorial Hospital	Sault Ste Marie	5.93%	236
Marquette General Hospital	Marquette	6.97%	545
Holland Community Hospital	Holland	7.07%	1231

NOTE: Hospital profiles are in alphabetical order by state, then city, then hospital within the city; Rankings are sorted by rate in descending order and exclude hospitals with less than 25 cases; (1) The number of cases is too small (n<25) for purposes of reliably predicting hospital performance; (2) Measure reflects the hospital's indication that its submission was based upon a sample of its relevant discharges; (3) Rate reflects fewer than the maximum possible quarters of data for the measure; (4) Inaccurate information submitted and suppressed for one or more quarters; (5) No data is available from the hospital for this measure; Please refer to the User's Guide for a full explanation of data

Bixby Medical Center

818 Riverside Avenue
Adrian, MI 49221
URL: www.promedica.org
Ownership: Voluntary non-profit - Other
Emergency Services: Yes
Phone: 517-265-0900
Fax: 517-265-0918
Accredited: Yes
Licensed Beds: 142

Key Personnel:

CEO. . . . . Randy Oostra
Director Medical/Surgical Nursing . . . . Kathy Greenlee
Director Medical/Surgical Nursing . . . . George Anterasian, MD
OB/GYN Womens Health. . . . . Arwana Reed
Chief Radiology . . . . John Berman, MD
Director Respiratory . . . . Charlene Oldeck

Measure	Cases	This Hospital	State Average	U.S. Average	Top Hospital
Heart Attack Care					
ACE Inhibitor or ARB for LVSD[1]	3	67%	86%	82%	100%
Aspirin at Arrival	39	92%	95%	92%	100%
Aspirin at Discharge[1]	20	80%	94%	90%	100%
Beta Blocker at Arrival	28	96%	90%	87%	100%
Beta Blocker at Discharge[1]	16	81%	93%	90%	100%
Fibrinolytic Medication Timing	0	-	28%	31%	100%
PCI Within 90 Minutes of Arrival	0	-	59%	54%	95%
Smoking Cessation Advice[1]	3	100%	93%	88%	100%
Heart Failure Care					
ACE Inhibitor or ARB for LVSD[1]	24	96%	84%	82%	100%
Discharge Instructions	54	74%	73%	61%	93%
Evaluation of LVS Function	68	93%	91%	83%	99%
Smoking Cessation Advice[1]	6	100%	86%	82%	100%
Pneumonia Care					
Appropriate Initial Antibiotic	74	95%	88%	83%	94%
Blood Culture Timing	76	89%	90%	90%	100%
Influenza Vaccine[1]	21	86%	73%	70%	100%
Initial Antibiotic Timing	112	78%	84%	80%	93%
Oxygenation Assessment	139	99%	100%	99%	100%
Pneumococcal Vaccine	96	91%	72%	69%	94%
Smoking Cessation Advice	28	82%	86%	80%	100%
Surgical Infection Prevention					
Prophylactic Antibiotic Given[2,3]	216	64%	82%	77%	95%
Prophylactic Antibiotic Selection[2]	73	88%	93%	90%	100%
Prophylactic Antibiotic Stopped[2,3]	209	83%	83%	72%	95%
Pregnancy Care					
Inpatient Neonatal Mortality	-	-	-	-	-
Third or Fourth Degree Laceration	-	-	2.62%	3.63%	3.27%

Allegan General Hospital

555 Linn Street
Allegan, MI 49010
Ownership: Voluntary non-profit - Private
Emergency Services: Yes
Phone: 269-673-8424
Fax: 269-673-4344
Accredited: No
Licensed Beds: 63

Key Personnel:

CEO. . . . . Gerald Barbins
Emergency Room . . . . Timothy Hall
Infection Control. . . . . Sandra Brenner
ICU . . . . Timothy Hall
Medical Surgical Nursing . . . . Tammy Niewenhais
OB/GYN. . . . . Jane Ward
Respiratory/Cardiopulmonary. . . . . Timothy Hall

Measure	Cases	This Hospital	State Average	U.S. Average	Top Hospital
Heart Attack Care					
ACE Inhibitor or ARB for LVSD	0	-	86%	82%	100%
Aspirin at Arrival[1]	10	60%	95%	92%	100%
Aspirin at Discharge[1]	6	50%	94%	90%	100%
Beta Blocker at Arrival[1]	10	60%	90%	87%	100%
Beta Blocker at Discharge[1]	6	50%	93%	90%	100%
Fibrinolytic Medication Timing	0	-	28%	31%	100%
PCI Within 90 Minutes of Arrival	0	-	59%	54%	95%
Smoking Cessation Advice[1]	1	100%	93%	88%	100%
Heart Failure Care					
ACE Inhibitor or ARB for LVSD[1]	15	67%	84%	82%	100%
Discharge Instructions	55	49%	73%	61%	93%
Evaluation of LVS Function	71	76%	91%	83%	99%
Smoking Cessation Advice[1]	5	60%	86%	82%	100%
Pneumonia Care					
Appropriate Initial Antibiotic	60	83%	88%	83%	94%
Blood Culture Timing	54	83%	90%	90%	100%
Influenza Vaccine[1]	13	62%	73%	70%	100%
Initial Antibiotic Timing	84	86%	84%	80%	93%
Oxygenation Assessment	89	97%	100%	99%	100%
Pneumococcal Vaccine	59	73%	72%	69%	94%
Smoking Cessation Advice[1]	17	82%	86%	80%	100%
Surgical Infection Prevention					
Prophylactic Antibiotic Given[3]	60	90%	82%	77%	95%
Prophylactic Antibiotic Selection	30	80%	93%	90%	100%
Prophylactic Antibiotic Stopped[3]	59	93%	83%	72%	95%
Pregnancy Care					
Inpatient Neonatal Mortality	-	-	-	-	-
Third or Fourth Degree Laceration	-	-	2.62%	3.63%	3.27%

Gratiot Medical Center

300 E Warwick Drive
Alma, MI 48801
URL: www.midmichigan.org
Ownership: Voluntary non-profit - Private
Emergency Services: Yes
Phone: 989-463-1101
Fax: 989-463-6948
Accredited: Yes
Licensed Beds: 142

Key Personnel:

President . . . . Tom Desauw
Manager Emergency Room . . . . Bob Peglow, RN
Director Infection Control . . . . Janet Davis, RN
Manager Radiology . . . . Bob Green
Respiratory Therapy. . . . . Jasmine Vanden

Measure	Cases	This Hospital	State Average	U.S. Average	Top Hospital
Heart Attack Care					
ACE Inhibitor or ARB for LVSD[1]	7	86%	86%	82%	100%
Aspirin at Arrival	51	92%	95%	92%	100%
Aspirin at Discharge[1]	24	96%	94%	90%	100%
Beta Blocker at Arrival	36	89%	90%	87%	100%
Beta Blocker at Discharge[1]	20	95%	93%	90%	100%
Fibrinolytic Medication Timing[1]	9	44%	28%	31%	100%
PCI Within 90 Minutes of Arrival	0	-	59%	54%	95%
Smoking Cessation Advice[1]	10	100%	93%	88%	100%
Heart Failure Care					
ACE Inhibitor or ARB for LVSD	51	76%	84%	82%	100%
Discharge Instructions	168	77%	73%	61%	93%
Evaluation of LVS Function	232	100%	91%	83%	99%
Smoking Cessation Advice	29	100%	86%	82%	100%
Pneumonia Care					
Appropriate Initial Antibiotic	109	88%	88%	83%	94%
Blood Culture Timing	134	96%	90%	90%	100%
Influenza Vaccine	32	94%	73%	70%	100%
Initial Antibiotic Timing	170	86%	84%	80%	93%
Oxygenation Assessment	219	100%	100%	99%	100%
Pneumococcal Vaccine	151	88%	72%	69%	94%
Smoking Cessation Advice	35	100%	86%	80%	100%
Surgical Infection Prevention					
Prophylactic Antibiotic Given[2,3]	143	82%	82%	77%	95%
Prophylactic Antibiotic Selection[2]	49	86%	93%	90%	100%
Prophylactic Antibiotic Stopped[2,3]	131	69%	83%	72%	95%
Pregnancy Care					
Inpatient Neonatal Mortality	656	0.30%	-	-	-
Third or Fourth Degree Laceration	446	3.36%	2.62%	3.63%	3.27%

Alpena Regional Medical Center

1501 W Chisholm Street
Alpena, MI 49707
E-mail: info@agh.org
URL: www.agh.org
Ownership: Government - Local
Emergency Services: Yes
Phone: 989-356-7390
Fax: 989-356-7773
Accredited: Yes
Licensed Beds: 146

Key Personnel:

CEO. . . . . John McVeety
Executive Director . . . . Richard McElroy
OB/GYN Women's Health . . . . Richard Bates, MD

NOTE: Hospital profiles are in alphabetical order by state, then city, then hospital within the city; Rankings are sorted by rate in descending order and exclude hospitals with less than 25 cases; (1) The number of cases is too small (n<25) for purposes of reliably predicting hospital performance; (2) Measure reflects the hospital's indication that its submission was based upon a sample of its relevant discharges; (3) Rate reflects fewer than the maximum possible quarters of data for the measure; (4) Inaccurate information submitted and suppressed for one or more quarters; (5) No data is available from the hospital for this measure; Please refer to the User's Guide for a full explanation of data

Measure	Cases	This Hospital	State Average	U.S. Average	Top Hospital
Heart Attack Care					
ACE Inhibitor or ARB for LVSD[1]	5	80%	86%	82%	100%
Aspirin at Arrival	69	99%	95%	92%	100%
Aspirin at Discharge	36	86%	94%	90%	100%
Beta Blocker at Arrival	52	96%	90%	87%	100%
Beta Blocker at Discharge	48	100%	93%	90%	100%
Fibrinolytic Medication Timing[1]	19	37%	28%	31%	100%
PCI Within 90 Minutes of Arrival	0	-	59%	54%	95%
Smoking Cessation Advice[1]	11	100%	93%	88%	100%
Heart Failure Care					
ACE Inhibitor or ARB for LVSD	81	78%	84%	82%	100%
Discharge Instructions	176	80%	73%	61%	93%
Evaluation of LVS Function	223	92%	91%	83%	99%
Smoking Cessation Advice[1]	24	92%	86%	82%	100%
Pneumonia Care					
Appropriate Initial Antibiotic	165	92%	88%	83%	94%
Blood Culture Timing	149	96%	90%	90%	100%
Influenza Vaccine	36	86%	73%	70%	100%
Initial Antibiotic Timing	205	87%	84%	80%	93%
Oxygenation Assessment	255	100%	100%	99%	100%
Pneumococcal Vaccine	181	91%	72%	69%	94%
Smoking Cessation Advice	51	88%	86%	80%	100%
Surgical Infection Prevention					
Prophylactic Antibiotic Given[2]	419	89%	82%	77%	95%
Prophylactic Antibiotic Selection[2]	110	98%	93%	90%	100%
Prophylactic Antibiotic Stopped[2]	406	93%	83%	72%	95%
Pregnancy Care					
Inpatient Neonatal Mortality	-	-	-	-	-
Third or Fourth Degree Laceration	-	-	2.62%	3.63%	3.27%

Saint Joseph Mercy Hospital

Alternate Name: Mercy Wood Hospital Unit
5301 E Huron River Drive — Phone: 734-712-3456
Ann Arbor, MI 48106 — Fax: 734-712-7133
Ownership: Voluntary non-profit - Church — Accredited: Yes
Emergency Services: Yes — Licensed Beds: 530

Key Personnel:
Administrator/President . . . . Gary Faja
Chief of Medical Staff . . . . Rossana DGrood
Emergency Room . . . . Mikheal Mikhail
Emergency Room . . . . John McCabe, MD

Measure	Cases	This Hospital	State Average	U.S. Average	Top Hospital
Heart Attack Care					
ACE Inhibitor or ARB for LVSD	163	98%	86%	82%	100%
Aspirin at Arrival	415	99%	95%	92%	100%
Aspirin at Discharge	642	99%	94%	90%	100%
Beta Blocker at Arrival	314	95%	90%	87%	100%
Beta Blocker at Discharge	640	99%	93%	90%	100%
Fibrinolytic Medication Timing	0	-	28%	31%	100%
PCI Within 90 Minutes of Arrival[1]	18	50%	59%	54%	95%
Smoking Cessation Advice	263	98%	93%	88%	100%
Heart Failure Care					
ACE Inhibitor or ARB for LVSD	330	93%	84%	82%	100%
Discharge Instructions	745	72%	73%	61%	93%
Evaluation of LVS Function	917	99%	91%	83%	99%
Smoking Cessation Advice	142	89%	86%	82%	100%
Pneumonia Care					
Appropriate Initial Antibiotic	301	90%	88%	83%	94%
Blood Culture Timing	370	97%	90%	90%	100%
Influenza Vaccine	104	67%	73%	70%	100%
Initial Antibiotic Timing	512	82%	84%	80%	93%
Oxygenation Assessment	655	100%	100%	99%	100%
Pneumococcal Vaccine	466	59%	72%	69%	94%
Smoking Cessation Advice	152	73%	86%	80%	100%
Surgical Infection Prevention					
Prophylactic Antibiotic Given[2]	374	91%	82%	77%	95%
Prophylactic Antibiotic Selection[2]	91	96%	93%	90%	100%
Prophylactic Antibiotic Stopped[2]	357	90%	83%	72%	95%
Pregnancy Care					
Inpatient Neonatal Mortality	-	-	-	-	-
Third or Fourth Degree Laceration	-	-	2.62%	3.63%	3.27%

University of Michigan Medical Center

1500 E Medical Center Drive — Phone: 734-936-4000
Ann Arbor, MI 48109
URL: www.med.umich.edu
Ownership: Govt - Hospital District or Authority — Accredited: Yes
Emergency Services: Yes — Licensed Beds: 86

Key Personnel:
Director/CEO . . . . Douglas L Strong, MBA
Chief Medical Staff . . . . David Spahlinger
Director Infection/Disease Control . . . . Candace Friedman, MPH
CCU Spvg. Nurse . . . . Stephanie Dillion
Director Medical/Surgical Nursing . . . . Francine Lundy
Chief Radiology . . . . N Reed Dunnick, MD
Respiratory/Cardiopulmonary . . . . K Bandy

Measure	Cases	This Hospital	State Average	U.S. Average	Top Hospital
Heart Attack Care					
ACE Inhibitor or ARB for LVSD	70	97%	86%	82%	100%
Aspirin at Arrival	273	100%	95%	92%	100%
Aspirin at Discharge	396	100%	94%	90%	100%
Beta Blocker at Arrival	240	99%	90%	87%	100%
Beta Blocker at Discharge	386	100%	93%	90%	100%
Fibrinolytic Medication Timing	0	-	28%	31%	100%
PCI Within 90 Minutes of Arrival[1]	8	100%	59%	54%	95%
Smoking Cessation Advice	125	98%	93%	88%	100%
Heart Failure Care					
ACE Inhibitor or ARB for LVSD	279	96%	84%	82%	100%
Discharge Instructions	569	96%	73%	61%	93%
Evaluation of LVS Function	634	100%	91%	83%	99%
Smoking Cessation Advice	120	96%	86%	82%	100%
Pneumonia Care					
Appropriate Initial Antibiotic	240	85%	88%	83%	94%
Blood Culture Timing	357	92%	90%	90%	100%
Influenza Vaccine	70	80%	73%	70%	100%
Initial Antibiotic Timing	397	73%	84%	80%	93%
Oxygenation Assessment	561	100%	100%	99%	100%
Pneumococcal Vaccine	293	83%	72%	69%	94%
Smoking Cessation Advice	110	90%	86%	80%	100%
Surgical Infection Prevention					
Prophylactic Antibiotic Given[3]	1,437	94%	82%	77%	95%
Prophylactic Antibiotic Selection	473	97%	93%	90%	100%
Prophylactic Antibiotic Stopped[3]	1,341	76%	83%	72%	95%
Pregnancy Care					
Inpatient Neonatal Mortality	-	-	-	-	-
Third or Fourth Degree Laceration	-	-	2.62%	3.63%	3.27%

Huron Medical Center

1100 S Van Dyke — Phone: 989-269-9521
Bad Axe, MI 48413 — Fax: 989-269-7948
URL: www.huronmedicalcenter.org
Ownership: Voluntary non-profit - Other — Accredited: No
Emergency Services: Yes — Licensed Beds: 64

Key Personnel:
President/CEO . . . . Kenneth Wilhelm
Emergency Room Director . . . . Rebecca O'Connor

Measure	Cases	This Hospital	State Average	U.S. Average	Top Hospital
Heart Attack Care					
ACE Inhibitor or ARB for LVSD[3]	0	-	86%	82%	100%
Aspirin at Arrival[3]	0	-	95%	92%	100%
Aspirin at Discharge[3]	0	-	94%	90%	100%
Beta Blocker at Arrival[3]	0	-	90%	87%	100%
Beta Blocker at Discharge[3]	0	-	93%	90%	100%
Fibrinolytic Medication Timing[3]	0	-	28%	31%	100%
PCI Within 90 Minutes of Arrival[5]	-	-	59%	54%	95%
Smoking Cessation Advice[3]	0	-	93%	88%	100%
Heart Failure Care					
ACE Inhibitor or ARB for LVSD[1]	16	44%	84%	82%	100%
Discharge Instructions	58	7%	73%	61%	93%

NOTE: Hospital profiles are in alphabetical order by state, then city, then hospital within the city; Rankings are sorted by rate in descending order and exclude hospitals with less than 25 cases; (1) The number of cases is too small (n<25) for purposes of reliably predicting hospital performance; (2) Measure reflects the hospital's indication that its submission was based upon a sample of its relevant discharges; (3) Rate reflects fewer than the maximum possible quarters of data for the measure; (4) Inaccurate information submitted and suppressed for one or more quarters; (5) No data is available from the hospital for this measure; Please refer to the User's Guide for a full explanation of data

Measure	Cases	This Hospital	State Average	U.S. Average	Top Hospital
Evaluation of LVS Function	77	57%	91%	83%	99%
Smoking Cessation Advice[1]	7	0%	86%	82%	100%
Pneumonia Care					
Appropriate Initial Antibiotic	67	70%	88%	83%	94%
Blood Culture Timing	50	58%	90%	90%	100%
Influenza Vaccine[1]	11	0%	73%	70%	100%
Initial Antibiotic Timing	79	92%	84%	80%	93%
Oxygenation Assessment	89	99%	100%	99%	100%
Pneumococcal Vaccine	61	3%	72%	69%	94%
Smoking Cessation Advice[1]	15	0%	86%	80%	100%
Surgical Infection Prevention					
Prophylactic Antibiotic Given[3]	110	45%	82%	77%	95%
Prophylactic Antibiotic Selection	41	100%	93%	90%	100%
Prophylactic Antibiotic Stopped[3]	107	79%	83%	72%	95%
Pregnancy Care					
Inpatient Neonatal Mortality	-	-	-	-	-
Third or Fourth Degree Laceration	-	-	2.62%	3.63%	3.27%

Battle Creek Health System

300 N Avenue
Battle Creek, MI 49017
URL: www.bchealth.com
Ownership: Voluntary non-profit - Church
Emergency Services: Yes
Phone: 269-966-8000
Fax: 269-966-8366
Accredited: Yes
Licensed Beds: 315

Key Personnel:

CEO . . . . Pat Garrett
ICU . . . . Annette Berning
Chief Radiology . . . . Steven Yuill, MD
Director of Pulmonary . . . . Joe McBribe

Measure	Cases	This Hospital	State Average	U.S. Average	Top Hospital
Heart Attack Care					
ACE Inhibitor or ARB for LVSD[1]	22	77%	86%	82%	100%
Aspirin at Arrival	105	93%	95%	92%	100%
Aspirin at Discharge	63	90%	94%	90%	100%
Beta Blocker at Arrival	57	93%	90%	87%	100%
Beta Blocker at Discharge	72	93%	93%	90%	100%
Fibrinolytic Medication Timing	0	-	28%	31%	100%
PCI Within 90 Minutes of Arrival	0	-	59%	54%	95%
Smoking Cessation Advice	29	97%	93%	88%	100%
Heart Failure Care					
ACE Inhibitor or ARB for LVSD	181	84%	84%	82%	100%
Discharge Instructions	350	55%	73%	61%	93%
Evaluation of LVS Function	437	97%	91%	83%	99%
Smoking Cessation Advice	114	97%	86%	82%	100%
Pneumonia Care					
Appropriate Initial Antibiotic	221	87%	88%	83%	94%
Blood Culture Timing	231	86%	90%	90%	100%
Influenza Vaccine[4,5]	-	-	73%	70%	100%
Initial Antibiotic Timing	326	80%	84%	80%	93%
Oxygenation Assessment	390	100%	100%	99%	100%
Pneumococcal Vaccine	238	86%	72%	69%	94%
Smoking Cessation Advice	120	95%	86%	80%	100%
Surgical Infection Prevention					
Prophylactic Antibiotic Given	715	81%	82%	77%	95%
Prophylactic Antibiotic Selection	164	100%	93%	90%	100%
Prophylactic Antibiotic Stopped	666	87%	83%	72%	95%
Pregnancy Care					
Inpatient Neonatal Mortality	1,067	0.28%	-	-	-
Third or Fourth Degree Laceration	857	2.80%	2.62%	3.63%	3.27%

Bay Regional Medical Center

1900 Columbus Avenue
Bay City, MI 48708
URL: www.baymed.org
Ownership: Voluntary non-profit - Other
Emergency Services: Yes
Phone: 989-894-3000
Fax: 989-894-4464
Accredited: Yes
Licensed Beds: 415

Key Personnel:

President/CEO . . . . Robert Wright
Chief Medical Staff . . . . Christopher Brueck, MD
Chief Catheterization Laboratory . . . . Willa Rousseau, MD
Emergency Room . . . . Pam Rau
Director Infection/Disease Control . . . . Karen Frahm, RN
Intensive/Coronary Care . . . . Willa Rousseau
Director Medical/Surgical Nursing . . . . Linda Szafranski
OB/GYN Womens Health . . . . Mary Schubert
Chief Radiology . . . . Dave Nall
Director Respiratory Therapy . . . . Ron Charter

Measure	Cases	This Hospital	State Average	U.S. Average	Top Hospital
Heart Attack Care					
ACE Inhibitor or ARB for LVSD	77	82%	86%	82%	100%
Aspirin at Arrival	213	93%	95%	92%	100%
Aspirin at Discharge	332	97%	94%	90%	100%
Beta Blocker at Arrival	208	88%	90%	87%	100%
Beta Blocker at Discharge	322	93%	93%	90%	100%
Fibrinolytic Medication Timing	0	-	28%	31%	100%
PCI Within 90 Minutes of Arrival[1]	14	71%	59%	54%	95%
Smoking Cessation Advice	122	99%	93%	88%	100%
Heart Failure Care					
ACE Inhibitor or ARB for LVSD	310	74%	84%	82%	100%
Discharge Instructions	686	94%	73%	61%	93%
Evaluation of LVS Function	803	97%	91%	83%	99%
Smoking Cessation Advice	116	99%	86%	82%	100%
Pneumonia Care					
Appropriate Initial Antibiotic	233	91%	88%	83%	94%
Blood Culture Timing	211	91%	90%	90%	100%
Influenza Vaccine	63	60%	73%	70%	100%
Initial Antibiotic Timing	354	86%	84%	80%	93%
Oxygenation Assessment	414	100%	100%	99%	100%
Pneumococcal Vaccine	291	76%	72%	69%	94%
Smoking Cessation Advice	84	98%	86%	80%	100%
Surgical Infection Prevention					
Prophylactic Antibiotic Given[2]	1,106	91%	82%	77%	95%
Prophylactic Antibiotic Selection[2]	244	96%	93%	90%	100%
Prophylactic Antibiotic Stopped[2]	1,065	90%	83%	72%	95%
Pregnancy Care					
Inpatient Neonatal Mortality	-	-	-	-	-
Third or Fourth Degree Laceration	-	-	2.62%	3.63%	3.27%

Mecosta County Medical Center

605 Oak Street
Big Rapids, MI 49307
URL: www.mcmc.br.com
Ownership: Government - Local
Emergency Services: Yes
Phone: 231-796-8691
Fax: 231-592-4462
Accredited: Yes
Licensed Beds: 74

Key Personnel:

CEO . . . . Thomas Daugherty
Chief Medical Staff . . . . Harold Moores, MD
Emergency Room . . . . Virginia Keusch, RN

Measure	Cases	This Hospital	State Average	U.S. Average	Top Hospital
Heart Attack Care					
ACE Inhibitor or ARB for LVSD[1]	2	50%	86%	82%	100%
Aspirin at Arrival	26	100%	95%	92%	100%
Aspirin at Discharge[1]	17	88%	94%	90%	100%
Beta Blocker at Arrival[1]	24	92%	90%	87%	100%
Beta Blocker at Discharge[1]	22	91%	93%	90%	100%
Fibrinolytic Medication Timing	0	-	28%	31%	100%
PCI Within 90 Minutes of Arrival	0	-	59%	54%	95%
Smoking Cessation Advice[1]	7	100%	93%	88%	100%
Heart Failure Care					
ACE Inhibitor or ARB for LVSD	25	92%	84%	82%	100%
Discharge Instructions	67	76%	73%	61%	93%
Evaluation of LVS Function	80	79%	91%	83%	99%
Smoking Cessation Advice[1]	15	80%	86%	82%	100%
Pneumonia Care					
Appropriate Initial Antibiotic	88	90%	88%	83%	94%
Blood Culture Timing	95	96%	90%	90%	100%
Influenza Vaccine[1]	20	85%	73%	70%	100%
Initial Antibiotic Timing	110	95%	84%	80%	93%
Oxygenation Assessment	137	100%	100%	99%	100%
Pneumococcal Vaccine	80	89%	72%	69%	94%
Smoking Cessation Advice	45	89%	86%	80%	100%
Surgical Infection Prevention					

NOTE: Hospital profiles are in alphabetical order by state, then city, then hospital within the city; Rankings are sorted by rate in descending order and exclude hospitals with less than 25 cases; (1) The number of cases is too small (n<25) for purposes of reliably predicting hospital performance; (2) Measure reflects the hospital's indication that its submission was based upon a sample of its relevant discharges; (3) Rate reflects fewer than the maximum possible quarters of data for the measure; (4) Inaccurate information submitted and suppressed for one or more quarters; (5) No data is available from the hospital for this measure; Please refer to the User's Guide for a full explanation of data

Measure	Cases	This Hospital	State Average	U.S. Average	Top Hospital
Prophylactic Antibiotic Given[2,3]	147	82%	82%	77%	95%
Prophylactic Antibiotic Selection[2]	56	89%	93%	90%	100%
Prophylactic Antibiotic Stopped[2,3]	142	75%	83%	72%	95%
Pregnancy Care					
Inpatient Neonatal Mortality	-	-	-	-	-
Third or Fourth Degree Laceration	-	-	2.62%	3.63%	3.27%

Brighton Hospital

12851 E Grand River Avenue
Brighton, MI 48116
Toll-Free: 888-215-2700
Phone: 810-227-1211
Fax: 810-227-1869

E-mail: info@brightonhospital.org
URL: www.stjohn.org/brighton
Ownership: Voluntary non-profit - Private
Accredited: Yes
Emergency Services: No
Licensed Beds: 63

Key Personnel:

President/CEO . . . . Denise Bertin-Epp
Chief of Medical Staff . . . . Michael Brooks, MD

Measure	Cases	This Hospital	State Average	U.S. Average	Top Hospital
Heart Attack Care					
ACE Inhibitor or ARB for LVSD[5]	-	-	86%	82%	100%
Aspirin at Arrival[5]	-	-	95%	92%	100%
Aspirin at Discharge[5]	-	-	94%	90%	100%
Beta Blocker at Arrival[5]	-	-	90%	87%	100%
Beta Blocker at Discharge[5]	-	-	93%	90%	100%
Fibrinolytic Medication Timing[5]	-	-	28%	31%	100%
PCI Within 90 Minutes of Arrival[5]	-	-	59%	54%	95%
Smoking Cessation Advice[5]	-	-	93%	88%	100%
Heart Failure Care					
ACE Inhibitor or ARB for LVSD[5]	-	-	84%	82%	100%
Discharge Instructions[5]	-	-	73%	61%	93%
Evaluation of LVS Function[5]	-	-	91%	83%	99%
Smoking Cessation Advice[5]	-	-	86%	82%	100%
Pneumonia Care					
Appropriate Initial Antibiotic[5]	-	-	88%	83%	94%
Blood Culture Timing[5]	-	-	90%	90%	100%
Influenza Vaccine[5]	-	-	73%	70%	100%
Initial Antibiotic Timing[5]	-	-	84%	80%	93%
Oxygenation Assessment[5]	-	-	100%	99%	100%
Pneumococcal Vaccine[5]	-	-	72%	69%	94%
Smoking Cessation Advice[5]	-	-	86%	80%	100%
Surgical Infection Prevention					
Prophylactic Antibiotic Given[5]	-	-	82%	77%	95%
Prophylactic Antibiotic Selection[5]	-	-	93%	90%	100%
Prophylactic Antibiotic Stopped[5]	-	-	83%	72%	95%
Pregnancy Care					
Inpatient Neonatal Mortality	-	-	-	-	-
Third or Fourth Degree Laceration	-	-	2.62%	3.63%	3.27%

Mercy Hospital

400 Hobart Street
Cadillac, MI 49601
Toll-Free: 800-336-3729
Phone: 231-876-7200
Fax: 231-876-7439

E-mail: mercycadillac@trinity-health.org
URL: www.mercycadillac.munsonhealthcare.org
Ownership: Voluntary non-profit - Church
Accredited: Yes
Emergency Services: Yes
Licensed Beds: 174

Key Personnel:

CEO . . . . John H Macleod
Emergency Room . . . . Teressa Hanson

Measure	Cases	This Hospital	State Average	U.S. Average	Top Hospital
Heart Attack Care					
ACE Inhibitor or ARB for LVSD[1]	5	100%	86%	82%	100%
Aspirin at Arrival	66	98%	95%	92%	100%
Aspirin at Discharge	26	88%	94%	90%	100%
Beta Blocker at Arrival	62	97%	90%	87%	100%
Beta Blocker at Discharge	27	100%	93%	90%	100%
Fibrinolytic Medication Timing[1]	1	100%	28%	31%	100%
PCI Within 90 Minutes of Arrival	0	-	59%	54%	95%
Smoking Cessation Advice[1]	2	100%	93%	88%	100%
Heart Failure Care					
ACE Inhibitor or ARB for LVSD	40	98%	84%	82%	100%
Discharge Instructions	79	96%	73%	61%	93%
Evaluation of LVS Function	99	95%	91%	83%	99%
Smoking Cessation Advice[1]	14	100%	86%	82%	100%
Pneumonia Care					
Appropriate Initial Antibiotic	116	91%	88%	83%	94%
Blood Culture Timing	102	86%	90%	90%	100%
Influenza Vaccine[4,5]	-	-	73%	70%	100%
Initial Antibiotic Timing	125	90%	84%	80%	93%
Oxygenation Assessment	160	99%	100%	99%	100%
Pneumococcal Vaccine	103	84%	72%	69%	94%
Smoking Cessation Advice	33	100%	86%	80%	100%
Surgical Infection Prevention					
Prophylactic Antibiotic Given[3]	213	90%	82%	77%	95%
Prophylactic Antibiotic Selection	60	98%	93%	90%	100%
Prophylactic Antibiotic Stopped[3]	213	100%	83%	72%	95%
Pregnancy Care					
Inpatient Neonatal Mortality	-	-	-	-	-
Third or Fourth Degree Laceration	-	-	2.62%	3.63%	3.27%

Carson City Hospital

406 E Elm Street
Box 879
Carson City, MI 48811
Phone: 989-584-3131
Fax: 989-584-6165
E-mail: bruce@carsoncityhospital.com
URL: www.carsoncityhospital.com
Ownership: Voluntary non-profit - Other
Accredited: Yes
Emergency Services: Yes
Licensed Beds: 77

Key Personnel:

President/CEO . . . . Bruce L Traverse
Chief Medical Staff . . . . H Chuck Wakefield, DO
Manager ER . . . . Shelly Whitcare, RN
Director Emergency Room . . . . Gregory Fuller, DO
Director Infection/Disease Control . . . . Judy Brown, RN
Ob/Gyn . . . . Michelle Becher, DO
Surgical Services . . . . Cheryl Young, RN
Chief Radiology . . . . Jim Newman, DO
Director Respiratory Therapy . . . . Joan Sweet

Measure	Cases	This Hospital	State Average	U.S. Average	Top Hospital
Heart Attack Care					
ACE Inhibitor or ARB for LVSD[1]	1	100%	86%	82%	100%
Aspirin at Arrival[1]	9	100%	95%	92%	100%
Aspirin at Discharge[1]	4	75%	94%	90%	100%
Beta Blocker at Arrival[1]	5	100%	90%	87%	100%
Beta Blocker at Discharge[1]	1	100%	93%	90%	100%
Fibrinolytic Medication Timing	0	-	28%	31%	100%
PCI Within 90 Minutes of Arrival	0	-	59%	54%	95%
Smoking Cessation Advice[1]	3	100%	93%	88%	100%
Heart Failure Care					
ACE Inhibitor or ARB for LVSD[1]	11	82%	84%	82%	100%
Discharge Instructions	30	83%	73%	61%	93%
Evaluation of LVS Function	39	97%	91%	83%	99%
Smoking Cessation Advice[1]	5	100%	86%	82%	100%
Pneumonia Care					
Appropriate Initial Antibiotic	53	92%	88%	83%	94%
Blood Culture Timing	26	92%	90%	90%	100%
Influenza Vaccine[1]	17	76%	73%	70%	100%
Initial Antibiotic Timing	54	85%	84%	80%	93%
Oxygenation Assessment	72	100%	100%	99%	100%
Pneumococcal Vaccine	43	79%	72%	69%	94%
Smoking Cessation Advice[1]	19	100%	86%	80%	100%
Surgical Infection Prevention					
Prophylactic Antibiotic Given	176	96%	82%	77%	95%
Prophylactic Antibiotic Selection	35	94%	93%	90%	100%
Prophylactic Antibiotic Stopped	172	94%	83%	72%	95%
Pregnancy Care					
Inpatient Neonatal Mortality	-	-	-	-	-
Third or Fourth Degree Laceration	-	-	2.62%	3.63%	3.27%

NOTE: Hospital profiles are in alphabetical order by state, then city, then hospital within the city; Rankings are sorted by rate in descending order and exclude hospitals with less than 25 cases; (1) The number of cases is too small (n<25) for purposes of reliably predicting hospital performance; (2) Measure reflects the hospital's indication that its submission was based upon a sample of its relevant discharges; (3) Rate reflects fewer than the maximum possible quarters of data for the measure; (4) Inaccurate information submitted and suppressed for one or more quarters; (5) No data is available from the hospital for this measure; Please refer to the User's Guide for a full explanation of data

Hills & Dales General Hospital

4675 Hill Street
Cass City, MI 48726
E-mail: publicinfo@hillsanddales.com
URL: www.hillsanddales.com
Ownership: Voluntary non-profit - Private
Emergency Services: Yes

Phone: 989-872-2121
Fax: 989-872-5376

Accredited: Yes
Licensed Beds: 65

Key Personnel:

President/CEO.......................... Dee McKrow
Cardiology............................ Jeffrey Carney, MD
OB/GYN................................ Gary Ritten, MD
Surgery............................... Francis Ozim, MD

Measure	Cases	This Hospital	State Average	U.S. Average	Top Hospital
Heart Attack Care					
ACE Inhibitor or ARB for LVSD[3]	0	-	86%	82%	100%
Aspirin at Arrival[1,3]	1	100%	95%	92%	100%
Aspirin at Discharge[1,3]	1	100%	94%	90%	100%
Beta Blocker at Arrival[1,3]	1	0%	90%	87%	100%
Beta Blocker at Discharge[1,3]	1	0%	93%	90%	100%
Fibrinolytic Medication Timing[3]	0	-	28%	31%	100%
PCI Within 90 Minutes of Arrival	0	-	59%	54%	95%
Smoking Cessation Advice[3]	0	-	93%	88%	100%
Heart Failure Care					
ACE Inhibitor or ARB for LVSD[1]	6	33%	84%	82%	100%
Discharge Instructions	30	40%	73%	61%	93%
Evaluation of LVS Function	42	24%	91%	83%	99%
Smoking Cessation Advice[1]	1	0%	86%	82%	100%
Pneumonia Care					
Appropriate Initial Antibiotic	36	78%	88%	83%	94%
Blood Culture Timing	29	83%	90%	90%	100%
Influenza Vaccine[1]	7	14%	73%	70%	100%
Initial Antibiotic Timing	44	93%	84%	80%	93%
Oxygenation Assessment	61	97%	100%	99%	100%
Pneumococcal Vaccine	38	13%	72%	69%	94%
Smoking Cessation Advice[1]	11	55%	86%	80%	100%
Surgical Infection Prevention					
Prophylactic Antibiotic Given[1]	8	50%	82%	77%	95%
Prophylactic Antibiotic Selection[1]	2	100%	93%	90%	100%
Prophylactic Antibiotic Stopped[1]	8	100%	83%	72%	95%
Pregnancy Care					
Inpatient Neonatal Mortality	-	-	-	-	-
Third or Fourth Degree Laceration	-	-	2.62%	3.63%	3.27%

Hayes Green Beach Memorial Hospital

321 E Harris Street
Charlotte, MI 48813
E-mail: mrush@hgbhealth.com
URL: www.hgbhealth.com
Ownership: Voluntary non-profit - Other
Emergency Services: Yes

Phone: 517-543-1050
Fax: 517-543-0875

Accredited: No
Licensed Beds: 45

Key Personnel:

President/CEO.......................... Matthew W Rush, CHE
Emergency Room......................... Sherman Horn
OB/GYN/Women's Health.................. Connie Herr
Respiratory Care....................... Frida Burke

Measure	Cases	This Hospital	State Average	U.S. Average	Top Hospital
Heart Attack Care					
ACE Inhibitor or ARB for LVSD[3]	0	-	86%	82%	100%
Aspirin at Arrival[1,3]	2	100%	95%	92%	100%
Aspirin at Discharge[1,3]	1	100%	94%	90%	100%
Beta Blocker at Arrival[1,3]	2	100%	90%	87%	100%
Beta Blocker at Discharge[1,3]	1	100%	93%	90%	100%
Fibrinolytic Medication Timing[3]	0	-	28%	31%	100%
PCI Within 90 Minutes of Arrival	0	-	59%	54%	95%
Smoking Cessation Advice[3]	0	-	93%	88%	100%
Heart Failure Care					
ACE Inhibitor or ARB for LVSD[1]	8	88%	84%	82%	100%
Discharge Instructions	45	60%	73%	61%	93%
Evaluation of LVS Function	57	82%	91%	83%	99%
Smoking Cessation Advice[1]	11	73%	86%	82%	100%
Pneumonia Care					
Appropriate Initial Antibiotic	56	88%	88%	83%	94%
Blood Culture Timing	30	90%	90%	90%	100%
Influenza Vaccine[1]	14	79%	73%	70%	100%
Initial Antibiotic Timing	58	78%	84%	80%	93%
Oxygenation Assessment	75	100%	100%	99%	100%
Pneumococcal Vaccine	46	37%	72%	69%	94%
Smoking Cessation Advice[1]	10	70%	86%	80%	100%
Surgical Infection Prevention					
Prophylactic Antibiotic Given[2,3]	68	62%	82%	77%	95%
Prophylactic Antibiotic Selection[1,2]	20	80%	93%	90%	100%
Prophylactic Antibiotic Stopped[2,3]	67	69%	83%	72%	95%
Pregnancy Care					
Inpatient Neonatal Mortality	-	-	-	-	-
Third or Fourth Degree Laceration	-	-	2.62%	3.63%	3.27%

Cheboygan Memorial Hospital

748 S Main Street
PO Box 419
Cheboygan, MI 49721
URL: www.cheboyganhospital.org
Ownership: Voluntary non-profit - Private
Emergency Services: Yes

Phone: 231-627-5601
Fax: 231-627-1471

Accredited: Yes
Licensed Beds: 92

Key Personnel:

President/CEO.......................... Barbara J Cliff
Emergency Medicine Director............ Kenneth Parada, MD
Women's/Children's Health Services..... Marvin K Coy

Measure	Cases	This Hospital	State Average	U.S. Average	Top Hospital
Heart Attack Care					
ACE Inhibitor or ARB for LVSD[1]	5	100%	86%	82%	100%
Aspirin at Arrival[1]	16	100%	95%	92%	100%
Aspirin at Discharge[1]	9	100%	94%	90%	100%
Beta Blocker at Arrival[1]	14	100%	90%	87%	100%
Beta Blocker at Discharge[1]	10	100%	93%	90%	100%
Fibrinolytic Medication Timing[1]	2	50%	28%	31%	100%
PCI Within 90 Minutes of Arrival	0	-	59%	54%	95%
Smoking Cessation Advice[1]	1	100%	93%	88%	100%
Heart Failure Care					
ACE Inhibitor or ARB for LVSD[1]	23	100%	84%	82%	100%
Discharge Instructions	65	100%	73%	61%	93%
Evaluation of LVS Function	79	99%	91%	83%	99%
Smoking Cessation Advice[1]	7	100%	86%	82%	100%
Pneumonia Care					
Appropriate Initial Antibiotic	64	92%	88%	83%	94%
Blood Culture Timing	64	97%	90%	90%	100%
Influenza Vaccine[1]	21	100%	73%	70%	100%
Initial Antibiotic Timing	96	81%	84%	80%	93%
Oxygenation Assessment	114	100%	100%	99%	100%
Pneumococcal Vaccine	72	94%	72%	69%	94%
Smoking Cessation Advice[1]	16	81%	86%	80%	100%
Surgical Infection Prevention					
Prophylactic Antibiotic Given	154	95%	82%	77%	95%
Prophylactic Antibiotic Selection	40	100%	93%	90%	100%
Prophylactic Antibiotic Stopped	148	98%	83%	72%	95%
Pregnancy Care					
Inpatient Neonatal Mortality	244	0.41%	-	-	-
Third or Fourth Degree Laceration	164	3.05%	2.62%	3.63%	3.27%

Chelsea Community Hospital

775 S Main Street
Chelsea, MI 48118
URL: www.cch.org
Ownership: Voluntary non-profit - Private
Emergency Services: No

Phone: 734-475-1311
Fax: 734-475-4066

Accredited: No
Licensed Beds: 113

Key Personnel:

CEO.................................... Kathleen Griffiths
Emergency Room......................... Nancy Fields

Measure	Cases	This Hospital	State Average	U.S. Average	Top Hospital
Heart Attack Care					
ACE Inhibitor or ARB for LVSD[1]	4	100%	86%	82%	100%
Aspirin at Arrival[1]	22	100%	95%	92%	100%

NOTE: Hospital profiles are in alphabetical order by state, then city, then hospital within the city; Rankings are sorted by rate in descending order and exclude hospitals with less than 25 cases; (1) The number of cases is too small (n<25) for purposes of reliably predicting hospital performance; (2) Measure reflects the hospital's indication that its submission was based upon a sample of its relevant discharges; (3) Rate reflects fewer than the maximum possible quarters of data for the measure; (4) Inaccurate information submitted and suppressed for one or more quarters; (5) No data is available from the hospital for this measure; Please refer to the User's Guide for a full explanation of data

Measure	Cases	This Hospital	State Average	U.S. Average	Top Hospital
Aspirin at Discharge[1]	15	100%	94%	90%	100%
Beta Blocker at Arrival[1]	21	90%	90%	87%	100%
Beta Blocker at Discharge[1]	18	100%	93%	90%	100%
Fibrinolytic Medication Timing	0	-	28%	31%	100%
PCI Within 90 Minutes of Arrival	0	-	59%	54%	95%
Smoking Cessation Advice[1]	1	100%	93%	88%	100%
Heart Failure Care					
ACE Inhibitor or ARB for LVSD[1]	18	100%	84%	82%	100%
Discharge Instructions	45	87%	73%	61%	93%
Evaluation of LVS Function	61	98%	91%	83%	99%
Smoking Cessation Advice[1]	5	100%	86%	82%	100%
Pneumonia Care					
Appropriate Initial Antibiotic	86	100%	88%	83%	94%
Blood Culture Timing	98	94%	90%	90%	100%
Influenza Vaccine[1]	22	100%	73%	70%	100%
Initial Antibiotic Timing	100	92%	84%	80%	93%
Oxygenation Assessment	127	100%	100%	99%	100%
Pneumococcal Vaccine	96	99%	72%	69%	94%
Smoking Cessation Advice	26	100%	86%	80%	100%
Surgical Infection Prevention					
Prophylactic Antibiotic Given	640	99%	82%	77%	95%
Prophylactic Antibiotic Selection	153	98%	93%	90%	100%
Prophylactic Antibiotic Stopped	628	96%	83%	72%	95%
Pregnancy Care					
Inpatient Neonatal Mortality	-	-	-	-	-
Third or Fourth Degree Laceration	-	-	2.62%	3.63%	3.27%

MidMichigan Medical Center-Clare

703 N McEwan Street — Phone: 989-802-5000
Clare, MI 48617 — Fax: 989-802-8895
URL: www.midmichigan.org
Ownership: Voluntary non-profit - Other — Accredited: Yes
Emergency Services: Yes — Licensed Beds: 64

Key Personnel:

Administrator . . . . Lawrence F Barco
Emergency Room . . . . Gregory Endres-Bercher, MD
Director Infection/Disease Control . . . . Bea Van Buskirk, RN
Coronary Care Unit Supervising Nurse . . . . Robert Briggs, RN
Director Medical/Surgical Nursing . . . . Bette Sheppard, RN
OB/GYN/Women's Health . . . . Deanna Puckingpaugh
Director Respiratory Therapy . . . . Wendy Bicknell

Measure	Cases	This Hospital	State Average	U.S. Average	Top Hospital
Heart Attack Care					
ACE Inhibitor or ARB for LVSD	0	-	86%	82%	100%
Aspirin at Arrival[1]	17	76%	95%	92%	100%
Aspirin at Discharge[1]	9	89%	94%	90%	100%
Beta Blocker at Arrival[1]	16	75%	90%	87%	100%
Beta Blocker at Discharge[1]	10	90%	93%	90%	100%
Fibrinolytic Medication Timing	0	-	28%	31%	100%
PCI Within 90 Minutes of Arrival	0	-	59%	54%	95%
Smoking Cessation Advice[1]	3	100%	93%	88%	100%
Heart Failure Care					
ACE Inhibitor or ARB for LVSD[1]	20	60%	84%	82%	100%
Discharge Instructions	116	73%	73%	61%	93%
Evaluation of LVS Function	126	84%	91%	83%	99%
Smoking Cessation Advice	26	73%	86%	82%	100%
Pneumonia Care					
Appropriate Initial Antibiotic	112	96%	88%	83%	94%
Blood Culture Timing	124	92%	90%	90%	100%
Influenza Vaccine	33	79%	73%	70%	100%
Initial Antibiotic Timing	159	89%	84%	80%	93%
Oxygenation Assessment	182	100%	100%	99%	100%
Pneumococcal Vaccine	122	72%	72%	69%	94%
Smoking Cessation Advice	44	82%	86%	80%	100%
Surgical Infection Prevention					
Prophylactic Antibiotic Given[3]	64	22%	82%	77%	95%
Prophylactic Antibiotic Selection[1]	17	35%	93%	90%	100%
Prophylactic Antibiotic Stopped[3]	63	54%	83%	72%	95%
Pregnancy Care					
Inpatient Neonatal Mortality	-	-	-	-	-
Third or Fourth Degree Laceration	-	-	2.62%	3.63%	3.27%

Saint Joseph's Healthcare

15855 Nineteen Mile Road — Phone: 586-263-2300
Clinton Township, MI 48038 — Fax: 586-263-2859
URL: www.stjoe-macomb.com
Ownership: Voluntary non-profit - Church — Accredited: Yes
Emergency Services: Yes — Licensed Beds: 435

Key Personnel:

President/CEO . . . . Barbara W Rossmann
Chief Medical Staff . . . . Richard Stone, MD
Chief Catheterization Laboratory . . . . Joseph Naoum, MD
Manager Infection Control . . . . Sharon Ritter
ICU Supervising Nurse . . . . Gary Plagens
Director Medical/Surgical Nursing . . . . Rose Mary Gaglio
Director Surgical Services . . . . Susan Assaf
Director Radiology . . . . Donna Moir
Supervisor Respiratory Care . . . . Doreen Shock

Measure	Cases	This Hospital	State Average	U.S. Average	Top Hospital
Heart Attack Care					
ACE Inhibitor or ARB for LVSD	54	100%	86%	82%	100%
Aspirin at Arrival	323	99%	95%	92%	100%
Aspirin at Discharge	308	99%	94%	90%	100%
Beta Blocker at Arrival	278	99%	90%	87%	100%
Beta Blocker at Discharge	305	100%	93%	90%	100%
Fibrinolytic Medication Timing[1]	1	0%	28%	31%	100%
PCI Within 90 Minutes of Arrival[1]	13	100%	59%	54%	95%
Smoking Cessation Advice	95	100%	93%	88%	100%
Heart Failure Care					
ACE Inhibitor or ARB for LVSD	158	99%	84%	82%	100%
Discharge Instructions	530	87%	73%	61%	93%
Evaluation of LVS Function	693	100%	91%	83%	99%
Smoking Cessation Advice	75	100%	86%	82%	100%
Pneumonia Care					
Appropriate Initial Antibiotic	292	91%	88%	83%	94%
Blood Culture Timing	301	60%	90%	90%	100%
Influenza Vaccine	68	87%	73%	70%	100%
Initial Antibiotic Timing	386	79%	84%	80%	93%
Oxygenation Assessment	447	100%	100%	99%	100%
Pneumococcal Vaccine	298	88%	72%	69%	94%
Smoking Cessation Advice	104	100%	86%	80%	100%
Surgical Infection Prevention					
Prophylactic Antibiotic Given[2]	1,270	94%	82%	77%	95%
Prophylactic Antibiotic Selection[2]	336	96%	93%	90%	100%
Prophylactic Antibiotic Stopped[2]	1,212	87%	83%	72%	95%
Pregnancy Care					
Inpatient Neonatal Mortality	-	-	-	-	-
Third or Fourth Degree Laceration	-	-	2.62%	3.63%	3.27%

Community Health Center of Branch County

274 E Chicago Street — Phone: 517-279-5400
Coldwater, MI 49036 — Fax: 517-279-5499
URL: www.chcbc.com
Ownership: Government - Local — Accredited: Yes
Emergency Services: Yes — Licensed Beds: 96

Key Personnel:

CEO . . . . Randy DeGroot
Medical Staff Services . . . . Cynthia Carpenter
Director Emergency Room . . . . Marion Labadee
Director Infection/Disease Control . . . . Connie Meyer
Director Medical Surgical Nursing . . . . Connie Meyer
OB/GYN Womens Health . . . . Helene Racey
Director Radiology . . . . Dei Dailey, MD
Director Respiratory Therapy . . . . Bruce Gregory

Measure	Cases	This Hospital	State Average	U.S. Average	Top Hospital
Heart Attack Care					
ACE Inhibitor or ARB for LVSD[1]	1	100%	86%	82%	100%
Aspirin at Arrival[1]	18	78%	95%	92%	100%
Aspirin at Discharge[1]	9	67%	94%	90%	100%
Beta Blocker at Arrival[1]	18	89%	90%	87%	100%
Beta Blocker at Discharge[1]	9	56%	93%	90%	100%
Fibrinolytic Medication Timing	0	-	28%	31%	100%
PCI Within 90 Minutes of Arrival	0	-	59%	54%	95%

NOTE: Hospital profiles are in alphabetical order by state, then city, then hospital within the city; Rankings are sorted by rate in descending order and exclude hospitals with less than 25 cases; (1) The number of cases is too small (n<25) for purposes of reliably predicting hospital performance; (2) Measure reflects the hospital's indication that its submission was based upon a sample of its relevant discharges; (3) Rate reflects fewer than the maximum possible quarters of data for the measure; (4) Inaccurate information submitted and suppressed for one or more quarters; (5) No data is available from the hospital for this measure; Please refer to the User's Guide for a full explanation of data

Smoking Cessation Advice[1]	1	0%	93%	88%	100%
Heart Failure Care					
ACE Inhibitor or ARB for LVSD[1]	21	67%	84%	82%	100%
Discharge Instructions	83	73%	73%	61%	93%
Evaluation of LVS Function	105	65%	91%	83%	99%
Smoking Cessation Advice[1]	6	83%	86%	82%	100%
Pneumonia Care					
Appropriate Initial Antibiotic	121	85%	88%	83%	94%
Blood Culture Timing	92	91%	90%	90%	100%
Influenza Vaccine	26	62%	73%	70%	100%
Initial Antibiotic Timing	115	84%	84%	80%	93%
Oxygenation Assessment	149	100%	100%	99%	100%
Pneumococcal Vaccine	90	47%	72%	69%	94%
Smoking Cessation Advice	38	71%	86%	80%	100%
Surgical Infection Prevention					
Prophylactic Antibiotic Given	285	88%	82%	77%	95%
Prophylactic Antibiotic Selection	65	88%	93%	90%	100%
Prophylactic Antibiotic Stopped	267	87%	83%	72%	95%
Pregnancy Care					
Inpatient Neonatal Mortality	-	-	-	-	-
Third or Fourth Degree Laceration	-	-	2.62%	3.63%	3.27%

Huron Valley-Sinai Hospital

1 William Carls Drive
Commerce Twp, MI 48382
URL: www.hvsh.org
Ownership: Voluntary non-profit - Other
Emergency Services: Yes

Phone: 248-937-3300
Fax: 248-937-5074
Accredited: Yes
Licensed Beds: 153

Key Personnel:
President . . . . Robert J Yellan
Chief of Medical Staff . . . . Marc P Bocknek

Measure	Cases	This Hospital	State Average	U.S. Average	Top Hospital
Heart Attack Care					
ACE Inhibitor or ARB for LVSD[1]	18	100%	86%	82%	100%
Aspirin at Arrival	100	94%	95%	92%	100%
Aspirin at Discharge	56	95%	94%	90%	100%
Beta Blocker at Arrival	76	96%	90%	87%	100%
Beta Blocker at Discharge	64	94%	93%	90%	100%
Fibrinolytic Medication Timing	0	-	28%	31%	100%
PCI Within 90 Minutes of Arrival	0	-	59%	54%	95%
Smoking Cessation Advice[1]	9	89%	93%	88%	100%
Heart Failure Care					
ACE Inhibitor or ARB for LVSD	68	85%	84%	82%	100%
Discharge Instructions	225	49%	73%	61%	93%
Evaluation of LVS Function	272	98%	91%	83%	99%
Smoking Cessation Advice	32	97%	86%	82%	100%
Pneumonia Care					
Appropriate Initial Antibiotic	107	86%	88%	83%	94%
Blood Culture Timing	107	92%	90%	90%	100%
Influenza Vaccine	26	69%	73%	70%	100%
Initial Antibiotic Timing	148	89%	84%	80%	93%
Oxygenation Assessment	190	100%	100%	99%	100%
Pneumococcal Vaccine	100	72%	72%	69%	94%
Smoking Cessation Advice	50	98%	86%	80%	100%
Surgical Infection Prevention					
Prophylactic Antibiotic Given[2]	625	95%	82%	77%	95%
Prophylactic Antibiotic Selection[2]	163	97%	93%	90%	100%
Prophylactic Antibiotic Stopped[2]	607	91%	83%	72%	95%
Pregnancy Care					
Inpatient Neonatal Mortality	-	-	-	-	-
Third or Fourth Degree Laceration	-	-	2.62%	3.63%	3.27%

Oakwood Hospital & Medical Center

18101 Oakwood Boulevard
PO Box 2500
Dearborn, MI 48124
E-mail: GUESTREL@oakwood.org
URL: www.oakwood.org
Ownership: Voluntary non-profit - Private
Emergency Services: Yes

Phone: 313-593-7000
Fax: 313-436-2038
Accredited: No
Licensed Beds: 632

Key Personnel:
President/CEO . . . . Jerry Fitzgerald

Measure	Cases	This Hospital	State Average	U.S. Average	Top Hospital
Heart Attack Care					
ACE Inhibitor or ARB for LVSD	339	92%	86%	82%	100%
Aspirin at Arrival	535	95%	95%	92%	100%
Aspirin at Discharge	861	98%	94%	90%	100%
Beta Blocker at Arrival	350	97%	90%	87%	100%
Beta Blocker at Discharge	995	98%	93%	90%	100%
Fibrinolytic Medication Timing[1]	2	0%	28%	31%	100%
PCI Within 90 Minutes of Arrival[1]	19	47%	59%	54%	95%
Smoking Cessation Advice	399	99%	93%	88%	100%
Heart Failure Care					
ACE Inhibitor or ARB for LVSD	563	90%	84%	82%	100%
Discharge Instructions	1,037	71%	73%	61%	93%
Evaluation of LVS Function	1,236	98%	91%	83%	99%
Smoking Cessation Advice	270	100%	86%	82%	100%
Pneumonia Care					
Appropriate Initial Antibiotic	432	93%	88%	83%	94%
Blood Culture Timing	515	95%	90%	90%	100%
Influenza Vaccine	94	85%	73%	70%	100%
Initial Antibiotic Timing	642	67%	84%	80%	93%
Oxygenation Assessment	803	100%	100%	99%	100%
Pneumococcal Vaccine	472	83%	72%	69%	94%
Smoking Cessation Advice	231	94%	86%	80%	100%
Surgical Infection Prevention					
Prophylactic Antibiotic Given[2]	1,503	93%	82%	77%	95%
Prophylactic Antibiotic Selection[2]	390	98%	93%	90%	100%
Prophylactic Antibiotic Stopped[2]	1,425	83%	83%	72%	95%
Pregnancy Care					
Inpatient Neonatal Mortality	-	-	-	-	-
Third or Fourth Degree Laceration	-	-	2.62%	3.63%	3.27%

Detroit Receiving Hosp & Univ Health Ctr

4201 Saint Antoine
Detroit, MI 48201
E-mail: lbowman@dmc.org
URL: www.drhuhc.org
Ownership: Voluntary non-profit - Other
Emergency Services: Yes

Phone: 313-745-3000
Fax: 313-966-7206
Accredited: Yes
Licensed Beds: 320

Key Personnel:
President . . . . Iris A Taylor, Ph.D RN
CEO . . . . Jeffrey H Dawkins
Chief Medical Staff . . . . Robert Wilson, MD
Executive Director Emergency Room . . . . Monica Marshall
Chief Emergency Medicine . . . . Padraic J Sweeny, MD
Coordinator Infection Control . . . . Beth Dziekan
ICU . . . . Sue Ellen Bennett, RN
Director Radiology . . . . Gail Alexander
Executive Director Respiratory . . . . Caaron Cook, PhD

Measure	Cases	This Hospital	State Average	U.S. Average	Top Hospital
Heart Attack Care					
ACE Inhibitor or ARB for LVSD	42	90%	86%	82%	100%
Aspirin at Arrival	196	98%	95%	92%	100%
Aspirin at Discharge	169	97%	94%	90%	100%
Beta Blocker at Arrival	186	97%	90%	87%	100%
Beta Blocker at Discharge	161	98%	93%	90%	100%
Fibrinolytic Medication Timing	0	-	28%	31%	100%
PCI Within 90 Minutes of Arrival[1]	5	60%	59%	54%	95%
Smoking Cessation Advice	86	94%	93%	88%	100%
Heart Failure Care					
ACE Inhibitor or ARB for LVSD	386	91%	84%	82%	100%
Discharge Instructions	672	83%	73%	61%	93%
Evaluation of LVS Function	720	98%	91%	83%	99%
Smoking Cessation Advice	323	93%	86%	82%	100%
Pneumonia Care					
Appropriate Initial Antibiotic	266	80%	88%	83%	94%
Blood Culture Timing	210	84%	90%	90%	100%
Influenza Vaccine	34	76%	73%	70%	100%
Initial Antibiotic Timing	322	65%	84%	80%	93%
Oxygenation Assessment	349	100%	100%	99%	100%
Pneumococcal Vaccine	76	59%	72%	69%	94%
Smoking Cessation Advice	183	83%	86%	80%	100%

NOTE: Hospital profiles are in alphabetical order by state, then city, then hospital within the city; Rankings are sorted by rate in descending order and exclude hospitals with less than 25 cases; (1) The number of cases is too small (n<25) for purposes of reliably predicting hospital performance; (2) Measure reflects the hospital's indication that its submission was based upon a sample of its relevant discharges; (3) Rate reflects fewer than the maximum possible quarters of data for the measure; (4) Inaccurate information submitted and suppressed for one or more quarters; (5) No data is available from the hospital for this measure; Please refer to the User's Guide for a full explanation of data

Measure	Cases	This Hospital	State Average	U.S. Average	Top Hospital
Surgical Infection Prevention					
Prophylactic Antibiotic Given[2]	96	85%	82%	77%	95%
Prophylactic Antibiotic Selection[2]	26	85%	93%	90%	100%
Prophylactic Antibiotic Stopped[2]	81	63%	83%	72%	95%
Pregnancy Care					
Inpatient Neonatal Mortality	-	-	-	-	-
Third or Fourth Degree Laceration	-	-	2.62%	3.63%	3.27%

Harper University Hospital

Alternate Name: Detroit Medical Center
3990 John R Street
Detroit, MI 48201
Phone: 313-745-8040
Fax: 313-745-1520
URL: www.harperhospital.org
Ownership: Voluntary non-profit - Private
Accredited: Yes
Emergency Services: No
Licensed Beds: 658

Key Personnel:

CEO . . . . Micheal Duggan
Chief Medical Staff . . . . Aguston Abulu, MD

Measure	Cases	This Hospital	State Average	U.S. Average	Top Hospital
Heart Attack Care					
ACE Inhibitor or ARB for LVSD	56	79%	86%	82%	100%
Aspirin at Arrival	83	98%	95%	92%	100%
Aspirin at Discharge	117	96%	94%	90%	100%
Beta Blocker at Arrival	72	92%	90%	87%	100%
Beta Blocker at Discharge	152	96%	93%	90%	100%
Fibrinolytic Medication Timing	0	-	28%	31%	100%
PCI Within 90 Minutes of Arrival[1]	2	50%	59%	54%	95%
Smoking Cessation Advice	63	92%	93%	88%	100%
Heart Failure Care					
ACE Inhibitor or ARB for LVSD	388	87%	84%	82%	100%
Discharge Instructions	813	69%	73%	61%	93%
Evaluation of LVS Function	872	99%	91%	83%	99%
Smoking Cessation Advice	185	97%	86%	82%	100%
Pneumonia Care					
Appropriate Initial Antibiotic	90	82%	88%	83%	94%
Blood Culture Timing	117	94%	90%	90%	100%
Influenza Vaccine	38	68%	73%	70%	100%
Initial Antibiotic Timing	196	63%	84%	80%	93%
Oxygenation Assessment	222	100%	100%	99%	100%
Pneumococcal Vaccine	90	69%	72%	69%	94%
Smoking Cessation Advice	53	92%	86%	80%	100%
Surgical Infection Prevention					
Prophylactic Antibiotic Given[2]	952	89%	82%	77%	95%
Prophylactic Antibiotic Selection[2]	203	84%	93%	90%	100%
Prophylactic Antibiotic Stopped[2]	908	70%	83%	72%	95%
Pregnancy Care					
Inpatient Neonatal Mortality	5,568	1.15%	-	-	-
Third or Fourth Degree Laceration	3,893	1.18%	2.62%	3.63%	3.27%

Henry Ford Hospital

2799 W Grand Boulevard
Detroit, MI 48202
Phone: 313-916-2600
Fax: 313-916-7236
URL: www.henryfordhealth.org
Ownership: Voluntary non-profit - Private
Accredited: Yes
Emergency Services: Yes
Licensed Beds: 903

Key Personnel:

CEO/COO . . . . Nancy Schlichting
Chief Medical Officer . . . . William Conway, MD
Director Catheterization Laboratory . . . . Phillip Kraft, MD
Emergency Room . . . . Michael Tomlanovich, MD
ICU Supervising Nurse . . . . Cheryl Simonetti
Director Medical/Surgical Nursing . . . . Rachael Hoffman
Director Pulmonary Medicine . . . . John Popovich, MD

Measure	Cases	This Hospital	State Average	U.S. Average	Top Hospital
Heart Attack Care					
ACE Inhibitor or ARB for LVSD[2]	68	96%	86%	82%	100%
Aspirin at Arrival[2]	236	99%	95%	92%	100%
Aspirin at Discharge[2]	316	99%	94%	90%	100%
Beta Blocker at Arrival[2]	197	99%	90%	87%	100%
Beta Blocker at Discharge[2]	315	99%	93%	90%	100%
Fibrinolytic Medication Timing[2]	0	-	28%	31%	100%
PCI Within 90 Minutes of Arrival[1,2]	5	80%	59%	54%	95%
Smoking Cessation Advice[2]	108	97%	93%	88%	100%
Heart Failure Care					
ACE Inhibitor or ARB for LVSD[2]	184	91%	84%	82%	100%
Discharge Instructions[2]	414	48%	73%	61%	93%
Evaluation of LVS Function[2]	466	98%	91%	83%	99%
Smoking Cessation Advice[2]	123	90%	86%	82%	100%
Pneumonia Care					
Appropriate Initial Antibiotic[2]	114	93%	88%	83%	94%
Blood Culture Timing[2]	134	87%	90%	90%	100%
Influenza Vaccine[1,2]	21	57%	73%	70%	100%
Initial Antibiotic Timing[2]	173	77%	84%	80%	93%
Oxygenation Assessment[2]	204	100%	100%	99%	100%
Pneumococcal Vaccine[2]	91	59%	72%	69%	94%
Smoking Cessation Advice[2]	49	86%	86%	80%	100%
Surgical Infection Prevention					
Prophylactic Antibiotic Given[2]	431	93%	82%	77%	95%
Prophylactic Antibiotic Selection[2]	111	96%	93%	90%	100%
Prophylactic Antibiotic Stopped[2]	417	89%	83%	72%	95%
Pregnancy Care					
Inpatient Neonatal Mortality	-	-	-	-	-
Third or Fourth Degree Laceration	-	-	2.62%	3.63%	3.27%

Karmanos Cancer Center

4100 John R
Detroit, MI 48201
Phone: 313-576-8660
Ownership: Proprietary
Accredited: Yes
Emergency Services: Yes

Measure	Cases	This Hospital	State Average	U.S. Average	Top Hospital
Heart Attack Care					
ACE Inhibitor or ARB for LVSD[3]	0	-	86%	82%	100%
Aspirin at Arrival[1,3]	1	100%	95%	92%	100%
Aspirin at Discharge[1,3]	1	100%	94%	90%	100%
Beta Blocker at Arrival[1,3]	1	100%	90%	87%	100%
Beta Blocker at Discharge[1,3]	1	100%	93%	90%	100%
Fibrinolytic Medication Timing[5]	-	-	28%	31%	100%
PCI Within 90 Minutes of Arrival[5]	-	-	59%	54%	95%
Smoking Cessation Advice[5]	-	-	93%	88%	100%
Heart Failure Care					
ACE Inhibitor or ARB for LVSD[1,3]	2	50%	84%	82%	100%
Discharge Instructions[1,3]	2	100%	73%	61%	93%
Evaluation of LVS Function[1,3]	9	67%	91%	83%	99%
Smoking Cessation Advice[3]	0	-	86%	82%	100%
Pneumonia Care					
Appropriate Initial Antibiotic[3]	0	-	88%	83%	94%
Blood Culture Timing[1,3]	12	92%	90%	90%	100%
Influenza Vaccine[5]	-	-	73%	70%	100%
Initial Antibiotic Timing[3]	43	65%	84%	80%	93%
Oxygenation Assessment[3]	49	100%	100%	99%	100%
Pneumococcal Vaccine[1,3]	10	40%	72%	69%	94%
Smoking Cessation Advice[1,3]	1	0%	86%	80%	100%
Surgical Infection Prevention					
Prophylactic Antibiotic Given[2,3]	44	98%	82%	77%	95%
Prophylactic Antibiotic Selection[2]	46	96%	93%	90%	100%
Prophylactic Antibiotic Stopped[2,3]	44	93%	83%	72%	95%
Pregnancy Care					
Inpatient Neonatal Mortality	-	-	-	-	-
Third or Fourth Degree Laceration	-	-	2.62%	3.63%	3.27%

Saint John Detroit Riverview Hospital

Alternate Name: Detroit Riverview Hospital
7733 E Jefferson Avenue
Detroit, MI 48214
Phone: 313-499-3000
Fax: 313-499-4197
URL: www.stjohn.org/detroitriverview
Ownership: Voluntary non-profit - Other
Accredited: Yes
Emergency Services: Yes
Licensed Beds: 262

Key Personnel:

President . . . . Anthony E Monroe
Chief Medical Staff . . . . Dhafer Salama, MD
Chief Medical Staff . . . . Charyl Gibbson

NOTE: Hospital profiles are in alphabetical order by state, then city, then hospital within the city; Rankings are sorted by rate in descending order and exclude hospitals with less than 25 cases; (1) The number of cases is too small (n<25) for purposes of reliably predicting hospital performance; (2) Measure reflects the hospital's indication that its submission was based upon a sample of its relevant discharges; (3) Rate reflects fewer than the maximum possible quarters of data for the measure; (4) Inaccurate information submitted and suppressed for one or more quarters; (5) No data is available from the hospital for this measure; Please refer to the User's Guide for a full explanation of data

Emergency Room . . . . John Baner, MD

Measure	Cases	This Hospital	State Average	U.S. Average	Top Hospital
Heart Attack Care					
ACE Inhibitor or ARB for LVSD[1]	4	75%	86%	82%	100%
Aspirin at Arrival	38	100%	95%	92%	100%
Aspirin at Discharge[1]	20	100%	94%	90%	100%
Beta Blocker at Arrival	34	100%	90%	87%	100%
Beta Blocker at Discharge[1]	18	100%	93%	90%	100%
Fibrinolytic Medication Timing	0	-	28%	31%	100%
PCI Within 90 Minutes of Arrival	0	-	59%	54%	95%
Smoking Cessation Advice[1]	4	75%	93%	88%	100%
Heart Failure Care					
ACE Inhibitor or ARB for LVSD	211	97%	84%	82%	100%
Discharge Instructions	447	81%	73%	61%	93%
Evaluation of LVS Function	531	99%	91%	83%	99%
Smoking Cessation Advice	183	95%	86%	82%	100%
Pneumonia Care					
Appropriate Initial Antibiotic	115	90%	88%	83%	94%
Blood Culture Timing	141	70%	90%	90%	100%
Influenza Vaccine	45	27%	73%	70%	100%
Initial Antibiotic Timing	199	80%	84%	80%	93%
Oxygenation Assessment	240	100%	100%	99%	100%
Pneumococcal Vaccine	90	76%	72%	69%	94%
Smoking Cessation Advice	79	87%	86%	80%	100%
Surgical Infection Prevention					
Prophylactic Antibiotic Given[2,3]	183	81%	82%	77%	95%
Prophylactic Antibiotic Selection[2]	69	96%	93%	90%	100%
Prophylactic Antibiotic Stopped[2,3]	175	53%	83%	72%	95%
Pregnancy Care					
Inpatient Neonatal Mortality	-	-	-	-	-
Third or Fourth Degree Laceration	-	-	2.62%	3.63%	3.27%

Saint John's Hospital and Medical Center

22101 Moross Road
Detroit, MI 48236
Ownership: Voluntary non-profit - Church
Emergency Services: Yes
Phone: 313-343-4000
Fax: 313-343-7468
Accredited: Yes
Licensed Beds: 607

Key Personnel:

CEO . . . . Mark Taylor
Head of Cardiology . . . . Juliet Gardin
Head of Emergency . . . . Patricia Mayne
Emergency Room . . . . Anthony Southall
OB/GYN Womens Health. . . . . Minuchehr Kashef, MD
Chief Radiology . . . . Kurt Tech, MD
Head of Respiratory Care. . . . . Janet Cobb

Measure	Cases	This Hospital	State Average	U.S. Average	Top Hospital
Heart Attack Care					
ACE Inhibitor or ARB for LVSD	147	95%	86%	82%	100%
Aspirin at Arrival	342	97%	95%	92%	100%
Aspirin at Discharge	508	98%	94%	90%	100%
Beta Blocker at Arrival	259	96%	90%	87%	100%
Beta Blocker at Discharge	570	98%	93%	90%	100%
Fibrinolytic Medication Timing	0	-	28%	31%	100%
PCI Within 90 Minutes of Arrival[1]	17	29%	59%	54%	95%
Smoking Cessation Advice	217	96%	93%	88%	100%
Heart Failure Care					
ACE Inhibitor or ARB for LVSD[2]	294	97%	84%	82%	100%
Discharge Instructions[2]	642	80%	73%	61%	93%
Evaluation of LVS Function[2]	729	98%	91%	83%	99%
Smoking Cessation Advice[2]	203	94%	86%	82%	100%
Pneumonia Care					
Appropriate Initial Antibiotic	394	92%	88%	83%	94%
Blood Culture Timing	419	86%	90%	90%	100%
Influenza Vaccine	85	74%	73%	70%	100%
Initial Antibiotic Timing	575	79%	84%	80%	93%
Oxygenation Assessment	666	100%	100%	99%	100%
Pneumococcal Vaccine	327	72%	72%	69%	94%
Smoking Cessation Advice	192	82%	86%	80%	100%
Surgical Infection Prevention					
Prophylactic Antibiotic Given[2,3]	1,006	97%	82%	77%	95%
Prophylactic Antibiotic Selection[2]	317	99%	93%	90%	100%
Prophylactic Antibiotic Stopped[2,3]	962	91%	83%	72%	95%
Pregnancy Care					
Inpatient Neonatal Mortality	-	-	-	-	-
Third or Fourth Degree Laceration	-	-	2.62%	3.63%	3.27%

Sinai-Grace Hospital

6071 W Outer Drive
Detroit, MI 48235
URL: www.sinaigrace.org
Ownership: Voluntary non-profit - Other
Emergency Services: Yes
Phone: 313-966-3300
Fax: 313-966-3546
Accredited: Yes
Licensed Beds: 404

Key Personnel:

President . . . . Patricia Maryland, DR PH
Chief Medical Staff. . . . . John Haapaniemi, DO
Cardiac Lab . . . . Diane Wehby
Director Emergency Services. . . . . Sheila Maine
Chief Emergency Services. . . . . Mark Brautigan, MD
Infection Control. . . . . Sheila Finch
Medical/Surgical Nursing . . . . Bonnie Reeves
Director OB/GYN Womens Health . . . . Brenda Nash
Director Radiology . . . . Terry Posa

Measure	Cases	This Hospital	State Average	U.S. Average	Top Hospital
Heart Attack Care					
ACE Inhibitor or ARB for LVSD	85	81%	86%	82%	100%
Aspirin at Arrival	391	95%	95%	92%	100%
Aspirin at Discharge	359	96%	94%	90%	100%
Beta Blocker at Arrival	311	93%	90%	87%	100%
Beta Blocker at Discharge	353	95%	93%	90%	100%
Fibrinolytic Medication Timing	0	-	28%	31%	100%
PCI Within 90 Minutes of Arrival[1]	6	33%	59%	54%	95%
Smoking Cessation Advice	147	93%	93%	88%	100%
Heart Failure Care					
ACE Inhibitor or ARB for LVSD	485	84%	84%	82%	100%
Discharge Instructions	931	92%	73%	61%	93%
Evaluation of LVS Function	1,083	99%	91%	83%	99%
Smoking Cessation Advice	406	93%	86%	82%	100%
Pneumonia Care					
Appropriate Initial Antibiotic	206	87%	88%	83%	94%
Blood Culture Timing	301	86%	90%	90%	100%
Influenza Vaccine	57	89%	73%	70%	100%
Initial Antibiotic Timing	434	77%	84%	80%	93%
Oxygenation Assessment	519	100%	100%	99%	100%
Pneumococcal Vaccine	203	69%	72%	69%	94%
Smoking Cessation Advice	146	82%	86%	80%	100%
Surgical Infection Prevention					
Prophylactic Antibiotic Given[2]	784	89%	82%	77%	95%
Prophylactic Antibiotic Selection[2]	198	98%	93%	90%	100%
Prophylactic Antibiotic Stopped[2]	718	92%	83%	72%	95%
Pregnancy Care					
Inpatient Neonatal Mortality	-	-	-	-	-
Third or Fourth Degree Laceration	-	-	2.62%	3.63%	3.27%

Borgess-Lee Memorial Hospital

420 W High Street
Dowagiac, MI 49047
Ownership: Voluntary non-profit - Church
Emergency Services: Yes
Phone: 269-783-3083
Fax: 269-783-3044
Accredited: Yes
Licensed Beds: 74

Key Personnel:

Chief Medical Staff. . . . . Mohammad Taqi
Emergency Room . . . . Paul Rehkepf, MD
Director Infection/Disease Control . . . . Sandy Claborn
Director Medical/Surgical Nursing/Peds . . . . Kande Haws
Director Surgery. . . . . Sandy Claborn
Chief Radiology . . . . Aquiles Lira, MD
Director Cardiopulmonary . . . . Shani Zinn

Measure	Cases	This Hospital	State Average	U.S. Average	Top Hospital
Heart Attack Care					
ACE Inhibitor or ARB for LVSD[1,2]	1	100%	86%	82%	100%
Aspirin at Arrival[1,2]	2	100%	95%	92%	100%
Aspirin at Discharge[1,2]	1	100%	94%	90%	100%

NOTE: Hospital profiles are in alphabetical order by state, then city, then hospital within the city; Rankings are sorted by rate in descending order and exclude hospitals with less than 25 cases; (1) The number of cases is too small (n<25) for purposes of reliably predicting hospital performance; (2) Measure reflects the hospital's indication that its submission was based upon a sample of its relevant discharges; (3) Rate reflects fewer than the maximum possible quarters of data for the measure; (4) Inaccurate information submitted and suppressed for one or more quarters; (5) No data is available from the hospital for this measure; Please refer to the User's Guide for a full explanation of data

Measure	Cases	This Hospital	State Average	U.S. Average	Top Hospital
Beta Blocker at Arrival[1,2]	3	67%	90%	87%	100%
Beta Blocker at Discharge[1,2]	1	100%	93%	90%	100%
Fibrinolytic Medication Timing[2]	0	-	28%	31%	100%
PCI Within 90 Minutes of Arrival[2]	0	-	59%	54%	95%
Smoking Cessation Advice[2]	0	-	93%	88%	100%
Heart Failure Care					
ACE Inhibitor or ARB for LVSD[2]	33	88%	84%	82%	100%
Discharge Instructions[2]	65	63%	73%	61%	93%
Evaluation of LVS Function[2]	71	76%	91%	83%	99%
Smoking Cessation Advice[1,2]	16	81%	86%	82%	100%
Pneumonia Care					
Appropriate Initial Antibiotic[2]	66	94%	88%	83%	94%
Blood Culture Timing[2]	57	88%	90%	90%	100%
Influenza Vaccine[1,2]	21	67%	73%	70%	100%
Initial Antibiotic Timing[2]	79	91%	84%	80%	93%
Oxygenation Assessment[2]	101	100%	100%	99%	100%
Pneumococcal Vaccine[2]	52	44%	72%	69%	94%
Smoking Cessation Advice[2]	26	69%	86%	80%	100%
Surgical Infection Prevention					
Prophylactic Antibiotic Given[1,2,3]	15	47%	82%	77%	95%
Prophylactic Antibiotic Selection[1,2]	3	100%	93%	90%	100%
Prophylactic Antibiotic Stopped[1,2,3]	14	86%	83%	72%	95%
Pregnancy Care					
Inpatient Neonatal Mortality	-	-	-	-	-
Third or Fourth Degree Laceration	-	-	2.62%	3.63%	3.27%

Saint John River District Hospital-East China

4100 River Road
East China Township, MI 48054
URL: www.stjohn.org
Ownership: Govt - Hospital District or Authority
Emergency Services: Yes

Phone: 810-329-7111
Fax: 810-329-8920
Accredited: Yes
Licensed Beds: 68

Key Personnel:
Chief Medical Staff. . . . . Eric Gloss, DO
Emergency Room . . . . Eric Gloss, DO
Director Infection/Disease Control . . . . Heidi Boadway, RN
Director Medical/Surgical Nursing . . . . Cheri Armstead, RN
OB/GYN Womens Health. . . . . Jose Peralta, MD
Chief Radiology . . . . Hernani Tansuche, MD
Director Respiratory Therapy . . . . Linda Delgoff, RRT

Measure	Cases	This Hospital	State Average	U.S. Average	Top Hospital
Heart Attack Care					
ACE Inhibitor or ARB for LVSD[1]	9	89%	86%	82%	100%
Aspirin at Arrival[1]	24	100%	95%	92%	100%
Aspirin at Discharge[1]	11	91%	94%	90%	100%
Beta Blocker at Arrival[1]	23	96%	90%	87%	100%
Beta Blocker at Discharge[1]	11	91%	93%	90%	100%
Fibrinolytic Medication Timing	0	-	28%	31%	100%
PCI Within 90 Minutes of Arrival	0	-	59%	54%	95%
Smoking Cessation Advice[1]	1	100%	93%	88%	100%
Heart Failure Care					
ACE Inhibitor or ARB for LVSD	47	98%	84%	82%	100%
Discharge Instructions	112	93%	73%	61%	93%
Evaluation of LVS Function	140	94%	91%	83%	99%
Smoking Cessation Advice[1]	10	70%	86%	82%	100%
Pneumonia Care					
Appropriate Initial Antibiotic	79	86%	88%	83%	94%
Blood Culture Timing	93	81%	90%	90%	100%
Influenza Vaccine[1]	17	71%	73%	70%	100%
Initial Antibiotic Timing	93	83%	84%	80%	93%
Oxygenation Assessment	124	97%	100%	99%	100%
Pneumococcal Vaccine	78	94%	72%	69%	94%
Smoking Cessation Advice[1]	13	92%	86%	80%	100%
Surgical Infection Prevention					
Prophylactic Antibiotic Given[3]	112	92%	82%	77%	95%
Prophylactic Antibiotic Selection	36	100%	93%	90%	100%
Prophylactic Antibiotic Stopped[3]	102	84%	83%	72%	95%
Pregnancy Care					
Inpatient Neonatal Mortality	-	-	-	-	-
Third or Fourth Degree Laceration	-	-	2.62%	3.63%	3.27%

Eaton Rapids Medical Center

1500 S Main Street
Eaton Rapids, MI 48827
URL: www.eatonrapidsmedicalcenter.org
Ownership: Voluntary non-profit - Private
Emergency Services: Yes

Phone: 517-663-2671
Fax: 517-663-4920
Accredited: Yes
Licensed Beds: 20

Key Personnel:
President/CEO. . . . . Jack Denton
Chief Medical Staff. . . . . Ashok Gupta, MD

Measure	Cases	This Hospital	State Average	U.S. Average	Top Hospital
Heart Attack Care					
ACE Inhibitor or ARB for LVSD[1]	1	100%	86%	82%	100%
Aspirin at Arrival[1]	7	100%	95%	92%	100%
Aspirin at Discharge[1]	2	100%	94%	90%	100%
Beta Blocker at Arrival[1]	6	83%	90%	87%	100%
Beta Blocker at Discharge[1]	1	100%	93%	90%	100%
Fibrinolytic Medication Timing	0	-	28%	31%	100%
PCI Within 90 Minutes of Arrival	0	-	59%	54%	95%
Smoking Cessation Advice	0	-	93%	88%	100%
Heart Failure Care					
ACE Inhibitor or ARB for LVSD[1]	11	82%	84%	82%	100%
Discharge Instructions	32	84%	73%	61%	93%
Evaluation of LVS Function	34	91%	91%	83%	99%
Smoking Cessation Advice[1]	4	75%	86%	82%	100%
Pneumonia Care					
Appropriate Initial Antibiotic[1]	20	95%	88%	83%	94%
Blood Culture Timing[1]	13	92%	90%	90%	100%
Influenza Vaccine[1]	4	75%	73%	70%	100%
Initial Antibiotic Timing	27	85%	84%	80%	93%
Oxygenation Assessment	31	100%	100%	99%	100%
Pneumococcal Vaccine[1]	16	94%	72%	69%	94%
Smoking Cessation Advice[1]	9	100%	86%	80%	100%
Surgical Infection Prevention					
Prophylactic Antibiotic Given[5]	-	-	82%	77%	95%
Prophylactic Antibiotic Selection[5]	-	-	93%	90%	100%
Prophylactic Antibiotic Stopped[5]	-	-	83%	72%	95%
Pregnancy Care					
Inpatient Neonatal Mortality	-	-	-	-	-
Third or Fourth Degree Laceration	-	-	2.62%	3.63%	3.27%

Saint Francis Hospital

3401 Ludington Street
Escanaba, MI 49829

Ownership: Voluntary non-profit - Church
Emergency Services: Yes

Toll-Free: 800-786-2040
Phone: 906-786-3311
Fax: 906-786-4004
Accredited: Yes
Licensed Beds: 110

Key Personnel:
CEO. . . . . Peter Jennings
Chief Medical Staff. . . . . Carol Krieg, MD
Emergency Room . . . . Shirley Parr

Measure	Cases	This Hospital	State Average	U.S. Average	Top Hospital
Heart Attack Care					
ACE Inhibitor or ARB for LVSD[1]	8	38%	86%	82%	100%
Aspirin at Arrival	32	94%	95%	92%	100%
Aspirin at Discharge[1]	24	96%	94%	90%	100%
Beta Blocker at Arrival	30	93%	90%	87%	100%
Beta Blocker at Discharge	25	88%	93%	90%	100%
Fibrinolytic Medication Timing	0	-	28%	31%	100%
PCI Within 90 Minutes of Arrival	0	-	59%	54%	95%
Smoking Cessation Advice[1]	2	100%	93%	88%	100%
Heart Failure Care					
ACE Inhibitor or ARB for LVSD	34	62%	84%	82%	100%
Discharge Instructions	86	78%	73%	61%	93%
Evaluation of LVS Function	102	95%	91%	83%	99%
Smoking Cessation Advice[1]	10	70%	86%	82%	100%
Pneumonia Care					
Appropriate Initial Antibiotic	104	79%	88%	83%	94%
Blood Culture Timing	113	95%	90%	90%	100%
Influenza Vaccine[1]	21	100%	73%	70%	100%
Initial Antibiotic Timing	156	90%	84%	80%	93%

NOTE: Hospital profiles are in alphabetical order by state, then city, then hospital within the city; Rankings are sorted by rate in descending order and exclude hospitals with less than 25 cases; (1) The number of cases is too small (n<25) for purposes of reliably predicting hospital performance; (2) Measure reflects the hospital's indication that its submission was based upon a sample of its relevant discharges; (3) Rate reflects fewer than the maximum possible quarters of data for the measure; (4) Inaccurate information submitted and suppressed for one or more quarters; (5) No data is available from the hospital for this measure; Please refer to the User's Guide for a full explanation of data

Measure	Cases	This Hospital	State Average	U.S. Average	Top Hospital
Oxygenation Assessment	194	100%	100%	99%	100%
Pneumococcal Vaccine	125	89%	72%	69%	94%
Smoking Cessation Advice	29	93%	86%	80%	100%
Surgical Infection Prevention					
Prophylactic Antibiotic Given	138	73%	82%	77%	95%
Prophylactic Antibiotic Selection	36	89%	93%	90%	100%
Prophylactic Antibiotic Stopped	120	75%	83%	72%	95%
Pregnancy Care					
Inpatient Neonatal Mortality	250	0.00%	-	-	-
Third or Fourth Degree Laceration	147	5.44%	2.62%	3.63%	3.27%

Botsford General Hospital

28050 Grand River Avenue
Farmington, MI 48336
URL: www.botsfordsystem.org
Ownership: Voluntary non-profit - Other
Emergency Services: Yes
Phone: 248-471-8000
Fax: 248-471-8807
Accredited: Yes
Licensed Beds: 336

Key Personnel:
CEO. . . . . Gerson I Cooper
Chief Medical Staff. . . . . David Susser, DO
OB/GYN Womens Health. . . . . Harvey Roth, DO
Director Respiratory Therapy . . . . Diane Scully

Measure	Cases	This Hospital	State Average	U.S. Average	Top Hospital
Heart Attack Care					
ACE Inhibitor or ARB for LVSD	48	92%	86%	82%	100%
Aspirin at Arrival	249	100%	95%	92%	100%
Aspirin at Discharge	168	92%	94%	90%	100%
Beta Blocker at Arrival	231	99%	90%	87%	100%
Beta Blocker at Discharge	174	97%	93%	90%	100%
Fibrinolytic Medication Timing	0	-	28%	31%	100%
PCI Within 90 Minutes of Arrival[1]	7	0%	59%	54%	95%
Smoking Cessation Advice	32	84%	93%	88%	100%
Heart Failure Care					
ACE Inhibitor or ARB for LVSD	200	92%	84%	82%	100%
Discharge Instructions	481	66%	73%	61%	93%
Evaluation of LVS Function	622	95%	91%	83%	99%
Smoking Cessation Advice	113	96%	86%	82%	100%
Pneumonia Care					
Appropriate Initial Antibiotic	243	86%	88%	83%	94%
Blood Culture Timing	306	87%	90%	90%	100%
Influenza Vaccine[4,5]	-	-	73%	70%	100%
Initial Antibiotic Timing	393	81%	84%	80%	93%
Oxygenation Assessment	475	100%	100%	99%	100%
Pneumococcal Vaccine	289	59%	72%	69%	94%
Smoking Cessation Advice	97	86%	86%	80%	100%
Surgical Infection Prevention					
Prophylactic Antibiotic Given[2]	396	89%	82%	77%	95%
Prophylactic Antibiotic Selection[2]	154	94%	93%	90%	100%
Prophylactic Antibiotic Stopped[2]	370	84%	83%	72%	95%
Pregnancy Care					
Inpatient Neonatal Mortality	-	-	-	-	-
Third or Fourth Degree Laceration	-	-	2.62%	3.63%	3.27%

Hurley Medical Center

1 Hurley Plaza
Flint, MI 48503
URL: www.hurleymc.com
Ownership: Voluntary non-profit - Private
Emergency Services: Yes
Phone: 810-257-9067
Fax: 810-257-9111
Accredited: Yes
Licensed Beds: 463

Key Personnel:
CEO. . . . . Andrea Price
OB/GYN Womens Health. . . . . John Herbert, MD
Director Respiratory Therapy . . . . Jeff Johnson

Measure	Cases	This Hospital	State Average	U.S. Average	Top Hospital
Heart Attack Care					
ACE Inhibitor or ARB for LVSD	26	88%	86%	82%	100%
Aspirin at Arrival	163	97%	95%	92%	100%
Aspirin at Discharge	99	98%	94%	90%	100%
Beta Blocker at Arrival	132	98%	90%	87%	100%
Beta Blocker at Discharge	107	95%	93%	90%	100%
Fibrinolytic Medication Timing	0	-	28%	31%	100%
PCI Within 90 Minutes of Arrival[1]	4	75%	59%	54%	95%
Smoking Cessation Advice	49	98%	93%	88%	100%
Heart Failure Care					
ACE Inhibitor or ARB for LVSD	209	83%	84%	82%	100%
Discharge Instructions	499	81%	73%	61%	93%
Evaluation of LVS Function	562	94%	91%	83%	99%
Smoking Cessation Advice	202	87%	86%	82%	100%
Pneumonia Care					
Appropriate Initial Antibiotic	239	87%	88%	83%	94%
Blood Culture Timing	230	90%	90%	90%	100%
Influenza Vaccine	36	78%	73%	70%	100%
Initial Antibiotic Timing	319	72%	84%	80%	93%
Oxygenation Assessment	374	99%	100%	99%	100%
Pneumococcal Vaccine	136	73%	72%	69%	94%
Smoking Cessation Advice	133	78%	86%	80%	100%
Surgical Infection Prevention					
Prophylactic Antibiotic Given[2]	495	84%	82%	77%	95%
Prophylactic Antibiotic Selection[2]	131	92%	93%	90%	100%
Prophylactic Antibiotic Stopped[2]	464	82%	83%	72%	95%
Pregnancy Care					
Inpatient Neonatal Mortality	-	-	-	-	-
Third or Fourth Degree Laceration	-	-	2.62%	3.63%	3.27%

McLaren Regional Medical Center

401 S Ballenger Highway
Flint, MI 48532
URL: www.mclaren.org
Ownership: Voluntary non-profit - Other
Emergency Services: Yes
Phone: 810-342-2000
Fax: 810-342-2428
Accredited: Yes
Licensed Beds: 452

Key Personnel:
President/CEO. . . . . Donald C Kooy
Chief Medical Staff. . . . . Jagdish Bhagat, MD
Infection Control Manager . . . . Janee Macklin
Department Chairman OB/GYN Womens Health JP Metz, MD
Director Surgical Services . . . . Debra Stephenson

Measure	Cases	This Hospital	State Average	U.S. Average	Top Hospital
Heart Attack Care					
ACE Inhibitor or ARB for LVSD[2]	86	63%	86%	82%	100%
Aspirin at Arrival[2]	299	97%	95%	92%	100%
Aspirin at Discharge[2]	386	93%	94%	90%	100%
Beta Blocker at Arrival[2]	190	93%	90%	87%	100%
Beta Blocker at Discharge[2]	396	92%	93%	90%	100%
Fibrinolytic Medication Timing[2]	0	-	28%	31%	100%
PCI Within 90 Minutes of Arrival[1,2]	9	89%	59%	54%	95%
Smoking Cessation Advice[2]	146	100%	93%	88%	100%
Heart Failure Care					
ACE Inhibitor or ARB for LVSD[2]	145	80%	84%	82%	100%
Discharge Instructions[2]	284	64%	73%	61%	93%
Evaluation of LVS Function[2]	338	86%	91%	83%	99%
Smoking Cessation Advice[2]	59	100%	86%	82%	100%
Pneumonia Care					
Appropriate Initial Antibiotic[2]	166	93%	88%	83%	94%
Blood Culture Timing[2]	186	92%	90%	90%	100%
Influenza Vaccine[2]	34	76%	73%	70%	100%
Initial Antibiotic Timing[2]	243	79%	84%	80%	93%
Oxygenation Assessment[2]	281	100%	100%	99%	100%
Pneumococcal Vaccine[2]	177	59%	72%	69%	94%
Smoking Cessation Advice[2]	53	92%	86%	80%	100%
Surgical Infection Prevention					
Prophylactic Antibiotic Given[2]	410	64%	82%	77%	95%
Prophylactic Antibiotic Selection[2]	123	91%	93%	90%	100%
Prophylactic Antibiotic Stopped[2]	389	61%	83%	72%	95%
Pregnancy Care					
Inpatient Neonatal Mortality	-	-	-	-	-
Third or Fourth Degree Laceration	-	-	2.62%	3.63%	3.27%

NOTE: Hospital profiles are in alphabetical order by state, then city, then hospital within the city; Rankings are sorted by rate in descending order and exclude hospitals with less than 25 cases; (1) The number of cases is too small (n<25) for purposes of reliably predicting hospital performance; (2) Measure reflects the hospital's indication that its submission was based upon a sample of its relevant discharges; (3) Rate reflects fewer than the maximum possible quarters of data for the measure; (4) Inaccurate information submitted and suppressed for one or more quarters; (5) No data is available from the hospital for this measure; Please refer to the User's Guide for a full explanation of data

Gerber Memorial Health Services

212 S Sullivan Street
Fremont, MI 49412
E-mail: hr@gmhs.org
URL: www.gmhs.org
Ownership: Voluntary non-profit - Other
Emergency Services: Yes

Phone: 231-924-3300
Fax: 231-924-1320

Accredited: Yes
Licensed Beds: 83

Key Personnel:

President . . . . Ned B Hughes Jr
Chief of Medical Staff. . . . . Chris Hudson
Director Emergency Room. . . . . Marianne Patton
Director Infection Control . . . . Gretchen Farinosi
Respiratory . . . . Scott Thumser

Measure	Cases	This Hospital	State Average	U.S. Average	Top Hospital
Heart Attack Care					
ACE Inhibitor or ARB for LVSD[1]	6	83%	86%	82%	100%
Aspirin at Arrival[1]	17	100%	95%	92%	100%
Aspirin at Discharge[1]	12	83%	94%	90%	100%
Beta Blocker at Arrival[1]	9	100%	90%	87%	100%
Beta Blocker at Discharge[1]	13	100%	93%	90%	100%
Fibrinolytic Medication Timing	0	-	28%	31%	100%
PCI Within 90 Minutes of Arrival	0	-	59%	54%	95%
Smoking Cessation Advice[1]	2	50%	93%	88%	100%
Heart Failure Care					
ACE Inhibitor or ARB for LVSD	28	89%	84%	82%	100%
Discharge Instructions	80	70%	73%	61%	93%
Evaluation of LVS Function	92	98%	91%	83%	99%
Smoking Cessation Advice[1]	13	100%	86%	82%	100%
Pneumonia Care					
Appropriate Initial Antibiotic	75	91%	88%	83%	94%
Blood Culture Timing	80	95%	90%	90%	100%
Influenza Vaccine[1]	15	87%	73%	70%	100%
Initial Antibiotic Timing	95	87%	84%	80%	93%
Oxygenation Assessment	122	100%	100%	99%	100%
Pneumococcal Vaccine	87	76%	72%	69%	94%
Smoking Cessation Advice	29	97%	86%	80%	100%
Surgical Infection Prevention					
Prophylactic Antibiotic Given	228	88%	82%	77%	95%
Prophylactic Antibiotic Selection	58	90%	93%	90%	100%
Prophylactic Antibiotic Stopped	218	94%	83%	72%	95%
Pregnancy Care					
Inpatient Neonatal Mortality	-	-	-	-	-
Third or Fourth Degree Laceration	-	-	2.62%	3.63%	3.27%

Garden City Hospital

6245 Inkster Road
Garden City, MI 48135
URL: www.gchosp.org
Ownership: Voluntary non-profit - Private
Emergency Services: Yes

Phone: 734-421-3300
Fax: 734-421-0593

Accredited: Yes
Licensed Beds: 323

Key Personnel:

President/CEO. . . . . Gary R Ley
Cardiology Services . . . . Debbie DeMatteis
Surgical Services . . . . Annette Krupa
Respiratory Care . . . . Debbie DeMatteis

Measure	Cases	This Hospital	State Average	U.S. Average	Top Hospital
Heart Attack Care					
ACE Inhibitor or ARB for LVSD	27	96%	86%	82%	100%
Aspirin at Arrival	148	99%	95%	92%	100%
Aspirin at Discharge	104	95%	94%	90%	100%
Beta Blocker at Arrival	94	100%	90%	87%	100%
Beta Blocker at Discharge	109	98%	93%	90%	100%
Fibrinolytic Medication Timing[1]	1	0%	28%	31%	100%
PCI Within 90 Minutes of Arrival[1]	8	100%	59%	54%	95%
Smoking Cessation Advice	48	94%	93%	88%	100%
Heart Failure Care					
ACE Inhibitor or ARB for LVSD	113	94%	84%	82%	100%
Discharge Instructions	346	79%	73%	61%	93%
Evaluation of LVS Function	438	96%	91%	83%	99%
Smoking Cessation Advice	72	90%	86%	82%	100%
Pneumonia Care					
Appropriate Initial Antibiotic	281	93%	88%	83%	94%
Blood Culture Timing	342	98%	90%	90%	100%
Influenza Vaccine	76	74%	73%	70%	100%
Initial Antibiotic Timing	385	87%	84%	80%	93%
Oxygenation Assessment	489	100%	100%	99%	100%
Pneumococcal Vaccine	312	70%	72%	69%	94%
Smoking Cessation Advice	96	73%	86%	80%	100%
Surgical Infection Prevention					
Prophylactic Antibiotic Given	411	96%	82%	77%	95%
Prophylactic Antibiotic Selection	96	99%	93%	90%	100%
Prophylactic Antibiotic Stopped	387	93%	83%	72%	95%
Pregnancy Care					
Inpatient Neonatal Mortality	-	-	-	-	-
Third or Fourth Degree Laceration	-	-	2.62%	3.63%	3.27%

Otsego Memorial Hospital

825 N Center Ave
Gaylord, MI 49735
E-mail: omh@otsegomemorialhospital.org
URL: otsegomemorialhospital.org
Ownership: Voluntary non-profit - Private
Emergency Services: Yes

Phone: 989-731-2100
Fax: 989-731-7792

Accredited: Yes
Licensed Beds: 53

Key Personnel:

Administrator/CEO. . . . . Thomas R Lemon
Chief Medical Staff. . . . . David Miner, MD
Emergency Room . . . . Laura Sincock, RN
Emergency Room . . . . David Hansmann, MD
Director Infection/Disease Control . . . . Lisa Stier, RN
Director Medical/Surgical Nursing . . . . Cindy Tallent
OB/GYN Womens Health. . . . . David Miner, MD
Chief Radiology . . . . Patrick McNamara
Director Respiratory Therapy . . . . Leah Gygan

Measure	Cases	This Hospital	State Average	U.S. Average	Top Hospital
Heart Attack Care					
ACE Inhibitor or ARB for LVSD	0	-	86%	82%	100%
Aspirin at Arrival[1]	7	100%	95%	92%	100%
Aspirin at Discharge[1]	3	100%	94%	90%	100%
Beta Blocker at Arrival[1]	7	86%	90%	87%	100%
Beta Blocker at Discharge[1]	3	67%	93%	90%	100%
Fibrinolytic Medication Timing[1]	1	0%	28%	31%	100%
PCI Within 90 Minutes of Arrival	0	-	59%	54%	95%
Smoking Cessation Advice	0	-	93%	88%	100%
Heart Failure Care					
ACE Inhibitor or ARB for LVSD	31	90%	84%	82%	100%
Discharge Instructions	65	89%	73%	61%	93%
Evaluation of LVS Function	76	91%	91%	83%	99%
Smoking Cessation Advice[1]	11	82%	86%	82%	100%
Pneumonia Care					
Appropriate Initial Antibiotic	59	93%	88%	83%	94%
Blood Culture Timing	61	92%	90%	90%	100%
Influenza Vaccine[1]	13	85%	73%	70%	100%
Initial Antibiotic Timing	73	88%	84%	80%	93%
Oxygenation Assessment	98	100%	100%	99%	100%
Pneumococcal Vaccine	60	90%	72%	69%	94%
Smoking Cessation Advice	30	97%	86%	80%	100%
Surgical Infection Prevention					
Prophylactic Antibiotic Given[2,3]	110	95%	82%	77%	95%
Prophylactic Antibiotic Selection[2]	37	97%	93%	90%	100%
Prophylactic Antibiotic Stopped[2,3]	110	91%	83%	72%	95%
Pregnancy Care					
Inpatient Neonatal Mortality	-	-	-	-	-
Third or Fourth Degree Laceration	-	-	2.62%	3.63%	3.27%

MidMichigan Medical Center-Gladwin

Alternate Name: Gladwin Hospital
515 Quarter Street
Gladwin, MI 48624
URL: www.midmichigan.org
Ownership: Voluntary non-profit - Private
Emergency Services: Yes

Phone: 989-426-9286
Fax: 989-246-6400

Accredited: Yes
Licensed Beds: 25

Key Personnel:

ER Manager. . . . . Georgette Walters

NOTE: Hospital profiles are in alphabetical order by state, then city, then hospital within the city; Rankings are sorted by rate in descending order and exclude hospitals with less than 25 cases; (1) The number of cases is too small (n<25) for purposes of reliably predicting hospital performance; (2) Measure reflects the hospital's indication that its submission was based upon a sample of its relevant discharges; (3) Rate reflects fewer than the maximum possible quarters of data for the measure; (4) Inaccurate information submitted and suppressed for one or more quarters; (5) No data is available from the hospital for this measure; Please refer to the User's Guide for a full explanation of data

Infection Control . . . . Sue Lennon
Medical Surgical Nursing . . . . Julie Wright

Measure	Cases	This Hospital	State Average	U.S. Average	Top Hospital
Heart Attack Care					
ACE Inhibitor or ARB for LVSD[1]	1	100%	86%	82%	100%
Aspirin at Arrival[1]	4	100%	95%	92%	100%
Aspirin at Discharge[1]	2	100%	94%	90%	100%
Beta Blocker at Arrival[1]	3	67%	90%	87%	100%
Beta Blocker at Discharge[1]	2	100%	93%	90%	100%
Fibrinolytic Medication Timing	0	-	28%	31%	100%
PCI Within 90 Minutes of Arrival	0	-	59%	54%	95%
Smoking Cessation Advice	0	-	93%	88%	100%
Heart Failure Care					
ACE Inhibitor or ARB for LVSD[1]	20	80%	84%	82%	100%
Discharge Instructions	56	88%	73%	61%	93%
Evaluation of LVS Function	76	97%	91%	83%	99%
Smoking Cessation Advice[1]	10	80%	86%	82%	100%
Pneumonia Care					
Appropriate Initial Antibiotic	46	91%	88%	83%	94%
Blood Culture Timing	76	92%	90%	90%	100%
Influenza Vaccine[1]	21	100%	73%	70%	100%
Initial Antibiotic Timing	103	82%	84%	80%	93%
Oxygenation Assessment	118	100%	100%	99%	100%
Pneumococcal Vaccine	79	100%	72%	69%	94%
Smoking Cessation Advice[1]	22	91%	86%	80%	100%
Surgical Infection Prevention					
Prophylactic Antibiotic Given[5]	-	-	82%	77%	95%
Prophylactic Antibiotic Selection[5]	-	-	93%	90%	100%
Prophylactic Antibiotic Stopped[5]	-	-	83%	72%	95%
Pregnancy Care					
Inpatient Neonatal Mortality	-	-	-	-	-
Third or Fourth Degree Laceration	-	-	2.62%	3.63%	3.27%

Genesys Regional Medical Center

One Genesys Parkway
Grand Blanc, MI 48439
Toll-Free: 888-606-6556
Phone: 810-606-5000
Fax: 810-606-6279

URL: www.genesys.org
Ownership: Voluntary non-profit - Church
Emergency Services: Yes
Accredited: Yes
Licensed Beds: 410

Key Personnel:
CEO . . . . Norma Hagenow
Medical Staff President . . . . Kenneth Steibel, MD
Cardiac Lab . . . . Paul Brown
Catheterization Lab . . . . Beverlee Smaka

Measure	Cases	This Hospital	State Average	U.S. Average	Top Hospital
Heart Attack Care					
ACE Inhibitor or ARB for LVSD	103	79%	86%	82%	100%
Aspirin at Arrival	651	98%	95%	92%	100%
Aspirin at Discharge	592	96%	94%	90%	100%
Beta Blocker at Arrival	508	95%	90%	87%	100%
Beta Blocker at Discharge	640	95%	93%	90%	100%
Fibrinolytic Medication Timing	0	-	28%	31%	100%
PCI Within 90 Minutes of Arrival	25	36%	59%	54%	95%
Smoking Cessation Advice	226	99%	93%	88%	100%
Heart Failure Care					
ACE Inhibitor or ARB for LVSD	206	80%	84%	82%	100%
Discharge Instructions	589	63%	73%	61%	93%
Evaluation of LVS Function	662	91%	91%	83%	99%
Smoking Cessation Advice	109	98%	86%	82%	100%
Pneumonia Care					
Appropriate Initial Antibiotic	294	93%	88%	83%	94%
Blood Culture Timing	376	85%	90%	90%	100%
Influenza Vaccine	130	38%	73%	70%	100%
Initial Antibiotic Timing	652	83%	84%	80%	93%
Oxygenation Assessment	784	100%	100%	99%	100%
Pneumococcal Vaccine	496	47%	72%	69%	94%
Smoking Cessation Advice	187	95%	86%	80%	100%
Surgical Infection Prevention					
Prophylactic Antibiotic Given[2,3]	517	89%	82%	77%	95%
Prophylactic Antibiotic Selection[2]	180	97%	93%	90%	100%
Prophylactic Antibiotic Stopped[2,3]	459	81%	83%	72%	95%
Pregnancy Care					
Inpatient Neonatal Mortality	-	-	-	-	-
Third or Fourth Degree Laceration	-	-	2.62%	3.63%	3.27%

North Ottawa Community Hospital

1309 Sheldon Road
Grand Haven, MI 49417
Phone: 616-842-3600
Fax: 616-847-5621
URL: www.noch.org
Ownership: Govt - Hospital District or Authority
Emergency Services: Yes
Accredited: Yes
Licensed Beds: 81

Key Personnel:
President/CEO . . . . Michael Payne
Chief Medical Staff . . . . M Gary Robertson, MD
Director Surgical Services . . . . John Oudshoorn
Director of Pulmonary . . . . Mark Ivey

Measure	Cases	This Hospital	State Average	U.S. Average	Top Hospital
Heart Attack Care					
ACE Inhibitor or ARB for LVSD[1]	2	100%	86%	82%	100%
Aspirin at Arrival[1]	10	60%	95%	92%	100%
Aspirin at Discharge[1]	7	71%	94%	90%	100%
Beta Blocker at Arrival[1]	14	86%	90%	87%	100%
Beta Blocker at Discharge[1]	8	88%	93%	90%	100%
Fibrinolytic Medication Timing	0	-	28%	31%	100%
PCI Within 90 Minutes of Arrival	0	-	59%	54%	95%
Smoking Cessation Advice[1]	2	50%	93%	88%	100%
Heart Failure Care					
ACE Inhibitor or ARB for LVSD[1]	10	70%	84%	82%	100%
Discharge Instructions	42	71%	73%	61%	93%
Evaluation of LVS Function	59	85%	91%	83%	99%
Smoking Cessation Advice[1]	1	100%	86%	82%	100%
Pneumonia Care					
Appropriate Initial Antibiotic	38	87%	88%	83%	94%
Blood Culture Timing	40	90%	90%	90%	100%
Influenza Vaccine[1]	8	88%	73%	70%	100%
Initial Antibiotic Timing	51	84%	84%	80%	93%
Oxygenation Assessment	63	100%	100%	99%	100%
Pneumococcal Vaccine	41	78%	72%	69%	94%
Smoking Cessation Advice[1]	7	57%	86%	80%	100%
Surgical Infection Prevention					
Prophylactic Antibiotic Given[3]	119	81%	82%	77%	95%
Prophylactic Antibiotic Selection	42	98%	93%	90%	100%
Prophylactic Antibiotic Stopped[3]	118	93%	83%	72%	95%
Pregnancy Care					
Inpatient Neonatal Mortality	-	-	-	-	-
Third or Fourth Degree Laceration	-	-	2.62%	3.63%	3.27%

Metro Health Hospital

1919 Boston SE
Grand Rapids, MI 49506
Toll-Free: 800-968-0051
Phone: 616-252-7200
Fax: 616-252-7478

URL: www.metrohealth.net
Ownership: Voluntary non-profit - Other
Emergency Services: Yes
Accredited: Yes
Licensed Beds: 208

Key Personnel:
President/CEO . . . . Michael Faas
Chief Medical Officer . . . . William Cunningham, MD
Director Heart/Vascular Services . . . . Dan Witt
Infection Control Supervisor . . . . Deborah Paul-Cheadle
Chief Medical Officer/Executive VP . . . . Dr. William Cunningham
Director Surgical Services . . . . Donna Rudy
Director Radiology . . . . Sylvia Huitsing

Measure	Cases	This Hospital	State Average	U.S. Average	Top Hospital
Heart Attack Care					
ACE Inhibitor or ARB for LVSD[1]	20	100%	86%	82%	100%
Aspirin at Arrival	103	100%	95%	92%	100%
Aspirin at Discharge	64	100%	94%	90%	100%
Beta Blocker at Arrival	91	99%	90%	87%	100%
Beta Blocker at Discharge	66	100%	93%	90%	100%
Fibrinolytic Medication Timing	0	-	28%	31%	100%

NOTE: Hospital profiles are in alphabetical order by state, then city, then hospital within the city; Rankings are sorted by rate in descending order and exclude hospitals with less than 25 cases; (1) The number of cases is too small (n<25) for purposes of reliably predicting hospital performance; (2) Measure reflects the hospital's indication that its submission was based upon a sample of its relevant discharges; (3) Rate reflects fewer than the maximum possible quarters of data for the measure; (4) Inaccurate information submitted and suppressed for one or more quarters; (5) No data is available from the hospital for this measure; Please refer to the User's Guide for a full explanation of data

PCI Within 90 Minutes of Arrival[1]	10	90%	59%	54%	95%
Smoking Cessation Advice[1]	22	100%	93%	88%	100%
Heart Failure Care					
ACE Inhibitor or ARB for LVSD	57	100%	84%	82%	100%
Discharge Instructions	122	96%	73%	61%	93%
Evaluation of LVS Function	157	97%	91%	83%	99%
Smoking Cessation Advice	25	100%	86%	82%	100%
Pneumonia Care					
Appropriate Initial Antibiotic	117	97%	88%	83%	94%
Blood Culture Timing	142	96%	90%	90%	100%
Influenza Vaccine[1]	23	87%	73%	70%	100%
Initial Antibiotic Timing	174	92%	84%	80%	93%
Oxygenation Assessment	210	100%	100%	99%	100%
Pneumococcal Vaccine	116	95%	72%	69%	94%
Smoking Cessation Advice	56	100%	86%	80%	100%
Surgical Infection Prevention					
Prophylactic Antibiotic Given[2]	253	79%	82%	77%	95%
Prophylactic Antibiotic Selection[2]	65	94%	93%	90%	100%
Prophylactic Antibiotic Stopped[2]	244	83%	83%	72%	95%
Pregnancy Care					
Inpatient Neonatal Mortality	-	-	-	-	-
Third or Fourth Degree Laceration	-	-	2.62%	3.63%	3.27%

Saint Mary's Health Care

200 Jefferson Street SE
Grand Rapids, MI 49503
URL: www.smhealthcare.org
Ownership: Voluntary non-profit - Church
Emergency Services: Yes
Phone: 616-752-6090
Fax: 616-732-3035
Accredited: No
Licensed Beds: 324

Key Personnel:

President/CEO . . . . Philip H McCorkle, Jr
Chief Medical Staff . . . . Dr Terrance Wrightn, MD
Administrative CEO . . . . Dr David Blair, MD
Emergency Room . . . . Dr Michael Olgren, MD
Infection Control Program Manager . . . . Mary Neuman, RN
Manager, Respiratory Care . . . . Laurie Tamminga

Measure	Cases	This Hospital	State Average	U.S. Average	Top Hospital
Heart Attack Care					
ACE Inhibitor or ARB for LVSD[1]	23	96%	86%	82%	100%
Aspirin at Arrival	145	96%	95%	92%	100%
Aspirin at Discharge	100	97%	94%	90%	100%
Beta Blocker at Arrival	110	98%	90%	87%	100%
Beta Blocker at Discharge	106	98%	93%	90%	100%
Fibrinolytic Medication Timing	0	-	28%	31%	100%
PCI Within 90 Minutes of Arrival[1]	9	56%	59%	54%	95%
Smoking Cessation Advice	29	97%	93%	88%	100%
Heart Failure Care					
ACE Inhibitor or ARB for LVSD	103	92%	84%	82%	100%
Discharge Instructions	267	54%	73%	61%	93%
Evaluation of LVS Function	338	97%	91%	83%	99%
Smoking Cessation Advice	71	96%	86%	82%	100%
Pneumonia Care					
Appropriate Initial Antibiotic	205	84%	88%	83%	94%
Blood Culture Timing	177	89%	90%	90%	100%
Influenza Vaccine	60	93%	73%	70%	100%
Initial Antibiotic Timing	328	77%	84%	80%	93%
Oxygenation Assessment	404	100%	100%	99%	100%
Pneumococcal Vaccine	225	74%	72%	69%	94%
Smoking Cessation Advice	110	92%	86%	80%	100%
Surgical Infection Prevention					
Prophylactic Antibiotic Given[2,3]	313	87%	82%	77%	95%
Prophylactic Antibiotic Selection[2]	97	94%	93%	90%	100%
Prophylactic Antibiotic Stopped[2,3]	300	86%	83%	72%	95%
Pregnancy Care					
Inpatient Neonatal Mortality	-	-	-	-	-
Third or Fourth Degree Laceration	-	-	2.62%	3.63%	3.27%

Spectrum Health

Alternate Name: Butterworth Hospital
100 Michigan Street NE
Grand Rapids, MI 49503
URL: www.spectrum-health.org
Ownership: Voluntary non-profit - Private
Emergency Services: Yes
Phone: 616-391-1700
Fax: 616-391-2780
Accredited: Yes
Licensed Beds: 529

Key Personnel:

CEO . . . . Richard C Breon
Chief Medical Staff . . . . Brian Roelof
Emergency Room . . . . Gwen Hoffman
Emergency Room . . . . Steven Holt
Director Infection/Disease Control . . . . Deb Paul
Director Medical/Surgical Nursing . . . . Jan Mathews
Chief Radiology . . . . Charles Luhenton
Director Respiratory Therapy . . . . Randy Kehr

Measure	Cases	This Hospital	State Average	U.S. Average	Top Hospital
Heart Attack Care					
ACE Inhibitor or ARB for LVSD	202	93%	86%	82%	100%
Aspirin at Arrival	508	100%	95%	92%	100%
Aspirin at Discharge	1,025	99%	94%	90%	100%
Beta Blocker at Arrival	414	99%	90%	87%	100%
Beta Blocker at Discharge	998	100%	93%	90%	100%
Fibrinolytic Medication Timing[1]	1	0%	28%	31%	100%
PCI Within 90 Minutes of Arrival	37	92%	59%	54%	95%
Smoking Cessation Advice	380	99%	93%	88%	100%
Heart Failure Care					
ACE Inhibitor or ARB for LVSD	335	94%	84%	82%	100%
Discharge Instructions	826	88%	73%	61%	93%
Evaluation of LVS Function	1,009	99%	91%	83%	99%
Smoking Cessation Advice	155	99%	86%	82%	100%
Pneumonia Care					
Appropriate Initial Antibiotic	593	97%	88%	83%	94%
Blood Culture Timing	728	86%	90%	90%	100%
Influenza Vaccine	150	91%	73%	70%	100%
Initial Antibiotic Timing	860	88%	84%	80%	93%
Oxygenation Assessment	1,061	100%	100%	99%	100%
Pneumococcal Vaccine	661	94%	72%	69%	94%
Smoking Cessation Advice	271	87%	86%	80%	100%
Surgical Infection Prevention					
Prophylactic Antibiotic Given[2,3]	372	86%	82%	77%	95%
Prophylactic Antibiotic Selection[2]	119	89%	93%	90%	100%
Prophylactic Antibiotic Stopped[2,3]	363	90%	83%	72%	95%
Pregnancy Care					
Inpatient Neonatal Mortality	8,861	0.49%	-	-	-
Third or Fourth Degree Laceration	5,726	2.15%	2.62%	3.63%	3.27%

Mercy Hospital-Grayling

1100 East Michigan Avenue
Grayling, MI 49738
URL: www.mercygrayling.munsonhealthcare.org
Ownership: Voluntary non-profit - Church
Emergency Services: Yes
Phone: 989-348-5461
Fax: 989-348-0485
Accredited: Yes
Licensed Beds: 130

Key Personnel:

CEO/President . . . . Stephen Reimer-Matuzsak
Chief of Medical Staff . . . . David Hunter
Director of Cardiology/Cardiac Lab . . . . Sue Boardman
Emergency Room . . . . D Gulow, MD

Measure	Cases	This Hospital	State Average	U.S. Average	Top Hospital
Heart Attack Care					
ACE Inhibitor or ARB for LVSD[1]	3	100%	86%	82%	100%
Aspirin at Arrival	29	100%	95%	92%	100%
Aspirin at Discharge[1]	15	93%	94%	90%	100%
Beta Blocker at Arrival	29	83%	90%	87%	100%
Beta Blocker at Discharge[1]	16	88%	93%	90%	100%
Fibrinolytic Medication Timing	0	-	28%	31%	100%
PCI Within 90 Minutes of Arrival	0	-	59%	54%	95%
Smoking Cessation Advice[1]	3	100%	93%	88%	100%
Heart Failure Care					
ACE Inhibitor or ARB for LVSD	26	85%	84%	82%	100%
Discharge Instructions	83	58%	73%	61%	93%
Evaluation of LVS Function	99	84%	91%	83%	99%
Smoking Cessation Advice[1]	19	37%	86%	82%	100%

NOTE: Hospital profiles are in alphabetical order by state, then city, then hospital within the city; Rankings are sorted by rate in descending order and exclude hospitals with less than 25 cases; (1) The number of cases is too small (n<25) for purposes of reliably predicting hospital performance; (2) Measure reflects the hospital's indication that its submission was based upon a sample of its relevant discharges; (3) Rate reflects fewer than the maximum possible quarters of data for the measure; (4) Inaccurate information submitted and suppressed for one or more quarters; (5) No data is available from the hospital for this measure; Please refer to the User's Guide for a full explanation of data

Measure	Cases	This Hospital	State Average	U.S. Average	Top Hospital
Pneumonia Care					
Appropriate Initial Antibiotic	193	91%	88%	83%	94%
Blood Culture Timing	152	88%	90%	90%	100%
Influenza Vaccine	48	54%	73%	70%	100%
Initial Antibiotic Timing	211	88%	84%	80%	93%
Oxygenation Assessment	272	100%	100%	99%	100%
Pneumococcal Vaccine	160	57%	72%	69%	94%
Smoking Cessation Advice	70	70%	86%	80%	100%
Surgical Infection Prevention					
Prophylactic Antibiotic Given	136	60%	82%	77%	95%
Prophylactic Antibiotic Selection	31	94%	93%	90%	100%
Prophylactic Antibiotic Stopped	122	84%	83%	72%	95%
Pregnancy Care					
Inpatient Neonatal Mortality	-	-	-	-	-
Third or Fourth Degree Laceration	-	-	2.62%	3.63%	3.27%

United Memorial Health Center

615 S Bower Street
Greenville, MI 48838

Toll-Free: 800-488-7560
Phone: 616-754-4691
Fax: 616-754-5054

E-mail: contactus@umha.org
URL: www.umha.org
Ownership: Voluntary non-profit - Other
Emergency Services: Yes
Accredited: Yes
Licensed Beds: 105

Key Personnel:
President/CEO. . . . . Paul Donir

Measure	Cases	This Hospital	State Average	U.S. Average	Top Hospital
Heart Attack Care					
ACE Inhibitor or ARB for LVSD[1]	1	100%	86%	82%	100%
Aspirin at Arrival[1]	22	86%	95%	92%	100%
Aspirin at Discharge[1]	9	100%	94%	90%	100%
Beta Blocker at Arrival[1]	18	100%	90%	87%	100%
Beta Blocker at Discharge[1]	9	100%	93%	90%	100%
Fibrinolytic Medication Timing	0	-	28%	31%	100%
PCI Within 90 Minutes of Arrival	0	-	59%	54%	95%
Smoking Cessation Advice[1]	1	100%	93%	88%	100%
Heart Failure Care					
ACE Inhibitor or ARB for LVSD[1]	14	100%	84%	82%	100%
Discharge Instructions	87	89%	73%	61%	93%
Evaluation of LVS Function	115	99%	91%	83%	99%
Smoking Cessation Advice[1]	14	100%	86%	82%	100%
Pneumonia Care					
Appropriate Initial Antibiotic	147	89%	88%	83%	94%
Blood Culture Timing	157	94%	90%	90%	100%
Influenza Vaccine	25	100%	73%	70%	100%
Initial Antibiotic Timing	195	94%	84%	80%	93%
Oxygenation Assessment	228	100%	100%	99%	100%
Pneumococcal Vaccine	133	93%	72%	69%	94%
Smoking Cessation Advice	59	95%	86%	80%	100%
Surgical Infection Prevention					
Prophylactic Antibiotic Given	146	97%	82%	77%	95%
Prophylactic Antibiotic Selection	43	100%	93%	90%	100%
Prophylactic Antibiotic Stopped	134	94%	83%	72%	95%
Pregnancy Care					
Inpatient Neonatal Mortality	-	-	-	-	-
Third or Fourth Degree Laceration	-	-	2.62%	3.63%	3.27%

Bon Secours Cottage Health Services

468 Cadieux Road
Grosse Point, MI 48230
URL: www.bonsecourscottage.org
Ownership: Voluntary non-profit - Church
Emergency Services: Yes

Phone: 313-343-1000
Fax: 313-343-1327
Accredited: Yes
Licensed Beds: 175

Key Personnel:
CEO. . . . . Richard VanLith
Catheterization Laboratory. . . . . Ken Brunell
Infection Control. . . . . Suzanne Gardner
Medical/Surgical Nursing . . . . Carol Greenberg
Respiratory Therapy. . . . . Scott Hoverman

Measure	Cases	This Hospital	State Average	U.S. Average	Top Hospital
Heart Attack Care					
ACE Inhibitor or ARB for LVSD[1]	21	86%	86%	82%	100%
Aspirin at Arrival	68	97%	95%	92%	100%
Aspirin at Discharge	48	100%	94%	90%	100%
Beta Blocker at Arrival	64	91%	90%	87%	100%
Beta Blocker at Discharge	57	98%	93%	90%	100%
Fibrinolytic Medication Timing	0	-	28%	31%	100%
PCI Within 90 Minutes of Arrival	0	-	59%	54%	95%
Smoking Cessation Advice[1]	7	71%	93%	88%	100%
Heart Failure Care					
ACE Inhibitor or ARB for LVSD	190	80%	84%	82%	100%
Discharge Instructions	474	61%	73%	61%	93%
Evaluation of LVS Function	549	92%	91%	83%	99%
Smoking Cessation Advice	62	65%	86%	82%	100%
Pneumonia Care					
Appropriate Initial Antibiotic	247	80%	88%	83%	94%
Blood Culture Timing	146	87%	90%	90%	100%
Influenza Vaccine	44	91%	73%	70%	100%
Initial Antibiotic Timing	246	73%	84%	80%	93%
Oxygenation Assessment	300	98%	100%	99%	100%
Pneumococcal Vaccine	178	77%	72%	69%	94%
Smoking Cessation Advice	74	84%	86%	80%	100%
Surgical Infection Prevention					
Prophylactic Antibiotic Given[3]	659	86%	82%	77%	95%
Prophylactic Antibiotic Selection	233	95%	93%	90%	100%
Prophylactic Antibiotic Stopped[3]	641	81%	83%	72%	95%
Pregnancy Care					
Inpatient Neonatal Mortality	-	-	-	-	-
Third or Fourth Degree Laceration	-	-	2.62%	3.63%	3.27%

Henry Ford Cottage Hospital

Alternate Name: Cottage Hospital of Grosse Pointe
159 Kercheval Avenue
Detroit, MI 48236
URL: www.henryfordhealth.org
Ownership: Voluntary non-profit - Other
Emergency Services: Yes

Phone: 313-640-1000
Fax: 313-640-2583
Accredited: Yes
Licensed Beds: 185

Key Personnel:
President/CEO. . . . . Anthony Armada

Measure	Cases	This Hospital	State Average	U.S. Average	Top Hospital
Heart Attack Care					
ACE Inhibitor or ARB for LVSD[5]	-	-	86%	82%	100%
Aspirin at Arrival[5]	-	-	95%	92%	100%
Aspirin at Discharge[5]	-	-	94%	90%	100%
Beta Blocker at Arrival[5]	-	-	90%	87%	100%
Beta Blocker at Discharge[5]	-	-	93%	90%	100%
Fibrinolytic Medication Timing[5]	-	-	28%	31%	100%
PCI Within 90 Minutes of Arrival[5]	-	-	59%	54%	95%
Smoking Cessation Advice[5]	-	-	93%	88%	100%
Heart Failure Care					
ACE Inhibitor or ARB for LVSD[5]	-	-	84%	82%	100%
Discharge Instructions[5]	-	-	73%	61%	93%
Evaluation of LVS Function[5]	-	-	91%	83%	99%
Smoking Cessation Advice[5]	-	-	86%	82%	100%
Pneumonia Care					
Appropriate Initial Antibiotic[5]	-	-	88%	83%	94%
Blood Culture Timing[5]	-	-	90%	90%	100%
Influenza Vaccine[5]	-	-	73%	70%	100%
Initial Antibiotic Timing[1,3]	1	100%	84%	80%	93%
Oxygenation Assessment[1,3]	1	100%	100%	99%	100%
Pneumococcal Vaccine[3]	0	-	72%	69%	94%
Smoking Cessation Advice[5]	-	-	86%	80%	100%
Surgical Infection Prevention					
Prophylactic Antibiotic Given[1,3]	5	80%	82%	77%	95%
Prophylactic Antibiotic Selection[5]	-	-	93%	90%	100%
Prophylactic Antibiotic Stopped[1,3]	5	100%	83%	72%	95%
Pregnancy Care					
Inpatient Neonatal Mortality	-	-	-	-	-
Third or Fourth Degree Laceration	-	-	2.62%	3.63%	3.27%

NOTE: Hospital profiles are in alphabetical order by state, then city, then hospital within the city; Rankings are sorted by rate in descending order and exclude hospitals with less than 25 cases; (1) The number of cases is too small (n<25) for purposes of reliably predicting hospital performance; (2) Measure reflects the hospital's indication that its submission was based upon a sample of its relevant discharges; (3) Rate reflects fewer than the maximum possible quarters of data for the measure; (4) Inaccurate information submitted and suppressed for one or more quarters; (5) No data is available from the hospital for this measure; Please refer to the User's Guide for a full explanation of data

Portage Health System

Alternate Name: Portage View Hospital
500 Campus Drive
Hancock, MI 49930

Toll-Free: 800-573-5001
Phone: 906-483-1000
Fax: 906-483-1521

E-mail: jsbigan@phsys.org
URL: www.portagehealth.org
Ownership: Voluntary non-profit - Other
Emergency Services: Yes

Accredited: Yes
Licensed Beds: 74

Key Personnel:
CEO. . . . . James Bogan
Medical Staff President . . . . David Kass, MD
Emergency Room . . . . Kirk Luskin
OB/GYN. . . . . Julie Meyer, DO
Director of Respiratory . . . . Dennis Jensen

Measure	Cases	This Hospital	State Average	U.S. Average	Top Hospital
Heart Attack Care					
ACE Inhibitor or ARB for LVSD[1]	3	67%	86%	82%	100%
Aspirin at Arrival[1]	18	100%	95%	92%	100%
Aspirin at Discharge[1]	11	91%	94%	90%	100%
Beta Blocker at Arrival[1]	16	100%	90%	87%	100%
Beta Blocker at Discharge[1]	12	92%	93%	90%	100%
Fibrinolytic Medication Timing	0	-	28%	31%	100%
PCI Within 90 Minutes of Arrival	0	-	59%	54%	95%
Smoking Cessation Advice[1]	1	100%	93%	88%	100%
Heart Failure Care					
ACE Inhibitor or ARB for LVSD[1]	11	82%	84%	82%	100%
Discharge Instructions[1]	23	61%	73%	61%	93%
Evaluation of LVS Function	30	93%	91%	83%	99%
Smoking Cessation Advice[1]	1	100%	86%	82%	100%
Pneumonia Care					
Appropriate Initial Antibiotic	59	88%	88%	83%	94%
Blood Culture Timing	37	97%	90%	90%	100%
Influenza Vaccine[1]	7	86%	73%	70%	100%
Initial Antibiotic Timing	69	90%	84%	80%	93%
Oxygenation Assessment	76	100%	100%	99%	100%
Pneumococcal Vaccine	54	69%	72%	69%	94%
Smoking Cessation Advice[1]	9	67%	86%	80%	100%
Surgical Infection Prevention					
Prophylactic Antibiotic Given[3]	77	75%	82%	77%	95%
Prophylactic Antibiotic Selection	27	93%	93%	90%	100%
Prophylactic Antibiotic Stopped[3]	65	57%	83%	72%	95%
Pregnancy Care					
Inpatient Neonatal Mortality	-	-	-	-	-
Third or Fourth Degree Laceration	-	-	2.62%	3.63%	3.27%

Saint John North Shores Hospital

26755 Ballard Road
Harrison Township, MI 48045

Phone: 586-465-5501
Fax: 586-466-5352

URL: www.stjohn.org
Ownership: Voluntary non-profit - Other
Emergency Services: Yes

Accredited: Yes
Licensed Beds: 96

Key Personnel:
Chief of Medical Staff. . . . . Anthony Southhall
Head of Emergency Room. . . . . Ted Kloks
Medical/Surgical Nursing . . . . Kathy Schroll, RN
Medical/Surgical Nursing . . . . Sue Peterfesa, RN
Manager Radiology . . . . Carol Porzondek
Manager Respiratory/Cardiopulmonary . . . . Paula Capo

Measure	Cases	This Hospital	State Average	U.S. Average	Top Hospital
Heart Attack Care					
ACE Inhibitor or ARB for LVSD[3]	0	-	86%	82%	100%
Aspirin at Arrival[3]	0	-	95%	92%	100%
Aspirin at Discharge[3]	0	-	94%	90%	100%
Beta Blocker at Arrival[3]	0	-	90%	87%	100%
Beta Blocker at Discharge[3]	0	-	93%	90%	100%
Fibrinolytic Medication Timing[3]	0	-	28%	31%	100%
PCI Within 90 Minutes of Arrival	0	-	59%	54%	95%
Smoking Cessation Advice[3]	0	-	93%	88%	100%
Heart Failure Care					
ACE Inhibitor or ARB for LVSD[1]	2	50%	84%	82%	100%
Discharge Instructions[1,3]	2	0%	73%	61%	93%
Evaluation of LVS Function[1]	14	50%	91%	83%	99%
Smoking Cessation Advice[3]	0	-	86%	82%	100%
Pneumonia Care					
Appropriate Initial Antibiotic[1,3]	3	67%	88%	83%	94%
Blood Culture Timing[1,3]	3	67%	90%	90%	100%
Influenza Vaccine[5]	-	-	73%	70%	100%
Initial Antibiotic Timing[1]	24	96%	84%	80%	93%
Oxygenation Assessment	26	100%	100%	99%	100%
Pneumococcal Vaccine[1]	11	55%	72%	69%	94%
Smoking Cessation Advice[1,3]	1	100%	86%	80%	100%
Surgical Infection Prevention					
Prophylactic Antibiotic Given[5]	-	-	82%	77%	95%
Prophylactic Antibiotic Selection[5]	-	-	93%	90%	100%
Prophylactic Antibiotic Stopped[5]	-	-	83%	72%	95%
Pregnancy Care					
Inpatient Neonatal Mortality	-	-	-	-	-
Third or Fourth Degree Laceration	-	-	2.62%	3.63%	3.27%

Pennock Hospital

1009 W Green Street
Hastings, MI 49058

Phone: 269-945-3451
Fax: 269-945-4130

E-mail: info@pennockhealth.com
URL: www.pennockhealth.com
Ownership: Voluntary non-profit - Other
Emergency Services: Yes

Accredited: Yes
Licensed Beds: 89

Key Personnel:
CEO. . . . . Harry Doele
Chief Medical Staff. . . . . Matt Garber, MD
Emergency Room . . . . Rosenne Woodliff
Director Infection/Disease Control . . . . Jeanne Pugh
Director Radiology . . . . Ron Martin
Cardiopulmonary . . . . Mark Homstead

Measure	Cases	This Hospital	State Average	U.S. Average	Top Hospital
Heart Attack Care					
ACE Inhibitor or ARB for LVSD[1]	4	100%	86%	82%	100%
Aspirin at Arrival	28	89%	95%	92%	100%
Aspirin at Discharge[1]	18	94%	94%	90%	100%
Beta Blocker at Arrival	25	96%	90%	87%	100%
Beta Blocker at Discharge[1]	17	88%	93%	90%	100%
Fibrinolytic Medication Timing	0	-	28%	31%	100%
PCI Within 90 Minutes of Arrival	0	-	59%	54%	95%
Smoking Cessation Advice[1]	2	100%	93%	88%	100%
Heart Failure Care					
ACE Inhibitor or ARB for LVSD	64	94%	84%	82%	100%
Discharge Instructions	109	70%	73%	61%	93%
Evaluation of LVS Function	146	98%	91%	83%	99%
Smoking Cessation Advice[1]	14	93%	86%	82%	100%
Pneumonia Care					
Appropriate Initial Antibiotic	105	86%	88%	83%	94%
Blood Culture Timing	93	99%	90%	90%	100%
Influenza Vaccine[1]	24	88%	73%	70%	100%
Initial Antibiotic Timing	152	87%	84%	80%	93%
Oxygenation Assessment	172	100%	100%	99%	100%
Pneumococcal Vaccine	102	94%	72%	69%	94%
Smoking Cessation Advice	34	88%	86%	80%	100%
Surgical Infection Prevention					
Prophylactic Antibiotic Given[2]	253	95%	82%	77%	95%
Prophylactic Antibiotic Selection[2]	54	96%	93%	90%	100%
Prophylactic Antibiotic Stopped[2]	244	94%	83%	72%	95%
Pregnancy Care					
Inpatient Neonatal Mortality	-	-	-	-	-
Third or Fourth Degree Laceration	-	-	2.62%	3.63%	3.27%

Hillsdale Community Health Center

168 S Howell Street
Hillsdale, MI 49242

Phone: 517-437-4451
Fax: 517-437-5215

URL: www.hchc.com
Ownership: Voluntary non-profit - Other
Emergency Services: Yes

Accredited: Yes
Licensed Beds: 65

Key Personnel:
Administrator/President . . . . Charles A Bianchi

NOTE: Hospital profiles are in alphabetical order by state, then city, then hospital within the city; Rankings are sorted by rate in descending order and exclude hospitals with less than 25 cases; (1) The number of cases is too small (n<25) for purposes of reliably predicting hospital performance; (2) Measure reflects the hospital's indication that its submission was based upon a sample of its relevant discharges; (3) Rate reflects fewer than the maximum possible quarters of data for the measure; (4) Inaccurate information submitted and suppressed for one or more quarters; (5) No data is available from the hospital for this measure; Please refer to the User's Guide for a full explanation of data

Chief Medical Staff. . . . . Pat Sudds
Emergency Room . . . . Keith Baron, MD
Director Infection/Disease Control . . . . Debra Shatelrow, RN
ICU . . . . Janice Gutowski
Intensive/Coronary Care . . . . Doris Whorley
Respiratory/Cardiopulmonary. . . . . Tom Candy

Measure	Cases	This Hospital	State Average	U.S. Average	Top Hospital
Heart Attack Care					
ACE Inhibitor or ARB for LVSD[1]	1	100%	86%	82%	100%
Aspirin at Arrival	29	100%	95%	92%	100%
Aspirin at Discharge[1]	11	100%	94%	90%	100%
Beta Blocker at Arrival	27	100%	90%	87%	100%
Beta Blocker at Discharge[1]	13	100%	93%	90%	100%
Fibrinolytic Medication Timing	0	-	28%	31%	100%
PCI Within 90 Minutes of Arrival	0	-	59%	54%	95%
Smoking Cessation Advice[1]	3	33%	93%	88%	100%
Heart Failure Care					
ACE Inhibitor or ARB for LVSD	40	98%	84%	82%	100%
Discharge Instructions	70	74%	73%	61%	93%
Evaluation of LVS Function	90	87%	91%	83%	99%
Smoking Cessation Advice[1]	7	86%	86%	82%	100%
Pneumonia Care					
Appropriate Initial Antibiotic	118	87%	88%	83%	94%
Blood Culture Timing	63	83%	90%	90%	100%
Influenza Vaccine	35	71%	73%	70%	100%
Initial Antibiotic Timing	124	74%	84%	80%	93%
Oxygenation Assessment	172	100%	100%	99%	100%
Pneumococcal Vaccine	112	72%	72%	69%	94%
Smoking Cessation Advice	48	83%	86%	80%	100%
Surgical Infection Prevention					
Prophylactic Antibiotic Given[3]	199	49%	82%	77%	95%
Prophylactic Antibiotic Selection	67	79%	93%	90%	100%
Prophylactic Antibiotic Stopped[3]	195	11%	83%	72%	95%
Pregnancy Care					
Inpatient Neonatal Mortality	-	-	-	-	-
Third or Fourth Degree Laceration	-	-	2.62%	3.63%	3.27%

Holland Community Hospital

602 Michigan Avenue
Holland, MI 49423
Phone: 616-392-5141
Fax: 616-394-3572
URL: www.hoho.org
Ownership: Voluntary non-profit - Private
Accredited: Yes
Emergency Services: Yes
Licensed Beds: 213

Key Personnel:

President/CEO. . . . . Dale Sowders
Chief Medical Officer . . . . Bob Bates, MD
Emergency Room . . . . Jan Culina, RN
Infection Control. . . . . Theresa Ellis, RN
ICU . . . . Todd Knight, RN
Medical/Surgical Nursing . . . . Carolyn Sehaeffer
OB/GYN Women's Health . . . . Kathy Austin, RN
Director Surgery. . . . . Sheila Lautenback, RN
Director Radiology . . . . Dennis Pacanowski

Measure	Cases	This Hospital	State Average	U.S. Average	Top Hospital
Heart Attack Care					
ACE Inhibitor or ARB for LVSD[1]	23	87%	86%	82%	100%
Aspirin at Arrival	128	99%	95%	92%	100%
Aspirin at Discharge	85	100%	94%	90%	100%
Beta Blocker at Arrival	96	95%	90%	87%	100%
Beta Blocker at Discharge	88	100%	93%	90%	100%
Fibrinolytic Medication Timing	0	-	28%	31%	100%
PCI Within 90 Minutes of Arrival[1]	6	100%	59%	54%	95%
Smoking Cessation Advice	27	100%	93%	88%	100%
Heart Failure Care					
ACE Inhibitor or ARB for LVSD	70	89%	84%	82%	100%
Discharge Instructions	137	94%	73%	61%	93%
Evaluation of LVS Function	180	99%	91%	83%	99%
Smoking Cessation Advice	26	100%	86%	82%	100%
Pneumonia Care					
Appropriate Initial Antibiotic	178	80%	88%	83%	94%
Blood Culture Timing	182	91%	90%	90%	100%
Influenza Vaccine	50	98%	73%	70%	100%
Initial Antibiotic Timing	245	82%	84%	80%	93%
Oxygenation Assessment	287	100%	100%	99%	100%
Pneumococcal Vaccine	182	92%	72%	69%	94%
Smoking Cessation Advice	69	93%	86%	80%	100%
Surgical Infection Prevention					
Prophylactic Antibiotic Given	543	91%	82%	77%	95%
Prophylactic Antibiotic Selection	139	91%	93%	90%	100%
Prophylactic Antibiotic Stopped	519	89%	83%	72%	95%
Pregnancy Care					
Inpatient Neonatal Mortality	1,788	0.11%	-	-	-
Third or Fourth Degree Laceration	1,231	7.07%	2.62%	3.63%	3.27%

Saint Joseph Mercy Livingston Hospital

620 Byron Road
Howell, MI 48843
Phone: 517-545-6000
Fax: 517-545-6192
URL: www.sjmh.com
Ownership: Voluntary non-profit - Other
Accredited: Yes
Emergency Services: Yes
Licensed Beds: 136

Key Personnel:

CEO. . . . . Garry Faja
Chief Medical Staff. . . . . Charles Kelly, DO
Emergency Room . . . . Pat Claffey, RN
Director Infection/Disease Control . . . . Charles Craig, MD
Director CCU . . . . Fran Rocheleau, RN
Director Medical/Surgical Nursing . . . . Fran Rocheleau, RN
OB/GYN Womens Health. . . . . Marvin Schrock, MD
Chief Radiology . . . . Allen Denton, DO
Director Respiratory Therapy . . . . Joe Shank

Measure	Cases	This Hospital	State Average	U.S. Average	Top Hospital
Heart Attack Care					
ACE Inhibitor or ARB for LVSD[1]	5	100%	86%	82%	100%
Aspirin at Arrival[1]	24	96%	95%	92%	100%
Aspirin at Discharge[1]	20	100%	94%	90%	100%
Beta Blocker at Arrival[1]	9	78%	90%	87%	100%
Beta Blocker at Discharge[1]	20	95%	93%	90%	100%
Fibrinolytic Medication Timing	0	-	28%	31%	100%
PCI Within 90 Minutes of Arrival	0	-	59%	54%	95%
Smoking Cessation Advice	0	-	93%	88%	100%
Heart Failure Care					
ACE Inhibitor or ARB for LVSD	41	88%	84%	82%	100%
Discharge Instructions	103	82%	73%	61%	93%
Evaluation of LVS Function	150	99%	91%	83%	99%
Smoking Cessation Advice[1]	9	100%	86%	82%	100%
Pneumonia Care					
Appropriate Initial Antibiotic	110	95%	88%	83%	94%
Blood Culture Timing	150	99%	90%	90%	100%
Influenza Vaccine	28	96%	73%	70%	100%
Initial Antibiotic Timing	166	89%	84%	80%	93%
Oxygenation Assessment	220	100%	100%	99%	100%
Pneumococcal Vaccine	145	94%	72%	69%	94%
Smoking Cessation Advice	38	82%	86%	80%	100%
Surgical Infection Prevention					
Prophylactic Antibiotic Given[2]	174	91%	82%	77%	95%
Prophylactic Antibiotic Selection[2]	44	98%	93%	90%	100%
Prophylactic Antibiotic Stopped[2]	168	85%	83%	72%	95%
Pregnancy Care					
Inpatient Neonatal Mortality	-	-	-	-	-
Third or Fourth Degree Laceration	-	-	2.62%	3.63%	3.27%

Ionia County Memorial Hospital

479 Lafayette Street
Ionia, MI 48846
Phone: 616-527-4200
Fax: 616-527-5731
E-mail: ltjalsma@ioniahoapitl.org
URL: www.ioniahospital.org
Ownership: Voluntary non-profit - Private
Accredited: Yes
Emergency Services: Yes
Licensed Beds: 25

Key Personnel:

Chief Medical Staff. . . . . Brian Thangamani, MD
Emergency Room . . . . Cheryl Koon, RN
Emergency Room . . . . Dr. Doyle Calley
Infection Control. . . . . Cheryl Koon, RN

NOTE: Hospital profiles are in alphabetical order by state, then city, then hospital within the city; Rankings are sorted by rate in descending order and exclude hospitals with less than 25 cases; (1) The number of cases is too small (n<25) for purposes of reliably predicting hospital performance; (2) Measure reflects the hospital's indication that its submission was based upon a sample of its relevant discharges; (3) Rate reflects fewer than the maximum possible quarters of data for the measure; (4) Inaccurate information submitted and suppressed for one or more quarters; (5) No data is available from the hospital for this measure; Please refer to the User's Guide for a full explanation of data

OB/GYN/Women's Health . . . . Sherill Billings, RN
Manager Radiology . . . . Ernest Heady
Respiratory Care Manager. . . . . Bob Neal, RT

Measure	Cases	This Hospital	State Average	U.S. Average	Top Hospital
Heart Attack Care					
ACE Inhibitor or ARB for LVSD[1]	2	100%	86%	82%	100%
Aspirin at Arrival[1]	5	100%	95%	92%	100%
Aspirin at Discharge[1]	2	100%	94%	90%	100%
Beta Blocker at Arrival[1]	4	100%	90%	87%	100%
Beta Blocker at Discharge[1]	1	100%	93%	90%	100%
Fibrinolytic Medication Timing	0	-	28%	31%	100%
PCI Within 90 Minutes of Arrival	0	-	59%	54%	95%
Smoking Cessation Advice[1]	1	100%	93%	88%	100%
Heart Failure Care					
ACE Inhibitor or ARB for LVSD[1]	8	88%	84%	82%	100%
Discharge Instructions	38	74%	73%	61%	93%
Evaluation of LVS Function	49	90%	91%	83%	99%
Smoking Cessation Advice[1]	6	83%	86%	82%	100%
Pneumonia Care					
Appropriate Initial Antibiotic	67	91%	88%	83%	94%
Blood Culture Timing	36	94%	90%	90%	100%
Influenza Vaccine[1]	16	25%	73%	70%	100%
Initial Antibiotic Timing	59	83%	84%	80%	93%
Oxygenation Assessment	72	100%	100%	99%	100%
Pneumococcal Vaccine	47	45%	72%	69%	94%
Smoking Cessation Advice[1]	15	87%	86%	80%	100%
Surgical Infection Prevention					
Prophylactic Antibiotic Given[1,3]	23	70%	82%	77%	95%
Prophylactic Antibiotic Selection[1]	4	100%	93%	90%	100%
Prophylactic Antibiotic Stopped[1,3]	21	100%	83%	72%	95%
Pregnancy Care					
Inpatient Neonatal Mortality	-	-	-	-	-
Third or Fourth Degree Laceration	-	-	2.62%	3.63%	3.27%

Dickinson County Healthcare System

1721 S Stephenson Avenue Phone: 906-776-5408
Iron Mountain, MI 49801 Fax: 906-776-5791
URL: www.dchs.org
Ownership: Government - Local Accredited: Yes
Emergency Services: Yes Licensed Beds: 96

Key Personnel:

Chief Medical Staff. . . . . Daniel Benishek

Measure	Cases	This Hospital	State Average	U.S. Average	Top Hospital
Heart Attack Care					
ACE Inhibitor or ARB for LVSD[1]	4	75%	86%	82%	100%
Aspirin at Arrival	38	95%	95%	92%	100%
Aspirin at Discharge	26	92%	94%	90%	100%
Beta Blocker at Arrival	29	83%	90%	87%	100%
Beta Blocker at Discharge	30	87%	93%	90%	100%
Fibrinolytic Medication Timing[1]	3	33%	28%	31%	100%
PCI Within 90 Minutes of Arrival	0	-	59%	54%	95%
Smoking Cessation Advice[1]	5	60%	93%	88%	100%
Heart Failure Care					
ACE Inhibitor or ARB for LVSD	25	76%	84%	82%	100%
Discharge Instructions	83	71%	73%	61%	93%
Evaluation of LVS Function	123	87%	91%	83%	99%
Smoking Cessation Advice[1]	6	100%	86%	82%	100%
Pneumonia Care					
Appropriate Initial Antibiotic	76	92%	88%	83%	94%
Blood Culture Timing	74	95%	90%	90%	100%
Influenza Vaccine[1]	19	68%	73%	70%	100%
Initial Antibiotic Timing	103	88%	84%	80%	93%
Oxygenation Assessment	147	100%	100%	99%	100%
Pneumococcal Vaccine	103	80%	72%	69%	94%
Smoking Cessation Advice	29	83%	86%	80%	100%
Surgical Infection Prevention					
Prophylactic Antibiotic Given	255	93%	82%	77%	95%
Prophylactic Antibiotic Selection	58	100%	93%	90%	100%
Prophylactic Antibiotic Stopped	247	89%	83%	72%	95%
Pregnancy Care					
Inpatient Neonatal Mortality	-	-	-	-	-
Third or Fourth Degree Laceration	-	-	2.62%	3.63%	3.27%

Iron County Community Hospitals

1400 W Ice Lake Road Phone: 906-265-6121
Iron River, MI 49935 Fax: 906-265-9793
URL: www.icch.org
Ownership: Voluntary non-profit - Private Accredited: No
Emergency Services: Yes Licensed Beds: 67

Key Personnel:

CEO. . . . . David Huff
Chief Medical Staff. . . . . Nase Rizkalla
Emergency Room . . . . James Grebner, MD
Director Infection/Disease Control . . . . Carolyn Dunlap
CCU Spvg. Nurse . . . . Mary Larson
Chief Radiology . . . . Lillian Simmons
Director Respiratory Therapy . . . . Mary Larson

Measure	Cases	This Hospital	State Average	U.S. Average	Top Hospital
Heart Attack Care					
ACE Inhibitor or ARB for LVSD[1]	3	67%	86%	82%	100%
Aspirin at Arrival[1]	7	71%	95%	92%	100%
Aspirin at Discharge[1]	4	50%	94%	90%	100%
Beta Blocker at Arrival[1]	6	100%	90%	87%	100%
Beta Blocker at Discharge[1]	3	100%	93%	90%	100%
Fibrinolytic Medication Timing[1]	1	0%	28%	31%	100%
PCI Within 90 Minutes of Arrival	0	-	59%	54%	95%
Smoking Cessation Advice	0	-	93%	88%	100%
Heart Failure Care					
ACE Inhibitor or ARB for LVSD[1]	10	100%	84%	82%	100%
Discharge Instructions	44	68%	73%	61%	93%
Evaluation of LVS Function	61	56%	91%	83%	99%
Smoking Cessation Advice[1]	6	33%	86%	82%	100%
Pneumonia Care					
Appropriate Initial Antibiotic	27	67%	88%	83%	94%
Blood Culture Timing	44	89%	90%	90%	100%
Influenza Vaccine[1]	7	100%	73%	70%	100%
Initial Antibiotic Timing	53	79%	84%	80%	93%
Oxygenation Assessment	79	100%	100%	99%	100%
Pneumococcal Vaccine	56	64%	72%	69%	94%
Smoking Cessation Advice[1]	11	55%	86%	80%	100%
Surgical Infection Prevention					
Prophylactic Antibiotic Given[5]	-	-	82%	77%	95%
Prophylactic Antibiotic Selection[5]	-	-	93%	90%	100%
Prophylactic Antibiotic Stopped[5]	-	-	83%	72%	95%
Pregnancy Care					
Inpatient Neonatal Mortality	-	-	-	-	-
Third or Fourth Degree Laceration	-	-	2.62%	3.63%	3.27%

Foote Health System

205 N East Avenue Phone: 517-788-4800
Jackson, MI 49201 Fax: 517-788-4829
URL: www.footehealth.org
Ownership: Voluntary non-profit - Other Accredited: Yes
Emergency Services: Yes Licensed Beds: 411

Key Personnel:

President . . . . Georgia Fojtasek
Chief Medical Staff. . . . . Ray King, MD

Measure	Cases	This Hospital	State Average	U.S. Average	Top Hospital
Heart Attack Care					
ACE Inhibitor or ARB for LVSD	38	87%	86%	82%	100%
Aspirin at Arrival	259	95%	95%	92%	100%
Aspirin at Discharge	137	96%	94%	90%	100%
Beta Blocker at Arrival	222	92%	90%	87%	100%
Beta Blocker at Discharge	168	98%	93%	90%	100%
Fibrinolytic Medication Timing[1]	10	30%	28%	31%	100%
PCI Within 90 Minutes of Arrival[1]	17	53%	59%	54%	95%
Smoking Cessation Advice	61	97%	93%	88%	100%
Heart Failure Care					
ACE Inhibitor or ARB for LVSD	138	89%	84%	82%	100%
Discharge Instructions	327	70%	73%	61%	93%

NOTE: Hospital profiles are in alphabetical order by state, then city, then hospital within the city; Rankings are sorted by rate in descending order and exclude hospitals with less than 25 cases; (1) The number of cases is too small (n<25) for purposes of reliably predicting hospital performance; (2) Measure reflects the hospital's indication that its submission was based upon a sample of its relevant discharges; (3) Rate reflects fewer than the maximum possible quarters of data for the measure; (4) Inaccurate information submitted and suppressed for one or more quarters; (5) No data is available from the hospital for this measure; Please refer to the User's Guide for a full explanation of data

Evaluation of LVS Function	401	95%	91%	83%	99%
Smoking Cessation Advice	70	97%	86%	82%	100%
Pneumonia Care					
Appropriate Initial Antibiotic[2]	128	90%	88%	83%	94%
Blood Culture Timing[2]	89	94%	90%	90%	100%
Influenza Vaccine[2]	30	90%	73%	70%	100%
Initial Antibiotic Timing[2]	169	78%	84%	80%	93%
Oxygenation Assessment[2]	202	100%	100%	99%	100%
Pneumococcal Vaccine[2]	117	87%	72%	69%	94%
Smoking Cessation Advice[2]	54	94%	86%	80%	100%
Surgical Infection Prevention					
Prophylactic Antibiotic Given[2,3]	190	90%	82%	77%	95%
Prophylactic Antibiotic Selection[2]	60	95%	93%	90%	100%
Prophylactic Antibiotic Stopped[2,3]	178	85%	83%	72%	95%
Pregnancy Care					
Inpatient Neonatal Mortality	-	-	-	-	-
Third or Fourth Degree Laceration	-	-	2.62%	3.63%	3.27%

Borgess Medical Center

1521 Gull Road
Suite 350
Kalamazoo, MI 49048
URL: www.borgess.com
Phone: 269-226-7000
Fax: 269-226-5966
Ownership: Voluntary non-profit - Other
Emergency Services: Yes
Accredited: Yes
Licensed Beds: 424

Key Personnel:

President/CEO. . . . . Randall Stasik
Chief Medical Staff. . . . . Dale Rowe, MD
Dir Cardiopulmonary/Cardiac Ultrasound . . . . . . Sharon Bedecsll, MD
Catheterization Lab . . . . William Campbell, MD
Director Emergency Room. . . . . Pat Mayne
Manager Infection Control . . . . Karen Miller
ICU . . . . Brad Gordon
Director Coronary Care/CSU Unit . . . . Steve Marzloff
Director Respiratory/Cardiopulmonary . . . . John Clark

Measure	Cases	This Hospital	State Average	U.S. Average	Top Hospital
Heart Attack Care					
ACE Inhibitor or ARB for LVSD[2]	59	78%	86%	82%	100%
Aspirin at Arrival[2]	89	97%	95%	92%	100%
Aspirin at Discharge[2]	275	98%	94%	90%	100%
Beta Blocker at Arrival[2]	73	92%	90%	87%	100%
Beta Blocker at Discharge[2]	273	96%	93%	90%	100%
Fibrinolytic Medication Timing[1,2]	1	0%	28%	31%	100%
PCI Within 90 Minutes of Arrival[1,2]	7	43%	59%	54%	95%
Smoking Cessation Advice[2]	99	99%	93%	88%	100%
Heart Failure Care					
ACE Inhibitor or ARB for LVSD[2]	137	82%	84%	82%	100%
Discharge Instructions[2]	240	76%	73%	61%	93%
Evaluation of LVS Function[2]	280	98%	91%	83%	99%
Smoking Cessation Advice[2]	53	94%	86%	82%	100%
Pneumonia Care					
Appropriate Initial Antibiotic[2]	81	90%	88%	83%	94%
Blood Culture Timing[2]	87	93%	90%	90%	100%
Influenza Vaccine[1,2]	21	86%	73%	70%	100%
Initial Antibiotic Timing[2]	110	87%	84%	80%	93%
Oxygenation Assessment[2]	139	100%	100%	99%	100%
Pneumococcal Vaccine[2]	95	86%	72%	69%	94%
Smoking Cessation Advice[2]	50	86%	86%	80%	100%
Surgical Infection Prevention					
Prophylactic Antibiotic Given[2]	347	82%	82%	77%	95%
Prophylactic Antibiotic Selection[2]	84	89%	93%	90%	100%
Prophylactic Antibiotic Stopped[2]	330	84%	83%	72%	95%
Pregnancy Care					
Inpatient Neonatal Mortality	-	-	-	-	-
Third or Fourth Degree Laceration	-	-	2.62%	3.63%	3.27%

Bronson Methodist Hospital

601 John Street
Box G
Kalamazoo, MI 49007
E-mail: bennettk@bronsonhg.org
URL: www.bronsonhealth.com
Phone: 269-341-7654
Fax: 269-341-8696
Ownership: Voluntary non-profit - Church
Emergency Services: Yes
Accredited: Yes
Licensed Beds: 343

Key Personnel:

President/CEO. . . . . Frank J Sardone

Measure	Cases	This Hospital	State Average	U.S. Average	Top Hospital
Heart Attack Care					
ACE Inhibitor or ARB for LVSD	124	80%	86%	82%	100%
Aspirin at Arrival	280	98%	95%	92%	100%
Aspirin at Discharge	388	98%	94%	90%	100%
Beta Blocker at Arrival	257	95%	90%	87%	100%
Beta Blocker at Discharge	428	98%	93%	90%	100%
Fibrinolytic Medication Timing[1]	1	0%	28%	31%	100%
PCI Within 90 Minutes of Arrival[1]	13	69%	59%	54%	95%
Smoking Cessation Advice	141	99%	93%	88%	100%
Heart Failure Care					
ACE Inhibitor or ARB for LVSD	190	88%	84%	82%	100%
Discharge Instructions	539	94%	73%	61%	93%
Evaluation of LVS Function	664	99%	91%	83%	99%
Smoking Cessation Advice	130	90%	86%	82%	100%
Pneumonia Care					
Appropriate Initial Antibiotic	222	97%	88%	83%	94%
Blood Culture Timing	280	91%	90%	90%	100%
Influenza Vaccine	71	77%	73%	70%	100%
Initial Antibiotic Timing	300	81%	84%	80%	93%
Oxygenation Assessment	426	100%	100%	99%	100%
Pneumococcal Vaccine	285	80%	72%	69%	94%
Smoking Cessation Advice	104	94%	86%	80%	100%
Surgical Infection Prevention					
Prophylactic Antibiotic Given[2]	1,653	96%	82%	77%	95%
Prophylactic Antibiotic Selection[2]	408	98%	93%	90%	100%
Prophylactic Antibiotic Stopped[2]	1,605	90%	83%	72%	95%
Pregnancy Care					
Inpatient Neonatal Mortality	-	-	-	-	-
Third or Fourth Degree Laceration	-	-	2.62%	3.63%	3.27%

Kelsey Memorial Hospital

418 Washington Avenue
Lakeview, MI 48850
URL: kelseymemorial.org
Phone: 989-352-7211
Fax: 616-754-5054
Ownership: Voluntary non-profit - Other
Emergency Services: Yes
Accredited: Yes
Licensed Beds: 94

Key Personnel:

CEO. . . . . Ken Cegner
Medical Staff . . . . M Dewys
Head of Respiratory Care. . . . . Marilyn Staton

Measure	Cases	This Hospital	State Average	U.S. Average	Top Hospital
Heart Attack Care					
ACE Inhibitor or ARB for LVSD[1,3]	1	100%	86%	82%	100%
Aspirin at Arrival[1,3]	2	100%	95%	92%	100%
Aspirin at Discharge[1,3]	3	100%	94%	90%	100%
Beta Blocker at Arrival[1,3]	3	100%	90%	87%	100%
Beta Blocker at Discharge[1,3]	3	100%	93%	90%	100%
Fibrinolytic Medication Timing[3]	0	-	28%	31%	100%
PCI Within 90 Minutes of Arrival	0	-	59%	54%	95%
Smoking Cessation Advice[3]	0	-	93%	88%	100%
Heart Failure Care					
ACE Inhibitor or ARB for LVSD[1]	7	100%	84%	82%	100%
Discharge Instructions	30	97%	73%	61%	93%
Evaluation of LVS Function	41	100%	91%	83%	99%
Smoking Cessation Advice[1]	3	100%	86%	82%	100%
Pneumonia Care					
Appropriate Initial Antibiotic	41	90%	88%	83%	94%
Blood Culture Timing	28	100%	90%	90%	100%
Influenza Vaccine[1]	12	100%	73%	70%	100%
Initial Antibiotic Timing	35	97%	84%	80%	93%

NOTE: Hospital profiles are in alphabetical order by state, then city, then hospital within the city; Rankings are sorted by rate in descending order and exclude hospitals with less than 25 cases; (1) The number of cases is too small (n<25) for purposes of reliably predicting hospital performance; (2) Measure reflects the hospital's indication that its submission was based upon a sample of its relevant discharges; (3) Rate reflects fewer than the maximum possible quarters of data for the measure; (4) Inaccurate information submitted and suppressed for one or more quarters; (5) No data is available from the hospital for this measure; Please refer to the User's Guide for a full explanation of data

Oxygenation Assessment	52	100%	100%	99%	100%
Pneumococcal Vaccine	33	100%	72%	69%	94%
Smoking Cessation Advice[1]	12	100%	86%	80%	100%
Surgical Infection Prevention					
Prophylactic Antibiotic Given[5]	-	-	82%	77%	95%
Prophylactic Antibiotic Selection[5]	-	-	93%	90%	100%
Prophylactic Antibiotic Stopped[5]	-	-	83%	72%	95%
Pregnancy Care					
Inpatient Neonatal Mortality	-	-	-	-	-
Third or Fourth Degree Laceration	-	-	2.62%	3.63%	3.27%

Ingham Regional Medical Center

401 W Greenlawn Ave
Lansing, MI 48910
Phone: 517-334-2967
Ownership: Voluntary non-profit - Private
Accredited: Yes
Emergency Services: Yes

Measure	Cases	This Hospital	State Average	U.S. Average	Top Hospital
Heart Attack Care					
ACE Inhibitor or ARB for LVSD	111	95%	86%	82%	100%
Aspirin at Arrival	290	99%	95%	92%	100%
Aspirin at Discharge	420	99%	94%	90%	100%
Beta Blocker at Arrival	211	95%	90%	87%	100%
Beta Blocker at Discharge	444	99%	93%	90%	100%
Fibrinolytic Medication Timing[1]	1	100%	28%	31%	100%
PCI Within 90 Minutes of Arrival[1]	15	33%	59%	54%	95%
Smoking Cessation Advice	157	100%	93%	88%	100%
Heart Failure Care					
ACE Inhibitor or ARB for LVSD	152	94%	84%	82%	100%
Discharge Instructions	454	98%	73%	61%	93%
Evaluation of LVS Function	515	97%	91%	83%	99%
Smoking Cessation Advice	90	100%	86%	82%	100%
Pneumonia Care					
Appropriate Initial Antibiotic	211	87%	88%	83%	94%
Blood Culture Timing	218	69%	90%	90%	100%
Influenza Vaccine	67	67%	73%	70%	100%
Initial Antibiotic Timing	296	83%	84%	80%	93%
Oxygenation Assessment	359	100%	100%	99%	100%
Pneumococcal Vaccine	217	54%	72%	69%	94%
Smoking Cessation Advice	78	97%	86%	80%	100%
Surgical Infection Prevention					
Prophylactic Antibiotic Given[2,3]	1,642	92%	82%	77%	95%
Prophylactic Antibiotic Selection[2]	519	92%	93%	90%	100%
Prophylactic Antibiotic Stopped[2,3]	1,539	87%	83%	72%	95%
Pregnancy Care					
Inpatient Neonatal Mortality	-	-	-	-	-
Third or Fourth Degree Laceration	-	-	2.62%	3.63%	3.27%

Sparrow Hospital

Alternate Name: Edward W Sparrow Hospital
1215 E Michigan Avenue
Lansing, MI 48912
Phone: 517-364-1000
Fax: 517-364-5050
URL: www.sparrow.org
Ownership: Voluntary non-profit - Other
Accredited: Yes
Emergency Services: Yes
Licensed Beds: 502
Key Personnel:
President/CEO. . . . . Joe Damore
Director Infection/Disease Control . . . . John Dyke, MD

Measure	Cases	This Hospital	State Average	U.S. Average	Top Hospital
Heart Attack Care					
ACE Inhibitor or ARB for LVSD	112	80%	86%	82%	100%
Aspirin at Arrival	245	98%	95%	92%	100%
Aspirin at Discharge	408	99%	94%	90%	100%
Beta Blocker at Arrival	211	93%	90%	87%	100%
Beta Blocker at Discharge	410	98%	93%	90%	100%
Fibrinolytic Medication Timing	0	-	28%	31%	100%
PCI Within 90 Minutes of Arrival[1]	19	21%	59%	54%	95%
Smoking Cessation Advice	145	93%	93%	88%	100%
Heart Failure Care					
ACE Inhibitor or ARB for LVSD	244	89%	84%	82%	100%
Discharge Instructions	493	61%	73%	61%	93%
Evaluation of LVS Function	588	91%	91%	83%	99%
Smoking Cessation Advice	87	83%	86%	82%	100%
Pneumonia Care					
Appropriate Initial Antibiotic	221	83%	88%	83%	94%
Blood Culture Timing	221	83%	90%	90%	100%
Influenza Vaccine	60	60%	73%	70%	100%
Initial Antibiotic Timing	328	73%	84%	80%	93%
Oxygenation Assessment	399	100%	100%	99%	100%
Pneumococcal Vaccine	249	64%	72%	69%	94%
Smoking Cessation Advice	106	76%	86%	80%	100%
Surgical Infection Prevention					
Prophylactic Antibiotic Given	1,523	75%	82%	77%	95%
Prophylactic Antibiotic Selection	354	88%	93%	90%	100%
Prophylactic Antibiotic Stopped	1,483	70%	83%	72%	95%
Pregnancy Care					
Inpatient Neonatal Mortality	-	-	-	-	-
Third or Fourth Degree Laceration	-	-	2.62%	3.63%	3.27%

Lapeer Regional Medical Center

1375 N Main Street
Lapeer, MI 48446
Phone: 810-667-5580
Fax: 810-667-5582
URL: www.lapeerregional.org
Ownership: Voluntary non-profit - Other
Accredited: Yes
Emergency Services: Yes
Licensed Beds: 185
Key Personnel:
President/CEO. . . . . Barton Buxton, EdD
Chief Medical Staff. . . . . Darlin David, MD
Director of Cardiology/Cardiac Lab. . . . . Jeff Haris
Director Emergency Room. . . . . Kim Parsons
Director Infection/Disease Control . . . . Florence Elston, RN
CCU Spvg. Nurse . . . . Jennifer Hanson, RN
Director Medical/Surgical Nursing . . . . Sue Baker
OB/GYN Womens Health. . . . . Jan Gromada, DO
Chief Radiology . . . . Kenneth Tarr, DO
Director of Pulmonary/Respiratory Care. . . . . . . Wael Al-Ameri

Measure	Cases	This Hospital	State Average	U.S. Average	Top Hospital
Heart Attack Care					
ACE Inhibitor or ARB for LVSD[1]	4	75%	86%	82%	100%
Aspirin at Arrival	85	94%	95%	92%	100%
Aspirin at Discharge	40	100%	94%	90%	100%
Beta Blocker at Arrival	80	92%	90%	87%	100%
Beta Blocker at Discharge	42	95%	93%	90%	100%
Fibrinolytic Medication Timing[1]	14	43%	28%	31%	100%
PCI Within 90 Minutes of Arrival	0	-	59%	54%	95%
Smoking Cessation Advice[1]	5	100%	93%	88%	100%
Heart Failure Care					
ACE Inhibitor or ARB for LVSD	70	87%	84%	82%	100%
Discharge Instructions	178	83%	73%	61%	93%
Evaluation of LVS Function	212	96%	91%	83%	99%
Smoking Cessation Advice	33	100%	86%	82%	100%
Pneumonia Care					
Appropriate Initial Antibiotic	159	94%	88%	83%	94%
Blood Culture Timing	198	94%	90%	90%	100%
Influenza Vaccine	49	96%	73%	70%	100%
Initial Antibiotic Timing	220	79%	84%	80%	93%
Oxygenation Assessment	254	100%	100%	99%	100%
Pneumococcal Vaccine	152	94%	72%	69%	94%
Smoking Cessation Advice	73	100%	86%	80%	100%
Surgical Infection Prevention					
Prophylactic Antibiotic Given[2]	404	92%	82%	77%	95%
Prophylactic Antibiotic Selection[2]	107	100%	93%	90%	100%
Prophylactic Antibiotic Stopped[2]	381	89%	83%	72%	95%
Pregnancy Care					
Inpatient Neonatal Mortality	-	-	-	-	-
Third or Fourth Degree Laceration	-	-	2.62%	3.63%	3.27%

NOTE: Hospital profiles are in alphabetical order by state, then city, then hospital within the city; Rankings are sorted by rate in descending order and exclude hospitals with less than 25 cases; (1) The number of cases is too small (n<25) for purposes of reliably predicting hospital performance; (2) Measure reflects the hospital's indication that its submission was based upon a sample of its relevant discharges; (3) Rate reflects fewer than the maximum possible quarters of data for the measure; (4) Inaccurate information submitted and suppressed for one or more quarters; (5) No data is available from the hospital for this measure; Please refer to the User's Guide for a full explanation of data

Saint Mary Mercy Hospital

36475 Five Mile Road
Livonia, MI 48154
Phone: 734-655-4800
Fax: 734-591-3854
URL: www.stmarymercy.org
Ownership: Voluntary non-profit - Church
Emergency Services: Yes
Accredited: Yes
Licensed Beds: 304

Key Personnel:
President/CEO . . . . David Spivey
Chief Medical Staff . . . . Prasad Mikkilineni, MD
Department Head Cardiovascular . . . . Freida Pruit-Craig
Catheterization Lab . . . . Freida Pruitt-Craig
Infection Control . . . . Jennifer L Furman
ICU . . . . Sandra Perez
Intensive/Coronary Care . . . . Butchi B Paidipaty
OB/GYN Womens Health . . . . Janet Sobo
Respiratory/Cardiopulmonary . . . . Jane Bon

Measure	Cases	This Hospital	State Average	U.S. Average	Top Hospital
Heart Attack Care					
ACE Inhibitor or ARB for LVSD	32	97%	86%	82%	100%
Aspirin at Arrival	230	99%	95%	92%	100%
Aspirin at Discharge	154	99%	94%	90%	100%
Beta Blocker at Arrival	216	99%	90%	87%	100%
Beta Blocker at Discharge	155	99%	93%	90%	100%
Fibrinolytic Medication Timing	0	-	28%	31%	100%
PCI Within 90 Minutes of Arrival[1]	10	70%	59%	54%	95%
Smoking Cessation Advice	36	100%	93%	88%	100%
Heart Failure Care					
ACE Inhibitor or ARB for LVSD	141	91%	84%	82%	100%
Discharge Instructions	343	47%	73%	61%	93%
Evaluation of LVS Function	533	97%	91%	83%	99%
Smoking Cessation Advice	44	98%	86%	82%	100%
Pneumonia Care					
Appropriate Initial Antibiotic	378	81%	88%	83%	94%
Blood Culture Timing	378	92%	90%	90%	100%
Influenza Vaccine[4,5]	-	-	73%	70%	100%
Initial Antibiotic Timing	550	81%	84%	80%	93%
Oxygenation Assessment	687	100%	100%	99%	100%
Pneumococcal Vaccine	500	49%	72%	69%	94%
Smoking Cessation Advice	83	92%	86%	80%	100%
Surgical Infection Prevention					
Prophylactic Antibiotic Given[3]	504	85%	82%	77%	95%
Prophylactic Antibiotic Selection	176	93%	93%	90%	100%
Prophylactic Antibiotic Stopped[3]	481	78%	83%	72%	95%
Pregnancy Care					
Inpatient Neonatal Mortality	711	0.14%	-	-	-
Third or Fourth Degree Laceration	992	2.22%	2.62%	3.63%	3.27%

Memorial Medical Center West Michigan

One Atkinson Drive
Ludington, MI 49431
Toll-Free: 888-742-7426
Phone: 231-843-2591
Fax: 231-845-1732
E-mail: bobm@mmcwm.com
URL: www.mmcwm.com
Ownership: Proprietary
Emergency Services: Yes
Accredited: No
Licensed Beds: 95

Key Personnel:
Administrator/President . . . . Robert C Marquardt
Chief Medical Staff . . . . Allan Nelson, MD
Medical Director/ER . . . . Steven Strbick, DO
Director Medical/Surgical Nursing . . . . Marilyn Hansberger, RN
Director Respiratory Therapy . . . . Greg Soper

Measure	Cases	This Hospital	State Average	U.S. Average	Top Hospital
Heart Attack Care					
ACE Inhibitor or ARB for LVSD[1]	2	50%	86%	82%	100%
Aspirin at Arrival[1]	15	93%	95%	92%	100%
Aspirin at Discharge[1]	6	100%	94%	90%	100%
Beta Blocker at Arrival[1]	6	100%	90%	87%	100%
Beta Blocker at Discharge[1]	7	100%	93%	90%	100%
Fibrinolytic Medication Timing	0	-	28%	31%	100%
PCI Within 90 Minutes of Arrival	0	-	59%	54%	95%
Smoking Cessation Advice	0	-	93%	88%	100%
Heart Failure Care					
ACE Inhibitor or ARB for LVSD[2]	45	87%	84%	82%	100%
Discharge Instructions[2]	79	42%	73%	61%	93%
Evaluation of LVS Function[2]	98	92%	91%	83%	99%
Smoking Cessation Advice[1,2]	16	81%	86%	82%	100%
Pneumonia Care					
Appropriate Initial Antibiotic[2]	60	83%	88%	83%	94%
Blood Culture Timing[2]	79	95%	90%	90%	100%
Influenza Vaccine[1]	12	83%	73%	70%	100%
Initial Antibiotic Timing[2]	89	89%	84%	80%	93%
Oxygenation Assessment[2]	110	100%	100%	99%	100%
Pneumococcal Vaccine[2]	81	81%	72%	69%	94%
Smoking Cessation Advice[1,2]	23	65%	86%	80%	100%
Surgical Infection Prevention					
Prophylactic Antibiotic Given	160	82%	82%	77%	95%
Prophylactic Antibiotic Selection	60	100%	93%	90%	100%
Prophylactic Antibiotic Stopped	148	89%	83%	72%	95%
Pregnancy Care					
Inpatient Neonatal Mortality	-	-	-	-	-
Third or Fourth Degree Laceration	-	-	2.62%	3.63%	3.27%

Saint John Oakland Hospital

Alternate Name: Oakland Saint John Health System Hospital
27351 Dequindre Road
Madison Heights, MI 48071
Toll-Free: 800-789-6334
Phone: 248-967-7000
Fax: 248-967-7794
URL: www.stjohn.org/oakland
Ownership: Voluntary non-profit - Other
Emergency Services: Yes
Accredited: Yes
Licensed Beds: 261

Key Personnel:
CEO . . . . Robert A Deputat
Chief of Medical Staff . . . . Gary Gerg
Emergency Room . . . . Robert Takla
Emergency Room . . . . Cherri Barnett, RN
Director Medical/Surgical Nursing . . . . Beverly Fletcher
Chief Radiology . . . . Charles Feinman, DO
Director Respiratory Therapy . . . . Jim Youngblood

Measure	Cases	This Hospital	State Average	U.S. Average	Top Hospital
Heart Attack Care					
ACE Inhibitor or ARB for LVSD[1]	6	67%	86%	82%	100%
Aspirin at Arrival	47	98%	95%	92%	100%
Aspirin at Discharge[1]	24	100%	94%	90%	100%
Beta Blocker at Arrival	38	97%	90%	87%	100%
Beta Blocker at Discharge	25	96%	93%	90%	100%
Fibrinolytic Medication Timing	0	-	28%	31%	100%
PCI Within 90 Minutes of Arrival	0	-	59%	54%	95%
Smoking Cessation Advice[1]	3	100%	93%	88%	100%
Heart Failure Care					
ACE Inhibitor or ARB for LVSD	127	98%	84%	82%	100%
Discharge Instructions	276	84%	73%	61%	93%
Evaluation of LVS Function	306	100%	91%	83%	99%
Smoking Cessation Advice	70	93%	86%	82%	100%
Pneumonia Care					
Appropriate Initial Antibiotic	75	93%	88%	83%	94%
Blood Culture Timing	124	97%	90%	90%	100%
Influenza Vaccine	25	24%	73%	70%	100%
Initial Antibiotic Timing	137	92%	84%	80%	93%
Oxygenation Assessment	175	100%	100%	99%	100%
Pneumococcal Vaccine	89	54%	72%	69%	94%
Smoking Cessation Advice	53	92%	86%	80%	100%
Surgical Infection Prevention					
Prophylactic Antibiotic Given[2,3]	107	93%	82%	77%	95%
Prophylactic Antibiotic Selection[2]	36	97%	93%	90%	100%
Prophylactic Antibiotic Stopped[2,3]	100	92%	83%	72%	95%
Pregnancy Care					
Inpatient Neonatal Mortality	-	-	-	-	-
Third or Fourth Degree Laceration	-	-	2.62%	3.63%	3.27%

West Shore Medical Center

Alternate Name: West Shore Hospital

NOTE: Hospital profiles are in alphabetical order by state, then city, then hospital within the city; Rankings are sorted by rate in descending order and exclude hospitals with less than 25 cases; (1) The number of cases is too small (n<25) for purposes of reliably predicting hospital performance; (2) Measure reflects the hospital's indication that its submission was based upon a sample of its relevant discharges; (3) Rate reflects fewer than the maximum possible quarters of data for the measure; (4) Inaccurate information submitted and suppressed for one or more quarters; (5) No data is available from the hospital for this measure; Please refer to the User's Guide for a full explanation of data

1465 E Parkdale Avenue
Manistee, MI 49660
URL: www.westshoremedcenter.org
Ownership: Proprietary
Emergency Services: Yes
Phone: 231-398-1000
Fax: 231-398-1098
Accredited: No

Key Personnel:
President . . . . Burton Parks
Manager Surgical Services . . . . Lori Schumacker

Measure	Cases	This Hospital	State Average	U.S. Average	Top Hospital
Heart Attack Care					
ACE Inhibitor or ARB for LVSD[1]	1	100%	86%	82%	100%
Aspirin at Arrival[1]	8	75%	95%	92%	100%
Aspirin at Discharge[1]	4	100%	94%	90%	100%
Beta Blocker at Arrival[1]	9	44%	90%	87%	100%
Beta Blocker at Discharge[1]	7	100%	93%	90%	100%
Fibrinolytic Medication Timing	0	-	28%	31%	100%
PCI Within 90 Minutes of Arrival	0	-	59%	54%	95%
Smoking Cessation Advice	0	-	93%	88%	100%
Heart Failure Care					
ACE Inhibitor or ARB for LVSD[1]	10	50%	84%	82%	100%
Discharge Instructions	32	75%	73%	61%	93%
Evaluation of LVS Function	46	72%	91%	83%	99%
Smoking Cessation Advice[1]	8	75%	86%	82%	100%
Pneumonia Care					
Appropriate Initial Antibiotic	76	95%	88%	83%	94%
Blood Culture Timing	62	95%	90%	90%	100%
Influenza Vaccine[1]	18	6%	73%	70%	100%
Initial Antibiotic Timing	90	93%	84%	80%	93%
Oxygenation Assessment	125	100%	100%	99%	100%
Pneumococcal Vaccine	80	20%	72%	69%	94%
Smoking Cessation Advice	35	86%	86%	80%	100%
Surgical Infection Prevention					
Prophylactic Antibiotic Given	106	86%	82%	77%	95%
Prophylactic Antibiotic Selection	31	97%	93%	90%	100%
Prophylactic Antibiotic Stopped	101	73%	83%	72%	95%
Pregnancy Care					
Inpatient Neonatal Mortality	-	-	-	-	-
Third or Fourth Degree Laceration	-	-	2.62%	3.63%	3.27%

Marlette Community Hospital

2770 Main Street
PO Box 307
Marlette, MI 48453
URL: www.marlettecommunityhospital.com
Ownership: Voluntary non-profit - Private
Emergency Services: Yes
Phone: 989-635-4000
Fax: 989-635-4027
Accredited: No
Licensed Beds: 97

Key Personnel:
Administrator/CEO . . . . David S McEwen
Chief Medical Staff . . . . William Starbird, MD
Manager Medical/Surgical Nursing . . . . Karen Bush
Director Respiratory Therapy . . . . Katrina Fritz

Measure	Cases	This Hospital	State Average	U.S. Average	Top Hospital
Heart Attack Care					
ACE Inhibitor or ARB for LVSD[3]	0	-	86%	82%	100%
Aspirin at Arrival[1,3]	3	67%	95%	92%	100%
Aspirin at Discharge[3]	0	-	94%	90%	100%
Beta Blocker at Arrival[1,3]	3	0%	90%	87%	100%
Beta Blocker at Discharge[3]	0	-	93%	90%	100%
Fibrinolytic Medication Timing[3]	0	-	28%	31%	100%
PCI Within 90 Minutes of Arrival[5]	-	-	59%	54%	95%
Smoking Cessation Advice[3]	0	-	93%	88%	100%
Heart Failure Care					
ACE Inhibitor or ARB for LVSD[1]	1	100%	84%	82%	100%
Discharge Instructions	25	68%	73%	61%	93%
Evaluation of LVS Function	26	62%	91%	83%	99%
Smoking Cessation Advice[1]	1	0%	86%	82%	100%
Pneumonia Care					
Appropriate Initial Antibiotic	30	87%	88%	83%	94%
Blood Culture Timing[1]	14	100%	90%	90%	100%
Influenza Vaccine[1]	7	43%	73%	70%	100%
Initial Antibiotic Timing[1]	23	74%	84%	80%	93%
Oxygenation Assessment	33	100%	100%	99%	100%
Pneumococcal Vaccine[1]	22	27%	72%	69%	94%
Smoking Cessation Advice[1]	4	100%	86%	80%	100%
Surgical Infection Prevention					
Prophylactic Antibiotic Given[3]	41	54%	82%	77%	95%
Prophylactic Antibiotic Selection[1]	15	93%	93%	90%	100%
Prophylactic Antibiotic Stopped[3]	40	95%	83%	72%	95%
Pregnancy Care					
Inpatient Neonatal Mortality	-	-	-	-	-
Third or Fourth Degree Laceration	-	-	2.62%	3.63%	3.27%

Marquette General Hospital

580 W College Avenue
Marquette, MI 49855
URL: www.mgh.org
Ownership: Voluntary non-profit - Private
Emergency Services: Yes
Phone: 906-228-9440
Fax: 906-225-3098
Accredited: Yes
Licensed Beds: 352

Key Personnel:
CEO . . . . Bill Nemacheck
Chief Medical Staff . . . . Dr Ken Davenport
Surgical Nurse . . . . Joanne Gwinn

Measure	Cases	This Hospital	State Average	U.S. Average	Top Hospital
Heart Attack Care					
ACE Inhibitor or ARB for LVSD	58	86%	86%	82%	100%
Aspirin at Arrival	92	99%	95%	92%	100%
Aspirin at Discharge	297	98%	94%	90%	100%
Beta Blocker at Arrival	65	88%	90%	87%	100%
Beta Blocker at Discharge	301	96%	93%	90%	100%
Fibrinolytic Medication Timing[1]	1	100%	28%	31%	100%
PCI Within 90 Minutes of Arrival[1]	4	0%	59%	54%	95%
Smoking Cessation Advice	112	99%	93%	88%	100%
Heart Failure Care					
ACE Inhibitor or ARB for LVSD	68	84%	84%	82%	100%
Discharge Instructions	145	73%	73%	61%	93%
Evaluation of LVS Function	168	95%	91%	83%	99%
Smoking Cessation Advice[1]	20	100%	86%	82%	100%
Pneumonia Care					
Appropriate Initial Antibiotic	83	90%	88%	83%	94%
Blood Culture Timing	92	100%	90%	90%	100%
Influenza Vaccine[1]	21	48%	73%	70%	100%
Initial Antibiotic Timing	133	79%	84%	80%	93%
Oxygenation Assessment	168	99%	100%	99%	100%
Pneumococcal Vaccine	111	54%	72%	69%	94%
Smoking Cessation Advice	54	100%	86%	80%	100%
Surgical Infection Prevention					
Prophylactic Antibiotic Given[2,3]	211	89%	82%	77%	95%
Prophylactic Antibiotic Selection[2]	67	96%	93%	90%	100%
Prophylactic Antibiotic Stopped[2,3]	206	54%	83%	72%	95%
Pregnancy Care					
Inpatient Neonatal Mortality	888	0.45%	-	-	-
Third or Fourth Degree Laceration	545	6.97%	2.62%	3.63%	3.27%

Oaklawn Hospital

200 N Madison Avenue
Marshall, MI 49068
URL: www.oaklawnhospital.org
Ownership: Voluntary non-profit - Other
Emergency Services: Yes
Phone: 269-781-4271
Fax: 269-781-7117
Accredited: Yes
Licensed Beds: 94

Key Personnel:
Administrator . . . . Rob Covert
Chief Medical Staff . . . . George Seifert, MD
Emergency Room . . . . David Komasara, MD
Director Infection/Disease Control . . . . Pat Jendryka, RN
Director Medical/Surgical Nursing . . . . Jody Wade, RN
OB/GYN Womens Health . . . . Neyca Bartlett, MD
Chief Radiology . . . . Rick Johnson, RRT
Director of Respiratory . . . . Alcides Gill, MD

Measure	Cases	This Hospital	State Average	U.S. Average	Top Hospital
Heart Attack Care					
ACE Inhibitor or ARB for LVSD	0	-	86%	82%	100%
Aspirin at Arrival[1]	10	100%	95%	92%	100%

NOTE: Hospital profiles are in alphabetical order by state, then city, then hospital within the city; Rankings are sorted by rate in descending order and exclude hospitals with less than 25 cases; (1) The number of cases is too small (n<25) for purposes of reliably predicting hospital performance; (2) Measure reflects the hospital's indication that its submission was based upon a sample of its relevant discharges; (3) Rate reflects fewer than the maximum possible quarters of data for the measure; (4) Inaccurate information submitted and suppressed for one or more quarters; (5) No data is available from the hospital for this measure; Please refer to the User's Guide for a full explanation of data

Measure	Cases	This Hospital	State Average	U.S. Average	Top Hospital
Aspirin at Discharge[1]	9	89%	94%	90%	100%
Beta Blocker at Arrival[1]	8	100%	90%	87%	100%
Beta Blocker at Discharge[1]	10	90%	93%	90%	100%
Fibrinolytic Medication Timing	0	-	28%	31%	100%
PCI Within 90 Minutes of Arrival	0	-	59%	54%	95%
Smoking Cessation Advice[1]	1	100%	93%	88%	100%
Heart Failure Care					
ACE Inhibitor or ARB for LVSD	33	94%	84%	82%	100%
Discharge Instructions	78	87%	73%	61%	93%
Evaluation of LVS Function	92	97%	91%	83%	99%
Smoking Cessation Advice[1]	13	100%	86%	82%	100%
Pneumonia Care					
Appropriate Initial Antibiotic	96	96%	88%	83%	94%
Blood Culture Timing	109	96%	90%	90%	100%
Influenza Vaccine	27	93%	73%	70%	100%
Initial Antibiotic Timing	146	94%	84%	80%	93%
Oxygenation Assessment	173	99%	100%	99%	100%
Pneumococcal Vaccine	116	93%	72%	69%	94%
Smoking Cessation Advice	44	93%	86%	80%	100%
Surgical Infection Prevention					
Prophylactic Antibiotic Given[2]	371	93%	82%	77%	95%
Prophylactic Antibiotic Selection[2]	110	99%	93%	90%	100%
Prophylactic Antibiotic Stopped[2]	362	95%	83%	72%	95%
Pregnancy Care					
Inpatient Neonatal Mortality	-	-	-	-	-
Third or Fourth Degree Laceration	-	-	2.62%	3.63%	3.27%

MidMichigan Medical Center

4005 Orchard Drive
Midland, MI 48670
Phone: 989-839-3000
Fax: 989-839-3307
URL: www.midmichigan.org
Ownership: Voluntary non-profit - Other
Accredited: Yes
Emergency Services: Yes
Licensed Beds: 250

Key Personnel:

CEO/President . . . . Rick Reynolds
Chief Medical Staff . . . . Walter Gruber, MD
Head of Emergency Room . . . . Diane Nold
Director Infection/Disease Control . . . . Brenda Dauer, RN
Chief OB/GYN . . . . Margie Kuhn, MD
Chief Radiology . . . . Rajnikant Mehta, MD
Manager Respiratory Therapy . . . . Carole Blahunka

Measure	Cases	This Hospital	State Average	U.S. Average	Top Hospital
Heart Attack Care					
ACE Inhibitor or ARB for LVSD[1]	24	88%	86%	82%	100%
Aspirin at Arrival	132	97%	95%	92%	100%
Aspirin at Discharge	92	98%	94%	90%	100%
Beta Blocker at Arrival	122	97%	90%	87%	100%
Beta Blocker at Discharge	94	100%	93%	90%	100%
Fibrinolytic Medication Timing[1]	2	0%	28%	31%	100%
PCI Within 90 Minutes of Arrival[1]	2	100%	59%	54%	95%
Smoking Cessation Advice[1]	21	100%	93%	88%	100%
Heart Failure Care					
ACE Inhibitor or ARB for LVSD	81	81%	84%	82%	100%
Discharge Instructions	224	87%	73%	61%	93%
Evaluation of LVS Function	266	97%	91%	83%	99%
Smoking Cessation Advice	30	83%	86%	82%	100%
Pneumonia Care					
Appropriate Initial Antibiotic	141	91%	88%	83%	94%
Blood Culture Timing	188	96%	90%	90%	100%
Influenza Vaccine	43	88%	73%	70%	100%
Initial Antibiotic Timing	262	84%	84%	80%	93%
Oxygenation Assessment	304	100%	100%	99%	100%
Pneumococcal Vaccine	218	91%	72%	69%	94%
Smoking Cessation Advice	56	89%	86%	80%	100%
Surgical Infection Prevention					
Prophylactic Antibiotic Given[2,3]	722	89%	82%	77%	95%
Prophylactic Antibiotic Selection[2]	214	74%	93%	90%	100%
Prophylactic Antibiotic Stopped[2,3]	701	92%	83%	72%	95%
Pregnancy Care					
Inpatient Neonatal Mortality	-	-	-	-	-
Third or Fourth Degree Laceration	-	-	2.62%	3.63%	3.27%

Mercy Memorial Hospital System

718 N Macomb Street
Monroe, MI 48162
Phone: 734-240-8400
Fax: 734-241-0032
URL: www.mercymemorial.org
Ownership: Voluntary non-profit - Other
Accredited: Yes
Emergency Services: Yes
Licensed Beds: 238

Key Personnel:

President/CEO . . . . Daniel L Wakeman
Cardiology . . . . David Rhodes
Emergency Room . . . . Lynn Lohner

Measure	Cases	This Hospital	State Average	U.S. Average	Top Hospital
Heart Attack Care					
ACE Inhibitor or ARB for LVSD[1]	16	62%	86%	82%	100%
Aspirin at Arrival	126	95%	95%	92%	100%
Aspirin at Discharge	47	89%	94%	90%	100%
Beta Blocker at Arrival	88	93%	90%	87%	100%
Beta Blocker at Discharge	55	95%	93%	90%	100%
Fibrinolytic Medication Timing[1]	6	33%	28%	31%	100%
PCI Within 90 Minutes of Arrival	0	-	59%	54%	95%
Smoking Cessation Advice[1]	6	67%	93%	88%	100%
Heart Failure Care					
ACE Inhibitor or ARB for LVSD	114	82%	84%	82%	100%
Discharge Instructions	338	66%	73%	61%	93%
Evaluation of LVS Function	438	84%	91%	83%	99%
Smoking Cessation Advice	69	90%	86%	82%	100%
Pneumonia Care					
Appropriate Initial Antibiotic	192	85%	88%	83%	94%
Blood Culture Timing	186	96%	90%	90%	100%
Influenza Vaccine	45	73%	73%	70%	100%
Initial Antibiotic Timing	231	79%	84%	80%	93%
Oxygenation Assessment	326	100%	100%	99%	100%
Pneumococcal Vaccine	166	80%	72%	69%	94%
Smoking Cessation Advice	97	85%	86%	80%	100%
Surgical Infection Prevention					
Prophylactic Antibiotic Given[2]	551	80%	82%	77%	95%
Prophylactic Antibiotic Selection[2]	146	92%	93%	90%	100%
Prophylactic Antibiotic Stopped[2]	533	77%	83%	72%	95%
Pregnancy Care					
Inpatient Neonatal Mortality	-	-	-	-	-
Third or Fourth Degree Laceration	-	-	2.62%	3.63%	3.27%

Mount Clemens Regional Medical Center

1000 Harrington Boulevard
Mount Clemens, MI 48043
Toll-Free: 800-779-7178
Phone: 586-493-8000
Fax: 586-741-4179
URL: www.mcrmc.org
Ownership: Voluntary non-profit - Other
Accredited: Yes
Emergency Services: Yes
Licensed Beds: 288

Key Personnel:

CEO . . . . Robert Milewski
Chief Medical Staff . . . . Michael Tawney, DO
Emergency Room . . . . Sue Durst, RN
Medical/Surgical Nursing . . . . Joan Simon
Chief Radiology . . . . Michele Blair, DO
Director Respiratory Therapy . . . . Linda Zimcosky

Measure	Cases	This Hospital	State Average	U.S. Average	Top Hospital
Heart Attack Care					
ACE Inhibitor or ARB for LVSD	65	69%	86%	82%	100%
Aspirin at Arrival	173	98%	95%	92%	100%
Aspirin at Discharge	143	97%	94%	90%	100%
Beta Blocker at Arrival	122	96%	90%	87%	100%
Beta Blocker at Discharge	168	97%	93%	90%	100%
Fibrinolytic Medication Timing	0	-	28%	31%	100%
PCI Within 90 Minutes of Arrival[1]	7	57%	59%	54%	95%
Smoking Cessation Advice	77	95%	93%	88%	100%
Heart Failure Care					
ACE Inhibitor or ARB for LVSD[2]	251	79%	84%	82%	100%
Discharge Instructions[2]	420	69%	73%	61%	93%
Evaluation of LVS Function[2]	488	98%	91%	83%	99%
Smoking Cessation Advice[2]	79	100%	86%	82%	100%
Pneumonia Care					

NOTE: Hospital profiles are in alphabetical order by state, then city, then hospital within the city; Rankings are sorted by rate in descending order and exclude hospitals with less than 25 cases; (1) The number of cases is too small (n<25) for purposes of reliably predicting hospital performance; (2) Measure reflects the hospital's indication that its submission was based upon a sample of its relevant discharges; (3) Rate reflects fewer than the maximum possible quarters of data for the measure; (4) Inaccurate information submitted and suppressed for one or more quarters; (5) No data is available from the hospital for this measure; Please refer to the User's Guide for a full explanation of data

Appropriate Initial Antibiotic[2]	154	91%	88%	83%	94%
Blood Culture Timing[2]	184	94%	90%	90%	100%
Influenza Vaccine	46	89%	73%	70%	100%
Initial Antibiotic Timing[2]	187	75%	84%	80%	93%
Oxygenation Assessment[2]	260	100%	100%	99%	100%
Pneumococcal Vaccine[2]	156	80%	72%	69%	94%
Smoking Cessation Advice[2]	76	95%	86%	80%	100%
Surgical Infection Prevention					
Prophylactic Antibiotic Given[2]	723	80%	82%	77%	95%
Prophylactic Antibiotic Selection[2]	175	88%	93%	90%	100%
Prophylactic Antibiotic Stopped[2]	698	70%	83%	72%	95%
Pregnancy Care					
Inpatient Neonatal Mortality	-	-	-	-	-
Third or Fourth Degree Laceration	-	-	2.62%	3.63%	3.27%

Central Michigan Community Hospital

1221 S Drive
Mount Pleasant, MI 48858
Phone: 989-772-6700
Fax: 989-772-1150
E-mail: mbousley@voyager.net
URL: www.cmch.org
Ownership: Voluntary non-profit - Other
Accredited: Yes
Emergency Services: Yes
Licensed Beds: 137

Key Personnel:

President/CEO . . . . Roger Kerr

Measure	Cases	This Hospital	State Average	U.S. Average	Top Hospital
Heart Attack Care					
ACE Inhibitor or ARB for LVSD[1]	4	100%	86%	82%	100%
Aspirin at Arrival	35	97%	95%	92%	100%
Aspirin at Discharge[1]	20	100%	94%	90%	100%
Beta Blocker at Arrival	36	86%	90%	87%	100%
Beta Blocker at Discharge[1]	22	82%	93%	90%	100%
Fibrinolytic Medication Timing[1]	4	50%	28%	31%	100%
PCI Within 90 Minutes of Arrival	0	-	59%	54%	95%
Smoking Cessation Advice[1]	8	50%	93%	88%	100%
Heart Failure Care					
ACE Inhibitor or ARB for LVSD	34	88%	84%	82%	100%
Discharge Instructions	103	90%	73%	61%	93%
Evaluation of LVS Function	141	94%	91%	83%	99%
Smoking Cessation Advice	27	93%	86%	82%	100%
Pneumonia Care					
Appropriate Initial Antibiotic	101	87%	88%	83%	94%
Blood Culture Timing	87	95%	90%	90%	100%
Influenza Vaccine[1]	21	86%	73%	70%	100%
Initial Antibiotic Timing	139	81%	84%	80%	93%
Oxygenation Assessment	172	100%	100%	99%	100%
Pneumococcal Vaccine	94	93%	72%	69%	94%
Smoking Cessation Advice	51	96%	86%	80%	100%
Surgical Infection Prevention					
Prophylactic Antibiotic Given	278	91%	82%	77%	95%
Prophylactic Antibiotic Selection	72	97%	93%	90%	100%
Prophylactic Antibiotic Stopped	275	89%	83%	72%	95%
Pregnancy Care					
Inpatient Neonatal Mortality	-	-	-	-	-
Third or Fourth Degree Laceration	-	-	2.62%	3.63%	3.27%

Hackley Hospital

1700 Clinton Street
Muskegon, MI 49442
Toll-Free: 800-825-4677
Phone: 231-726-3511
Fax: 231-726-2232
URL: www.hackley.org
Ownership: Voluntary non-profit - Private
Accredited: Yes
Emergency Services: Yes
Licensed Beds: 181

Key Personnel:

CEO . . . . Gordon A Mudler
Chief Medical Staff . . . . Herbert Miller, MD
OB/GYN Womens Health . . . . Thomas Yetman, DO
Director Respiratory Therapy . . . . Jane Otrhalek

Measure	Cases	This Hospital	State Average	U.S. Average	Top Hospital
Heart Attack Care					
ACE Inhibitor or ARB for LVSD[1]	8	100%	86%	82%	100%
Aspirin at Arrival	62	100%	95%	92%	100%
Aspirin at Discharge	28	96%	94%	90%	100%
Beta Blocker at Arrival	61	98%	90%	87%	100%
Beta Blocker at Discharge	26	96%	93%	90%	100%
Fibrinolytic Medication Timing	0	-	28%	31%	100%
PCI Within 90 Minutes of Arrival	0	-	59%	54%	95%
Smoking Cessation Advice[1]	2	100%	93%	88%	100%
Heart Failure Care					
ACE Inhibitor or ARB for LVSD	48	96%	84%	82%	100%
Discharge Instructions	121	83%	73%	61%	93%
Evaluation of LVS Function	153	97%	91%	83%	99%
Smoking Cessation Advice[1]	22	91%	86%	82%	100%
Pneumonia Care					
Appropriate Initial Antibiotic	119	87%	88%	83%	94%
Blood Culture Timing	94	86%	90%	90%	100%
Influenza Vaccine[4,5]	-	-	73%	70%	100%
Initial Antibiotic Timing	127	96%	84%	80%	93%
Oxygenation Assessment	175	100%	100%	99%	100%
Pneumococcal Vaccine	109	94%	72%	69%	94%
Smoking Cessation Advice	39	95%	86%	80%	100%
Surgical Infection Prevention					
Prophylactic Antibiotic Given[3]	466	91%	82%	77%	95%
Prophylactic Antibiotic Selection	161	97%	93%	90%	100%
Prophylactic Antibiotic Stopped[3]	457	91%	83%	72%	95%
Pregnancy Care					
Inpatient Neonatal Mortality	-	-	-	-	-
Third or Fourth Degree Laceration	-	-	2.62%	3.63%	3.27%

Mercy General Health Partners

Alternate Name: MGHP
1500 E Sherman Boulevard
Muskegon, MI 49444
Phone: 231-672-2000
Fax: 231-672-3854
URL: www.mghp.com
Ownership: Voluntary non-profit - Other
Accredited: Yes
Emergency Services: Yes
Licensed Beds: 282

Key Personnel:

President/CEO . . . . Roger W Spoelman
VP/Chief Medical Officer . . . . F Remington Sprague, MD
Cardiac Lab . . . . Leon Conklin
Manager Catheterization Lab . . . . Carol Robinson
Infection Control . . . . Kurt Atton
ICU . . . . Jill VanLente
Intensive Coronary Care . . . . Rick Denaie
Director Medical/Surgical Services . . . . Kim Maguire
Director Women's/Children's Services . . . . Elaine Skinner
Executive Director . . . . Linda Bailey
Respiratory/Cardio-Pulmonary Services . . . . Leon Conklin

Measure	Cases	This Hospital	State Average	U.S. Average	Top Hospital
Heart Attack Care					
ACE Inhibitor or ARB for LVSD	126	94%	86%	82%	100%
Aspirin at Arrival	229	100%	95%	92%	100%
Aspirin at Discharge	406	100%	94%	90%	100%
Beta Blocker at Arrival	187	99%	90%	87%	100%
Beta Blocker at Discharge	406	99%	93%	90%	100%
Fibrinolytic Medication Timing[3]	0	-	28%	31%	100%
PCI Within 90 Minutes of Arrival[1]	15	27%	59%	54%	95%
Smoking Cessation Advice[3]	36	100%	93%	88%	100%
Heart Failure Care					
ACE Inhibitor or ARB for LVSD	100	91%	84%	82%	100%
Discharge Instructions[3]	75	77%	73%	61%	93%
Evaluation of LVS Function	306	98%	91%	83%	99%
Smoking Cessation Advice[1,3]	18	100%	86%	82%	100%
Pneumonia Care					
Appropriate Initial Antibiotic[1,3]	13	100%	88%	83%	94%
Blood Culture Timing[3]	29	100%	90%	90%	100%
Influenza Vaccine[5]	-	-	73%	70%	100%
Initial Antibiotic Timing	150	84%	84%	80%	93%
Oxygenation Assessment	195	100%	100%	99%	100%
Pneumococcal Vaccine	111	81%	72%	69%	94%
Smoking Cessation Advice[1,3]	6	100%	86%	80%	100%
Surgical Infection Prevention					
Prophylactic Antibiotic Given[2,3]	199	83%	82%	77%	95%

NOTE: Hospital profiles are in alphabetical order by state, then city, then hospital within the city; Rankings are sorted by rate in descending order and exclude hospitals with less than 25 cases; (1) The number of cases is too small (n<25) for purposes of reliably predicting hospital performance; (2) Measure reflects the hospital's indication that its submission was based upon a sample of its relevant discharges; (3) Rate reflects fewer than the maximum possible quarters of data for the measure; (4) Inaccurate information submitted and suppressed for one or more quarters; (5) No data is available from the hospital for this measure; Please refer to the User's Guide for a full explanation of data

Measure	Cases	This Hospital	State Average	U.S. Average	Top Hospital
Prophylactic Antibiotic Selection[5]	-	-	93%	90%	100%
Prophylactic Antibiotic Stopped[2,3]	193	80%	83%	72%	95%
Pregnancy Care					
Inpatient Neonatal Mortality	-	-	-	-	-
Third or Fourth Degree Laceration	-	-	2.62%	3.63%	3.27%

Memorial Healthcare Center

Alternate Name: Memorial Hospital
826 W King Street
Owosso, MI 48867

Toll-Free: 800-206-8706
Phone: 989-723-5211
Fax: 989-725-8937

URL: www.memorialhealthcare.org
Ownership: Voluntary non-profit - Other
Emergency Services: Yes

Accredited: Yes
Licensed Beds: 143

Key Personnel:
President . . . . Cheryl Peterson
Chief Medical Staff. . . . . Michael Schmidt, DO
Cardiac Laboratory. . . . . Kathy Whal
Manager Emergency Room . . . . Vicki Watkins
Infection Control. . . . . Lynn Howes
OB/GYN Womens Health. . . . . Janet Johnston
Director Radiology . . . . Marge Thompson
Respiratory Therapy. . . . . Doug Rowden

Measure	Cases	This Hospital	State Average	U.S. Average	Top Hospital
Heart Attack Care					
ACE Inhibitor or ARB for LVSD[1]	4	100%	86%	82%	100%
Aspirin at Arrival	34	88%	95%	92%	100%
Aspirin at Discharge[1]	19	95%	94%	90%	100%
Beta Blocker at Arrival[1]	23	87%	90%	87%	100%
Beta Blocker at Discharge[1]	19	89%	93%	90%	100%
Fibrinolytic Medication Timing[1]	1	0%	28%	31%	100%
PCI Within 90 Minutes of Arrival	0	-	59%	54%	95%
Smoking Cessation Advice[1]	4	75%	93%	88%	100%
Heart Failure Care					
ACE Inhibitor or ARB for LVSD	39	74%	84%	82%	100%
Discharge Instructions	88	82%	73%	61%	93%
Evaluation of LVS Function	113	88%	91%	83%	99%
Smoking Cessation Advice[1]	14	64%	86%	82%	100%
Pneumonia Care					
Appropriate Initial Antibiotic	121	79%	88%	83%	94%
Blood Culture Timing	76	82%	90%	90%	100%
Influenza Vaccine[1]	22	91%	73%	70%	100%
Initial Antibiotic Timing	136	75%	84%	80%	93%
Oxygenation Assessment	166	100%	100%	99%	100%
Pneumococcal Vaccine	92	93%	72%	69%	94%
Smoking Cessation Advice	37	86%	86%	80%	100%
Surgical Infection Prevention					
Prophylactic Antibiotic Given[2,3]	238	89%	82%	77%	95%
Prophylactic Antibiotic Selection[2]	72	93%	93%	90%	100%
Prophylactic Antibiotic Stopped[2,3]	222	77%	83%	72%	95%
Pregnancy Care					
Inpatient Neonatal Mortality	-	-	-	-	-
Third or Fourth Degree Laceration	-	-	2.62%	3.63%	3.27%

Northern Michigan Hospital

416 Connable Avenue
Petoskey, MI 49770
URL: www.northernhealth.org
Ownership: Voluntary non-profit - Other
Emergency Services: Yes

Phone: 231-487-4000
Fax: 231-487-7798

Accredited: Yes
Licensed Beds: 243

Key Personnel:
President/CEO. . . . . Thomas Mroczkowski
Director Respiratory Therapy . . . . Mick Stoddard

Measure	Cases	This Hospital	State Average	U.S. Average	Top Hospital
Heart Attack Care					
ACE Inhibitor or ARB for LVSD	61	85%	86%	82%	100%
Aspirin at Arrival	95	98%	95%	92%	100%
Aspirin at Discharge	253	100%	94%	90%	100%
Beta Blocker at Arrival	76	96%	90%	87%	100%
Beta Blocker at Discharge	304	99%	93%	90%	100%
Fibrinolytic Medication Timing	0	-	28%	31%	100%
PCI Within 90 Minutes of Arrival[1]	5	60%	59%	54%	95%
Smoking Cessation Advice	112	100%	93%	88%	100%
Heart Failure Care					
ACE Inhibitor or ARB for LVSD	105	91%	84%	82%	100%
Discharge Instructions	217	79%	73%	61%	93%
Evaluation of LVS Function	236	93%	91%	83%	99%
Smoking Cessation Advice	37	97%	86%	82%	100%
Pneumonia Care					
Appropriate Initial Antibiotic	67	85%	88%	83%	94%
Blood Culture Timing	73	96%	90%	90%	100%
Influenza Vaccine[1]	12	100%	73%	70%	100%
Initial Antibiotic Timing	96	88%	84%	80%	93%
Oxygenation Assessment	122	100%	100%	99%	100%
Pneumococcal Vaccine	84	80%	72%	69%	94%
Smoking Cessation Advice[1]	24	33%	86%	80%	100%
Surgical Infection Prevention					
Prophylactic Antibiotic Given[2,3]	192	71%	82%	77%	95%
Prophylactic Antibiotic Selection[2]	67	97%	93%	90%	100%
Prophylactic Antibiotic Stopped[2,3]	196	82%	83%	72%	95%
Pregnancy Care					
Inpatient Neonatal Mortality	-	-	-	-	-
Third or Fourth Degree Laceration	-	-	2.62%	3.63%	3.27%

North Oakland Medical Center

Alternate Name: Pontiac General Hospital
461 W Huron
Pontiac, MI 48341
URL: www.nomc.org
Ownership: Voluntary non-profit - Private
Emergency Services: Yes

Phone: 248-857-7200
Fax: 248-857-6801

Accredited: Yes
Licensed Beds: 380

Key Personnel:
CEO/President. . . . . Robert Davis
Chief of Medical Staff. Bruce Lessien
Emergency Room . . . . Derrek McCallmont, MD
Director Infection/Disease Control . . . . Luretta Pandya, RN
OB/GYN Womens Health. . . . . W Hill
Director Respiratory Therapy . . . . Eliezer Basse

Measure	Cases	This Hospital	State Average	U.S. Average	Top Hospital
Heart Attack Care					
ACE Inhibitor or ARB for LVSD[1]	1	100%	86%	82%	100%
Aspirin at Arrival	31	100%	95%	92%	100%
Aspirin at Discharge[1]	11	100%	94%	90%	100%
Beta Blocker at Arrival	25	100%	90%	87%	100%
Beta Blocker at Discharge[1]	8	100%	93%	90%	100%
Fibrinolytic Medication Timing[3]	0	-	28%	31%	100%
PCI Within 90 Minutes of Arrival	0	-	59%	54%	95%
Smoking Cessation Advice[3]	0	-	93%	88%	100%
Heart Failure Care					
ACE Inhibitor or ARB for LVSD	63	86%	84%	82%	100%
Discharge Instructions[3]	40	80%	73%	61%	93%
Evaluation of LVS Function	221	96%	91%	83%	99%
Smoking Cessation Advice[1,3]	16	81%	86%	82%	100%
Pneumonia Care					
Appropriate Initial Antibiotic[1,3]	23	91%	88%	83%	94%
Blood Culture Timing[3]	25	88%	90%	90%	100%
Influenza Vaccine[5]	-	-	73%	70%	100%
Initial Antibiotic Timing	162	68%	84%	80%	93%
Oxygenation Assessment	193	99%	100%	99%	100%
Pneumococcal Vaccine	93	74%	72%	69%	94%
Smoking Cessation Advice[1,3]	7	100%	86%	80%	100%
Surgical Infection Prevention					
Prophylactic Antibiotic Given[2,3]	67	84%	82%	77%	95%
Prophylactic Antibiotic Selection[5]	-	-	93%	90%	100%
Prophylactic Antibiotic Stopped[2,3]	63	92%	83%	72%	95%
Pregnancy Care					
Inpatient Neonatal Mortality[2]	511	0.59%	-	-	-
Third or Fourth Degree Laceration[2]	982	3.97%	2.62%	3.63%	3.27%

POH Medical Center

Alternate Name: Pontiac Osteopathic Hospital

NOTE: Hospital profiles are in alphabetical order by state, then city, then hospital within the city; Rankings are sorted by rate in descending order and exclude hospitals with less than 25 cases; (1) The number of cases is too small (n<25) for purposes of reliably predicting hospital performance; (2) Measure reflects the hospital's indication that its submission was based upon a sample of its relevant discharges; (3) Rate reflects fewer than the maximum possible quarters of data for the measure; (4) Inaccurate information submitted and suppressed for one or more quarters; (5) No data is available from the hospital for this measure; Please refer to the User's Guide for a full explanation of data

50 N Perry Street
Pontiac, MI 48342
URL: www.pohmedical.org
Ownership: Voluntary non-profit - Other
Emergency Services: Yes
Phone: 248-338-5000
Fax: 248-338-5667
Accredited: Yes
Licensed Beds: 308

Key Personnel:
CEO. . . . . Patrick Lamberti
Chief Medical Staff. . . . . Steve Calkin
Chief Catheterization Laboratory . . . . John Q Dickey, Jr, DO
Head of Emergency Room. . . . . D Gardner
Director Infection/Disease Control . . . . MO Doyle, DO
Chief Radiology . . . . DA Kellam, DO
Director of Pulmonary/Respiratory . . . . John Rossertto

Measure	Cases	This Hospital	State Average	U.S. Average	Top Hospital
Heart Attack Care					
ACE Inhibitor or ARB for LVSD[1]	19	89%	86%	82%	100%
Aspirin at Arrival	71	94%	95%	92%	100%
Aspirin at Discharge	35	69%	94%	90%	100%
Beta Blocker at Arrival	69	91%	90%	87%	100%
Beta Blocker at Discharge	37	84%	93%	90%	100%
Fibrinolytic Medication Timing	0	-	28%	31%	100%
PCI Within 90 Minutes of Arrival	0	-	59%	54%	95%
Smoking Cessation Advice[1]	11	64%	93%	88%	100%
Heart Failure Care					
ACE Inhibitor or ARB for LVSD	131	73%	84%	82%	100%
Discharge Instructions	198	26%	73%	61%	93%
Evaluation of LVS Function	251	98%	91%	83%	99%
Smoking Cessation Advice	76	72%	86%	82%	100%
Pneumonia Care					
Appropriate Initial Antibiotic	122	95%	88%	83%	94%
Blood Culture Timing	112	47%	90%	90%	100%
Influenza Vaccine[1]	21	24%	73%	70%	100%
Initial Antibiotic Timing	150	89%	84%	80%	93%
Oxygenation Assessment	186	100%	100%	99%	100%
Pneumococcal Vaccine	69	42%	72%	69%	94%
Smoking Cessation Advice	82	77%	86%	80%	100%
Surgical Infection Prevention					
Prophylactic Antibiotic Given[2]	179	83%	82%	77%	95%
Prophylactic Antibiotic Selection[2]	39	92%	93%	90%	100%
Prophylactic Antibiotic Stopped[2]	166	70%	83%	72%	95%
Pregnancy Care					
Inpatient Neonatal Mortality	-	-	-	-	-
Third or Fourth Degree Laceration	-	-	2.62%	3.63%	3.27%

Saint Joseph Mercy Oakland

44405 Woodward Avenue
Pontiac, MI 48341
URL: www.stjoesoakland.org
Ownership: Voluntary non-profit - Church
Emergency Services: Yes
Phone: 248-858-3000
Fax: 248-858-3068
Accredited: Yes
Licensed Beds: 428

Key Personnel:
CEO/President. . . . . Jack Weiner
Chief Medical Staff. . . . . Herold Portnoy
Emergency Room . . . . Mery Jo Malafa
Emergency Room . . . . Thomas Petinga, DO
Director Infection/Disease Control . . . . Sue Fin
Chief Radiology . . . . Robert Steele, MD
Director Respiratory Therapy . . . . Marie Stock

Measure	Cases	This Hospital	State Average	U.S. Average	Top Hospital
Heart Attack Care					
ACE Inhibitor or ARB for LVSD	97	100%	86%	82%	100%
Aspirin at Arrival	280	100%	95%	92%	100%
Aspirin at Discharge	409	100%	94%	90%	100%
Beta Blocker at Arrival	248	99%	90%	87%	100%
Beta Blocker at Discharge	398	99%	93%	90%	100%
Fibrinolytic Medication Timing	0	-	28%	31%	100%
PCI Within 90 Minutes of Arrival[1]	9	78%	59%	54%	95%
Smoking Cessation Advice	136	100%	93%	88%	100%
Heart Failure Care					
ACE Inhibitor or ARB for LVSD	261	100%	84%	82%	100%
Discharge Instructions	585	87%	73%	61%	93%
Evaluation of LVS Function	685	100%	91%	83%	99%
Smoking Cessation Advice	105	100%	86%	82%	100%
Pneumonia Care					
Appropriate Initial Antibiotic	186	95%	88%	83%	94%
Blood Culture Timing	303	90%	90%	90%	100%
Influenza Vaccine	72	85%	73%	70%	100%
Initial Antibiotic Timing	380	86%	84%	80%	93%
Oxygenation Assessment	469	100%	100%	99%	100%
Pneumococcal Vaccine	293	84%	72%	69%	94%
Smoking Cessation Advice	124	90%	86%	80%	100%
Surgical Infection Prevention					
Prophylactic Antibiotic Given[2]	1,264	99%	82%	77%	95%
Prophylactic Antibiotic Selection[2]	312	99%	93%	90%	100%
Prophylactic Antibiotic Stopped[2]	1,175	95%	83%	72%	95%
Pregnancy Care					
Inpatient Neonatal Mortality	-	-	-	-	-
Third or Fourth Degree Laceration	-	-	2.62%	3.63%	3.27%

Mercy Hospital

2601 Electric Avenue
Port Huron, MI 48060
URL: www.mercyporthuron.com
Ownership: Voluntary non-profit - Church
Emergency Services: Yes
Phone: 810-985-1500
Fax: 810-985-1508
Accredited: Yes
Licensed Beds: 119

Key Personnel:
President/CEO. . . . . Peter Karadjoff
Emergency Room . . . . Jere Baldwin, MD
Director Infection/Disease Control . . . . D Heide

Measure	Cases	This Hospital	State Average	U.S. Average	Top Hospital
Heart Attack Care					
ACE Inhibitor or ARB for LVSD[1]	8	75%	86%	82%	100%
Aspirin at Arrival	37	95%	95%	92%	100%
Aspirin at Discharge[1]	20	80%	94%	90%	100%
Beta Blocker at Arrival	34	97%	90%	87%	100%
Beta Blocker at Discharge	25	88%	93%	90%	100%
Fibrinolytic Medication Timing[1]	1	0%	28%	31%	100%
PCI Within 90 Minutes of Arrival	0	-	59%	54%	95%
Smoking Cessation Advice[1]	5	100%	93%	88%	100%
Heart Failure Care					
ACE Inhibitor or ARB for LVSD	55	73%	84%	82%	100%
Discharge Instructions	162	93%	73%	61%	93%
Evaluation of LVS Function	193	95%	91%	83%	99%
Smoking Cessation Advice	36	100%	86%	82%	100%
Pneumonia Care					
Appropriate Initial Antibiotic	122	89%	88%	83%	94%
Blood Culture Timing	88	84%	90%	90%	100%
Influenza Vaccine	29	79%	73%	70%	100%
Initial Antibiotic Timing	151	81%	84%	80%	93%
Oxygenation Assessment	195	100%	100%	99%	100%
Pneumococcal Vaccine	118	69%	72%	69%	94%
Smoking Cessation Advice	55	98%	86%	80%	100%
Surgical Infection Prevention					
Prophylactic Antibiotic Given[3]	499	92%	82%	77%	95%
Prophylactic Antibiotic Selection	178	97%	93%	90%	100%
Prophylactic Antibiotic Stopped[3]	425	65%	83%	72%	95%
Pregnancy Care					
Inpatient Neonatal Mortality	-	-	-	-	-
Third or Fourth Degree Laceration	-	-	2.62%	3.63%	3.27%

Port Huron Hospital

1221 Pine Grove Avenue
Port Huron, MI 48060
E-mail: phhwebmaster@porthuronhosp.org
URL: www.porthuronhospital.org
Ownership: Voluntary non-profit - Other
Emergency Services: Yes
Phone: 810-987-5000
Fax: 810-985-2675
Accredited: Yes
Licensed Beds: 186

Key Personnel:
President/CEO. . . . . Brian M Connolly
Chief Medical Staff. . . . . Daniel Anceti, DO
Cardiac Lab . . . . Pat Roberts
Catheterization Lab . . . . Pat Roberts
Emergency Room . . . . Paul Britz

NOTE: Hospital profiles are in alphabetical order by state, then city, then hospital within the city; Rankings are sorted by rate in descending order and exclude hospitals with less than 25 cases; (1) The number of cases is too small (n<25) for purposes of reliably predicting hospital performance; (2) Measure reflects the hospital's indication that its submission was based upon a sample of its relevant discharges; (3) Rate reflects fewer than the maximum possible quarters of data for the measure; (4) Inaccurate information submitted and suppressed for one or more quarters; (5) No data is available from the hospital for this measure; Please refer to the User's Guide for a full explanation of data

Emergency Room . . . . Thabit Bahhur, MD
OB/GYN Womens Health. . . . . Kathy Smith
Respiratory/Cardiopulmonary. . . . . Chris Babcock

Measure	Cases	This Hospital	State Average	U.S. Average	Top Hospital
Heart Attack Care					
ACE Inhibitor or ARB for LVSD	52	85%	86%	82%	100%
Aspirin at Arrival	206	95%	95%	92%	100%
Aspirin at Discharge	289	97%	94%	90%	100%
Beta Blocker at Arrival	187	91%	90%	87%	100%
Beta Blocker at Discharge	291	98%	93%	90%	100%
Fibrinolytic Medication Timing	0	-	28%	31%	100%
PCI Within 90 Minutes of Arrival[1]	5	40%	59%	54%	95%
Smoking Cessation Advice	89	96%	93%	88%	100%
Heart Failure Care					
ACE Inhibitor or ARB for LVSD	127	89%	84%	82%	100%
Discharge Instructions	302	81%	73%	61%	93%
Evaluation of LVS Function	370	95%	91%	83%	99%
Smoking Cessation Advice	64	97%	86%	82%	100%
Pneumonia Care					
Appropriate Initial Antibiotic	215	93%	88%	83%	94%
Blood Culture Timing	162	93%	90%	90%	100%
Influenza Vaccine	49	76%	73%	70%	100%
Initial Antibiotic Timing	266	83%	84%	80%	93%
Oxygenation Assessment	318	100%	100%	99%	100%
Pneumococcal Vaccine	196	79%	72%	69%	94%
Smoking Cessation Advice	83	100%	86%	80%	100%
Surgical Infection Prevention					
Prophylactic Antibiotic Given	640	83%	82%	77%	95%
Prophylactic Antibiotic Selection	142	97%	93%	90%	100%
Prophylactic Antibiotic Stopped	624	86%	83%	72%	95%
Pregnancy Care					
Inpatient Neonatal Mortality	-	-	-	-	-
Third or Fourth Degree Laceration	-	-	2.62%	3.63%	3.27%

Spectrum Health-Reed City Campus

Alternate Name: Reed City Hospital
300 N Patterson Road
PO Box 75
Reed City, MI 49677
Phone: 231-832-3271
Fax: 231-832-1817
URL: www.spectrum-health.org
Ownership: Voluntary non-profit - Private
Accredited: Yes
Emergency Services: Yes
Licensed Beds: 106

Key Personnel:
CEO. . . . . Tom Kauffman

Measure	Cases	This Hospital	State Average	U.S. Average	Top Hospital
Heart Attack Care					
ACE Inhibitor or ARB for LVSD[1]	2	100%	86%	82%	100%
Aspirin at Arrival[1]	7	100%	95%	92%	100%
Aspirin at Discharge[1]	3	100%	94%	90%	100%
Beta Blocker at Arrival[1]	7	100%	90%	87%	100%
Beta Blocker at Discharge[1]	2	100%	93%	90%	100%
Fibrinolytic Medication Timing	0	-	28%	31%	100%
PCI Within 90 Minutes of Arrival	0	-	59%	54%	95%
Smoking Cessation Advice[1]	1	100%	93%	88%	100%
Heart Failure Care					
ACE Inhibitor or ARB for LVSD	28	89%	84%	82%	100%
Discharge Instructions	59	95%	73%	61%	93%
Evaluation of LVS Function	69	100%	91%	83%	99%
Smoking Cessation Advice[1]	14	100%	86%	82%	100%
Pneumonia Care					
Appropriate Initial Antibiotic	63	89%	88%	83%	94%
Blood Culture Timing	66	98%	90%	90%	100%
Influenza Vaccine[1]	13	92%	73%	70%	100%
Initial Antibiotic Timing	94	94%	84%	80%	93%
Oxygenation Assessment	99	100%	100%	99%	100%
Pneumococcal Vaccine	62	98%	72%	69%	94%
Smoking Cessation Advice	30	100%	86%	80%	100%
Surgical Infection Prevention					
Prophylactic Antibiotic Given	38	100%	82%	77%	95%
Prophylactic Antibiotic Selection[1]	8	100%	93%	90%	100%
Prophylactic Antibiotic Stopped	38	100%	83%	72%	95%
Pregnancy Care					
Inpatient Neonatal Mortality	-	-	-	-	-
Third or Fourth Degree Laceration	-	-	2.62%	3.63%	3.27%

Crittenton Hospital Medical Center

1101 W University Drive
Rochester, MI 48307
Phone: 248-652-5000
Fax: 248-650-0353
URL: www.crittenton.com
Ownership: Voluntary non-profit - Private
Accredited: Yes
Emergency Services: Yes
Licensed Beds: 290

Key Personnel:
President/CEO. . . . . Lynn C Orfgen
Chief Medical Staff. . . . . Bradford Merrelli, MD
Chief Medical Officer . . . . Frank D Sottile, MD

Measure	Cases	This Hospital	State Average	U.S. Average	Top Hospital
Heart Attack Care					
ACE Inhibitor or ARB for LVSD[1]	15	100%	86%	82%	100%
Aspirin at Arrival	90	98%	95%	92%	100%
Aspirin at Discharge	81	99%	94%	90%	100%
Beta Blocker at Arrival	68	91%	90%	87%	100%
Beta Blocker at Discharge	81	95%	93%	90%	100%
Fibrinolytic Medication Timing	0	-	28%	31%	100%
PCI Within 90 Minutes of Arrival[1]	3	67%	59%	54%	95%
Smoking Cessation Advice	26	100%	93%	88%	100%
Heart Failure Care					
ACE Inhibitor or ARB for LVSD	113	88%	84%	82%	100%
Discharge Instructions	281	67%	73%	61%	93%
Evaluation of LVS Function	343	98%	91%	83%	99%
Smoking Cessation Advice	42	98%	86%	82%	100%
Pneumonia Care					
Appropriate Initial Antibiotic	167	88%	88%	83%	94%
Blood Culture Timing	179	93%	90%	90%	100%
Influenza Vaccine	48	50%	73%	70%	100%
Initial Antibiotic Timing	225	84%	84%	80%	93%
Oxygenation Assessment	287	100%	100%	99%	100%
Pneumococcal Vaccine	212	42%	72%	69%	94%
Smoking Cessation Advice	43	95%	86%	80%	100%
Surgical Infection Prevention					
Prophylactic Antibiotic Given[2,3]	456	87%	82%	77%	95%
Prophylactic Antibiotic Selection[2]	148	97%	93%	90%	100%
Prophylactic Antibiotic Stopped[2,3]	447	78%	83%	72%	95%
Pregnancy Care					
Inpatient Neonatal Mortality	-	-	-	-	-
Third or Fourth Degree Laceration	-	-	2.62%	3.63%	3.27%

William Beaumont Hospital

3601 West Thirteen Mile Road
Royal Oak, MI 48073
Phone: 248-898-5000
Fax: 248-551-0854
URL: www.beaumonthospitals.com
Ownership: Proprietary
Accredited: No
Emergency Services: Yes
Licensed Beds: 997

Key Personnel:
President/CEO. . . . . Ted Wasson
Executive VP/Chief Medical Officer . . . . Ronald B Irwin, MD
Emergency Room . . . . Andrew Wilson, MD
Infection Control. . . . . Jeffrey Bond, MD

Measure	Cases	This Hospital	State Average	U.S. Average	Top Hospital
Heart Attack Care					
ACE Inhibitor or ARB for LVSD[2]	128	91%	86%	82%	100%
Aspirin at Arrival[2]	356	97%	95%	92%	100%
Aspirin at Discharge[2]	409	99%	94%	90%	100%
Beta Blocker at Arrival[2]	298	95%	90%	87%	100%
Beta Blocker at Discharge[2]	478	99%	93%	90%	100%
Fibrinolytic Medication Timing[2]	0	-	28%	31%	100%
PCI Within 90 Minutes of Arrival[1,2]	14	93%	59%	54%	95%
Smoking Cessation Advice[2]	163	99%	93%	88%	100%
Heart Failure Care					
ACE Inhibitor or ARB for LVSD[2]	225	93%	84%	82%	100%
Discharge Instructions[2]	476	64%	73%	61%	93%

NOTE: Hospital profiles are in alphabetical order by state, then city, then hospital within the city; Rankings are sorted by rate in descending order and exclude hospitals with less than 25 cases; (1) The number of cases is too small (n<25) for purposes of reliably predicting hospital performance; (2) Measure reflects the hospital's indication that its submission was based upon a sample of its relevant discharges; (3) Rate reflects fewer than the maximum possible quarters of data for the measure; (4) Inaccurate information submitted and suppressed for one or more quarters; (5) No data is available from the hospital for this measure; Please refer to the User's Guide for a full explanation of data

Measure	Cases	This Hospital	State Average	U.S. Average	Top Hospital
Evaluation of LVS Function[2]	592	100%	91%	83%	99%
Smoking Cessation Advice[2]	78	95%	86%	82%	100%
Pneumonia Care					
Appropriate Initial Antibiotic[2]	242	93%	88%	83%	94%
Blood Culture Timing[2]	271	93%	90%	90%	100%
Influenza Vaccine[2]	61	13%	73%	70%	100%
Initial Antibiotic Timing[2]	379	68%	84%	80%	93%
Oxygenation Assessment[2]	501	100%	100%	99%	100%
Pneumococcal Vaccine[2]	333	46%	72%	69%	94%
Smoking Cessation Advice[2]	93	90%	86%	80%	100%
Surgical Infection Prevention					
Prophylactic Antibiotic Given[2]	478	92%	82%	77%	95%
Prophylactic Antibiotic Selection[2]	119	92%	93%	90%	100%
Prophylactic Antibiotic Stopped[2]	465	90%	83%	72%	95%
Pregnancy Care					
Inpatient Neonatal Mortality	-	-	-	-	-
Third or Fourth Degree Laceration	-	-	2.62%	3.63%	3.27%

Covenant Medical Center

1447 N Harrison St
Saginaw, MI 48602
URL: www.covenanthealthcare.com
Ownership: Voluntary non-profit - Other
Emergency Services: Yes

Phone: 989-583-0000
Fax: 989-583-6457
Accredited: Yes
Licensed Beds: 709

Key Personnel:

CEO . . . . Spencer T Maidlow
Director Cardiovascular Services . . . . Bob Kin
Manager Emergency Room . . . . Sherri Alisoglu, RN
Chief Emergency Medicine Section . . . . Joesph C Spadafore, MD
OB/GYN Women's Health Director. . . . . Connie Reynolds, RN
Director Surgical Services . . . . John Germain
Manager Respiratory/Cardiopulmonary . . . . Rod Conklin

Measure	Cases	This Hospital	State Average	U.S. Average	Top Hospital
Heart Attack Care					
ACE Inhibitor or ARB for LVSD	145	80%	86%	82%	100%
Aspirin at Arrival	296	96%	95%	92%	100%
Aspirin at Discharge	338	94%	94%	90%	100%
Beta Blocker at Arrival	224	88%	90%	87%	100%
Beta Blocker at Discharge	454	95%	93%	90%	100%
Fibrinolytic Medication Timing[1]	1	0%	28%	31%	100%
PCI Within 90 Minutes of Arrival[1]	8	38%	59%	54%	95%
Smoking Cessation Advice	199	100%	93%	88%	100%
Heart Failure Care					
ACE Inhibitor or ARB for LVSD	360	73%	84%	82%	100%
Discharge Instructions	691	74%	73%	61%	93%
Evaluation of LVS Function	808	98%	91%	83%	99%
Smoking Cessation Advice	180	97%	86%	82%	100%
Pneumonia Care					
Appropriate Initial Antibiotic	290	90%	88%	83%	94%
Blood Culture Timing	351	90%	90%	90%	100%
Influenza Vaccine	68	87%	73%	70%	100%
Initial Antibiotic Timing	427	83%	84%	80%	93%
Oxygenation Assessment	541	100%	100%	99%	100%
Pneumococcal Vaccine	320	88%	72%	69%	94%
Smoking Cessation Advice	148	98%	86%	80%	100%
Surgical Infection Prevention					
Prophylactic Antibiotic Given[2]	583	83%	82%	77%	95%
Prophylactic Antibiotic Selection[2]	143	96%	93%	90%	100%
Prophylactic Antibiotic Stopped[2]	559	66%	83%	72%	95%
Pregnancy Care					
Inpatient Neonatal Mortality	-	-	-	-	-
Third or Fourth Degree Laceration	-	-	2.62%	3.63%	3.27%

HealthSource Saginaw

Alternate Name: Saginaw Community Hosptial
3340 Hospital Road
Saginaw, MI 48603
Ownership: Voluntary non-profit - Other
Emergency Services: Yes

Phone: 989-790-7700
Fax: 989-790-9297
Accredited: Yes
Licensed Beds: 317

Key Personnel:

Administrator/CEO . . . . Lester Heybor Jr
Chief of Medical Staff. D Kuligowsky, MD
Director Infection/Disease Control . . . . Sherry Baker

Measure	Cases	This Hospital	State Average	U.S. Average	Top Hospital
Heart Attack Care					
ACE Inhibitor or ARB for LVSD[5]	-	-	86%	82%	100%
Aspirin at Arrival[5]	-	-	95%	92%	100%
Aspirin at Discharge[5]	-	-	94%	90%	100%
Beta Blocker at Arrival[5]	-	-	90%	87%	100%
Beta Blocker at Discharge[5]	-	-	93%	90%	100%
Fibrinolytic Medication Timing[5]	-	-	28%	31%	100%
PCI Within 90 Minutes of Arrival[5]	-	-	59%	54%	95%
Smoking Cessation Advice[5]	-	-	93%	88%	100%
Heart Failure Care					
ACE Inhibitor or ARB for LVSD[5]	-	-	84%	82%	100%
Discharge Instructions[5]	-	-	73%	61%	93%
Evaluation of LVS Function[5]	-	-	91%	83%	99%
Smoking Cessation Advice[5]	-	-	86%	82%	100%
Pneumonia Care					
Appropriate Initial Antibiotic[5]	-	-	88%	83%	94%
Blood Culture Timing[5]	-	-	90%	90%	100%
Influenza Vaccine[5]	-	-	73%	70%	100%
Initial Antibiotic Timing[5]	-	-	84%	80%	93%
Oxygenation Assessment[5]	-	-	100%	99%	100%
Pneumococcal Vaccine[5]	-	-	72%	69%	94%
Smoking Cessation Advice[5]	-	-	86%	80%	100%
Surgical Infection Prevention					
Prophylactic Antibiotic Given[5]	-	-	82%	77%	95%
Prophylactic Antibiotic Selection[5]	-	-	93%	90%	100%
Prophylactic Antibiotic Stopped[5]	-	-	83%	72%	95%
Pregnancy Care					
Inpatient Neonatal Mortality	-	-	-	-	-
Third or Fourth Degree Laceration	-	-	2.62%	3.63%	3.27%

Saint Mary's of Michigan

Alternate Name: Saint Mary's of Michigan Medical Center
800 S Washington Avenue
Saginaw, MI 48601
URL: www.stmarysofmichigan.org
Ownership: Voluntary non-profit - Church
Emergency Services: Yes

Phone: 989-907-8000
Fax: 989-907-8141
Accredited: Yes
Licensed Beds: 268

Key Personnel:

President . . . . Fleury Yelvingpon
Chief Medical Staff. . . . . Dr Mark Lester
Emergency Room . . . . Shane Hunt
Chief Nurse Cardiology . . . . Judy Johnson
Respiratory Therapy. . . . . Pam Hair

Measure	Cases	This Hospital	State Average	U.S. Average	Top Hospital
Heart Attack Care					
ACE Inhibitor or ARB for LVSD[2]	71	68%	86%	82%	100%
Aspirin at Arrival[2]	94	96%	95%	92%	100%
Aspirin at Discharge[2]	235	97%	94%	90%	100%
Beta Blocker at Arrival[2]	79	91%	90%	87%	100%
Beta Blocker at Discharge[2]	255	96%	93%	90%	100%
Fibrinolytic Medication Timing[2]	0	-	28%	31%	100%
PCI Within 90 Minutes of Arrival[1,2]	6	67%	59%	54%	95%
Smoking Cessation Advice[2]	110	89%	93%	88%	100%
Heart Failure Care					
ACE Inhibitor or ARB for LVSD[2]	131	81%	84%	82%	100%
Discharge Instructions[2]	268	80%	73%	61%	93%
Evaluation of LVS Function[2]	314	98%	91%	83%	99%
Smoking Cessation Advice[2]	70	80%	86%	82%	100%
Pneumonia Care					
Appropriate Initial Antibiotic[2]	103	92%	88%	83%	94%
Blood Culture Timing[2]	139	87%	90%	90%	100%
Influenza Vaccine[2]	26	58%	73%	70%	100%
Initial Antibiotic Timing[2]	161	81%	84%	80%	93%
Oxygenation Assessment[2]	208	100%	100%	99%	100%
Pneumococcal Vaccine[2]	128	72%	72%	69%	94%
Smoking Cessation Advice[2]	50	70%	86%	80%	100%
Surgical Infection Prevention					
Prophylactic Antibiotic Given[2,3]	258	82%	82%	77%	95%

NOTE: Hospital profiles are in alphabetical order by state, then city, then hospital within the city; Rankings are sorted by rate in descending order and exclude hospitals with less than 25 cases; (1) The number of cases is too small (n<25) for purposes of reliably predicting hospital performance; (2) Measure reflects the hospital's indication that its submission was based upon a sample of its relevant discharges; (3) Rate reflects fewer than the maximum possible quarters of data for the measure; (4) Inaccurate information submitted and suppressed for one or more quarters; (5) No data is available from the hospital for this measure; Please refer to the User's Guide for a full explanation of data

Measure	Cases	This Hospital	State Average	U.S. Average	Top Hospital
Prophylactic Antibiotic Selection[2]	91	97%	93%	90%	100%
Prophylactic Antibiotic Stopped[2,3]	252	77%	83%	72%	95%
Pregnancy Care					
Inpatient Neonatal Mortality	-	-	-	-	-
Third or Fourth Degree Laceration	-	-	2.62%	3.63%	3.27%

Clinton Memorial Hospital

805 S Oakland Street
Saint Johns, MI 48879
URL: www.clintonmemorial.org
Ownership: Proprietary
Emergency Services: Yes

Phone: 989-224-6881
Fax: 989-227-3347

Accredited: No
Licensed Beds: 28

Key Personnel:
President/CEO.......................... Ed Brunn
Chief of Medical Staff..................... Paul David Minnick
Emergency Room .... Diane Simon
Infection Control......................... Ricki Burk
Respiratory/Cardiopulmonary............... Jim Gunther

Measure	Cases	This Hospital	State Average	U.S. Average	Top Hospital
Heart Attack Care					
ACE Inhibitor or ARB for LVSD[3]	0	-	86%	82%	100%
Aspirin at Arrival[1,3]	4	100%	95%	92%	100%
Aspirin at Discharge[1,3]	4	100%	94%	90%	100%
Beta Blocker at Arrival[1,3]	4	100%	90%	87%	100%
Beta Blocker at Discharge[1,3]	3	100%	93%	90%	100%
Fibrinolytic Medication Timing[3]	0	-	28%	31%	100%
PCI Within 90 Minutes of Arrival	0	-	59%	54%	95%
Smoking Cessation Advice[3]	0	-	93%	88%	100%
Heart Failure Care					
ACE Inhibitor or ARB for LVSD[1,3]	10	70%	84%	82%	100%
Discharge Instructions[3]	30	43%	73%	61%	93%
Evaluation of LVS Function[3]	33	85%	91%	83%	99%
Smoking Cessation Advice[1,3]	4	100%	86%	82%	100%
Pneumonia Care					
Appropriate Initial Antibiotic	34	79%	88%	83%	94%
Blood Culture Timing[1]	20	95%	90%	90%	100%
Influenza Vaccine[1]	12	25%	73%	70%	100%
Initial Antibiotic Timing	31	84%	84%	80%	93%
Oxygenation Assessment	40	100%	100%	99%	100%
Pneumococcal Vaccine	25	72%	72%	69%	94%
Smoking Cessation Advice[1]	11	91%	86%	80%	100%
Surgical Infection Prevention					
Prophylactic Antibiotic Given[5]	-	-	82%	77%	95%
Prophylactic Antibiotic Selection[5]	-	-	93%	90%	100%
Prophylactic Antibiotic Stopped[5]	-	-	83%	72%	95%
Pregnancy Care					
Inpatient Neonatal Mortality	-	-	-	-	-
Third or Fourth Degree Laceration	-	-	2.62%	3.63%	3.27%

Lakeland Hospital-Saint Joseph

1234 Napier Avenue
Saint Joseph, MI 49085
URL: www.lakelandhealth.org
Ownership: Voluntary non-profit - Other
Emergency Services: Yes

Phone: 269-983-8300
Fax: 269-982-4855

Accredited: Yes
Licensed Beds: 254

Key Personnel:
CEO/President.......................... Joseph Wasserman
Chief Medical Staff....................... Ken Edwards, MD
Director of Cardiology/Cardiac Lab........... Bart Btrndt
Emergency Room .... John Elsner
Emergency Room .... Laurie Fleming
OB/GYN Womens Health.................. Daniel Lewis, MD
Chief Radiology .... William Leahey, MD
Director Respiratory Therapy .... Jim Hightower

Measure	Cases	This Hospital	State Average	U.S. Average	Top Hospital
Heart Attack Care					
ACE Inhibitor or ARB for LVSD	72	79%	86%	82%	100%
Aspirin at Arrival	303	96%	95%	92%	100%
Aspirin at Discharge	298	97%	94%	90%	100%
Beta Blocker at Arrival	266	96%	90%	87%	100%
Beta Blocker at Discharge	302	95%	93%	90%	100%
Fibrinolytic Medication Timing[1]	2	0%	28%	31%	100%
PCI Within 90 Minutes of Arrival[1]	9	56%	59%	54%	95%
Smoking Cessation Advice	109	98%	93%	88%	100%
Heart Failure Care					
ACE Inhibitor or ARB for LVSD	199	88%	84%	82%	100%
Discharge Instructions	416	82%	73%	61%	93%
Evaluation of LVS Function	469	94%	91%	83%	99%
Smoking Cessation Advice	74	99%	86%	82%	100%
Pneumonia Care					
Appropriate Initial Antibiotic	223	84%	88%	83%	94%
Blood Culture Timing	200	94%	90%	90%	100%
Influenza Vaccine	43	86%	73%	70%	100%
Initial Antibiotic Timing	280	81%	84%	80%	93%
Oxygenation Assessment	329	100%	100%	99%	100%
Pneumococcal Vaccine	192	74%	72%	69%	94%
Smoking Cessation Advice	65	95%	86%	80%	100%
Surgical Infection Prevention					
Prophylactic Antibiotic Given[2,3]	272	70%	82%	77%	95%
Prophylactic Antibiotic Selection[2]	88	86%	93%	90%	100%
Prophylactic Antibiotic Stopped[2,3]	267	60%	83%	72%	95%
Pregnancy Care					
Inpatient Neonatal Mortality	-	-	-	-	-
Third or Fourth Degree Laceration	-	-	2.62%	3.63%	3.27%

Saint Joseph Mercy Saline Hospital

400 W Russell Street
Saline, MI 48176
URL: www.sjmh.com/who/saline
Ownership: Voluntary non-profit - Church
Emergency Services: Yes

Phone: 734-429-1500
Fax: 734-429-4662

Accredited: Yes
Licensed Beds: 82

Key Personnel:
President/CEO.......................... Stacey Breedveld
Chief Medical Staff....................... Renee Kinch
Emergency Room .... Robert McCurdy, MD
Chief Radiology .... Raymond Whiteman, MD

Measure	Cases	This Hospital	State Average	U.S. Average	Top Hospital
Heart Attack Care					
ACE Inhibitor or ARB for LVSD	0	-	86%	82%	100%
Aspirin at Arrival[1]	8	100%	95%	92%	100%
Aspirin at Discharge[1]	4	100%	94%	90%	100%
Beta Blocker at Arrival[1]	5	80%	90%	87%	100%
Beta Blocker at Discharge[1]	5	80%	93%	90%	100%
Fibrinolytic Medication Timing	0	-	28%	31%	100%
PCI Within 90 Minutes of Arrival	0	-	59%	54%	95%
Smoking Cessation Advice	0	-	93%	88%	100%
Heart Failure Care					
ACE Inhibitor or ARB for LVSD[1]	11	100%	84%	82%	100%
Discharge Instructions	40	82%	73%	61%	93%
Evaluation of LVS Function	60	95%	91%	83%	99%
Smoking Cessation Advice[1]	2	100%	86%	82%	100%
Pneumonia Care					
Appropriate Initial Antibiotic	41	90%	88%	83%	94%
Blood Culture Timing	50	96%	90%	90%	100%
Influenza Vaccine[1]	13	85%	73%	70%	100%
Initial Antibiotic Timing	68	94%	84%	80%	93%
Oxygenation Assessment	78	100%	100%	99%	100%
Pneumococcal Vaccine	61	85%	72%	69%	94%
Smoking Cessation Advice[1]	12	92%	86%	80%	100%
Surgical Infection Prevention					
Prophylactic Antibiotic Given[2]	35	91%	82%	77%	95%
Prophylactic Antibiotic Selection[1,2]	10	100%	93%	90%	100%
Prophylactic Antibiotic Stopped[2]	35	89%	83%	72%	95%
Pregnancy Care					
Inpatient Neonatal Mortality	-	-	-	-	-
Third or Fourth Degree Laceration	-	-	2.62%	3.63%	3.27%

NOTE: Hospital profiles are in alphabetical order by state, then city, then hospital within the city; Rankings are sorted by rate in descending order and exclude hospitals with less than 25 cases; (1) The number of cases is too small (n<25) for purposes of reliably predicting hospital performance; (2) Measure reflects the hospital's indication that its submission was based upon a sample of its relevant discharges; (3) Rate reflects fewer than the maximum possible quarters of data for the measure; (4) Inaccurate information submitted and suppressed for one or more quarters; (5) No data is available from the hospital for this measure; Please refer to the User's Guide for a full explanation of data

McKenzie Memorial Hospital

120 Delaware Street
Sandusky, MI 48471
URL: www.mckenziehospital.com
Ownership: Voluntary non-profit - Private
Emergency Services: Yes

Phone: 810-648-3770
Fax: 810-648-4204
Accredited: No
Licensed Beds: 25

Key Personnel:

President/CEO. . . . . JoAnn Hall
Chief Medical Staff. . . . . Balu Kamalapurkar, MD
Emergency Room Supervisor . . . . Konni Phillips, RN
Infection Control. . . . . Janet Herbert, RN
Surgical Services Director . . . . Tammy Cliff, RN
Respiratory/Cardiopulmonary. . . . . Veronica Longton

Measure	Cases	This Hospital	State Average	U.S. Average	Top Hospital
Heart Attack Care					
ACE Inhibitor or ARB for LVSD[3]	0	-	86%	82%	100%
Aspirin at Arrival[1,3]	2	100%	95%	92%	100%
Aspirin at Discharge[1,3]	2	100%	94%	90%	100%
Beta Blocker at Arrival[1,3]	2	50%	90%	87%	100%
Beta Blocker at Discharge[1,3]	2	100%	93%	90%	100%
Fibrinolytic Medication Timing[3]	0	-	28%	31%	100%
PCI Within 90 Minutes of Arrival[5]	-	-	59%	54%	95%
Smoking Cessation Advice[3]	0	-	93%	88%	100%
Heart Failure Care					
ACE Inhibitor or ARB for LVSD[5]	-	-	84%	82%	100%
Discharge Instructions[5]	-	-	73%	61%	93%
Evaluation of LVS Function[5]	-	-	91%	83%	99%
Smoking Cessation Advice[5]	-	-	86%	82%	100%
Pneumonia Care					
Appropriate Initial Antibiotic[1,3]	16	94%	88%	83%	94%
Blood Culture Timing[1]	6	83%	90%	90%	100%
Influenza Vaccine[1]	7	57%	73%	70%	100%
Initial Antibiotic Timing[1,3]	22	91%	84%	80%	93%
Oxygenation Assessment[1,3]	23	100%	100%	99%	100%
Pneumococcal Vaccine[1,3]	12	33%	72%	69%	94%
Smoking Cessation Advice[1,3]	4	100%	86%	80%	100%
Surgical Infection Prevention					
Prophylactic Antibiotic Given[1,3]	16	69%	82%	77%	95%
Prophylactic Antibiotic Selection[1]	8	50%	93%	90%	100%
Prophylactic Antibiotic Stopped[1,3]	15	100%	83%	72%	95%
Pregnancy Care					
Inpatient Neonatal Mortality	-	-	-	-	-
Third or Fourth Degree Laceration	-	-	2.62%	3.63%	3.27%

Chippewa County War Memorial Hospital

Alternate Name: War Memorial Hospital
500 Osborn Boulevard
Sault Ste Marie, MI 49783
Ownership: Voluntary non-profit - Other
Emergency Services: Yes

Phone: 906-635-4460
Fax: 906-635-4467
Accredited: Yes

Key Personnel:

CEO. . . . . David Jahn
Chief Medical Staff. . . . . Dr Tetcalfs
Emergency Room . . . . Jane McLeod, RN

Measure	Cases	This Hospital	State Average	U.S. Average	Top Hospital
Heart Attack Care					
ACE Inhibitor or ARB for LVSD[1]	3	33%	86%	82%	100%
Aspirin at Arrival	27	85%	95%	92%	100%
Aspirin at Discharge[1]	17	65%	94%	90%	100%
Beta Blocker at Arrival	30	87%	90%	87%	100%
Beta Blocker at Discharge[1]	21	76%	93%	90%	100%
Fibrinolytic Medication Timing[1]	1	100%	28%	31%	100%
PCI Within 90 Minutes of Arrival	0	-	59%	54%	95%
Smoking Cessation Advice[1]	5	80%	93%	88%	100%
Heart Failure Care					
ACE Inhibitor or ARB for LVSD	30	43%	84%	82%	100%
Discharge Instructions	85	13%	73%	61%	93%
Evaluation of LVS Function	108	84%	91%	83%	99%
Smoking Cessation Advice[1]	11	18%	86%	82%	100%
Pneumonia Care					
Appropriate Initial Antibiotic	119	64%	88%	83%	94%
Blood Culture Timing	78	95%	90%	90%	100%
Influenza Vaccine[1]	11	45%	73%	70%	100%
Initial Antibiotic Timing	132	79%	84%	80%	93%
Oxygenation Assessment	149	93%	100%	99%	100%
Pneumococcal Vaccine	90	36%	72%	69%	94%
Smoking Cessation Advice	26	31%	86%	80%	100%
Surgical Infection Prevention					
Prophylactic Antibiotic Given[3]	107	21%	82%	77%	95%
Prophylactic Antibiotic Selection	31	90%	93%	90%	100%
Prophylactic Antibiotic Stopped[3]	99	61%	83%	72%	95%
Pregnancy Care					
Inpatient Neonatal Mortality	333	0.30%	-	-	-
Third or Fourth Degree Laceration	236	5.93%	2.62%	3.63%	3.27%

South Haven Community Hospital

955 S Bailey Avenue
South Haven, MI 49090
E-mail: info@shch.org
URL: www.shch.org
Ownership: Govt - Hospital District or Authority
Emergency Services: Yes

Phone: 269-637-5271
Fax: 269-639-1208
Accredited: Yes
Licensed Beds: 82

Key Personnel:

President/CEO. . . . . Craig Marks
Chief Medical Staff. . . . . Karen Janson, MD
Director Cardiology . . . . Tom Bauer
Director Emergency Services. . . . . Paul Wahby, DO
Director Infection/Disease Control . . . . Teresa Horan
Director Medical/Surgical Nursing . . . . Barbara Lute, RN
OB/GYN. . . . . Kara Cockfield, MD
Chief Radiology . . . . Edward Maas, MD
Director Respiratory Therapy. . . . . Mike Musgrove

Measure	Cases	This Hospital	State Average	U.S. Average	Top Hospital
Heart Attack Care					
ACE Inhibitor or ARB for LVSD[3]	0	-	86%	82%	100%
Aspirin at Arrival[1,3]	5	100%	95%	92%	100%
Aspirin at Discharge[1,3]	2	50%	94%	90%	100%
Beta Blocker at Arrival[1,3]	7	71%	90%	87%	100%
Beta Blocker at Discharge[1,3]	3	67%	93%	90%	100%
Fibrinolytic Medication Timing[3]	0	-	28%	31%	100%
PCI Within 90 Minutes of Arrival[5]	-	-	59%	54%	95%
Smoking Cessation Advice[3]	0	-	93%	88%	100%
Heart Failure Care					
ACE Inhibitor or ARB for LVSD[1]	10	100%	84%	82%	100%
Discharge Instructions	33	61%	73%	61%	93%
Evaluation of LVS Function	38	76%	91%	83%	99%
Smoking Cessation Advice[1]	7	43%	86%	82%	100%
Pneumonia Care					
Appropriate Initial Antibiotic	71	70%	88%	83%	94%
Blood Culture Timing	46	93%	90%	90%	100%
Influenza Vaccine[1]	11	55%	73%	70%	100%
Initial Antibiotic Timing	75	72%	84%	80%	93%
Oxygenation Assessment	87	100%	100%	99%	100%
Pneumococcal Vaccine	45	49%	72%	69%	94%
Smoking Cessation Advice[1]	20	80%	86%	80%	100%
Surgical Infection Prevention					
Prophylactic Antibiotic Given[3]	73	74%	82%	77%	95%
Prophylactic Antibiotic Selection	30	83%	93%	90%	100%
Prophylactic Antibiotic Stopped[3]	72	89%	83%	72%	95%
Pregnancy Care					
Inpatient Neonatal Mortality	430	0.00%	-	-	-
Third or Fourth Degree Laceration	342	0.29%	2.62%	3.63%	3.27%

Providence Hospital

16001 West 9 Mile Road
Southfield, MI 48075
URL: www.stjohn.org/Providence
Ownership: Voluntary non-profit - Church
Emergency Services: Yes

Phone: 248-849-3000
Fax: 248-849-3035
Accredited: Yes
Licensed Beds: 459

Key Personnel:

CEO. . . . . Brian Connolly
Emergency Room . . . . John McCabe, MD
Chief Radiology . . . . James Karo, MD

NOTE: Hospital profiles are in alphabetical order by state, then city, then hospital within the city; Rankings are sorted by rate in descending order and exclude hospitals with less than 25 cases; (1) The number of cases is too small (n<25) for purposes of reliably predicting hospital performance; (2) Measure reflects the hospital's indication that its submission was based upon a sample of its relevant discharges; (3) Rate reflects fewer than the maximum possible quarters of data for the measure; (4) Inaccurate information submitted and suppressed for one or more quarters; (5) No data is available from the hospital for this measure; Please refer to the User's Guide for a full explanation of data

Measure	Cases	This Hospital	State Average	U.S. Average	Top Hospital
Heart Attack Care					
ACE Inhibitor or ARB for LVSD	112	97%	86%	82%	100%
Aspirin at Arrival	319	98%	95%	92%	100%
Aspirin at Discharge	471	98%	94%	90%	100%
Beta Blocker at Arrival	280	96%	90%	87%	100%
Beta Blocker at Discharge	477	98%	93%	90%	100%
Fibrinolytic Medication Timing	0	-	28%	31%	100%
PCI Within 90 Minutes of Arrival[1]	10	40%	59%	54%	95%
Smoking Cessation Advice	135	96%	93%	88%	100%
Heart Failure Care					
ACE Inhibitor or ARB for LVSD	403	98%	84%	82%	100%
Discharge Instructions	893	77%	73%	61%	93%
Evaluation of LVS Function	1,046	97%	91%	83%	99%
Smoking Cessation Advice	188	87%	86%	82%	100%
Pneumonia Care					
Appropriate Initial Antibiotic	374	94%	88%	83%	94%
Blood Culture Timing	358	85%	90%	90%	100%
Influenza Vaccine	80	74%	73%	70%	100%
Initial Antibiotic Timing	507	90%	84%	80%	93%
Oxygenation Assessment	591	100%	100%	99%	100%
Pneumococcal Vaccine	340	65%	72%	69%	94%
Smoking Cessation Advice	118	89%	86%	80%	100%
Surgical Infection Prevention					
Prophylactic Antibiotic Given[2,3]	624	95%	82%	77%	95%
Prophylactic Antibiotic Selection[2]	279	98%	93%	90%	100%
Prophylactic Antibiotic Stopped[2,3]	577	89%	83%	72%	95%
Pregnancy Care					
Inpatient Neonatal Mortality	-	-	-	-	-
Third or Fourth Degree Laceration	-	-	2.62%	3.63%	3.27%

Straith Hospital for Special Surgery

23901 Lahser
Southfield, MI 48033
Phone: 248-357-3360
Ownership: Voluntary non-profit - Other
Accredited: Yes
Emergency Services: No

Measure	Cases	This Hospital	State Average	U.S. Average	Top Hospital
Heart Attack Care					
ACE Inhibitor or ARB for LVSD[5]	-	-	86%	82%	100%
Aspirin at Arrival[5]	-	-	95%	92%	100%
Aspirin at Discharge[5]	-	-	94%	90%	100%
Beta Blocker at Arrival[5]	-	-	90%	87%	100%
Beta Blocker at Discharge[5]	-	-	93%	90%	100%
Fibrinolytic Medication Timing[5]	-	-	28%	31%	100%
PCI Within 90 Minutes of Arrival[5]	-	-	59%	54%	95%
Smoking Cessation Advice[5]	-	-	93%	88%	100%
Heart Failure Care					
ACE Inhibitor or ARB for LVSD[5]	-	-	84%	82%	100%
Discharge Instructions[5]	-	-	73%	61%	93%
Evaluation of LVS Function[5]	-	-	91%	83%	99%
Smoking Cessation Advice[5]	-	-	86%	82%	100%
Pneumonia Care					
Appropriate Initial Antibiotic[5]	-	-	88%	83%	94%
Blood Culture Timing[5]	-	-	90%	90%	100%
Influenza Vaccine[5]	-	-	73%	70%	100%
Initial Antibiotic Timing[5]	-	-	84%	80%	93%
Oxygenation Assessment[5]	-	-	100%	99%	100%
Pneumococcal Vaccine[5]	-	-	72%	69%	94%
Smoking Cessation Advice[5]	-	-	86%	80%	100%
Surgical Infection Prevention					
Prophylactic Antibiotic Given[5]	-	-	82%	77%	95%
Prophylactic Antibiotic Selection[5]	-	-	93%	90%	100%
Prophylactic Antibiotic Stopped[5]	-	-	83%	72%	95%
Pregnancy Care					
Inpatient Neonatal Mortality	-	-	-	-	-
Third or Fourth Degree Laceration	-	-	2.62%	3.63%	3.27%

Sturgis Hospital

916 Myrtle Avenue
Sturgis, MI 49091
Phone: 269-651-7824
Fax: 269-659-6713
URL: www.sturgishospital.com
Ownership: Government - Local
Accredited: Yes
Emergency Services: Yes
Licensed Beds: 94

Key Personnel:

CEO . . . . Robert L LaBarge
Chief of Medical Staff . . . . Edward Griffin, MD
Cardiac Lab . . . . Shirley Betts
Emergency Room . . . . Martie Gillespie
Infection Control . . . . Sarah Hagen
Surgical/Medical/ICU . . . . Shirley Betts
Respiratory Therapy . . . . Shirley Betts

Measure	Cases	This Hospital	State Average	U.S. Average	Top Hospital
Heart Attack Care					
ACE Inhibitor or ARB for LVSD[3]	0	-	86%	82%	100%
Aspirin at Arrival[1,3]	4	100%	95%	92%	100%
Aspirin at Discharge[1,3]	5	100%	94%	90%	100%
Beta Blocker at Arrival[1,3]	4	75%	90%	87%	100%
Beta Blocker at Discharge[1,3]	4	100%	93%	90%	100%
Fibrinolytic Medication Timing[3]	0	-	28%	31%	100%
PCI Within 90 Minutes of Arrival	0	-	59%	54%	95%
Smoking Cessation Advice[1,3]	1	100%	93%	88%	100%
Heart Failure Care					
ACE Inhibitor or ARB for LVSD	25	76%	84%	82%	100%
Discharge Instructions	94	81%	73%	61%	93%
Evaluation of LVS Function	119	93%	91%	83%	99%
Smoking Cessation Advice[1]	11	73%	86%	82%	100%
Pneumonia Care					
Appropriate Initial Antibiotic	67	76%	88%	83%	94%
Blood Culture Timing	46	98%	90%	90%	100%
Influenza Vaccine[1]	13	8%	73%	70%	100%
Initial Antibiotic Timing	65	75%	84%	80%	93%
Oxygenation Assessment	81	100%	100%	99%	100%
Pneumococcal Vaccine	53	6%	72%	69%	94%
Smoking Cessation Advice[1]	17	71%	86%	80%	100%
Surgical Infection Prevention					
Prophylactic Antibiotic Given[3]	99	63%	82%	77%	95%
Prophylactic Antibiotic Selection	36	94%	93%	90%	100%
Prophylactic Antibiotic Stopped[3]	97	86%	83%	72%	95%
Pregnancy Care					
Inpatient Neonatal Mortality	424	0.24%	-	-	-
Third or Fourth Degree Laceration	293	4.78%	2.62%	3.63%	3.27%

Saint Joseph Health System

200 Hemlock Street
PO Box 659
Tawas City, MI 48764
Phone: 989-362-3411
Fax: 989-362-9376
URL: www.sjhsys.org
Ownership: Voluntary non-profit - Other
Accredited: Yes
Emergency Services: Yes
Licensed Beds: 49

Key Personnel:

President/CEO . . . . Patrick J Murtha
Director Surgical Services . . . . Pat Visscher

Measure	Cases	This Hospital	State Average	U.S. Average	Top Hospital
Heart Attack Care					
ACE Inhibitor or ARB for LVSD[1]	2	0%	86%	82%	100%
Aspirin at Arrival[1]	6	100%	95%	92%	100%
Aspirin at Discharge[1]	6	100%	94%	90%	100%
Beta Blocker at Arrival[1]	9	100%	90%	87%	100%
Beta Blocker at Discharge[1]	5	100%	93%	90%	100%
Fibrinolytic Medication Timing	0	-	28%	31%	100%
PCI Within 90 Minutes of Arrival	0	-	59%	54%	95%
Smoking Cessation Advice	0	-	93%	88%	100%
Heart Failure Care					
ACE Inhibitor or ARB for LVSD	35	80%	84%	82%	100%
Discharge Instructions	94	95%	73%	61%	93%
Evaluation of LVS Function	106	92%	91%	83%	99%
Smoking Cessation Advice[1]	15	93%	86%	82%	100%
Pneumonia Care					

NOTE: Hospital profiles are in alphabetical order by state, then city, then hospital within the city; Rankings are sorted by rate in descending order and exclude hospitals with less than 25 cases; (1) The number of cases is too small (n<25) for purposes of reliably predicting hospital performance; (2) Measure reflects the hospital's indication that its submission was based upon a sample of its relevant discharges; (3) Rate reflects fewer than the maximum possible quarters of data for the measure; (4) Inaccurate information submitted and suppressed for one or more quarters; (5) No data is available from the hospital for this measure; Please refer to the User's Guide for a full explanation of data

Appropriate Initial Antibiotic	73	92%	88%	83%	94%
Blood Culture Timing	67	88%	90%	90%	100%
Influenza Vaccine[1]	20	100%	73%	70%	100%
Initial Antibiotic Timing	78	92%	84%	80%	93%
Oxygenation Assessment	115	100%	100%	99%	100%
Pneumococcal Vaccine	80	90%	72%	69%	94%
Smoking Cessation Advice[1]	23	96%	86%	80%	100%
Surgical Infection Prevention					
Prophylactic Antibiotic Given[2]	188	93%	82%	77%	95%
Prophylactic Antibiotic Selection[2]	45	98%	93%	90%	100%
Prophylactic Antibiotic Stopped[2]	173	99%	83%	72%	95%
Pregnancy Care					
Inpatient Neonatal Mortality	-	-	-	-	-
Third or Fourth Degree Laceration	-	-	2.62%	3.63%	3.27%

Oakwood Heritage Hospital

Alternate Name: Heritage Hospital
10000 Telegraph
Taylor, MI 48180
Phone: 313-295-5000
Fax: 313-295-5205
URL: www.oakwod.org
Ownership: Govt - Hospital District or Authority
Accredited: Yes
Emergency Services: Yes
Licensed Beds: 233

Key Personnel:

CEO. . . . . Rick Hillbom
Chief Medical Staff. . . . . Vijay Khanna, MD
Emergency Room . . . . Deb Vogel, RN
Cardiology . . . . Abil Karamali
Chief Radiology . . . . Jamie Herdt
Director Respiratory Therapy . . . . Troy Adamon

Measure	Cases	This Hospital	State Average	U.S. Average	Top Hospital
Heart Attack Care					
ACE Inhibitor or ARB for LVSD[1]	12	100%	86%	82%	100%
Aspirin at Arrival	56	98%	95%	92%	100%
Aspirin at Discharge	26	100%	94%	90%	100%
Beta Blocker at Arrival	31	100%	90%	87%	100%
Beta Blocker at Discharge	37	97%	93%	90%	100%
Fibrinolytic Medication Timing	0	-	28%	31%	100%
PCI Within 90 Minutes of Arrival	0	-	59%	54%	95%
Smoking Cessation Advice[1]	10	100%	93%	88%	100%
Heart Failure Care					
ACE Inhibitor or ARB for LVSD	80	99%	84%	82%	100%
Discharge Instructions	132	97%	73%	61%	93%
Evaluation of LVS Function	216	100%	91%	83%	99%
Smoking Cessation Advice	44	100%	86%	82%	100%
Pneumonia Care					
Appropriate Initial Antibiotic	131	95%	88%	83%	94%
Blood Culture Timing	239	97%	90%	90%	100%
Influenza Vaccine	58	100%	73%	70%	100%
Initial Antibiotic Timing	262	86%	84%	80%	93%
Oxygenation Assessment	327	100%	100%	99%	100%
Pneumococcal Vaccine	192	99%	72%	69%	94%
Smoking Cessation Advice	92	100%	86%	80%	100%
Surgical Infection Prevention					
Prophylactic Antibiotic Given	156	94%	82%	77%	95%
Prophylactic Antibiotic Selection	30	100%	93%	90%	100%
Prophylactic Antibiotic Stopped	150	93%	83%	72%	95%
Pregnancy Care					
Inpatient Neonatal Mortality	-	-	-	-	-
Third or Fourth Degree Laceration	-	-	2.62%	3.63%	3.27%

Herrick Memorial Hospital

500 E Pottawatamie Street
Tecumseh, MI 49286
Phone: 517-423-2141
Fax: 517-424-3900
Ownership: Government - Federal
Accredited: Yes
Emergency Services: Yes
Licensed Beds: 100

Key Personnel:

CEO. . . . . John Robertstad
Chief Medical Staff. . . . . David Kaisler, MD
Emergency Room . . . . Rosalie Turek, MD
Director Infection/Disease Control . . . . Claudette Bryan
CCU Spvg. Nurse . . . . Christine Mathis
OB/GYN Womens Health. . . . . Donald Samuel, MD
Chief Radiology . . . . Nancy Newlin, MD
Director Respiratory Therapy . . . . James Justus

Measure	Cases	This Hospital	State Average	U.S. Average	Top Hospital
Heart Attack Care					
ACE Inhibitor or ARB for LVSD[1]	1	100%	86%	82%	100%
Aspirin at Arrival[1]	10	90%	95%	92%	100%
Aspirin at Discharge[1]	5	100%	94%	90%	100%
Beta Blocker at Arrival[1]	8	75%	90%	87%	100%
Beta Blocker at Discharge[1]	5	80%	93%	90%	100%
Fibrinolytic Medication Timing	0	-	28%	31%	100%
PCI Within 90 Minutes of Arrival	0	-	59%	54%	95%
Smoking Cessation Advice[1]	1	100%	93%	88%	100%
Heart Failure Care					
ACE Inhibitor or ARB for LVSD[1]	6	100%	84%	82%	100%
Discharge Instructions	25	48%	73%	61%	93%
Evaluation of LVS Function	31	87%	91%	83%	99%
Smoking Cessation Advice[1]	4	75%	86%	82%	100%
Pneumonia Care					
Appropriate Initial Antibiotic	50	90%	88%	83%	94%
Blood Culture Timing	39	95%	90%	90%	100%
Influenza Vaccine[1]	9	78%	73%	70%	100%
Initial Antibiotic Timing	45	96%	84%	80%	93%
Oxygenation Assessment	64	98%	100%	99%	100%
Pneumococcal Vaccine	45	84%	72%	69%	94%
Smoking Cessation Advice[1]	10	100%	86%	80%	100%
Surgical Infection Prevention					
Prophylactic Antibiotic Given[5]	-	-	82%	77%	95%
Prophylactic Antibiotic Selection[5]	-	-	93%	90%	100%
Prophylactic Antibiotic Stopped[5]	-	-	83%	72%	95%
Pregnancy Care					
Inpatient Neonatal Mortality	-	-	-	-	-
Third or Fourth Degree Laceration	-	-	2.62%	3.63%	3.27%

Three Rivers Area Hospital

701 South Health Parkway
Three Rivers, MI 49093
Phone: 269-278-1145
Fax: 269-273-9611
E-mail: info@threerivershealth.org
URL: www.threerivershealth.org
Ownership: Govt - Hospital District or Authority
Accredited: Yes
Emergency Services: Yes
Licensed Beds: 60

Key Personnel:

Administrator/President . . . . Matt Chambers
Emergency Room . . . . Brian Bowdich, MD
Director Medical/Surgical Nursing . . . . Nancy Buscher

Measure	Cases	This Hospital	State Average	U.S. Average	Top Hospital
Heart Attack Care					
ACE Inhibitor or ARB for LVSD	0	-	86%	82%	100%
Aspirin at Arrival[1]	11	73%	95%	92%	100%
Aspirin at Discharge[1]	8	62%	94%	90%	100%
Beta Blocker at Arrival[1]	11	73%	90%	87%	100%
Beta Blocker at Discharge[1]	8	100%	93%	90%	100%
Fibrinolytic Medication Timing	0	-	28%	31%	100%
PCI Within 90 Minutes of Arrival	0	-	59%	54%	95%
Smoking Cessation Advice[1]	2	100%	93%	88%	100%
Heart Failure Care					
ACE Inhibitor or ARB for LVSD[1]	14	50%	84%	82%	100%
Discharge Instructions	46	65%	73%	61%	93%
Evaluation of LVS Function	60	82%	91%	83%	99%
Smoking Cessation Advice[1]	12	83%	86%	82%	100%
Pneumonia Care					
Appropriate Initial Antibiotic	77	88%	88%	83%	94%
Blood Culture Timing	73	86%	90%	90%	100%
Influenza Vaccine[1]	16	81%	73%	70%	100%
Initial Antibiotic Timing	91	84%	84%	80%	93%
Oxygenation Assessment	102	100%	100%	99%	100%
Pneumococcal Vaccine	60	72%	72%	69%	94%
Smoking Cessation Advice	28	89%	86%	80%	100%
Surgical Infection Prevention					
Prophylactic Antibiotic Given[3]	41	24%	82%	77%	95%
Prophylactic Antibiotic Selection	27	81%	93%	90%	100%

NOTE: Hospital profiles are in alphabetical order by state, then city, then hospital within the city; Rankings are sorted by rate in descending order and exclude hospitals with less than 25 cases; (1) The number of cases is too small (n<25) for purposes of reliably predicting hospital performance; (2) Measure reflects the hospital's indication that its submission was based upon a sample of its relevant discharges; (3) Rate reflects fewer than the maximum possible quarters of data for the measure; (4) Inaccurate information submitted and suppressed for one or more quarters; (5) No data is available from the hospital for this measure; Please refer to the User's Guide for a full explanation of data

Prophylactic Antibiotic Stopped[3]	40	100%	83%	72%	95%
Pregnancy Care					
Inpatient Neonatal Mortality	347	0.00%	-	-	-
Third or Fourth Degree Laceration	278	0.00%	2.62%	3.63%	3.27%

Munson Medical Center

1105 6th Street
Traverse City, MI 49684

Toll-Free: 800-468-6766
Phone: 231-935-5000
Fax: 231-935-6548

E-mail: contact@mhc.net
URL: www.munsonhealthcare.org
Ownership: Voluntary non-profit - Other
Emergency Services: Yes

Accredited: Yes
Licensed Beds: 391

Key Personnel:
President/CEO . . . . Edwin A Ness

Measure	Cases	This Hospital	State Average	U.S. Average	Top Hospital
Heart Attack Care					
ACE Inhibitor or ARB for LVSD	220	90%	86%	82%	100%
Aspirin at Arrival	348	97%	95%	92%	100%
Aspirin at Discharge	713	99%	94%	90%	100%
Beta Blocker at Arrival	272	93%	90%	87%	100%
Beta Blocker at Discharge	779	98%	93%	90%	100%
Fibrinolytic Medication Timing[1]	1	0%	28%	31%	100%
PCI Within 90 Minutes of Arrival[1]	14	29%	59%	54%	95%
Smoking Cessation Advice	280	99%	93%	88%	100%
Heart Failure Care					
ACE Inhibitor or ARB for LVSD	170	87%	84%	82%	100%
Discharge Instructions	357	87%	73%	61%	93%
Evaluation of LVS Function	403	97%	91%	83%	99%
Smoking Cessation Advice	55	93%	86%	82%	100%
Pneumonia Care					
Appropriate Initial Antibiotic	184	98%	88%	83%	94%
Blood Culture Timing	215	94%	90%	90%	100%
Influenza Vaccine	48	88%	73%	70%	100%
Initial Antibiotic Timing	266	86%	84%	80%	93%
Oxygenation Assessment	341	99%	100%	99%	100%
Pneumococcal Vaccine	246	93%	72%	69%	94%
Smoking Cessation Advice	82	96%	86%	80%	100%
Surgical Infection Prevention					
Prophylactic Antibiotic Given[2]	612	91%	82%	77%	95%
Prophylactic Antibiotic Selection[2]	154	99%	93%	90%	100%
Prophylactic Antibiotic Stopped[2]	591	87%	83%	72%	95%
Pregnancy Care					
Inpatient Neonatal Mortality	-	-	-	-	-
Third or Fourth Degree Laceration	-	-	2.62%	3.63%	3.27%

Oakwood Southshore Medical Center

5450 Fort Street
Trenton, MI 48183
Ownership: Govt - Hospital District or Authority
Emergency Services: Yes

Phone: 734-671-3802
Fax: 734-671-3891
Accredited: Yes
Licensed Beds: 183

Key Personnel:
President/CEO . . . . Gerald Fitzgerald
Chief Medical Staff . . . . Malcolm Henochmd
Infection Control Specialist . . . . Susan Ottosen
Chief OB/GYN . . . . Deeb Shalhoub, MD
Asst Director, Surgical Services . . . . Kathy Young
Chief of Radiology . . . . Bruno Borin, DO
Director Respiratory Therapy . . . . Troy Adamen

Measure	Cases	This Hospital	State Average	U.S. Average	Top Hospital
Heart Attack Care					
ACE Inhibitor or ARB for LVSD[1]	22	95%	86%	82%	100%
Aspirin at Arrival	115	97%	95%	92%	100%
Aspirin at Discharge	58	93%	94%	90%	100%
Beta Blocker at Arrival	82	100%	90%	87%	100%
Beta Blocker at Discharge	74	99%	93%	90%	100%
Fibrinolytic Medication Timing	0	-	28%	31%	100%
PCI Within 90 Minutes of Arrival	0	-	59%	54%	95%
Smoking Cessation Advice[1]	8	100%	93%	88%	100%
Heart Failure Care					
ACE Inhibitor or ARB for LVSD	121	83%	84%	82%	100%
Discharge Instructions	244	75%	73%	61%	93%
Evaluation of LVS Function	324	93%	91%	83%	99%
Smoking Cessation Advice	65	97%	86%	82%	100%
Pneumonia Care					
Appropriate Initial Antibiotic	179	96%	88%	83%	94%
Blood Culture Timing	234	98%	90%	90%	100%
Influenza Vaccine	60	85%	73%	70%	100%
Initial Antibiotic Timing	287	90%	84%	80%	93%
Oxygenation Assessment	353	100%	100%	99%	100%
Pneumococcal Vaccine	230	89%	72%	69%	94%
Smoking Cessation Advice	87	97%	86%	80%	100%
Surgical Infection Prevention					
Prophylactic Antibiotic Given	270	91%	82%	77%	95%
Prophylactic Antibiotic Selection	71	99%	93%	90%	100%
Prophylactic Antibiotic Stopped	248	86%	83%	72%	95%
Pregnancy Care					
Inpatient Neonatal Mortality	-	-	-	-	-
Third or Fourth Degree Laceration	-	-	2.62%	3.63%	3.27%

William Beaumont Hospital

44201 Dequindre Road
Troy, MI 48085
URL: www.beaumonthospitals.com
Ownership: Voluntary non-profit - Other
Emergency Services: Yes

Phone: 248-964-5000
Fax: 248-964-8842

Accredited: Yes
Licensed Beds: 226

Key Personnel:
Chief Medical Staff . . . . Richardpher Herbert, DO
Cardiac Lab . . . . Terry Wagner
Chief Catheterization Laboratory . . . . David Forst, MD
Emergency Room . . . . William Anderson, MD
Director Infection/Disease Control . . . . Doris Neumeyer
CCU Supervising Nurse . . . . Debbie Guido Allen, RN
Director Medical/Surgical Nursing . . . . Nancy Susick
OB/GYN Womens Health . . . . Thomas P Wolf, MD
Chief Radiology . . . . Thomas Verhelle, MD
Director Respiratory Therapy . . . . Thomas Buday

Measure	Cases	This Hospital	State Average	U.S. Average	Top Hospital
Heart Attack Care					
ACE Inhibitor or ARB for LVSD	90	93%	86%	82%	100%
Aspirin at Arrival	296	95%	95%	92%	100%
Aspirin at Discharge	252	100%	94%	90%	100%
Beta Blocker at Arrival	216	94%	90%	87%	100%
Beta Blocker at Discharge	273	99%	93%	90%	100%
Fibrinolytic Medication Timing	0	-	28%	31%	100%
PCI Within 90 Minutes of Arrival[1]	13	38%	59%	54%	95%
Smoking Cessation Advice	85	100%	93%	88%	100%
Heart Failure Care					
ACE Inhibitor or ARB for LVSD	260	80%	84%	82%	100%
Discharge Instructions	543	45%	73%	61%	93%
Evaluation of LVS Function	666	99%	91%	83%	99%
Smoking Cessation Advice	62	100%	86%	82%	100%
Pneumonia Care					
Appropriate Initial Antibiotic	262	95%	88%	83%	94%
Blood Culture Timing	295	94%	90%	90%	100%
Influenza Vaccine	71	82%	73%	70%	100%
Initial Antibiotic Timing	381	69%	84%	80%	93%
Oxygenation Assessment	496	100%	100%	99%	100%
Pneumococcal Vaccine	320	83%	72%	69%	94%
Smoking Cessation Advice	100	99%	86%	80%	100%
Surgical Infection Prevention					
Prophylactic Antibiotic Given[2]	712	91%	82%	77%	95%
Prophylactic Antibiotic Selection[2]	187	98%	93%	90%	100%
Prophylactic Antibiotic Stopped[2]	662	89%	83%	72%	95%
Pregnancy Care					
Inpatient Neonatal Mortality	-	-	-	-	-
Third or Fourth Degree Laceration	-	-	2.62%	3.63%	3.27%

NOTE: Hospital profiles are in alphabetical order by state, then city, then hospital within the city; Rankings are sorted by rate in descending order and exclude hospitals with less than 25 cases; (1) The number of cases is too small (n<25) for purposes of reliably predicting hospital performance; (2) Measure reflects the hospital's indication that its submission was based upon a sample of its relevant discharges; (3) Rate reflects fewer than the maximum possible quarters of data for the measure; (4) Inaccurate information submitted and suppressed for one or more quarters; (5) No data is available from the hospital for this measure; Please refer to the User's Guide for a full explanation of data

Bronson Vicksburg Hospital

13326 N Boulevard
Vicksburg, MI 49097
URL: www.bronsonhealth.com
Ownership: Voluntary non-profit - Other
Emergency Services: Yes

Phone: 269-649-2321
Fax: 269-649-2905
Accredited: Yes
Licensed Beds: 41

Key Personnel:

Administrator . . . . Laura Howard
President/CEO . . . . Frank Sardone
Chief Medical Staff . . . . James Simonds Jr, CPM
VP . . . . Cheryl Knapp
Emergency Room . . . . Gerald Friedman, MD
Chief Surgery . . . . Daniel Stewart, MD
Infection Control . . . . Cindy Gentz, RN
Chief Medicine . . . . Gerald Friedman, MD

Measure	Cases	This Hospital	State Average	U.S. Average	Top Hospital
Heart Attack Care					
ACE Inhibitor or ARB for LVSD[5]	-	-	86%	82%	100%
Aspirin at Arrival[5]	-	-	95%	92%	100%
Aspirin at Discharge[5]	-	-	94%	90%	100%
Beta Blocker at Arrival[5]	-	-	90%	87%	100%
Beta Blocker at Discharge[5]	-	-	93%	90%	100%
Fibrinolytic Medication Timing[5]	-	-	28%	31%	100%
PCI Within 90 Minutes of Arrival[5]	-	-	59%	54%	95%
Smoking Cessation Advice[5]	-	-	93%	88%	100%
Heart Failure Care					
ACE Inhibitor or ARB for LVSD[5]	-	-	84%	82%	100%
Discharge Instructions[5]	-	-	73%	61%	93%
Evaluation of LVS Function[5]	-	-	91%	83%	99%
Smoking Cessation Advice[5]	-	-	86%	82%	100%
Pneumonia Care					
Appropriate Initial Antibiotic[5]	-	-	88%	83%	94%
Blood Culture Timing[5]	-	-	90%	90%	100%
Influenza Vaccine[5]	-	-	73%	70%	100%
Initial Antibiotic Timing[5]	-	-	84%	80%	93%
Oxygenation Assessment[5]	-	-	100%	99%	100%
Pneumococcal Vaccine[5]	-	-	72%	69%	94%
Smoking Cessation Advice[5]	-	-	86%	80%	100%
Surgical Infection Prevention					
Prophylactic Antibiotic Given[5]	-	-	82%	77%	95%
Prophylactic Antibiotic Selection[5]	-	-	93%	90%	100%
Prophylactic Antibiotic Stopped[5]	-	-	83%	72%	95%
Pregnancy Care					
Inpatient Neonatal Mortality	-	-	-	-	-
Third or Fourth Degree Laceration	-	-	2.62%	3.63%	3.27%

Henry Ford Bi-County Hospital

13355 E Ten Mile Road
Warren, MI 48089
URL: www.henryfordhealth.org
Ownership: Voluntary non-profit - Private
Emergency Services: Yes

Phone: 586-759-7444
Fax: 586-759-7489
Accredited: No
Licensed Beds: 231

Key Personnel:

Chief Medical Officer . . . . Gary L Moorman, DO

Measure	Cases	This Hospital	State Average	U.S. Average	Top Hospital
Heart Attack Care					
ACE Inhibitor or ARB for LVSD[1]	16	75%	86%	82%	100%
Aspirin at Arrival	88	95%	95%	92%	100%
Aspirin at Discharge	46	87%	94%	90%	100%
Beta Blocker at Arrival	58	97%	90%	87%	100%
Beta Blocker at Discharge	46	93%	93%	90%	100%
Fibrinolytic Medication Timing	0	-	28%	31%	100%
PCI Within 90 Minutes of Arrival	0	-	59%	54%	95%
Smoking Cessation Advice[1]	16	88%	93%	88%	100%
Heart Failure Care					
ACE Inhibitor or ARB for LVSD	94	67%	84%	82%	100%
Discharge Instructions	268	37%	73%	61%	93%
Evaluation of LVS Function	319	97%	91%	83%	99%
Smoking Cessation Advice	45	73%	86%	82%	100%
Pneumonia Care					
Appropriate Initial Antibiotic	140	86%	88%	83%	94%
Blood Culture Timing	157	96%	90%	90%	100%
Influenza Vaccine	33	52%	73%	70%	100%
Initial Antibiotic Timing	207	75%	84%	80%	93%
Oxygenation Assessment	244	99%	100%	99%	100%
Pneumococcal Vaccine	128	42%	72%	69%	94%
Smoking Cessation Advice	71	82%	86%	80%	100%
Surgical Infection Prevention					
Prophylactic Antibiotic Given[2]	253	99%	82%	77%	95%
Prophylactic Antibiotic Selection[2]	54	100%	93%	90%	100%
Prophylactic Antibiotic Stopped[2]	241	90%	83%	72%	95%
Pregnancy Care					
Inpatient Neonatal Mortality	-	-	-	-	-
Third or Fourth Degree Laceration	-	-	2.62%	3.63%	3.27%

Saint John Macomb Hospital

Alternate Name: Macomb Hospital Center
11800 E 12 Mile
Warren, MI 48093
URL: www.stjohn.org
Ownership: Voluntary non-profit - Other
Emergency Services: Yes

Phone: 586-573-5000
Fax: 586-573-5199
Accredited: Yes
Licensed Beds: 376

Key Personnel:

President/CEO . . . . John E Knox
Chief Medical Staff . . . . Suraj Nighoon, MD
Chief Catheterization Laboratory . . . . Lingareddy Devireddy, MD
Emergency Room . . . . John Bauer, MD
Director Infection/Disease Control . . . . Richard Pokriefka, D.O.
Director Medical/Surgical Nursing . . . . Kim Knight, RN
OB/GYN Womens Health . . . . Andres Santiviago, MD
Chief Radiology . . . . Jay Zeskino, MD
Director Respiratory Therapy . . . . Valerie Dornan

Measure	Cases	This Hospital	State Average	U.S. Average	Top Hospital
Heart Attack Care					
ACE Inhibitor or ARB for LVSD	105	97%	86%	82%	100%
Aspirin at Arrival	310	98%	95%	92%	100%
Aspirin at Discharge	341	97%	94%	90%	100%
Beta Blocker at Arrival	244	94%	90%	87%	100%
Beta Blocker at Discharge	330	98%	93%	90%	100%
Fibrinolytic Medication Timing	0	-	28%	31%	100%
PCI Within 90 Minutes of Arrival[1]	16	75%	59%	54%	95%
Smoking Cessation Advice	122	98%	93%	88%	100%
Heart Failure Care					
ACE Inhibitor or ARB for LVSD	227	95%	84%	82%	100%
Discharge Instructions	579	82%	73%	61%	93%
Evaluation of LVS Function	714	95%	91%	83%	99%
Smoking Cessation Advice	102	83%	86%	82%	100%
Pneumonia Care					
Appropriate Initial Antibiotic	317	87%	88%	83%	94%
Blood Culture Timing	382	90%	90%	90%	100%
Influenza Vaccine	90	70%	73%	70%	100%
Initial Antibiotic Timing	481	88%	84%	80%	93%
Oxygenation Assessment	551	99%	100%	99%	100%
Pneumococcal Vaccine	393	72%	72%	69%	94%
Smoking Cessation Advice	108	68%	86%	80%	100%
Surgical Infection Prevention					
Prophylactic Antibiotic Given[2,3]	429	78%	82%	77%	95%
Prophylactic Antibiotic Selection[2]	257	89%	93%	90%	100%
Prophylactic Antibiotic Stopped[2,3]	401	81%	83%	72%	95%
Pregnancy Care					
Inpatient Neonatal Mortality	-	-	-	-	-
Third or Fourth Degree Laceration	-	-	2.62%	3.63%	3.27%

Southeast Michigan Surgical Hospital

21230 Dequindre
Warren, MI 48091
URL: www.smshinc.com
Ownership: Voluntary non-profit - Private
Emergency Services: No

Phone: 586-427-1000
Fax: 586-759-0237
Accredited: Yes
Licensed Beds: 20

Key Personnel:

CEO . . . . Larry Belenke
Chief Medical Staff . . . . John D'Alessandro, DO
Medical/Surgical Nursing . . . . Julie Lugartos, RN

NOTE: Hospital profiles are in alphabetical order by state, then city, then hospital within the city; Rankings are sorted by rate in descending order and exclude hospitals with less than 25 cases; (1) The number of cases is too small (n<25) for purposes of reliably predicting hospital performance; (2) Measure reflects the hospital's indication that its submission was based upon a sample of its relevant discharges; (3) Rate reflects fewer than the maximum possible quarters of data for the measure; (4) Inaccurate information submitted and suppressed for one or more quarters; (5) No data is available from the hospital for this measure; Please refer to the User's Guide for a full explanation of data

Measure	Cases	This Hospital	State Average	U.S. Average	Top Hospital
Heart Attack Care					
ACE Inhibitor or ARB for LVSD[5]	-	-	86%	82%	100%
Aspirin at Arrival[5]	-	-	95%	92%	100%
Aspirin at Discharge[5]	-	-	94%	90%	100%
Beta Blocker at Arrival[5]	-	-	90%	87%	100%
Beta Blocker at Discharge[5]	-	-	93%	90%	100%
Fibrinolytic Medication Timing[5]	-	-	28%	31%	100%
PCI Within 90 Minutes of Arrival[5]	-	-	59%	54%	95%
Smoking Cessation Advice[5]	-	-	93%	88%	100%
Heart Failure Care					
ACE Inhibitor or ARB for LVSD[5]	-	-	84%	82%	100%
Discharge Instructions[5]	-	-	73%	61%	93%
Evaluation of LVS Function[5]	-	-	91%	83%	99%
Smoking Cessation Advice[5]	-	-	86%	82%	100%
Pneumonia Care					
Appropriate Initial Antibiotic[5]	-	-	88%	83%	94%
Blood Culture Timing[5]	-	-	90%	90%	100%
Influenza Vaccine[5]	-	-	73%	70%	100%
Initial Antibiotic Timing[5]	-	-	84%	80%	93%
Oxygenation Assessment[5]	-	-	100%	99%	100%
Pneumococcal Vaccine[5]	-	-	72%	69%	94%
Smoking Cessation Advice[5]	-	-	86%	80%	100%
Surgical Infection Prevention					
Prophylactic Antibiotic Given[1,3]	1	0%	82%	77%	95%
Prophylactic Antibiotic Selection[5]	-	-	93%	90%	100%
Prophylactic Antibiotic Stopped[1,3]	1	100%	83%	72%	95%
Pregnancy Care					
Inpatient Neonatal Mortality	-	-	-	-	-
Third or Fourth Degree Laceration	-	-	2.62%	3.63%	3.27%

Community Hospital Watervliet

400 Medical Park Drive
Watervliet, MI 49098
Toll-Free: 800-463-1164
Phone: 269-463-3111
Fax: 269-463-4452

URL: www.communityhospitalwatervliet.com
Ownership: Voluntary non-profit - Private
Emergency Services: Yes
Accredited: Yes
Licensed Beds: 70

Key Personnel:
CEO/Administration . . . . Fritz Fahrenbacher
Director of Cardiology/Cardiac Lab. . . . . Donald Brooks
Emergency Room Director. . . . . Milt Bulles
Emergency Department . . . . Kathy Davis
Infection Control. . . . . Theda Koshar
Surgery . . . . Edythe Hedman
Obstetrics. . . . . Jean Litaker
Respiratory Therapy. . . . . Dorothy Messinger

Measure	Cases	This Hospital	State Average	U.S. Average	Top Hospital
Heart Attack Care					
ACE Inhibitor or ARB for LVSD	0	-	86%	82%	100%
Aspirin at Arrival[1]	12	83%	95%	92%	100%
Aspirin at Discharge[1]	5	100%	94%	90%	100%
Beta Blocker at Arrival[1]	11	55%	90%	87%	100%
Beta Blocker at Discharge[1]	3	67%	93%	90%	100%
Fibrinolytic Medication Timing	0	-	28%	31%	100%
PCI Within 90 Minutes of Arrival	0	-	59%	54%	95%
Smoking Cessation Advice	0	-	93%	88%	100%
Heart Failure Care					
ACE Inhibitor or ARB for LVSD[1]	18	50%	84%	82%	100%
Discharge Instructions[1,3]	12	92%	73%	61%	93%
Evaluation of LVS Function	84	64%	91%	83%	99%
Smoking Cessation Advice[1]	8	38%	86%	82%	100%
Pneumonia Care					
Appropriate Initial Antibiotic[1,3]	20	90%	88%	83%	94%
Blood Culture Timing[1,3]	15	87%	90%	90%	100%
Influenza Vaccine[5]	-	-	73%	70%	100%
Initial Antibiotic Timing	74	89%	84%	80%	93%
Oxygenation Assessment	94	99%	100%	99%	100%
Pneumococcal Vaccine	63	70%	72%	69%	94%
Smoking Cessation Advice[1]	23	70%	86%	80%	100%
Surgical Infection Prevention					
Prophylactic Antibiotic Given	152	93%	82%	77%	95%
Prophylactic Antibiotic Selection	41	98%	93%	90%	100%
Prophylactic Antibiotic Stopped	151	89%	83%	72%	95%
Pregnancy Care					
Inpatient Neonatal Mortality	-	-	-	-	-
Third or Fourth Degree Laceration	-	-	2.62%	3.63%	3.27%

Oakwood Annapolis Hospital

Alternate Name: Oakwood Hospital-Annapolis Center
33155 Annapolis Avenue
Wayne, MI 48184
Phone: 734-467-4000
Fax: 734-467-4017
URL: www.oakwood.org
Ownership: Govt - Hospital District or Authority
Emergency Services: Yes
Accredited: Yes
Licensed Beds: 296

Key Personnel:
CEO. . . . . Tom Kochis
Emergency Room . . . . Charles Ceeter
OB/GYN Womens Health. . . . . Franklin Castillo, MD
Director Respiratory Therapy . . . . Betty Ferris

Measure	Cases	This Hospital	State Average	U.S. Average	Top Hospital
Heart Attack Care					
ACE Inhibitor or ARB for LVSD	33	88%	86%	82%	100%
Aspirin at Arrival	118	97%	95%	92%	100%
Aspirin at Discharge	65	97%	94%	90%	100%
Beta Blocker at Arrival	87	98%	90%	87%	100%
Beta Blocker at Discharge	77	100%	93%	90%	100%
Fibrinolytic Medication Timing	0	-	28%	31%	100%
PCI Within 90 Minutes of Arrival[1]	12	50%	59%	54%	95%
Smoking Cessation Advice	26	100%	93%	88%	100%
Heart Failure Care					
ACE Inhibitor or ARB for LVSD	173	82%	84%	82%	100%
Discharge Instructions	381	66%	73%	61%	93%
Evaluation of LVS Function	475	96%	91%	83%	99%
Smoking Cessation Advice	127	100%	86%	82%	100%
Pneumonia Care					
Appropriate Initial Antibiotic	215	95%	88%	83%	94%
Blood Culture Timing	307	98%	90%	90%	100%
Influenza Vaccine	74	92%	73%	70%	100%
Initial Antibiotic Timing	403	85%	84%	80%	93%
Oxygenation Assessment	475	100%	100%	99%	100%
Pneumococcal Vaccine	260	93%	72%	69%	94%
Smoking Cessation Advice	160	98%	86%	80%	100%
Surgical Infection Prevention					
Prophylactic Antibiotic Given[2]	344	94%	82%	77%	95%
Prophylactic Antibiotic Selection[2]	99	94%	93%	90%	100%
Prophylactic Antibiotic Stopped[2]	325	78%	83%	72%	95%
Pregnancy Care					
Inpatient Neonatal Mortality	-	-	-	-	-
Third or Fourth Degree Laceration	-	-	2.62%	3.63%	3.27%

West Branch Regional Medical Center

Alternate Name: Tolfree Memorial Hospital
2463 South M-30
West Branch, MI 48661
Phone: 989-345-3660
Fax: 989-343-3113
URL: www.wbrmc.org
Ownership: Government - Local
Emergency Services: Yes
Accredited: Yes
Licensed Beds: 88

Key Personnel:
CEO. . . . . Douglas E Pattullo
Chief Medical Staff. . . . . Wilfredo Abesamis, MD
Director Infection/Disease Control . . . . Kathleen DeHaan, RN
CCU Spvg. Nurse . . . . Judy Maass, RN
Director Medical/Surgical Nursing . . . . Noreen Connolly
OB/GYN Womens Health. . . . . Mario Toledo, MD
Chief Radiology . . . . Stephen Brown, MD
Director Respiratory Therapy . . . . Joseph Bell

Measure	Cases	This Hospital	State Average	U.S. Average	Top Hospital
Heart Attack Care					
ACE Inhibitor or ARB for LVSD[1]	5	100%	86%	82%	100%
Aspirin at Arrival	57	95%	95%	92%	100%
Aspirin at Discharge[1]	21	95%	94%	90%	100%

NOTE: Hospital profiles are in alphabetical order by state, then city, then hospital within the city; Rankings are sorted by rate in descending order and exclude hospitals with less than 25 cases; (1) The number of cases is too small (n<25) for purposes of reliably predicting hospital performance; (2) Measure reflects the hospital's indication that its submission was based upon a sample of its relevant discharges; (3) Rate reflects fewer than the maximum possible quarters of data for the measure; (4) Inaccurate information submitted and suppressed for one or more quarters; (5) No data is available from the hospital for this measure; Please refer to the User's Guide for a full explanation of data

Beta Blocker at Arrival	60	98%	90%	87%	100%
Beta Blocker at Discharge	28	100%	93%	90%	100%
Fibrinolytic Medication Timing[1]	5	60%	28%	31%	100%
PCI Within 90 Minutes of Arrival	0	-	59%	54%	95%
Smoking Cessation Advice[1]	4	100%	93%	88%	100%
Heart Failure Care					
ACE Inhibitor or ARB for LVSD	52	94%	84%	82%	100%
Discharge Instructions	159	69%	73%	61%	93%
Evaluation of LVS Function	184	91%	91%	83%	99%
Smoking Cessation Advice[1]	24	92%	86%	82%	100%
Pneumonia Care					
Appropriate Initial Antibiotic	108	80%	88%	83%	94%
Blood Culture Timing	102	94%	90%	90%	100%
Influenza Vaccine	27	63%	73%	70%	100%
Initial Antibiotic Timing	132	70%	84%	80%	93%
Oxygenation Assessment	161	100%	100%	99%	100%
Pneumococcal Vaccine	85	51%	72%	69%	94%
Smoking Cessation Advice	40	75%	86%	80%	100%
Surgical Infection Prevention					
Prophylactic Antibiotic Given[3]	223	65%	82%	77%	95%
Prophylactic Antibiotic Selection	68	97%	93%	90%	100%
Prophylactic Antibiotic Stopped[3]	217	45%	83%	72%	95%
Pregnancy Care					
Inpatient Neonatal Mortality	-	-	-	-	-
Third or Fourth Degree Laceration	-	-	2.62%	3.63%	3.27%

Henry Ford Wyandotte Hospital

Alternate Name: Henry Ford Health System
2333 Biddle Avenue
Wyandotte, MI 48192

Toll-Free: 800-436-7936
Phone: 734-246-6000
Fax: 734-246-8795

URL: www.henryfordwyandotte.com
Ownership: Voluntary non-profit - Private
Emergency Services: Yes

Accredited: Yes
Licensed Beds: 162

Key Personnel:
CEO. . . . . Thomas Caulfield
Chief Medical Staff. . . . . Malcolm E Williamson, DO
Emergency Room . . . . Paula Lane, RN
Medical/Surgical Nursing . . . . Felecia Williams
OB/GYN Womens Health. . . . . Denise Morton
Director Respiratory Therapy . . . . Roland Leal

Measure	Cases	This Hospital	State Average	U.S. Average	Top Hospital
Heart Attack Care					
ACE Inhibitor or ARB for LVSD	54	72%	86%	82%	100%
Aspirin at Arrival	273	93%	95%	92%	100%
Aspirin at Discharge	180	87%	94%	90%	100%
Beta Blocker at Arrival	290	90%	90%	87%	100%
Beta Blocker at Discharge	205	86%	93%	90%	100%
Fibrinolytic Medication Timing[1]	1	0%	28%	31%	100%
PCI Within 90 Minutes of Arrival[1]	14	64%	59%	54%	95%
Smoking Cessation Advice	53	100%	93%	88%	100%
Heart Failure Care					
ACE Inhibitor or ARB for LVSD[2]	101	86%	84%	82%	100%
Discharge Instructions[2]	227	48%	73%	61%	93%
Evaluation of LVS Function[2]	285	89%	91%	83%	99%
Smoking Cessation Advice[2]	40	98%	86%	82%	100%
Pneumonia Care					
Appropriate Initial Antibiotic[2]	113	83%	88%	83%	94%
Blood Culture Timing[2]	124	85%	90%	90%	100%
Influenza Vaccine[4,5]	-	-	73%	70%	100%
Initial Antibiotic Timing[2]	172	86%	84%	80%	93%
Oxygenation Assessment[2]	180	100%	100%	99%	100%
Pneumococcal Vaccine[2]	123	54%	72%	69%	94%
Smoking Cessation Advice[2]	47	98%	86%	80%	100%
Surgical Infection Prevention					
Prophylactic Antibiotic Given[2,3]	213	78%	82%	77%	95%
Prophylactic Antibiotic Selection[2]	72	86%	93%	90%	100%
Prophylactic Antibiotic Stopped[2,3]	157	97%	83%	72%	95%
Pregnancy Care					
Inpatient Neonatal Mortality	-	-	-	-	-
Third or Fourth Degree Laceration	-	-	2.62%	3.63%	3.27%

Zeeland Community Hospital

8333 Felch St
Zeeland, MI 49464
E-mail: parnoldink@zch.org
URL: www.zch.org
Ownership: Voluntary non-profit - Private
Emergency Services: Yes

Phone: 616-772-4644
Fax: 616-748-2828

Accredited: Yes
Licensed Beds: 57

Key Personnel:
President/CEO. . . . . Henry A Veenstra
Chief Medical Staff. . . . . Dr Duane Saxton
Manager Catheterization . . . . Larry McMullin
Manager Emergency Room. . . . . Marlene Holstine
Infection Control. . . . . Pat VanOmen, RN
Medical/Surgical Nursing Manager. . . . . Julianne Carey
Manager OB/GYN/Women's Health. . . . . Juliane Carey
Manager Radiology . . . . Scott Weenum
Manager Respiratory/Cardiopulmonary . . . . Lawrence McMullin

Measure	Cases	This Hospital	State Average	U.S. Average	Top Hospital
Heart Attack Care					
ACE Inhibitor or ARB for LVSD[1]	2	50%	86%	82%	100%
Aspirin at Arrival[1]	15	100%	95%	92%	100%
Aspirin at Discharge[1]	7	100%	94%	90%	100%
Beta Blocker at Arrival[1]	13	85%	90%	87%	100%
Beta Blocker at Discharge[1]	8	88%	93%	90%	100%
Fibrinolytic Medication Timing	0	-	28%	31%	100%
PCI Within 90 Minutes of Arrival	0	-	59%	54%	95%
Smoking Cessation Advice[1]	1	100%	93%	88%	100%
Heart Failure Care					
ACE Inhibitor or ARB for LVSD	26	92%	84%	82%	100%
Discharge Instructions	54	94%	73%	61%	93%
Evaluation of LVS Function	78	92%	91%	83%	99%
Smoking Cessation Advice[1]	10	100%	86%	82%	100%
Pneumonia Care					
Appropriate Initial Antibiotic	64	95%	88%	83%	94%
Blood Culture Timing	76	97%	90%	90%	100%
Influenza Vaccine[1]	16	100%	73%	70%	100%
Initial Antibiotic Timing	88	95%	84%	80%	93%
Oxygenation Assessment	108	100%	100%	99%	100%
Pneumococcal Vaccine	77	97%	72%	69%	94%
Smoking Cessation Advice[1]	8	100%	86%	80%	100%
Surgical Infection Prevention					
Prophylactic Antibiotic Given[2]	221	92%	82%	77%	95%
Prophylactic Antibiotic Selection[2]	59	88%	93%	90%	100%
Prophylactic Antibiotic Stopped[2]	218	91%	83%	72%	95%
Pregnancy Care					
Inpatient Neonatal Mortality	-	-	-	-	-
Third or Fourth Degree Laceration	-	-	2.62%	3.63%	3.27%

NOTE: Hospital profiles are in alphabetical order by state, then city, then hospital within the city; Rankings are sorted by rate in descending order and exclude hospitals with less than 25 cases; (1) The number of cases is too small (n<25) for purposes of reliably predicting hospital performance; (2) Measure reflects the hospital's indication that its submission was based upon a sample of its relevant discharges; (3) Rate reflects fewer than the maximum possible quarters of data for the measure; (4) Inaccurate information submitted and suppressed for one or more quarters; (5) No data is available from the hospital for this measure; Please refer to the User's Guide for a full explanation of data

Heart Attack Care

1. ACE Inhibitor or ARB for LVSD

Hospital Name	City	Rate	Cases
Fairview Southdale Hospital	Edina	98%	138
Hennepin County Medical Center	Minneapolis	98%	42
Methodist Hospital	Saint Louis Park	96%	72
Saint Joseph's Hospital	Saint Paul	94%	50
Saint mary's Medical Center	Duluth	94%	179
Saint Lukes Hospital	Duluth	91%	56
Regions Hospital	Saint Paul	89%	87
United Hospital	Saint Paul	89%	74
Mercy Hospital	Coon Rapids	88%	83
Saint Cloud Hospital	Saint Cloud	88%	113
Abbott-Northwestern Hospital	Minneapolis	87%	190
North Memorial Health Care	Robbinsdale	87%	155
Saint Marys Hospital	Rochester	87%	62
University of Minnesota Med Ctr-Fairview	Minneapolis	77%	47

2. Aspirin at Arrival

Hospital Name	City	Rate	Cases
Austin Medical Center	Austin	100%	27
Fairview Ridges Hospital	Burnsville	100%	38
Immanuel Saint Joseph's-Mayo Health System	Mankato	100%	105
Methodist Hospital	Saint Louis Park	100%	273
North Country Regional Hospital	Bemidji	100%	35
Saint John's Hospital	Maplewood	100%	77
Saint Marys Hospital	Rochester	100%	124
Saint mary's Medical Center	Duluth	100%	216
Fairview Southdale Hospital	Edina	99%	364
Hennepin County Medical Center	Minneapolis	99%	191
Mercy Hospital	Coon Rapids	99%	327
North Memorial Health Care	Robbinsdale	99%	495
Regions Hospital	Saint Paul	99%	251
Saint Cloud Hospital	Saint Cloud	99%	211
Saint Joseph's Hospital	Saint Paul	99%	152
Albert Lea Medical Center-Mayo Health System	Albert Lea	98%	43
Saint Joseph's Medical Center	Brainerd	98%	43
Saint Lukes Hospital	Duluth	98%	128
United Hospital	Saint Paul	98%	288
University of Minnesota Med Ctr-Fairview	Minneapolis	97%	95
Abbott-Northwestern Hospital	Minneapolis	96%	245
Lake Region Healthcare Corporation	Fergus Falls	96%	27
Grand Itasca Clinic and Hospital	Grand Rapids	95%	40
Unity Hospital	Fridley	95%	62
University Medical Center-Mesabi	Hibbing	93%	28

3. Aspirin at Discharge

Hospital Name	City	Rate	Cases
Fairview Southdale Hospital	Edina	100%	547
Immanuel Saint Joseph's-Mayo Health System	Mankato	100%	115
Mercy Hospital	Coon Rapids	100%	463
Saint Joseph's Hospital	Saint Paul	100%	253
Methodist Hospital	Saint Louis Park	99%	318
Saint Cloud Hospital	Saint Cloud	99%	570
Saint Lukes Hospital	Duluth	99%	164
Saint Marys Hospital	Rochester	99%	233
Saint mary's Medical Center	Duluth	99%	501
University of Minnesota Med Ctr-Fairview	Minneapolis	99%	142
Abbott-Northwestern Hospital	Minneapolis	98%	803
Hennepin County Medical Center	Minneapolis	98%	178
North Memorial Health Care	Robbinsdale	98%	500
Regions Hospital	Saint Paul	98%	336
United Hospital	Saint Paul	98%	462
Saint John's Hospital	Maplewood	93%	41
Albert Lea Medical Center-Mayo Health System	Albert Lea	92%	37
Unity Hospital	Fridley	92%	39
Grand Itasca Clinic and Hospital	Grand Rapids	84%	25

4. Beta Blocker at Arrival

Hospital Name	City	Rate	Cases
Albert Lea Medical Center-Mayo Health System	Albert Lea	100%	43
Fairview Ridges Hospital	Burnsville	100%	38
Fairview Southdale Hospital	Edina	100%	340
Hennepin County Medical Center	Minneapolis	99%	170
Immanuel Saint Joseph's-Mayo Health System	Mankato	99%	98
Saint Marys Hospital	Rochester	99%	103
Saint John's Hospital	Maplewood	98%	48
Saint mary's Medical Center	Duluth	98%	166
Regions Hospital	Saint Paul	97%	217
Saint Joseph's Medical Center	Brainerd	97%	33
Methodist Hospital	Saint Louis Park	96%	199
North Memorial Health Care	Robbinsdale	96%	447
Saint Cloud Hospital	Saint Cloud	96%	168
Saint Joseph's Hospital	Saint Paul	96%	96
United Hospital	Saint Paul	96%	228
University of Minnesota Med Ctr-Fairview	Minneapolis	96%	81
Grand Itasca Clinic and Hospital	Grand Rapids	95%	40
Mercy Hospital	Coon Rapids	95%	239
Abbott-Northwestern Hospital	Minneapolis	94%	220
Saint Lukes Hospital	Duluth	94%	124
Lake Region Healthcare Corporation	Fergus Falls	93%	28
University Medical Center-Mesabi	Hibbing	93%	30
Unity Hospital	Fridley	89%	45

5. Beta Blocker at Discharge

Hospital Name	City	Rate	Cases
Albert Lea Medical Center-Mayo Health System	Albert Lea	100%	39
Fairview Southdale Hospital	Edina	100%	545
Mercy Hospital	Coon Rapids	100%	489
Methodist Hospital	Saint Louis Park	99%	329
Saint Cloud Hospital	Saint Cloud	99%	604
Saint Lukes Hospital	Duluth	99%	190
Saint Marys Hospital	Rochester	99%	269
Saint mary's Medical Center	Duluth	99%	589
Abbott-Northwestern Hospital	Minneapolis	98%	923
North Memorial Health Care	Robbinsdale	98%	506
Regions Hospital	Saint Paul	98%	350
Saint Joseph's Hospital	Saint Paul	98%	218
United Hospital	Saint Paul	98%	499
University of Minnesota Med Ctr-Fairview	Minneapolis	98%	133
Grand Itasca Clinic and Hospital	Grand Rapids	97%	29
Hennepin County Medical Center	Minneapolis	97%	155
Immanuel Saint Joseph's-Mayo Health System	Mankato	96%	107
Unity Hospital	Fridley	95%	43

7. PCI Within 90 Minutes of Arrival

Hospital Name	City	Rate	Cases
North Memorial Health Care	Robbinsdale	92%	26
Mercy Hospital	Coon Rapids	64%	28

8. Smoking Cessation Advice

Hospital Name	City	Rate	Cases
Fairview Southdale Hospital	Edina	100%	158
Immanuel Saint Joseph's-Mayo Health System	Mankato	100%	30
Mercy Hospital	Coon Rapids	99%	197
Saint Marys Hospital	Rochester	99%	75
United Hospital	Saint Paul	99%	170
Regions Hospital	Saint Paul	98%	118
Saint mary's Medical Center	Duluth	98%	224
University of Minnesota Med Ctr-Fairview	Minneapolis	98%	49
North Memorial Health Care	Robbinsdale	97%	145
Saint Joseph's Hospital	Saint Paul	97%	101
Hennepin County Medical Center	Minneapolis	96%	83
Methodist Hospital	Saint Louis Park	95%	94
Saint Cloud Hospital	Saint Cloud	95%	213
Abbott-Northwestern Hospital	Minneapolis	94%	348
Saint Lukes Hospital	Duluth	88%	50

Heart Failure Care

9. ACE Inhibitor or ARB for LVSD

Hospital Name	City	Rate	Cases
Fairmont Medical Center	Fairmont	100%	26
Ridgeview Medical Center	Waconia	98%	51
Community Memorial Hospital	Winona	97%	29
Fairview Lakes Health Services	Wyoming	96%	27
Fairview Ridges Hospital	Burnsville	93%	44
University Medical Center-Mesabi	Hibbing	92%	60
Fairview Southdale Hospital	Edina	91%	171
Saint Lukes Hospital	Duluth	91%	97
Methodist Hospital	Saint Louis Park	90%	203
North Country Regional Hospital	Bemidji	90%	49
Regions Hospital	Saint Paul	90%	165
Albert Lea Medical Center-Mayo Health System	Albert Lea	89%	28
Saint Joseph's Hospital	Saint Paul	89%	137
Saint Marys Hospital	Rochester	89%	135
Abbott-Northwestern Hospital	Minneapolis	88%	394
Austin Medical Center	Austin	88%	26
Lake Region Healthcare Corporation	Fergus Falls	88%	34
Saint mary's Medical Center	Duluth	87%	217
North Memorial Health Care	Robbinsdale	85%	242
Saint Cloud Hospital	Saint Cloud	85%	256
Douglas County Hospital	Alexandria	84%	49

NOTE: Hospital profiles are in alphabetical order by state, then city, then hospital within the city; Rankings are sorted by rate in descending order and exclude hospitals with less than 25 cases; (1) The number of cases is too small (n<25) for purposes of reliably predicting hospital performance; (2) Measure reflects the hospital's indication that its submission was based upon a sample of its relevant discharges; (3) Rate reflects fewer than the maximum possible quarters of data for the measure; (4) Inaccurate information submitted and suppressed for one or more quarters; (5) No data is available from the hospital for this measure; Please refer to the User's Guide for a full explanation of data

Hospital Name	City	Rate	Cases
Fairview Red Wing Hospital	Red Wing	84%	25
Hennepin County Medical Center	Minneapolis	84%	219
Saint John's Hospital	Maplewood	84%	94
Unity Hospital	Fridley	83%	76
University of Minnesota Med Ctr-Fairview	Minneapolis	83%	158
Immanuel Saint Joseph's-Mayo Health System	Mankato	82%	79
Saint Francis Regional Medical Center	Shakopee	82%	34
Mercy Hospital	Coon Rapids	81%	169
United Hospital	Saint Paul	76%	272
Saint Joseph's Medical Center	Brainerd	74%	53
Buffalo Hospital	Buffalo	63%	27

10. Discharge Instructions

Hospital Name	City	Rate	Cases
Owatonna Hospital	Owatonna	98%	51
Austin Medical Center	Austin	96%	78
Fairview Northland Regional Health Care	Princeton	94%	53
University Medical Center-Mesabi	Hibbing	94%	115
Fairview Southdale Hospital	Edina	92%	333
Fairview Ridges Hospital	Burnsville	91%	103
Ridgeview Medical Center	Waconia	91%	66
Unity Hospital	Fridley	88%	207
Saint Joseph's Hospital	Saint Paul	87%	234
Fairmont Medical Center	Fairmont	86%	58
Mercy Hospital	Coon Rapids	86%	368
Immanuel Saint Joseph's-Mayo Health System	Mankato	85%	138
Saint Marys Hospital	Rochester	85%	247
Saint John's Hospital	Maplewood	82%	174
Lakeview Hospital	Stillwater	76%	50
Cambridge Medical Center	Cambridge	75%	51
Douglas County Hospital	Alexandria	75%	76
Kanabec Hospital	Mora	75%	48
Saint Cloud Hospital	Saint Cloud	75%	430
Fairview Red Wing Hospital	Red Wing	74%	47
United Hospital	Saint Paul	74%	404
North Country Regional Hospital	Bemidji	73%	86
Regions Hospital	Saint Paul	73%	266
Methodist Hospital	Saint Louis Park	72%	409
Woodwinds Health Campus	Woodbury	72%	40
New Ulm Medical Center	New Ulm	68%	25
University of Minnesota Med Ctr-Fairview	Minneapolis	68%	241
Abbott-Northwestern Hospital	Minneapolis	67%	681
Albert Lea Medical Center-Mayo Health System	Albert Lea	67%	52
Virginia Regional Medical Center	Virginia	67%	54
Lake Region Healthcare Corporation	Fergus Falls	66%	71
Riverwood HealthCare Center	Aitkin	66%	29
Saint Joseph's Medical Center	Brainerd	64%	203
Avera Marshall Regional Medical Center	Marshall	63%	30
Saint Lukes Hospital	Duluth	63%	204
Saint mary's Medical Center	Duluth	62%	301
Hutchinson Area Health Care	Hutchinson	60%	43
Mille Lacs Health System	Onamia	58%	33
North Memorial Health Care	Robbinsdale	58%	452
Riverview Health	Crookston	56%	34
Saint Francis Regional Medical Center	Shakopee	56%	62
Rochester Methodist Hospital	Rochester	53%	34
Hennepin County Medical Center	Minneapolis	47%	341
Regina Medical Center	Hastings	46%	46
Buffalo Hospital	Buffalo	41%	41
Fairview Lakes Health Services	Wyoming	40%	72
Northfield Hospital	Northfield	39%	49
District One Hospital	Faribault	36%	36
Northwest Medical Center	Thief River Falls	36%	36
Rice Memorial Hospital	Willmar	32%	74
Glencoe Regional Health Services	Glencoe	31%	36
Saint Mary's Regional Health Center	Detroit Lakes	30%	37
Mercy Hospital & Health Care Center	Moose Lake	24%	25
Monticello-Big Lake Community Hospital	Monticello	24%	34
Deer River Healthcare Center	Deer River	19%	32
Community Memorial Hospital Association	Cloquet	15%	34
Falls Memorial Hospital	Int'l Falls	11%	28

11. Evaluation of LVS Function

Hospital Name	City	Rate	Cases
Austin Medical Center	Austin	100%	113
Fairview Lakes Health Services	Wyoming	100%	94
Fairview Northland Regional Health Care	Princeton	100%	72
Fairview Southdale Hospital	Edina	100%	441
Owatonna Hospital	Owatonna	100%	62
Saint Marys Hospital	Rochester	100%	329
Methodist Hospital	Saint Louis Park	99%	536
Abbott-Northwestern Hospital	Minneapolis	98%	844
Hennepin County Medical Center	Minneapolis	98%	422
Mercy Hospital	Coon Rapids	98%	441
Regions Hospital	Saint Paul	98%	383
Ridgeview Medical Center	Waconia	98%	99
Rochester Methodist Hospital	Rochester	98%	44
Unity Hospital	Fridley	98%	272
University of Minnesota Med Ctr-Fairview	Minneapolis	98%	284
Albert Lea Medical Center-Mayo Health System	Albert Lea	97%	74
Douglas County Hospital	Alexandria	97%	112
North Country Regional Hospital	Bemidji	97%	111
Saint Cloud Hospital	Saint Cloud	97%	556
Fairview Red Wing Hospital	Red Wing	96%	68
Saint John's Hospital	Maplewood	96%	248
Saint Joseph's Hospital	Saint Paul	96%	314
Woodwinds Health Campus	Woodbury	96%	49
Community Memorial Hospital	Winona	95%	86
Fairmont Medical Center	Fairmont	94%	96
Lakeview Hospital	Stillwater	94%	68
Saint mary's Medical Center	Duluth	93%	395
Hutchinson Area Health Care	Hutchinson	92%	60
United Hospital	Saint Paul	92%	544
University Medical Center-Mesabi	Hibbing	92%	160
North Memorial Health Care	Robbinsdale	91%	580
Saint Lukes Hospital	Duluth	91%	250
Buffalo Hospital	Buffalo	90%	59
Cambridge Medical Center	Cambridge	90%	77
Fairview Ridges Hospital	Burnsville	90%	156
Immanuel Saint Joseph's-Mayo Health System	Mankato	90%	181
Saint Joseph's Area Health Services	Park Rapids	90%	31
First Care Medical Services	Fosston	89%	28
New Ulm Medical Center	New Ulm	88%	59
Northfield Hospital	Northfield	88%	77
Saint Francis Regional Medical Center	Shakopee	87%	90
Lake Region Healthcare Corporation	Fergus Falls	86%	120
Olmsted Medical Center Hospital	Rochester	86%	37
Regina Medical Center	Hastings	86%	69
Virginia Regional Medical Center	Virginia	86%	115
Rice Memorial Hospital	Willmar	85%	96
Grand Itasca Clinic and Hospital	Grand Rapids	84%	50
Queen of Peace Hospital	New Prague	84%	31
Saint Joseph's Medical Center	Brainerd	84%	243
Waseca Medical Center-Mayo Health System	Waseca	84%	25
Riverwood HealthCare Center	Aitkin	82%	33
Monticello-Big Lake Community Hospital	Monticello	80%	41
Swift County-Benson Hospital	Benson	80%	25
Avera Marshall Regional Medical Center	Marshall	79%	42
Community Memorial Hospital Association	Cloquet	79%	52
Worthington Regional Hospital	Worthington	79%	29
Deer River Healthcare Center	Deer River	76%	38
United Hospital District	Blue Earth	75%	28
Glencoe Regional Health Services	Glencoe	74%	72
Kanabec Hospital	Mora	73%	63
Saint Gabriel's Hospital	Little Falls	73%	26
Mille Lacs Health System	Onamia	69%	39
Meeker County Memorial Hospital	Litchfield	65%	31
Saint Peter Community Hospital	Saint Peter	65%	26
Northwest Medical Center	Thief River Falls	63%	52
District One Hospital	Faribault	60%	52
Saint Mary's Regional Health Center	Detroit Lakes	56%	57
Riverview Health	Crookston	48%	50
Lakewood Health System Hospital	Staples	47%	34
Mercy Hospital & Health Care Center	Moose Lake	47%	34
Roseau Area Hospital & Homes	Roseau	45%	29
Saint Francis Medical Center	Breckenridge	41%	37
Chippewa County Montevideo Hospital	Montevideo	39%	36
Falls Memorial Hospital	Int'l Falls	0%	38

12. Smoking Cessation Advice

Hospital Name	City	Rate	Cases
Fairview Southdale Hospital	Edina	100%	44
Regions Hospital	Saint Paul	99%	98
Mercy Hospital	Coon Rapids	97%	64
University of Minnesota Med Ctr-Fairview	Minneapolis	96%	48
Saint Joseph's Hospital	Saint Paul	92%	49
Unity Hospital	Fridley	92%	38
Saint mary's Medical Center	Duluth	88%	51
United Hospital	Saint Paul	88%	73
Methodist Hospital	Saint Louis Park	85%	54
Saint John's Hospital	Maplewood	85%	26
University Medical Center-Mesabi	Hibbing	84%	25
Saint Marys Hospital	Rochester	83%	30
Abbott-Northwestern Hospital	Minneapolis	81%	135
Saint Cloud Hospital	Saint Cloud	75%	73
Hennepin County Medical Center	Minneapolis	70%	151
North Memorial Health Care	Robbinsdale	68%	92
Saint Lukes Hospital	Duluth	62%	26

NOTE: Hospital profiles are in alphabetical order by state, then city, then hospital within the city; Rankings are sorted by rate in descending order and exclude hospitals with less than 25 cases; (1) The number of cases is too small (n<25) for purposes of reliably predicting hospital performance; (2) Measure reflects the hospital's indication that its submission was based upon a sample of its relevant discharges; (3) Rate reflects fewer than the maximum possible quarters of data for the measure; (4) Inaccurate information submitted and suppressed for one or more quarters; (5) No data is available from the hospital for this measure; Please refer to the User's Guide for a full explanation of data

Pneumonia Care

13. Appropriate Initial Antibiotic

Hospital Name	City	Rate	Cases
Fairmont Medical Center	Fairmont	96%	71
Waseca Medical Center-Mayo Health System	Waseca	96%	26
Owatonna Hospital	Owatonna	95%	84
Lakeview Hospital	Stillwater	93%	57
Cambridge Medical Center	Cambridge	92%	80
North Country Regional Hospital	Bemidji	92%	91
Saint Cloud Hospital	Saint Cloud	92%	209
Woodwinds Health Campus	Woodbury	92%	37
Fairview Southdale Hospital	Edina	91%	139
Saint Joseph's Medical Center	Brainerd	91%	146
Fairview Red Wing Hospital	Red Wing	90%	78
Mercy Hospital & Health Care Center	Moose Lake	90%	41
Methodist Hospital	Saint Louis Park	90%	289
Saint Joseph's Hospital	Saint Paul	90%	81
Saint Marys Hospital	Rochester	90%	73
Albert Lea Medical Center-Mayo Health System	Albert Lea	89%	54
Austin Medical Center	Austin	89%	84
Buffalo Hospital	Buffalo	89%	74
Douglas County Hospital	Alexandria	89%	84
Fairview Lakes Health Services	Wyoming	89%	116
Ridgeview Medical Center	Waconia	89%	79
Saint mary's Medical Center	Duluth	88%	117
Fairview Northland Regional Health Care	Princeton	87%	61
Glencoe Regional Health Services	Glencoe	87%	38
Monticello-Big Lake Community Hospital	Monticello	87%	46
North Memorial Health Care	Robbinsdale	87%	308
Abbott-Northwestern Hospital	Minneapolis	86%	236
Fairview Ridges Hospital	Burnsville	86%	174
Regina Medical Center	Hastings	86%	36
Rice Memorial Hospital	Willmar	86%	87
Northfield Hospital	Northfield	84%	68
Regions Hospital	Saint Paul	84%	193
Saint Francis Regional Medical Center	Shakopee	84%	62
Saint Joseph's Area Health Services	Park Rapids	84%	55
Lake Region Healthcare Corporation	Fergus Falls	83%	48
Mercy Hospital	Coon Rapids	82%	173
Saint Francis Medical Center	Breckenridge	82%	33
Unity Hospital	Fridley	82%	176
Hennepin County Medical Center	Minneapolis	81%	187
Saint John's Hospital	Maplewood	81%	139
Sioux Valley Luverne Hospital	Luverne	81%	27
Tri-County Hospital	Wadena	81%	80
District One Hospital	Faribault	80%	50
Immanuel Saint Joseph's-Mayo Health System	Mankato	80%	75
University Medical Center-Mesabi	Hibbing	80%	102
Virginia Regional Medical Center	Virginia	80%	49
Albany Area Hospital	Albany	79%	29
Community Memorial Hospital Association	Cloquet	79%	52
Riverview Health	Crookston	79%	28
United Hospital	Saint Paul	79%	225
New Ulm Medical Center	New Ulm	78%	32
Saint Lukes Hospital	Duluth	78%	101
Saint Gabriel's Hospital	Little Falls	77%	43
Saint Mary's Regional Health Center	Detroit Lakes	77%	74
Deer River Healthcare Center	Deer River	76%	29
Hutchinson Area Health Care	Hutchinson	76%	34
Northwest Medical Center	Thief River Falls	76%	25
Avera Marshall Regional Medical Center	Marshall	73%	44
Falls Memorial Hospital	Int'l Falls	72%	25
University of Minnesota Med Ctr-Fairview	Minneapolis	71%	125
Chippewa County Montevideo Hospital	Montevideo	69%	32
Swift County-Benson Hospital	Benson	69%	29
Kanabec Hospital	Mora	64%	50
Lakewood Health System Hospital	Staples	61%	36
Perham Memorial Hospital and Home	Perham	56%	32

14. Blood Culture Timing

Hospital Name	City	Rate	Cases
Fairmont Medical Center	Fairmont	100%	82
Saint Gabriel's Hospital	Little Falls	100%	30
Fairview Northland Regional Health Care	Princeton	99%	72
Fairview Southdale Hospital	Edina	98%	185
Owatonna Hospital	Owatonna	98%	62
Saint Joseph's Area Health Services	Park Rapids	98%	49
Fairview Red Wing Hospital	Red Wing	97%	61
Fairview Ridges Hospital	Burnsville	97%	146
Lakeview Hospital	Stillwater	97%	34
Douglas County Hospital	Alexandria	96%	92
Saint Cloud Hospital	Saint Cloud	96%	226
Saint Francis Regional Medical Center	Shakopee	96%	56
Saint Joseph's Medical Center	Brainerd	96%	161
Austin Medical Center	Austin	95%	99
Hutchinson Area Health Care	Hutchinson	95%	37
New Ulm Medical Center	New Ulm	94%	31
Ridgeview Medical Center	Waconia	94%	143
Saint Marys Hospital	Rochester	94%	72
Saint mary's Medical Center	Duluth	94%	109
University Medical Center-Mesabi	Hibbing	94%	83
Albert Lea Medical Center-Mayo Health System	Albert Lea	93%	59
Fairview Lakes Health Services	Wyoming	93%	103
Saint Lukes Hospital	Duluth	93%	70
Cambridge Medical Center	Cambridge	92%	48
Lake Region Healthcare Corporation	Fergus Falls	92%	51
Methodist Hospital	Saint Louis Park	92%	269
Rice Memorial Hospital	Willmar	92%	74
Tri-County Hospital	Wadena	92%	25
North Country Regional Hospital	Bemidji	91%	89
North Memorial Health Care	Robbinsdale	91%	184
Virginia Regional Medical Center	Virginia	91%	47
District One Hospital	Faribault	90%	42
Saint John's Hospital	Maplewood	90%	89
Abbott-Northwestern Hospital	Minneapolis	89%	201
Regina Medical Center	Hastings	88%	41
Unity Hospital	Fridley	88%	140
Regions Hospital	Saint Paul	87%	181
United Hospital	Saint Paul	87%	176
Mercy Hospital	Coon Rapids	86%	118
Woodwinds Health Campus	Woodbury	84%	37
University of Minnesota Med Ctr-Fairview	Minneapolis	82%	115
Immanuel Saint Joseph's-Mayo Health System	Mankato	80%	66
Saint Joseph's Hospital	Saint Paul	79%	70
Buffalo Hospital	Buffalo	77%	66
Community Memorial Hospital Association	Cloquet	77%	30
Hennepin County Medical Center	Minneapolis	75%	205
Saint Mary's Regional Health Center	Detroit Lakes	75%	28

15. Influenza Vaccine

Hospital Name	City	Rate	Cases
North Country Regional Hospital	Bemidji	100%	25
Ridgeview Medical Center	Waconia	100%	37
Fairmont Medical Center	Fairmont	96%	27
Fairview Ridges Hospital	Burnsville	96%	46
Austin Medical Center	Austin	94%	31
Douglas County Hospital	Alexandria	94%	32
Saint John's Hospital	Maplewood	93%	29
Fairview Southdale Hospital	Edina	92%	59
Saint Cloud Hospital	Saint Cloud	90%	63
University of Minnesota Med Ctr-Fairview	Minneapolis	88%	48
Unity Hospital	Fridley	85%	47
Saint Lukes Hospital	Duluth	83%	30
Mercy Hospital	Coon Rapids	79%	42
North Memorial Health Care	Robbinsdale	77%	74
Saint Joseph's Medical Center	Brainerd	77%	44
Saint mary's Medical Center	Duluth	77%	35
Tri-County Hospital	Wadena	77%	26
University Medical Center-Mesabi	Hibbing	76%	33
Saint Joseph's Hospital	Saint Paul	74%	27
Abbott-Northwestern Hospital	Minneapolis	73%	67
Methodist Hospital	Saint Louis Park	73%	97
United Hospital	Saint Paul	70%	47
Immanuel Saint Joseph's-Mayo Health System	Mankato	69%	26
Virginia Regional Medical Center	Virginia	60%	25
Regions Hospital	Saint Paul	54%	67
Hennepin County Medical Center	Minneapolis	30%	70

16. Initial Antibiotic Timing

Hospital Name	City	Rate	Cases
Stevens Community Medical Center	Morris	100%	29
Fairview Northland Regional Health Care	Princeton	99%	81
Albany Area Hospital	Albany	96%	27
Lake Region Healthcare Corporation	Fergus Falls	96%	82
Saint Francis Regional Medical Center	Shakopee	96%	110
Hutchinson Area Health Care	Hutchinson	95%	58
Woodwinds Health Campus	Woodbury	95%	63
Buffalo Hospital	Buffalo	94%	89
Community Memorial Hospital	Winona	94%	98
Regina Medical Center	Hastings	94%	51
Albert Lea Medical Center-Mayo Health System	Albert Lea	93%	83
Douglas County Hospital	Alexandria	93%	136
Fairview Lakes Health Services	Wyoming	93%	144
Owatonna Hospital	Owatonna	93%	81
Fairmont Medical Center	Fairmont	92%	118
Lakeview Hospital	Stillwater	92%	84
Lakewood Health System Hospital	Staples	91%	43

NOTE: Hospital profiles are in alphabetical order by state, then city, then hospital within the city; Rankings are sorted by rate in descending order and exclude hospitals with less than 25 cases; (1) The number of cases is too small (n<25) for purposes of reliably predicting hospital performance; (2) Measure reflects the hospital's indication that its submission was based upon a sample of its relevant discharges; (3) Rate reflects fewer than the maximum possible quarters of data for the measure; (4) Inaccurate information submitted and suppressed for one or more quarters; (5) No data is available from the hospital for this measure; Please refer to the User's Guide for a full explanation of data

Saint John's Hospital	Maplewood	91%	179
Saint Joseph's Area Health Services	Park Rapids	91%	86
Saint Joseph's Hospital	Saint Paul	91%	159
District One Hospital	Faribault	90%	68
Fairview Red Wing Hospital	Red Wing	90%	88
North Memorial Health Care	Robbinsdale	90%	387
Ridgeview Medical Center	Waconia	90%	123
Saint Francis Medical Center	Breckenridge	90%	41
Tri-County Hospital	Wadena	90%	109
Madison Hospital	Madison	89%	28
Northfield Hospital	Northfield	89%	53
Waseca Medical Center-Mayo Health System	Waseca	89%	28
Chippewa County Montevideo Hospital	Montevideo	88%	40
North Country Regional Hospital	Bemidji	88%	155
Perham Memorial Hospital and Home	Perham	88%	48
Sioux Valley Luverne Hospital	Luverne	88%	41
United Hospital District	Blue Earth	88%	26
Austin Medical Center	Austin	87%	149
Cambridge Medical Center	Cambridge	87%	111
Municipal Hospital and Granite Manor	Granite Falls	87%	31
Saint Cloud Hospital	Saint Cloud	87%	314
Saint Joseph's Medical Center	Brainerd	86%	235
Immanuel Saint Joseph's-Mayo Health System	Mankato	85%	81
Riverview Health	Crookston	85%	34
Saint Marys Hospital	Rochester	85%	124
Saint Peter Community Hospital	Saint Peter	85%	27
Swift County-Benson Hospital	Benson	85%	34
Worthington Regional Hospital	Worthington	84%	57
Methodist Hospital	Saint Louis Park	83%	431
Rice Memorial Hospital	Willmar	83%	126
Saint Gabriel's Hospital	Little Falls	83%	72
Fairview Southdale Hospital	Edina	82%	262
Saint Mary's Regional Health Center	Detroit Lakes	82%	77
Northwest Medical Center	Thief River Falls	81%	32
University Medical Center-Mesabi	Hibbing	81%	167
Fairview Ridges Hospital	Burnsville	80%	214
Grand Itasca Clinic and Hospital	Grand Rapids	80%	107
Saint mary's Medical Center	Duluth	80%	170
Deer River Healthcare Center	Deer River	79%	34
Kanabec Hospital	Mora	78%	79
Mille Lacs Health System	Onamia	78%	45
Regions Hospital	Saint Paul	76%	336
Roseau Area Hospital & Homes	Roseau	76%	25
Community Memorial Hospital Association	Cloquet	75%	55
Unity Hospital	Fridley	75%	239
Abbott-Northwestern Hospital	Minneapolis	74%	341
Avera Marshall Regional Medical Center	Marshall	73%	30
Mercy Hospital	Coon Rapids	72%	228
Monticello-Big Lake Community Hospital	Monticello	72%	50
Mercy Hospital & Health Care Center	Moose Lake	70%	46
United Hospital	Saint Paul	70%	287
New Ulm Medical Center	New Ulm	69%	42
Olmsted Medical Center Hospital	Rochester	68%	47
Falls Memorial Hospital	Int'l Falls	66%	35
Saint Lukes Hospital	Duluth	66%	154
Virginia Regional Medical Center	Virginia	66%	82
Hennepin County Medical Center	Minneapolis	61%	417
University of Minnesota Med Ctr-Fairview	Minneapolis	60%	212

17. Oxygenation Assessment

Hospital Name	City	Rate	Cases
Abbott-Northwestern Hospital	Minneapolis	100%	451
Albert Lea Medical Center-Mayo Health System	Albert Lea	100%	97
Austin Medical Center	Austin	100%	172
Bigfork Valley Hospital	Bigfork	100%	25
Buffalo Hospital	Buffalo	100%	123
Cambridge Medical Center	Cambridge	100%	149
Chippewa County Montevideo Hospital	Montevideo	100%	42
Community Memorial Hospital	Winona	100%	124
Community Memorial Hospital Association	Cloquet	100%	63
Deer River Healthcare Center	Deer River	100%	38
District One Hospital	Faribault	100%	74
Douglas County Hospital	Alexandria	100%	184
Fairmont Medical Center	Fairmont	100%	150
Fairview Lakes Health Services	Wyoming	100%	168
Fairview Northland Regional Health Care	Princeton	100%	101
Fairview Red Wing Hospital	Red Wing	100%	110
Fairview Southdale Hospital	Edina	100%	296
Falls Memorial Hospital	Int'l Falls	100%	44
Glencoe Regional Health Services	Glencoe	100%	60
Grand Itasca Clinic and Hospital	Grand Rapids	100%	123
Hutchinson Area Health Care	Hutchinson	100%	68
Kanabec Hospital	Mora	100%	81
Lake Region Healthcare Corporation	Fergus Falls	100%	102
Lakeview Hospital	Stillwater	100%	103
Lakewood Health System Hospital	Staples	100%	53
Madison Hospital	Madison	100%	30
Mercy Hospital	Coon Rapids	100%	267
Mercy Hospital & Health Care Center	Moose Lake	100%	58
Methodist Hospital	Saint Louis Park	100%	566
Mille Lacs Health System	Onamia	100%	49
Municipal Hospital and Granite Manor	Granite Falls	100%	38
New Ulm Medical Center	New Ulm	100%	52
North Country Regional Hospital	Bemidji	100%	181
North Memorial Health Care	Robbinsdale	100%	471
Northfield Hospital	Northfield	100%	72
Northwest Medical Center	Thief River Falls	100%	42
Owatonna Hospital	Owatonna	100%	94
Redwood Area Hospital	Redwood Falls	100%	25
Regina Medical Center	Hastings	100%	65
Regions Hospital	Saint Paul	100%	428
Rice Memorial Hospital	Willmar	100%	144
Ridgeview Medical Center	Waconia	100%	227
Riverview Health	Crookston	100%	43
Saint Cloud Hospital	Saint Cloud	100%	390
Saint Francis Medical Center	Breckenridge	100%	57
Saint Francis Regional Medical Center	Shakopee	100%	134
Saint Gabriel's Hospital	Little Falls	100%	85
Saint John's Hospital	Maplewood	100%	221
Saint Joseph's Area Health Services	Park Rapids	100%	111
Saint Joseph's Hospital	Saint Paul	100%	190
Saint Joseph's Medical Center	Brainerd	100%	261
Saint Lukes Hospital	Duluth	100%	187
Saint Mary's Regional Health Center	Detroit Lakes	100%	100
Saint Marys Hospital	Rochester	100%	167
Saint Peter Community Hospital	Saint Peter	100%	35
Saint mary's Medical Center	Duluth	100%	209
Sioux Valley Luverne Hospital	Luverne	100%	49
Stevens Community Medical Center	Morris	100%	29
Swift County-Benson Hospital	Benson	100%	44
United Hospital District	Blue Earth	100%	30
Unity Hospital	Fridley	100%	280
University Medical Center-Mesabi	Hibbing	100%	191
University of Minnesota Med Ctr-Fairview	Minneapolis	100%	274
Waseca Medical Center-Mayo Health System	Waseca	100%	36
Woodwinds Health Campus	Woodbury	100%	83
Worthington Regional Hospital	Worthington	100%	69
Fairview Ridges Hospital	Burnsville	99%	270
Hennepin County Medical Center	Minneapolis	99%	492
Tri-County Hospital	Wadena	99%	148
United Hospital	Saint Paul	99%	340
Avera Marshall Regional Medical Center	Marshall	98%	49
Olmsted Medical Center Hospital	Rochester	98%	62
Perham Memorial Hospital and Home	Perham	98%	54
Rochester Methodist Hospital	Rochester	98%	40
Roseau Area Hospital & Homes	Roseau	98%	42
Albany Area Hospital	Albany	97%	31
Virginia Regional Medical Center	Virginia	97%	100
Immanuel Saint Joseph's-Mayo Health System	Mankato	95%	133
Meeker County Memorial Hospital	Litchfield	94%	35
Monticello-Big Lake Community Hospital	Monticello	89%	71

18. Pneumococcal Vaccine

Hospital Name	City	Rate	Cases
Waseca Medical Center-Mayo Health System	Waseca	100%	26
Fairmont Medical Center	Fairmont	99%	120
Ridgeview Medical Center	Waconia	99%	166
Cambridge Medical Center	Cambridge	98%	88
Austin Medical Center	Austin	97%	149
Rice Memorial Hospital	Willmar	97%	109
Lakeview Hospital	Stillwater	96%	77
North Country Regional Hospital	Bemidji	96%	120
Woodwinds Health Campus	Woodbury	96%	54
Douglas County Hospital	Alexandria	95%	142
Fairview Northland Regional Health Care	Princeton	95%	66
New Ulm Medical Center	New Ulm	95%	40
Owatonna Hospital	Owatonna	94%	78
Fairview Southdale Hospital	Edina	93%	219
Saint Francis Medical Center	Breckenridge	93%	45
Rochester Methodist Hospital	Rochester	92%	78
Saint Cloud Hospital	Saint Cloud	92%	287
Worthington Regional Hospital	Worthington	92%	52
Kanabec Hospital	Mora	91%	58
Saint John's Hospital	Maplewood	90%	140
Saint Marys Hospital	Rochester	90%	134
Community Memorial Hospital	Winona	89%	87
Fairview Red Wing Hospital	Red Wing	88%	76
Fairview Ridges Hospital	Burnsville	86%	161

NOTE: Hospital profiles are in alphabetical order by state, then city, then hospital within the city; Rankings are sorted by rate in descending order and exclude hospitals with less than 25 cases; (1) The number of cases is too small (n<25) for purposes of reliably predicting hospital performance; (2) Measure reflects the hospital's indication that its submission was based upon a sample of its relevant discharges; (3) Rate reflects fewer than the maximum possible quarters of data for the measure; (4) Inaccurate information submitted and suppressed for one or more quarters; (5) No data is available from the hospital for this measure; Please refer to the User's Guide for a full explanation of data

Hospital Name	City	Rate	Cases
Saint mary's Medical Center	Duluth	84%	148
Grand Itasca Clinic and Hospital	Grand Rapids	83%	99
Saint Joseph's Area Health Services	Park Rapids	83%	82
Saint Joseph's Hospital	Saint Paul	83%	106
Fairview Lakes Health Services	Wyoming	82%	102
Perham Memorial Hospital and Home	Perham	82%	38
Albert Lea Medical Center-Mayo Health System	Albert Lea	81%	78
Sioux Valley Luverne Hospital	Luverne	80%	41
Avera Marshall Regional Medical Center	Marshall	79%	38
Methodist Hospital	Saint Louis Park	79%	377
Northwest Medical Center	Thief River Falls	79%	28
Roseau Area Hospital & Homes	Roseau	79%	28
University of Minnesota Med Ctr-Fairview	Minneapolis	79%	113
Hutchinson Area Health Care	Hutchinson	77%	48
Olmsted Medical Center Hospital	Rochester	77%	39
Saint Lukes Hospital	Duluth	77%	113
Lake Region Healthcare Corporation	Fergus Falls	76%	76
Northfield Hospital	Northfield	76%	49
Riverview Health	Crookston	75%	28
Saint Joseph's Medical Center	Brainerd	75%	189
Community Memorial Hospital Association	Cloquet	74%	39
Deer River Healthcare Center	Deer River	73%	26
Mercy Hospital	Coon Rapids	73%	164
Unity Hospital	Fridley	73%	191
Buffalo Hospital	Buffalo	72%	82
University Medical Center-Mesabi	Hibbing	72%	115
Saint Francis Regional Medical Center	Shakopee	71%	85
Regions Hospital	Saint Paul	70%	257
Glencoe Regional Health Services	Glencoe	69%	36
Immanuel Saint Joseph's-Mayo Health System	Mankato	68%	109
Tri-County Hospital	Wadena	68%	104
Saint Mary's Regional Health Center	Detroit Lakes	66%	70
Falls Memorial Hospital	Int'l Falls	64%	33
North Memorial Health Care	Robbinsdale	64%	285
Abbott-Northwestern Hospital	Minneapolis	63%	287
Saint Gabriel's Hospital	Little Falls	60%	67
Virginia Regional Medical Center	Virginia	60%	73
Mille Lacs Health System	Onamia	59%	37
Swift County-Benson Hospital	Benson	59%	34
United Hospital	Saint Paul	59%	197
District One Hospital	Faribault	55%	51
Mercy Hospital & Health Care Center	Moose Lake	50%	44
Monticello-Big Lake Community Hospital	Monticello	46%	39
Regina Medical Center	Hastings	35%	46
Chippewa County Montevideo Hospital	Montevideo	30%	30
Hennepin County Medical Center	Minneapolis	19%	151
Lakewood Health System Hospital	Staples	19%	37

19. Smoking Cessation Advice

Hospital Name	City	Rate	Cases
Cambridge Medical Center	Cambridge	100%	30
Douglas County Hospital	Alexandria	100%	25
Fairview Southdale Hospital	Edina	100%	53
University of Minnesota Med Ctr-Fairview	Minneapolis	99%	76
Ridgeview Medical Center	Waconia	97%	29
Saint Francis Regional Medical Center	Shakopee	97%	29
Fairview Northland Regional Health Care	Princeton	96%	28
Regions Hospital	Saint Paul	93%	128
Saint Lukes Hospital	Duluth	93%	44
Rochester Methodist Hospital	Rochester	92%	25
North Memorial Health Care	Robbinsdale	85%	111
United Hospital	Saint Paul	84%	80
Saint mary's Medical Center	Duluth	81%	64
Mercy Hospital	Coon Rapids	80%	64
Saint Cloud Hospital	Saint Cloud	80%	87
Fairview Ridges Hospital	Burnsville	79%	57
Methodist Hospital	Saint Louis Park	79%	117
North Country Regional Hospital	Bemidji	77%	43
Abbott-Northwestern Hospital	Minneapolis	73%	90
Saint Joseph's Medical Center	Brainerd	73%	51
Fairview Lakes Health Services	Wyoming	72%	29
Unity Hospital	Fridley	71%	52
University Medical Center-Mesabi	Hibbing	70%	37
Buffalo Hospital	Buffalo	65%	26
Saint Joseph's Hospital	Saint Paul	58%	40
Hennepin County Medical Center	Minneapolis	56%	213
Saint John's Hospital	Maplewood	44%	34

Surgical Infection Prevention

20. Prophylactic Antibiotic Given

Hospital Name	City	Rate	Cases
Kanabec Hospital	Mora	98%	47
Methodist Hospital	Saint Louis Park	97%	236
Saint Joseph's Medical Center	Brainerd	97%	278
Fairview Southdale Hospital	Edina	96%	243
Rochester Methodist Hospital	Rochester	96%	511
Virginia Regional Medical Center	Virginia	96%	55
Austin Medical Center	Austin	94%	144
Fairview Lakes Health Services	Wyoming	94%	118
Saint Marys Hospital	Rochester	94%	494
Fairview Red Wing Hospital	Red Wing	93%	206
Regina Medical Center	Hastings	93%	151
University of Minnesota Med Ctr-Fairview	Minneapolis	93%	191
Buffalo Hospital	Buffalo	92%	64
Lakewood Health System Hospital	Staples	92%	39
North Country Regional Hospital	Bemidji	92%	454
Ridgeview Medical Center	Waconia	92%	407
Albert Lea Medical Center-Mayo Health System	Albert Lea	91%	206
Douglas County Hospital	Alexandria	91%	297
Fairmont Medical Center	Fairmont	90%	125
Mercy Hospital	Coon Rapids	89%	176
Mercy Hospital & Health Care Center	Moose Lake	89%	37
Miller Dwan Medical Center	Duluth	89%	36
Northfield Hospital	Northfield	89%	141
Northwest Medical Center	Thief River Falls	89%	147
Saint mary's Medical Center	Duluth	89%	95
Fairview Ridges Hospital	Burnsville	88%	125
Hutchinson Area Health Care	Hutchinson	88%	138
Owatonna Hospital	Owatonna	88%	78
Regions Hospital	Saint Paul	88%	960
Community Memorial Hospital	Winona	87%	30
Fairview Northland Regional Health Care	Princeton	87%	90
Lakeview Hospital	Stillwater	87%	261
Saint Mary's Regional Health Center	Detroit Lakes	86%	87
Lake Region Healthcare Corporation	Fergus Falls	84%	179
Saint Francis Regional Medical Center	Shakopee	84%	75
Cambridge Medical Center	Cambridge	83%	63
Abbott-Northwestern Hospital	Minneapolis	82%	173
Unity Hospital	Fridley	82%	94
District One Hospital	Faribault	81%	75
Immanuel Saint Joseph's-Mayo Health System	Mankato	79%	135
Grand Itasca Clinic and Hospital	Grand Rapids	78%	49
Olmsted Medical Center Hospital	Rochester	78%	40
Saint John's Hospital	Maplewood	77%	739
Rice Memorial Hospital	Willmar	76%	399
New Ulm Medical Center	New Ulm	74%	42
University Medical Center-Mesabi	Hibbing	73%	117
Hennepin County Medical Center	Minneapolis	72%	362
Woodwinds Health Campus	Woodbury	71%	645
Saint Lukes Hospital	Duluth	70%	224
Tri-County Hospital	Wadena	69%	29
Glencoe Regional Health Services	Glencoe	65%	40
North Memorial Health Care	Robbinsdale	62%	93
Saint Cloud Hospital	Saint Cloud	60%	436
Saint Joseph's Hospital	Saint Paul	59%	533
Community Memorial Hospital Association	Cloquet	55%	73
Meeker County Memorial Hospital	Litchfield	50%	38
United Hospital	Saint Paul	46%	171

21. Prophylactic Antibiotic Selection

Hospital Name	City	Rate	Cases
Albert Lea Medical Center-Mayo Health System	Albert Lea	100%	51
District One Hospital	Faribault	100%	29
Fairview Lakes Health Services	Wyoming	100%	39
Lakeview Hospital	Stillwater	100%	64
Regina Medical Center	Hastings	100%	40
Saint Joseph's Medical Center	Brainerd	100%	62
Woodwinds Health Campus	Woodbury	99%	217
North Memorial Health Care	Robbinsdale	98%	92
Rochester Methodist Hospital	Rochester	98%	93
Saint Joseph's Hospital	Saint Paul	98%	152
Saint Lukes Hospital	Duluth	98%	107
Abbott-Northwestern Hospital	Minneapolis	97%	98
Fairmont Medical Center	Fairmont	97%	31
Fairview Red Wing Hospital	Red Wing	97%	72
New Ulm Medical Center	New Ulm	97%	38
Saint Francis Regional Medical Center	Shakopee	97%	35
Saint Marys Hospital	Rochester	97%	105
University of Minnesota Med Ctr-Fairview	Minneapolis	97%	66
Mercy Hospital	Coon Rapids	96%	106
Northfield Hospital	Northfield	96%	28
United Hospital	Saint Paul	96%	94
Fairview Ridges Hospital	Burnsville	95%	41
Fairview Southdale Hospital	Edina	95%	86
Lake Region Healthcare Corporation	Fergus Falls	95%	83
North Country Regional Hospital	Bemidji	95%	128
Northwest Medical Center	Thief River Falls	95%	38

NOTE: Hospital profiles are in alphabetical order by state, then city, then hospital within the city; Rankings are sorted by rate in descending order and exclude hospitals with less than 25 cases; (1) The number of cases is too small (n<25) for purposes of reliably predicting hospital performance; (2) Measure reflects the hospital's indication that its submission was based upon a sample of its relevant discharges; (3) Rate reflects fewer than the maximum possible quarters of data for the measure; (4) Inaccurate information submitted and suppressed for one or more quarters; (5) No data is available from the hospital for this measure; Please refer to the User's Guide for a full explanation of data

Hospital Name	City	Rate	Cases
Regions Hospital	Saint Paul	95%	237
Saint Cloud Hospital	Saint Cloud	95%	86
Saint John's Hospital	Maplewood	95%	229
Douglas County Hospital	Alexandria	94%	49
Hutchinson Area Health Care	Hutchinson	94%	36
Immanuel Saint Joseph's-Mayo Health System	Mankato	92%	49
Saint mary's Medical Center	Duluth	92%	97
Buffalo Hospital	Buffalo	91%	35
Cambridge Medical Center	Cambridge	91%	35
Owatonna Hospital	Owatonna	91%	47
Methodist Hospital	Saint Louis Park	89%	82
Austin Medical Center	Austin	88%	26
Rice Memorial Hospital	Willmar	88%	100
Ridgeview Medical Center	Waconia	87%	54
Unity Hospital	Fridley	84%	49
Hennepin County Medical Center	Minneapolis	83%	100
Community Memorial Hospital	Winona	37%	30

22. Prophylactic Antibiotic Stopped

Hospital Name	City	Rate	Cases
Saint Mary's Regional Health Center	Detroit Lakes	100%	86
Kanabec Hospital	Mora	98%	45
Austin Medical Center	Austin	97%	136
Meeker County Memorial Hospital	Litchfield	97%	36
New Ulm Medical Center	New Ulm	97%	38
Community Memorial Hospital Association	Cloquet	96%	72
Fairview Northland Regional Health Care	Princeton	94%	84
Lakeview Hospital	Stillwater	94%	247
Northfield Hospital	Northfield	94%	134
Northwest Medical Center	Thief River Falls	94%	142
Saint mary's Medical Center	Duluth	93%	89
Albert Lea Medical Center-Mayo Health System	Albert Lea	92%	194
Mercy Hospital	Coon Rapids	92%	171
Fairview Southdale Hospital	Edina	91%	235
Hutchinson Area Health Care	Hutchinson	91%	134
Methodist Hospital	Saint Louis Park	91%	232
Abbott-Northwestern Hospital	Minneapolis	90%	166
District One Hospital	Faribault	90%	71
Grand Itasca Clinic and Hospital	Grand Rapids	90%	48
Douglas County Hospital	Alexandria	89%	271
Regina Medical Center	Hastings	89%	150
University of Minnesota Med Ctr-Fairview	Minneapolis	89%	185
Immanuel Saint Joseph's-Mayo Health System	Mankato	88%	129
North Country Regional Hospital	Bemidji	88%	434
Rochester Methodist Hospital	Rochester	87%	502
Saint Lukes Hospital	Duluth	87%	220
Cambridge Medical Center	Cambridge	86%	63
Fairview Red Wing Hospital	Red Wing	85%	198
Fairview Ridges Hospital	Burnsville	83%	120
Saint Francis Regional Medical Center	Shakopee	83%	72
Woodwinds Health Campus	Woodbury	83%	636
Rice Memorial Hospital	Willmar	82%	391
Fairmont Medical Center	Fairmont	80%	122
Miller Dwan Medical Center	Duluth	80%	35
Glencoe Regional Health Services	Glencoe	79%	39
Lake Region Healthcare Corporation	Fergus Falls	79%	174
North Memorial Health Care	Robbinsdale	79%	89
Saint Joseph's Hospital	Saint Paul	78%	511
Regions Hospital	Saint Paul	77%	892
Saint John's Hospital	Maplewood	77%	737
Lakewood Health System Hospital	Staples	76%	37
Saint Cloud Hospital	Saint Cloud	76%	418
Mercy Hospital & Health Care Center	Moose Lake	75%	36
Hennepin County Medical Center	Minneapolis	74%	346
United Hospital	Saint Paul	73%	168
Unity Hospital	Fridley	70%	94
Fairview Lakes Health Services	Wyoming	69%	116
Buffalo Hospital	Buffalo	67%	63
University Medical Center-Mesabi	Hibbing	64%	111
Community Memorial Hospital	Winona	63%	30
Saint Marys Hospital	Rochester	63%	483
Saint Joseph's Medical Center	Brainerd	59%	278
Tri-County Hospital	Wadena	57%	28
Ridgeview Medical Center	Waconia	55%	400
Olmsted Medical Center Hospital	Rochester	54%	39
Owatonna Hospital	Owatonna	38%	73
Virginia Regional Medical Center	Virginia	34%	53

Pregnancy Care

23. Inpatient Neonatal Mortality

Hospital Name	City	Rate	Cases
Fairview Southdale Hospital	Edina	0.00%	3643
Rice Memorial Hospital	Willmar	0.00%	248
Saint Joseph's Medical Center	Brainerd	0.00%	665
Woodwinds Health Campus	Woodbury	0.00%	1508
Saint John's Hospital	Maplewood	0.07%	3000
Methodist Hospital	Saint Louis Park	0.08%	3814
Lakeview Hospital	Stillwater	0.14%	717
Fairview Ridges Hospital	Burnsville	0.19%	3088
Saint Joseph's Hospital	Saint Paul	0.19%	1038
Rochester Methodist Hospital	Rochester	0.23%	444
Saint Lukes Hospital	Duluth	0.37%	819
Hennepin County Medical Center	Minneapolis	0.52%	3080
University Medical Center-Mesabi	Hibbing	0.52%	383
Monticello-Big Lake Community Hospital	Monticello	0.55%	550
University of Minnesota Med Ctr-Fairview	Minneapolis	1.11%	2873

24. Third or Fourth Degree Laceration

Hospital Name	City	Rate	Cases
University Medical Center-Mesabi	Hibbing	2.14%	234
Rochester Methodist Hospital	Rochester	2.58%	1589
Saint Joseph's Hospital	Saint Paul	2.64%	910
Saint Joseph's Medical Center	Brainerd	3.23%	620
Saint John's Hospital	Maplewood	3.24%	2343
Rice Memorial Hospital	Willmar	3.30%	666
Hennepin County Medical Center	Minneapolis	3.59%	2371
Methodist Hospital	Saint Louis Park	4.03%	2801
Woodwinds Health Campus	Woodbury	4.49%	1137
University of Minnesota Med Ctr-Fairview	Minneapolis	4.53%	1878
Lakeview Hospital	Stillwater	4.55%	549
Saint Lukes Hospital	Duluth	4.78%	523
Fairview Ridges Hospital	Burnsville	5.96%	2216
Fairview Southdale Hospital	Edina	7.12%	2403
Monticello-Big Lake Community Hospital	Monticello	8.68%	484

NOTE: Hospital profiles are in alphabetical order by state, then city, then hospital within the city; Rankings are sorted by rate in descending order and exclude hospitals with less than 25 cases; (1) The number of cases is too small (n<25) for purposes of reliably predicting hospital performance; (2) Measure reflects the hospital's indication that its submission was based upon a sample of its relevant discharges; (3) Rate reflects fewer than the maximum possible quarters of data for the measure; (4) Inaccurate information submitted and suppressed for one or more quarters; (5) No data is available from the hospital for this measure; Please refer to the User's Guide for a full explanation of data

Riverwood HealthCare Center

200 Bunker Hill Drive
Aitkin, MN 56431
Phone: 218-927-2121
Fax: 218-927-5575
URL: www.riverwoodhealthcare.com
Ownership: Voluntary non-profit - Private
Accredited: No
Emergency Services: Yes
Licensed Beds: 36

Key Personnel:
CEO. . . . . Michael Hagem
Chief Medical Staff. . . . . James Harris, MD
Director Emergency Room. . . . . James Harris
Infection Control. . . . . Linda Chantland, RN

Measure	Cases	This Hospital	State Average	U.S. Average	Top Hospital
Heart Attack Care					
ACE Inhibitor or ARB for LVSD[1]	4	100%	89%	82%	100%
Aspirin at Arrival[1]	8	100%	92%	92%	100%
Aspirin at Discharge[1]	7	100%	93%	90%	100%
Beta Blocker at Arrival[1]	7	100%	88%	87%	100%
Beta Blocker at Discharge[1]	6	83%	95%	90%	100%
Fibrinolytic Medication Timing[1]	1	0%	40%	31%	100%
PCI Within 90 Minutes of Arrival	0	-	77%	54%	95%
Smoking Cessation Advice	0	-	68%	88%	100%
Heart Failure Care					
ACE Inhibitor or ARB for LVSD[1]	17	100%	85%	82%	100%
Discharge Instructions	29	66%	54%	61%	93%
Evaluation of LVS Function	33	82%	77%	83%	99%
Smoking Cessation Advice[1]	6	33%	67%	82%	100%
Pneumonia Care					
Appropriate Initial Antibiotic[1,3]	1	0%	80%	83%	94%
Blood Culture Timing[1,3]	1	100%	94%	90%	100%
Influenza Vaccine	0	-	76%	70%	100%
Initial Antibiotic Timing[3]	0	-	85%	80%	93%
Oxygenation Assessment[1,3]	1	100%	99%	99%	100%
Pneumococcal Vaccine[1,3]	1	100%	73%	69%	94%
Smoking Cessation Advice[3]	0	-	70%	80%	100%
Surgical Infection Prevention					
Prophylactic Antibiotic Given[5]	-	-	78%	77%	95%
Prophylactic Antibiotic Selection[5]	-	-	94%	90%	100%
Prophylactic Antibiotic Stopped[5]	-	-	82%	72%	95%
Pregnancy Care					
Inpatient Neonatal Mortality	-	-	-	-	-
Third or Fourth Degree Laceration	-	-	4.42%	3.63%	3.27%

Albany Area Hospital

300 3rd Avenue
Albany, MN 56307
Phone: 320-845-2121
Fax: 320-845-4707
E-mail: mgoebel@means.net
URL: www.albanyareahospital.com
Ownership: Voluntary non-profit - Church
Accredited: No
Emergency Services: Yes
Licensed Beds: 17

Key Personnel:
Administrator . . . . Ben Koppelman
Chief Medical Staff. . . . . Daron Gersch
Emergency Room . . . . Daron Gersch
Director Infection/Disease Control . . . . Bernita Hinnenkamp
Chief Radiology . . . . Marilyn Bergmann

Measure	Cases	This Hospital	State Average	U.S. Average	Top Hospital
Heart Attack Care					
ACE Inhibitor or ARB for LVSD[3]	0	-	89%	82%	100%
Aspirin at Arrival[3]	0	-	92%	92%	100%
Aspirin at Discharge[3]	0	-	93%	90%	100%
Beta Blocker at Arrival[3]	0	-	88%	87%	100%
Beta Blocker at Discharge[1,3]	1	100%	95%	90%	100%
Fibrinolytic Medication Timing[1,3]	1	0%	40%	31%	100%
PCI Within 90 Minutes of Arrival[5]	-	-	77%	54%	95%
Smoking Cessation Advice[3]	0	-	68%	88%	100%
Heart Failure Care					
ACE Inhibitor or ARB for LVSD	0	-	85%	82%	100%
Discharge Instructions[1]	6	17%	54%	61%	93%
Evaluation of LVS Function[1]	10	50%	77%	83%	99%
Smoking Cessation Advice[1]	2	50%	67%	82%	100%
Pneumonia Care					
Appropriate Initial Antibiotic	29	79%	80%	83%	94%
Blood Culture Timing[1]	3	100%	94%	90%	100%
Influenza Vaccine[1]	4	50%	76%	70%	100%
Initial Antibiotic Timing	27	96%	85%	80%	93%
Oxygenation Assessment	31	97%	99%	99%	100%
Pneumococcal Vaccine[1]	24	46%	73%	69%	94%
Smoking Cessation Advice[1]	5	20%	70%	80%	100%
Surgical Infection Prevention					
Prophylactic Antibiotic Given[1,3]	3	33%	78%	77%	95%
Prophylactic Antibiotic Selection[1]	1	100%	94%	90%	100%
Prophylactic Antibiotic Stopped[1,3]	2	100%	82%	72%	95%
Pregnancy Care					
Inpatient Neonatal Mortality	-	-	-	-	-
Third or Fourth Degree Laceration	-	-	4.42%	3.63%	3.27%

Albert Lea Medical Center-Mayo Health System

Alternate Name: Naeve Hospital-Albert Lea Medical Center
404 Fountain Street
Albert Lea, MN 56007
Phone: 507-373-2384
Fax: 507-377-6248
Ownership: Voluntary non-profit - Private
Accredited: Yes
Emergency Services: Yes
Licensed Beds: 119

Key Personnel:
CEO. . . . . Mark Ciota, MD
Chief Medical Staff. . . . . John Grzybowski, MD
Emergency Room . . . . Michael Ulrich, MD
Infection Control. . . . . Tammy Williams
ICU . . . . Nancy Christensen
Medical/Surgical Nursing . . . . Nancy Christensen
OB/GYN Womens Health. . . . . Joy Shaft

Measure	Cases	This Hospital	State Average	U.S. Average	Top Hospital
Heart Attack Care					
ACE Inhibitor or ARB for LVSD[1]	7	100%	89%	82%	100%
Aspirin at Arrival	43	98%	92%	92%	100%
Aspirin at Discharge	37	92%	93%	90%	100%
Beta Blocker at Arrival	43	100%	88%	87%	100%
Beta Blocker at Discharge	39	100%	95%	90%	100%
Fibrinolytic Medication Timing	0	-	40%	31%	100%
PCI Within 90 Minutes of Arrival	0	-	77%	54%	95%
Smoking Cessation Advice[1]	9	100%	68%	88%	100%
Heart Failure Care					
ACE Inhibitor or ARB for LVSD	28	89%	85%	82%	100%
Discharge Instructions	52	67%	54%	61%	93%
Evaluation of LVS Function	74	97%	77%	83%	99%
Smoking Cessation Advice[1]	6	100%	67%	82%	100%
Pneumonia Care					
Appropriate Initial Antibiotic	54	89%	80%	83%	94%
Blood Culture Timing	59	93%	94%	90%	100%
Influenza Vaccine[1]	15	73%	76%	70%	100%
Initial Antibiotic Timing	83	93%	85%	80%	93%
Oxygenation Assessment	97	100%	99%	99%	100%
Pneumococcal Vaccine	78	81%	73%	69%	94%
Smoking Cessation Advice[1]	21	86%	70%	80%	100%
Surgical Infection Prevention					
Prophylactic Antibiotic Given[3]	206	91%	78%	77%	95%
Prophylactic Antibiotic Selection	51	100%	94%	90%	100%
Prophylactic Antibiotic Stopped[3]	194	92%	82%	72%	95%
Pregnancy Care					
Inpatient Neonatal Mortality	-	-	-	-	-
Third or Fourth Degree Laceration	-	-	4.42%	3.63%	3.27%

Douglas County Hospital

111 17th Avenue East
Alexandria, MN 56308
Phone: 320-762-1511
Fax: 320-762-6034
E-mail: hr@dchospital.com
URL: www.dchospital.com
Ownership: Government - Local
Accredited: Yes
Emergency Services: Yes
Licensed Beds: 127

Key Personnel:
Administrator . . . . William G Flaig
Emergency Room . . . . Kevin Wedman, RN
Director Infection/Disease Control . . . . Bonnie Freudenberg
Clinical Director ICU/CCU . . . . Lois Nelson, RN

NOTE: Hospital profiles are in alphabetical order by state, then city, then hospital within the city; Rankings are sorted by rate in descending order and exclude hospitals with less than 25 cases; (1) The number of cases is too small (n<25) for purposes of reliably predicting hospital performance; (2) Measure reflects the hospital's indication that its submission was based upon a sample of its relevant discharges; (3) Rate reflects fewer than the maximum possible quarters of data for the measure; (4) Inaccurate information submitted and suppressed for one or more quarters; (5) No data is available from the hospital for this measure; Please refer to the User's Guide for a full explanation of data

Chief Radiology . . . . Linda Kalb
Respiratory Care Coordinator. . . . . David Holm

Measure	Cases	This Hospital	State Average	U.S. Average	Top Hospital
Heart Attack Care					
ACE Inhibitor or ARB for LVSD[1]	2	100%	89%	82%	100%
Aspirin at Arrival[1]	10	100%	92%	92%	100%
Aspirin at Discharge[1]	3	100%	93%	90%	100%
Beta Blocker at Arrival[1]	3	67%	88%	87%	100%
Beta Blocker at Discharge[1]	1	100%	95%	90%	100%
Fibrinolytic Medication Timing	0	-	40%	31%	100%
PCI Within 90 Minutes of Arrival	0	-	77%	54%	95%
Smoking Cessation Advice	0	-	68%	88%	100%
Heart Failure Care					
ACE Inhibitor or ARB for LVSD	49	84%	85%	82%	100%
Discharge Instructions	76	75%	54%	61%	93%
Evaluation of LVS Function	112	97%	77%	83%	99%
Smoking Cessation Advice[1]	11	100%	67%	82%	100%
Pneumonia Care					
Appropriate Initial Antibiotic	84	89%	80%	83%	94%
Blood Culture Timing	92	96%	94%	90%	100%
Influenza Vaccine	32	94%	76%	70%	100%
Initial Antibiotic Timing	136	93%	85%	80%	93%
Oxygenation Assessment	184	100%	99%	99%	100%
Pneumococcal Vaccine	142	95%	73%	69%	94%
Smoking Cessation Advice	25	100%	70%	80%	100%
Surgical Infection Prevention					
Prophylactic Antibiotic Given[2,3]	297	91%	78%	77%	95%
Prophylactic Antibiotic Selection[2]	49	94%	94%	90%	100%
Prophylactic Antibiotic Stopped[2,3]	271	89%	82%	72%	95%
Pregnancy Care					
Inpatient Neonatal Mortality	-	-	-	-	-
Third or Fourth Degree Laceration	-	-	4.42%	3.63%	3.27%

Austin Medical Center

1000 First Drive Northwest
Austin, MN 55912
Ownership: Voluntary non-profit - Other
Emergency Services: Yes
Phone: 507-433-7351
Accredited: Yes

Measure	Cases	This Hospital	State Average	U.S. Average	Top Hospital
Heart Attack Care					
ACE Inhibitor or ARB for LVSD[1]	9	100%	89%	82%	100%
Aspirin at Arrival	27	100%	92%	92%	100%
Aspirin at Discharge[1]	14	100%	93%	90%	100%
Beta Blocker at Arrival[1]	22	100%	88%	87%	100%
Beta Blocker at Discharge[1]	11	100%	95%	90%	100%
Fibrinolytic Medication Timing	0	-	40%	31%	100%
PCI Within 90 Minutes of Arrival	0	-	77%	54%	95%
Smoking Cessation Advice[1]	1	100%	68%	88%	100%
Heart Failure Care					
ACE Inhibitor or ARB for LVSD	26	88%	85%	82%	100%
Discharge Instructions	78	96%	54%	61%	93%
Evaluation of LVS Function	113	100%	77%	83%	99%
Smoking Cessation Advice[1]	7	71%	67%	82%	100%
Pneumonia Care					
Appropriate Initial Antibiotic	84	89%	80%	83%	94%
Blood Culture Timing	99	95%	94%	90%	100%
Influenza Vaccine	31	94%	76%	70%	100%
Initial Antibiotic Timing	149	87%	85%	80%	93%
Oxygenation Assessment	172	100%	99%	99%	100%
Pneumococcal Vaccine	149	97%	73%	69%	94%
Smoking Cessation Advice[1]	14	100%	70%	80%	100%
Surgical Infection Prevention					
Prophylactic Antibiotic Given	144	94%	78%	77%	95%
Prophylactic Antibiotic Selection	26	88%	94%	90%	100%
Prophylactic Antibiotic Stopped	136	97%	82%	72%	95%
Pregnancy Care					
Inpatient Neonatal Mortality	-	-	-	-	-
Third or Fourth Degree Laceration	-	-	4.42%	3.63%	3.27%

Lakewood Health Center

Alternate Name: Lakewood Health Care Center
600 Main Avenue S
Baudette, MN 56623
Ownership: Voluntary non-profit - Church
Emergency Services: Yes
Phone: 218-634-2120
Fax: 218-634-1307
Accredited: No
Licensed Beds: 65

Key Personnel:
CEO. . . . . Shar Ray Palm
Chief Medical Staff. . . . . Robert Rayer, MD

Measure	Cases	This Hospital	State Average	U.S. Average	Top Hospital
Heart Attack Care					
ACE Inhibitor or ARB for LVSD[3]	0	-	89%	82%	100%
Aspirin at Arrival[1,3]	1	100%	92%	92%	100%
Aspirin at Discharge[1,3]	1	100%	93%	90%	100%
Beta Blocker at Arrival[1,3]	1	100%	88%	87%	100%
Beta Blocker at Discharge[1,3]	1	100%	95%	90%	100%
Fibrinolytic Medication Timing[3]	0	-	40%	31%	100%
PCI Within 90 Minutes of Arrival	0	-	77%	54%	95%
Smoking Cessation Advice[3]	0	-	68%	88%	100%
Heart Failure Care					
ACE Inhibitor or ARB for LVSD[1]	1	100%	85%	82%	100%
Discharge Instructions[1]	8	50%	54%	61%	93%
Evaluation of LVS Function[1]	8	25%	77%	83%	99%
Smoking Cessation Advice	0	-	67%	82%	100%
Pneumonia Care					
Appropriate Initial Antibiotic[1]	10	90%	80%	83%	94%
Blood Culture Timing[1]	1	100%	94%	90%	100%
Influenza Vaccine[1]	4	100%	76%	70%	100%
Initial Antibiotic Timing[1]	11	100%	85%	80%	93%
Oxygenation Assessment[1]	13	100%	99%	99%	100%
Pneumococcal Vaccine[1]	10	80%	73%	69%	94%
Smoking Cessation Advice[1]	1	100%	70%	80%	100%
Surgical Infection Prevention					
Prophylactic Antibiotic Given[5]	-	-	78%	77%	95%
Prophylactic Antibiotic Selection[5]	-	-	94%	90%	100%
Prophylactic Antibiotic Stopped[5]	-	-	82%	72%	95%
Pregnancy Care					
Inpatient Neonatal Mortality	-	-	-	-	-
Third or Fourth Degree Laceration	-	-	4.42%	3.63%	3.27%

North Country Regional Hospital

1300 Anne Street NW
Bemidji, MN 56601
URL: www.nchs.com
Ownership: Voluntary non-profit - Private
Emergency Services: Yes
Phone: 218-751-5430
Fax: 218-333-5880
Accredited: No
Licensed Beds: 184

Key Personnel:
President/CEO. . . . . James F Hanko
Chief Medical Staff. . . . . Maria Statton
Infection Control. . . . . Wendy Gullicksrad
ICU . . . . Nancy Mickelberg
Intensive/Coronary Care . . . . Kathryn Edwards-Olson
Medical/Surgical Nursing . . . . Monica Wells
OB/GYN Womens Health. . . . . Shannon Rankin, RN
Respiratory/Cardiopulmonary. . . . . Gary Johnson

Measure	Cases	This Hospital	State Average	U.S. Average	Top Hospital
Heart Attack Care					
ACE Inhibitor or ARB for LVSD[1]	5	80%	89%	82%	100%
Aspirin at Arrival	35	100%	92%	92%	100%
Aspirin at Discharge[1]	16	94%	93%	90%	100%
Beta Blocker at Arrival[1]	18	100%	88%	87%	100%
Beta Blocker at Discharge[1]	16	94%	95%	90%	100%
Fibrinolytic Medication Timing[1]	4	25%	40%	31%	100%
PCI Within 90 Minutes of Arrival	0	-	77%	54%	95%
Smoking Cessation Advice[1]	3	100%	68%	88%	100%
Heart Failure Care					
ACE Inhibitor or ARB for LVSD	49	90%	85%	82%	100%
Discharge Instructions	86	73%	54%	61%	93%
Evaluation of LVS Function	111	97%	77%	83%	99%
Smoking Cessation Advice[1]	17	94%	67%	82%	100%
Pneumonia Care					

NOTE: Hospital profiles are in alphabetical order by state, then city, then hospital within the city; Rankings are sorted by rate in descending order and exclude hospitals with less than 25 cases; (1) The number of cases is too small (n<25) for purposes of reliably predicting hospital performance; (2) Measure reflects the hospital's indication that its submission was based upon a sample of its relevant discharges; (3) Rate reflects fewer than the maximum possible quarters of data for the measure; (4) Inaccurate information submitted and suppressed for one or more quarters; (5) No data is available from the hospital for this measure; Please refer to the User's Guide for a full explanation of data

Appropriate Initial Antibiotic	91	92%	80%	83%	94%
Blood Culture Timing	89	91%	94%	90%	100%
Influenza Vaccine	25	100%	76%	70%	100%
Initial Antibiotic Timing	155	88%	85%	80%	93%
Oxygenation Assessment	181	100%	99%	99%	100%
Pneumococcal Vaccine	120	96%	73%	69%	94%
Smoking Cessation Advice	43	77%	70%	80%	100%
Surgical Infection Prevention					
Prophylactic Antibiotic Given	454	92%	78%	77%	95%
Prophylactic Antibiotic Selection	128	95%	94%	90%	100%
Prophylactic Antibiotic Stopped	434	88%	82%	72%	95%
Pregnancy Care					
Inpatient Neonatal Mortality	-	-	-	-	-
Third or Fourth Degree Laceration	-	-	4.42%	3.63%	3.27%

Swift County-Benson Hospital

1815 Wisconsin Avenue
Benson, MN 56215

Toll-Free: 800-324-0787
Phone: 320-843-4232
Fax: 320-843-4172

URL: www.scbh.org
Ownership: Govt - Hospital District or Authority
Emergency Services: Yes
Accredited: No
Licensed Beds: 31

Key Personnel:

CEO . . . . Frank Lawatsch
Emergency Room . . . . Roberta Carter
Director Infection/Disease Control . . . . Holly Rodahl, RN
Director Medical/Surgical Nursing . . . . Roberta Carter, RN
Director Radiology . . . . Jackie Carmina, RRT

Measure	Cases	This Hospital	State Average	U.S. Average	Top Hospital
Heart Attack Care					
ACE Inhibitor or ARB for LVSD[3]	0	-	89%	82%	100%
Aspirin at Arrival[1,3]	3	100%	92%	92%	100%
Aspirin at Discharge[1,3]	3	100%	93%	90%	100%
Beta Blocker at Arrival[1,3]	3	100%	88%	87%	100%
Beta Blocker at Discharge[1,3]	3	100%	95%	90%	100%
Fibrinolytic Medication Timing[3]	0	-	40%	31%	100%
PCI Within 90 Minutes of Arrival	0	-	77%	54%	95%
Smoking Cessation Advice[3]	0	-	68%	88%	100%
Heart Failure Care					
ACE Inhibitor or ARB for LVSD[1]	6	100%	85%	82%	100%
Discharge Instructions[1]	15	87%	54%	61%	93%
Evaluation of LVS Function	25	80%	77%	83%	99%
Smoking Cessation Advice[1]	1	0%	67%	82%	100%
Pneumonia Care					
Appropriate Initial Antibiotic	29	69%	80%	83%	94%
Blood Culture Timing[1]	9	89%	94%	90%	100%
Influenza Vaccine[1]	12	100%	76%	70%	100%
Initial Antibiotic Timing	34	85%	85%	80%	93%
Oxygenation Assessment	44	100%	99%	99%	100%
Pneumococcal Vaccine	34	59%	73%	69%	94%
Smoking Cessation Advice[1]	10	0%	70%	80%	100%
Surgical Infection Prevention					
Prophylactic Antibiotic Given[5]	-	-	78%	77%	95%
Prophylactic Antibiotic Selection[5]	-	-	94%	90%	100%
Prophylactic Antibiotic Stopped[5]	-	-	82%	72%	95%
Pregnancy Care					
Inpatient Neonatal Mortality	-	-	-	-	-
Third or Fourth Degree Laceration	-	-	4.42%	3.63%	3.27%

Bigfork Valley Hospital

258 Pine Tree Drive
PO Box 258
Bigfork, MN 56628
E-mail: wecare@bigforkvalley.org
URL: www.bigforkvalley.org

Phone: 218-743-3177
Fax: 218-743-3559

Ownership: Govt - Hospital District or Authority
Emergency Services: Yes
Accredited: No
Licensed Beds: 20

Key Personnel:

Administrator . . . . Dan Odegaard
Chief Medical Staff . . . . George Rounds

Measure	Cases	This Hospital	State Average	U.S. Average	Top Hospital
Heart Attack Care					
ACE Inhibitor or ARB for LVSD[5]	-	-	89%	82%	100%
Aspirin at Arrival[5]	-	-	92%	92%	100%
Aspirin at Discharge[5]	-	-	93%	90%	100%
Beta Blocker at Arrival[5]	-	-	88%	87%	100%
Beta Blocker at Discharge[5]	-	-	95%	90%	100%
Fibrinolytic Medication Timing[5]	-	-	40%	31%	100%
PCI Within 90 Minutes of Arrival[5]	-	-	77%	54%	95%
Smoking Cessation Advice[5]	-	-	68%	88%	100%
Heart Failure Care					
ACE Inhibitor or ARB for LVSD[1,3]	2	50%	85%	82%	100%
Discharge Instructions[1,3]	2	0%	54%	61%	93%
Evaluation of LVS Function[1,3]	7	43%	77%	83%	99%
Smoking Cessation Advice[3]	0	-	67%	82%	100%
Pneumonia Care					
Appropriate Initial Antibiotic[1,3]	16	88%	80%	83%	94%
Blood Culture Timing[1]	5	60%	94%	90%	100%
Influenza Vaccine[1]	7	57%	76%	70%	100%
Initial Antibiotic Timing[1,3]	18	100%	85%	80%	93%
Oxygenation Assessment[3]	25	100%	99%	99%	100%
Pneumococcal Vaccine[1,3]	19	58%	73%	69%	94%
Smoking Cessation Advice[1,3]	7	71%	70%	80%	100%
Surgical Infection Prevention					
Prophylactic Antibiotic Given[5]	-	-	78%	77%	95%
Prophylactic Antibiotic Selection[5]	-	-	94%	90%	100%
Prophylactic Antibiotic Stopped[5]	-	-	82%	72%	95%
Pregnancy Care					
Inpatient Neonatal Mortality	-	-	-	-	-
Third or Fourth Degree Laceration	-	-	4.42%	3.63%	3.27%

United Hospital District

515 South Moore
PO Box 160
Blue Earth, MN 56013
URL: www.uhd.org

Phone: 507-526-3273
Fax: 507-526-3621

Ownership: Govt - Hospital District or Authority
Emergency Services: Yes
Accredited: Yes
Licensed Beds: 43

Key Personnel:

Administrator . . . . Jeff Lang
Chief Medical Staff . . . . Terry Cahill, MD
Emergency Room . . . . Joseph Tempel, MD
Infection Control . . . . Pam Manzke

Measure	Cases	This Hospital	State Average	U.S. Average	Top Hospital
Heart Attack Care					
ACE Inhibitor or ARB for LVSD[1]	1	100%	89%	82%	100%
Aspirin at Arrival[1]	5	80%	92%	92%	100%
Aspirin at Discharge[1]	4	75%	93%	90%	100%
Beta Blocker at Arrival[1]	6	100%	88%	87%	100%
Beta Blocker at Discharge[1]	3	67%	95%	90%	100%
Fibrinolytic Medication Timing	0	-	40%	31%	100%
PCI Within 90 Minutes of Arrival	0	-	77%	54%	95%
Smoking Cessation Advice	0	-	68%	88%	100%
Heart Failure Care					
ACE Inhibitor or ARB for LVSD[1]	13	85%	85%	82%	100%
Discharge Instructions[1]	19	68%	54%	61%	93%
Evaluation of LVS Function	28	75%	77%	83%	99%
Smoking Cessation Advice[1]	1	0%	67%	82%	100%
Pneumonia Care					
Appropriate Initial Antibiotic[1]	22	86%	80%	83%	94%
Blood Culture Timing[1]	4	100%	94%	90%	100%
Influenza Vaccine[1]	3	100%	76%	70%	100%
Initial Antibiotic Timing	26	88%	85%	80%	93%
Oxygenation Assessment	30	100%	99%	99%	100%
Pneumococcal Vaccine[1]	23	65%	73%	69%	94%
Smoking Cessation Advice[1]	2	0%	70%	80%	100%
Surgical Infection Prevention					
Prophylactic Antibiotic Given[1,3]	12	67%	78%	77%	95%
Prophylactic Antibiotic Selection[1]	12	100%	94%	90%	100%
Prophylactic Antibiotic Stopped[1,3]	12	100%	82%	72%	95%
Pregnancy Care					
Inpatient Neonatal Mortality	-	-	-	-	-

NOTE: Hospital profiles are in alphabetical order by state, then city, then hospital within the city; Rankings are sorted by rate in descending order and exclude hospitals with less than 25 cases; (1) The number of cases is too small (n<25) for purposes of reliably predicting hospital performance; (2) Measure reflects the hospital's indication that its submission was based upon a sample of its relevant discharges; (3) Rate reflects fewer than the maximum possible quarters of data for the measure; (4) Inaccurate information submitted and suppressed for one or more quarters; (5) No data is available from the hospital for this measure; Please refer to the User's Guide for a full explanation of data

Third or Fourth Degree Laceration	-	-	4.42%	3.63%	3.27%

Saint Joseph's Medical Center

523 N 3rd Street
Brainerd, MN 56401
URL: www.sjmcmn.org
Ownership: Voluntary non-profit - Church
Emergency Services: Yes
Phone: 218-829-2861
Fax: 218-828-3103
Accredited: Yes
Licensed Beds: 162

Key Personnel:
President/CEO. . . . . Jani Wiebolt

Measure	Cases	This Hospital	State Average	U.S. Average	Top Hospital
Heart Attack Care					
ACE Inhibitor or ARB for LVSD[1]	6	83%	89%	82%	100%
Aspirin at Arrival	43	98%	92%	92%	100%
Aspirin at Discharge[1]	19	79%	93%	90%	100%
Beta Blocker at Arrival	33	97%	88%	87%	100%
Beta Blocker at Discharge[1]	21	81%	95%	90%	100%
Fibrinolytic Medication Timing	0	-	40%	31%	100%
PCI Within 90 Minutes of Arrival	0	-	77%	54%	95%
Smoking Cessation Advice	0	-	68%	88%	100%
Heart Failure Care					
ACE Inhibitor or ARB for LVSD	53	74%	85%	82%	100%
Discharge Instructions	203	64%	54%	61%	93%
Evaluation of LVS Function	243	84%	77%	83%	99%
Smoking Cessation Advice[1]	21	81%	67%	82%	100%
Pneumonia Care					
Appropriate Initial Antibiotic	146	91%	80%	83%	94%
Blood Culture Timing	161	96%	94%	90%	100%
Influenza Vaccine	44	77%	76%	70%	100%
Initial Antibiotic Timing	235	86%	85%	80%	93%
Oxygenation Assessment	261	100%	99%	99%	100%
Pneumococcal Vaccine	189	75%	73%	69%	94%
Smoking Cessation Advice	51	73%	70%	80%	100%
Surgical Infection Prevention					
Prophylactic Antibiotic Given[2,3]	278	97%	78%	77%	95%
Prophylactic Antibiotic Selection[2]	62	100%	94%	90%	100%
Prophylactic Antibiotic Stopped[2,3]	278	59%	82%	72%	95%
Pregnancy Care					
Inpatient Neonatal Mortality	665	0.00%	-	-	-
Third or Fourth Degree Laceration	620	3.23%	4.42%	3.63%	3.27%

Saint Francis Medical Center

2400 Saint Francis Drive
Breckenridge, MN 56520
URL: www.sfcare.org
Ownership: Voluntary non-profit - Church
Emergency Services: Yes
Phone: 218-643-3000
Fax: 218-643-7502
Accredited: No
Licensed Beds: 42

Key Personnel:
CEO. . . . . David Nelson
Director Medical/Surgical Nursing . . . . Nancy Norwick
Chief Radiology . . . . Larry Licht, MD

Measure	Cases	This Hospital	State Average	U.S. Average	Top Hospital
Heart Attack Care					
ACE Inhibitor or ARB for LVSD[3]	0	-	89%	82%	100%
Aspirin at Arrival[1,3]	7	86%	92%	92%	100%
Aspirin at Discharge[1,3]	4	75%	93%	90%	100%
Beta Blocker at Arrival[1,3]	5	80%	88%	87%	100%
Beta Blocker at Discharge[1,3]	3	100%	95%	90%	100%
Fibrinolytic Medication Timing[1,3]	2	0%	40%	31%	100%
PCI Within 90 Minutes of Arrival[5]	-	-	77%	54%	95%
Smoking Cessation Advice[3]	0	-	68%	88%	100%
Heart Failure Care					
ACE Inhibitor or ARB for LVSD[1]	4	100%	85%	82%	100%
Discharge Instructions[1]	19	58%	54%	61%	93%
Evaluation of LVS Function	37	41%	77%	83%	99%
Smoking Cessation Advice[1]	4	75%	67%	82%	100%
Pneumonia Care					
Appropriate Initial Antibiotic	33	82%	80%	83%	94%
Blood Culture Timing[1]	1	100%	94%	90%	100%
Influenza Vaccine[1]	6	83%	76%	70%	100%
Initial Antibiotic Timing	41	90%	85%	80%	93%
Oxygenation Assessment	57	100%	99%	99%	100%
Pneumococcal Vaccine	45	93%	73%	69%	94%
Smoking Cessation Advice[1]	10	80%	70%	80%	100%
Surgical Infection Prevention					
Prophylactic Antibiotic Given[5]	-	-	78%	77%	95%
Prophylactic Antibiotic Selection[5]	-	-	94%	90%	100%
Prophylactic Antibiotic Stopped[5]	-	-	82%	72%	95%
Pregnancy Care					
Inpatient Neonatal Mortality	-	-	-	-	-
Third or Fourth Degree Laceration	-	-	4.42%	3.63%	3.27%

Buffalo Hospital

Alternate Name: Allina Hospitals & Clinics
303 Catlin Street
Buffalo, MN 55313
URL: www.buffalohospital.org
Ownership: Voluntary non-profit - Other
Emergency Services: Yes
Phone: 763-682-1212
Fax: 763-684-7104
Accredited: Yes
Licensed Beds: 65

Key Personnel:
President/CEO. . . . . Steve Hatkin
Chief Medical Staff. . . . . Dr Charles Yancey
Supervising Nurse CCU/Dir Med/Surg Nurse . . . Gretchen Frederick
Nurse Manager, Surgical Services. . . . . Julianne Wagner
Chief Radiology . . . . Kurt Scheurer, MD
Director Respiratory Therapy . . . . Kris Rowe

Measure	Cases	This Hospital	State Average	U.S. Average	Top Hospital
Heart Attack Care					
ACE Inhibitor or ARB for LVSD[1]	3	100%	89%	82%	100%
Aspirin at Arrival[1]	9	89%	92%	92%	100%
Aspirin at Discharge[1]	5	60%	93%	90%	100%
Beta Blocker at Arrival[1]	9	78%	88%	87%	100%
Beta Blocker at Discharge[1]	9	100%	95%	90%	100%
Fibrinolytic Medication Timing	0	-	40%	31%	100%
PCI Within 90 Minutes of Arrival	0	-	77%	54%	95%
Smoking Cessation Advice	0	-	68%	88%	100%
Heart Failure Care					
ACE Inhibitor or ARB for LVSD	27	63%	85%	82%	100%
Discharge Instructions	41	41%	54%	61%	93%
Evaluation of LVS Function	59	90%	77%	83%	99%
Smoking Cessation Advice[1]	6	67%	67%	82%	100%
Pneumonia Care					
Appropriate Initial Antibiotic	74	89%	80%	83%	94%
Blood Culture Timing	66	77%	94%	90%	100%
Influenza Vaccine[1]	19	79%	76%	70%	100%
Initial Antibiotic Timing	89	94%	85%	80%	93%
Oxygenation Assessment	123	100%	99%	99%	100%
Pneumococcal Vaccine	82	72%	73%	69%	94%
Smoking Cessation Advice	26	65%	70%	80%	100%
Surgical Infection Prevention					
Prophylactic Antibiotic Given[2,3]	64	92%	78%	77%	95%
Prophylactic Antibiotic Selection[2]	35	91%	94%	90%	100%
Prophylactic Antibiotic Stopped[2,3]	63	67%	82%	72%	95%
Pregnancy Care					
Inpatient Neonatal Mortality	-	-	-	-	-
Third or Fourth Degree Laceration	-	-	4.42%	3.63%	3.27%

Fairview Ridges Hospital

201 E Nicollet Boulevard
Burnsville, MN 55337
URL: www.fairview.org
Ownership: Voluntary non-profit - Church
Emergency Services: Yes
Phone: 952-892-2000
Fax: 952-892-2107
Accredited: Yes
Licensed Beds: 150

Key Personnel:
President/CEO. . . . . Sara Criger

Measure	Cases	This Hospital	State Average	U.S. Average	Top Hospital
Heart Attack Care					
ACE Inhibitor or ARB for LVSD[1]	4	100%	89%	82%	100%
Aspirin at Arrival	38	100%	92%	92%	100%
Aspirin at Discharge[1]	17	94%	93%	90%	100%

NOTE: Hospital profiles are in alphabetical order by state, then city, then hospital within the city; Rankings are sorted by rate in descending order and exclude hospitals with less than 25 cases; (1) The number of cases is too small (n<25) for purposes of reliably predicting hospital performance; (2) Measure reflects the hospital's indication that its submission was based upon a sample of its relevant discharges; (3) Rate reflects fewer than the maximum possible quarters of data for the measure; (4) Inaccurate information submitted and suppressed for one or more quarters; (5) No data is available from the hospital for this measure; Please refer to the User's Guide for a full explanation of data

Measure	Cases	This Hospital	State Average	U.S. Average	Top Hospital
Beta Blocker at Arrival	38	100%	88%	87%	100%
Beta Blocker at Discharge[1]	18	100%	95%	90%	100%
Fibrinolytic Medication Timing	0	-	40%	31%	100%
PCI Within 90 Minutes of Arrival	0	-	77%	54%	95%
Smoking Cessation Advice[1]	1	100%	68%	88%	100%
Heart Failure Care					
ACE Inhibitor or ARB for LVSD	44	93%	85%	82%	100%
Discharge Instructions	103	91%	54%	61%	93%
Evaluation of LVS Function	156	90%	77%	83%	99%
Smoking Cessation Advice[1]	19	58%	67%	82%	100%
Pneumonia Care					
Appropriate Initial Antibiotic	174	86%	80%	83%	94%
Blood Culture Timing	146	97%	94%	90%	100%
Influenza Vaccine	46	96%	76%	70%	100%
Initial Antibiotic Timing	214	80%	85%	80%	93%
Oxygenation Assessment	270	99%	99%	99%	100%
Pneumococcal Vaccine	161	86%	73%	69%	94%
Smoking Cessation Advice	57	79%	70%	80%	100%
Surgical Infection Prevention					
Prophylactic Antibiotic Given[2,3]	125	88%	78%	77%	95%
Prophylactic Antibiotic Selection[2]	41	95%	94%	90%	100%
Prophylactic Antibiotic Stopped[2,3]	120	83%	82%	72%	95%
Pregnancy Care					
Inpatient Neonatal Mortality	3,088	0.19%	-	-	-
Third or Fourth Degree Laceration	2,216	5.96%	4.42%	3.63%	3.27%

Cambridge Medical Center

701 South Dellwood
Cambridge, MN 55008
Phone: 763-689-7700
Ownership: Voluntary non-profit - Other
Accredited: Yes
Emergency Services: Yes

Measure	Cases	This Hospital	State Average	U.S. Average	Top Hospital
Heart Attack Care					
ACE Inhibitor or ARB for LVSD[1]	3	67%	89%	82%	100%
Aspirin at Arrival[1]	15	93%	92%	92%	100%
Aspirin at Discharge[1]	7	100%	93%	90%	100%
Beta Blocker at Arrival[1]	11	82%	88%	87%	100%
Beta Blocker at Discharge[1]	8	88%	95%	90%	100%
Fibrinolytic Medication Timing	0	-	40%	31%	100%
PCI Within 90 Minutes of Arrival	0	-	77%	54%	95%
Smoking Cessation Advice	0	-	68%	88%	100%
Heart Failure Care					
ACE Inhibitor or ARB for LVSD[1]	20	90%	85%	82%	100%
Discharge Instructions	51	75%	54%	61%	93%
Evaluation of LVS Function	77	90%	77%	83%	99%
Smoking Cessation Advice[1]	8	100%	67%	82%	100%
Pneumonia Care					
Appropriate Initial Antibiotic	80	92%	80%	83%	94%
Blood Culture Timing	48	92%	94%	90%	100%
Influenza Vaccine[1]	20	100%	76%	70%	100%
Initial Antibiotic Timing	111	87%	85%	80%	93%
Oxygenation Assessment	149	100%	99%	99%	100%
Pneumococcal Vaccine	88	98%	73%	69%	94%
Smoking Cessation Advice	30	100%	70%	80%	100%
Surgical Infection Prevention					
Prophylactic Antibiotic Given[2,3]	63	83%	78%	77%	95%
Prophylactic Antibiotic Selection[2]	35	91%	94%	90%	100%
Prophylactic Antibiotic Stopped[2,3]	63	86%	82%	72%	95%
Pregnancy Care					
Inpatient Neonatal Mortality	-	-	-	-	-
Third or Fourth Degree Laceration	-	-	4.42%	3.63%	3.27%

Sanford Canby Medical Center

112 Saint Olaf Avenue S
Canby, MN 56220
Phone: 507-223-7277
Fax: 507-223-7465
URL: www.sanfordcanby.org
Ownership: Voluntary non-profit - Private
Accredited: No
Emergency Services: Yes
Licensed Beds: 102
Key Personnel:
CEO. . . . . Robert Foreman

Measure	Cases	This Hospital	State Average	U.S. Average	Top Hospital
Heart Attack Care					
ACE Inhibitor or ARB for LVSD[3]	0	-	89%	82%	100%
Aspirin at Arrival[3]	0	-	92%	92%	100%
Aspirin at Discharge[3]	0	-	93%	90%	100%
Beta Blocker at Arrival[1,3]	1	100%	88%	87%	100%
Beta Blocker at Discharge[1,3]	1	100%	95%	90%	100%
Fibrinolytic Medication Timing[1,3]	1	100%	40%	31%	100%
PCI Within 90 Minutes of Arrival[5]	-	-	77%	54%	95%
Smoking Cessation Advice[3]	0	-	68%	88%	100%
Heart Failure Care					
ACE Inhibitor or ARB for LVSD[1]	3	100%	85%	82%	100%
Discharge Instructions[1]	6	33%	54%	61%	93%
Evaluation of LVS Function[1]	16	69%	77%	83%	99%
Smoking Cessation Advice[1]	1	0%	67%	82%	100%
Pneumonia Care					
Appropriate Initial Antibiotic[1,3]	10	50%	80%	83%	94%
Blood Culture Timing[1]	1	100%	94%	90%	100%
Influenza Vaccine[1]	5	80%	76%	70%	100%
Initial Antibiotic Timing[1,3]	19	84%	85%	80%	93%
Oxygenation Assessment[1,3]	23	100%	99%	99%	100%
Pneumococcal Vaccine[1,3]	14	57%	73%	69%	94%
Smoking Cessation Advice[1,3]	1	100%	70%	80%	100%
Surgical Infection Prevention					
Prophylactic Antibiotic Given[1,3]	1	0%	78%	77%	95%
Prophylactic Antibiotic Selection	0	-	94%	90%	100%
Prophylactic Antibiotic Stopped[1,3]	1	100%	82%	72%	95%
Pregnancy Care					
Inpatient Neonatal Mortality	-	-	-	-	-
Third or Fourth Degree Laceration	-	-	4.42%	3.63%	3.27%

Community Memorial Hospital Association

512 Skyline Boulevard
Cloquet, MN 55720
Phone: 218-879-4641
Fax: 218-879-9167
Ownership: Voluntary non-profit - Private
Accredited: No
Emergency Services: Yes
Licensed Beds: 36
Key Personnel:
Administrator . . . . Rick Breuer
Chief Medical Staff. . . . . Victoria Heren
Director of Cardiology/Cardiac Lab. . . . . Linda Vittperner
Emergency Room . . . . Les Riess, MD
Director Infection/Disease Control . . . . Andrea Peterson
Medical/Surgical Nursing . . . . Tom Gauthier
OB/GYN Womens Health. . . . . Arne Vainio
Director Respiratory Therapy . . . . Jack Reynolds

Measure	Cases	This Hospital	State Average	U.S. Average	Top Hospital
Heart Attack Care					
ACE Inhibitor or ARB for LVSD	0	-	89%	82%	100%
Aspirin at Arrival[1]	11	100%	92%	92%	100%
Aspirin at Discharge[1]	9	89%	93%	90%	100%
Beta Blocker at Arrival[1]	13	100%	88%	87%	100%
Beta Blocker at Discharge[1]	10	100%	95%	90%	100%
Fibrinolytic Medication Timing	0	-	40%	31%	100%
PCI Within 90 Minutes of Arrival	0	-	77%	54%	95%
Smoking Cessation Advice[1]	2	0%	68%	88%	100%
Heart Failure Care					
ACE Inhibitor or ARB for LVSD[1]	18	72%	85%	82%	100%
Discharge Instructions	34	15%	54%	61%	93%
Evaluation of LVS Function	52	79%	77%	83%	99%
Smoking Cessation Advice[1]	7	43%	67%	82%	100%
Pneumonia Care					
Appropriate Initial Antibiotic	52	79%	80%	83%	94%
Blood Culture Timing	30	77%	94%	90%	100%
Influenza Vaccine[1]	10	20%	76%	70%	100%
Initial Antibiotic Timing	55	75%	85%	80%	93%
Oxygenation Assessment	63	100%	99%	99%	100%
Pneumococcal Vaccine	39	74%	73%	69%	94%
Smoking Cessation Advice[1]	17	47%	70%	80%	100%
Surgical Infection Prevention					
Prophylactic Antibiotic Given	73	55%	78%	77%	95%
Prophylactic Antibiotic Selection[1]	14	93%	94%	90%	100%

NOTE: Hospital profiles are in alphabetical order by state, then city, then hospital within the city; Rankings are sorted by rate in descending order and exclude hospitals with less than 25 cases; (1) The number of cases is too small (n<25) for purposes of reliably predicting hospital performance; (2) Measure reflects the hospital's indication that its submission was based upon a sample of its relevant discharges; (3) Rate reflects fewer than the maximum possible quarters of data for the measure; (4) Inaccurate information submitted and suppressed for one or more quarters; (5) No data is available from the hospital for this measure; Please refer to the User's Guide for a full explanation of data

Measure	Cases	This Hospital	State Average	U.S. Average	Top Hospital
Prophylactic Antibiotic Stopped	72	96%	82%	72%	95%
Pregnancy Care					
Inpatient Neonatal Mortality	-	-	-	-	-
Third or Fourth Degree Laceration	-	-	4.42%	3.63%	3.27%

Mercy Hospital

4050 Coon Rapids Boulevard
Coon Rapids, MN 55433
URL: www.mercy-unity.com
Ownership: Voluntary non-profit - Private
Emergency Services: Yes
Phone: 763-236-6000
Fax: 763-236-8124
Accredited: Yes
Licensed Beds: 271

Key Personnel:
President . . . . Venetia HM Kudrle
Chief Medical Staff . . . . Donald Collins
Director Cardiology . . . . Steven Remole
Director Emergency Room . . . . Allen Fuller

Measure	Cases	This Hospital	State Average	U.S. Average	Top Hospital
Heart Attack Care					
ACE Inhibitor or ARB for LVSD	83	88%	89%	82%	100%
Aspirin at Arrival	327	99%	92%	92%	100%
Aspirin at Discharge	463	100%	93%	90%	100%
Beta Blocker at Arrival	239	95%	88%	87%	100%
Beta Blocker at Discharge	489	100%	95%	90%	100%
Fibrinolytic Medication Timing	0	-	40%	31%	100%
PCI Within 90 Minutes of Arrival	28	64%	77%	54%	95%
Smoking Cessation Advice	197	99%	68%	88%	100%
Heart Failure Care					
ACE Inhibitor or ARB for LVSD	169	81%	85%	82%	100%
Discharge Instructions	368	86%	54%	61%	93%
Evaluation of LVS Function	441	98%	77%	83%	99%
Smoking Cessation Advice	64	97%	67%	82%	100%
Pneumonia Care					
Appropriate Initial Antibiotic	173	82%	80%	83%	94%
Blood Culture Timing	118	86%	94%	90%	100%
Influenza Vaccine	42	79%	76%	70%	100%
Initial Antibiotic Timing	228	72%	85%	80%	93%
Oxygenation Assessment	267	100%	99%	99%	100%
Pneumococcal Vaccine	164	73%	73%	69%	94%
Smoking Cessation Advice	64	80%	70%	80%	100%
Surgical Infection Prevention					
Prophylactic Antibiotic Given[2,3]	176	89%	78%	77%	95%
Prophylactic Antibiotic Selection[2]	106	96%	94%	90%	100%
Prophylactic Antibiotic Stopped[2,3]	171	92%	82%	72%	95%
Pregnancy Care					
Inpatient Neonatal Mortality	-	-	-	-	-
Third or Fourth Degree Laceration	-	-	4.42%	3.63%	3.27%

Riverview Health

323 S Minnesota Street
Crookston, MN 56716
URL: www.riverviewhealth.org
Ownership: Voluntary non-profit - Private
Emergency Services: Yes
Phone: 218-281-9200
Fax: 218-281-9222
Accredited: No
Licensed Beds: 49

Key Personnel:
President/CEO . . . . Debra Boardman
Chief Medical Staff . . . . Dr Erik Kanten, MD
Emergency Room Supervisor . . . . Mary Pufall
Infection Control . . . . Dee Dee Wielsma
Medical/Surgical Nursing . . . . Merleen Knott
Respiratory/Cardiopulmonary . . . . Mary Ann Boushee

Measure	Cases	This Hospital	State Average	U.S. Average	Top Hospital
Heart Attack Care					
ACE Inhibitor or ARB for LVSD[1]	2	50%	89%	82%	100%
Aspirin at Arrival[1]	18	89%	92%	92%	100%
Aspirin at Discharge[1]	12	75%	93%	90%	100%
Beta Blocker at Arrival[1]	19	79%	88%	87%	100%
Beta Blocker at Discharge[1]	16	75%	95%	90%	100%
Fibrinolytic Medication Timing	0	-	40%	31%	100%
PCI Within 90 Minutes of Arrival	0	-	77%	54%	95%
Smoking Cessation Advice	0	-	68%	88%	100%
Heart Failure Care					
ACE Inhibitor or ARB for LVSD[1]	16	56%	85%	82%	100%
Discharge Instructions	34	56%	54%	61%	93%
Evaluation of LVS Function	50	48%	77%	83%	99%
Smoking Cessation Advice[1]	6	17%	67%	82%	100%
Pneumonia Care					
Appropriate Initial Antibiotic	28	79%	80%	83%	94%
Blood Culture Timing[1]	13	100%	94%	90%	100%
Influenza Vaccine[1]	8	50%	76%	70%	100%
Initial Antibiotic Timing	34	85%	85%	80%	93%
Oxygenation Assessment	43	100%	99%	99%	100%
Pneumococcal Vaccine	28	75%	73%	69%	94%
Smoking Cessation Advice[1]	6	83%	70%	80%	100%
Surgical Infection Prevention					
Prophylactic Antibiotic Given[1]	24	88%	78%	77%	95%
Prophylactic Antibiotic Selection[1]	8	100%	94%	90%	100%
Prophylactic Antibiotic Stopped[1]	23	65%	82%	72%	95%
Pregnancy Care					
Inpatient Neonatal Mortality	-	-	-	-	-
Third or Fourth Degree Laceration	-	-	4.42%	3.63%	3.27%

Deer River Healthcare Center

Alternate Name: Community Memorial Hospital
1002 Comstock Drive
Deer River, MN 56636
URL: www.drhc.org
Ownership: Voluntary non-profit - Private
Emergency Services: Yes
Phone: 218-246-2900
Fax: 218-246-3013
Accredited: No
Licensed Beds: 20

Key Personnel:
CEO . . . . Jeffrey Stampohar
Chief Medical Staff . . . . David Goodall, MD
Cardiac Lab . . . . Angie Olson, RN
Emergency Room . . . . Kelly Skelly, RN
Director Infection/Disease Control . . . . Christine Adams
Medical Surgical Nursing . . . . Kelly Skelly, RN

Measure	Cases	This Hospital	State Average	U.S. Average	Top Hospital
Heart Attack Care					
ACE Inhibitor or ARB for LVSD[2]	0	-	89%	82%	100%
Aspirin at Arrival[1,2]	6	83%	92%	92%	100%
Aspirin at Discharge[1,2]	6	83%	93%	90%	100%
Beta Blocker at Arrival[1,2]	7	86%	88%	87%	100%
Beta Blocker at Discharge[1,2]	6	100%	95%	90%	100%
Fibrinolytic Medication Timing[2,3]	0	-	40%	31%	100%
PCI Within 90 Minutes of Arrival[5]	-	-	77%	54%	95%
Smoking Cessation Advice[1,2]	2	0%	68%	88%	100%
Heart Failure Care					
ACE Inhibitor or ARB for LVSD[1,2]	3	67%	85%	82%	100%
Discharge Instructions[2]	32	19%	54%	61%	93%
Evaluation of LVS Function[2]	38	76%	77%	83%	99%
Smoking Cessation Advice[1,2]	8	25%	67%	82%	100%
Pneumonia Care					
Appropriate Initial Antibiotic[2]	29	76%	80%	83%	94%
Blood Culture Timing[1,2]	8	100%	94%	90%	100%
Influenza Vaccine[1,2]	5	80%	76%	70%	100%
Initial Antibiotic Timing[2]	34	79%	85%	80%	93%
Oxygenation Assessment[2]	38	100%	99%	99%	100%
Pneumococcal Vaccine[2]	26	73%	73%	69%	94%
Smoking Cessation Advice[1,2]	7	43%	70%	80%	100%
Surgical Infection Prevention					
Prophylactic Antibiotic Given[2,3]	0	-	78%	77%	95%
Prophylactic Antibiotic Selection[5]	-	-	94%	90%	100%
Prophylactic Antibiotic Stopped[2,3]	0	-	82%	72%	95%
Pregnancy Care					
Inpatient Neonatal Mortality	-	-	-	-	-
Third or Fourth Degree Laceration	-	-	4.42%	3.63%	3.27%

NOTE: Hospital profiles are in alphabetical order by state, then city, then hospital within the city; Rankings are sorted by rate in descending order and exclude hospitals with less than 25 cases; (1) The number of cases is too small (n<25) for purposes of reliably predicting hospital performance; (2) Measure reflects the hospital's indication that its submission was based upon a sample of its relevant discharges; (3) Rate reflects fewer than the maximum possible quarters of data for the measure; (4) Inaccurate information submitted and suppressed for one or more quarters; (5) No data is available from the hospital for this measure; Please refer to the User's Guide for a full explanation of data

Saint Mary's Regional Health Center

1027 Washington Avenue
Detroit Lakes, MN 56501
URL: www.smrhc.com
Ownership: Voluntary non-profit - Church
Emergency Services: Yes
Phone: 218-847-5611
Fax: 218-847-7674
Accredited: Yes
Licensed Beds: 187

Key Personnel:
President/CEO . . . . . Thomas R Thompson
Chief Medical Staff . . . . . Knute Thorsgard, MD
Emergency Room . . . . . Peg Severson
Director Infection/Disease Control . . . . . Jackie Nordick
OB/GYN Womens Health . . . . . Mary Groth, MD
Chief Radiology . . . . . Gary Gran, MD
Director Respiratory Therapy . . . . . Laurie Olson

Measure	Cases	This Hospital	State Average	U.S. Average	Top Hospital
Heart Attack Care					
ACE Inhibitor or ARB for LVSD[1]	3	67%	89%	82%	100%
Aspirin at Arrival[1]	24	79%	92%	92%	100%
Aspirin at Discharge[1]	13	85%	93%	90%	100%
Beta Blocker at Arrival[1]	22	82%	88%	87%	100%
Beta Blocker at Discharge[1]	14	100%	95%	90%	100%
Fibrinolytic Medication Timing[1]	1	0%	40%	31%	100%
PCI Within 90 Minutes of Arrival	0	-	77%	54%	95%
Smoking Cessation Advice[1]	1	0%	68%	88%	100%
Heart Failure Care					
ACE Inhibitor or ARB for LVSD[1]	16	75%	85%	82%	100%
Discharge Instructions	37	30%	54%	61%	93%
Evaluation of LVS Function	57	56%	77%	83%	99%
Smoking Cessation Advice[1]	8	75%	67%	82%	100%
Pneumonia Care					
Appropriate Initial Antibiotic	74	77%	80%	83%	94%
Blood Culture Timing	28	75%	94%	90%	100%
Influenza Vaccine[1]	20	65%	76%	70%	100%
Initial Antibiotic Timing	77	82%	85%	80%	93%
Oxygenation Assessment	100	100%	99%	99%	100%
Pneumococcal Vaccine	70	66%	73%	69%	94%
Smoking Cessation Advice[1]	14	86%	70%	80%	100%
Surgical Infection Prevention					
Prophylactic Antibiotic Given[2,3]	87	86%	78%	77%	95%
Prophylactic Antibiotic Selection[1,2]	5	60%	94%	90%	100%
Prophylactic Antibiotic Stopped[2,3]	86	100%	82%	72%	95%
Pregnancy Care					
Inpatient Neonatal Mortality	-	-	-	-	-
Third or Fourth Degree Laceration	-	-	4.42%	3.63%	3.27%

Miller Dwan Medical Center

502 E Second St
Duluth, MN 55805
Ownership: Voluntary non-profit - Private
Emergency Services: No
Phone: 218-786-2646
Accredited: Yes

Measure	Cases	This Hospital	State Average	U.S. Average	Top Hospital
Heart Attack Care					
ACE Inhibitor or ARB for LVSD[3]	0	-	89%	82%	100%
Aspirin at Arrival[3]	0	-	92%	92%	100%
Aspirin at Discharge[1,3]	1	100%	93%	90%	100%
Beta Blocker at Arrival[3]	0	-	88%	87%	100%
Beta Blocker at Discharge[1,3]	1	100%	95%	90%	100%
Fibrinolytic Medication Timing[5]	-	-	40%	31%	100%
PCI Within 90 Minutes of Arrival[5]	-	-	77%	54%	95%
Smoking Cessation Advice[5]	-	-	68%	88%	100%
Heart Failure Care					
ACE Inhibitor or ARB for LVSD[1]	9	44%	85%	82%	100%
Discharge Instructions[1,3]	5	0%	54%	61%	93%
Evaluation of LVS Function[1]	18	56%	77%	83%	99%
Smoking Cessation Advice[1,3]	2	50%	67%	82%	100%
Pneumonia Care					
Appropriate Initial Antibiotic[3]	0	-	80%	83%	94%
Blood Culture Timing[3]	0	-	94%	90%	100%
Influenza Vaccine[5]	-	-	76%	70%	100%
Initial Antibiotic Timing[1]	3	100%	85%	80%	93%
Oxygenation Assessment[1]	7	100%	99%	99%	100%
Pneumococcal Vaccine[1]	11	73%	73%	69%	94%
Smoking Cessation Advice[1,3]	1	100%	70%	80%	100%
Surgical Infection Prevention					
Prophylactic Antibiotic Given[2,3]	36	89%	78%	77%	95%
Prophylactic Antibiotic Selection[5]	-	-	94%	90%	100%
Prophylactic Antibiotic Stopped[2,3]	35	80%	82%	72%	95%
Pregnancy Care					
Inpatient Neonatal Mortality	-	-	-	-	-
Third or Fourth Degree Laceration	-	-	4.42%	3.63%	3.27%

Saint Lukes Hospital

915 E 1st St
Duluth, MN 55805
Ownership: Voluntary non-profit - Private
Emergency Services: Yes
Phone: 218-249-5555
Accredited: Yes

Measure	Cases	This Hospital	State Average	U.S. Average	Top Hospital
Heart Attack Care					
ACE Inhibitor or ARB for LVSD	56	91%	89%	82%	100%
Aspirin at Arrival	128	98%	92%	92%	100%
Aspirin at Discharge	164	99%	93%	90%	100%
Beta Blocker at Arrival	124	94%	88%	87%	100%
Beta Blocker at Discharge	190	99%	95%	90%	100%
Fibrinolytic Medication Timing	0	-	40%	31%	100%
PCI Within 90 Minutes of Arrival[1]	4	75%	77%	54%	95%
Smoking Cessation Advice	50	88%	68%	88%	100%
Heart Failure Care					
ACE Inhibitor or ARB for LVSD[2]	97	91%	85%	82%	100%
Discharge Instructions[2]	204	63%	54%	61%	93%
Evaluation of LVS Function[2]	250	91%	77%	83%	99%
Smoking Cessation Advice[2]	26	62%	67%	82%	100%
Pneumonia Care					
Appropriate Initial Antibiotic	101	78%	80%	83%	94%
Blood Culture Timing	70	93%	94%	90%	100%
Influenza Vaccine	30	83%	76%	70%	100%
Initial Antibiotic Timing	154	66%	85%	80%	93%
Oxygenation Assessment	187	100%	99%	99%	100%
Pneumococcal Vaccine	113	77%	73%	69%	94%
Smoking Cessation Advice	44	93%	70%	80%	100%
Surgical Infection Prevention					
Prophylactic Antibiotic Given[2,3]	224	70%	78%	77%	95%
Prophylactic Antibiotic Selection[2]	107	98%	94%	90%	100%
Prophylactic Antibiotic Stopped[2,3]	220	87%	82%	72%	95%
Pregnancy Care					
Inpatient Neonatal Mortality[2]	819	0.37%	-	-	-
Third or Fourth Degree Laceration[2]	523	4.78%	4.42%	3.63%	3.27%

Saint mary's Medical Center

407 E 3rd St
Duluth, MN 55805
URL: www.smdc.org
Ownership: Voluntary non-profit - Church
Emergency Services: Yes
Phone: 218-786-4000
Accredited: Yes
Licensed Beds: 690

Key Personnel:
CEO . . . . . Peter E Pearson
Chief of Medical Staff . . . . . Hugh Renierd
VP . . . . . Mike Motley
VP Surgical Specialties . . . . . Thurza Bender
Head of Emergency Room . . . . . Linda Waigh
VP . . . . . Harvey Anderson
VP Surgery/Operative/Diagnosic Services . . . . . Thurza Bender
VP . . . . . Robert Bender
VP . . . . . Joanne Cirillo
Chief Medical Officer . . . . . Thomas Nelson, MD
VP . . . . . Ann Bussey
Chief of Respiratory Care . . . . . Sherry Mlodovyniec

Measure	Cases	This Hospital	State Average	U.S. Average	Top Hospital
Heart Attack Care					
ACE Inhibitor or ARB for LVSD	179	94%	89%	82%	100%
Aspirin at Arrival	216	100%	92%	92%	100%

NOTE: Hospital profiles are in alphabetical order by state, then city, then hospital within the city; Rankings are sorted by rate in descending order and exclude hospitals with less than 25 cases; (1) The number of cases is too small (n<25) for purposes of reliably predicting hospital performance; (2) Measure reflects the hospital's indication that its submission was based upon a sample of its relevant discharges; (3) Rate reflects fewer than the maximum possible quarters of data for the measure; (4) Inaccurate information submitted and suppressed for one or more quarters; (5) No data is available from the hospital for this measure; Please refer to the User's Guide for a full explanation of data

Aspirin at Discharge	501	99%	93%	90%	100%
Beta Blocker at Arrival	166	98%	88%	87%	100%
Beta Blocker at Discharge	589	99%	95%	90%	100%
Fibrinolytic Medication Timing	0	-	40%	31%	100%
PCI Within 90 Minutes of Arrival[1]	13	69%	77%	54%	95%
Smoking Cessation Advice	224	98%	68%	88%	100%
Heart Failure Care					
ACE Inhibitor or ARB for LVSD	217	87%	85%	82%	100%
Discharge Instructions	301	62%	54%	61%	93%
Evaluation of LVS Function	395	93%	77%	83%	99%
Smoking Cessation Advice	51	88%	67%	82%	100%
Pneumonia Care					
Appropriate Initial Antibiotic	117	88%	80%	83%	94%
Blood Culture Timing	109	94%	94%	90%	100%
Influenza Vaccine	35	77%	76%	70%	100%
Initial Antibiotic Timing	170	80%	85%	80%	93%
Oxygenation Assessment	209	100%	99%	99%	100%
Pneumococcal Vaccine	148	84%	73%	69%	94%
Smoking Cessation Advice	64	81%	70%	80%	100%
Surgical Infection Prevention					
Prophylactic Antibiotic Given[2,3]	95	89%	78%	77%	95%
Prophylactic Antibiotic Selection[2]	97	92%	94%	90%	100%
Prophylactic Antibiotic Stopped[2,3]	89	93%	82%	72%	95%
Pregnancy Care					
Inpatient Neonatal Mortality	-	-	-	-	-
Third or Fourth Degree Laceration	-	-	4.42%	3.63%	3.27%

Fairview Southdale Hospital

6401 France Avenue S
Edina, MN 55435
Phone: 952-924-5000
Fax: 952-924-5970
URL: www.fairview.org
Ownership: Voluntary non-profit - Private
Accredited: Yes
Emergency Services: Yes
Licensed Beds: 390

Key Personnel:

President/CEO. . . . . Gary Strong
Chief Medical Staff. . . . . James Bishop, MD
Cardiac Laboratory. . . . . Cheri Hammer
ICU . . . . Lisa Winship, RN
Cardiac Care Nurse Manager . . . . Joy Wilde, RN
Manager Medical/Surgical Nursing. . . . . Kathleen Jahr, RN
Director Medical/Surgical Nursing . . . . James Bishop, MD
Director Radiology . . . . Judy Sager

Measure	Cases	This Hospital	State Average	U.S. Average	Top Hospital
Heart Attack Care					
ACE Inhibitor or ARB for LVSD	138	98%	89%	82%	100%
Aspirin at Arrival	364	99%	92%	92%	100%
Aspirin at Discharge	547	100%	93%	90%	100%
Beta Blocker at Arrival	340	100%	88%	87%	100%
Beta Blocker at Discharge	545	100%	95%	90%	100%
Fibrinolytic Medication Timing	0	-	40%	31%	100%
PCI Within 90 Minutes of Arrival[1]	23	96%	77%	54%	95%
Smoking Cessation Advice	158	100%	68%	88%	100%
Heart Failure Care					
ACE Inhibitor or ARB for LVSD	171	91%	85%	82%	100%
Discharge Instructions	333	92%	54%	61%	93%
Evaluation of LVS Function	441	100%	77%	83%	99%
Smoking Cessation Advice	44	100%	67%	82%	100%
Pneumonia Care					
Appropriate Initial Antibiotic	139	91%	80%	83%	94%
Blood Culture Timing	185	98%	94%	90%	100%
Influenza Vaccine	59	92%	76%	70%	100%
Initial Antibiotic Timing	262	82%	85%	80%	93%
Oxygenation Assessment	296	100%	99%	99%	100%
Pneumococcal Vaccine	219	93%	73%	69%	94%
Smoking Cessation Advice	53	100%	70%	80%	100%
Surgical Infection Prevention					
Prophylactic Antibiotic Given[2,3]	243	96%	78%	77%	95%
Prophylactic Antibiotic Selection[2]	86	95%	94%	90%	100%
Prophylactic Antibiotic Stopped[2,3]	235	91%	82%	72%	95%
Pregnancy Care					
Inpatient Neonatal Mortality	3,643	0.00%	-	-	-
Third or Fourth Degree Laceration	2,403	7.12%	4.42%	3.63%	3.27%

Fairmont Medical Center

800 Medical Center Drive
PO Box 800
Fairmont, MN 56031
Phone: 507-238-8100
Fax: 507-238-8686
URL: www.fairmontmedicalcenter.org
Ownership: Voluntary non-profit - Other
Accredited: Yes
Emergency Services: Yes
Licensed Beds: 94

Key Personnel:

CEO. . . . . Barbara Allen, MD
Chief of Medical Staff. Timothy Bachenberg
Emergency Room . . . . Cheryl Martinson
Emergency Room . . . . Carol Shukla
Director Infection/Disease Control . . . . Roger Drahota
ICU . . . . Carol Shukla
Medical Surgical Nursing . . . . Carol Shukla
Director Radiology . . . . Chris Ward
Director Respiratory Therapy . . . . Herald Herfendal

Measure	Cases	This Hospital	State Average	U.S. Average	Top Hospital
Heart Attack Care					
ACE Inhibitor or ARB for LVSD[1]	5	100%	89%	82%	100%
Aspirin at Arrival[1]	23	100%	92%	92%	100%
Aspirin at Discharge[1]	17	100%	93%	90%	100%
Beta Blocker at Arrival[1]	21	95%	88%	87%	100%
Beta Blocker at Discharge[1]	18	100%	95%	90%	100%
Fibrinolytic Medication Timing	0	-	40%	31%	100%
PCI Within 90 Minutes of Arrival	0	-	77%	54%	95%
Smoking Cessation Advice[1]	1	100%	68%	88%	100%
Heart Failure Care					
ACE Inhibitor or ARB for LVSD	26	100%	85%	82%	100%
Discharge Instructions	58	86%	54%	61%	93%
Evaluation of LVS Function	96	94%	77%	83%	99%
Smoking Cessation Advice[1]	4	100%	67%	82%	100%
Pneumonia Care					
Appropriate Initial Antibiotic	71	96%	80%	83%	94%
Blood Culture Timing	82	100%	94%	90%	100%
Influenza Vaccine	27	96%	76%	70%	100%
Initial Antibiotic Timing	118	92%	85%	80%	93%
Oxygenation Assessment	150	100%	99%	99%	100%
Pneumococcal Vaccine	120	99%	73%	69%	94%
Smoking Cessation Advice[1]	14	100%	70%	80%	100%
Surgical Infection Prevention					
Prophylactic Antibiotic Given[3]	125	90%	78%	77%	95%
Prophylactic Antibiotic Selection	31	97%	94%	90%	100%
Prophylactic Antibiotic Stopped[3]	122	80%	82%	72%	95%
Pregnancy Care					
Inpatient Neonatal Mortality	-	-	-	-	-
Third or Fourth Degree Laceration	-	-	4.42%	3.63%	3.27%

District One Hospital

200 State Street
Faribault, MN 55021
Phone: 507-334-6451
Fax: 507-332-4848
E-mail: doh@districtonehospital.com
URL: www.districtonehospital.com
Ownership: Govt - Hospital District or Authority
Accredited: Yes
Emergency Services: Yes
Licensed Beds: 99

Key Personnel:

CEO. . . . . James Wolf
Manager Emergency . . . . Cheryl Arnold
Manager Nurse Surgical Services . . . . Kris Bauer
Manager Emergency Services. . . . . Cheryl Arnold
Nurse Manager Ed/Infection Control . . . . Rae Ormsby
Nurse Manager Surgical Services . . . . Kris Bauer
Manager Respiratory Care. . . . . James Rothmann

Measure	Cases	This Hospital	State Average	U.S. Average	Top Hospital
Heart Attack Care					
ACE Inhibitor or ARB for LVSD[1]	1	100%	89%	82%	100%
Aspirin at Arrival[1]	7	71%	92%	92%	100%
Aspirin at Discharge[1]	3	67%	93%	90%	100%
Beta Blocker at Arrival[1]	7	43%	88%	87%	100%

NOTE: Hospital profiles are in alphabetical order by state, then city, then hospital within the city; Rankings are sorted by rate in descending order and exclude hospitals with less than 25 cases; (1) The number of cases is too small (n<25) for purposes of reliably predicting hospital performance; (2) Measure reflects the hospital's indication that its submission was based upon a sample of its relevant discharges; (3) Rate reflects fewer than the maximum possible quarters of data for the measure; (4) Inaccurate information submitted and suppressed for one or more quarters; (5) No data is available from the hospital for this measure; Please refer to the User's Guide for a full explanation of data

Measure	Cases	This Hospital	State Average	U.S. Average	Top Hospital
Beta Blocker at Discharge[1]	3	67%	95%	90%	100%
Fibrinolytic Medication Timing	0	-	40%	31%	100%
PCI Within 90 Minutes of Arrival	0	-	77%	54%	95%
Smoking Cessation Advice[1]	1	0%	68%	88%	100%
Heart Failure Care					
ACE Inhibitor or ARB for LVSD[1]	12	83%	85%	82%	100%
Discharge Instructions	36	36%	54%	61%	93%
Evaluation of LVS Function	52	60%	77%	83%	99%
Smoking Cessation Advice[1]	1	0%	67%	82%	100%
Pneumonia Care					
Appropriate Initial Antibiotic	50	80%	80%	83%	94%
Blood Culture Timing	42	90%	94%	90%	100%
Influenza Vaccine[1]	12	25%	76%	70%	100%
Initial Antibiotic Timing	68	90%	85%	80%	93%
Oxygenation Assessment	74	100%	99%	99%	100%
Pneumococcal Vaccine	51	55%	73%	69%	94%
Smoking Cessation Advice[1]	12	50%	70%	80%	100%
Surgical Infection Prevention					
Prophylactic Antibiotic Given[3]	75	81%	78%	77%	95%
Prophylactic Antibiotic Selection	29	100%	94%	90%	100%
Prophylactic Antibiotic Stopped[3]	71	90%	82%	72%	95%
Pregnancy Care					
Inpatient Neonatal Mortality	-	-	-	-	-
Third or Fourth Degree Laceration	-	-	4.42%	3.63%	3.27%

Lake Region Healthcare Corporation

712 Cascade Street South — Phone: 218-736-8000
Fergus Falls, MN 56537 — Fax: 218-736-8765
URL: www.lrhc.org
Ownership: Voluntary non-profit - Private — Accredited: Yes
Emergency Services: Yes — Licensed Beds: 108

Key Personnel:

President/CEO. . . . . Ed Mehl
Chief Medical Staff. . . . . D Traiser, MD
Manager Emergency Room . . . . Else Malbraaten
Infection Control. . . . . JoAnn Bowman, RN
Intensive Coronary. . . . . Rick Dean
Surgical Nursing Manager . . . . Kathy Mattson
Manager Respiratory . . . . Molly Leinen

Measure	Cases	This Hospital	State Average	U.S. Average	Top Hospital
Heart Attack Care					
ACE Inhibitor or ARB for LVSD[1]	5	100%	89%	82%	100%
Aspirin at Arrival	27	96%	92%	92%	100%
Aspirin at Discharge[1]	15	93%	93%	90%	100%
Beta Blocker at Arrival	28	93%	88%	87%	100%
Beta Blocker at Discharge[1]	14	93%	95%	90%	100%
Fibrinolytic Medication Timing[1]	12	83%	40%	31%	100%
PCI Within 90 Minutes of Arrival	0	-	77%	54%	95%
Smoking Cessation Advice[1]	2	100%	68%	88%	100%
Heart Failure Care					
ACE Inhibitor or ARB for LVSD	34	88%	85%	82%	100%
Discharge Instructions	71	66%	54%	61%	93%
Evaluation of LVS Function	120	86%	77%	83%	99%
Smoking Cessation Advice[1]	5	0%	67%	82%	100%
Pneumonia Care					
Appropriate Initial Antibiotic	48	83%	80%	83%	94%
Blood Culture Timing	51	92%	94%	90%	100%
Influenza Vaccine[1]	10	80%	76%	70%	100%
Initial Antibiotic Timing	82	96%	85%	80%	93%
Oxygenation Assessment	102	100%	99%	99%	100%
Pneumococcal Vaccine	76	76%	73%	69%	94%
Smoking Cessation Advice[1]	12	58%	70%	80%	100%
Surgical Infection Prevention					
Prophylactic Antibiotic Given[3]	179	84%	78%	77%	95%
Prophylactic Antibiotic Selection	83	95%	94%	90%	100%
Prophylactic Antibiotic Stopped[3]	174	79%	82%	72%	95%
Pregnancy Care					
Inpatient Neonatal Mortality	-	-	-	-	-
Third or Fourth Degree Laceration	-	-	4.42%	3.63%	3.27%

First Care Medical Services

900 Hilligoss Boulevard Se — Phone: 218-435-1133
Fosston, MN 56542
Ownership: Voluntary non-profit - Private — Accredited: No
Emergency Services: Yes

Key Personnel:

CEO. . . . . Patricia Wangler

Measure	Cases	This Hospital	State Average	U.S. Average	Top Hospital
Heart Attack Care					
ACE Inhibitor or ARB for LVSD[1]	4	100%	89%	82%	100%
Aspirin at Arrival[1]	13	100%	92%	92%	100%
Aspirin at Discharge[1]	7	100%	93%	90%	100%
Beta Blocker at Arrival[1]	12	92%	88%	87%	100%
Beta Blocker at Discharge[1]	7	100%	95%	90%	100%
Fibrinolytic Medication Timing	0	-	40%	31%	100%
PCI Within 90 Minutes of Arrival	0	-	77%	54%	95%
Smoking Cessation Advice[1]	1	0%	68%	88%	100%
Heart Failure Care					
ACE Inhibitor or ARB for LVSD[1]	7	100%	85%	82%	100%
Discharge Instructions[1]	12	100%	54%	61%	93%
Evaluation of LVS Function	28	89%	77%	83%	99%
Smoking Cessation Advice[1]	6	83%	67%	82%	100%
Pneumonia Care					
Appropriate Initial Antibiotic[1]	12	75%	80%	83%	94%
Blood Culture Timing[1]	2	100%	94%	90%	100%
Influenza Vaccine[1]	4	100%	76%	70%	100%
Initial Antibiotic Timing[1]	14	93%	85%	80%	93%
Oxygenation Assessment[1]	23	100%	99%	99%	100%
Pneumococcal Vaccine[1]	16	94%	73%	69%	94%
Smoking Cessation Advice[1]	3	100%	70%	80%	100%
Surgical Infection Prevention					
Prophylactic Antibiotic Given[1,3]	13	100%	78%	77%	95%
Prophylactic Antibiotic Selection[1]	2	100%	94%	90%	100%
Prophylactic Antibiotic Stopped[1,3]	13	85%	82%	72%	95%
Pregnancy Care					
Inpatient Neonatal Mortality	-	-	-	-	-
Third or Fourth Degree Laceration	-	-	4.42%	3.63%	3.27%

Unity Hospital

550 Osborne Road — Phone: 763-236-5000
Fridley, MN 55432 — Fax: 763-236-3516
URL: www.allina.com
Ownership: Voluntary non-profit - Other — Accredited: Yes
Emergency Services: Yes — Licensed Beds: 275

Key Personnel:

President . . . . Venetia H M Kudrle

Measure	Cases	This Hospital	State Average	U.S. Average	Top Hospital
Heart Attack Care					
ACE Inhibitor or ARB for LVSD[1]	7	86%	89%	82%	100%
Aspirin at Arrival	62	95%	92%	92%	100%
Aspirin at Discharge	39	92%	93%	90%	100%
Beta Blocker at Arrival	45	89%	88%	87%	100%
Beta Blocker at Discharge	43	95%	95%	90%	100%
Fibrinolytic Medication Timing	0	-	40%	31%	100%
PCI Within 90 Minutes of Arrival	0	-	77%	54%	95%
Smoking Cessation Advice[1]	9	89%	68%	88%	100%
Heart Failure Care					
ACE Inhibitor or ARB for LVSD	76	83%	85%	82%	100%
Discharge Instructions	207	88%	54%	61%	93%
Evaluation of LVS Function	272	98%	77%	83%	99%
Smoking Cessation Advice	38	92%	67%	82%	100%
Pneumonia Care					
Appropriate Initial Antibiotic	176	82%	80%	83%	94%
Blood Culture Timing	140	88%	94%	90%	100%
Influenza Vaccine	47	85%	76%	70%	100%
Initial Antibiotic Timing	239	75%	85%	80%	93%
Oxygenation Assessment	280	100%	99%	99%	100%
Pneumococcal Vaccine	191	73%	73%	69%	94%
Smoking Cessation Advice	52	71%	70%	80%	100%
Surgical Infection Prevention					

NOTE: Hospital profiles are in alphabetical order by state, then city, then hospital within the city; Rankings are sorted by rate in descending order and exclude hospitals with less than 25 cases; (1) The number of cases is too small (n<25) for purposes of reliably predicting hospital performance; (2) Measure reflects the hospital's indication that its submission was based upon a sample of its relevant discharges; (3) Rate reflects fewer than the maximum possible quarters of data for the measure; (4) Inaccurate information submitted and suppressed for one or more quarters; (5) No data is available from the hospital for this measure; Please refer to the User's Guide for a full explanation of data

Measure	Cases	This Hospital	State Average	U.S. Average	Top Hospital
Prophylactic Antibiotic Given[2,3]	94	82%	78%	77%	95%
Prophylactic Antibiotic Selection[2]	49	84%	94%	90%	100%
Prophylactic Antibiotic Stopped[2,3]	94	70%	82%	72%	95%
Pregnancy Care					
Inpatient Neonatal Mortality	-	-	-	-	-
Third or Fourth Degree Laceration	-	-	4.42%	3.63%	3.27%

Glencoe Regional Health Services

1805 Hennepin Avenue N
Glencoe, MN 55336
Phone: 320-864-3121
Fax: 320-864-7887
URL: www.grhsonline.org
Ownership: Voluntary non-profit - Private
Accredited: No
Emergency Services: Yes
Licensed Beds: 25

Key Personnel:

President/CEO . . . . John D Braband
Chief Medical Staff . . . . Dennis Jacobson, MD
Emergency Room . . . . Phyllis Brinkman, RN
Infection Control . . . . Rhonda Buerkle
CCU Spvg. Nurse . . . . Barb Magnuson, RN
Medical Surgical Nursing . . . . Karen Ruckentin, RN
Director Radiology . . . . Brian Thieman
Director Respiratory Therapy . . . . Dan Werth

Measure	Cases	This Hospital	State Average	U.S. Average	Top Hospital
Heart Attack Care					
ACE Inhibitor or ARB for LVSD[3]	0	-	89%	82%	100%
Aspirin at Arrival[1,3]	4	75%	92%	92%	100%
Aspirin at Discharge[1,3]	3	67%	93%	90%	100%
Beta Blocker at Arrival[1,3]	4	75%	88%	87%	100%
Beta Blocker at Discharge[1,3]	3	100%	95%	90%	100%
Fibrinolytic Medication Timing[1,3]	1	0%	40%	31%	100%
PCI Within 90 Minutes of Arrival	0	-	77%	54%	95%
Smoking Cessation Advice[1,3]	1	0%	68%	88%	100%
Heart Failure Care					
ACE Inhibitor or ARB for LVSD[1]	24	79%	85%	82%	100%
Discharge Instructions	36	31%	54%	61%	93%
Evaluation of LVS Function	72	74%	77%	83%	99%
Smoking Cessation Advice[1]	1	0%	67%	82%	100%
Pneumonia Care					
Appropriate Initial Antibiotic	38	87%	80%	83%	94%
Blood Culture Timing[1]	14	100%	94%	90%	100%
Influenza Vaccine[1]	5	40%	76%	70%	100%
Initial Antibiotic Timing[1]	23	83%	85%	80%	93%
Oxygenation Assessment	60	100%	99%	99%	100%
Pneumococcal Vaccine	36	69%	73%	69%	94%
Smoking Cessation Advice[1]	5	20%	70%	80%	100%
Surgical Infection Prevention					
Prophylactic Antibiotic Given[3]	40	65%	78%	77%	95%
Prophylactic Antibiotic Selection[1]	15	100%	94%	90%	100%
Prophylactic Antibiotic Stopped[3]	39	79%	82%	72%	95%
Pregnancy Care					
Inpatient Neonatal Mortality	-	-	-	-	-
Third or Fourth Degree Laceration	-	-	4.42%	3.63%	3.27%

Glacial Ridge Hospital

10 4th Avenue SE
Glenwood, MN 56334
Toll-Free: 866-667-4747
Phone: 320-634-4521
Fax: 320-634-2253
URL: www.glacialridge.org
Ownership: Govt - Hospital District or Authority
Accredited: No
Emergency Services: Yes
Licensed Beds: 19

Key Personnel:

CEO . . . . Kirk Stensrud
Chief Medical Staff . . . . D Eric Westberg, MD
Chief Radiology . . . . Jean Mattson

Measure	Cases	This Hospital	State Average	U.S. Average	Top Hospital
Heart Attack Care					
ACE Inhibitor or ARB for LVSD[5]	-	-	89%	82%	100%
Aspirin at Arrival[5]	-	-	92%	92%	100%
Aspirin at Discharge[5]	-	-	93%	90%	100%
Beta Blocker at Arrival[5]	-	-	88%	87%	100%
Beta Blocker at Discharge[5]	-	-	95%	90%	100%
Fibrinolytic Medication Timing[5]	-	-	40%	31%	100%
PCI Within 90 Minutes of Arrival[5]	-	-	77%	54%	95%
Smoking Cessation Advice[5]	-	-	68%	88%	100%
Heart Failure Care					
ACE Inhibitor or ARB for LVSD[5]	-	-	85%	82%	100%
Discharge Instructions[5]	-	-	54%	61%	93%
Evaluation of LVS Function[5]	-	-	77%	83%	99%
Smoking Cessation Advice[5]	-	-	67%	82%	100%
Pneumonia Care					
Appropriate Initial Antibiotic[5]	-	-	80%	83%	94%
Blood Culture Timing[5]	-	-	94%	90%	100%
Influenza Vaccine[5]	-	-	76%	70%	100%
Initial Antibiotic Timing[5]	-	-	85%	80%	93%
Oxygenation Assessment[5]	-	-	99%	99%	100%
Pneumococcal Vaccine[5]	-	-	73%	69%	94%
Smoking Cessation Advice[5]	-	-	70%	80%	100%
Surgical Infection Prevention					
Prophylactic Antibiotic Given[5]	-	-	78%	77%	95%
Prophylactic Antibiotic Selection[5]	-	-	94%	90%	100%
Prophylactic Antibiotic Stopped[5]	-	-	82%	72%	95%
Pregnancy Care					
Inpatient Neonatal Mortality	-	-	-	-	-
Third or Fourth Degree Laceration	-	-	4.42%	3.63%	3.27%

Grand Itasca Clinic and Hospital

1601 Golf Course Road
Grand Rapids, MN 55744
Phone: 218-326-3401
Fax: 218-999-1514
E-mail: info@granditasca.org
URL: www.granditasca.org
Ownership: Voluntary non-profit - Private
Accredited: Yes
Emergency Services: Yes

Key Personnel:

President/CEO . . . . Dan McCormick
Chief Medical Officer . . . . Jack Carlisle, MD
Chief Emergency Medicine . . . . Tom Lorenz, MD
Chief Surgery . . . . John Kole, MD
Chief Radiology . . . . Bill Johnson, MD

Measure	Cases	This Hospital	State Average	U.S. Average	Top Hospital
Heart Attack Care					
ACE Inhibitor or ARB for LVSD[1]	7	100%	89%	82%	100%
Aspirin at Arrival	40	95%	92%	92%	100%
Aspirin at Discharge	25	84%	93%	90%	100%
Beta Blocker at Arrival	40	95%	88%	87%	100%
Beta Blocker at Discharge	29	97%	95%	90%	100%
Fibrinolytic Medication Timing[3]	0	-	40%	31%	100%
PCI Within 90 Minutes of Arrival	0	-	77%	54%	95%
Smoking Cessation Advice[3]	0	-	68%	88%	100%
Heart Failure Care					
ACE Inhibitor or ARB for LVSD[1]	17	94%	85%	82%	100%
Discharge Instructions[1,3]	11	27%	54%	61%	93%
Evaluation of LVS Function	50	84%	77%	83%	99%
Smoking Cessation Advice[3]	0	-	67%	82%	100%
Pneumonia Care					
Appropriate Initial Antibiotic[1,3]	15	87%	80%	83%	94%
Blood Culture Timing[1,3]	9	89%	94%	90%	100%
Influenza Vaccine[5]	-	-	76%	70%	100%
Initial Antibiotic Timing	107	80%	85%	80%	93%
Oxygenation Assessment	123	100%	99%	99%	100%
Pneumococcal Vaccine	99	83%	73%	69%	94%
Smoking Cessation Advice[1,3]	4	100%	70%	80%	100%
Surgical Infection Prevention					
Prophylactic Antibiotic Given[2,3]	49	78%	78%	77%	95%
Prophylactic Antibiotic Selection[5]	-	-	94%	90%	100%
Prophylactic Antibiotic Stopped[2,3]	48	90%	82%	72%	95%
Pregnancy Care					
Inpatient Neonatal Mortality	-	-	-	-	-
Third or Fourth Degree Laceration	-	-	4.42%	3.63%	3.27%

NOTE: Hospital profiles are in alphabetical order by state, then city, then hospital within the city; Rankings are sorted by rate in descending order and exclude hospitals with less than 25 cases; (1) The number of cases is too small (n<25) for purposes of reliably predicting hospital performance; (2) Measure reflects the hospital's indication that its submission was based upon a sample of its relevant discharges; (3) Rate reflects fewer than the maximum possible quarters of data for the measure; (4) Inaccurate information submitted and suppressed for one or more quarters; (5) No data is available from the hospital for this measure; Please refer to the User's Guide for a full explanation of data

Municipal Hospital and Granite Manor

345 Tenth Avenue
Granite Falls, MN 56241
Phone: 320-564-3111
Ownership: Government - Local
Accredited: No
Emergency Services: Yes

Measure	Cases	This Hospital	State Average	U.S. Average	Top Hospital
Heart Attack Care					
ACE Inhibitor or ARB for LVSD[1]	1	0%	89%	82%	100%
Aspirin at Arrival[1]	8	88%	92%	92%	100%
Aspirin at Discharge[1]	6	83%	93%	90%	100%
Beta Blocker at Arrival[1]	4	75%	88%	87%	100%
Beta Blocker at Discharge[1]	8	88%	95%	90%	100%
Fibrinolytic Medication Timing	0	-	40%	31%	100%
PCI Within 90 Minutes of Arrival	0	-	77%	54%	95%
Smoking Cessation Advice[1]	2	0%	68%	88%	100%
Heart Failure Care					
ACE Inhibitor or ARB for LVSD[1]	6	83%	85%	82%	100%
Discharge Instructions[1]	9	56%	54%	61%	93%
Evaluation of LVS Function[1]	13	85%	77%	83%	99%
Smoking Cessation Advice[1]	2	50%	67%	82%	100%
Pneumonia Care					
Appropriate Initial Antibiotic[1]	21	57%	80%	83%	94%
Blood Culture Timing[1]	3	100%	94%	90%	100%
Influenza Vaccine[1]	4	75%	76%	70%	100%
Initial Antibiotic Timing	31	87%	85%	80%	93%
Oxygenation Assessment	38	100%	99%	99%	100%
Pneumococcal Vaccine[1]	20	75%	73%	69%	94%
Smoking Cessation Advice[1]	7	0%	70%	80%	100%
Surgical Infection Prevention					
Prophylactic Antibiotic Given[1,3]	3	33%	78%	77%	95%
Prophylactic Antibiotic Selection	0	-	94%	90%	100%
Prophylactic Antibiotic Stopped[1,3]	2	100%	82%	72%	95%
Pregnancy Care					
Inpatient Neonatal Mortality	-	-	-	-	-
Third or Fourth Degree Laceration	-	-	4.42%	3.63%	3.27%

Kittson Memorial Health Care Center

Alternate Name: Kittson Memorial Hospital
1010 S Birch
Hallock, MN 56728
Toll-Free: 800-843-6016
Phone: 218-843-3612
Fax: 218-843-2311
Ownership: Voluntary non-profit - Private
Accredited: No
Emergency Services: Yes
Licensed Beds: 15

Key Personnel:

Administrator . . . . Rick Failing
Chief Medical Staff. . . . . Roland Larter, MD
Emergency Room . . . . Ginger Ledoux

Measure	Cases	This Hospital	State Average	U.S. Average	Top Hospital
Heart Attack Care					
ACE Inhibitor or ARB for LVSD[5]	-	-	89%	82%	100%
Aspirin at Arrival[5]	-	-	92%	92%	100%
Aspirin at Discharge[5]	-	-	93%	90%	100%
Beta Blocker at Arrival[5]	-	-	88%	87%	100%
Beta Blocker at Discharge[5]	-	-	95%	90%	100%
Fibrinolytic Medication Timing[5]	-	-	40%	31%	100%
PCI Within 90 Minutes of Arrival[5]	-	-	77%	54%	95%
Smoking Cessation Advice[5]	-	-	68%	88%	100%
Heart Failure Care					
ACE Inhibitor or ARB for LVSD[5]	-	-	85%	82%	100%
Discharge Instructions[5]	-	-	54%	61%	93%
Evaluation of LVS Function[5]	-	-	77%	83%	99%
Smoking Cessation Advice[5]	-	-	67%	82%	100%
Pneumonia Care					
Appropriate Initial Antibiotic[1,2]	16	25%	80%	83%	94%
Blood Culture Timing[1,2]	2	100%	94%	90%	100%
Influenza Vaccine[1]	3	100%	76%	70%	100%
Initial Antibiotic Timing[1,2]	5	100%	85%	80%	93%
Oxygenation Assessment[1,2]	19	100%	99%	99%	100%
Pneumococcal Vaccine[1,2]	18	33%	73%	69%	94%
Smoking Cessation Advice[2]	0	-	70%	80%	100%
Surgical Infection Prevention					
Prophylactic Antibiotic Given[5]	-	-	78%	77%	95%
Prophylactic Antibiotic Selection[5]	-	-	94%	90%	100%
Prophylactic Antibiotic Stopped[5]	-	-	82%	72%	95%
Pregnancy Care					
Inpatient Neonatal Mortality	-	-	-	-	-
Third or Fourth Degree Laceration	-	-	4.42%	3.63%	3.27%

Regina Medical Center

1175 Nininger Road
Hastings, MN 55033
Phone: 651-480-4100
Fax: 651-480-4212
URL: www.reginamedical.org
Ownership: Voluntary non-profit - Church
Accredited: Yes
Emergency Services: Yes
Licensed Beds: 57

Key Personnel:

President/CEO. . . . . Mark Wilson
Chief of Medical Staff. . . . . Lon Peterson
Emergency Room . . . . Mary Tobias
Infection Control. . . . . Pam Fox
ICU . . . . Mary Jo Huppert
Medical Surgical Nursing . . . . Mary Jo Huppert
Surgery Center Manager . . . . Barb Kendall
Respiratory/Cardiopulmonary. . . . . Michael Schweitzer, CRT

Measure	Cases	This Hospital	State Average	U.S. Average	Top Hospital
Heart Attack Care					
ACE Inhibitor or ARB for LVSD[1]	2	100%	89%	82%	100%
Aspirin at Arrival[1]	6	83%	92%	92%	100%
Aspirin at Discharge[1]	5	60%	93%	90%	100%
Beta Blocker at Arrival[1]	9	89%	88%	87%	100%
Beta Blocker at Discharge[1]	8	100%	95%	90%	100%
Fibrinolytic Medication Timing	0	-	40%	31%	100%
PCI Within 90 Minutes of Arrival	0	-	77%	54%	95%
Smoking Cessation Advice[1]	3	33%	68%	88%	100%
Heart Failure Care					
ACE Inhibitor or ARB for LVSD[1]	21	95%	85%	82%	100%
Discharge Instructions	46	46%	54%	61%	93%
Evaluation of LVS Function	69	86%	77%	83%	99%
Smoking Cessation Advice[1]	7	71%	67%	82%	100%
Pneumonia Care					
Appropriate Initial Antibiotic	36	86%	80%	83%	94%
Blood Culture Timing	41	88%	94%	90%	100%
Influenza Vaccine[1]	7	71%	76%	70%	100%
Initial Antibiotic Timing	51	94%	85%	80%	93%
Oxygenation Assessment	65	100%	99%	99%	100%
Pneumococcal Vaccine	46	35%	73%	69%	94%
Smoking Cessation Advice[1]	9	44%	70%	80%	100%
Surgical Infection Prevention					
Prophylactic Antibiotic Given[2]	151	93%	78%	77%	95%
Prophylactic Antibiotic Selection[2]	40	100%	94%	90%	100%
Prophylactic Antibiotic Stopped[2]	150	89%	82%	72%	95%
Pregnancy Care					
Inpatient Neonatal Mortality	-	-	-	-	-
Third or Fourth Degree Laceration	-	-	4.42%	3.63%	3.27%

University Medical Center-Mesabi

Alternate Name: Mesabi Regional Medical Center
750 E 34th Street
Hibbing, MN 55746
Phone: 218-262-4881
Fax: 218-362-6619
Ownership: Voluntary non-profit - Other
Accredited: Yes
Emergency Services: Yes
Licensed Beds: 175

Key Personnel:

President/CEO. . . . . Larry Pfaff
Chief Medical Staff. . . . . Ann Steciw, MD
Emergency Room . . . . Paul Kindamo, MD
Director Infection/Disease Control . . . . Char Pulling
CCU Spvg. Nurse . . . . Linda Olson
Director Medical/Surgical Nursing . . . . Linda Olson
OB/GYN Womens Health. . . . . Bruce Neiger, MD
Chief Radiology . . . . Daniel Vechell, MD
Director Respiratory Therapy . . . . Carmen Bodle

Measure	Cases	This Hospital	State Average	U.S. Average	Top Hospital

NOTE: Hospital profiles are in alphabetical order by state, then city, then hospital within the city; Rankings are sorted by rate in descending order and exclude hospitals with less than 25 cases; (1) The number of cases is too small (n<25) for purposes of reliably predicting hospital performance; (2) Measure reflects the hospital's indication that its submission was based upon a sample of its relevant discharges; (3) Rate reflects fewer than the maximum possible quarters of data for the measure; (4) Inaccurate information submitted and suppressed for one or more quarters; (5) No data is available from the hospital for this measure; Please refer to the User's Guide for a full explanation of data

Heart Attack Care					
ACE Inhibitor or ARB for LVSD[1]	4	100%	89%	82%	100%
Aspirin at Arrival	28	93%	92%	92%	100%
Aspirin at Discharge[1]	13	100%	93%	90%	100%
Beta Blocker at Arrival	30	93%	88%	87%	100%
Beta Blocker at Discharge[1]	18	100%	95%	90%	100%
Fibrinolytic Medication Timing[1]	7	43%	40%	31%	100%
PCI Within 90 Minutes of Arrival	0	-	77%	54%	95%
Smoking Cessation Advice[1]	6	100%	68%	88%	100%
Heart Failure Care					
ACE Inhibitor or ARB for LVSD	60	92%	85%	82%	100%
Discharge Instructions	115	94%	54%	61%	93%
Evaluation of LVS Function	160	92%	77%	83%	99%
Smoking Cessation Advice	25	84%	67%	82%	100%
Pneumonia Care					
Appropriate Initial Antibiotic	102	80%	80%	83%	94%
Blood Culture Timing	83	94%	94%	90%	100%
Influenza Vaccine	33	76%	76%	70%	100%
Initial Antibiotic Timing	167	81%	85%	80%	93%
Oxygenation Assessment	191	100%	99%	99%	100%
Pneumococcal Vaccine	115	72%	73%	69%	94%
Smoking Cessation Advice	37	70%	70%	80%	100%
Surgical Infection Prevention					
Prophylactic Antibiotic Given	117	73%	78%	77%	95%
Prophylactic Antibiotic Selection[1]	17	82%	94%	90%	100%
Prophylactic Antibiotic Stopped	111	64%	82%	72%	95%
Pregnancy Care					
Inpatient Neonatal Mortality	383	0.52%	-	-	-
Third or Fourth Degree Laceration	234	2.14%	4.42%	3.63%	3.27%

Hutchinson Area Health Care

1095 Highway 15 S
Hutchinson, MN 55350

Toll-Free: 800-454-3903
Phone: 320-234-5000
Fax: 320-587-3340

URL: www.hahc-hmc.com
Ownership: Government - Local
Emergency Services: Yes

Accredited: Yes
Licensed Beds: 66

Key Personnel:
Administrator . . . . Phillip Graves
Emergency Room . . . . George Gordon
Director Infection/Disease Control . . . . Linette Wendlandt

Measure	Cases	This Hospital	State Average	U.S. Average	Top Hospital
Heart Attack Care					
ACE Inhibitor or ARB for LVSD	0	-	89%	82%	100%
Aspirin at Arrival[1]	6	100%	92%	92%	100%
Aspirin at Discharge[1]	5	100%	93%	90%	100%
Beta Blocker at Arrival[1]	6	100%	88%	87%	100%
Beta Blocker at Discharge[1]	4	100%	95%	90%	100%
Fibrinolytic Medication Timing	0	-	40%	31%	100%
PCI Within 90 Minutes of Arrival	0	-	77%	54%	95%
Smoking Cessation Advice	0	-	68%	88%	100%
Heart Failure Care					
ACE Inhibitor or ARB for LVSD[1]	19	79%	85%	82%	100%
Discharge Instructions	43	60%	54%	61%	93%
Evaluation of LVS Function	60	92%	77%	83%	99%
Smoking Cessation Advice[1]	8	100%	67%	82%	100%
Pneumonia Care					
Appropriate Initial Antibiotic	34	76%	80%	83%	94%
Blood Culture Timing	37	95%	94%	90%	100%
Influenza Vaccine[1]	11	73%	76%	70%	100%
Initial Antibiotic Timing	58	95%	85%	80%	93%
Oxygenation Assessment	68	100%	99%	99%	100%
Pneumococcal Vaccine	48	77%	73%	69%	94%
Smoking Cessation Advice[1]	9	100%	70%	80%	100%
Surgical Infection Prevention					
Prophylactic Antibiotic Given[3]	138	88%	78%	77%	95%
Prophylactic Antibiotic Selection	36	94%	94%	90%	100%
Prophylactic Antibiotic Stopped[3]	134	91%	82%	72%	95%
Pregnancy Care					
Inpatient Neonatal Mortality	-	-	-	-	-
Third or Fourth Degree Laceration	-	-	4.42%	3.63%	3.27%

Falls Memorial Hospital

Alternate Name: Int'l Falls Memorial Hospital
1400 Highway 71
Int'l Falls, MN 56649
URL: www.fmh-mn.com
Ownership: Voluntary non-profit - Private
Emergency Services: Yes

Phone: 218-283-4481
Fax: 218-283-2281

Accredited: Yes
Licensed Beds: 25

Key Personnel:
CEO. . . . . Ty Erickson
Chief Medical Staff. . . . . Morgan Althoen, MD
Director Emergency Services. . . . . Morgan Althoen, MD
Director Infection Control . . . . Douglas Johnson, MD
Director Intensive Coronary Care. . . . . Daniel Ramquist, MD
Director Radiology . . . . Daniel Courneya, MD

Measure	Cases	This Hospital	State Average	U.S. Average	Top Hospital
Heart Attack Care					
ACE Inhibitor or ARB for LVSD[3]	0	-	89%	82%	100%
Aspirin at Arrival[1,3]	8	88%	92%	92%	100%
Aspirin at Discharge[1,3]	3	100%	93%	90%	100%
Beta Blocker at Arrival[1,3]	8	88%	88%	87%	100%
Beta Blocker at Discharge[1,3]	3	100%	95%	90%	100%
Fibrinolytic Medication Timing[1,3]	4	25%	40%	31%	100%
PCI Within 90 Minutes of Arrival[5]	-	-	77%	54%	95%
Smoking Cessation Advice[3]	0	-	68%	88%	100%
Heart Failure Care					
ACE Inhibitor or ARB for LVSD	0	-	85%	82%	100%
Discharge Instructions	28	11%	54%	61%	93%
Evaluation of LVS Function	38	0%	77%	83%	99%
Smoking Cessation Advice[1]	2	100%	67%	82%	100%
Pneumonia Care					
Appropriate Initial Antibiotic	25	72%	80%	83%	94%
Blood Culture Timing[1]	19	100%	94%	90%	100%
Influenza Vaccine[1]	6	100%	76%	70%	100%
Initial Antibiotic Timing	35	66%	85%	80%	93%
Oxygenation Assessment	44	100%	99%	99%	100%
Pneumococcal Vaccine	33	64%	73%	69%	94%
Smoking Cessation Advice[1]	6	83%	70%	80%	100%
Surgical Infection Prevention					
Prophylactic Antibiotic Given[5]	-	-	78%	77%	95%
Prophylactic Antibiotic Selection[5]	-	-	94%	90%	100%
Prophylactic Antibiotic Stopped[5]	-	-	82%	72%	95%
Pregnancy Care					
Inpatient Neonatal Mortality	-	-	-	-	-
Third or Fourth Degree Laceration	-	-	4.42%	3.63%	3.27%

Lake City Medical Center Mayo Health System

500 West Grant Street
Lake City, MN 55041
Ownership: Voluntary non-profit - Private
Emergency Services: Yes

Phone: 651-345-1114

Accredited: Yes

Measure	Cases	This Hospital	State Average	U.S. Average	Top Hospital
Heart Attack Care					
ACE Inhibitor or ARB for LVSD[1,3]	2	100%	89%	82%	100%
Aspirin at Arrival[1,3]	8	75%	92%	92%	100%
Aspirin at Discharge[1,3]	7	100%	93%	90%	100%
Beta Blocker at Arrival[1,3]	8	88%	88%	87%	100%
Beta Blocker at Discharge[1,3]	6	100%	95%	90%	100%
Fibrinolytic Medication Timing[1,3]	3	33%	40%	31%	100%
PCI Within 90 Minutes of Arrival[5]	-	-	77%	54%	95%
Smoking Cessation Advice[1,3]	1	100%	68%	88%	100%
Heart Failure Care					
ACE Inhibitor or ARB for LVSD[1]	4	75%	85%	82%	100%
Discharge Instructions[1]	10	30%	54%	61%	93%
Evaluation of LVS Function[1]	9	67%	77%	83%	99%
Smoking Cessation Advice	0	-	67%	82%	100%
Pneumonia Care					
Appropriate Initial Antibiotic[1]	11	91%	80%	83%	94%
Blood Culture Timing	0	-	94%	90%	100%
Influenza Vaccine	0	-	76%	70%	100%
Initial Antibiotic Timing[1]	9	89%	85%	80%	93%

NOTE: Hospital profiles are in alphabetical order by state, then city, then hospital within the city; Rankings are sorted by rate in descending order and exclude hospitals with less than 25 cases; (1) The number of cases is too small (n<25) for purposes of reliably predicting hospital performance; (2) Measure reflects the hospital's indication that its submission was based upon a sample of its relevant discharges; (3) Rate reflects fewer than the maximum possible quarters of data for the measure; (4) Inaccurate information submitted and suppressed for one or more quarters; (5) No data is available from the hospital for this measure; Please refer to the User's Guide for a full explanation of data

Oxygenation Assessment[1]	15	100%	99%	99%	100%
Pneumococcal Vaccine[1]	10	70%	73%	69%	94%
Smoking Cessation Advice[1]	2	50%	70%	80%	100%
Surgical Infection Prevention					
Prophylactic Antibiotic Given[1,3]	22	73%	78%	77%	95%
Prophylactic Antibiotic Selection[1]	6	100%	94%	90%	100%
Prophylactic Antibiotic Stopped[1,3]	20	30%	82%	72%	95%
Pregnancy Care					
Inpatient Neonatal Mortality	-	-	-	-	-
Third or Fourth Degree Laceration	-	-	4.42%	3.63%	3.27%

Minnesota Valley Memorial Hospital

Alternate Name: Minnesota Valley Health Center
621 S 4th Street
Le Sueur, MN 56058
E-mail: mvhc@mnic.net
Phone: 507-665-3375
Fax: 507-665-2191
Ownership: Voluntary non-profit - Private
Emergency Services: Yes
Accredited: No
Licensed Beds: 109

Key Personnel:
Administrator . . . . Jerry Boerboom
Chief of Medical Staff. . . . . John N Taylor
Director of Cardiology Department . . . . John Bernhardson
Director of Emergency Room . . . . Pam William

Measure	Cases	This Hospital	State Average	U.S. Average	Top Hospital
Heart Attack Care					
ACE Inhibitor or ARB for LVSD[5]	-	-	89%	82%	100%
Aspirin at Arrival[5]	-	-	92%	92%	100%
Aspirin at Discharge[5]	-	-	93%	90%	100%
Beta Blocker at Arrival[5]	-	-	88%	87%	100%
Beta Blocker at Discharge[5]	-	-	95%	90%	100%
Fibrinolytic Medication Timing[5]	-	-	40%	31%	100%
PCI Within 90 Minutes of Arrival[5]	-	-	77%	54%	95%
Smoking Cessation Advice[5]	-	-	68%	88%	100%
Heart Failure Care					
ACE Inhibitor or ARB for LVSD[5]	-	-	85%	82%	100%
Discharge Instructions[5]	-	-	54%	61%	93%
Evaluation of LVS Function[5]	-	-	77%	83%	99%
Smoking Cessation Advice[5]	-	-	67%	82%	100%
Pneumonia Care					
Appropriate Initial Antibiotic[1]	7	86%	80%	83%	94%
Blood Culture Timing[1]	1	100%	94%	90%	100%
Influenza Vaccine[1]	3	100%	76%	70%	100%
Initial Antibiotic Timing[1]	10	100%	85%	80%	93%
Oxygenation Assessment[1]	12	100%	99%	99%	100%
Pneumococcal Vaccine[1]	12	75%	73%	69%	94%
Smoking Cessation Advice	0	-	70%	80%	100%
Surgical Infection Prevention					
Prophylactic Antibiotic Given[5]	-	-	78%	77%	95%
Prophylactic Antibiotic Selection[5]	-	-	94%	90%	100%
Prophylactic Antibiotic Stopped[5]	-	-	82%	72%	95%
Pregnancy Care					
Inpatient Neonatal Mortality	-	-	-	-	-
Third or Fourth Degree Laceration	-	-	4.42%	3.63%	3.27%

Meeker County Memorial Hospital

612 South Sibley Avenue
Litchfield, MN 55355
URL: www.mcmh-litchfield.org
Phone: 320-693-3242
Fax: 320-693-4567
Ownership: Government - Local
Emergency Services: No
Accredited: No
Licensed Beds: 38

Key Personnel:
President/CEO. . . . . Michael Schramm
Chief Medical Staff. . . . . Debra Peterson, MD
Emergency Room . . . . Sharon Then
Infection Control. . . . . Joyce Carlson, RN
ICU . . . . Angie Dietel
Medical/Surgical Nursing . . . . Angie Dietel, RN
OB/GYN/Women's Health . . . . Angie Dietel

Measure	Cases	This Hospital	State Average	U.S. Average	Top Hospital
Heart Attack Care					
ACE Inhibitor or ARB for LVSD[1]	2	100%	89%	82%	100%
Aspirin at Arrival[1]	9	100%	92%	92%	100%
Aspirin at Discharge[1]	7	100%	93%	90%	100%
Beta Blocker at Arrival[1]	10	90%	88%	87%	100%
Beta Blocker at Discharge[1]	7	86%	95%	90%	100%
Fibrinolytic Medication Timing	0	-	40%	31%	100%
PCI Within 90 Minutes of Arrival	0	-	77%	54%	95%
Smoking Cessation Advice	0	-	68%	88%	100%
Heart Failure Care					
ACE Inhibitor or ARB for LVSD[1]	7	57%	85%	82%	100%
Discharge Instructions[1]	16	6%	54%	61%	93%
Evaluation of LVS Function	31	65%	77%	83%	99%
Smoking Cessation Advice	0	-	67%	82%	100%
Pneumonia Care					
Appropriate Initial Antibiotic[1]	24	54%	80%	83%	94%
Blood Culture Timing[1]	6	100%	94%	90%	100%
Influenza Vaccine[1]	5	0%	76%	70%	100%
Initial Antibiotic Timing[1]	13	54%	85%	80%	93%
Oxygenation Assessment	35	94%	99%	99%	100%
Pneumococcal Vaccine[1]	24	8%	73%	69%	94%
Smoking Cessation Advice[1]	6	50%	70%	80%	100%
Surgical Infection Prevention					
Prophylactic Antibiotic Given	38	50%	78%	77%	95%
Prophylactic Antibiotic Selection[1]	5	80%	94%	90%	100%
Prophylactic Antibiotic Stopped	36	97%	82%	72%	95%
Pregnancy Care					
Inpatient Neonatal Mortality	-	-	-	-	-
Third or Fourth Degree Laceration	-	-	4.42%	3.63%	3.27%

Saint Gabriel's Hospital

815 Southeast 2nd Street
Little Falls, MN 56345
URL: www.stgabriels.com
Phone: 320-632-5441
Fax: 320-632-1190
Ownership: Voluntary non-profit - Private
Emergency Services: Yes
Accredited: No
Licensed Beds: 49

Key Personnel:
President/CEO. . . . . Carl Vaagenes
Surgical Services Manager . . . . Mary Bauer
Emergency Room Manager . . . . Jane Smalley
Infection Control Coordinator . . . . Susan Newkirk
Intensive/Coronary Care Manager . . . . Jane Smalley
Respiratory/Cardiopulmonary Supervisor. . . . . . Kim Borgstrom

Measure	Cases	This Hospital	State Average	U.S. Average	Top Hospital
Heart Attack Care					
ACE Inhibitor or ARB for LVSD[1]	1	100%	89%	82%	100%
Aspirin at Arrival[1]	6	83%	92%	92%	100%
Aspirin at Discharge[1]	4	100%	93%	90%	100%
Beta Blocker at Arrival[1]	4	100%	88%	87%	100%
Beta Blocker at Discharge[1]	7	100%	95%	90%	100%
Fibrinolytic Medication Timing	0	-	40%	31%	100%
PCI Within 90 Minutes of Arrival	0	-	77%	54%	95%
Smoking Cessation Advice[1]	2	50%	68%	88%	100%
Heart Failure Care					
ACE Inhibitor or ARB for LVSD[1]	5	80%	85%	82%	100%
Discharge Instructions[1]	14	14%	54%	61%	93%
Evaluation of LVS Function	26	73%	77%	83%	99%
Smoking Cessation Advice[1]	1	100%	67%	82%	100%
Pneumonia Care					
Appropriate Initial Antibiotic	43	77%	80%	83%	94%
Blood Culture Timing	30	100%	94%	90%	100%
Influenza Vaccine[1]	21	52%	76%	70%	100%
Initial Antibiotic Timing	72	83%	85%	80%	93%
Oxygenation Assessment	85	100%	99%	99%	100%
Pneumococcal Vaccine	67	60%	73%	69%	94%
Smoking Cessation Advice[1]	14	57%	70%	80%	100%
Surgical Infection Prevention					
Prophylactic Antibiotic Given[5]	-	-	78%	77%	95%
Prophylactic Antibiotic Selection[5]	-	-	94%	90%	100%
Prophylactic Antibiotic Stopped[5]	-	-	82%	72%	95%
Pregnancy Care					
Inpatient Neonatal Mortality	-	-	-	-	-
Third or Fourth Degree Laceration	-	-	4.42%	3.63%	3.27%

NOTE: Hospital profiles are in alphabetical order by state, then city, then hospital within the city; Rankings are sorted by rate in descending order and exclude hospitals with less than 25 cases; (1) The number of cases is too small (n<25) for purposes of reliably predicting hospital performance; (2) Measure reflects the hospital's indication that its submission was based upon a sample of its relevant discharges; (3) Rate reflects fewer than the maximum possible quarters of data for the measure; (4) Inaccurate information submitted and suppressed for one or more quarters; (5) No data is available from the hospital for this measure; Please refer to the User's Guide for a full explanation of data

Sioux Valley Luverne Hospital

1600 North Kniss Avenue
PO Box 1019
Luverne, MN 56156
Phone: 507-283-2321
Fax: 507-283-2091
E-mail: info@siouxvalleyluverne.org
URL: www.siouxvalleyluverne.org
Ownership: Voluntary non-profit - Private
Accredited: No
Emergency Services: Yes
Licensed Beds: 28

Key Personnel:

CEO. . . . . Mark A Henke
Emergency Department Manager . . . . Lynn DeBerg, RN
Surgery Manager. . . . . Mary O'Toole-Hemme, RN
Infection Control Officer . . . . Kristin Peterson
Medical/Surgical Patient Manager . . . . Sharon Fraser, RN
Respiratory Care Manager. . . . . Julia Silvrants

Measure	Cases	This Hospital	State Average	U.S. Average	Top Hospital
Heart Attack Care					
ACE Inhibitor or ARB for LVSD	0	-	89%	82%	100%
Aspirin at Arrival[1]	5	80%	92%	92%	100%
Aspirin at Discharge[1]	4	100%	93%	90%	100%
Beta Blocker at Arrival[1]	6	83%	88%	87%	100%
Beta Blocker at Discharge[1]	3	100%	95%	90%	100%
Fibrinolytic Medication Timing[1]	1	0%	40%	31%	100%
PCI Within 90 Minutes of Arrival	0	-	77%	54%	95%
Smoking Cessation Advice	0	-	68%	88%	100%
Heart Failure Care					
ACE Inhibitor or ARB for LVSD[1]	3	67%	85%	82%	100%
Discharge Instructions[1]	13	31%	54%	61%	93%
Evaluation of LVS Function[1]	21	33%	77%	83%	99%
Smoking Cessation Advice[1]	2	50%	67%	82%	100%
Pneumonia Care					
Appropriate Initial Antibiotic	27	81%	80%	83%	94%
Blood Culture Timing[1]	2	100%	94%	90%	100%
Influenza Vaccine[1]	8	75%	76%	70%	100%
Initial Antibiotic Timing	41	88%	85%	80%	93%
Oxygenation Assessment	49	100%	99%	99%	100%
Pneumococcal Vaccine	41	80%	73%	69%	94%
Smoking Cessation Advice[1]	3	33%	70%	80%	100%
Surgical Infection Prevention					
Prophylactic Antibiotic Given[1]	22	36%	78%	77%	95%
Prophylactic Antibiotic Selection[1]	3	100%	94%	90%	100%
Prophylactic Antibiotic Stopped[1]	22	91%	82%	72%	95%
Pregnancy Care					
Inpatient Neonatal Mortality	-	-	-	-	-
Third or Fourth Degree Laceration	-	-	4.42%	3.63%	3.27%

Madison Hospital

900 2nd Avenue
Madison, MN 56256
Phone: 320-598-7536
Fax: 320-598-3923
URL: www.madisonlutheranhome.com
Ownership: Voluntary non-profit - Church
Accredited: No
Emergency Services: Yes
Licensed Beds: 21

Key Personnel:

Chief of Medical Staff. . . . . D Gromg, MD
Director Infection/Disease Control . . . . Mary Woodrich
Director Radiology . . . . Jill Mortenson

Measure	Cases	This Hospital	State Average	U.S. Average	Top Hospital
Heart Attack Care					
ACE Inhibitor or ARB for LVSD[5]	-	-	89%	82%	100%
Aspirin at Arrival[5]	-	-	92%	92%	100%
Aspirin at Discharge[5]	-	-	93%	90%	100%
Beta Blocker at Arrival[5]	-	-	88%	87%	100%
Beta Blocker at Discharge[5]	-	-	95%	90%	100%
Fibrinolytic Medication Timing[5]	-	-	40%	31%	100%
PCI Within 90 Minutes of Arrival[5]	-	-	77%	54%	95%
Smoking Cessation Advice[5]	-	-	68%	88%	100%
Heart Failure Care					
ACE Inhibitor or ARB for LVSD[1]	5	100%	85%	82%	100%
Discharge Instructions[1]	11	9%	54%	61%	93%
Evaluation of LVS Function[1]	18	44%	77%	83%	99%
Smoking Cessation Advice[1]	1	0%	67%	82%	100%
Pneumonia Care					
Appropriate Initial Antibiotic[1]	15	60%	80%	83%	94%
Blood Culture Timing	0	-	94%	90%	100%
Influenza Vaccine[1]	7	57%	76%	70%	100%
Initial Antibiotic Timing	28	89%	85%	80%	93%
Oxygenation Assessment	30	100%	99%	99%	100%
Pneumococcal Vaccine[1]	24	50%	73%	69%	94%
Smoking Cessation Advice[1]	7	29%	70%	80%	100%
Surgical Infection Prevention					
Prophylactic Antibiotic Given[5]	-	-	78%	77%	95%
Prophylactic Antibiotic Selection[5]	-	-	94%	90%	100%
Prophylactic Antibiotic Stopped[5]	-	-	82%	72%	95%
Pregnancy Care					
Inpatient Neonatal Mortality	-	-	-	-	-
Third or Fourth Degree Laceration	-	-	4.42%	3.63%	3.27%

Immanuel Saint Joseph's-Mayo Health System

1025 Marsh Street
PO Box 8673
Mankato, MN 56002
Toll-Free: 800-327-3721
Phone: 507-625-4031
Fax: 507-385-2908
E-mail: isjinfo@mayo.edu
URL: www.isj-mhs.org
Ownership: Voluntary non-profit - Private
Accredited: Yes
Emergency Services: Yes
Licensed Beds: 272

Key Personnel:

CEO. . . . . William C Rupp, MD
Chief Medical Staff. . . . . Michael Wolf, MD
Director Radiology . . . . Anne Chapman
Director Respiratory Therapy . . . . Lisa Hamel

Measure	Cases	This Hospital	State Average	U.S. Average	Top Hospital
Heart Attack Care					
ACE Inhibitor or ARB for LVSD[1]	20	100%	89%	82%	100%
Aspirin at Arrival	105	100%	92%	92%	100%
Aspirin at Discharge	115	100%	93%	90%	100%
Beta Blocker at Arrival	98	99%	88%	87%	100%
Beta Blocker at Discharge	107	96%	95%	90%	100%
Fibrinolytic Medication Timing[1]	1	100%	40%	31%	100%
PCI Within 90 Minutes of Arrival[1]	6	67%	77%	54%	95%
Smoking Cessation Advice	30	100%	68%	88%	100%
Heart Failure Care					
ACE Inhibitor or ARB for LVSD	79	82%	85%	82%	100%
Discharge Instructions	138	85%	54%	61%	93%
Evaluation of LVS Function	181	90%	77%	83%	99%
Smoking Cessation Advice[1]	12	75%	67%	82%	100%
Pneumonia Care					
Appropriate Initial Antibiotic	75	80%	80%	83%	94%
Blood Culture Timing	66	80%	94%	90%	100%
Influenza Vaccine	26	69%	76%	70%	100%
Initial Antibiotic Timing	81	85%	85%	80%	93%
Oxygenation Assessment	133	95%	99%	99%	100%
Pneumococcal Vaccine	109	68%	73%	69%	94%
Smoking Cessation Advice[1]	17	94%	70%	80%	100%
Surgical Infection Prevention					
Prophylactic Antibiotic Given[3]	135	79%	78%	77%	95%
Prophylactic Antibiotic Selection	49	92%	94%	90%	100%
Prophylactic Antibiotic Stopped[3]	129	88%	82%	72%	95%
Pregnancy Care					
Inpatient Neonatal Mortality	-	-	-	-	-
Third or Fourth Degree Laceration	-	-	4.42%	3.63%	3.27%

Saint John's Hospital

1575 Beam Avenue
Maplewood, MN 55109
Phone: 651-232-7000
Fax: 651-232-7240
URL: www.stjohnshospital-mn.org
Ownership: Voluntary non-profit - Private
Accredited: Yes
Emergency Services: Yes
Licensed Beds: 184

Key Personnel:

CEO. . . . . Scott L North
Emergency Room . . . . Patrick Marabella, MD
Director Infection/Disease Control . . . . Kathy Miller, RN
Director Medical/Surgical Nursing . . . . Jan Kuklok, RN
OB/GYN Womens Health. . . . . Ron Mjanger, MD

NOTE: Hospital profiles are in alphabetical order by state, then city, then hospital within the city; Rankings are sorted by rate in descending order and exclude hospitals with less than 25 cases; (1) The number of cases is too small (n<25) for purposes of reliably predicting hospital performance; (2) Measure reflects the hospital's indication that its submission was based upon a sample of its relevant discharges; (3) Rate reflects fewer than the maximum possible quarters of data for the measure; (4) Inaccurate information submitted and suppressed for one or more quarters; (5) No data is available from the hospital for this measure; Please refer to the User's Guide for a full explanation of data

Chief Radiology . . . . Clifford Leach, MD
Director Respiratory Therapy . . . . Jerry Leis

Measure	Cases	This Hospital	State Average	U.S. Average	Top Hospital
Heart Attack Care					
ACE Inhibitor or ARB for LVSD[1]	15	80%	89%	82%	100%
Aspirin at Arrival	77	100%	92%	92%	100%
Aspirin at Discharge	41	93%	93%	90%	100%
Beta Blocker at Arrival	48	98%	88%	87%	100%
Beta Blocker at Discharge[1]	23	96%	95%	90%	100%
Fibrinolytic Medication Timing	0	-	40%	31%	100%
PCI Within 90 Minutes of Arrival	0	-	77%	54%	95%
Smoking Cessation Advice[1]	4	50%	68%	88%	100%
Heart Failure Care					
ACE Inhibitor or ARB for LVSD[2]	94	84%	85%	82%	100%
Discharge Instructions[2]	174	82%	54%	61%	93%
Evaluation of LVS Function[2]	248	96%	77%	83%	99%
Smoking Cessation Advice[2]	26	85%	67%	82%	100%
Pneumonia Care					
Appropriate Initial Antibiotic[2]	139	81%	80%	83%	94%
Blood Culture Timing[2]	89	90%	94%	90%	100%
Influenza Vaccine	29	93%	76%	70%	100%
Initial Antibiotic Timing[2]	179	91%	85%	80%	93%
Oxygenation Assessment[2]	221	100%	99%	99%	100%
Pneumococcal Vaccine[2]	140	90%	73%	69%	94%
Smoking Cessation Advice[2]	34	44%	70%	80%	100%
Surgical Infection Prevention					
Prophylactic Antibiotic Given[2,3]	739	77%	78%	77%	95%
Prophylactic Antibiotic Selection[2]	229	95%	94%	90%	100%
Prophylactic Antibiotic Stopped[2,3]	737	77%	82%	72%	95%
Pregnancy Care					
Inpatient Neonatal Mortality	3,000	0.07%	-	-	-
Third or Fourth Degree Laceration	2,343	3.24%	4.42%	3.63%	3.27%

Avera Marshall Regional Medical Center

300 S Bruce Street
Marshall, MN 56258
Phone: 507-532-9661
Fax: 507-537-9053
E-mail: info@averamarshall.org
URL: www.averamarshall.org
Ownership: Government - Local
Accredited: Yes
Emergency Services: Yes
Licensed Beds: 49

Key Personnel:

CEO. . . . . M Burmam
Chief Medical Staff. . . . . Joe Willett
Cardiac Rehabilitation Coordinator. . . . . Monica Senden
Emergency Room . . . . T Odland, MD
Director Surgical Services . . . . Donna Erbes
Director Respiratory Therapy . . . . Roger Holbeck

Measure	Cases	This Hospital	State Average	U.S. Average	Top Hospital
Heart Attack Care					
ACE Inhibitor or ARB for LVSD	0	-	89%	82%	100%
Aspirin at Arrival[1]	3	100%	92%	92%	100%
Aspirin at Discharge[1]	2	50%	93%	90%	100%
Beta Blocker at Arrival[1]	2	100%	88%	87%	100%
Beta Blocker at Discharge[1]	2	100%	95%	90%	100%
Fibrinolytic Medication Timing	0	-	40%	31%	100%
PCI Within 90 Minutes of Arrival	0	-	77%	54%	95%
Smoking Cessation Advice[1]	1	0%	68%	88%	100%
Heart Failure Care					
ACE Inhibitor or ARB for LVSD[1]	10	90%	85%	82%	100%
Discharge Instructions	30	63%	54%	61%	93%
Evaluation of LVS Function	42	79%	77%	83%	99%
Smoking Cessation Advice[1]	1	100%	67%	82%	100%
Pneumonia Care					
Appropriate Initial Antibiotic	44	73%	80%	83%	94%
Blood Culture Timing[1]	12	100%	94%	90%	100%
Influenza Vaccine[1]	5	100%	76%	70%	100%
Initial Antibiotic Timing	30	73%	85%	80%	93%
Oxygenation Assessment	49	98%	99%	99%	100%
Pneumococcal Vaccine	38	79%	73%	69%	94%
Smoking Cessation Advice[1]	5	80%	70%	80%	100%
Surgical Infection Prevention					
Prophylactic Antibiotic Given[1,3]	5	40%	78%	77%	95%
Prophylactic Antibiotic Selection[1]	5	100%	94%	90%	100%
Prophylactic Antibiotic Stopped[1,3]	5	100%	82%	72%	95%
Pregnancy Care					
Inpatient Neonatal Mortality	-	-	-	-	-
Third or Fourth Degree Laceration	-	-	4.42%	3.63%	3.27%

Abbott-Northwestern Hospital

800 E 28th Street
Minneapolis, MN 55407
Phone: 612-863-4000
Fax: 612-863-3658
URL: www.abbottnorthwestern.com
Ownership: Voluntary non-profit - Private
Accredited: Yes
Emergency Services: Yes
Licensed Beds: 958

Key Personnel:

President . . . . Jeff Peterson
President Medical Staff . . . . Michael Tedford, MD
Director Cardiology . . . . Robert Hauser, MD
Emergency Department. . . . . Lee Arostegui, MD
Director OB/GYN . . . . Ronald Peterson, MD
Director Surgery. . . . . Mark Migliori, MD
Director Radiology . . . . Wendy Nazarian, MD

Measure	Cases	This Hospital	State Average	U.S. Average	Top Hospital
Heart Attack Care					
ACE Inhibitor or ARB for LVSD	190	87%	89%	82%	100%
Aspirin at Arrival	245	96%	92%	92%	100%
Aspirin at Discharge	803	98%	93%	90%	100%
Beta Blocker at Arrival	220	94%	88%	87%	100%
Beta Blocker at Discharge	923	98%	95%	90%	100%
Fibrinolytic Medication Timing[1]	1	100%	40%	31%	100%
PCI Within 90 Minutes of Arrival[1]	11	73%	77%	54%	95%
Smoking Cessation Advice	348	94%	68%	88%	100%
Heart Failure Care					
ACE Inhibitor or ARB for LVSD	394	88%	85%	82%	100%
Discharge Instructions	681	67%	54%	61%	93%
Evaluation of LVS Function	844	98%	77%	83%	99%
Smoking Cessation Advice	135	81%	67%	82%	100%
Pneumonia Care					
Appropriate Initial Antibiotic	236	86%	80%	83%	94%
Blood Culture Timing	201	89%	94%	90%	100%
Influenza Vaccine	67	73%	76%	70%	100%
Initial Antibiotic Timing	341	74%	85%	80%	93%
Oxygenation Assessment	451	100%	99%	99%	100%
Pneumococcal Vaccine	287	63%	73%	69%	94%
Smoking Cessation Advice	90	73%	70%	80%	100%
Surgical Infection Prevention					
Prophylactic Antibiotic Given[2,3]	173	82%	78%	77%	95%
Prophylactic Antibiotic Selection[2]	98	97%	94%	90%	100%
Prophylactic Antibiotic Stopped[2,3]	166	90%	82%	72%	95%
Pregnancy Care					
Inpatient Neonatal Mortality	-	-	-	-	-
Third or Fourth Degree Laceration	-	-	4.42%	3.63%	3.27%

Hennepin County Medical Center

Alternate Name: HCMC
701 Park Avenue
Minneapolis, MN 55415
Phone: 612-873-2338
Fax: 612-904-4214
URL: www.hcmc.org
Ownership: Government - Local
Accredited: Yes
Emergency Services: Yes
Licensed Beds: 910

Key Personnel:

CEO. . . . . Jeff Spartz
Manager Cardiac Lab. Nancy Zender
Manager Catheterization Lab . . . . Dee Gaiser
Manager Emergency Room . . . . Carol Halley
Director Infection Control . . . . Mary Ellen Bennett
Manager Intensive/Coronary Care . . . . Karen McCampbell
Associate Administrator Women's Health. . . . . . Chris Wolohan
Director Radiology . . . . Diane Kelly
Director Respiratory/Cardiopulmonary . . . . Judy Hannigan

Measure	Cases	This Hospital	State Average	U.S. Average	Top Hospital

NOTE: Hospital profiles are in alphabetical order by state, then city, then hospital within the city; Rankings are sorted by rate in descending order and exclude hospitals with less than 25 cases; (1) The number of cases is too small (n<25) for purposes of reliably predicting hospital performance; (2) Measure reflects the hospital's indication that its submission was based upon a sample of its relevant discharges; (3) Rate reflects fewer than the maximum possible quarters of data for the measure; (4) Inaccurate information submitted and suppressed for one or more quarters; (5) No data is available from the hospital for this measure; Please refer to the User's Guide for a full explanation of data

Heart Attack Care					
ACE Inhibitor or ARB for LVSD	42	98%	89%	82%	100%
Aspirin at Arrival	191	99%	92%	92%	100%
Aspirin at Discharge	178	98%	93%	90%	100%
Beta Blocker at Arrival	170	99%	88%	87%	100%
Beta Blocker at Discharge	155	97%	95%	90%	100%
Fibrinolytic Medication Timing[1]	1	0%	40%	31%	100%
PCI Within 90 Minutes of Arrival[1]	15	60%	77%	54%	95%
Smoking Cessation Advice	83	96%	68%	88%	100%
Heart Failure Care					
ACE Inhibitor or ARB for LVSD	219	84%	85%	82%	100%
Discharge Instructions	341	47%	54%	61%	93%
Evaluation of LVS Function	422	98%	77%	83%	99%
Smoking Cessation Advice	151	70%	67%	82%	100%
Pneumonia Care					
Appropriate Initial Antibiotic	187	81%	80%	83%	94%
Blood Culture Timing	205	75%	94%	90%	100%
Influenza Vaccine	70	30%	76%	70%	100%
Initial Antibiotic Timing	417	61%	85%	80%	93%
Oxygenation Assessment	492	99%	99%	99%	100%
Pneumococcal Vaccine	151	19%	73%	69%	94%
Smoking Cessation Advice	213	56%	70%	80%	100%
Surgical Infection Prevention					
Prophylactic Antibiotic Given[2]	362	72%	78%	77%	95%
Prophylactic Antibiotic Selection[2]	100	83%	94%	90%	100%
Prophylactic Antibiotic Stopped[2]	346	74%	82%	72%	95%
Pregnancy Care					
Inpatient Neonatal Mortality	3,080	0.52%	-	-	-
Third or Fourth Degree Laceration	2,371	3.59%	4.42%	3.63%	3.27%

Phillips Eye Institute

2215 Park Avenue South
Minneapolis, MN 55404
Phone: 612-775-8800
Ownership: Voluntary non-profit - Other
Accredited: Yes
Emergency Services: Yes

Measure	Cases	This Hospital	State Average	U.S. Average	Top Hospital
Heart Attack Care					
ACE Inhibitor or ARB for LVSD[5]	-	-	89%	82%	100%
Aspirin at Arrival[5]	-	-	92%	92%	100%
Aspirin at Discharge[5]	-	-	93%	90%	100%
Beta Blocker at Arrival[5]	-	-	88%	87%	100%
Beta Blocker at Discharge[5]	-	-	95%	90%	100%
Fibrinolytic Medication Timing[5]	-	-	40%	31%	100%
PCI Within 90 Minutes of Arrival[5]	-	-	77%	54%	95%
Smoking Cessation Advice[5]	-	-	68%	88%	100%
Heart Failure Care					
ACE Inhibitor or ARB for LVSD[5]	-	-	85%	82%	100%
Discharge Instructions[5]	-	-	54%	61%	93%
Evaluation of LVS Function[5]	-	-	77%	83%	99%
Smoking Cessation Advice[5]	-	-	67%	82%	100%
Pneumonia Care					
Appropriate Initial Antibiotic[5]	-	-	80%	83%	94%
Blood Culture Timing[5]	-	-	94%	90%	100%
Influenza Vaccine[5]	-	-	76%	70%	100%
Initial Antibiotic Timing[5]	-	-	85%	80%	93%
Oxygenation Assessment[5]	-	-	99%	99%	100%
Pneumococcal Vaccine[5]	-	-	73%	69%	94%
Smoking Cessation Advice[5]	-	-	70%	80%	100%
Surgical Infection Prevention					
Prophylactic Antibiotic Given[5]	-	-	78%	77%	95%
Prophylactic Antibiotic Selection[5]	-	-	94%	90%	100%
Prophylactic Antibiotic Stopped[5]	-	-	82%	72%	95%
Pregnancy Care					
Inpatient Neonatal Mortality	-	-	-	-	-
Third or Fourth Degree Laceration	-	-	4.42%	3.63%	3.27%

University of Minnesota Med Ctr-Fairview

500 Harvard Street
Minneapolis, MN 55455
Phone: 612-626-3000
Fax: 612-672-7186
URL: www.fairview.org
Ownership: Voluntary non-profit - Private
Accredited: Yes
Emergency Services: Yes
Licensed Beds: 1,868

Key Personnel:

President/CEO . . . . David R Page
Emergency Room . . . . Charles Andres, MD
Director Infection/Disease Control . . . . Frank Rhame, MD
Director Medical/Surgical Nursing . . . . Joanne Disch
OB/GYN Womens Health. . . . . Les Twigga, MD
Chief Radiology . . . . William Thompson, MD
Director Respiratory Therapy . . . . Michael Boyle

Measure	Cases	This Hospital	State Average	U.S. Average	Top Hospital
Heart Attack Care					
ACE Inhibitor or ARB for LVSD	47	77%	89%	82%	100%
Aspirin at Arrival	95	97%	92%	92%	100%
Aspirin at Discharge	142	99%	93%	90%	100%
Beta Blocker at Arrival	81	96%	88%	87%	100%
Beta Blocker at Discharge	133	98%	95%	90%	100%
Fibrinolytic Medication Timing	0	-	40%	31%	100%
PCI Within 90 Minutes of Arrival[1]	3	67%	77%	54%	95%
Smoking Cessation Advice	49	98%	68%	88%	100%
Heart Failure Care					
ACE Inhibitor or ARB for LVSD	158	83%	85%	82%	100%
Discharge Instructions	241	68%	54%	61%	93%
Evaluation of LVS Function	284	98%	77%	83%	99%
Smoking Cessation Advice	48	96%	67%	82%	100%
Pneumonia Care					
Appropriate Initial Antibiotic	125	71%	80%	83%	94%
Blood Culture Timing	115	82%	94%	90%	100%
Influenza Vaccine	48	88%	76%	70%	100%
Initial Antibiotic Timing	212	60%	85%	80%	93%
Oxygenation Assessment	274	100%	99%	99%	100%
Pneumococcal Vaccine	113	79%	73%	69%	94%
Smoking Cessation Advice	76	99%	70%	80%	100%
Surgical Infection Prevention					
Prophylactic Antibiotic Given[2,3]	191	93%	78%	77%	95%
Prophylactic Antibiotic Selection[2]	66	97%	94%	90%	100%
Prophylactic Antibiotic Stopped[2,3]	185	89%	82%	72%	95%
Pregnancy Care					
Inpatient Neonatal Mortality	2,873	1.11%	-	-	-
Third or Fourth Degree Laceration	1,878	4.53%	4.42%	3.63%	3.27%

Chippewa County Montevideo Hospital

824 N 11th Street
Montevideo, MN 56265
Phone: 320-269-8878
Fax: 320-269-8186
Ownership: Government - Local
Accredited: No
Emergency Services: Yes
Licensed Beds: 35

Measure	Cases	This Hospital	State Average	U.S. Average	Top Hospital
Heart Attack Care					
ACE Inhibitor or ARB for LVSD[1]	2	100%	89%	82%	100%
Aspirin at Arrival[1]	9	89%	92%	92%	100%
Aspirin at Discharge[1]	8	100%	93%	90%	100%
Beta Blocker at Arrival[1]	9	89%	88%	87%	100%
Beta Blocker at Discharge[1]	7	86%	95%	90%	100%
Fibrinolytic Medication Timing	0	-	40%	31%	100%
PCI Within 90 Minutes of Arrival	0	-	77%	54%	95%
Smoking Cessation Advice	0	-	68%	88%	100%
Heart Failure Care					
ACE Inhibitor or ARB for LVSD[1]	7	57%	85%	82%	100%
Discharge Instructions[1]	23	0%	54%	61%	93%
Evaluation of LVS Function	36	39%	77%	83%	99%
Smoking Cessation Advice[1]	1	0%	67%	82%	100%
Pneumonia Care					
Appropriate Initial Antibiotic	32	69%	80%	83%	94%
Blood Culture Timing[1]	7	100%	94%	90%	100%
Influenza Vaccine[1]	7	57%	76%	70%	100%
Initial Antibiotic Timing	40	88%	85%	80%	93%

NOTE: Hospital profiles are in alphabetical order by state, then city, then hospital within the city; Rankings are sorted by rate in descending order and exclude hospitals with less than 25 cases; (1) The number of cases is too small (n<25) for purposes of reliably predicting hospital performance; (2) Measure reflects the hospital's indication that its submission was based upon a sample of its relevant discharges; (3) Rate reflects fewer than the maximum possible quarters of data for the measure; (4) Inaccurate information submitted and suppressed for one or more quarters; (5) No data is available from the hospital for this measure; Please refer to the User's Guide for a full explanation of data

Oxygenation Assessment	42	100%	99%	99%	100%
Pneumococcal Vaccine	30	30%	73%	69%	94%
Smoking Cessation Advice[1]	4	25%	70%	80%	100%
Surgical Infection Prevention					
Prophylactic Antibiotic Given[5]	-	-	78%	77%	95%
Prophylactic Antibiotic Selection[5]	-	-	94%	90%	100%
Prophylactic Antibiotic Stopped[5]	-	-	82%	72%	95%
Pregnancy Care					
Inpatient Neonatal Mortality	-	-	-	-	-
Third or Fourth Degree Laceration	-	-	4.42%	3.63%	3.27%

Monticello-Big Lake Community Hospital

1013 Hart Boulevard
Monticello, MN 55362
URL: www.mblch.com
Phone: 763-295-2945
Fax: 763-295-4593
Ownership: Govt - Hospital District or Authority
Emergency Services: Yes
Accredited: Yes
Licensed Beds: 39

Key Personnel:
Chief Medical Staff....................... William Scheig, MD

Measure	Cases	This Hospital	State Average	U.S. Average	Top Hospital
Heart Attack Care					
ACE Inhibitor or ARB for LVSD	0	-	89%	82%	100%
Aspirin at Arrival[1]	4	75%	92%	92%	100%
Aspirin at Discharge[1]	5	100%	93%	90%	100%
Beta Blocker at Arrival[1]	4	50%	88%	87%	100%
Beta Blocker at Discharge[1]	5	60%	95%	90%	100%
Fibrinolytic Medication Timing	0	-	40%	31%	100%
PCI Within 90 Minutes of Arrival	0	-	77%	54%	95%
Smoking Cessation Advice	0	-	68%	88%	100%
Heart Failure Care					
ACE Inhibitor or ARB for LVSD[1,2]	12	92%	85%	82%	100%
Discharge Instructions[2]	34	24%	54%	61%	93%
Evaluation of LVS Function[2]	41	80%	77%	83%	99%
Smoking Cessation Advice[1,2]	9	56%	67%	82%	100%
Pneumonia Care					
Appropriate Initial Antibiotic	46	87%	80%	83%	94%
Blood Culture Timing[1]	24	83%	94%	90%	100%
Influenza Vaccine[1]	12	42%	76%	70%	100%
Initial Antibiotic Timing	50	72%	85%	80%	93%
Oxygenation Assessment	71	89%	99%	99%	100%
Pneumococcal Vaccine	39	46%	73%	69%	94%
Smoking Cessation Advice[1]	22	41%	70%	80%	100%
Surgical Infection Prevention					
Prophylactic Antibiotic Given[1,3]	14	86%	78%	77%	95%
Prophylactic Antibiotic Selection[1]	14	100%	94%	90%	100%
Prophylactic Antibiotic Stopped[1,3]	14	43%	82%	72%	95%
Pregnancy Care					
Inpatient Neonatal Mortality	550	0.55%	-	-	-
Third or Fourth Degree Laceration	484	8.68%	4.42%	3.63%	3.27%

Mercy Hospital & Health Care Center

710 S Kenwood Avenue
Moose Lake, MN 55767
URL: www.mercymooselake.org
Phone: 218-485-4481
Fax: 218-485-5855
Ownership: Govt - Hospital District or Authority
Emergency Services: No
Accredited: No
Licensed Beds: 25

Key Personnel:
CEO................................. Jason Douglas
Director Infection/Disease Control .... Sally Behn

Measure	Cases	This Hospital	State Average	U.S. Average	Top Hospital
Heart Attack Care					
ACE Inhibitor or ARB for LVSD[3]	0	-	89%	82%	100%
Aspirin at Arrival[1,3]	5	60%	92%	92%	100%
Aspirin at Discharge[1,3]	4	100%	93%	90%	100%
Beta Blocker at Arrival[1,3]	3	100%	88%	87%	100%
Beta Blocker at Discharge[1,3]	5	100%	95%	90%	100%
Fibrinolytic Medication Timing[3]	0	-	40%	31%	100%
PCI Within 90 Minutes of Arrival	0	-	77%	54%	95%
Smoking Cessation Advice[3]	0	-	68%	88%	100%
Heart Failure Care					
ACE Inhibitor or ARB for LVSD[1]	5	60%	85%	82%	100%
Discharge Instructions	25	24%	54%	61%	93%
Evaluation of LVS Function	34	47%	77%	83%	99%
Smoking Cessation Advice[1]	5	80%	67%	82%	100%
Pneumonia Care					
Appropriate Initial Antibiotic	41	90%	80%	83%	94%
Blood Culture Timing[1]	21	90%	94%	90%	100%
Influenza Vaccine[1]	6	67%	76%	70%	100%
Initial Antibiotic Timing	46	70%	85%	80%	93%
Oxygenation Assessment	58	100%	99%	99%	100%
Pneumococcal Vaccine	44	50%	73%	69%	94%
Smoking Cessation Advice[1]	11	91%	70%	80%	100%
Surgical Infection Prevention					
Prophylactic Antibiotic Given[3]	37	89%	78%	77%	95%
Prophylactic Antibiotic Selection[1]	10	100%	94%	90%	100%
Prophylactic Antibiotic Stopped[3]	36	75%	82%	72%	95%
Pregnancy Care					
Inpatient Neonatal Mortality	-	-	-	-	-
Third or Fourth Degree Laceration	-	-	4.42%	3.63%	3.27%

Kanabec Hospital

301 S Hwy 65
Mora, MN 55051
Toll-Free: 800-245-5671
Phone: 320-679-1212
Fax: 320-225-3613
Ownership: Government - Local
Emergency Services: Yes
Accredited: Yes
Licensed Beds: 49

Key Personnel:
CEO................................. Randy Ulseth
Chief Medical Staff....................... Randy Bostrom, MD
Emergency Room .... Dorothy Kohl, RN
Infection Control Coordinator .... Barry Vermilyea
Respiratory Therapy...................... Brian Dewitt

Measure	Cases	This Hospital	State Average	U.S. Average	Top Hospital
Heart Attack Care					
ACE Inhibitor or ARB for LVSD[3]	0	-	89%	82%	100%
Aspirin at Arrival[1,3]	2	100%	92%	92%	100%
Aspirin at Discharge[1,3]	1	100%	93%	90%	100%
Beta Blocker at Arrival[1,3]	2	100%	88%	87%	100%
Beta Blocker at Discharge[1,3]	1	100%	95%	90%	100%
Fibrinolytic Medication Timing[3]	0	-	40%	31%	100%
PCI Within 90 Minutes of Arrival[5]	-	-	77%	54%	95%
Smoking Cessation Advice[3]	0	-	68%	88%	100%
Heart Failure Care					
ACE Inhibitor or ARB for LVSD[1]	9	100%	85%	82%	100%
Discharge Instructions	48	75%	54%	61%	93%
Evaluation of LVS Function	63	73%	77%	83%	99%
Smoking Cessation Advice[1]	5	100%	67%	82%	100%
Pneumonia Care					
Appropriate Initial Antibiotic	50	64%	80%	83%	94%
Blood Culture Timing[1]	11	100%	94%	90%	100%
Influenza Vaccine[1]	14	100%	76%	70%	100%
Initial Antibiotic Timing	79	78%	85%	80%	93%
Oxygenation Assessment	81	100%	99%	99%	100%
Pneumococcal Vaccine	58	91%	73%	69%	94%
Smoking Cessation Advice[1]	14	100%	70%	80%	100%
Surgical Infection Prevention					
Prophylactic Antibiotic Given[3]	47	98%	78%	77%	95%
Prophylactic Antibiotic Selection[1]	17	100%	94%	90%	100%
Prophylactic Antibiotic Stopped[3]	45	98%	82%	72%	95%
Pregnancy Care					
Inpatient Neonatal Mortality	-	-	-	-	-
Third or Fourth Degree Laceration	-	-	4.42%	3.63%	3.27%

Stevens Community Medical Center

400 East First Street
PO Box 660
Morris, MN 56267
URL: www.scmcmorris.com
Phone: 320-589-1313
Fax: 320-589-1065
Ownership: Voluntary non-profit - Private
Emergency Services: Yes
Accredited: No
Licensed Beds: 54

Key Personnel:
President/CEO.......................... John Rau

NOTE: Hospital profiles are in alphabetical order by state, then city, then hospital within the city; Rankings are sorted by rate in descending order and exclude hospitals with less than 25 cases; (1) The number of cases is too small (n<25) for purposes of reliably predicting hospital performance; (2) Measure reflects the hospital's indication that its submission was based upon a sample of its relevant discharges; (3) Rate reflects fewer than the maximum possible quarters of data for the measure; (4) Inaccurate information submitted and suppressed for one or more quarters; (5) No data is available from the hospital for this measure; Please refer to the User's Guide for a full explanation of data

Chief Medical Staff . . . . Joan Krajen Radcliffe, MD
Emergency Room . . . . Gaither Bynum, MD
ICU . . . . Suzie Eklund, RN
Medical/Surgical Nursing . . . . Kathy O'Keefe, RN
Director Radiology . . . . Corryn Schoenherr

Measure	Cases	This Hospital	State Average	U.S. Average	Top Hospital
Heart Attack Care					
ACE Inhibitor or ARB for LVSD[3]	0	-	89%	82%	100%
Aspirin at Arrival[1,3]	2	50%	92%	92%	100%
Aspirin at Discharge[1,3]	1	100%	93%	90%	100%
Beta Blocker at Arrival[1,3]	2	50%	88%	87%	100%
Beta Blocker at Discharge[1,3]	1	100%	95%	90%	100%
Fibrinolytic Medication Timing[3]	0	-	40%	31%	100%
PCI Within 90 Minutes of Arrival[5]	-	-	77%	54%	95%
Smoking Cessation Advice[3]	0	-	68%	88%	100%
Heart Failure Care					
ACE Inhibitor or ARB for LVSD[3]	0	-	85%	82%	100%
Discharge Instructions[1,3]	5	80%	54%	61%	93%
Evaluation of LVS Function[1,3]	7	86%	77%	83%	99%
Smoking Cessation Advice[1,3]	1	100%	67%	82%	100%
Pneumonia Care					
Appropriate Initial Antibiotic[1,3]	12	92%	80%	83%	94%
Blood Culture Timing[5]	-	-	94%	90%	100%
Influenza Vaccine[5]	-	-	76%	70%	100%
Initial Antibiotic Timing[3]	29	100%	85%	80%	93%
Oxygenation Assessment[3]	29	100%	99%	99%	100%
Pneumococcal Vaccine[1,3]	21	62%	73%	69%	94%
Smoking Cessation Advice[1,3]	4	75%	70%	80%	100%
Surgical Infection Prevention					
Prophylactic Antibiotic Given[5]	-	-	78%	77%	95%
Prophylactic Antibiotic Selection[5]	-	-	94%	90%	100%
Prophylactic Antibiotic Stopped[5]	-	-	82%	72%	95%
Pregnancy Care					
Inpatient Neonatal Mortality	-	-	-	-	-
Third or Fourth Degree Laceration	-	-	4.42%	3.63%	3.27%

Queen of Peace Hospital

301 2nd Street NE
New Prague, MN 56071
Toll-Free: 800-584-6667
Phone: 952-758-4431
Fax: 952-758-5009
E-mail: info@qofp.org
URL: www.queenofpeacehospital.com
Ownership: Voluntary non-profit - Private
Accredited: No
Emergency Services: Yes
Licensed Beds: 25

Key Personnel:
Chief Medical Staff . . . . Dan Berg, MD
Cardiac Lab . . . . Deb Murry, RN
Emergency Room . . . . Michael Wilcox, MD
ICU Supervising Nurse . . . . Claudia Hollom, RN
Intensive/Coronary Care . . . . Claudia Hollom, RN
Director Radiology . . . . Chacko Thomas
Director Respiratory Therapy . . . . Greg Koch

Measure	Cases	This Hospital	State Average	U.S. Average	Top Hospital
Heart Attack Care					
ACE Inhibitor or ARB for LVSD[3]	0	-	89%	82%	100%
Aspirin at Arrival[1,3]	2	100%	92%	92%	100%
Aspirin at Discharge[1,3]	2	50%	93%	90%	100%
Beta Blocker at Arrival[1,3]	3	67%	88%	87%	100%
Beta Blocker at Discharge[1,3]	3	67%	95%	90%	100%
Fibrinolytic Medication Timing[3]	0	-	40%	31%	100%
PCI Within 90 Minutes of Arrival	0	-	77%	54%	95%
Smoking Cessation Advice[3]	0	-	68%	88%	100%
Heart Failure Care					
ACE Inhibitor or ARB for LVSD[1,3]	5	100%	85%	82%	100%
Discharge Instructions[1,3]	20	95%	54%	61%	93%
Evaluation of LVS Function[3]	31	84%	77%	83%	99%
Smoking Cessation Advice[1,3]	1	0%	67%	82%	100%
Pneumonia Care					
Appropriate Initial Antibiotic[1,3]	15	93%	80%	83%	94%
Blood Culture Timing[1,3]	11	91%	94%	90%	100%
Influenza Vaccine[5]	-	-	76%	70%	100%
Initial Antibiotic Timing[1,3]	23	65%	85%	80%	93%
Oxygenation Assessment[1,3]	24	100%	99%	99%	100%
Pneumococcal Vaccine[1,3]	19	11%	73%	69%	94%
Smoking Cessation Advice[1,3]	3	100%	70%	80%	100%
Surgical Infection Prevention					
Prophylactic Antibiotic Given[5]	-	-	78%	77%	95%
Prophylactic Antibiotic Selection[5]	-	-	94%	90%	100%
Prophylactic Antibiotic Stopped[5]	-	-	82%	72%	95%
Pregnancy Care					
Inpatient Neonatal Mortality	-	-	-	-	-
Third or Fourth Degree Laceration	-	-	4.42%	3.63%	3.27%

New Ulm Medical Center

1324 Fifth Street North
PO Box 577
New Ulm, MN 56073
Toll-Free: 800-795-1211
Phone: 507-233-1000
Fax: 507-233-1552
URL: www.newulmmedicalcenter.com
Ownership: Voluntary non-profit - Private
Accredited: Yes
Emergency Services: Yes
Licensed Beds: 62

Key Personnel:
Administrator . . . . Lori Wightman
Chief Medical Staff . . . . John Krikavar, MD
Emergency Room Manager . . . . Julie Halvorson
Manager Med/Surg/CCU . . . . Marilyn Swan
Manager Respiratory Therapy . . . . Kathleen Bauer

Measure	Cases	This Hospital	State Average	U.S. Average	Top Hospital
Heart Attack Care					
ACE Inhibitor or ARB for LVSD[1]	4	75%	89%	82%	100%
Aspirin at Arrival[1]	12	83%	92%	92%	100%
Aspirin at Discharge[1]	9	67%	93%	90%	100%
Beta Blocker at Arrival[1]	12	92%	88%	87%	100%
Beta Blocker at Discharge[1]	12	83%	95%	90%	100%
Fibrinolytic Medication Timing	0	-	40%	31%	100%
PCI Within 90 Minutes of Arrival[5]	-	-	77%	54%	95%
Smoking Cessation Advice[1]	1	100%	68%	88%	100%
Heart Failure Care					
ACE Inhibitor or ARB for LVSD[1]	14	93%	85%	82%	100%
Discharge Instructions	25	68%	54%	61%	93%
Evaluation of LVS Function	59	88%	77%	83%	99%
Smoking Cessation Advice[1]	5	80%	67%	82%	100%
Pneumonia Care					
Appropriate Initial Antibiotic	32	78%	80%	83%	94%
Blood Culture Timing	31	94%	94%	90%	100%
Influenza Vaccine[1]	7	71%	76%	70%	100%
Initial Antibiotic Timing	42	69%	85%	80%	93%
Oxygenation Assessment	52	100%	99%	99%	100%
Pneumococcal Vaccine	40	95%	73%	69%	94%
Smoking Cessation Advice[1]	5	60%	70%	80%	100%
Surgical Infection Prevention					
Prophylactic Antibiotic Given[2,3]	42	74%	78%	77%	95%
Prophylactic Antibiotic Selection[2]	38	97%	94%	90%	100%
Prophylactic Antibiotic Stopped[2,3]	38	97%	82%	72%	95%
Pregnancy Care					
Inpatient Neonatal Mortality	-	-	-	-	-
Third or Fourth Degree Laceration	-	-	4.42%	3.63%	3.27%

Northfield Hospital

801 West 1st Street
Northfield, MN 55057
Phone: 507-646-1000
Fax: 507-646-1392
E-mail: richardsons@northfieldhospital.org
URL: www.northfieldhospital.org
Ownership: Government - Local
Accredited: Yes
Emergency Services: Yes
Licensed Beds: 37

Key Personnel:
CEO . . . . Ken Bank
Emergency Room . . . . Deb Maestri
Emergency Room . . . . Doris Ertekeson
Director Infection Control . . . . Bernice Pulja
Cardiology Director . . . . Margi Henry
Director Surgery . . . . Karen Geiger
Respiratory Care Chief . . . . Stacy Zell

NOTE: Hospital profiles are in alphabetical order by state, then city, then hospital within the city; Rankings are sorted by rate in descending order and exclude hospitals with less than 25 cases; (1) The number of cases is too small (n<25) for purposes of reliably predicting hospital performance; (2) Measure reflects the hospital's indication that its submission was based upon a sample of its relevant discharges; (3) Rate reflects fewer than the maximum possible quarters of data for the measure; (4) Inaccurate information submitted and suppressed for one or more quarters; (5) No data is available from the hospital for this measure; Please refer to the User's Guide for a full explanation of data

Measure	Cases	This Hospital	State Average	U.S. Average	Top Hospital
Heart Attack Care					
ACE Inhibitor or ARB for LVSD[1]	3	100%	89%	82%	100%
Aspirin at Arrival[1]	9	89%	92%	92%	100%
Aspirin at Discharge[1]	8	100%	93%	90%	100%
Beta Blocker at Arrival[1]	10	100%	88%	87%	100%
Beta Blocker at Discharge[1]	7	100%	95%	90%	100%
Fibrinolytic Medication Timing	0	-	40%	31%	100%
PCI Within 90 Minutes of Arrival	0	-	77%	54%	95%
Smoking Cessation Advice	0	-	68%	88%	100%
Heart Failure Care					
ACE Inhibitor or ARB for LVSD[1,2]	16	69%	85%	82%	100%
Discharge Instructions[2]	49	39%	54%	61%	93%
Evaluation of LVS Function[2]	77	88%	77%	83%	99%
Smoking Cessation Advice[1,2]	2	100%	67%	82%	100%
Pneumonia Care					
Appropriate Initial Antibiotic	68	84%	80%	83%	94%
Blood Culture Timing[1]	21	95%	94%	90%	100%
Influenza Vaccine[1]	11	55%	76%	70%	100%
Initial Antibiotic Timing	53	89%	85%	80%	93%
Oxygenation Assessment	72	100%	99%	99%	100%
Pneumococcal Vaccine	49	76%	73%	69%	94%
Smoking Cessation Advice[1]	9	56%	70%	80%	100%
Surgical Infection Prevention					
Prophylactic Antibiotic Given	141	89%	78%	77%	95%
Prophylactic Antibiotic Selection	28	96%	94%	90%	100%
Prophylactic Antibiotic Stopped	134	94%	82%	72%	95%
Pregnancy Care					
Inpatient Neonatal Mortality	-	-	-	-	-
Third or Fourth Degree Laceration	-	-	4.42%	3.63%	3.27%

Mille Lacs Health System

Alternate Name: Mille Lacs Hospital
200 N Elm Street
Box A
Onamia, MN 56359
Phone: 320-532-3154
Fax: 320-532-3111
Ownership: Voluntary non-profit - Private
Emergency Services: No
Accredited: No
Licensed Beds: 108

Key Personnel:

CEO . . . . Dan Reiner
Chief of Medical Staff . . . . Tom Bracken, MD
Surgical Services . . . . Linda Heinrich

Measure	Cases	This Hospital	State Average	U.S. Average	Top Hospital
Heart Attack Care					
ACE Inhibitor or ARB for LVSD[1,3]	3	33%	89%	82%	100%
Aspirin at Arrival[1,3]	9	67%	92%	92%	100%
Aspirin at Discharge[1,3]	7	71%	93%	90%	100%
Beta Blocker at Arrival[1,3]	7	57%	88%	87%	100%
Beta Blocker at Discharge[1,3]	7	86%	95%	90%	100%
Fibrinolytic Medication Timing[3]	0	-	40%	31%	100%
PCI Within 90 Minutes of Arrival	0	-	77%	54%	95%
Smoking Cessation Advice[1,3]	1	0%	68%	88%	100%
Heart Failure Care					
ACE Inhibitor or ARB for LVSD[1]	12	92%	85%	82%	100%
Discharge Instructions	33	58%	54%	61%	93%
Evaluation of LVS Function	39	69%	77%	83%	99%
Smoking Cessation Advice[1]	5	80%	67%	82%	100%
Pneumonia Care					
Appropriate Initial Antibiotic[1]	23	87%	80%	83%	94%
Blood Culture Timing[1]	18	100%	94%	90%	100%
Influenza Vaccine[1]	6	67%	76%	70%	100%
Initial Antibiotic Timing	45	78%	85%	80%	93%
Oxygenation Assessment	49	100%	99%	99%	100%
Pneumococcal Vaccine	37	59%	73%	69%	94%
Smoking Cessation Advice[1]	10	70%	70%	80%	100%
Surgical Infection Prevention					
Prophylactic Antibiotic Given[1]	7	29%	78%	77%	95%
Prophylactic Antibiotic Selection[1]	3	100%	94%	90%	100%
Prophylactic Antibiotic Stopped[1]	7	57%	82%	72%	95%
Pregnancy Care					
Inpatient Neonatal Mortality	-	-	-	-	-
Third or Fourth Degree Laceration	-	-	4.42%	3.63%	3.27%

Ortonville Area Health Services

450 Eastvold Avenue
Ortonville, MN 56278
Phone: 320-839-2502
Fax: 320-839-4107
E-mail: lillehak@oahs.us
URL: www.oahs.us
Ownership: Government - Local
Emergency Services: Yes
Accredited: No
Licensed Beds: 105

Key Personnel:

Administrator/CEO . . . . Richard Ash
Chief Medical Staff . . . . Bryan S Delage, MD
Emergency Room . . . . Linda Sis
Infection Control Nurse . . . . Kristine Meyer
Medical Surgical Nursing . . . . Colleen McCabe, DON

Measure	Cases	This Hospital	State Average	U.S. Average	Top Hospital
Heart Attack Care					
ACE Inhibitor or ARB for LVSD[1,3]	2	50%	89%	82%	100%
Aspirin at Arrival[1,3]	12	92%	92%	92%	100%
Aspirin at Discharge[1,3]	8	88%	93%	90%	100%
Beta Blocker at Arrival[1,3]	12	75%	88%	87%	100%
Beta Blocker at Discharge[1,3]	11	82%	95%	90%	100%
Fibrinolytic Medication Timing[1,3]	1	0%	40%	31%	100%
PCI Within 90 Minutes of Arrival	0	-	77%	54%	95%
Smoking Cessation Advice[3]	0	-	68%	88%	100%
Heart Failure Care					
ACE Inhibitor or ARB for LVSD[1,3]	3	100%	85%	82%	100%
Discharge Instructions[1,3]	11	18%	54%	61%	93%
Evaluation of LVS Function[1,3]	14	50%	77%	83%	99%
Smoking Cessation Advice[1,3]	3	33%	67%	82%	100%
Pneumonia Care					
Appropriate Initial Antibiotic[1,3]	12	33%	80%	83%	94%
Blood Culture Timing[3]	0	-	94%	90%	100%
Influenza Vaccine[1]	5	0%	76%	70%	100%
Initial Antibiotic Timing[1,3]	13	100%	85%	80%	93%
Oxygenation Assessment[1,3]	14	86%	99%	99%	100%
Pneumococcal Vaccine[1,3]	10	0%	73%	69%	94%
Smoking Cessation Advice[1,3]	3	0%	70%	80%	100%
Surgical Infection Prevention					
Prophylactic Antibiotic Given[5]	-	-	78%	77%	95%
Prophylactic Antibiotic Selection[5]	-	-	94%	90%	100%
Prophylactic Antibiotic Stopped[5]	-	-	82%	72%	95%
Pregnancy Care					
Inpatient Neonatal Mortality	-	-	-	-	-
Third or Fourth Degree Laceration	-	-	4.42%	3.63%	3.27%

Owatonna Hospital

903 S Oak Avenue
Owatonna, MN 55060
Phone: 507-451-3850
Fax: 507-444-6053
URL: www.owatonnahospital.com
Ownership: Voluntary non-profit - Other
Emergency Services: Yes
Accredited: Yes
Licensed Beds: 48

Key Personnel:

Emergency Room . . . . Anne Draeger
Infection Control . . . . Pam Schultz
ICU . . . . Kathy Meier
Intensive Coronary . . . . Sharon Kopp
Medical/Surgical Nursing . . . . Sharon Kapp
OB/GYN Womens Health . . . . Sharon Kapp
Director of Pulmonary/Respiratory Care . . . . . . Ross Kientz

Measure	Cases	This Hospital	State Average	U.S. Average	Top Hospital
Heart Attack Care					
ACE Inhibitor or ARB for LVSD[1]	3	67%	89%	82%	100%
Aspirin at Arrival[1]	12	92%	92%	92%	100%
Aspirin at Discharge[1]	10	100%	93%	90%	100%
Beta Blocker at Arrival[1]	9	89%	88%	87%	100%
Beta Blocker at Discharge[1]	9	100%	95%	90%	100%
Fibrinolytic Medication Timing	0	-	40%	31%	100%
PCI Within 90 Minutes of Arrival	0	-	77%	54%	95%
Smoking Cessation Advice[1]	2	100%	68%	88%	100%

NOTE: Hospital profiles are in alphabetical order by state, then city, then hospital within the city; Rankings are sorted by rate in descending order and exclude hospitals with less than 25 cases; (1) The number of cases is too small (n<25) for purposes of reliably predicting hospital performance; (2) Measure reflects the hospital's indication that its submission was based upon a sample of its relevant discharges; (3) Rate reflects fewer than the maximum possible quarters of data for the measure; (4) Inaccurate information submitted and suppressed for one or more quarters; (5) No data is available from the hospital for this measure; Please refer to the User's Guide for a full explanation of data

Measure	Cases	This Hospital	State Average	U.S. Average	Top Hospital
Heart Failure Care					
ACE Inhibitor or ARB for LVSD[1]	15	100%	85%	82%	100%
Discharge Instructions	51	98%	54%	61%	93%
Evaluation of LVS Function	62	100%	77%	83%	99%
Smoking Cessation Advice[1]	4	100%	67%	82%	100%
Pneumonia Care					
Appropriate Initial Antibiotic	84	95%	80%	83%	94%
Blood Culture Timing	62	98%	94%	90%	100%
Influenza Vaccine[1]	16	75%	76%	70%	100%
Initial Antibiotic Timing	81	93%	85%	80%	93%
Oxygenation Assessment	94	100%	99%	99%	100%
Pneumococcal Vaccine	78	94%	73%	69%	94%
Smoking Cessation Advice[1]	13	100%	70%	80%	100%
Surgical Infection Prevention					
Prophylactic Antibiotic Given[2,3]	78	88%	78%	77%	95%
Prophylactic Antibiotic Selection[2]	47	91%	94%	90%	100%
Prophylactic Antibiotic Stopped[2,3]	73	38%	82%	72%	95%
Pregnancy Care					
Inpatient Neonatal Mortality	-	-	-	-	-
Third or Fourth Degree Laceration	-	-	4.42%	3.63%	3.27%

Saint Joseph's Area Health Services

Alternate Name: Saint Joseph's Hospital
600 Pleasant Avenue
Park Rapids, MN 56470
Phone: 218-732-3311
Fax: 218-732-1368
URL: www.sjahs.org
Ownership: Voluntary non-profit - Church
Accredited: No
Emergency Services: Yes
Licensed Beds: 50

Key Personnel:

President/CEO . . . . Peter Jacobson
Emergency Room Manager . . . . Brenda Huwe
ICU . . . . Bob Sauser
Medical Surgical Nursing Supervisor . . . . Peggy Pearson
Surgery Manager . . . . Paulette Goldammer

Measure	Cases	This Hospital	State Average	U.S. Average	Top Hospital
Heart Attack Care					
ACE Inhibitor or ARB for LVSD[1]	1	100%	89%	82%	100%
Aspirin at Arrival[1]	18	100%	92%	92%	100%
Aspirin at Discharge[1]	5	100%	93%	90%	100%
Beta Blocker at Arrival[1]	17	88%	88%	87%	100%
Beta Blocker at Discharge[1]	6	83%	95%	90%	100%
Fibrinolytic Medication Timing[1]	1	0%	40%	31%	100%
PCI Within 90 Minutes of Arrival	0	-	77%	54%	95%
Smoking Cessation Advice[1]	2	0%	68%	88%	100%
Heart Failure Care					
ACE Inhibitor or ARB for LVSD[1]	11	55%	85%	82%	100%
Discharge Instructions[1]	23	65%	54%	61%	93%
Evaluation of LVS Function	31	90%	77%	83%	99%
Smoking Cessation Advice[1]	4	50%	67%	82%	100%
Pneumonia Care					
Appropriate Initial Antibiotic	55	84%	80%	83%	94%
Blood Culture Timing	49	98%	94%	90%	100%
Influenza Vaccine[1]	8	75%	76%	70%	100%
Initial Antibiotic Timing	86	91%	85%	80%	93%
Oxygenation Assessment	111	100%	99%	99%	100%
Pneumococcal Vaccine	82	83%	73%	69%	94%
Smoking Cessation Advice[1]	24	79%	70%	80%	100%
Surgical Infection Prevention					
Prophylactic Antibiotic Given[5]	-	-	78%	77%	95%
Prophylactic Antibiotic Selection[5]	-	-	94%	90%	100%
Prophylactic Antibiotic Stopped[5]	-	-	82%	72%	95%
Pregnancy Care					
Inpatient Neonatal Mortality	-	-	-	-	-
Third or Fourth Degree Laceration	-	-	4.42%	3.63%	3.27%

Paynesville Area Health Care System

Alternate Name: Paynesville Area Hospital
200 W 1st Street
Paynesville, MN 56362
Toll-Free: 800-242-3767
Phone: 320-243-3779
Fax: 320-243-6707
URL: www.pahcs.com
Ownership: Govt - Hospital District or Authority
Accredited: No
Emergency Services: Yes
Licensed Beds: 94

Key Personnel:

CEO . . . . Steven T Moburg
Infection Control . . . . Karen Schlangen

Measure	Cases	This Hospital	State Average	U.S. Average	Top Hospital
Heart Attack Care					
ACE Inhibitor or ARB for LVSD[5]	-	-	89%	82%	100%
Aspirin at Arrival[5]	-	-	92%	92%	100%
Aspirin at Discharge[5]	-	-	93%	90%	100%
Beta Blocker at Arrival[5]	-	-	88%	87%	100%
Beta Blocker at Discharge[5]	-	-	95%	90%	100%
Fibrinolytic Medication Timing[5]	-	-	40%	31%	100%
PCI Within 90 Minutes of Arrival[5]	-	-	77%	54%	95%
Smoking Cessation Advice[5]	-	-	68%	88%	100%
Heart Failure Care					
ACE Inhibitor or ARB for LVSD[1]	4	100%	85%	82%	100%
Discharge Instructions[1]	13	31%	54%	61%	93%
Evaluation of LVS Function[1]	20	70%	77%	83%	99%
Smoking Cessation Advice[1]	3	33%	67%	82%	100%
Pneumonia Care					
Appropriate Initial Antibiotic[1]	16	94%	80%	83%	94%
Blood Culture Timing[1]	3	100%	94%	90%	100%
Influenza Vaccine[1]	2	50%	76%	70%	100%
Initial Antibiotic Timing[1]	20	90%	85%	80%	93%
Oxygenation Assessment[1]	22	100%	99%	99%	100%
Pneumococcal Vaccine[1]	14	64%	73%	69%	94%
Smoking Cessation Advice[1]	4	25%	70%	80%	100%
Surgical Infection Prevention					
Prophylactic Antibiotic Given[5]	-	-	78%	77%	95%
Prophylactic Antibiotic Selection[5]	-	-	94%	90%	100%
Prophylactic Antibiotic Stopped[5]	-	-	82%	72%	95%
Pregnancy Care					
Inpatient Neonatal Mortality	-	-	-	-	-
Third or Fourth Degree Laceration	-	-	4.42%	3.63%	3.27%

Perham Memorial Hospital and Home

665 3rd Street SW
Perham, MN 56573
Phone: 218-346-4500
Fax: 218-346-4540
E-mail: information@pmhh.com
URL: www.pmhh.com
Ownership: Govt - Hospital District or Authority
Accredited: No
Emergency Services: Yes
Licensed Beds: 25

Key Personnel:

Administrator . . . . Chuck Hofius
Chief Medical Staff . . . . J Blickenstaff, MD
Director Infection/Disease Control . . . . Nancy Fehrenbach
Director Medical/Surgical Nursing . . . . Bonnie Johnson
Chief Radiology . . . . Loren Cavalier

Measure	Cases	This Hospital	State Average	U.S. Average	Top Hospital
Heart Attack Care					
ACE Inhibitor or ARB for LVSD[1,3]	1	100%	89%	82%	100%
Aspirin at Arrival[1,3]	4	100%	92%	92%	100%
Aspirin at Discharge[1,3]	4	75%	93%	90%	100%
Beta Blocker at Arrival[1,3]	7	71%	88%	87%	100%
Beta Blocker at Discharge[1,3]	5	100%	95%	90%	100%
Fibrinolytic Medication Timing[3]	0	-	40%	31%	100%
PCI Within 90 Minutes of Arrival	0	-	77%	54%	95%
Smoking Cessation Advice[1,3]	1	100%	68%	88%	100%
Heart Failure Care					
ACE Inhibitor or ARB for LVSD[2]	0	-	85%	82%	100%
Discharge Instructions[1,2]	14	57%	54%	61%	93%
Evaluation of LVS Function[1,2]	13	31%	77%	83%	99%
Smoking Cessation Advice[1,2]	3	33%	67%	82%	100%
Pneumonia Care					
Appropriate Initial Antibiotic	32	56%	80%	83%	94%
Blood Culture Timing[1]	4	100%	94%	90%	100%

NOTE: Hospital profiles are in alphabetical order by state, then city, then hospital within the city; Rankings are sorted by rate in descending order and exclude hospitals with less than 25 cases; (1) The number of cases is too small (n<25) for purposes of reliably predicting hospital performance; (2) Measure reflects the hospital's indication that its submission was based upon a sample of its relevant discharges; (3) Rate reflects fewer than the maximum possible quarters of data for the measure; (4) Inaccurate information submitted and suppressed for one or more quarters; (5) No data is available from the hospital for this measure; Please refer to the User's Guide for a full explanation of data

Measure	Cases	This Hospital	State Average	U.S. Average	Top Hospital
Influenza Vaccine[1]	9	100%	76%	70%	100%
Initial Antibiotic Timing	48	88%	85%	80%	93%
Oxygenation Assessment	54	98%	99%	99%	100%
Pneumococcal Vaccine	38	82%	73%	69%	94%
Smoking Cessation Advice[1]	5	80%	70%	80%	100%
Surgical Infection Prevention					
Prophylactic Antibiotic Given[1]	22	73%	78%	77%	95%
Prophylactic Antibiotic Selection[1]	1	100%	94%	90%	100%
Prophylactic Antibiotic Stopped[1]	22	100%	82%	72%	95%
Pregnancy Care					
Inpatient Neonatal Mortality	-	-	-	-	-
Third or Fourth Degree Laceration	-	-	4.42%	3.63%	3.27%

Lakeside Hospital

129 6th Ave Se
Pine City, MN 55063
Ownership: Proprietary
Emergency Services: No
Phone: 320-629-2542
Accredited: No

Measure	Cases	This Hospital	State Average	U.S. Average	Top Hospital
Heart Attack Care					
ACE Inhibitor or ARB for LVSD[5]	-	-	89%	82%	100%
Aspirin at Arrival[5]	-	-	92%	92%	100%
Aspirin at Discharge[5]	-	-	93%	90%	100%
Beta Blocker at Arrival[5]	-	-	88%	87%	100%
Beta Blocker at Discharge[5]	-	-	95%	90%	100%
Fibrinolytic Medication Timing[5]	-	-	40%	31%	100%
PCI Within 90 Minutes of Arrival[5]	-	-	77%	54%	95%
Smoking Cessation Advice[5]	-	-	68%	88%	100%
Heart Failure Care					
ACE Inhibitor or ARB for LVSD[1]	1	100%	85%	82%	100%
Discharge Instructions[3]	0	-	54%	61%	93%
Evaluation of LVS Function[1]	5	40%	77%	83%	99%
Smoking Cessation Advice[3]	0	-	67%	82%	100%
Pneumonia Care					
Appropriate Initial Antibiotic[1,3]	2	0%	80%	83%	94%
Blood Culture Timing[3]	0	-	94%	90%	100%
Influenza Vaccine[5]	-	-	76%	70%	100%
Initial Antibiotic Timing[1,3]	8	100%	85%	80%	93%
Oxygenation Assessment[1,3]	9	100%	99%	99%	100%
Pneumococcal Vaccine[1,3]	8	100%	73%	69%	94%
Smoking Cessation Advice[3]	0	-	70%	80%	100%
Surgical Infection Prevention					
Prophylactic Antibiotic Given[5]	-	-	78%	77%	95%
Prophylactic Antibiotic Selection[5]	-	-	94%	90%	100%
Prophylactic Antibiotic Stopped[5]	-	-	82%	72%	95%
Pregnancy Care					
Inpatient Neonatal Mortality	-	-	-	-	-
Third or Fourth Degree Laceration	-	-	4.42%	3.63%	3.27%

Fairview Northland Regional Health Care

Alternate Name: Fariview Princeton and Milaca Hospital
911 Northland Drive
Princeton, MN 55371
Ownership: Voluntary non-profit - Other
Emergency Services: Yes
Phone: 763-389-1313
Fax: 763-389-6306
Accredited: Yes
Licensed Beds: 41

Key Personnel:
President . . . . Michael Youso

Measure	Cases	This Hospital	State Average	U.S. Average	Top Hospital
Heart Attack Care					
ACE Inhibitor or ARB for LVSD[1]	3	100%	89%	82%	100%
Aspirin at Arrival[1]	20	100%	92%	92%	100%
Aspirin at Discharge[1]	10	100%	93%	90%	100%
Beta Blocker at Arrival[1]	14	100%	88%	87%	100%
Beta Blocker at Discharge[1]	11	100%	95%	90%	100%
Fibrinolytic Medication Timing	0	-	40%	31%	100%
PCI Within 90 Minutes of Arrival	0	-	77%	54%	95%
Smoking Cessation Advice[1]	2	100%	68%	88%	100%
Heart Failure Care					
ACE Inhibitor or ARB for LVSD[1]	20	100%	85%	82%	100%
Discharge Instructions	53	94%	54%	61%	93%
Evaluation of LVS Function	72	100%	77%	83%	99%
Smoking Cessation Advice[1]	16	100%	67%	82%	100%
Pneumonia Care					
Appropriate Initial Antibiotic	61	87%	80%	83%	94%
Blood Culture Timing	72	99%	94%	90%	100%
Influenza Vaccine[1]	12	100%	76%	70%	100%
Initial Antibiotic Timing	81	99%	85%	80%	93%
Oxygenation Assessment	101	100%	99%	99%	100%
Pneumococcal Vaccine	66	95%	73%	69%	94%
Smoking Cessation Advice	28	96%	70%	80%	100%
Surgical Infection Prevention					
Prophylactic Antibiotic Given[2,3]	90	87%	78%	77%	95%
Prophylactic Antibiotic Selection[1,2]	22	100%	94%	90%	100%
Prophylactic Antibiotic Stopped[2,3]	84	94%	82%	72%	95%
Pregnancy Care					
Inpatient Neonatal Mortality	-	-	-	-	-
Third or Fourth Degree Laceration	-	-	4.42%	3.63%	3.27%

Fairview Red Wing Hospital

1407 West 4th Street
Red Wing, MN 55066
URL: www.redwing.fairview.org
Ownership: Voluntary non-profit - Private
Emergency Services: Yes
Phone: 651-267-5000
Fax: 651-385-3304
Accredited: Yes
Licensed Beds: 96

Key Personnel:
Administrator . . . . Scott Wordelman
Chief Medical Staff . . . . Jack Alexander
Emergency Room . . . . Jane Gisslen
Manager Respiratory Therapy . . . . Jeff Norton

Measure	Cases	This Hospital	State Average	U.S. Average	Top Hospital
Heart Attack Care					
ACE Inhibitor or ARB for LVSD[1]	4	75%	89%	82%	100%
Aspirin at Arrival[1]	12	92%	92%	92%	100%
Aspirin at Discharge[1]	9	89%	93%	90%	100%
Beta Blocker at Arrival[1]	11	91%	88%	87%	100%
Beta Blocker at Discharge[1]	8	88%	95%	90%	100%
Fibrinolytic Medication Timing	0	-	40%	31%	100%
PCI Within 90 Minutes of Arrival	0	-	77%	54%	95%
Smoking Cessation Advice[1]	1	0%	68%	88%	100%
Heart Failure Care					
ACE Inhibitor or ARB for LVSD	25	84%	85%	82%	100%
Discharge Instructions	47	74%	54%	61%	93%
Evaluation of LVS Function	68	96%	77%	83%	99%
Smoking Cessation Advice[1]	9	78%	67%	82%	100%
Pneumonia Care					
Appropriate Initial Antibiotic	78	90%	80%	83%	94%
Blood Culture Timing	61	97%	94%	90%	100%
Influenza Vaccine[1]	12	83%	76%	70%	100%
Initial Antibiotic Timing	88	90%	85%	80%	93%
Oxygenation Assessment	110	100%	99%	99%	100%
Pneumococcal Vaccine	76	88%	73%	69%	94%
Smoking Cessation Advice[1]	10	60%	70%	80%	100%
Surgical Infection Prevention					
Prophylactic Antibiotic Given[3]	206	93%	78%	77%	95%
Prophylactic Antibiotic Selection	72	97%	94%	90%	100%
Prophylactic Antibiotic Stopped[3]	198	85%	82%	72%	95%
Pregnancy Care					
Inpatient Neonatal Mortality	-	-	-	-	-
Third or Fourth Degree Laceration	-	-	4.42%	3.63%	3.27%

Red Lake Comprehensive Health Services

PO Box 249
Redlake, MN 56671
Ownership: Government - Federal
Emergency Services: Yes
Phone: 218-679-3316
Fax: 218-679-3990
Accredited: Yes
Licensed Beds: 23

Key Personnel:
CEO . . . . Tony James
Chief Medical Staff . . . . John Robinson
Emergency Room . . . . Joyce Kennedy

Measure	Cases	This Hospital	State Average	U.S. Average	Top Hospital

NOTE: Hospital profiles are in alphabetical order by state, then city, then hospital within the city; Rankings are sorted by rate in descending order and exclude hospitals with less than 25 cases; (1) The number of cases is too small (n<25) for purposes of reliably predicting hospital performance; (2) Measure reflects the hospital's indication that its submission was based upon a sample of its relevant discharges; (3) Rate reflects fewer than the maximum possible quarters of data for the measure; (4) Inaccurate information submitted and suppressed for one or more quarters; (5) No data is available from the hospital for this measure; Please refer to the User's Guide for a full explanation of data

Heart Attack Care					
ACE Inhibitor or ARB for LVSD[3]	0	-	89%	82%	100%
Aspirin at Arrival[1,3]	1	0%	92%	92%	100%
Aspirin at Discharge[3]	0	-	93%	90%	100%
Beta Blocker at Arrival[1,3]	1	0%	88%	87%	100%
Beta Blocker at Discharge[3]	0	-	95%	90%	100%
Fibrinolytic Medication Timing[3]	0	-	40%	31%	100%
PCI Within 90 Minutes of Arrival	0	-	77%	54%	95%
Smoking Cessation Advice[3]	0	-	68%	88%	100%
Heart Failure Care					
ACE Inhibitor or ARB for LVSD[1]	1	100%	85%	82%	100%
Discharge Instructions[1,3]	2	0%	54%	61%	93%
Evaluation of LVS Function[1]	7	86%	77%	83%	99%
Smoking Cessation Advice[3]	0	-	67%	82%	100%
Pneumonia Care					
Appropriate Initial Antibiotic[1,3]	1	100%	80%	83%	94%
Blood Culture Timing[1,3]	1	100%	94%	90%	100%
Influenza Vaccine[5]	-	-	76%	70%	100%
Initial Antibiotic Timing[1]	10	70%	85%	80%	93%
Oxygenation Assessment[1]	13	100%	99%	99%	100%
Pneumococcal Vaccine[1]	2	100%	73%	69%	94%
Smoking Cessation Advice[1,3]	1	0%	70%	80%	100%
Surgical Infection Prevention					
Prophylactic Antibiotic Given[5]	-	-	78%	77%	95%
Prophylactic Antibiotic Selection[5]	-	-	94%	90%	100%
Prophylactic Antibiotic Stopped[5]	-	-	82%	72%	95%
Pregnancy Care					
Inpatient Neonatal Mortality	-	-	-	-	-
Third or Fourth Degree Laceration	-	-	4.42%	3.63%	3.27%

Redwood Area Hospital

100 Fallwood Road
Redwood Falls, MN 56283
Phone: 507-637-4500
Fax: 507-697-6000
E-mail: jim.schulte@redwoodareahospital.org
URL: www.RedwoodAreaHospital.org
Ownership: Government - Local
Accredited: No
Emergency Services: Yes
Licensed Beds: 25

Key Personnel:

Administrator . . . . James E Schulte
Chief of Cardiac Lab . . . . Lori Highty
Director Infection/Disease Control . . . . Julie Fiala, RN
Chief Radiology . . . . Lynn Juell, RRT
Director Respiratory Therapy . . . . Lance Lothert

Measure	Cases	This Hospital	State Average	U.S. Average	Top Hospital
Heart Attack Care					
ACE Inhibitor or ARB for LVSD[1,3]	1	100%	89%	82%	100%
Aspirin at Arrival[1,3]	3	67%	92%	92%	100%
Aspirin at Discharge[1,3]	1	100%	93%	90%	100%
Beta Blocker at Arrival[1,3]	4	75%	88%	87%	100%
Beta Blocker at Discharge[1,3]	1	100%	95%	90%	100%
Fibrinolytic Medication Timing[3]	0	-	40%	31%	100%
PCI Within 90 Minutes of Arrival[5]	-	-	77%	54%	95%
Smoking Cessation Advice[3]	0	-	68%	88%	100%
Heart Failure Care					
ACE Inhibitor or ARB for LVSD[1]	3	100%	85%	82%	100%
Discharge Instructions[1]	11	36%	54%	61%	93%
Evaluation of LVS Function[1]	24	79%	77%	83%	99%
Smoking Cessation Advice[1]	2	100%	67%	82%	100%
Pneumonia Care					
Appropriate Initial Antibiotic[1]	9	89%	80%	83%	94%
Blood Culture Timing[1]	3	100%	94%	90%	100%
Influenza Vaccine[1]	6	50%	76%	70%	100%
Initial Antibiotic Timing[1]	20	90%	85%	80%	93%
Oxygenation Assessment	25	100%	99%	99%	100%
Pneumococcal Vaccine[1]	13	69%	73%	69%	94%
Smoking Cessation Advice[1]	3	100%	70%	80%	100%
Surgical Infection Prevention					
Prophylactic Antibiotic Given[1,3]	1	100%	78%	77%	95%
Prophylactic Antibiotic Selection[5]	-	-	94%	90%	100%
Prophylactic Antibiotic Stopped[1,3]	1	100%	82%	72%	95%
Pregnancy Care					

Inpatient Neonatal Mortality	-	-	-	-	-
Third or Fourth Degree Laceration	-	-	4.42%	3.63%	3.27%

North Memorial Health Care

3300 Oakdale N
Robbinsdale, MN 55422
Phone: 763-520-5200
Fax: 763-520-5006
URL: www.northmemorial.com
Ownership: Voluntary non-profit - Private
Accredited: Yes
Emergency Services: Yes
Licensed Beds: 518

Key Personnel:

CEO . . . . David Cress
Chief Medical Staff . . . . Bruce Adams, MD
Emergency Room . . . . David Roberts, MD
Director Infection/Disease Control . . . . CG Schrock, MD
CCU Spvg. Nurse . . . . Julie Burkhardt
OB/GYN Womens Health . . . . James Krause, MD
Director Respiratory Therapy . . . . Nick Kuhnley

Measure	Cases	This Hospital	State Average	U.S. Average	Top Hospital
Heart Attack Care					
ACE Inhibitor or ARB for LVSD	155	87%	89%	82%	100%
Aspirin at Arrival	495	99%	92%	92%	100%
Aspirin at Discharge	500	98%	93%	90%	100%
Beta Blocker at Arrival	447	96%	88%	87%	100%
Beta Blocker at Discharge	506	98%	95%	90%	100%
Fibrinolytic Medication Timing[1]	1	100%	40%	31%	100%
PCI Within 90 Minutes of Arrival	26	92%	77%	54%	95%
Smoking Cessation Advice	145	97%	68%	88%	100%
Heart Failure Care					
ACE Inhibitor or ARB for LVSD	242	85%	85%	82%	100%
Discharge Instructions	452	58%	54%	61%	93%
Evaluation of LVS Function	580	91%	77%	83%	99%
Smoking Cessation Advice	92	68%	67%	82%	100%
Pneumonia Care					
Appropriate Initial Antibiotic	308	87%	80%	83%	94%
Blood Culture Timing	184	91%	94%	90%	100%
Influenza Vaccine	74	77%	76%	70%	100%
Initial Antibiotic Timing	387	90%	85%	80%	93%
Oxygenation Assessment	471	100%	99%	99%	100%
Pneumococcal Vaccine	285	64%	73%	69%	94%
Smoking Cessation Advice	111	85%	70%	80%	100%
Surgical Infection Prevention					
Prophylactic Antibiotic Given[3]	93	62%	78%	77%	95%
Prophylactic Antibiotic Selection	92	98%	94%	90%	100%
Prophylactic Antibiotic Stopped[3]	89	79%	82%	72%	95%
Pregnancy Care					
Inpatient Neonatal Mortality	-	-	-	-	-
Third or Fourth Degree Laceration	-	-	4.42%	3.63%	3.27%

Olmsted Medical Center Hospital

1650 4th Street SE
Rochester, MN 55904
Phone: 507-529-6600
Fax: 507-529-6622
URL: www.olmsteadmedicalcenter.org
Ownership: Voluntary non-profit - Private
Accredited: No
Emergency Services: Yes
Licensed Beds: 45

Key Personnel:

President . . . . Noel Peterson, MD
Chief Medical Staff . . . . David Westgard, MD
Emergency Room . . . . Jay Myers
Infection Control . . . . Vicky Shultz
Manager Surgery . . . . Ben Riker
Manager Radiology . . . . Scott Van Benschoten

Measure	Cases	This Hospital	State Average	U.S. Average	Top Hospital
Heart Attack Care					
ACE Inhibitor or ARB for LVSD[1]	2	100%	89%	82%	100%
Aspirin at Arrival[1]	7	100%	92%	92%	100%
Aspirin at Discharge[1]	5	100%	93%	90%	100%
Beta Blocker at Arrival[1]	4	75%	88%	87%	100%
Beta Blocker at Discharge[1]	7	86%	95%	90%	100%
Fibrinolytic Medication Timing[3]	0	-	40%	31%	100%
PCI Within 90 Minutes of Arrival	0	-	77%	54%	95%
Smoking Cessation Advice[3]	0	-	68%	88%	100%

NOTE: Hospital profiles are in alphabetical order by state, then city, then hospital within the city; Rankings are sorted by rate in descending order and exclude hospitals with less than 25 cases; (1) The number of cases is too small (n<25) for purposes of reliably predicting hospital performance; (2) Measure reflects the hospital's indication that its submission was based upon a sample of its relevant discharges; (3) Rate reflects fewer than the maximum possible quarters of data for the measure; (4) Inaccurate information submitted and suppressed for one or more quarters; (5) No data is available from the hospital for this measure; Please refer to the User's Guide for a full explanation of data

Measure	Cases	This Hospital	State Average	U.S. Average	Top Hospital
Heart Failure Care					
ACE Inhibitor or ARB for LVSD[1]	12	83%	85%	82%	100%
Discharge Instructions[1,3]	7	86%	54%	61%	93%
Evaluation of LVS Function	37	86%	77%	83%	99%
Smoking Cessation Advice[3]	0	-	67%	82%	100%
Pneumonia Care					
Appropriate Initial Antibiotic[1,3]	10	80%	80%	83%	94%
Blood Culture Timing[1,3]	8	88%	94%	90%	100%
Influenza Vaccine[5]	-	-	76%	70%	100%
Initial Antibiotic Timing	47	68%	85%	80%	93%
Oxygenation Assessment	62	98%	99%	99%	100%
Pneumococcal Vaccine	39	77%	73%	69%	94%
Smoking Cessation Advice[1,3]	4	100%	70%	80%	100%
Surgical Infection Prevention					
Prophylactic Antibiotic Given[3]	40	78%	78%	77%	95%
Prophylactic Antibiotic Selection[5]	-	-	94%	90%	100%
Prophylactic Antibiotic Stopped[3]	39	54%	82%	72%	95%
Pregnancy Care					
Inpatient Neonatal Mortality	-	-	-	-	-
Third or Fourth Degree Laceration	-	-	4.42%	3.63%	3.27%

Rochester Methodist Hospital

201 West Center Street
Rochester, MN 55905
URL: www.mayoclinic.org/contact
Ownership: Voluntary non-profit - Private
Emergency Services: No

Phone: 507-266-7890
Fax: 507-284-0161
Accredited: Yes
Licensed Beds: 794

Key Personnel:
Director Infection/Disease Control . . . . Rodney Thompson, MD
CCU Spvg. Nurse . . . . Mary Ann Healey
OB/GYN Womens Health. . . . . Karl Podratz, MD

Measure	Cases	This Hospital	State Average	U.S. Average	Top Hospital
Heart Attack Care					
ACE Inhibitor or ARB for LVSD[3]	0	-	89%	82%	100%
Aspirin at Arrival[1,3]	1	100%	92%	92%	100%
Aspirin at Discharge[1,3]	1	100%	93%	90%	100%
Beta Blocker at Arrival[1,3]	1	100%	88%	87%	100%
Beta Blocker at Discharge[1,3]	2	100%	95%	90%	100%
Fibrinolytic Medication Timing[3]	0	-	40%	31%	100%
PCI Within 90 Minutes of Arrival	0	-	77%	54%	95%
Smoking Cessation Advice[3]	0	-	68%	88%	100%
Heart Failure Care					
ACE Inhibitor or ARB for LVSD[1]	14	79%	85%	82%	100%
Discharge Instructions	34	53%	54%	61%	93%
Evaluation of LVS Function	44	98%	77%	83%	99%
Smoking Cessation Advice[1]	1	100%	67%	82%	100%
Pneumonia Care					
Appropriate Initial Antibiotic[1,2]	9	89%	80%	83%	94%
Blood Culture Timing[1,2]	2	100%	94%	90%	100%
Influenza Vaccine[1,2]	22	100%	76%	70%	100%
Initial Antibiotic Timing[1,2]	23	61%	85%	80%	93%
Oxygenation Assessment[2]	40	98%	99%	99%	100%
Pneumococcal Vaccine[2]	78	92%	73%	69%	94%
Smoking Cessation Advice[2]	25	92%	70%	80%	100%
Surgical Infection Prevention					
Prophylactic Antibiotic Given[2]	511	96%	78%	77%	95%
Prophylactic Antibiotic Selection[2]	93	98%	94%	90%	100%
Prophylactic Antibiotic Stopped[2]	502	87%	82%	72%	95%
Pregnancy Care					
Inpatient Neonatal Mortality[2]	444	0.23%	-	-	-
Third or Fourth Degree Laceration[2]	1,589	2.58%	4.42%	3.63%	3.27%

Saint Marys Hospital

1216 2nd Saint Sw
Rochester, MN 55902
Ownership: Voluntary non-profit - Church
Emergency Services: Yes

Phone: 507-255-5123
Accredited: Yes

Measure	Cases	This Hospital	State Average	U.S. Average	Top Hospital
Heart Attack Care					
ACE Inhibitor or ARB for LVSD[2]	62	87%	89%	82%	100%
Aspirin at Arrival[2]	124	100%	92%	92%	100%
Aspirin at Discharge[2]	233	99%	93%	90%	100%
Beta Blocker at Arrival[2]	103	99%	88%	87%	100%
Beta Blocker at Discharge[2]	269	99%	95%	90%	100%
Fibrinolytic Medication Timing[2]	0	-	40%	31%	100%
PCI Within 90 Minutes of Arrival[1,2]	10	70%	77%	54%	95%
Smoking Cessation Advice[2]	75	99%	68%	88%	100%
Heart Failure Care					
ACE Inhibitor or ARB for LVSD[2]	135	89%	85%	82%	100%
Discharge Instructions[2]	247	85%	54%	61%	93%
Evaluation of LVS Function[2]	329	100%	77%	83%	99%
Smoking Cessation Advice[2]	30	83%	67%	82%	100%
Pneumonia Care					
Appropriate Initial Antibiotic[2]	73	90%	80%	83%	94%
Blood Culture Timing[2]	72	94%	94%	90%	100%
Influenza Vaccine[1,2]	23	87%	76%	70%	100%
Initial Antibiotic Timing[2]	124	85%	85%	80%	93%
Oxygenation Assessment[2]	167	100%	99%	99%	100%
Pneumococcal Vaccine[2]	134	90%	73%	69%	94%
Smoking Cessation Advice[1,2]	19	79%	70%	80%	100%
Surgical Infection Prevention					
Prophylactic Antibiotic Given[2]	494	94%	78%	77%	95%
Prophylactic Antibiotic Selection[2]	105	97%	94%	90%	100%
Prophylactic Antibiotic Stopped[2]	483	63%	82%	72%	95%
Pregnancy Care					
Inpatient Neonatal Mortality	-	-	-	-	-
Third or Fourth Degree Laceration	-	-	4.42%	3.63%	3.27%

Roseau Area Hospital & Homes

Alternate Name: Roseau Area Hospital
715 Delmore Drive
Roseau, MN 56751
URL: www.rahhinc.com
Ownership: Voluntary non-profit - Private
Emergency Services: Yes

Phone: 218-463-2500
Fax: 218-463-1266
Accredited: Yes
Licensed Beds: 25

Key Personnel:
CEO. . . . . Keith Okeson
Chief Medical Staff. . . . . Ron Brummer, MD
Director Infection/Disease Control . . . . Jane Hirst, RN
Director Medical/Surgical Nursing . . . . Roxanne Fabian
Director Respiratory Therapy . . . . Chris Berger

Measure	Cases	This Hospital	State Average	U.S. Average	Top Hospital
Heart Attack Care					
ACE Inhibitor or ARB for LVSD[1]	1	100%	89%	82%	100%
Aspirin at Arrival[1]	6	100%	92%	92%	100%
Aspirin at Discharge[1]	7	100%	93%	90%	100%
Beta Blocker at Arrival[1]	6	67%	88%	87%	100%
Beta Blocker at Discharge[1]	5	100%	95%	90%	100%
Fibrinolytic Medication Timing[1]	1	100%	40%	31%	100%
PCI Within 90 Minutes of Arrival	0	-	77%	54%	95%
Smoking Cessation Advice	0	-	68%	88%	100%
Heart Failure Care					
ACE Inhibitor or ARB for LVSD[1]	6	83%	85%	82%	100%
Discharge Instructions[1]	18	22%	54%	61%	93%
Evaluation of LVS Function	29	45%	77%	83%	99%
Smoking Cessation Advice[1]	1	100%	67%	82%	100%
Pneumonia Care					
Appropriate Initial Antibiotic[1]	24	88%	80%	83%	94%
Blood Culture Timing[1]	14	86%	94%	90%	100%
Influenza Vaccine[1]	9	78%	76%	70%	100%
Initial Antibiotic Timing	25	76%	85%	80%	93%
Oxygenation Assessment	42	98%	99%	99%	100%
Pneumococcal Vaccine	28	79%	73%	69%	94%
Smoking Cessation Advice[1]	4	75%	70%	80%	100%
Surgical Infection Prevention					
Prophylactic Antibiotic Given[5]	-	-	78%	77%	95%
Prophylactic Antibiotic Selection[5]	-	-	94%	90%	100%
Prophylactic Antibiotic Stopped[5]	-	-	82%	72%	95%
Pregnancy Care					
Inpatient Neonatal Mortality	-	-	-	-	-

NOTE: Hospital profiles are in alphabetical order by state, then city, then hospital within the city; Rankings are sorted by rate in descending order and exclude hospitals with less than 25 cases; (1) The number of cases is too small (n<25) for purposes of reliably predicting hospital performance; (2) Measure reflects the hospital's indication that its submission was based upon a sample of its relevant discharges; (3) Rate reflects fewer than the maximum possible quarters of data for the measure; (4) Inaccurate information submitted and suppressed for one or more quarters; (5) No data is available from the hospital for this measure; Please refer to the User's Guide for a full explanation of data

Third or Fourth Degree Laceration	-	-	4.42%	3.63%	3.27%

Saint Cloud Hospital

1406 Sixth Avenue North
Saint Cloud, MN 56303
Toll-Free: 800-835-6652
Phone: 320-251-2700
Fax: 320-255-5711
URL: www.centracare.com
Ownership: Voluntary non-profit - Private
Accredited: Yes
Emergency Services: Yes
Licensed Beds: 489

Key Personnel:

CEO. . . . . Craig Broman
Chief Medical Staff. . . . . Paul Dorsher, MD
Emergency Room . . . . Peter Charvat
Emergency Room . . . . Jack Stinolgel, DO
OB/GYN Womens Health. . . . . Janell Strom, MD
Manager Radiology . . . . Mary Super

Measure	Cases	This Hospital	State Average	U.S. Average	Top Hospital
Heart Attack Care					
ACE Inhibitor or ARB for LVSD[2]	113	88%	89%	82%	100%
Aspirin at Arrival[2]	211	99%	92%	92%	100%
Aspirin at Discharge[2]	570	99%	93%	90%	100%
Beta Blocker at Arrival[2]	168	96%	88%	87%	100%
Beta Blocker at Discharge[2]	604	99%	95%	90%	100%
Fibrinolytic Medication Timing[2]	0	-	40%	31%	100%
PCI Within 90 Minutes of Arrival[1,2]	11	82%	77%	54%	95%
Smoking Cessation Advice[2]	213	95%	68%	88%	100%
Heart Failure Care					
ACE Inhibitor or ARB for LVSD[2]	256	85%	85%	82%	100%
Discharge Instructions[2]	430	75%	54%	61%	93%
Evaluation of LVS Function[2]	556	97%	77%	83%	99%
Smoking Cessation Advice[2]	73	75%	67%	82%	100%
Pneumonia Care					
Appropriate Initial Antibiotic	209	92%	80%	83%	94%
Blood Culture Timing	226	96%	94%	90%	100%
Influenza Vaccine	63	90%	76%	70%	100%
Initial Antibiotic Timing	314	87%	85%	80%	93%
Oxygenation Assessment	390	100%	99%	99%	100%
Pneumococcal Vaccine	287	92%	73%	69%	94%
Smoking Cessation Advice	87	80%	70%	80%	100%
Surgical Infection Prevention					
Prophylactic Antibiotic Given[2]	436	60%	78%	77%	95%
Prophylactic Antibiotic Selection[2]	86	95%	94%	90%	100%
Prophylactic Antibiotic Stopped[2]	418	76%	82%	72%	95%
Pregnancy Care					
Inpatient Neonatal Mortality	-	-	-	-	-
Third or Fourth Degree Laceration	-	-	4.42%	3.63%	3.27%

Saint James Health Services

1207 6th Avenue South
Saint James, MN 56081
Phone: 507-375-3261
Fax: 507-375-8605
URL: www.stjmc.org
Ownership: Voluntary non-profit - Other
Accredited: Yes
Emergency Services: Yes
Licensed Beds: 31

Key Personnel:

Administrator . . . . Lee Holter
Emergency Room . . . . Linda Winkleman
Director Infection/Disease Control . . . . Sue Piper

Measure	Cases	This Hospital	State Average	U.S. Average	Top Hospital
Heart Attack Care					
ACE Inhibitor or ARB for LVSD[5]	-	-	89%	82%	100%
Aspirin at Arrival[5]	-	-	92%	92%	100%
Aspirin at Discharge[5]	-	-	93%	90%	100%
Beta Blocker at Arrival[5]	-	-	88%	87%	100%
Beta Blocker at Discharge[5]	-	-	95%	90%	100%
Fibrinolytic Medication Timing[5]	-	-	40%	31%	100%
PCI Within 90 Minutes of Arrival[5]	-	-	77%	54%	95%
Smoking Cessation Advice[5]	-	-	68%	88%	100%
Heart Failure Care					
ACE Inhibitor or ARB for LVSD[1]	5	80%	85%	82%	100%
Discharge Instructions[1]	8	38%	54%	61%	93%
Evaluation of LVS Function[1]	13	54%	77%	83%	99%
Smoking Cessation Advice[1]	2	0%	67%	82%	100%
Pneumonia Care					
Appropriate Initial Antibiotic[1]	10	50%	80%	83%	94%
Blood Culture Timing	0	-	94%	90%	100%
Influenza Vaccine[1]	1	0%	76%	70%	100%
Initial Antibiotic Timing[1]	12	92%	85%	80%	93%
Oxygenation Assessment[1]	14	100%	99%	99%	100%
Pneumococcal Vaccine[1]	11	27%	73%	69%	94%
Smoking Cessation Advice[1]	2	100%	70%	80%	100%
Surgical Infection Prevention					
Prophylactic Antibiotic Given[5]	-	-	78%	77%	95%
Prophylactic Antibiotic Selection[5]	-	-	94%	90%	100%
Prophylactic Antibiotic Stopped[5]	-	-	82%	72%	95%
Pregnancy Care					
Inpatient Neonatal Mortality	-	-	-	-	-
Third or Fourth Degree Laceration	-	-	4.42%	3.63%	3.27%

Methodist Hospital

6500 Excelsior Boulevard
Saint Louis Park, MN 55426
Phone: 952-993-5000
Fax: 952-993-1638
URL: www.parknicollet.com/methodist
Ownership: Voluntary non-profit - Private
Accredited: Yes
Emergency Services: Yes
Licensed Beds: 426

Key Personnel:

President/CEO. . . . . David Wessner

Measure	Cases	This Hospital	State Average	U.S. Average	Top Hospital
Heart Attack Care					
ACE Inhibitor or ARB for LVSD	72	96%	89%	82%	100%
Aspirin at Arrival	273	100%	92%	92%	100%
Aspirin at Discharge	318	99%	93%	90%	100%
Beta Blocker at Arrival	199	96%	88%	87%	100%
Beta Blocker at Discharge	329	99%	95%	90%	100%
Fibrinolytic Medication Timing	0	-	40%	31%	100%
PCI Within 90 Minutes of Arrival[1]	13	85%	77%	54%	95%
Smoking Cessation Advice	94	95%	68%	88%	100%
Heart Failure Care					
ACE Inhibitor or ARB for LVSD	203	90%	85%	82%	100%
Discharge Instructions	409	72%	54%	61%	93%
Evaluation of LVS Function	536	99%	77%	83%	99%
Smoking Cessation Advice	54	85%	67%	82%	100%
Pneumonia Care					
Appropriate Initial Antibiotic	289	90%	80%	83%	94%
Blood Culture Timing	269	92%	94%	90%	100%
Influenza Vaccine	97	73%	76%	70%	100%
Initial Antibiotic Timing	431	83%	85%	80%	93%
Oxygenation Assessment	566	100%	99%	99%	100%
Pneumococcal Vaccine	377	79%	73%	69%	94%
Smoking Cessation Advice	117	79%	70%	80%	100%
Surgical Infection Prevention					
Prophylactic Antibiotic Given[2,3]	236	97%	78%	77%	95%
Prophylactic Antibiotic Selection[2]	82	89%	94%	90%	100%
Prophylactic Antibiotic Stopped[2,3]	232	91%	82%	72%	95%
Pregnancy Care					
Inpatient Neonatal Mortality	3,814	0.08%	-	-	-
Third or Fourth Degree Laceration	2,801	4.03%	4.42%	3.63%	3.27%

Regions Hospital

640 Jackson Street
Saint Paul, MN 55101
Phone: 651-254-3456
Fax: 651-254-2836
URL: www.regionshospital.com
Ownership: Govt - Hospital District or Authority
Accredited: Yes
Emergency Services: Yes
Licensed Beds: 427

Key Personnel:

Administrator/President . . . . Terri Finzen
Chief Medical Staff. . . . . Sue Freeman, MD
Chief Catheterization Laboratory . . . . Deb McKane
Emergency Room . . . . Wayne Hass, MD
CCU Spvg. Nurse . . . . Shirley Hubenette
OB/GYN Womens Health. . . . . Dennis Bealka, MD
Chief Radiology . . . . Joseph Tashjiam, MD
Director Respiratory Therapy . . . . Sandy Presnail

NOTE: Hospital profiles are in alphabetical order by state, then city, then hospital within the city; Rankings are sorted by rate in descending order and exclude hospitals with less than 25 cases; (1) The number of cases is too small (n<25) for purposes of reliably predicting hospital performance; (2) Measure reflects the hospital's indication that its submission was based upon a sample of its relevant discharges; (3) Rate reflects fewer than the maximum possible quarters of data for the measure; (4) Inaccurate information submitted and suppressed for one or more quarters; (5) No data is available from the hospital for this measure; Please refer to the User's Guide for a full explanation of data

Measure	Cases	This Hospital	State Average	U.S. Average	Top Hospital
Heart Attack Care					
ACE Inhibitor or ARB for LVSD	87	89%	89%	82%	100%
Aspirin at Arrival	251	99%	92%	92%	100%
Aspirin at Discharge	336	98%	93%	90%	100%
Beta Blocker at Arrival	217	97%	88%	87%	100%
Beta Blocker at Discharge	350	98%	95%	90%	100%
Fibrinolytic Medication Timing[1]	1	100%	40%	31%	100%
PCI Within 90 Minutes of Arrival[1]	11	100%	77%	54%	95%
Smoking Cessation Advice	118	98%	68%	88%	100%
Heart Failure Care					
ACE Inhibitor or ARB for LVSD	165	90%	85%	82%	100%
Discharge Instructions	266	73%	54%	61%	93%
Evaluation of LVS Function	383	98%	77%	83%	99%
Smoking Cessation Advice	98	99%	67%	82%	100%
Pneumonia Care					
Appropriate Initial Antibiotic	193	84%	80%	83%	94%
Blood Culture Timing	181	87%	94%	90%	100%
Influenza Vaccine	67	54%	76%	70%	100%
Initial Antibiotic Timing	336	76%	85%	80%	93%
Oxygenation Assessment	428	100%	99%	99%	100%
Pneumococcal Vaccine	257	70%	73%	69%	94%
Smoking Cessation Advice	128	93%	70%	80%	100%
Surgical Infection Prevention					
Prophylactic Antibiotic Given[2]	960	88%	78%	77%	95%
Prophylactic Antibiotic Selection[2]	237	95%	94%	90%	100%
Prophylactic Antibiotic Stopped[2]	892	77%	82%	72%	95%
Pregnancy Care					
Inpatient Neonatal Mortality	-	-	-	-	-
Third or Fourth Degree Laceration	-	-	4.42%	3.63%	3.27%

Saint Joseph's Hospital

Alternate Name: HealthEast Saint Joseph's Hospital
69 W Exchange Street
Saint Paul, MN 55102
Phone: 651-232-3000
Fax: 651-232-3601
Ownership: Voluntary non-profit - Private
Accredited: Yes
Emergency Services: Yes
Licensed Beds: 401

Key Personnel:

CEO . . . . Soett Batulif
Chief Medical Staff . . . . Ken Hoj, MD
Chief Catheterization Laboratory . . . . Randall Johnson, MD
Emergency Room . . . . Patrick Marabella, MD
Director Infection/Disease Control . . . . Luis Villar, MD
CCU Spvg. Nurse . . . . Colleen Nadeau
Director Medical/Surgical Nursing . . . . Barb Miller-Maclin
OB/GYN Womens Health . . . . R Mjanger, MD
Director Respiratory Therapy . . . . Scott Sapp

Measure	Cases	This Hospital	State Average	U.S. Average	Top Hospital
Heart Attack Care					
ACE Inhibitor or ARB for LVSD[2]	50	94%	89%	82%	100%
Aspirin at Arrival[2]	152	99%	92%	92%	100%
Aspirin at Discharge[2]	253	100%	93%	90%	100%
Beta Blocker at Arrival[2]	96	96%	88%	87%	100%
Beta Blocker at Discharge[2]	218	98%	95%	90%	100%
Fibrinolytic Medication Timing[2]	0	-	40%	31%	100%
PCI Within 90 Minutes of Arrival[1,2]	10	60%	77%	54%	95%
Smoking Cessation Advice[2]	101	97%	68%	88%	100%
Heart Failure Care					
ACE Inhibitor or ARB for LVSD[2]	137	89%	85%	82%	100%
Discharge Instructions[2]	234	87%	54%	61%	93%
Evaluation of LVS Function[2]	314	96%	77%	83%	99%
Smoking Cessation Advice[2]	49	92%	67%	82%	100%
Pneumonia Care					
Appropriate Initial Antibiotic	81	90%	80%	83%	94%
Blood Culture Timing	70	79%	94%	90%	100%
Influenza Vaccine	27	74%	76%	70%	100%
Initial Antibiotic Timing	159	91%	85%	80%	93%
Oxygenation Assessment	190	100%	99%	99%	100%
Pneumococcal Vaccine	106	83%	73%	69%	94%
Smoking Cessation Advice	40	58%	70%	80%	100%
Surgical Infection Prevention					
Prophylactic Antibiotic Given[2,3]	533	59%	78%	77%	95%
Prophylactic Antibiotic Selection[2]	152	98%	94%	90%	100%
Prophylactic Antibiotic Stopped[2,3]	511	78%	82%	72%	95%
Pregnancy Care					
Inpatient Neonatal Mortality	1,038	0.19%	-	-	-
Third or Fourth Degree Laceration	910	2.64%	4.42%	3.63%	3.27%

United Hospital

333 N Smith Avenue
Saint Paul, MN 55102
Phone: 651-241-8000
Fax: 651-241-8118
Ownership: Voluntary non-profit - Private
Accredited: Yes
Emergency Services: Yes
Licensed Beds: 572

Key Personnel:

CEO/President . . . . Mark Mishek
Chief Medical Staff . . . . Daniel Foley, MD
Director Infection/Disease Control . . . . Anita Romani
CCU Spvg. Nurse . . . . Julianne Deutsch

Measure	Cases	This Hospital	State Average	U.S. Average	Top Hospital
Heart Attack Care					
ACE Inhibitor or ARB for LVSD	74	89%	89%	82%	100%
Aspirin at Arrival	288	98%	92%	92%	100%
Aspirin at Discharge	462	98%	93%	90%	100%
Beta Blocker at Arrival	228	96%	88%	87%	100%
Beta Blocker at Discharge	499	98%	95%	90%	100%
Fibrinolytic Medication Timing[1]	1	0%	40%	31%	100%
PCI Within 90 Minutes of Arrival[1]	22	100%	77%	54%	95%
Smoking Cessation Advice	170	99%	68%	88%	100%
Heart Failure Care					
ACE Inhibitor or ARB for LVSD	272	76%	85%	82%	100%
Discharge Instructions	404	74%	54%	61%	93%
Evaluation of LVS Function	544	92%	77%	83%	99%
Smoking Cessation Advice	73	88%	67%	82%	100%
Pneumonia Care					
Appropriate Initial Antibiotic	225	79%	80%	83%	94%
Blood Culture Timing	176	87%	94%	90%	100%
Influenza Vaccine	47	70%	76%	70%	100%
Initial Antibiotic Timing	287	70%	85%	80%	93%
Oxygenation Assessment	340	99%	99%	99%	100%
Pneumococcal Vaccine	197	59%	73%	69%	94%
Smoking Cessation Advice	80	84%	70%	80%	100%
Surgical Infection Prevention					
Prophylactic Antibiotic Given[2,3]	171	46%	78%	77%	95%
Prophylactic Antibiotic Selection[2]	94	96%	94%	90%	100%
Prophylactic Antibiotic Stopped[2,3]	168	73%	82%	72%	95%
Pregnancy Care					
Inpatient Neonatal Mortality	-	-	-	-	-
Third or Fourth Degree Laceration	-	-	4.42%	3.63%	3.27%

Saint Peter Community Hospital

1900 Sunrise Drive
Saint Peter, MN 56082
Phone: 507-931-2200
Fax: 507-934-7651
URL: www.stpeterhealth.org
Ownership: Government - Local
Accredited: No
Emergency Services: No

Key Personnel:

CEO . . . . Jeanne Johnson
Chief Medical Staff . . . . Paulette Redman
Director Infection/Disease Control . . . . Jan Wimpsett
Director Medical/Surgical Nursing . . . . Marcia Narveson
Chief Radiology . . . . Judy Hahn

Measure	Cases	This Hospital	State Average	U.S. Average	Top Hospital
Heart Attack Care					
ACE Inhibitor or ARB for LVSD[3]	0	-	89%	82%	100%
Aspirin at Arrival[1,3]	3	100%	92%	92%	100%
Aspirin at Discharge[1,3]	2	100%	93%	90%	100%
Beta Blocker at Arrival[1,3]	4	75%	88%	87%	100%
Beta Blocker at Discharge[1,3]	3	100%	95%	90%	100%
Fibrinolytic Medication Timing[3]	0	-	40%	31%	100%
PCI Within 90 Minutes of Arrival[5]	-	-	77%	54%	95%
Smoking Cessation Advice[3]	0	-	68%	88%	100%

NOTE: Hospital profiles are in alphabetical order by state, then city, then hospital within the city; Rankings are sorted by rate in descending order and exclude hospitals with less than 25 cases; (1) The number of cases is too small (n<25) for purposes of reliably predicting hospital performance; (2) Measure reflects the hospital's indication that its submission was based upon a sample of its relevant discharges; (3) Rate reflects fewer than the maximum possible quarters of data for the measure; (4) Inaccurate information submitted and suppressed for one or more quarters; (5) No data is available from the hospital for this measure; Please refer to the User's Guide for a full explanation of data

Heart Failure Care					
ACE Inhibitor or ARB for LVSD[1]	8	50%	85%	82%	100%
Discharge Instructions[1]	13	8%	54%	61%	93%
Evaluation of LVS Function	26	65%	77%	83%	99%
Smoking Cessation Advice[1]	5	0%	67%	82%	100%
Pneumonia Care					
Appropriate Initial Antibiotic[1]	23	96%	80%	83%	94%
Blood Culture Timing[1]	14	100%	94%	90%	100%
Influenza Vaccine[1]	9	89%	76%	70%	100%
Initial Antibiotic Timing	27	85%	85%	80%	93%
Oxygenation Assessment	35	100%	99%	99%	100%
Pneumococcal Vaccine[1]	24	83%	73%	69%	94%
Smoking Cessation Advice[1]	3	33%	70%	80%	100%
Surgical Infection Prevention					
Prophylactic Antibiotic Given[5]	-	-	78%	77%	95%
Prophylactic Antibiotic Selection[5]	-	-	94%	90%	100%
Prophylactic Antibiotic Stopped[5]	-	-	82%	72%	95%
Pregnancy Care					
Inpatient Neonatal Mortality	-	-	-	-	-
Third or Fourth Degree Laceration	-	-	4.42%	3.63%	3.27%

Saint Michael's Hospital & Nursing Home

425 N Elm Street — Phone: 320-352-2221
Sauk Centre, MN 56378 — Fax: 320-352-5150
E-mail: andreaf@stmichaelshospital.org
URL: www.stmichaelshospital.org
Ownership: Proprietary — Accredited: No
Emergency Services: Yes — Licensed Beds: 28

Key Personnel:
CEO. . . . . Del Christianson
Chief Medical Staff. . . . . Keith Olson, MD
Director Radiology . . . . Marie George

Measure	Cases	This Hospital	State Average	U.S. Average	Top Hospital
Heart Attack Care					
ACE Inhibitor or ARB for LVSD[5]	-	-	89%	82%	100%
Aspirin at Arrival[5]	-	-	92%	92%	100%
Aspirin at Discharge[5]	-	-	93%	90%	100%
Beta Blocker at Arrival[5]	-	-	88%	87%	100%
Beta Blocker at Discharge[5]	-	-	95%	90%	100%
Fibrinolytic Medication Timing[5]	-	-	40%	31%	100%
PCI Within 90 Minutes of Arrival[5]	-	-	77%	54%	95%
Smoking Cessation Advice[5]	-	-	68%	88%	100%
Heart Failure Care					
ACE Inhibitor or ARB for LVSD[1]	1	100%	85%	82%	100%
Discharge Instructions[1]	4	0%	54%	61%	93%
Evaluation of LVS Function[1]	6	100%	77%	83%	99%
Smoking Cessation Advice[1]	1	0%	67%	82%	100%
Pneumonia Care					
Appropriate Initial Antibiotic[1]	13	85%	80%	83%	94%
Blood Culture Timing[1]	6	100%	94%	90%	100%
Influenza Vaccine[1]	1	100%	76%	70%	100%
Initial Antibiotic Timing[1]	19	100%	85%	80%	93%
Oxygenation Assessment[1]	20	100%	99%	99%	100%
Pneumococcal Vaccine[1]	14	50%	73%	69%	94%
Smoking Cessation Advice[1]	2	50%	70%	80%	100%
Surgical Infection Prevention					
Prophylactic Antibiotic Given[1]	10	80%	78%	77%	95%
Prophylactic Antibiotic Selection[1]	2	100%	94%	90%	100%
Prophylactic Antibiotic Stopped[1]	10	100%	82%	72%	95%
Pregnancy Care					
Inpatient Neonatal Mortality	-	-	-	-	-
Third or Fourth Degree Laceration	-	-	4.42%	3.63%	3.27%

Saint Francis Regional Medical Center

1455 Saint Francis Avenue — Phone: 952-403-3000
Shakopee, MN 55379 — Fax: 952-403-2767
Ownership: Voluntary non-profit - Church — Accredited: Yes
Emergency Services: Yes — Licensed Beds: 70

Key Personnel:
President . . . . Thomas O'Connor

Measure	Cases	This Hospital	State Average	U.S. Average	Top Hospital
Heart Attack Care					
ACE Inhibitor or ARB for LVSD	0	-	89%	82%	100%
Aspirin at Arrival[1]	11	82%	92%	92%	100%
Aspirin at Discharge[1]	3	100%	93%	90%	100%
Beta Blocker at Arrival[1]	10	60%	88%	87%	100%
Beta Blocker at Discharge[1]	2	100%	95%	90%	100%
Fibrinolytic Medication Timing	0	-	40%	31%	100%
PCI Within 90 Minutes of Arrival	0	-	77%	54%	95%
Smoking Cessation Advice	0	-	68%	88%	100%
Heart Failure Care					
ACE Inhibitor or ARB for LVSD	34	82%	85%	82%	100%
Discharge Instructions	62	56%	54%	61%	93%
Evaluation of LVS Function	90	87%	77%	83%	99%
Smoking Cessation Advice[1]	7	86%	67%	82%	100%
Pneumonia Care					
Appropriate Initial Antibiotic	62	84%	80%	83%	94%
Blood Culture Timing	56	96%	94%	90%	100%
Influenza Vaccine[1]	23	74%	76%	70%	100%
Initial Antibiotic Timing	110	96%	85%	80%	93%
Oxygenation Assessment	134	100%	99%	99%	100%
Pneumococcal Vaccine	85	71%	73%	69%	94%
Smoking Cessation Advice	29	97%	70%	80%	100%
Surgical Infection Prevention					
Prophylactic Antibiotic Given[2,3]	75	84%	78%	77%	95%
Prophylactic Antibiotic Selection[2]	35	97%	94%	90%	100%
Prophylactic Antibiotic Stopped[2,3]	72	83%	82%	72%	95%
Pregnancy Care					
Inpatient Neonatal Mortality	-	-	-	-	-
Third or Fourth Degree Laceration	-	-	4.42%	3.63%	3.27%

Springfield Medical Center

625 N Jackson — Phone: 507-723-6201
Springfield, MN 56087 — Fax: 507-723-6447
URL: www.mayohealthsystem.org
Ownership: Voluntary non-profit - Private — Accredited: Yes
Emergency Services: Yes — Licensed Beds: 24

Key Personnel:
Administrator . . . . Scott Thoreson
Chief Medical Staff. . . . . Margo Woodford
Emergency Room . . . . Margo Woodford, RN
Director Infection/Disease Control . . . . Janet Redman
Chief Radiology . . . . Denise Reiner

Measure	Cases	This Hospital	State Average	U.S. Average	Top Hospital
Heart Attack Care					
ACE Inhibitor or ARB for LVSD[1,3]	1	100%	89%	82%	100%
Aspirin at Arrival[1,3]	2	100%	92%	92%	100%
Aspirin at Discharge[1,3]	1	100%	93%	90%	100%
Beta Blocker at Arrival[1,3]	2	100%	88%	87%	100%
Beta Blocker at Discharge[1,3]	2	100%	95%	90%	100%
Fibrinolytic Medication Timing[3]	0	-	40%	31%	100%
PCI Within 90 Minutes of Arrival[5]	-	-	77%	54%	95%
Smoking Cessation Advice[3]	0	-	68%	88%	100%
Heart Failure Care					
ACE Inhibitor or ARB for LVSD[1]	2	100%	85%	82%	100%
Discharge Instructions[1]	10	100%	54%	61%	93%
Evaluation of LVS Function[1]	18	83%	77%	83%	99%
Smoking Cessation Advice	0	-	67%	82%	100%
Pneumonia Care					
Appropriate Initial Antibiotic[1]	12	100%	80%	83%	94%
Blood Culture Timing[1]	1	100%	94%	90%	100%
Influenza Vaccine[1]	2	100%	76%	70%	100%
Initial Antibiotic Timing[1]	15	93%	85%	80%	93%
Oxygenation Assessment[1]	20	100%	99%	99%	100%
Pneumococcal Vaccine[1]	12	67%	73%	69%	94%
Smoking Cessation Advice[1]	3	100%	70%	80%	100%
Surgical Infection Prevention					
Prophylactic Antibiotic Given[1]	12	58%	78%	77%	95%
Prophylactic Antibiotic Selection[1]	1	100%	94%	90%	100%
Prophylactic Antibiotic Stopped[1]	10	70%	82%	72%	95%
Pregnancy Care					

NOTE: Hospital profiles are in alphabetical order by state, then city, then hospital within the city; Rankings are sorted by rate in descending order and exclude hospitals with less than 25 cases; (1) The number of cases is too small (n<25) for purposes of reliably predicting hospital performance; (2) Measure reflects the hospital's indication that its submission was based upon a sample of its relevant discharges; (3) Rate reflects fewer than the maximum possible quarters of data for the measure; (4) Inaccurate information submitted and suppressed for one or more quarters; (5) No data is available from the hospital for this measure; Please refer to the User's Guide for a full explanation of data

Inpatient Neonatal Mortality	-	-	-	-	-
Third or Fourth Degree Laceration	-	-	4.42%	3.63%	3.27%

Lakewood Health System Hospital

49725 County 83
Staples, MN 56479
Phone: 218-894-1515
Fax: 218-894-8355
E-mail: janetjacobson@lakewoodhealthsystem.com
URL: www.lakewoodhealthsystem.com
Ownership: Voluntary non-profit - Private
Accredited: No
Emergency Services: Yes
Licensed Beds: 140

Key Personnel:
CEO. . . . . Tim Rice
Chief Medical Staff. . . . . John Halfen, MD
Emergency Room . . . . Laurie Bach, MD

Measure	Cases	This Hospital	State Average	U.S. Average	Top Hospital
Heart Attack Care					
ACE Inhibitor or ARB for LVSD[3]	0	-	89%	82%	100%
Aspirin at Arrival[1,3]	2	100%	92%	92%	100%
Aspirin at Discharge[1,3]	1	100%	93%	90%	100%
Beta Blocker at Arrival[1,3]	2	100%	88%	87%	100%
Beta Blocker at Discharge[1,3]	1	100%	95%	90%	100%
Fibrinolytic Medication Timing[3]	0	-	40%	31%	100%
PCI Within 90 Minutes of Arrival	0	-	77%	54%	95%
Smoking Cessation Advice[1,3]	1	0%	68%	88%	100%
Heart Failure Care					
ACE Inhibitor or ARB for LVSD[1]	5	100%	85%	82%	100%
Discharge Instructions[1]	24	4%	54%	61%	93%
Evaluation of LVS Function	34	47%	77%	83%	99%
Smoking Cessation Advice[1]	6	17%	67%	82%	100%
Pneumonia Care					
Appropriate Initial Antibiotic	36	61%	80%	83%	94%
Blood Culture Timing[1]	4	100%	94%	90%	100%
Influenza Vaccine[1]	7	29%	76%	70%	100%
Initial Antibiotic Timing	43	91%	85%	80%	93%
Oxygenation Assessment	53	100%	99%	99%	100%
Pneumococcal Vaccine	37	19%	73%	69%	94%
Smoking Cessation Advice[1]	9	22%	70%	80%	100%
Surgical Infection Prevention					
Prophylactic Antibiotic Given	39	92%	78%	77%	95%
Prophylactic Antibiotic Selection[1]	8	100%	94%	90%	100%
Prophylactic Antibiotic Stopped	37	76%	82%	72%	95%
Pregnancy Care					
Inpatient Neonatal Mortality	-	-	-	-	-
Third or Fourth Degree Laceration	-	-	4.42%	3.63%	3.27%

Lakeview Hospital

927 Churchill Street West
Stillwater, MN 55082
Toll-Free: 800-423-7212
Phone: 651-439-4556
Fax: 651-430-4528

URL: www.lakeview.org
Ownership: Voluntary non-profit - Private
Accredited: Yes
Emergency Services: Yes
Licensed Beds: 98

Key Personnel:
CEO. . . . . Jeff Robertson
Emergency Room . . . . Di Anne, RN

Measure	Cases	This Hospital	State Average	U.S. Average	Top Hospital
Heart Attack Care					
ACE Inhibitor or ARB for LVSD[1]	3	100%	89%	82%	100%
Aspirin at Arrival[1]	20	85%	92%	92%	100%
Aspirin at Discharge[1]	14	93%	93%	90%	100%
Beta Blocker at Arrival[1]	11	100%	88%	87%	100%
Beta Blocker at Discharge[1]	16	100%	95%	90%	100%
Fibrinolytic Medication Timing	0	-	40%	31%	100%
PCI Within 90 Minutes of Arrival	0	-	77%	54%	95%
Smoking Cessation Advice[1]	1	100%	68%	88%	100%
Heart Failure Care					
ACE Inhibitor or ARB for LVSD[1]	14	93%	85%	82%	100%
Discharge Instructions	50	76%	54%	61%	93%
Evaluation of LVS Function	68	94%	77%	83%	99%
Smoking Cessation Advice[1]	4	100%	67%	82%	100%
Pneumonia Care					
Appropriate Initial Antibiotic	57	93%	80%	83%	94%
Blood Culture Timing	34	97%	94%	90%	100%
Influenza Vaccine[1]	22	95%	76%	70%	100%
Initial Antibiotic Timing	84	92%	85%	80%	93%
Oxygenation Assessment	103	100%	99%	99%	100%
Pneumococcal Vaccine	77	96%	73%	69%	94%
Smoking Cessation Advice[1]	11	82%	70%	80%	100%
Surgical Infection Prevention					
Prophylactic Antibiotic Given[2]	261	87%	78%	77%	95%
Prophylactic Antibiotic Selection[2]	64	100%	94%	90%	100%
Prophylactic Antibiotic Stopped[2]	247	94%	82%	72%	95%
Pregnancy Care					
Inpatient Neonatal Mortality	717	0.14%	-	-	-
Third or Fourth Degree Laceration	549	4.55%	4.42%	3.63%	3.27%

Northwest Medical Center

120 LaBree Avenue South
PO Box 531
Thief River Falls, MN 56701
Phone: 218-681-4240
Fax: 218-681-5614
E-mail: nwmc@nwmc.org
URL: www.nwmc.org
Ownership: Voluntary non-profit - Private
Accredited: No
Emergency Services: Yes
Licensed Beds: 99

Key Personnel:
CEO. . . . . Chris Harff
Director Infection/Disease Control . . . . Sharon Jorde, RN
OB/GYN Womens Health. . . . . Juho Kropp, MD

Measure	Cases	This Hospital	State Average	U.S. Average	Top Hospital
Heart Attack Care					
ACE Inhibitor or ARB for LVSD[1]	1	100%	89%	82%	100%
Aspirin at Arrival[1]	10	100%	92%	92%	100%
Aspirin at Discharge[1]	5	100%	93%	90%	100%
Beta Blocker at Arrival[1]	9	100%	88%	87%	100%
Beta Blocker at Discharge[1]	5	80%	95%	90%	100%
Fibrinolytic Medication Timing[1]	2	50%	40%	31%	100%
PCI Within 90 Minutes of Arrival	0	-	77%	54%	95%
Smoking Cessation Advice	0	-	68%	88%	100%
Heart Failure Care					
ACE Inhibitor or ARB for LVSD[1]	11	36%	85%	82%	100%
Discharge Instructions	36	36%	54%	61%	93%
Evaluation of LVS Function	52	63%	77%	83%	99%
Smoking Cessation Advice[1]	3	67%	67%	82%	100%
Pneumonia Care					
Appropriate Initial Antibiotic	25	76%	80%	83%	94%
Blood Culture Timing[1]	8	88%	94%	90%	100%
Influenza Vaccine[1]	2	100%	76%	70%	100%
Initial Antibiotic Timing	32	81%	85%	80%	93%
Oxygenation Assessment	42	100%	99%	99%	100%
Pneumococcal Vaccine	28	79%	73%	69%	94%
Smoking Cessation Advice[1]	6	50%	70%	80%	100%
Surgical Infection Prevention					
Prophylactic Antibiotic Given	147	89%	78%	77%	95%
Prophylactic Antibiotic Selection	38	95%	94%	90%	100%
Prophylactic Antibiotic Stopped	142	94%	82%	72%	95%
Pregnancy Care					
Inpatient Neonatal Mortality	-	-	-	-	-
Third or Fourth Degree Laceration	-	-	4.42%	3.63%	3.27%

Sanford Tracy Medical Center

251 5th Street E
Tracy, MN 56175
Phone: 507-629-3200
Fax: 507-629-3202
URL: www.sanfordtracy.org
Ownership: Voluntary non-profit - Private
Accredited: No
Emergency Services: Yes
Licensed Beds: 37

Key Personnel:
President/CEO. . . . . Rick Nordahl
Chief Medical Staff. . . . . Jared Fazal, MD
Director Infection/Disease Control . . . . Sue Swan, RN

Measure	Cases	This Hospital	State Average	U.S. Average	Top Hospital

NOTE: Hospital profiles are in alphabetical order by state, then city, then hospital within the city; Rankings are sorted by rate in descending order and exclude hospitals with less than 25 cases; (1) The number of cases is too small (n<25) for purposes of reliably predicting hospital performance; (2) Measure reflects the hospital's indication that its submission was based upon a sample of its relevant discharges; (3) Rate reflects fewer than the maximum possible quarters of data for the measure; (4) Inaccurate information submitted and suppressed for one or more quarters; (5) No data is available from the hospital for this measure; Please refer to the User's Guide for a full explanation of data

Measure	Cases	This Hospital	State Average	U.S. Average	Top Hospital
Heart Attack Care					
ACE Inhibitor or ARB for LVSD[3]	0	-	89%	82%	100%
Aspirin at Arrival[1,3]	1	100%	92%	92%	100%
Aspirin at Discharge[1,3]	1	100%	93%	90%	100%
Beta Blocker at Arrival[1,3]	1	100%	88%	87%	100%
Beta Blocker at Discharge[1,3]	1	100%	95%	90%	100%
Fibrinolytic Medication Timing[3]	0	-	40%	31%	100%
PCI Within 90 Minutes of Arrival	0	-	77%	54%	95%
Smoking Cessation Advice[3]	0	-	68%	88%	100%
Heart Failure Care					
ACE Inhibitor or ARB for LVSD[1,3]	3	67%	85%	82%	100%
Discharge Instructions[1,3]	4	25%	54%	61%	93%
Evaluation of LVS Function[1,3]	8	75%	77%	83%	99%
Smoking Cessation Advice[3]	0	-	67%	82%	100%
Pneumonia Care					
Appropriate Initial Antibiotic[1,3]	4	100%	80%	83%	94%
Blood Culture Timing[1,3]	2	100%	94%	90%	100%
Influenza Vaccine[5]	-	-	76%	70%	100%
Initial Antibiotic Timing[1,3]	7	86%	85%	80%	93%
Oxygenation Assessment[1,3]	8	88%	99%	99%	100%
Pneumococcal Vaccine[1,3]	7	86%	73%	69%	94%
Smoking Cessation Advice[1,3]	1	0%	70%	80%	100%
Surgical Infection Prevention					
Prophylactic Antibiotic Given[5]	-	-	78%	77%	95%
Prophylactic Antibiotic Selection[5]	-	-	94%	90%	100%
Prophylactic Antibiotic Stopped[5]	-	-	82%	72%	95%
Pregnancy Care					
Inpatient Neonatal Mortality	-	-	-	-	-
Third or Fourth Degree Laceration	-	-	4.42%	3.63%	3.27%

Virginia Regional Medical Center

901 9th Street North
Virginia, MN 55792

Toll-Free: 866-441-3340
Phone: 218-741-3340
Fax: 218-749-9448

E-mail: marketing@vrmc.org
URL: www.vrmc.org
Ownership: Government - Local
Emergency Services: Yes

Accredited: Yes
Licensed Beds: 83

Key Personnel:
Administrator . . . . Keith Harvey
Cardiac Rehab Program Coordinator . . . . Heather Parenteau
Director Infection/Disease Control . . . . Jan Jonassen
Respiratory/Cardiopulmonary . . . . Alan Garrison

Measure	Cases	This Hospital	State Average	U.S. Average	Top Hospital
Heart Attack Care					
ACE Inhibitor or ARB for LVSD[1]	3	100%	89%	82%	100%
Aspirin at Arrival[1]	16	94%	92%	92%	100%
Aspirin at Discharge[1]	10	100%	93%	90%	100%
Beta Blocker at Arrival[1]	17	88%	88%	87%	100%
Beta Blocker at Discharge[1]	10	100%	95%	90%	100%
Fibrinolytic Medication Timing[1]	2	100%	40%	31%	100%
PCI Within 90 Minutes of Arrival	0	-	77%	54%	95%
Smoking Cessation Advice	0	-	68%	88%	100%
Heart Failure Care					
ACE Inhibitor or ARB for LVSD[1]	24	96%	85%	82%	100%
Discharge Instructions	54	67%	54%	61%	93%
Evaluation of LVS Function	115	86%	77%	83%	99%
Smoking Cessation Advice[1]	8	75%	67%	82%	100%
Pneumonia Care					
Appropriate Initial Antibiotic	49	80%	80%	83%	94%
Blood Culture Timing	47	91%	94%	90%	100%
Influenza Vaccine	25	60%	76%	70%	100%
Initial Antibiotic Timing	82	66%	85%	80%	93%
Oxygenation Assessment	100	97%	99%	99%	100%
Pneumococcal Vaccine	73	60%	73%	69%	94%
Smoking Cessation Advice[1]	14	79%	70%	80%	100%
Surgical Infection Prevention					
Prophylactic Antibiotic Given[2,3]	55	96%	78%	77%	95%
Prophylactic Antibiotic Selection[1,2]	21	100%	94%	90%	100%
Prophylactic Antibiotic Stopped[2,3]	53	34%	82%	72%	95%
Pregnancy Care					
Inpatient Neonatal Mortality	-	-	-	-	-
Third or Fourth Degree Laceration	-	-	4.42%	3.63%	3.27%

Saint Elizabeth Medical Center

Alternate Name: Saint Elizabeth Medical Center
1200 5th Grant Boulevard West
Wabasha, MN 55981
URL: www.stelizabethswabasha.org
Ownership: Voluntary non-profit - Church
Emergency Services: Yes

Phone: 651-565-4531
Fax: 651-565-2482

Accredited: No
Licensed Beds: 31

Key Personnel:
President/CEO . . . . Thomas Crowley
Chief Medical Staff . . . . Rob Taylor, DO
Emergency Room . . . . Meresa Hager

Measure	Cases	This Hospital	State Average	U.S. Average	Top Hospital
Heart Attack Care					
ACE Inhibitor or ARB for LVSD[3]	0	-	89%	82%	100%
Aspirin at Arrival[1,3]	1	100%	92%	92%	100%
Aspirin at Discharge[1,3]	2	100%	93%	90%	100%
Beta Blocker at Arrival[1,3]	1	100%	88%	87%	100%
Beta Blocker at Discharge[1,3]	2	100%	95%	90%	100%
Fibrinolytic Medication Timing[3]	0	-	40%	31%	100%
PCI Within 90 Minutes of Arrival	0	-	77%	54%	95%
Smoking Cessation Advice[3]	0	-	68%	88%	100%
Heart Failure Care					
ACE Inhibitor or ARB for LVSD[3]	0	-	85%	82%	100%
Discharge Instructions[1,3]	1	100%	54%	61%	93%
Evaluation of LVS Function[1,3]	5	20%	77%	83%	99%
Smoking Cessation Advice[3]	0	-	67%	82%	100%
Pneumonia Care					
Appropriate Initial Antibiotic[1,3]	8	100%	80%	83%	94%
Blood Culture Timing[1,3]	2	100%	94%	90%	100%
Influenza Vaccine[5]	-	-	76%	70%	100%
Initial Antibiotic Timing[1,3]	10	90%	85%	80%	93%
Oxygenation Assessment[1,3]	10	100%	99%	99%	100%
Pneumococcal Vaccine[1,3]	6	83%	73%	69%	94%
Smoking Cessation Advice[1,3]	1	100%	70%	80%	100%
Surgical Infection Prevention					
Prophylactic Antibiotic Given[1,2]	13	77%	78%	77%	95%
Prophylactic Antibiotic Selection[1,2]	3	67%	94%	90%	100%
Prophylactic Antibiotic Stopped[1,2]	13	69%	82%	72%	95%
Pregnancy Care					
Inpatient Neonatal Mortality	-	-	-	-	-
Third or Fourth Degree Laceration	-	-	4.42%	3.63%	3.27%

Ridgeview Medical Center

500 S Maple Street
Waconia, MN 55387

Toll-Free: 800-967-4620
Phone: 952-442-2191
Fax: 952-442-6529

E-mail: info@ridgeviewmedical.org
URL: www.ridgeviewmedical.org
Ownership: Voluntary non-profit - Private
Emergency Services: Yes

Accredited: Yes
Licensed Beds: 129

Key Personnel:
President/CEO . . . . Robert Stevens

Measure	Cases	This Hospital	State Average	U.S. Average	Top Hospital
Heart Attack Care					
ACE Inhibitor or ARB for LVSD[1]	3	67%	89%	82%	100%
Aspirin at Arrival[1]	17	100%	92%	92%	100%
Aspirin at Discharge[1]	8	100%	93%	90%	100%
Beta Blocker at Arrival[1]	18	100%	88%	87%	100%
Beta Blocker at Discharge[1]	11	100%	95%	90%	100%
Fibrinolytic Medication Timing	0	-	40%	31%	100%
PCI Within 90 Minutes of Arrival	0	-	77%	54%	95%
Smoking Cessation Advice	0	-	68%	88%	100%
Heart Failure Care					
ACE Inhibitor or ARB for LVSD	51	98%	85%	82%	100%
Discharge Instructions	66	91%	54%	61%	93%
Evaluation of LVS Function	99	98%	77%	83%	99%
Smoking Cessation Advice[1]	3	100%	67%	82%	100%

NOTE: Hospital profiles are in alphabetical order by state, then city, then hospital within the city; Rankings are sorted by rate in descending order and exclude hospitals with less than 25 cases; (1) The number of cases is too small (n<25) for purposes of reliably predicting hospital performance; (2) Measure reflects the hospital's indication that its submission was based upon a sample of its relevant discharges; (3) Rate reflects fewer than the maximum possible quarters of data for the measure; (4) Inaccurate information submitted and suppressed for one or more quarters; (5) No data is available from the hospital for this measure; Please refer to the User's Guide for a full explanation of data

Pneumonia Care					
Appropriate Initial Antibiotic	79	89%	80%	83%	94%
Blood Culture Timing	143	94%	94%	90%	100%
Influenza Vaccine	37	100%	76%	70%	100%
Initial Antibiotic Timing	123	90%	85%	80%	93%
Oxygenation Assessment	227	100%	99%	99%	100%
Pneumococcal Vaccine	166	99%	73%	69%	94%
Smoking Cessation Advice	29	97%	70%	80%	100%
Surgical Infection Prevention					
Prophylactic Antibiotic Given[2,3]	407	92%	78%	77%	95%
Prophylactic Antibiotic Selection[2]	54	87%	94%	90%	100%
Prophylactic Antibiotic Stopped[2,3]	400	55%	82%	72%	95%
Pregnancy Care					
Inpatient Neonatal Mortality	-	-	-	-	-
Third or Fourth Degree Laceration	-	-	4.42%	3.63%	3.27%

Tri-County Hospital

415 N Jefferson Street
Wadena, MN 56482

Toll-Free: 800-631-1811
Phone: 218-631-3510
Fax: 218-631-7496

E-mail: contact@tricountyhospital.org
URL: www.tricountyhospital.org
Ownership: Voluntary non-profit - Other
Emergency Services: Yes

Accredited: Yes
Licensed Beds: 49

Key Personnel:
CEO. . . . . Dennis Miley
Chief Medical Staff. . . . . Shaneen Schmidt, MD
Cardiac Lab . . . . Lois Miller
Emergency Room . . . . Robin Klemek
Director Infection/Disease Control . . . . Corrinne Neisess
Director Medical/Surgical Nursing . . . . Maureen Ideker
OB/GYN Womens Health. . . . . Kris Wallgren
Chief Radiology . . . . Carol Windels
Director Respiratory Therapy . . . . Pat Malvin

Measure	Cases	This Hospital	State Average	U.S. Average	Top Hospital
Heart Attack Care					
ACE Inhibitor or ARB for LVSD[3]	0	-	89%	82%	100%
Aspirin at Arrival[1,3]	1	100%	92%	92%	100%
Aspirin at Discharge[1,3]	1	100%	93%	90%	100%
Beta Blocker at Arrival[1,3]	1	100%	88%	87%	100%
Beta Blocker at Discharge[1,3]	1	100%	95%	90%	100%
Fibrinolytic Medication Timing[3]	0	-	40%	31%	100%
PCI Within 90 Minutes of Arrival[5]	-	-	77%	54%	95%
Smoking Cessation Advice[3]	0	-	68%	88%	100%
Heart Failure Care					
ACE Inhibitor or ARB for LVSD[1]	13	92%	85%	82%	100%
Discharge Instructions[5]	-	-	54%	61%	93%
Evaluation of LVS Function[5]	-	-	77%	83%	99%
Smoking Cessation Advice[5]	-	-	67%	82%	100%
Pneumonia Care					
Appropriate Initial Antibiotic	80	81%	80%	83%	94%
Blood Culture Timing	25	92%	94%	90%	100%
Influenza Vaccine	26	77%	76%	70%	100%
Initial Antibiotic Timing	109	90%	85%	80%	93%
Oxygenation Assessment	148	99%	99%	99%	100%
Pneumococcal Vaccine	104	68%	73%	69%	94%
Smoking Cessation Advice[1]	22	86%	70%	80%	100%
Surgical Infection Prevention					
Prophylactic Antibiotic Given	29	69%	78%	77%	95%
Prophylactic Antibiotic Selection[1]	5	80%	94%	90%	100%
Prophylactic Antibiotic Stopped	28	57%	82%	72%	95%
Pregnancy Care					
Inpatient Neonatal Mortality	-	-	-	-	-
Third or Fourth Degree Laceration	-	-	4.42%	3.63%	3.27%

Waseca Medical Center-Mayo Health System

Alternate Name: Waseca Area Memorial Hospital

501 N State Street
Waseca, MN 56093
Ownership: Voluntary non-profit - Private
Emergency Services: Yes

Phone: 507-835-1210
Fax: 507-837-4280
Accredited: Yes
Licensed Beds: 35

Key Personnel:
Associate Administrator . . . . Cheryl Pratt
Surgery Manager . . . . Marian Keller

Measure	Cases	This Hospital	State Average	U.S. Average	Top Hospital
Heart Attack Care					
ACE Inhibitor or ARB for LVSD	0	-	89%	82%	100%
Aspirin at Arrival[1]	4	100%	92%	92%	100%
Aspirin at Discharge[1]	2	100%	93%	90%	100%
Beta Blocker at Arrival[1]	5	80%	88%	87%	100%
Beta Blocker at Discharge[1]	3	67%	95%	90%	100%
Fibrinolytic Medication Timing	0	-	40%	31%	100%
PCI Within 90 Minutes of Arrival	0	-	77%	54%	95%
Smoking Cessation Advice[1]	1	100%	68%	88%	100%
Heart Failure Care					
ACE Inhibitor or ARB for LVSD[1]	7	100%	85%	82%	100%
Discharge Instructions[1]	14	64%	54%	61%	93%
Evaluation of LVS Function	25	84%	77%	83%	99%
Smoking Cessation Advice[1]	1	100%	67%	82%	100%
Pneumonia Care					
Appropriate Initial Antibiotic	26	96%	80%	83%	94%
Blood Culture Timing[1]	12	100%	94%	90%	100%
Influenza Vaccine[1]	7	100%	76%	70%	100%
Initial Antibiotic Timing	28	89%	85%	80%	93%
Oxygenation Assessment	36	100%	99%	99%	100%
Pneumococcal Vaccine	26	100%	73%	69%	94%
Smoking Cessation Advice[1]	8	62%	70%	80%	100%
Surgical Infection Prevention					
Prophylactic Antibiotic Given[1,3]	2	50%	78%	77%	95%
Prophylactic Antibiotic Selection[1]	1	100%	94%	90%	100%
Prophylactic Antibiotic Stopped[1,3]	2	100%	82%	72%	95%
Pregnancy Care					
Inpatient Neonatal Mortality	-	-	-	-	-
Third or Fourth Degree Laceration	-	-	4.42%	3.63%	3.27%

Westbrook Health Center

Alternate Name: Schmidt Memorial Hospital
PO Box 188
Westbrook, MN 56183
Ownership: Voluntary non-profit - Private
Emergency Services: Yes

Phone: 507-274-6121
Fax: 507-274-5671
Accredited: No
Licensed Beds: 13

Key Personnel:
CEO. . . . . Rick Nordahl
Chief Medical Staff. . . . . JC Cassel, MD
Emergency Room . . . . Priscilla Comnick
Director Infection/Disease Control . . . . Karen Fay

Measure	Cases	This Hospital	State Average	U.S. Average	Top Hospital
Heart Attack Care					
ACE Inhibitor or ARB for LVSD[5]	-	-	89%	82%	100%
Aspirin at Arrival[5]	-	-	92%	92%	100%
Aspirin at Discharge[5]	-	-	93%	90%	100%
Beta Blocker at Arrival[5]	-	-	88%	87%	100%
Beta Blocker at Discharge[5]	-	-	95%	90%	100%
Fibrinolytic Medication Timing[5]	-	-	40%	31%	100%
PCI Within 90 Minutes of Arrival[5]	-	-	77%	54%	95%
Smoking Cessation Advice[5]	-	-	68%	88%	100%
Heart Failure Care					
ACE Inhibitor or ARB for LVSD[3]	0	-	85%	82%	100%
Discharge Instructions[1,3]	1	0%	54%	61%	93%
Evaluation of LVS Function[1,3]	1	0%	77%	83%	99%
Smoking Cessation Advice[3]	0	-	67%	82%	100%
Pneumonia Care					
Appropriate Initial Antibiotic[1,3]	4	50%	80%	83%	94%
Blood Culture Timing[3]	0	-	94%	90%	100%
Influenza Vaccine[5]	-	-	76%	70%	100%
Initial Antibiotic Timing[1,3]	5	80%	85%	80%	93%
Oxygenation Assessment[1,3]	5	100%	99%	99%	100%

NOTE: Hospital profiles are in alphabetical order by state, then city, then hospital within the city; Rankings are sorted by rate in descending order and exclude hospitals with less than 25 cases; (1) The number of cases is too small (n<25) for purposes of reliably predicting hospital performance; (2) Measure reflects the hospital's indication that its submission was based upon a sample of its relevant discharges; (3) Rate reflects fewer than the maximum possible quarters of data for the measure; (4) Inaccurate information submitted and suppressed for one or more quarters; (5) No data is available from the hospital for this measure; Please refer to the User's Guide for a full explanation of data

Pneumococcal Vaccine[1,3]	2	100%	73%	69%	94%
Smoking Cessation Advice[3]	0	-	70%	80%	100%
Surgical Infection Prevention					
Prophylactic Antibiotic Given[5]	-	-	78%	77%	95%
Prophylactic Antibiotic Selection[5]	-	-	94%	90%	100%
Prophylactic Antibiotic Stopped[5]	-	-	82%	72%	95%
Pregnancy Care					
Inpatient Neonatal Mortality	-	-	-	-	-
Third or Fourth Degree Laceration	-	-	4.42%	3.63%	3.27%

Rice Memorial Hospital

301 Becker Avenue SW
Willmar, MN 56201
Ownership: Government - Local
Emergency Services: Yes

Phone: 320-235-4543
Fax: 320-231-4869
Accredited: Yes
Licensed Beds: 136

Key Personnel:
CEO. . . . . Lawrence J Massa
Chief Medical Staff. . . . . Janae Bell, MD
Emergency Room . . . . John Moran
Director Infection/Disease Control . . . . Barb Piasecki
CCU Spvg. Nurse . . . . Kathy Dillox, RN
Director Medical/Surgical Nursing . . . . Kathy Dillon
OB/GYN Womens Health. . . . . Glenn Buchanan, MD
Director Radiology . . . . Tony Rime
Director Respiratory Therapy . . . . Brent Hanson

Measure	Cases	This Hospital	State Average	U.S. Average	Top Hospital
Heart Attack Care					
ACE Inhibitor or ARB for LVSD[1]	6	100%	89%	82%	100%
Aspirin at Arrival[1]	17	100%	92%	92%	100%
Aspirin at Discharge[1]	11	91%	93%	90%	100%
Beta Blocker at Arrival[1]	15	87%	88%	87%	100%
Beta Blocker at Discharge[1]	15	87%	95%	90%	100%
Fibrinolytic Medication Timing	0	-	40%	31%	100%
PCI Within 90 Minutes of Arrival	0	-	77%	54%	95%
Smoking Cessation Advice	0	-	68%	88%	100%
Heart Failure Care					
ACE Inhibitor or ARB for LVSD[1]	17	88%	85%	82%	100%
Discharge Instructions	74	32%	54%	61%	93%
Evaluation of LVS Function	96	85%	77%	83%	99%
Smoking Cessation Advice[1]	4	100%	67%	82%	100%
Pneumonia Care					
Appropriate Initial Antibiotic	87	86%	80%	83%	94%
Blood Culture Timing	74	92%	94%	90%	100%
Influenza Vaccine[1]	23	96%	76%	70%	100%
Initial Antibiotic Timing	126	83%	85%	80%	93%
Oxygenation Assessment	144	100%	99%	99%	100%
Pneumococcal Vaccine	109	97%	73%	69%	94%
Smoking Cessation Advice[1]	19	95%	70%	80%	100%
Surgical Infection Prevention					
Prophylactic Antibiotic Given	399	76%	78%	77%	95%
Prophylactic Antibiotic Selection	100	88%	94%	90%	100%
Prophylactic Antibiotic Stopped	391	82%	82%	72%	95%
Pregnancy Care					
Inpatient Neonatal Mortality[2]	248	0.00%	-	-	-
Third or Fourth Degree Laceration	666	3.30%	4.42%	3.63%	3.27%

Windom Area Hospital

2150 Hospital Drive
PO Box 339
Windom, MN 56101
E-mail: contactus@windomareahospital.com
URL: www.windomareahospital.com
Ownership: Government - Local
Emergency Services: Yes

Phone: 507-831-2400
Fax: 507-831-5749
Accredited: No
Licensed Beds: 35

Key Personnel:
CEO. . . . . Gerri Burmeister
Chief Medical Staff. . . . . Rod Dynes, MD
Emergency Room . . . . Patty Hinkeldey, RN
Infection Control. . . . . Marcia Fast, RN
Medical Surgical Nursing . . . . Kari Witte, RN

Measure	Cases	This Hospital	State Average	U.S. Average	Top Hospital
Heart Attack Care					
ACE Inhibitor or ARB for LVSD[3]	0	-	89%	82%	100%
Aspirin at Arrival[3]	0	-	92%	92%	100%
Aspirin at Discharge[3]	0	-	93%	90%	100%
Beta Blocker at Arrival[3]	0	-	88%	87%	100%
Beta Blocker at Discharge[3]	0	-	95%	90%	100%
Fibrinolytic Medication Timing[1,3]	1	0%	40%	31%	100%
PCI Within 90 Minutes of Arrival[5]	-	-	77%	54%	95%
Smoking Cessation Advice[3]	0	-	68%	88%	100%
Heart Failure Care					
ACE Inhibitor or ARB for LVSD[1,2]	4	100%	85%	82%	100%
Discharge Instructions[1,2]	12	33%	54%	61%	93%
Evaluation of LVS Function[1,2]	17	71%	77%	83%	99%
Smoking Cessation Advice[2]	0	-	67%	82%	100%
Pneumonia Care					
Appropriate Initial Antibiotic[1]	18	39%	80%	83%	94%
Blood Culture Timing[1]	1	100%	94%	90%	100%
Influenza Vaccine[1]	3	100%	76%	70%	100%
Initial Antibiotic Timing[1]	16	94%	85%	80%	93%
Oxygenation Assessment[1]	18	100%	99%	99%	100%
Pneumococcal Vaccine[1]	12	83%	73%	69%	94%
Smoking Cessation Advice[1]	5	80%	70%	80%	100%
Surgical Infection Prevention					
Prophylactic Antibiotic Given[1,3]	6	67%	78%	77%	95%
Prophylactic Antibiotic Selection[5]	-	-	94%	90%	100%
Prophylactic Antibiotic Stopped[1,3]	6	100%	82%	72%	95%
Pregnancy Care					
Inpatient Neonatal Mortality	-	-	-	-	-
Third or Fourth Degree Laceration	-	-	4.42%	3.63%	3.27%

Community Memorial Hospital

Alternate Name: Winona Health
855 Mankato Avenue
Winona, MN 55987

Toll-Free: 800-944-3960
Phone: 507-454-3650
Fax: 507-457-4413

URL: www.winonahealth.org
Ownership: Voluntary non-profit - Private
Emergency Services: Yes

Accredited: No
Licensed Beds: 99

Key Personnel:
Administrator/President/CEO . . . . Rachelle Schultz
Chief Medical Staff. . . . . Charles Shepard
Emergency Room . . . . Marc Dummit, MD
Director Infection/Disease Control . . . . Linda Pozanc
OB/GYN Womens Health. . . . . Scott Birdsall, MD
Chief Radiology . . . . James Erwin, MD
Director Respiratory Therapy . . . . Gary Haggerty

Measure	Cases	This Hospital	State Average	U.S. Average	Top Hospital
Heart Attack Care					
ACE Inhibitor or ARB for LVSD[1]	4	100%	89%	82%	100%
Aspirin at Arrival[1]	23	100%	92%	92%	100%
Aspirin at Discharge[1]	16	100%	93%	90%	100%
Beta Blocker at Arrival[1]	23	100%	88%	87%	100%
Beta Blocker at Discharge[1]	17	100%	95%	90%	100%
Fibrinolytic Medication Timing[3]	0	-	40%	31%	100%
PCI Within 90 Minutes of Arrival	0	-	77%	54%	95%
Smoking Cessation Advice[3]	0	-	68%	88%	100%
Heart Failure Care					
ACE Inhibitor or ARB for LVSD	29	97%	85%	82%	100%
Discharge Instructions[1,3]	15	93%	54%	61%	93%
Evaluation of LVS Function	86	95%	77%	83%	99%
Smoking Cessation Advice[1,3]	2	100%	67%	82%	100%
Pneumonia Care					
Appropriate Initial Antibiotic[1,3]	23	83%	80%	83%	94%
Blood Culture Timing[1,3]	24	100%	94%	90%	100%
Influenza Vaccine[5]	-	-	76%	70%	100%
Initial Antibiotic Timing	98	94%	85%	80%	93%
Oxygenation Assessment	124	100%	99%	99%	100%
Pneumococcal Vaccine	87	89%	73%	69%	94%
Smoking Cessation Advice[1,3]	7	86%	70%	80%	100%
Surgical Infection Prevention					
Prophylactic Antibiotic Given[3]	30	87%	78%	77%	95%
Prophylactic Antibiotic Selection	30	37%	94%	90%	100%

NOTE: Hospital profiles are in alphabetical order by state, then city, then hospital within the city; Rankings are sorted by rate in descending order and exclude hospitals with less than 25 cases; (1) The number of cases is too small (n<25) for purposes of reliably predicting hospital performance; (2) Measure reflects the hospital's indication that its submission was based upon a sample of its relevant discharges; (3) Rate reflects fewer than the maximum possible quarters of data for the measure; (4) Inaccurate information submitted and suppressed for one or more quarters; (5) No data is available from the hospital for this measure; Please refer to the User's Guide for a full explanation of data

Prophylactic Antibiotic Stopped[3]	30	63%	82%	72%	95%
Pregnancy Care					
Inpatient Neonatal Mortality	-	-	-	-	-
Third or Fourth Degree Laceration	-	-	4.42%	3.63%	3.27%

Woodwinds Health Campus

1925 Woodwinds Drive
Woodbury, MN 55125
URL: www.woodwinds.org
Ownership: Voluntary non-profit - Private
Emergency Services: Yes
Phone: 651-232-0228
Fax: 651-232-2551
Accredited: Yes
Licensed Beds: 70

Key Personnel:
CEO. . . . . Julie Schmidt

Measure	Cases	This Hospital	State Average	U.S. Average	Top Hospital
Heart Attack Care					
ACE Inhibitor or ARB for LVSD[1]	5	80%	89%	82%	100%
Aspirin at Arrival[1]	23	100%	92%	92%	100%
Aspirin at Discharge[1]	7	86%	93%	90%	100%
Beta Blocker at Arrival[1]	13	77%	88%	87%	100%
Beta Blocker at Discharge[1]	4	75%	95%	90%	100%
Fibrinolytic Medication Timing	0	-	40%	31%	100%
PCI Within 90 Minutes of Arrival	0	-	77%	54%	95%
Smoking Cessation Advice[1]	1	100%	68%	88%	100%
Heart Failure Care					
ACE Inhibitor or ARB for LVSD[1]	12	92%	85%	82%	100%
Discharge Instructions	40	72%	54%	61%	93%
Evaluation of LVS Function	49	96%	77%	83%	99%
Smoking Cessation Advice[1]	4	75%	67%	82%	100%
Pneumonia Care					
Appropriate Initial Antibiotic	37	92%	80%	83%	94%
Blood Culture Timing	37	84%	94%	90%	100%
Influenza Vaccine[1]	12	92%	76%	70%	100%
Initial Antibiotic Timing	63	95%	85%	80%	93%
Oxygenation Assessment	83	100%	99%	99%	100%
Pneumococcal Vaccine	54	96%	73%	69%	94%
Smoking Cessation Advice[1]	18	67%	70%	80%	100%
Surgical Infection Prevention					
Prophylactic Antibiotic Given[2,3]	645	71%	78%	77%	95%
Prophylactic Antibiotic Selection[2]	217	99%	94%	90%	100%
Prophylactic Antibiotic Stopped[2,3]	636	83%	82%	72%	95%
Pregnancy Care					
Inpatient Neonatal Mortality	1,508	0.00%	-	-	-
Third or Fourth Degree Laceration	1,137	4.49%	4.42%	3.63%	3.27%

Worthington Regional Hospital

1018 6th Avenue
Worthington, MN 56187
Ownership: Government - Local
Emergency Services: Yes
Phone: 507-372-2941
Fax: 507-372-7686
Accredited: No
Licensed Beds: 93

Key Personnel:
Administrator . . . . Melvin J Platt
Chief Medical Staff. . . . . Mell Platt
Emergency Room . . . . Charles Fitch, MD
Director Infection/Disease Control . . . . LaVonne Foss
CCU Spvg. Nurse . . . . Diane Zandstra

Measure	Cases	This Hospital	State Average	U.S. Average	Top Hospital
Heart Attack Care					
ACE Inhibitor or ARB for LVSD	0	-	89%	82%	100%
Aspirin at Arrival[1]	8	88%	92%	92%	100%
Aspirin at Discharge[1]	6	100%	93%	90%	100%
Beta Blocker at Arrival[1]	8	88%	88%	87%	100%
Beta Blocker at Discharge[1]	7	100%	95%	90%	100%
Fibrinolytic Medication Timing[3]	0	-	40%	31%	100%
PCI Within 90 Minutes of Arrival	0	-	77%	54%	95%
Smoking Cessation Advice[3]	0	-	68%	88%	100%
Heart Failure Care					
ACE Inhibitor or ARB for LVSD[1]	7	71%	85%	82%	100%
Discharge Instructions[1,3]	5	40%	54%	61%	93%
Evaluation of LVS Function	29	79%	77%	83%	99%
Smoking Cessation Advice[3]	0	-	67%	82%	100%
Pneumonia Care					
Appropriate Initial Antibiotic[1,3]	7	100%	80%	83%	94%
Blood Culture Timing[1,3]	3	100%	94%	90%	100%
Influenza Vaccine[5]	-	-	76%	70%	100%
Initial Antibiotic Timing	57	84%	85%	80%	93%
Oxygenation Assessment	69	100%	99%	99%	100%
Pneumococcal Vaccine	52	92%	73%	69%	94%
Smoking Cessation Advice[1,3]	2	50%	70%	80%	100%
Surgical Infection Prevention					
Prophylactic Antibiotic Given[1,3]	14	86%	78%	77%	95%
Prophylactic Antibiotic Selection[1]	14	100%	94%	90%	100%
Prophylactic Antibiotic Stopped[1,3]	14	86%	82%	72%	95%
Pregnancy Care					
Inpatient Neonatal Mortality	-	-	-	-	-
Third or Fourth Degree Laceration	-	-	4.42%	3.63%	3.27%

Fairview Lakes Health Services

5200 Fairview Boulevard
Wyoming, MN 55092
Ownership: Voluntary non-profit - Private
Emergency Services: Yes
Phone: 651-982-7000
Accredited: Yes

Measure	Cases	This Hospital	State Average	U.S. Average	Top Hospital
Heart Attack Care					
ACE Inhibitor or ARB for LVSD[1]	3	100%	89%	82%	100%
Aspirin at Arrival[1]	17	100%	92%	92%	100%
Aspirin at Discharge[1]	10	100%	93%	90%	100%
Beta Blocker at Arrival[1]	16	100%	88%	87%	100%
Beta Blocker at Discharge[1]	11	100%	95%	90%	100%
Fibrinolytic Medication Timing	0	-	40%	31%	100%
PCI Within 90 Minutes of Arrival	0	-	77%	54%	95%
Smoking Cessation Advice[1]	1	0%	68%	88%	100%
Heart Failure Care					
ACE Inhibitor or ARB for LVSD	27	96%	85%	82%	100%
Discharge Instructions	72	40%	54%	61%	93%
Evaluation of LVS Function	94	100%	77%	83%	99%
Smoking Cessation Advice[1]	14	79%	67%	82%	100%
Pneumonia Care					
Appropriate Initial Antibiotic	116	89%	80%	83%	94%
Blood Culture Timing	103	93%	94%	90%	100%
Influenza Vaccine[1]	14	100%	76%	70%	100%
Initial Antibiotic Timing	144	93%	85%	80%	93%
Oxygenation Assessment	168	100%	99%	99%	100%
Pneumococcal Vaccine	102	82%	73%	69%	94%
Smoking Cessation Advice	29	72%	70%	80%	100%
Surgical Infection Prevention					
Prophylactic Antibiotic Given[2,3]	118	94%	78%	77%	95%
Prophylactic Antibiotic Selection[2]	39	100%	94%	90%	100%
Prophylactic Antibiotic Stopped[2,3]	116	69%	82%	72%	95%
Pregnancy Care					
Inpatient Neonatal Mortality	-	-	-	-	-
Third or Fourth Degree Laceration	-	-	4.42%	3.63%	3.27%

NOTE: Hospital profiles are in alphabetical order by state, then city, then hospital within the city; Rankings are sorted by rate in descending order and exclude hospitals with less than 25 cases; (1) The number of cases is too small (n<25) for purposes of reliably predicting hospital performance; (2) Measure reflects the hospital's indication that its submission was based upon a sample of its relevant discharges; (3) Rate reflects fewer than the maximum possible quarters of data for the measure; (4) Inaccurate information submitted and suppressed for one or more quarters; (5) No data is available from the hospital for this measure; Please refer to the User's Guide for a full explanation of data

Heart Attack Care

1. ACE Inhibitor or ARB for LVSD

Hospital Name	City	Rate	Cases
Saint Joseph Health Center	Kansas City	100%	97
University of Missouri Hospital and Clinics	Columbia	100%	40
Des Peres Hospital	Saint Louis	98%	51
Saint John's Regional Health Center	Springfield	97%	186
Barnes-Jewish Saint Peters Hospital	Saint Peters	96%	27
Boone Hospital Center	Columbia	95%	152
Saint Francis Medical Center	Cape Girardeau	95%	60
Cox Med Ctrs-North and South & Walnut Lawn	Springfield	93%	100
Research Medical Center	Kansas City	93%	68
Missouri Baptist Medical Center	Saint Louis	92%	96
Saint John's Mercy Medical Center	Saint Louis	92%	165
Saint Mary's Health Center	Saint Louis	92%	52
North Kansas City Hospital	North Kansas City	91%	122
Barnes-Jewish Hospital	Saint Louis	90%	180
Christian Hospital Northeast	Saint Louis	90%	107
Saint Luke's Hospital	Chesterfield	90%	67
Saint Joseph Health Center-Saint Charles	Saint Charles	89%	134
Heartland Health	Saint Joseph	88%	84
Saint Joseph Hospital of Kirkwood	Saint Louis	88%	40
Saint Luke's Hospital of Kansas City	Kansas City	88%	132
Southeast Missouri Hospital	Cape Girardeau	86%	64
DePaul Health Center	Bridgeton	84%	104
Lake Regional Health Systems	Osage Beach	84%	43
SLUCare	Saint Louis	84%	90
Saint Anthony's Medical Center	Saint Louis	84%	68
Saint John's Regional Medical Center	Joplin	84%	122
Freeman Health System	Joplin	81%	64
Centerpoint Medical Center of Independence	Independence	80%	92
Skaggs Community Health Center	Branson	68%	31
Jefferson Memorial Hospital	Crystal City	66%	58

2. Aspirin at Arrival

Hospital Name	City	Rate	Cases
Audrain Medical Center	Mexico	100%	50
Capital Region Medical Center	Jefferson City	100%	77
Hannibal Regional Hospital	Hannibal	100%	36
Saint Joseph Health Center	Kansas City	100%	221
Saint Joseph Health Center-Saint Charles	Saint Charles	100%	222
Saint Luke's Northland Hospital	Kansas City	100%	26
Saint Mary's Medical Center	Blue Springs	100%	54
Southeast Missouri Hospital	Cape Girardeau	100%	126
University of Missouri Hospital and Clinics	Columbia	100%	77
Boone Hospital Center	Columbia	99%	186
Des Peres Hospital	Saint Louis	99%	99
Lee's Summit Hospital	Lee's Summit	99%	81
Skaggs Community Health Center	Branson	99%	190
Barnes-Jewish Saint Peters Hospital	Saint Peters	98%	165
Christian Hospital Northeast	Saint Louis	98%	347
Cox Med Ctrs-North and South & Walnut Lawn	Springfield	98%	412
Liberty Hospital	Liberty	98%	46
Medical Center of Independence	Independence	98%	89
Missouri Baptist Medical Center	Saint Louis	98%	179
Ozarks Medical Center	West Plains	98%	53
Research Medical Center	Kansas City	98%	162
Saint John's Mercy Medical Center	Saint Louis	98%	356
Saint John's Regional Health Center	Springfield	98%	397
Saint Joseph Hospital of Kirkwood	Saint Louis	98%	137
Saint Luke's Hospital of Kansas City	Kansas City	98%	175
Saint Mary's Health Center	Saint Louis	98%	201
Saint Marys Health Center	Jefferson City	98%	111
Jefferson Memorial Hospital	Crystal City	97%	147
North Kansas City Hospital	North Kansas City	97%	234
Saint Anthony's Medical Center	Saint Louis	97%	314
Saint Joseph Hospital West	Lake Saint Louis	97%	58
Truman Medical Centers	Kansas City	97%	36
Barnes-Jewish Hospital	Saint Louis	96%	450
DePaul Health Center	Bridgeton	96%	264
Forest Park Hospital	Saint Louis	96%	48
Freeman Health System	Joplin	96%	209
Missouri Southern Healthcare	Dexter	96%	45
SLUCare	Saint Louis	96%	127
Saint Alexius Hospital	Saint Louis	96%	47
Saint Francis Medical Center	Cape Girardeau	96%	176
Saint John's Regional Medical Center	Joplin	96%	199
Saint Luke's Hospital	Chesterfield	96%	199
Lake Regional Health Systems	Osage Beach	95%	178
Bothwell Regional Health Center	Sedalia	94%	65
Heartland Health	Saint Joseph	94%	261
Missouri Delta Medical Center	Sikeston	94%	31
Poplar Bluff Regional Medical Center	Poplar Bluff	94%	95
Saint John's Mercy Hospital	Washington	94%	85
Centerpoint Medical Center of Independence	Independence	93%	190
Phelps County Regional Medical Center	Rolla	89%	91
Mineral Area Regional Medical Center	Farmington	70%	33

3. Aspirin at Discharge

Hospital Name	City	Rate	Cases
Audrain Medical Center	Mexico	100%	49
Lee's Summit Hospital	Lee's Summit	100%	70
Medical Center of Independence	Independence	100%	74
North Kansas City Hospital	North Kansas City	100%	303
SLUCare	Saint Louis	100%	167
Saint Joseph Health Center	Kansas City	100%	391
Saint Marys Health Center	Jefferson City	100%	105
Truman Medical Centers	Kansas City	100%	26
University of Missouri Hospital and Clinics	Columbia	100%	221
Barnes-Jewish Hospital	Saint Louis	99%	624
Boone Hospital Center	Columbia	99%	498
Capital Region Medical Center	Jefferson City	99%	76
DePaul Health Center	Bridgeton	99%	267
Research Medical Center	Kansas City	99%	279
Saint Joseph Health Center-Saint Charles	Saint Charles	99%	351
Saint Luke's Hospital of Kansas City	Kansas City	99%	563
Des Peres Hospital	Saint Louis	98%	255
Freeman Health System	Joplin	98%	364
Heartland Health	Saint Joseph	98%	261
Missouri Baptist Medical Center	Saint Louis	98%	367
Saint John's Mercy Medical Center	Saint Louis	98%	523
Saint John's Regional Health Center	Springfield	98%	617
Saint Mary's Health Center	Saint Louis	98%	257
Centerpoint Medical Center of Independence	Independence	97%	220
Saint Joseph Hospital of Kirkwood	Saint Louis	97%	150
Saint Luke's Hospital	Chesterfield	97%	242
Skaggs Community Health Center	Branson	97%	182
Cox Med Ctrs-North and South & Walnut Lawn	Springfield	96%	542
Lake Regional Health Systems	Osage Beach	96%	164
Saint Anthony's Medical Center	Saint Louis	96%	297
Saint John's Regional Medical Center	Joplin	96%	304
Saint Mary's Medical Center	Blue Springs	96%	27
Southeast Missouri Hospital	Cape Girardeau	96%	248
Ozarks Medical Center	West Plains	95%	40
Saint Francis Medical Center	Cape Girardeau	95%	245
Barnes-Jewish Saint Peters Hospital	Saint Peters	94%	142
Christian Hospital Northeast	Saint Louis	94%	376
Jefferson Memorial Hospital	Crystal City	93%	181
Missouri Southern Healthcare	Dexter	93%	30
Forest Park Hospital	Saint Louis	91%	58
Liberty Hospital	Liberty	90%	30
Saint John's Mercy Hospital	Washington	90%	60
Phelps County Regional Medical Center	Rolla	88%	56
Bothwell Regional Health Center	Sedalia	84%	25
Poplar Bluff Regional Medical Center	Poplar Bluff	83%	98

4. Beta Blocker at Arrival

Hospital Name	City	Rate	Cases
Audrain Medical Center	Mexico	100%	33
Forest Park Hospital	Saint Louis	100%	50
Saint Joseph Health Center-Saint Charles	Saint Charles	100%	222
Saint Joseph Health Center	Kansas City	99%	180
Saint Joseph Hospital of Kirkwood	Saint Louis	99%	105
University of Missouri Hospital and Clinics	Columbia	99%	84
Capital Region Medical Center	Jefferson City	98%	62
Cox Med Ctrs-North and South & Walnut Lawn	Springfield	98%	366
Des Peres Hospital	Saint Louis	98%	98
Heartland Health	Saint Joseph	98%	163
North Kansas City Hospital	North Kansas City	98%	209
Saint Joseph Hospital West	Lake Saint Louis	98%	64
Saint Mary's Medical Center	Blue Springs	98%	48
Research Medical Center	Kansas City	97%	121
Saint Luke's Hospital	Chesterfield	97%	153
Missouri Baptist Medical Center	Saint Louis	96%	160
Saint Luke's Hospital of Kansas City	Kansas City	96%	135
Barnes-Jewish Hospital	Saint Louis	95%	443
SLUCare	Saint Louis	95%	98
Saint Francis Medical Center	Cape Girardeau	95%	130
Saint John's Mercy Medical Center	Saint Louis	95%	298
Hannibal Regional Hospital	Hannibal	94%	35
Saint Anthony's Medical Center	Saint Louis	94%	215
Saint John's Regional Health Center	Springfield	94%	272
Saint Mary's Health Center	Saint Louis	94%	173
Skaggs Community Health Center	Branson	94%	164
Barnes-Jewish Saint Peters Hospital	Saint Peters	92%	160
Boone Hospital Center	Columbia	92%	178
Phelps County Regional Medical Center	Rolla	92%	78

NOTE: Hospital profiles are in alphabetical order by state, then city, then hospital within the city; Rankings are sorted by rate in descending order and exclude hospitals with less than 25 cases; (1) The number of cases is too small (n<25) for purposes of reliably predicting hospital performance; (2) Measure reflects the hospital's indication that its submission was based upon a sample of its relevant discharges; (3) Rate reflects fewer than the maximum possible quarters of data for the measure; (4) Inaccurate information submitted and suppressed for one or more quarters; (5) No data is available from the hospital for this measure; Please refer to the User's Guide for a full explanation of data

Hospital Name	City	Rate	Cases
Saint Marys Health Center	Jefferson City	92%	95
Southeast Missouri Hospital	Cape Girardeau	92%	91
Christian Hospital Northeast	Saint Louis	91%	330
Lee's Summit Hospital	Lee's Summit	91%	66
Liberty Hospital	Liberty	91%	33
Missouri Southern Healthcare	Dexter	91%	35
Centerpoint Medical Center of Independence	Independence	90%	154
DePaul Health Center	Bridgeton	90%	189
Freeman Health System	Joplin	90%	143
Jefferson Memorial Hospital	Crystal City	90%	141
Poplar Bluff Regional Medical Center	Poplar Bluff	89%	96
Truman Medical Centers	Kansas City	89%	38
Ozarks Medical Center	West Plains	88%	48
Saint Alexius Hospital	Saint Louis	88%	34
Saint John's Regional Medical Center	Joplin	88%	162
Saint John's Mercy Hospital	Washington	87%	55
Lake Regional Health Systems	Osage Beach	82%	133
Bothwell Regional Health Center	Sedalia	80%	61
Medical Center of Independence	Independence	76%	63

5. Beta Blocker at Discharge

Hospital Name	City	Rate	Cases
Audrain Medical Center	Mexico	100%	48
Lee's Summit Hospital	Lee's Summit	100%	67
North Kansas City Hospital	North Kansas City	100%	319
Saint Joseph Health Center	Kansas City	100%	357
Saint Mary's Medical Center	Blue Springs	100%	26
University of Missouri Hospital and Clinics	Columbia	100%	232
Capital Region Medical Center	Jefferson City	99%	79
SLUCare	Saint Louis	99%	189
Saint Joseph Health Center-Saint Charles	Saint Charles	99%	368
Saint Luke's Hospital of Kansas City	Kansas City	99%	595
Boone Hospital Center	Columbia	98%	523
Cox Med Ctrs-North and South & Walnut Lawn	Springfield	98%	559
Missouri Baptist Medical Center	Saint Louis	98%	375
Research Medical Center	Kansas City	98%	266
Saint John's Mercy Medical Center	Saint Louis	98%	535
Saint John's Regional Health Center	Springfield	98%	587
Saint Joseph Hospital of Kirkwood	Saint Louis	98%	154
Southeast Missouri Hospital	Cape Girardeau	98%	254
Des Peres Hospital	Saint Louis	97%	256
Heartland Health	Saint Joseph	97%	318
Liberty Hospital	Liberty	97%	32
Saint Francis Medical Center	Cape Girardeau	97%	235
Barnes-Jewish Hospital	Saint Louis	96%	689
Barnes-Jewish Saint Peters Hospital	Saint Peters	96%	146
Centerpoint Medical Center of Independence	Independence	96%	223
Christian Hospital Northeast	Saint Louis	96%	398
Freeman Health System	Joplin	96%	296
Saint Alexius Hospital	Saint Louis	96%	25
Saint Mary's Health Center	Saint Louis	96%	264
DePaul Health Center	Bridgeton	95%	283
Forest Park Hospital	Saint Louis	95%	59
Phelps County Regional Medical Center	Rolla	95%	73
Saint Marys Health Center	Jefferson City	95%	110
Medical Center of Independence	Independence	94%	68
Saint Anthony's Medical Center	Saint Louis	94%	319
Saint John's Regional Medical Center	Joplin	94%	355
Saint Luke's Hospital	Chesterfield	94%	252
Hannibal Regional Hospital	Hannibal	93%	29
Saint Joseph Hospital West	Lake Saint Louis	93%	29
Jefferson Memorial Hospital	Crystal City	92%	184
Skaggs Community Health Center	Branson	92%	172
Truman Medical Centers	Kansas City	92%	25
Missouri Southern Healthcare	Dexter	91%	34
Lake Regional Health Systems	Osage Beach	90%	161
Ozarks Medical Center	West Plains	88%	41
Bothwell Regional Health Center	Sedalia	86%	29
Saint John's Mercy Hospital	Washington	86%	43
Poplar Bluff Regional Medical Center	Poplar Bluff	82%	100

6. Fibrinolytic Medication Timing

Hospital Name	City	Rate	Cases
Bothwell Regional Health Center	Sedalia	4%	26

7. PCI Within 90 Minutes of Arrival

Hospital Name	City	Rate	Cases
Saint John's Regional Health Center	Springfield	49%	39

8. Smoking Cessation Advice

Hospital Name	City	Rate	Cases
DePaul Health Center	Bridgeton	100%	125
Lee's Summit Hospital	Lee's Summit	100%	27
Medical Center of Independence	Independence	100%	26
Saint Francis Medical Center	Cape Girardeau	100%	107
Saint John's Mercy Medical Center	Saint Louis	100%	171
Saint John's Regional Health Center	Springfield	100%	262
Saint Joseph Health Center	Kansas City	100%	143
Saint Joseph Hospital of Kirkwood	Saint Louis	100%	38
Saint Marys Health Center	Jefferson City	100%	43
Skaggs Community Health Center	Branson	100%	56
Southeast Missouri Hospital	Cape Girardeau	100%	114
Boone Hospital Center	Columbia	99%	206
Christian Hospital Northeast	Saint Louis	99%	144
Des Peres Hospital	Saint Louis	99%	106
Lake Regional Health Systems	Osage Beach	99%	70
Missouri Baptist Medical Center	Saint Louis	99%	131
SLUCare	Saint Louis	99%	92
Saint Anthony's Medical Center	Saint Louis	99%	130
Barnes-Jewish Saint Peters Hospital	Saint Peters	98%	54
Freeman Health System	Joplin	98%	165
Heartland Health	Saint Joseph	98%	125
North Kansas City Hospital	North Kansas City	98%	134
Saint Joseph Health Center-Saint Charles	Saint Charles	98%	128
Saint Luke's Hospital	Chesterfield	98%	64
Saint Luke's Hospital of Kansas City	Kansas City	98%	250
Saint Mary's Health Center	Saint Louis	98%	105
Capital Region Medical Center	Jefferson City	97%	32
Cox Med Ctrs-North and South & Walnut Lawn	Springfield	97%	234
Research Medical Center	Kansas City	97%	97
University of Missouri Hospital and Clinics	Columbia	97%	110
Centerpoint Medical Center of Independence	Independence	96%	112
Barnes-Jewish Hospital	Saint Louis	95%	224
Saint John's Regional Medical Center	Joplin	94%	159
Poplar Bluff Regional Medical Center	Poplar Bluff	90%	52
Jefferson Memorial Hospital	Crystal City	71%	73

Heart Failure Care

9. ACE Inhibitor or ARB for LVSD

Hospital Name	City	Rate	Cases
Moberly Regional Medical Center	Moberly	100%	27
Saint Joseph Health Center	Kansas City	99%	160
Capital Region Medical Center	Jefferson City	98%	62
Audrain Medical Center	Mexico	96%	78
Saint John's Mercy Hospital	Washington	96%	79
Saint Joseph Hospital of Kirkwood	Saint Louis	96%	73
Saint Luke's Hospital	Chesterfield	96%	198
Saint Luke's Hospital of Kansas City	Kansas City	95%	275
Saint Francis Medical Center	Cape Girardeau	94%	119
University of Missouri Hospital and Clinics	Columbia	94%	90
Boone Hospital Center	Columbia	93%	339
Saint Marys Health Center	Jefferson City	93%	75
Barnes-Jewish Hospital	Saint Louis	92%	430
Freeman Health System	Joplin	92%	105
Saint John's Regional Health Center	Springfield	92%	355
Saint Mary's Health Center	Saint Louis	92%	250
Cox Med Ctrs-North and South & Walnut Lawn	Springfield	91%	140
Hannibal Regional Hospital	Hannibal	91%	54
Des Peres Hospital	Saint Louis	90%	149
Saint John's Mercy Medical Center	Saint Louis	90%	262
Truman Medical Centers	Kansas City	90%	198
Research Medical Center	Kansas City	88%	249
Saint Mary's Medical Center	Blue Springs	88%	42
Missouri Delta Medical Center	Sikeston	87%	85
North Kansas City Hospital	North Kansas City	87%	134
Heartland Health	Saint Joseph	86%	220
Missouri Baptist Medical Center	Saint Louis	86%	293
Christian Hospital Northeast	Saint Louis	85%	325
Phelps County Regional Medical Center	Rolla	85%	68
Saint Joseph Health Center-Saint Charles	Saint Charles	85%	134
Truman Medical Center-Lakewood	Kansas City	85%	34
Forest Park Hospital	Saint Louis	84%	112
SLUCare	Saint Louis	84%	260
Saint Joseph Hospital West	Lake Saint Louis	84%	56
Mineral Area Regional Medical Center	Farmington	83%	35
Barnes-Jewish Saint Peters Hospital	Saint Peters	82%	50
Lee's Summit Hospital	Lee's Summit	82%	45
Parkland Health Center	Farmington	82%	72
Columbia Regional Hospital	Columbia	81%	36
Ozarks Medical Center	West Plains	81%	48
Saint Alexius Hospital	Saint Louis	81%	78
Centerpoint Medical Center of Independence	Independence	80%	100
DePaul Health Center	Bridgeton	80%	265
Lake Regional Health Systems	Osage Beach	79%	81
Skaggs Community Health Center	Branson	78%	65
Southeast Missouri Hospital	Cape Girardeau	78%	105

NOTE: Hospital profiles are in alphabetical order by state, then city, then hospital within the city; Rankings are sorted by rate in descending order and exclude hospitals with less than 25 cases; (1) The number of cases is too small (n<25) for purposes of reliably predicting hospital performance; (2) Measure reflects the hospital's indication that its submission was based upon a sample of its relevant discharges; (3) Rate reflects fewer than the maximum possible quarters of data for the measure; (4) Inaccurate information submitted and suppressed for one or more quarters; (5) No data is available from the hospital for this measure; Please refer to the User's Guide for a full explanation of data

Bothwell Regional Health Center	Sedalia	77%	108
Jefferson Memorial Hospital	Crystal City	77%	126
Saint John's Regional Medical Center	Joplin	75%	167
Saint Anthony's Medical Center	Saint Louis	74%	166
Twin Rivers Regional Medical Center	Kennett	68%	44
Golden Valley Memorial Hospital	Clinton	66%	41
Liberty Hospital	Liberty	64%	94
Medical Center of Independence	Independence	64%	55
Poplar Bluff Regional Medical Center	Poplar Bluff	62%	119
Northeast Regional Medical Center	Kirksville	58%	26
Pemiscot Memorial Hospital	Hayti	54%	28

10. Discharge Instructions

Hospital Name	City	Rate	Cases
Saint Joseph Health Center	Kansas City	100%	310
Twin Rivers Regional Medical Center	Kennett	100%	89
Lafayette Regional Health Center	Lexington	97%	32
Freeman Neosho Hospital	Neosho	96%	27
Saint Luke's Hospital	Chesterfield	96%	393
Southeast Missouri Hospital	Cape Girardeau	96%	248
Saint Francis Hospital & Health Services	Maryville	94%	31
Saint Francis Medical Center	Cape Girardeau	92%	272
Saint Marys Health Center	Jefferson City	91%	172
Audrain Medical Center	Mexico	90%	148
SLUCare	Saint Louis	90%	358
Cooper County Memorial Hospital	Boonville	89%	28
Hannibal Regional Hospital	Hannibal	89%	112
Saint John's Mercy Hospital	Washington	89%	197
Capital Region Medical Center	Jefferson City	88%	161
Des Peres Hospital	Saint Louis	88%	329
Missouri Baptist Hospital Sullivan	Sullivan	87%	53
Saint Mary's Medical Center	Blue Springs	87%	94
Truman Medical Centers	Kansas City	87%	299
Lake Regional Health Systems	Osage Beach	86%	189
Missouri Delta Medical Center	Sikeston	86%	188
University of Missouri Hospital and Clinics	Columbia	86%	156
Boone Hospital Center	Columbia	85%	498
Heartland Health	Saint Joseph	85%	469
Moberly Regional Medical Center	Moberly	85%	62
Parkland Health Center	Farmington	85%	105
Pike County Memorial Hospital	Louisiana	85%	26
Saint John's Regional Health Center	Springfield	82%	574
Barnes-Jewish Hospital	Saint Louis	81%	715
Jefferson Memorial Hospital	Crystal City	81%	280
Phelps County Regional Medical Center	Rolla	80%	133
Saint John's Mercy Medical Center	Saint Louis	80%	471
Cox Med Ctrs-North and South & Walnut Lawn	Springfield	78%	306
Research Medical Center	Kansas City	77%	448
Barnes-Jewish West County Hospital	Saint Louis	74%	43
DePaul Health Center	Bridgeton	72%	551
Saint Joseph Hospital of Kirkwood	Saint Louis	71%	208
Saint Mary's Health Center	Saint Louis	71%	644
Christian Hospital Northeast	Saint Louis	70%	655
Saint John's Hospital at Lebanon	Lebanon	69%	71
Saint Luke's Northland Hospital	Kansas City	67%	57
Freeman Health System	Joplin	66%	209
Medical Center of Independence	Independence	66%	143
Saint Luke's Hospital of Kansas City	Kansas City	66%	421
Bates County Memorial Hospital	Butler	64%	81
Centerpoint Medical Center of Independence	Independence	64%	207
Northeast Regional Medical Center	Kirksville	64%	50
Northwest Medical Center	Albany	64%	25
Liberty Hospital	Liberty	63%	211
Missouri Baptist Medical Center	Saint Louis	63%	551
Ste Genevieve County Memorial Hospital	Sainte Genevieve	63%	35
Poplar Bluff Regional Medical Center	Poplar Bluff	62%	252
Lee's Summit Hospital	Lee's Summit	61%	79
North Kansas City Hospital	North Kansas City	60%	299
Saint Anthony's Medical Center	Saint Louis	60%	303
Saint Joseph Health Center-Saint Charles	Saint Charles	60%	264
Golden Valley Memorial Hospital	Clinton	59%	108
Ripley County Memorial Hospital	Doniphan	59%	54
Bothwell Regional Health Center	Sedalia	58%	139
Saint John's Regional Medical Center	Joplin	57%	336
Saint Joseph Hospital West	Lake Saint Louis	57%	137
Barnes-Jewish Saint Peters Hospital	Saint Peters	56%	121
Nevada Regional Medical Center	Nevada	56%	34
Citizens Memorial Hospital	Bolivar	55%	53
Columbia Regional Hospital	Columbia	52%	46
McCune-Brooks Hospital	Carthage	45%	40
Saint Luke's East Lee's Summit Hospital	Lees Summit	43%	30
Forest Park Hospital	Saint Louis	42%	242
Ozarks Medical Center	West Plains	37%	89
Wright Memorial Hospital	Trenton	37%	27

Skaggs Community Health Center	Branson	35%	155
Cameron Regional Medical Center	Cameron	32%	31
Saint Alexius Hospital	Saint Louis	28%	193
Mineral Area Regional Medical Center	Farmington	27%	81
Fitzgibbon Memorial Hospital	Marshall	25%	56
Western Missouri Medical Center	Warrensburg	22%	67
Ray County Memorial Hospital	Richmond	19%	31
Pemiscot Memorial Hospital	Hayti	9%	150
Texas County Memorial Hospital	Houston	2%	45
Sac-Osage Hospital	Osceola	0%	30

11. Evaluation of LVS Function

Hospital Name	City	Rate	Cases
Saint Luke's Hospital	Chesterfield	100%	521
Boone Hospital Center	Columbia	99%	573
Missouri Baptist Hospital Sullivan	Sullivan	99%	71
Saint John's Mercy Hospital	Washington	99%	231
Saint John's Regional Health Center	Springfield	99%	690
Saint Joseph Health Center	Kansas City	99%	385
University of Missouri Hospital and Clinics	Columbia	99%	186
Barnes-Jewish West County Hospital	Saint Louis	98%	53
Capital Region Medical Center	Jefferson City	98%	209
Freeman Health System	Joplin	98%	246
Northeast Regional Medical Center	Kirksville	98%	87
SLUCare	Saint Louis	98%	394
Saint Francis Hospital & Health Services	Maryville	98%	58
Saint Francis Medical Center	Cape Girardeau	98%	341
Saint John's Mercy Medical Center	Saint Louis	98%	555
Saint Joseph Health Center-Saint Charles	Saint Charles	98%	321
Saint Luke's Hospital of Kansas City	Kansas City	98%	490
Saint Mary's Health Center	Saint Louis	98%	775
Saint Marys Health Center	Jefferson City	98%	217
Audrain Medical Center	Mexico	97%	196
Barnes-Jewish Hospital	Saint Louis	97%	842
North Kansas City Hospital	North Kansas City	97%	343
Parkland Health Center	Farmington	97%	186
Saint Joseph Hospital of Kirkwood	Saint Louis	97%	291
Saint Luke's Northland Hospital	Kansas City	97%	72
Truman Medical Centers	Kansas City	97%	318
Heartland Health	Saint Joseph	96%	569
Missouri Baptist Medical Center	Saint Louis	96%	701
Saint Joseph Hospital West	Lake Saint Louis	96%	159
Barnes-Jewish Saint Peters Hospital	Saint Peters	95%	144
Freeman Neosho Hospital	Neosho	95%	42
Research Medical Center	Kansas City	95%	535
Saint Alexius Hospital	Saint Louis	95%	255
Skaggs Community Health Center	Branson	95%	183
Des Peres Hospital	Saint Louis	94%	405
Lee's Summit Hospital	Lee's Summit	94%	126
Moberly Regional Medical Center	Moberly	94%	101
Phelps County Regional Medical Center	Rolla	94%	187
Saint Anthony's Medical Center	Saint Louis	94%	397
Christian Hospital Northeast	Saint Louis	93%	839
DePaul Health Center	Bridgeton	93%	686
Pike County Memorial Hospital	Louisiana	92%	53
Poplar Bluff Regional Medical Center	Poplar Bluff	92%	308
Saint Luke's East Lee's Summit Hospital	Lees Summit	92%	36
Saint Mary's Medical Center	Blue Springs	92%	130
Cox Med Ctrs-North and South & Walnut Lawn	Springfield	91%	407
Lincoln County Medical Center	Troy	91%	32
Medical Center of Independence	Independence	91%	176
Bothwell Regional Health Center	Sedalia	90%	182
Columbia Regional Hospital	Columbia	90%	58
Liberty Hospital	Liberty	90%	266
Twin Rivers Regional Medical Center	Kennett	90%	119
Callaway Community Hospital	Fulton	89%	37
Saint John's Hospital of Aurora	Aurora	89%	36
Forest Park Hospital	Saint Louis	88%	299
Hannibal Regional Hospital	Hannibal	88%	162
Truman Medical Center-Lakewood	Kansas City	87%	67
Mineral Area Regional Medical Center	Farmington	85%	128
Missouri Delta Medical Center	Sikeston	85%	234
Southeast Missouri Hospital	Cape Girardeau	85%	302
Wright Memorial Hospital	Trenton	85%	41
Centerpoint Medical Center of Independence	Independence	84%	294
Doctors Hospital of Springfield	Springfield	84%	38
Saint John's Regional Medical Center	Joplin	84%	402
Citizens Memorial Hospital	Bolivar	83%	75
Research Belton Hospital	Belton	83%	63
Lafayette Regional Health Center	Lexington	82%	57
Nevada Regional Medical Center	Nevada	82%	40
Jefferson Memorial Hospital	Crystal City	81%	349
Ozarks Medical Center	West Plains	80%	140
McCune-Brooks Hospital	Carthage	78%	69

NOTE: Hospital profiles are in alphabetical order by state, then city, then hospital within the city; Rankings are sorted by rate in descending order and exclude hospitals with less than 25 cases; (1) The number of cases is too small (n<25) for purposes of reliably predicting hospital performance; (2) Measure reflects the hospital's indication that its submission was based upon a sample of its relevant discharges; (3) Rate reflects fewer than the maximum possible quarters of data for the measure; (4) Inaccurate information submitted and suppressed for one or more quarters; (5) No data is available from the hospital for this measure; Please refer to the User's Guide for a full explanation of data

Ste Genevieve County Memorial Hospital	Sainte Genevieve	78%	65
Golden Valley Memorial Hospital	Clinton	77%	187
Lake Regional Health Systems	Osage Beach	77%	224
Cooper County Memorial Hospital	Boonville	76%	41
Cameron Regional Medical Center	Cameron	75%	63
Hedrick Medical Center	Chillicothe	75%	44
Northwest Medical Center	Albany	73%	41
Saint John's Hospital at Lebanon	Lebanon	73%	83
Cass Medical Center	Harrisonville	68%	28
Community Hospital Association	Fairfax	64%	25
Fitzgibbon Memorial Hospital	Marshall	62%	89
Texas County Memorial Hospital	Houston	62%	66
Saint Francis Hospital	Mountain View	60%	25
Western Missouri Medical Center	Warrensburg	52%	98
Ripley County Memorial Hospital	Doniphan	49%	67
Pemiscot Memorial Hospital	Hayti	48%	179
Carroll County Memorial Hospital	Carrollton	44%	59
Missouri Southern Healthcare	Dexter	44%	123
Cox Monett Hospital	Monett	42%	36
Ray County Memorial Hospital	Richmond	36%	55
Bates County Memorial Hospital	Butler	11%	109
General JJ Pershing Memorial Hospital	Brookfield	0%	46
Sac-Osage Hospital	Osceola	0%	38

12. Smoking Cessation Advice

Hospital Name	City	Rate	Cases
Bothwell Regional Health Center	Sedalia	100%	29
Freeman Health System	Joplin	100%	48
Missouri Delta Medical Center	Sikeston	100%	63
Saint Francis Medical Center	Cape Girardeau	100%	62
Saint John's Mercy Hospital	Washington	100%	36
Saint John's Mercy Medical Center	Saint Louis	100%	76
Saint John's Regional Health Center	Springfield	100%	107
Saint Joseph Health Center	Kansas City	100%	51
Christian Hospital Northeast	Saint Louis	99%	160
DePaul Health Center	Bridgeton	99%	150
Des Peres Hospital	Saint Louis	99%	67
Heartland Health	Saint Joseph	99%	89
Research Medical Center	Kansas City	99%	118
SLUCare	Saint Louis	99%	136
Saint Alexius Hospital	Saint Louis	99%	70
Saint Mary's Health Center	Saint Louis	99%	173
Saint Luke's Hospital of Kansas City	Kansas City	98%	119
Liberty Hospital	Liberty	97%	36
Medical Center of Independence	Independence	97%	29
Missouri Baptist Medical Center	Saint Louis	97%	71
Saint Anthony's Medical Center	Saint Louis	97%	67
Saint Luke's Hospital	Chesterfield	97%	39
Saint Marys Health Center	Jefferson City	97%	32
Skaggs Community Health Center	Branson	97%	36
Barnes-Jewish Hospital	Saint Louis	96%	184
Truman Medical Centers	Kansas City	96%	139
Capital Region Medical Center	Jefferson City	95%	44
Phelps County Regional Medical Center	Rolla	94%	34
University of Missouri Hospital and Clinics	Columbia	94%	48
Boone Hospital Center	Columbia	93%	76
Saint Joseph Health Center-Saint Charles	Saint Charles	93%	58
Southeast Missouri Hospital	Cape Girardeau	93%	59
Cox Med Ctrs-North and South & Walnut Lawn	Springfield	90%	87
Parkland Health Center	Farmington	90%	30
Centerpoint Medical Center of Independence	Independence	89%	63
Lake Regional Health Systems	Osage Beach	89%	38
North Kansas City Hospital	North Kansas City	88%	59
Poplar Bluff Regional Medical Center	Poplar Bluff	86%	65
Ozarks Medical Center	West Plains	84%	25
Saint Joseph Hospital of Kirkwood	Saint Louis	84%	25
Saint John's Regional Medical Center	Joplin	80%	76
Golden Valley Memorial Hospital	Clinton	74%	39
Jefferson Memorial Hospital	Crystal City	58%	45
Forest Park Hospital	Saint Louis	49%	73

Pneumonia Care

13. Appropriate Initial Antibiotic

Hospital Name	City	Rate	Cases
Saint Francis Hospital & Health Services	Maryville	98%	49
Freeman Neosho Hospital	Neosho	97%	73
Missouri Baptist Hospital Sullivan	Sullivan	97%	89
Saint Francis Hospital	Mountain View	97%	33
Saint John's Hospital of Aurora	Aurora	97%	69
Saint John's Hospital-Caseville	Cassville	97%	34
Barnes-Jewish West County Hospital	Saint Louis	94%	54
Barnes-Jewish Saint Peters Hospital	Saint Peters	93%	156
Capital Region Medical Center	Jefferson City	92%	130
McCune-Brooks Hospital	Carthage	92%	48
Parkland Health Center	Farmington	92%	99
Perry County Memorial Hospital	Perryville	92%	26
SLUCare	Saint Louis	91%	129
Saint Francis Medical Center	Cape Girardeau	90%	102
Saint Luke's Northland Hospital	Kansas City	90%	82
Cameron Regional Medical Center	Cameron	89%	65
Freeman Health System	Joplin	89%	298
Lake Regional Health Systems	Osage Beach	89%	160
Saint John's Regional Health Center	Springfield	89%	412
Saint Luke's Hospital	Chesterfield	89%	243
Audrain Medical Center	Mexico	88%	97
Doctors Hospital of Springfield	Springfield	88%	40
Harrison County Community Hospital	Bethany	88%	43
Truman Medical Centers	Kansas City	88%	99
Washington County Memorial Hospital	Potosi	88%	68
Centerpoint Medical Center of Independence	Independence	87%	140
DePaul Health Center	Bridgeton	87%	235
Medical Center of Independence	Independence	87%	102
Ozarks Medical Center	West Plains	87%	115
Saint Alexius Hospital	Saint Louis	87%	119
University of Missouri Hospital and Clinics	Columbia	87%	75
Des Peres Hospital	Saint Louis	86%	192
Heartland Health	Saint Joseph	86%	322
Lee's Summit Hospital	Lee's Summit	86%	99
Saint Anthony's Medical Center	Saint Louis	86%	186
Saint John's Mercy Hospital	Washington	86%	183
Saint Mary's Health Center	Saint Louis	86%	241
Callaway Community Hospital	Fulton	85%	40
Missouri Delta Medical Center	Sikeston	85%	115
Saint John's Regional Medical Center	Joplin	85%	263
Columbia Regional Hospital	Columbia	84%	38
Fitzgibbon Memorial Hospital	Marshall	84%	90
Golden Valley Memorial Hospital	Clinton	84%	80
Hedrick Medical Center	Chillicothe	84%	44
Moberly Regional Medical Center	Moberly	84%	98
Pike County Memorial Hospital	Louisiana	84%	38
Saint John's Mercy Medical Center	Saint Louis	84%	302
Christian Hospital Northeast	Saint Louis	83%	223
Phelps County Regional Medical Center	Rolla	83%	193
Saint Joseph Health Center-Saint Charles	Saint Charles	83%	156
Saint Joseph Hospital West	Lake Saint Louis	83%	175
Saint Marys Health Center	Jefferson City	83%	131
Liberty Hospital	Liberty	82%	219
Mineral Area Regional Medical Center	Farmington	82%	117
Research Medical Center	Kansas City	82%	118
Saint Joseph Health Center	Kansas City	82%	203
Western Missouri Medical Center	Warrensburg	82%	74
Hannibal Regional Hospital	Hannibal	81%	171
Northeast Regional Medical Center	Kirksville	81%	59
Saint Joseph Hospital of Kirkwood	Saint Louis	81%	189
Barnes-Jewish Hospital	Saint Louis	80%	237
Boone Hospital Center	Columbia	80%	143
Saint Luke's Hospital of Kansas City	Kansas City	80%	125
Missouri Baptist Medical Center	Saint Louis	79%	312
Cooper County Memorial Hospital	Boonville	78%	72
Jefferson Memorial Hospital	Crystal City	78%	215
Southeast Missouri Hospital	Cape Girardeau	78%	152
Lincoln County Medical Center	Troy	77%	31
Texas County Memorial Hospital	Houston	77%	95
Citizens Memorial Hospital	Bolivar	76%	91
Cox Med Ctrs-North and South & Walnut Lawn	Springfield	75%	457
Nevada Regional Medical Center	Nevada	75%	32
Cass Medical Center	Harrisonville	74%	61
Saint John's Hospital at Lebanon	Lebanon	74%	116
Saint Luke's East Lee's Summit Hospital	Lees Summit	74%	31
Saint Mary's Medical Center	Blue Springs	74%	156
Bothwell Regional Health Center	Sedalia	73%	134
Lafayette Regional Health Center	Lexington	73%	71
Wright Memorial Hospital	Trenton	72%	36
General JJ Pershing Memorial Hospital	Brookfield	71%	70
Twin Rivers Regional Medical Center	Kennett	71%	70
Ripley County Memorial Hospital	Doniphan	70%	47
Ste Genevieve County Memorial Hospital	Sainte Genevieve	70%	43
North Kansas City Hospital	North Kansas City	68%	200
Poplar Bluff Regional Medical Center	Poplar Bluff	68%	261
Skaggs Community Health Center	Branson	67%	151
Cox Monett Hospital	Monett	66%	56
Ray County Memorial Hospital	Richmond	66%	32
Northwest Medical Center	Albany	62%	32
Pemiscot Memorial Hospital	Hayti	55%	42
Bates County Memorial Hospital	Butler	52%	66
Forest Park Hospital	Saint Louis	51%	100
Sac-Osage Hospital	Osceola	51%	43
Community Hospital Association	Fairfax	20%	35

NOTE: Hospital profiles are in alphabetical order by state, then city, then hospital within the city; Rankings are sorted by rate in descending order and exclude hospitals with less than 25 cases; (1) The number of cases is too small (n<25) for purposes of reliably predicting hospital performance; (2) Measure reflects the hospital's indication that its submission was based upon a sample of its relevant discharges; (3) Rate reflects fewer than the maximum possible quarters of data for the measure; (4) Inaccurate information submitted and suppressed for one or more quarters; (5) No data is available from the hospital for this measure; Please refer to the User's Guide for a full explanation of data

14. Blood Culture Timing

Hospital Name	City	Rate	Cases
Barnes-Jewish West County Hospital	Saint Louis	100%	36
Freeman Neosho Hospital	Neosho	99%	84
Saint Luke's Northland Hospital	Kansas City	99%	70
Boone Hospital Center	Columbia	98%	124
Fitzgibbon Memorial Hospital	Marshall	98%	43
Missouri Baptist Hospital Sullivan	Sullivan	98%	80
Saint John's Mercy Hospital	Washington	98%	129
Audrain Medical Center	Mexico	97%	126
Northeast Regional Medical Center	Kirksville	97%	74
Saint Francis Medical Center	Cape Girardeau	97%	151
Saint John's Regional Health Center	Springfield	97%	435
Southeast Missouri Hospital	Cape Girardeau	97%	155
Ste Genevieve County Memorial Hospital	Sainte Genevieve	97%	35
DePaul Health Center	Bridgeton	96%	280
Forest Park Hospital	Saint Louis	96%	82
Barnes-Jewish Saint Peters Hospital	Saint Peters	95%	161
Freeman Health System	Joplin	95%	300
Hannibal Regional Hospital	Hannibal	95%	202
Saint Joseph Hospital West	Lake Saint Louis	95%	172
Texas County Memorial Hospital	Houston	95%	55
Liberty Hospital	Liberty	94%	205
Missouri Baptist Medical Center	Saint Louis	94%	317
Nevada Regional Medical Center	Nevada	94%	36
Saint Francis Hospital	Mountain View	94%	36
Saint John's Hospital at Lebanon	Lebanon	94%	47
Saint John's Hospital of Aurora	Aurora	94%	66
Saint Joseph Hospital of Kirkwood	Saint Louis	94%	192
Saint Luke's Hospital	Chesterfield	94%	191
Bothwell Regional Health Center	Sedalia	93%	97
Centerpoint Medical Center of Independence	Independence	93%	156
Citizens Memorial Hospital	Bolivar	93%	70
Des Peres Hospital	Saint Louis	93%	180
McCune-Brooks Hospital	Carthage	93%	46
Moberly Regional Medical Center	Moberly	93%	85
Saint Alexius Hospital	Saint Louis	93%	118
Saint John's Mercy Medical Center	Saint Louis	93%	251
Capital Region Medical Center	Jefferson City	92%	123
Cox Med Ctrs-North and South & Walnut Lawn	Springfield	92%	363
Lake Regional Health Systems	Osage Beach	92%	131
Lee's Summit Hospital	Lee's Summit	92%	89
Parkland Health Center	Farmington	92%	83
Poplar Bluff Regional Medical Center	Poplar Bluff	92%	171
SLUCare	Saint Louis	92%	126
Saint Anthony's Medical Center	Saint Louis	92%	230
Saint Mary's Health Center	Saint Louis	92%	295
Bates County Memorial Hospital	Butler	91%	44
Cox Monett Hospital	Monett	91%	43
Lafayette Regional Health Center	Lexington	91%	32
Medical Center of Independence	Independence	91%	101
Missouri Delta Medical Center	Sikeston	91%	107
University of Missouri Hospital and Clinics	Columbia	91%	85
Christian Hospital Northeast	Saint Louis	90%	247
Golden Valley Memorial Hospital	Clinton	90%	83
Heartland Health	Saint Joseph	90%	311
Ozarks Medical Center	West Plains	90%	120
Saint Francis Hospital & Health Services	Maryville	90%	29
Saint Joseph Health Center-Saint Charles	Saint Charles	90%	203
Cass Medical Center	Harrisonville	89%	28
Mineral Area Regional Medical Center	Farmington	89%	99
Research Medical Center	Kansas City	89%	89
Saint Joseph Health Center	Kansas City	89%	162
Skaggs Community Health Center	Branson	89%	132
Saint John's Regional Medical Center	Joplin	88%	274
Saint Luke's Hospital of Kansas City	Kansas City	88%	115
Truman Medical Centers	Kansas City	88%	128
Western Missouri Medical Center	Warrensburg	88%	59
Pike County Memorial Hospital	Louisiana	87%	52
Barnes-Jewish Hospital	Saint Louis	86%	208
Saint Mary's Medical Center	Blue Springs	86%	118
Cooper County Memorial Hospital	Boonville	85%	26
Doctors Hospital of Springfield	Springfield	84%	38
North Kansas City Hospital	North Kansas City	83%	126
Saint Marys Health Center	Jefferson City	82%	124
Washington County Memorial Hospital	Potosi	82%	55
Cameron Regional Medical Center	Cameron	81%	84
Phelps County Regional Medical Center	Rolla	80%	175
Twin Rivers Regional Medical Center	Kennett	75%	53
Jefferson Memorial Hospital	Crystal City	72%	103
Saint Luke's East Lee's Summit Hospital	Lees Summit	71%	35

15. Influenza Vaccine

Hospital Name	City	Rate	Cases
Freeman Neosho Hospital	Neosho	100%	26
Parkland Health Center	Farmington	100%	27
Freeman Health System	Joplin	97%	98
Heartland Health	Saint Joseph	97%	95
Saint Luke's Hospital	Chesterfield	97%	72
Saint Marys Health Center	Jefferson City	97%	39
Saint John's Hospital at Lebanon	Lebanon	96%	27
Saint John's Regional Health Center	Springfield	96%	164
Lake Regional Health Systems	Osage Beach	95%	44
Audrain Medical Center	Mexico	94%	34
Saint Francis Medical Center	Cape Girardeau	94%	47
Saint Luke's Northland Hospital	Kansas City	92%	26
Saint Anthony's Medical Center	Saint Louis	89%	45
Skaggs Community Health Center	Branson	87%	38
Saint John's Mercy Hospital	Washington	86%	58
Saint John's Mercy Medical Center	Saint Louis	85%	85
Capital Region Medical Center	Jefferson City	84%	44
DePaul Health Center	Bridgeton	84%	69
Christian Hospital Northeast	Saint Louis	81%	78
Saint Alexius Hospital	Saint Louis	81%	31
Saint Luke's Hospital of Kansas City	Kansas City	80%	41
Missouri Baptist Medical Center	Saint Louis	78%	96
Ozarks Medical Center	West Plains	78%	32
Saint Joseph Hospital of Kirkwood	Saint Louis	77%	61
Moberly Regional Medical Center	Moberly	75%	32
Barnes-Jewish Saint Peters Hospital	Saint Peters	74%	35
Phelps County Regional Medical Center	Rolla	68%	47
Citizens Memorial Hospital	Bolivar	67%	30
Saint John's Regional Medical Center	Joplin	66%	140
Saint Joseph Health Center	Kansas City	63%	41
Forest Park Hospital	Saint Louis	62%	34
Barnes-Jewish Hospital	Saint Louis	61%	56
Bothwell Regional Health Center	Sedalia	61%	33
Hannibal Regional Hospital	Hannibal	61%	57
Boone Hospital Center	Columbia	60%	45
Saint Joseph Hospital West	Lake Saint Louis	60%	50
Centerpoint Medical Center of Independence	Independence	59%	51
Cameron Regional Medical Center	Cameron	58%	26
Liberty Hospital	Liberty	57%	68
Poplar Bluff Regional Medical Center	Poplar Bluff	57%	61
SLUCare	Saint Louis	57%	28
Saint Mary's Medical Center	Blue Springs	57%	49
Research Medical Center	Kansas City	55%	33
Saint Joseph Health Center-Saint Charles	Saint Charles	52%	60
North Kansas City Hospital	North Kansas City	51%	43
Lee's Summit Hospital	Lee's Summit	48%	40
Saint Mary's Health Center	Saint Louis	48%	54
University of Missouri Hospital and Clinics	Columbia	23%	39
Jefferson Memorial Hospital	Crystal City	8%	48

16. Initial Antibiotic Timing

Hospital Name	City	Rate	Cases
Freeman Neosho Hospital	Neosho	100%	112
Saint John's Hospital-Caseville	Cassville	97%	34
Harrison County Community Hospital	Bethany	96%	48
Nevada Regional Medical Center	Nevada	96%	55
Audrain Medical Center	Mexico	95%	154
Pike County Memorial Hospital	Louisiana	94%	79
Missouri Baptist Hospital Sullivan	Sullivan	93%	104
Cameron Regional Medical Center	Cameron	92%	129
Carroll County Memorial Hospital	Carrollton	92%	60
Western Missouri Medical Center	Warrensburg	92%	96
Wright Memorial Hospital	Trenton	92%	48
Boone Hospital Center	Columbia	91%	186
Capital Region Medical Center	Jefferson City	91%	184
Golden Valley Memorial Hospital	Clinton	91%	142
Lake Regional Health Systems	Osage Beach	91%	196
Parkland Health Center	Farmington	91%	144
Research Belton Hospital	Belton	91%	45
Community Hospital Association	Fairfax	90%	39
Hermann Area District Hospital	Hermann	90%	29
Moberly Regional Medical Center	Moberly	90%	144
Saint Francis Hospital & Health Services	Maryville	90%	61
Saint Francis Medical Center	Cape Girardeau	90%	168
Barnes-Jewish Saint Peters Hospital	Saint Peters	89%	204
Barnes-Jewish West County Hospital	Saint Louis	89%	66
Bates County Memorial Hospital	Butler	89%	80
Freeman Health System	Joplin	89%	409
Liberty Hospital	Liberty	89%	322
McCune-Brooks Hospital	Carthage	89%	87
Saint John's Hospital of Aurora	Aurora	89%	74
Saint Luke's East Lee's Summit Hospital	Lees Summit	89%	44

NOTE: Hospital profiles are in alphabetical order by state, then city, then hospital within the city; Rankings are sorted by rate in descending order and exclude hospitals with less than 25 cases; (1) The number of cases is too small (n<25) for purposes of reliably predicting hospital performance; (2) Measure reflects the hospital's indication that its submission was based upon a sample of its relevant discharges; (3) Rate reflects fewer than the maximum possible quarters of data for the measure; (4) Inaccurate information submitted and suppressed for one or more quarters; (5) No data is available from the hospital for this measure; Please refer to the User's Guide for a full explanation of data

Centerpoint Medical Center of Independence	Independence	88%	216
Perry County Memorial Hospital	Perryville	88%	33
Saint John's Regional Medical Center	Joplin	88%	413
Saint Mary's Medical Center	Blue Springs	88%	189
Saint Alexius Hospital	Saint Louis	87%	179
Saint Joseph Hospital West	Lake Saint Louis	87%	206
Washington County Memorial Hospital	Potosi	87%	79
Cooper County Memorial Hospital	Boonville	86%	94
Northeast Regional Medical Center	Kirksville	86%	105
Saint John's Regional Health Center	Springfield	86%	501
Saint Luke's Northland Hospital	Kansas City	86%	101
Advanced Healthcare Medical Center	Ellington	85%	26
Lee's Summit Hospital	Lee's Summit	85%	171
Saint John's Mercy Hospital	Washington	85%	222
Des Peres Hospital	Saint Louis	84%	261
Hedrick Medical Center	Chillicothe	84%	62
Saint Joseph Hospital of Kirkwood	Saint Louis	84%	231
Ste Genevieve County Memorial Hospital	Sainte Genevieve	84%	58
Lincoln County Medical Center	Troy	83%	36
Saint Luke's Hospital	Chesterfield	83%	375
Bothwell Regional Health Center	Sedalia	82%	221
Cass Medical Center	Harrisonville	82%	55
Fitzgibbon Memorial Hospital	Marshall	82%	125
Medical Center of Independence	Independence	82%	127
Mineral Area Regional Medical Center	Farmington	82%	174
Northwest Medical Center	Albany	82%	44
Saint John's Mercy Medical Center	Saint Louis	82%	470
Saint Joseph Health Center	Kansas City	82%	222
Lafayette Regional Health Center	Lexington	81%	94
Saint Francis Hospital	Mountain View	81%	57
Christian Hospital Northeast	Saint Louis	80%	352
Hannibal Regional Hospital	Hannibal	80%	259
Heartland Health	Saint Joseph	80%	412
North Kansas City Hospital	North Kansas City	80%	265
Ripley County Memorial Hospital	Doniphan	80%	76
Saint John's Hospital at Lebanon	Lebanon	80%	127
Missouri Baptist Medical Center	Saint Louis	79%	476
Missouri Delta Medical Center	Sikeston	79%	173
Ozarks Medical Center	West Plains	79%	163
Phelps County Regional Medical Center	Rolla	79%	266
Saint Marys Health Center	Jefferson City	79%	224
Missouri Southern Healthcare	Dexter	78%	106
Research Medical Center	Kansas City	77%	193
Saint Joseph Health Center-Saint Charles	Saint Charles	77%	260
Texas County Memorial Hospital	Houston	77%	111
Saint Anthony's Medical Center	Saint Louis	76%	289
Saint Luke's Hospital of Kansas City	Kansas City	76%	206
DePaul Health Center	Bridgeton	75%	345
Doctors Hospital of Springfield	Springfield	75%	60
SLUCare	Saint Louis	75%	212
Citizens Memorial Hospital	Bolivar	74%	117
Twin Rivers Regional Medical Center	Kennett	74%	95
Columbia Regional Hospital	Columbia	73%	30
Cox Med Ctrs-North and South & Walnut Lawn	Springfield	73%	576
Saint Mary's Health Center	Saint Louis	72%	349
Skaggs Community Health Center	Branson	71%	180
Cox Monett Hospital	Monett	70%	64
Southeast Missouri Hospital	Cape Girardeau	69%	196
University of Missouri Hospital and Clinics	Columbia	69%	142
Forest Park Hospital	Saint Louis	68%	122
General JJ Pershing Memorial Hospital	Brookfield	68%	77
Truman Medical Center-Lakewood	Kansas City	68%	53
Poplar Bluff Regional Medical Center	Poplar Bluff	67%	281
Barnes-Jewish Hospital	Saint Louis	65%	401
Callaway Community Hospital	Fulton	62%	42
Pemiscot Memorial Hospital	Hayti	60%	43
Truman Medical Centers	Kansas City	60%	164
Jefferson Memorial Hospital	Crystal City	59%	267
Sac-Osage Hospital	Osceola	59%	39
Ray County Memorial Hospital	Richmond	48%	33

17. Oxygenation Assessment

Hospital Name	City	Rate	Cases
Advanced Healthcare Medical Center	Ellington	100%	31
Audrain Medical Center	Mexico	100%	195
Barnes-Jewish Hospital	Saint Louis	100%	459
Barnes-Jewish Saint Peters Hospital	Saint Peters	100%	224
Barnes-Jewish West County Hospital	Saint Louis	100%	72
Bates County Memorial Hospital	Butler	100%	89
Boone Hospital Center	Columbia	100%	236
Bothwell Regional Health Center	Sedalia	100%	243
Callaway Community Hospital	Fulton	100%	51
Capital Region Medical Center	Jefferson City	100%	217
Cass Medical Center	Harrisonville	100%	61
Christian Hospital Northeast	Saint Louis	100%	393
Citizens Memorial Hospital	Bolivar	100%	147
Columbia Regional Hospital	Columbia	100%	48
Community Hospital Association	Fairfax	100%	56
Cox Med Ctrs-North and South & Walnut Lawn	Springfield	100%	693
Cox Monett Hospital	Monett	100%	76
DePaul Health Center	Bridgeton	100%	459
Des Peres Hospital	Saint Louis	100%	318
Doctors Hospital of Springfield	Springfield	100%	77
Fitzgibbon Memorial Hospital	Marshall	100%	137
Forest Park Hospital	Saint Louis	100%	171
Freeman Health System	Joplin	100%	476
Freeman Neosho Hospital	Neosho	100%	128
Golden Valley Memorial Hospital	Clinton	100%	165
Hannibal Regional Hospital	Hannibal	100%	353
Heartland Health	Saint Joseph	100%	511
Hedrick Medical Center	Chillicothe	100%	68
Hermann Area District Hospital	Hermann	100%	34
Lafayette Regional Health Center	Lexington	100%	111
Lake Regional Health Systems	Osage Beach	100%	231
Lee's Summit Hospital	Lee's Summit	100%	197
Liberty Hospital	Liberty	100%	415
Lincoln County Medical Center	Troy	100%	46
McCune-Brooks Hospital	Carthage	100%	92
Medical Center of Independence	Independence	100%	165
Mineral Area Regional Medical Center	Farmington	100%	201
Missouri Baptist Hospital Sullivan	Sullivan	100%	123
Missouri Baptist Medical Center	Saint Louis	100%	560
Missouri Delta Medical Center	Sikeston	100%	224
Missouri Southern Healthcare	Dexter	100%	137
Moberly Regional Medical Center	Moberly	100%	189
Nevada Regional Medical Center	Nevada	100%	69
Northwest Medical Center	Albany	100%	50
Ozarks Medical Center	West Plains	100%	204
Perry County Memorial Hospital	Perryville	100%	45
Phelps County Regional Medical Center	Rolla	100%	284
Pike County Memorial Hospital	Louisiana	100%	93
Putnam County Memorial Hospital	Unionville	100%	27
Research Medical Center	Kansas City	100%	235
Ripley County Memorial Hospital	Doniphan	100%	77
SLUCare	Saint Louis	100%	236
Saint Alexius Hospital	Saint Louis	100%	219
Saint Anthony's Medical Center	Saint Louis	100%	347
Saint Francis Hospital	Mountain View	100%	74
Saint Francis Hospital & Health Services	Maryville	100%	76
Saint Francis Medical Center	Cape Girardeau	100%	234
Saint John's Hospital at Lebanon	Lebanon	100%	168
Saint John's Hospital of Aurora	Aurora	100%	93
Saint John's Hospital-Caseville	Cassville	100%	43
Saint John's Mercy Hospital	Washington	100%	294
Saint John's Mercy Medical Center	Saint Louis	100%	500
Saint John's Regional Health Center	Springfield	100%	726
Saint Joseph Health Center	Kansas City	100%	278
Saint Joseph Health Center-Saint Charles	Saint Charles	100%	336
Saint Joseph Hospital West	Lake Saint Louis	100%	268
Saint Joseph Hospital of Kirkwood	Saint Louis	100%	277
Saint Luke's East Lee's Summit Hospital	Lees Summit	100%	48
Saint Luke's Hospital	Chesterfield	100%	480
Saint Luke's Hospital of Kansas City	Kansas City	100%	271
Saint Luke's Northland Hospital	Kansas City	100%	121
Saint Mary's Health Center	Saint Louis	100%	433
Saint Marys Health Center	Jefferson City	100%	243
Skaggs Community Health Center	Branson	100%	235
Southeast Missouri Hospital	Cape Girardeau	100%	252
Ste Genevieve County Memorial Hospital	Sainte Genevieve	100%	83
Sullivan County Memorial Hospital	Milan	100%	26
Truman Medical Center-Lakewood	Kansas City	100%	80
Truman Medical Centers	Kansas City	100%	181
University of Missouri Hospital and Clinics	Columbia	100%	177
Washington County Memorial Hospital	Potosi	100%	100
Wright Memorial Hospital	Trenton	100%	54
Cameron Regional Medical Center	Cameron	99%	161
Centerpoint Medical Center of Independence	Independence	99%	269
Cooper County Memorial Hospital	Boonville	99%	102
North Kansas City Hospital	North Kansas City	99%	322
Poplar Bluff Regional Medical Center	Poplar Bluff	99%	383
Saint John's Regional Medical Center	Joplin	99%	494
Saint Mary's Medical Center	Blue Springs	99%	214
Texas County Memorial Hospital	Houston	99%	139
Northeast Regional Medical Center	Kirksville	98%	131
Parkland Health Center	Farmington	98%	157
Ray County Memorial Hospital	Richmond	98%	41
Research Belton Hospital	Belton	98%	61
Western Missouri Medical Center	Warrensburg	98%	129
Carroll County Memorial Hospital	Carrollton	97%	79

NOTE: Hospital profiles are in alphabetical order by state, then city, then hospital within the city; Rankings are sorted by rate in descending order and exclude hospitals with less than 25 cases; (1) The number of cases is too small (n<25) for purposes of reliably predicting hospital performance; (2) Measure reflects the hospital's indication that its submission was based upon a sample of its relevant discharges; (3) Rate reflects fewer than the maximum possible quarters of data for the measure; (4) Inaccurate information submitted and suppressed for one or more quarters; (5) No data is available from the hospital for this measure; Please refer to the User's Guide for a full explanation of data

Harrison County Community Hospital	Bethany	97%	60
Jefferson Memorial Hospital	Crystal City	97%	314
Twin Rivers Regional Medical Center	Kennett	97%	128
General JJ Pershing Memorial Hospital	Brookfield	93%	88
Sac-Osage Hospital	Osceola	80%	44
Pemiscot Memorial Hospital	Hayti	72%	47

18. Pneumococcal Vaccine

Hospital Name	City	Rate	Cases
Freeman Neosho Hospital	Neosho	100%	76
Saint Francis Hospital & Health Services	Maryville	100%	61
Pike County Memorial Hospital	Louisiana	98%	59
Audrain Medical Center	Mexico	97%	118
Perry County Memorial Hospital	Perryville	97%	38
Saint John's Hospital-Caseville	Cassville	97%	29
Cooper County Memorial Hospital	Boonville	96%	67
Freeman Health System	Joplin	96%	281
Missouri Baptist Hospital Sullivan	Sullivan	95%	83
Saint Francis Medical Center	Cape Girardeau	95%	159
Saint John's Regional Health Center	Springfield	95%	497
Saint Luke's Hospital	Chesterfield	95%	359
Hedrick Medical Center	Chillicothe	94%	48
Barnes-Jewish West County Hospital	Saint Louis	92%	51
Boone Hospital Center	Columbia	92%	166
Capital Region Medical Center	Jefferson City	92%	145
Heartland Health	Saint Joseph	91%	318
Saint Luke's Northland Hospital	Kansas City	91%	77
Liberty Hospital	Liberty	90%	247
Saint John's Hospital at Lebanon	Lebanon	90%	101
Saint John's Mercy Hospital	Washington	90%	180
Saint John's Mercy Medical Center	Saint Louis	89%	297
Saint Luke's Hospital of Kansas City	Kansas City	89%	171
Cass Medical Center	Harrisonville	88%	42
Saint Joseph Health Center-Saint Charles	Saint Charles	88%	236
Medical Center of Independence	Independence	86%	98
Nevada Regional Medical Center	Nevada	86%	42
Saint John's Hospital of Aurora	Aurora	86%	64
Saint Marys Health Center	Jefferson City	86%	170
Bothwell Regional Health Center	Sedalia	85%	163
Parkland Health Center	Farmington	85%	101
Saint Joseph Hospital of Kirkwood	Saint Louis	85%	188
DePaul Health Center	Bridgeton	84%	258
Wright Memorial Hospital	Trenton	84%	38
Community Hospital Association	Fairfax	83%	47
Lake Regional Health Systems	Osage Beach	83%	145
Moberly Regional Medical Center	Moberly	82%	124
Saint Anthony's Medical Center	Saint Louis	82%	226
Research Belton Hospital	Belton	80%	41
Saint Mary's Medical Center	Blue Springs	80%	132
Lincoln County Medical Center	Troy	79%	29
Hannibal Regional Hospital	Hannibal	78%	240
Saint Mary's Health Center	Saint Louis	78%	262
Skaggs Community Health Center	Branson	78%	155
Des Peres Hospital	Saint Louis	77%	213
Phelps County Regional Medical Center	Rolla	77%	175
Saint Joseph Health Center	Kansas City	77%	183
Doctors Hospital of Springfield	Springfield	76%	50
Lee's Summit Hospital	Lee's Summit	76%	135
Missouri Baptist Medical Center	Saint Louis	76%	404
Missouri Delta Medical Center	Sikeston	76%	132
Ozarks Medical Center	West Plains	76%	118
Saint Alexius Hospital	Saint Louis	76%	105
Barnes-Jewish Saint Peters Hospital	Saint Peters	75%	130
North Kansas City Hospital	North Kansas City	75%	193
Northeast Regional Medical Center	Kirksville	75%	92
Saint Francis Hospital	Mountain View	74%	54
Research Medical Center	Kansas City	73%	154
Truman Medical Centers	Kansas City	73%	44
Christian Hospital Northeast	Saint Louis	72%	222
Saint Joseph Hospital West	Lake Saint Louis	72%	169
SLUCare	Saint Louis	71%	114
Ste Genevieve County Memorial Hospital	Sainte Genevieve	71%	52
Twin Rivers Regional Medical Center	Kennett	71%	52
Golden Valley Memorial Hospital	Clinton	67%	104
McCune-Brooks Hospital	Carthage	66%	59
Cox Monett Hospital	Monett	63%	43
Cameron Regional Medical Center	Cameron	62%	108
Citizens Memorial Hospital	Bolivar	62%	93
Centerpoint Medical Center of Independence	Independence	61%	193
Cox Med Ctrs-North and South & Walnut Lawn	Springfield	60%	345
Southeast Missouri Hospital	Cape Girardeau	60%	156
Forest Park Hospital	Saint Louis	59%	96
Missouri Southern Healthcare	Dexter	59%	83
Bates County Memorial Hospital	Butler	58%	55
University of Missouri Hospital and Clinics	Columbia	58%	79
Lafayette Regional Health Center	Lexington	57%	65
Saint John's Regional Medical Center	Joplin	57%	323
Fitzgibbon Memorial Hospital	Marshall	56%	82
Columbia Regional Hospital	Columbia	55%	29
Barnes-Jewish Hospital	Saint Louis	54%	161
Washington County Memorial Hospital	Potosi	54%	50
General JJ Pershing Memorial Hospital	Brookfield	53%	59
Poplar Bluff Regional Medical Center	Poplar Bluff	51%	243
Carroll County Memorial Hospital	Carrollton	49%	43
Callaway Community Hospital	Fulton	48%	27
Mineral Area Regional Medical Center	Farmington	46%	125
Truman Medical Center-Lakewood	Kansas City	46%	26
Hermann Area District Hospital	Hermann	44%	27
Harrison County Community Hospital	Bethany	41%	34
Texas County Memorial Hospital	Houston	38%	97
Sac-Osage Hospital	Osceola	32%	28
Western Missouri Medical Center	Warrensburg	30%	80
Ripley County Memorial Hospital	Doniphan	24%	45
Jefferson Memorial Hospital	Crystal City	18%	176

19. Smoking Cessation Advice

Hospital Name	City	Rate	Cases
Freeman Neosho Hospital	Neosho	100%	36
Lee's Summit Hospital	Lee's Summit	100%	36
Liberty Hospital	Liberty	100%	144
Missouri Delta Medical Center	Sikeston	100%	76
Saint Francis Medical Center	Cape Girardeau	100%	45
Saint Joseph Health Center	Kansas City	100%	49
Christian Hospital Northeast	Saint Louis	99%	92
Saint Anthony's Medical Center	Saint Louis	99%	83
Saint John's Mercy Hospital	Washington	99%	71
Saint Joseph Health Center-Saint Charles	Saint Charles	99%	70
Saint Luke's Hospital of Kansas City	Kansas City	99%	68
DePaul Health Center	Bridgeton	98%	137
Missouri Baptist Medical Center	Saint Louis	98%	119
Saint John's Mercy Medical Center	Saint Louis	98%	105
Twin Rivers Regional Medical Center	Kennett	98%	50
Bothwell Regional Health Center	Sedalia	97%	59
Des Peres Hospital	Saint Louis	97%	73
Freeman Health System	Joplin	97%	132
Heartland Health	Saint Joseph	97%	159
Moberly Regional Medical Center	Moberly	97%	39
Saint John's Hospital at Lebanon	Lebanon	97%	35
Saint John's Regional Health Center	Springfield	97%	216
Saint Mary's Health Center	Saint Louis	97%	115
Audrain Medical Center	Mexico	96%	50
Boone Hospital Center	Columbia	96%	45
Medical Center of Independence	Independence	96%	49
Saint Alexius Hospital	Saint Louis	96%	82
Saint Marys Health Center	Jefferson City	96%	47
Phelps County Regional Medical Center	Rolla	94%	81
Barnes-Jewish Saint Peters Hospital	Saint Peters	93%	44
Capital Region Medical Center	Jefferson City	93%	60
SLUCare	Saint Louis	93%	83
Saint Mary's Medical Center	Blue Springs	93%	58
Cameron Regional Medical Center	Cameron	92%	36
Cooper County Memorial Hospital	Boonville	92%	26
Truman Medical Centers	Kansas City	92%	95
Centerpoint Medical Center of Independence	Independence	91%	64
Research Medical Center	Kansas City	91%	67
Hannibal Regional Hospital	Hannibal	90%	68
Saint Joseph Hospital of Kirkwood	Saint Louis	90%	60
Saint Luke's Hospital	Chesterfield	90%	69
Southeast Missouri Hospital	Cape Girardeau	90%	52
Lake Regional Health Systems	Osage Beach	89%	66
Citizens Memorial Hospital	Bolivar	88%	40
Saint Joseph Hospital West	Lake Saint Louis	88%	65
Skaggs Community Health Center	Branson	88%	66
Mineral Area Regional Medical Center	Farmington	87%	52
Fitzgibbon Memorial Hospital	Marshall	86%	35
Barnes-Jewish Hospital	Saint Louis	85%	152
Parkland Health Center	Farmington	83%	41
North Kansas City Hospital	North Kansas City	82%	77
Golden Valley Memorial Hospital	Clinton	81%	59
Saint John's Regional Medical Center	Joplin	81%	167
Saint Luke's Northland Hospital	Kansas City	81%	36
Cox Med Ctrs-North and South & Walnut Lawn	Springfield	77%	194
Poplar Bluff Regional Medical Center	Poplar Bluff	75%	102
University of Missouri Hospital and Clinics	Columbia	75%	75
Jefferson Memorial Hospital	Crystal City	68%	92
Ozarks Medical Center	West Plains	67%	58
Western Missouri Medical Center	Warrensburg	63%	35
Forest Park Hospital	Saint Louis	62%	48

NOTE: Hospital profiles are in alphabetical order by state, then city, then hospital within the city; Rankings are sorted by rate in descending order and exclude hospitals with less than 25 cases; (1) The number of cases is too small (n<25) for purposes of reliably predicting hospital performance; (2) Measure reflects the hospital's indication that its submission was based upon a sample of its relevant discharges; (3) Rate reflects fewer than the maximum possible quarters of data for the measure; (4) Inaccurate information submitted and suppressed for one or more quarters; (5) No data is available from the hospital for this measure; Please refer to the User's Guide for a full explanation of data

Hospital Name	City	Rate	Cases
Washington County Memorial Hospital	Potosi	58%	26
Texas County Memorial Hospital	Houston	52%	31

Surgical Infection Prevention

20. Prophylactic Antibiotic Given

Hospital Name	City	Rate	Cases
Saint Joseph Health Center	Kansas City	97%	159
Saint Luke's Hospital of Kansas City	Kansas City	97%	763
Truman Medical Center-Lakewood	Kansas City	97%	61
Boone Hospital Center	Columbia	96%	804
Parkland Health Center	Farmington	96%	112
Barnes-Jewish West County Hospital	Saint Louis	95%	710
Doctors Hospital of Springfield	Springfield	95%	37
Missouri Baptist Hospital Sullivan	Sullivan	95%	37
Missouri Baptist Medical Center	Saint Louis	95%	773
Saint Francis Hospital & Health Services	Maryville	95%	125
Saint Marys Health Center	Jefferson City	95%	475
Twin Rivers Regional Medical Center	Kennett	95%	86
DePaul Health Center	Bridgeton	94%	1224
Saint John's Mercy Hospital	Washington	94%	354
Saint John's Mercy Medical Center	Saint Louis	94%	1001
Saint Mary's Health Center	Saint Louis	94%	1024
Barnes-Jewish Hospital	Saint Louis	93%	715
Barnes-Jewish Saint Peters Hospital	Saint Peters	93%	357
Freeman Health System	Joplin	93%	337
Heartland Health	Saint Joseph	93%	323
Audrain Medical Center	Mexico	92%	193
Christian Hospital Northeast	Saint Louis	92%	588
Saint Francis Medical Center	Cape Girardeau	91%	410
Saint John's Regional Health Center	Springfield	91%	360
Saint Joseph Hospital West	Lake Saint Louis	90%	381
Hannibal Regional Hospital	Hannibal	89%	310
Skaggs Community Health Center	Branson	89%	260
Capital Region Medical Center	Jefferson City	87%	428
Centerpoint Medical Center of Independence	Independence	87%	191
Research Medical Center	Kansas City	87%	278
Saint Anthony's Medical Center	Saint Louis	87%	639
Saint Joseph Health Center-Saint Charles	Saint Charles	87%	724
Saint Joseph Hospital of Kirkwood	Saint Louis	87%	643
Nevada Regional Medical Center	Nevada	86%	81
Saint John's Regional Medical Center	Joplin	86%	998
Ste Genevieve County Memorial Hospital	Sainte Genevieve	86%	42
Lee's Summit Hospital	Lee's Summit	85%	143
Saint Mary's Medical Center	Blue Springs	85%	86
Saint Luke's Northland Hospital	Kansas City	84%	159
Truman Medical Centers	Kansas City	84%	175
University of Missouri Hospital and Clinics	Columbia	84%	228
Phelps County Regional Medical Center	Rolla	83%	106
Cox Med Ctrs-North and South & Walnut Lawn	Springfield	82%	706
Citizens Memorial Hospital	Bolivar	81%	113
Liberty Hospital	Liberty	80%	369
Western Missouri Medical Center	Warrensburg	80%	61
Southeast Missouri Hospital	Cape Girardeau	79%	592
Des Peres Hospital	Saint Louis	77%	342
SLUCare	Saint Louis	77%	237
Cox Monett Hospital	Monett	76%	78
Lake Regional Health Systems	Osage Beach	76%	247
Columbia Regional Hospital	Columbia	74%	177
Saint Alexius Hospital	Saint Louis	74%	72
Fitzgibbon Memorial Hospital	Marshall	73%	88
Golden Valley Memorial Hospital	Clinton	73%	59
Saint Luke's East Lee's Summit Hospital	Lees Summit	73%	161
Saint Luke's Hospital	Chesterfield	73%	171
McCune-Brooks Hospital	Carthage	70%	54
Mineral Area Regional Medical Center	Farmington	69%	70
North Kansas City Hospital	North Kansas City	69%	480
Poplar Bluff Regional Medical Center	Poplar Bluff	69%	597
Jefferson Memorial Hospital	Crystal City	66%	244
Medical Center of Independence	Independence	66%	77
Cameron Regional Medical Center	Cameron	65%	51
Saint John's Hospital at Lebanon	Lebanon	62%	52
Forest Park Hospital	Saint Louis	61%	105
Bothwell Regional Health Center	Sedalia	59%	237
Moberly Regional Medical Center	Moberly	57%	53
Bates County Memorial Hospital	Butler	56%	39
Lincoln County Medical Center	Troy	56%	39
Ozarks Medical Center	West Plains	56%	156
Missouri Delta Medical Center	Sikeston	52%	86
Northeast Regional Medical Center	Kirksville	50%	149
Research Belton Hospital	Belton	30%	27

21. Prophylactic Antibiotic Selection

Hospital Name	City	Rate	Cases
Golden Valley Memorial Hospital	Clinton	100%	25
Saint Francis Hospital & Health Services	Maryville	100%	44
Barnes-Jewish West County Hospital	Saint Louis	99%	197
Hannibal Regional Hospital	Hannibal	99%	100
Cox Med Ctrs-North and South & Walnut Lawn	Springfield	98%	547
Freeman Health System	Joplin	98%	114
Jefferson Memorial Hospital	Crystal City	98%	94
Audrain Medical Center	Mexico	97%	68
Citizens Memorial Hospital	Bolivar	97%	58
DePaul Health Center	Bridgeton	97%	312
North Kansas City Hospital	North Kansas City	97%	125
Barnes-Jewish Hospital	Saint Louis	96%	160
Barnes-Jewish Saint Peters Hospital	Saint Peters	96%	74
Missouri Baptist Medical Center	Saint Louis	96%	167
Saint John's Mercy Medical Center	Saint Louis	96%	255
Saint John's Regional Health Center	Springfield	96%	96
Saint Joseph Hospital West	Lake Saint Louis	96%	108
Western Missouri Medical Center	Warrensburg	96%	56
Boone Hospital Center	Columbia	95%	164
Heartland Health	Saint Joseph	95%	250
Liberty Hospital	Liberty	95%	136
Northeast Regional Medical Center	Kirksville	95%	55
Saint John's Regional Medical Center	Joplin	95%	259
Saint Joseph Health Center-Saint Charles	Saint Charles	95%	195
Saint Joseph Hospital of Kirkwood	Saint Louis	95%	224
Saint John's Hospital at Lebanon	Lebanon	94%	50
Saint Mary's Health Center	Saint Louis	94%	253
SLUCare	Saint Louis	93%	54
Capital Region Medical Center	Jefferson City	92%	125
Saint Anthony's Medical Center	Saint Louis	92%	215
Saint John's Mercy Hospital	Washington	92%	36
Skaggs Community Health Center	Branson	92%	72
Southeast Missouri Hospital	Cape Girardeau	92%	140
Truman Medical Centers	Kansas City	92%	48
Bothwell Regional Health Center	Sedalia	91%	81
Saint Francis Medical Center	Cape Girardeau	91%	205
Saint Joseph Health Center	Kansas City	90%	71
Centerpoint Medical Center of Independence	Independence	89%	83
Research Medical Center	Kansas City	89%	139
Saint Luke's East Lee's Summit Hospital	Lees Summit	89%	72
Phelps County Regional Medical Center	Rolla	88%	103
Des Peres Hospital	Saint Louis	86%	92
Ozarks Medical Center	West Plains	85%	54
Saint Marys Health Center	Jefferson City	85%	96
Saint Luke's Northland Hospital	Kansas City	84%	51
Saint Mary's Medical Center	Blue Springs	84%	38
Christian Hospital Northeast	Saint Louis	82%	138
Poplar Bluff Regional Medical Center	Poplar Bluff	82%	102
Saint Luke's Hospital of Kansas City	Kansas City	81%	170
Lee's Summit Hospital	Lee's Summit	78%	58
Lake Regional Health Systems	Osage Beach	77%	88
Missouri Delta Medical Center	Sikeston	77%	31
Saint Luke's Hospital	Chesterfield	75%	105
University of Missouri Hospital and Clinics	Columbia	70%	74
Columbia Regional Hospital	Columbia	63%	65

22. Prophylactic Antibiotic Stopped

Hospital Name	City	Rate	Cases
Missouri Baptist Hospital Sullivan	Sullivan	100%	35
Ste Genevieve County Memorial Hospital	Sainte Genevieve	100%	41
Fitzgibbon Memorial Hospital	Marshall	99%	88
Saint Francis Hospital & Health Services	Maryville	98%	121
Saint John's Mercy Hospital	Washington	98%	341
Parkland Health Center	Farmington	97%	101
Moberly Regional Medical Center	Moberly	96%	51
Barnes-Jewish West County Hospital	Saint Louis	94%	703
DePaul Health Center	Bridgeton	93%	1135
Saint Joseph Health Center	Kansas City	92%	158
Saint Joseph Health Center-Saint Charles	Saint Charles	92%	701
Boone Hospital Center	Columbia	90%	757
Jefferson Memorial Hospital	Crystal City	89%	238
Saint John's Regional Health Center	Springfield	89%	354
Saint Joseph Hospital of Kirkwood	Saint Louis	89%	633
Twin Rivers Regional Medical Center	Kennett	89%	74
Barnes-Jewish Saint Peters Hospital	Saint Peters	88%	351
Heartland Health	Saint Joseph	87%	312
Saint Mary's Health Center	Saint Louis	87%	997
Capital Region Medical Center	Jefferson City	86%	420
Doctors Hospital of Springfield	Springfield	86%	35
Christian Hospital Northeast	Saint Louis	85%	536
Liberty Hospital	Liberty	84%	359
Saint Joseph Hospital West	Lake Saint Louis	84%	375

NOTE: Hospital profiles are in alphabetical order by state, then city, then hospital within the city; Rankings are sorted by rate in descending order and exclude hospitals with less than 25 cases; (1) The number of cases is too small (n<25) for purposes of reliably predicting hospital performance; (2) Measure reflects the hospital's indication that its submission was based upon a sample of its relevant discharges; (3) Rate reflects fewer than the maximum possible quarters of data for the measure; (4) Inaccurate information submitted and suppressed for one or more quarters; (5) No data is available from the hospital for this measure; Please refer to the User's Guide for a full explanation of data

Hannibal Regional Hospital	Hannibal	83%	299
Missouri Delta Medical Center	Sikeston	83%	78
Phelps County Regional Medical Center	Rolla	83%	101
Barnes-Jewish Hospital	Saint Louis	82%	636
Missouri Baptist Medical Center	Saint Louis	82%	723
Saint Francis Medical Center	Cape Girardeau	82%	384
Bothwell Regional Health Center	Sedalia	81%	230
Cox Med Ctrs-North and South & Walnut Lawn	Springfield	80%	691
Lee's Summit Hospital	Lee's Summit	80%	137
Mineral Area Regional Medical Center	Farmington	80%	69
Forest Park Hospital	Saint Louis	79%	99
Saint Luke's East Lee's Summit Hospital	Lees Summit	79%	160
Saint John's Mercy Medical Center	Saint Louis	78%	958
Saint Luke's Northland Hospital	Kansas City	78%	152
Golden Valley Memorial Hospital	Clinton	76%	59
University of Missouri Hospital and Clinics	Columbia	76%	214
Audrain Medical Center	Mexico	75%	189
North Kansas City Hospital	North Kansas City	74%	469
Saint Luke's Hospital of Kansas City	Kansas City	71%	737
Saint Alexius Hospital	Saint Louis	69%	71
Saint John's Regional Medical Center	Joplin	69%	986
Saint Marys Health Center	Jefferson City	69%	463
Truman Medical Centers	Kansas City	69%	174
Saint Anthony's Medical Center	Saint Louis	67%	606
Southeast Missouri Hospital	Cape Girardeau	65%	592
Columbia Regional Hospital	Columbia	64%	162
Northeast Regional Medical Center	Kirksville	64%	134
Ozarks Medical Center	West Plains	63%	131
Freeman Health System	Joplin	61%	321
Lake Regional Health Systems	Osage Beach	61%	246
Saint Luke's Hospital	Chesterfield	60%	164
Saint Mary's Medical Center	Blue Springs	58%	74
Skaggs Community Health Center	Branson	58%	260
Poplar Bluff Regional Medical Center	Poplar Bluff	57%	577
Cameron Regional Medical Center	Cameron	55%	51
Citizens Memorial Hospital	Bolivar	52%	112
Des Peres Hospital	Saint Louis	52%	338
Nevada Regional Medical Center	Nevada	52%	79
Cox Monett Hospital	Monett	50%	74
Medical Center of Independence	Independence	49%	70
Research Medical Center	Kansas City	42%	272
SLUCare	Saint Louis	42%	229
Western Missouri Medical Center	Warrensburg	42%	53
Bates County Memorial Hospital	Butler	37%	38
Lincoln County Medical Center	Troy	36%	39
Centerpoint Medical Center of Independence	Independence	31%	186
McCune-Brooks Hospital	Carthage	29%	52
Saint John's Hospital at Lebanon	Lebanon	16%	49
Truman Medical Center-Lakewood	Kansas City	16%	58

Pregnancy Care

23. Inpatient Neonatal Mortality

Hospital Name	City	Rate	Cases
Perry County Memorial Hospital	Perryville	0.00%	144
Missouri Baptist Medical Center	Saint Louis	0.07%	4228
Saint Mary's Medical Center	Blue Springs	0.08%	1252
Western Missouri Medical Center	Warrensburg	0.13%	797
Saint Joseph Health Center	Kansas City	0.23%	1297
Saint Anthony's Medical Center	Saint Louis	0.24%	1661
Saint John's Regional Medical Center	Joplin	0.33%	896
Columbia Regional Hospital	Columbia	1.37%	1894

24. Third or Fourth Degree Laceration

Hospital Name	City	Rate	Cases
Western Missouri Medical Center	Warrensburg	2.23%	629
Saint John's Regional Medical Center	Joplin	3.79%	633
Saint Joseph Health Center	Kansas City	3.79%	896
Missouri Baptist Medical Center	Saint Louis	4.24%	2785
Perry County Memorial Hospital	Perryville	5.08%	118
Saint Anthony's Medical Center	Saint Louis	5.46%	1080
Saint Mary's Medical Center	Blue Springs	5.61%	909
Columbia Regional Hospital	Columbia	5.85%	1163

NOTE: Hospital profiles are in alphabetical order by state, then city, then hospital within the city; Rankings are sorted by rate in descending order and exclude hospitals with less than 25 cases; (1) The number of cases is too small (n<25) for purposes of reliably predicting hospital performance; (2) Measure reflects the hospital's indication that its submission was based upon a sample of its relevant discharges; (3) Rate reflects fewer than the maximum possible quarters of data for the measure; (4) Inaccurate information submitted and suppressed for one or more quarters; (5) No data is available from the hospital for this measure; Please refer to the User's Guide for a full explanation of data

Northwest Medical Center

705 N College
Albany, MO 64402
URL: www.gcmh.org
Ownership: Voluntary non-profit - Private
Emergency Services: Yes
Phone: 660-756-3941
Fax: 660-726-3647
Accredited: No
Licensed Beds: 45

Key Personnel:
President . . . . Arturo Tenorio, MD

Measure	Cases	This Hospital	State Average	U.S. Average	Top Hospital
Heart Attack Care					
ACE Inhibitor or ARB for LVSD[1]	2	50%	76%	82%	100%
Aspirin at Arrival[1]	10	90%	92%	92%	100%
Aspirin at Discharge[1]	8	75%	87%	90%	100%
Beta Blocker at Arrival[1]	10	80%	83%	87%	100%
Beta Blocker at Discharge[1]	8	100%	87%	90%	100%
Fibrinolytic Medication Timing	0	-	26%	31%	100%
PCI Within 90 Minutes of Arrival	0	-	61%	54%	95%
Smoking Cessation Advice[1]	1	100%	92%	88%	100%
Heart Failure Care					
ACE Inhibitor or ARB for LVSD[1]	5	60%	84%	82%	100%
Discharge Instructions	25	64%	62%	61%	93%
Evaluation of LVS Function	41	73%	79%	83%	99%
Smoking Cessation Advice[1]	6	50%	80%	82%	100%
Pneumonia Care					
Appropriate Initial Antibiotic	32	62%	81%	83%	94%
Blood Culture Timing[1]	7	86%	92%	90%	100%
Influenza Vaccine[1]	5	80%	70%	70%	100%
Initial Antibiotic Timing	44	82%	81%	80%	93%
Oxygenation Assessment	50	100%	99%	99%	100%
Pneumococcal Vaccine[1]	24	75%	70%	69%	94%
Smoking Cessation Advice[1]	14	71%	83%	80%	100%
Surgical Infection Prevention					
Prophylactic Antibiotic Given[1,3]	5	80%	78%	77%	95%
Prophylactic Antibiotic Selection[5]	-	-	91%	90%	100%
Prophylactic Antibiotic Stopped[1,3]	5	40%	72%	72%	95%
Pregnancy Care					
Inpatient Neonatal Mortality	-	-	-	-	-
Third or Fourth Degree Laceration	-	-	-	3.63%	3.27%

Saint John's Hospital of Aurora

500 Porter Avenue
Aurora, MO 65605
E-mail: ach@achmo.com
URL: www.achmo.com
Ownership: Voluntary non-profit - Private
Emergency Services: Yes
Phone: 417-678-2122
Fax: 417-678-7877
Accredited: Yes
Licensed Beds: 59

Key Personnel:
Administrator . . . . Garry Jordan
Administrator & COO . . . . Don Buchanan
Chief Medical Staff. . . . . Joseph Bizek
Emergency Room . . . . Kent Stringer
Director Infection/Disease Control . . . . Debbie Nelson
Director Medical/Surgical Nursing . . . . Karen Sheperd
OB/GYN Womens Health. . . . . Brian Basham
Director Respiratory Therapy . . . . Rick Machmuller

Measure	Cases	This Hospital	State Average	U.S. Average	Top Hospital
Heart Attack Care					
ACE Inhibitor or ARB for LVSD[5]	-	-	76%	82%	100%
Aspirin at Arrival[5]	-	-	92%	92%	100%
Aspirin at Discharge[5]	-	-	87%	90%	100%
Beta Blocker at Arrival[5]	-	-	83%	87%	100%
Beta Blocker at Discharge[5]	-	-	87%	90%	100%
Fibrinolytic Medication Timing[5]	-	-	26%	31%	100%
PCI Within 90 Minutes of Arrival[5]	-	-	61%	54%	95%
Smoking Cessation Advice[5]	-	-	92%	88%	100%
Heart Failure Care					
ACE Inhibitor or ARB for LVSD[1,2]	8	88%	84%	82%	100%
Discharge Instructions[1,2]	22	55%	62%	61%	93%
Evaluation of LVS Function[2]	36	89%	79%	83%	99%
Smoking Cessation Advice[1,2]	8	88%	80%	82%	100%
Pneumonia Care					
Appropriate Initial Antibiotic[2]	69	97%	81%	83%	94%
Blood Culture Timing[2]	66	94%	92%	90%	100%
Influenza Vaccine[1]	21	86%	70%	70%	100%
Initial Antibiotic Timing[2]	74	89%	81%	80%	93%
Oxygenation Assessment[2]	93	100%	99%	99%	100%
Pneumococcal Vaccine[2]	64	86%	70%	69%	94%
Smoking Cessation Advice[1,2]	23	100%	83%	80%	100%
Surgical Infection Prevention					
Prophylactic Antibiotic Given[5]	-	-	78%	77%	95%
Prophylactic Antibiotic Selection[5]	-	-	91%	90%	100%
Prophylactic Antibiotic Stopped[5]	-	-	72%	72%	95%
Pregnancy Care					
Inpatient Neonatal Mortality	-	-	-	-	-
Third or Fourth Degree Laceration	-	-	-	3.63%	3.27%

Research Belton Hospital

17065 S 71 Highway
Belton, MO 64012
Ownership: Voluntary non-profit - Private
Emergency Services: Yes
Phone: 816-348-1200
Fax: 816-348-1293
Accredited: Yes
Licensed Beds: 75

Key Personnel:
CEO. . . . . Steve Newton
Chief Medical Staff. . . . . Kirk Barnett
Emergency Room . . . . Carol Creek, RN
Director Infection/Disease Control . . . . Cheryl Davis
Supervisor Respiratory Therapy. . . . . Gary Skiles

Measure	Cases	This Hospital	State Average	U.S. Average	Top Hospital
Heart Attack Care					
ACE Inhibitor or ARB for LVSD[1]	2	50%	76%	82%	100%
Aspirin at Arrival[1]	9	100%	92%	92%	100%
Aspirin at Discharge[1]	7	86%	87%	90%	100%
Beta Blocker at Arrival[1]	7	71%	83%	87%	100%
Beta Blocker at Discharge[1]	6	67%	87%	90%	100%
Fibrinolytic Medication Timing[3]	0	-	26%	31%	100%
PCI Within 90 Minutes of Arrival	0	-	61%	54%	95%
Smoking Cessation Advice[3]	0	-	92%	88%	100%
Heart Failure Care					
ACE Inhibitor or ARB for LVSD[1]	17	82%	84%	82%	100%
Discharge Instructions[1,3]	6	50%	62%	61%	93%
Evaluation of LVS Function	63	83%	79%	83%	99%
Smoking Cessation Advice[1,3]	1	100%	80%	82%	100%
Pneumonia Care					
Appropriate Initial Antibiotic[1,3]	4	100%	81%	83%	94%
Blood Culture Timing[1,3]	5	80%	92%	90%	100%
Influenza Vaccine[5]	-	-	70%	70%	100%
Initial Antibiotic Timing	45	91%	81%	80%	93%
Oxygenation Assessment	61	98%	99%	99%	100%
Pneumococcal Vaccine	41	80%	70%	69%	94%
Smoking Cessation Advice[1,3]	2	100%	83%	80%	100%
Surgical Infection Prevention					
Prophylactic Antibiotic Given[2,3]	27	30%	78%	77%	95%
Prophylactic Antibiotic Selection[5]	-	-	91%	90%	100%
Prophylactic Antibiotic Stopped[1,2,3]	24	50%	72%	72%	95%
Pregnancy Care					
Inpatient Neonatal Mortality	-	-	-	-	-
Third or Fourth Degree Laceration	-	-	-	3.63%	3.27%

Harrison County Community Hospital

Alternate Name: Noll Memorial Hospital
2600 Miller Street
Bethany, MO 64424
Ownership: Govt - Hospital District or Authority
Emergency Services: Yes
Phone: 660-425-2211
Fax: 660-425-2366
Accredited: No
Licensed Beds: 23

Key Personnel:
Administrator . . . . Rich Hamilton
Chief Medical Staff. . . . . Natu Patel
Emergency Room . . . . Crystal Hicks
Respiratory Care . . . . Marry Elfberr

Measure	Cases	This Hospital	State Average	U.S. Average	Top Hospital
Heart Attack Care					

NOTE: Hospital profiles are in alphabetical order by state, then city, then hospital within the city; Rankings are sorted by rate in descending order and exclude hospitals with less than 25 cases; (1) The number of cases is too small (n<25) for purposes of reliably predicting hospital performance; (2) Measure reflects the hospital's indication that its submission was based upon a sample of its relevant discharges; (3) Rate reflects fewer than the maximum possible quarters of data for the measure; (4) Inaccurate information submitted and suppressed for one or more quarters; (5) No data is available from the hospital for this measure; Please refer to the User's Guide for a full explanation of data

ACE Inhibitor or ARB for LVSD[5]	-	-	76%	82%	100%
Aspirin at Arrival[5]	-	-	92%	92%	100%
Aspirin at Discharge[5]	-	-	87%	90%	100%
Beta Blocker at Arrival[5]	-	-	83%	87%	100%
Beta Blocker at Discharge[5]	-	-	87%	90%	100%
Fibrinolytic Medication Timing[5]	-	-	26%	31%	100%
PCI Within 90 Minutes of Arrival[5]	-	-	61%	54%	95%
Smoking Cessation Advice[5]	-	-	92%	88%	100%
Heart Failure Care					
ACE Inhibitor or ARB for LVSD[1,2]	1	100%	84%	82%	100%
Discharge Instructions[1,2]	5	0%	62%	61%	93%
Evaluation of LVS Function[1,2]	13	46%	79%	83%	99%
Smoking Cessation Advice[1,2]	1	0%	80%	82%	100%
Pneumonia Care					
Appropriate Initial Antibiotic[2]	43	88%	81%	83%	94%
Blood Culture Timing[1,2]	13	100%	92%	90%	100%
Influenza Vaccine[1]	10	40%	70%	70%	100%
Initial Antibiotic Timing[2]	48	96%	81%	80%	93%
Oxygenation Assessment[2]	60	97%	99%	99%	100%
Pneumococcal Vaccine[2]	34	41%	70%	69%	94%
Smoking Cessation Advice[1,2]	15	13%	83%	80%	100%
Surgical Infection Prevention					
Prophylactic Antibiotic Given[5]	-	-	78%	77%	95%
Prophylactic Antibiotic Selection[5]	-	-	91%	90%	100%
Prophylactic Antibiotic Stopped[5]	-	-	72%	72%	95%
Pregnancy Care					
Inpatient Neonatal Mortality	-	-	-	-	-
Third or Fourth Degree Laceration	-	-	-	3.63%	3.27%

Saint Mary's Medical Center

201 W RD Mize Road
Blue Springs, MO 64014
Phone: 816-228-5900
Fax: 816-655-5649
Ownership: Voluntary non-profit - Church
Accredited: Yes
Emergency Services: Yes
Licensed Beds: 143

Key Personnel:

President/CEO. . . . . Gordon Docking
Chief of Medical Staff. . . . . Steve Sanders
Emergency Room . . . . Judy Avise
Director of Pulmonary/Respiratory Care. . . . . . . Laera Foster

Measure	Cases	This Hospital	State Average	U.S. Average	Top Hospital
Heart Attack Care					
ACE Inhibitor or ARB for LVSD[1]	9	89%	76%	82%	100%
Aspirin at Arrival	54	100%	92%	92%	100%
Aspirin at Discharge	27	96%	87%	90%	100%
Beta Blocker at Arrival	48	98%	83%	87%	100%
Beta Blocker at Discharge	26	100%	87%	90%	100%
Fibrinolytic Medication Timing	0	-	26%	31%	100%
PCI Within 90 Minutes of Arrival	0	-	61%	54%	95%
Smoking Cessation Advice[1]	3	100%	92%	88%	100%
Heart Failure Care					
ACE Inhibitor or ARB for LVSD	42	88%	84%	82%	100%
Discharge Instructions	94	87%	62%	61%	93%
Evaluation of LVS Function	130	92%	79%	83%	99%
Smoking Cessation Advice[1]	20	100%	80%	82%	100%
Pneumonia Care					
Appropriate Initial Antibiotic	156	74%	81%	83%	94%
Blood Culture Timing	118	86%	92%	90%	100%
Influenza Vaccine	49	57%	70%	70%	100%
Initial Antibiotic Timing	189	88%	81%	80%	93%
Oxygenation Assessment	214	99%	99%	99%	100%
Pneumococcal Vaccine	132	80%	70%	69%	94%
Smoking Cessation Advice	58	93%	83%	80%	100%
Surgical Infection Prevention					
Prophylactic Antibiotic Given[2,3]	86	85%	78%	77%	95%
Prophylactic Antibiotic Selection[2]	38	84%	91%	90%	100%
Prophylactic Antibiotic Stopped[2,3]	74	58%	72%	72%	95%
Pregnancy Care					
Inpatient Neonatal Mortality	1,252	0.08%	-	-	-
Third or Fourth Degree Laceration	909	5.61%	-	3.63%	3.27%

Citizens Memorial Hospital

1500 N Oakland
Bolivar, MO 65613
Phone: 417-326-6000
Fax: 417-326-0338
URL: www.citizensmemorial.com
Ownership: Govt - Hospital District or Authority
Accredited: Yes
Emergency Services: Yes
Licensed Beds: 74

Key Personnel:

CEO. . . . . Donald J Babb
Chief Medical Staff. . . . . Dennis Boeke, DO
Director Surgery/Outpatient Services . . . . Nancy Nickos
Emergency Room . . . . Jeffrey Smieshek, DO
Director Infection/Disease Control . . . . Helen Molchan, RN
Director Medical/Surgical Nursing . . . . Missy Davis
Director Radiology . . . . Greg Elliott
Director Respiratory Care. . . . . Allen Morris

Measure	Cases	This Hospital	State Average	U.S. Average	Top Hospital
Heart Attack Care					
ACE Inhibitor or ARB for LVSD[1]	2	100%	76%	82%	100%
Aspirin at Arrival[1]	13	100%	92%	92%	100%
Aspirin at Discharge[1]	12	92%	87%	90%	100%
Beta Blocker at Arrival[1]	17	88%	83%	87%	100%
Beta Blocker at Discharge[1]	13	85%	87%	90%	100%
Fibrinolytic Medication Timing	0	-	26%	31%	100%
PCI Within 90 Minutes of Arrival	0	-	61%	54%	95%
Smoking Cessation Advice	0	-	92%	88%	100%
Heart Failure Care					
ACE Inhibitor or ARB for LVSD[1]	15	93%	84%	82%	100%
Discharge Instructions	53	55%	62%	61%	93%
Evaluation of LVS Function	75	83%	79%	83%	99%
Smoking Cessation Advice[1]	9	78%	80%	82%	100%
Pneumonia Care					
Appropriate Initial Antibiotic	91	76%	81%	83%	94%
Blood Culture Timing	70	93%	92%	90%	100%
Influenza Vaccine	30	67%	70%	70%	100%
Initial Antibiotic Timing	117	74%	81%	80%	93%
Oxygenation Assessment	147	100%	99%	99%	100%
Pneumococcal Vaccine	93	62%	70%	69%	94%
Smoking Cessation Advice	40	88%	83%	80%	100%
Surgical Infection Prevention					
Prophylactic Antibiotic Given[3]	113	81%	78%	77%	95%
Prophylactic Antibiotic Selection	58	97%	91%	90%	100%
Prophylactic Antibiotic Stopped[3]	112	52%	72%	72%	95%
Pregnancy Care					
Inpatient Neonatal Mortality	-	-	-	-	-
Third or Fourth Degree Laceration	-	-	-	3.63%	3.27%

Cooper County Memorial Hospital

17651 B Highway
Boonville, MO 65233
Phone: 660-882-7461
Fax: 660-882-6093
Ownership: Government - Local
Accredited: No
Emergency Services: No
Licensed Beds: 70

Key Personnel:

CEO. . . . . Matt Waterman

Measure	Cases	This Hospital	State Average	U.S. Average	Top Hospital
Heart Attack Care					
ACE Inhibitor or ARB for LVSD[2]	0	-	76%	82%	100%
Aspirin at Arrival[1,2]	6	100%	92%	92%	100%
Aspirin at Discharge[1,2]	4	75%	87%	90%	100%
Beta Blocker at Arrival[1,2]	8	100%	83%	87%	100%
Beta Blocker at Discharge[1,2]	6	100%	87%	90%	100%
Fibrinolytic Medication Timing[2]	0	-	26%	31%	100%
PCI Within 90 Minutes of Arrival[2]	0	-	61%	54%	95%
Smoking Cessation Advice[2]	0	-	92%	88%	100%
Heart Failure Care					
ACE Inhibitor or ARB for LVSD[1,2]	5	60%	84%	82%	100%
Discharge Instructions[2]	28	89%	62%	61%	93%
Evaluation of LVS Function[2]	41	76%	79%	83%	99%
Smoking Cessation Advice[1,2]	8	88%	80%	82%	100%
Pneumonia Care					
Appropriate Initial Antibiotic[2]	72	78%	81%	83%	94%
Blood Culture Timing[2]	26	85%	92%	90%	100%

NOTE: Hospital profiles are in alphabetical order by state, then city, then hospital within the city; Rankings are sorted by rate in descending order and exclude hospitals with less than 25 cases; (1) The number of cases is too small (n<25) for purposes of reliably predicting hospital performance; (2) Measure reflects the hospital's indication that its submission was based upon a sample of its relevant discharges; (3) Rate reflects fewer than the maximum possible quarters of data for the measure; (4) Inaccurate information submitted and suppressed for one or more quarters; (5) No data is available from the hospital for this measure; Please refer to the User's Guide for a full explanation of data

Measure	Cases	This Hospital	State Average	U.S. Average	Top Hospital
Influenza Vaccine[1]	17	88%	70%	70%	100%
Initial Antibiotic Timing[2]	94	86%	81%	80%	93%
Oxygenation Assessment[2]	102	99%	99%	99%	100%
Pneumococcal Vaccine[2]	67	96%	70%	69%	94%
Smoking Cessation Advice[2]	26	92%	83%	80%	100%
Surgical Infection Prevention					
Prophylactic Antibiotic Given[5]	-	-	78%	77%	95%
Prophylactic Antibiotic Selection[5]	-	-	91%	90%	100%
Prophylactic Antibiotic Stopped[5]	-	-	72%	72%	95%
Pregnancy Care					
Inpatient Neonatal Mortality	-	-	-	-	-
Third or Fourth Degree Laceration	-	-	-	3.63%	3.27%

Skaggs Community Health Center

Alternate Name: Skaggs Community Hospital
PO Box 650 Phone: 417-335-7000
Branson, MO 65615 Fax: 417-334-1505
URL: www.skaggs.net
Ownership: Voluntary non-profit - Private Accredited: Yes
Emergency Services: Yes Licensed Beds: 177

Key Personnel:

Administrator/CEO . . . . Stephen M Erixson, MHA
Cardiac Lab . . . . Jon Jenkins
Emergency Room . . . . Bob Denton
Infection Control . . . . Ann Erving
ICU . . . . Angilee McPathe
OB/GYN/Women's Health . . . . Carrie Holloway
Respiratory/Cardiopulmonary . . . . Paula Fortson

Measure	Cases	This Hospital	State Average	U.S. Average	Top Hospital
Heart Attack Care					
ACE Inhibitor or ARB for LVSD[2]	31	68%	76%	82%	100%
Aspirin at Arrival[2]	190	99%	92%	92%	100%
Aspirin at Discharge[2]	182	97%	87%	90%	100%
Beta Blocker at Arrival[2]	164	94%	83%	87%	100%
Beta Blocker at Discharge[2]	172	92%	87%	90%	100%
Fibrinolytic Medication Timing[2]	0	-	26%	31%	100%
PCI Within 90 Minutes of Arrival[1,2]	11	73%	61%	54%	95%
Smoking Cessation Advice[2]	56	100%	92%	88%	100%
Heart Failure Care					
ACE Inhibitor or ARB for LVSD[2]	65	78%	84%	82%	100%
Discharge Instructions[2]	155	35%	62%	61%	93%
Evaluation of LVS Function[2]	183	95%	79%	83%	99%
Smoking Cessation Advice[2]	36	97%	80%	82%	100%
Pneumonia Care					
Appropriate Initial Antibiotic[2]	151	67%	81%	83%	94%
Blood Culture Timing[2]	132	89%	92%	90%	100%
Influenza Vaccine	38	87%	70%	70%	100%
Initial Antibiotic Timing[2]	180	71%	81%	80%	93%
Oxygenation Assessment[2]	235	100%	99%	99%	100%
Pneumococcal Vaccine[2]	155	78%	70%	69%	94%
Smoking Cessation Advice[2]	66	88%	83%	80%	100%
Surgical Infection Prevention					
Prophylactic Antibiotic Given[3]	260	89%	78%	77%	95%
Prophylactic Antibiotic Selection	72	92%	91%	90%	100%
Prophylactic Antibiotic Stopped[3]	260	58%	72%	72%	95%
Pregnancy Care					
Inpatient Neonatal Mortality	-	-	-	-	-
Third or Fourth Degree Laceration	-	-	-	3.63%	3.27%

DePaul Health Center

12303 DePaul Drive Phone: 314-344-6000
Bridgeton, MO 63044 Fax: 314-344-6840
URL: www.ssmdepaul.com
Ownership: Voluntary non-profit - Church Accredited: Yes
Emergency Services: Yes Licensed Beds: 538

Key Personnel:

Chief Medical Staff . . . . Kevin Johnson, MD
Director of Cardiology/Cardiac Lab . . . . Mindy Manley
Emergency Room . . . . Clare Mir

Measure	Cases	This Hospital	State Average	U.S. Average	Top Hospital
Heart Attack Care					
ACE Inhibitor or ARB for LVSD	104	84%	76%	82%	100%
Aspirin at Arrival	264	96%	92%	92%	100%
Aspirin at Discharge	267	99%	87%	90%	100%
Beta Blocker at Arrival	189	90%	83%	87%	100%
Beta Blocker at Discharge	283	95%	87%	90%	100%
Fibrinolytic Medication Timing[1]	2	50%	26%	31%	100%
PCI Within 90 Minutes of Arrival[1]	14	57%	61%	54%	95%
Smoking Cessation Advice	125	100%	92%	88%	100%
Heart Failure Care					
ACE Inhibitor or ARB for LVSD	265	80%	84%	82%	100%
Discharge Instructions	551	72%	62%	61%	93%
Evaluation of LVS Function	686	93%	79%	83%	99%
Smoking Cessation Advice	150	99%	80%	82%	100%
Pneumonia Care					
Appropriate Initial Antibiotic	235	87%	81%	83%	94%
Blood Culture Timing	280	96%	92%	90%	100%
Influenza Vaccine	69	84%	70%	70%	100%
Initial Antibiotic Timing	345	75%	81%	80%	93%
Oxygenation Assessment	459	100%	99%	99%	100%
Pneumococcal Vaccine	258	84%	70%	69%	94%
Smoking Cessation Advice	137	98%	83%	80%	100%
Surgical Infection Prevention					
Prophylactic Antibiotic Given	1,224	94%	78%	77%	95%
Prophylactic Antibiotic Selection	312	97%	91%	90%	100%
Prophylactic Antibiotic Stopped	1,135	93%	72%	72%	95%
Pregnancy Care					
Inpatient Neonatal Mortality	-	-	-	-	-
Third or Fourth Degree Laceration	-	-	-	3.63%	3.27%

General JJ Pershing Memorial Hospital

130 E Lockling Avenue Phone: 660-258-2222
Brookfield, MO 64628 Fax: 660-258-5668
Ownership: Voluntary non-profit - Private Accredited: No
Emergency Services: Yes Licensed Beds: 57

Key Personnel:

Administrator/CEO . . . . Phil Hamilton
Chief Medical Staff . . . . BD Howell, MD
Emergency Room . . . . PC Rivera, MD
Respiratory Therapy . . . . Terry Brosemer

Measure	Cases	This Hospital	State Average	U.S. Average	Top Hospital
Heart Attack Care					
ACE Inhibitor or ARB for LVSD[3]	0	-	76%	82%	100%
Aspirin at Arrival[1,3]	2	100%	92%	92%	100%
Aspirin at Discharge[1,3]	2	0%	87%	90%	100%
Beta Blocker at Arrival[1,3]	2	100%	83%	87%	100%
Beta Blocker at Discharge[1,3]	2	0%	87%	90%	100%
Fibrinolytic Medication Timing[3]	0	-	26%	31%	100%
PCI Within 90 Minutes of Arrival	0	-	61%	54%	95%
Smoking Cessation Advice[3]	0	-	92%	88%	100%
Heart Failure Care					
ACE Inhibitor or ARB for LVSD	0	-	84%	82%	100%
Discharge Instructions[1]	18	67%	62%	61%	93%
Evaluation of LVS Function	46	0%	79%	83%	99%
Smoking Cessation Advice[1]	4	25%	80%	82%	100%
Pneumonia Care					
Appropriate Initial Antibiotic	70	71%	81%	83%	94%
Blood Culture Timing[1]	17	100%	92%	90%	100%
Influenza Vaccine[1]	23	70%	70%	70%	100%
Initial Antibiotic Timing	77	68%	81%	80%	93%
Oxygenation Assessment	88	93%	99%	99%	100%
Pneumococcal Vaccine	59	53%	70%	69%	94%
Smoking Cessation Advice[1]	13	8%	83%	80%	100%
Surgical Infection Prevention					
Prophylactic Antibiotic Given[5]	-	-	78%	77%	95%
Prophylactic Antibiotic Selection[5]	-	-	91%	90%	100%
Prophylactic Antibiotic Stopped[5]	-	-	72%	72%	95%
Pregnancy Care					
Inpatient Neonatal Mortality	-	-	-	-	-
Third or Fourth Degree Laceration	-	-	-	3.63%	3.27%

NOTE: Hospital profiles are in alphabetical order by state, then city, then hospital within the city; Rankings are sorted by rate in descending order and exclude hospitals with less than 25 cases; (1) The number of cases is too small (n<25) for purposes of reliably predicting hospital performance; (2) Measure reflects the hospital's indication that its submission was based upon a sample of its relevant discharges; (3) Rate reflects fewer than the maximum possible quarters of data for the measure; (4) Inaccurate information submitted and suppressed for one or more quarters; (5) No data is available from the hospital for this measure; Please refer to the User's Guide for a full explanation of data

Bates County Memorial Hospital

615 W Nursery Street
Butler, MO 64730
URL: www.bcmhospital.com
Ownership: Government - Local
Emergency Services: Yes

Phone: 660-200-7000
Fax: 660-200-7016

Accredited: No
Licensed Beds: 60

Key Personnel:

President/CEO . . . . Gaylon C Lowery, CHE
Chief Medical Staff . . . . Jim Miller, DO
Emergency Room . . . . Kelly Phillips
Infection Control . . . . Carmen Matter, RN
ICU . . . . Donna Short, RN
Medical/Surgical Nursing . . . . Donna Short, RN
Respiratory/Cardiopulmonary . . . . Wayne Rives

Measure	Cases	This Hospital	State Average	U.S. Average	Top Hospital
Heart Attack Care					
ACE Inhibitor or ARB for LVSD[2]	0	-	76%	82%	100%
Aspirin at Arrival[1,2]	15	87%	92%	92%	100%
Aspirin at Discharge[1,2]	7	86%	87%	90%	100%
Beta Blocker at Arrival[1,2]	12	75%	83%	87%	100%
Beta Blocker at Discharge[1,2]	8	38%	87%	90%	100%
Fibrinolytic Medication Timing[2]	0	-	26%	31%	100%
PCI Within 90 Minutes of Arrival[2]	0	-	61%	54%	95%
Smoking Cessation Advice[1,2]	3	67%	92%	88%	100%
Heart Failure Care					
ACE Inhibitor or ARB for LVSD[1,2]	4	75%	84%	82%	100%
Discharge Instructions[2]	81	64%	62%	61%	93%
Evaluation of LVS Function[2]	109	11%	79%	83%	99%
Smoking Cessation Advice[1,2]	11	55%	80%	82%	100%
Pneumonia Care					
Appropriate Initial Antibiotic[2]	66	52%	81%	83%	94%
Blood Culture Timing[2]	44	91%	92%	90%	100%
Influenza Vaccine[1]	19	58%	70%	70%	100%
Initial Antibiotic Timing[2]	80	89%	81%	80%	93%
Oxygenation Assessment[2]	89	100%	99%	99%	100%
Pneumococcal Vaccine[2]	55	58%	70%	69%	94%
Smoking Cessation Advice[1,2]	22	59%	83%	80%	100%
Surgical Infection Prevention					
Prophylactic Antibiotic Given[2,3]	39	56%	78%	77%	95%
Prophylactic Antibiotic Selection[1,2]	17	100%	91%	90%	100%
Prophylactic Antibiotic Stopped[2,3]	38	37%	72%	72%	95%
Pregnancy Care					
Inpatient Neonatal Mortality	-	-	-	-	-
Third or Fourth Degree Laceration	-	-	-	3.63%	3.27%

Cameron Regional Medical Center

1600 East Evergreen
PO Box 557
Cameron, MO 64429
URL: www.cameronregional.org
Ownership: Voluntary non-profit - Private
Emergency Services: Yes

Phone: 816-632-2101
Fax: 816-649-3206

Accredited: No
Licensed Beds: 57

Key Personnel:

CEO . . . . Joseph F Abrutz, Jr
Chief Medical Staff . . . . Frederick Kiehl, DO
Emergency Room . . . . Fred Kiehl, DO
Director Infection/Disease Control . . . . Ginger Graham, RN
Director Medical/Surgical Nursing . . . . Barbara Lee, RN
Surgical Services . . . . Marla Cowell, RN
Director Radiology . . . . Vernon Boswell
Director Respiratory Therapy . . . . Cheryl Calvert, RRT

Measure	Cases	This Hospital	State Average	U.S. Average	Top Hospital
Heart Attack Care					
ACE Inhibitor or ARB for LVSD[1,3]	1	100%	76%	82%	100%
Aspirin at Arrival[1,3]	12	92%	92%	92%	100%
Aspirin at Discharge[1,3]	7	71%	87%	90%	100%
Beta Blocker at Arrival[1,3]	16	94%	83%	87%	100%
Beta Blocker at Discharge[1,3]	12	92%	87%	90%	100%
Fibrinolytic Medication Timing[3]	0	-	26%	31%	100%
PCI Within 90 Minutes of Arrival[5]	-	-	61%	54%	95%
Smoking Cessation Advice[1,3]	1	100%	92%	88%	100%
Heart Failure Care					
ACE Inhibitor or ARB for LVSD[1,2]	15	80%	84%	82%	100%
Discharge Instructions[2]	31	32%	62%	61%	93%
Evaluation of LVS Function[2]	63	75%	79%	83%	99%
Smoking Cessation Advice[1,2]	10	90%	80%	82%	100%
Pneumonia Care					
Appropriate Initial Antibiotic[2]	65	89%	81%	83%	94%
Blood Culture Timing[2]	84	81%	92%	90%	100%
Influenza Vaccine	26	58%	70%	70%	100%
Initial Antibiotic Timing[2]	129	92%	81%	80%	93%
Oxygenation Assessment[2]	161	99%	99%	99%	100%
Pneumococcal Vaccine[2]	108	62%	70%	69%	94%
Smoking Cessation Advice[2]	36	92%	83%	80%	100%
Surgical Infection Prevention					
Prophylactic Antibiotic Given[2,3]	51	65%	78%	77%	95%
Prophylactic Antibiotic Selection[1,2]	20	100%	91%	90%	100%
Prophylactic Antibiotic Stopped[2,3]	51	55%	72%	72%	95%
Pregnancy Care					
Inpatient Neonatal Mortality	-	-	-	-	-
Third or Fourth Degree Laceration	-	-	-	3.63%	3.27%

Saint Francis Medical Center

211 Saint Francis Drive
Cape Girardeau, MO 63703
URL: www.sfmc.net
Ownership: Voluntary non-profit - Church
Emergency Services: Yes

Phone: 573-331-3000
Fax: 573-331-5031

Accredited: Yes
Licensed Beds: 264

Key Personnel:

CEO . . . . Stephen Bjlich
Chief Medical Staff . . . . Billy Hammond, MD
Director of Cardiology/Cardiac Lab . . . . Savid Stagner
Emergency Room . . . . Marcia Abernathy
OB/GYN Womens Health . . . . Ann Behrend-Uhls, MD
Chief Radiology . . . . WJ Stoecker, MD
Director of Pulmonary/Respiratory Care . . . . Lisa Newcomer

Measure	Cases	This Hospital	State Average	U.S. Average	Top Hospital
Heart Attack Care					
ACE Inhibitor or ARB for LVSD	60	95%	76%	82%	100%
Aspirin at Arrival	176	96%	92%	92%	100%
Aspirin at Discharge	245	95%	87%	90%	100%
Beta Blocker at Arrival	130	95%	83%	87%	100%
Beta Blocker at Discharge	235	97%	87%	90%	100%
Fibrinolytic Medication Timing	0	-	26%	31%	100%
PCI Within 90 Minutes of Arrival[1]	12	33%	61%	54%	95%
Smoking Cessation Advice	107	100%	92%	88%	100%
Heart Failure Care					
ACE Inhibitor or ARB for LVSD	119	94%	84%	82%	100%
Discharge Instructions	272	92%	62%	61%	93%
Evaluation of LVS Function	341	98%	79%	83%	99%
Smoking Cessation Advice	62	100%	80%	82%	100%
Pneumonia Care					
Appropriate Initial Antibiotic	102	90%	81%	83%	94%
Blood Culture Timing	151	97%	92%	90%	100%
Influenza Vaccine	47	94%	70%	70%	100%
Initial Antibiotic Timing	168	90%	81%	80%	93%
Oxygenation Assessment	234	100%	99%	99%	100%
Pneumococcal Vaccine	159	95%	70%	69%	94%
Smoking Cessation Advice	45	100%	83%	80%	100%
Surgical Infection Prevention					
Prophylactic Antibiotic Given[3]	410	91%	78%	77%	95%
Prophylactic Antibiotic Selection	205	91%	91%	90%	100%
Prophylactic Antibiotic Stopped[3]	384	82%	72%	72%	95%
Pregnancy Care					
Inpatient Neonatal Mortality	-	-	-	-	-
Third or Fourth Degree Laceration	-	-	-	3.63%	3.27%

NOTE: Hospital profiles are in alphabetical order by state, then city, then hospital within the city; Rankings are sorted by rate in descending order and exclude hospitals with less than 25 cases; (1) The number of cases is too small (n<25) for purposes of reliably predicting hospital performance; (2) Measure reflects the hospital's indication that its submission was based upon a sample of its relevant discharges; (3) Rate reflects fewer than the maximum possible quarters of data for the measure; (4) Inaccurate information submitted and suppressed for one or more quarters; (5) No data is available from the hospital for this measure; Please refer to the User's Guide for a full explanation of data

Southeast Missouri Hospital

1701 Lacey Street
Cape Girardeau, MO 63701
URL: www.southeastmissourihospital.com
Ownership: Voluntary non-profit - Other
Emergency Services: Yes
Phone: 573-334-4822
Fax: 573-651-5850
Accredited: Yes
Licensed Beds: 269

Key Personnel:
CEO. . . . . James W Wente
Chief of Medical Staff. . . . . Lee Taylor, MD

Measure	Cases	This Hospital	State Average	U.S. Average	Top Hospital
Heart Attack Care					
ACE Inhibitor or ARB for LVSD	64	86%	76%	82%	100%
Aspirin at Arrival	126	100%	92%	92%	100%
Aspirin at Discharge	248	96%	87%	90%	100%
Beta Blocker at Arrival	91	92%	83%	87%	100%
Beta Blocker at Discharge	254	98%	87%	90%	100%
Fibrinolytic Medication Timing	0	-	26%	31%	100%
PCI Within 90 Minutes of Arrival[1]	7	71%	61%	54%	95%
Smoking Cessation Advice	114	100%	92%	88%	100%
Heart Failure Care					
ACE Inhibitor or ARB for LVSD	105	78%	84%	82%	100%
Discharge Instructions	248	96%	62%	61%	93%
Evaluation of LVS Function	302	85%	79%	83%	99%
Smoking Cessation Advice	59	93%	80%	82%	100%
Pneumonia Care					
Appropriate Initial Antibiotic	152	78%	81%	83%	94%
Blood Culture Timing	155	97%	92%	90%	100%
Influenza Vaccine[4,5]	-	-	70%	70%	100%
Initial Antibiotic Timing	196	69%	81%	80%	93%
Oxygenation Assessment	252	100%	99%	99%	100%
Pneumococcal Vaccine	156	60%	70%	69%	94%
Smoking Cessation Advice	52	90%	83%	80%	100%
Surgical Infection Prevention					
Prophylactic Antibiotic Given	592	79%	78%	77%	95%
Prophylactic Antibiotic Selection	140	92%	91%	90%	100%
Prophylactic Antibiotic Stopped	592	65%	72%	72%	95%
Pregnancy Care					
Inpatient Neonatal Mortality	-	-	-	-	-
Third or Fourth Degree Laceration	-	-	-	3.63%	3.27%

Carroll County Memorial Hospital

1502 North Jefferson Street
Carrollton, MO 64633
URL: www.kcdawn.com/CCMH
Ownership: Proprietary
Emergency Services: Yes
Phone: 660-542-1695
Fax: 660-542-0363
Accredited: No
Licensed Beds: 77

Key Personnel:
President/CEO. . . . . Jerry Dover
Chief Medical Staff. . . . . Marvin E Ross, DO
Emergency Room . . . . Alex Dymek, MD
Emergency Room . . . . Barbara Hines, RN
Infection Control. . . . . Vicki Lyon, RN
Medical Surgical Nursing . . . . Vicki Lyon, RN
Respiratory/Cardiopulmonary. . . . . Shannon Jordan, CRRT

Measure	Cases	This Hospital	State Average	U.S. Average	Top Hospital
Heart Attack Care					
ACE Inhibitor or ARB for LVSD[3]	0	-	76%	82%	100%
Aspirin at Arrival[1,3]	2	100%	92%	92%	100%
Aspirin at Discharge[1,3]	2	50%	87%	90%	100%
Beta Blocker at Arrival[1,3]	3	67%	83%	87%	100%
Beta Blocker at Discharge[1,3]	2	100%	87%	90%	100%
Fibrinolytic Medication Timing[5]	-	-	26%	31%	100%
PCI Within 90 Minutes of Arrival[5]	-	-	61%	54%	95%
Smoking Cessation Advice[5]	-	-	92%	88%	100%
Heart Failure Care					
ACE Inhibitor or ARB for LVSD[1]	3	67%	84%	82%	100%
Discharge Instructions[5]	-	-	62%	61%	93%
Evaluation of LVS Function	59	44%	79%	83%	99%
Smoking Cessation Advice[5]	-	-	80%	82%	100%
Pneumonia Care					
Appropriate Initial Antibiotic[5]	-	-	81%	83%	94%
Blood Culture Timing[5]	-	-	92%	90%	100%
Influenza Vaccine[5]	-	-	70%	70%	100%
Initial Antibiotic Timing	60	92%	81%	80%	93%
Oxygenation Assessment	79	97%	99%	99%	100%
Pneumococcal Vaccine	43	49%	70%	69%	94%
Smoking Cessation Advice[5]	-	-	83%	80%	100%
Surgical Infection Prevention					
Prophylactic Antibiotic Given[5]	-	-	78%	77%	95%
Prophylactic Antibiotic Selection[5]	-	-	91%	90%	100%
Prophylactic Antibiotic Stopped[5]	-	-	72%	72%	95%
Pregnancy Care					
Inpatient Neonatal Mortality	-	-	-	-	-
Third or Fourth Degree Laceration	-	-	-	3.63%	3.27%

McCune-Brooks Hospital

627 W Centennial Street
Carthage, MO 64836
E-mail: mbhhr1@ipa.net
URL: www.mccunebrooks.org
Ownership: Government - Local
Emergency Services: Yes
Phone: 417-358-8121
Fax: 417-359-2522
Accredited: No
Licensed Beds: 54

Key Personnel:
CEO/President. . . . . Robert Copeland
Chief Medical Staff. . . . . Keathe Dillird, MD
Emergency Room . . . . Joseph T Quay Jr, DO
Director Infection/Disease Control . . . . Pat Bearden
Chief Radiology . . . . Wayne E Putnam, DO
Director Respiratory Therapy . . . . Chalaine Bell, RRT

Measure	Cases	This Hospital	State Average	U.S. Average	Top Hospital
Heart Attack Care					
ACE Inhibitor or ARB for LVSD[1]	2	50%	76%	82%	100%
Aspirin at Arrival[1]	11	55%	92%	92%	100%
Aspirin at Discharge[1]	6	83%	87%	90%	100%
Beta Blocker at Arrival[1]	6	50%	83%	87%	100%
Beta Blocker at Discharge[1]	6	67%	87%	90%	100%
Fibrinolytic Medication Timing	0	-	26%	31%	100%
PCI Within 90 Minutes of Arrival	0	-	61%	54%	95%
Smoking Cessation Advice	0	-	92%	88%	100%
Heart Failure Care					
ACE Inhibitor or ARB for LVSD[1]	14	86%	84%	82%	100%
Discharge Instructions	40	45%	62%	61%	93%
Evaluation of LVS Function	69	78%	79%	83%	99%
Smoking Cessation Advice[1]	10	80%	80%	82%	100%
Pneumonia Care					
Appropriate Initial Antibiotic	48	92%	81%	83%	94%
Blood Culture Timing	46	93%	92%	90%	100%
Influenza Vaccine[1]	12	75%	70%	70%	100%
Initial Antibiotic Timing	87	89%	81%	80%	93%
Oxygenation Assessment	92	100%	99%	99%	100%
Pneumococcal Vaccine	59	66%	70%	69%	94%
Smoking Cessation Advice[1]	19	79%	83%	80%	100%
Surgical Infection Prevention					
Prophylactic Antibiotic Given	54	70%	78%	77%	95%
Prophylactic Antibiotic Selection[1]	15	100%	91%	90%	100%
Prophylactic Antibiotic Stopped	52	29%	72%	72%	95%
Pregnancy Care					
Inpatient Neonatal Mortality	-	-	-	-	-
Third or Fourth Degree Laceration	-	-	-	3.63%	3.27%

Saint John's Hospital-Caseville

94 Main Street
Cassville, MO 65625
URL: southbarrycountyhospital.com
Ownership: Voluntary non-profit - Church
Emergency Services: Yes
Phone: 417-847-6000
Fax: 417-847-6047
Accredited: Yes
Licensed Beds: 18

Key Personnel:
President . . . . Gary Jordan
Chief Medical Staff. . . . . K Duane Cox, MD
Emergency Room . . . . Victor Mangler
Emergency Room . . . . Jerry Jumper
Infection Control. . . . . Joyce Noland, RN
Director of Pulmonary/Respiratory Care. . . . . . . Tam Hill

NOTE: Hospital profiles are in alphabetical order by state, then city, then hospital within the city; Rankings are sorted by rate in descending order and exclude hospitals with less than 25 cases; (1) The number of cases is too small (n<25) for purposes of reliably predicting hospital performance; (2) Measure reflects the hospital's indication that its submission was based upon a sample of its relevant discharges; (3) Rate reflects fewer than the maximum possible quarters of data for the measure; (4) Inaccurate information submitted and suppressed for one or more quarters; (5) No data is available from the hospital for this measure; Please refer to the User's Guide for a full explanation of data

Measure	Cases	This Hospital	State Average	U.S. Average	Top Hospital
Heart Attack Care					
ACE Inhibitor or ARB for LVSD[5]	-	-	76%	82%	100%
Aspirin at Arrival[5]	-	-	92%	92%	100%
Aspirin at Discharge[5]	-	-	87%	90%	100%
Beta Blocker at Arrival[5]	-	-	83%	87%	100%
Beta Blocker at Discharge[5]	-	-	87%	90%	100%
Fibrinolytic Medication Timing[5]	-	-	26%	31%	100%
PCI Within 90 Minutes of Arrival[5]	-	-	61%	54%	95%
Smoking Cessation Advice[5]	-	-	92%	88%	100%
Heart Failure Care					
ACE Inhibitor or ARB for LVSD[1,2]	1	100%	84%	82%	100%
Discharge Instructions[1,2]	5	60%	62%	61%	93%
Evaluation of LVS Function[1,2]	5	60%	79%	83%	99%
Smoking Cessation Advice[1,2]	1	100%	80%	82%	100%
Pneumonia Care					
Appropriate Initial Antibiotic[2]	34	97%	81%	83%	94%
Blood Culture Timing[1,2]	18	83%	92%	90%	100%
Influenza Vaccine[1]	9	89%	70%	70%	100%
Initial Antibiotic Timing[2]	34	97%	81%	80%	93%
Oxygenation Assessment[2]	43	100%	99%	99%	100%
Pneumococcal Vaccine[2]	29	97%	70%	69%	94%
Smoking Cessation Advice[1,2]	12	75%	83%	80%	100%
Surgical Infection Prevention					
Prophylactic Antibiotic Given[5]	-	-	78%	77%	95%
Prophylactic Antibiotic Selection[5]	-	-	91%	90%	100%
Prophylactic Antibiotic Stopped[5]	-	-	72%	72%	95%
Pregnancy Care					
Inpatient Neonatal Mortality	-	-	-	-	-
Third or Fourth Degree Laceration	-	-	-	3.63%	3.27%

Saint Luke's Hospital

232 S Woods Mill Road
Chesterfield, MO 63017
Phone: 314-434-1500
Fax: 314-205-6865
URL: www.goodhealthmatters.com
Ownership: Voluntary non-profit - Private
Emergency Services: Yes
Accredited: Yes
Licensed Beds: 493

Key Personnel:

President/CEO. . . . . Gary Olson, MD
Chief Medical Staff. . . . . Paul A Mennes, MD
Emergency Room . . . . Michael Meinzen, MD
Director Infection/Disease Control . . . . Leon Robison, MD
Director Respiratory Therapy . . . . Jackie Holloman

Measure	Cases	This Hospital	State Average	U.S. Average	Top Hospital
Heart Attack Care					
ACE Inhibitor or ARB for LVSD	67	90%	76%	82%	100%
Aspirin at Arrival	199	96%	92%	92%	100%
Aspirin at Discharge	242	97%	87%	90%	100%
Beta Blocker at Arrival	153	97%	83%	87%	100%
Beta Blocker at Discharge	252	94%	87%	90%	100%
Fibrinolytic Medication Timing	0	-	26%	31%	100%
PCI Within 90 Minutes of Arrival[1]	10	20%	61%	54%	95%
Smoking Cessation Advice	64	98%	92%	88%	100%
Heart Failure Care					
ACE Inhibitor or ARB for LVSD[2]	198	96%	84%	82%	100%
Discharge Instructions[2]	393	96%	62%	61%	93%
Evaluation of LVS Function[2]	521	100%	79%	83%	99%
Smoking Cessation Advice[2]	39	97%	80%	82%	100%
Pneumonia Care					
Appropriate Initial Antibiotic	243	89%	81%	83%	94%
Blood Culture Timing	191	94%	92%	90%	100%
Influenza Vaccine	72	97%	70%	70%	100%
Initial Antibiotic Timing	375	83%	81%	80%	93%
Oxygenation Assessment	480	100%	99%	99%	100%
Pneumococcal Vaccine	359	95%	70%	69%	94%
Smoking Cessation Advice	69	90%	83%	80%	100%
Surgical Infection Prevention					
Prophylactic Antibiotic Given[3]	171	73%	78%	77%	95%
Prophylactic Antibiotic Selection	105	75%	91%	90%	100%
Prophylactic Antibiotic Stopped[3]	164	60%	72%	72%	95%
Pregnancy Care					
Inpatient Neonatal Mortality	-	-	-	-	-
Third or Fourth Degree Laceration	-	-	-	3.63%	3.27%

Hedrick Medical Center

100 Central Street
Chillicothe, MO 64601
Phone: 660-646-1480
Fax: 660-646-6024
URL: www.saintlukeshealthsystem.org
Ownership: Government - Local
Emergency Services: Yes
Accredited: No
Licensed Beds: 49

Key Personnel:

CEO. . . . . James K Johnson

Measure	Cases	This Hospital	State Average	U.S. Average	Top Hospital
Heart Attack Care					
ACE Inhibitor or ARB for LVSD	0	-	76%	82%	100%
Aspirin at Arrival[1]	5	80%	92%	92%	100%
Aspirin at Discharge[1]	3	100%	87%	90%	100%
Beta Blocker at Arrival[1]	3	100%	83%	87%	100%
Beta Blocker at Discharge[1]	3	100%	87%	90%	100%
Fibrinolytic Medication Timing	0	-	26%	31%	100%
PCI Within 90 Minutes of Arrival	0	-	61%	54%	95%
Smoking Cessation Advice	0	-	92%	88%	100%
Heart Failure Care					
ACE Inhibitor or ARB for LVSD[1]	7	100%	84%	82%	100%
Discharge Instructions[1]	22	82%	62%	61%	93%
Evaluation of LVS Function	44	75%	79%	83%	99%
Smoking Cessation Advice[1]	1	0%	80%	82%	100%
Pneumonia Care					
Appropriate Initial Antibiotic	44	84%	81%	83%	94%
Blood Culture Timing[1]	21	95%	92%	90%	100%
Influenza Vaccine[1]	12	92%	70%	70%	100%
Initial Antibiotic Timing	62	84%	81%	80%	93%
Oxygenation Assessment	68	100%	99%	99%	100%
Pneumococcal Vaccine	48	94%	70%	69%	94%
Smoking Cessation Advice[1]	14	86%	83%	80%	100%
Surgical Infection Prevention					
Prophylactic Antibiotic Given[1,3]	5	60%	78%	77%	95%
Prophylactic Antibiotic Selection[1]	2	100%	91%	90%	100%
Prophylactic Antibiotic Stopped[1,3]	5	100%	72%	72%	95%
Pregnancy Care					
Inpatient Neonatal Mortality	-	-	-	-	-
Third or Fourth Degree Laceration	-	-	-	3.63%	3.27%

Golden Valley Memorial Hospital

1600 N 2nd Street
Clinton, MO 64735
Phone: 660-885-2253
Fax: 660-885-5012
Ownership: Govt - Hospital District or Authority
Emergency Services: Yes
Accredited: Yes
Licensed Beds: 106

Key Personnel:

Administrator/CEO. . . . . Randy S Wertz
Chief of Medical Staff. Bruce Bellmay, MD
Emergency Room . . . . Gial Brown
Director Infection/Disease Control . . . . Claudia Gibson
Director Radiology . . . . Chuck Collins
Director Respiratory Therapy . . . . Jim Witteman

Measure	Cases	This Hospital	State Average	U.S. Average	Top Hospital
Heart Attack Care					
ACE Inhibitor or ARB for LVSD[1,2]	1	0%	76%	82%	100%
Aspirin at Arrival[1,2]	14	79%	92%	92%	100%
Aspirin at Discharge[1,2]	8	88%	87%	90%	100%
Beta Blocker at Arrival[1,2]	14	50%	83%	87%	100%
Beta Blocker at Discharge[1,2]	9	44%	87%	90%	100%
Fibrinolytic Medication Timing[2]	0	-	26%	31%	100%
PCI Within 90 Minutes of Arrival[2]	0	-	61%	54%	95%
Smoking Cessation Advice[1,2]	2	100%	92%	88%	100%
Heart Failure Care					
ACE Inhibitor or ARB for LVSD[2]	41	66%	84%	82%	100%
Discharge Instructions[2]	108	59%	62%	61%	93%
Evaluation of LVS Function[2]	187	77%	79%	83%	99%
Smoking Cessation Advice[2]	39	74%	80%	82%	100%
Pneumonia Care					

NOTE: Hospital profiles are in alphabetical order by state, then city, then hospital within the city; Rankings are sorted by rate in descending order and exclude hospitals with less than 25 cases; (1) The number of cases is too small (n<25) for purposes of reliably predicting hospital performance; (2) Measure reflects the hospital's indication that its submission was based upon a sample of its relevant discharges; (3) Rate reflects fewer than the maximum possible quarters of data for the measure; (4) Inaccurate information submitted and suppressed for one or more quarters; (5) No data is available from the hospital for this measure; Please refer to the User's Guide for a full explanation of data

Appropriate Initial Antibiotic[2]	80	84%	81%	83%	94%
Blood Culture Timing[2]	83	90%	92%	90%	100%
Influenza Vaccine[4,5]	-	-	70%	70%	100%
Initial Antibiotic Timing[2]	142	91%	81%	80%	93%
Oxygenation Assessment[2]	165	100%	99%	99%	100%
Pneumococcal Vaccine[2]	104	67%	70%	69%	94%
Smoking Cessation Advice[2]	59	81%	83%	80%	100%
Surgical Infection Prevention					
Prophylactic Antibiotic Given[3]	59	73%	78%	77%	95%
Prophylactic Antibiotic Selection	25	100%	91%	90%	100%
Prophylactic Antibiotic Stopped[3]	59	76%	72%	72%	95%
Pregnancy Care					
Inpatient Neonatal Mortality	-	-	-	-	-
Third or Fourth Degree Laceration	-	-	-	3.63%	3.27%

Boone Hospital Center

1600 E Broadway
Columbia, MO 65201
Phone: 573-815-8000
Ownership: Voluntary non-profit - Private
Accredited: Yes
Emergency Services: Yes

Measure	Cases	This Hospital	State Average	U.S. Average	Top Hospital
Heart Attack Care					
ACE Inhibitor or ARB for LVSD	152	95%	76%	82%	100%
Aspirin at Arrival	186	99%	92%	92%	100%
Aspirin at Discharge	498	99%	87%	90%	100%
Beta Blocker at Arrival	178	92%	83%	87%	100%
Beta Blocker at Discharge	523	98%	87%	90%	100%
Fibrinolytic Medication Timing	0	-	26%	31%	100%
PCI Within 90 Minutes of Arrival[1]	12	92%	61%	54%	95%
Smoking Cessation Advice	206	99%	92%	88%	100%
Heart Failure Care					
ACE Inhibitor or ARB for LVSD	339	93%	84%	82%	100%
Discharge Instructions	498	85%	62%	61%	93%
Evaluation of LVS Function	573	99%	79%	83%	99%
Smoking Cessation Advice	76	93%	80%	82%	100%
Pneumonia Care					
Appropriate Initial Antibiotic	143	80%	81%	83%	94%
Blood Culture Timing	124	98%	92%	90%	100%
Influenza Vaccine	45	60%	70%	70%	100%
Initial Antibiotic Timing	186	91%	81%	80%	93%
Oxygenation Assessment	236	100%	99%	99%	100%
Pneumococcal Vaccine	166	92%	70%	69%	94%
Smoking Cessation Advice	45	96%	83%	80%	100%
Surgical Infection Prevention					
Prophylactic Antibiotic Given	804	96%	78%	77%	95%
Prophylactic Antibiotic Selection	164	95%	91%	90%	100%
Prophylactic Antibiotic Stopped	757	90%	72%	72%	95%
Pregnancy Care					
Inpatient Neonatal Mortality	-	-	-	-	-
Third or Fourth Degree Laceration	-	-	-	3.63%	3.27%

Columbia Regional Hospital

404 Keene Street
Columbia, MO 65201
Phone: 573-875-9200
Fax: 573-875-9869
Ownership: Voluntary non-profit - Private
Accredited: Yes
Emergency Services: Yes
Licensed Beds: 255

Key Personnel:

CEO. . . . . Jim Poehling
Director Medical/Surgical Nursing . . . . Mary Halliburton
Director Respiratory Therapy . . . . Janeanne Miller

Measure	Cases	This Hospital	State Average	U.S. Average	Top Hospital
Heart Attack Care					
ACE Inhibitor or ARB for LVSD[3]	0	-	76%	82%	100%
Aspirin at Arrival[1,3]	3	100%	92%	92%	100%
Aspirin at Discharge[1,3]	4	100%	87%	90%	100%
Beta Blocker at Arrival[1,3]	2	50%	83%	87%	100%
Beta Blocker at Discharge[1,3]	3	67%	87%	90%	100%
Fibrinolytic Medication Timing[3]	0	-	26%	31%	100%
PCI Within 90 Minutes of Arrival	0	-	61%	54%	95%
Smoking Cessation Advice[1,3]	1	100%	92%	88%	100%

Heart Failure Care					
ACE Inhibitor or ARB for LVSD	36	81%	84%	82%	100%
Discharge Instructions	46	52%	62%	61%	93%
Evaluation of LVS Function	58	90%	79%	83%	99%
Smoking Cessation Advice[1]	21	62%	80%	82%	100%
Pneumonia Care					
Appropriate Initial Antibiotic	38	84%	81%	83%	94%
Blood Culture Timing[1]	21	90%	92%	90%	100%
Influenza Vaccine[1]	6	83%	70%	70%	100%
Initial Antibiotic Timing	30	73%	81%	80%	93%
Oxygenation Assessment	48	100%	99%	99%	100%
Pneumococcal Vaccine	29	55%	70%	69%	94%
Smoking Cessation Advice[1]	18	83%	83%	80%	100%
Surgical Infection Prevention					
Prophylactic Antibiotic Given[3]	177	74%	78%	77%	95%
Prophylactic Antibiotic Selection	65	63%	91%	90%	100%
Prophylactic Antibiotic Stopped[3]	162	64%	72%	72%	95%
Pregnancy Care					
Inpatient Neonatal Mortality	1,894	1.37%	-	-	-
Third or Fourth Degree Laceration	1,163	5.85%	-	3.63%	3.27%

University of Missouri Hospital and Clinics

One Hospital Drive
Columbia, MO 65212
Phone: 573-882-4141
Fax: 573-884-7470
URL: www.missouri.edu
Ownership: Government - State
Accredited: Yes
Emergency Services: Yes
Licensed Beds: 495

Key Personnel:

President/CEO. . . . . Patsy J Hart
Chief Medical Staff. . . . . Karl Weber, MD
Chief Catheterization Laboratory . . . . Donald Voelker, MD
Emergency Room . . . . Gwen Burley
Director Infection/Disease Control . . . . E Dale Everett
OB/GYN Womens Health. . . . . William Griffin, MD
Manager Radiology . . . . Larry Kirschner
Director Respiratory Therapy . . . . Mark Jackson

Measure	Cases	This Hospital	State Average	U.S. Average	Top Hospital
Heart Attack Care					
ACE Inhibitor or ARB for LVSD	40	100%	76%	82%	100%
Aspirin at Arrival	77	100%	92%	92%	100%
Aspirin at Discharge	221	100%	87%	90%	100%
Beta Blocker at Arrival	84	99%	83%	87%	100%
Beta Blocker at Discharge	232	100%	87%	90%	100%
Fibrinolytic Medication Timing	0	-	26%	31%	100%
PCI Within 90 Minutes of Arrival[1]	5	80%	61%	54%	95%
Smoking Cessation Advice	110	97%	92%	88%	100%
Heart Failure Care					
ACE Inhibitor or ARB for LVSD	90	94%	84%	82%	100%
Discharge Instructions	156	86%	62%	61%	93%
Evaluation of LVS Function	186	99%	79%	83%	99%
Smoking Cessation Advice	48	94%	80%	82%	100%
Pneumonia Care					
Appropriate Initial Antibiotic	75	87%	81%	83%	94%
Blood Culture Timing	85	91%	92%	90%	100%
Influenza Vaccine	39	23%	70%	70%	100%
Initial Antibiotic Timing	142	69%	81%	80%	93%
Oxygenation Assessment	177	100%	99%	99%	100%
Pneumococcal Vaccine	79	58%	70%	69%	94%
Smoking Cessation Advice	75	75%	83%	80%	100%
Surgical Infection Prevention					
Prophylactic Antibiotic Given[3]	228	84%	78%	77%	95%
Prophylactic Antibiotic Selection	74	70%	91%	90%	100%
Prophylactic Antibiotic Stopped[3]	214	76%	72%	72%	95%
Pregnancy Care					
Inpatient Neonatal Mortality	-	-	-	-	-
Third or Fourth Degree Laceration	-	-	-	3.63%	3.27%

Barnes-Jewish West County Hospital

Alternate Name: Barnes West County Hospital

NOTE: Hospital profiles are in alphabetical order by state, then city, then hospital within the city; Rankings are sorted by rate in descending order and exclude hospitals with less than 25 cases; (1) The number of cases is too small (n<25) for purposes of reliably predicting hospital performance; (2) Measure reflects the hospital's indication that its submission was based upon a sample of its relevant discharges; (3) Rate reflects fewer than the maximum possible quarters of data for the measure; (4) Inaccurate information submitted and suppressed for one or more quarters; (5) No data is available from the hospital for this measure; Please refer to the User's Guide for a full explanation of data

12634 Olive Boulevard
Saint Louis, MO 63141
Ownership: Voluntary non-profit - Private
Emergency Services: Yes

Phone: 314-996-8000
Fax: 314-286-0305
Accredited: Yes
Licensed Beds: 113

Key Personnel:

CEO. . . . . Pat Mohrman
Chief Medical Staff. . . . . Ram Voltzky, MD
Chief Medical Staff. . . . . Allan Londe
Emergency Room . . . . Thomas Phill
Emergency Room . . . . Ren Kozikowski
Director Respiratory Therapy . . . . Marnell Dickson

Measure	Cases	This Hospital	State Average	U.S. Average	Top Hospital
Heart Attack Care					
ACE Inhibitor or ARB for LVSD[2,3]	0	-	76%	82%	100%
Aspirin at Arrival[1,2,3]	1	100%	92%	92%	100%
Aspirin at Discharge[1,2,3]	1	100%	87%	90%	100%
Beta Blocker at Arrival[2,3]	0	-	83%	87%	100%
Beta Blocker at Discharge[1,2,3]	1	0%	87%	90%	100%
Fibrinolytic Medication Timing[2,3]	0	-	26%	31%	100%
PCI Within 90 Minutes of Arrival[2]	0	-	61%	54%	95%
Smoking Cessation Advice[2,3]	0	-	92%	88%	100%
Heart Failure Care					
ACE Inhibitor or ARB for LVSD[1]	14	100%	84%	82%	100%
Discharge Instructions	43	74%	62%	61%	93%
Evaluation of LVS Function	53	98%	79%	83%	99%
Smoking Cessation Advice[1]	2	100%	80%	82%	100%
Pneumonia Care					
Appropriate Initial Antibiotic	54	94%	81%	83%	94%
Blood Culture Timing	36	100%	92%	90%	100%
Influenza Vaccine[1]	10	70%	70%	70%	100%
Initial Antibiotic Timing	66	89%	81%	80%	93%
Oxygenation Assessment	72	100%	99%	99%	100%
Pneumococcal Vaccine	51	92%	70%	69%	94%
Smoking Cessation Advice[1]	7	86%	83%	80%	100%
Surgical Infection Prevention					
Prophylactic Antibiotic Given	710	95%	78%	77%	95%
Prophylactic Antibiotic Selection	197	99%	91%	90%	100%
Prophylactic Antibiotic Stopped	703	94%	72%	72%	95%
Pregnancy Care					
Inpatient Neonatal Mortality	-	-	-	-	-
Third or Fourth Degree Laceration	-	-	-	3.63%	3.27%

Jefferson Memorial Hospital

1400 US Highway 61 S
PO Box 350
Crystal City, MO 63019
E-mail: info@jeffersonmemorial.org
URL: www.jeffersonmemorial.org
Ownership: Voluntary non-profit - Private
Emergency Services: Yes

Phone: 636-933-1000
Fax: 636-933-1119
Accredited: Yes
Licensed Beds: 210

Key Personnel:

President . . . . Dennis Gannon
Chief Medical Staff. . . . . Indu Patel
Cardiac Lab . . . . Shelia Julian
Catheterization Lab . . . . Shelia Julian
Emergency Room . . . . Sandy Conn
Emergency Room . . . . Tobey Harris, MD
Manager Infection/Disease Control . . . . Linda Ferrara
ICU . . . . Chere Belknap
Respiratory/Cardiopulmonary. . . . . Jeoff Williams

Measure	Cases	This Hospital	State Average	U.S. Average	Top Hospital
Heart Attack Care					
ACE Inhibitor or ARB for LVSD	58	66%	76%	82%	100%
Aspirin at Arrival	147	97%	92%	92%	100%
Aspirin at Discharge	181	93%	87%	90%	100%
Beta Blocker at Arrival	141	90%	83%	87%	100%
Beta Blocker at Discharge	184	92%	87%	90%	100%
Fibrinolytic Medication Timing[1]	1	100%	26%	31%	100%
PCI Within 90 Minutes of Arrival[1]	2	0%	61%	54%	95%
Smoking Cessation Advice	73	71%	92%	88%	100%
Heart Failure Care					
ACE Inhibitor or ARB for LVSD	126	77%	84%	82%	100%
Discharge Instructions	280	81%	62%	61%	93%
Evaluation of LVS Function	349	81%	79%	83%	99%
Smoking Cessation Advice	45	58%	80%	82%	100%
Pneumonia Care					
Appropriate Initial Antibiotic	215	78%	81%	83%	94%
Blood Culture Timing	103	72%	92%	90%	100%
Influenza Vaccine	48	8%	70%	70%	100%
Initial Antibiotic Timing	267	59%	81%	80%	93%
Oxygenation Assessment	314	97%	99%	99%	100%
Pneumococcal Vaccine	176	18%	70%	69%	94%
Smoking Cessation Advice	92	68%	83%	80%	100%
Surgical Infection Prevention					
Prophylactic Antibiotic Given[3]	244	66%	78%	77%	95%
Prophylactic Antibiotic Selection	94	98%	91%	90%	100%
Prophylactic Antibiotic Stopped[3]	238	89%	72%	72%	95%
Pregnancy Care					
Inpatient Neonatal Mortality	-	-	-	-	-
Third or Fourth Degree Laceration	-	-	-	3.63%	3.27%

Missouri Southern Healthcare

1200 N One Mile Road
Dexter, MO 63841
Ownership: Proprietary
Emergency Services: No

Phone: 573-624-5566
Fax: 573-624-6265
Accredited: No
Licensed Beds: 50

Key Personnel:

President/CEO. . . . . John Graves
Chief Medical Staff. . . . . Reza Jalal, MD
Emergency Room . . . . Cathy Hawthorne
Infection Control. . . . . Christine Neuber
ICU . . . . Christie DeArmen
Medical/Surgical Nursing . . . . Amy Akers
Respiratory/Cardiopulmonary. . . . . Patti Elders

Measure	Cases	This Hospital	State Average	U.S. Average	Top Hospital
Heart Attack Care					
ACE Inhibitor or ARB for LVSD[1]	2	100%	76%	82%	100%
Aspirin at Arrival	45	96%	92%	92%	100%
Aspirin at Discharge	30	93%	87%	90%	100%
Beta Blocker at Arrival	35	91%	83%	87%	100%
Beta Blocker at Discharge	34	91%	87%	90%	100%
Fibrinolytic Medication Timing[3]	0	-	26%	31%	100%
PCI Within 90 Minutes of Arrival	0	-	61%	54%	95%
Smoking Cessation Advice[1,3]	1	100%	92%	88%	100%
Heart Failure Care					
ACE Inhibitor or ARB for LVSD[1]	15	67%	84%	82%	100%
Discharge Instructions[1,3]	16	6%	62%	61%	93%
Evaluation of LVS Function	123	44%	79%	83%	99%
Smoking Cessation Advice[1,3]	3	67%	80%	82%	100%
Pneumonia Care					
Appropriate Initial Antibiotic[1,3]	15	60%	81%	83%	94%
Blood Culture Timing[1,3]	15	93%	92%	90%	100%
Influenza Vaccine[5]	-	-	70%	70%	100%
Initial Antibiotic Timing	106	78%	81%	80%	93%
Oxygenation Assessment	137	100%	99%	99%	100%
Pneumococcal Vaccine	83	59%	70%	69%	94%
Smoking Cessation Advice[1,3]	12	75%	83%	80%	100%
Surgical Infection Prevention					
Prophylactic Antibiotic Given[1,3]	1	100%	78%	77%	95%
Prophylactic Antibiotic Selection[5]	-	-	91%	90%	100%
Prophylactic Antibiotic Stopped[1,3]	1	100%	72%	72%	95%
Pregnancy Care					
Inpatient Neonatal Mortality	-	-	-	-	-
Third or Fourth Degree Laceration	-	-	-	3.63%	3.27%

Ripley County Memorial Hospital

109 Plum Street
Doniphan, MO 63935
Ownership: Voluntary non-profit - Other
Emergency Services: Yes

Phone: 573-996-2141
Fax: 573-996-3949
Accredited: No
Licensed Beds: 30

Key Personnel:

CEO/President. . . . . Ray Freeman
Chief of Medical Staff. . . . . Gary Ward

NOTE: Hospital profiles are in alphabetical order by state, then city, then hospital within the city; Rankings are sorted by rate in descending order and exclude hospitals with less than 25 cases; (1) The number of cases is too small (n<25) for purposes of reliably predicting hospital performance; (2) Measure reflects the hospital's indication that its submission was based upon a sample of its relevant discharges; (3) Rate reflects fewer than the maximum possible quarters of data for the measure; (4) Inaccurate information submitted and suppressed for one or more quarters; (5) No data is available from the hospital for this measure; Please refer to the User's Guide for a full explanation of data

Emergency Room . . . . Tamy Ryan
Director Radiology . . . . Karen Glaze
Director Respiratory Therapy . . . . Rick Lane

Measure	Cases	This Hospital	State Average	U.S. Average	Top Hospital
Heart Attack Care					
ACE Inhibitor or ARB for LVSD[3]	0	-	76%	82%	100%
Aspirin at Arrival[1,3]	3	67%	92%	92%	100%
Aspirin at Discharge[1,3]	2	100%	87%	90%	100%
Beta Blocker at Arrival[1,3]	3	67%	83%	87%	100%
Beta Blocker at Discharge[1,3]	1	100%	87%	90%	100%
Fibrinolytic Medication Timing[3]	0	-	26%	31%	100%
PCI Within 90 Minutes of Arrival	0	-	61%	54%	95%
Smoking Cessation Advice[3]	0	-	92%	88%	100%
Heart Failure Care					
ACE Inhibitor or ARB for LVSD[1,2]	10	20%	84%	82%	100%
Discharge Instructions[2]	54	59%	62%	61%	93%
Evaluation of LVS Function[2]	67	49%	79%	83%	99%
Smoking Cessation Advice[1,2]	15	73%	80%	82%	100%
Pneumonia Care					
Appropriate Initial Antibiotic	47	70%	81%	83%	94%
Blood Culture Timing[1]	8	100%	92%	90%	100%
Influenza Vaccine[1]	13	31%	70%	70%	100%
Initial Antibiotic Timing	76	80%	81%	80%	93%
Oxygenation Assessment	77	100%	99%	99%	100%
Pneumococcal Vaccine	45	24%	70%	69%	94%
Smoking Cessation Advice[1]	14	86%	83%	80%	100%
Surgical Infection Prevention					
Prophylactic Antibiotic Given[5]	-	-	78%	77%	95%
Prophylactic Antibiotic Selection[5]	-	-	91%	90%	100%
Prophylactic Antibiotic Stopped[5]	-	-	72%	72%	95%
Pregnancy Care					
Inpatient Neonatal Mortality	-	-	-	-	-
Third or Fourth Degree Laceration	-	-	-	3.63%	3.27%

Advanced Healthcare Medical Center

Highway 21 South
Ellington, MO 63638
Ownership: Voluntary non-profit - Private
Emergency Services: Yes
Phone: 573-663-2511
Fax: 573-663-7264
Accredited: No
Licensed Beds: 25

Key Personnel:

CEO . . . . Greg Carda
Chief Medical Staff . . . . Tirso Albana
Chief Medical Staff . . . . Tual Rains
Emergency Room . . . . Cherri Barton
Respiratory Care . . . . Mark Dragon

Measure	Cases	This Hospital	State Average	U.S. Average	Top Hospital
Heart Attack Care					
ACE Inhibitor or ARB for LVSD[5]	-	-	76%	82%	100%
Aspirin at Arrival[5]	-	-	92%	92%	100%
Aspirin at Discharge[5]	-	-	87%	90%	100%
Beta Blocker at Arrival[5]	-	-	83%	87%	100%
Beta Blocker at Discharge[5]	-	-	87%	90%	100%
Fibrinolytic Medication Timing[5]	-	-	26%	31%	100%
PCI Within 90 Minutes of Arrival[5]	-	-	61%	54%	95%
Smoking Cessation Advice[5]	-	-	92%	88%	100%
Heart Failure Care					
ACE Inhibitor or ARB for LVSD[2]	0	-	84%	82%	100%
Discharge Instructions[1,2]	13	0%	62%	61%	93%
Evaluation of LVS Function[1,2]	15	7%	79%	83%	99%
Smoking Cessation Advice[1,2]	4	50%	80%	82%	100%
Pneumonia Care					
Appropriate Initial Antibiotic[1,2]	23	70%	81%	83%	94%
Blood Culture Timing[2]	0	-	92%	90%	100%
Influenza Vaccine[1]	5	40%	70%	70%	100%
Initial Antibiotic Timing[2]	26	85%	81%	80%	93%
Oxygenation Assessment[2]	31	100%	99%	99%	100%
Pneumococcal Vaccine[1,2]	14	14%	70%	69%	94%
Smoking Cessation Advice[1,2]	9	89%	83%	80%	100%
Surgical Infection Prevention					
Prophylactic Antibiotic Given[5]	-	-	78%	77%	95%
Prophylactic Antibiotic Selection[5]	-	-	91%	90%	100%
Prophylactic Antibiotic Stopped[5]	-	-	72%	72%	95%
Pregnancy Care					
Inpatient Neonatal Mortality	-	-	-	-	-
Third or Fourth Degree Laceration	-	-	-	3.63%	3.27%

Community Hospital Association

Alternate Name: Fairfax Community Hospital
405 E Main
PO Box 107
Fairfax, MO 64446
Ownership: Voluntary non-profit - Private
Emergency Services: No
Phone: 660-686-2211
Fax: 660-686-2618
Accredited: No
Licensed Beds: 25

Key Personnel:

Administrator . . . . Myra Evans
Chief Medical Staff . . . . James Humphrey, MD
Emergency Room . . . . Teresa Oylear, FNP
Infection Control . . . . Linda Winkelman, RN
Medical/Surgical Nursing . . . . Rhonda Evans, RN, CCM
Coordinator Surgery . . . . Betty Goins, RN
Director Radiology . . . . Beth Mackey
Director Cardiopulmonary Care . . . . Jackie Martin, RN

Measure	Cases	This Hospital	State Average	U.S. Average	Top Hospital
Heart Attack Care					
ACE Inhibitor or ARB for LVSD[5]	-	-	76%	82%	100%
Aspirin at Arrival[5]	-	-	92%	92%	100%
Aspirin at Discharge[5]	-	-	87%	90%	100%
Beta Blocker at Arrival[5]	-	-	83%	87%	100%
Beta Blocker at Discharge[5]	-	-	87%	90%	100%
Fibrinolytic Medication Timing[5]	-	-	26%	31%	100%
PCI Within 90 Minutes of Arrival[5]	-	-	61%	54%	95%
Smoking Cessation Advice[5]	-	-	92%	88%	100%
Heart Failure Care					
ACE Inhibitor or ARB for LVSD[1,2]	2	100%	84%	82%	100%
Discharge Instructions[1,2]	17	59%	62%	61%	93%
Evaluation of LVS Function[2]	25	64%	79%	83%	99%
Smoking Cessation Advice[1,2]	3	0%	80%	82%	100%
Pneumonia Care					
Appropriate Initial Antibiotic	35	20%	81%	83%	94%
Blood Culture Timing[1]	1	100%	92%	90%	100%
Influenza Vaccine[1]	8	75%	70%	70%	100%
Initial Antibiotic Timing	39	90%	81%	80%	93%
Oxygenation Assessment	56	100%	99%	99%	100%
Pneumococcal Vaccine	47	83%	70%	69%	94%
Smoking Cessation Advice[1]	11	64%	83%	80%	100%
Surgical Infection Prevention					
Prophylactic Antibiotic Given[5]	-	-	78%	77%	95%
Prophylactic Antibiotic Selection[5]	-	-	91%	90%	100%
Prophylactic Antibiotic Stopped[5]	-	-	72%	72%	95%
Pregnancy Care					
Inpatient Neonatal Mortality	-	-	-	-	-
Third or Fourth Degree Laceration	-	-	-	3.63%	3.27%

Mineral Area Regional Medical Center

Alternate Name: Mineral Area Osteopathic Hospital
1212 Weber Road
Farmington, MO 63640
URL: www.marmc.org
Ownership: Voluntary non-profit - Private
Emergency Services: Yes
Phone: 573-756-4581
Fax: 573-756-5834
Accredited: Yes
Licensed Beds: 141

Key Personnel:

CEO . . . . Stephen L Crain
Chief Staff . . . . Henry Steele
Emergency Room . . . . Beth Skaggs
Director Infection/Disease Control . . . . Jack Marler
Director Radiology . . . . Jeff Pigg
Director Respiratory Therapy . . . . Gay Wilkinson

Measure	Cases	This Hospital	State Average	U.S. Average	Top Hospital
Heart Attack Care					
ACE Inhibitor or ARB for LVSD[1]	4	75%	76%	82%	100%
Aspirin at Arrival	33	70%	92%	92%	100%

NOTE: Hospital profiles are in alphabetical order by state, then city, then hospital within the city; Rankings are sorted by rate in descending order and exclude hospitals with less than 25 cases; (1) The number of cases is too small (n<25) for purposes of reliably predicting hospital performance; (2) Measure reflects the hospital's indication that its submission was based upon a sample of its relevant discharges; (3) Rate reflects fewer than the maximum possible quarters of data for the measure; (4) Inaccurate information submitted and suppressed for one or more quarters; (5) No data is available from the hospital for this measure; Please refer to the User's Guide for a full explanation of data

Aspirin at Discharge[1]	15	60%	87%	90%	100%
Beta Blocker at Arrival[1]	22	68%	83%	87%	100%
Beta Blocker at Discharge[1]	16	50%	87%	90%	100%
Fibrinolytic Medication Timing	0	-	26%	31%	100%
PCI Within 90 Minutes of Arrival	0	-	61%	54%	95%
Smoking Cessation Advice[1]	7	100%	92%	88%	100%
Heart Failure Care					
ACE Inhibitor or ARB for LVSD	35	83%	84%	82%	100%
Discharge Instructions	81	27%	62%	61%	93%
Evaluation of LVS Function	128	85%	79%	83%	99%
Smoking Cessation Advice[1]	20	90%	80%	82%	100%
Pneumonia Care					
Appropriate Initial Antibiotic	117	82%	81%	83%	94%
Blood Culture Timing	99	89%	92%	90%	100%
Influenza Vaccine[4,5]	-	-	70%	70%	100%
Initial Antibiotic Timing	174	82%	81%	80%	93%
Oxygenation Assessment	201	100%	99%	99%	100%
Pneumococcal Vaccine	125	46%	70%	69%	94%
Smoking Cessation Advice	52	87%	83%	80%	100%
Surgical Infection Prevention					
Prophylactic Antibiotic Given[2]	70	69%	78%	77%	95%
Prophylactic Antibiotic Selection[1,2]	11	91%	91%	90%	100%
Prophylactic Antibiotic Stopped[2]	69	80%	72%	72%	95%
Pregnancy Care					
Inpatient Neonatal Mortality	-	-	-	-	-
Third or Fourth Degree Laceration	-	-	-	3.63%	3.27%

Parkland Health Center

Alternate Name: Bonne Terre Hospital
1101 W Liberty Street
Farmington, MO 63640
Phone: 573-760-8175
Fax: 573-760-8171
E-mail: ssg.2352@bjc.org
URL: www.bjc.org
Ownership: Voluntary non-profit - Private
Accredited: Yes
Emergency Services: Yes
Licensed Beds: 130

Key Personnel:

CEO. . . . . Richard Conklin
Chief of Medical Staff. . . . . Gary Grix
Emergency Room . . . . Dana Day
Respiratory Care . . . . Mark Bailey

Measure	Cases	This Hospital	State Average	U.S. Average	Top Hospital
Heart Attack Care					
ACE Inhibitor or ARB for LVSD[1]	2	50%	76%	82%	100%
Aspirin at Arrival[1]	14	93%	92%	92%	100%
Aspirin at Discharge[1]	12	100%	87%	90%	100%
Beta Blocker at Arrival[1]	15	73%	83%	87%	100%
Beta Blocker at Discharge[1]	13	92%	87%	90%	100%
Fibrinolytic Medication Timing[1]	1	0%	26%	31%	100%
PCI Within 90 Minutes of Arrival	0	-	61%	54%	95%
Smoking Cessation Advice[1]	5	100%	92%	88%	100%
Heart Failure Care					
ACE Inhibitor or ARB for LVSD	72	82%	84%	82%	100%
Discharge Instructions	105	85%	62%	61%	93%
Evaluation of LVS Function	186	97%	79%	83%	99%
Smoking Cessation Advice	30	90%	80%	82%	100%
Pneumonia Care					
Appropriate Initial Antibiotic	99	92%	81%	83%	94%
Blood Culture Timing	83	92%	92%	90%	100%
Influenza Vaccine	27	100%	70%	70%	100%
Initial Antibiotic Timing	144	91%	81%	80%	93%
Oxygenation Assessment	157	98%	99%	99%	100%
Pneumococcal Vaccine	101	85%	70%	69%	94%
Smoking Cessation Advice	41	83%	83%	80%	100%
Surgical Infection Prevention					
Prophylactic Antibiotic Given	112	96%	78%	77%	95%
Prophylactic Antibiotic Selection[1]	21	100%	91%	90%	100%
Prophylactic Antibiotic Stopped	101	97%	72%	72%	95%
Pregnancy Care					
Inpatient Neonatal Mortality	-	-	-	-	-
Third or Fourth Degree Laceration	-	-	-	3.63%	3.27%

Christian Hospital Northwest

1225 Graham Road
Florissant, MO 63031
Phone: 314-653-5000
Fax: 314-653-4141
URL: www.bjc.org/chnenw.html
Ownership: Voluntary non-profit - Private
Accredited: Yes
Emergency Services: Yes
Licensed Beds: 223

Key Personnel:

President/CEO. . . . . Paul Macek
Chief of Medical Staff. . . . . Steven Hadvina
Emergency Room . . . . Jeane Arana
ICU . . . . John Gloss
OB/GYN Womens Health. . . . . Aaron Pile
Director Radiology . . . . Walt DeLaney
Director of Respiratory . . . . Neil Hattler

Measure	Cases	This Hospital	State Average	U.S. Average	Top Hospital
Heart Attack Care					
ACE Inhibitor or ARB for LVSD[5]	-	-	76%	82%	100%
Aspirin at Arrival[5]	-	-	92%	92%	100%
Aspirin at Discharge[5]	-	-	87%	90%	100%
Beta Blocker at Arrival[5]	-	-	83%	87%	100%
Beta Blocker at Discharge[5]	-	-	87%	90%	100%
Fibrinolytic Medication Timing[5]	-	-	26%	31%	100%
PCI Within 90 Minutes of Arrival[5]	-	-	61%	54%	95%
Smoking Cessation Advice[5]	-	-	92%	88%	100%
Heart Failure Care					
ACE Inhibitor or ARB for LVSD[5]	-	-	84%	82%	100%
Discharge Instructions[5]	-	-	62%	61%	93%
Evaluation of LVS Function[5]	-	-	79%	83%	99%
Smoking Cessation Advice[5]	-	-	80%	82%	100%
Pneumonia Care					
Appropriate Initial Antibiotic[5]	-	-	81%	83%	94%
Blood Culture Timing[5]	-	-	92%	90%	100%
Influenza Vaccine[5]	-	-	70%	70%	100%
Initial Antibiotic Timing[5]	-	-	81%	80%	93%
Oxygenation Assessment[5]	-	-	99%	99%	100%
Pneumococcal Vaccine[5]	-	-	70%	69%	94%
Smoking Cessation Advice[5]	-	-	83%	80%	100%
Surgical Infection Prevention					
Prophylactic Antibiotic Given[5]	-	-	78%	77%	95%
Prophylactic Antibiotic Selection[5]	-	-	91%	90%	100%
Prophylactic Antibiotic Stopped[5]	-	-	72%	72%	95%
Pregnancy Care					
Inpatient Neonatal Mortality	-	-	-	-	-
Third or Fourth Degree Laceration	-	-	-	3.63%	3.27%

Callaway Community Hospital

10 South Hospital Drive
Fulton, MO 65251
Phone: 573-642-3376
Fax: 573-592-6679
URL: www.cchfulton.com
Ownership: Proprietary
Accredited: Yes
Emergency Services: Yes
Licensed Beds: 53

Key Personnel:

CEO. . . . . John T Graves
Chief Medical Staff. . . . . Michael Wilson, MD
Emergency Room . . . . Riley Selby
Director Infection/Disease Control . . . . Terri Herold
Director Medical/Surgical Nursing . . . . Dawn Moore
Director Respiratory Therapy . . . . Kathy Green

Measure	Cases	This Hospital	State Average	U.S. Average	Top Hospital
Heart Attack Care					
ACE Inhibitor or ARB for LVSD[1,2]	1	0%	76%	82%	100%
Aspirin at Arrival[1,2]	5	100%	92%	92%	100%
Aspirin at Discharge[1,2]	5	100%	87%	90%	100%
Beta Blocker at Arrival[1,2]	5	100%	83%	87%	100%
Beta Blocker at Discharge[1,2]	5	100%	87%	90%	100%
Fibrinolytic Medication Timing[2]	0	-	26%	31%	100%
PCI Within 90 Minutes of Arrival[2]	0	-	61%	54%	95%
Smoking Cessation Advice[1,2]	1	100%	92%	88%	100%
Heart Failure Care					
ACE Inhibitor or ARB for LVSD[1,2]	10	70%	84%	82%	100%
Discharge Instructions[1,2]	14	57%	62%	61%	93%

NOTE: Hospital profiles are in alphabetical order by state, then city, then hospital within the city; Rankings are sorted by rate in descending order and exclude hospitals with less than 25 cases; (1) The number of cases is too small (n<25) for purposes of reliably predicting hospital performance; (2) Measure reflects the hospital's indication that its submission was based upon a sample of its relevant discharges; (3) Rate reflects fewer than the maximum possible quarters of data for the measure; (4) Inaccurate information submitted and suppressed for one or more quarters; (5) No data is available from the hospital for this measure; Please refer to the User's Guide for a full explanation of data

Measure	Cases	This Hospital	State Average	U.S. Average	Top Hospital
Evaluation of LVS Function[2]	37	89%	79%	83%	99%
Smoking Cessation Advice[1,2]	11	91%	80%	82%	100%
Pneumonia Care					
Appropriate Initial Antibiotic[2]	40	85%	81%	83%	94%
Blood Culture Timing[1,2]	17	100%	92%	90%	100%
Influenza Vaccine[1]	4	25%	70%	70%	100%
Initial Antibiotic Timing[2]	42	62%	81%	80%	93%
Oxygenation Assessment[2]	51	100%	99%	99%	100%
Pneumococcal Vaccine[2]	27	48%	70%	69%	94%
Smoking Cessation Advice[1,2]	16	88%	83%	80%	100%
Surgical Infection Prevention					
Prophylactic Antibiotic Given[1,2,3]	3	67%	78%	77%	95%
Prophylactic Antibiotic Selection[1,2]	3	100%	91%	90%	100%
Prophylactic Antibiotic Stopped[1,2,3]	3	67%	72%	72%	95%
Pregnancy Care					
Inpatient Neonatal Mortality	-	-	-	-	-
Third or Fourth Degree Laceration	-	-	-	3.63%	3.27%

Hannibal Regional Hospital

Alternate Name: Hannibal Regional Healthcare System
Highway 36 W
PO Box 551
Hannibal, MO 63401
Phone: 573-248-1300
Fax: 573-248-5264
E-mail: webmaster@hrhonline.org
URL: www.hrhonline.org
Ownership: Voluntary non-profit - Private
Accredited: Yes
Emergency Services: Yes
Licensed Beds: 105

Key Personnel:

President . . . . John Grossmeier
Chief Medical Staff . . . . E Meidl, MD
Director Emergency Services . . . . Diane Boewe
Infection Control . . . . Leanna Darnold
Intensive Coronary Care . . . . Laura Miller, RN
OB/GYN Womens Health . . . . Lynn Walley, MD
Chief Radiology . . . . Joel Hasslen, MD
Director Respiratory Therapy . . . . Robert Crawford

Measure	Cases	This Hospital	State Average	U.S. Average	Top Hospital
Heart Attack Care					
ACE Inhibitor or ARB for LVSD[1,2]	6	100%	76%	82%	100%
Aspirin at Arrival[2]	36	100%	92%	92%	100%
Aspirin at Discharge[1,2]	22	91%	87%	90%	100%
Beta Blocker at Arrival[2]	35	94%	83%	87%	100%
Beta Blocker at Discharge[2]	29	93%	87%	90%	100%
Fibrinolytic Medication Timing[1,2]	2	50%	26%	31%	100%
PCI Within 90 Minutes of Arrival[2]	0	-	61%	54%	95%
Smoking Cessation Advice[1,2]	6	83%	92%	88%	100%
Heart Failure Care					
ACE Inhibitor or ARB for LVSD[2]	54	91%	84%	82%	100%
Discharge Instructions[2]	112	89%	62%	61%	93%
Evaluation of LVS Function[2]	162	88%	79%	83%	99%
Smoking Cessation Advice[1,2]	23	83%	80%	82%	100%
Pneumonia Care					
Appropriate Initial Antibiotic[2]	171	81%	81%	83%	94%
Blood Culture Timing[2]	202	95%	92%	90%	100%
Influenza Vaccine	57	61%	70%	70%	100%
Initial Antibiotic Timing[2]	259	80%	81%	80%	93%
Oxygenation Assessment[2]	353	100%	99%	99%	100%
Pneumococcal Vaccine[2]	240	78%	70%	69%	94%
Smoking Cessation Advice[2]	68	90%	83%	80%	100%
Surgical Infection Prevention					
Prophylactic Antibiotic Given[2,3]	310	89%	78%	77%	95%
Prophylactic Antibiotic Selection[2]	100	99%	91%	90%	100%
Prophylactic Antibiotic Stopped[2,3]	299	83%	72%	72%	95%
Pregnancy Care					
Inpatient Neonatal Mortality	-	-	-	-	-
Third or Fourth Degree Laceration	-	-	-	3.63%	3.27%

Cass Medical Center

1800 E Mechanic Street
Harrisonville, MO 64701
Phone: 816-380-3474
Fax: 816-380-4639
E-mail: apeters@cassmed.org
URL: www.cassmedicalcenter.com
Ownership: Voluntary non-profit - Other
Accredited: No
Emergency Services: Yes
Licensed Beds: 49

Key Personnel:

CEO . . . . Chris Lang
CNO . . . . Glenda Percival, RN
Chief Medical Staff . . . . Christopher Maxwell
Emergency Room . . . . Violet Warren
Infection Control . . . . Melinda Flanner
Medical Surgical Nursing . . . . Kaye Markham
Respiratory/Cardiopulmonary . . . . Melissa Jennings

Measure	Cases	This Hospital	State Average	U.S. Average	Top Hospital
Heart Attack Care					
ACE Inhibitor or ARB for LVSD[2,3]	0	-	76%	82%	100%
Aspirin at Arrival[1,2,3]	4	50%	92%	92%	100%
Aspirin at Discharge[1,2,3]	4	50%	87%	90%	100%
Beta Blocker at Arrival[1,2,3]	6	67%	83%	87%	100%
Beta Blocker at Discharge[1,2,3]	4	75%	87%	90%	100%
Fibrinolytic Medication Timing[2,3]	0	-	26%	31%	100%
PCI Within 90 Minutes of Arrival[2]	0	-	61%	54%	95%
Smoking Cessation Advice[2,3]	0	-	92%	88%	100%
Heart Failure Care					
ACE Inhibitor or ARB for LVSD[1,2]	7	86%	84%	82%	100%
Discharge Instructions[1,2]	22	59%	62%	61%	93%
Evaluation of LVS Function[2]	28	68%	79%	83%	99%
Smoking Cessation Advice[1,2]	4	100%	80%	82%	100%
Pneumonia Care					
Appropriate Initial Antibiotic[2]	61	74%	81%	83%	94%
Blood Culture Timing[2]	28	89%	92%	90%	100%
Influenza Vaccine[1]	6	50%	70%	70%	100%
Initial Antibiotic Timing[2]	55	82%	81%	80%	93%
Oxygenation Assessment[2]	61	100%	99%	99%	100%
Pneumococcal Vaccine[2]	42	88%	70%	69%	94%
Smoking Cessation Advice[1,2]	20	70%	83%	80%	100%
Surgical Infection Prevention					
Prophylactic Antibiotic Given[5]	-	-	78%	77%	95%
Prophylactic Antibiotic Selection[5]	-	-	91%	90%	100%
Prophylactic Antibiotic Stopped[5]	-	-	72%	72%	95%
Pregnancy Care					
Inpatient Neonatal Mortality	-	-	-	-	-
Third or Fourth Degree Laceration	-	-	-	3.63%	3.27%

Pemiscot Memorial Hospital

Alternate Name: Pemiscot Memorial Hospital
Highway 61 and Reed
Hayti, MO 63851
Phone: 573-359-1372
Fax: 573-359-3601
Ownership: Voluntary non-profit - Other
Accredited: No
Emergency Services: Yes
Licensed Beds: 245

Key Personnel:

Administrator . . . . Daryl Jean
Chief Medical Staff . . . . Jafer Gheraibeh, MD
Director Infection/Disease Control . . . . Micky Wilkerson, RN
Director Respiratory Therapy . . . . Sharon Baucom

Measure	Cases	This Hospital	State Average	U.S. Average	Top Hospital
Heart Attack Care					
ACE Inhibitor or ARB for LVSD[1]	1	0%	76%	82%	100%
Aspirin at Arrival[1]	6	67%	92%	92%	100%
Aspirin at Discharge[1]	5	80%	87%	90%	100%
Beta Blocker at Arrival[1]	7	57%	83%	87%	100%
Beta Blocker at Discharge[1]	5	80%	87%	90%	100%
Fibrinolytic Medication Timing	0	-	26%	31%	100%
PCI Within 90 Minutes of Arrival	0	-	61%	54%	95%
Smoking Cessation Advice[1]	4	25%	92%	88%	100%
Heart Failure Care					
ACE Inhibitor or ARB for LVSD	28	54%	84%	82%	100%
Discharge Instructions	150	9%	62%	61%	93%
Evaluation of LVS Function	179	48%	79%	83%	99%

NOTE: Hospital profiles are in alphabetical order by state, then city, then hospital within the city; Rankings are sorted by rate in descending order and exclude hospitals with less than 25 cases; (1) The number of cases is too small (n<25) for purposes of reliably predicting hospital performance; (2) Measure reflects the hospital's indication that its submission was based upon a sample of its relevant discharges; (3) Rate reflects fewer than the maximum possible quarters of data for the measure; (4) Inaccurate information submitted and suppressed for one or more quarters; (5) No data is available from the hospital for this measure; Please refer to the User's Guide for a full explanation of data

Measure	Cases	This Hospital	State Average	U.S. Average	Top Hospital
Smoking Cessation Advice[1]	22	32%	80%	82%	100%
Pneumonia Care					
Appropriate Initial Antibiotic	42	55%	81%	83%	94%
Blood Culture Timing[1]	18	83%	92%	90%	100%
Influenza Vaccine[1]	8	50%	70%	70%	100%
Initial Antibiotic Timing	43	60%	81%	80%	93%
Oxygenation Assessment	47	72%	99%	99%	100%
Pneumococcal Vaccine[1]	18	22%	70%	69%	94%
Smoking Cessation Advice[1]	13	38%	83%	80%	100%
Surgical Infection Prevention					
Prophylactic Antibiotic Given[1,3]	5	20%	78%	77%	95%
Prophylactic Antibiotic Selection[1]	4	25%	91%	90%	100%
Prophylactic Antibiotic Stopped[1,3]	4	100%	72%	72%	95%
Pregnancy Care					
Inpatient Neonatal Mortality	-	-	-	-	-
Third or Fourth Degree Laceration	-	-	-	3.63%	3.27%

Hermann Area District Hospital

509 W 18th Street
Hermann, MO 65041
Phone: 573-486-2191
Fax: 573-486-3743
E-mail: hadh@ktif.net
Ownership: Govt - Hospital District or Authority
Accredited: No
Emergency Services: Yes
Licensed Beds: 44

Key Personnel:

President/CEO . . . . Gene E Bock
Chief Medical Staff . . . . Dale F Dierberg, MD
Emergency Room . . . . James W Keith, DO
Medical Director Infection/Disease . . . . James T Shaw, MD
Director Medical/Surgical Nursing . . . . Rhonda Polly, RN, M
Director Pulmonary Services . . . . Thomas W Schneider, MD

Measure	Cases	This Hospital	State Average	U.S. Average	Top Hospital
Heart Attack Care					
ACE Inhibitor or ARB for LVSD[5]	-	-	76%	82%	100%
Aspirin at Arrival[5]	-	-	92%	92%	100%
Aspirin at Discharge[5]	-	-	87%	90%	100%
Beta Blocker at Arrival[5]	-	-	83%	87%	100%
Beta Blocker at Discharge[5]	-	-	87%	90%	100%
Fibrinolytic Medication Timing[5]	-	-	26%	31%	100%
PCI Within 90 Minutes of Arrival[5]	-	-	61%	54%	95%
Smoking Cessation Advice[5]	-	-	92%	88%	100%
Heart Failure Care					
ACE Inhibitor or ARB for LVSD[1,2]	1	100%	84%	82%	100%
Discharge Instructions[1,2]	10	80%	62%	61%	93%
Evaluation of LVS Function[1,2]	19	26%	79%	83%	99%
Smoking Cessation Advice[1,2]	3	33%	80%	82%	100%
Pneumonia Care					
Appropriate Initial Antibiotic[1,2]	19	89%	81%	83%	94%
Blood Culture Timing[1,2]	6	83%	92%	90%	100%
Influenza Vaccine[1]	4	50%	70%	70%	100%
Initial Antibiotic Timing[2]	29	90%	81%	80%	93%
Oxygenation Assessment[2]	34	100%	99%	99%	100%
Pneumococcal Vaccine[2]	27	44%	70%	69%	94%
Smoking Cessation Advice[1,2]	4	75%	83%	80%	100%
Surgical Infection Prevention					
Prophylactic Antibiotic Given[5]	-	-	78%	77%	95%
Prophylactic Antibiotic Selection[5]	-	-	91%	90%	100%
Prophylactic Antibiotic Stopped[5]	-	-	72%	72%	95%
Pregnancy Care					
Inpatient Neonatal Mortality	-	-	-	-	-
Third or Fourth Degree Laceration	-	-	-	3.63%	3.27%

Texas County Memorial Hospital

1333 Sam Houston Boulevard
Houston, MO 65483
Toll-Free: 866-967-3311
Phone: 417-967-3311
Fax: 417-967-1234
URL: www.tcmh.org
Ownership: Voluntary non-profit - Other
Accredited: No
Emergency Services: Yes
Licensed Beds: 66

Key Personnel:

President/CEO . . . . Wes Murray
Infection Control . . . . Colette Briggs, LPN
Infection Control . . . . Tasaduq Fazili, MD
Surgical Services . . . . Kim Jordan, RN
Director Respiratory Therapy . . . . Harry Willis, RCP CRT

Measure	Cases	This Hospital	State Average	U.S. Average	Top Hospital
Heart Attack Care					
ACE Inhibitor or ARB for LVSD[1]	3	33%	76%	82%	100%
Aspirin at Arrival[1]	14	93%	92%	92%	100%
Aspirin at Discharge[1]	12	92%	87%	90%	100%
Beta Blocker at Arrival[1]	16	75%	83%	87%	100%
Beta Blocker at Discharge[1]	15	73%	87%	90%	100%
Fibrinolytic Medication Timing[1]	1	0%	26%	31%	100%
PCI Within 90 Minutes of Arrival	0	-	61%	54%	95%
Smoking Cessation Advice[1]	1	0%	92%	88%	100%
Heart Failure Care					
ACE Inhibitor or ARB for LVSD[1]	11	73%	84%	82%	100%
Discharge Instructions	45	2%	62%	61%	93%
Evaluation of LVS Function	66	62%	79%	83%	99%
Smoking Cessation Advice[1]	11	55%	80%	82%	100%
Pneumonia Care					
Appropriate Initial Antibiotic	95	77%	81%	83%	94%
Blood Culture Timing	55	95%	92%	90%	100%
Influenza Vaccine[1]	18	50%	70%	70%	100%
Initial Antibiotic Timing	111	77%	81%	80%	93%
Oxygenation Assessment	139	99%	99%	99%	100%
Pneumococcal Vaccine	97	38%	70%	69%	94%
Smoking Cessation Advice	31	52%	83%	80%	100%
Surgical Infection Prevention					
Prophylactic Antibiotic Given[1,3]	12	75%	78%	77%	95%
Prophylactic Antibiotic Selection[1]	5	100%	91%	90%	100%
Prophylactic Antibiotic Stopped[1,3]	11	73%	72%	72%	95%
Pregnancy Care					
Inpatient Neonatal Mortality	-	-	-	-	-
Third or Fourth Degree Laceration	-	-	-	3.63%	3.27%

Centerpoint Medical Center of Independence

19600 East 39th Street
Independence, MO 64057
Phone: 816-698-7000
Ownership: Voluntary non-profit - Private
Accredited: Yes
Emergency Services: Yes

Measure	Cases	This Hospital	State Average	U.S. Average	Top Hospital
Heart Attack Care					
ACE Inhibitor or ARB for LVSD	92	80%	76%	82%	100%
Aspirin at Arrival	190	93%	92%	92%	100%
Aspirin at Discharge	220	97%	87%	90%	100%
Beta Blocker at Arrival	154	90%	83%	87%	100%
Beta Blocker at Discharge	223	96%	87%	90%	100%
Fibrinolytic Medication Timing	0	-	26%	31%	100%
PCI Within 90 Minutes of Arrival[1]	11	82%	61%	54%	95%
Smoking Cessation Advice	112	96%	92%	88%	100%
Heart Failure Care					
ACE Inhibitor or ARB for LVSD	100	80%	84%	82%	100%
Discharge Instructions	207	64%	62%	61%	93%
Evaluation of LVS Function	294	84%	79%	83%	99%
Smoking Cessation Advice	63	89%	80%	82%	100%
Pneumonia Care					
Appropriate Initial Antibiotic	140	87%	81%	83%	94%
Blood Culture Timing	156	93%	92%	90%	100%
Influenza Vaccine	51	59%	70%	70%	100%
Initial Antibiotic Timing	216	88%	81%	80%	93%
Oxygenation Assessment	269	99%	99%	99%	100%
Pneumococcal Vaccine	193	61%	70%	69%	94%
Smoking Cessation Advice	64	91%	83%	80%	100%
Surgical Infection Prevention					
Prophylactic Antibiotic Given[2,3]	191	87%	78%	77%	95%
Prophylactic Antibiotic Selection[2]	83	89%	91%	90%	100%
Prophylactic Antibiotic Stopped[2,3]	186	31%	72%	72%	95%
Pregnancy Care					
Inpatient Neonatal Mortality	-	-	-	-	-
Third or Fourth Degree Laceration	-	-	-	3.63%	3.27%

NOTE: Hospital profiles are in alphabetical order by state, then city, then hospital within the city; Rankings are sorted by rate in descending order and exclude hospitals with less than 25 cases; (1) The number of cases is too small (n<25) for purposes of reliably predicting hospital performance; (2) Measure reflects the hospital's indication that its submission was based upon a sample of its relevant discharges; (3) Rate reflects fewer than the maximum possible quarters of data for the measure; (4) Inaccurate information submitted and suppressed for one or more quarters; (5) No data is available from the hospital for this measure; Please refer to the User's Guide for a full explanation of data

Medical Center of Independence

17203 E 23rd Street
Independence, MO 64057
Ownership: Voluntary non-profit - Private
Emergency Services: Yes
Phone: 816-478-5000
Fax: 816-478-5578
Accredited: Yes
Licensed Beds: 205

Key Personnel:
CEO . . . . J Kent Howard
Chief Medical Staff . . . . Robert Meyer, MD
Emergency Room . . . . Pete Wembleton, RN
Director Medical/Surgical Nursing . . . . Nancy Dycus, RN
Director Radiology . . . . HP Fritz

Measure	Cases	This Hospital	State Average	U.S. Average	Top Hospital
Heart Attack Care					
ACE Inhibitor or ARB for LVSD[1]	18	50%	76%	82%	100%
Aspirin at Arrival	89	98%	92%	92%	100%
Aspirin at Discharge	74	100%	87%	90%	100%
Beta Blocker at Arrival	63	76%	83%	87%	100%
Beta Blocker at Discharge	68	94%	87%	90%	100%
Fibrinolytic Medication Timing	0	-	26%	31%	100%
PCI Within 90 Minutes of Arrival[1]	7	71%	61%	54%	95%
Smoking Cessation Advice	26	100%	92%	88%	100%
Heart Failure Care					
ACE Inhibitor or ARB for LVSD	55	64%	84%	82%	100%
Discharge Instructions	143	66%	62%	61%	93%
Evaluation of LVS Function	176	91%	79%	83%	99%
Smoking Cessation Advice	29	97%	80%	82%	100%
Pneumonia Care					
Appropriate Initial Antibiotic	102	87%	81%	83%	94%
Blood Culture Timing	101	91%	92%	90%	100%
Influenza Vaccine[1]	22	77%	70%	70%	100%
Initial Antibiotic Timing	127	82%	81%	80%	93%
Oxygenation Assessment	165	100%	99%	99%	100%
Pneumococcal Vaccine	98	86%	70%	69%	94%
Smoking Cessation Advice	49	96%	83%	80%	100%
Surgical Infection Prevention					
Prophylactic Antibiotic Given[2,3]	77	66%	78%	77%	95%
Prophylactic Antibiotic Selection[1,2]	23	83%	91%	90%	100%
Prophylactic Antibiotic Stopped[2,3]	70	49%	72%	72%	95%
Pregnancy Care					
Inpatient Neonatal Mortality	-	-	-	-	-
Third or Fourth Degree Laceration	-	-	-	3.63%	3.27%

Capital Region Medical Center

1125 Madison Street
Jefferson City, MO 65102
E-mail: info@mail.crmc.org
URL: www.crmc.org
Ownership: Voluntary non-profit - Private
Emergency Services: Yes
Phone: 573-632-5000
Fax: 573-632-5880
Accredited: Yes
Licensed Beds: 134

Key Personnel:
President . . . . Ed Farnsworth
Chief Medical Staff . . . . Doug Wheeler, DO
Director Surgical Services . . . . Nancy Jo Wirman
Manager Radiology . . . . Kristy Trent
Respiratory . . . . Anita Smith

Measure	Cases	This Hospital	State Average	U.S. Average	Top Hospital
Heart Attack Care					
ACE Inhibitor or ARB for LVSD[1]	11	100%	76%	82%	100%
Aspirin at Arrival	77	100%	92%	92%	100%
Aspirin at Discharge	76	99%	87%	90%	100%
Beta Blocker at Arrival	62	98%	83%	87%	100%
Beta Blocker at Discharge	79	99%	87%	90%	100%
Fibrinolytic Medication Timing[1]	2	0%	26%	31%	100%
PCI Within 90 Minutes of Arrival[1]	5	100%	61%	54%	95%
Smoking Cessation Advice	32	97%	92%	88%	100%
Heart Failure Care					
ACE Inhibitor or ARB for LVSD	62	98%	84%	82%	100%
Discharge Instructions	161	88%	62%	61%	93%
Evaluation of LVS Function	209	98%	79%	83%	99%
Smoking Cessation Advice	44	95%	80%	82%	100%
Pneumonia Care					
Appropriate Initial Antibiotic	130	92%	81%	83%	94%
Blood Culture Timing	123	92%	92%	90%	100%
Influenza Vaccine	44	84%	70%	70%	100%
Initial Antibiotic Timing	184	91%	81%	80%	93%
Oxygenation Assessment	217	100%	99%	99%	100%
Pneumococcal Vaccine	145	92%	70%	69%	94%
Smoking Cessation Advice	60	93%	83%	80%	100%
Surgical Infection Prevention					
Prophylactic Antibiotic Given	428	87%	78%	77%	95%
Prophylactic Antibiotic Selection	125	92%	91%	90%	100%
Prophylactic Antibiotic Stopped	420	86%	72%	72%	95%
Pregnancy Care					
Inpatient Neonatal Mortality	-	-	-	-	-
Third or Fourth Degree Laceration	-	-	-	3.63%	3.27%

Saint Marys Health Center

100 Saint Mary's Medical Plaza
Jefferson City, MO 65101
URL: www.stmarys-jeffcity.com
Ownership: Proprietary
Emergency Services: Yes
Phone: 573-761-7000
Fax: 573-636-5733
Accredited: Yes
Licensed Beds: 167

Key Personnel:
President/CEO . . . . Elizabeth Aderholdt
Chief Medical Staff . . . . John Lucia
Cardiac Laboratory . . . . Dinah Scearce
Catheterization Laboratory . . . . Tim Carter
Emergency Room . . . . Cowen Douglas
Infection Control . . . . Kathy Kormann
ICU . . . . Gwen Douglas
Intensive/Coronary Care . . . . Gwen Douglas
Medical Surgical Nursing . . . . Chris Brandel
OB/GYN/Womens Health . . . . Jennie Thomas
Respiratory/Cardiopulmonary . . . . Dinah Scearce

Measure	Cases	This Hospital	State Average	U.S. Average	Top Hospital
Heart Attack Care					
ACE Inhibitor or ARB for LVSD[1]	15	87%	76%	82%	100%
Aspirin at Arrival	111	98%	92%	92%	100%
Aspirin at Discharge	105	100%	87%	90%	100%
Beta Blocker at Arrival	95	92%	83%	87%	100%
Beta Blocker at Discharge	110	95%	87%	90%	100%
Fibrinolytic Medication Timing[1]	5	60%	26%	31%	100%
PCI Within 90 Minutes of Arrival[1]	8	100%	61%	54%	95%
Smoking Cessation Advice	43	100%	92%	88%	100%
Heart Failure Care					
ACE Inhibitor or ARB for LVSD	75	93%	84%	82%	100%
Discharge Instructions	172	91%	62%	61%	93%
Evaluation of LVS Function	217	98%	79%	83%	99%
Smoking Cessation Advice	32	97%	80%	82%	100%
Pneumonia Care					
Appropriate Initial Antibiotic[2]	131	83%	81%	83%	94%
Blood Culture Timing[2]	124	82%	92%	90%	100%
Influenza Vaccine	39	97%	70%	70%	100%
Initial Antibiotic Timing[2]	224	79%	81%	80%	93%
Oxygenation Assessment[2]	243	100%	99%	99%	100%
Pneumococcal Vaccine[2]	170	86%	70%	69%	94%
Smoking Cessation Advice[2]	47	96%	83%	80%	100%
Surgical Infection Prevention					
Prophylactic Antibiotic Given	475	95%	78%	77%	95%
Prophylactic Antibiotic Selection	96	85%	91%	90%	100%
Prophylactic Antibiotic Stopped	463	69%	72%	72%	95%
Pregnancy Care					
Inpatient Neonatal Mortality	-	-	-	-	-
Third or Fourth Degree Laceration	-	-	-	3.63%	3.27%

Freeman Health System

Alternate Name: Oak Hill Hospital
1102 W 32nd Street
Joplin, MO 64804
Ownership: Voluntary non-profit - Other
Emergency Services: Yes
Phone: 417-623-2801
Fax: 417-647-3716
Accredited: Yes
Licensed Beds: 203

Key Personnel:
Administrator . . . . Gary Duncan

NOTE: Hospital profiles are in alphabetical order by state, then city, then hospital within the city; Rankings are sorted by rate in descending order and exclude hospitals with less than 25 cases; (1) The number of cases is too small (n<25) for purposes of reliably predicting hospital performance; (2) Measure reflects the hospital's indication that its submission was based upon a sample of its relevant discharges; (3) Rate reflects fewer than the maximum possible quarters of data for the measure; (4) Inaccurate information submitted and suppressed for one or more quarters; (5) No data is available from the hospital for this measure; Please refer to the User's Guide for a full explanation of data

Chief Medical Staff. . . . . Christopher Andrew, MD
Emergency Room . . . . JW Pyron, DO
Coordinator Infection Control . . . . Madonna Briley
Director Medical/Surgical Nursing . . . . Karen Wells
OB/GYN Womens Health. . . . . Jeffrey L Cox, MD
Director Radiology . . . . Shawn Snider
Director Respiratory Therapy . . . . Kathy Hutchinson

Measure	Cases	This Hospital	State Average	U.S. Average	Top Hospital
Heart Attack Care					
ACE Inhibitor or ARB for LVSD	64	81%	76%	82%	100%
Aspirin at Arrival	209	96%	92%	92%	100%
Aspirin at Discharge	364	98%	87%	90%	100%
Beta Blocker at Arrival	143	90%	83%	87%	100%
Beta Blocker at Discharge	296	96%	87%	90%	100%
Fibrinolytic Medication Timing[1]	1	0%	26%	31%	100%
PCI Within 90 Minutes of Arrival[1]	13	92%	61%	54%	95%
Smoking Cessation Advice	165	98%	92%	88%	100%
Heart Failure Care					
ACE Inhibitor or ARB for LVSD	105	92%	84%	82%	100%
Discharge Instructions	209	66%	62%	61%	93%
Evaluation of LVS Function	246	98%	79%	83%	99%
Smoking Cessation Advice	48	100%	80%	82%	100%
Pneumonia Care					
Appropriate Initial Antibiotic	298	89%	81%	83%	94%
Blood Culture Timing	300	95%	92%	90%	100%
Influenza Vaccine	98	97%	70%	70%	100%
Initial Antibiotic Timing	409	89%	81%	80%	93%
Oxygenation Assessment	476	100%	99%	99%	100%
Pneumococcal Vaccine	281	96%	70%	69%	94%
Smoking Cessation Advice	132	97%	83%	80%	100%
Surgical Infection Prevention					
Prophylactic Antibiotic Given	337	93%	78%	77%	95%
Prophylactic Antibiotic Selection	114	98%	91%	90%	100%
Prophylactic Antibiotic Stopped	321	61%	72%	72%	95%
Pregnancy Care					
Inpatient Neonatal Mortality	-	-	-	-	-
Third or Fourth Degree Laceration	-	-	-	3.63%	3.27%

Saint John's Regional Medical Center

2727 McClelland Boulevard
Joplin, MO 64804
URL: www.stj.com
Ownership: Voluntary non-profit - Church
Emergency Services: Yes
Phone: 417-781-2727
Fax: 417-625-2910
Accredited: Yes
Licensed Beds: 367

Key Personnel:

President/CEO. . . . . Gary Rowe
Chief Medical Staff. . . . . J Marhnez, MD
Chief Catheterization Laboratory . . . . FH Corcoran, MD
Director Infection/Disease Control . . . . Donna Stokes
OB/GYN Womens Health. . . . . R Boice, DO
Chief Radiology . . . . Curtis Hammerman, MD
Director Respiratory Therapy . . . . Michael O'Leary

Measure	Cases	This Hospital	State Average	U.S. Average	Top Hospital
Heart Attack Care					
ACE Inhibitor or ARB for LVSD	122	84%	76%	82%	100%
Aspirin at Arrival	199	96%	92%	92%	100%
Aspirin at Discharge	304	96%	87%	90%	100%
Beta Blocker at Arrival	162	88%	83%	87%	100%
Beta Blocker at Discharge	355	94%	87%	90%	100%
Fibrinolytic Medication Timing[1]	14	64%	26%	31%	100%
PCI Within 90 Minutes of Arrival[1]	7	29%	61%	54%	95%
Smoking Cessation Advice	159	94%	92%	88%	100%
Heart Failure Care					
ACE Inhibitor or ARB for LVSD	167	75%	84%	82%	100%
Discharge Instructions	336	57%	62%	61%	93%
Evaluation of LVS Function	402	84%	79%	83%	99%
Smoking Cessation Advice	76	80%	80%	82%	100%
Pneumonia Care					
Appropriate Initial Antibiotic	263	85%	81%	83%	94%
Blood Culture Timing	274	88%	92%	90%	100%
Influenza Vaccine	140	66%	70%	70%	100%
Initial Antibiotic Timing	413	88%	81%	80%	93%
Oxygenation Assessment	494	99%	99%	99%	100%
Pneumococcal Vaccine	323	57%	70%	69%	94%
Smoking Cessation Advice	167	81%	83%	80%	100%
Surgical Infection Prevention					
Prophylactic Antibiotic Given	998	86%	78%	77%	95%
Prophylactic Antibiotic Selection	259	95%	91%	90%	100%
Prophylactic Antibiotic Stopped	986	69%	72%	72%	95%
Pregnancy Care					
Inpatient Neonatal Mortality	896	0.33%	-	-	-
Third or Fourth Degree Laceration	633	3.79%	-	3.63%	3.27%

Research Medical Center

2316 E Meyer Boulevard
Kansas City, MO 64132
Ownership: Proprietary
Emergency Services: Yes
Phone: 816-276-4000
Fax: 816-276-3571
Accredited: Yes
Licensed Beds: 536

Key Personnel:

Administrator/CEO . . . . Steven Newton
Chief Medical Staff. . . . . J Stephen Scherer, MD
Emergency Room . . . . Gregg Minion, MD
Director Infection/Disease Control . . . . David McKinsey, MD
OB/GYN Womens Health. . . . . Bradley Sullivan, MD
Chief Radiology . . . . Mark Idstrom, MD
Director Pulmonary Services . . . . Karen Mitchel

Measure	Cases	This Hospital	State Average	U.S. Average	Top Hospital
Heart Attack Care					
ACE Inhibitor or ARB for LVSD	68	93%	76%	82%	100%
Aspirin at Arrival	162	98%	92%	92%	100%
Aspirin at Discharge	279	99%	87%	90%	100%
Beta Blocker at Arrival	121	97%	83%	87%	100%
Beta Blocker at Discharge	266	98%	87%	90%	100%
Fibrinolytic Medication Timing	0	-	26%	31%	100%
PCI Within 90 Minutes of Arrival[1]	8	88%	61%	54%	95%
Smoking Cessation Advice	97	97%	92%	88%	100%
Heart Failure Care					
ACE Inhibitor or ARB for LVSD	249	88%	84%	82%	100%
Discharge Instructions	448	77%	62%	61%	93%
Evaluation of LVS Function	535	95%	79%	83%	99%
Smoking Cessation Advice	118	99%	80%	82%	100%
Pneumonia Care					
Appropriate Initial Antibiotic	118	82%	81%	83%	94%
Blood Culture Timing	89	89%	92%	90%	100%
Influenza Vaccine	33	55%	70%	70%	100%
Initial Antibiotic Timing	193	77%	81%	80%	93%
Oxygenation Assessment	235	100%	99%	99%	100%
Pneumococcal Vaccine	154	73%	70%	69%	94%
Smoking Cessation Advice	67	91%	83%	80%	100%
Surgical Infection Prevention					
Prophylactic Antibiotic Given[2,3]	278	87%	78%	77%	95%
Prophylactic Antibiotic Selection[2]	139	89%	91%	90%	100%
Prophylactic Antibiotic Stopped[2,3]	272	42%	72%	72%	95%
Pregnancy Care					
Inpatient Neonatal Mortality	-	-	-	-	-
Third or Fourth Degree Laceration	-	-	-	3.63%	3.27%

Saint Joseph Health Center

1000 Carondelet Drive
Kansas City, MO 64114
Ownership: Voluntary non-profit - Church
Emergency Services: Yes
Phone: 816-942-4400
Fax: 816-943-2840
Accredited: Yes
Licensed Beds: 300

Key Personnel:

CEO. . . . . Bruce Van Cleave, MD
Emergency Room . . . . Lily Averson
Chief Radiology . . . . John MacPhail
Director Respiratory Therapy . . . . Joe McDonald

Measure	Cases	This Hospital	State Average	U.S. Average	Top Hospital
Heart Attack Care					
ACE Inhibitor or ARB for LVSD	97	100%	76%	82%	100%
Aspirin at Arrival	221	100%	92%	92%	100%

NOTE: Hospital profiles are in alphabetical order by state, then city, then hospital within the city; Rankings are sorted by rate in descending order and exclude hospitals with less than 25 cases; (1) The number of cases is too small (n<25) for purposes of reliably predicting hospital performance; (2) Measure reflects the hospital's indication that its submission was based upon a sample of its relevant discharges; (3) Rate reflects fewer than the maximum possible quarters of data for the measure; (4) Inaccurate information submitted and suppressed for one or more quarters; (5) No data is available from the hospital for this measure; Please refer to the User's Guide for a full explanation of data

Aspirin at Discharge	391	100%	87%	90%	100%
Beta Blocker at Arrival	180	99%	83%	87%	100%
Beta Blocker at Discharge	357	100%	87%	90%	100%
Fibrinolytic Medication Timing	0	-	26%	31%	100%
PCI Within 90 Minutes of Arrival[1]	9	67%	61%	54%	95%
Smoking Cessation Advice	143	100%	92%	88%	100%
Heart Failure Care					
ACE Inhibitor or ARB for LVSD	160	99%	84%	82%	100%
Discharge Instructions	310	100%	62%	61%	93%
Evaluation of LVS Function	385	99%	79%	83%	99%
Smoking Cessation Advice	51	100%	80%	82%	100%
Pneumonia Care					
Appropriate Initial Antibiotic	203	82%	81%	83%	94%
Blood Culture Timing	162	89%	92%	90%	100%
Influenza Vaccine	41	63%	70%	70%	100%
Initial Antibiotic Timing	222	82%	81%	80%	93%
Oxygenation Assessment	278	100%	99%	99%	100%
Pneumococcal Vaccine	183	77%	70%	69%	94%
Smoking Cessation Advice	49	100%	83%	80%	100%
Surgical Infection Prevention					
Prophylactic Antibiotic Given[2,3]	159	97%	78%	77%	95%
Prophylactic Antibiotic Selection[2]	71	90%	91%	90%	100%
Prophylactic Antibiotic Stopped[2,3]	158	92%	72%	72%	95%
Pregnancy Care					
Inpatient Neonatal Mortality	1,297	0.23%	-	-	-
Third or Fourth Degree Laceration	896	3.79%	-	3.63%	3.27%

Saint Luke's Hospital of Kansas City

4401 Wornall Road
Kansas City, MO 64111
URL: www.staintlukeshealthsystem.org
Ownership: Voluntary non-profit - Other
Emergency Services: Yes
Phone: 816-932-2000
Fax: 816-932-3599
Accredited: Yes
Licensed Beds: 629

Key Personnel:
CEO. . . . . Rich Hastings
Director Emergency Room. . . . . Denise Kintigh

Measure	Cases	This Hospital	State Average	U.S. Average	Top Hospital
Heart Attack Care					
ACE Inhibitor or ARB for LVSD	132	88%	76%	82%	100%
Aspirin at Arrival	175	98%	92%	92%	100%
Aspirin at Discharge	563	99%	87%	90%	100%
Beta Blocker at Arrival	135	96%	83%	87%	100%
Beta Blocker at Discharge	595	99%	87%	90%	100%
Fibrinolytic Medication Timing[1]	1	0%	26%	31%	100%
PCI Within 90 Minutes of Arrival[1]	7	57%	61%	54%	95%
Smoking Cessation Advice	250	98%	92%	88%	100%
Heart Failure Care					
ACE Inhibitor or ARB for LVSD	275	95%	84%	82%	100%
Discharge Instructions	421	66%	62%	61%	93%
Evaluation of LVS Function	490	98%	79%	83%	99%
Smoking Cessation Advice	119	98%	80%	82%	100%
Pneumonia Care					
Appropriate Initial Antibiotic	125	80%	81%	83%	94%
Blood Culture Timing	115	88%	92%	90%	100%
Influenza Vaccine	41	80%	70%	70%	100%
Initial Antibiotic Timing	206	76%	81%	80%	93%
Oxygenation Assessment	271	100%	99%	99%	100%
Pneumococcal Vaccine	171	89%	70%	69%	94%
Smoking Cessation Advice	68	99%	83%	80%	100%
Surgical Infection Prevention					
Prophylactic Antibiotic Given[3]	763	97%	78%	77%	95%
Prophylactic Antibiotic Selection	170	81%	91%	90%	100%
Prophylactic Antibiotic Stopped[3]	737	71%	72%	72%	95%
Pregnancy Care					
Inpatient Neonatal Mortality	-	-	-	-	-
Third or Fourth Degree Laceration	-	-	-	3.63%	3.27%

Saint Luke's Northland Hospital

5830 N W Barry Road
Kansas City, MO 64154
URL: www.saintlukeshealthsystem.org
Ownership: Voluntary non-profit - Other
Emergency Services: Yes
Phone: 816-891-6000
Fax: 816-880-6155
Accredited: Yes
Licensed Beds: 58

Key Personnel:
CEO. . . . . Don Sipes
President . . . . N Gary Wages

Measure	Cases	This Hospital	State Average	U.S. Average	Top Hospital
Heart Attack Care					
ACE Inhibitor or ARB for LVSD[1]	2	50%	76%	82%	100%
Aspirin at Arrival	26	100%	92%	92%	100%
Aspirin at Discharge[1]	13	92%	87%	90%	100%
Beta Blocker at Arrival[1]	16	94%	83%	87%	100%
Beta Blocker at Discharge[1]	12	92%	87%	90%	100%
Fibrinolytic Medication Timing	0	-	26%	31%	100%
PCI Within 90 Minutes of Arrival	0	-	61%	54%	95%
Smoking Cessation Advice[1]	1	100%	92%	88%	100%
Heart Failure Care					
ACE Inhibitor or ARB for LVSD[1]	21	90%	84%	82%	100%
Discharge Instructions	57	67%	62%	61%	93%
Evaluation of LVS Function	72	97%	79%	83%	99%
Smoking Cessation Advice[1]	9	89%	80%	82%	100%
Pneumonia Care					
Appropriate Initial Antibiotic	82	90%	81%	83%	94%
Blood Culture Timing	70	99%	92%	90%	100%
Influenza Vaccine	26	92%	70%	70%	100%
Initial Antibiotic Timing	101	86%	81%	80%	93%
Oxygenation Assessment	121	100%	99%	99%	100%
Pneumococcal Vaccine	77	91%	70%	69%	94%
Smoking Cessation Advice	36	81%	83%	80%	100%
Surgical Infection Prevention					
Prophylactic Antibiotic Given[3]	159	84%	78%	77%	95%
Prophylactic Antibiotic Selection	51	84%	91%	90%	100%
Prophylactic Antibiotic Stopped[3]	152	78%	72%	72%	95%
Pregnancy Care					
Inpatient Neonatal Mortality	-	-	-	-	-
Third or Fourth Degree Laceration	-	-	-	3.63%	3.27%

Saint Lukes Cancer Institute

4401 Wornall Road
Kansas City, MO 64111
Ownership: Voluntary non-profit - Private
Emergency Services: No
Phone: 816-932-2823
Accredited: No

Measure	Cases	This Hospital	State Average	U.S. Average	Top Hospital
Heart Attack Care					
ACE Inhibitor or ARB for LVSD[5]	-	-	76%	82%	100%
Aspirin at Arrival[5]	-	-	92%	92%	100%
Aspirin at Discharge[5]	-	-	87%	90%	100%
Beta Blocker at Arrival[5]	-	-	83%	87%	100%
Beta Blocker at Discharge[5]	-	-	87%	90%	100%
Fibrinolytic Medication Timing[5]	-	-	26%	31%	100%
PCI Within 90 Minutes of Arrival[5]	-	-	61%	54%	95%
Smoking Cessation Advice[5]	-	-	92%	88%	100%
Heart Failure Care					
ACE Inhibitor or ARB for LVSD[1,3]	1	100%	84%	82%	100%
Discharge Instructions[1,3]	3	0%	62%	61%	93%
Evaluation of LVS Function[1,3]	3	100%	79%	83%	99%
Smoking Cessation Advice[1,3]	2	50%	80%	82%	100%
Pneumonia Care					
Appropriate Initial Antibiotic[1]	1	100%	81%	83%	94%
Blood Culture Timing[1]	7	100%	92%	90%	100%
Influenza Vaccine[1]	3	67%	70%	70%	100%
Initial Antibiotic Timing[1]	5	80%	81%	80%	93%
Oxygenation Assessment[1]	16	100%	99%	99%	100%
Pneumococcal Vaccine[1]	5	40%	70%	69%	94%
Smoking Cessation Advice[1]	4	75%	83%	80%	100%
Surgical Infection Prevention					
Prophylactic Antibiotic Given[1,3]	19	100%	78%	77%	95%

NOTE: Hospital profiles are in alphabetical order by state, then city, then hospital within the city; Rankings are sorted by rate in descending order and exclude hospitals with less than 25 cases; (1) The number of cases is too small (n<25) for purposes of reliably predicting hospital performance; (2) Measure reflects the hospital's indication that its submission was based upon a sample of its relevant discharges; (3) Rate reflects fewer than the maximum possible quarters of data for the measure; (4) Inaccurate information submitted and suppressed for one or more quarters; (5) No data is available from the hospital for this measure; Please refer to the User's Guide for a full explanation of data

Prophylactic Antibiotic Selection[1]	19	84%	91%	90%	100%
Prophylactic Antibiotic Stopped[1,3]	17	41%	72%	72%	95%
Pregnancy Care					
Inpatient Neonatal Mortality	-	-	-	-	-
Third or Fourth Degree Laceration	-	-	-	3.63%	3.27%

Truman Medical Center-Lakewood

7900 Lee's Summit Road
Kansas City, MO 64139
URL: www.trumed.org
Ownership: Voluntary non-profit - Private
Emergency Services: Yes
Phone: 816-404-7000
Fax: 816-404-8038
Accredited: Yes
Licensed Beds: 304

Key Personnel:
CEO. . . . . Harold Siglar
Chief Medical Officer . . . . Mark Steele
Emergency Room . . . . Gloria Field
Emergency Room . . . . Dana Basara, RN

Measure	Cases	This Hospital	State Average	U.S. Average	Top Hospital
Heart Attack Care					
ACE Inhibitor or ARB for LVSD[1]	1	100%	76%	82%	100%
Aspirin at Arrival[1]	3	100%	92%	92%	100%
Aspirin at Discharge[1]	2	50%	87%	90%	100%
Beta Blocker at Arrival[1]	5	80%	83%	87%	100%
Beta Blocker at Discharge[1]	3	67%	87%	90%	100%
Fibrinolytic Medication Timing[3]	0	-	26%	31%	100%
PCI Within 90 Minutes of Arrival	0	-	61%	54%	95%
Smoking Cessation Advice[1,3]	1	100%	92%	88%	100%
Heart Failure Care					
ACE Inhibitor or ARB for LVSD	34	85%	84%	82%	100%
Discharge Instructions[1,3]	11	100%	62%	61%	93%
Evaluation of LVS Function	67	87%	79%	83%	99%
Smoking Cessation Advice[1,3]	4	100%	80%	82%	100%
Pneumonia Care					
Appropriate Initial Antibiotic[1,3]	19	79%	81%	83%	94%
Blood Culture Timing[1,3]	11	100%	92%	90%	100%
Influenza Vaccine[5]	-	-	70%	70%	100%
Initial Antibiotic Timing	53	68%	81%	80%	93%
Oxygenation Assessment	80	100%	99%	99%	100%
Pneumococcal Vaccine	26	46%	70%	69%	94%
Smoking Cessation Advice[1,3]	11	82%	83%	80%	100%
Surgical Infection Prevention					
Prophylactic Antibiotic Given[2,3]	61	97%	78%	77%	95%
Prophylactic Antibiotic Selection[5]	-	-	91%	90%	100%
Prophylactic Antibiotic Stopped[2,3]	58	16%	72%	72%	95%
Pregnancy Care					
Inpatient Neonatal Mortality	-	-	-	-	-
Third or Fourth Degree Laceration	-	-	-	3.63%	3.27%

Truman Medical Centers

2301 Holmes Street
Kansas City, MO 64108
URL: www.trumed.org
Ownership: Voluntary non-profit - Private
Emergency Services: Yes
Phone: 816-404-1000
Fax: 816-404-3779
Accredited: Yes
Licensed Beds: 651

Key Personnel:
President/CEO. . . . . John Blueford
Chief Medical Staff. . . . . Mark Steele, MD
ER Chair . . . . Robert Schwab, MD
OB/GYN Womens Health. . . . . James Youngblood, MD
Chief Radiology . . . . Gerald Finke, MD
Respiratory/Cardiopulmonary. . . . . Gary Salzman, MD

Measure	Cases	This Hospital	State Average	U.S. Average	Top Hospital
Heart Attack Care					
ACE Inhibitor or ARB for LVSD[1]	11	91%	76%	82%	100%
Aspirin at Arrival	36	97%	92%	92%	100%
Aspirin at Discharge	26	100%	87%	90%	100%
Beta Blocker at Arrival	38	89%	83%	87%	100%
Beta Blocker at Discharge	25	92%	87%	90%	100%
Fibrinolytic Medication Timing[1]	1	0%	26%	31%	100%
PCI Within 90 Minutes of Arrival	0	-	61%	54%	95%
Smoking Cessation Advice[1]	16	100%	92%	88%	100%
Heart Failure Care					
ACE Inhibitor or ARB for LVSD[2]	198	90%	84%	82%	100%
Discharge Instructions[2]	299	87%	62%	61%	93%
Evaluation of LVS Function[2]	318	97%	79%	83%	99%
Smoking Cessation Advice[2]	139	96%	80%	82%	100%
Pneumonia Care					
Appropriate Initial Antibiotic[2]	99	88%	81%	83%	94%
Blood Culture Timing[2]	128	88%	92%	90%	100%
Influenza Vaccine[1,2]	19	68%	70%	70%	100%
Initial Antibiotic Timing[2]	164	60%	81%	80%	93%
Oxygenation Assessment[2]	181	100%	99%	99%	100%
Pneumococcal Vaccine[2]	44	73%	70%	69%	94%
Smoking Cessation Advice[2]	95	92%	83%	80%	100%
Surgical Infection Prevention					
Prophylactic Antibiotic Given[2,3]	175	84%	78%	77%	95%
Prophylactic Antibiotic Selection[2]	48	92%	91%	90%	100%
Prophylactic Antibiotic Stopped[2,3]	174	69%	72%	72%	95%
Pregnancy Care					
Inpatient Neonatal Mortality	-	-	-	-	-
Third or Fourth Degree Laceration	-	-	-	3.63%	3.27%

Twin Rivers Regional Medical Center

1301 1st Street
Kennett, MO 63857
URL: www.twinrivermedcenter.com
Ownership: Voluntary non-profit - Private
Emergency Services: Yes
Phone: 573-888-4522
Fax: 573-888-5525
Accredited: Yes
Licensed Beds: 116

Key Personnel:
Administrator/CEO. . . . . John McClellan
Chief Medical Staff. . . . . Maynard Sisler, MD
Emergency Room . . . . Bobby Sibbens, DO
Director Infection/Disease Control . . . . Joanne Burton, RN
Director Radiology . . . . Larry Sando
Director Respiratory Therapy. . . . . Jill Midkiff

Measure	Cases	This Hospital	State Average	U.S. Average	Top Hospital
Heart Attack Care					
ACE Inhibitor or ARB for LVSD[1]	4	75%	76%	82%	100%
Aspirin at Arrival[1]	18	83%	92%	92%	100%
Aspirin at Discharge[1]	13	54%	87%	90%	100%
Beta Blocker at Arrival[1]	18	67%	83%	87%	100%
Beta Blocker at Discharge[1]	15	67%	87%	90%	100%
Fibrinolytic Medication Timing	0	-	26%	31%	100%
PCI Within 90 Minutes of Arrival	0	-	61%	54%	95%
Smoking Cessation Advice[1]	5	100%	92%	88%	100%
Heart Failure Care					
ACE Inhibitor or ARB for LVSD	44	68%	84%	82%	100%
Discharge Instructions	89	100%	62%	61%	93%
Evaluation of LVS Function	119	90%	79%	83%	99%
Smoking Cessation Advice[1]	22	100%	80%	82%	100%
Pneumonia Care					
Appropriate Initial Antibiotic	70	71%	81%	83%	94%
Blood Culture Timing	53	75%	92%	90%	100%
Influenza Vaccine[1]	12	67%	70%	70%	100%
Initial Antibiotic Timing	95	74%	81%	80%	93%
Oxygenation Assessment	128	97%	99%	99%	100%
Pneumococcal Vaccine	52	71%	70%	69%	94%
Smoking Cessation Advice	50	98%	83%	80%	100%
Surgical Infection Prevention					
Prophylactic Antibiotic Given[2]	86	95%	78%	77%	95%
Prophylactic Antibiotic Selection[1,2]	21	100%	91%	90%	100%
Prophylactic Antibiotic Stopped[2]	74	89%	72%	72%	95%
Pregnancy Care					
Inpatient Neonatal Mortality	-	-	-	-	-
Third or Fourth Degree Laceration	-	-	-	3.63%	3.27%

Northeast Regional Medical Center

Alternate Name: Grim-Smith Hospital and Clinic

NOTE: Hospital profiles are in alphabetical order by state, then city, then hospital within the city; Rankings are sorted by rate in descending order and exclude hospitals with less than 25 cases; (1) The number of cases is too small (n<25) for purposes of reliably predicting hospital performance; (2) Measure reflects the hospital's indication that its submission was based upon a sample of its relevant discharges; (3) Rate reflects fewer than the maximum possible quarters of data for the measure; (4) Inaccurate information submitted and suppressed for one or more quarters; (5) No data is available from the hospital for this measure; Please refer to the User's Guide for a full explanation of data

315 S Osteopathy	Toll-Free: 888-785-7770
PO Box C8502	Phone: 660-785-1000
Kirksville, MO 63501	Fax: 660-785-1110
URL: www.nermc.com	
Ownership: Proprietary	Accredited: Yes
Emergency Services: Yes	Licensed Beds: 109

Key Personnel:
CEO. . . . . Ranee Brayton
Chief Medical Staff. . . . . Ronald Phillips, MD
Emergency Room . . . . Jerry L Wait, DO
Director Infection/Disease Control . . . . Nita Coale, RN
CNO. . . . . Peg Ernst, RN
OB/GYN Womens Health. . . . . Ralph Boling, DO
Director Respiratory Therapy . . . . Don Miller

Measure	Cases	This Hospital	State Average	U.S. Average	Top Hospital
Heart Attack Care					
ACE Inhibitor or ARB for LVSD[1]	3	67%	76%	82%	100%
Aspirin at Arrival[1]	15	100%	92%	92%	100%
Aspirin at Discharge[1]	13	100%	87%	90%	100%
Beta Blocker at Arrival[1]	17	100%	83%	87%	100%
Beta Blocker at Discharge[1]	17	94%	87%	90%	100%
Fibrinolytic Medication Timing[1]	1	0%	26%	31%	100%
PCI Within 90 Minutes of Arrival	0	-	61%	54%	95%
Smoking Cessation Advice[1]	1	100%	92%	88%	100%
Heart Failure Care					
ACE Inhibitor or ARB for LVSD	26	58%	84%	82%	100%
Discharge Instructions	50	64%	62%	61%	93%
Evaluation of LVS Function	87	98%	79%	83%	99%
Smoking Cessation Advice[1]	12	100%	80%	82%	100%
Pneumonia Care					
Appropriate Initial Antibiotic[2]	59	81%	81%	83%	94%
Blood Culture Timing[2]	74	97%	92%	90%	100%
Influenza Vaccine[1,2]	18	67%	70%	70%	100%
Initial Antibiotic Timing[2]	105	86%	81%	80%	93%
Oxygenation Assessment[2]	131	98%	99%	99%	100%
Pneumococcal Vaccine[2]	92	75%	70%	69%	94%
Smoking Cessation Advice[1,2]	24	88%	83%	80%	100%
Surgical Infection Prevention					
Prophylactic Antibiotic Given[2,3]	149	50%	78%	77%	95%
Prophylactic Antibiotic Selection[2]	55	95%	91%	90%	100%
Prophylactic Antibiotic Stopped[2,3]	134	64%	72%	72%	95%
Pregnancy Care					
Inpatient Neonatal Mortality	-	-	-	-	-
Third or Fourth Degree Laceration	-	-	-	3.63%	3.27%

Saint Joseph Hospital West

100 Medical Plaza	Toll-Free: 800-362-2993
Lake Saint Louis, MO 63367	Phone: 636-625-5200
	Fax: 636-625-5314
Ownership: Voluntary non-profit - Church	Accredited: Yes
Emergency Services: Yes	Licensed Beds: 100

Key Personnel:
CEO. . . . . Kevin Kast
Chief Medical Staff. . . . . James Freeman, MD
Emergency Room . . . . Tim Thompson, MD

Measure	Cases	This Hospital	State Average	U.S. Average	Top Hospital
Heart Attack Care					
ACE Inhibitor or ARB for LVSD[1]	8	88%	76%	82%	100%
Aspirin at Arrival	58	97%	92%	92%	100%
Aspirin at Discharge[1]	23	87%	87%	90%	100%
Beta Blocker at Arrival	64	98%	83%	87%	100%
Beta Blocker at Discharge	29	93%	87%	90%	100%
Fibrinolytic Medication Timing[1]	7	86%	26%	31%	100%
PCI Within 90 Minutes of Arrival	0	-	61%	54%	95%
Smoking Cessation Advice[1]	8	88%	92%	88%	100%
Heart Failure Care					
ACE Inhibitor or ARB for LVSD	56	84%	84%	82%	100%
Discharge Instructions	137	57%	62%	61%	93%
Evaluation of LVS Function	159	96%	79%	83%	99%
Smoking Cessation Advice[1]	15	93%	80%	82%	100%
Pneumonia Care					
Appropriate Initial Antibiotic	175	83%	81%	83%	94%
Blood Culture Timing	172	95%	92%	90%	100%
Influenza Vaccine	50	60%	70%	70%	100%
Initial Antibiotic Timing	206	87%	81%	80%	93%
Oxygenation Assessment	268	100%	99%	99%	100%
Pneumococcal Vaccine	169	72%	70%	69%	94%
Smoking Cessation Advice	65	88%	83%	80%	100%
Surgical Infection Prevention					
Prophylactic Antibiotic Given	381	90%	78%	77%	95%
Prophylactic Antibiotic Selection	108	96%	91%	90%	100%
Prophylactic Antibiotic Stopped	375	84%	72%	72%	95%
Pregnancy Care					
Inpatient Neonatal Mortality	-	-	-	-	-
Third or Fourth Degree Laceration	-	-	-	3.63%	3.27%

Barton County Memorial Hospital

Second & Gulf Street	Phone: 417-682-6081
Lamar, MO 64759	Fax: 417-682-2138
Ownership: Government - Local	Accredited: No
Emergency Services: No	Licensed Beds: 49

Key Personnel:
CEO. . . . . Rudy Snedigar
Chief Medical Staff. . . . . Joseph Wilson
Emergency Room . . . . Kate Mallumian
Respiratory/Cardiopulmonary. . . . . Carrie Whitesell

Measure	Cases	This Hospital	State Average	U.S. Average	Top Hospital
Heart Attack Care					
ACE Inhibitor or ARB for LVSD[3]	0	-	76%	82%	100%
Aspirin at Arrival[1,3]	2	100%	92%	92%	100%
Aspirin at Discharge[1,3]	1	0%	87%	90%	100%
Beta Blocker at Arrival[1,3]	2	100%	83%	87%	100%
Beta Blocker at Discharge[1,3]	1	100%	87%	90%	100%
Fibrinolytic Medication Timing[3]	0	-	26%	31%	100%
PCI Within 90 Minutes of Arrival[5]	-	-	61%	54%	95%
Smoking Cessation Advice[3]	0	-	92%	88%	100%
Heart Failure Care					
ACE Inhibitor or ARB for LVSD[1,2,3]	1	100%	84%	82%	100%
Discharge Instructions[1,2,3]	10	0%	62%	61%	93%
Evaluation of LVS Function[1,2,3]	11	18%	79%	83%	99%
Smoking Cessation Advice[1,2,3]	1	0%	80%	82%	100%
Pneumonia Care					
Appropriate Initial Antibiotic[1,3]	7	71%	81%	83%	94%
Blood Culture Timing[1,3]	4	100%	92%	90%	100%
Influenza Vaccine[1]	1	0%	70%	70%	100%
Initial Antibiotic Timing[1,3]	8	75%	81%	80%	93%
Oxygenation Assessment[1,3]	8	100%	99%	99%	100%
Pneumococcal Vaccine[1,3]	5	0%	70%	69%	94%
Smoking Cessation Advice[3]	0	-	83%	80%	100%
Surgical Infection Prevention					
Prophylactic Antibiotic Given[5]	-	-	78%	77%	95%
Prophylactic Antibiotic Selection[5]	-	-	91%	90%	100%
Prophylactic Antibiotic Stopped[5]	-	-	72%	72%	95%
Pregnancy Care					
Inpatient Neonatal Mortality	-	-	-	-	-
Third or Fourth Degree Laceration	-	-	-	3.63%	3.27%

Saint John's Hospital at Lebanon

100 Hospital Drive	Phone: 417-533-6100
Lebanon, MO 65536	Fax: 417-533-6040
E-mail: rttinshaw@sprg.smhs.com	
Ownership: Voluntary non-profit - Church	Accredited: Yes
Emergency Services: Yes	Licensed Beds: 41

Key Personnel:
President/CEO. . . . . Gary Pulsipher
Medical/Surgical Nursing . . . . D D Irish, RN
OB/GYN Womens Health. . . . . Mary Brewer, RN
Respiratory/Cardiopulmonary. . . . . Kent Wapelhorst

Measure	Cases	This Hospital	State Average	U.S. Average	Top Hospital
Heart Attack Care					
ACE Inhibitor or ARB for LVSD[1]	4	75%	76%	82%	100%

NOTE: Hospital profiles are in alphabetical order by state, then city, then hospital within the city; Rankings are sorted by rate in descending order and exclude hospitals with less than 25 cases; (1) The number of cases is too small (n<25) for purposes of reliably predicting hospital performance; (2) Measure reflects the hospital's indication that its submission was based upon a sample of its relevant discharges; (3) Rate reflects fewer than the maximum possible quarters of data for the measure; (4) Inaccurate information submitted and suppressed for one or more quarters; (5) No data is available from the hospital for this measure; Please refer to the User's Guide for a full explanation of data

Measure	Cases	This Hospital	State Average	U.S. Average	Top Hospital
Aspirin at Arrival[1]	23	87%	92%	92%	100%
Aspirin at Discharge[1]	16	81%	87%	90%	100%
Beta Blocker at Arrival[1]	22	91%	83%	87%	100%
Beta Blocker at Discharge[1]	17	94%	87%	90%	100%
Fibrinolytic Medication Timing	0	-	26%	31%	100%
PCI Within 90 Minutes of Arrival	0	-	61%	54%	95%
Smoking Cessation Advice[1]	1	100%	92%	88%	100%
Heart Failure Care					
ACE Inhibitor or ARB for LVSD[1]	18	89%	84%	82%	100%
Discharge Instructions	71	69%	62%	61%	93%
Evaluation of LVS Function	83	73%	79%	83%	99%
Smoking Cessation Advice[1]	9	100%	80%	82%	100%
Pneumonia Care					
Appropriate Initial Antibiotic	116	74%	81%	83%	94%
Blood Culture Timing	47	94%	92%	90%	100%
Influenza Vaccine	27	96%	70%	70%	100%
Initial Antibiotic Timing	127	80%	81%	80%	93%
Oxygenation Assessment	168	100%	99%	99%	100%
Pneumococcal Vaccine	101	90%	70%	69%	94%
Smoking Cessation Advice	35	97%	83%	80%	100%
Surgical Infection Prevention					
Prophylactic Antibiotic Given[3]	52	62%	78%	77%	95%
Prophylactic Antibiotic Selection	50	94%	91%	90%	100%
Prophylactic Antibiotic Stopped[3]	49	16%	72%	72%	95%
Pregnancy Care					
Inpatient Neonatal Mortality	-	-	-	-	-
Third or Fourth Degree Laceration	-	-	-	3.63%	3.27%

Lee's Summit Hospital

530 NW Murray Road
Lee's Summit, MO 64081
URL: www.leessummithospital.com
Ownership: Proprietary
Emergency Services: Yes
Phone: 816-969-6000
Fax: 816-969-6523
Accredited: Yes
Licensed Beds: 83

Key Personnel:

President/CEO. . . . . Carolyn W Caldwell
President Medical Staff . . . . Andrew S Pavlovich, MD

Measure	Cases	This Hospital	State Average	U.S. Average	Top Hospital
Heart Attack Care					
ACE Inhibitor or ARB for LVSD[1]	16	100%	76%	82%	100%
Aspirin at Arrival	81	99%	92%	92%	100%
Aspirin at Discharge	70	100%	87%	90%	100%
Beta Blocker at Arrival	66	91%	83%	87%	100%
Beta Blocker at Discharge	67	100%	87%	90%	100%
Fibrinolytic Medication Timing[1]	1	100%	26%	31%	100%
PCI Within 90 Minutes of Arrival[1]	4	75%	61%	54%	95%
Smoking Cessation Advice	27	100%	92%	88%	100%
Heart Failure Care					
ACE Inhibitor or ARB for LVSD	45	82%	84%	82%	100%
Discharge Instructions	79	61%	62%	61%	93%
Evaluation of LVS Function	126	94%	79%	83%	99%
Smoking Cessation Advice[1]	6	100%	80%	82%	100%
Pneumonia Care					
Appropriate Initial Antibiotic	99	86%	81%	83%	94%
Blood Culture Timing	89	92%	92%	90%	100%
Influenza Vaccine	40	48%	70%	70%	100%
Initial Antibiotic Timing	171	85%	81%	80%	93%
Oxygenation Assessment	197	100%	99%	99%	100%
Pneumococcal Vaccine	135	76%	70%	69%	94%
Smoking Cessation Advice	36	100%	83%	80%	100%
Surgical Infection Prevention					
Prophylactic Antibiotic Given[2,3]	143	85%	78%	77%	95%
Prophylactic Antibiotic Selection[2]	58	78%	91%	90%	100%
Prophylactic Antibiotic Stopped[2,3]	137	80%	72%	72%	95%
Pregnancy Care					
Inpatient Neonatal Mortality	-	-	-	-	-
Third or Fourth Degree Laceration	-	-	-	3.63%	3.27%

Saint Luke's East Lee's Summit Hospital

100 N E Saint Luke's Boulevard
Lees Summit, MO 64086
Ownership: Voluntary non-profit - Private
Emergency Services: Yes
Phone: 816-347-5000
Accredited: Yes

Measure	Cases	This Hospital	State Average	U.S. Average	Top Hospital
Heart Attack Care					
ACE Inhibitor or ARB for LVSD[1,3]	1	0%	76%	82%	100%
Aspirin at Arrival[1,3]	4	100%	92%	92%	100%
Aspirin at Discharge[1,3]	3	67%	87%	90%	100%
Beta Blocker at Arrival[1,3]	3	67%	83%	87%	100%
Beta Blocker at Discharge[1,3]	3	100%	87%	90%	100%
Fibrinolytic Medication Timing[3]	0	-	26%	31%	100%
PCI Within 90 Minutes of Arrival	0	-	61%	54%	95%
Smoking Cessation Advice[3]	0	-	92%	88%	100%
Heart Failure Care					
ACE Inhibitor or ARB for LVSD[1,3]	15	73%	84%	82%	100%
Discharge Instructions[3]	30	43%	62%	61%	93%
Evaluation of LVS Function[3]	36	92%	79%	83%	99%
Smoking Cessation Advice[1,3]	5	60%	80%	82%	100%
Pneumonia Care					
Appropriate Initial Antibiotic[3]	31	74%	81%	83%	94%
Blood Culture Timing	35	71%	92%	90%	100%
Influenza Vaccine[1]	4	50%	70%	70%	100%
Initial Antibiotic Timing[3]	44	89%	81%	80%	93%
Oxygenation Assessment[3]	48	100%	99%	99%	100%
Pneumococcal Vaccine[1,3]	21	71%	70%	69%	94%
Smoking Cessation Advice[1,3]	16	56%	83%	80%	100%
Surgical Infection Prevention					
Prophylactic Antibiotic Given[3]	161	73%	78%	77%	95%
Prophylactic Antibiotic Selection	72	89%	91%	90%	100%
Prophylactic Antibiotic Stopped[3]	160	79%	72%	72%	95%
Pregnancy Care					
Inpatient Neonatal Mortality	-	-	-	-	-
Third or Fourth Degree Laceration	-	-	-	3.63%	3.27%

Lafayette Regional Health Center

1500 State Street
Lexington, MO 64067
URL: lafayetteregionalhealthcenter.com
Ownership: Proprietary
Emergency Services: Yes
Phone: 660-259-2203
Fax: 660-259-6833
Accredited: Yes
Licensed Beds: 49

Key Personnel:

President/CEO. . . . . Bret Kolmant
Chief Medical Staff. . . . . Roger Sacry, MD
Emergency Room . . . . Terri Elliott, RN
Infection Control. . . . . Gini Summers, RN
ICU . . . . Dena Stark, RN
Medical/Surgical Nursing . . . . Kim Leakey, RN
Respiratory/Cardiopulmonary. . . . . Stephen Skinner

Measure	Cases	This Hospital	State Average	U.S. Average	Top Hospital
Heart Attack Care					
ACE Inhibitor or ARB for LVSD[1]	2	50%	76%	82%	100%
Aspirin at Arrival[1]	6	100%	92%	92%	100%
Aspirin at Discharge[1]	5	80%	87%	90%	100%
Beta Blocker at Arrival[1]	7	71%	83%	87%	100%
Beta Blocker at Discharge[1]	4	75%	87%	90%	100%
Fibrinolytic Medication Timing	0	-	26%	31%	100%
PCI Within 90 Minutes of Arrival	0	-	61%	54%	95%
Smoking Cessation Advice[1]	1	100%	92%	88%	100%
Heart Failure Care					
ACE Inhibitor or ARB for LVSD[1]	16	81%	84%	82%	100%
Discharge Instructions	32	97%	62%	61%	93%
Evaluation of LVS Function	57	82%	79%	83%	99%
Smoking Cessation Advice[1]	7	86%	80%	82%	100%
Pneumonia Care					
Appropriate Initial Antibiotic	71	73%	81%	83%	94%
Blood Culture Timing	32	91%	92%	90%	100%
Influenza Vaccine[1]	20	70%	70%	70%	100%
Initial Antibiotic Timing	94	81%	81%	80%	93%

NOTE: Hospital profiles are in alphabetical order by state, then city, then hospital within the city; Rankings are sorted by rate in descending order and exclude hospitals with less than 25 cases; (1) The number of cases is too small (n<25) for purposes of reliably predicting hospital performance; (2) Measure reflects the hospital's indication that its submission was based upon a sample of its relevant discharges; (3) Rate reflects fewer than the maximum possible quarters of data for the measure; (4) Inaccurate information submitted and suppressed for one or more quarters; (5) No data is available from the hospital for this measure; Please refer to the User's Guide for a full explanation of data

Oxygenation Assessment	111	100%	99%	99%	100%
Pneumococcal Vaccine	65	57%	70%	69%	94%
Smoking Cessation Advice[1]	20	95%	83%	80%	100%
Surgical Infection Prevention					
Prophylactic Antibiotic Given[1,2,3]	6	17%	78%	77%	95%
Prophylactic Antibiotic Selection[1,2]	2	100%	91%	90%	100%
Prophylactic Antibiotic Stopped[1,2,3]	2	50%	72%	72%	95%
Pregnancy Care					
Inpatient Neonatal Mortality	-	-	-	-	-
Third or Fourth Degree Laceration	-	-	-	3.63%	3.27%

Liberty Hospital

2525 Glenn Hendren Drive
PO Box 1002
Liberty, MO 64069
URL: www.libertyhospital.org
Phone: 816-781-7200
Fax: 816-792-7117
Ownership: Govt - Hospital District or Authority
Emergency Services: Yes
Accredited: Yes
Licensed Beds: 202

Key Personnel:

CEO/President. . . . . Joe Crossett
Chief Medical Staff. . . . . Steve Starr, MD
Director of Cardiology/Cardiac Lab. . . . . Georgia Solovic
Emergency Room . . . . Brian Robb, DO
Director Infection/Disease Control . . . . Maggie Hagan, MD
CCU Spvg. Nurse . . . . Kathy Taylor
Director Medical/Surgical Nursing . . . . Jan Osborne
Director Radiology . . . . Tom Brown
Director Respiratory Therapy . . . . Vicky Foster

Measure	Cases	This Hospital	State Average	U.S. Average	Top Hospital
Heart Attack Care					
ACE Inhibitor or ARB for LVSD[1]	15	87%	76%	82%	100%
Aspirin at Arrival	46	98%	92%	92%	100%
Aspirin at Discharge	30	90%	87%	90%	100%
Beta Blocker at Arrival	33	91%	83%	87%	100%
Beta Blocker at Discharge	32	97%	87%	90%	100%
Fibrinolytic Medication Timing	0	-	26%	31%	100%
PCI Within 90 Minutes of Arrival	0	-	61%	54%	95%
Smoking Cessation Advice[1]	11	100%	92%	88%	100%
Heart Failure Care					
ACE Inhibitor or ARB for LVSD	94	64%	84%	82%	100%
Discharge Instructions	211	63%	62%	61%	93%
Evaluation of LVS Function	266	90%	79%	83%	99%
Smoking Cessation Advice	36	97%	80%	82%	100%
Pneumonia Care					
Appropriate Initial Antibiotic	219	82%	81%	83%	94%
Blood Culture Timing	205	94%	92%	90%	100%
Influenza Vaccine	68	57%	70%	70%	100%
Initial Antibiotic Timing	322	89%	81%	80%	93%
Oxygenation Assessment	415	100%	99%	99%	100%
Pneumococcal Vaccine	247	90%	70%	69%	94%
Smoking Cessation Advice	144	100%	83%	80%	100%
Surgical Infection Prevention					
Prophylactic Antibiotic Given[3]	369	80%	78%	77%	95%
Prophylactic Antibiotic Selection	136	95%	91%	90%	100%
Prophylactic Antibiotic Stopped[3]	359	84%	72%	72%	95%
Pregnancy Care					
Inpatient Neonatal Mortality	-	-	-	-	-
Third or Fourth Degree Laceration	-	-	-	3.63%	3.27%

Pike County Memorial Hospital

2305 W Georgia Street
Louisiana, MO 63353
URL: www.pcmh-mo.org
Phone: 573-754-5531
Fax: 573-754-5874
Ownership: Government - Local
Emergency Services: Yes
Accredited: Yes
Licensed Beds: 45

Key Personnel:

CEO/President. . . . . Lorraine Harness
Chief Medical Staff. . . . . Phillip Pitney, MD
Emergency Room Director. . . . . Katy Scott
Director Infection Control . . . . Paulette Powelson, RN
Director Surgical Services . . . . Dianne Oliver
Director Radiology . . . . Rebekka Thornton
Director Respiratory/Cardiopulmonary . . . . Judy Prater

Measure	Cases	This Hospital	State Average	U.S. Average	Top Hospital
Heart Attack Care					
ACE Inhibitor or ARB for LVSD[1,2]	2	50%	76%	82%	100%
Aspirin at Arrival[1,2]	8	62%	92%	92%	100%
Aspirin at Discharge[1,2]	3	33%	87%	90%	100%
Beta Blocker at Arrival[1,2]	6	17%	83%	87%	100%
Beta Blocker at Discharge[1,2]	5	20%	87%	90%	100%
Fibrinolytic Medication Timing[2]	0	-	26%	31%	100%
PCI Within 90 Minutes of Arrival[2]	0	-	61%	54%	95%
Smoking Cessation Advice[2]	0	-	92%	88%	100%
Heart Failure Care					
ACE Inhibitor or ARB for LVSD[1,2]	13	77%	84%	82%	100%
Discharge Instructions[2]	26	85%	62%	61%	93%
Evaluation of LVS Function[2]	53	92%	79%	83%	99%
Smoking Cessation Advice[1,2]	6	100%	80%	82%	100%
Pneumonia Care					
Appropriate Initial Antibiotic[2]	38	84%	81%	83%	94%
Blood Culture Timing[2]	52	87%	92%	90%	100%
Influenza Vaccine[1]	16	94%	70%	70%	100%
Initial Antibiotic Timing[2]	79	94%	81%	80%	93%
Oxygenation Assessment[2]	93	100%	99%	99%	100%
Pneumococcal Vaccine[2]	59	98%	70%	69%	94%
Smoking Cessation Advice[1,2]	24	100%	83%	80%	100%
Surgical Infection Prevention					
Prophylactic Antibiotic Given[5]	-	-	78%	77%	95%
Prophylactic Antibiotic Selection[5]	-	-	91%	90%	100%
Prophylactic Antibiotic Stopped[5]	-	-	72%	72%	95%
Pregnancy Care					
Inpatient Neonatal Mortality	-	-	-	-	-
Third or Fourth Degree Laceration	-	-	-	3.63%	3.27%

Fitzgibbon Memorial Hospital

2305 S Highway 65
Marshall, MO 65340
E-mail: snewman@murlin.com
Phone: 660-886-7431
Fax: 660-886-9001
Ownership: Voluntary non-profit - Other
Emergency Services: No
Accredited: No
Licensed Beds: 60

Key Personnel:

CEO. . . . . Ronald A Ott
Chief Medical Staff. . . . . Roy Elsrink
Director Infection/Disease Control . . . . Linda Cook, RN
Director Medical/Surgical Nursing . . . . Lynne Ott, RN, B
OB/GYN Womens Health. . . . . William J Smith, MD
Chief Radiology . . . . Greg Dixon
Director Respiratory Therapy . . . . Jo Banks

Measure	Cases	This Hospital	State Average	U.S. Average	Top Hospital
Heart Attack Care					
ACE Inhibitor or ARB for LVSD[1]	1	0%	76%	82%	100%
Aspirin at Arrival[1]	7	86%	92%	92%	100%
Aspirin at Discharge[1]	3	100%	87%	90%	100%
Beta Blocker at Arrival[1]	5	20%	83%	87%	100%
Beta Blocker at Discharge[1]	2	50%	87%	90%	100%
Fibrinolytic Medication Timing[1]	1	0%	26%	31%	100%
PCI Within 90 Minutes of Arrival	0	-	61%	54%	95%
Smoking Cessation Advice	0	-	92%	88%	100%
Heart Failure Care					
ACE Inhibitor or ARB for LVSD[1]	23	70%	84%	82%	100%
Discharge Instructions	56	25%	62%	61%	93%
Evaluation of LVS Function	89	62%	79%	83%	99%
Smoking Cessation Advice[1]	4	50%	80%	82%	100%
Pneumonia Care					
Appropriate Initial Antibiotic	90	84%	81%	83%	94%
Blood Culture Timing	43	98%	92%	90%	100%
Influenza Vaccine[1]	23	74%	70%	70%	100%
Initial Antibiotic Timing	125	82%	81%	80%	93%
Oxygenation Assessment	137	100%	99%	99%	100%
Pneumococcal Vaccine	82	56%	70%	69%	94%
Smoking Cessation Advice	35	86%	83%	80%	100%
Surgical Infection Prevention					

NOTE: Hospital profiles are in alphabetical order by state, then city, then hospital within the city; Rankings are sorted by rate in descending order and exclude hospitals with less than 25 cases; (1) The number of cases is too small (n<25) for purposes of reliably predicting hospital performance; (2) Measure reflects the hospital's indication that its submission was based upon a sample of its relevant discharges; (3) Rate reflects fewer than the maximum possible quarters of data for the measure; (4) Inaccurate information submitted and suppressed for one or more quarters; (5) No data is available from the hospital for this measure; Please refer to the User's Guide for a full explanation of data

Measure	Cases	This Hospital	State Average	U.S. Average	Top Hospital
Prophylactic Antibiotic Given	88	73%	78%	77%	95%
Prophylactic Antibiotic Selection[1]	22	100%	91%	90%	100%
Prophylactic Antibiotic Stopped	88	99%	72%	72%	95%
Pregnancy Care					
Inpatient Neonatal Mortality	-	-	-	-	-
Third or Fourth Degree Laceration	-	-	-	3.63%	3.27%

Saint Francis Hospital & Health Services

Alternate Name: Saint Francis Hospital
2016 S Main Street
Maryville, MO 64468
URL: www.stfrancismaryville.com
Ownership: Voluntary non-profit - Church
Emergency Services: Yes
Phone: 660-562-2600
Fax: 660-562-7911
Accredited: Yes
Licensed Beds: 81
Key Personnel:
President/CEO. . . . . Mike Baumgartner

Measure	Cases	This Hospital	State Average	U.S. Average	Top Hospital
Heart Attack Care					
ACE Inhibitor or ARB for LVSD	0	-	76%	82%	100%
Aspirin at Arrival[1]	7	100%	92%	92%	100%
Aspirin at Discharge[1]	6	67%	87%	90%	100%
Beta Blocker at Arrival[1]	5	100%	83%	87%	100%
Beta Blocker at Discharge[1]	6	100%	87%	90%	100%
Fibrinolytic Medication Timing	0	-	26%	31%	100%
PCI Within 90 Minutes of Arrival	0	-	61%	54%	95%
Smoking Cessation Advice[1]	1	100%	92%	88%	100%
Heart Failure Care					
ACE Inhibitor or ARB for LVSD[1]	12	92%	84%	82%	100%
Discharge Instructions	31	94%	62%	61%	93%
Evaluation of LVS Function	58	98%	79%	83%	99%
Smoking Cessation Advice[1]	5	100%	80%	82%	100%
Pneumonia Care					
Appropriate Initial Antibiotic	49	98%	81%	83%	94%
Blood Culture Timing	29	90%	92%	90%	100%
Influenza Vaccine[1]	9	100%	70%	70%	100%
Initial Antibiotic Timing	61	90%	81%	80%	93%
Oxygenation Assessment	76	100%	99%	99%	100%
Pneumococcal Vaccine	61	100%	70%	69%	94%
Smoking Cessation Advice[1]	9	100%	83%	80%	100%
Surgical Infection Prevention					
Prophylactic Antibiotic Given[3]	125	95%	78%	77%	95%
Prophylactic Antibiotic Selection	44	100%	91%	90%	100%
Prophylactic Antibiotic Stopped[3]	121	98%	72%	72%	95%
Pregnancy Care					
Inpatient Neonatal Mortality	-	-	-	-	-
Third or Fourth Degree Laceration	-	-	-	3.63%	3.27%

Scotland County Memorial Hospital

Sigler Street
RR 1, Box 53
Memphis, MO 63555
Ownership: Govt - Hospital District or Authority
Emergency Services: Yes
Phone: 660-465-8511
Fax: 660-465-2513
Accredited: No
Licensed Beds: 40
Key Personnel:
CEO. . . . . Marcia R Dial
Chief of Medical Staff. . . . . Robert Snyder
Director Emergency Room. . . . . Berna Harcrow

Measure	Cases	This Hospital	State Average	U.S. Average	Top Hospital
Heart Attack Care					
ACE Inhibitor or ARB for LVSD[5]	-	-	76%	82%	100%
Aspirin at Arrival[5]	-	-	92%	92%	100%
Aspirin at Discharge[5]	-	-	87%	90%	100%
Beta Blocker at Arrival[5]	-	-	83%	87%	100%
Beta Blocker at Discharge[5]	-	-	87%	90%	100%
Fibrinolytic Medication Timing[5]	-	-	26%	31%	100%
PCI Within 90 Minutes of Arrival[5]	-	-	61%	54%	95%
Smoking Cessation Advice[5]	-	-	92%	88%	100%
Heart Failure Care					
ACE Inhibitor or ARB for LVSD[1,3]	7	100%	84%	82%	100%
Discharge Instructions[1,3]	5	100%	62%	61%	93%
Evaluation of LVS Function[1,3]	13	62%	79%	83%	99%
Smoking Cessation Advice[1,3]	3	0%	80%	82%	100%
Pneumonia Care					
Appropriate Initial Antibiotic[1,3]	11	73%	81%	83%	94%
Blood Culture Timing[3]	0	-	92%	90%	100%
Influenza Vaccine[5]	-	-	70%	70%	100%
Initial Antibiotic Timing[1,3]	2	50%	81%	80%	93%
Oxygenation Assessment[1,3]	13	100%	99%	99%	100%
Pneumococcal Vaccine[1,3]	8	62%	70%	69%	94%
Smoking Cessation Advice[1,3]	3	100%	83%	80%	100%
Surgical Infection Prevention					
Prophylactic Antibiotic Given[5]	-	-	78%	77%	95%
Prophylactic Antibiotic Selection[5]	-	-	91%	90%	100%
Prophylactic Antibiotic Stopped[5]	-	-	72%	72%	95%
Pregnancy Care					
Inpatient Neonatal Mortality	-	-	-	-	-
Third or Fourth Degree Laceration	-	-	-	3.63%	3.27%

Audrain Medical Center

620 E Monroe
Mexico, MO 65265
URL: www.audrainmedicalcenter.com
Ownership: Voluntary non-profit - Private
Emergency Services: Yes
Phone: 573-582-5000
Fax: 573-582-3700
Accredited: Yes
Licensed Beds: 107
Key Personnel:
President/CEO. . . . . David Neuendorf

Measure	Cases	This Hospital	State Average	U.S. Average	Top Hospital
Heart Attack Care					
ACE Inhibitor or ARB for LVSD[1,2]	10	100%	76%	82%	100%
Aspirin at Arrival[2]	50	100%	92%	92%	100%
Aspirin at Discharge[2]	49	100%	87%	90%	100%
Beta Blocker at Arrival[2]	33	100%	83%	87%	100%
Beta Blocker at Discharge[2]	48	100%	87%	90%	100%
Fibrinolytic Medication Timing[1,2]	1	0%	26%	31%	100%
PCI Within 90 Minutes of Arrival[1,2]	3	67%	61%	54%	95%
Smoking Cessation Advice[1,2]	20	100%	92%	88%	100%
Heart Failure Care					
ACE Inhibitor or ARB for LVSD	78	96%	84%	82%	100%
Discharge Instructions	148	90%	62%	61%	93%
Evaluation of LVS Function	196	97%	79%	83%	99%
Smoking Cessation Advice[1]	19	89%	80%	82%	100%
Pneumonia Care					
Appropriate Initial Antibiotic[2]	97	88%	81%	83%	94%
Blood Culture Timing[2]	126	97%	92%	90%	100%
Influenza Vaccine	34	94%	70%	70%	100%
Initial Antibiotic Timing[2]	154	95%	81%	80%	93%
Oxygenation Assessment[2]	195	100%	99%	99%	100%
Pneumococcal Vaccine[2]	118	97%	70%	69%	94%
Smoking Cessation Advice[2]	50	96%	83%	80%	100%
Surgical Infection Prevention					
Prophylactic Antibiotic Given	193	92%	78%	77%	95%
Prophylactic Antibiotic Selection	68	97%	91%	90%	100%
Prophylactic Antibiotic Stopped	189	75%	72%	72%	95%
Pregnancy Care					
Inpatient Neonatal Mortality	-	-	-	-	-
Third or Fourth Degree Laceration	-	-	-	3.63%	3.27%

Sullivan County Memorial Hospital

Alternate Name: SCMH
630 W 3rd Street
Milan, MO 63556
Ownership: Government - Local
Emergency Services: No
Phone: 660-265-4212
Fax: 660-265-3609
Accredited: No
Licensed Beds: 39
Key Personnel:
CEO. . . . . Martha Gragg
Chief Medical Staff. . . . . Tom Williams
Emergency Room . . . . Lisa Stafford, RN
Infection Control. . . . . Kim Ray, RN
Med Surg Nursing/Director Pat Clin Serv . . . . . . Carol Foldyce, CRN
Manager Cardiac Rehabilitation/Pulmonary . . . . Dixie Cooley, CRN

NOTE: Hospital profiles are in alphabetical order by state, then city, then hospital within the city; Rankings are sorted by rate in descending order and exclude hospitals with less than 25 cases; (1) The number of cases is too small (n<25) for purposes of reliably predicting hospital performance; (2) Measure reflects the hospital's indication that its submission was based upon a sample of its relevant discharges; (3) Rate reflects fewer than the maximum possible quarters of data for the measure; (4) Inaccurate information submitted and suppressed for one or more quarters; (5) No data is available from the hospital for this measure; Please refer to the User's Guide for a full explanation of data

Measure	Cases	This Hospital	State Average	U.S. Average	Top Hospital
Heart Attack Care					
ACE Inhibitor or ARB for LVSD[3]	0	-	76%	82%	100%
Aspirin at Arrival[3]	0	-	92%	92%	100%
Aspirin at Discharge[3]	0	-	87%	90%	100%
Beta Blocker at Arrival[3]	0	-	83%	87%	100%
Beta Blocker at Discharge[3]	0	-	87%	90%	100%
Fibrinolytic Medication Timing[1,3]	1	0%	26%	31%	100%
PCI Within 90 Minutes of Arrival[5]	-	-	61%	54%	95%
Smoking Cessation Advice[3]	0	-	92%	88%	100%
Heart Failure Care					
ACE Inhibitor or ARB for LVSD	0	-	84%	82%	100%
Discharge Instructions[1]	11	0%	62%	61%	93%
Evaluation of LVS Function[1]	9	11%	79%	83%	99%
Smoking Cessation Advice	0	-	80%	82%	100%
Pneumonia Care					
Appropriate Initial Antibiotic[1,3]	14	79%	81%	83%	94%
Blood Culture Timing[3]	0	-	92%	90%	100%
Influenza Vaccine[1]	2	50%	70%	70%	100%
Initial Antibiotic Timing[1,3]	20	90%	81%	80%	93%
Oxygenation Assessment[3]	26	100%	99%	99%	100%
Pneumococcal Vaccine[1,3]	16	25%	70%	69%	94%
Smoking Cessation Advice[1,3]	5	60%	83%	80%	100%
Surgical Infection Prevention					
Prophylactic Antibiotic Given[5]	-	-	78%	77%	95%
Prophylactic Antibiotic Selection[5]	-	-	91%	90%	100%
Prophylactic Antibiotic Stopped[5]	-	-	72%	72%	95%
Pregnancy Care					
Inpatient Neonatal Mortality	-	-	-	-	-
Third or Fourth Degree Laceration	-	-	-	3.63%	3.27%

Moberly Regional Medical Center

1515 Union Avenue
Moberly, MO 65270
URL: www.moberlyhospital.com
Ownership: Proprietary
Emergency Services: Yes
Phone: 660-263-8400
Fax: 660-269-3091
Accredited: Yes
Licensed Beds: 114

Key Personnel:

Interim CEO. . . . . Jay Hodges
Chief Medical Staff. . . . . Ahmed Habib, MD
Director Cardiology . . . . Ahmed Habib, MD
Infection Control. . . . . Roanetta Bodgers
Director Medical Surgical Nursing . . . . Ann Wadle, RN
Director OB/GYN Womens Health . . . . Sally Walker, RN
Director Radiology . . . . Donald Sanders
Director of Pulmonary . . . . Chuck Johnson

Measure	Cases	This Hospital	State Average	U.S. Average	Top Hospital
Heart Attack Care					
ACE Inhibitor or ARB for LVSD[1]	4	100%	76%	82%	100%
Aspirin at Arrival[1]	21	100%	92%	92%	100%
Aspirin at Discharge[1]	14	100%	87%	90%	100%
Beta Blocker at Arrival[1]	17	88%	83%	87%	100%
Beta Blocker at Discharge[1]	17	100%	87%	90%	100%
Fibrinolytic Medication Timing	0	-	26%	31%	100%
PCI Within 90 Minutes of Arrival	0	-	61%	54%	95%
Smoking Cessation Advice[1]	6	83%	92%	88%	100%
Heart Failure Care					
ACE Inhibitor or ARB for LVSD	27	100%	84%	82%	100%
Discharge Instructions	62	85%	62%	61%	93%
Evaluation of LVS Function	101	94%	79%	83%	99%
Smoking Cessation Advice[1]	18	100%	80%	82%	100%
Pneumonia Care					
Appropriate Initial Antibiotic	98	84%	81%	83%	94%
Blood Culture Timing	85	93%	92%	90%	100%
Influenza Vaccine	32	75%	70%	70%	100%
Initial Antibiotic Timing	144	90%	81%	80%	93%
Oxygenation Assessment	189	100%	99%	99%	100%
Pneumococcal Vaccine	124	82%	70%	69%	94%
Smoking Cessation Advice	39	97%	83%	80%	100%
Surgical Infection Prevention					
Prophylactic Antibiotic Given[2,3]	53	57%	78%	77%	95%
Prophylactic Antibiotic Selection[1,2]	22	95%	91%	90%	100%
Prophylactic Antibiotic Stopped[2,3]	51	96%	72%	72%	95%
Pregnancy Care					
Inpatient Neonatal Mortality	-	-	-	-	-
Third or Fourth Degree Laceration	-	-	-	3.63%	3.27%

Cox Monett Hospital

Alternate Name: Saint Vincent's Hospital
801 Lincoln Avenue
Monett, MO 65708
Ownership: Voluntary non-profit - Private
Emergency Services: Yes
Phone: 417-235-3144
Fax: 417-354-1412
Accredited: No
Licensed Beds: 78

Key Personnel:

CEO. . . . . Gregory Johnson
Chief of Medical Staff. . . . . Amber Ecomomu, MD
Director Emergency Room. . . . . Dennis Hughs, MD

Measure	Cases	This Hospital	State Average	U.S. Average	Top Hospital
Heart Attack Care					
ACE Inhibitor or ARB for LVSD[1,2,3]	1	0%	76%	82%	100%
Aspirin at Arrival[1,2,3]	4	50%	92%	92%	100%
Aspirin at Discharge[1,2,3]	2	50%	87%	90%	100%
Beta Blocker at Arrival[1,2,3]	5	60%	83%	87%	100%
Beta Blocker at Discharge[1,2,3]	3	100%	87%	90%	100%
Fibrinolytic Medication Timing[2,3]	0	-	26%	31%	100%
PCI Within 90 Minutes of Arrival[2]	0	-	61%	54%	95%
Smoking Cessation Advice[2,3]	0	-	92%	88%	100%
Heart Failure Care					
ACE Inhibitor or ARB for LVSD[1,2]	8	75%	84%	82%	100%
Discharge Instructions[1,2]	23	65%	62%	61%	93%
Evaluation of LVS Function[2]	36	42%	79%	83%	99%
Smoking Cessation Advice[1,2]	7	14%	80%	82%	100%
Pneumonia Care					
Appropriate Initial Antibiotic[2]	56	66%	81%	83%	94%
Blood Culture Timing[2]	43	91%	92%	90%	100%
Influenza Vaccine[4,5]	-	-	70%	70%	100%
Initial Antibiotic Timing[2]	64	70%	81%	80%	93%
Oxygenation Assessment[2]	76	100%	99%	99%	100%
Pneumococcal Vaccine[2]	43	63%	70%	69%	94%
Smoking Cessation Advice[1,2]	19	63%	83%	80%	100%
Surgical Infection Prevention					
Prophylactic Antibiotic Given[2]	78	76%	78%	77%	95%
Prophylactic Antibiotic Selection[1,2]	19	100%	91%	90%	100%
Prophylactic Antibiotic Stopped[2]	74	50%	72%	72%	95%
Pregnancy Care					
Inpatient Neonatal Mortality	-	-	-	-	-
Third or Fourth Degree Laceration	-	-	-	3.63%	3.27%

Saint Francis Hospital

100 W Highway 60
Mountain View, MO 65548
Ownership: Voluntary non-profit - Private
Emergency Services: No
Phone: 417-934-2246
Fax: 417-934-6024
Accredited: No
Licensed Beds: 42

Key Personnel:

President . . . . Don Swafford
Chief Medical Staff. . . . . Mohammed Tabibi, DO
Emergency Room . . . . Ernest L Carampatan, MD
Infection Control. . . . . Jill Mundt, MT ASCP
Medical Surgical Nursing . . . . Kurtis Abbey, RN
Respiratory/Cardiopulmonary. . . . . Pam Cygal, RRT

Measure	Cases	This Hospital	State Average	U.S. Average	Top Hospital
Heart Attack Care					
ACE Inhibitor or ARB for LVSD[3]	0	-	76%	82%	100%
Aspirin at Arrival[1,3]	1	100%	92%	92%	100%
Aspirin at Discharge[3]	0	-	87%	90%	100%
Beta Blocker at Arrival[3]	0	-	83%	87%	100%
Beta Blocker at Discharge[3]	0	-	87%	90%	100%
Fibrinolytic Medication Timing[3]	0	-	26%	31%	100%
PCI Within 90 Minutes of Arrival[5]	-	-	61%	54%	95%
Smoking Cessation Advice[3]	0	-	92%	88%	100%
Heart Failure Care					

NOTE: Hospital profiles are in alphabetical order by state, then city, then hospital within the city; Rankings are sorted by rate in descending order and exclude hospitals with less than 25 cases; (1) The number of cases is too small (n<25) for purposes of reliably predicting hospital performance; (2) Measure reflects the hospital's indication that its submission was based upon a sample of its relevant discharges; (3) Rate reflects fewer than the maximum possible quarters of data for the measure; (4) Inaccurate information submitted and suppressed for one or more quarters; (5) No data is available from the hospital for this measure; Please refer to the User's Guide for a full explanation of data

Measure	Cases	This Hospital	State Average	U.S. Average	Top Hospital
ACE Inhibitor or ARB for LVSD[1,2]	2	100%	84%	82%	100%
Discharge Instructions[1,2]	10	50%	62%	61%	93%
Evaluation of LVS Function[2]	25	60%	79%	83%	99%
Smoking Cessation Advice[1,2]	2	50%	80%	82%	100%
Pneumonia Care					
Appropriate Initial Antibiotic[2]	33	97%	81%	83%	94%
Blood Culture Timing[2]	36	94%	92%	90%	100%
Influenza Vaccine[1]	16	88%	70%	70%	100%
Initial Antibiotic Timing[2]	57	81%	81%	80%	93%
Oxygenation Assessment[2]	74	100%	99%	99%	100%
Pneumococcal Vaccine[2]	54	74%	70%	69%	94%
Smoking Cessation Advice[1,2]	12	67%	83%	80%	100%
Surgical Infection Prevention					
Prophylactic Antibiotic Given[5]	-	-	78%	77%	95%
Prophylactic Antibiotic Selection[5]	-	-	91%	90%	100%
Prophylactic Antibiotic Stopped[5]	-	-	72%	72%	95%
Pregnancy Care					
Inpatient Neonatal Mortality	-	-	-	-	-
Third or Fourth Degree Laceration	-	-	-	3.63%	3.27%

Freeman Neosho Hospital

113 W Hickory
Neosho, MO 64850
URL: www.freemanhealth.com
Ownership: Voluntary non-profit - Private
Emergency Services: Yes
Phone: 417-451-1234
Fax: 417-347-3716
Accredited: No
Licensed Beds: 67

Key Personnel:

President/CEO . . . . Gary Duncan

Measure	Cases	This Hospital	State Average	U.S. Average	Top Hospital
Heart Attack Care					
ACE Inhibitor or ARB for LVSD[1]	1	100%	76%	82%	100%
Aspirin at Arrival[1]	12	100%	92%	92%	100%
Aspirin at Discharge[1]	6	100%	87%	90%	100%
Beta Blocker at Arrival[1]	6	100%	83%	87%	100%
Beta Blocker at Discharge[1]	6	100%	87%	90%	100%
Fibrinolytic Medication Timing	0	-	26%	31%	100%
PCI Within 90 Minutes of Arrival	0	-	61%	54%	95%
Smoking Cessation Advice	0	-	92%	88%	100%
Heart Failure Care					
ACE Inhibitor or ARB for LVSD[1]	15	100%	84%	82%	100%
Discharge Instructions	27	96%	62%	61%	93%
Evaluation of LVS Function	42	95%	79%	83%	99%
Smoking Cessation Advice[1]	6	100%	80%	82%	100%
Pneumonia Care					
Appropriate Initial Antibiotic	73	97%	81%	83%	94%
Blood Culture Timing	84	99%	92%	90%	100%
Influenza Vaccine	26	100%	70%	70%	100%
Initial Antibiotic Timing	112	100%	81%	80%	93%
Oxygenation Assessment	128	100%	99%	99%	100%
Pneumococcal Vaccine	76	100%	70%	69%	94%
Smoking Cessation Advice	36	100%	83%	80%	100%
Surgical Infection Prevention					
Prophylactic Antibiotic Given[5]	-	-	78%	77%	95%
Prophylactic Antibiotic Selection[5]	-	-	91%	90%	100%
Prophylactic Antibiotic Stopped[5]	-	-	72%	72%	95%
Pregnancy Care					
Inpatient Neonatal Mortality	-	-	-	-	-
Third or Fourth Degree Laceration	-	-	-	3.63%	3.27%

Nevada Regional Medical Center

Alternate Name: Nevada City Hospital
800 South Ash Street
Nevada, MO 64772
URL: www.nrmchealth.com
Ownership: Government - Local
Emergency Services: Yes
Phone: 417-667-3355
Fax: 417-448-3848
Accredited: Yes
Licensed Beds: 53

Key Personnel:

President/CEO . . . . Judy Feuquay
Emergency Room . . . . Holly Busher, RN
Same Day Surgery . . . . Joy Jefferies

Measure	Cases	This Hospital	State Average	U.S. Average	Top Hospital
Heart Attack Care					
ACE Inhibitor or ARB for LVSD[1,2,3]	2	100%	76%	82%	100%
Aspirin at Arrival[1,2,3]	6	83%	92%	92%	100%
Aspirin at Discharge[1,2,3]	6	83%	87%	90%	100%
Beta Blocker at Arrival[1,2,3]	3	67%	83%	87%	100%
Beta Blocker at Discharge[1,2,3]	6	100%	87%	90%	100%
Fibrinolytic Medication Timing[2,3]	0	-	26%	31%	100%
PCI Within 90 Minutes of Arrival[2]	0	-	61%	54%	95%
Smoking Cessation Advice[1,2,3]	1	100%	92%	88%	100%
Heart Failure Care					
ACE Inhibitor or ARB for LVSD[1,2]	10	80%	84%	82%	100%
Discharge Instructions[2]	34	56%	62%	61%	93%
Evaluation of LVS Function[2]	40	82%	79%	83%	99%
Smoking Cessation Advice[1,2]	5	80%	80%	82%	100%
Pneumonia Care					
Appropriate Initial Antibiotic[2]	32	75%	81%	83%	94%
Blood Culture Timing[2]	36	94%	92%	90%	100%
Influenza Vaccine[1]	11	100%	70%	70%	100%
Initial Antibiotic Timing[2]	55	96%	81%	80%	93%
Oxygenation Assessment[2]	69	100%	99%	99%	100%
Pneumococcal Vaccine[2]	42	86%	70%	69%	94%
Smoking Cessation Advice[1,2]	14	100%	83%	80%	100%
Surgical Infection Prevention					
Prophylactic Antibiotic Given[2]	81	86%	78%	77%	95%
Prophylactic Antibiotic Selection[1,2]	18	83%	91%	90%	100%
Prophylactic Antibiotic Stopped[2]	79	52%	72%	72%	95%
Pregnancy Care					
Inpatient Neonatal Mortality	-	-	-	-	-
Third or Fourth Degree Laceration	-	-	-	3.63%	3.27%

North Kansas City Hospital

2800 Clay Edwards Drive
North Kansas City, MO 64116
URL: www.nkch.org
Ownership: Government - Local
Emergency Services: Yes
Phone: 816-691-2000
Fax: 816-346-7020
Accredited: Yes
Licensed Beds: 351

Key Personnel:

President/CEO . . . . David Carpenter
Chief Medical Staff . . . . Leslie Thomas, MD
Emergency Room Manager . . . . Cathy Menninga
VP . . . . Marion Cunningham

Measure	Cases	This Hospital	State Average	U.S. Average	Top Hospital
Heart Attack Care					
ACE Inhibitor or ARB for LVSD	122	91%	76%	82%	100%
Aspirin at Arrival	234	97%	92%	92%	100%
Aspirin at Discharge	303	100%	87%	90%	100%
Beta Blocker at Arrival	209	98%	83%	87%	100%
Beta Blocker at Discharge	319	100%	87%	90%	100%
Fibrinolytic Medication Timing	0	-	26%	31%	100%
PCI Within 90 Minutes of Arrival[1]	21	76%	61%	54%	95%
Smoking Cessation Advice	134	98%	92%	88%	100%
Heart Failure Care					
ACE Inhibitor or ARB for LVSD	134	87%	84%	82%	100%
Discharge Instructions	299	60%	62%	61%	93%
Evaluation of LVS Function	343	97%	79%	83%	99%
Smoking Cessation Advice	59	88%	80%	82%	100%
Pneumonia Care					
Appropriate Initial Antibiotic	200	68%	81%	83%	94%
Blood Culture Timing	126	83%	92%	90%	100%
Influenza Vaccine	43	51%	70%	70%	100%
Initial Antibiotic Timing	265	80%	81%	80%	93%
Oxygenation Assessment	322	99%	99%	99%	100%
Pneumococcal Vaccine	193	75%	70%	69%	94%
Smoking Cessation Advice	77	82%	83%	80%	100%
Surgical Infection Prevention					
Prophylactic Antibiotic Given[3]	480	69%	78%	77%	95%
Prophylactic Antibiotic Selection	125	97%	91%	90%	100%
Prophylactic Antibiotic Stopped[3]	469	74%	72%	72%	95%
Pregnancy Care					
Inpatient Neonatal Mortality	-	-	-	-	-

NOTE: Hospital profiles are in alphabetical order by state, then city, then hospital within the city; Rankings are sorted by rate in descending order and exclude hospitals with less than 25 cases; (1) The number of cases is too small (n<25) for purposes of reliably predicting hospital performance; (2) Measure reflects the hospital's indication that its submission was based upon a sample of its relevant discharges; (3) Rate reflects fewer than the maximum possible quarters of data for the measure; (4) Inaccurate information submitted and suppressed for one or more quarters; (5) No data is available from the hospital for this measure; Please refer to the User's Guide for a full explanation of data

Third or Fourth Degree Laceration	-	-	-	3.63%	3.27%

Lake Regional Health Systems

54 Hospital Drive
Osage Beach, MO 65065
E-mail: dwakeford@socket.net
URL: www.lakeregional.com
Phone: 573-348-8000
Fax: 573-348-8268
Ownership: Voluntary non-profit - Other
Emergency Services: Yes
Accredited: Yes
Licensed Beds: 140

Key Personnel:

Administrator/CEO . . . . Michael E Henze
Chief Medical Staff. . . . . Grant Barnum, MD
Director of Cardiology/Cardiac Lab. . . . . Tonnie Rugen
Emergency Room Director. . . . . Mellisa Hunter
Chief Radiology . . . . Steve Groteweil
Director Respiratory Therapy . . . . Scott Steinmetz

Measure	Cases	This Hospital	State Average	U.S. Average	Top Hospital
Heart Attack Care					
ACE Inhibitor or ARB for LVSD	43	84%	76%	82%	100%
Aspirin at Arrival	178	95%	92%	92%	100%
Aspirin at Discharge	164	96%	87%	90%	100%
Beta Blocker at Arrival	133	82%	83%	87%	100%
Beta Blocker at Discharge	161	90%	87%	90%	100%
Fibrinolytic Medication Timing	0	-	26%	31%	100%
PCI Within 90 Minutes of Arrival[1]	8	62%	61%	54%	95%
Smoking Cessation Advice	70	99%	92%	88%	100%
Heart Failure Care					
ACE Inhibitor or ARB for LVSD	81	79%	84%	82%	100%
Discharge Instructions	189	86%	62%	61%	93%
Evaluation of LVS Function	224	77%	79%	83%	99%
Smoking Cessation Advice	38	89%	80%	82%	100%
Pneumonia Care					
Appropriate Initial Antibiotic	160	89%	81%	83%	94%
Blood Culture Timing	131	92%	92%	90%	100%
Influenza Vaccine	44	95%	70%	70%	100%
Initial Antibiotic Timing	196	91%	81%	80%	93%
Oxygenation Assessment	231	100%	99%	99%	100%
Pneumococcal Vaccine	145	83%	70%	69%	94%
Smoking Cessation Advice	66	89%	83%	80%	100%
Surgical Infection Prevention					
Prophylactic Antibiotic Given[3]	247	76%	78%	77%	95%
Prophylactic Antibiotic Selection	88	77%	91%	90%	100%
Prophylactic Antibiotic Stopped[3]	246	61%	72%	72%	95%
Pregnancy Care					
Inpatient Neonatal Mortality	-	-	-	-	-
Third or Fourth Degree Laceration	-	-	-	3.63%	3.27%

Sac-Osage Hospital

PO Box 426
Osceola, MO 64776
Phone: 417-646-8181
Fax: 417-646-8416
Ownership: Govt - Hospital District or Authority
Emergency Services: No
Accredited: No
Licensed Beds: 47

Key Personnel:

Chief of Medical Staff. Wayne L. Morton, MD
Director Respiratory . . . . Tracy Fletcher

Measure	Cases	This Hospital	State Average	U.S. Average	Top Hospital
Heart Attack Care					
ACE Inhibitor or ARB for LVSD[3]	0	-	76%	82%	100%
Aspirin at Arrival[1,3]	3	100%	92%	92%	100%
Aspirin at Discharge[1,3]	2	50%	87%	90%	100%
Beta Blocker at Arrival[1,3]	3	33%	83%	87%	100%
Beta Blocker at Discharge[1,3]	2	50%	87%	90%	100%
Fibrinolytic Medication Timing[3]	0	-	26%	31%	100%
PCI Within 90 Minutes of Arrival[5]	-	-	61%	54%	95%
Smoking Cessation Advice[1,3]	1	0%	92%	88%	100%
Heart Failure Care					
ACE Inhibitor or ARB for LVSD	0	-	84%	82%	100%
Discharge Instructions	30	0%	62%	61%	93%
Evaluation of LVS Function	38	0%	79%	83%	99%
Smoking Cessation Advice[1]	12	17%	80%	82%	100%
Pneumonia Care					
Appropriate Initial Antibiotic	43	51%	81%	83%	94%
Blood Culture Timing[1]	8	100%	92%	90%	100%
Influenza Vaccine[1]	7	29%	70%	70%	100%
Initial Antibiotic Timing	39	59%	81%	80%	93%
Oxygenation Assessment	44	80%	99%	99%	100%
Pneumococcal Vaccine	28	32%	70%	69%	94%
Smoking Cessation Advice[1]	15	27%	83%	80%	100%
Surgical Infection Prevention					
Prophylactic Antibiotic Given[5]	-	-	78%	77%	95%
Prophylactic Antibiotic Selection[5]	-	-	91%	90%	100%
Prophylactic Antibiotic Stopped[5]	-	-	72%	72%	95%
Pregnancy Care					
Inpatient Neonatal Mortality	-	-	-	-	-
Third or Fourth Degree Laceration	-	-	-	3.63%	3.27%

Perry County Memorial Hospital

Alternate Name: Perry County Health System
434 N West Street
Perryville, MO 63775
URL: www.pchmo.org
Phone: 573-547-2536
Fax: 573-547-3776
Ownership: Government - Local
Emergency Services: Yes
Accredited: Yes
Licensed Beds: 51

Key Personnel:

President/CEO. . . . . Patrick Carron
Chief Medical Staff. . . . . Mohammad Moaddabi
Emergency Room . . . . Barb Ernst
Infection Control Nurse. . . . . Katie Godsey
OB/GYN/Women's Health . . . . Tanya Mero, MD
Director Radiology . . . . Christopher Wibbenmeyer
Director Pulmonary Therapy . . . . Cheryl Westrich

Measure	Cases	This Hospital	State Average	U.S. Average	Top Hospital
Heart Attack Care					
ACE Inhibitor or ARB for LVSD[3]	0	-	76%	82%	100%
Aspirin at Arrival[1,3]	3	67%	92%	92%	100%
Aspirin at Discharge[1,3]	2	50%	87%	90%	100%
Beta Blocker at Arrival[1,3]	3	100%	83%	87%	100%
Beta Blocker at Discharge[1,3]	2	100%	87%	90%	100%
Fibrinolytic Medication Timing[3]	0	-	26%	31%	100%
PCI Within 90 Minutes of Arrival[5]	-	-	61%	54%	95%
Smoking Cessation Advice[3]	0	-	92%	88%	100%
Heart Failure Care					
ACE Inhibitor or ARB for LVSD[1,2]	2	100%	84%	82%	100%
Discharge Instructions[1,2]	9	100%	62%	61%	93%
Evaluation of LVS Function[1,2]	18	89%	79%	83%	99%
Smoking Cessation Advice[1,2]	5	100%	80%	82%	100%
Pneumonia Care					
Appropriate Initial Antibiotic[2]	26	92%	81%	83%	94%
Blood Culture Timing[1,2]	22	86%	92%	90%	100%
Influenza Vaccine[1]	7	100%	70%	70%	100%
Initial Antibiotic Timing[2]	33	88%	81%	80%	93%
Oxygenation Assessment[2]	45	100%	99%	99%	100%
Pneumococcal Vaccine[2]	38	97%	70%	69%	94%
Smoking Cessation Advice[1,2]	8	88%	83%	80%	100%
Surgical Infection Prevention					
Prophylactic Antibiotic Given[1,2]	11	82%	78%	77%	95%
Prophylactic Antibiotic Selection[1,2]	3	100%	91%	90%	100%
Prophylactic Antibiotic Stopped[1,2]	11	91%	72%	72%	95%
Pregnancy Care					
Inpatient Neonatal Mortality	144	0.00%	-	-	-
Third or Fourth Degree Laceration	118	5.08%	-	3.63%	3.27%

Poplar Bluff Regional Medical Center

2620 N Westwood Boulevard
Poplar Bluff, MO 63901
E-mail: info@pbrmc.hma-corp.com
URL: www.poplarbluffregional.com
Phone: 573-785-7721
Fax: 573-686-5388
Ownership: Voluntary non-profit - Private
Emergency Services: Yes
Accredited: Yes
Licensed Beds: 423

Key Personnel:

CEO. . . . . Bruce Eady

NOTE: Hospital profiles are in alphabetical order by state, then city, then hospital within the city; Rankings are sorted by rate in descending order and exclude hospitals with less than 25 cases; (1) The number of cases is too small (n<25) for purposes of reliably predicting hospital performance; (2) Measure reflects the hospital's indication that its submission was based upon a sample of its relevant discharges; (3) Rate reflects fewer than the maximum possible quarters of data for the measure; (4) Inaccurate information submitted and suppressed for one or more quarters; (5) No data is available from the hospital for this measure; Please refer to the User's Guide for a full explanation of data

Measure	Cases	This Hospital	State Average	U.S. Average	Top Hospital
Heart Attack Care					
ACE Inhibitor or ARB for LVSD[1]	15	53%	76%	82%	100%
Aspirin at Arrival	95	94%	92%	92%	100%
Aspirin at Discharge	98	83%	87%	90%	100%
Beta Blocker at Arrival	96	89%	83%	87%	100%
Beta Blocker at Discharge	100	82%	87%	90%	100%
Fibrinolytic Medication Timing[1]	11	9%	26%	31%	100%
PCI Within 90 Minutes of Arrival[1]	2	50%	61%	54%	95%
Smoking Cessation Advice	52	90%	92%	88%	100%
Heart Failure Care					
ACE Inhibitor or ARB for LVSD	119	62%	84%	82%	100%
Discharge Instructions	252	62%	62%	61%	93%
Evaluation of LVS Function	308	92%	79%	83%	99%
Smoking Cessation Advice	65	86%	80%	82%	100%
Pneumonia Care					
Appropriate Initial Antibiotic[2]	261	68%	81%	83%	94%
Blood Culture Timing[2]	171	92%	92%	90%	100%
Influenza Vaccine	61	57%	70%	70%	100%
Initial Antibiotic Timing[2]	281	67%	81%	80%	93%
Oxygenation Assessment[2]	383	99%	99%	99%	100%
Pneumococcal Vaccine[2]	243	51%	70%	69%	94%
Smoking Cessation Advice[2]	102	75%	83%	80%	100%
Surgical Infection Prevention					
Prophylactic Antibiotic Given[2]	597	69%	78%	77%	95%
Prophylactic Antibiotic Selection[2]	102	82%	91%	90%	100%
Prophylactic Antibiotic Stopped[2]	577	57%	72%	72%	95%
Pregnancy Care					
Inpatient Neonatal Mortality	-	-	-	-	-
Third or Fourth Degree Laceration	-	-	-	3.63%	3.27%

Washington County Memorial Hospital

300 Health Way
Potosi, MO 63664
E-mail: wcmhadm@mail.potosi.k12.mo.us
URL: www.wcmhosp.org
Phone: 573-438-5451
Fax: 573-438-2399
Ownership: Government - Local
Emergency Services: Yes
Accredited: No
Licensed Beds: 42

Key Personnel:
CEO. . . . . H Clark Duncan
Chief Medical Staff. . . . . Frezerick Fyat, Dr
Head of Emergency Room. . . . . A Minichuck

Measure	Cases	This Hospital	State Average	U.S. Average	Top Hospital
Heart Attack Care					
ACE Inhibitor or ARB for LVSD[2,3]	0	-	76%	82%	100%
Aspirin at Arrival[1,2,3]	5	80%	92%	92%	100%
Aspirin at Discharge[1,2,3]	4	75%	87%	90%	100%
Beta Blocker at Arrival[1,2,3]	5	60%	83%	87%	100%
Beta Blocker at Discharge[1,2,3]	4	50%	87%	90%	100%
Fibrinolytic Medication Timing[2,3]	0	-	26%	31%	100%
PCI Within 90 Minutes of Arrival[2]	0	-	61%	54%	95%
Smoking Cessation Advice[2,3]	0	-	92%	88%	100%
Heart Failure Care					
ACE Inhibitor or ARB for LVSD[1,2]	1	100%	84%	82%	100%
Discharge Instructions[1,2]	16	19%	62%	61%	93%
Evaluation of LVS Function[1,2]	20	30%	79%	83%	99%
Smoking Cessation Advice[1,2]	1	100%	80%	82%	100%
Pneumonia Care					
Appropriate Initial Antibiotic[2]	68	88%	81%	83%	94%
Blood Culture Timing[2]	55	82%	92%	90%	100%
Influenza Vaccine[1]	11	55%	70%	70%	100%
Initial Antibiotic Timing[2]	79	87%	81%	80%	93%
Oxygenation Assessment[2]	100	100%	99%	99%	100%
Pneumococcal Vaccine[2]	50	54%	70%	69%	94%
Smoking Cessation Advice[2]	26	58%	83%	80%	100%
Surgical Infection Prevention					
Prophylactic Antibiotic Given[5]	-	-	78%	77%	95%
Prophylactic Antibiotic Selection[5]	-	-	91%	90%	100%
Prophylactic Antibiotic Stopped[5]	-	-	72%	72%	95%
Pregnancy Care					
Inpatient Neonatal Mortality	-	-	-	-	-
Third or Fourth Degree Laceration	-	-	-	3.63%	3.27%

Ray County Memorial Hospital

904 Wollard Boulevard
Richmond, MO 64085
Phone: 816-470-5432
Fax: 816-470-8382
Ownership: Government - Local
Emergency Services: No
Accredited: No
Licensed Beds: 63

Key Personnel:
Administrator . . . . Tommy Hicks
CNO. . . . . Donna Lamar, RN
Chief Medical Staff. . . . . Daniel M Rosak, MD
Coordinator Infection Control . . . . Jackie Devaul, RN
Manager Radiology . . . . Jenny Riey
Director Respiratory Therapy . . . . Paul Hayes

Measure	Cases	This Hospital	State Average	U.S. Average	Top Hospital
Heart Attack Care					
ACE Inhibitor or ARB for LVSD[3]	0	-	76%	82%	100%
Aspirin at Arrival[1,3]	2	0%	92%	92%	100%
Aspirin at Discharge[1,3]	2	50%	87%	90%	100%
Beta Blocker at Arrival[1,3]	3	33%	83%	87%	100%
Beta Blocker at Discharge[1,3]	2	50%	87%	90%	100%
Fibrinolytic Medication Timing[1,3]	1	0%	26%	31%	100%
PCI Within 90 Minutes of Arrival	0	-	61%	54%	95%
Smoking Cessation Advice[3]	0	-	92%	88%	100%
Heart Failure Care					
ACE Inhibitor or ARB for LVSD[1]	6	83%	84%	82%	100%
Discharge Instructions	31	19%	62%	61%	93%
Evaluation of LVS Function	55	36%	79%	83%	99%
Smoking Cessation Advice[1]	2	50%	80%	82%	100%
Pneumonia Care					
Appropriate Initial Antibiotic	32	66%	81%	83%	94%
Blood Culture Timing[1]	7	100%	92%	90%	100%
Influenza Vaccine[1]	8	62%	70%	70%	100%
Initial Antibiotic Timing	33	48%	81%	80%	93%
Oxygenation Assessment	41	98%	99%	99%	100%
Pneumococcal Vaccine[1]	24	42%	70%	69%	94%
Smoking Cessation Advice[1]	4	25%	83%	80%	100%
Surgical Infection Prevention					
Prophylactic Antibiotic Given[5]	-	-	78%	77%	95%
Prophylactic Antibiotic Selection[5]	-	-	91%	90%	100%
Prophylactic Antibiotic Stopped[5]	-	-	72%	72%	95%
Pregnancy Care					
Inpatient Neonatal Mortality	-	-	-	-	-
Third or Fourth Degree Laceration	-	-	-	3.63%	3.27%

Saint Mary's Health Center

6420 Clayton Road
Saint Louis, MO 63117
Phone: 314-768-8000
Fax: 314-768-7131
Ownership: Voluntary non-profit - Church
Emergency Services: Yes
Accredited: Yes
Licensed Beds: 622

Key Personnel:
President/CEO. . . . . Susan Scholl
Director Infection/Disease Control . . . . Theresa Grattan
Director Respiratory Therapy . . . . Micheal Emerson

Measure	Cases	This Hospital	State Average	U.S. Average	Top Hospital
Heart Attack Care					
ACE Inhibitor or ARB for LVSD	52	92%	76%	82%	100%
Aspirin at Arrival	201	98%	92%	92%	100%
Aspirin at Discharge	257	98%	87%	90%	100%
Beta Blocker at Arrival	173	94%	83%	87%	100%
Beta Blocker at Discharge	264	96%	87%	90%	100%
Fibrinolytic Medication Timing	0	-	26%	31%	100%
PCI Within 90 Minutes of Arrival[1]	9	67%	61%	54%	95%
Smoking Cessation Advice	105	98%	92%	88%	100%
Heart Failure Care					
ACE Inhibitor or ARB for LVSD	250	92%	84%	82%	100%
Discharge Instructions	644	71%	62%	61%	93%
Evaluation of LVS Function	775	98%	79%	83%	99%
Smoking Cessation Advice	173	99%	80%	82%	100%

NOTE: Hospital profiles are in alphabetical order by state, then city, then hospital within the city; Rankings are sorted by rate in descending order and exclude hospitals with less than 25 cases; (1) The number of cases is too small (n<25) for purposes of reliably predicting hospital performance; (2) Measure reflects the hospital's indication that its submission was based upon a sample of its relevant discharges; (3) Rate reflects fewer than the maximum possible quarters of data for the measure; (4) Inaccurate information submitted and suppressed for one or more quarters; (5) No data is available from the hospital for this measure; Please refer to the User's Guide for a full explanation of data

Pneumonia Care					
Appropriate Initial Antibiotic	241	86%	81%	83%	94%
Blood Culture Timing	295	92%	92%	90%	100%
Influenza Vaccine	54	48%	70%	70%	100%
Initial Antibiotic Timing	349	72%	81%	80%	93%
Oxygenation Assessment	433	100%	99%	99%	100%
Pneumococcal Vaccine	262	78%	70%	69%	94%
Smoking Cessation Advice	115	97%	83%	80%	100%
Surgical Infection Prevention					
Prophylactic Antibiotic Given	1,024	94%	78%	77%	95%
Prophylactic Antibiotic Selection	253	94%	91%	90%	100%
Prophylactic Antibiotic Stopped	997	87%	72%	72%	95%
Pregnancy Care					
Inpatient Neonatal Mortality	-	-	-	-	-
Third or Fourth Degree Laceration	-	-	-	3.63%	3.27%

Phelps County Regional Medical Center

1000 W 10th Street
Rolla, MO 65401
Phone: 573-364-8899
Fax: 573-458-8413
E-mail: bharvey@rollanet.org
URL: www.rollanet.org/~pcrmc
Ownership: Government - Local
Emergency Services: Yes
Accredited: Yes
Licensed Beds: 232

Key Personnel:

CEO. . . . . David Ross
Director of Medical Staff. . . . . Jay Crump
Emergency Room . . . . . Adella Schultz
Emergency Room . . . . . Jeff Folhein
Director Medical/Surgical Nursing . . . . . Barbara Marcus, RN
OB/GYN Womens Health. . . . . Angela Buontempo, DO
Chief Radiology . . . . . A Riaz, MD
Director Respiratory Therapy . . . . . Gerard Kilroy

Measure	Cases	This Hospital	State Average	U.S. Average	Top Hospital
Heart Attack Care					
ACE Inhibitor or ARB for LVSD[1,2]	13	92%	76%	82%	100%
Aspirin at Arrival[2]	91	89%	92%	92%	100%
Aspirin at Discharge[2]	56	88%	87%	90%	100%
Beta Blocker at Arrival[2]	78	92%	83%	87%	100%
Beta Blocker at Discharge[2]	73	95%	87%	90%	100%
Fibrinolytic Medication Timing[2]	0	-	26%	31%	100%
PCI Within 90 Minutes of Arrival[2]	0	-	61%	54%	95%
Smoking Cessation Advice[1,2]	21	95%	92%	88%	100%
Heart Failure Care					
ACE Inhibitor or ARB for LVSD[2]	68	85%	84%	82%	100%
Discharge Instructions[2]	133	80%	62%	61%	93%
Evaluation of LVS Function[2]	187	94%	79%	83%	99%
Smoking Cessation Advice[2]	34	94%	80%	82%	100%
Pneumonia Care					
Appropriate Initial Antibiotic[2]	193	83%	81%	83%	94%
Blood Culture Timing[2]	175	80%	92%	90%	100%
Influenza Vaccine	47	68%	70%	70%	100%
Initial Antibiotic Timing[2]	266	79%	81%	80%	93%
Oxygenation Assessment[2]	284	100%	99%	99%	100%
Pneumococcal Vaccine[2]	175	77%	70%	69%	94%
Smoking Cessation Advice[2]	81	94%	83%	80%	100%
Surgical Infection Prevention					
Prophylactic Antibiotic Given[2,3]	106	83%	78%	77%	95%
Prophylactic Antibiotic Selection[2]	103	88%	91%	90%	100%
Prophylactic Antibiotic Stopped[2,3]	101	83%	72%	72%	95%
Pregnancy Care					
Inpatient Neonatal Mortality	-	-	-	-	-
Third or Fourth Degree Laceration	-	-	-	3.63%	3.27%

Saint Joseph Health Center-Saint Charles

Alternate Name: Saint Joseph Health Center
300 1st Capitol Drive
Saint Charles, MO 63301
Toll-Free: 800-835-1212
Phone: 636-947-5000
Fax: 636-947-5609
E-mail: mblamy@ssmhc.com
Ownership: Voluntary non-profit - Private
Emergency Services: Yes
Accredited: Yes
Licensed Beds: 342

Key Personnel:

CEO. . . . . Sherlyn Hailstone
Chief of Medical Staff. . . . . Fil Ferrigni, MD
Emergency Room Director. . . . . Alan Umbright
OB/GYN Womens Health. . . . . Scott Williams
Surgical Services . . . . . Joseph Seger
Chief Radiology . . . . . Lewis Halberson
Director Respiratory Therapy . . . . . Steven Conway

Measure	Cases	This Hospital	State Average	U.S. Average	Top Hospital
Heart Attack Care					
ACE Inhibitor or ARB for LVSD	134	89%	76%	82%	100%
Aspirin at Arrival	222	100%	92%	92%	100%
Aspirin at Discharge	351	99%	87%	90%	100%
Beta Blocker at Arrival	222	100%	83%	87%	100%
Beta Blocker at Discharge	368	99%	87%	90%	100%
Fibrinolytic Medication Timing[1]	5	60%	26%	31%	100%
PCI Within 90 Minutes of Arrival[1]	18	78%	61%	54%	95%
Smoking Cessation Advice	128	98%	92%	88%	100%
Heart Failure Care					
ACE Inhibitor or ARB for LVSD	134	85%	84%	82%	100%
Discharge Instructions	264	60%	62%	61%	93%
Evaluation of LVS Function	321	98%	79%	83%	99%
Smoking Cessation Advice	58	93%	80%	82%	100%
Pneumonia Care					
Appropriate Initial Antibiotic	156	83%	81%	83%	94%
Blood Culture Timing	203	90%	92%	90%	100%
Influenza Vaccine	60	52%	70%	70%	100%
Initial Antibiotic Timing	260	77%	81%	80%	93%
Oxygenation Assessment	336	100%	99%	99%	100%
Pneumococcal Vaccine	236	88%	70%	69%	94%
Smoking Cessation Advice	70	99%	83%	80%	100%
Surgical Infection Prevention					
Prophylactic Antibiotic Given	724	87%	78%	77%	95%
Prophylactic Antibiotic Selection	195	95%	91%	90%	100%
Prophylactic Antibiotic Stopped	701	92%	72%	72%	95%
Pregnancy Care					
Inpatient Neonatal Mortality	-	-	-	-	-
Third or Fourth Degree Laceration	-	-	-	3.63%	3.27%

Heartland Health

Alternate Name: Heartland Regional Medical Center
5325 Faraon Street
Saint Joseph, MO 64506
Phone: 816-271-6000
Fax: 816-271-6656
URL: www.heartland-health.com
Ownership: Voluntary non-profit - Other
Emergency Services: Yes
Accredited: Yes
Licensed Beds: 690

Key Personnel:

President/CEO. . . . . Lowell C Kruse
Chief Medical Officer . . . . . Dr Robert Permut, MD
Chief Catheterization Laboratory . . . . . Steven K Rowe, MD
Emergency Room . . . . . Raman J Patel, MD
Director Infection/Disease Control . . . . . Betty Shellenberder
CCU Spvg. Nurse . . . . . Susan Ide
Director Medical/Surgical Nursing . . . . . Lisa Michaelis
OB/GYN Womens Health. . . . . Robert L Corder, MD
Director Radiology . . . . . Cindy Wise
Director Respiratory Therapy . . . . . Don Hutchin

Measure	Cases	This Hospital	State Average	U.S. Average	Top Hospital
Heart Attack Care					
ACE Inhibitor or ARB for LVSD	84	88%	76%	82%	100%
Aspirin at Arrival	261	94%	92%	92%	100%
Aspirin at Discharge	261	98%	87%	90%	100%
Beta Blocker at Arrival	163	98%	83%	87%	100%
Beta Blocker at Discharge	318	97%	87%	90%	100%
Fibrinolytic Medication Timing[1]	2	0%	26%	31%	100%

NOTE: Hospital profiles are in alphabetical order by state, then city, then hospital within the city; Rankings are sorted by rate in descending order and exclude hospitals with less than 25 cases; (1) The number of cases is too small (n<25) for purposes of reliably predicting hospital performance; (2) Measure reflects the hospital's indication that its submission was based upon a sample of its relevant discharges; (3) Rate reflects fewer than the maximum possible quarters of data for the measure; (4) Inaccurate information submitted and suppressed for one or more quarters; (5) No data is available from the hospital for this measure; Please refer to the User's Guide for a full explanation of data

Measure	Cases	This Hospital	State Average	U.S. Average	Top Hospital
PCI Within 90 Minutes of Arrival[1]	8	62%	61%	54%	95%
Smoking Cessation Advice	125	98%	92%	88%	100%
Heart Failure Care					
ACE Inhibitor or ARB for LVSD	220	86%	84%	82%	100%
Discharge Instructions	469	85%	62%	61%	93%
Evaluation of LVS Function	569	96%	79%	83%	99%
Smoking Cessation Advice	89	99%	80%	82%	100%
Pneumonia Care					
Appropriate Initial Antibiotic	322	86%	81%	83%	94%
Blood Culture Timing	311	90%	92%	90%	100%
Influenza Vaccine	95	97%	70%	70%	100%
Initial Antibiotic Timing	412	80%	81%	80%	93%
Oxygenation Assessment	511	100%	99%	99%	100%
Pneumococcal Vaccine	318	91%	70%	69%	94%
Smoking Cessation Advice	159	97%	83%	80%	100%
Surgical Infection Prevention					
Prophylactic Antibiotic Given[2,3]	323	93%	78%	77%	95%
Prophylactic Antibiotic Selection[2]	250	95%	91%	90%	100%
Prophylactic Antibiotic Stopped[2,3]	312	87%	72%	72%	95%
Pregnancy Care					
Inpatient Neonatal Mortality	-	-	-	-	-
Third or Fourth Degree Laceration	-	-	-	3.63%	3.27%

Barnes-Jewish Hospital

One Barnes-Jewish Hospital Plaza
Saint Louis, MO 63110
Toll-Free: 800-451-4892
Phone: 314-747-3000
Fax: 314-362-3421
URL: www.barnesjewish.org
Ownership: Voluntary non-profit - Other
Accredited: Yes
Emergency Services: Yes
Licensed Beds: 1,371

Key Personnel:

President/CEO . . . . Ronald G Evens, MD
Chief Medical Staff . . . . Steve Miller, MD CMO
VP . . . . Lincoln Scott
OB/GYN Women's Health . . . . Judy Paull, RN
Director Radiology . . . . Gary Brink
Director Respiratory Therapy . . . . Darnetta Clinkscale

Measure	Cases	This Hospital	State Average	U.S. Average	Top Hospital
Heart Attack Care					
ACE Inhibitor or ARB for LVSD	180	90%	76%	82%	100%
Aspirin at Arrival	450	96%	92%	92%	100%
Aspirin at Discharge	624	99%	87%	90%	100%
Beta Blocker at Arrival	443	95%	83%	87%	100%
Beta Blocker at Discharge	689	96%	87%	90%	100%
Fibrinolytic Medication Timing[1]	16	69%	26%	31%	100%
PCI Within 90 Minutes of Arrival[1]	11	100%	61%	54%	95%
Smoking Cessation Advice	224	95%	92%	88%	100%
Heart Failure Care					
ACE Inhibitor or ARB for LVSD	430	92%	84%	82%	100%
Discharge Instructions	715	81%	62%	61%	93%
Evaluation of LVS Function	842	97%	79%	83%	99%
Smoking Cessation Advice	184	96%	80%	82%	100%
Pneumonia Care					
Appropriate Initial Antibiotic	237	80%	81%	83%	94%
Blood Culture Timing	208	86%	92%	90%	100%
Influenza Vaccine	56	61%	70%	70%	100%
Initial Antibiotic Timing	401	65%	81%	80%	93%
Oxygenation Assessment	459	100%	99%	99%	100%
Pneumococcal Vaccine	161	54%	70%	69%	94%
Smoking Cessation Advice	152	85%	83%	80%	100%
Surgical Infection Prevention					
Prophylactic Antibiotic Given	715	93%	78%	77%	95%
Prophylactic Antibiotic Selection	160	96%	91%	90%	100%
Prophylactic Antibiotic Stopped	636	82%	72%	72%	95%
Pregnancy Care					
Inpatient Neonatal Mortality	-	-	-	-	-
Third or Fourth Degree Laceration	-	-	-	3.63%	3.27%

Christian Hospital Northeast

11133 Dunn Road
Saint Louis, MO 63136
Phone: 314-653-5000
Fax: 314-653-4130
URL: www.christianhospital.org
Ownership: Voluntary non-profit - Private
Accredited: Yes
Emergency Services: Yes
Licensed Beds: 493

Key Personnel:

President . . . . Ron McMullen
Chief Medical Staff . . . . Stephen Hazama
Emergency Room . . . . William Svancarek, MD
Chief of Radiology . . . . Hilton Price, MD
Respiratory Care . . . . Neil Hittler

Measure	Cases	This Hospital	State Average	U.S. Average	Top Hospital
Heart Attack Care					
ACE Inhibitor or ARB for LVSD	107	90%	76%	82%	100%
Aspirin at Arrival	347	98%	92%	92%	100%
Aspirin at Discharge	376	94%	87%	90%	100%
Beta Blocker at Arrival	330	91%	83%	87%	100%
Beta Blocker at Discharge	398	96%	87%	90%	100%
Fibrinolytic Medication Timing[1]	5	40%	26%	31%	100%
PCI Within 90 Minutes of Arrival[1]	6	67%	61%	54%	95%
Smoking Cessation Advice	144	99%	92%	88%	100%
Heart Failure Care					
ACE Inhibitor or ARB for LVSD	325	85%	84%	82%	100%
Discharge Instructions	655	70%	62%	61%	93%
Evaluation of LVS Function	839	93%	79%	83%	99%
Smoking Cessation Advice	160	99%	80%	82%	100%
Pneumonia Care					
Appropriate Initial Antibiotic	223	83%	81%	83%	94%
Blood Culture Timing	247	90%	92%	90%	100%
Influenza Vaccine	78	81%	70%	70%	100%
Initial Antibiotic Timing	352	80%	81%	80%	93%
Oxygenation Assessment	393	100%	99%	99%	100%
Pneumococcal Vaccine	222	72%	70%	69%	94%
Smoking Cessation Advice	92	99%	83%	80%	100%
Surgical Infection Prevention					
Prophylactic Antibiotic Given	588	92%	78%	77%	95%
Prophylactic Antibiotic Selection	138	82%	91%	90%	100%
Prophylactic Antibiotic Stopped	536	85%	72%	72%	95%
Pregnancy Care					
Inpatient Neonatal Mortality	-	-	-	-	-
Third or Fourth Degree Laceration	-	-	-	3.63%	3.27%

Forest Park Hospital

Alternate Name: Deaconess Hospital
6150 Oakland Avenue
Saint Louis, MO 63139
Phone: 314-768-3000
Fax: 314-768-3990
Ownership: Proprietary
Accredited: Yes
Emergency Services: Yes
Licensed Beds: 527

Key Personnel:

President/CEO . . . . John Hirsch, MD
Chief Medical Staff . . . . M Robert Hill, MD
Emergency Room . . . . Horacio Marafioti, MD
Director Medical/Surgical Nursing . . . . Gay Cunningham, RN
Director Pulmonary Therapy . . . . Korgi Hedde

Measure	Cases	This Hospital	State Average	U.S. Average	Top Hospital
Heart Attack Care					
ACE Inhibitor or ARB for LVSD[1]	16	81%	76%	82%	100%
Aspirin at Arrival	48	96%	92%	92%	100%
Aspirin at Discharge	58	91%	87%	90%	100%
Beta Blocker at Arrival	50	100%	83%	87%	100%
Beta Blocker at Discharge	59	95%	87%	90%	100%
Fibrinolytic Medication Timing[1]	3	0%	26%	31%	100%
PCI Within 90 Minutes of Arrival	0	-	61%	54%	95%
Smoking Cessation Advice[1]	20	65%	92%	88%	100%
Heart Failure Care					
ACE Inhibitor or ARB for LVSD	112	84%	84%	82%	100%
Discharge Instructions	242	42%	62%	61%	93%
Evaluation of LVS Function	299	88%	79%	83%	99%
Smoking Cessation Advice	73	49%	80%	82%	100%
Pneumonia Care					

NOTE: Hospital profiles are in alphabetical order by state, then city, then hospital within the city; Rankings are sorted by rate in descending order and exclude hospitals with less than 25 cases; (1) The number of cases is too small (n<25) for purposes of reliably predicting hospital performance; (2) Measure reflects the hospital's indication that its submission was based upon a sample of its relevant discharges; (3) Rate reflects fewer than the maximum possible quarters of data for the measure; (4) Inaccurate information submitted and suppressed for one or more quarters; (5) No data is available from the hospital for this measure; Please refer to the User's Guide for a full explanation of data

Appropriate Initial Antibiotic	100	51%	81%	83%	94%
Blood Culture Timing	82	96%	92%	90%	100%
Influenza Vaccine	34	62%	70%	70%	100%
Initial Antibiotic Timing	122	68%	81%	80%	93%
Oxygenation Assessment	171	100%	99%	99%	100%
Pneumococcal Vaccine	96	59%	70%	69%	94%
Smoking Cessation Advice	48	62%	83%	80%	100%
Surgical Infection Prevention					
Prophylactic Antibiotic Given[3]	105	61%	78%	77%	95%
Prophylactic Antibiotic Selection[1]	9	89%	91%	90%	100%
Prophylactic Antibiotic Stopped[3]	99	79%	72%	72%	95%
Pregnancy Care					
Inpatient Neonatal Mortality	-	-	-	-	-
Third or Fourth Degree Laceration	-	-	-	3.63%	3.27%

Saint Alexius Hospital

3933 South Broadway
Saint Louis, MO 63118
URL: www.stalexiushospital.com
Ownership: Proprietary
Emergency Services: Yes

Phone: 314-865-7000
Fax: 314-865-7938

Accredited: Yes
Licensed Beds: 203

Key Personnel:
CEO. . . . . David Seifert
Chief Medical Staff. . . . . Patrick Durbin, MD
Emergency Room . . . . Dawn Bassett-McLean, RN
OB/GYN Womens Health. . . . . Louis Ojascastro, MD
Chief Radiology . . . . Jonathan Dehner, MD

Measure	Cases	This Hospital	State Average	U.S. Average	Top Hospital
Heart Attack Care					
ACE Inhibitor or ARB for LVSD[1]	11	100%	76%	82%	100%
Aspirin at Arrival	47	96%	92%	92%	100%
Aspirin at Discharge[1]	22	100%	87%	90%	100%
Beta Blocker at Arrival	34	88%	83%	87%	100%
Beta Blocker at Discharge	25	96%	87%	90%	100%
Fibrinolytic Medication Timing[1]	2	0%	26%	31%	100%
PCI Within 90 Minutes of Arrival	0	-	61%	54%	95%
Smoking Cessation Advice[1]	7	100%	92%	88%	100%
Heart Failure Care					
ACE Inhibitor or ARB for LVSD	78	81%	84%	82%	100%
Discharge Instructions	193	28%	62%	61%	93%
Evaluation of LVS Function	255	95%	79%	83%	99%
Smoking Cessation Advice	70	99%	80%	82%	100%
Pneumonia Care					
Appropriate Initial Antibiotic	119	87%	81%	83%	94%
Blood Culture Timing	118	93%	92%	90%	100%
Influenza Vaccine	31	81%	70%	70%	100%
Initial Antibiotic Timing	179	87%	81%	80%	93%
Oxygenation Assessment	219	100%	99%	99%	100%
Pneumococcal Vaccine	105	76%	70%	69%	94%
Smoking Cessation Advice	82	96%	83%	80%	100%
Surgical Infection Prevention					
Prophylactic Antibiotic Given	72	74%	78%	77%	95%
Prophylactic Antibiotic Selection[1]	20	90%	91%	90%	100%
Prophylactic Antibiotic Stopped	71	69%	72%	72%	95%
Pregnancy Care					
Inpatient Neonatal Mortality	-	-	-	-	-
Third or Fourth Degree Laceration	-	-	-	3.63%	3.27%

Saint Anthony's Medical Center

10010 Kennerly Road
Saint Louis, MO 63128
E-mail: webmaster@samcstl.org
URL: www.stanthonysmedicalcenter.com
Ownership: Voluntary non-profit - Church
Emergency Services: Yes

Phone: 314-525-1000
Fax: 314-525-4040

Accredited: Yes
Licensed Beds: 767

Key Personnel:
CEO. . . . . Tom Rockerf

Measure	Cases	This Hospital	State Average	U.S. Average	Top Hospital
Heart Attack Care					
ACE Inhibitor or ARB for LVSD[2]	68	84%	76%	82%	100%
Aspirin at Arrival[2]	314	97%	92%	92%	100%
Aspirin at Discharge[2]	297	96%	87%	90%	100%
Beta Blocker at Arrival[2]	215	94%	83%	87%	100%
Beta Blocker at Discharge[2]	319	94%	87%	90%	100%
Fibrinolytic Medication Timing[2]	0	-	26%	31%	100%
PCI Within 90 Minutes of Arrival[1,2]	21	52%	61%	54%	95%
Smoking Cessation Advice[2]	130	99%	92%	88%	100%
Heart Failure Care					
ACE Inhibitor or ARB for LVSD[2]	166	74%	84%	82%	100%
Discharge Instructions[2]	303	60%	62%	61%	93%
Evaluation of LVS Function[2]	397	94%	79%	83%	99%
Smoking Cessation Advice[2]	67	97%	80%	82%	100%
Pneumonia Care					
Appropriate Initial Antibiotic[2]	186	86%	81%	83%	94%
Blood Culture Timing[2]	230	92%	92%	90%	100%
Influenza Vaccine[2]	45	89%	70%	70%	100%
Initial Antibiotic Timing[2]	289	76%	81%	80%	93%
Oxygenation Assessment[2]	347	100%	99%	99%	100%
Pneumococcal Vaccine[2]	226	82%	70%	69%	94%
Smoking Cessation Advice[2]	83	99%	83%	80%	100%
Surgical Infection Prevention					
Prophylactic Antibiotic Given[2,3]	639	87%	78%	77%	95%
Prophylactic Antibiotic Selection[2]	215	92%	91%	90%	100%
Prophylactic Antibiotic Stopped[2,3]	606	67%	72%	72%	95%
Pregnancy Care					
Inpatient Neonatal Mortality[2]	1,661	0.24%	-	-	-
Third or Fourth Degree Laceration[2]	1,080	5.46%	-	3.63%	3.27%

Saint John's Mercy Medical Center

615 S New Ballas Road
Saint Louis, MO 63141
URL: www.stjohnsmercy.org
Ownership: Voluntary non-profit - Church
Emergency Services: Yes

Phone: 314-251-6000
Fax: 314-251-4719

Accredited: Yes
Licensed Beds: 979

Key Personnel:
Co-President . . . . Mark Stauder
Co-President . . . . John Sullivan
Chief of Medical Staff. . . . . Martin Bell
Director Pulmonary Therapy . . . . Paul Bast

Measure	Cases	This Hospital	State Average	U.S. Average	Top Hospital
Heart Attack Care					
ACE Inhibitor or ARB for LVSD	165	92%	76%	82%	100%
Aspirin at Arrival	356	98%	92%	92%	100%
Aspirin at Discharge	523	98%	87%	90%	100%
Beta Blocker at Arrival	298	95%	83%	87%	100%
Beta Blocker at Discharge	535	98%	87%	90%	100%
Fibrinolytic Medication Timing	0	-	26%	31%	100%
PCI Within 90 Minutes of Arrival[1]	14	36%	61%	54%	95%
Smoking Cessation Advice	171	100%	92%	88%	100%
Heart Failure Care					
ACE Inhibitor or ARB for LVSD	262	90%	84%	82%	100%
Discharge Instructions	471	80%	62%	61%	93%
Evaluation of LVS Function	555	98%	79%	83%	99%
Smoking Cessation Advice	76	100%	80%	82%	100%
Pneumonia Care					
Appropriate Initial Antibiotic[2]	302	84%	81%	83%	94%
Blood Culture Timing[2]	251	93%	92%	90%	100%
Influenza Vaccine[2]	85	85%	70%	70%	100%
Initial Antibiotic Timing[2]	470	82%	81%	80%	93%
Oxygenation Assessment[2]	500	100%	99%	99%	100%
Pneumococcal Vaccine[2]	297	89%	70%	69%	94%
Smoking Cessation Advice[2]	105	98%	83%	80%	100%
Surgical Infection Prevention					
Prophylactic Antibiotic Given[2]	1,001	94%	78%	77%	95%
Prophylactic Antibiotic Selection[2]	255	96%	91%	90%	100%
Prophylactic Antibiotic Stopped[2]	958	78%	72%	72%	95%
Pregnancy Care					
Inpatient Neonatal Mortality	-	-	-	-	-
Third or Fourth Degree Laceration	-	-	-	3.63%	3.27%

NOTE: Hospital profiles are in alphabetical order by state, then city, then hospital within the city; Rankings are sorted by rate in descending order and exclude hospitals with less than 25 cases; (1) The number of cases is too small (n<25) for purposes of reliably predicting hospital performance; (2) Measure reflects the hospital's indication that its submission was based upon a sample of its relevant discharges; (3) Rate reflects fewer than the maximum possible quarters of data for the measure; (4) Inaccurate information submitted and suppressed for one or more quarters; (5) No data is available from the hospital for this measure; Please refer to the User's Guide for a full explanation of data

SLUCare

Alternate Name: St. Louis University Hospital
3635 Vista Avenue at Grand Boulevard
PO Box 15250
Saint Louis, MO 63110
E-mail: slucare@slu.edu
URL: www.slucare.edu/clinical
Ownership: Proprietary
Emergency Services: Yes

Toll-Free: 866-977-4440
Phone: 314-977-4440
Fax: 314-577-8825

Accredited: Yes
Licensed Beds: 356

Key Personnel:
CEO/Executive Director . . . . James Kimmny
Chief Medical Staff. . . . . Coy Fitch, MD
Director Infection/Disease Control . . . . Donald J Kennedy, MD
Director Radiology . . . . Ben Frey
Director Respiratory Therapy . . . . John Hemkens

Measure	Cases	This Hospital	State Average	U.S. Average	Top Hospital
Heart Attack Care					
ACE Inhibitor or ARB for LVSD	90	84%	76%	82%	100%
Aspirin at Arrival	127	96%	92%	92%	100%
Aspirin at Discharge	167	100%	87%	90%	100%
Beta Blocker at Arrival	98	95%	83%	87%	100%
Beta Blocker at Discharge	189	99%	87%	90%	100%
Fibrinolytic Medication Timing	0	-	26%	31%	100%
PCI Within 90 Minutes of Arrival[1]	12	75%	61%	54%	95%
Smoking Cessation Advice	92	99%	92%	88%	100%
Heart Failure Care					
ACE Inhibitor or ARB for LVSD	260	84%	84%	82%	100%
Discharge Instructions	358	90%	62%	61%	93%
Evaluation of LVS Function	394	98%	79%	83%	99%
Smoking Cessation Advice	136	99%	80%	82%	100%
Pneumonia Care					
Appropriate Initial Antibiotic	129	91%	81%	83%	94%
Blood Culture Timing	126	92%	92%	90%	100%
Influenza Vaccine	28	57%	70%	70%	100%
Initial Antibiotic Timing	212	75%	81%	80%	93%
Oxygenation Assessment	236	100%	99%	99%	100%
Pneumococcal Vaccine	114	71%	70%	69%	94%
Smoking Cessation Advice	83	93%	83%	80%	100%
Surgical Infection Prevention					
Prophylactic Antibiotic Given[2]	237	77%	78%	77%	95%
Prophylactic Antibiotic Selection[2]	54	93%	91%	90%	100%
Prophylactic Antibiotic Stopped[2]	229	42%	72%	72%	95%
Pregnancy Care					
Inpatient Neonatal Mortality	-	-	-	-	-
Third or Fourth Degree Laceration	-	-	-	3.63%	3.27%

Barnes-Jewish Saint Peters Hospital

Alternate Name: Barnes Saint Peters Hospital
10 Hospital Drive
Saint Peters, MO 63376
URL: www.bjsph.org
Ownership: Voluntary non-profit - Other
Emergency Services: Yes

Phone: 636-916-9000
Fax: 636-916-9127

Accredited: Yes
Licensed Beds: 111

Key Personnel:
CEO. . . . . David Ross
Chief Medical Staff. . . . . Phil Brick
Emergency Room . . . . Scott Carruth
Manager Infection/Disease Control . . . . Janice Setzer
OB/GYN Womens Health. . . . . Lora Mills
Chief Radiology . . . . William Dawson, MD
Respiratory Therapy. . . . . Maria Ftiffler

Measure	Cases	This Hospital	State Average	U.S. Average	Top Hospital
Heart Attack Care					
ACE Inhibitor or ARB for LVSD	27	96%	76%	82%	100%
Aspirin at Arrival	165	98%	92%	92%	100%
Aspirin at Discharge	142	94%	87%	90%	100%
Beta Blocker at Arrival	160	92%	83%	87%	100%
Beta Blocker at Discharge	146	96%	87%	90%	100%
Fibrinolytic Medication Timing	0	-	26%	31%	100%
PCI Within 90 Minutes of Arrival[1]	4	25%	61%	54%	95%
Smoking Cessation Advice	54	98%	92%	88%	100%
Heart Failure Care					
ACE Inhibitor or ARB for LVSD	50	82%	84%	82%	100%
Discharge Instructions	121	56%	62%	61%	93%
Evaluation of LVS Function	144	95%	79%	83%	99%
Smoking Cessation Advice[1]	19	95%	80%	82%	100%
Pneumonia Care					
Appropriate Initial Antibiotic	156	93%	81%	83%	94%
Blood Culture Timing	161	95%	92%	90%	100%
Influenza Vaccine	35	74%	70%	70%	100%
Initial Antibiotic Timing	204	89%	81%	80%	93%
Oxygenation Assessment	224	100%	99%	99%	100%
Pneumococcal Vaccine	130	75%	70%	69%	94%
Smoking Cessation Advice	44	93%	83%	80%	100%
Surgical Infection Prevention					
Prophylactic Antibiotic Given	357	93%	78%	77%	95%
Prophylactic Antibiotic Selection	74	96%	91%	90%	100%
Prophylactic Antibiotic Stopped	351	88%	72%	72%	95%
Pregnancy Care					
Inpatient Neonatal Mortality	-	-	-	-	-
Third or Fourth Degree Laceration	-	-	-	3.63%	3.27%

Ste Genevieve County Memorial Hospital

800 Ste Genevieve Drive, PO Box 468
Sainte Genevieve, MO 63670
Ownership: Voluntary non-profit - Other
Emergency Services: No

Phone: 573-883-2751

Accredited: No

Measure	Cases	This Hospital	State Average	U.S. Average	Top Hospital
Heart Attack Care					
ACE Inhibitor or ARB for LVSD	0	-	76%	82%	100%
Aspirin at Arrival[1]	3	100%	92%	92%	100%
Aspirin at Discharge[1]	1	100%	87%	90%	100%
Beta Blocker at Arrival[1]	3	67%	83%	87%	100%
Beta Blocker at Discharge[1]	1	100%	87%	90%	100%
Fibrinolytic Medication Timing	0	-	26%	31%	100%
PCI Within 90 Minutes of Arrival	0	-	61%	54%	95%
Smoking Cessation Advice	0	-	92%	88%	100%
Heart Failure Care					
ACE Inhibitor or ARB for LVSD[1]	5	60%	84%	82%	100%
Discharge Instructions	35	63%	62%	61%	93%
Evaluation of LVS Function	65	78%	79%	83%	99%
Smoking Cessation Advice[1]	3	67%	80%	82%	100%
Pneumonia Care					
Appropriate Initial Antibiotic	43	70%	81%	83%	94%
Blood Culture Timing	35	97%	92%	90%	100%
Influenza Vaccine[1]	15	93%	70%	70%	100%
Initial Antibiotic Timing	58	84%	81%	80%	93%
Oxygenation Assessment	83	100%	99%	99%	100%
Pneumococcal Vaccine	52	71%	70%	69%	94%
Smoking Cessation Advice[1]	14	50%	83%	80%	100%
Surgical Infection Prevention					
Prophylactic Antibiotic Given	42	86%	78%	77%	95%
Prophylactic Antibiotic Selection[1]	11	82%	91%	90%	100%
Prophylactic Antibiotic Stopped	41	100%	72%	72%	95%
Pregnancy Care					
Inpatient Neonatal Mortality	-	-	-	-	-
Third or Fourth Degree Laceration	-	-	-	3.63%	3.27%

Salem Memorial District Hospital

Highway 72 N
Salem, MO 65560
Ownership: Government - Local
Emergency Services: No

Phone: 573-729-6626
Fax: 573-729-4511
Accredited: No
Licensed Beds: 59

Key Personnel:
Administrator . . . . Dennis P Pryor
Emergency Room . . . . Brenda Gott
Director Infection/Disease Control . . . . Cliff Free
OB/GYN Womens Health. . . . . Yvonne Prince

Measure	Cases	This Hospital	State Average	U.S. Average	Top Hospital
Heart Attack Care					
ACE Inhibitor or ARB for LVSD[5]	-	-	76%	82%	100%

NOTE: Hospital profiles are in alphabetical order by state, then city, then hospital within the city; Rankings are sorted by rate in descending order and exclude hospitals with less than 25 cases; (1) The number of cases is too small (n<25) for purposes of reliably predicting hospital performance; (2) Measure reflects the hospital's indication that its submission was based upon a sample of its relevant discharges; (3) Rate reflects fewer than the maximum possible quarters of data for the measure; (4) Inaccurate information submitted and suppressed for one or more quarters; (5) No data is available from the hospital for this measure; Please refer to the User's Guide for a full explanation of data

Measure	Cases	This Hospital	State Average	U.S. Average	Top Hospital
Aspirin at Arrival[5]	-	-	92%	92%	100%
Aspirin at Discharge[5]	-	-	87%	90%	100%
Beta Blocker at Arrival[5]	-	-	83%	87%	100%
Beta Blocker at Discharge[5]	-	-	87%	90%	100%
Fibrinolytic Medication Timing[5]	-	-	26%	31%	100%
PCI Within 90 Minutes of Arrival[5]	-	-	61%	54%	95%
Smoking Cessation Advice[5]	-	-	92%	88%	100%
Heart Failure Care					
ACE Inhibitor or ARB for LVSD[1,2,3]	4	100%	84%	82%	100%
Discharge Instructions[1,2,3]	7	0%	62%	61%	93%
Evaluation of LVS Function[1,2,3]	10	90%	79%	83%	99%
Smoking Cessation Advice[1,2,3]	2	100%	80%	82%	100%
Pneumonia Care					
Appropriate Initial Antibiotic[1,2,3]	10	80%	81%	83%	94%
Blood Culture Timing[1,2,3]	5	100%	92%	90%	100%
Influenza Vaccine[5]	-	-	70%	70%	100%
Initial Antibiotic Timing[1,2,3]	13	62%	81%	80%	93%
Oxygenation Assessment[1,2,3]	14	100%	99%	99%	100%
Pneumococcal Vaccine[1,2,3]	10	60%	70%	69%	94%
Smoking Cessation Advice[1,2,3]	2	100%	83%	80%	100%
Surgical Infection Prevention					
Prophylactic Antibiotic Given[5]	-	-	78%	77%	95%
Prophylactic Antibiotic Selection[5]	-	-	91%	90%	100%
Prophylactic Antibiotic Stopped[5]	-	-	72%	72%	95%
Pregnancy Care					
Inpatient Neonatal Mortality	-	-	-	-	-
Third or Fourth Degree Laceration	-	-	-	3.63%	3.27%

Bothwell Regional Health Center

601 E 14th Street
Sedalia, MO 65301
Phone: 660-826-8833
Fax: 660-827-6784
Ownership: Government - Local
Accredited: Yes
Emergency Services: Yes
Licensed Beds: 170

Key Personnel:

CEO . . . . John Dawes
Chief of Medical Staff . . . . Phillip Horneospel
Director of Emergency Room . . . . Richard Beamon
Emergency Room . . . . Karen Toy
OB/GYN Womens Health . . . . Elmer Van Dyke
Chief Radiology . . . . David Roehars, MD
Director Respiratory Therapy . . . . Brian Carr

Measure	Cases	This Hospital	State Average	U.S. Average	Top Hospital
Heart Attack Care					
ACE Inhibitor or ARB for LVSD[1,2]	9	89%	76%	82%	100%
Aspirin at Arrival[2]	65	94%	92%	92%	100%
Aspirin at Discharge[2]	25	84%	87%	90%	100%
Beta Blocker at Arrival[2]	61	80%	83%	87%	100%
Beta Blocker at Discharge[2]	29	86%	87%	90%	100%
Fibrinolytic Medication Timing[2]	26	4%	26%	31%	100%
PCI Within 90 Minutes of Arrival[2]	0	-	61%	54%	95%
Smoking Cessation Advice[1,2]	3	100%	92%	88%	100%
Heart Failure Care					
ACE Inhibitor or ARB for LVSD[2]	108	77%	84%	82%	100%
Discharge Instructions[2]	139	58%	62%	61%	93%
Evaluation of LVS Function[2]	182	90%	79%	83%	99%
Smoking Cessation Advice[2]	29	100%	80%	82%	100%
Pneumonia Care					
Appropriate Initial Antibiotic[2]	134	73%	81%	83%	94%
Blood Culture Timing[2]	97	93%	92%	90%	100%
Influenza Vaccine	33	61%	70%	70%	100%
Initial Antibiotic Timing[2]	221	82%	81%	80%	93%
Oxygenation Assessment[2]	243	100%	99%	99%	100%
Pneumococcal Vaccine[2]	163	85%	70%	69%	94%
Smoking Cessation Advice[2]	59	97%	83%	80%	100%
Surgical Infection Prevention					
Prophylactic Antibiotic Given[2,3]	237	59%	78%	77%	95%
Prophylactic Antibiotic Selection[2]	81	91%	91%	90%	100%
Prophylactic Antibiotic Stopped[2,3]	230	81%	72%	72%	95%
Pregnancy Care					
Inpatient Neonatal Mortality	-	-	-	-	-
Third or Fourth Degree Laceration	-	-	-	3.63%	3.27%

Missouri Delta Medical Center

Alternate Name: Missouri Delta Community Hospital
1008 N Main Street
Sikeston, MO 63801
Phone: 573-471-1600
Fax: 573-472-7606
URL: www.missouridelta.com
Ownership: Voluntary non-profit - Other
Accredited: Yes
Emergency Services: Yes
Licensed Beds: 188

Key Personnel:

Administrator/President . . . . Charles D Ancell
Chief Medical Staff . . . . Mowaffaq Said, MD
Cardiology . . . . Cindy Shands
Chief Catheterization Laboratory . . . . Frank Kroetz, MD
Emergency Room . . . . Darline Brown, RN
Director Infection/Disease Control . . . . Joy Cauthorn
CCU Spvg. Nurse . . . . Angie Friend
Director Medical/Surgical Nursing . . . . Brend LaBrot
OB/GYN Womens Health . . . . Tony Poole, MD
Director Radiology . . . . Debbie Norville
Director Respiratory Therapy . . . . Norma Jamerson

Measure	Cases	This Hospital	State Average	U.S. Average	Top Hospital
Heart Attack Care					
ACE Inhibitor or ARB for LVSD[1,2]	3	33%	76%	82%	100%
Aspirin at Arrival[2]	31	94%	92%	92%	100%
Aspirin at Discharge[1,2]	15	87%	87%	90%	100%
Beta Blocker at Arrival[1,2]	16	88%	83%	87%	100%
Beta Blocker at Discharge[1,2]	14	93%	87%	90%	100%
Fibrinolytic Medication Timing[2]	0	-	26%	31%	100%
PCI Within 90 Minutes of Arrival[2]	0	-	61%	54%	95%
Smoking Cessation Advice[1,2]	2	100%	92%	88%	100%
Heart Failure Care					
ACE Inhibitor or ARB for LVSD[2]	85	87%	84%	82%	100%
Discharge Instructions[2]	188	86%	62%	61%	93%
Evaluation of LVS Function[2]	234	85%	79%	83%	99%
Smoking Cessation Advice[2]	63	100%	80%	82%	100%
Pneumonia Care					
Appropriate Initial Antibiotic[2]	115	85%	81%	83%	94%
Blood Culture Timing[2]	107	91%	92%	90%	100%
Influenza Vaccine[4,5]	-	-	70%	70%	100%
Initial Antibiotic Timing[2]	173	79%	81%	80%	93%
Oxygenation Assessment[2]	224	100%	99%	99%	100%
Pneumococcal Vaccine[2]	132	76%	70%	69%	94%
Smoking Cessation Advice[2]	76	100%	83%	80%	100%
Surgical Infection Prevention					
Prophylactic Antibiotic Given[2,3]	86	52%	78%	77%	95%
Prophylactic Antibiotic Selection[2]	31	77%	91%	90%	100%
Prophylactic Antibiotic Stopped[2,3]	78	83%	72%	72%	95%
Pregnancy Care					
Inpatient Neonatal Mortality	-	-	-	-	-
Third or Fourth Degree Laceration	-	-	-	3.63%	3.27%

Cox Med Ctrs-North and South & Walnut Lawn

1423 N Jefferson Street
Springfield, MO 65802
Phone: 417-269-3000
Fax: 417-269-4104
URL: www.coxhealth.com
Ownership: Voluntary non-profit - Church
Accredited: Yes
Emergency Services: Yes
Licensed Beds: 800

Key Personnel:

President/CEO . . . . Robert Benzanson
Acting Director ER . . . . Drew Alexander
Emergency Room . . . . Mark Ross, MD
Director Infection/Disease Control . . . . Susan Soetaert
OB/GYN/Women's Health . . . . Kathleen Graves, MD
Director Radiology . . . . Shawn Snider
Director Respiratory Therapy . . . . David Tucker

Measure	Cases	This Hospital	State Average	U.S. Average	Top Hospital
Heart Attack Care					
ACE Inhibitor or ARB for LVSD	100	93%	76%	82%	100%
Aspirin at Arrival	412	98%	92%	92%	100%
Aspirin at Discharge	542	96%	87%	90%	100%
Beta Blocker at Arrival	366	98%	83%	87%	100%
Beta Blocker at Discharge	559	98%	87%	90%	100%

NOTE: Hospital profiles are in alphabetical order by state, then city, then hospital within the city; Rankings are sorted by rate in descending order and exclude hospitals with less than 25 cases; (1) The number of cases is too small (n<25) for purposes of reliably predicting hospital performance; (2) Measure reflects the hospital's indication that its submission was based upon a sample of its relevant discharges; (3) Rate reflects fewer than the maximum possible quarters of data for the measure; (4) Inaccurate information submitted and suppressed for one or more quarters; (5) No data is available from the hospital for this measure; Please refer to the User's Guide for a full explanation of data

Measure	Cases	This Hospital	State Average	U.S. Average	Top Hospital
Fibrinolytic Medication Timing[1]	12	33%	26%	31%	100%
PCI Within 90 Minutes of Arrival[1]	17	35%	61%	54%	95%
Smoking Cessation Advice	234	97%	92%	88%	100%
Heart Failure Care					
ACE Inhibitor or ARB for LVSD	140	91%	84%	82%	100%
Discharge Instructions	306	78%	62%	61%	93%
Evaluation of LVS Function	407	91%	79%	83%	99%
Smoking Cessation Advice	87	90%	80%	82%	100%
Pneumonia Care					
Appropriate Initial Antibiotic	457	75%	81%	83%	94%
Blood Culture Timing	363	92%	92%	90%	100%
Influenza Vaccine[4,5]	-	-	70%	70%	100%
Initial Antibiotic Timing	576	73%	81%	80%	93%
Oxygenation Assessment	693	100%	99%	99%	100%
Pneumococcal Vaccine	345	60%	70%	69%	94%
Smoking Cessation Advice	194	77%	83%	80%	100%
Surgical Infection Prevention					
Prophylactic Antibiotic Given[3]	706	82%	78%	77%	95%
Prophylactic Antibiotic Selection	547	98%	91%	90%	100%
Prophylactic Antibiotic Stopped[3]	691	80%	72%	72%	95%
Pregnancy Care					
Inpatient Neonatal Mortality	-	-	-	-	-
Third or Fourth Degree Laceration	-	-	-	3.63%	3.27%

Doctors Hospital of Springfield

2828 North National
Springfield, MO 65803
Phone: 417-837-4000
Ownership: Proprietary
Accredited: Yes
Emergency Services: Yes

Measure	Cases	This Hospital	State Average	U.S. Average	Top Hospital
Heart Attack Care					
ACE Inhibitor or ARB for LVSD[1,3]	1	100%	76%	82%	100%
Aspirin at Arrival[1,3]	1	100%	92%	92%	100%
Aspirin at Discharge[1,3]	1	100%	87%	90%	100%
Beta Blocker at Arrival[1,3]	1	0%	83%	87%	100%
Beta Blocker at Discharge[1,3]	1	100%	87%	90%	100%
Fibrinolytic Medication Timing[3]	0	-	26%	31%	100%
PCI Within 90 Minutes of Arrival	0	-	61%	54%	95%
Smoking Cessation Advice[3]	0	-	92%	88%	100%
Heart Failure Care					
ACE Inhibitor or ARB for LVSD[1]	11	100%	84%	82%	100%
Discharge Instructions[1]	17	35%	62%	61%	93%
Evaluation of LVS Function	38	84%	79%	83%	99%
Smoking Cessation Advice[1]	6	83%	80%	82%	100%
Pneumonia Care					
Appropriate Initial Antibiotic	40	88%	81%	83%	94%
Blood Culture Timing	38	84%	92%	90%	100%
Influenza Vaccine[1]	2	100%	70%	70%	100%
Initial Antibiotic Timing	60	75%	81%	80%	93%
Oxygenation Assessment	77	100%	99%	99%	100%
Pneumococcal Vaccine	50	76%	70%	69%	94%
Smoking Cessation Advice[1]	19	63%	83%	80%	100%
Surgical Infection Prevention					
Prophylactic Antibiotic Given	37	95%	78%	77%	95%
Prophylactic Antibiotic Selection[1]	9	100%	91%	90%	100%
Prophylactic Antibiotic Stopped	35	86%	72%	72%	95%
Pregnancy Care					
Inpatient Neonatal Mortality	-	-	-	-	-
Third or Fourth Degree Laceration	-	-	-	3.63%	3.27%

Saint John's Regional Health Center

1235 E Cherokee
Springfield, MO 65804
Phone: 417-885-2000
Fax: 417-820-6996
URL: www.stjohns.com
Ownership: Voluntary non-profit - Church
Accredited: Yes
Emergency Services: Yes
Licensed Beds: 866

Key Personnel:

President/CEO . . . . Allen L Shockley
Chief Medical Staff. . . . . J Kent Dexter, MD
Emergency Room Head. . . . . Constant Donovan
Emergency Room . . . . Ted McMurry, MD
Director Infection/Disease Control . . . . Patti Reynolds
OB/GYN Womens Health. . . . . Al Bonebrake, MD
Director Radiology . . . . Eddie Terrill
Director Respiratory Therapy . . . . Jim Pattinson

Measure	Cases	This Hospital	State Average	U.S. Average	Top Hospital
Heart Attack Care					
ACE Inhibitor or ARB for LVSD	186	97%	76%	82%	100%
Aspirin at Arrival	397	98%	92%	92%	100%
Aspirin at Discharge	617	98%	87%	90%	100%
Beta Blocker at Arrival	272	94%	83%	87%	100%
Beta Blocker at Discharge	587	98%	87%	90%	100%
Fibrinolytic Medication Timing[1]	1	100%	26%	31%	100%
PCI Within 90 Minutes of Arrival	39	49%	61%	54%	95%
Smoking Cessation Advice	262	100%	92%	88%	100%
Heart Failure Care					
ACE Inhibitor or ARB for LVSD	355	92%	84%	82%	100%
Discharge Instructions	574	82%	62%	61%	93%
Evaluation of LVS Function	690	99%	79%	83%	99%
Smoking Cessation Advice	107	100%	80%	82%	100%
Pneumonia Care					
Appropriate Initial Antibiotic	412	89%	81%	83%	94%
Blood Culture Timing	435	97%	92%	90%	100%
Influenza Vaccine	164	96%	70%	70%	100%
Initial Antibiotic Timing	501	86%	81%	80%	93%
Oxygenation Assessment	726	100%	99%	99%	100%
Pneumococcal Vaccine	497	95%	70%	69%	94%
Smoking Cessation Advice	216	97%	83%	80%	100%
Surgical Infection Prevention					
Prophylactic Antibiotic Given[2]	360	91%	78%	77%	95%
Prophylactic Antibiotic Selection[2]	96	96%	91%	90%	100%
Prophylactic Antibiotic Stopped[2]	354	89%	72%	72%	95%
Pregnancy Care					
Inpatient Neonatal Mortality	-	-	-	-	-
Third or Fourth Degree Laceration	-	-	-	3.63%	3.27%

Missouri Baptist Hospital Sullivan

751 Sappington Bridge Road
Sullivan, MO 63080
Phone: 573-468-4186
Fax: 573-860-2696
URL: www.missouribaptistsullivan.org
Ownership: Voluntary non-profit - Private
Accredited: No
Emergency Services: Yes
Licensed Beds: 46

Key Personnel:

President . . . . Tony Schwarm
Director Emergency Department . . . . Jerry Fitzgerald, DO

Measure	Cases	This Hospital	State Average	U.S. Average	Top Hospital
Heart Attack Care					
ACE Inhibitor or ARB for LVSD	0	-	76%	82%	100%
Aspirin at Arrival[1]	8	100%	92%	92%	100%
Aspirin at Discharge[1]	1	100%	87%	90%	100%
Beta Blocker at Arrival[1]	8	100%	83%	87%	100%
Beta Blocker at Discharge[1]	1	100%	87%	90%	100%
Fibrinolytic Medication Timing	0	-	26%	31%	100%
PCI Within 90 Minutes of Arrival	0	-	61%	54%	95%
Smoking Cessation Advice	0	-	92%	88%	100%
Heart Failure Care					
ACE Inhibitor or ARB for LVSD[1]	23	96%	84%	82%	100%
Discharge Instructions	53	87%	62%	61%	93%
Evaluation of LVS Function	71	99%	79%	83%	99%
Smoking Cessation Advice[1]	12	100%	80%	82%	100%
Pneumonia Care					
Appropriate Initial Antibiotic	89	97%	81%	83%	94%
Blood Culture Timing	80	98%	92%	90%	100%
Influenza Vaccine[1]	20	100%	70%	70%	100%
Initial Antibiotic Timing	104	93%	81%	80%	93%
Oxygenation Assessment	123	100%	99%	99%	100%
Pneumococcal Vaccine	83	95%	70%	69%	94%
Smoking Cessation Advice[1]	21	100%	83%	80%	100%
Surgical Infection Prevention					
Prophylactic Antibiotic Given	37	95%	78%	77%	95%
Prophylactic Antibiotic Selection[1]	6	67%	91%	90%	100%

NOTE: Hospital profiles are in alphabetical order by state, then city, then hospital within the city; Rankings are sorted by rate in descending order and exclude hospitals with less than 25 cases; (1) The number of cases is too small (n<25) for purposes of reliably predicting hospital performance; (2) Measure reflects the hospital's indication that its submission was based upon a sample of its relevant discharges; (3) Rate reflects fewer than the maximum possible quarters of data for the measure; (4) Inaccurate information submitted and suppressed for one or more quarters; (5) No data is available from the hospital for this measure; Please refer to the User's Guide for a full explanation of data

Prophylactic Antibiotic Stopped	35	100%	72%	72%	95%
Pregnancy Care					
Inpatient Neonatal Mortality	-	-	-	-	-
Third or Fourth Degree Laceration	-	-	-	3.63%	3.27%

Des Peres Hospital

2345 Dougherty Ferry Road
Saint Louis, MO 63122

Toll-Free: 877-752-1139
Phone: 314-966-9100
Fax: 314-966-9274

Ownership: Proprietary
Emergency Services: Yes

Accredited: Yes
Licensed Beds: 167

Key Personnel:
Administrator/CEO . . . . Michele Meyer
Chief Medical Staff . . . . Micheal Chablt
Emergency Room . . . . Pam Stingle
Chief Radiology . . . . James Mulkey, MD

Measure	Cases	This Hospital	State Average	U.S. Average	Top Hospital
Heart Attack Care					
ACE Inhibitor or ARB for LVSD	51	98%	76%	82%	100%
Aspirin at Arrival	99	99%	92%	92%	100%
Aspirin at Discharge	255	98%	87%	90%	100%
Beta Blocker at Arrival	98	98%	83%	87%	100%
Beta Blocker at Discharge	256	97%	87%	90%	100%
Fibrinolytic Medication Timing[1]	1	0%	26%	31%	100%
PCI Within 90 Minutes of Arrival[1]	4	50%	61%	54%	95%
Smoking Cessation Advice	106	99%	92%	88%	100%
Heart Failure Care					
ACE Inhibitor or ARB for LVSD	149	90%	84%	82%	100%
Discharge Instructions	329	88%	62%	61%	93%
Evaluation of LVS Function	405	94%	79%	83%	99%
Smoking Cessation Advice	67	99%	80%	82%	100%
Pneumonia Care					
Appropriate Initial Antibiotic	192	86%	81%	83%	94%
Blood Culture Timing	180	93%	92%	90%	100%
Influenza Vaccine[4,5]	-	-	70%	70%	100%
Initial Antibiotic Timing	261	84%	81%	80%	93%
Oxygenation Assessment	318	100%	99%	99%	100%
Pneumococcal Vaccine	213	77%	70%	69%	94%
Smoking Cessation Advice	73	97%	83%	80%	100%
Surgical Infection Prevention					
Prophylactic Antibiotic Given[2]	342	77%	78%	77%	95%
Prophylactic Antibiotic Selection[2]	92	86%	91%	90%	100%
Prophylactic Antibiotic Stopped[2]	338	52%	72%	72%	95%
Pregnancy Care					
Inpatient Neonatal Mortality	-	-	-	-	-
Third or Fourth Degree Laceration	-	-	-	3.63%	3.27%

Missouri Baptist Medical Center

3015 N Ballas Road
Saint Louis, MO 63131
URL: www.bjc.org

Phone: 314-996-5000
Fax: 314-432-1024

Ownership: Voluntary non-profit - Private
Emergency Services: Yes

Accredited: Yes
Licensed Beds: 379

Key Personnel:
President . . . . Carm Moceri
Chief Medical Staff . . . . Harry Wartsworth, MD
Director Cardiac Services . . . . Douglas Sohn
Catheterization Services Manager . . . . Jennifer Francis
Emergency Room Manager . . . . Patti Kelly
OB/GYN Womens Health . . . . Ingrid Pokinghorme
Director Respiratory Therapy . . . . Frank Caruso

Measure	Cases	This Hospital	State Average	U.S. Average	Top Hospital
Heart Attack Care					
ACE Inhibitor or ARB for LVSD	96	92%	76%	82%	100%
Aspirin at Arrival	179	98%	92%	92%	100%
Aspirin at Discharge	367	98%	87%	90%	100%
Beta Blocker at Arrival	160	96%	83%	87%	100%
Beta Blocker at Discharge	375	98%	87%	90%	100%
Fibrinolytic Medication Timing	0	-	26%	31%	100%
PCI Within 90 Minutes of Arrival[1]	5	80%	61%	54%	95%
Smoking Cessation Advice	131	99%	92%	88%	100%
Heart Failure Care					
ACE Inhibitor or ARB for LVSD	293	86%	84%	82%	100%
Discharge Instructions	551	63%	62%	61%	93%
Evaluation of LVS Function	701	96%	79%	83%	99%
Smoking Cessation Advice	71	97%	80%	82%	100%
Pneumonia Care					
Appropriate Initial Antibiotic	312	79%	81%	83%	94%
Blood Culture Timing	317	94%	92%	90%	100%
Influenza Vaccine	96	78%	70%	70%	100%
Initial Antibiotic Timing	476	79%	81%	80%	93%
Oxygenation Assessment	560	100%	99%	99%	100%
Pneumococcal Vaccine	404	76%	70%	69%	94%
Smoking Cessation Advice	119	98%	83%	80%	100%
Surgical Infection Prevention					
Prophylactic Antibiotic Given	773	95%	78%	77%	95%
Prophylactic Antibiotic Selection	167	96%	91%	90%	100%
Prophylactic Antibiotic Stopped	723	82%	72%	72%	95%
Pregnancy Care					
Inpatient Neonatal Mortality	4,228	0.07%	-	-	-
Third or Fourth Degree Laceration	2,785	4.24%	-	3.63%	3.27%

Wright Memorial Hospital

701 East First Street
Trenton, MO 64683

Phone: 660-359-5621

Ownership: Government - Local
Emergency Services: Yes

Accredited: No

Measure	Cases	This Hospital	State Average	U.S. Average	Top Hospital
Heart Attack Care					
ACE Inhibitor or ARB for LVSD[1,3]	2	50%	76%	82%	100%
Aspirin at Arrival[1,3]	3	100%	92%	92%	100%
Aspirin at Discharge[1,3]	1	100%	87%	90%	100%
Beta Blocker at Arrival[1,3]	6	100%	83%	87%	100%
Beta Blocker at Discharge[1,3]	3	100%	87%	90%	100%
Fibrinolytic Medication Timing[1,3]	1	0%	26%	31%	100%
PCI Within 90 Minutes of Arrival[5]	-	-	61%	54%	95%
Smoking Cessation Advice[3]	0	-	92%	88%	100%
Heart Failure Care					
ACE Inhibitor or ARB for LVSD[1,2]	11	91%	84%	82%	100%
Discharge Instructions[2]	27	37%	62%	61%	93%
Evaluation of LVS Function[2]	41	85%	79%	83%	99%
Smoking Cessation Advice[1,2]	5	100%	80%	82%	100%
Pneumonia Care					
Appropriate Initial Antibiotic[2]	36	72%	81%	83%	94%
Blood Culture Timing[1,2]	18	94%	92%	90%	100%
Influenza Vaccine[1]	10	80%	70%	70%	100%
Initial Antibiotic Timing[2]	48	92%	81%	80%	93%
Oxygenation Assessment[2]	54	100%	99%	99%	100%
Pneumococcal Vaccine[2]	38	84%	70%	69%	94%
Smoking Cessation Advice[1,2]	12	100%	83%	80%	100%
Surgical Infection Prevention					
Prophylactic Antibiotic Given[1,2,3]	1	0%	78%	77%	95%
Prophylactic Antibiotic Selection[2]	0	-	91%	90%	100%
Prophylactic Antibiotic Stopped[1,2,3]	1	100%	72%	72%	95%
Pregnancy Care					
Inpatient Neonatal Mortality	-	-	-	-	-
Third or Fourth Degree Laceration	-	-	-	3.63%	3.27%

Lincoln County Medical Center

1000 East Cherry Street
Troy, MO 63379

Phone: 636-528-8551

Ownership: Government - Local
Emergency Services: Yes

Accredited: No

Measure	Cases	This Hospital	State Average	U.S. Average	Top Hospital
Heart Attack Care					
ACE Inhibitor or ARB for LVSD[2]	0	-	76%	82%	100%
Aspirin at Arrival[1,2]	2	50%	92%	92%	100%
Aspirin at Discharge[2]	0	-	87%	90%	100%
Beta Blocker at Arrival[2]	0	-	83%	87%	100%
Beta Blocker at Discharge[2]	0	-	87%	90%	100%
Fibrinolytic Medication Timing[2]	0	-	26%	31%	100%

NOTE: Hospital profiles are in alphabetical order by state, then city, then hospital within the city; Rankings are sorted by rate in descending order and exclude hospitals with less than 25 cases; (1) The number of cases is too small (n<25) for purposes of reliably predicting hospital performance; (2) Measure reflects the hospital's indication that its submission was based upon a sample of its relevant discharges; (3) Rate reflects fewer than the maximum possible quarters of data for the measure; (4) Inaccurate information submitted and suppressed for one or more quarters; (5) No data is available from the hospital for this measure; Please refer to the User's Guide for a full explanation of data

PCI Within 90 Minutes of Arrival[2]	0	-	61%	54%	95%
Smoking Cessation Advice[2]	0	-	92%	88%	100%
Heart Failure Care					
ACE Inhibitor or ARB for LVSD[1,2]	13	92%	84%	82%	100%
Discharge Instructions[1,2]	21	71%	62%	61%	93%
Evaluation of LVS Function[2]	32	91%	79%	83%	99%
Smoking Cessation Advice[1,2]	9	78%	80%	82%	100%
Pneumonia Care					
Appropriate Initial Antibiotic[2]	31	77%	81%	83%	94%
Blood Culture Timing[1,2]	20	100%	92%	90%	100%
Influenza Vaccine[1]	12	83%	70%	70%	100%
Initial Antibiotic Timing[2]	36	83%	81%	80%	93%
Oxygenation Assessment[2]	46	100%	99%	99%	100%
Pneumococcal Vaccine[2]	29	79%	70%	69%	94%
Smoking Cessation Advice[1,2]	10	50%	83%	80%	100%
Surgical Infection Prevention					
Prophylactic Antibiotic Given[2,3]	39	56%	78%	77%	95%
Prophylactic Antibiotic Selection[1,2]	17	88%	91%	90%	100%
Prophylactic Antibiotic Stopped[2,3]	39	36%	72%	72%	95%
Pregnancy Care					
Inpatient Neonatal Mortality	-	-	-	-	-
Third or Fourth Degree Laceration	-	-	-	3.63%	3.27%

Putnam County Memorial Hospital

1926 Oak Street
Unionville, MO 63565
E-mail: rmagers@istlaplata.net
Phone: 660-947-2411
Fax: 660-947-3825
Ownership: Government - Local
Emergency Services: No
Accredited: No
Licensed Beds: 40

Key Personnel:

CEO. . . . . Ray Magers
Chief Medical Staff. . . . . W Stephen Casady
Emergency Room . . . . James Pigg
Infection Control. . . . . Deb Smith, RN
Respiratory . . . . Gayla Webber

Measure	Cases	This Hospital	State Average	U.S. Average	Top Hospital
Heart Attack Care					
ACE Inhibitor or ARB for LVSD[3]	0	-	76%	82%	100%
Aspirin at Arrival[3]	0	-	92%	92%	100%
Aspirin at Discharge[3]	0	-	87%	90%	100%
Beta Blocker at Arrival[3]	0	-	83%	87%	100%
Beta Blocker at Discharge[3]	0	-	87%	90%	100%
Fibrinolytic Medication Timing[3]	0	-	26%	31%	100%
PCI Within 90 Minutes of Arrival	0	-	61%	54%	95%
Smoking Cessation Advice[3]	0	-	92%	88%	100%
Heart Failure Care					
ACE Inhibitor or ARB for LVSD[1,3]	1	100%	84%	82%	100%
Discharge Instructions[1,3]	5	40%	62%	61%	93%
Evaluation of LVS Function[1,3]	10	70%	79%	83%	99%
Smoking Cessation Advice[1,3]	1	0%	80%	82%	100%
Pneumonia Care					
Appropriate Initial Antibiotic[1]	17	94%	81%	83%	94%
Blood Culture Timing	0	-	92%	90%	100%
Influenza Vaccine[1]	6	67%	70%	70%	100%
Initial Antibiotic Timing[1]	23	96%	81%	80%	93%
Oxygenation Assessment	27	100%	99%	99%	100%
Pneumococcal Vaccine[1]	21	62%	70%	69%	94%
Smoking Cessation Advice[1]	6	100%	83%	80%	100%
Surgical Infection Prevention					
Prophylactic Antibiotic Given[5]	-	-	78%	77%	95%
Prophylactic Antibiotic Selection[5]	-	-	91%	90%	100%
Prophylactic Antibiotic Stopped[5]	-	-	72%	72%	95%
Pregnancy Care					
Inpatient Neonatal Mortality	-	-	-	-	-
Third or Fourth Degree Laceration	-	-	-	3.63%	3.27%

Western Missouri Medical Center

403 Burkarth Road
Warrensburg, MO 64093
Phone: 660-747-2500
Fax: 660-747-8455
Ownership: Govt - Hospital District or Authority
Emergency Services: Yes
Accredited: Yes
Licensed Beds: 92

Key Personnel:

President/CEO. . . . . Gregory B Vinardi
Medical Staff President . . . . Linda Pal, MD
Surgery Director. . . . . Judy Kratz
Emergency Room Medical Director . . . . Mike Misko, MD
Emergency Room Director. . . . . Laura Pinson, RN
Infection Control. . . . . Carol Kientzy, RN
ICU . . . . Rosemary Zelazek, RN
OB/GYN/Womens Health. . . . . Renee Schwermer, RN
Respiratory/Cardiopulmonary. . . . . Joe Stockton

Measure	Cases	This Hospital	State Average	U.S. Average	Top Hospital
Heart Attack Care					
ACE Inhibitor or ARB for LVSD[2]	0	-	76%	82%	100%
Aspirin at Arrival[1,2]	5	100%	92%	92%	100%
Aspirin at Discharge[1,2]	2	100%	87%	90%	100%
Beta Blocker at Arrival[1,2]	3	67%	83%	87%	100%
Beta Blocker at Discharge[1,2]	2	50%	87%	90%	100%
Fibrinolytic Medication Timing[2]	0	-	26%	31%	100%
PCI Within 90 Minutes of Arrival[2]	0	-	61%	54%	95%
Smoking Cessation Advice[2]	0	-	92%	88%	100%
Heart Failure Care					
ACE Inhibitor or ARB for LVSD[1,2]	17	65%	84%	82%	100%
Discharge Instructions[2]	67	22%	62%	61%	93%
Evaluation of LVS Function[2]	98	52%	79%	83%	99%
Smoking Cessation Advice[1,2]	16	56%	80%	82%	100%
Pneumonia Care					
Appropriate Initial Antibiotic[2]	74	82%	81%	83%	94%
Blood Culture Timing[2]	59	88%	92%	90%	100%
Influenza Vaccine[1]	21	29%	70%	70%	100%
Initial Antibiotic Timing[2]	96	92%	81%	80%	93%
Oxygenation Assessment[2]	129	98%	99%	99%	100%
Pneumococcal Vaccine[2]	80	30%	70%	69%	94%
Smoking Cessation Advice[2]	35	63%	83%	80%	100%
Surgical Infection Prevention					
Prophylactic Antibiotic Given[2,3]	61	80%	78%	77%	95%
Prophylactic Antibiotic Selection[2]	56	96%	91%	90%	100%
Prophylactic Antibiotic Stopped[2,3]	53	42%	72%	72%	95%
Pregnancy Care					
Inpatient Neonatal Mortality	797	0.13%	-	-	-
Third or Fourth Degree Laceration	629	2.23%	-	3.63%	3.27%

Saint Joseph Hospital of Kirkwood

525 Couch Avenue
Saint Louis, MO 63122
URL: www.stjosephkirkwood.com
Phone: 314-966-1500
Fax: 314-633-4195
Ownership: Voluntary non-profit - Church
Emergency Services: Yes
Accredited: Yes
Licensed Beds: 269

Key Personnel:

President . . . . Sherry Hausmann
Chief of Medical Staff. . . . . Dr Timothy Pratt
Emergency Room . . . . Donna Robinson
Infection Control. . . . . Linda Maly
OB/GYN Womens Health. . . . . Mary Brobst
Director Respiratory Therapy . . . . Warner Buerke

Measure	Cases	This Hospital	State Average	U.S. Average	Top Hospital
Heart Attack Care					
ACE Inhibitor or ARB for LVSD	40	88%	76%	82%	100%
Aspirin at Arrival	137	98%	92%	92%	100%
Aspirin at Discharge	150	97%	87%	90%	100%
Beta Blocker at Arrival	105	99%	83%	87%	100%
Beta Blocker at Discharge	154	98%	87%	90%	100%
Fibrinolytic Medication Timing	0	-	26%	31%	100%
PCI Within 90 Minutes of Arrival[1]	2	50%	61%	54%	95%
Smoking Cessation Advice	38	100%	92%	88%	100%
Heart Failure Care					
ACE Inhibitor or ARB for LVSD	73	96%	84%	82%	100%

NOTE: Hospital profiles are in alphabetical order by state, then city, then hospital within the city; Rankings are sorted by rate in descending order and exclude hospitals with less than 25 cases; (1) The number of cases is too small (n<25) for purposes of reliably predicting hospital performance; (2) Measure reflects the hospital's indication that its submission was based upon a sample of its relevant discharges; (3) Rate reflects fewer than the maximum possible quarters of data for the measure; (4) Inaccurate information submitted and suppressed for one or more quarters; (5) No data is available from the hospital for this measure; Please refer to the User's Guide for a full explanation of data

Discharge Instructions	208	71%	62%	61%	93%
Evaluation of LVS Function	291	97%	79%	83%	99%
Smoking Cessation Advice	25	84%	80%	82%	100%
Pneumonia Care					
Appropriate Initial Antibiotic	189	81%	81%	83%	94%
Blood Culture Timing	192	94%	92%	90%	100%
Influenza Vaccine	61	77%	70%	70%	100%
Initial Antibiotic Timing	231	84%	81%	80%	93%
Oxygenation Assessment	277	100%	99%	99%	100%
Pneumococcal Vaccine	188	85%	70%	69%	94%
Smoking Cessation Advice	60	90%	83%	80%	100%
Surgical Infection Prevention					
Prophylactic Antibiotic Given[3]	643	87%	78%	77%	95%
Prophylactic Antibiotic Selection	224	95%	91%	90%	100%
Prophylactic Antibiotic Stopped[3]	633	89%	72%	72%	95%
Pregnancy Care					
Inpatient Neonatal Mortality	-	-	-	-	-
Third or Fourth Degree Laceration	-	-	-	3.63%	3.27%

Saint John's Mercy Hospital

200 Madison Avenue
Washington, MO 63090
URL: www.stjohnsmercy.org
Ownership: Voluntary non-profit - Church
Emergency Services: Yes
Phone: 636-239-8000
Fax: 314-569-6733
Accredited: Yes
Licensed Beds: 187

Key Personnel:

President/CEO . . . . Michael Zilm
Chief Medical Staff . . . . Thomas B Riechers, MD
Emergency Room . . . . Alan DuMontier
Emergency Room . . . . Robert Mecker, MD
Director Infection/Disease Control . . . . Phyllis Cassette, RN
Director Medical/Surgical Nursing . . . . Vera Haney, RN
OB/GYN Womens Health . . . . Ann Dean
Director of Pulmonary Therapy . . . . Michael Boudimet

Measure	Cases	This Hospital	State Average	U.S. Average	Top Hospital
Heart Attack Care					
ACE Inhibitor or ARB for LVSD[1]	19	84%	76%	82%	100%
Aspirin at Arrival	85	94%	92%	92%	100%
Aspirin at Discharge	60	90%	87%	90%	100%
Beta Blocker at Arrival	55	87%	83%	87%	100%
Beta Blocker at Discharge	43	86%	87%	90%	100%
Fibrinolytic Medication Timing[1]	1	0%	26%	31%	100%
PCI Within 90 Minutes of Arrival	0	-	61%	54%	95%
Smoking Cessation Advice[1]	10	100%	92%	88%	100%
Heart Failure Care					
ACE Inhibitor or ARB for LVSD	79	96%	84%	82%	100%
Discharge Instructions	197	89%	62%	61%	93%
Evaluation of LVS Function	231	99%	79%	83%	99%
Smoking Cessation Advice	36	100%	80%	82%	100%
Pneumonia Care					
Appropriate Initial Antibiotic[2]	183	86%	81%	83%	94%
Blood Culture Timing[2]	129	98%	92%	90%	100%
Influenza Vaccine[2]	58	86%	70%	70%	100%
Initial Antibiotic Timing[2]	222	85%	81%	80%	93%
Oxygenation Assessment[2]	294	100%	99%	99%	100%
Pneumococcal Vaccine[2]	180	90%	70%	69%	94%
Smoking Cessation Advice[2]	71	99%	83%	80%	100%
Surgical Infection Prevention					
Prophylactic Antibiotic Given[2]	354	94%	78%	77%	95%
Prophylactic Antibiotic Selection[2]	36	92%	91%	90%	100%
Prophylactic Antibiotic Stopped[2]	341	98%	72%	72%	95%
Pregnancy Care					
Inpatient Neonatal Mortality	-	-	-	-	-
Third or Fourth Degree Laceration	-	-	-	3.63%	3.27%

Ozarks Medical Center

1100 Kentucky Avenue
West Plains, MO 65775
URL: www.ozarksmedical.com
Ownership: Voluntary non-profit - Other
Emergency Services: Yes
Phone: 417-256-9111
Fax: 417-257-6770
Accredited: Yes
Licensed Beds: 114

Key Personnel:

President/CEO . . . . Philip Bagby
Chief Medical Staff . . . . Jeffrey Roylance, MD
Cardiac Lab . . . . Liz Palomino, RN
Emergency Room . . . . Dennise Lawson, RN
Infection Control . . . . Jill Tate, RN
Manager Medical/Surgical Nursing . . . . Bonnie Sanders, RN
Womens Health Manager . . . . Joanna Patillo, RN
Director Radiology . . . . Stephanie Kernodle
Director Cardiopulmonary Services . . . . Bill Windell

Measure	Cases	This Hospital	State Average	U.S. Average	Top Hospital
Heart Attack Care					
ACE Inhibitor or ARB for LVSD[1]	8	75%	76%	82%	100%
Aspirin at Arrival	53	98%	92%	92%	100%
Aspirin at Discharge	40	95%	87%	90%	100%
Beta Blocker at Arrival	48	88%	83%	87%	100%
Beta Blocker at Discharge	41	88%	87%	90%	100%
Fibrinolytic Medication Timing[1]	4	0%	26%	31%	100%
PCI Within 90 Minutes of Arrival[1]	1	0%	61%	54%	95%
Smoking Cessation Advice[1]	8	62%	92%	88%	100%
Heart Failure Care					
ACE Inhibitor or ARB for LVSD	48	81%	84%	82%	100%
Discharge Instructions	89	37%	62%	61%	93%
Evaluation of LVS Function	140	80%	79%	83%	99%
Smoking Cessation Advice	25	84%	80%	82%	100%
Pneumonia Care					
Appropriate Initial Antibiotic	115	87%	81%	83%	94%
Blood Culture Timing	120	90%	92%	90%	100%
Influenza Vaccine	32	78%	70%	70%	100%
Initial Antibiotic Timing	163	79%	81%	80%	93%
Oxygenation Assessment	204	100%	99%	99%	100%
Pneumococcal Vaccine	118	76%	70%	69%	94%
Smoking Cessation Advice	58	67%	83%	80%	100%
Surgical Infection Prevention					
Prophylactic Antibiotic Given[3]	156	56%	78%	77%	95%
Prophylactic Antibiotic Selection	54	85%	91%	90%	100%
Prophylactic Antibiotic Stopped[3]	131	63%	72%	72%	95%
Pregnancy Care					
Inpatient Neonatal Mortality	-	-	-	-	-
Third or Fourth Degree Laceration	-	-	-	3.63%	3.27%

NOTE: Hospital profiles are in alphabetical order by state, then city, then hospital within the city; Rankings are sorted by rate in descending order and exclude hospitals with less than 25 cases; (1) The number of cases is too small (n<25) for purposes of reliably predicting hospital performance; (2) Measure reflects the hospital's indication that its submission was based upon a sample of its relevant discharges; (3) Rate reflects fewer than the maximum possible quarters of data for the measure; (4) Inaccurate information submitted and suppressed for one or more quarters; (5) No data is available from the hospital for this measure; Please refer to the User's Guide for a full explanation of data

Heart Attack Care

1. ACE Inhibitor or ARB for LVSD

Hospital Name	City	Rate	Cases
Immanuel Medical Center	Omaha	97%	35
Creighton University Medical Center	Omaha	93%	67
Nebraska Heart Hospital	Lincoln	92%	75
Nebraska Medical Center	Omaha	90%	58
Faith Regional Health Services-East Campus	Norfolk	88%	26
Saint Francis Med Ctr/Memorial Health Center	Grand Island	88%	25
Alegent Health Bergen Mercy Medical Center	Omaha	87%	46
Methodist Hospital	Omaha	87%	46
Saint Elizabeth Regional Medical Center	Lincoln	84%	32
Good Samaritan	Kearney	82%	28
BryanLGH Medical Center	Lincoln	81%	78

2. Aspirin at Arrival

Hospital Name	City	Rate	Cases
Alegent Health Bergen Mercy Medical Center	Omaha	100%	166
Alegent Health Lakeside Hospital	Omaha	100%	77
Fremont Area Medical Center	Fremont	100%	36
Immanuel Medical Center	Omaha	100%	106
Alegent Health-Midlands Hospital	Papillion	99%	85
Saint Elizabeth Regional Medical Center	Lincoln	99%	82
Saint Francis Med Ctr/Memorial Health Center	Grand Island	99%	84
Creighton University Medical Center	Omaha	97%	101
Good Samaritan	Kearney	97%	75
Great Plains Regional Medical Center	North Platte	97%	32
Nebraska Medical Center	Omaha	97%	186
Regional West Medical Center	Scottsbluff	97%	32
Methodist Hospital	Omaha	96%	163
BryanLGH Medical Center	Lincoln	95%	164
Faith Regional Health Services-East Campus	Norfolk	95%	57
Mary Lanning Memorial Hospital	Hastings	94%	32

3. Aspirin at Discharge

Hospital Name	City	Rate	Cases
Alegent Health Bergen Mercy Medical Center	Omaha	100%	197
Alegent Health Lakeside Hospital	Omaha	100%	61
Creighton University Medical Center	Omaha	100%	241
Fremont Area Medical Center	Fremont	100%	28
Alegent Health-Midlands Hospital	Papillion	99%	74
Faith Regional Health Services-East Campus	Norfolk	99%	77
Good Samaritan	Kearney	99%	121
Immanuel Medical Center	Omaha	99%	160
Methodist Hospital	Omaha	99%	170
Nebraska Medical Center	Omaha	99%	244
Saint Elizabeth Regional Medical Center	Lincoln	99%	87
Nebraska Heart Hospital	Lincoln	98%	324
BryanLGH Medical Center	Lincoln	97%	325
Saint Francis Med Ctr/Memorial Health Center	Grand Island	97%	73

4. Beta Blocker at Arrival

Hospital Name	City	Rate	Cases
Alegent Health Lakeside Hospital	Omaha	100%	66
Fremont Area Medical Center	Fremont	100%	32
Alegent Health-Midlands Hospital	Papillion	99%	69
Creighton University Medical Center	Omaha	99%	100
Immanuel Medical Center	Omaha	99%	94
Faith Regional Health Services-East Campus	Norfolk	98%	48
Nebraska Medical Center	Omaha	98%	172
Alegent Health Bergen Mercy Medical Center	Omaha	97%	130
BryanLGH Medical Center	Lincoln	97%	118
Saint Elizabeth Regional Medical Center	Lincoln	97%	65
Saint Francis Med Ctr/Memorial Health Center	Grand Island	97%	62
Methodist Hospital	Omaha	94%	137
Good Samaritan	Kearney	84%	58
Mary Lanning Memorial Hospital	Hastings	72%	32

5. Beta Blocker at Discharge

Hospital Name	City	Rate	Cases
Alegent Health Lakeside Hospital	Omaha	100%	66
Creighton University Medical Center	Omaha	100%	288
Faith Regional Health Services-East Campus	Norfolk	100%	88
Fremont Area Medical Center	Fremont	100%	32
Immanuel Medical Center	Omaha	100%	181
Nebraska Medical Center	Omaha	100%	249
Alegent Health Bergen Mercy Medical Center	Omaha	99%	203
Alegent Health-Midlands Hospital	Papillion	99%	71
Good Samaritan	Kearney	98%	134
Methodist Hospital	Omaha	98%	188
Saint Elizabeth Regional Medical Center	Lincoln	98%	85
Nebraska Heart Hospital	Lincoln	97%	310
Saint Francis Med Ctr/Memorial Health Center	Grand Island	96%	72
BryanLGH Medical Center	Lincoln	95%	353

8. Smoking Cessation Advice

Hospital Name	City	Rate	Cases
Alegent Health Bergen Mercy Medical Center	Omaha	100%	71
Alegent Health-Midlands Hospital	Papillion	100%	37
Faith Regional Health Services-East Campus	Norfolk	100%	27
Immanuel Medical Center	Omaha	100%	61
Methodist Hospital	Omaha	100%	49
Nebraska Medical Center	Omaha	99%	105
Creighton University Medical Center	Omaha	98%	80
Good Samaritan	Kearney	98%	57
Saint Elizabeth Regional Medical Center	Lincoln	97%	29
Saint Francis Med Ctr/Memorial Health Center	Grand Island	97%	35
Nebraska Heart Hospital	Lincoln	93%	111
BryanLGH Medical Center	Lincoln	92%	126

Heart Failure Care

9. ACE Inhibitor or ARB for LVSD

Hospital Name	City	Rate	Cases
Alegent Health Lakeside Hospital	Omaha	100%	27
Immanuel Medical Center	Omaha	99%	84
Alegent Health-Midlands Hospital	Papillion	95%	59
Creighton University Medical Center	Omaha	93%	149
Alegent Health Bergen Mercy Medical Center	Omaha	92%	130
Good Samaritan	Kearney	88%	48
Nebraska Heart Hospital	Lincoln	88%	292
Saint Elizabeth Regional Medical Center	Lincoln	88%	60
Methodist Hospital	Omaha	86%	183
Saint Francis Med Ctr/Memorial Health Center	Grand Island	86%	44
BryanLGH Medical Center	Lincoln	85%	278
Faith Regional Health Services-East Campus	Norfolk	83%	66
Nebraska Medical Center	Omaha	79%	177
Great Plains Regional Medical Center	North Platte	77%	31
Mary Lanning Memorial Hospital	Hastings	52%	63

10. Discharge Instructions

Hospital Name	City	Rate	Cases
Alegent Health Lakeside Hospital	Omaha	96%	55
Immanuel Medical Center	Omaha	95%	123
Alegent Health-Midlands Hospital	Papillion	94%	113
Saint Elizabeth Regional Medical Center	Lincoln	91%	95
Alegent Health Bergen Mercy Medical Center	Omaha	89%	276
Box Butte General Hospital	Alliance	89%	35
Saint Francis Med Ctr/Memorial Health Center	Grand Island	87%	107
Creighton University Medical Center	Omaha	86%	271
BryanLGH Medical Center	Lincoln	84%	403
Fremont Area Medical Center	Fremont	82%	39
Nebraska Heart Hospital	Lincoln	82%	323
Great Plains Regional Medical Center	North Platte	78%	91
Methodist Hospital	Omaha	77%	296
Columbus Community Hospital	Columbus	71%	28
Faith Regional Health Services-East Campus	Norfolk	71%	92
Good Samaritan	Kearney	62%	119
Mary Lanning Memorial Hospital	Hastings	59%	95
Nebraska Medical Center	Omaha	59%	271
Regional West Medical Center	Scottsbluff	52%	62
Memorial Hospital	Seward	0%	25

11. Evaluation of LVS Function

Hospital Name	City	Rate	Cases
Alegent Health Lakeside Hospital	Omaha	100%	72
Fremont Area Medical Center	Fremont	100%	68
Howard County Community Hospital	Saint Paul	100%	28
Nebraska Medical Center	Omaha	100%	327
Alegent Health Bergen Mercy Medical Center	Omaha	99%	335
Alegent Health-Midlands Hospital	Papillion	99%	147
Creighton University Medical Center	Omaha	99%	303
Immanuel Medical Center	Omaha	99%	181
Nebraska Heart Hospital	Lincoln	99%	364
Saint Francis Med Ctr/Memorial Health Center	Grand Island	98%	154
Beatrice Community Hospital & Health Center	Beatrice	97%	30
Methodist Hospital	Omaha	97%	374
BryanLGH Medical Center	Lincoln	96%	514
Faith Regional Health Services-East Campus	Norfolk	96%	134
Saint Elizabeth Regional Medical Center	Lincoln	96%	142
Tri-Valley Health System	Cambridge	96%	28
Mary Lanning Memorial Hospital	Hastings	93%	153
Ogallala Community Hospital	Ogallala	93%	28

NOTE: Hospital profiles are in alphabetical order by state, then city, then hospital within the city; Rankings are sorted by rate in descending order and exclude hospitals with less than 25 cases; (1) The number of cases is too small (n<25) for purposes of reliably predicting hospital performance; (2) Measure reflects the hospital's indication that its submission was based upon a sample of its relevant discharges; (3) Rate reflects fewer than the maximum possible quarters of data for the measure; (4) Inaccurate information submitted and suppressed for one or more quarters; (5) No data is available from the hospital for this measure; Please refer to the User's Guide for a full explanation of data

Hospital Name	City	Rate	Cases
Great Plains Regional Medical Center	North Platte	91%	113
Columbus Community Hospital	Columbus	90%	49
Saint Francis Memorial Hospital	West Point	90%	41
Good Samaritan	Kearney	89%	168
Regional West Medical Center	Scottsbluff	84%	88
Jennie M Melham Memorial Medical Center	Broken Bow	83%	29
Tri-County Area Hospital District	Lexington	81%	31
Memorial Hospital	Seward	61%	36
Box Butte General Hospital	Alliance	45%	60

12. Smoking Cessation Advice

Hospital Name	City	Rate	Cases
Alegent Health Bergen Mercy Medical Center	Omaha	100%	49
Alegent Health-Midlands Hospital	Papillion	100%	36
Immanuel Medical Center	Omaha	100%	30
Methodist Hospital	Omaha	100%	46
Creighton University Medical Center	Omaha	96%	75
BryanLGH Medical Center	Lincoln	94%	66
Great Plains Regional Medical Center	North Platte	92%	26
Good Samaritan	Kearney	91%	35
Nebraska Medical Center	Omaha	89%	63
Saint Francis Med Ctr/Memorial Health Center	Grand Island	84%	25
Nebraska Heart Hospital	Lincoln	80%	51

Pneumonia Care

13. Appropriate Initial Antibiotic

Hospital Name	City	Rate	Cases
Harlan County Hospital	Alma	100%	26
Phelps Memorial Health Center	Holdrege	100%	25
Avera Saint Anthony's Hospital	O'Neill	97%	36
Tri-Valley Health System	Cambridge	97%	32
Alegent Health-Midlands Hospital	Papillion	96%	111
Box Butte General Hospital	Alliance	95%	38
Ogallala Community Hospital	Ogallala	95%	41
Alegent Health Bergen Mercy Medical Center	Omaha	94%	171
Alegent Health Lakeside Hospital	Omaha	93%	54
Columbus Community Hospital	Columbus	93%	30
Good Samaritan	Kearney	93%	97
Saint Elizabeth Regional Medical Center	Lincoln	93%	134
Immanuel Medical Center	Omaha	92%	101
Nebraska Medical Center	Omaha	92%	61
Tri-County Area Hospital District	Lexington	92%	48
Community Hospital	McCook	91%	45
Faith Regional Health Services-East Campus	Norfolk	91%	70
Jennie M Melham Memorial Medical Center	Broken Bow	91%	55
Boone County Health Center	Albion	90%	39
Beatrice Community Hospital & Health Center	Beatrice	88%	26
BryanLGH Medical Center	Lincoln	88%	133
Methodist Hospital	Omaha	88%	268
Fremont Area Medical Center	Fremont	87%	95
Mary Lanning Memorial Hospital	Hastings	87%	106
Creighton University Medical Center	Omaha	86%	70
Saint Francis Med Ctr/Memorial Health Center	Grand Island	86%	156
Creighton Area Health Services	Creighton	85%	34
Great Plains Regional Medical Center	North Platte	81%	116
Memorial Hospital	Seward	81%	37
York General Hospital	York	81%	26
Regional West Medical Center	Scottsbluff	80%	66
Memorial Community Hospital	Blair	72%	25

14. Blood Culture Timing

Hospital Name	City	Rate	Cases
Alegent Health Lakeside Hospital	Omaha	100%	53
Faith Regional Health Services-East Campus	Norfolk	100%	71
Memorial Community Hospital	Blair	100%	26
Immanuel Medical Center	Omaha	99%	119
Alegent Health Bergen Mercy Medical Center	Omaha	98%	191
Alegent Health-Midlands Hospital	Papillion	98%	105
Fremont Area Medical Center	Fremont	98%	82
Columbus Community Hospital	Columbus	97%	35
Great Plains Regional Medical Center	North Platte	97%	76
Mary Lanning Memorial Hospital	Hastings	96%	104
BryanLGH Medical Center	Lincoln	95%	149
Creighton University Medical Center	Omaha	94%	96
Saint Francis Med Ctr/Memorial Health Center	Grand Island	93%	165
Good Samaritan	Kearney	92%	60
Methodist Hospital	Omaha	92%	243
Nebraska Medical Center	Omaha	92%	79
Saint Elizabeth Regional Medical Center	Lincoln	90%	101
Regional West Medical Center	Scottsbluff	88%	57
Beatrice Community Hospital & Health Center	Beatrice	78%	27

15. Influenza Vaccine

Hospital Name	City	Rate	Cases
Alegent Health-Midlands Hospital	Papillion	100%	36
Alegent Health Bergen Mercy Medical Center	Omaha	98%	64
Immanuel Medical Center	Omaha	97%	34
BryanLGH Medical Center	Lincoln	92%	61
Jennie M Melham Memorial Medical Center	Broken Bow	85%	27
Fremont Area Medical Center	Fremont	84%	31
Regional West Medical Center	Scottsbluff	82%	34
Great Plains Regional Medical Center	North Platte	81%	36
Mary Lanning Memorial Hospital	Hastings	73%	44
Saint Francis Med Ctr/Memorial Health Center	Grand Island	64%	66
Good Samaritan	Kearney	58%	36

16. Initial Antibiotic Timing

Hospital Name	City	Rate	Cases
Creighton Area Health Services	Creighton	100%	43
Memorial Community Hospital	Blair	100%	31
Saint Francis Memorial Hospital	West Point	100%	26
Valley County Hospital	Ord	100%	36
Jennie M Melham Memorial Medical Center	Broken Bow	99%	86
Alegent Health-Midlands Hospital	Papillion	97%	133
Tri-Valley Health System	Cambridge	97%	32
Alegent Health Lakeside Hospital	Omaha	96%	71
Columbus Community Hospital	Columbus	96%	50
Harlan County Hospital	Alma	96%	28
Jefferson Community Health Center	Fairbury	96%	28
Alegent Health Bergen Mercy Medical Center	Omaha	95%	242
Saint Francis Med Ctr/Memorial Health Center	Grand Island	95%	244
Saunders Medical Center	Wahoo	95%	38
Immanuel Medical Center	Omaha	94%	177
Litzenberg Memorial County Hospital	Central City	94%	32
Boone County Health Center	Albion	93%	57
Gordon Memorial Hospital District	Gordon	93%	27
Memorial Hospital	Seward	92%	51
Thayer County Health Services	Hebron	92%	26
Faith Regional Health Services-East Campus	Norfolk	91%	106
Fremont Area Medical Center	Fremont	91%	122
Ogallala Community Hospital	Ogallala	91%	35
Regional West Medical Center	Scottsbluff	91%	97
Tri-County Area Hospital District	Lexington	91%	75
Community Hospital	McCook	90%	61
Beatrice Community Hospital & Health Center	Beatrice	89%	37
Great Plains Regional Medical Center	North Platte	89%	158
Memorial Hospital	Schuyler	89%	27
Phelps Memorial Health Center	Holdrege	89%	53
Avera Saint Anthony's Hospital	O'Neill	88%	51
Nemaha County Hospital	Auburn	88%	26
York General Hospital	York	88%	25
Good Samaritan	Kearney	87%	136
Saint Elizabeth Regional Medical Center	Lincoln	86%	166
BryanLGH Medical Center	Lincoln	84%	228
Nebraska Medical Center	Omaha	83%	115
Creighton University Medical Center	Omaha	81%	134
Mary Lanning Memorial Hospital	Hastings	80%	172
Memorial Hospital	Aurora	79%	28
Methodist Hospital	Omaha	78%	353
Box Butte General Hospital	Alliance	75%	53
Memorial Health Center	Sidney	68%	28

17. Oxygenation Assessment

Hospital Name	City	Rate	Cases
Alegent Health Bergen Mercy Medical Center	Omaha	100%	328
Alegent Health Lakeside Hospital	Omaha	100%	90
Alegent Health-Midlands Hospital	Papillion	100%	157
Avera Saint Anthony's Hospital	O'Neill	100%	58
Beatrice Community Hospital & Health Center	Beatrice	100%	43
Boone County Health Center	Albion	100%	84
Box Butte General Hospital	Alliance	100%	57
BryanLGH Medical Center	Lincoln	100%	306
Columbus Community Hospital	Columbus	100%	72
Community Hospital	Falls City	100%	25
Community Hospital	McCook	100%	75
Creighton Area Health Services	Creighton	100%	59
Creighton University Medical Center	Omaha	100%	158
Faith Regional Health Services-East Campus	Norfolk	100%	137
Fremont Area Medical Center	Fremont	100%	172
Good Samaritan	Kearney	100%	190
Gordon Memorial Hospital District	Gordon	100%	34
Great Plains Regional Medical Center	North Platte	100%	192
Harlan County Hospital	Alma	100%	30
Howard County Community Hospital	Saint Paul	100%	27
Immanuel Medical Center	Omaha	100%	206

NOTE: Hospital profiles are in alphabetical order by state, then city, then hospital within the city; Rankings are sorted by rate in descending order and exclude hospitals with less than 25 cases; (1) The number of cases is too small (n<25) for purposes of reliably predicting hospital performance; (2) Measure reflects the hospital's indication that its submission was based upon a sample of its relevant discharges; (3) Rate reflects fewer than the maximum possible quarters of data for the measure; (4) Inaccurate information submitted and suppressed for one or more quarters; (5) No data is available from the hospital for this measure; Please refer to the User's Guide for a full explanation of data

Hospital Name	City	Rate	Cases
Jefferson Community Health Center	Fairbury	100%	33
Jennie M Melham Memorial Medical Center	Broken Bow	100%	123
Memorial Community Hospital	Blair	100%	44
Memorial Health Center	Sidney	100%	32
Memorial Hospital	Schuyler	100%	33
Memorial Hospital	Seward	100%	62
Nebraska Medical Center	Omaha	100%	149
Nemaha County Hospital	Auburn	100%	33
Ogallala Community Hospital	Ogallala	100%	45
Perkins County Health Services	Grant	100%	26
Phelps Memorial Health Center	Holdrege	100%	62
Regional West Medical Center	Scottsbluff	100%	121
Saint Elizabeth Regional Medical Center	Lincoln	100%	199
Saint Francis Med Ctr/Memorial Health Center	Grand Island	100%	330
Saint Francis Memorial Hospital	West Point	100%	32
Saunders Medical Center	Wahoo	100%	44
Thayer County Health Services	Hebron	100%	32
Tri-Valley Health System	Cambridge	100%	47
Valley County Hospital	Ord	100%	42
Webster County Community Hospital	Red Cloud	100%	40
York General Hospital	York	100%	35
Mary Lanning Memorial Hospital	Hastings	99%	221
Methodist Hospital	Omaha	99%	473
Tri-County Area Hospital District	Lexington	99%	90
Memorial Hospital	Aurora	97%	33
Litzenberg Memorial County Hospital	Central City	94%	34

18. Pneumococcal Vaccine

Hospital Name	City	Rate	Cases
Alegent Health-Midlands Hospital	Papillion	100%	100
Jefferson Community Health Center	Fairbury	100%	28
Alegent Health Bergen Mercy Medical Center	Omaha	99%	216
Alegent Health Lakeside Hospital	Omaha	98%	57
Faith Regional Health Services-East Campus	Norfolk	98%	101
Immanuel Medical Center	Omaha	98%	133
Beatrice Community Hospital & Health Center	Beatrice	97%	29
Saunders Medical Center	Wahoo	97%	35
Jennie M Melham Memorial Medical Center	Broken Bow	96%	92
York General Hospital	York	96%	26
BryanLGH Medical Center	Lincoln	92%	226
Saint Francis Memorial Hospital	West Point	92%	26
Columbus Community Hospital	Columbus	91%	54
Regional West Medical Center	Scottsbluff	89%	80
Saint Elizabeth Regional Medical Center	Lincoln	89%	138
Perkins County Health Services	Grant	88%	25
Tri-County Area Hospital District	Lexington	87%	61
Gordon Memorial Hospital District	Gordon	86%	28
Creighton University Medical Center	Omaha	85%	71
Good Samaritan	Kearney	85%	137
Memorial Community Hospital	Blair	84%	32
Saint Francis Med Ctr/Memorial Health Center	Grand Island	83%	207
Phelps Memorial Health Center	Holdrege	82%	38
Ogallala Community Hospital	Ogallala	81%	26
Boone County Health Center	Albion	80%	60
Memorial Hospital	Schuyler	76%	25
Community Hospital	McCook	75%	56
Methodist Hospital	Omaha	75%	317
Great Plains Regional Medical Center	North Platte	72%	130
Litzenberg Memorial County Hospital	Central City	72%	25
Creighton Area Health Services	Creighton	70%	50
Fremont Area Medical Center	Fremont	70%	115
Valley County Hospital	Ord	69%	35
Mary Lanning Memorial Hospital	Hastings	67%	159
Avera Saint Anthony's Hospital	O'Neill	62%	37
Tri-Valley Health System	Cambridge	62%	37
Webster County Community Hospital	Red Cloud	57%	30
Nebraska Medical Center	Omaha	55%	78
Box Butte General Hospital	Alliance	20%	40
Memorial Hospital	Seward	7%	42

19. Smoking Cessation Advice

Hospital Name	City	Rate	Cases
Alegent Health Bergen Mercy Medical Center	Omaha	100%	61
Alegent Health-Midlands Hospital	Papillion	100%	38
Great Plains Regional Medical Center	North Platte	100%	45
Immanuel Medical Center	Omaha	98%	58
Creighton University Medical Center	Omaha	97%	61
Good Samaritan	Kearney	92%	52
Saint Francis Med Ctr/Memorial Health Center	Grand Island	92%	52
Methodist Hospital	Omaha	91%	78
Fremont Area Medical Center	Fremont	89%	35
BryanLGH Medical Center	Lincoln	85%	62
Faith Regional Health Services-East Campus	Norfolk	76%	29
Nebraska Medical Center	Omaha	74%	35
Saint Elizabeth Regional Medical Center	Lincoln	69%	45
Regional West Medical Center	Scottsbluff	68%	28
Mary Lanning Memorial Hospital	Hastings	62%	26

Surgical Infection Prevention

20. Prophylactic Antibiotic Given

Hospital Name	City	Rate	Cases
Jefferson Community Health Center	Fairbury	98%	46
York General Hospital	York	98%	52
Fremont Area Medical Center	Fremont	97%	231
Nebraska Heart Hospital	Lincoln	95%	85
Alegent Health Bergen Mercy Medical Center	Omaha	94%	814
Columbus Community Hospital	Columbus	94%	205
Immanuel Medical Center	Omaha	94%	367
Nebraska Orthopaedic Hospital	Omaha	94%	194
Saint Francis Med Ctr/Memorial Health Center	Grand Island	94%	598
BryanLGH Medical Center	Lincoln	93%	843
Alegent Health Lakeside Hospital	Omaha	92%	146
Good Samaritan	Kearney	91%	686
Methodist Hospital	Omaha	91%	408
Alegent Health-Midlands Hospital	Papillion	90%	112
Faith Regional Health Services-East Campus	Norfolk	90%	472
Saint Francis Memorial Hospital	West Point	89%	47
Tri-County Area Hospital District	Lexington	89%	36
Beatrice Community Hospital & Health Center	Beatrice	88%	85
Great Plains Regional Medical Center	North Platte	88%	170
Lincoln Surgical Hospital	Lincoln	87%	157
Saint Elizabeth Regional Medical Center	Lincoln	86%	1123
Creighton University Medical Center	Omaha	84%	453
Nebraska Medical Center	Omaha	80%	544
Community Hospital	McCook	75%	99
Phelps Memorial Health Center	Holdrege	75%	61
Mary Lanning Memorial Hospital	Hastings	73%	324
Regional West Medical Center	Scottsbluff	72%	381
Boone County Health Center	Albion	57%	28

21. Prophylactic Antibiotic Selection

Hospital Name	City	Rate	Cases
Alegent Health Bergen Mercy Medical Center	Omaha	100%	79
Community Hospital	McCook	100%	27
Methodist Hospital	Omaha	100%	101
Nebraska Heart Hospital	Lincoln	100%	35
Nebraska Orthopaedic Hospital	Omaha	100%	33
Regional West Medical Center	Scottsbluff	100%	116
Faith Regional Health Services-East Campus	Norfolk	99%	152
Great Plains Regional Medical Center	North Platte	98%	54
Lincoln Surgical Hospital	Lincoln	98%	54
Alegent Health-Midlands Hospital	Papillion	97%	30
Good Samaritan	Kearney	97%	209
Nebraska Medical Center	Omaha	96%	75
Saint Francis Med Ctr/Memorial Health Center	Grand Island	96%	151
Columbus Community Hospital	Columbus	95%	39
Fremont Area Medical Center	Fremont	94%	80
Immanuel Medical Center	Omaha	94%	65
Saint Elizabeth Regional Medical Center	Lincoln	94%	375
Mary Lanning Memorial Hospital	Hastings	93%	111
BryanLGH Medical Center	Lincoln	90%	225
Alegent Health Lakeside Hospital	Omaha	89%	28
Creighton University Medical Center	Omaha	86%	86

22. Prophylactic Antibiotic Stopped

Hospital Name	City	Rate	Cases
Jefferson Community Health Center	Fairbury	98%	43
York General Hospital	York	98%	51
Boone County Health Center	Albion	96%	26
Saint Francis Memorial Hospital	West Point	96%	45
Alegent Health Bergen Mercy Medical Center	Omaha	94%	785
Mary Lanning Memorial Hospital	Hastings	94%	310
Alegent Health-Midlands Hospital	Papillion	93%	107
Alegent Health Lakeside Hospital	Omaha	92%	142
Community Hospital	McCook	92%	97
Immanuel Medical Center	Omaha	92%	353
Columbus Community Hospital	Columbus	91%	198
Nebraska Medical Center	Omaha	91%	523
Faith Regional Health Services-East Campus	Norfolk	89%	453
Fremont Area Medical Center	Fremont	88%	231
Methodist Hospital	Omaha	88%	392
Nebraska Heart Hospital	Lincoln	88%	81
Nebraska Orthopaedic Hospital	Omaha	88%	190
Saint Elizabeth Regional Medical Center	Lincoln	86%	1090
BryanLGH Medical Center	Lincoln	84%	803
Lincoln Surgical Hospital	Lincoln	82%	157

NOTE: Hospital profiles are in alphabetical order by state, then city, then hospital within the city; Rankings are sorted by rate in descending order and exclude hospitals with less than 25 cases; (1) The number of cases is too small (n<25) for purposes of reliably predicting hospital performance; (2) Measure reflects the hospital's indication that its submission was based upon a sample of its relevant discharges; (3) Rate reflects fewer than the maximum possible quarters of data for the measure; (4) Inaccurate information submitted and suppressed for one or more quarters; (5) No data is available from the hospital for this measure; Please refer to the User's Guide for a full explanation of data

Good Samaritan	Kearney	78%	671
Regional West Medical Center	Scottsbluff	75%	375
Saint Francis Med Ctr/Memorial Health Center	Grand Island	71%	579
Phelps Memorial Health Center	Holdrege	69%	59
Great Plains Regional Medical Center	North Platte	60%	167
Creighton University Medical Center	Omaha	59%	448
Tri-County Area Hospital District	Lexington	49%	35
Beatrice Community Hospital & Health Center	Beatrice	44%	85

Pregnancy Care

23. Inpatient Neonatal Mortality

Hospital Name	City	Rate	Cases
Regional West Medical Center	Scottsbluff	0.00%	845
Methodist Hospital	Omaha	0.36%	1682
Nebraska Medical Center	Omaha	0.51%	590

24. Third or Fourth Degree Laceration

Hospital Name	City	Rate	Cases
Regional West Medical Center	Scottsbluff	2.69%	668
Nebraska Medical Center	Omaha	2.87%	2023
Methodist Hospital	Omaha	5.76%	2447

NOTE: Hospital profiles are in alphabetical order by state, then city, then hospital within the city; Rankings are sorted by rate in descending order and exclude hospitals with less than 25 cases; (1) The number of cases is too small (n<25) for purposes of reliably predicting hospital performance; (2) Measure reflects the hospital's indication that its submission was based upon a sample of its relevant discharges; (3) Rate reflects fewer than the maximum possible quarters of data for the measure; (4) Inaccurate information submitted and suppressed for one or more quarters; (5) No data is available from the hospital for this measure; Please refer to the User's Guide for a full explanation of data

Brown County Hospital

945 E Zero Street
Ainsworth, NE 69210
Ownership: Government - Local
Emergency Services: Yes
Phone: 402-387-2800
Fax: 402-387-2804
Accredited: No
Licensed Beds: 25

Key Personnel:
Chief Medical Staff . . . . Shobha Dixit, MD
Infection Control . . . . Maureen Jackman

Measure	Cases	This Hospital	State Average	U.S. Average	Top Hospital
Heart Attack Care					
ACE Inhibitor or ARB for LVSD[5]	-	-	90%	82%	100%
Aspirin at Arrival[5]	-	-	88%	92%	100%
Aspirin at Discharge[5]	-	-	90%	90%	100%
Beta Blocker at Arrival[5]	-	-	81%	87%	100%
Beta Blocker at Discharge[5]	-	-	95%	90%	100%
Fibrinolytic Medication Timing[5]	-	-	25%	31%	100%
PCI Within 90 Minutes of Arrival[5]	-	-	83%	54%	95%
Smoking Cessation Advice[5]	-	-	84%	88%	100%
Heart Failure Care					
ACE Inhibitor or ARB for LVSD[3]	0	-	76%	82%	100%
Discharge Instructions[1,3]	2	0%	54%	61%	93%
Evaluation of LVS Function[1,3]	2	0%	72%	83%	99%
Smoking Cessation Advice[3]	0	-	62%	82%	100%
Pneumonia Care					
Appropriate Initial Antibiotic[1]	11	91%	90%	83%	94%
Blood Culture Timing[1]	1	100%	96%	90%	100%
Influenza Vaccine[1]	3	100%	77%	70%	100%
Initial Antibiotic Timing[1]	15	87%	91%	80%	93%
Oxygenation Assessment[1]	19	100%	97%	99%	100%
Pneumococcal Vaccine[1]	15	40%	70%	69%	94%
Smoking Cessation Advice[1]	4	50%	64%	80%	100%
Surgical Infection Prevention					
Prophylactic Antibiotic Given[5]	-	-	79%	77%	95%
Prophylactic Antibiotic Selection[5]	-	-	94%	90%	100%
Prophylactic Antibiotic Stopped[5]	-	-	83%	72%	95%
Pregnancy Care					
Inpatient Neonatal Mortality	-	-	-	-	-
Third or Fourth Degree Laceration	-	-	-	3.63%	3.27%

Boone County Health Center

Alternate Name: Boone County Community Hospital
723 W Fairview
Albion, NE 68620
Ownership: Government - Local
Emergency Services: Yes
Phone: 402-395-2191
Fax: 402-395-5165
Accredited: No
Licensed Beds: 34

Key Personnel:
Administrator . . . . Gayle Primrose
Chief Medical Staff . . . . Bradley Hupp, MD
Director Respiratory Therapy . . . . Betty Schwalm

Measure	Cases	This Hospital	State Average	U.S. Average	Top Hospital
Heart Attack Care					
ACE Inhibitor or ARB for LVSD[1]	2	100%	90%	82%	100%
Aspirin at Arrival[1]	7	86%	88%	92%	100%
Aspirin at Discharge[1]	7	86%	90%	90%	100%
Beta Blocker at Arrival[1]	10	90%	81%	87%	100%
Beta Blocker at Discharge[1]	7	100%	95%	90%	100%
Fibrinolytic Medication Timing	0	-	25%	31%	100%
PCI Within 90 Minutes of Arrival	0	-	83%	54%	95%
Smoking Cessation Advice[1]	1	100%	84%	88%	100%
Heart Failure Care					
ACE Inhibitor or ARB for LVSD[1]	9	89%	76%	82%	100%
Discharge Instructions[1]	13	8%	54%	61%	93%
Evaluation of LVS Function[1]	24	83%	72%	83%	99%
Smoking Cessation Advice[1]	1	0%	62%	82%	100%
Pneumonia Care					
Appropriate Initial Antibiotic	39	90%	90%	83%	94%
Blood Culture Timing[1]	11	100%	96%	90%	100%
Influenza Vaccine[1]	16	75%	77%	70%	100%
Initial Antibiotic Timing	57	93%	91%	80%	93%
Oxygenation Assessment	84	100%	97%	99%	100%
Pneumococcal Vaccine	60	80%	70%	69%	94%
Smoking Cessation Advice[1]	11	64%	64%	80%	100%
Surgical Infection Prevention					
Prophylactic Antibiotic Given	28	57%	79%	77%	95%
Prophylactic Antibiotic Selection[1]	5	100%	94%	90%	100%
Prophylactic Antibiotic Stopped	26	96%	83%	72%	95%
Pregnancy Care					
Inpatient Neonatal Mortality	-	-	-	-	-
Third or Fourth Degree Laceration	-	-	-	3.63%	3.27%

Box Butte General Hospital

2101 Box Butte Avenue
PO Box 810
Alliance, NE 69301
E-mail: boxbutte@btigate.com
URL: www.bbgh.org
Ownership: Government - Local
Emergency Services: Yes
Phone: 308-762-6660
Fax: 308-762-1923
Accredited: Yes
Licensed Beds: 44

Key Personnel:
CEO . . . . Dan Griess
ER Coordinator . . . . Larry Steele, RN
Director Infection/Disease Control . . . . Mary Mockerman
Director Medical/Surgical Nursing . . . . Ellen Murray
Respiratory Therapy Manager . . . . Robyn Larvie, RRT

Measure	Cases	This Hospital	State Average	U.S. Average	Top Hospital
Heart Attack Care					
ACE Inhibitor or ARB for LVSD[3]	0	-	90%	82%	100%
Aspirin at Arrival[1,3]	5	80%	88%	92%	100%
Aspirin at Discharge[1,3]	5	80%	90%	90%	100%
Beta Blocker at Arrival[1,3]	3	33%	81%	87%	100%
Beta Blocker at Discharge[1,3]	5	40%	95%	90%	100%
Fibrinolytic Medication Timing[3]	0	-	25%	31%	100%
PCI Within 90 Minutes of Arrival[5]	-	-	83%	54%	95%
Smoking Cessation Advice[1,3]	1	0%	84%	88%	100%
Heart Failure Care					
ACE Inhibitor or ARB for LVSD[1]	4	75%	76%	82%	100%
Discharge Instructions	35	89%	54%	61%	93%
Evaluation of LVS Function	60	45%	72%	83%	99%
Smoking Cessation Advice[1]	6	33%	62%	82%	100%
Pneumonia Care					
Appropriate Initial Antibiotic	38	95%	90%	83%	94%
Blood Culture Timing[1]	11	100%	96%	90%	100%
Influenza Vaccine[1]	15	13%	77%	70%	100%
Initial Antibiotic Timing	53	75%	91%	80%	93%
Oxygenation Assessment	57	100%	97%	99%	100%
Pneumococcal Vaccine	40	20%	70%	69%	94%
Smoking Cessation Advice[1]	11	18%	64%	80%	100%
Surgical Infection Prevention					
Prophylactic Antibiotic Given[5]	-	-	79%	77%	95%
Prophylactic Antibiotic Selection[5]	-	-	94%	90%	100%
Prophylactic Antibiotic Stopped[5]	-	-	83%	72%	95%
Pregnancy Care					
Inpatient Neonatal Mortality	-	-	-	-	-
Third or Fourth Degree Laceration	-	-	-	3.63%	3.27%

Harlan County Hospital

717 N Brown
Alma, NE 68920
Ownership: Government - Local
Emergency Services: No
Phone: 308-928-2151
Fax: 308-928-2774
Accredited: No
Licensed Beds: 25

Key Personnel:
Administrator . . . . Allen VanDriel
Director Infection/Disease Control . . . . Sharee Ring, RN

Measure	Cases	This Hospital	State Average	U.S. Average	Top Hospital
Heart Attack Care					
ACE Inhibitor or ARB for LVSD[3]	0	-	90%	82%	100%
Aspirin at Arrival[1,3]	2	50%	88%	92%	100%
Aspirin at Discharge[3]	0	-	90%	90%	100%
Beta Blocker at Arrival[1,3]	2	0%	81%	87%	100%
Beta Blocker at Discharge[3]	0	-	95%	90%	100%

NOTE: Hospital profiles are in alphabetical order by state, then city, then hospital within the city; Rankings are sorted by rate in descending order and exclude hospitals with less than 25 cases; (1) The number of cases is too small (n<25) for purposes of reliably predicting hospital performance; (2) Measure reflects the hospital's indication that its submission was based upon a sample of its relevant discharges; (3) Rate reflects fewer than the maximum possible quarters of data for the measure; (4) Inaccurate information submitted and suppressed for one or more quarters; (5) No data is available from the hospital for this measure; Please refer to the User's Guide for a full explanation of data

Fibrinolytic Medication Timing[3]	0	-	25%	31%	100%
PCI Within 90 Minutes of Arrival[5]	-	-	83%	54%	95%
Smoking Cessation Advice[3]	0	-	84%	88%	100%
Heart Failure Care					
ACE Inhibitor or ARB for LVSD	0	-	76%	82%	100%
Discharge Instructions[1]	3	33%	54%	61%	93%
Evaluation of LVS Function[1]	3	33%	72%	83%	99%
Smoking Cessation Advice[1]	1	0%	62%	82%	100%
Pneumonia Care					
Appropriate Initial Antibiotic	26	100%	90%	83%	94%
Blood Culture Timing[1]	4	75%	96%	90%	100%
Influenza Vaccine[1]	9	44%	77%	70%	100%
Initial Antibiotic Timing	28	96%	91%	80%	93%
Oxygenation Assessment	30	100%	97%	99%	100%
Pneumococcal Vaccine[1]	23	35%	70%	69%	94%
Smoking Cessation Advice[1]	7	0%	64%	80%	100%
Surgical Infection Prevention					
Prophylactic Antibiotic Given[5]	-	-	79%	77%	95%
Prophylactic Antibiotic Selection[5]	-	-	94%	90%	100%
Prophylactic Antibiotic Stopped[5]	-	-	83%	72%	95%
Pregnancy Care					
Inpatient Neonatal Mortality	-	-	-	-	-
Third or Fourth Degree Laceration	-	-	-	3.63%	3.27%

Nemaha County Hospital

2022 13th Street
Auburn, NE 68305
E-mail: nc00123@navix.net
Ownership: Government - Local
Emergency Services: Yes

Phone: 402-274-4366
Fax: 402-274-4399
Accredited: No
Licensed Beds: 32

Key Personnel:

CEO. . . . . Martin Fattig
Chief Medical Staff. . . . . Mike Zaruba
Director Infection/Disease Control . . . . Pam John
CCU Spvg. Nurse . . . . Susan Joy
Director Medical/Surgical Nursing . . . . Kermit Moore
Chief Radiology . . . . Ken Rogge
Director Respiratory Therapy . . . . Ken Rogge

Measure	Cases	This Hospital	State Average	U.S. Average	Top Hospital
Heart Attack Care					
ACE Inhibitor or ARB for LVSD[5]	-	-	90%	82%	100%
Aspirin at Arrival[5]	-	-	88%	92%	100%
Aspirin at Discharge[5]	-	-	90%	90%	100%
Beta Blocker at Arrival[5]	-	-	81%	87%	100%
Beta Blocker at Discharge[5]	-	-	95%	90%	100%
Fibrinolytic Medication Timing[5]	-	-	25%	31%	100%
PCI Within 90 Minutes of Arrival[5]	-	-	83%	54%	95%
Smoking Cessation Advice[5]	-	-	84%	88%	100%
Heart Failure Care					
ACE Inhibitor or ARB for LVSD[1]	2	100%	76%	82%	100%
Discharge Instructions[1]	6	33%	54%	61%	93%
Evaluation of LVS Function[1]	7	86%	72%	83%	99%
Smoking Cessation Advice[1]	1	100%	62%	82%	100%
Pneumonia Care					
Appropriate Initial Antibiotic[1]	11	91%	90%	83%	94%
Blood Culture Timing[1]	3	100%	96%	90%	100%
Influenza Vaccine[1]	7	86%	77%	70%	100%
Initial Antibiotic Timing	26	88%	91%	80%	93%
Oxygenation Assessment	33	100%	97%	99%	100%
Pneumococcal Vaccine[1]	20	50%	70%	69%	94%
Smoking Cessation Advice[1]	4	25%	64%	80%	100%
Surgical Infection Prevention					
Prophylactic Antibiotic Given[1,3]	5	80%	79%	77%	95%
Prophylactic Antibiotic Selection[1]	4	100%	94%	90%	100%
Prophylactic Antibiotic Stopped[1,3]	5	80%	83%	72%	95%
Pregnancy Care					
Inpatient Neonatal Mortality	-	-	-	-	-
Third or Fourth Degree Laceration	-	-	-	3.63%	3.27%

Memorial Hospital

Alternate Name: Memorial Community Health

1423 7th Street
Aurora, NE 68818
URL: www.memorialcommunityhealth.net
Ownership: Voluntary non-profit - Private
Emergency Services: Yes

Phone: 402-694-3171
Fax: 402-694-3177
Accredited: No
Licensed Beds: 75

Key Personnel:

CEO. . . . . Diane Keller
Chief Medical Staff. . . . . John Wilcox, MD
Director Emergency Room. . . . . Chaeryl Ericson
Infection Control. . . . . Laurie Andrews
Medical Surgical Nursing . . . . Cheryl Erickson
OB/GYN/Women's Health . . . . Ann Oswald
Director of Pulmonary . . . . Glenda Schepers

Measure	Cases	This Hospital	State Average	U.S. Average	Top Hospital
Heart Attack Care					
ACE Inhibitor or ARB for LVSD[3]	0	-	90%	82%	100%
Aspirin at Arrival[1,3]	1	100%	88%	92%	100%
Aspirin at Discharge[3]	0	-	90%	90%	100%
Beta Blocker at Arrival[1,3]	3	33%	81%	87%	100%
Beta Blocker at Discharge[1,3]	3	67%	95%	90%	100%
Fibrinolytic Medication Timing[3]	0	-	25%	31%	100%
PCI Within 90 Minutes of Arrival	0	-	83%	54%	95%
Smoking Cessation Advice[3]	0	-	84%	88%	100%
Heart Failure Care					
ACE Inhibitor or ARB for LVSD[1]	7	86%	76%	82%	100%
Discharge Instructions[1]	8	75%	54%	61%	93%
Evaluation of LVS Function[1]	14	86%	72%	83%	99%
Smoking Cessation Advice[1]	2	0%	62%	82%	100%
Pneumonia Care					
Appropriate Initial Antibiotic[1]	17	88%	90%	83%	94%
Blood Culture Timing[1]	2	100%	96%	90%	100%
Influenza Vaccine[1]	4	100%	77%	70%	100%
Initial Antibiotic Timing	28	79%	91%	80%	93%
Oxygenation Assessment	33	97%	97%	99%	100%
Pneumococcal Vaccine[1]	19	95%	70%	69%	94%
Smoking Cessation Advice[1]	5	100%	64%	80%	100%
Surgical Infection Prevention					
Prophylactic Antibiotic Given[1]	8	100%	79%	77%	95%
Prophylactic Antibiotic Selection[1]	2	50%	94%	90%	100%
Prophylactic Antibiotic Stopped[1]	8	88%	83%	72%	95%
Pregnancy Care					
Inpatient Neonatal Mortality	-	-	-	-	-
Third or Fourth Degree Laceration	-	-	-	3.63%	3.27%

Rock County Hospital

HC 75
Box 300
Bassett, NE 68714
E-mail: rch@huntel.net
Ownership: Govt - Hospital District or Authority
Emergency Services: Yes

Phone: 402-684-3366
Fax: 402-684-3677
Accredited: No
Licensed Beds: 17

Key Personnel:

Administrator . . . . Stacey A Knox
Chief Medical Staff. . . . . John Cherry, MD
Emergency Room . . . . Teresa Patrick, RN, MSN
Director Infection/Disease Control . . . . Barb Kaup
Director Radiology . . . . Marilyn Luna

Measure	Cases	This Hospital	State Average	U.S. Average	Top Hospital
Heart Attack Care					
ACE Inhibitor or ARB for LVSD[5]	-	-	90%	82%	100%
Aspirin at Arrival[5]	-	-	88%	92%	100%
Aspirin at Discharge[5]	-	-	90%	90%	100%
Beta Blocker at Arrival[5]	-	-	81%	87%	100%
Beta Blocker at Discharge[5]	-	-	95%	90%	100%
Fibrinolytic Medication Timing[5]	-	-	25%	31%	100%
PCI Within 90 Minutes of Arrival[5]	-	-	83%	54%	95%
Smoking Cessation Advice[5]	-	-	84%	88%	100%
Heart Failure Care					
ACE Inhibitor or ARB for LVSD[5]	-	-	76%	82%	100%
Discharge Instructions[5]	-	-	54%	61%	93%
Evaluation of LVS Function[5]	-	-	72%	83%	99%

NOTE: Hospital profiles are in alphabetical order by state, then city, then hospital within the city; Rankings are sorted by rate in descending order and exclude hospitals with less than 25 cases; (1) The number of cases is too small (n<25) for purposes of reliably predicting hospital performance; (2) Measure reflects the hospital's indication that its submission was based upon a sample of its relevant discharges; (3) Rate reflects fewer than the maximum possible quarters of data for the measure; (4) Inaccurate information submitted and suppressed for one or more quarters; (5) No data is available from the hospital for this measure; Please refer to the User's Guide for a full explanation of data

Smoking Cessation Advice[5]	-	-	62%	82%	100%
Pneumonia Care					
Appropriate Initial Antibiotic[1,3]	1	100%	90%	83%	94%
Blood Culture Timing[3]	0	-	96%	90%	100%
Influenza Vaccine[5]	-	-	77%	70%	100%
Initial Antibiotic Timing[1,3]	2	100%	91%	80%	93%
Oxygenation Assessment[1,3]	2	50%	97%	99%	100%
Pneumococcal Vaccine[1,3]	1	0%	70%	69%	94%
Smoking Cessation Advice[3]	0	-	64%	80%	100%
Surgical Infection Prevention					
Prophylactic Antibiotic Given[5]	-	-	79%	77%	95%
Prophylactic Antibiotic Selection[5]	-	-	94%	90%	100%
Prophylactic Antibiotic Stopped[5]	-	-	83%	72%	95%
Pregnancy Care					
Inpatient Neonatal Mortality	-	-	-	-	-
Third or Fourth Degree Laceration	-	-	-	3.63%	3.27%

Beatrice Community Hospital & Health Center

1110 N 10th Street
Beatrice, NE 68310
Phone: 402-228-3344
Fax: 402-223-7299
E-mail: info@bchhc.org
URL: www.beatricecommunityhospital.com
Ownership: Voluntary non-profit - Private
Accredited: Yes
Emergency Services: Yes
Licensed Beds: 47

Key Personnel:

CEO. . . . . Thomas Sommers
Chief Medical Staff. . . . . Darin Hoffman
Director Emergency Room. . . . . Jay Crowder, MD
Director Infection Control . . . . Rose Wischmeir
ICU . . . . Sue Schouboe, RN
Intensive Coronary. . . . . Sue Schouboe
OB/GYN Women's Health . . . . Ruth Claassen, RN
CEO. . . . . Larry Emerson
Respiratory/Cardiopulmonary. . . . . Keith Luedders

Measure	Cases	This Hospital	State Average	U.S. Average	Top Hospital
Heart Attack Care					
ACE Inhibitor or ARB for LVSD[3]	0	-	90%	82%	100%
Aspirin at Arrival[1,3]	1	100%	88%	92%	100%
Aspirin at Discharge[1,3]	1	100%	90%	90%	100%
Beta Blocker at Arrival[3]	0	-	81%	87%	100%
Beta Blocker at Discharge[1,3]	1	100%	95%	90%	100%
Fibrinolytic Medication Timing[3]	0	-	25%	31%	100%
PCI Within 90 Minutes of Arrival[5]	-	-	83%	54%	95%
Smoking Cessation Advice[3]	0	-	84%	88%	100%
Heart Failure Care					
ACE Inhibitor or ARB for LVSD[1]	8	88%	76%	82%	100%
Discharge Instructions[1]	22	86%	54%	61%	93%
Evaluation of LVS Function	30	97%	72%	83%	99%
Smoking Cessation Advice[1]	5	60%	62%	82%	100%
Pneumonia Care					
Appropriate Initial Antibiotic	26	88%	90%	83%	94%
Blood Culture Timing	27	78%	96%	90%	100%
Influenza Vaccine[1]	10	100%	77%	70%	100%
Initial Antibiotic Timing	37	89%	91%	80%	93%
Oxygenation Assessment	43	100%	97%	99%	100%
Pneumococcal Vaccine	29	97%	70%	69%	94%
Smoking Cessation Advice[1]	5	40%	64%	80%	100%
Surgical Infection Prevention					
Prophylactic Antibiotic Given	85	88%	79%	77%	95%
Prophylactic Antibiotic Selection[1]	15	93%	94%	90%	100%
Prophylactic Antibiotic Stopped	85	44%	83%	72%	95%
Pregnancy Care					
Inpatient Neonatal Mortality	-	-	-	-	-
Third or Fourth Degree Laceration	-	-	-	3.63%	3.27%

Beatrice State Developmental Center

3000 Lincoln Boulevard
PO Box 808
Beatrice, NE 68310
Toll-Free: 800-430-5755
Phone: 402-223-6600
Fax: 402-223-6150
URL: www.hhs.state.ne.us
Ownership: Government - State
Accredited: No
Emergency Services: No
Licensed Beds: 31

Key Personnel:

CEO. . . . . Nancy Montanez
Chief Medical Staff. . . . . Hal Thaut

Measure	Cases	This Hospital	State Average	U.S. Average	Top Hospital
Heart Attack Care					
ACE Inhibitor or ARB for LVSD[5]	-	-	90%	82%	100%
Aspirin at Arrival[5]	-	-	88%	92%	100%
Aspirin at Discharge[5]	-	-	90%	90%	100%
Beta Blocker at Arrival[5]	-	-	81%	87%	100%
Beta Blocker at Discharge[5]	-	-	95%	90%	100%
Fibrinolytic Medication Timing[5]	-	-	25%	31%	100%
PCI Within 90 Minutes of Arrival[5]	-	-	83%	54%	95%
Smoking Cessation Advice[5]	-	-	84%	88%	100%
Heart Failure Care					
ACE Inhibitor or ARB for LVSD[5]	-	-	76%	82%	100%
Discharge Instructions[5]	-	-	54%	61%	93%
Evaluation of LVS Function[5]	-	-	72%	83%	99%
Smoking Cessation Advice[5]	-	-	62%	82%	100%
Pneumonia Care					
Appropriate Initial Antibiotic[5]	-	-	90%	83%	94%
Blood Culture Timing[5]	-	-	96%	90%	100%
Influenza Vaccine[5]	-	-	77%	70%	100%
Initial Antibiotic Timing[5]	-	-	91%	80%	93%
Oxygenation Assessment[5]	-	-	97%	99%	100%
Pneumococcal Vaccine[5]	-	-	70%	69%	94%
Smoking Cessation Advice[5]	-	-	64%	80%	100%
Surgical Infection Prevention					
Prophylactic Antibiotic Given[5]	-	-	79%	77%	95%
Prophylactic Antibiotic Selection[5]	-	-	94%	90%	100%
Prophylactic Antibiotic Stopped[5]	-	-	83%	72%	95%
Pregnancy Care					
Inpatient Neonatal Mortality	-	-	-	-	-
Third or Fourth Degree Laceration	-	-	-	3.63%	3.27%

Dundy County Hospital

1313 N Cheyenne Street
Benkelman, NE 69021
Phone: 308-423-2204
Fax: 308-423-2298
URL: www.bwtelcom.net/dch
Ownership: Government - Local
Accredited: No
Emergency Services: Yes
Licensed Beds: 14

Key Personnel:

Administrator . . . . Rita Jones
Chief Staff . . . . Shiuvoun Torres, MD
Emergency Room . . . . Teresa Sander, RN
Emergency Room . . . . Kellie Minor, RN
Infection Control. . . . . Jennifer Hansen
Medical/Surgical Nursing . . . . Tammi Cawthra, RN
OB/GYN Women's Health . . . . Carla Burdy, RN
Respiratory/Cardiopulmonary. . . . . Jason Erhart, RT

Measure	Cases	This Hospital	State Average	U.S. Average	Top Hospital
Heart Attack Care					
ACE Inhibitor or ARB for LVSD[3]	0	-	90%	82%	100%
Aspirin at Arrival[1,3]	1	100%	88%	92%	100%
Aspirin at Discharge[3]	0	-	90%	90%	100%
Beta Blocker at Arrival[1,3]	1	100%	81%	87%	100%
Beta Blocker at Discharge[3]	0	-	95%	90%	100%
Fibrinolytic Medication Timing[3]	0	-	25%	31%	100%
PCI Within 90 Minutes of Arrival[5]	-	-	83%	54%	95%
Smoking Cessation Advice[3]	0	-	84%	88%	100%
Heart Failure Care					
ACE Inhibitor or ARB for LVSD	0	-	76%	82%	100%
Discharge Instructions[1]	3	33%	54%	61%	93%
Evaluation of LVS Function[1]	4	25%	72%	83%	99%
Smoking Cessation Advice	0	-	62%	82%	100%

NOTE: Hospital profiles are in alphabetical order by state, then city, then hospital within the city; Rankings are sorted by rate in descending order and exclude hospitals with less than 25 cases; (1) The number of cases is too small (n<25) for purposes of reliably predicting hospital performance; (2) Measure reflects the hospital's indication that its submission was based upon a sample of its relevant discharges; (3) Rate reflects fewer than the maximum possible quarters of data for the measure; (4) Inaccurate information submitted and suppressed for one or more quarters; (5) No data is available from the hospital for this measure; Please refer to the User's Guide for a full explanation of data

Measure	Cases	This Hospital	State Average	U.S. Average	Top Hospital
Pneumonia Care					
Appropriate Initial Antibiotic[1]	6	50%	90%	83%	94%
Blood Culture Timing[1]	1	100%	96%	90%	100%
Influenza Vaccine[1]	1	100%	77%	70%	100%
Initial Antibiotic Timing[1]	7	100%	91%	80%	93%
Oxygenation Assessment[1]	8	100%	97%	99%	100%
Pneumococcal Vaccine[1]	7	29%	70%	69%	94%
Smoking Cessation Advice[1]	2	0%	64%	80%	100%
Surgical Infection Prevention					
Prophylactic Antibiotic Given[1,3]	1	0%	79%	77%	95%
Prophylactic Antibiotic Selection[5]	-	-	94%	90%	100%
Prophylactic Antibiotic Stopped[1,3]	1	0%	83%	72%	95%
Pregnancy Care					
Inpatient Neonatal Mortality	-	-	-	-	-
Third or Fourth Degree Laceration	-	-	-	3.63%	3.27%

Memorial Community Hospital

810 N 22nd Street
Blair, NE 68008
E-mail: jtriplett@mchhs.org
URL: www.mchhs.org
Ownership: Voluntary non-profit - Other
Emergency Services: Yes

Phone: 402-426-1172
Fax: 402-426-1439

Accredited: No
Licensed Beds: 29

Key Personnel:
President/CEO . . . . Sally Harvey
Chief of Medical Staff . . . . Brad Sawtule, MD
Infection Control Nurse. Annette Spooner

Measure	Cases	This Hospital	State Average	U.S. Average	Top Hospital
Heart Attack Care					
ACE Inhibitor or ARB for LVSD[3]	0	-	90%	82%	100%
Aspirin at Arrival[1,3]	2	100%	88%	92%	100%
Aspirin at Discharge[1,3]	1	100%	90%	90%	100%
Beta Blocker at Arrival[1,3]	2	100%	81%	87%	100%
Beta Blocker at Discharge[1,3]	1	100%	95%	90%	100%
Fibrinolytic Medication Timing[3]	0	-	25%	31%	100%
PCI Within 90 Minutes of Arrival[5]	-	-	83%	54%	95%
Smoking Cessation Advice[3]	0	-	84%	88%	100%
Heart Failure Care					
ACE Inhibitor or ARB for LVSD[1]	4	100%	76%	82%	100%
Discharge Instructions[1]	12	83%	54%	61%	93%
Evaluation of LVS Function[1]	21	90%	72%	83%	99%
Smoking Cessation Advice	0	-	62%	82%	100%
Pneumonia Care					
Appropriate Initial Antibiotic	25	72%	90%	83%	94%
Blood Culture Timing	26	100%	96%	90%	100%
Influenza Vaccine[1]	11	91%	77%	70%	100%
Initial Antibiotic Timing	31	100%	91%	80%	93%
Oxygenation Assessment	44	100%	97%	99%	100%
Pneumococcal Vaccine	32	84%	70%	69%	94%
Smoking Cessation Advice[1]	9	78%	64%	80%	100%
Surgical Infection Prevention					
Prophylactic Antibiotic Given[1,3]	5	80%	79%	77%	95%
Prophylactic Antibiotic Selection[1]	2	100%	94%	90%	100%
Prophylactic Antibiotic Stopped[1,3]	5	80%	83%	72%	95%
Pregnancy Care					
Inpatient Neonatal Mortality	-	-	-	-	-
Third or Fourth Degree Laceration	-	-	-	3.63%	3.27%

Jennie M Melham Memorial Medical Center

145 Memorial Drive
Broken Bow, NE 68822
URL: www.brokenbow-ne.com/community/healthcare/melham.htm
Ownership: Voluntary non-profit - Private
Emergency Services: Yes

Phone: 308-872-6891
Fax: 308-872-6116

Accredited: No
Licensed Beds: 39

Key Personnel:
President/CEO . . . . Michael Steckler
Infection Control . . . . Steve Osborn
Respiratory/Cardiopulmonary. . . . . Glenda Mackey

Measure	Cases	This Hospital	State Average	U.S. Average	Top Hospital
Heart Attack Care					
ACE Inhibitor or ARB for LVSD[3]	0	-	90%	82%	100%
Aspirin at Arrival[1,3]	4	75%	88%	92%	100%
Aspirin at Discharge[1,3]	2	100%	90%	90%	100%
Beta Blocker at Arrival[1,3]	3	100%	81%	87%	100%
Beta Blocker at Discharge[1,3]	2	100%	95%	90%	100%
Fibrinolytic Medication Timing[1,3]	1	0%	25%	31%	100%
PCI Within 90 Minutes of Arrival[5]	-	-	83%	54%	95%
Smoking Cessation Advice[3]	0	-	84%	88%	100%
Heart Failure Care					
ACE Inhibitor or ARB for LVSD[1]	12	75%	76%	82%	100%
Discharge Instructions[1]	16	62%	54%	61%	93%
Evaluation of LVS Function	29	83%	72%	83%	99%
Smoking Cessation Advice[1]	3	100%	62%	82%	100%
Pneumonia Care					
Appropriate Initial Antibiotic	55	91%	90%	83%	94%
Blood Culture Timing[1]	3	100%	96%	90%	100%
Influenza Vaccine	27	85%	77%	70%	100%
Initial Antibiotic Timing	86	99%	91%	80%	93%
Oxygenation Assessment	123	100%	97%	99%	100%
Pneumococcal Vaccine	92	96%	70%	69%	94%
Smoking Cessation Advice[1]	13	77%	64%	80%	100%
Surgical Infection Prevention					
Prophylactic Antibiotic Given[1,3]	1	0%	79%	77%	95%
Prophylactic Antibiotic Selection[5]	-	-	94%	90%	100%
Prophylactic Antibiotic Stopped[3]	0	-	83%	72%	95%
Pregnancy Care					
Inpatient Neonatal Mortality	-	-	-	-	-
Third or Fourth Degree Laceration	-	-	-	3.63%	3.27%

Callaway District Hospital

211 Kimball Street
PO Box 100
Callaway, NE 68825
URL: www.callaway-ne.com/hospital
Ownership: Govt - Hospital District or Authority
Emergency Services: Yes

Phone: 308-836-2228
Fax: 308-836-2733

Accredited: No

Key Personnel:
Administrator . . . . Marvin Neth

Measure	Cases	This Hospital	State Average	U.S. Average	Top Hospital
Heart Attack Care					
ACE Inhibitor or ARB for LVSD[5]	-	-	90%	82%	100%
Aspirin at Arrival[5]	-	-	88%	92%	100%
Aspirin at Discharge[5]	-	-	90%	90%	100%
Beta Blocker at Arrival[5]	-	-	81%	87%	100%
Beta Blocker at Discharge[5]	-	-	95%	90%	100%
Fibrinolytic Medication Timing[5]	-	-	25%	31%	100%
PCI Within 90 Minutes of Arrival[5]	-	-	83%	54%	95%
Smoking Cessation Advice[5]	-	-	84%	88%	100%
Heart Failure Care					
ACE Inhibitor or ARB for LVSD[3]	0	-	76%	82%	100%
Discharge Instructions[3]	0	-	54%	61%	93%
Evaluation of LVS Function[3]	0	-	72%	83%	99%
Smoking Cessation Advice[3]	0	-	62%	82%	100%
Pneumonia Care					
Appropriate Initial Antibiotic[3]	0	-	90%	83%	94%
Blood Culture Timing[1,3]	2	100%	96%	90%	100%
Influenza Vaccine[5]	-	-	77%	70%	100%
Initial Antibiotic Timing[1,3]	4	100%	91%	80%	93%
Oxygenation Assessment[1,3]	7	100%	97%	99%	100%
Pneumococcal Vaccine[1,3]	6	33%	70%	69%	94%
Smoking Cessation Advice[3]	0	-	64%	80%	100%
Surgical Infection Prevention					
Prophylactic Antibiotic Given[5]	-	-	79%	77%	95%
Prophylactic Antibiotic Selection[5]	-	-	94%	90%	100%
Prophylactic Antibiotic Stopped[5]	-	-	83%	72%	95%
Pregnancy Care					
Inpatient Neonatal Mortality	-	-	-	-	-
Third or Fourth Degree Laceration	-	-	-	3.63%	3.27%

NOTE: Hospital profiles are in alphabetical order by state, then city, then hospital within the city; Rankings are sorted by rate in descending order and exclude hospitals with less than 25 cases; (1) The number of cases is too small (n<25) for purposes of reliably predicting hospital performance; (2) Measure reflects the hospital's indication that its submission was based upon a sample of its relevant discharges; (3) Rate reflects fewer than the maximum possible quarters of data for the measure; (4) Inaccurate information submitted and suppressed for one or more quarters; (5) No data is available from the hospital for this measure; Please refer to the User's Guide for a full explanation of data

Tri-Valley Health System

PO Box 488
Cambridge, NE 69022
URL: www.trivalleyhealth.com
Ownership: Government - Local
Emergency Services: Yes
Phone: 308-697-3329
Fax: 308-697-4918
Accredited: No
Licensed Beds: 25

Key Personnel:

CEO. . . . . Lynn Milnes
Chief of Medical Staff. . . . . Lennis Deaver, MD
Emergency Room . . . . Rhonda Sherman
Infection Control. . . . . Shelly Shellabarger
Medical Surgical Nursing . . . . Judy Hayes, RN
Director Respiratory Therapy . . . . Kathy Weaver

Measure	Cases	This Hospital	State Average	U.S. Average	Top Hospital
Heart Attack Care					
ACE Inhibitor or ARB for LVSD[3]	0	-	90%	82%	100%
Aspirin at Arrival[1,3]	1	0%	88%	92%	100%
Aspirin at Discharge[3]	0	-	90%	90%	100%
Beta Blocker at Arrival[1,3]	1	100%	81%	87%	100%
Beta Blocker at Discharge[3]	0	-	95%	90%	100%
Fibrinolytic Medication Timing[1,3]	1	0%	25%	31%	100%
PCI Within 90 Minutes of Arrival	0	-	83%	54%	95%
Smoking Cessation Advice[3]	0	-	84%	88%	100%
Heart Failure Care					
ACE Inhibitor or ARB for LVSD[1]	10	90%	76%	82%	100%
Discharge Instructions[1]	23	48%	54%	61%	93%
Evaluation of LVS Function	28	96%	72%	83%	99%
Smoking Cessation Advice[1]	3	67%	62%	82%	100%
Pneumonia Care					
Appropriate Initial Antibiotic	32	97%	90%	83%	94%
Blood Culture Timing[1]	2	100%	96%	90%	100%
Influenza Vaccine[4,5]	-	-	77%	70%	100%
Initial Antibiotic Timing	32	97%	91%	80%	93%
Oxygenation Assessment	47	100%	97%	99%	100%
Pneumococcal Vaccine	37	62%	70%	69%	94%
Smoking Cessation Advice[1]	4	75%	64%	80%	100%
Surgical Infection Prevention					
Prophylactic Antibiotic Given[1,3]	2	0%	79%	77%	95%
Prophylactic Antibiotic Selection[5]	-	-	94%	90%	100%
Prophylactic Antibiotic Stopped[1,3]	2	100%	83%	72%	95%
Pregnancy Care					
Inpatient Neonatal Mortality	-	-	-	-	-
Third or Fourth Degree Laceration	-	-	-	3.63%	3.27%

Litzenberg Memorial County Hospital

RR 2
Box 1
Central City, NE 68826
Ownership: Government - Local
Emergency Services: Yes
Phone: 308-946-3015
Fax: 308-946-2633
Accredited: No
Licensed Beds: 79

Key Personnel:

CEO. . . . . Mike Bowlman
Chief Medical Staff. . . . . Gerome Dackey
Emergency Room . . . . Diane Schoch
Director Infection/Disease Control . . . . Lavonne Solomon, L.P.N.
Director Respiratory Therapy . . . . Candy Zyweic

Measure	Cases	This Hospital	State Average	U.S. Average	Top Hospital
Heart Attack Care					
ACE Inhibitor or ARB for LVSD[3]	0	-	90%	82%	100%
Aspirin at Arrival[1,3]	1	100%	88%	92%	100%
Aspirin at Discharge[1,3]	1	100%	90%	90%	100%
Beta Blocker at Arrival[1,3]	1	100%	81%	87%	100%
Beta Blocker at Discharge[1,3]	1	100%	95%	90%	100%
Fibrinolytic Medication Timing[3]	0	-	25%	31%	100%
PCI Within 90 Minutes of Arrival[5]	-	-	83%	54%	95%
Smoking Cessation Advice[3]	0	-	84%	88%	100%
Heart Failure Care					
ACE Inhibitor or ARB for LVSD[1]	3	67%	76%	82%	100%
Discharge Instructions[1]	10	50%	54%	61%	93%
Evaluation of LVS Function[1]	18	39%	72%	83%	99%
Smoking Cessation Advice	0	-	62%	82%	100%
Pneumonia Care					
Appropriate Initial Antibiotic[1]	12	100%	90%	83%	94%
Blood Culture Timing[1]	5	100%	96%	90%	100%
Influenza Vaccine[1]	6	100%	77%	70%	100%
Initial Antibiotic Timing	32	94%	91%	80%	93%
Oxygenation Assessment	34	94%	97%	99%	100%
Pneumococcal Vaccine	25	72%	70%	69%	94%
Smoking Cessation Advice[1]	1	100%	64%	80%	100%
Surgical Infection Prevention					
Prophylactic Antibiotic Given[1]	9	89%	79%	77%	95%
Prophylactic Antibiotic Selection[1]	3	100%	94%	90%	100%
Prophylactic Antibiotic Stopped[1]	8	88%	83%	72%	95%
Pregnancy Care					
Inpatient Neonatal Mortality	-	-	-	-	-
Third or Fourth Degree Laceration	-	-	-	3.63%	3.27%

Chadron Community Hospital

821 Morehead Street
Chadron, NE 69337
Ownership: Voluntary non-profit - Private
Emergency Services: Yes
Phone: 308-432-5586
Fax: 308-432-2737
Accredited: No
Licensed Beds: 42

Key Personnel:

CEO. . . . . Harold Kruger
Chief Medical Staff. . . . . Catherine Satera
Chief of Medical Staff. . . . . Jeffrey Lias
Emergency Room . . . . Sandra Ingwersen

Measure	Cases	This Hospital	State Average	U.S. Average	Top Hospital
Heart Attack Care					
ACE Inhibitor or ARB for LVSD[3]	0	-	90%	82%	100%
Aspirin at Arrival[3]	0	-	88%	92%	100%
Aspirin at Discharge[3]	0	-	90%	90%	100%
Beta Blocker at Arrival[3]	0	-	81%	87%	100%
Beta Blocker at Discharge[3]	0	-	95%	90%	100%
Fibrinolytic Medication Timing[1,3]	1	0%	25%	31%	100%
PCI Within 90 Minutes of Arrival	0	-	83%	54%	95%
Smoking Cessation Advice[3]	0	-	84%	88%	100%
Heart Failure Care					
ACE Inhibitor or ARB for LVSD	0	-	76%	82%	100%
Discharge Instructions[1]	2	100%	54%	61%	93%
Evaluation of LVS Function[1]	7	29%	72%	83%	99%
Smoking Cessation Advice	0	-	62%	82%	100%
Pneumonia Care					
Appropriate Initial Antibiotic[1]	13	62%	90%	83%	94%
Blood Culture Timing[1]	2	100%	96%	90%	100%
Influenza Vaccine[1]	4	100%	77%	70%	100%
Initial Antibiotic Timing[1]	17	94%	91%	80%	93%
Oxygenation Assessment[1]	18	100%	97%	99%	100%
Pneumococcal Vaccine[1]	14	64%	70%	69%	94%
Smoking Cessation Advice[1]	1	0%	64%	80%	100%
Surgical Infection Prevention					
Prophylactic Antibiotic Given[5]	-	-	79%	77%	95%
Prophylactic Antibiotic Selection[5]	-	-	94%	90%	100%
Prophylactic Antibiotic Stopped[5]	-	-	83%	72%	95%
Pregnancy Care					
Inpatient Neonatal Mortality	-	-	-	-	-
Third or Fourth Degree Laceration	-	-	-	3.63%	3.27%

Columbus Community Hospital

4600 38th Street
PO Box 1800
Columbus, NE 68602
E-mail: info@columbushosp.org
URL: www.columbushosp.org
Ownership: Voluntary non-profit - Other
Emergency Services: Yes
Phone: 402-564-7118
Fax: 402-563-3267
Accredited: Yes
Licensed Beds: 81

Key Personnel:

President/CEO. . . . . Donald Zornes
Emergency Room . . . . Cathy Hare
Director Infection/Disease Control . . . . Cookie Walsh
OB/GYN Womens Health. . . . . Diane Ward, MD

NOTE: Hospital profiles are in alphabetical order by state, then city, then hospital within the city; Rankings are sorted by rate in descending order and exclude hospitals with less than 25 cases; (1) The number of cases is too small (n<25) for purposes of reliably predicting hospital performance; (2) Measure reflects the hospital's indication that its submission was based upon a sample of its relevant discharges; (3) Rate reflects fewer than the maximum possible quarters of data for the measure; (4) Inaccurate information submitted and suppressed for one or more quarters; (5) No data is available from the hospital for this measure; Please refer to the User's Guide for a full explanation of data

Measure	Cases	This Hospital	State Average	U.S. Average	Top Hospital
Heart Attack Care					
ACE Inhibitor or ARB for LVSD[1]	2	100%	90%	82%	100%
Aspirin at Arrival[1]	9	100%	88%	92%	100%
Aspirin at Discharge[1]	6	100%	90%	90%	100%
Beta Blocker at Arrival[1]	9	89%	81%	87%	100%
Beta Blocker at Discharge[1]	7	100%	95%	90%	100%
Fibrinolytic Medication Timing	0	-	25%	31%	100%
PCI Within 90 Minutes of Arrival	0	-	83%	54%	95%
Smoking Cessation Advice	0	-	84%	88%	100%
Heart Failure Care					
ACE Inhibitor or ARB for LVSD[1]	19	95%	76%	82%	100%
Discharge Instructions	28	71%	54%	61%	93%
Evaluation of LVS Function	49	90%	72%	83%	99%
Smoking Cessation Advice[1]	6	100%	62%	82%	100%
Pneumonia Care					
Appropriate Initial Antibiotic	30	93%	90%	83%	94%
Blood Culture Timing	35	97%	96%	90%	100%
Influenza Vaccine[1]	13	92%	77%	70%	100%
Initial Antibiotic Timing	50	96%	91%	80%	93%
Oxygenation Assessment	72	100%	97%	99%	100%
Pneumococcal Vaccine	54	91%	70%	69%	94%
Smoking Cessation Advice[1]	8	88%	64%	80%	100%
Surgical Infection Prevention					
Prophylactic Antibiotic Given[2]	205	94%	79%	77%	95%
Prophylactic Antibiotic Selection[2]	39	95%	94%	90%	100%
Prophylactic Antibiotic Stopped[2]	198	91%	83%	72%	95%
Pregnancy Care					
Inpatient Neonatal Mortality	-	-	-	-	-
Third or Fourth Degree Laceration	-	-	-	3.63%	3.27%

Cozad Community Hospital

300 E 12th
Cozad, NE 69130
Ownership: Voluntary non-profit - Other
Emergency Services: Yes

Phone: 308-784-2261
Fax: 308-784-4691
Accredited: No
Licensed Beds: 30

Key Personnel:
Administrator . . . . Lyle Davis
Emergency Room . . . . Tammy McMichael
Emergency Room . . . . Marilyn Bergman
Director Infection/Disease Control . . . . Jo Griffith
Director Medical/Surgical Nursing . . . . Marilyn Bergman
Chief Radiology . . . . Shirley Heidebrink
Director Respiratory Therapy . . . . Cindy Benjamin

Measure	Cases	This Hospital	State Average	U.S. Average	Top Hospital
Heart Attack Care					
ACE Inhibitor or ARB for LVSD[5]	-	-	90%	82%	100%
Aspirin at Arrival[5]	-	-	88%	92%	100%
Aspirin at Discharge[5]	-	-	90%	90%	100%
Beta Blocker at Arrival[5]	-	-	81%	87%	100%
Beta Blocker at Discharge[5]	-	-	95%	90%	100%
Fibrinolytic Medication Timing[5]	-	-	25%	31%	100%
PCI Within 90 Minutes of Arrival[5]	-	-	83%	54%	95%
Smoking Cessation Advice[5]	-	-	84%	88%	100%
Heart Failure Care					
ACE Inhibitor or ARB for LVSD[3]	0	-	76%	82%	100%
Discharge Instructions[1,3]	3	33%	54%	61%	93%
Evaluation of LVS Function[1,3]	5	60%	72%	83%	99%
Smoking Cessation Advice[1,3]	1	100%	62%	82%	100%
Pneumonia Care					
Appropriate Initial Antibiotic[1]	14	64%	90%	83%	94%
Blood Culture Timing[1]	1	100%	96%	90%	100%
Influenza Vaccine[1]	3	100%	77%	70%	100%
Initial Antibiotic Timing[1]	11	73%	91%	80%	93%
Oxygenation Assessment[1]	16	100%	97%	99%	100%
Pneumococcal Vaccine[1]	12	58%	70%	69%	94%
Smoking Cessation Advice	0	-	64%	80%	100%
Surgical Infection Prevention					
Prophylactic Antibiotic Given[5]	-	-	79%	77%	95%
Prophylactic Antibiotic Selection[5]	-	-	94%	90%	100%
Prophylactic Antibiotic Stopped[5]	-	-	83%	72%	95%

Measure	Cases	This Hospital	State Average	U.S. Average	Top Hospital
Pregnancy Care					
Inpatient Neonatal Mortality	-	-	-	-	-
Third or Fourth Degree Laceration	-	-	-	3.63%	3.27%

Creighton Area Health Services

Alternate Name: Centre/Verdigre Clinic
1503 Main Street
PO Box 186
Creighton, NE 68729
E-mail: marketing@cahs-ne.org
Ownership: Government - Local
Emergency Services: Yes

Phone: 402-358-5700
Fax: 402-358-5769
Accredited: No
Licensed Beds: 69

Key Personnel:
CEO. . . . . Jeffrey A Lingerfelt
Chief Medical Staff. . . . . Ron Morris
Medical Surgical Nursing . . . . Jean Henes, DON
Respiratory . . . . Chad Thompson

Measure	Cases	This Hospital	State Average	U.S. Average	Top Hospital
Heart Attack Care					
ACE Inhibitor or ARB for LVSD[3]	0	-	90%	82%	100%
Aspirin at Arrival[1,3]	4	50%	88%	92%	100%
Aspirin at Discharge[1,3]	3	67%	90%	90%	100%
Beta Blocker at Arrival[1,3]	4	50%	81%	87%	100%
Beta Blocker at Discharge[1,3]	3	100%	95%	90%	100%
Fibrinolytic Medication Timing[3]	0	-	25%	31%	100%
PCI Within 90 Minutes of Arrival[5]	-	-	83%	54%	95%
Smoking Cessation Advice[3]	0	-	84%	88%	100%
Heart Failure Care					
ACE Inhibitor or ARB for LVSD[5]	-	-	76%	82%	100%
Discharge Instructions[5]	-	-	54%	61%	93%
Evaluation of LVS Function[5]	-	-	72%	83%	99%
Smoking Cessation Advice[5]	-	-	62%	82%	100%
Pneumonia Care					
Appropriate Initial Antibiotic	34	85%	90%	83%	94%
Blood Culture Timing	0	-	96%	90%	100%
Influenza Vaccine[1]	14	79%	77%	70%	100%
Initial Antibiotic Timing	43	100%	91%	80%	93%
Oxygenation Assessment	59	100%	97%	99%	100%
Pneumococcal Vaccine	50	70%	70%	69%	94%
Smoking Cessation Advice[1]	7	29%	64%	80%	100%
Surgical Infection Prevention					
Prophylactic Antibiotic Given[5]	-	-	79%	77%	95%
Prophylactic Antibiotic Selection[5]	-	-	94%	90%	100%
Prophylactic Antibiotic Stopped[5]	-	-	83%	72%	95%
Pregnancy Care					
Inpatient Neonatal Mortality	-	-	-	-	-
Third or Fourth Degree Laceration	-	-	-	3.63%	3.27%

Crete Area Medical Center

1540 Grove Street
Box 220
Crete, NE 68333
URL: www.creteareamedicalcenter.com
Ownership: Voluntary non-profit - Private
Emergency Services: Yes

Phone: 402-826-2154
Fax: 402-826-7950
Accredited: No
Licensed Beds: 57

Key Personnel:
Administrator . . . . Joseph W Lohrman

Measure	Cases	This Hospital	State Average	U.S. Average	Top Hospital
Heart Attack Care					
ACE Inhibitor or ARB for LVSD[3]	0	-	90%	82%	100%
Aspirin at Arrival[3]	0	-	88%	92%	100%
Aspirin at Discharge[3]	0	-	90%	90%	100%
Beta Blocker at Arrival[3]	0	-	81%	87%	100%
Beta Blocker at Discharge[3]	0	-	95%	90%	100%
Fibrinolytic Medication Timing[3]	0	-	25%	31%	100%
PCI Within 90 Minutes of Arrival	0	-	83%	54%	95%
Smoking Cessation Advice[3]	0	-	84%	88%	100%
Heart Failure Care					
ACE Inhibitor or ARB for LVSD[1]	2	100%	76%	82%	100%
Discharge Instructions[1]	2	50%	54%	61%	93%

NOTE: Hospital profiles are in alphabetical order by state, then city, then hospital within the city; Rankings are sorted by rate in descending order and exclude hospitals with less than 25 cases; (1) The number of cases is too small (n<25) for purposes of reliably predicting hospital performance; (2) Measure reflects the hospital's indication that its submission was based upon a sample of its relevant discharges; (3) Rate reflects fewer than the maximum possible quarters of data for the measure; (4) Inaccurate information submitted and suppressed for one or more quarters; (5) No data is available from the hospital for this measure; Please refer to the User's Guide for a full explanation of data

Evaluation of LVS Function[1]	8	62%	72%	83%	99%
Smoking Cessation Advice[1]	2	50%	62%	82%	100%
Pneumonia Care					
Appropriate Initial Antibiotic[1]	8	88%	90%	83%	94%
Blood Culture Timing[1]	3	100%	96%	90%	100%
Influenza Vaccine[1]	8	88%	77%	70%	100%
Initial Antibiotic Timing[1]	16	69%	91%	80%	93%
Oxygenation Assessment[1]	20	95%	97%	99%	100%
Pneumococcal Vaccine[1]	17	82%	70%	69%	94%
Smoking Cessation Advice[1]	4	50%	64%	80%	100%
Surgical Infection Prevention					
Prophylactic Antibiotic Given[5]	-	-	79%	77%	95%
Prophylactic Antibiotic Selection[5]	-	-	94%	90%	100%
Prophylactic Antibiotic Stopped[5]	-	-	83%	72%	95%
Pregnancy Care					
Inpatient Neonatal Mortality	-	-	-	-	-
Third or Fourth Degree Laceration	-	-	-	3.63%	3.27%

Butler County Health Care Center

372 S 9th Street
David City, NE 68632
URL: www.bchccnet.org
Ownership: Government - Local
Emergency Services: Yes

Phone: 402-367-1200
Fax: 402-367-1350
Accredited: No
Licensed Beds: 25

Key Personnel:
Administrator/CEO . . . . Donald T Naiberk
Chief Medical Staff. . . . . V Thoendel, MD
Emergency Department. . . . . Joyce Jelinek, RN
Emergency Room . . . . J Witter, MD
Infection Control Coordinator . . . . Connie Janicek, RN
Director Medical/Surgical Nursing . . . . Sue Birkel, RN
Surgery . . . . Joyce Jelinek, RN
Director Respiratory Therapy . . . . Wes Stephens

Measure	Cases	This Hospital	State Average	U.S. Average	Top Hospital
Heart Attack Care					
ACE Inhibitor or ARB for LVSD[3]	0	-	90%	82%	100%
Aspirin at Arrival[3]	0	-	88%	92%	100%
Aspirin at Discharge[3]	0	-	90%	90%	100%
Beta Blocker at Arrival[3]	0	-	81%	87%	100%
Beta Blocker at Discharge[3]	0	-	95%	90%	100%
Fibrinolytic Medication Timing[1,3]	5	20%	25%	31%	100%
PCI Within 90 Minutes of Arrival[5]	-	-	83%	54%	95%
Smoking Cessation Advice[3]	0	-	84%	88%	100%
Heart Failure Care					
ACE Inhibitor or ARB for LVSD[1,3]	1	100%	76%	82%	100%
Discharge Instructions[1,3]	5	100%	54%	61%	93%
Evaluation of LVS Function[1,3]	7	57%	72%	83%	99%
Smoking Cessation Advice[3]	0	-	62%	82%	100%
Pneumonia Care					
Appropriate Initial Antibiotic[1]	16	69%	90%	83%	94%
Blood Culture Timing[1]	1	100%	96%	90%	100%
Influenza Vaccine[1]	6	83%	77%	70%	100%
Initial Antibiotic Timing[1]	16	88%	91%	80%	93%
Oxygenation Assessment[1]	20	100%	97%	99%	100%
Pneumococcal Vaccine[1]	17	65%	70%	69%	94%
Smoking Cessation Advice[1]	3	67%	64%	80%	100%
Surgical Infection Prevention					
Prophylactic Antibiotic Given[1]	22	73%	79%	77%	95%
Prophylactic Antibiotic Selection[1]	4	75%	94%	90%	100%
Prophylactic Antibiotic Stopped[1]	22	95%	83%	72%	95%
Pregnancy Care					
Inpatient Neonatal Mortality	-	-	-	-	-
Third or Fourth Degree Laceration	-	-	-	3.63%	3.27%

Jefferson Community Health Center

Alternate Name: Jefferson County Memorial Hospital

PO Box 277
Fairbury, NE 68352
E-mail: lana.likens@jchc.us
URL: www.jchc.us
Ownership: Voluntary non-profit - Private
Emergency Services: Yes

Phone: 402-729-3351
Fax: 402-729-2102
Accredited: No
Licensed Beds: 33

Key Personnel:
CEO. . . . . Bill Welch
Chief Medical Staff. . . . . Craig Shumard, MD
Emergency Room . . . . Judy McGee, CNE
Director Infection/Disease Control . . . . Mary Heidemann
Director Medical/Surgical Nursing . . . . Judy McGee, CNE
OB/GYN/Women's Health . . . . Judy McGee, CNE
Surgical Supervisor . . . . Ermel Heuer, RN
Director Respiratory Therapy . . . . Jack Pollock

Measure	Cases	This Hospital	State Average	U.S. Average	Top Hospital
Heart Attack Care					
ACE Inhibitor or ARB for LVSD[1,3]	1	100%	90%	82%	100%
Aspirin at Arrival[1,3]	1	0%	88%	92%	100%
Aspirin at Discharge[1,3]	1	0%	90%	90%	100%
Beta Blocker at Arrival[3]	0	-	81%	87%	100%
Beta Blocker at Discharge[1,3]	1	100%	95%	90%	100%
Fibrinolytic Medication Timing[3]	0	-	25%	31%	100%
PCI Within 90 Minutes of Arrival[5]	-	-	83%	54%	95%
Smoking Cessation Advice[3]	0	-	84%	88%	100%
Heart Failure Care					
ACE Inhibitor or ARB for LVSD[1]	3	100%	76%	82%	100%
Discharge Instructions[1]	5	100%	54%	61%	93%
Evaluation of LVS Function[1]	7	100%	72%	83%	99%
Smoking Cessation Advice	0	-	62%	82%	100%
Pneumonia Care					
Appropriate Initial Antibiotic[1]	21	100%	90%	83%	94%
Blood Culture Timing[1]	9	100%	96%	90%	100%
Influenza Vaccine[1]	12	83%	77%	70%	100%
Initial Antibiotic Timing	28	96%	91%	80%	93%
Oxygenation Assessment	33	100%	97%	99%	100%
Pneumococcal Vaccine	28	100%	70%	69%	94%
Smoking Cessation Advice[1]	2	100%	64%	80%	100%
Surgical Infection Prevention					
Prophylactic Antibiotic Given	46	98%	79%	77%	95%
Prophylactic Antibiotic Selection[1]	8	100%	94%	90%	100%
Prophylactic Antibiotic Stopped	43	98%	83%	72%	95%
Pregnancy Care					
Inpatient Neonatal Mortality	-	-	-	-	-
Third or Fourth Degree Laceration	-	-	-	3.63%	3.27%

Community Hospital

2307 Barada Street
Falls City, NE 68355
URL: www.hhs.state.ne.us/index.htm
Ownership: Voluntary non-profit - Private
Emergency Services: Yes

Phone: 402-245-2428
Fax: 402-245-4841
Accredited: No
Licensed Beds: 35

Measure	Cases	This Hospital	State Average	U.S. Average	Top Hospital
Heart Attack Care					
ACE Inhibitor or ARB for LVSD[1,3]	1	100%	90%	82%	100%
Aspirin at Arrival[1,3]	1	100%	88%	92%	100%
Aspirin at Discharge[1,3]	1	100%	90%	90%	100%
Beta Blocker at Arrival[3]	0	-	81%	87%	100%
Beta Blocker at Discharge[3]	0	-	95%	90%	100%
Fibrinolytic Medication Timing[1,3]	3	67%	25%	31%	100%
PCI Within 90 Minutes of Arrival[5]	-	-	83%	54%	95%
Smoking Cessation Advice[3]	0	-	84%	88%	100%
Heart Failure Care					
ACE Inhibitor or ARB for LVSD[1]	4	100%	76%	82%	100%
Discharge Instructions[1]	9	67%	54%	61%	93%
Evaluation of LVS Function[1]	21	67%	72%	83%	99%
Smoking Cessation Advice[1]	2	100%	62%	82%	100%
Pneumonia Care					
Appropriate Initial Antibiotic[1]	12	75%	90%	83%	94%
Blood Culture Timing[1]	2	100%	96%	90%	100%
Influenza Vaccine[1]	6	100%	77%	70%	100%

NOTE: Hospital profiles are in alphabetical order by state, then city, then hospital within the city; Rankings are sorted by rate in descending order and exclude hospitals with less than 25 cases; (1) The number of cases is too small (n<25) for purposes of reliably predicting hospital performance; (2) Measure reflects the hospital's indication that its submission was based upon a sample of its relevant discharges; (3) Rate reflects fewer than the maximum possible quarters of data for the measure; (4) Inaccurate information submitted and suppressed for one or more quarters; (5) No data is available from the hospital for this measure; Please refer to the User's Guide for a full explanation of data

Initial Antibiotic Timing[1]	16	94%	91%	80%	93%
Oxygenation Assessment	25	100%	97%	99%	100%
Pneumococcal Vaccine[1]	22	77%	70%	69%	94%
Smoking Cessation Advice[1]	6	83%	64%	80%	100%
Surgical Infection Prevention					
Prophylactic Antibiotic Given[1]	11	91%	79%	77%	95%
Prophylactic Antibiotic Selection[1]	1	100%	94%	90%	100%
Prophylactic Antibiotic Stopped[1]	11	100%	83%	72%	95%
Pregnancy Care					
Inpatient Neonatal Mortality	-	-	-	-	-
Third or Fourth Degree Laceration	-	-	-	3.63%	3.27%

Franklin County Memorial Hospital

1406 Q Street
PO Box 315
Franklin, NE 68939
URL: www.franklincountymemorialhospital.org
Ownership: Voluntary non-profit - Other
Emergency Services: Yes

Toll-Free: 800-753-2479
Phone: 308-425-6221
Fax: 308-425-3164

Accredited: No
Licensed Beds: 12

Key Personnel:
President/CEO. . . . . Jerrell F Gerdes, FACHE
Chief Medical Staff. . . . . Linda Mazour
Cardiac Lab . . . . Gaylene Wentworth

Measure	Cases	This Hospital	State Average	U.S. Average	Top Hospital
Heart Attack Care					
ACE Inhibitor or ARB for LVSD[5]	-	-	90%	82%	100%
Aspirin at Arrival[5]	-	-	88%	92%	100%
Aspirin at Discharge[5]	-	-	90%	90%	100%
Beta Blocker at Arrival[5]	-	-	81%	87%	100%
Beta Blocker at Discharge[5]	-	-	95%	90%	100%
Fibrinolytic Medication Timing[5]	-	-	25%	31%	100%
PCI Within 90 Minutes of Arrival[5]	-	-	83%	54%	95%
Smoking Cessation Advice[5]	-	-	84%	88%	100%
Heart Failure Care					
ACE Inhibitor or ARB for LVSD[3]	0	-	76%	82%	100%
Discharge Instructions[1,3]	3	0%	54%	61%	93%
Evaluation of LVS Function[1,3]	9	11%	72%	83%	99%
Smoking Cessation Advice[3]	0	-	62%	82%	100%
Pneumonia Care					
Appropriate Initial Antibiotic[1,3]	8	100%	90%	83%	94%
Blood Culture Timing	0	-	96%	90%	100%
Influenza Vaccine[1]	4	100%	77%	70%	100%
Initial Antibiotic Timing[1,3]	11	100%	91%	80%	93%
Oxygenation Assessment[1,3]	14	100%	97%	99%	100%
Pneumococcal Vaccine[1,3]	10	70%	70%	69%	94%
Smoking Cessation Advice[1,3]	2	100%	64%	80%	100%
Surgical Infection Prevention					
Prophylactic Antibiotic Given[5]	-	-	79%	77%	95%
Prophylactic Antibiotic Selection[5]	-	-	94%	90%	100%
Prophylactic Antibiotic Stopped[5]	-	-	83%	72%	95%
Pregnancy Care					
Inpatient Neonatal Mortality	-	-	-	-	-
Third or Fourth Degree Laceration	-	-	-	3.63%	3.27%

Fremont Area Medical Center

Alternate Name: Memorial Hospital of Dodge County
450 E 23rd Street
Fremont, NE 68025
Ownership: Government - Local
Emergency Services: Yes

Phone: 402-721-1610
Fax: 402-727-3433
Accredited: Yes
Licensed Beds: 262

Key Personnel:
President/CEO. . . . . Michael Leibert
Cardiology . . . . Brian Brodd
Emergency Room . . . . Brian K Elliott, MD
Infection Control. . . . . Gerri Means
Surgical Services . . . . Don Tricarico
Chief Radiology . . . . Duane Krause, MD
Respiratory . . . . Brian Brodd

Measure	Cases	This Hospital	State Average	U.S. Average	Top Hospital
Heart Attack Care					
ACE Inhibitor or ARB for LVSD[1]	5	100%	90%	82%	100%
Aspirin at Arrival	36	100%	88%	92%	100%
Aspirin at Discharge	28	100%	90%	90%	100%
Beta Blocker at Arrival	32	100%	81%	87%	100%
Beta Blocker at Discharge	32	100%	95%	90%	100%
Fibrinolytic Medication Timing	0	-	25%	31%	100%
PCI Within 90 Minutes of Arrival[1]	1	100%	83%	54%	95%
Smoking Cessation Advice[1]	9	78%	84%	88%	100%
Heart Failure Care					
ACE Inhibitor or ARB for LVSD[1]	17	94%	76%	82%	100%
Discharge Instructions	39	82%	54%	61%	93%
Evaluation of LVS Function	68	100%	72%	83%	99%
Smoking Cessation Advice[1]	8	88%	62%	82%	100%
Pneumonia Care					
Appropriate Initial Antibiotic	95	87%	90%	83%	94%
Blood Culture Timing	82	98%	96%	90%	100%
Influenza Vaccine	31	84%	77%	70%	100%
Initial Antibiotic Timing	122	91%	91%	80%	93%
Oxygenation Assessment	172	100%	97%	99%	100%
Pneumococcal Vaccine	115	70%	70%	69%	94%
Smoking Cessation Advice	35	89%	64%	80%	100%
Surgical Infection Prevention					
Prophylactic Antibiotic Given[3]	231	97%	79%	77%	95%
Prophylactic Antibiotic Selection	80	94%	94%	90%	100%
Prophylactic Antibiotic Stopped[3]	231	88%	83%	72%	95%
Pregnancy Care					
Inpatient Neonatal Mortality	-	-	-	-	-
Third or Fourth Degree Laceration	-	-	-	3.63%	3.27%

Warren Memorial Hospital

905 2nd Street
Friend, NE 68359
URL: www.warrenmemorialhospital.org
Ownership: Government - Local
Emergency Services: Yes

Phone: 402-947-2541
Fax: 402-947-2881

Accredited: No
Licensed Beds: 15

Key Personnel:
President/CEO. . . . . Amy Fish
Chief of Medical Staff. . . . . Darin Gregory
Infection Control. . . . . Trish Ricenbaw
Medical Surgical Nursing . . . . Fran Prokop

Measure	Cases	This Hospital	State Average	U.S. Average	Top Hospital
Heart Attack Care					
ACE Inhibitor or ARB for LVSD[5]	-	-	90%	82%	100%
Aspirin at Arrival[5]	-	-	88%	92%	100%
Aspirin at Discharge[5]	-	-	90%	90%	100%
Beta Blocker at Arrival[5]	-	-	81%	87%	100%
Beta Blocker at Discharge[5]	-	-	95%	90%	100%
Fibrinolytic Medication Timing[5]	-	-	25%	31%	100%
PCI Within 90 Minutes of Arrival[5]	-	-	83%	54%	95%
Smoking Cessation Advice[5]	-	-	84%	88%	100%
Heart Failure Care					
ACE Inhibitor or ARB for LVSD[3]	0	-	76%	82%	100%
Discharge Instructions[1,3]	1	0%	54%	61%	93%
Evaluation of LVS Function[1,3]	1	100%	72%	83%	99%
Smoking Cessation Advice[3]	0	-	62%	82%	100%
Pneumonia Care					
Appropriate Initial Antibiotic[1,3]	3	100%	90%	83%	94%
Blood Culture Timing[1,3]	1	100%	96%	90%	100%
Influenza Vaccine[5]	-	-	77%	70%	100%
Initial Antibiotic Timing[1,3]	3	100%	91%	80%	93%
Oxygenation Assessment[1,3]	4	100%	97%	99%	100%
Pneumococcal Vaccine[1,3]	4	50%	70%	69%	94%
Smoking Cessation Advice[1,3]	1	0%	64%	80%	100%
Surgical Infection Prevention					
Prophylactic Antibiotic Given[5]	-	-	79%	77%	95%
Prophylactic Antibiotic Selection[5]	-	-	94%	90%	100%
Prophylactic Antibiotic Stopped[5]	-	-	83%	72%	95%
Pregnancy Care					
Inpatient Neonatal Mortality	-	-	-	-	-
Third or Fourth Degree Laceration	-	-	-	3.63%	3.27%

NOTE: Hospital profiles are in alphabetical order by state, then city, then hospital within the city; Rankings are sorted by rate in descending order and exclude hospitals with less than 25 cases; (1) The number of cases is too small (n<25) for purposes of reliably predicting hospital performance; (2) Measure reflects the hospital's indication that its submission was based upon a sample of its relevant discharges; (3) Rate reflects fewer than the maximum possible quarters of data for the measure; (4) Inaccurate information submitted and suppressed for one or more quarters; (5) No data is available from the hospital for this measure; Please refer to the User's Guide for a full explanation of data

Fillmore County Hospital

1325 H Street
Geneva, NE 68361

Toll-Free: 877-277-9771
Phone: 402-759-3167
Fax: 402-759-3093

Ownership: Government - Local
Emergency Services: Yes

Accredited: No
Licensed Beds: 33

Key Personnel:
President/CEO . . . . Larry Eichelberger

Measure	Cases	This Hospital	State Average	U.S. Average	Top Hospital
Heart Attack Care					
ACE Inhibitor or ARB for LVSD[3]	0	-	90%	82%	100%
Aspirin at Arrival[1,3]	1	100%	88%	92%	100%
Aspirin at Discharge[1,3]	1	100%	90%	90%	100%
Beta Blocker at Arrival[1,3]	1	100%	81%	87%	100%
Beta Blocker at Discharge[1,3]	2	100%	95%	90%	100%
Fibrinolytic Medication Timing[3]	0	-	25%	31%	100%
PCI Within 90 Minutes of Arrival	0	-	83%	54%	95%
Smoking Cessation Advice[3]	0	-	84%	88%	100%
Heart Failure Care					
ACE Inhibitor or ARB for LVSD[1,3]	3	33%	76%	82%	100%
Discharge Instructions[1,3]	1	0%	54%	61%	93%
Evaluation of LVS Function[1,3]	9	44%	72%	83%	99%
Smoking Cessation Advice[1,3]	1	0%	62%	82%	100%
Pneumonia Care					
Appropriate Initial Antibiotic[1,2]	4	75%	90%	83%	94%
Blood Culture Timing[2]	0	-	96%	90%	100%
Influenza Vaccine[1]	2	50%	77%	70%	100%
Initial Antibiotic Timing[1,2]	4	100%	91%	80%	93%
Oxygenation Assessment[1,2]	10	100%	97%	99%	100%
Pneumococcal Vaccine[1,2]	6	50%	70%	69%	94%
Smoking Cessation Advice[1,2]	2	100%	64%	80%	100%
Surgical Infection Prevention					
Prophylactic Antibiotic Given[1,2,3]	9	33%	79%	77%	95%
Prophylactic Antibiotic Selection[1,2]	4	100%	94%	90%	100%
Prophylactic Antibiotic Stopped[1,2,3]	9	100%	83%	72%	95%
Pregnancy Care					
Inpatient Neonatal Mortality	-	-	-	-	-
Third or Fourth Degree Laceration	-	-	-	3.63%	3.27%

Gordon Memorial Hospital District

300 E 8th Street
Gordon, NE 69343
URL: www.gordonhospital.org

Phone: 308-282-0401
Fax: 308-282-0431

Ownership: Govt - Hospital District or Authority
Emergency Services: Yes

Accredited: No
Licensed Beds: 25

Key Personnel:
President/CEO . . . . Kay Garcia
Chief Medical Staff . . . . J F Hutchins, MD
Infection Control . . . . Kathie King
Respiratory/Cardiopulmonary . . . . Jan Fairhead

Measure	Cases	This Hospital	State Average	U.S. Average	Top Hospital
Heart Attack Care					
ACE Inhibitor or ARB for LVSD[5]	-	-	90%	82%	100%
Aspirin at Arrival[5]	-	-	88%	92%	100%
Aspirin at Discharge[5]	-	-	90%	90%	100%
Beta Blocker at Arrival[5]	-	-	81%	87%	100%
Beta Blocker at Discharge[5]	-	-	95%	90%	100%
Fibrinolytic Medication Timing[5]	-	-	25%	31%	100%
PCI Within 90 Minutes of Arrival[5]	-	-	83%	54%	95%
Smoking Cessation Advice[5]	-	-	84%	88%	100%
Heart Failure Care					
ACE Inhibitor or ARB for LVSD[5]	-	-	76%	82%	100%
Discharge Instructions[5]	-	-	54%	61%	93%
Evaluation of LVS Function[5]	-	-	72%	83%	99%
Smoking Cessation Advice[5]	-	-	62%	82%	100%
Pneumonia Care					
Appropriate Initial Antibiotic[1]	24	96%	90%	83%	94%
Blood Culture Timing[1]	2	100%	96%	90%	100%
Influenza Vaccine[1]	12	92%	77%	70%	100%
Initial Antibiotic Timing	27	93%	91%	80%	93%
Oxygenation Assessment	34	100%	97%	99%	100%
Pneumococcal Vaccine	28	86%	70%	69%	94%
Smoking Cessation Advice[1]	10	50%	64%	80%	100%
Surgical Infection Prevention					
Prophylactic Antibiotic Given[5]	-	-	79%	77%	95%
Prophylactic Antibiotic Selection[5]	-	-	94%	90%	100%
Prophylactic Antibiotic Stopped[5]	-	-	83%	72%	95%
Pregnancy Care					
Inpatient Neonatal Mortality	-	-	-	-	-
Third or Fourth Degree Laceration	-	-	-	3.63%	3.27%

Gothenburg Memorial Hospital

PO Box 469
Gothenburg, NE 69138
Ownership: Govt - Hospital District or Authority
Emergency Services: Yes

Phone: 308-537-3661
Fax: 308-537-3074
Accredited: No
Licensed Beds: 12

Key Personnel:
Administrator . . . . Roger Heidebrink

Measure	Cases	This Hospital	State Average	U.S. Average	Top Hospital
Heart Attack Care					
ACE Inhibitor or ARB for LVSD[5]	-	-	90%	82%	100%
Aspirin at Arrival[5]	-	-	88%	92%	100%
Aspirin at Discharge[5]	-	-	90%	90%	100%
Beta Blocker at Arrival[5]	-	-	81%	87%	100%
Beta Blocker at Discharge[5]	-	-	95%	90%	100%
Fibrinolytic Medication Timing[5]	-	-	25%	31%	100%
PCI Within 90 Minutes of Arrival[5]	-	-	83%	54%	95%
Smoking Cessation Advice[5]	-	-	84%	88%	100%
Heart Failure Care					
ACE Inhibitor or ARB for LVSD[3]	0	-	76%	82%	100%
Discharge Instructions[1,3]	1	100%	54%	61%	93%
Evaluation of LVS Function[1,3]	2	50%	72%	83%	99%
Smoking Cessation Advice[3]	0	-	62%	82%	100%
Pneumonia Care					
Appropriate Initial Antibiotic[1]	12	92%	90%	83%	94%
Blood Culture Timing[1]	4	100%	96%	90%	100%
Influenza Vaccine[1]	3	100%	77%	70%	100%
Initial Antibiotic Timing[1]	14	93%	91%	80%	93%
Oxygenation Assessment[1]	17	100%	97%	99%	100%
Pneumococcal Vaccine[1]	15	87%	70%	69%	94%
Smoking Cessation Advice[1]	2	100%	64%	80%	100%
Surgical Infection Prevention					
Prophylactic Antibiotic Given[5]	-	-	79%	77%	95%
Prophylactic Antibiotic Selection[5]	-	-	94%	90%	100%
Prophylactic Antibiotic Stopped[5]	-	-	83%	72%	95%
Pregnancy Care					
Inpatient Neonatal Mortality	-	-	-	-	-
Third or Fourth Degree Laceration	-	-	-	3.63%	3.27%

Saint Francis Med Ctr/Memorial Health Center

Alternate Name: Saint Francis Medical Center
2620 W Faidley Avenue
Grand Island, NE 68803

Toll-Free: 800-353-4896
Phone: 308-384-4600
Fax: 308-398-5589

URL: www.saintfrancisgi.org
Ownership: Voluntary non-profit - Church
Emergency Services: Yes

Accredited: Yes
Licensed Beds: 200

Key Personnel:
President/CEO . . . . Michael R Gloor, FACHE
Director Surgery . . . . Dee Donaldson, RN
Director Maternal Child . . . . Jan Spale
Director Radiology . . . . Jacqueline Huldt
Director Cardiology . . . . Karen Riva

Measure	Cases	This Hospital	State Average	U.S. Average	Top Hospital
Heart Attack Care					
ACE Inhibitor or ARB for LVSD	25	88%	90%	82%	100%
Aspirin at Arrival	84	99%	88%	92%	100%
Aspirin at Discharge	73	97%	90%	90%	100%
Beta Blocker at Arrival	62	97%	81%	87%	100%
Beta Blocker at Discharge	72	96%	95%	90%	100%

NOTE: Hospital profiles are in alphabetical order by state, then city, then hospital within the city; Rankings are sorted by rate in descending order and exclude hospitals with less than 25 cases; (1) The number of cases is too small (n<25) for purposes of reliably predicting hospital performance; (2) Measure reflects the hospital's indication that its submission was based upon a sample of its relevant discharges; (3) Rate reflects fewer than the maximum possible quarters of data for the measure; (4) Inaccurate information submitted and suppressed for one or more quarters; (5) No data is available from the hospital for this measure; Please refer to the User's Guide for a full explanation of data

Measure	Cases	This Hospital	State Average	U.S. Average	Top Hospital
Fibrinolytic Medication Timing[1]	6	50%	25%	31%	100%
PCI Within 90 Minutes of Arrival[1]	2	100%	83%	54%	95%
Smoking Cessation Advice	35	97%	84%	88%	100%
Heart Failure Care					
ACE Inhibitor or ARB for LVSD	44	86%	76%	82%	100%
Discharge Instructions	107	87%	54%	61%	93%
Evaluation of LVS Function	154	98%	72%	83%	99%
Smoking Cessation Advice	25	84%	62%	82%	100%
Pneumonia Care					
Appropriate Initial Antibiotic	156	86%	90%	83%	94%
Blood Culture Timing	165	93%	96%	90%	100%
Influenza Vaccine	66	64%	77%	70%	100%
Initial Antibiotic Timing	244	95%	91%	80%	93%
Oxygenation Assessment	330	100%	97%	99%	100%
Pneumococcal Vaccine	207	83%	70%	69%	94%
Smoking Cessation Advice	52	92%	64%	80%	100%
Surgical Infection Prevention					
Prophylactic Antibiotic Given	598	94%	79%	77%	95%
Prophylactic Antibiotic Selection	151	96%	94%	90%	100%
Prophylactic Antibiotic Stopped	579	71%	83%	72%	95%
Pregnancy Care					
Inpatient Neonatal Mortality	-	-	-	-	-
Third or Fourth Degree Laceration	-	-	-	3.63%	3.27%

Perkins County Health Services

Alternate Name: Perkins County Community Hospital
900 Lincoln Avenue
Grant, NE 69140
Ownership: Govt - Hospital District or Authority
Emergency Services: Yes
Phone: 308-352-7200
Fax: 308-352-7290
Accredited: No
Licensed Beds: 20

Measure	Cases	This Hospital	State Average	U.S. Average	Top Hospital
Heart Attack Care					
ACE Inhibitor or ARB for LVSD[3]	0	-	90%	82%	100%
Aspirin at Arrival[1,3]	2	100%	88%	92%	100%
Aspirin at Discharge[1,3]	2	100%	90%	90%	100%
Beta Blocker at Arrival[1,3]	1	100%	81%	87%	100%
Beta Blocker at Discharge[1,3]	2	100%	95%	90%	100%
Fibrinolytic Medication Timing[3]	0	-	25%	31%	100%
PCI Within 90 Minutes of Arrival[5]	-	-	83%	54%	95%
Smoking Cessation Advice[3]	0	-	84%	88%	100%
Heart Failure Care					
ACE Inhibitor or ARB for LVSD[1,3]	3	33%	76%	82%	100%
Discharge Instructions[1,3]	5	0%	54%	61%	93%
Evaluation of LVS Function[1,3]	8	88%	72%	83%	99%
Smoking Cessation Advice[3]	0	-	62%	82%	100%
Pneumonia Care					
Appropriate Initial Antibiotic[1]	17	100%	90%	83%	94%
Blood Culture Timing[1]	3	67%	96%	90%	100%
Influenza Vaccine[1]	13	100%	77%	70%	100%
Initial Antibiotic Timing[1]	21	95%	91%	80%	93%
Oxygenation Assessment	26	100%	97%	99%	100%
Pneumococcal Vaccine	25	88%	70%	69%	94%
Smoking Cessation Advice[1]	2	0%	64%	80%	100%
Surgical Infection Prevention					
Prophylactic Antibiotic Given[5]	-	-	79%	77%	95%
Prophylactic Antibiotic Selection[5]	-	-	94%	90%	100%
Prophylactic Antibiotic Stopped[5]	-	-	83%	72%	95%
Pregnancy Care					
Inpatient Neonatal Mortality	-	-	-	-	-
Third or Fourth Degree Laceration	-	-	-	3.63%	3.27%

Mary Lanning Memorial Hospital

715 N Saint Joseph Avenue
Hastings, NE 68901
Ownership: Voluntary non-profit - Private
Emergency Services: Yes
Phone: 402-463-4521
Fax: 402-461-5321
Accredited: Yes
Licensed Beds: 183

Key Personnel:
CEO . . . . W Michael Kearney
Chief Medical Staff . . . . Gary Caingren
Emergency Room . . . . Ronda Ehly
Infection Control . . . . Connie Hyde

Measure	Cases	This Hospital	State Average	U.S. Average	Top Hospital
Heart Attack Care					
ACE Inhibitor or ARB for LVSD[1]	4	25%	90%	82%	100%
Aspirin at Arrival	32	94%	88%	92%	100%
Aspirin at Discharge[1]	19	89%	90%	90%	100%
Beta Blocker at Arrival	32	72%	81%	87%	100%
Beta Blocker at Discharge[1]	20	70%	95%	90%	100%
Fibrinolytic Medication Timing[1]	6	50%	25%	31%	100%
PCI Within 90 Minutes of Arrival	0	-	83%	54%	95%
Smoking Cessation Advice[1]	8	75%	84%	88%	100%
Heart Failure Care					
ACE Inhibitor or ARB for LVSD	63	52%	76%	82%	100%
Discharge Instructions	95	59%	54%	61%	93%
Evaluation of LVS Function	153	93%	72%	83%	99%
Smoking Cessation Advice[1]	7	29%	62%	82%	100%
Pneumonia Care					
Appropriate Initial Antibiotic	106	87%	90%	83%	94%
Blood Culture Timing	104	96%	96%	90%	100%
Influenza Vaccine	44	73%	77%	70%	100%
Initial Antibiotic Timing	172	80%	91%	80%	93%
Oxygenation Assessment	221	99%	97%	99%	100%
Pneumococcal Vaccine	159	67%	70%	69%	94%
Smoking Cessation Advice	26	62%	64%	80%	100%
Surgical Infection Prevention					
Prophylactic Antibiotic Given[3]	324	73%	79%	77%	95%
Prophylactic Antibiotic Selection	111	93%	94%	90%	100%
Prophylactic Antibiotic Stopped[3]	310	94%	83%	72%	95%
Pregnancy Care					
Inpatient Neonatal Mortality	-	-	-	-	-
Third or Fourth Degree Laceration	-	-	-	3.63%	3.27%

Thayer County Health Services

Alternate Name: Thayer County Memorial Hospital
120 Park Avenue
Hebron, NE 68370
E-mail: tach@allpl.net
Ownership: Government - Local
Emergency Services: Yes
Phone: 402-768-4614
Fax: 402-768-4669
Accredited: No
Licensed Beds: 14

Key Personnel:
President/CEO . . . . Mark Lisa, FACHE
Chief Medical Staff . . . . Timothy J Sullivan, MD
Infection Control . . . . Marla Heitmann, RN
ICU . . . . Jolynn Hacker, RN
Medical Surgical Nursing . . . . Mary Ann Kasl

Measure	Cases	This Hospital	State Average	U.S. Average	Top Hospital
Heart Attack Care					
ACE Inhibitor or ARB for LVSD[3]	0	-	90%	82%	100%
Aspirin at Arrival[3]	0	-	88%	92%	100%
Aspirin at Discharge[3]	0	-	90%	90%	100%
Beta Blocker at Arrival[1,3]	1	0%	81%	87%	100%
Beta Blocker at Discharge[3]	0	-	95%	90%	100%
Fibrinolytic Medication Timing[1,3]	1	0%	25%	31%	100%
PCI Within 90 Minutes of Arrival[5]	-	-	83%	54%	95%
Smoking Cessation Advice[3]	0	-	84%	88%	100%
Heart Failure Care					
ACE Inhibitor or ARB for LVSD[1,3]	4	75%	76%	82%	100%
Discharge Instructions[1,3]	9	0%	54%	61%	93%
Evaluation of LVS Function[1,3]	18	44%	72%	83%	99%
Smoking Cessation Advice[3]	0	-	62%	82%	100%
Pneumonia Care					
Appropriate Initial Antibiotic[1,3]	11	91%	90%	83%	94%
Blood Culture Timing[1,3]	2	100%	96%	90%	100%
Influenza Vaccine	0	-	77%	70%	100%
Initial Antibiotic Timing	26	92%	91%	80%	93%
Oxygenation Assessment	32	100%	97%	99%	100%
Pneumococcal Vaccine[1,3]	12	17%	70%	69%	94%
Smoking Cessation Advice[1,3]	1	0%	64%	80%	100%
Surgical Infection Prevention					
Prophylactic Antibiotic Given[5]	-	-	79%	77%	95%
Prophylactic Antibiotic Selection[5]	-	-	94%	90%	100%
Prophylactic Antibiotic Stopped[5]	-	-	83%	72%	95%

NOTE: Hospital profiles are in alphabetical order by state, then city, then hospital within the city; Rankings are sorted by rate in descending order and exclude hospitals with less than 25 cases; (1) The number of cases is too small (n<25) for purposes of reliably predicting hospital performance; (2) Measure reflects the hospital's indication that its submission was based upon a sample of its relevant discharges; (3) Rate reflects fewer than the maximum possible quarters of data for the measure; (4) Inaccurate information submitted and suppressed for one or more quarters; (5) No data is available from the hospital for this measure; Please refer to the User's Guide for a full explanation of data

Pregnancy Care					
Inpatient Neonatal Mortality	-	-	-	-	-
Third or Fourth Degree Laceration	-	-	-	3.63%	3.27%

Henderson Health Care Services

Alternate Name: Henderson Community Hospital
1621 Front Street
Henderson, NE 68371
Phone: 402-723-4512
Fax: 402-723-4520
Ownership: Voluntary non-profit - Private
Accredited: No
Emergency Services: Yes
Licensed Beds: 59

Key Personnel:

Administrator . . . . Calvin Graber
Chief Medical Staff. . . . . Robet J Wochner, MD
Director Medical/Surgical Nursing . . . . Darlene Janzen
Chief Radiology . . . . Tyrone Seeger

Measure	Cases	This Hospital	State Average	U.S. Average	Top Hospital
Heart Attack Care					
ACE Inhibitor or ARB for LVSD[5]	-	-	90%	82%	100%
Aspirin at Arrival[5]	-	-	88%	92%	100%
Aspirin at Discharge[5]	-	-	90%	90%	100%
Beta Blocker at Arrival[5]	-	-	81%	87%	100%
Beta Blocker at Discharge[5]	-	-	95%	90%	100%
Fibrinolytic Medication Timing[5]	-	-	25%	31%	100%
PCI Within 90 Minutes of Arrival[5]	-	-	83%	54%	95%
Smoking Cessation Advice[5]	-	-	84%	88%	100%
Heart Failure Care					
ACE Inhibitor or ARB for LVSD[5]	-	-	76%	82%	100%
Discharge Instructions[5]	-	-	54%	61%	93%
Evaluation of LVS Function[5]	-	-	72%	83%	99%
Smoking Cessation Advice[5]	-	-	62%	82%	100%
Pneumonia Care					
Appropriate Initial Antibiotic[1,3]	2	100%	90%	83%	94%
Blood Culture Timing[3]	0	-	96%	90%	100%
Influenza Vaccine[5]	-	-	77%	70%	100%
Initial Antibiotic Timing[1,3]	3	100%	91%	80%	93%
Oxygenation Assessment[1,3]	3	100%	97%	99%	100%
Pneumococcal Vaccine[1,3]	3	100%	70%	69%	94%
Smoking Cessation Advice[3]	0	-	64%	80%	100%
Surgical Infection Prevention					
Prophylactic Antibiotic Given[5]	-	-	79%	77%	95%
Prophylactic Antibiotic Selection[5]	-	-	94%	90%	100%
Prophylactic Antibiotic Stopped[5]	-	-	83%	72%	95%
Pregnancy Care					
Inpatient Neonatal Mortality	-	-	-	-	-
Third or Fourth Degree Laceration	-	-	-	3.63%	3.27%

Phelps Memorial Health Center

1215 Tibbals Street
Holdrege, NE 68949
Phone: 308-995-2211
Fax: 308-995-3333
URL: www.phelpsmemorial.com
Ownership: Voluntary non-profit - Other
Accredited: Yes
Emergency Services: Yes
Licensed Beds: 49

Key Personnel:

Administrator/CEO. . . . . Joyce Grove Hein
Chief Medical Staff. . . . . Stuart Embury, MD
Infection Control. . . . . Laurie Raboin
Unit Manager Intensive Coronary. . . . . Susan Rieker
Unit Manager OB/GYN Womens Health . . . . . . Miki Nichols
Respiratory Therapy. . . . . Tracie Elliott

Measure	Cases	This Hospital	State Average	U.S. Average	Top Hospital
Heart Attack Care					
ACE Inhibitor or ARB for LVSD[3]	0	-	90%	82%	100%
Aspirin at Arrival[1,3]	3	67%	88%	92%	100%
Aspirin at Discharge[1,3]	1	100%	90%	90%	100%
Beta Blocker at Arrival[1,3]	2	100%	81%	87%	100%
Beta Blocker at Discharge[1,3]	2	100%	95%	90%	100%
Fibrinolytic Medication Timing[1,3]	2	50%	25%	31%	100%
PCI Within 90 Minutes of Arrival	0	-	83%	54%	95%
Smoking Cessation Advice[3]	0	-	84%	88%	100%
Heart Failure Care					
ACE Inhibitor or ARB for LVSD[1]	2	100%	76%	82%	100%
Discharge Instructions[1]	10	70%	54%	61%	93%
Evaluation of LVS Function[1]	20	70%	72%	83%	99%
Smoking Cessation Advice[1]	3	33%	62%	82%	100%
Pneumonia Care					
Appropriate Initial Antibiotic	25	100%	90%	83%	94%
Blood Culture Timing[1]	2	100%	96%	90%	100%
Influenza Vaccine[1]	14	100%	77%	70%	100%
Initial Antibiotic Timing	53	89%	91%	80%	93%
Oxygenation Assessment	62	100%	97%	99%	100%
Pneumococcal Vaccine	38	82%	70%	69%	94%
Smoking Cessation Advice[1]	11	91%	64%	80%	100%
Surgical Infection Prevention					
Prophylactic Antibiotic Given	61	75%	79%	77%	95%
Prophylactic Antibiotic Selection[1]	19	95%	94%	90%	100%
Prophylactic Antibiotic Stopped	59	69%	83%	72%	95%
Pregnancy Care					
Inpatient Neonatal Mortality	-	-	-	-	-
Third or Fourth Degree Laceration	-	-	-	3.63%	3.27%

Chase County Hospital

600 W 12th Street
Imperial, NE 69033
Phone: 308-882-7111
Fax: 308-882-5950
E-mail: ccch@chase30co.com
Ownership: Government - Local
Accredited: No
Emergency Services: Yes
Licensed Beds: 26

Key Personnel:

CEO. . . . . Julie Sharp
Chief Medical Staff. . . . . Lola Jones, DO

Measure	Cases	This Hospital	State Average	U.S. Average	Top Hospital
Heart Attack Care					
ACE Inhibitor or ARB for LVSD[5]	-	-	90%	82%	100%
Aspirin at Arrival[5]	-	-	88%	92%	100%
Aspirin at Discharge[5]	-	-	90%	90%	100%
Beta Blocker at Arrival[5]	-	-	81%	87%	100%
Beta Blocker at Discharge[5]	-	-	95%	90%	100%
Fibrinolytic Medication Timing[5]	-	-	25%	31%	100%
PCI Within 90 Minutes of Arrival[5]	-	-	83%	54%	95%
Smoking Cessation Advice[5]	-	-	84%	88%	100%
Heart Failure Care					
ACE Inhibitor or ARB for LVSD[3]	0	-	76%	82%	100%
Discharge Instructions[1,3]	1	0%	54%	61%	93%
Evaluation of LVS Function[1,3]	1	0%	72%	83%	99%
Smoking Cessation Advice[3]	0	-	62%	82%	100%
Pneumonia Care					
Appropriate Initial Antibiotic[1]	11	100%	90%	83%	94%
Blood Culture Timing	0	-	96%	90%	100%
Influenza Vaccine[1]	4	25%	77%	70%	100%
Initial Antibiotic Timing[1]	13	92%	91%	80%	93%
Oxygenation Assessment[1]	15	100%	97%	99%	100%
Pneumococcal Vaccine[1]	11	36%	70%	69%	94%
Smoking Cessation Advice[1]	1	100%	64%	80%	100%
Surgical Infection Prevention					
Prophylactic Antibiotic Given[5]	-	-	79%	77%	95%
Prophylactic Antibiotic Selection[5]	-	-	94%	90%	100%
Prophylactic Antibiotic Stopped[5]	-	-	83%	72%	95%
Pregnancy Care					
Inpatient Neonatal Mortality	-	-	-	-	-
Third or Fourth Degree Laceration	-	-	-	3.63%	3.27%

Good Samaritan

10 East 31st Street
Kearney, NE 68847
Phone: 308-865-7100
Fax: 308-865-2924
URL: www.gshs.org
Ownership: Voluntary non-profit - Church
Accredited: Yes
Emergency Services: Yes
Licensed Beds: 287

Key Personnel:

President/CEO. . . . . John W Allen
Emergency Services Director. . . . . Paul O'Connell
ICU Director . . . . Valerie Fredericksen
Surgery Director. . . . . Ron Langford
Respiratory Therapy Director . . . . Bill Bonner

NOTE: Hospital profiles are in alphabetical order by state, then city, then hospital within the city; Rankings are sorted by rate in descending order and exclude hospitals with less than 25 cases; (1) The number of cases is too small (n<25) for purposes of reliably predicting hospital performance; (2) Measure reflects the hospital's indication that its submission was based upon a sample of its relevant discharges; (3) Rate reflects fewer than the maximum possible quarters of data for the measure; (4) Inaccurate information submitted and suppressed for one or more quarters; (5) No data is available from the hospital for this measure; Please refer to the User's Guide for a full explanation of data

Measure	Cases	This Hospital	State Average	U.S. Average	Top Hospital
Heart Attack Care					
ACE Inhibitor or ARB for LVSD	28	82%	90%	82%	100%
Aspirin at Arrival	75	97%	88%	92%	100%
Aspirin at Discharge	121	99%	90%	90%	100%
Beta Blocker at Arrival	58	84%	81%	87%	100%
Beta Blocker at Discharge	134	98%	95%	90%	100%
Fibrinolytic Medication Timing[1]	1	100%	25%	31%	100%
PCI Within 90 Minutes of Arrival[1]	6	50%	83%	54%	95%
Smoking Cessation Advice	57	98%	84%	88%	100%
Heart Failure Care					
ACE Inhibitor or ARB for LVSD	48	88%	76%	82%	100%
Discharge Instructions	119	62%	54%	61%	93%
Evaluation of LVS Function	168	89%	72%	83%	99%
Smoking Cessation Advice	35	91%	62%	82%	100%
Pneumonia Care					
Appropriate Initial Antibiotic	97	93%	90%	83%	94%
Blood Culture Timing	60	92%	96%	90%	100%
Influenza Vaccine	36	58%	77%	70%	100%
Initial Antibiotic Timing	136	87%	91%	80%	93%
Oxygenation Assessment	190	100%	97%	99%	100%
Pneumococcal Vaccine	137	85%	70%	69%	94%
Smoking Cessation Advice	52	92%	64%	80%	100%
Surgical Infection Prevention					
Prophylactic Antibiotic Given[3]	686	91%	79%	77%	95%
Prophylactic Antibiotic Selection	209	97%	94%	90%	100%
Prophylactic Antibiotic Stopped[3]	671	78%	83%	72%	95%
Pregnancy Care					
Inpatient Neonatal Mortality	-	-	-	-	-
Third or Fourth Degree Laceration	-	-	-	3.63%	3.27%

Tri-County Area Hospital District

1201 Erie Street
PO Box 980
Lexington, NE 68850
E-mail: tch_carolynm@webco.net
URL: www.tricountyhospital.com
Ownership: Govt - Hospital District or Authority
Emergency Services: Yes

Phone: 308-324-5651
Fax: 308-324-8359
Accredited: No
Licensed Beds: 40

Key Personnel:
CEO. . . . . Calvin Hiner
Chief Medical Staff. . . . . Fran Acosta-Carlson, MD
Emergency Room . . . . John Ford, MD
Emergency Room . . . . Brooke Naputi, RN
Infection Control. . . . . Kathy Gorache, RN
Director Radiology . . . . Jolene Swartz
Director Respiratory Therapy . . . . Tom Grooms

Measure	Cases	This Hospital	State Average	U.S. Average	Top Hospital
Heart Attack Care					
ACE Inhibitor or ARB for LVSD[5]	-	-	90%	82%	100%
Aspirin at Arrival[5]	-	-	88%	92%	100%
Aspirin at Discharge[5]	-	-	90%	90%	100%
Beta Blocker at Arrival[5]	-	-	81%	87%	100%
Beta Blocker at Discharge[5]	-	-	95%	90%	100%
Fibrinolytic Medication Timing[5]	-	-	25%	31%	100%
PCI Within 90 Minutes of Arrival[5]	-	-	83%	54%	95%
Smoking Cessation Advice[5]	-	-	84%	88%	100%
Heart Failure Care					
ACE Inhibitor or ARB for LVSD[1]	7	100%	76%	82%	100%
Discharge Instructions[1]	24	50%	54%	61%	93%
Evaluation of LVS Function	31	81%	72%	83%	99%
Smoking Cessation Advice[1]	3	33%	62%	82%	100%
Pneumonia Care					
Appropriate Initial Antibiotic	48	92%	90%	83%	94%
Blood Culture Timing[1]	11	100%	96%	90%	100%
Influenza Vaccine[1]	13	69%	77%	70%	100%
Initial Antibiotic Timing	75	91%	91%	80%	93%
Oxygenation Assessment	90	99%	97%	99%	100%
Pneumococcal Vaccine	61	87%	70%	69%	94%
Smoking Cessation Advice[1]	19	79%	64%	80%	100%
Surgical Infection Prevention					
Prophylactic Antibiotic Given	36	89%	79%	77%	95%
Prophylactic Antibiotic Selection[1]	7	86%	94%	90%	100%
Prophylactic Antibiotic Stopped	35	49%	83%	72%	95%
Pregnancy Care					
Inpatient Neonatal Mortality	-	-	-	-	-
Third or Fourth Degree Laceration	-	-	-	3.63%	3.27%

BryanLGH Medical Center

1600 S 48th Street
Lincoln, NE 68506
URL: www.bryanlgh.org
Ownership: Voluntary non-profit - Private
Emergency Services: Yes

Phone: 402-489-0200
Fax: 402-481-8306
Accredited: Yes
Licensed Beds: 316

Key Personnel:
President/CEO. . . . . Craig Ames
Chief Medical Staff. . . . . Jeffrey Marple, MD
Chief Catheterization Laboratory . . . . Su Eells
Emergency Room . . . . Terry Rounsborg, MD
Director Infection/Disease Control . . . . Larry Krebsbach
CCU Spvg. Nurse . . . . Louis Lemon
Director Medical/Surgical Nursing . . . . Denise Linder
OB/GYN Womens Health. . . . . Deanna Hutchins, MD
Chief Radiology . . . . Janet Matthes, MD
Director Respiratory Therapy . . . . Steve Steinkuehler

Measure	Cases	This Hospital	State Average	U.S. Average	Top Hospital
Heart Attack Care					
ACE Inhibitor or ARB for LVSD	78	81%	90%	82%	100%
Aspirin at Arrival	164	95%	88%	92%	100%
Aspirin at Discharge	325	97%	90%	90%	100%
Beta Blocker at Arrival	118	97%	81%	87%	100%
Beta Blocker at Discharge	353	95%	95%	90%	100%
Fibrinolytic Medication Timing	0	-	25%	31%	100%
PCI Within 90 Minutes of Arrival[1]	6	100%	83%	54%	95%
Smoking Cessation Advice	126	92%	84%	88%	100%
Heart Failure Care					
ACE Inhibitor or ARB for LVSD	278	85%	76%	82%	100%
Discharge Instructions	403	84%	54%	61%	93%
Evaluation of LVS Function	514	96%	72%	83%	99%
Smoking Cessation Advice	66	94%	62%	82%	100%
Pneumonia Care					
Appropriate Initial Antibiotic	133	88%	90%	83%	94%
Blood Culture Timing	149	95%	96%	90%	100%
Influenza Vaccine	61	92%	77%	70%	100%
Initial Antibiotic Timing	228	84%	91%	80%	93%
Oxygenation Assessment	306	100%	97%	99%	100%
Pneumococcal Vaccine	226	92%	70%	69%	94%
Smoking Cessation Advice	62	85%	64%	80%	100%
Surgical Infection Prevention					
Prophylactic Antibiotic Given	843	93%	79%	77%	95%
Prophylactic Antibiotic Selection	225	90%	94%	90%	100%
Prophylactic Antibiotic Stopped	803	84%	83%	72%	95%
Pregnancy Care					
Inpatient Neonatal Mortality	-	-	-	-	-
Third or Fourth Degree Laceration	-	-	-	3.63%	3.27%

Lincoln Surgical Hospital

1710 South 70th St, Suite 200
Lincoln, NE 68506
Ownership: Proprietary
Emergency Services: No

Phone: 402-483-1550
Accredited: No

Measure	Cases	This Hospital	State Average	U.S. Average	Top Hospital
Heart Attack Care					
ACE Inhibitor or ARB for LVSD[5]	-	-	90%	82%	100%
Aspirin at Arrival[5]	-	-	88%	92%	100%
Aspirin at Discharge[5]	-	-	90%	90%	100%
Beta Blocker at Arrival[5]	-	-	81%	87%	100%
Beta Blocker at Discharge[5]	-	-	95%	90%	100%
Fibrinolytic Medication Timing[5]	-	-	25%	31%	100%
PCI Within 90 Minutes of Arrival[5]	-	-	83%	54%	95%
Smoking Cessation Advice[5]	-	-	84%	88%	100%

NOTE: Hospital profiles are in alphabetical order by state, then city, then hospital within the city; Rankings are sorted by rate in descending order and exclude hospitals with less than 25 cases; (1) The number of cases is too small (n<25) for purposes of reliably predicting hospital performance; (2) Measure reflects the hospital's indication that its submission was based upon a sample of its relevant discharges; (3) Rate reflects fewer than the maximum possible quarters of data for the measure; (4) Inaccurate information submitted and suppressed for one or more quarters; (5) No data is available from the hospital for this measure; Please refer to the User's Guide for a full explanation of data

Measure	Cases	This Hospital	State Average	U.S. Average	Top Hospital
Heart Failure Care					
ACE Inhibitor or ARB for LVSD[5]	-	-	76%	82%	100%
Discharge Instructions[5]	-	-	54%	61%	93%
Evaluation of LVS Function[5]	-	-	72%	83%	99%
Smoking Cessation Advice[5]	-	-	62%	82%	100%
Pneumonia Care					
Appropriate Initial Antibiotic[5]	-	-	90%	83%	94%
Blood Culture Timing[5]	-	-	96%	90%	100%
Influenza Vaccine[5]	-	-	77%	70%	100%
Initial Antibiotic Timing[5]	-	-	91%	80%	93%
Oxygenation Assessment[5]	-	-	97%	99%	100%
Pneumococcal Vaccine[5]	-	-	70%	69%	94%
Smoking Cessation Advice[5]	-	-	64%	80%	100%
Surgical Infection Prevention					
Prophylactic Antibiotic Given[3]	157	87%	79%	77%	95%
Prophylactic Antibiotic Selection	54	98%	94%	90%	100%
Prophylactic Antibiotic Stopped[3]	157	82%	83%	72%	95%
Pregnancy Care					
Inpatient Neonatal Mortality	-	-	-	-	-
Third or Fourth Degree Laceration	-	-	-	3.63%	3.27%

Nebraska Heart Hospital

7500 S 91st St
Lincoln, NE 68526

Toll-Free: 800-644-3627
Phone: 402-327-2700
Fax: 402-328-3010

E-mail: info@neheart.com
URL: www.neheart.com
Ownership: Proprietary
Emergency Services: No

Accredited: No
Licensed Beds: 63

Key Personnel:
CEO. . . . . Sheryl D Dodds

Measure	Cases	This Hospital	State Average	U.S. Average	Top Hospital
Heart Attack Care					
ACE Inhibitor or ARB for LVSD	75	92%	90%	82%	100%
Aspirin at Arrival[1]	23	87%	88%	92%	100%
Aspirin at Discharge	324	98%	90%	90%	100%
Beta Blocker at Arrival[1]	23	61%	81%	87%	100%
Beta Blocker at Discharge	310	97%	95%	90%	100%
Fibrinolytic Medication Timing	0	-	25%	31%	100%
PCI Within 90 Minutes of Arrival	0	-	83%	54%	95%
Smoking Cessation Advice	111	93%	84%	88%	100%
Heart Failure Care					
ACE Inhibitor or ARB for LVSD	292	88%	76%	82%	100%
Discharge Instructions	323	82%	54%	61%	93%
Evaluation of LVS Function	364	99%	72%	83%	99%
Smoking Cessation Advice	51	80%	62%	82%	100%
Pneumonia Care					
Appropriate Initial Antibiotic[1]	1	100%	90%	83%	94%
Blood Culture Timing[1]	1	100%	96%	90%	100%
Influenza Vaccine[1]	2	50%	77%	70%	100%
Initial Antibiotic Timing[1]	2	100%	91%	80%	93%
Oxygenation Assessment[1]	3	100%	97%	99%	100%
Pneumococcal Vaccine[1]	4	100%	70%	69%	94%
Smoking Cessation Advice[1]	5	100%	64%	80%	100%
Surgical Infection Prevention					
Prophylactic Antibiotic Given[2,3]	85	95%	79%	77%	95%
Prophylactic Antibiotic Selection[2]	35	100%	94%	90%	100%
Prophylactic Antibiotic Stopped[2,3]	81	88%	83%	72%	95%
Pregnancy Care					
Inpatient Neonatal Mortality	-	-	-	-	-
Third or Fourth Degree Laceration	-	-	-	3.63%	3.27%

Saint Elizabeth Regional Medical Center

555 S 70th Street
Lincoln, NE 68510
URL: www.stelizabethonline.com
Ownership: Voluntary non-profit - Church
Emergency Services: Yes

Phone: 402-489-7181
Fax: 402-219-7673

Accredited: Yes
Licensed Beds: 197

Key Personnel:
President/CEO. . . . . Robert J Lanik
Chief Medical Staff. . . . . Dr. Greg Heidrick
OB/GYN Womens Health. . . . . Dr. Sean Kenney
Director Respiratory Therapy . . . . Jay Snyder

Measure	Cases	This Hospital	State Average	U.S. Average	Top Hospital
Heart Attack Care					
ACE Inhibitor or ARB for LVSD	32	84%	90%	82%	100%
Aspirin at Arrival	82	99%	88%	92%	100%
Aspirin at Discharge	87	99%	90%	90%	100%
Beta Blocker at Arrival	65	97%	81%	87%	100%
Beta Blocker at Discharge	85	98%	95%	90%	100%
Fibrinolytic Medication Timing	0	-	25%	31%	100%
PCI Within 90 Minutes of Arrival[1]	10	80%	83%	54%	95%
Smoking Cessation Advice	29	97%	84%	88%	100%
Heart Failure Care					
ACE Inhibitor or ARB for LVSD	60	88%	76%	82%	100%
Discharge Instructions	95	91%	54%	61%	93%
Evaluation of LVS Function	142	96%	72%	83%	99%
Smoking Cessation Advice[1]	11	64%	62%	82%	100%
Pneumonia Care					
Appropriate Initial Antibiotic	134	93%	90%	83%	94%
Blood Culture Timing	101	90%	96%	90%	100%
Influenza Vaccine[1]	24	88%	77%	70%	100%
Initial Antibiotic Timing	166	86%	91%	80%	93%
Oxygenation Assessment	199	100%	97%	99%	100%
Pneumococcal Vaccine	138	89%	70%	69%	94%
Smoking Cessation Advice	45	69%	64%	80%	100%
Surgical Infection Prevention					
Prophylactic Antibiotic Given[3]	1,123	86%	79%	77%	95%
Prophylactic Antibiotic Selection	375	94%	94%	90%	100%
Prophylactic Antibiotic Stopped[3]	1,090	86%	83%	72%	95%
Pregnancy Care					
Inpatient Neonatal Mortality	-	-	-	-	-
Third or Fourth Degree Laceration	-	-	-	3.63%	3.27%

Niobrara Valley Hospital

401 S 5th Street
Lynch, NE 68746
Ownership: Voluntary non-profit - Private
Emergency Services: Yes

Phone: 402-569-2451
Fax: 402-569-2474
Accredited: No
Licensed Beds: 20

Key Personnel:
CEO. . . . . Bruce Purviance
Director Infection/Disease Control . . . . Barb Hart, RN
Director Medical/Surgical Nursing . . . . April Micanek
Chief Radiology . . . . Daniel Melkus, MD

Measure	Cases	This Hospital	State Average	U.S. Average	Top Hospital
Heart Attack Care					
ACE Inhibitor or ARB for LVSD[5]	-	-	90%	82%	100%
Aspirin at Arrival[5]	-	-	88%	92%	100%
Aspirin at Discharge[5]	-	-	90%	90%	100%
Beta Blocker at Arrival[5]	-	-	81%	87%	100%
Beta Blocker at Discharge[5]	-	-	95%	90%	100%
Fibrinolytic Medication Timing[5]	-	-	25%	31%	100%
PCI Within 90 Minutes of Arrival[5]	-	-	83%	54%	95%
Smoking Cessation Advice[5]	-	-	84%	88%	100%
Heart Failure Care					
ACE Inhibitor or ARB for LVSD[5]	-	-	76%	82%	100%
Discharge Instructions[5]	-	-	54%	61%	93%
Evaluation of LVS Function[5]	-	-	72%	83%	99%
Smoking Cessation Advice[5]	-	-	62%	82%	100%
Pneumonia Care					
Appropriate Initial Antibiotic[1,3]	2	100%	90%	83%	94%
Blood Culture Timing[1,3]	1	100%	96%	90%	100%
Influenza Vaccine[1]	1	100%	77%	70%	100%
Initial Antibiotic Timing[1,3]	3	67%	91%	80%	93%
Oxygenation Assessment[1,3]	3	100%	97%	99%	100%
Pneumococcal Vaccine[1,3]	3	33%	70%	69%	94%
Smoking Cessation Advice[3]	0	-	64%	80%	100%
Surgical Infection Prevention					
Prophylactic Antibiotic Given[5]	-	-	79%	77%	95%
Prophylactic Antibiotic Selection[5]	-	-	94%	90%	100%
Prophylactic Antibiotic Stopped[5]	-	-	83%	72%	95%
Pregnancy Care					

NOTE: Hospital profiles are in alphabetical order by state, then city, then hospital within the city; Rankings are sorted by rate in descending order and exclude hospitals with less than 25 cases; (1) The number of cases is too small (n<25) for purposes of reliably predicting hospital performance; (2) Measure reflects the hospital's indication that its submission was based upon a sample of its relevant discharges; (3) Rate reflects fewer than the maximum possible quarters of data for the measure; (4) Inaccurate information submitted and suppressed for one or more quarters; (5) No data is available from the hospital for this measure; Please refer to the User's Guide for a full explanation of data

Inpatient Neonatal Mortality	-	-	-	-	-
Third or Fourth Degree Laceration	-	-	-	3.63%	3.27%

Community Hospital

1301 E H Street
McCook, NE 69001
Ownership: Voluntary non-profit - Other
Emergency Services: Yes
Phone: 308-345-2650
Fax: 308-345-8358
Accredited: Yes
Licensed Beds: 44

Measure	Cases	This Hospital	State Average	U.S. Average	Top Hospital
Heart Attack Care					
ACE Inhibitor or ARB for LVSD[1]	3	100%	90%	82%	100%
Aspirin at Arrival[1]	4	75%	88%	92%	100%
Aspirin at Discharge[1]	2	50%	90%	90%	100%
Beta Blocker at Arrival[1]	5	40%	81%	87%	100%
Beta Blocker at Discharge[1]	2	100%	95%	90%	100%
Fibrinolytic Medication Timing	0	-	25%	31%	100%
PCI Within 90 Minutes of Arrival	0	-	83%	54%	95%
Smoking Cessation Advice	0	-	84%	88%	100%
Heart Failure Care					
ACE Inhibitor or ARB for LVSD[1]	1	100%	76%	82%	100%
Discharge Instructions[1]	14	79%	54%	61%	93%
Evaluation of LVS Function[1]	16	56%	72%	83%	99%
Smoking Cessation Advice[1]	1	0%	62%	82%	100%
Pneumonia Care					
Appropriate Initial Antibiotic	45	91%	90%	83%	94%
Blood Culture Timing[1]	12	100%	96%	90%	100%
Influenza Vaccine[1]	15	87%	77%	70%	100%
Initial Antibiotic Timing	61	90%	91%	80%	93%
Oxygenation Assessment	75	100%	97%	99%	100%
Pneumococcal Vaccine	56	75%	70%	69%	94%
Smoking Cessation Advice[1]	17	65%	64%	80%	100%
Surgical Infection Prevention					
Prophylactic Antibiotic Given	99	75%	79%	77%	95%
Prophylactic Antibiotic Selection	27	100%	94%	90%	100%
Prophylactic Antibiotic Stopped	97	92%	83%	72%	95%
Pregnancy Care					
Inpatient Neonatal Mortality	-	-	-	-	-
Third or Fourth Degree Laceration	-	-	-	3.63%	3.27%

Kearney County Health Services

727 E First Street
Minden, NE 08959
URL: www.kchs.org
Ownership: Government - Local
Emergency Services: Yes
Phone: 308-832-3400
Fax: 308-832-3417
Accredited: No
Licensed Beds: 15

Key Personnel:
CEO. . . . . John Rainey
Chief of Medical Staff. . . . . John Grove, MD

Measure	Cases	This Hospital	State Average	U.S. Average	Top Hospital
Heart Attack Care					
ACE Inhibitor or ARB for LVSD[5]	-	-	90%	82%	100%
Aspirin at Arrival[5]	-	-	88%	92%	100%
Aspirin at Discharge[5]	-	-	90%	90%	100%
Beta Blocker at Arrival[5]	-	-	81%	87%	100%
Beta Blocker at Discharge[5]	-	-	95%	90%	100%
Fibrinolytic Medication Timing[5]	-	-	25%	31%	100%
PCI Within 90 Minutes of Arrival[5]	-	-	83%	54%	95%
Smoking Cessation Advice[5]	-	-	84%	88%	100%
Heart Failure Care					
ACE Inhibitor or ARB for LVSD[2,3]	0	-	76%	82%	100%
Discharge Instructions[2,3]	0	-	54%	61%	93%
Evaluation of LVS Function[1,2,3]	1	100%	72%	83%	99%
Smoking Cessation Advice[2,3]	0	-	62%	82%	100%
Pneumonia Care					
Appropriate Initial Antibiotic[1,3]	8	100%	90%	83%	94%
Blood Culture Timing[1,3]	1	100%	96%	90%	100%
Influenza Vaccine[5]	-	-	77%	70%	100%
Initial Antibiotic Timing[3]	0	-	91%	80%	93%
Oxygenation Assessment[1,3]	9	100%	97%	99%	100%
Pneumococcal Vaccine[1,3]	6	83%	70%	69%	94%
Smoking Cessation Advice[1,3]	1	0%	64%	80%	100%
Surgical Infection Prevention					
Prophylactic Antibiotic Given[5]	-	-	79%	77%	95%
Prophylactic Antibiotic Selection[5]	-	-	94%	90%	100%
Prophylactic Antibiotic Stopped[5]	-	-	83%	72%	95%
Pregnancy Care					
Inpatient Neonatal Mortality	-	-	-	-	-
Third or Fourth Degree Laceration	-	-	-	3.63%	3.27%

Antelope Memorial Hospital

102 W 9th Street
Neligh, NE 68756
E-mail: dmtr@bloomnet.com
Ownership: Voluntary non-profit - Private
Emergency Services: Yes
Phone: 402-887-4151
Fax: 402-887-4092
Accredited: No
Licensed Beds: 45

Key Personnel:
CEO. . . . . Jack Greene

Measure	Cases	This Hospital	State Average	U.S. Average	Top Hospital
Heart Attack Care					
ACE Inhibitor or ARB for LVSD[1,3]	1	100%	90%	82%	100%
Aspirin at Arrival[1,3]	2	100%	88%	92%	100%
Aspirin at Discharge[1,3]	2	100%	90%	90%	100%
Beta Blocker at Arrival[1,3]	2	100%	81%	87%	100%
Beta Blocker at Discharge[1,3]	2	100%	95%	90%	100%
Fibrinolytic Medication Timing[3]	0	-	25%	31%	100%
PCI Within 90 Minutes of Arrival[5]	-	-	83%	54%	95%
Smoking Cessation Advice[3]	0	-	84%	88%	100%
Heart Failure Care					
ACE Inhibitor or ARB for LVSD[1]	2	0%	76%	82%	100%
Discharge Instructions[1]	6	17%	54%	61%	93%
Evaluation of LVS Function[1]	14	21%	72%	83%	99%
Smoking Cessation Advice	0	-	62%	82%	100%
Pneumonia Care					
Appropriate Initial Antibiotic[1]	6	83%	90%	83%	94%
Blood Culture Timing[1]	1	100%	96%	90%	100%
Influenza Vaccine[1]	2	50%	77%	70%	100%
Initial Antibiotic Timing[1]	10	90%	91%	80%	93%
Oxygenation Assessment[1]	14	100%	97%	99%	100%
Pneumococcal Vaccine[1]	12	50%	70%	69%	94%
Smoking Cessation Advice[1]	5	40%	64%	80%	100%
Surgical Infection Prevention					
Prophylactic Antibiotic Given[5]	-	-	79%	77%	95%
Prophylactic Antibiotic Selection[5]	-	-	94%	90%	100%
Prophylactic Antibiotic Stopped[5]	-	-	83%	72%	95%
Pregnancy Care					
Inpatient Neonatal Mortality	-	-	-	-	-
Third or Fourth Degree Laceration	-	-	-	3.63%	3.27%

Faith Regional Health Services-East Campus

1500 Koenigstein Avenue
Norfolk, NE 68701
URL: www.frhs.org
Ownership: Voluntary non-profit - Other
Emergency Services: Yes
Phone: 402-371-4800
Fax: 402-644-7324
Accredited: Yes
Licensed Beds: 166

Key Personnel:
CEO. . . . . Robert Driewer
Chief Medical Staff. . . . . Tim Davy
ICU Supervising Nurse. Linda Douglas
Medical/Surgical Nursing Director . . . . Brenda Hokamp
Surgery Director. . . . . Mick Pick
Respiratory Therapy Director . . . . Terry Woockman

Measure	Cases	This Hospital	State Average	U.S. Average	Top Hospital
Heart Attack Care					
ACE Inhibitor or ARB for LVSD	26	88%	90%	82%	100%
Aspirin at Arrival	57	95%	88%	92%	100%
Aspirin at Discharge	77	99%	90%	90%	100%
Beta Blocker at Arrival	48	98%	81%	87%	100%
Beta Blocker at Discharge	88	100%	95%	90%	100%
Fibrinolytic Medication Timing	0	-	25%	31%	100%
PCI Within 90 Minutes of Arrival[1]	4	50%	83%	54%	95%

NOTE: Hospital profiles are in alphabetical order by state, then city, then hospital within the city; Rankings are sorted by rate in descending order and exclude hospitals with less than 25 cases; (1) The number of cases is too small (n<25) for purposes of reliably predicting hospital performance; (2) Measure reflects the hospital's indication that its submission was based upon a sample of its relevant discharges; (3) Rate reflects fewer than the maximum possible quarters of data for the measure; (4) Inaccurate information submitted and suppressed for one or more quarters; (5) No data is available from the hospital for this measure; Please refer to the User's Guide for a full explanation of data

Measure	Cases	This Hospital	State Average	U.S. Average	Top Hospital
Smoking Cessation Advice	27	100%	84%	88%	100%
Heart Failure Care					
ACE Inhibitor or ARB for LVSD	66	83%	76%	82%	100%
Discharge Instructions	92	71%	54%	61%	93%
Evaluation of LVS Function	134	96%	72%	83%	99%
Smoking Cessation Advice[1]	19	95%	62%	82%	100%
Pneumonia Care					
Appropriate Initial Antibiotic	70	91%	90%	83%	94%
Blood Culture Timing	71	100%	96%	90%	100%
Influenza Vaccine[1]	20	95%	77%	70%	100%
Initial Antibiotic Timing	106	91%	91%	80%	93%
Oxygenation Assessment	137	100%	97%	99%	100%
Pneumococcal Vaccine	101	98%	70%	69%	94%
Smoking Cessation Advice	29	76%	64%	80%	100%
Surgical Infection Prevention					
Prophylactic Antibiotic Given[3]	472	90%	79%	77%	95%
Prophylactic Antibiotic Selection	152	99%	94%	90%	100%
Prophylactic Antibiotic Stopped[3]	453	89%	83%	72%	95%
Pregnancy Care					
Inpatient Neonatal Mortality	-	-	-	-	-
Third or Fourth Degree Laceration	-	-	-	3.63%	3.27%

Great Plains Regional Medical Center

601 W Leota St
PO Box 1167
North Platte, NE 69101
Phone: 308-696-8000
Fax: 308-535-3410
Ownership: Voluntary non-profit - Private
Accredited: Yes
Emergency Services: Yes
Licensed Beds: 116

Key Personnel:
President/CEO . . . . Lucinda A Bradley
Chief Medical Staff . . . . Dr. Clint Schafer
Director Infection/Disease Control . . . . Teresa Mowak
ICU Director . . . . Stephanie Jacobson
Women's Services Director . . . . Karen Hipwell
Cardiopulmonary Imaging Director . . . . Gil Smith

Measure	Cases	This Hospital	State Average	U.S. Average	Top Hospital
Heart Attack Care					
ACE Inhibitor or ARB for LVSD[1]	6	83%	90%	82%	100%
Aspirin at Arrival	32	97%	88%	92%	100%
Aspirin at Discharge[1]	19	100%	90%	90%	100%
Beta Blocker at Arrival[1]	21	86%	81%	87%	100%
Beta Blocker at Discharge[1]	19	95%	95%	90%	100%
Fibrinolytic Medication Timing[1]	3	33%	25%	31%	100%
PCI Within 90 Minutes of Arrival	0	-	83%	54%	95%
Smoking Cessation Advice[1]	4	100%	84%	88%	100%
Heart Failure Care					
ACE Inhibitor or ARB for LVSD	31	77%	76%	82%	100%
Discharge Instructions	91	78%	54%	61%	93%
Evaluation of LVS Function	113	91%	72%	83%	99%
Smoking Cessation Advice	26	92%	62%	82%	100%
Pneumonia Care					
Appropriate Initial Antibiotic	116	81%	90%	83%	94%
Blood Culture Timing	76	97%	96%	90%	100%
Influenza Vaccine	36	81%	77%	70%	100%
Initial Antibiotic Timing	158	89%	91%	80%	93%
Oxygenation Assessment	192	100%	97%	99%	100%
Pneumococcal Vaccine	130	72%	70%	69%	94%
Smoking Cessation Advice	45	100%	64%	80%	100%
Surgical Infection Prevention					
Prophylactic Antibiotic Given[3]	170	88%	79%	77%	95%
Prophylactic Antibiotic Selection	54	98%	94%	90%	100%
Prophylactic Antibiotic Stopped[3]	167	60%	83%	72%	95%
Pregnancy Care					
Inpatient Neonatal Mortality	-	-	-	-	-
Third or Fourth Degree Laceration	-	-	-	3.63%	3.27%

Avera Saint Anthony's Hospital

Alternate Name: Saint Anthony's Hospital
300 N 2nd Street
O'Neill, NE 68763
URL: www.avera-sta.org
Phone: 402-336-2611
Fax: 402-336-5145
Ownership: Voluntary non-profit - Church
Accredited: No
Emergency Services: Yes
Licensed Beds: 25

Key Personnel:
President/CEO . . . . Ronald J Cork
Chief Medical Staff . . . . Robi Singh, MD
Emergency Room . . . . Mark J Ptacek, MD
Director Infection/Disease Control . . . . Val Wecker, RN
Director Radiology . . . . Jason Hofer
Director Respiratory Therapy . . . . Bonnie Heimes

Measure	Cases	This Hospital	State Average	U.S. Average	Top Hospital
Heart Attack Care					
ACE Inhibitor or ARB for LVSD[5]	-	-	90%	82%	100%
Aspirin at Arrival[5]	-	-	88%	92%	100%
Aspirin at Discharge[5]	-	-	90%	90%	100%
Beta Blocker at Arrival[5]	-	-	81%	87%	100%
Beta Blocker at Discharge[5]	-	-	95%	90%	100%
Fibrinolytic Medication Timing[5]	-	-	25%	31%	100%
PCI Within 90 Minutes of Arrival[5]	-	-	83%	54%	95%
Smoking Cessation Advice[5]	-	-	84%	88%	100%
Heart Failure Care					
ACE Inhibitor or ARB for LVSD[1]	10	100%	76%	82%	100%
Discharge Instructions[1]	14	50%	54%	61%	93%
Evaluation of LVS Function[1]	24	75%	72%	83%	99%
Smoking Cessation Advice[1]	2	50%	62%	82%	100%
Pneumonia Care					
Appropriate Initial Antibiotic	36	97%	90%	83%	94%
Blood Culture Timing	0	-	96%	90%	100%
Influenza Vaccine[1]	10	80%	77%	70%	100%
Initial Antibiotic Timing	51	88%	91%	80%	93%
Oxygenation Assessment	58	100%	97%	99%	100%
Pneumococcal Vaccine	37	62%	70%	69%	94%
Smoking Cessation Advice[1]	11	36%	64%	80%	100%
Surgical Infection Prevention					
Prophylactic Antibiotic Given[5]	-	-	79%	77%	95%
Prophylactic Antibiotic Selection[5]	-	-	94%	90%	100%
Prophylactic Antibiotic Stopped[5]	-	-	83%	72%	95%
Pregnancy Care					
Inpatient Neonatal Mortality	-	-	-	-	-
Third or Fourth Degree Laceration	-	-	-	3.63%	3.27%

Oakland Memorial Hospital

601 E Second Avenue
Oakland, NE 68045
Phone: 402-685-5601
Fax: 402-685-6223
Ownership: Voluntary non-profit - Other
Accredited: No
Emergency Services: Yes
Licensed Beds: 23

Key Personnel:
Administrator . . . . Karen Vlach
Chief Medical Staff . . . . Tracy Martin
Emergency Room . . . . GE Petersons
Director Infection/Disease Control . . . . Mary Fran Bacon

Measure	Cases	This Hospital	State Average	U.S. Average	Top Hospital
Heart Attack Care					
ACE Inhibitor or ARB for LVSD[5]	-	-	90%	82%	100%
Aspirin at Arrival[5]	-	-	88%	92%	100%
Aspirin at Discharge[5]	-	-	90%	90%	100%
Beta Blocker at Arrival[5]	-	-	81%	87%	100%
Beta Blocker at Discharge[5]	-	-	95%	90%	100%
Fibrinolytic Medication Timing[5]	-	-	25%	31%	100%
PCI Within 90 Minutes of Arrival[5]	-	-	83%	54%	95%
Smoking Cessation Advice[5]	-	-	84%	88%	100%
Heart Failure Care					
ACE Inhibitor or ARB for LVSD[1]	3	33%	76%	82%	100%
Discharge Instructions[1]	7	86%	54%	61%	93%
Evaluation of LVS Function[1]	10	70%	72%	83%	99%
Smoking Cessation Advice[1]	4	25%	62%	82%	100%
Pneumonia Care					
Appropriate Initial Antibiotic[1,3]	8	88%	90%	83%	94%
Blood Culture Timing[1,3]	1	100%	96%	90%	100%

NOTE: Hospital profiles are in alphabetical order by state, then city, then hospital within the city; Rankings are sorted by rate in descending order and exclude hospitals with less than 25 cases; (1) The number of cases is too small (n<25) for purposes of reliably predicting hospital performance; (2) Measure reflects the hospital's indication that its submission was based upon a sample of its relevant discharges; (3) Rate reflects fewer than the maximum possible quarters of data for the measure; (4) Inaccurate information submitted and suppressed for one or more quarters; (5) No data is available from the hospital for this measure; Please refer to the User's Guide for a full explanation of data

Measure	Cases	This Hospital	State Average	U.S. Average	Top Hospital
Influenza Vaccine[1]	4	50%	77%	70%	100%
Initial Antibiotic Timing[1,3]	10	70%	91%	80%	93%
Oxygenation Assessment[1,3]	10	100%	97%	99%	100%
Pneumococcal Vaccine[1,3]	7	71%	70%	69%	94%
Smoking Cessation Advice[1,3]	1	0%	64%	80%	100%
Surgical Infection Prevention					
Prophylactic Antibiotic Given[5]	-	-	79%	77%	95%
Prophylactic Antibiotic Selection[5]	-	-	94%	90%	100%
Prophylactic Antibiotic Stopped[5]	-	-	83%	72%	95%
Pregnancy Care					
Inpatient Neonatal Mortality	-	-	-	-	-
Third or Fourth Degree Laceration	-	-	-	3.63%	3.27%

Ogallala Community Hospital

2601 N Spruce Street
Ogallala, NE 69153
Ownership: Voluntary non-profit - Private
Emergency Services: Yes
Phone: 308-284-4011
Fax: 308-284-7262
Accredited: No
Licensed Beds: 18

Key Personnel:

CEO. . . . . Margie Molitor
Emergency Room . . . . Aric DeYoung
Infection Control. . . . . Stacy Olea
Chief Radiology . . . . Stacy Olea
Respiratory Therapist. . . . . Terry Folk

Measure	Cases	This Hospital	State Average	U.S. Average	Top Hospital
Heart Attack Care					
ACE Inhibitor or ARB for LVSD[3]	0	-	90%	82%	100%
Aspirin at Arrival[1,3]	1	100%	88%	92%	100%
Aspirin at Discharge[3]	0	-	90%	90%	100%
Beta Blocker at Arrival[1,3]	2	100%	81%	87%	100%
Beta Blocker at Discharge[1,3]	1	100%	95%	90%	100%
Fibrinolytic Medication Timing[3]	0	-	25%	31%	100%
PCI Within 90 Minutes of Arrival[5]	-	-	83%	54%	95%
Smoking Cessation Advice[1,3]	1	0%	84%	88%	100%
Heart Failure Care					
ACE Inhibitor or ARB for LVSD[1]	10	90%	76%	82%	100%
Discharge Instructions[1]	16	62%	54%	61%	93%
Evaluation of LVS Function	28	93%	72%	83%	99%
Smoking Cessation Advice[1]	2	0%	62%	82%	100%
Pneumonia Care					
Appropriate Initial Antibiotic	41	95%	90%	83%	94%
Blood Culture Timing[1]	5	80%	96%	90%	100%
Influenza Vaccine[1]	7	86%	77%	70%	100%
Initial Antibiotic Timing	35	91%	91%	80%	93%
Oxygenation Assessment	45	100%	97%	99%	100%
Pneumococcal Vaccine	26	81%	70%	69%	94%
Smoking Cessation Advice[1]	7	71%	64%	80%	100%
Surgical Infection Prevention					
Prophylactic Antibiotic Given[1,3]	8	88%	79%	77%	95%
Prophylactic Antibiotic Selection[1]	8	100%	94%	90%	100%
Prophylactic Antibiotic Stopped[1,3]	8	100%	83%	72%	95%
Pregnancy Care					
Inpatient Neonatal Mortality	-	-	-	-	-
Third or Fourth Degree Laceration	-	-	-	3.63%	3.27%

Alegent Health Bergen Mercy Medical Center

Alternate Name: Bergen Mercy Medical Center
7500 Mercy Road
Omaha, NE 68124
URL: www.alegent.com
Ownership: Voluntary non-profit - Church
Emergency Services: Yes
Phone: 402-398-6060
Fax: 402-398-6032
Accredited: Yes
Licensed Beds: 400

Key Personnel:

President/CEO. . . . . Richard A Hachten II
CEO. . . . . Charles Brummund
Chief Medical Staff. . . . . Joseph A Jarzobski
Chief Catheterization Laboratory . . . Randy Reddell
Emergency Room . . . . Thomas Dunbar, MD
Director Infection/Disease Control . . Peggy Leubbert
ICU . . . . Diana Nielsen
OB/GYN. . . . . Thomas M Besse, MD
Pediatric Surgery . . . . Shahab F Abdessalam, MD
Chief Radiology . . . . Kimberly A Apker, MD

Measure	Cases	This Hospital	State Average	U.S. Average	Top Hospital
Heart Attack Care					
ACE Inhibitor or ARB for LVSD	46	87%	90%	82%	100%
Aspirin at Arrival	166	100%	88%	92%	100%
Aspirin at Discharge	197	100%	90%	90%	100%
Beta Blocker at Arrival	130	97%	81%	87%	100%
Beta Blocker at Discharge	203	99%	95%	90%	100%
Fibrinolytic Medication Timing	0	-	25%	31%	100%
PCI Within 90 Minutes of Arrival[1]	5	100%	83%	54%	95%
Smoking Cessation Advice	71	100%	84%	88%	100%
Heart Failure Care					
ACE Inhibitor or ARB for LVSD	130	92%	76%	82%	100%
Discharge Instructions	276	89%	54%	61%	93%
Evaluation of LVS Function	335	99%	72%	83%	99%
Smoking Cessation Advice	49	100%	62%	82%	100%
Pneumonia Care					
Appropriate Initial Antibiotic	171	94%	90%	83%	94%
Blood Culture Timing	191	98%	96%	90%	100%
Influenza Vaccine	64	98%	77%	70%	100%
Initial Antibiotic Timing	242	95%	91%	80%	93%
Oxygenation Assessment	328	100%	97%	99%	100%
Pneumococcal Vaccine	216	99%	70%	69%	94%
Smoking Cessation Advice	61	100%	64%	80%	100%
Surgical Infection Prevention					
Prophylactic Antibiotic Given[2,3]	814	94%	79%	77%	95%
Prophylactic Antibiotic Selection[2]	79	100%	94%	90%	100%
Prophylactic Antibiotic Stopped[2,3]	785	94%	83%	72%	95%
Pregnancy Care					
Inpatient Neonatal Mortality	-	-	-	-	-
Third or Fourth Degree Laceration	-	-	-	3.63%	3.27%

Alegent Health Lakeside Hospital

16901 Lakeside Hills Ct
Omaha, NE 68130
Ownership: Voluntary non-profit - Church
Emergency Services: Yes
Phone: 402-717-8000
Accredited: No

Measure	Cases	This Hospital	State Average	U.S. Average	Top Hospital
Heart Attack Care					
ACE Inhibitor or ARB for LVSD[1]	10	100%	90%	82%	100%
Aspirin at Arrival	77	100%	88%	92%	100%
Aspirin at Discharge	61	100%	90%	90%	100%
Beta Blocker at Arrival	66	100%	81%	87%	100%
Beta Blocker at Discharge	66	100%	95%	90%	100%
Fibrinolytic Medication Timing	0	-	25%	31%	100%
PCI Within 90 Minutes of Arrival[1]	7	100%	83%	54%	95%
Smoking Cessation Advice[1]	20	100%	84%	88%	100%
Heart Failure Care					
ACE Inhibitor or ARB for LVSD	27	100%	76%	82%	100%
Discharge Instructions	55	96%	54%	61%	93%
Evaluation of LVS Function	72	100%	72%	83%	99%
Smoking Cessation Advice[1]	9	100%	62%	82%	100%
Pneumonia Care					
Appropriate Initial Antibiotic	54	93%	90%	83%	94%
Blood Culture Timing	53	100%	96%	90%	100%
Influenza Vaccine[1]	10	100%	77%	70%	100%
Initial Antibiotic Timing	71	96%	91%	80%	93%
Oxygenation Assessment	90	100%	97%	99%	100%
Pneumococcal Vaccine	57	98%	70%	69%	94%
Smoking Cessation Advice[1]	18	100%	64%	80%	100%
Surgical Infection Prevention					
Prophylactic Antibiotic Given[2,3]	146	92%	79%	77%	95%
Prophylactic Antibiotic Selection[2]	28	89%	94%	90%	100%
Prophylactic Antibiotic Stopped[2,3]	142	92%	83%	72%	95%
Pregnancy Care					
Inpatient Neonatal Mortality	-	-	-	-	-
Third or Fourth Degree Laceration	-	-	-	3.63%	3.27%

NOTE: Hospital profiles are in alphabetical order by state, then city, then hospital within the city; Rankings are sorted by rate in descending order and exclude hospitals with less than 25 cases; (1) The number of cases is too small (n<25) for purposes of reliably predicting hospital performance; (2) Measure reflects the hospital's indication that its submission was based upon a sample of its relevant discharges; (3) Rate reflects fewer than the maximum possible quarters of data for the measure; (4) Inaccurate information submitted and suppressed for one or more quarters; (5) No data is available from the hospital for this measure; Please refer to the User's Guide for a full explanation of data

Creighton University Medical Center

601 N 30th Street
Omaha, NE 68131
URL: www.creightonhospital.com
Ownership: Proprietary
Emergency Services: Yes

Phone: 402-449-4000
Fax: 402-449-5020
Accredited: Yes
Licensed Beds: 404

Key Personnel:

President/CEO . . . . Matthew A Kurs
Chief Medical Staff . . . . Eugene Rich, MD
Chief Catheterization Laboratory . . . . Syed M Mohiuddin, MD
Emergency Room . . . . Wes Grigsby, MD
Director Infection/Disease Control . . . . Ann Lorenzen
CCU Spvg. Nurse . . . . Anita Larsen, RN
Director Medical/Surgical Nursing . . . . Anita Larsen
OB/GYN Womens Health . . . . Alfred Fleming
Chief Radiology . . . . Charles Lerner, MD

Measure	Cases	This Hospital	State Average	U.S. Average	Top Hospital
Heart Attack Care					
ACE Inhibitor or ARB for LVSD	67	93%	90%	82%	100%
Aspirin at Arrival	101	97%	88%	92%	100%
Aspirin at Discharge	241	100%	90%	90%	100%
Beta Blocker at Arrival	100	99%	81%	87%	100%
Beta Blocker at Discharge	288	100%	95%	90%	100%
Fibrinolytic Medication Timing	0	-	25%	31%	100%
PCI Within 90 Minutes of Arrival[1]	8	62%	83%	54%	95%
Smoking Cessation Advice	80	98%	84%	88%	100%
Heart Failure Care					
ACE Inhibitor or ARB for LVSD	149	93%	76%	82%	100%
Discharge Instructions	271	86%	54%	61%	93%
Evaluation of LVS Function	303	99%	72%	83%	99%
Smoking Cessation Advice	75	96%	62%	82%	100%
Pneumonia Care					
Appropriate Initial Antibiotic	70	86%	90%	83%	94%
Blood Culture Timing	96	94%	96%	90%	100%
Influenza Vaccine[1]	18	78%	77%	70%	100%
Initial Antibiotic Timing	134	81%	91%	80%	93%
Oxygenation Assessment	158	100%	97%	99%	100%
Pneumococcal Vaccine	71	85%	70%	69%	94%
Smoking Cessation Advice	61	97%	64%	80%	100%
Surgical Infection Prevention					
Prophylactic Antibiotic Given[2]	453	84%	79%	77%	95%
Prophylactic Antibiotic Selection[2]	86	86%	94%	90%	100%
Prophylactic Antibiotic Stopped[2]	448	59%	83%	72%	95%
Pregnancy Care					
Inpatient Neonatal Mortality	-	-	-	-	-
Third or Fourth Degree Laceration	-	-	-	3.63%	3.27%

Immanuel Medical Center

6901 N 72nd Street
Omaha, NE 68122
URL: www.alegent.com
Ownership: Voluntary non-profit - Church
Emergency Services: Yes

Phone: 402-572-2121
Fax: 402-572-2268
Accredited: Yes
Licensed Beds: 601

Key Personnel:

Administrator . . . . Barbara Goodrich
Manager Respiratory Therapy . . . . Kevin Miller

Measure	Cases	This Hospital	State Average	U.S. Average	Top Hospital
Heart Attack Care					
ACE Inhibitor or ARB for LVSD	35	97%	90%	82%	100%
Aspirin at Arrival	106	100%	88%	92%	100%
Aspirin at Discharge	160	99%	90%	90%	100%
Beta Blocker at Arrival	94	99%	81%	87%	100%
Beta Blocker at Discharge	181	100%	95%	90%	100%
Fibrinolytic Medication Timing[1]	1	0%	25%	31%	100%
PCI Within 90 Minutes of Arrival[1]	7	100%	83%	54%	95%
Smoking Cessation Advice	61	100%	84%	88%	100%
Heart Failure Care					
ACE Inhibitor or ARB for LVSD	84	99%	76%	82%	100%
Discharge Instructions	123	95%	54%	61%	93%
Evaluation of LVS Function	181	99%	72%	83%	99%
Smoking Cessation Advice	30	100%	62%	82%	100%
Pneumonia Care					
Appropriate Initial Antibiotic	101	92%	90%	83%	94%
Blood Culture Timing	119	99%	96%	90%	100%
Influenza Vaccine	34	97%	77%	70%	100%
Initial Antibiotic Timing	177	94%	91%	80%	93%
Oxygenation Assessment	206	100%	97%	99%	100%
Pneumococcal Vaccine	133	98%	70%	69%	94%
Smoking Cessation Advice	58	98%	64%	80%	100%
Surgical Infection Prevention					
Prophylactic Antibiotic Given[2,3]	367	94%	79%	77%	95%
Prophylactic Antibiotic Selection[2]	65	94%	94%	90%	100%
Prophylactic Antibiotic Stopped[2,3]	353	92%	83%	72%	95%
Pregnancy Care					
Inpatient Neonatal Mortality	-	-	-	-	-
Third or Fourth Degree Laceration	-	-	-	3.63%	3.27%

Methodist Hospital

8303 Dodge Street
Omaha, NE 68114
URL: www.bestcare.org
Ownership: Voluntary non-profit - Private
Emergency Services: Yes

Phone: 402-390-4000
Fax: 402-354-8735
Accredited: Yes
Licensed Beds: 430

Key Personnel:

CEO/President . . . . John Fraser
Chief Medical Staff . . . . C Lee Retelsdorf, MD
Director of Cardiology/Cardiac Lab. . . . . Chuck Olson
Emergency Room . . . . Brad Lockee, MD
Director Medical/Surgical Nursing . . . . Toddy Manson
Director of Pulmonary . . . . Tracey Dorheim

Measure	Cases	This Hospital	State Average	U.S. Average	Top Hospital
Heart Attack Care					
ACE Inhibitor or ARB for LVSD	46	87%	90%	82%	100%
Aspirin at Arrival	163	96%	88%	92%	100%
Aspirin at Discharge	170	99%	90%	90%	100%
Beta Blocker at Arrival	137	94%	81%	87%	100%
Beta Blocker at Discharge	188	98%	95%	90%	100%
Fibrinolytic Medication Timing	0	-	25%	31%	100%
PCI Within 90 Minutes of Arrival[1]	14	64%	83%	54%	95%
Smoking Cessation Advice	49	100%	84%	88%	100%
Heart Failure Care					
ACE Inhibitor or ARB for LVSD	183	86%	76%	82%	100%
Discharge Instructions	296	77%	54%	61%	93%
Evaluation of LVS Function	374	97%	72%	83%	99%
Smoking Cessation Advice	46	100%	62%	82%	100%
Pneumonia Care					
Appropriate Initial Antibiotic	268	88%	90%	83%	94%
Blood Culture Timing	243	92%	96%	90%	100%
Influenza Vaccine[4,5]	-	-	77%	70%	100%
Initial Antibiotic Timing	353	78%	91%	80%	93%
Oxygenation Assessment	473	99%	97%	99%	100%
Pneumococcal Vaccine	317	75%	70%	69%	94%
Smoking Cessation Advice	78	91%	64%	80%	100%
Surgical Infection Prevention					
Prophylactic Antibiotic Given[2]	408	91%	79%	77%	95%
Prophylactic Antibiotic Selection[2]	101	100%	94%	90%	100%
Prophylactic Antibiotic Stopped[2]	392	88%	83%	72%	95%
Pregnancy Care					
Inpatient Neonatal Mortality	1,682	0.36%	-	-	-
Third or Fourth Degree Laceration	2,447	5.76%	-	3.63%	3.27%

Nebraska Medical Center

Alternate Name: Clarkson Hospital
987400 Nebraska Medical Center
Omaha, NE 68198
URL: www.nebraskamed.com
Ownership: Voluntary non-profit - Private
Emergency Services: Yes

Phone: 402-559-2000
Fax: 402-595-1091
Accredited: Yes
Licensed Beds: 735

Key Personnel:

Administrator/CEO . . . . Glenn Fosdick
Chief Medical Staff . . . . Stephen Smith, MD
Director Cardiology . . . . Lynette Wheeler
Director Emergency Room . . . . Shelly Schwedhelm, RN

NOTE: Hospital profiles are in alphabetical order by state, then city, then hospital within the city; Rankings are sorted by rate in descending order and exclude hospitals with less than 25 cases; (1) The number of cases is too small (n<25) for purposes of reliably predicting hospital performance; (2) Measure reflects the hospital's indication that its submission was based upon a sample of its relevant discharges; (3) Rate reflects fewer than the maximum possible quarters of data for the measure; (4) Inaccurate information submitted and suppressed for one or more quarters; (5) No data is available from the hospital for this measure; Please refer to the User's Guide for a full explanation of data

Emergency Room . . . . Joseph M Sippel, MD
Director Infection/Disease Control . . . . Theresa Franco
Director Intensive Coronary . . . . Maureen Kelpe
Director Medical/Surgical Nursing . . . . Connie Ogden, RN
Director Medical/Surgical Nursing . . . . Terry Patterson
Director OB/GYN Womens Health . . . . Susan Adams, RN

Measure	Cases	This Hospital	State Average	U.S. Average	Top Hospital
Heart Attack Care					
ACE Inhibitor or ARB for LVSD[2]	58	90%	90%	82%	100%
Aspirin at Arrival[2]	186	97%	88%	92%	100%
Aspirin at Discharge[2]	244	99%	90%	90%	100%
Beta Blocker at Arrival[2]	172	98%	81%	87%	100%
Beta Blocker at Discharge[2]	249	100%	95%	90%	100%
Fibrinolytic Medication Timing[1,2]	1	0%	25%	31%	100%
PCI Within 90 Minutes of Arrival[1,2]	9	67%	83%	54%	95%
Smoking Cessation Advice[2]	105	99%	84%	88%	100%
Heart Failure Care					
ACE Inhibitor or ARB for LVSD[2]	177	79%	76%	82%	100%
Discharge Instructions[2]	271	59%	54%	61%	93%
Evaluation of LVS Function[2]	327	100%	72%	83%	99%
Smoking Cessation Advice[2]	63	89%	62%	82%	100%
Pneumonia Care					
Appropriate Initial Antibiotic[2]	61	92%	90%	83%	94%
Blood Culture Timing[2]	79	92%	96%	90%	100%
Influenza Vaccine[1,2]	15	60%	77%	70%	100%
Initial Antibiotic Timing[2]	115	83%	91%	80%	93%
Oxygenation Assessment[2]	149	100%	97%	99%	100%
Pneumococcal Vaccine[2]	78	55%	70%	69%	94%
Smoking Cessation Advice[2]	35	74%	64%	80%	100%
Surgical Infection Prevention					
Prophylactic Antibiotic Given[2]	544	80%	79%	77%	95%
Prophylactic Antibiotic Selection[2]	75	96%	94%	90%	100%
Prophylactic Antibiotic Stopped[2]	523	91%	83%	72%	95%
Pregnancy Care					
Inpatient Neonatal Mortality[2]	590	0.51%	-	-	-
Third or Fourth Degree Laceration	2,023	2.87%	-	3.63%	3.27%

Nebraska Orthopaedic Hospital

2808 South 143rd Plz
Omaha, NE 68144
Ownership: Proprietary
Emergency Services: No
Phone: 402-637-0600
Accredited: No

Measure	Cases	This Hospital	State Average	U.S. Average	Top Hospital
Heart Attack Care					
ACE Inhibitor or ARB for LVSD[5]	-	-	90%	82%	100%
Aspirin at Arrival[5]	-	-	88%	92%	100%
Aspirin at Discharge[5]	-	-	90%	90%	100%
Beta Blocker at Arrival[5]	-	-	81%	87%	100%
Beta Blocker at Discharge[5]	-	-	95%	90%	100%
Fibrinolytic Medication Timing[5]	-	-	25%	31%	100%
PCI Within 90 Minutes of Arrival[5]	-	-	83%	54%	95%
Smoking Cessation Advice[5]	-	-	84%	88%	100%
Heart Failure Care					
ACE Inhibitor or ARB for LVSD[5]	-	-	76%	82%	100%
Discharge Instructions[5]	-	-	54%	61%	93%
Evaluation of LVS Function[5]	-	-	72%	83%	99%
Smoking Cessation Advice[5]	-	-	62%	82%	100%
Pneumonia Care					
Appropriate Initial Antibiotic[5]	-	-	90%	83%	94%
Blood Culture Timing[5]	-	-	96%	90%	100%
Influenza Vaccine[5]	-	-	77%	70%	100%
Initial Antibiotic Timing[5]	-	-	91%	80%	93%
Oxygenation Assessment[5]	-	-	97%	99%	100%
Pneumococcal Vaccine[5]	-	-	70%	69%	94%
Smoking Cessation Advice[5]	-	-	64%	80%	100%
Surgical Infection Prevention					
Prophylactic Antibiotic Given[2]	194	94%	79%	77%	95%
Prophylactic Antibiotic Selection[2]	33	100%	94%	90%	100%
Prophylactic Antibiotic Stopped[2]	190	88%	83%	72%	95%
Pregnancy Care					
Inpatient Neonatal Mortality	-	-	-	-	-
Third or Fourth Degree Laceration	-	-	-	3.63%	3.27%

Valley County Hospital

217 Westridge Drive
Ord, NE 68862
Ownership: Government - Local
Emergency Services: Yes
Phone: 308-728-3211
Fax: 308-728-7809
Accredited: No
Licensed Beds: 26

Key Personnel:
CEO. . . . . Neelam Bhardwaj
Chief of Medical Staff. . . . . Jennifer Bengston

Measure	Cases	This Hospital	State Average	U.S. Average	Top Hospital
Heart Attack Care					
ACE Inhibitor or ARB for LVSD[3]	0	-	90%	82%	100%
Aspirin at Arrival[3]	0	-	88%	92%	100%
Aspirin at Discharge[3]	0	-	90%	90%	100%
Beta Blocker at Arrival[3]	0	-	81%	87%	100%
Beta Blocker at Discharge[3]	0	-	95%	90%	100%
Fibrinolytic Medication Timing[1,3]	1	0%	25%	31%	100%
PCI Within 90 Minutes of Arrival[5]	-	-	83%	54%	95%
Smoking Cessation Advice[3]	0	-	84%	88%	100%
Heart Failure Care					
ACE Inhibitor or ARB for LVSD[1]	1	0%	76%	82%	100%
Discharge Instructions[1]	7	71%	54%	61%	93%
Evaluation of LVS Function[1]	14	29%	72%	83%	99%
Smoking Cessation Advice[1]	4	75%	62%	82%	100%
Pneumonia Care					
Appropriate Initial Antibiotic[1]	22	95%	90%	83%	94%
Blood Culture Timing[1]	16	100%	96%	90%	100%
Influenza Vaccine[1]	10	40%	77%	70%	100%
Initial Antibiotic Timing	36	100%	91%	80%	93%
Oxygenation Assessment	42	100%	97%	99%	100%
Pneumococcal Vaccine	35	69%	70%	69%	94%
Smoking Cessation Advice[1]	2	100%	64%	80%	100%
Surgical Infection Prevention					
Prophylactic Antibiotic Given[5]	-	-	79%	77%	95%
Prophylactic Antibiotic Selection[5]	-	-	94%	90%	100%
Prophylactic Antibiotic Stopped[5]	-	-	83%	72%	95%
Pregnancy Care					
Inpatient Neonatal Mortality	-	-	-	-	-
Third or Fourth Degree Laceration	-	-	-	3.63%	3.27%

Annie Jeffrey Memorial County Health Center

Alternate Name: Annie Jeffrey Memorial County Hospital
PO Box 428
Osceola, NE 68651
E-mail: aj70907@alltel.net
Ownership: Government - Local
Emergency Services: Yes
Phone: 402-747-2031
Fax: 402-747-1405
Accredited: No
Licensed Beds: 21

Key Personnel:
Administrator/CEO . . . . Carol E Jones
Director Medical/Surgical Nursing . . . . Chris Gabel
OB/GYN Womens Health. . . . . Kent Siemers
Chief Radiology . . . . Greg Foote, MD

Measure	Cases	This Hospital	State Average	U.S. Average	Top Hospital
Heart Attack Care					
ACE Inhibitor or ARB for LVSD[5]	-	-	90%	82%	100%
Aspirin at Arrival[5]	-	-	88%	92%	100%
Aspirin at Discharge[5]	-	-	90%	90%	100%
Beta Blocker at Arrival[5]	-	-	81%	87%	100%
Beta Blocker at Discharge[5]	-	-	95%	90%	100%
Fibrinolytic Medication Timing[5]	-	-	25%	31%	100%
PCI Within 90 Minutes of Arrival[5]	-	-	83%	54%	95%
Smoking Cessation Advice[5]	-	-	84%	88%	100%
Heart Failure Care					
ACE Inhibitor or ARB for LVSD[5]	-	-	76%	82%	100%
Discharge Instructions[5]	-	-	54%	61%	93%
Evaluation of LVS Function[5]	-	-	72%	83%	99%
Smoking Cessation Advice[5]	-	-	62%	82%	100%
Pneumonia Care					

NOTE: Hospital profiles are in alphabetical order by state, then city, then hospital within the city; Rankings are sorted by rate in descending order and exclude hospitals with less than 25 cases; (1) The number of cases is too small (n<25) for purposes of reliably predicting hospital performance; (2) Measure reflects the hospital's indication that its submission was based upon a sample of its relevant discharges; (3) Rate reflects fewer than the maximum possible quarters of data for the measure; (4) Inaccurate information submitted and suppressed for one or more quarters; (5) No data is available from the hospital for this measure; Please refer to the User's Guide for a full explanation of data

Measure	Cases	This Hospital	State Average	U.S. Average	Top Hospital
Appropriate Initial Antibiotic[1,3]	4	100%	90%	83%	94%
Blood Culture Timing[1,3]	2	100%	96%	90%	100%
Influenza Vaccine[5]	-	-	77%	70%	100%
Initial Antibiotic Timing[1,3]	4	100%	91%	80%	93%
Oxygenation Assessment[1,3]	6	100%	97%	99%	100%
Pneumococcal Vaccine[1,3]	5	80%	70%	69%	94%
Smoking Cessation Advice[1,3]	1	100%	64%	80%	100%
Surgical Infection Prevention					
Prophylactic Antibiotic Given[5]	-	-	79%	77%	95%
Prophylactic Antibiotic Selection[5]	-	-	94%	90%	100%
Prophylactic Antibiotic Stopped[5]	-	-	83%	72%	95%
Pregnancy Care					
Inpatient Neonatal Mortality	-	-	-	-	-
Third or Fourth Degree Laceration	-	-	-	3.63%	3.27%

Garden County Hospital

1100 W Second
Oshkosh, NE 69154
E-mail: gchadmin@lakemac.net
Ownership: Government - Local
Emergency Services: Yes

Phone: 308-772-3283
Fax: 308-772-3189

Accredited: No
Licensed Beds: 56

Key Personnel:

CEO. . . . . Diana Steven
Chief Medical Staff. . . . . Pawel Szczykutowizz
Chief Medical Staff. . . . . Saurabh Sheel
Emergency Room . . . . Julie Transmeir

Measure	Cases	This Hospital	State Average	U.S. Average	Top Hospital
Heart Attack Care					
ACE Inhibitor or ARB for LVSD[5]	-	-	90%	82%	100%
Aspirin at Arrival[5]	-	-	88%	92%	100%
Aspirin at Discharge[5]	-	-	90%	90%	100%
Beta Blocker at Arrival[5]	-	-	81%	87%	100%
Beta Blocker at Discharge[5]	-	-	95%	90%	100%
Fibrinolytic Medication Timing[5]	-	-	25%	31%	100%
PCI Within 90 Minutes of Arrival[5]	-	-	83%	54%	95%
Smoking Cessation Advice[5]	-	-	84%	88%	100%
Heart Failure Care					
ACE Inhibitor or ARB for LVSD[3]	0	-	76%	82%	100%
Discharge Instructions[1,3]	2	50%	54%	61%	93%
Evaluation of LVS Function[1,3]	3	33%	72%	83%	99%
Smoking Cessation Advice[3]	0	-	62%	82%	100%
Pneumonia Care					
Appropriate Initial Antibiotic[1,3]	2	100%	90%	83%	94%
Blood Culture Timing[5]	-	-	96%	90%	100%
Influenza Vaccine[5]	-	-	77%	70%	100%
Initial Antibiotic Timing[1,3]	2	100%	91%	80%	93%
Oxygenation Assessment[1,3]	2	100%	97%	99%	100%
Pneumococcal Vaccine[1,3]	2	50%	70%	69%	94%
Smoking Cessation Advice[3]	0	-	64%	80%	100%
Surgical Infection Prevention					
Prophylactic Antibiotic Given[5]	-	-	79%	77%	95%
Prophylactic Antibiotic Selection[5]	-	-	94%	90%	100%
Prophylactic Antibiotic Stopped[5]	-	-	83%	72%	95%
Pregnancy Care					
Inpatient Neonatal Mortality	-	-	-	-	-
Third or Fourth Degree Laceration	-	-	-	3.63%	3.27%

Osmond General Hospital

402 North Maple Street
Osmond, NE 68765
URL: www.osmondhospital.com
Ownership: Voluntary non-profit - Private
Emergency Services: Yes

Phone: 402-748-3393
Fax: 402-748-3349

Accredited: No
Licensed Beds: 37

Key Personnel:

CEO. . . . . Celine Mlady
Infection Control. . . . . Lynn Riedmiller

Measure	Cases	This Hospital	State Average	U.S. Average	Top Hospital
Heart Attack Care					
ACE Inhibitor or ARB for LVSD[5]	-	-	90%	82%	100%
Aspirin at Arrival[5]	-	-	88%	92%	100%
Aspirin at Discharge[5]	-	-	90%	90%	100%
Beta Blocker at Arrival[5]	-	-	81%	87%	100%
Beta Blocker at Discharge[5]	-	-	95%	90%	100%
Fibrinolytic Medication Timing[5]	-	-	25%	31%	100%
PCI Within 90 Minutes of Arrival[5]	-	-	83%	54%	95%
Smoking Cessation Advice[5]	-	-	84%	88%	100%
Heart Failure Care					
ACE Inhibitor or ARB for LVSD[5]	-	-	76%	82%	100%
Discharge Instructions[5]	-	-	54%	61%	93%
Evaluation of LVS Function[5]	-	-	72%	83%	99%
Smoking Cessation Advice[5]	-	-	62%	82%	100%
Pneumonia Care					
Appropriate Initial Antibiotic[1,3]	1	100%	90%	83%	94%
Blood Culture Timing[1,3]	1	100%	96%	90%	100%
Influenza Vaccine[5]	-	-	77%	70%	100%
Initial Antibiotic Timing[1,3]	1	100%	91%	80%	93%
Oxygenation Assessment[1,3]	1	0%	97%	99%	100%
Pneumococcal Vaccine[3]	0	-	70%	69%	94%
Smoking Cessation Advice[3]	0	-	64%	80%	100%
Surgical Infection Prevention					
Prophylactic Antibiotic Given[5]	-	-	79%	77%	95%
Prophylactic Antibiotic Selection[5]	-	-	94%	90%	100%
Prophylactic Antibiotic Stopped[5]	-	-	83%	72%	95%
Pregnancy Care					
Inpatient Neonatal Mortality	-	-	-	-	-
Third or Fourth Degree Laceration	-	-	-	3.63%	3.27%

Alegent Health-Midlands Hospital

Alternate Name: Midlands Community Hospital
11111 S 84th Street
Papillion, NE 68046
URL: www.alegent.com
Ownership: Voluntary non-profit - Church
Emergency Services: Yes

Phone: 402-593-3100
Fax: 402-593-3117

Accredited: Yes
Licensed Beds: 150

Key Personnel:

Cardiac Lab . . . . Georgia Blobaum
ICU . . . . Tami Field
Medical Surgical Nursing . . . . Lisa Campbell
Surgical Services . . . . Lisa Campbell

Measure	Cases	This Hospital	State Average	U.S. Average	Top Hospital
Heart Attack Care					
ACE Inhibitor or ARB for LVSD[1]	16	100%	90%	82%	100%
Aspirin at Arrival	85	99%	88%	92%	100%
Aspirin at Discharge	74	99%	90%	90%	100%
Beta Blocker at Arrival	69	99%	81%	87%	100%
Beta Blocker at Discharge	71	99%	95%	90%	100%
Fibrinolytic Medication Timing	0	-	25%	31%	100%
PCI Within 90 Minutes of Arrival[1]	5	100%	83%	54%	95%
Smoking Cessation Advice	37	100%	84%	88%	100%
Heart Failure Care					
ACE Inhibitor or ARB for LVSD	59	95%	76%	82%	100%
Discharge Instructions	113	94%	54%	61%	93%
Evaluation of LVS Function	147	99%	72%	83%	99%
Smoking Cessation Advice	36	100%	62%	82%	100%
Pneumonia Care					
Appropriate Initial Antibiotic	111	96%	90%	83%	94%
Blood Culture Timing	105	98%	96%	90%	100%
Influenza Vaccine	36	100%	77%	70%	100%
Initial Antibiotic Timing	133	97%	91%	80%	93%
Oxygenation Assessment	157	100%	97%	99%	100%
Pneumococcal Vaccine	100	100%	70%	69%	94%
Smoking Cessation Advice	38	100%	64%	80%	100%
Surgical Infection Prevention					
Prophylactic Antibiotic Given[2,3]	112	90%	79%	77%	95%
Prophylactic Antibiotic Selection[2]	30	97%	94%	90%	100%
Prophylactic Antibiotic Stopped[2,3]	107	93%	83%	72%	95%
Pregnancy Care					
Inpatient Neonatal Mortality	-	-	-	-	-
Third or Fourth Degree Laceration	-	-	-	3.63%	3.27%

NOTE: Hospital profiles are in alphabetical order by state, then city, then hospital within the city; Rankings are sorted by rate in descending order and exclude hospitals with less than 25 cases; (1) The number of cases is too small (n<25) for purposes of reliably predicting hospital performance; (2) Measure reflects the hospital's indication that its submission was based upon a sample of its relevant discharges; (3) Rate reflects fewer than the maximum possible quarters of data for the measure; (4) Inaccurate information submitted and suppressed for one or more quarters; (5) No data is available from the hospital for this measure; Please refer to the User's Guide for a full explanation of data

Pawnee County Memorial Hospital

600 I Street
Pawnee City, NE 68420
Ownership: Government - Local
Emergency Services: Yes

Phone: 402-852-2231
Fax: 402-852-2098
Accredited: No
Licensed Beds: 21

Key Personnel:
Chief of Medical Staff.................... Richard Jackson
Director Medical/Surgical Nursing .... Betty Thomas, RN
Chief Radiology.......................... Tom Campbell

Measure	Cases	This Hospital	State Average	U.S. Average	Top Hospital
Heart Attack Care					
ACE Inhibitor or ARB for LVSD[5]	-	-	90%	82%	100%
Aspirin at Arrival[5]	-	-	88%	92%	100%
Aspirin at Discharge[5]	-	-	90%	90%	100%
Beta Blocker at Arrival[5]	-	-	81%	87%	100%
Beta Blocker at Discharge[5]	-	-	95%	90%	100%
Fibrinolytic Medication Timing[5]	-	-	25%	31%	100%
PCI Within 90 Minutes of Arrival[5]	-	-	83%	54%	95%
Smoking Cessation Advice[5]	-	-	84%	88%	100%
Heart Failure Care					
ACE Inhibitor or ARB for LVSD[1,3]	3	67%	76%	82%	100%
Discharge Instructions[1,3]	5	40%	54%	61%	93%
Evaluation of LVS Function[1,3]	7	57%	72%	83%	99%
Smoking Cessation Advice[1,3]	1	100%	62%	82%	100%
Pneumonia Care					
Appropriate Initial Antibiotic[1,3]	4	100%	90%	83%	94%
Blood Culture Timing[1,3]	2	100%	96%	90%	100%
Influenza Vaccine[1]	3	67%	77%	70%	100%
Initial Antibiotic Timing[1,3]	15	100%	91%	80%	93%
Oxygenation Assessment[1,3]	16	100%	97%	99%	100%
Pneumococcal Vaccine[1,3]	14	71%	70%	69%	94%
Smoking Cessation Advice[1,3]	2	100%	64%	80%	100%
Surgical Infection Prevention					
Prophylactic Antibiotic Given[5]	-	-	79%	77%	95%
Prophylactic Antibiotic Selection[5]	-	-	94%	90%	100%
Prophylactic Antibiotic Stopped[5]	-	-	83%	72%	95%
Pregnancy Care					
Inpatient Neonatal Mortality	-	-	-	-	-
Third or Fourth Degree Laceration	-	-	-	3.63%	3.27%

Pender Community Hospital

603 Earl Street
Pender, NE 68047
URL: www.pendercommunityhospital.com
Ownership: Govt - Hospital District or Authority
Emergency Services: Yes

Phone: 402-385-3083
Fax: 402-385-2155
Accredited: No
Licensed Beds: 47

Key Personnel:
CEO/Administrator...................... Michael Hansen, FACHE
Chief Medical Staff...................... David Hollting
Emergency Room .... Dee Moeller
Surgery Supervisor .... Sue Hansen, RN

Measure	Cases	This Hospital	State Average	U.S. Average	Top Hospital
Heart Attack Care					
ACE Inhibitor or ARB for LVSD[5]	-	-	90%	82%	100%
Aspirin at Arrival[5]	-	-	88%	92%	100%
Aspirin at Discharge[5]	-	-	90%	90%	100%
Beta Blocker at Arrival[5]	-	-	81%	87%	100%
Beta Blocker at Discharge[5]	-	-	95%	90%	100%
Fibrinolytic Medication Timing[5]	-	-	25%	31%	100%
PCI Within 90 Minutes of Arrival[5]	-	-	83%	54%	95%
Smoking Cessation Advice[5]	-	-	84%	88%	100%
Heart Failure Care					
ACE Inhibitor or ARB for LVSD[5]	-	-	76%	82%	100%
Discharge Instructions[5]	-	-	54%	61%	93%
Evaluation of LVS Function[5]	-	-	72%	83%	99%
Smoking Cessation Advice[5]	-	-	62%	82%	100%
Pneumonia Care					
Appropriate Initial Antibiotic[1,3]	3	67%	90%	83%	94%
Blood Culture Timing[3]	0	-	96%	90%	100%
Influenza Vaccine[5]	-	-	77%	70%	100%
Initial Antibiotic Timing[1,3]	4	100%	91%	80%	93%
Oxygenation Assessment[1,3]	5	60%	97%	99%	100%
Pneumococcal Vaccine[1,3]	2	50%	70%	69%	94%
Smoking Cessation Advice[3]	0	-	64%	80%	100%
Surgical Infection Prevention					
Prophylactic Antibiotic Given[5]	-	-	79%	77%	95%
Prophylactic Antibiotic Selection[5]	-	-	94%	90%	100%
Prophylactic Antibiotic Stopped[5]	-	-	83%	72%	95%
Pregnancy Care					
Inpatient Neonatal Mortality	-	-	-	-	-
Third or Fourth Degree Laceration	-	-	-	3.63%	3.27%

Plainview Public Hospital

Alternate Name: Plainview Area Health System
704 N 3rd Street
Plainview, NE 68769
Ownership: Government - Local
Emergency Services: Yes

Phone: 402-582-4245
Fax: 402-582-3940
Accredited: No
Licensed Beds: 19

Key Personnel:
President/CEO.......................... Bryan Roby
Chief Medical Staff...................... Edward Botha, MD
Cardiac Lab .... Jill Anson, RN
Emergency Room .... Deb Rutledge, RN
Infection Control......................... Mary Scranton, LPN
Respiratory/Cardiopulmonary............... Elaine Hulse, RT

Measure	Cases	This Hospital	State Average	U.S. Average	Top Hospital
Heart Attack Care					
ACE Inhibitor or ARB for LVSD[3]	0	-	90%	82%	100%
Aspirin at Arrival[1,3]	1	100%	88%	92%	100%
Aspirin at Discharge[1,3]	1	100%	90%	90%	100%
Beta Blocker at Arrival[1,3]	1	100%	81%	87%	100%
Beta Blocker at Discharge[1,3]	1	100%	95%	90%	100%
Fibrinolytic Medication Timing[3]	0	-	25%	31%	100%
PCI Within 90 Minutes of Arrival[5]	-	-	83%	54%	95%
Smoking Cessation Advice[3]	0	-	84%	88%	100%
Heart Failure Care					
ACE Inhibitor or ARB for LVSD[1]	1	0%	76%	82%	100%
Discharge Instructions[1]	13	85%	54%	61%	93%
Evaluation of LVS Function[1]	20	40%	72%	83%	99%
Smoking Cessation Advice	0	-	62%	82%	100%
Pneumonia Care					
Appropriate Initial Antibiotic[1]	9	100%	90%	83%	94%
Blood Culture Timing[1]	4	75%	96%	90%	100%
Influenza Vaccine[1]	2	50%	77%	70%	100%
Initial Antibiotic Timing[1]	15	100%	91%	80%	93%
Oxygenation Assessment[1]	16	100%	97%	99%	100%
Pneumococcal Vaccine[1]	12	50%	70%	69%	94%
Smoking Cessation Advice[1]	1	0%	64%	80%	100%
Surgical Infection Prevention					
Prophylactic Antibiotic Given[5]	-	-	79%	77%	95%
Prophylactic Antibiotic Selection[5]	-	-	94%	90%	100%
Prophylactic Antibiotic Stopped[5]	-	-	83%	72%	95%
Pregnancy Care					
Inpatient Neonatal Mortality	-	-	-	-	-
Third or Fourth Degree Laceration	-	-	-	3.63%	3.27%

Webster County Community Hospital

6th & Franklin
Red Cloud, NE 68970
Ownership: Government - Local
Emergency Services: Yes

Phone: 402-746-2291
Fax: 402-746-2910
Accredited: No
Licensed Beds: 16

Key Personnel:
CEO/President.......................... Robert Sheckler
Chief of Medical Staff..................... Della Chan
Director Infection/Disease Control .... Diane Hoffman
Chief Radiology .... Carol Morris

Measure	Cases	This Hospital	State Average	U.S. Average	Top Hospital
Heart Attack Care					
ACE Inhibitor or ARB for LVSD[5]	-	-	90%	82%	100%
Aspirin at Arrival[5]	-	-	88%	92%	100%

NOTE: Hospital profiles are in alphabetical order by state, then city, then hospital within the city; Rankings are sorted by rate in descending order and exclude hospitals with less than 25 cases; (1) The number of cases is too small (n<25) for purposes of reliably predicting hospital performance; (2) Measure reflects the hospital's indication that its submission was based upon a sample of its relevant discharges; (3) Rate reflects fewer than the maximum possible quarters of data for the measure; (4) Inaccurate information submitted and suppressed for one or more quarters; (5) No data is available from the hospital for this measure; Please refer to the User's Guide for a full explanation of data

Measure	Cases	This Hospital	State Average	U.S. Average	Top Hospital
Aspirin at Discharge[5]	-	-	90%	90%	100%
Beta Blocker at Arrival[5]	-	-	81%	87%	100%
Beta Blocker at Discharge[5]	-	-	95%	90%	100%
Fibrinolytic Medication Timing[5]	-	-	25%	31%	100%
PCI Within 90 Minutes of Arrival[5]	-	-	83%	54%	95%
Smoking Cessation Advice[5]	-	-	84%	88%	100%
Heart Failure Care					
ACE Inhibitor or ARB for LVSD[1]	1	0%	76%	82%	100%
Discharge Instructions[1]	3	0%	54%	61%	93%
Evaluation of LVS Function[1]	5	60%	72%	83%	99%
Smoking Cessation Advice[1]	3	33%	62%	82%	100%
Pneumonia Care					
Appropriate Initial Antibiotic[1,2]	13	77%	90%	83%	94%
Blood Culture Timing[1,2]	13	77%	96%	90%	100%
Influenza Vaccine[1,2]	10	80%	77%	70%	100%
Initial Antibiotic Timing[1,2]	22	91%	91%	80%	93%
Oxygenation Assessment[2]	40	100%	97%	99%	100%
Pneumococcal Vaccine[2]	30	57%	70%	69%	94%
Smoking Cessation Advice[1,2]	4	0%	64%	80%	100%
Surgical Infection Prevention					
Prophylactic Antibiotic Given[5]	-	-	79%	77%	95%
Prophylactic Antibiotic Selection[5]	-	-	94%	90%	100%
Prophylactic Antibiotic Stopped[5]	-	-	83%	72%	95%
Pregnancy Care					
Inpatient Neonatal Mortality	-	-	-	-	-
Third or Fourth Degree Laceration	-	-	-	3.63%	3.27%

Howard County Community Hospital

1113 Sherman Street
Saint Paul, NE 68873
Ownership: Proprietary
Emergency Services: Yes
Phone: 308-754-4421
Fax: 308-754-4429
Accredited: No
Licensed Beds: 25

Key Personnel:
CEO. . . . . Arthur Frable

Measure	Cases	This Hospital	State Average	U.S. Average	Top Hospital
Heart Attack Care					
ACE Inhibitor or ARB for LVSD[1]	1	100%	90%	82%	100%
Aspirin at Arrival[1]	5	80%	88%	92%	100%
Aspirin at Discharge[1]	5	60%	90%	90%	100%
Beta Blocker at Arrival[1]	5	100%	81%	87%	100%
Beta Blocker at Discharge[1]	4	100%	95%	90%	100%
Fibrinolytic Medication Timing	0	-	25%	31%	100%
PCI Within 90 Minutes of Arrival	0	-	83%	54%	95%
Smoking Cessation Advice	0	-	84%	88%	100%
Heart Failure Care					
ACE Inhibitor or ARB for LVSD[1]	5	80%	76%	82%	100%
Discharge Instructions[1]	17	35%	54%	61%	93%
Evaluation of LVS Function	28	100%	72%	83%	99%
Smoking Cessation Advice[1]	3	67%	62%	82%	100%
Pneumonia Care					
Appropriate Initial Antibiotic[1]	14	86%	90%	83%	94%
Blood Culture Timing[1]	4	100%	96%	90%	100%
Influenza Vaccine[1]	5	80%	77%	70%	100%
Initial Antibiotic Timing[1]	14	93%	91%	80%	93%
Oxygenation Assessment	27	100%	97%	99%	100%
Pneumococcal Vaccine[1]	21	100%	70%	69%	94%
Smoking Cessation Advice[1]	4	100%	64%	80%	100%
Surgical Infection Prevention					
Prophylactic Antibiotic Given[1,3]	9	89%	79%	77%	95%
Prophylactic Antibiotic Selection[1]	4	100%	94%	90%	100%
Prophylactic Antibiotic Stopped[1,3]	9	89%	83%	72%	95%
Pregnancy Care					
Inpatient Neonatal Mortality	-	-	-	-	-
Third or Fourth Degree Laceration	-	-	-	3.63%	3.27%

Memorial Hospital

104 W 17th Street
Schuyler, NE 68661
URL: www.algent.com
Ownership: Voluntary non-profit - Private
Emergency Services: Yes
Phone: 402-352-2441
Fax: 402-352-2643
Accredited: No

Key Personnel:
President/CEO. . . . . Larry Jensen
Chief Medical Staff. . . . . James Martin, MD
Emergency Room . . . . Rita Zelda, RN
Director Infection/Disease Control . . . . Rose Neuhaus, RN
Director Medical/Surgical Nursing . . . . Rita Zelda, RN
Chief Radiology . . . . Cathy Krzycki

Measure	Cases	This Hospital	State Average	U.S. Average	Top Hospital
Heart Attack Care					
ACE Inhibitor or ARB for LVSD[3]	0	-	90%	82%	100%
Aspirin at Arrival[1,3]	1	100%	88%	92%	100%
Aspirin at Discharge[1,3]	1	100%	90%	90%	100%
Beta Blocker at Arrival[1,3]	1	0%	81%	87%	100%
Beta Blocker at Discharge[1,3]	1	100%	95%	90%	100%
Fibrinolytic Medication Timing[3]	0	-	25%	31%	100%
PCI Within 90 Minutes of Arrival[5]	-	-	83%	54%	95%
Smoking Cessation Advice[3]	0	-	84%	88%	100%
Heart Failure Care					
ACE Inhibitor or ARB for LVSD[1]	1	100%	76%	82%	100%
Discharge Instructions[1]	13	31%	54%	61%	93%
Evaluation of LVS Function[1]	14	71%	72%	83%	99%
Smoking Cessation Advice	0	-	62%	82%	100%
Pneumonia Care					
Appropriate Initial Antibiotic[1]	17	88%	90%	83%	94%
Blood Culture Timing	0	-	96%	90%	100%
Influenza Vaccine[1]	5	40%	77%	70%	100%
Initial Antibiotic Timing	27	89%	91%	80%	93%
Oxygenation Assessment	33	100%	97%	99%	100%
Pneumococcal Vaccine	25	76%	70%	69%	94%
Smoking Cessation Advice[1]	2	50%	64%	80%	100%
Surgical Infection Prevention					
Prophylactic Antibiotic Given[5]	-	-	79%	77%	95%
Prophylactic Antibiotic Selection[5]	-	-	94%	90%	100%
Prophylactic Antibiotic Stopped[5]	-	-	83%	72%	95%
Pregnancy Care					
Inpatient Neonatal Mortality	-	-	-	-	-
Third or Fourth Degree Laceration	-	-	-	3.63%	3.27%

Regional West Medical Center

4021 Avenue B
Scottsbluff, NE 69361
URL: www.rwmc.net
Ownership: Voluntary non-profit - Private
Emergency Services: Yes
Phone: 308-635-3711
Fax: 308-630-1815
Accredited: Yes
Licensed Beds: 203

Key Personnel:
President/CEO. . . . . Todd S Sorensen, MD
Chief Medical Staff. . . . . Diane Gilles, MD
Catheterization Lab . . . . Mike Smith
Emergency Room . . . . Shirley Barlow
Director Infection/Disease Control . . . . Marsha Meyer
Intensive/Coronary Care . . . . Shirley Barlow
Medical/Surgical Nursing . . . . Susan Wilson
Ob/Gyn . . . . Linda Armstrong
Director Cardio-Pulmonary Services . . . . Mike Smith

Measure	Cases	This Hospital	State Average	U.S. Average	Top Hospital
Heart Attack Care					
ACE Inhibitor or ARB for LVSD[1]	4	50%	90%	82%	100%
Aspirin at Arrival	32	97%	88%	92%	100%
Aspirin at Discharge[1]	21	81%	90%	90%	100%
Beta Blocker at Arrival[1]	24	88%	81%	87%	100%
Beta Blocker at Discharge[1]	13	77%	95%	90%	100%
Fibrinolytic Medication Timing[1]	3	33%	25%	31%	100%
PCI Within 90 Minutes of Arrival	0	-	83%	54%	95%
Smoking Cessation Advice[1]	3	33%	84%	88%	100%
Heart Failure Care					

NOTE: Hospital profiles are in alphabetical order by state, then city, then hospital within the city; Rankings are sorted by rate in descending order and exclude hospitals with less than 25 cases; (1) The number of cases is too small (n<25) for purposes of reliably predicting hospital performance; (2) Measure reflects the hospital's indication that its submission was based upon a sample of its relevant discharges; (3) Rate reflects fewer than the maximum possible quarters of data for the measure; (4) Inaccurate information submitted and suppressed for one or more quarters; (5) No data is available from the hospital for this measure; Please refer to the User's Guide for a full explanation of data

ACE Inhibitor or ARB for LVSD[1]	21	86%	76%	82%	100%
Discharge Instructions	62	52%	54%	61%	93%
Evaluation of LVS Function	88	84%	72%	83%	99%
Smoking Cessation Advice[1]	16	62%	62%	82%	100%
Pneumonia Care					
Appropriate Initial Antibiotic	66	80%	90%	83%	94%
Blood Culture Timing	57	88%	96%	90%	100%
Influenza Vaccine	34	82%	77%	70%	100%
Initial Antibiotic Timing	97	91%	91%	80%	93%
Oxygenation Assessment	121	100%	97%	99%	100%
Pneumococcal Vaccine	80	89%	70%	69%	94%
Smoking Cessation Advice	28	68%	64%	80%	100%
Surgical Infection Prevention					
Prophylactic Antibiotic Given[3]	381	72%	79%	77%	95%
Prophylactic Antibiotic Selection	116	100%	94%	90%	100%
Prophylactic Antibiotic Stopped[3]	375	75%	83%	72%	95%
Pregnancy Care					
Inpatient Neonatal Mortality	845	0.00%	-	-	-
Third or Fourth Degree Laceration	668	2.69%	-	3.63%	3.27%

Memorial Hospital

300 N Columbia Avenue
Seward, NE 68434
E-mail: rwaltz@navix.net
URL: www.mhcs-seward.org
Ownership: Voluntary non-profit - Private
Emergency Services: Yes

Phone: 402-643-2971
Fax: 402-646-4639

Accredited: No
Licensed Beds: 34

Key Personnel:
Administrator/CEO . . . . Ronald D Waltz
Chief Medical Staff. . . . . Kari Eskens
Director Infection/Disease Control . . . . Jan Lucas
Director Respiratory Therapy . . . . Sharol Forsythe

Measure	Cases	This Hospital	State Average	U.S. Average	Top Hospital
Heart Attack Care					
ACE Inhibitor or ARB for LVSD[1,3]	1	100%	90%	82%	100%
Aspirin at Arrival[1,3]	4	75%	88%	92%	100%
Aspirin at Discharge[1,3]	3	100%	90%	90%	100%
Beta Blocker at Arrival[1,3]	5	60%	81%	87%	100%
Beta Blocker at Discharge[1,3]	3	67%	95%	90%	100%
Fibrinolytic Medication Timing[3]	0	-	25%	31%	100%
PCI Within 90 Minutes of Arrival	0	-	83%	54%	95%
Smoking Cessation Advice[3]	0	-	84%	88%	100%
Heart Failure Care					
ACE Inhibitor or ARB for LVSD[1]	9	78%	76%	82%	100%
Discharge Instructions	25	0%	54%	61%	93%
Evaluation of LVS Function	36	61%	72%	83%	99%
Smoking Cessation Advice[1]	3	0%	62%	82%	100%
Pneumonia Care					
Appropriate Initial Antibiotic	37	81%	90%	83%	94%
Blood Culture Timing[1]	3	100%	96%	90%	100%
Influenza Vaccine[1]	7	0%	77%	70%	100%
Initial Antibiotic Timing	51	92%	91%	80%	93%
Oxygenation Assessment	62	100%	97%	99%	100%
Pneumococcal Vaccine	42	7%	70%	69%	94%
Smoking Cessation Advice[1]	12	0%	64%	80%	100%
Surgical Infection Prevention					
Prophylactic Antibiotic Given[5]	-	-	79%	77%	95%
Prophylactic Antibiotic Selection[5]	-	-	94%	90%	100%
Prophylactic Antibiotic Stopped[5]	-	-	83%	72%	95%
Pregnancy Care					
Inpatient Neonatal Mortality	-	-	-	-	-
Third or Fourth Degree Laceration	-	-	-	3.63%	3.27%

Memorial Health Center

645 Osage Street
Sidney, NE 69162
E-mail: mhchk@wheatbelt.com
URL: www.memorialhealthcenter.org
Ownership: Voluntary non-profit - Other
Emergency Services: Yes

Phone: 308-254-5825
Fax: 308-254-2300

Accredited: No

Key Personnel:
CEO. . . . . Danielle L Gearhart
Chief of Staff . . . . Michael Matthews, MD
Director Medical/Surgical Nursing . . . . Tammy Williams
Respiratory/Cardiopulmonary. . . . . Janet Franzen

Measure	Cases	This Hospital	State Average	U.S. Average	Top Hospital
Heart Attack Care					
ACE Inhibitor or ARB for LVSD[3]	0	-	90%	82%	100%
Aspirin at Arrival[1,3]	3	100%	88%	92%	100%
Aspirin at Discharge[1,3]	1	100%	90%	90%	100%
Beta Blocker at Arrival[1,3]	3	67%	81%	87%	100%
Beta Blocker at Discharge[1,3]	1	100%	95%	90%	100%
Fibrinolytic Medication Timing[1,3]	4	25%	25%	31%	100%
PCI Within 90 Minutes of Arrival	0	-	83%	54%	95%
Smoking Cessation Advice[3]	0	-	84%	88%	100%
Heart Failure Care					
ACE Inhibitor or ARB for LVSD[1,3]	4	100%	76%	82%	100%
Discharge Instructions[1,3]	16	0%	54%	61%	93%
Evaluation of LVS Function[1,3]	22	77%	72%	83%	99%
Smoking Cessation Advice[1,3]	5	80%	62%	82%	100%
Pneumonia Care					
Appropriate Initial Antibiotic[1,3]	21	86%	90%	83%	94%
Blood Culture Timing[1]	4	100%	96%	90%	100%
Influenza Vaccine[1]	7	43%	77%	70%	100%
Initial Antibiotic Timing[3]	28	68%	91%	80%	93%
Oxygenation Assessment[3]	32	100%	97%	99%	100%
Pneumococcal Vaccine[1,3]	23	57%	70%	69%	94%
Smoking Cessation Advice[1,3]	6	100%	64%	80%	100%
Surgical Infection Prevention					
Prophylactic Antibiotic Given[5]	-	-	79%	77%	95%
Prophylactic Antibiotic Selection[5]	-	-	94%	90%	100%
Prophylactic Antibiotic Stopped[5]	-	-	83%	72%	95%
Pregnancy Care					
Inpatient Neonatal Mortality	-	-	-	-	-
Third or Fourth Degree Laceration	-	-	-	3.63%	3.27%

Brodstone Memorial Nuckolls County Hospital

520 E 10th Street
PO Box 187
Superior, NE 68978
Ownership: Voluntary non-profit - Private
Emergency Services: Yes

Phone: 402-879-3281
Fax: 402-879-3401

Accredited: No
Licensed Beds: 25

Key Personnel:
CEO. . . . . John Keelan
Chief Medical Staff. . . . . Robert Leibel
Emergency Room . . . . Dordas Judy, MD
Infection Control. . . . . Pam Bower
Medical/Surgical Nursing . . . . Dorcas Judy
Respiratory Care . . . . Carla Ost

Measure	Cases	This Hospital	State Average	U.S. Average	Top Hospital
Heart Attack Care					
ACE Inhibitor or ARB for LVSD[3]	0	-	90%	82%	100%
Aspirin at Arrival[1,3]	3	67%	88%	92%	100%
Aspirin at Discharge[1,3]	3	67%	90%	90%	100%
Beta Blocker at Arrival[1,3]	3	67%	81%	87%	100%
Beta Blocker at Discharge[1,3]	3	100%	95%	90%	100%
Fibrinolytic Medication Timing[3]	0	-	25%	31%	100%
PCI Within 90 Minutes of Arrival	0	-	83%	54%	95%
Smoking Cessation Advice[1,3]	1	100%	84%	88%	100%
Heart Failure Care					
ACE Inhibitor or ARB for LVSD[1]	2	0%	76%	82%	100%
Discharge Instructions[1]	15	53%	54%	61%	93%
Evaluation of LVS Function[1]	21	90%	72%	83%	99%
Smoking Cessation Advice	0	-	62%	82%	100%
Pneumonia Care					
Appropriate Initial Antibiotic[1]	15	93%	90%	83%	94%
Blood Culture Timing[1]	4	100%	96%	90%	100%
Influenza Vaccine[1]	6	100%	77%	70%	100%
Initial Antibiotic Timing[1]	17	71%	91%	80%	93%
Oxygenation Assessment[1]	23	91%	97%	99%	100%
Pneumococcal Vaccine[1]	17	71%	70%	69%	94%
Smoking Cessation Advice[1]	3	67%	64%	80%	100%

NOTE: Hospital profiles are in alphabetical order by state, then city, then hospital within the city; Rankings are sorted by rate in descending order and exclude hospitals with less than 25 cases; (1) The number of cases is too small (n<25) for purposes of reliably predicting hospital performance; (2) Measure reflects the hospital's indication that its submission was based upon a sample of its relevant discharges; (3) Rate reflects fewer than the maximum possible quarters of data for the measure; (4) Inaccurate information submitted and suppressed for one or more quarters; (5) No data is available from the hospital for this measure; Please refer to the User's Guide for a full explanation of data

Measure	Cases	This Hospital	State Average	U.S. Average	Top Hospital
Surgical Infection Prevention					
Prophylactic Antibiotic Given[1,3]	1	100%	79%	77%	95%
Prophylactic Antibiotic Selection[5]	-	-	94%	90%	100%
Prophylactic Antibiotic Stopped[1,3]	1	100%	83%	72%	95%
Pregnancy Care					
Inpatient Neonatal Mortality	-	-	-	-	-
Third or Fourth Degree Laceration	-	-	-	3.63%	3.27%

Community Memorial Hospital

1579 Midland Street
Syracuse, NE 68446
URL: www.syracusecmh.org
Ownership: Govt - Hospital District or Authority
Emergency Services: Yes

Phone: 402-269-2011
Fax: 402-269-2795
Accredited: No
Licensed Beds: 18

Key Personnel:
President/CEO . . . . Allleen Klaasmeyer
Chief Medical Staff . . . . Erin Haubschman, MD
Respiratory Therapy . . . . Karen Teten

Measure	Cases	This Hospital	State Average	U.S. Average	Top Hospital
Heart Attack Care					
ACE Inhibitor or ARB for LVSD[5]	-	-	90%	82%	100%
Aspirin at Arrival[5]	-	-	88%	92%	100%
Aspirin at Discharge[5]	-	-	90%	90%	100%
Beta Blocker at Arrival[5]	-	-	81%	87%	100%
Beta Blocker at Discharge[5]	-	-	95%	90%	100%
Fibrinolytic Medication Timing[5]	-	-	25%	31%	100%
PCI Within 90 Minutes of Arrival[5]	-	-	83%	54%	95%
Smoking Cessation Advice[5]	-	-	84%	88%	100%
Heart Failure Care					
ACE Inhibitor or ARB for LVSD[1,2,3]	1	100%	76%	82%	100%
Discharge Instructions[1,2,3]	3	0%	54%	61%	93%
Evaluation of LVS Function[1,2,3]	4	25%	72%	83%	99%
Smoking Cessation Advice[2,3]	0	-	62%	82%	100%
Pneumonia Care					
Appropriate Initial Antibiotic[1,2,3]	1	100%	90%	83%	94%
Blood Culture Timing[2,3]	0	-	96%	90%	100%
Influenza Vaccine[5]	-	-	77%	70%	100%
Initial Antibiotic Timing[1,2,3]	1	100%	91%	80%	93%
Oxygenation Assessment[1,2,3]	1	100%	97%	99%	100%
Pneumococcal Vaccine[1,2,3]	1	0%	70%	69%	94%
Smoking Cessation Advice[2,3]	0	-	64%	80%	100%
Surgical Infection Prevention					
Prophylactic Antibiotic Given[5]	-	-	79%	77%	95%
Prophylactic Antibiotic Selection[5]	-	-	94%	90%	100%
Prophylactic Antibiotic Stopped[5]	-	-	83%	72%	95%
Pregnancy Care					
Inpatient Neonatal Mortality	-	-	-	-	-
Third or Fourth Degree Laceration	-	-	-	3.63%	3.27%

Johnson County Hospital

202 High Street
Tecumseh, NE 68450
Ownership: Government - Local
Emergency Services: Yes

Phone: 402-335-3361
Fax: 402-335-6342
Accredited: No
Licensed Beds: 19

Key Personnel:
Administrator/CEO . . . . Dianne Newman
Chief Medical Staff . . . . Stacey Goodrich
Emergency Room . . . . Ruth Bossung, RN
Director Infection/Disease Control . . . . Janice Gerdes
Director Medical/Surgical Nursing . . . . Ruth Bossung, RN/B
Director Respiratory Therapy . . . . Janice Gerdes

Measure	Cases	This Hospital	State Average	U.S. Average	Top Hospital
Heart Attack Care					
ACE Inhibitor or ARB for LVSD[3]	0	-	90%	82%	100%
Aspirin at Arrival[1,3]	1	100%	88%	92%	100%
Aspirin at Discharge[3]	0	-	90%	90%	100%
Beta Blocker at Arrival[1,3]	1	100%	81%	87%	100%
Beta Blocker at Discharge[3]	0	-	95%	90%	100%
Fibrinolytic Medication Timing[3]	0	-	25%	31%	100%
PCI Within 90 Minutes of Arrival[5]	-	-	83%	54%	95%
Smoking Cessation Advice[3]	0	-	84%	88%	100%
Heart Failure Care					
ACE Inhibitor or ARB for LVSD[1,3]	2	100%	76%	82%	100%
Discharge Instructions[1,3]	6	83%	54%	61%	93%
Evaluation of LVS Function[1,3]	11	82%	72%	83%	99%
Smoking Cessation Advice[3]	0	-	62%	82%	100%
Pneumonia Care					
Appropriate Initial Antibiotic[1,3]	6	100%	90%	83%	94%
Blood Culture Timing[1]	2	100%	96%	90%	100%
Influenza Vaccine[1]	3	67%	77%	70%	100%
Initial Antibiotic Timing[1,3]	9	100%	91%	80%	93%
Oxygenation Assessment[1,3]	11	100%	97%	99%	100%
Pneumococcal Vaccine[1,3]	8	88%	70%	69%	94%
Smoking Cessation Advice[1,3]	2	50%	64%	80%	100%
Surgical Infection Prevention					
Prophylactic Antibiotic Given[1,3]	8	100%	79%	77%	95%
Prophylactic Antibiotic Selection[1]	2	50%	94%	90%	100%
Prophylactic Antibiotic Stopped[1,3]	8	62%	83%	72%	95%
Pregnancy Care					
Inpatient Neonatal Mortality	-	-	-	-	-
Third or Fourth Degree Laceration	-	-	-	3.63%	3.27%

Tilden Community Hospital

308 W 2nd and Pine Street
Tilden, NE 68781
E-mail: info@tildenhospital.org
URL: www.tildenhospital.org
Ownership: Government - Local
Emergency Services: Yes

Phone: 402-368-5343
Fax: 402-368-7746
Accredited: No
Licensed Beds: 20

Key Personnel:
Administrator . . . . LuAnn Brandt

Measure	Cases	This Hospital	State Average	U.S. Average	Top Hospital
Heart Attack Care					
ACE Inhibitor or ARB for LVSD[5]	-	-	90%	82%	100%
Aspirin at Arrival[5]	-	-	88%	92%	100%
Aspirin at Discharge[5]	-	-	90%	90%	100%
Beta Blocker at Arrival[5]	-	-	81%	87%	100%
Beta Blocker at Discharge[5]	-	-	95%	90%	100%
Fibrinolytic Medication Timing[5]	-	-	25%	31%	100%
PCI Within 90 Minutes of Arrival[5]	-	-	83%	54%	95%
Smoking Cessation Advice[5]	-	-	84%	88%	100%
Heart Failure Care					
ACE Inhibitor or ARB for LVSD[3]	0	-	76%	82%	100%
Discharge Instructions[1,3]	1	0%	54%	61%	93%
Evaluation of LVS Function[1,3]	1	100%	72%	83%	99%
Smoking Cessation Advice[3]	0	-	62%	82%	100%
Pneumonia Care					
Appropriate Initial Antibiotic[1]	5	80%	90%	83%	94%
Blood Culture Timing[1]	3	100%	96%	90%	100%
Influenza Vaccine[1]	1	0%	77%	70%	100%
Initial Antibiotic Timing[1]	5	100%	91%	80%	93%
Oxygenation Assessment[1]	9	100%	97%	99%	100%
Pneumococcal Vaccine[1]	5	80%	70%	69%	94%
Smoking Cessation Advice[1]	6	50%	64%	80%	100%
Surgical Infection Prevention					
Prophylactic Antibiotic Given[5]	-	-	79%	77%	95%
Prophylactic Antibiotic Selection[5]	-	-	94%	90%	100%
Prophylactic Antibiotic Stopped[5]	-	-	83%	72%	95%
Pregnancy Care					
Inpatient Neonatal Mortality	-	-	-	-	-
Third or Fourth Degree Laceration	-	-	-	3.63%	3.27%

Cherry County Hospital

Highway 12 & Green Street
Valentine, NE 69201
Ownership: Govt - Hospital District or Authority
Emergency Services: Yes

Phone: 402-376-2525
Fax: 402-376-1627
Accredited: No
Licensed Beds: 36

Key Personnel:
Administrator . . . . Brent A Peterson
Emergency Room . . . . Becky Peterson
Director Infection/Disease Control . . . . Darlene Myer

NOTE: Hospital profiles are in alphabetical order by state, then city, then hospital within the city; Rankings are sorted by rate in descending order and exclude hospitals with less than 25 cases; (1) The number of cases is too small (n<25) for purposes of reliably predicting hospital performance; (2) Measure reflects the hospital's indication that its submission was based upon a sample of its relevant discharges; (3) Rate reflects fewer than the maximum possible quarters of data for the measure; (4) Inaccurate information submitted and suppressed for one or more quarters; (5) No data is available from the hospital for this measure; Please refer to the User's Guide for a full explanation of data

Measure	Cases	This Hospital	State Average	U.S. Average	Top Hospital
Heart Attack Care					
ACE Inhibitor or ARB for LVSD[3]	0	-	90%	82%	100%
Aspirin at Arrival[3]	0	-	88%	92%	100%
Aspirin at Discharge[3]	0	-	90%	90%	100%
Beta Blocker at Arrival[3]	0	-	81%	87%	100%
Beta Blocker at Discharge[3]	0	-	95%	90%	100%
Fibrinolytic Medication Timing[3]	0	-	25%	31%	100%
PCI Within 90 Minutes of Arrival[5]	-	-	83%	54%	95%
Smoking Cessation Advice[3]	0	-	84%	88%	100%
Heart Failure Care					
ACE Inhibitor or ARB for LVSD[3]	0	-	76%	82%	100%
Discharge Instructions[1,3]	1	0%	54%	61%	93%
Evaluation of LVS Function[1,3]	2	100%	72%	83%	99%
Smoking Cessation Advice[3]	0	-	62%	82%	100%
Pneumonia Care					
Appropriate Initial Antibiotic[1,3]	6	100%	90%	83%	94%
Blood Culture Timing[1,3]	2	100%	96%	90%	100%
Influenza Vaccine[1]	4	50%	77%	70%	100%
Initial Antibiotic Timing[1,3]	14	79%	91%	80%	93%
Oxygenation Assessment[1,3]	17	100%	97%	99%	100%
Pneumococcal Vaccine[1,3]	15	60%	70%	69%	94%
Smoking Cessation Advice[1,3]	1	100%	64%	80%	100%
Surgical Infection Prevention					
Prophylactic Antibiotic Given[5]	-	-	79%	77%	95%
Prophylactic Antibiotic Selection[5]	-	-	94%	90%	100%
Prophylactic Antibiotic Stopped[5]	-	-	83%	72%	95%
Pregnancy Care					
Inpatient Neonatal Mortality	-	-	-	-	-
Third or Fourth Degree Laceration	-	-	-	3.63%	3.27%

Saunders Medical Center

805 West 10th Street
Wahoo, NE 68086
E-mail: info@saunders-health.org
URL: www.saunders-health.org
Ownership: Voluntary non-profit - Other
Emergency Services: Yes
Phone: 402-443-4191
Fax: 402-443-1401
Accredited: No

Key Personnel:
Chief Medical Staff . . . . Leo Meduna, MD
Emergency Room . . . . Leo Meduna, MD
Director Infection/Disease Control . . . . Bev Janacek, RN
Director Respiratory Therapy . . . . Nila Haroon

Measure	Cases	This Hospital	State Average	U.S. Average	Top Hospital
Heart Attack Care					
ACE Inhibitor or ARB for LVSD[3]	0	-	90%	82%	100%
Aspirin at Arrival[1,3]	1	100%	88%	92%	100%
Aspirin at Discharge[3]	0	-	90%	90%	100%
Beta Blocker at Arrival[1,3]	1	100%	81%	87%	100%
Beta Blocker at Discharge[3]	0	-	95%	90%	100%
Fibrinolytic Medication Timing[3]	0	-	25%	31%	100%
PCI Within 90 Minutes of Arrival[5]	-	-	83%	54%	95%
Smoking Cessation Advice[3]	0	-	84%	88%	100%
Heart Failure Care					
ACE Inhibitor or ARB for LVSD[1]	5	80%	76%	82%	100%
Discharge Instructions[1]	9	44%	54%	61%	93%
Evaluation of LVS Function[1]	20	90%	72%	83%	99%
Smoking Cessation Advice[1]	2	0%	62%	82%	100%
Pneumonia Care					
Appropriate Initial Antibiotic[1]	21	95%	90%	83%	94%
Blood Culture Timing[1]	10	100%	96%	90%	100%
Influenza Vaccine[1]	9	89%	77%	70%	100%
Initial Antibiotic Timing	38	95%	91%	80%	93%
Oxygenation Assessment	44	100%	97%	99%	100%
Pneumococcal Vaccine	35	97%	70%	69%	94%
Smoking Cessation Advice[1]	2	50%	64%	80%	100%
Surgical Infection Prevention					
Prophylactic Antibiotic Given[5]	-	-	79%	77%	95%
Prophylactic Antibiotic Selection[5]	-	-	94%	90%	100%
Prophylactic Antibiotic Stopped[5]	-	-	83%	72%	95%
Pregnancy Care					
Inpatient Neonatal Mortality	-	-	-	-	-
Third or Fourth Degree Laceration	-	-	-	3.63%	3.27%

Providence Medical Center

1200 Providence Road
Wayne, NE 68787
URL: www.providencemedical.com
Ownership: Voluntary non-profit - Church
Emergency Services: Yes
Phone: 402-375-3800
Fax: 402-375-7989
Accredited: No
Licensed Beds: 25

Key Personnel:
Administrator . . . . Marcile Thomas
Infection Control Nurse. Kathy Hillier
Director Surgery. . . . . Karlene Maler
Director Radiology . . . . Terri McCraney
Director of Respiratory Therapy . . . . Theresa Beva

Measure	Cases	This Hospital	State Average	U.S. Average	Top Hospital
Heart Attack Care					
ACE Inhibitor or ARB for LVSD[1,3]	1	100%	90%	82%	100%
Aspirin at Arrival[1,3]	3	100%	88%	92%	100%
Aspirin at Discharge[1,3]	2	50%	90%	90%	100%
Beta Blocker at Arrival[1,3]	3	67%	81%	87%	100%
Beta Blocker at Discharge[1,3]	2	100%	95%	90%	100%
Fibrinolytic Medication Timing[3]	0	-	25%	31%	100%
PCI Within 90 Minutes of Arrival	0	-	83%	54%	95%
Smoking Cessation Advice[3]	0	-	84%	88%	100%
Heart Failure Care					
ACE Inhibitor or ARB for LVSD[1]	6	100%	76%	82%	100%
Discharge Instructions[1]	8	75%	54%	61%	93%
Evaluation of LVS Function[1]	22	68%	72%	83%	99%
Smoking Cessation Advice[1]	1	100%	62%	82%	100%
Pneumonia Care					
Appropriate Initial Antibiotic[1]	13	69%	90%	83%	94%
Blood Culture Timing	0	-	96%	90%	100%
Influenza Vaccine[1]	2	100%	77%	70%	100%
Initial Antibiotic Timing[1]	14	100%	91%	80%	93%
Oxygenation Assessment[1]	21	100%	97%	99%	100%
Pneumococcal Vaccine[1]	19	79%	70%	69%	94%
Smoking Cessation Advice[1]	2	50%	64%	80%	100%
Surgical Infection Prevention					
Prophylactic Antibiotic Given[1]	9	11%	79%	77%	95%
Prophylactic Antibiotic Selection[1]	3	100%	94%	90%	100%
Prophylactic Antibiotic Stopped[1]	8	88%	83%	72%	95%
Pregnancy Care					
Inpatient Neonatal Mortality	-	-	-	-	-
Third or Fourth Degree Laceration	-	-	-	3.63%	3.27%

Saint Francis Memorial Hospital

430 N Monitor Street
West Point, NE 68788
E-mail: jmeiergerd@fcswp.org
URL: www.fcswp.org/sfmh
Ownership: Voluntary non-profit - Church
Emergency Services: Yes
Phone: 402-372-2404
Fax: 402-372-2360
Accredited: No
Licensed Beds: 25

Key Personnel:
President/CEO. . . . . Ron Briggs
Director Infection/Disease Control . . . . Karen Spenner, RN
Director Radiology . . . . Brenda Jennelle, RT

Measure	Cases	This Hospital	State Average	U.S. Average	Top Hospital
Heart Attack Care					
ACE Inhibitor or ARB for LVSD[3]	0	-	90%	82%	100%
Aspirin at Arrival[1,3]	5	100%	88%	92%	100%
Aspirin at Discharge[1,3]	3	100%	90%	90%	100%
Beta Blocker at Arrival[1,3]	4	100%	81%	87%	100%
Beta Blocker at Discharge[1,3]	1	100%	95%	90%	100%
Fibrinolytic Medication Timing[1,3]	1	0%	25%	31%	100%
PCI Within 90 Minutes of Arrival[5]	-	-	83%	54%	95%
Smoking Cessation Advice[3]	0	-	84%	88%	100%
Heart Failure Care					
ACE Inhibitor or ARB for LVSD[1]	13	69%	76%	82%	100%
Discharge Instructions[1]	21	81%	54%	61%	93%

NOTE: Hospital profiles are in alphabetical order by state, then city, then hospital within the city; Rankings are sorted by rate in descending order and exclude hospitals with less than 25 cases; (1) The number of cases is too small (n<25) for purposes of reliably predicting hospital performance; (2) Measure reflects the hospital's indication that its submission was based upon a sample of its relevant discharges; (3) Rate reflects fewer than the maximum possible quarters of data for the measure; (4) Inaccurate information submitted and suppressed for one or more quarters; (5) No data is available from the hospital for this measure; Please refer to the User's Guide for a full explanation of data

Evaluation of LVS Function	41	90%	72%	83%	99%
Smoking Cessation Advice[1]	3	67%	62%	82%	100%
Pneumonia Care					
Appropriate Initial Antibiotic[1]	19	89%	90%	83%	94%
Blood Culture Timing[1]	3	100%	96%	90%	100%
Influenza Vaccine[1]	4	75%	77%	70%	100%
Initial Antibiotic Timing	26	100%	91%	80%	93%
Oxygenation Assessment	32	100%	97%	99%	100%
Pneumococcal Vaccine	26	92%	70%	69%	94%
Smoking Cessation Advice[1]	4	50%	64%	80%	100%
Surgical Infection Prevention					
Prophylactic Antibiotic Given	47	89%	79%	77%	95%
Prophylactic Antibiotic Selection[1]	8	100%	94%	90%	100%
Prophylactic Antibiotic Stopped	45	96%	83%	72%	95%
Pregnancy Care					
Inpatient Neonatal Mortality	-	-	-	-	-
Third or Fourth Degree Laceration	-	-	-	3.63%	3.27%

Winnebago Hospital

Alternate Name: PHS Indian Hospital
Highway 77/75
Winnebago, NE 68071
URL: www.ihs.gov
Phone: 402-878-2231
Fax: 402-878-2535
Ownership: Government - Federal
Emergency Services: Yes
Accredited: Yes
Licensed Beds: 57

Key Personnel:

CEO . . . . Linus Everling
Chief of Medical Staff . . . . Anwar Mohammed
Emergency Room . . . . Deb Saunsoci
Director Infection/Disease Control . . . . Sharon Wacker
Director Medical/Surgical Nursing . . . . Melinda Balderas
Chief Radiology . . . . Sherrill Svoboda
Respiratory Care . . . . Sophie Chao

Measure	Cases	This Hospital	State Average	U.S. Average	Top Hospital
Heart Attack Care					
ACE Inhibitor or ARB for LVSD[5]	-	-	90%	82%	100%
Aspirin at Arrival[5]	-	-	88%	92%	100%
Aspirin at Discharge[5]	-	-	90%	90%	100%
Beta Blocker at Arrival[5]	-	-	81%	87%	100%
Beta Blocker at Discharge[5]	-	-	95%	90%	100%
Fibrinolytic Medication Timing[5]	-	-	25%	31%	100%
PCI Within 90 Minutes of Arrival[5]	-	-	83%	54%	95%
Smoking Cessation Advice[5]	-	-	84%	88%	100%
Heart Failure Care					
ACE Inhibitor or ARB for LVSD[1,3]	1	0%	76%	82%	100%
Discharge Instructions[1,3]	5	40%	54%	61%	93%
Evaluation of LVS Function[1,3]	5	60%	72%	83%	99%
Smoking Cessation Advice[1,3]	2	0%	62%	82%	100%
Pneumonia Care					
Appropriate Initial Antibiotic[5]	-	-	90%	83%	94%
Blood Culture Timing[5]	-	-	96%	90%	100%
Influenza Vaccine[5]	-	-	77%	70%	100%
Initial Antibiotic Timing[5]	-	-	91%	80%	93%
Oxygenation Assessment[5]	-	-	97%	99%	100%
Pneumococcal Vaccine[5]	-	-	70%	69%	94%
Smoking Cessation Advice[5]	-	-	64%	80%	100%
Surgical Infection Prevention					
Prophylactic Antibiotic Given[5]	-	-	79%	77%	95%
Prophylactic Antibiotic Selection[5]	-	-	94%	90%	100%
Prophylactic Antibiotic Stopped[5]	-	-	83%	72%	95%
Pregnancy Care					
Inpatient Neonatal Mortality	-	-	-	-	-
Third or Fourth Degree Laceration	-	-	-	3.63%	3.27%

York General Hospital

2222 Lincoln Avenue
York, NE 68467
E-mail: yorkgenhosp@navix.net
URL: www.yorkhospital.org
Phone: 402-362-6671
Fax: 402-362-0499
Ownership: Voluntary non-profit - Private
Emergency Services: Yes
Accredited: No
Licensed Beds: 48

Key Personnel:

CEO . . . . Charles Schulz

Measure	Cases	This Hospital	State Average	U.S. Average	Top Hospital
Heart Attack Care					
ACE Inhibitor or ARB for LVSD[5]	-	-	90%	82%	100%
Aspirin at Arrival[5]	-	-	88%	92%	100%
Aspirin at Discharge[5]	-	-	90%	90%	100%
Beta Blocker at Arrival[5]	-	-	81%	87%	100%
Beta Blocker at Discharge[5]	-	-	95%	90%	100%
Fibrinolytic Medication Timing[5]	-	-	25%	31%	100%
PCI Within 90 Minutes of Arrival[5]	-	-	83%	54%	95%
Smoking Cessation Advice[5]	-	-	84%	88%	100%
Heart Failure Care					
ACE Inhibitor or ARB for LVSD[5]	-	-	76%	82%	100%
Discharge Instructions[5]	-	-	54%	61%	93%
Evaluation of LVS Function[5]	-	-	72%	83%	99%
Smoking Cessation Advice[5]	-	-	62%	82%	100%
Pneumonia Care					
Appropriate Initial Antibiotic	26	81%	90%	83%	94%
Blood Culture Timing[1]	12	92%	96%	90%	100%
Influenza Vaccine[1]	7	100%	77%	70%	100%
Initial Antibiotic Timing	25	88%	91%	80%	93%
Oxygenation Assessment	35	100%	97%	99%	100%
Pneumococcal Vaccine	26	96%	70%	69%	94%
Smoking Cessation Advice[1]	2	100%	64%	80%	100%
Surgical Infection Prevention					
Prophylactic Antibiotic Given[2]	52	98%	79%	77%	95%
Prophylactic Antibiotic Selection[1,2]	16	100%	94%	90%	100%
Prophylactic Antibiotic Stopped[2]	51	98%	83%	72%	95%
Pregnancy Care					
Inpatient Neonatal Mortality	-	-	-	-	-
Third or Fourth Degree Laceration	-	-	-	3.63%	3.27%

NOTE: Hospital profiles are in alphabetical order by state, then city, then hospital within the city; Rankings are sorted by rate in descending order and exclude hospitals with less than 25 cases; (1) The number of cases is too small (n<25) for purposes of reliably predicting hospital performance; (2) Measure reflects the hospital's indication that its submission was based upon a sample of its relevant discharges; (3) Rate reflects fewer than the maximum possible quarters of data for the measure; (4) Inaccurate information submitted and suppressed for one or more quarters; (5) No data is available from the hospital for this measure; Please refer to the User's Guide for a full explanation of data

Heart Attack Care

1. ACE Inhibitor or ARB for LVSD

Hospital Name	City	Rate	Cases
Trinity Health	Minot	100%	27
MeritCare Medical Center	Fargo	97%	103
Altru Hospital	Grand Forks	95%	39
Innovis Health	Fargo	82%	39

2. Aspirin at Arrival

Hospital Name	City	Rate	Cases
Altru Hospital	Grand Forks	100%	101
Saint Alexius Medical Center	Bismarck	100%	100
Medcenter One	Bismarck	99%	89
MeritCare Medical Center	Fargo	99%	193
Trinity Health	Minot	99%	126
Innovis Health	Fargo	93%	81
Saint Joseph's Hospital & Health Center	Dickinson	88%	32

3. Aspirin at Discharge

Hospital Name	City	Rate	Cases
Altru Hospital	Grand Forks	100%	215
Medcenter One	Bismarck	99%	129
MeritCare Medical Center	Fargo	99%	506
Trinity Health	Minot	99%	178
Saint Alexius Medical Center	Bismarck	98%	199
Innovis Health	Fargo	95%	190

4. Beta Blocker at Arrival

Hospital Name	City	Rate	Cases
Trinity Health	Minot	100%	91
Altru Hospital	Grand Forks	98%	85
MeritCare Medical Center	Fargo	98%	175
Saint Alexius Medical Center	Bismarck	98%	99
Medcenter One	Bismarck	95%	82
Innovis Health	Fargo	89%	66

5. Beta Blocker at Discharge

Hospital Name	City	Rate	Cases
MeritCare Medical Center	Fargo	100%	499
Altru Hospital	Grand Forks	99%	202
Trinity Health	Minot	99%	204
Medcenter One	Bismarck	98%	113
Saint Alexius Medical Center	Bismarck	98%	196
Saint Joseph's Hospital & Health Center	Dickinson	96%	25
Innovis Health	Fargo	93%	182

8. Smoking Cessation Advice

Hospital Name	City	Rate	Cases
Medcenter One	Bismarck	100%	36
Saint Alexius Medical Center	Bismarck	99%	68
Altru Hospital	Grand Forks	98%	86
MeritCare Medical Center	Fargo	98%	167
Innovis Health	Fargo	93%	68

Heart Failure Care

9. ACE Inhibitor or ARB for LVSD

Hospital Name	City	Rate	Cases
Trinity Health	Minot	94%	89
Altru Hospital	Grand Forks	91%	53
Saint Alexius Medical Center	Bismarck	90%	97
Medcenter One	Bismarck	86%	85
Innovis Health	Fargo	82%	44
MeritCare Medical Center	Fargo	73%	118

10. Discharge Instructions

Hospital Name	City	Rate	Cases
Medcenter One	Bismarck	95%	141
Saint Alexius Medical Center	Bismarck	95%	203
Trinity Health	Minot	82%	40
Jamestown Hospital	Jamestown	80%	40
Mercy Medical Center	Williston	80%	25
Altru Hospital	Grand Forks	78%	137
Mercy Hospital	Devils Lake	77%	26
MeritCare Medical Center	Fargo	77%	201
Saint Joseph's Hospital & Health Center	Dickinson	70%	53
West River Regional Medical Center	Hettinger	67%	46
Innovis Health	Fargo	63%	107

11. Evaluation of LVS Function

Hospital Name	City	Rate	Cases
Medcenter One	Bismarck	99%	198
MeritCare Medical Center	Fargo	99%	278
Trinity Health	Minot	99%	249
Saint Alexius Medical Center	Bismarck	98%	244
Mercy Medical Center	Williston	92%	39
Innovis Health	Fargo	90%	133
Altru Hospital	Grand Forks	88%	181
West River Regional Medical Center	Hettinger	78%	69
Saint Joseph's Hospital & Health Center	Dickinson	75%	85
Jamestown Hospital	Jamestown	70%	57
Mercy Hospital	Devils Lake	67%	36
Linton Hospital	Linton	16%	32
Quentin N Burdick Mem Healthcare Facility	Belcourt	0%	29

12. Smoking Cessation Advice

Hospital Name	City	Rate	Cases
Medcenter One	Bismarck	100%	28
Saint Alexius Medical Center	Bismarck	96%	26
MeritCare Medical Center	Fargo	70%	37

Pneumonia Care

13. Appropriate Initial Antibiotic

Hospital Name	City	Rate	Cases
Jamestown Hospital	Jamestown	98%	54
Innovis Health	Fargo	96%	56
MeritCare Medical Center	Fargo	89%	139
Medcenter One	Bismarck	88%	85
Altru Hospital	Grand Forks	87%	117
Saint Alexius Medical Center	Bismarck	87%	85
Mercy Medical Center	Williston	85%	52
Saint Joseph's Hospital & Health Center	Dickinson	80%	30
Mercy Hospital	Devils Lake	77%	65
Linton Hospital	Linton	19%	31

14. Blood Culture Timing

Hospital Name	City	Rate	Cases
Mercy Hospital	Devils Lake	100%	36
Jamestown Hospital	Jamestown	97%	63
Saint Alexius Medical Center	Bismarck	97%	60
Medcenter One	Bismarck	95%	79
Mercy Medical Center	Williston	93%	46
MeritCare Medical Center	Fargo	93%	129
Altru Hospital	Grand Forks	92%	143
Saint Joseph's Hospital & Health Center	Dickinson	92%	38
Innovis Health	Fargo	90%	51

15. Influenza Vaccine

Hospital Name	City	Rate	Cases
Altru Hospital	Grand Forks	88%	40
Saint Alexius Medical Center	Bismarck	88%	25
MeritCare Medical Center	Fargo	77%	52

16. Initial Antibiotic Timing

Hospital Name	City	Rate	Cases
Heart of America Medical Center	Rugby	100%	39
Hillsboro Medical Center	Hillsboro	100%	25
West River Regional Medical Center	Hettinger	98%	64
Linton Hospital	Linton	94%	36
Medcenter One	Bismarck	94%	121
Wishek Community Hospital	Wishek	94%	33
Saint Joseph's Hospital & Health Center	Dickinson	92%	53
Jamestown Hospital	Jamestown	91%	91
Trinity Health	Minot	89%	192
Innovis Health	Fargo	86%	66
Mercy Hospital	Devils Lake	81%	57
Saint Alexius Medical Center	Bismarck	81%	106
MeritCare Medical Center	Fargo	80%	234
Altru Hospital	Grand Forks	79%	193
Mercy Medical Center	Williston	78%	64
Quentin N Burdick Mem Healthcare Facility	Belcourt	70%	50

17. Oxygenation Assessment

Hospital Name	City	Rate	Cases
Altru Hospital	Grand Forks	100%	250
Heart of America Medical Center	Rugby	100%	49
Hillsboro Medical Center	Hillsboro	100%	31
Innovis Health	Fargo	100%	87

NOTE: Hospital profiles are in alphabetical order by state, then city, then hospital within the city; Rankings are sorted by rate in descending order and exclude hospitals with less than 25 cases; (1) The number of cases is too small (n<25) for purposes of reliably predicting hospital performance; (2) Measure reflects the hospital's indication that its submission was based upon a sample of its relevant discharges; (3) Rate reflects fewer than the maximum possible quarters of data for the measure; (4) Inaccurate information submitted and suppressed for one or more quarters; (5) No data is available from the hospital for this measure; Please refer to the User's Guide for a full explanation of data

Hospital Name	City	Rate	Cases
Jamestown Hospital	Jamestown	100%	118
Linton Hospital	Linton	100%	43
Medcenter One	Bismarck	100%	146
Mercy Hospital	Devils Lake	100%	97
Mercy Medical Center	Williston	100%	85
MeritCare Medical Center	Fargo	100%	276
Pembina County Memorial Hospital	Cavalier	100%	27
Quentin N Burdick Mem Healthcare Facility	Belcourt	100%	58
Saint Alexius Medical Center	Bismarck	100%	147
Saint Joseph's Hospital & Health Center	Dickinson	100%	67
Trinity Health	Minot	100%	238
Wishek Community Hospital	Wishek	100%	40
West River Regional Medical Center	Hettinger	97%	77

18. Pneumococcal Vaccine

Hospital Name	City	Rate	Cases
Hillsboro Medical Center	Hillsboro	97%	29
Saint Alexius Medical Center	Bismarck	97%	117
Mercy Medical Center	Williston	94%	65
Altru Hospital	Grand Forks	92%	181
Trinity Health	Minot	92%	172
Medcenter One	Bismarck	90%	98
Saint Joseph's Hospital & Health Center	Dickinson	85%	48
West River Regional Medical Center	Hettinger	85%	73
MeritCare Medical Center	Fargo	84%	205
Heart of America Medical Center	Rugby	82%	40
Innovis Health	Fargo	80%	64
Jamestown Hospital	Jamestown	75%	84
Wishek Community Hospital	Wishek	72%	40
Linton Hospital	Linton	59%	37
Mercy Hospital	Devils Lake	48%	58
Quentin N Burdick Mem Healthcare Facility	Belcourt	26%	31

19. Smoking Cessation Advice

Hospital Name	City	Rate	Cases
Altru Hospital	Grand Forks	94%	63
Saint Alexius Medical Center	Bismarck	92%	40
Medcenter One	Bismarck	85%	34
MeritCare Medical Center	Fargo	74%	53
Mercy Hospital	Devils Lake	52%	27

Surgical Infection Prevention

20. Prophylactic Antibiotic Given

Hospital Name	City	Rate	Cases
MeritCare Medical Center	Fargo	93%	326
Mercy Medical Center	Williston	91%	172
Saint Joseph's Hospital & Health Center	Dickinson	91%	165
Innovis Health	Fargo	90%	167
Jamestown Hospital	Jamestown	90%	63
Altru Hospital	Grand Forks	89%	312
Saint Alexius Medical Center	Bismarck	89%	1204
Medcenter One	Bismarck	88%	197
Trinity Health	Minot	87%	134

21. Prophylactic Antibiotic Selection

Hospital Name	City	Rate	Cases
Saint Joseph's Hospital & Health Center	Dickinson	100%	40
Innovis Health	Fargo	97%	60
Medcenter One	Bismarck	97%	102
Altru Hospital	Grand Forks	95%	81
Saint Alexius Medical Center	Bismarck	95%	263
Mercy Medical Center	Williston	94%	36
MeritCare Medical Center	Fargo	87%	86

22. Prophylactic Antibiotic Stopped

Hospital Name	City	Rate	Cases
MeritCare Medical Center	Fargo	88%	313
Trinity Health	Minot	85%	133
Medcenter One	Bismarck	83%	196
Jamestown Hospital	Jamestown	81%	59
Saint Joseph's Hospital & Health Center	Dickinson	81%	167
Mercy Medical Center	Williston	80%	172
Innovis Health	Fargo	79%	159
Altru Hospital	Grand Forks	67%	299
Saint Alexius Medical Center	Bismarck	60%	1170

Pregnancy Care

23. Inpatient Neonatal Mortality

Hospital Name	City	Rate	Cases
Mercy Hospital	Devils Lake	0.00%	310
Mercy Medical Center	Williston	0.00%	364
Saint Joseph's Hospital & Health Center	Dickinson	0.00%	319
Saint Alexius Medical Center	Bismarck	0.39%	1290

24. Third or Fourth Degree Laceration

Hospital Name	City	Rate	Cases
Mercy Medical Center	Williston	2.46%	284
Saint Joseph's Hospital & Health Center	Dickinson	3.64%	220
Mercy Hospital	Devils Lake	5.00%	220
Saint Alexius Medical Center	Bismarck	6.05%	893

NOTE: Hospital profiles are in alphabetical order by state, then city, then hospital within the city; Rankings are sorted by rate in descending order and exclude hospitals with less than 25 cases; (1) The number of cases is too small (n<25) for purposes of reliably predicting hospital performance; (2) Measure reflects the hospital's indication that its submission was based upon a sample of its relevant discharges; (3) Rate reflects fewer than the maximum possible quarters of data for the measure; (4) Inaccurate information submitted and suppressed for one or more quarters; (5) No data is available from the hospital for this measure; Please refer to the User's Guide for a full explanation of data

Quentin N Burdick Mem Healthcare Facility

Alternate Name: Quentin N Burdick Comprehensive Health Facility
PO Box 160
Belcourt, ND 58316
Ownership: Government - Federal
Emergency Services: Yes
Phone: 701-477-6111
Fax: 701-477-8410
Accredited: Yes
Licensed Beds: 29

Key Personnel:
CEO. . . . . Levern Parker
Chief Medical Staff. . . . . Penny Wilkie, MD
Emergency Room . . . . Cheryl LaVallie
Director Infection/Disease Control . . . . . Virginia Thomas
CCU Spvg. Nurse . . . . Cheryl LaVallie
Director Medical/Surgical Nursing . . . . . Cheryl LaVallie
Respiratory Therapy. . . . . Lisa Davidson

Measure	Cases	This Hospital	State Average	U.S. Average	Top Hospital
Heart Attack Care					
ACE Inhibitor or ARB for LVSD[5]	-	-	83%	82%	100%
Aspirin at Arrival[5]	-	-	92%	92%	100%
Aspirin at Discharge[5]	-	-	91%	90%	100%
Beta Blocker at Arrival[5]	-	-	84%	87%	100%
Beta Blocker at Discharge[5]	-	-	95%	90%	100%
Fibrinolytic Medication Timing[5]	-	-	28%	31%	100%
PCI Within 90 Minutes of Arrival[5]	-	-	78%	54%	95%
Smoking Cessation Advice[5]	-	-	74%	88%	100%
Heart Failure Care					
ACE Inhibitor or ARB for LVSD	0	-	72%	82%	100%
Discharge Instructions[3]	0	-	63%	61%	93%
Evaluation of LVS Function	29	0%	67%	83%	99%
Smoking Cessation Advice[3]	0	-	67%	82%	100%
Pneumonia Care					
Appropriate Initial Antibiotic[1,3]	9	11%	75%	83%	94%
Blood Culture Timing[1,3]	5	80%	95%	90%	100%
Influenza Vaccine[4,5]	-	-	77%	70%	100%
Initial Antibiotic Timing	50	70%	90%	80%	93%
Oxygenation Assessment	58	100%	100%	99%	100%
Pneumococcal Vaccine	31	26%	74%	69%	94%
Smoking Cessation Advice[1,3]	5	20%	63%	80%	100%
Surgical Infection Prevention					
Prophylactic Antibiotic Given[1,3]	2	0%	81%	77%	95%
Prophylactic Antibiotic Selection[5]	-	-	96%	90%	100%
Prophylactic Antibiotic Stopped[1,3]	2	100%	79%	72%	95%
Pregnancy Care					
Inpatient Neonatal Mortality	-	-	-	-	-
Third or Fourth Degree Laceration	-	-	-	3.63%	3.27%

Medcenter One

300 N 7th Street
PO Box 5525
Bismarck, ND 58506
Ownership: Voluntary non-profit - Private
Emergency Services: Yes
Phone: 701-323-6000
Fax: 701-323-5221
Accredited: Yes
Licensed Beds: 238

Key Personnel:
CEO. . . . . James C Cooper
Chief Medical Staff. . . . . Dr. Les Rainwater
Catheterization Lab . . . . Wade Miller
Emergency Room . . . . Dr. Craig Lambrecht
Emergency Room . . . . Ardys Olson
Infection Control. . . . . Jodi Barnum
ICU . . . . Connie Stewart
Director Medical Surgical Nursing . . . . . Ione Eckroth
OB/GYN Womens Health. . . . . Kathy Schaefer, MD

Measure	Cases	This Hospital	State Average	U.S. Average	Top Hospital
Heart Attack Care					
ACE Inhibitor or ARB for LVSD[1]	23	96%	83%	82%	100%
Aspirin at Arrival	89	99%	92%	92%	100%
Aspirin at Discharge	129	99%	91%	90%	100%
Beta Blocker at Arrival	82	95%	84%	87%	100%
Beta Blocker at Discharge	113	98%	95%	90%	100%
Fibrinolytic Medication Timing[1]	5	20%	28%	31%	100%
PCI Within 90 Minutes of Arrival[1]	4	25%	78%	54%	95%
Smoking Cessation Advice	36	100%	74%	88%	100%
Heart Failure Care					
ACE Inhibitor or ARB for LVSD[2]	85	86%	72%	82%	100%
Discharge Instructions[2]	141	95%	63%	61%	93%
Evaluation of LVS Function[2]	198	99%	67%	83%	99%
Smoking Cessation Advice[2]	28	100%	67%	82%	100%
Pneumonia Care					
Appropriate Initial Antibiotic	85	88%	75%	83%	94%
Blood Culture Timing	79	95%	95%	90%	100%
Influenza Vaccine[1]	22	100%	77%	70%	100%
Initial Antibiotic Timing	121	94%	90%	80%	93%
Oxygenation Assessment	146	100%	100%	99%	100%
Pneumococcal Vaccine	98	90%	74%	69%	94%
Smoking Cessation Advice	34	85%	63%	80%	100%
Surgical Infection Prevention					
Prophylactic Antibiotic Given[3]	197	88%	81%	77%	95%
Prophylactic Antibiotic Selection	102	97%	96%	90%	100%
Prophylactic Antibiotic Stopped[3]	196	83%	79%	72%	95%
Pregnancy Care					
Inpatient Neonatal Mortality	-	-	-	-	-
Third or Fourth Degree Laceration	-	-	-	3.63%	3.27%

Saint Alexius Medical Center

900 East Broadway Avenue
Bismarck, ND 58501
Ownership: Voluntary non-profit - Church
Emergency Services: Yes
Phone: 701-530-7000
Fax: 701-530-7161
Accredited: Yes
Licensed Beds: 307

Key Personnel:
CEO. . . . . Richard A Tschider
Emergency Room . . . . Kathy Seidel
Director Medical/Surgical Nursing . . . . . Donna Gage
OB/GYN Womens Health. . . . . Jerry Obritsch
Chief Radiology . . . . Doug Peterson
Director Respiratory Therapy . . . . . . Mike Range

Measure	Cases	This Hospital	State Average	U.S. Average	Top Hospital
Heart Attack Care					
ACE Inhibitor or ARB for LVSD[1]	17	94%	83%	82%	100%
Aspirin at Arrival	100	100%	92%	92%	100%
Aspirin at Discharge	199	98%	91%	90%	100%
Beta Blocker at Arrival	99	98%	84%	87%	100%
Beta Blocker at Discharge	196	98%	95%	90%	100%
Fibrinolytic Medication Timing[1]	5	60%	28%	31%	100%
PCI Within 90 Minutes of Arrival[1]	7	100%	78%	54%	95%
Smoking Cessation Advice	68	99%	74%	88%	100%
Heart Failure Care					
ACE Inhibitor or ARB for LVSD	97	90%	72%	82%	100%
Discharge Instructions	203	95%	63%	61%	93%
Evaluation of LVS Function	244	98%	67%	83%	99%
Smoking Cessation Advice	26	96%	67%	82%	100%
Pneumonia Care					
Appropriate Initial Antibiotic	85	87%	75%	83%	94%
Blood Culture Timing	60	97%	95%	90%	100%
Influenza Vaccine	25	88%	77%	70%	100%
Initial Antibiotic Timing	106	81%	90%	80%	93%
Oxygenation Assessment	147	100%	100%	99%	100%
Pneumococcal Vaccine	117	97%	74%	69%	94%
Smoking Cessation Advice	40	92%	63%	80%	100%
Surgical Infection Prevention					
Prophylactic Antibiotic Given	1,204	89%	81%	77%	95%
Prophylactic Antibiotic Selection	263	95%	96%	90%	100%
Prophylactic Antibiotic Stopped	1,170	60%	79%	72%	95%
Pregnancy Care					
Inpatient Neonatal Mortality	1,290	0.39%	-	-	-
Third or Fourth Degree Laceration	893	6.05%	-	3.63%	3.27%

Saint Andrews Health Center

Alternate Name: Saint Andrews Hospital

NOTE: Hospital profiles are in alphabetical order by state, then city, then hospital within the city; Rankings are sorted by rate in descending order and exclude hospitals with less than 25 cases; (1) The number of cases is too small (n<25) for purposes of reliably predicting hospital performance; (2) Measure reflects the hospital's indication that its submission was based upon a sample of its relevant discharges; (3) Rate reflects fewer than the maximum possible quarters of data for the measure; (4) Inaccurate information submitted and suppressed for one or more quarters; (5) No data is available from the hospital for this measure; Please refer to the User's Guide for a full explanation of data

316 Ohmer Street
Bottineau, ND 58318
E-mail: sahc@utma.com
URL: www.standrewshealth.us
Ownership: Voluntary non-profit - Church
Emergency Services: Yes
Phone: 701-228-9300
Fax: 701-228-9384
Accredited: No
Licensed Beds: 25

Key Personnel:
Administrator/CEO . . . . Jodi Atkinson
Chief Medical Staff . . . . Dinesh Agnihotri, MD
Emergency Room . . . . Gwen Wall

Measure	Cases	This Hospital	State Average	U.S. Average	Top Hospital
Heart Attack Care					
ACE Inhibitor or ARB for LVSD[1,3]	1	0%	83%	82%	100%
Aspirin at Arrival[1,3]	1	100%	92%	92%	100%
Aspirin at Discharge[1,3]	1	100%	91%	90%	100%
Beta Blocker at Arrival[1,3]	1	100%	84%	87%	100%
Beta Blocker at Discharge[1,3]	1	100%	95%	90%	100%
Fibrinolytic Medication Timing[3]	0	-	28%	31%	100%
PCI Within 90 Minutes of Arrival[5]	-	-	78%	54%	95%
Smoking Cessation Advice[3]	0	-	74%	88%	100%
Heart Failure Care					
ACE Inhibitor or ARB for LVSD[1]	2	0%	72%	82%	100%
Discharge Instructions[1]	7	57%	63%	61%	93%
Evaluation of LVS Function[1]	9	78%	67%	83%	99%
Smoking Cessation Advice[1]	1	0%	67%	82%	100%
Pneumonia Care					
Appropriate Initial Antibiotic[1]	13	100%	75%	83%	94%
Blood Culture Timing[1]	6	100%	95%	90%	100%
Influenza Vaccine[1]	1	0%	77%	70%	100%
Initial Antibiotic Timing[1]	18	89%	90%	80%	93%
Oxygenation Assessment[1]	24	100%	100%	99%	100%
Pneumococcal Vaccine[1]	20	55%	74%	69%	94%
Smoking Cessation Advice[1]	3	0%	63%	80%	100%
Surgical Infection Prevention					
Prophylactic Antibiotic Given[5]	-	-	81%	77%	95%
Prophylactic Antibiotic Selection[5]	-	-	96%	90%	100%
Prophylactic Antibiotic Stopped[5]	-	-	79%	72%	95%
Pregnancy Care					
Inpatient Neonatal Mortality	-	-	-	-	-
Third or Fourth Degree Laceration	-	-	-	3.63%	3.27%

Towner County Medical Center

PO Box 688
Cando, ND 58324
Toll-Free: 800-943-3337
Phone: 701-968-4411
Fax: 701-968-2519
E-mail: tcmc@tcmedcenter.com
URL: www.tcmedcetner.com
Ownership: Government - Local
Emergency Services: Yes
Accredited: No
Licensed Beds: 32

Key Personnel:
CEO. . . . . Timothy Tracy
Chief Medical Staff. . . . . Russell Petty, MD
Director Infection/Disease Control . . . . Kristi Lee-Weyrauch
Director Respiratory Therapy . . . . Carol Lang

Measure	Cases	This Hospital	State Average	U.S. Average	Top Hospital
Heart Attack Care					
ACE Inhibitor or ARB for LVSD[3]	0	-	83%	82%	100%
Aspirin at Arrival[1,3]	1	100%	92%	92%	100%
Aspirin at Discharge[3]	0	-	91%	90%	100%
Beta Blocker at Arrival[1,3]	1	0%	84%	87%	100%
Beta Blocker at Discharge[3]	0	-	95%	90%	100%
Fibrinolytic Medication Timing[3]	0	-	28%	31%	100%
PCI Within 90 Minutes of Arrival[5]	-	-	78%	54%	95%
Smoking Cessation Advice[3]	0	-	74%	88%	100%
Heart Failure Care					
ACE Inhibitor or ARB for LVSD[1,3]	3	33%	72%	82%	100%
Discharge Instructions[1,3]	3	0%	63%	61%	93%
Evaluation of LVS Function[1,3]	7	43%	67%	83%	99%
Smoking Cessation Advice[3]	0	-	67%	82%	100%
Pneumonia Care					
Appropriate Initial Antibiotic[1]	2	50%	75%	83%	94%
Blood Culture Timing[1]	3	100%	95%	90%	100%
Influenza Vaccine[1]	2	50%	77%	70%	100%
Initial Antibiotic Timing[1]	5	80%	90%	80%	93%
Oxygenation Assessment[1]	11	100%	100%	99%	100%
Pneumococcal Vaccine[1]	9	44%	74%	69%	94%
Smoking Cessation Advice[1]	1	0%	63%	80%	100%
Surgical Infection Prevention					
Prophylactic Antibiotic Given[5]	-	-	81%	77%	95%
Prophylactic Antibiotic Selection[5]	-	-	96%	90%	100%
Prophylactic Antibiotic Stopped[5]	-	-	79%	72%	95%
Pregnancy Care					
Inpatient Neonatal Mortality	-	-	-	-	-
Third or Fourth Degree Laceration	-	-	-	3.63%	3.27%

Carrington Health Center

Alternate Name: Carrington Hospital
800 N 4th Street
Carrington, ND 58421
URL: www.carringtonhealthcenter.com
Ownership: Voluntary non-profit - Private
Emergency Services: Yes
Phone: 701-652-3141
Fax: 701-652-2884
Accredited: No
Licensed Beds: 25

Key Personnel:
Administrator/CEO . . . . Johnson Smith
Director Infection/Disease Control . . . . Bernardine Anderson

Measure	Cases	This Hospital	State Average	U.S. Average	Top Hospital
Heart Attack Care					
ACE Inhibitor or ARB for LVSD[1,3]	1	100%	83%	82%	100%
Aspirin at Arrival[1,3]	1	100%	92%	92%	100%
Aspirin at Discharge[1,3]	1	100%	91%	90%	100%
Beta Blocker at Arrival[1,3]	1	100%	84%	87%	100%
Beta Blocker at Discharge[1,3]	1	100%	95%	90%	100%
Fibrinolytic Medication Timing[3]	0	-	28%	31%	100%
PCI Within 90 Minutes of Arrival[5]	-	-	78%	54%	95%
Smoking Cessation Advice[3]	0	-	74%	88%	100%
Heart Failure Care					
ACE Inhibitor or ARB for LVSD[1,3]	2	100%	72%	82%	100%
Discharge Instructions[1,3]	13	15%	63%	61%	93%
Evaluation of LVS Function[1,3]	20	55%	67%	83%	99%
Smoking Cessation Advice[1,3]	1	0%	67%	82%	100%
Pneumonia Care					
Appropriate Initial Antibiotic[1,3]	15	80%	75%	83%	94%
Blood Culture Timing[1,3]	1	100%	95%	90%	100%
Influenza Vaccine[1]	5	60%	77%	70%	100%
Initial Antibiotic Timing[1,3]	17	94%	90%	80%	93%
Oxygenation Assessment[1,3]	21	100%	100%	99%	100%
Pneumococcal Vaccine[1,3]	19	68%	74%	69%	94%
Smoking Cessation Advice[1,3]	2	100%	63%	80%	100%
Surgical Infection Prevention					
Prophylactic Antibiotic Given[5]	-	-	81%	77%	95%
Prophylactic Antibiotic Selection[5]	-	-	96%	90%	100%
Prophylactic Antibiotic Stopped[5]	-	-	79%	72%	95%
Pregnancy Care					
Inpatient Neonatal Mortality	-	-	-	-	-
Third or Fourth Degree Laceration	-	-	-	3.63%	3.27%

Pembina County Memorial Hospital

PO Box 380
Cavalier, ND 58220
Ownership: Voluntary non-profit - Private
Emergency Services: Yes
Phone: 701-265-8461
Fax: 701-265-8752
Accredited: No
Licensed Beds: 29

Key Personnel:
CEO. . . . . Sarah Boss
Chief of Medical Staff . . . . Susan Thompson
Emergency Room . . . . Kathelen Duff

Measure	Cases	This Hospital	State Average	U.S. Average	Top Hospital
Heart Attack Care					
ACE Inhibitor or ARB for LVSD[2]	0	-	83%	82%	100%
Aspirin at Arrival[2]	0	-	92%	92%	100%
Aspirin at Discharge[2]	0	-	91%	90%	100%
Beta Blocker at Arrival[2]	0	-	84%	87%	100%

NOTE: Hospital profiles are in alphabetical order by state, then city, then hospital within the city; Rankings are sorted by rate in descending order and exclude hospitals with less than 25 cases; (1) The number of cases is too small (n<25) for purposes of reliably predicting hospital performance; (2) Measure reflects the hospital's indication that its submission was based upon a sample of its relevant discharges; (3) Rate reflects fewer than the maximum possible quarters of data for the measure; (4) Inaccurate information submitted and suppressed for one or more quarters; (5) No data is available from the hospital for this measure; Please refer to the User's Guide for a full explanation of data

Measure	Cases	This Hospital	State Average	U.S. Average	Top Hospital
Beta Blocker at Discharge[2]	0	-	95%	90%	100%
Fibrinolytic Medication Timing[2]	0	-	28%	31%	100%
PCI Within 90 Minutes of Arrival[2]	0	-	78%	54%	95%
Smoking Cessation Advice[2]	0	-	74%	88%	100%
Heart Failure Care					
ACE Inhibitor or ARB for LVSD[1,2]	2	50%	72%	82%	100%
Discharge Instructions[1,2]	9	100%	63%	61%	93%
Evaluation of LVS Function[1,2]	13	38%	67%	83%	99%
Smoking Cessation Advice[1,2]	1	100%	67%	82%	100%
Pneumonia Care					
Appropriate Initial Antibiotic[1,2,3]	18	72%	75%	83%	94%
Blood Culture Timing[2]	0	-	95%	90%	100%
Influenza Vaccine[4,5]	-	-	77%	70%	100%
Initial Antibiotic Timing[1,2,3]	20	90%	90%	80%	93%
Oxygenation Assessment[2,3]	27	100%	100%	99%	100%
Pneumococcal Vaccine[1,2,3]	16	81%	74%	69%	94%
Smoking Cessation Advice[1,2,3]	7	100%	63%	80%	100%
Surgical Infection Prevention					
Prophylactic Antibiotic Given[5]	-	-	81%	77%	95%
Prophylactic Antibiotic Selection[5]	-	-	96%	90%	100%
Prophylactic Antibiotic Stopped[5]	-	-	79%	72%	95%
Pregnancy Care					
Inpatient Neonatal Mortality	-	-	-	-	-
Third or Fourth Degree Laceration	-	-	-	3.63%	3.27%

Mercy Hospital

1031 7th Street NE
Devils Lake, ND 58301
URL: www.MercyHospitalDL.com
Ownership: Voluntary non-profit - Church
Emergency Services: Yes

Phone: 701-662-2131
Fax: 701-662-9651
Accredited: Yes
Licensed Beds: 50

Key Personnel:

CEO. . . . . Marlene Krein
Senior VP. . . . . Jerry Lindell
Chief Medical Staff. . . . . Roberto Moraleda, MD
Emergency Room . . . . Anthony Rayer
Director Infection/Disease Control . . . . Maribeth Bradley
Director Radiology . . . . Roxanne Hawley
Director Respiratory Therapy . . . . Rick Morse

Measure	Cases	This Hospital	State Average	U.S. Average	Top Hospital
Heart Attack Care					
ACE Inhibitor or ARB for LVSD[1]	1	100%	83%	82%	100%
Aspirin at Arrival[1]	11	91%	92%	92%	100%
Aspirin at Discharge[1]	6	83%	91%	90%	100%
Beta Blocker at Arrival[1]	15	80%	84%	87%	100%
Beta Blocker at Discharge[1]	7	86%	95%	90%	100%
Fibrinolytic Medication Timing[1]	1	0%	28%	31%	100%
PCI Within 90 Minutes of Arrival	0	-	78%	54%	95%
Smoking Cessation Advice	0	-	74%	88%	100%
Heart Failure Care					
ACE Inhibitor or ARB for LVSD[1]	7	43%	72%	82%	100%
Discharge Instructions	26	77%	63%	61%	93%
Evaluation of LVS Function	36	67%	67%	83%	99%
Smoking Cessation Advice[1]	1	100%	67%	82%	100%
Pneumonia Care					
Appropriate Initial Antibiotic	65	77%	75%	83%	94%
Blood Culture Timing	36	100%	95%	90%	100%
Influenza Vaccine[1]	13	54%	77%	70%	100%
Initial Antibiotic Timing	57	81%	90%	80%	93%
Oxygenation Assessment	97	100%	100%	99%	100%
Pneumococcal Vaccine	58	48%	74%	69%	94%
Smoking Cessation Advice	27	52%	63%	80%	100%
Surgical Infection Prevention					
Prophylactic Antibiotic Given[1]	7	86%	81%	77%	95%
Prophylactic Antibiotic Selection[1]	2	100%	96%	90%	100%
Prophylactic Antibiotic Stopped[1]	7	57%	79%	72%	95%
Pregnancy Care					
Inpatient Neonatal Mortality	310	0.00%	-	-	-
Third or Fourth Degree Laceration	220	5.00%	-	3.63%	3.27%

Saint Joseph's Hospital & Health Center

30 7th Street W
Dickinson, ND 58601
Ownership: Voluntary non-profit - Church
Emergency Services: Yes

Phone: 701-456-4000
Fax: 701-456-4800
Accredited: Yes
Licensed Beds: 109

Key Personnel:

President/CEO. . . . . Allan Sonduck
Chief Medical Staff. . . . . Amy Okasa, MD
Emergency Room . . . . Becky Elkins
Infection Control. . . . . Tavia Voll
ICU . . . . Denette Lothspeich
Respiratory/Cardiopulmonary. . . . . Bev Berger

Measure	Cases	This Hospital	State Average	U.S. Average	Top Hospital
Heart Attack Care					
ACE Inhibitor or ARB for LVSD[1]	3	100%	83%	82%	100%
Aspirin at Arrival	32	88%	92%	92%	100%
Aspirin at Discharge[1]	21	95%	91%	90%	100%
Beta Blocker at Arrival[1]	22	100%	84%	87%	100%
Beta Blocker at Discharge	25	96%	95%	90%	100%
Fibrinolytic Medication Timing[1]	5	40%	28%	31%	100%
PCI Within 90 Minutes of Arrival	0	-	78%	54%	95%
Smoking Cessation Advice[1]	1	0%	74%	88%	100%
Heart Failure Care					
ACE Inhibitor or ARB for LVSD[1]	13	85%	72%	82%	100%
Discharge Instructions	53	70%	63%	61%	93%
Evaluation of LVS Function	85	75%	67%	83%	99%
Smoking Cessation Advice[1]	8	50%	67%	82%	100%
Pneumonia Care					
Appropriate Initial Antibiotic	30	80%	75%	83%	94%
Blood Culture Timing	38	92%	95%	90%	100%
Influenza Vaccine[1]	12	100%	77%	70%	100%
Initial Antibiotic Timing	53	92%	90%	80%	93%
Oxygenation Assessment	67	100%	100%	99%	100%
Pneumococcal Vaccine	48	85%	74%	69%	94%
Smoking Cessation Advice[1]	14	71%	63%	80%	100%
Surgical Infection Prevention					
Prophylactic Antibiotic Given	165	91%	81%	77%	95%
Prophylactic Antibiotic Selection	40	100%	96%	90%	100%
Prophylactic Antibiotic Stopped	167	81%	79%	72%	95%
Pregnancy Care					
Inpatient Neonatal Mortality	319	0.00%	-	-	-
Third or Fourth Degree Laceration	220	3.64%	-	3.63%	3.27%

Jacobson Memorial Hospital Care Center

601 E Street N
Elgin, ND 58533
Ownership: Voluntary non-profit - Other
Emergency Services: Yes

Phone: 701-584-2792
Fax: 701-584-3348
Accredited: No
Licensed Beds: 50

Key Personnel:

President/CEO. . . . . Douglas W Wamack
Chief Medical Staff. . . . . Dakshina Walgampaya, MD
Emergency Room . . . . Marcy Dawson, RN
Director Infection/Disease Control . . . . Nadia Tymkowych
Surgical Services . . . . Thomas Matheson, MD
Chief Radiology . . . . Tanya Elmer

Measure	Cases	This Hospital	State Average	U.S. Average	Top Hospital
Heart Attack Care					
ACE Inhibitor or ARB for LVSD[3]	0	-	83%	82%	100%
Aspirin at Arrival[1,3]	3	100%	92%	92%	100%
Aspirin at Discharge[1,3]	2	100%	91%	90%	100%
Beta Blocker at Arrival[1,3]	2	50%	84%	87%	100%
Beta Blocker at Discharge[1,3]	1	100%	95%	90%	100%
Fibrinolytic Medication Timing[1,3]	1	0%	28%	31%	100%
PCI Within 90 Minutes of Arrival[5]	-	-	78%	54%	95%
Smoking Cessation Advice[1,3]	1	100%	74%	88%	100%
Heart Failure Care					
ACE Inhibitor or ARB for LVSD[5]	-	-	72%	82%	100%
Discharge Instructions[5]	-	-	63%	61%	93%
Evaluation of LVS Function[5]	-	-	67%	83%	99%
Smoking Cessation Advice[5]	-	-	67%	82%	100%
Pneumonia Care					

NOTE: Hospital profiles are in alphabetical order by state, then city, then hospital within the city; Rankings are sorted by rate in descending order and exclude hospitals with less than 25 cases; (1) The number of cases is too small (n<25) for purposes of reliably predicting hospital performance; (2) Measure reflects the hospital's indication that its submission was based upon a sample of its relevant discharges; (3) Rate reflects fewer than the maximum possible quarters of data for the measure; (4) Inaccurate information submitted and suppressed for one or more quarters; (5) No data is available from the hospital for this measure; Please refer to the User's Guide for a full explanation of data

Appropriate Initial Antibiotic[1]	5	100%	75%	83%	94%
Blood Culture Timing[1]	6	100%	95%	90%	100%
Influenza Vaccine[1]	5	80%	77%	70%	100%
Initial Antibiotic Timing[1]	11	100%	90%	80%	93%
Oxygenation Assessment[1]	12	100%	100%	99%	100%
Pneumococcal Vaccine[1]	12	92%	74%	69%	94%
Smoking Cessation Advice[1]	1	0%	63%	80%	100%
Surgical Infection Prevention					
Prophylactic Antibiotic Given[5]	-	-	81%	77%	95%
Prophylactic Antibiotic Selection[5]	-	-	96%	90%	100%
Prophylactic Antibiotic Stopped[5]	-	-	79%	72%	95%
Pregnancy Care					
Inpatient Neonatal Mortality	-	-	-	-	-
Third or Fourth Degree Laceration	-	-	-	3.63%	3.27%

Innovis Health

3000 32nd Avenue South
Fargo, ND 58103
URL: www.innovishealth.com
Ownership: Voluntary non-profit - Private
Emergency Services: Yes

Phone: 701-364-8044
Fax: 701-364-8078
Accredited: No
Licensed Beds: 74

Key Personnel:
CEO. . . . . Paul Wilson
Chief Medical Staff. . . . . Michael Priggs
Director Respiratory Care. . . . . Kete Fteinke

Measure	Cases	This Hospital	State Average	U.S. Average	Top Hospital
Heart Attack Care					
ACE Inhibitor or ARB for LVSD	39	82%	83%	82%	100%
Aspirin at Arrival	81	93%	92%	92%	100%
Aspirin at Discharge	190	95%	91%	90%	100%
Beta Blocker at Arrival	66	89%	84%	87%	100%
Beta Blocker at Discharge	182	93%	95%	90%	100%
Fibrinolytic Medication Timing	0	-	28%	31%	100%
PCI Within 90 Minutes of Arrival[1]	5	60%	78%	54%	95%
Smoking Cessation Advice	68	93%	74%	88%	100%
Heart Failure Care					
ACE Inhibitor or ARB for LVSD	44	82%	72%	82%	100%
Discharge Instructions	107	63%	63%	61%	93%
Evaluation of LVS Function	133	90%	67%	83%	99%
Smoking Cessation Advice[1]	18	78%	67%	82%	100%
Pneumonia Care					
Appropriate Initial Antibiotic	56	96%	75%	83%	94%
Blood Culture Timing	51	90%	95%	90%	100%
Influenza Vaccine[1]	16	81%	77%	70%	100%
Initial Antibiotic Timing	66	86%	90%	80%	93%
Oxygenation Assessment	87	100%	100%	99%	100%
Pneumococcal Vaccine	64	80%	74%	69%	94%
Smoking Cessation Advice[1]	15	87%	63%	80%	100%
Surgical Infection Prevention					
Prophylactic Antibiotic Given[2,3]	167	90%	81%	77%	95%
Prophylactic Antibiotic Selection[2]	60	97%	96%	90%	100%
Prophylactic Antibiotic Stopped[2,3]	159	79%	79%	72%	95%
Pregnancy Care					
Inpatient Neonatal Mortality	-	-	-	-	-
Third or Fourth Degree Laceration	-	-	-	3.63%	3.27%

MeritCare Medical Center

Alternate Name: MeritCare Hospital
720 4th Street N
Fargo, ND 58122
E-mail: feedback@meritcare.com
URL: www.meritcare.com
Ownership: Voluntary non-profit - Private
Emergency Services: Yes

Phone: 701-234-2000
Fax: 701-234-6979
Accredited: Yes
Licensed Beds: 583

Key Personnel:
President/CEO. . . . . Roger Gilbertson, MD
Chief Medical Staff. . . . . Gregory Post, MD
Cardiac Lab . . . . Randy Werlinger
Catheterization Lab . . . . David Gausman
Emergency Room . . . . Mary Jagim
Emergency Room . . . . Greg Bjerke, MD
Infection Control. . . . . Joan Cook
ICU . . . . Cheryl Anderson
CCU Spvg. Nurse . . . . Kate Fragodt
Medical Surgical Nursing . . . . Barb LeDoux
OB/GYN/Women's Health . . . . Thomas Herzog, MD
Respiratory/Cardiopulmonary. . . . . Gary Lee

Measure	Cases	This Hospital	State Average	U.S. Average	Top Hospital
Heart Attack Care					
ACE Inhibitor or ARB for LVSD	103	97%	83%	82%	100%
Aspirin at Arrival	193	99%	92%	92%	100%
Aspirin at Discharge	506	99%	91%	90%	100%
Beta Blocker at Arrival	175	98%	84%	87%	100%
Beta Blocker at Discharge	499	100%	95%	90%	100%
Fibrinolytic Medication Timing	0	-	28%	31%	100%
PCI Within 90 Minutes of Arrival[1]	12	83%	78%	54%	95%
Smoking Cessation Advice	167	98%	74%	88%	100%
Heart Failure Care					
ACE Inhibitor or ARB for LVSD	118	73%	72%	82%	100%
Discharge Instructions	201	77%	63%	61%	93%
Evaluation of LVS Function	278	99%	67%	83%	99%
Smoking Cessation Advice	37	70%	67%	82%	100%
Pneumonia Care					
Appropriate Initial Antibiotic	139	89%	75%	83%	94%
Blood Culture Timing	129	93%	95%	90%	100%
Influenza Vaccine	52	77%	77%	70%	100%
Initial Antibiotic Timing	234	80%	90%	80%	93%
Oxygenation Assessment	276	100%	100%	99%	100%
Pneumococcal Vaccine	205	84%	74%	69%	94%
Smoking Cessation Advice	53	74%	63%	80%	100%
Surgical Infection Prevention					
Prophylactic Antibiotic Given	326	93%	81%	77%	95%
Prophylactic Antibiotic Selection	86	87%	96%	90%	100%
Prophylactic Antibiotic Stopped	313	88%	79%	72%	95%
Pregnancy Care					
Inpatient Neonatal Mortality	-	-	-	-	-
Third or Fourth Degree Laceration	-	-	-	3.63%	3.27%

PHS Indian Hospital at Fort Yates

PO Box J
Fort Yates, ND 58538
Ownership: Government - Federal
Emergency Services: Yes

Phone: 701-854-3831
Fax: 701-854-7399
Accredited: Yes
Licensed Beds: 12

Key Personnel:
CEO. . . . . Tim Yellow
Chief Medical Staff. . . . . Jackie Quisno, MD

Measure	Cases	This Hospital	State Average	U.S. Average	Top Hospital
Heart Attack Care					
ACE Inhibitor or ARB for LVSD[5]	-	-	83%	82%	100%
Aspirin at Arrival[5]	-	-	92%	92%	100%
Aspirin at Discharge[5]	-	-	91%	90%	100%
Beta Blocker at Arrival[5]	-	-	84%	87%	100%
Beta Blocker at Discharge[5]	-	-	95%	90%	100%
Fibrinolytic Medication Timing[5]	-	-	28%	31%	100%
PCI Within 90 Minutes of Arrival[5]	-	-	78%	54%	95%
Smoking Cessation Advice[5]	-	-	74%	88%	100%
Heart Failure Care					
ACE Inhibitor or ARB for LVSD[5]	-	-	72%	82%	100%
Discharge Instructions[5]	-	-	63%	61%	93%
Evaluation of LVS Function[5]	-	-	67%	83%	99%
Smoking Cessation Advice[5]	-	-	67%	82%	100%
Pneumonia Care					
Appropriate Initial Antibiotic[1,3]	1	0%	75%	83%	94%
Blood Culture Timing[3]	0	-	95%	90%	100%
Influenza Vaccine[5]	-	-	77%	70%	100%
Initial Antibiotic Timing[1,3]	1	100%	90%	80%	93%
Oxygenation Assessment[3]	0	-	100%	99%	100%
Pneumococcal Vaccine[3]	0	-	74%	69%	94%
Smoking Cessation Advice[3]	0	-	63%	80%	100%
Surgical Infection Prevention					
Prophylactic Antibiotic Given[5]	-	-	81%	77%	95%
Prophylactic Antibiotic Selection[5]	-	-	96%	90%	100%

NOTE: Hospital profiles are in alphabetical order by state, then city, then hospital within the city; Rankings are sorted by rate in descending order and exclude hospitals with less than 25 cases; (1) The number of cases is too small (n<25) for purposes of reliably predicting hospital performance; (2) Measure reflects the hospital's indication that its submission was based upon a sample of its relevant discharges; (3) Rate reflects fewer than the maximum possible quarters of data for the measure; (4) Inaccurate information submitted and suppressed for one or more quarters; (5) No data is available from the hospital for this measure; Please refer to the User's Guide for a full explanation of data

Prophylactic Antibiotic Stopped[5]	-	-	79%	72%	95%
Pregnancy Care					
Inpatient Neonatal Mortality	-	-	-	-	-
Third or Fourth Degree Laceration	-	-	-	3.63%	3.27%

Altru Hospital

1200 South Columbia Road
PO Box 6002
Grand Forks, ND 58206
E-mail: contactus@altru.org
URL: www.altru.org
Phone: 701-780-5000
Fax: 701-780-1093
Ownership: Voluntary non-profit - Other
Emergency Services: Yes
Accredited: Yes
Licensed Beds: 352

Key Personnel:
President . . . . Casey Ryan, MD
Chief Medical Staff . . . . Norman Byers, MD
Manager Emergency Room . . . . Tom Alinder
Manager Medical & Surgical Nursing . . . . Bill Woods
OB/GYN Womens Health. . . . . Renee Axtman
Manager Radiology . . . . Steve Metcaff
Manager Respiratory/Cardiopulmonary . . . . Erin Dionne

Measure	Cases	This Hospital	State Average	U.S. Average	Top Hospital
Heart Attack Care					
ACE Inhibitor or ARB for LVSD	39	95%	83%	82%	100%
Aspirin at Arrival	101	100%	92%	92%	100%
Aspirin at Discharge	215	100%	91%	90%	100%
Beta Blocker at Arrival	85	98%	84%	87%	100%
Beta Blocker at Discharge	202	99%	95%	90%	100%
Fibrinolytic Medication Timing	0	-	28%	31%	100%
PCI Within 90 Minutes of Arrival[1]	2	100%	78%	54%	95%
Smoking Cessation Advice	86	98%	74%	88%	100%
Heart Failure Care					
ACE Inhibitor or ARB for LVSD	53	91%	72%	82%	100%
Discharge Instructions	137	78%	63%	61%	93%
Evaluation of LVS Function	181	88%	67%	83%	99%
Smoking Cessation Advice[1]	23	96%	67%	82%	100%
Pneumonia Care					
Appropriate Initial Antibiotic	117	87%	75%	83%	94%
Blood Culture Timing	143	92%	95%	90%	100%
Influenza Vaccine	40	88%	77%	70%	100%
Initial Antibiotic Timing	193	79%	90%	80%	93%
Oxygenation Assessment	250	100%	100%	99%	100%
Pneumococcal Vaccine	181	92%	74%	69%	94%
Smoking Cessation Advice	63	94%	63%	80%	100%
Surgical Infection Prevention					
Prophylactic Antibiotic Given	312	89%	81%	77%	95%
Prophylactic Antibiotic Selection	81	95%	96%	90%	100%
Prophylactic Antibiotic Stopped	299	67%	79%	72%	95%
Pregnancy Care					
Inpatient Neonatal Mortality	-	-	-	-	-
Third or Fourth Degree Laceration	-	-	-	3.63%	3.27%

West River Regional Medical Center

1000 Highway 12
Hettinger, ND 58639
E-mail: jiml@wrhs.com
URL: www.wrhs.com
Phone: 701-567-4561
Fax: 701-567-6364
Ownership: Voluntary non-profit - Private
Emergency Services: Yes
Accredited: No
Licensed Beds: 46

Key Personnel:
Administrator/CEO . . . . James K Long

Measure	Cases	This Hospital	State Average	U.S. Average	Top Hospital
Heart Attack Care					
ACE Inhibitor or ARB for LVSD	0	-	83%	82%	100%
Aspirin at Arrival[1]	12	92%	92%	92%	100%
Aspirin at Discharge[1]	8	88%	91%	90%	100%
Beta Blocker at Arrival[1]	9	89%	84%	87%	100%
Beta Blocker at Discharge[1]	9	78%	95%	90%	100%
Fibrinolytic Medication Timing[1]	6	67%	28%	31%	100%
PCI Within 90 Minutes of Arrival	0	-	78%	54%	95%
Smoking Cessation Advice	0	-	74%	88%	100%
Heart Failure Care					
ACE Inhibitor or ARB for LVSD[1]	14	86%	72%	82%	100%
Discharge Instructions	46	67%	63%	61%	93%
Evaluation of LVS Function	69	78%	67%	83%	99%
Smoking Cessation Advice[1]	2	100%	67%	82%	100%
Pneumonia Care					
Appropriate Initial Antibiotic[1]	22	77%	75%	83%	94%
Blood Culture Timing[1]	10	100%	95%	90%	100%
Influenza Vaccine[1]	12	100%	77%	70%	100%
Initial Antibiotic Timing	64	98%	90%	80%	93%
Oxygenation Assessment	77	97%	100%	99%	100%
Pneumococcal Vaccine	73	85%	74%	69%	94%
Smoking Cessation Advice[1]	6	100%	63%	80%	100%
Surgical Infection Prevention					
Prophylactic Antibiotic Given[1]	11	82%	81%	77%	95%
Prophylactic Antibiotic Selection[1]	1	100%	96%	90%	100%
Prophylactic Antibiotic Stopped[1]	10	90%	79%	72%	95%
Pregnancy Care					
Inpatient Neonatal Mortality	-	-	-	-	-
Third or Fourth Degree Laceration	-	-	-	3.63%	3.27%

Hillsboro Medical Center

12 3rd Street SE
Hillsboro, ND 58045
E-mail: darleneswanson@meritcare.com
Phone: 701-636-450l
Fax: 701-636-3206
Ownership: Voluntary non-profit - Other
Emergency Services: Yes
Accredited: No
Licensed Beds: 20

Key Personnel:
Administrator . . . . Bruce Bowersox
Chief Medical Staff. . . . . Charles Breen
Director Infection/Disease Control . . . . Julieeen Rosenberg
Director Medical/Surgical Nursing . . . . Julie Rosenberg

Measure	Cases	This Hospital	State Average	U.S. Average	Top Hospital
Heart Attack Care					
ACE Inhibitor or ARB for LVSD[3]	0	-	83%	82%	100%
Aspirin at Arrival[3]	0	-	92%	92%	100%
Aspirin at Discharge[3]	0	-	91%	90%	100%
Beta Blocker at Arrival[3]	0	-	84%	87%	100%
Beta Blocker at Discharge[3]	0	-	95%	90%	100%
Fibrinolytic Medication Timing[3]	0	-	28%	31%	100%
PCI Within 90 Minutes of Arrival[5]	-	-	78%	54%	95%
Smoking Cessation Advice[3]	0	-	74%	88%	100%
Heart Failure Care					
ACE Inhibitor or ARB for LVSD	0	-	72%	82%	100%
Discharge Instructions	0	-	63%	61%	93%
Evaluation of LVS Function[1]	4	75%	67%	83%	99%
Smoking Cessation Advice	0	-	67%	82%	100%
Pneumonia Care					
Appropriate Initial Antibiotic[1]	16	81%	75%	83%	94%
Blood Culture Timing[1]	7	86%	95%	90%	100%
Influenza Vaccine[1]	3	100%	77%	70%	100%
Initial Antibiotic Timing	25	100%	90%	80%	93%
Oxygenation Assessment	31	100%	100%	99%	100%
Pneumococcal Vaccine	29	97%	74%	69%	94%
Smoking Cessation Advice[1]	4	75%	63%	80%	100%
Surgical Infection Prevention					
Prophylactic Antibiotic Given[5]	-	-	81%	77%	95%
Prophylactic Antibiotic Selection[5]	-	-	96%	90%	100%
Prophylactic Antibiotic Stopped[5]	-	-	79%	72%	95%
Pregnancy Care					
Inpatient Neonatal Mortality	-	-	-	-	-
Third or Fourth Degree Laceration	-	-	-	3.63%	3.27%

Jamestown Hospital

419 5th Street NE
Jamestown, ND 58401
URL: www.jamestownhospital.com
Phone: 701-252-1050
Fax: 701-952-3270
Ownership: Voluntary non-profit - Other
Emergency Services: Yes
Accredited: Yes
Licensed Beds: 56

Key Personnel:
President/CEO. . . . . Martin I Richman
Chief Medical Staff. . . . . David M Muhs, MD

NOTE: Hospital profiles are in alphabetical order by state, then city, then hospital within the city; Rankings are sorted by rate in descending order and exclude hospitals with less than 25 cases; (1) The number of cases is too small (n<25) for purposes of reliably predicting hospital performance; (2) Measure reflects the hospital's indication that its submission was based upon a sample of its relevant discharges; (3) Rate reflects fewer than the maximum possible quarters of data for the measure; (4) Inaccurate information submitted and suppressed for one or more quarters; (5) No data is available from the hospital for this measure; Please refer to the User's Guide for a full explanation of data

Emergency Room . . . . Donna Gullickson
Infection Control . . . . Laura Sanary
Manager Respiratory Therapy . . . . Vicki Brown

Measure	Cases	This Hospital	State Average	U.S. Average	Top Hospital
Heart Attack Care					
ACE Inhibitor or ARB for LVSD	0	-	83%	82%	100%
Aspirin at Arrival[1]	22	95%	92%	92%	100%
Aspirin at Discharge[1]	9	78%	91%	90%	100%
Beta Blocker at Arrival[1]	22	91%	84%	87%	100%
Beta Blocker at Discharge[1]	9	100%	95%	90%	100%
Fibrinolytic Medication Timing[1]	1	0%	28%	31%	100%
PCI Within 90 Minutes of Arrival	0	-	78%	54%	95%
Smoking Cessation Advice[1]	2	50%	74%	88%	100%
Heart Failure Care					
ACE Inhibitor or ARB for LVSD[1]	15	87%	72%	82%	100%
Discharge Instructions	40	80%	63%	61%	93%
Evaluation of LVS Function	57	70%	67%	83%	99%
Smoking Cessation Advice[1]	10	90%	67%	82%	100%
Pneumonia Care					
Appropriate Initial Antibiotic	54	98%	75%	83%	94%
Blood Culture Timing	63	97%	95%	90%	100%
Influenza Vaccine[1]	19	79%	77%	70%	100%
Initial Antibiotic Timing	91	91%	90%	80%	93%
Oxygenation Assessment	118	100%	100%	99%	100%
Pneumococcal Vaccine	84	75%	74%	69%	94%
Smoking Cessation Advice[1]	11	82%	63%	80%	100%
Surgical Infection Prevention					
Prophylactic Antibiotic Given[3]	63	90%	81%	77%	95%
Prophylactic Antibiotic Selection[1]	20	90%	96%	90%	100%
Prophylactic Antibiotic Stopped[3]	59	81%	79%	72%	95%
Pregnancy Care					
Inpatient Neonatal Mortality	-	-	-	-	-
Third or Fourth Degree Laceration	-	-	-	3.63%	3.27%

Linton Hospital

518 N Broadway
Linton, ND 58552
E-mail: linthosp@bentel.com
Ownership: Government - Local
Emergency Services: Yes
Phone: 701-254-4511
Fax: 701-254-4578
Accredited: No
Licensed Beds: 25

Key Personnel:
President/CEO . . . . Jay Jahnig
Chief Medical Staff . . . . Donald Grinz
Infection Control . . . . Melanie Jangula, RN

Measure	Cases	This Hospital	State Average	U.S. Average	Top Hospital
Heart Attack Care					
ACE Inhibitor or ARB for LVSD[1,3]	1	100%	83%	82%	100%
Aspirin at Arrival[1,3]	1	0%	92%	92%	100%
Aspirin at Discharge[1,3]	1	0%	91%	90%	100%
Beta Blocker at Arrival[1,3]	1	0%	84%	87%	100%
Beta Blocker at Discharge[1,3]	2	50%	95%	90%	100%
Fibrinolytic Medication Timing[3]	0	-	28%	31%	100%
PCI Within 90 Minutes of Arrival[5]	-	-	78%	54%	95%
Smoking Cessation Advice[3]	0	-	74%	88%	100%
Heart Failure Care					
ACE Inhibitor or ARB for LVSD[1]	1	0%	72%	82%	100%
Discharge Instructions[1]	11	45%	63%	61%	93%
Evaluation of LVS Function	32	16%	67%	83%	99%
Smoking Cessation Advice[1]	2	0%	67%	82%	100%
Pneumonia Care					
Appropriate Initial Antibiotic	31	19%	75%	83%	94%
Blood Culture Timing[1]	5	100%	95%	90%	100%
Influenza Vaccine[1]	8	88%	77%	70%	100%
Initial Antibiotic Timing	36	94%	90%	80%	93%
Oxygenation Assessment	43	100%	100%	99%	100%
Pneumococcal Vaccine	37	59%	74%	69%	94%
Smoking Cessation Advice[1]	1	0%	63%	80%	100%
Surgical Infection Prevention					
Prophylactic Antibiotic Given[5]	-	-	81%	77%	95%
Prophylactic Antibiotic Selection[5]	-	-	96%	90%	100%
Prophylactic Antibiotic Stopped[5]	-	-	79%	72%	95%
Pregnancy Care					
Inpatient Neonatal Mortality	-	-	-	-	-
Third or Fourth Degree Laceration	-	-	-	3.63%	3.27%

Union Hospital

42 6th Avenue SE
Mayville, ND 58257
Ownership: Voluntary non-profit - Private
Emergency Services: Yes
Phone: 701-786-3800
Fax: 701-788-2145
Accredited: No
Licensed Beds: 25

Key Personnel:
President/CEO . . . . Roger Baier
Chief Medical Staff . . . . Marsha Lange, MD
Director Medical/Surgical Nursing . . . . Doris Vigen, RN
Director Respiratory Therapy . . . . Cynthia Thompson

Measure	Cases	This Hospital	State Average	U.S. Average	Top Hospital
Heart Attack Care					
ACE Inhibitor or ARB for LVSD[1,3]	1	100%	83%	82%	100%
Aspirin at Arrival[1,3]	7	100%	92%	92%	100%
Aspirin at Discharge[1,3]	4	100%	91%	90%	100%
Beta Blocker at Arrival[1,3]	11	100%	84%	87%	100%
Beta Blocker at Discharge[1,3]	8	100%	95%	90%	100%
Fibrinolytic Medication Timing[3]	0	-	28%	31%	100%
PCI Within 90 Minutes of Arrival[5]	-	-	78%	54%	95%
Smoking Cessation Advice[3]	0	-	74%	88%	100%
Heart Failure Care					
ACE Inhibitor or ARB for LVSD[1]	4	75%	72%	82%	100%
Discharge Instructions[1]	6	67%	63%	61%	93%
Evaluation of LVS Function[1]	13	69%	67%	83%	99%
Smoking Cessation Advice	0	-	67%	82%	100%
Pneumonia Care					
Appropriate Initial Antibiotic[1]	11	82%	75%	83%	94%
Blood Culture Timing[1]	3	100%	95%	90%	100%
Influenza Vaccine[1]	3	100%	77%	70%	100%
Initial Antibiotic Timing[1]	19	84%	90%	80%	93%
Oxygenation Assessment[1]	22	100%	100%	99%	100%
Pneumococcal Vaccine[1]	20	70%	74%	69%	94%
Smoking Cessation Advice	0	-	63%	80%	100%
Surgical Infection Prevention					
Prophylactic Antibiotic Given[5]	-	-	81%	77%	95%
Prophylactic Antibiotic Selection[5]	-	-	96%	90%	100%
Prophylactic Antibiotic Stopped[5]	-	-	79%	72%	95%
Pregnancy Care					
Inpatient Neonatal Mortality	-	-	-	-	-
Third or Fourth Degree Laceration	-	-	-	3.63%	3.27%

Trinity Health

One West Burdick Expressway
PO Box 5020
Minot, ND 58702
E-mail: info@trinityhealth.org
URL: www.trinityhealth.org
Ownership: Voluntary non-profit - Other
Emergency Services: Yes
Toll-Free: 800-862-0005
Phone: 701-857-5000
Fax: 701-857-5408
Accredited: Yes
Licensed Beds: 441

Key Personnel:
Chief Medical Staff . . . . Sharleen Larson
Director Infection/Disease Control . . . . Brenda Lokken
Director Medical/Surgical Nursing . . . . Corrine Semmen
Director Respiratory Therapy . . . . Joan Groves

Measure	Cases	This Hospital	State Average	U.S. Average	Top Hospital
Heart Attack Care					
ACE Inhibitor or ARB for LVSD	27	100%	83%	82%	100%
Aspirin at Arrival	126	99%	92%	92%	100%
Aspirin at Discharge	178	99%	91%	90%	100%
Beta Blocker at Arrival	91	100%	84%	87%	100%
Beta Blocker at Discharge	204	99%	95%	90%	100%
Fibrinolytic Medication Timing[3]	0	-	28%	31%	100%
PCI Within 90 Minutes of Arrival[1]	8	100%	78%	54%	95%
Smoking Cessation Advice[1,3]	24	100%	74%	88%	100%
Heart Failure Care					

NOTE: Hospital profiles are in alphabetical order by state, then city, then hospital within the city; Rankings are sorted by rate in descending order and exclude hospitals with less than 25 cases; (1) The number of cases is too small (n<25) for purposes of reliably predicting hospital performance; (2) Measure reflects the hospital's indication that its submission was based upon a sample of its relevant discharges; (3) Rate reflects fewer than the maximum possible quarters of data for the measure; (4) Inaccurate information submitted and suppressed for one or more quarters; (5) No data is available from the hospital for this measure; Please refer to the User's Guide for a full explanation of data

ACE Inhibitor or ARB for LVSD	89	94%	72%	82%	100%
Discharge Instructions[3]	40	82%	63%	61%	93%
Evaluation of LVS Function	249	99%	67%	83%	99%
Smoking Cessation Advice[1,3]	6	100%	67%	82%	100%
Pneumonia Care					
Appropriate Initial Antibiotic[1,3]	19	95%	75%	83%	94%
Blood Culture Timing[1,3]	23	100%	95%	90%	100%
Influenza Vaccine[5]	-	-	77%	70%	100%
Initial Antibiotic Timing	192	89%	90%	80%	93%
Oxygenation Assessment	238	100%	100%	99%	100%
Pneumococcal Vaccine	172	92%	74%	69%	94%
Smoking Cessation Advice[1,3]	5	100%	63%	80%	100%
Surgical Infection Prevention					
Prophylactic Antibiotic Given[3]	134	87%	81%	77%	95%
Prophylactic Antibiotic Selection[5]	-	-	96%	90%	100%
Prophylactic Antibiotic Stopped[3]	133	85%	79%	72%	95%
Pregnancy Care					
Inpatient Neonatal Mortality	-	-	-	-	-
Third or Fourth Degree Laceration	-	-	-	3.63%	3.27%

Presentation Medical Center

213 2nd Avenue NE
Rolla, ND 58367
URL: www.pmc-rolla.com
Ownership: Voluntary non-profit - Church
Emergency Services: Yes

Phone: 701-477-3161
Fax: 701-477-5564
Accredited: No
Licensed Beds: 25

Key Personnel:
President/CEO . . . . Kimber L Wraalstad, CHE
Emergency Room . . . . Bonnie McDougall
Infection Control . . . . Bonnie McDougall, RN
CCU Supervisor . . . . Peggy McPougall
Medical/Surgical Nursing . . . . Peggy McDougall, RN
Respiratory/Cardiopulmonary . . . . Kathleen Longon, CRTT

Measure	Cases	This Hospital	State Average	U.S. Average	Top Hospital
Heart Attack Care					
ACE Inhibitor or ARB for LVSD[5]	-	-	83%	82%	100%
Aspirin at Arrival[5]	-	-	92%	92%	100%
Aspirin at Discharge[5]	-	-	91%	90%	100%
Beta Blocker at Arrival[5]	-	-	84%	87%	100%
Beta Blocker at Discharge[5]	-	-	95%	90%	100%
Fibrinolytic Medication Timing[5]	-	-	28%	31%	100%
PCI Within 90 Minutes of Arrival[5]	-	-	78%	54%	95%
Smoking Cessation Advice[5]	-	-	74%	88%	100%
Heart Failure Care					
ACE Inhibitor or ARB for LVSD	0	-	72%	82%	100%
Discharge Instructions[1]	5	20%	63%	61%	93%
Evaluation of LVS Function[1]	7	86%	67%	83%	99%
Smoking Cessation Advice[1]	1	100%	67%	82%	100%
Pneumonia Care					
Appropriate Initial Antibiotic[1]	7	100%	75%	83%	94%
Blood Culture Timing[1]	8	100%	95%	90%	100%
Influenza Vaccine[1]	3	100%	77%	70%	100%
Initial Antibiotic Timing[1]	18	94%	90%	80%	93%
Oxygenation Assessment[1]	20	100%	100%	99%	100%
Pneumococcal Vaccine[1]	18	100%	74%	69%	94%
Smoking Cessation Advice[1]	7	86%	63%	80%	100%
Surgical Infection Prevention					
Prophylactic Antibiotic Given[5]	-	-	81%	77%	95%
Prophylactic Antibiotic Selection[5]	-	-	96%	90%	100%
Prophylactic Antibiotic Stopped[5]	-	-	79%	72%	95%
Pregnancy Care					
Inpatient Neonatal Mortality	-	-	-	-	-
Third or Fourth Degree Laceration	-	-	-	3.63%	3.27%

Heart of America Medical Center

Alternate Name: Good Samaritan Hospital Association
800 S Main
Rugby, ND 58368
E-mail: admin@hamc.com
URL: www.hamc.com
Ownership: Voluntary non-profit - Other
Emergency Services: Yes

Phone: 701-776-5261
Fax: 701-776-5448
Accredited: No
Licensed Beds: 38

Key Personnel:
Administrator/CEO . . . . Jerry E Jurena
Chief Medical Staff . . . . Ron Skipper
Director Infection/Disease Control . . . . Mary Haugen
Director Medical/Surgical Nursing . . . . Julie Baustad
Director Respiratory Therapy . . . . Allan Meckle

Measure	Cases	This Hospital	State Average	U.S. Average	Top Hospital
Heart Attack Care					
ACE Inhibitor or ARB for LVSD	0	-	83%	82%	100%
Aspirin at Arrival[1]	6	83%	92%	92%	100%
Aspirin at Discharge[1]	5	80%	91%	90%	100%
Beta Blocker at Arrival[1]	6	100%	84%	87%	100%
Beta Blocker at Discharge[1]	5	100%	95%	90%	100%
Fibrinolytic Medication Timing	0	-	28%	31%	100%
PCI Within 90 Minutes of Arrival	0	-	78%	54%	95%
Smoking Cessation Advice	0	-	74%	88%	100%
Heart Failure Care					
ACE Inhibitor or ARB for LVSD	0	-	72%	82%	100%
Discharge Instructions[1]	12	75%	63%	61%	93%
Evaluation of LVS Function[1]	23	35%	67%	83%	99%
Smoking Cessation Advice	0	-	67%	82%	100%
Pneumonia Care					
Appropriate Initial Antibiotic[1]	23	87%	75%	83%	94%
Blood Culture Timing[1]	12	100%	95%	90%	100%
Influenza Vaccine[1]	9	89%	77%	70%	100%
Initial Antibiotic Timing	39	100%	90%	80%	93%
Oxygenation Assessment	49	100%	100%	99%	100%
Pneumococcal Vaccine	40	82%	74%	69%	94%
Smoking Cessation Advice[1]	3	100%	63%	80%	100%
Surgical Infection Prevention					
Prophylactic Antibiotic Given[3]	0	-	81%	77%	95%
Prophylactic Antibiotic Selection	0	-	96%	90%	100%
Prophylactic Antibiotic Stopped[3]	0	-	79%	72%	95%
Pregnancy Care					
Inpatient Neonatal Mortality	-	-	-	-	-
Third or Fourth Degree Laceration	-	-	-	3.63%	3.27%

Mountrail County Medical Center

Alternate Name: Stanley Community Hospital
502 3rd Street SE
Stanley, ND 58784
URL: www.stanleyhealth.org
Ownership: Voluntary non-profit - Private
Emergency Services: Yes

Phone: 701-628-2424
Fax: 701-628-3274
Accredited: No
Licensed Beds: 25

Key Personnel:
CEO . . . . Mitch Luepp
Cardiac Lab . . . . Judy Hove
Respiratory Care . . . . Mark Andrews

Measure	Cases	This Hospital	State Average	U.S. Average	Top Hospital
Heart Attack Care					
ACE Inhibitor or ARB for LVSD[5]	-	-	83%	82%	100%
Aspirin at Arrival[5]	-	-	92%	92%	100%
Aspirin at Discharge[5]	-	-	91%	90%	100%
Beta Blocker at Arrival[5]	-	-	84%	87%	100%
Beta Blocker at Discharge[5]	-	-	95%	90%	100%
Fibrinolytic Medication Timing[5]	-	-	28%	31%	100%
PCI Within 90 Minutes of Arrival[5]	-	-	78%	54%	95%
Smoking Cessation Advice[5]	-	-	74%	88%	100%
Heart Failure Care					
ACE Inhibitor or ARB for LVSD[5]	-	-	72%	82%	100%
Discharge Instructions[5]	-	-	63%	61%	93%
Evaluation of LVS Function[5]	-	-	67%	83%	99%
Smoking Cessation Advice[5]	-	-	67%	82%	100%
Pneumonia Care					
Appropriate Initial Antibiotic[1]	13	100%	75%	83%	94%

NOTE: Hospital profiles are in alphabetical order by state, then city, then hospital within the city; Rankings are sorted by rate in descending order and exclude hospitals with less than 25 cases; (1) The number of cases is too small (n<25) for purposes of reliably predicting hospital performance; (2) Measure reflects the hospital's indication that its submission was based upon a sample of its relevant discharges; (3) Rate reflects fewer than the maximum possible quarters of data for the measure; (4) Inaccurate information submitted and suppressed for one or more quarters; (5) No data is available from the hospital for this measure; Please refer to the User's Guide for a full explanation of data

Measure	Cases	This Hospital	State Average	U.S. Average	Top Hospital
Blood Culture Timing[1]	2	100%	95%	90%	100%
Influenza Vaccine[1]	2	100%	77%	70%	100%
Initial Antibiotic Timing[1]	18	94%	90%	80%	93%
Oxygenation Assessment[1]	20	100%	100%	99%	100%
Pneumococcal Vaccine[1]	18	72%	74%	69%	94%
Smoking Cessation Advice[1]	4	50%	63%	80%	100%
Surgical Infection Prevention					
Prophylactic Antibiotic Given[5]	-	-	81%	77%	95%
Prophylactic Antibiotic Selection[5]	-	-	96%	90%	100%
Prophylactic Antibiotic Stopped[5]	-	-	79%	72%	95%
Pregnancy Care					
Inpatient Neonatal Mortality	-	-	-	-	-
Third or Fourth Degree Laceration	-	-	-	3.63%	3.27%

Tioga Medical Center

PO Box 159
Tioga, ND 58852
Ownership: Voluntary non-profit - Other
Emergency Services: Yes

Phone: 701-664-3305
Fax: 701-664-3644
Accredited: No
Licensed Beds: 29

Key Personnel:

CEO. . . . . Randy Paderson
Chief Medical Staff. . . . . MV Patel, MD
Director Infection/Disease Control . . . . Shelley Eide, RN
Director Respiratory Therapy . . . . Curtis Hawkinson

Measure	Cases	This Hospital	State Average	U.S. Average	Top Hospital
Heart Attack Care					
ACE Inhibitor or ARB for LVSD[3]	0	-	83%	82%	100%
Aspirin at Arrival[1,3]	1	100%	92%	92%	100%
Aspirin at Discharge[1,3]	1	100%	91%	90%	100%
Beta Blocker at Arrival[1,3]	1	100%	84%	87%	100%
Beta Blocker at Discharge[1,3]	1	100%	95%	90%	100%
Fibrinolytic Medication Timing[3]	0	-	28%	31%	100%
PCI Within 90 Minutes of Arrival[5]	-	-	78%	54%	95%
Smoking Cessation Advice[3]	0	-	74%	88%	100%
Heart Failure Care					
ACE Inhibitor or ARB for LVSD[1]	1	100%	72%	82%	100%
Discharge Instructions[1]	2	50%	63%	61%	93%
Evaluation of LVS Function[1]	5	100%	67%	83%	99%
Smoking Cessation Advice	0	-	67%	82%	100%
Pneumonia Care					
Appropriate Initial Antibiotic[1]	12	58%	75%	83%	94%
Blood Culture Timing[1]	1	100%	95%	90%	100%
Influenza Vaccine[1]	4	75%	77%	70%	100%
Initial Antibiotic Timing[1]	13	92%	90%	80%	93%
Oxygenation Assessment[1]	17	100%	100%	99%	100%
Pneumococcal Vaccine[1]	12	75%	74%	69%	94%
Smoking Cessation Advice[1]	2	100%	63%	80%	100%
Surgical Infection Prevention					
Prophylactic Antibiotic Given[5]	-	-	81%	77%	95%
Prophylactic Antibiotic Selection[5]	-	-	96%	90%	100%
Prophylactic Antibiotic Stopped[5]	-	-	79%	72%	95%
Pregnancy Care					
Inpatient Neonatal Mortality	-	-	-	-	-
Third or Fourth Degree Laceration	-	-	-	3.63%	3.27%

McKenzie County Memorial Hospital

516 N Main Street
Watford City, ND 58854
Ownership: Voluntary non-profit - Other
Emergency Services: Yes

Phone: 701-842-3000
Fax: 701-842-6248
Accredited: No
Licensed Beds: 24

Key Personnel:

Administrator . . . . Colette Anderson
CEO. . . . . Kris Pacheo

Measure	Cases	This Hospital	State Average	U.S. Average	Top Hospital
Heart Attack Care					
ACE Inhibitor or ARB for LVSD[3]	0	-	83%	82%	100%
Aspirin at Arrival[1,3]	1	100%	92%	92%	100%
Aspirin at Discharge[1,3]	1	100%	91%	90%	100%
Beta Blocker at Arrival[1,3]	1	100%	84%	87%	100%
Beta Blocker at Discharge[1,3]	1	100%	95%	90%	100%
Fibrinolytic Medication Timing[3]	0	-	28%	31%	100%
PCI Within 90 Minutes of Arrival[5]	-	-	78%	54%	95%
Smoking Cessation Advice[3]	0	-	74%	88%	100%
Heart Failure Care					
ACE Inhibitor or ARB for LVSD[1,3]	1	100%	72%	82%	100%
Discharge Instructions[1,3]	7	0%	63%	61%	93%
Evaluation of LVS Function[1,3]	15	47%	67%	83%	99%
Smoking Cessation Advice[3]	0	-	67%	82%	100%
Pneumonia Care					
Appropriate Initial Antibiotic[1,3]	20	75%	75%	83%	94%
Blood Culture Timing[1]	2	50%	95%	90%	100%
Influenza Vaccine[1]	1	0%	77%	70%	100%
Initial Antibiotic Timing[1,3]	18	100%	90%	80%	93%
Oxygenation Assessment[1,3]	24	100%	100%	99%	100%
Pneumococcal Vaccine[1,3]	16	6%	74%	69%	94%
Smoking Cessation Advice[1,3]	3	33%	63%	80%	100%
Surgical Infection Prevention					
Prophylactic Antibiotic Given[5]	-	-	81%	77%	95%
Prophylactic Antibiotic Selection[5]	-	-	96%	90%	100%
Prophylactic Antibiotic Stopped[5]	-	-	79%	72%	95%
Pregnancy Care					
Inpatient Neonatal Mortality	-	-	-	-	-
Third or Fourth Degree Laceration	-	-	-	3.63%	3.27%

Mercy Medical Center

1301 15th Avenue West
Williston, ND 58801

Toll-Free: 800-544-3579
Phone: 701-774-7400
Fax: 701-774-7479

URL: www.mercy-williston.org
Ownership: Voluntary non-profit - Church
Emergency Services: Yes

Accredited: Yes
Licensed Beds: 87

Key Personnel:

President/CEO. . . . . Kim Miller
Chief Medical Staff. . . . . M A Olson, MD
Director Anesthesiology/Surgical Service. . . . . . Lynette Nygaard
Cardiac Rehabilitation . . . . Gloria Fenster
ER/Director Inpatient Clinical Practice . . . . Karen Bercier, RN
Infection Control. . . . . VeAnna Selid, RN
ICU . . . . Tami Peterson
Medical/Surgical Unit . . . . Tami Peterson
Obstetrical/Gynecological Unit . . . . Cami Knapkewicz
Respiratory Therapy. . . . . Lori Potts

Measure	Cases	This Hospital	State Average	U.S. Average	Top Hospital
Heart Attack Care					
ACE Inhibitor or ARB for LVSD[1]	1	0%	83%	82%	100%
Aspirin at Arrival[1]	7	100%	92%	92%	100%
Aspirin at Discharge[1]	5	100%	91%	90%	100%
Beta Blocker at Arrival[1]	6	83%	84%	87%	100%
Beta Blocker at Discharge[1]	5	100%	95%	90%	100%
Fibrinolytic Medication Timing	0	-	28%	31%	100%
PCI Within 90 Minutes of Arrival	0	-	78%	54%	95%
Smoking Cessation Advice[1]	1	0%	74%	88%	100%
Heart Failure Care					
ACE Inhibitor or ARB for LVSD[1]	7	71%	72%	82%	100%
Discharge Instructions	25	80%	63%	61%	93%
Evaluation of LVS Function	39	92%	67%	83%	99%
Smoking Cessation Advice[1]	3	0%	67%	82%	100%
Pneumonia Care					
Appropriate Initial Antibiotic	52	85%	75%	83%	94%
Blood Culture Timing	46	93%	95%	90%	100%
Influenza Vaccine[1]	16	88%	77%	70%	100%
Initial Antibiotic Timing	64	78%	90%	80%	93%
Oxygenation Assessment	85	100%	100%	99%	100%
Pneumococcal Vaccine	65	94%	74%	69%	94%
Smoking Cessation Advice[1]	16	69%	63%	80%	100%
Surgical Infection Prevention					
Prophylactic Antibiotic Given	172	91%	81%	77%	95%
Prophylactic Antibiotic Selection	36	94%	96%	90%	100%
Prophylactic Antibiotic Stopped	172	80%	79%	72%	95%
Pregnancy Care					
Inpatient Neonatal Mortality	364	0.00%	-	-	-
Third or Fourth Degree Laceration	284	2.46%	-	3.63%	3.27%

NOTE: Hospital profiles are in alphabetical order by state, then city, then hospital within the city; Rankings are sorted by rate in descending order and exclude hospitals with less than 25 cases; (1) The number of cases is too small (n<25) for purposes of reliably predicting hospital performance; (2) Measure reflects the hospital's indication that its submission was based upon a sample of its relevant discharges; (3) Rate reflects fewer than the maximum possible quarters of data for the measure; (4) Inaccurate information submitted and suppressed for one or more quarters; (5) No data is available from the hospital for this measure; Please refer to the User's Guide for a full explanation of data

Wishek Community Hospital

1007 4th Avenue S
PO Box 647
Wishek, ND 58495
E-mail: wchcbek@bektel.com
URL: www.wishekhospital.com
Toll-Free: 800-492-2364
Phone: 701-452-2326
Fax: 701-452-2392
Ownership: Voluntary non-profit - Other
Emergency Services: Yes
Accredited: No
Licensed Beds: 24

Key Personnel:
Chief Medical Staff. . . . . Alan R Lindemann, MD
Head of Radiology . . . . J Vilhauer

Measure	Cases	This Hospital	State Average	U.S. Average	Top Hospital
Heart Attack Care					
ACE Inhibitor or ARB for LVSD[1]	2	100%	83%	82%	100%
Aspirin at Arrival[1]	7	100%	92%	92%	100%
Aspirin at Discharge[1]	7	100%	91%	90%	100%
Beta Blocker at Arrival[1]	7	86%	84%	87%	100%
Beta Blocker at Discharge[1]	7	100%	95%	90%	100%
Fibrinolytic Medication Timing[1]	3	33%	28%	31%	100%
PCI Within 90 Minutes of Arrival	0	-	78%	54%	95%
Smoking Cessation Advice	0	-	74%	88%	100%
Heart Failure Care					
ACE Inhibitor or ARB for LVSD[1,3]	1	100%	72%	82%	100%
Discharge Instructions[1,3]	6	100%	63%	61%	93%
Evaluation of LVS Function[1,3]	8	12%	67%	83%	99%
Smoking Cessation Advice[3]	0	-	67%	82%	100%
Pneumonia Care					
Appropriate Initial Antibiotic[1,3]	13	46%	75%	83%	94%
Blood Culture Timing[1]	3	100%	95%	90%	100%
Influenza Vaccine[1]	9	78%	77%	70%	100%
Initial Antibiotic Timing	33	94%	90%	80%	93%
Oxygenation Assessment	40	100%	100%	99%	100%
Pneumococcal Vaccine	40	72%	74%	69%	94%
Smoking Cessation Advice[1,3]	2	0%	63%	80%	100%
Surgical Infection Prevention					
Prophylactic Antibiotic Given[5]	-	-	81%	77%	95%
Prophylactic Antibiotic Selection[5]	-	-	96%	90%	100%
Prophylactic Antibiotic Stopped[5]	-	-	79%	72%	95%
Pregnancy Care					
Inpatient Neonatal Mortality	-	-	-	-	-
Third or Fourth Degree Laceration	-	-	-	3.63%	3.27%

NOTE: Hospital profiles are in alphabetical order by state, then city, then hospital within the city; Rankings are sorted by rate in descending order and exclude hospitals with less than 25 cases; (1) The number of cases is too small (n<25) for purposes of reliably predicting hospital performance; (2) Measure reflects the hospital's indication that its submission was based upon a sample of its relevant discharges; (3) Rate reflects fewer than the maximum possible quarters of data for the measure; (4) Inaccurate information submitted and suppressed for one or more quarters; (5) No data is available from the hospital for this measure; Please refer to the User's Guide for a full explanation of data

Heart Attack Care

1. ACE Inhibitor or ARB for LVSD

Hospital Name	City	Rate	Cases
Integris Baptist Medical Center	Oklahoma City	100%	100
Oklahoma Heart Hospital	Oklahoma City	100%	55
Hillcrest Medical Center	Tulsa	97%	69
O U Medical Center	Oklahoma City	96%	26
Jane Phillips Medical Center	Bartlesville	95%	37
Norman Regional Hospital	Norman	94%	31
Saint Anthony Hospital	Oklahoma City	92%	37
Saint Francis Hospital	Tulsa	90%	115
Saint John Medical Center	Tulsa	90%	125
Midwest Regional Medical Center	Midwest City	89%	71
Comanche County Memorial Hospital	Lawton	88%	59
Deaconess Hospital	Oklahoma City	88%	40
Mercy Memorial Health Center	Ardmore	87%	30
Saint Francis Heart Hospital	Tulsa	86%	109
Oklahoma State University Medical Center	Tulsa	83%	75
Integris Southwest Medical Center	Oklahoma City	78%	65

2. Aspirin at Arrival

Hospital Name	City	Rate	Cases
O U Medical Center	Oklahoma City	100%	121
Oklahoma Heart Hospital	Oklahoma City	100%	65
Stillwater Medical Center	Stillwater	100%	40
Hillcrest Medical Center	Tulsa	99%	211
Integris Baptist Medical Center	Oklahoma City	99%	251
Integris Bass Baptist Health Center	Enid	99%	69
Integris Southwest Medical Center	Oklahoma City	99%	228
Jane Phillips Medical Center	Bartlesville	99%	135
Norman Regional Hospital	Norman	99%	165
Southcrest Hospital	Tulsa	99%	94
Medical Center of Southeastern Oklahoma	Durant	98%	54
Saint Anthony Hospital	Oklahoma City	98%	172
Comanche County Memorial Hospital	Lawton	97%	177
Edmond Medical Center	Edmond	97%	34
Saint Francis Hospital	Tulsa	97%	472
Saint John Medical Center	Tulsa	97%	415
Muskogee Regional Medical Center	Muskogee	96%	130
Duncan Regional Hospital	Duncan	95%	38
Integris Grove General Hospital	Grove	95%	37
Midwest Regional Medical Center	Midwest City	95%	301
Oklahoma State University Medical Center	Tulsa	94%	125
Unity Health Center	Shawnee	94%	67
Deaconess Hospital	Oklahoma City	93%	91
Mercy Memorial Health Center	Ardmore	93%	142
Saint Mary's Regional Medical Center	Enid	93%	71
Valley View Regional Hospital	Ada	92%	36
Saint Francis Heart Hospital	Tulsa	90%	136
Ponca City Medical Center	Ponca City	85%	47
McAlester Regional Health Center	McAlester	83%	42

3. Aspirin at Discharge

Hospital Name	City	Rate	Cases
Integris Baptist Medical Center	Oklahoma City	100%	525
Medical Center of Southeastern Oklahoma	Durant	100%	35
Southcrest Hospital	Tulsa	100%	118
O U Medical Center	Oklahoma City	99%	152
Oklahoma Heart Hospital	Oklahoma City	99%	302
Comanche County Memorial Hospital	Lawton	98%	301
Hillcrest Medical Center	Tulsa	98%	327
Jane Phillips Medical Center	Bartlesville	98%	161
Saint Anthony Hospital	Oklahoma City	98%	223
Saint Francis Heart Hospital	Tulsa	98%	507
Saint John Medical Center	Tulsa	98%	532
Saint Francis Hospital	Tulsa	97%	492
Norman Regional Hospital	Norman	96%	170
Deaconess Hospital	Oklahoma City	95%	92
Mercy Memorial Health Center	Ardmore	95%	131
Oklahoma State University Medical Center	Tulsa	94%	206
Integris Bass Baptist Health Center	Enid	92%	74
Integris Southwest Medical Center	Oklahoma City	91%	236
Muskogee Regional Medical Center	Muskogee	91%	57
Unity Health Center	Shawnee	90%	29
Midwest Regional Medical Center	Midwest City	89%	319
Saint Mary's Regional Medical Center	Enid	86%	72
Integris Grove General Hospital	Grove	84%	31

4. Beta Blocker at Arrival

Hospital Name	City	Rate	Cases
Southcrest Hospital	Tulsa	100%	83
O U Medical Center	Oklahoma City	99%	104
Saint John Medical Center	Tulsa	99%	350
Medical Center of Southeastern Oklahoma	Durant	98%	42
Muskogee Regional Medical Center	Muskogee	98%	107
Oklahoma Heart Hospital	Oklahoma City	98%	57
Duncan Regional Hospital	Duncan	97%	30
Hillcrest Medical Center	Tulsa	97%	187
Integris Southwest Medical Center	Oklahoma City	97%	181
Norman Regional Hospital	Norman	97%	122
Unity Health Center	Shawnee	97%	34
Comanche County Memorial Hospital	Lawton	96%	157
Integris Baptist Medical Center	Oklahoma City	96%	153
Jane Phillips Medical Center	Bartlesville	94%	125
Saint Anthony Hospital	Oklahoma City	94%	140
Integris Bass Baptist Health Center	Enid	93%	60
Integris Grove General Hospital	Grove	91%	32
Mercy Memorial Health Center	Ardmore	90%	90
Saint Francis Hospital	Tulsa	90%	316
Saint Francis Heart Hospital	Tulsa	86%	118
Valley View Regional Hospital	Ada	85%	26
Oklahoma State University Medical Center	Tulsa	84%	106
Edmond Medical Center	Edmond	83%	30
Deaconess Hospital	Oklahoma City	82%	44
Midwest Regional Medical Center	Midwest City	81%	258
Saint Mary's Regional Medical Center	Enid	77%	56
Jackson County Memorial Hospital	Altus	74%	27
Ponca City Medical Center	Ponca City	69%	42
McAlester Regional Health Center	McAlester	66%	38

5. Beta Blocker at Discharge

Hospital Name	City	Rate	Cases
Medical Center of Southeastern Oklahoma	Durant	100%	29
Oklahoma Heart Hospital	Oklahoma City	100%	296
Southcrest Hospital	Tulsa	100%	114
Integris Baptist Medical Center	Oklahoma City	99%	474
Norman Regional Hospital	Norman	99%	172
Saint John Medical Center	Tulsa	99%	520
Comanche County Memorial Hospital	Lawton	98%	291
Hillcrest Medical Center	Tulsa	98%	347
Saint Anthony Hospital	Oklahoma City	98%	205
Deaconess Hospital	Oklahoma City	97%	99
Jane Phillips Medical Center	Bartlesville	97%	148
O U Medical Center	Oklahoma City	97%	147
Saint Francis Heart Hospital	Tulsa	97%	510
Saint Francis Hospital	Tulsa	97%	479
Mercy Memorial Health Center	Ardmore	95%	131
Muskogee Regional Medical Center	Muskogee	95%	74
Integris Grove General Hospital	Grove	94%	31
Oklahoma State University Medical Center	Tulsa	93%	201
Integris Southwest Medical Center	Oklahoma City	92%	223
Unity Health Center	Shawnee	90%	29
Midwest Regional Medical Center	Midwest City	89%	285
Integris Bass Baptist Health Center	Enid	87%	71
Edmond Medical Center	Edmond	85%	26
Saint Mary's Regional Medical Center	Enid	84%	69

8. Smoking Cessation Advice

Hospital Name	City	Rate	Cases
Deaconess Hospital	Oklahoma City	100%	35
Integris Baptist Medical Center	Oklahoma City	100%	219
Integris Bass Baptist Health Center	Enid	100%	35
Norman Regional Hospital	Norman	100%	74
O U Medical Center	Oklahoma City	100%	68
Oklahoma Heart Hospital	Oklahoma City	100%	120
Saint Francis Hospital	Tulsa	100%	208
Saint John Medical Center	Tulsa	100%	214
Comanche County Memorial Hospital	Lawton	99%	130
Jane Phillips Medical Center	Bartlesville	98%	47
Mercy Memorial Health Center	Ardmore	98%	46
Integris Southwest Medical Center	Oklahoma City	97%	127
Saint Francis Heart Hospital	Tulsa	96%	277
Hillcrest Medical Center	Tulsa	94%	147
Oklahoma State University Medical Center	Tulsa	94%	98
Southcrest Hospital	Tulsa	94%	35
Midwest Regional Medical Center	Midwest City	92%	123
Saint Anthony Hospital	Oklahoma City	92%	92

Heart Failure Care

9. ACE Inhibitor or ARB for LVSD

Hospital Name	City	Rate	Cases
Duncan Regional Hospital	Duncan	100%	34
Medical Center of Southeastern Oklahoma	Durant	100%	76

NOTE: Hospital profiles are in alphabetical order by state, then city, then hospital within the city; Rankings are sorted by rate in descending order and exclude hospitals with less than 25 cases; (1) The number of cases is too small (n<25) for purposes of reliably predicting hospital performance; (2) Measure reflects the hospital's indication that its submission was based upon a sample of its relevant discharges; (3) Rate reflects fewer than the maximum possible quarters of data for the measure; (4) Inaccurate information submitted and suppressed for one or more quarters; (5) No data is available from the hospital for this measure; Please refer to the User's Guide for a full explanation of data

Hospital Name	City	Rate	Cases
Southcrest Hospital	Tulsa	100%	98
Integris Baptist Medical Center	Oklahoma City	99%	310
Oklahoma Heart Hospital	Oklahoma City	99%	192
Hillcrest Medical Center	Tulsa	98%	214
Mercy Health Center	Oklahoma City	97%	38
Integris Clinton Regional Hospital	Clinton	94%	50
Norman Regional Hospital	Norman	93%	87
Muskogee Regional Medical Center	Muskogee	92%	83
Comanche County Memorial Hospital	Lawton	91%	135
O U Medical Center	Oklahoma City	90%	208
Saint Francis Heart Hospital	Tulsa	90%	116
Jackson County Memorial Hospital	Altus	89%	65
Jane Phillips Medical Center	Bartlesville	89%	80
Great Plains Regional Medical Center	Elk City	88%	34
Memorial Hospital of Stillwell	Stillwell	88%	41
Saint Francis Hospital	Tulsa	88%	276
Tahlequah City Hospital	Tahlequah	88%	42
Integris Baptist Regional Health Center	Miami	87%	45
Saint John Medical Center	Tulsa	87%	336
Midwest Regional Medical Center	Midwest City	86%	201
Oklahoma State University Medical Center	Tulsa	86%	153
Deaconess Hospital	Oklahoma City	85%	61
Mercy Memorial Health Center	Ardmore	85%	82
Saint Anthony Hospital	Oklahoma City	85%	259
Integris Southwest Medical Center	Oklahoma City	84%	215
Southwestern Medical Center	Lawton	82%	34
Unity Health Center	Shawnee	82%	72
Edmond Medical Center	Edmond	81%	26
McAlester Regional Health Center	McAlester	79%	58
Valley View Regional Hospital	Ada	72%	39
Eastern Oklahoma Medical Center	Poteau	62%	45
Saint Mary's Regional Medical Center	Enid	62%	55

10. Discharge Instructions

Hospital Name	City	Rate	Cases
Medical Center of Southeastern Oklahoma	Durant	100%	190
Oklahoma Heart Hospital	Oklahoma City	100%	295
Woodward Hospital and Health Center	Woodward	100%	44
Integris Mayes County Medical Center	Pryor	97%	31
Duncan Regional Hospital	Duncan	95%	99
Saint Mary's Regional Medical Center	Enid	95%	149
Southcrest Hospital	Tulsa	95%	198
Integris Bass Baptist Health Center	Enid	94%	67
Integris Grove General Hospital	Grove	93%	70
O U Medical Center	Oklahoma City	93%	377
Ponca City Medical Center	Ponca City	92%	66
Pushmataha Hospital	Antlers	92%	40
Integris Clinton Regional Hospital	Clinton	91%	65
Norman Regional Hospital	Norman	91%	214
Grady Memorial Hospital	Chickasha	90%	71
Integris Canadian Valley Regional Hospital	Yukon	90%	70
Integris Baptist Medical Center	Oklahoma City	89%	494
Integris Baptist Regional Health Center	Miami	89%	129
Pauls Valley General Hospital	Pauls Valley	88%	49
Claremore Regional Hospital	Claremore	86%	43
Unity Health Center	Shawnee	86%	131
Muskogee Regional Medical Center	Muskogee	84%	194
Midwest Regional Medical Center	Midwest City	80%	400
Saint Francis Hospital	Broken Arrow	80%	35
Stillwater Medical Center	Stillwater	80%	66
Saint Francis Heart Hospital	Tulsa	79%	137
Integris Blackwell Regional Hospital	Blackwell	78%	51
PHS Indian Hospital	Claremore	74%	39
Saint John Medical Center	Tulsa	74%	627
Mercy Health Center	Oklahoma City	73%	89
Hillcrest Medical Center	Tulsa	72%	527
Integris Southwest Medical Center	Oklahoma City	71%	355
Memorial Hospital of Stillwell	Stillwell	71%	72
Mercy Memorial Health Center	Ardmore	70%	205
Jackson County Memorial Hospital	Altus	69%	98
Henryetta Medical Center	Henryetta	67%	30
Holdenville General Hospital	Holdenville	66%	29
Integris Marshall County Medical Center	Madill	65%	26
Craig General Hospital	Vinita	64%	44
Purcell Municipal Hospital	Purcell	63%	52
Comanche County Memorial Hospital	Lawton	62%	278
Saint Anthony Hospital	Oklahoma City	62%	441
Eastern Oklahoma Medical Center	Poteau	61%	171
Sequoyah Memorial Hospital	Sallisaw	61%	41
Valley View Regional Hospital	Ada	58%	120
Great Plains Regional Medical Center	Elk City	55%	58
Saint Francis Hospital	Tulsa	54%	542
Tahlequah City Hospital	Tahlequah	51%	68
Sayre Memorial Hospital	Sayre	50%	26
McCurtain Memorial Hospital	Idabel	48%	48
Saint John Sapulpa Hospital	Sapulpa	48%	46
Deaconess Hospital	Oklahoma City	45%	113
Edmond Medical Center	Edmond	45%	55
Choctaw Memorial Hospital	Hugo	40%	67
McAlester Regional Health Center	McAlester	38%	146
Haskell County Healthcare System	Stigler	37%	30
Jane Phillips Medical Center	Bartlesville	36%	159
Oklahoma State University Medical Center	Tulsa	28%	304
Southwestern Medical Center	Lawton	21%	86
Okmulgee Memorial Hospital	Okmulgee	18%	33
Cushing Regional Hospital	Cushing	11%	61
Moore Medical Center	Moore	11%	28
Kingfisher Regional	Kingfisher	0%	25
W W Hastings Indian Hospital	Tahlequah	0%	33

11. Evaluation of LVS Function

Hospital Name	City	Rate	Cases
Integris Baptist Medical Center	Oklahoma City	100%	575
Integris Baptist Regional Health Center	Miami	100%	150
Integris Clinton Regional Hospital	Clinton	100%	82
Medical Center of Southeastern Oklahoma	Durant	100%	287
Memorial Hospital	Frederick	100%	37
Norman Regional Hospital	Norman	100%	267
Oklahoma Heart Hospital	Oklahoma City	100%	312
Integris Blackwell Regional Hospital	Blackwell	99%	77
O U Medical Center	Oklahoma City	99%	405
Claremore Regional Hospital	Claremore	98%	66
Mercy Health Center	Oklahoma City	98%	128
Saint John Medical Center	Tulsa	98%	725
Duncan Regional Hospital	Duncan	97%	144
Southcrest Hospital	Tulsa	97%	227
Comanche County Memorial Hospital	Lawton	96%	304
Saint Anthony Hospital	Oklahoma City	96%	492
Saint Francis Hospital	Broken Arrow	96%	52
Saint Francis Hospital	Tulsa	95%	646
Woodward Hospital and Health Center	Woodward	95%	63
Great Plains Regional Medical Center	Elk City	94%	82
Hillcrest Medical Center	Tulsa	94%	608
Integris Mayes County Medical Center	Pryor	94%	52
Midwest Regional Medical Center	Midwest City	94%	464
Saint Francis Heart Hospital	Tulsa	94%	93
Muskogee Regional Medical Center	Muskogee	93%	256
Stillwater Medical Center	Stillwater	93%	84
Unity Health Center	Shawnee	93%	158
Integris Southwest Medical Center	Oklahoma City	92%	415
Memorial Hospital of Stillwell	Stillwell	92%	88
Mercy Memorial Health Center	Ardmore	92%	248
PHS Indian Hospital	Claremore	92%	40
Deaconess Hospital	Oklahoma City	91%	150
Integris Canadian Valley Regional Hospital	Yukon	91%	95
Integris Grove General Hospital	Grove	91%	103
Oklahoma State University Medical Center	Tulsa	91%	333
Moore Medical Center	Moore	90%	30
Share Medical Center	Alva	90%	30
Valley View Regional Hospital	Ada	90%	143
Integris Bass Baptist Health Center	Enid	89%	110
Jackson County Memorial Hospital	Altus	87%	132
Jane Phillips Medical Center	Bartlesville	87%	175
Tahlequah City Hospital	Tahlequah	87%	93
Craig General Hospital	Vinita	86%	51
Pushmataha Hospital	Antlers	86%	50
Sequoyah Memorial Hospital	Sallisaw	86%	44
Grady Memorial Hospital	Chickasha	84%	86
Integris Marshall County Medical Center	Madill	84%	38
Edmond Medical Center	Edmond	80%	71
Kingfisher Regional	Kingfisher	79%	33
Logan Medical Center	Guthrie	79%	39
W W Hastings Indian Hospital	Tahlequah	78%	32
McCurtain Memorial Hospital	Idabel	76%	54
Southwestern Medical Center	Lawton	76%	105
Henryetta Medical Center	Henryetta	73%	41
Mary Hurley Hospital	Coalgate	72%	32
Pauls Valley General Hospital	Pauls Valley	70%	67
Ponca City Medical Center	Ponca City	70%	81
Holdenville General Hospital	Holdenville	68%	40
McAlester Regional Health Center	McAlester	67%	202
Saint Mary's Regional Medical Center	Enid	67%	212
Perry Memorial Hospital	Perry	65%	31
Saint John Sapulpa Hospital	Sapulpa	62%	53
Purcell Municipal Hospital	Purcell	55%	64
Eastern Oklahoma Medical Center	Poteau	53%	196
Wagoner Hospital	Wagoner	52%	27
Cushing Regional Hospital	Cushing	43%	81

NOTE: Hospital profiles are in alphabetical order by state, then city, then hospital within the city; Rankings are sorted by rate in descending order and exclude hospitals with less than 25 cases; (1) The number of cases is too small (n<25) for purposes of reliably predicting hospital performance; (2) Measure reflects the hospital's indication that its submission was based upon a sample of its relevant discharges; (3) Rate reflects fewer than the maximum possible quarters of data for the measure; (4) Inaccurate information submitted and suppressed for one or more quarters; (5) No data is available from the hospital for this measure; Please refer to the User's Guide for a full explanation of data

Hospital Name	City	Rate	Cases
Haskell County Healthcare System	Stigler	40%	43
Okmulgee Memorial Hospital	Okmulgee	36%	47
Johnston Memorial Hospital	Tishomingo	35%	51
Pawnee Municipal Hospital	Pawnee	32%	25
Choctaw Memorial Hospital	Hugo	27%	95
Harmon Memorial Hospital	Hollis	22%	32
Sayre Memorial Hospital	Sayre	19%	27
Carnegie Tri-County Municipal Hospital	Carnegie	8%	36

12. Smoking Cessation Advice

Hospital Name	City	Rate	Cases
Comanche County Memorial Hospital	Lawton	100%	76
Integris Baptist Regional Health Center	Miami	100%	27
Integris Grove General Hospital	Grove	100%	26
Jackson County Memorial Hospital	Altus	100%	25
McAlester Regional Health Center	McAlester	100%	51
Medical Center of Southeastern Oklahoma	Durant	100%	62
Muskogee Regional Medical Center	Muskogee	100%	49
Oklahoma Heart Hospital	Oklahoma City	100%	65
Saint Anthony Hospital	Oklahoma City	100%	137
Unity Health Center	Shawnee	100%	27
Integris Baptist Medical Center	Oklahoma City	99%	111
Midwest Regional Medical Center	Midwest City	99%	97
Saint Francis Hospital	Tulsa	99%	149
Integris Southwest Medical Center	Oklahoma City	98%	120
Norman Regional Hospital	Norman	98%	51
Deaconess Hospital	Oklahoma City	97%	31
Saint John Medical Center	Tulsa	97%	156
Southcrest Hospital	Tulsa	97%	30
Saint Francis Heart Hospital	Tulsa	96%	25
Valley View Regional Hospital	Ada	96%	27
Eastern Oklahoma Medical Center	Poteau	95%	40
Mercy Memorial Health Center	Ardmore	95%	73
O U Medical Center	Oklahoma City	95%	155
Oklahoma State University Medical Center	Tulsa	94%	122
Jane Phillips Medical Center	Bartlesville	87%	30
Hillcrest Medical Center	Tulsa	86%	153

Pneumonia Care

13. Appropriate Initial Antibiotic

Hospital Name	City	Rate	Cases
Elkview General Hospital	Hobart	100%	32
Integris Clinton Regional Hospital	Clinton	99%	68
Norman Regional Hospital	Norman	99%	219
Okmulgee Memorial Hospital	Okmulgee	98%	41
Integris Marshall County Medical Center	Madill	97%	103
Integris Mayes County Medical Center	Pryor	97%	67
Saint Francis Hospital	Broken Arrow	97%	103
Bristow Medical Center	Bristow	95%	37
Pauls Valley General Hospital	Pauls Valley	95%	64
Sayre Memorial Hospital	Sayre	95%	83
Claremore Regional Hospital	Claremore	94%	87
Holdenville General Hospital	Holdenville	94%	35
Integris Southwest Medical Center	Oklahoma City	94%	249
Craig General Hospital	Vinita	92%	73
Deaconess Hospital	Oklahoma City	92%	119
Fairfax Memorial Hospital	Fairfax	92%	26
Oklahoma State University Medical Center	Tulsa	92%	151
Seminole Medical Center	Seminole	92%	40
Sequoyah Memorial Hospital	Sallisaw	92%	49
Duncan Regional Hospital	Duncan	91%	138
Integris Blackwell Regional Hospital	Blackwell	91%	90
Muskogee Regional Medical Center	Muskogee	91%	87
Perry Memorial Hospital	Perry	91%	35
Pushmataha Hospital	Antlers	91%	56
Saint Anthony Hospital	Oklahoma City	90%	182
Southcrest Hospital	Tulsa	90%	105
Stillwater Medical Center	Stillwater	90%	102
Henryetta Medical Center	Henryetta	89%	56
Integris Baptist Medical Center	Oklahoma City	89%	238
McCurtain Memorial Hospital	Idabel	89%	74
O U Medical Center	Oklahoma City	89%	128
Haskell County Healthcare System	Stigler	88%	57
Logan Medical Center	Guthrie	88%	40
Saint Francis Hospital	Tulsa	88%	637
Southwestern Medical Center	Lawton	88%	97
Grady Memorial Hospital	Chickasha	87%	117
PHS Indian Hospital	Claremore	87%	46
Saint John Medical Center	Tulsa	87%	351
W W Hastings Indian Hospital	Tahlequah	87%	75
Integris Baptist Regional Health Center	Miami	86%	174
Integris Canadian Valley Regional Hospital	Yukon	86%	180
Integris Grove General Hospital	Grove	86%	118
Mercy Health Center	Oklahoma City	86%	143
Saint Mary's Regional Medical Center	Enid	86%	92
Unity Health Center	Shawnee	86%	182
Ponca City Medical Center	Ponca City	85%	92
Saint John Sapulpa Hospital	Sapulpa	85%	65
Chickasaw Nation Health System	Ada	84%	64
Choctaw Memorial Hospital	Hugo	84%	64
Choctaw Nation Health Care Center	Talihina	84%	25
Comanche County Memorial Hospital	Lawton	84%	185
Hillcrest Medical Center	Tulsa	84%	241
Jackson County Memorial Hospital	Altus	84%	116
Valley View Regional Hospital	Ada	84%	114
Cleveland Area Hospital	Cleveland	83%	29
Integris Bass Baptist Health Center	Enid	83%	105
Woodward Hospital and Health Center	Woodward	83%	48
Kingfisher Regional	Kingfisher	81%	48
Lindsay Municipal Hospital	Lindsay	81%	27
Tahlequah City Hospital	Tahlequah	80%	54
Eastern Oklahoma Medical Center	Poteau	79%	107
Mercy Memorial Health Center	Ardmore	79%	228
Great Plains Regional Medical Center	Elk City	78%	68
Wagoner Hospital	Wagoner	78%	41
Memorial Hospital	Frederick	76%	25
Parkview Hospital	El Reno	76%	58
Cushing Regional Hospital	Cushing	75%	91
Purcell Municipal Hospital	Purcell	75%	81
Stroud Regional Medical Center	Stroud	74%	34
Edmond Medical Center	Edmond	73%	71
Jane Phillips Medical Center	Bartlesville	73%	257
Medical Center of Southeastern Oklahoma	Durant	72%	166
Midwest Regional Medical Center	Midwest City	71%	216
Moore Medical Center	Moore	71%	52
Atoka Memorial Hospital	Atoka	69%	26
McAlester Regional Health Center	McAlester	69%	108
Memorial Hospital of Texas County	Guymon	65%	88
Drumright Regional Hospital	Drumright	62%	55
Harmon Memorial Hospital	Hollis	60%	40
Johnston Memorial Hospital	Tishomingo	56%	36
Weatherford Regional Hospital	Weatherford	55%	66
Lawton Indian Hospital	Lawton	53%	32
Mary Hurley Hospital	Coalgate	52%	29

14. Blood Culture Timing

Hospital Name	City	Rate	Cases
Holdenville General Hospital	Holdenville	100%	42
Medical Center of Southeastern Oklahoma	Durant	100%	142
Pauls Valley General Hospital	Pauls Valley	100%	41
Integris Blackwell Regional Hospital	Blackwell	99%	71
Integris Clinton Regional Hospital	Clinton	99%	82
Norman Regional Hospital	Norman	99%	303
Mercy Memorial Health Center	Ardmore	98%	126
Stillwater Medical Center	Stillwater	98%	102
Unity Health Center	Shawnee	97%	203
Henryetta Medical Center	Henryetta	96%	71
Jackson County Memorial Hospital	Altus	96%	70
Logan Medical Center	Guthrie	96%	28
Saint Francis Hospital	Broken Arrow	96%	113
Saint Mary's Regional Medical Center	Enid	96%	74
Southcrest Hospital	Tulsa	96%	98
Chickasaw Nation Health System	Ada	95%	44
Duncan Regional Hospital	Duncan	95%	147
Integris Baptist Medical Center	Oklahoma City	95%	214
Integris Grove General Hospital	Grove	95%	117
Integris Mayes County Medical Center	Pryor	95%	56
Sequoyah Memorial Hospital	Sallisaw	95%	44
Woodward Hospital and Health Center	Woodward	95%	55
Deaconess Hospital	Oklahoma City	94%	154
Edmond Medical Center	Edmond	94%	64
Integris Marshall County Medical Center	Madill	94%	50
Grady Memorial Hospital	Chickasha	93%	60
Great Plains Regional Medical Center	Elk City	93%	68
Integris Canadian Valley Regional Hospital	Yukon	93%	104
Integris Southwest Medical Center	Oklahoma City	93%	267
Jane Phillips Medical Center	Bartlesville	93%	175
McAlester Regional Health Center	McAlester	93%	94
McCurtain Memorial Hospital	Idabel	93%	68
Mercy Health Center	Oklahoma City	93%	163
Okmulgee Memorial Hospital	Okmulgee	93%	27
Purcell Municipal Hospital	Purcell	93%	42
Saint Anthony Hospital	Oklahoma City	93%	195
Saint Francis Hospital	Tulsa	93%	661
Claremore Regional Hospital	Claremore	92%	90
Ponca City Medical Center	Ponca City	92%	60
Tahlequah City Hospital	Tahlequah	92%	50

NOTE: Hospital profiles are in alphabetical order by state, then city, then hospital within the city; Rankings are sorted by rate in descending order and exclude hospitals with less than 25 cases; (1) The number of cases is too small (n<25) for purposes of reliably predicting hospital performance; (2) Measure reflects the hospital's indication that its submission was based upon a sample of its relevant discharges; (3) Rate reflects fewer than the maximum possible quarters of data for the measure; (4) Inaccurate information submitted and suppressed for one or more quarters; (5) No data is available from the hospital for this measure; Please refer to the User's Guide for a full explanation of data

Hospital Name	City	Rate	Cases
Hillcrest Medical Center	Tulsa	91%	149
Moore Medical Center	Moore	91%	34
Saint John Medical Center	Tulsa	91%	255
Southwestern Medical Center	Lawton	91%	67
O U Medical Center	Oklahoma City	90%	156
Midwest Regional Medical Center	Midwest City	89%	178
Cushing Regional Hospital	Cushing	88%	60
Muskogee Regional Medical Center	Muskogee	88%	86
Saint John Sapulpa Hospital	Sapulpa	87%	55
W W Hastings Indian Hospital	Tahlequah	87%	52
Integris Bass Baptist Health Center	Enid	86%	95
Parkview Hospital	El Reno	85%	33
Comanche County Memorial Hospital	Lawton	84%	173
Integris Baptist Regional Health Center	Miami	82%	108
Oklahoma State University Medical Center	Tulsa	81%	131
Pushmataha Hospital	Antlers	81%	57
Valley View Regional Hospital	Ada	81%	116
Choctaw Memorial Hospital	Hugo	79%	38
Eastern Oklahoma Medical Center	Poteau	77%	48
PHS Indian Hospital	Claremore	68%	38

15. Influenza Vaccine

Hospital Name	City	Rate	Cases
Integris Blackwell Regional Hospital	Blackwell	100%	33
Medical Center of Southeastern Oklahoma	Durant	100%	66
Norman Regional Hospital	Norman	100%	98
Saint Francis Hospital	Broken Arrow	100%	29
Unity Health Center	Shawnee	98%	54
Craig General Hospital	Vinita	96%	25
Integris Baptist Regional Health Center	Miami	96%	50
Saint John Medical Center	Tulsa	96%	92
Woodward Hospital and Health Center	Woodward	96%	28
Mercy Health Center	Oklahoma City	95%	73
Memorial Hospital of Texas County	Guymon	93%	28
Saint Anthony Hospital	Oklahoma City	93%	57
Integris Bass Baptist Health Center	Enid	92%	37
Claremore Regional Hospital	Claremore	91%	34
Comanche County Memorial Hospital	Lawton	91%	46
Integris Marshall County Medical Center	Madill	90%	31
Deaconess Hospital	Oklahoma City	88%	69
Edmond Medical Center	Edmond	88%	25
Duncan Regional Hospital	Duncan	87%	53
Southcrest Hospital	Tulsa	87%	31
Integris Clinton Regional Hospital	Clinton	86%	35
Stillwater Medical Center	Stillwater	84%	38
Integris Grove General Hospital	Grove	83%	52
Saint Francis Hospital	Tulsa	83%	197
Saint Mary's Regional Medical Center	Enid	83%	48
Muskogee Regional Medical Center	Muskogee	80%	25
Integris Baptist Medical Center	Oklahoma City	79%	80
Valley View Regional Hospital	Ada	78%	37
Henryetta Medical Center	Henryetta	77%	31
Sayre Memorial Hospital	Sayre	76%	37
Purcell Municipal Hospital	Purcell	73%	37
Midwest Regional Medical Center	Midwest City	72%	58
Southwestern Medical Center	Lawton	69%	39
Integris Southwest Medical Center	Oklahoma City	68%	76
Jane Phillips Medical Center	Bartlesville	67%	61
O U Medical Center	Oklahoma City	64%	33
McCurtain Memorial Hospital	Idabel	52%	31
Cushing Regional Hospital	Cushing	49%	35
Mercy Memorial Health Center	Ardmore	46%	67
Oklahoma State University Medical Center	Tulsa	46%	52
Hillcrest Medical Center	Tulsa	41%	37
Eastern Oklahoma Medical Center	Poteau	31%	26

16. Initial Antibiotic Timing

Hospital Name	City	Rate	Cases
Craig General Hospital	Vinita	98%	82
Henryetta Medical Center	Henryetta	98%	80
Share Medical Center	Alva	98%	48
Medical Center of Southeastern Oklahoma	Durant	97%	219
Fairfax Memorial Hospital	Fairfax	96%	28
Norman Regional Hospital	Norman	96%	367
Perry Memorial Hospital	Perry	96%	55
Holdenville General Hospital	Holdenville	95%	65
McAlester Regional Health Center	McAlester	94%	145
Pushmataha Hospital	Antlers	94%	63
Saint Francis Hospital	Broken Arrow	94%	129
Sayre Memorial Hospital	Sayre	94%	120
Stillwater Medical Center	Stillwater	94%	142
Integris Mayes County Medical Center	Pryor	93%	75
Integris Southwest Medical Center	Oklahoma City	93%	352
Jackson County Memorial Hospital	Altus	93%	147
Logan Medical Center	Guthrie	93%	45
Moore Medical Center	Moore	93%	43
Bristow Medical Center	Bristow	92%	40
Cushing Regional Hospital	Cushing	92%	113
Integris Bass Baptist Health Center	Enid	92%	119
Elkview General Hospital	Hobart	91%	35
Integris Blackwell Regional Hospital	Blackwell	91%	141
Integris Grove General Hospital	Grove	91%	183
Unity Health Center	Shawnee	91%	253
Woodward Hospital and Health Center	Woodward	91%	101
Integris Canadian Valley Regional Hospital	Yukon	90%	163
Integris Clinton Regional Hospital	Clinton	90%	132
Jane Phillips Medical Center	Bartlesville	90%	250
Claremore Regional Hospital	Claremore	89%	124
Pauls Valley General Hospital	Pauls Valley	89%	76
Seminole Medical Center	Seminole	89%	44
Integris Baptist Regional Health Center	Miami	88%	252
Parkview Hospital	El Reno	88%	76
Duncan Regional Hospital	Duncan	87%	196
Saint Anthony Hospital	Oklahoma City	87%	258
Integris Marshall County Medical Center	Madill	86%	141
Johnston Memorial Hospital	Tishomingo	86%	51
Southcrest Hospital	Tulsa	86%	139
Southwestern Medical Center	Lawton	86%	135
Tahlequah City Hospital	Tahlequah	86%	88
Saint Mary's Regional Medical Center	Enid	85%	162
Grady Memorial Hospital	Chickasha	84%	115
Haskell County Healthcare System	Stigler	84%	64
McCurtain Memorial Hospital	Idabel	84%	99
Memorial Hospital	Frederick	84%	31
Okmulgee Memorial Hospital	Okmulgee	84%	50
Arbuckle Memorial Hospital	Sulphur	83%	29
PHS Indian Hospital	Claremore	83%	52
Memorial Hospital of Stillwell	Stillwell	82%	45
Mercy Health Center	Oklahoma City	82%	251
Choctaw Nation Health Care Center	Talihina	81%	27
Drumright Regional Hospital	Drumright	81%	67
Hillcrest Medical Center	Tulsa	81%	243
Ponca City Medical Center	Ponca City	81%	99
Saint John Sapulpa Hospital	Sapulpa	81%	83
Harmon Memorial Hospital	Hollis	80%	85
Valley View Regional Hospital	Ada	80%	147
Choctaw Memorial Hospital	Hugo	79%	87
Purcell Municipal Hospital	Purcell	79%	143
Great Plains Regional Medical Center	Elk City	78%	115
Oklahoma State University Medical Center	Tulsa	78%	225
Stroud Regional Medical Center	Stroud	78%	36
Deaconess Hospital	Oklahoma City	77%	189
Saint John Medical Center	Tulsa	77%	425
Sequoyah Memorial Hospital	Sallisaw	77%	66
Comanche County Memorial Hospital	Lawton	76%	257
Eastern Oklahoma Medical Center	Poteau	76%	144
Edmond Medical Center	Edmond	76%	97
Mercy Memorial Health Center	Ardmore	76%	322
Midwest Regional Medical Center	Midwest City	74%	309
Muskogee Regional Medical Center	Muskogee	74%	143
Chickasaw Nation Health System	Ada	73%	70
Saint Francis Hospital	Tulsa	73%	754
Healdton Municipal Hospital	Healdton	71%	28
Wagoner Hospital	Wagoner	69%	36
Integris Baptist Medical Center	Oklahoma City	68%	372
Weatherford Regional Hospital	Weatherford	67%	63
Cleveland Area Hospital	Cleveland	66%	29
O U Medical Center	Oklahoma City	65%	209
Memorial Hospital of Texas County	Guymon	64%	59
W W Hastings Indian Hospital	Tahlequah	61%	80
Mary Hurley Hospital	Coalgate	60%	52
Lawton Indian Hospital	Lawton	54%	37

17. Oxygenation Assessment

Hospital Name	City	Rate	Cases
Arbuckle Memorial Hospital	Sulphur	100%	40
Bristow Medical Center	Bristow	100%	47
Chickasaw Nation Health System	Ada	100%	91
Choctaw Memorial Hospital	Hugo	100%	97
Choctaw Nation Health Care Center	Talihina	100%	29
Claremore Regional Hospital	Claremore	100%	149
Cleveland Area Hospital	Cleveland	100%	34
Comanche County Memorial Hospital	Lawton	100%	317
Craig General Hospital	Vinita	100%	96
Cushing Regional Hospital	Cushing	100%	151
Deaconess Hospital	Oklahoma City	100%	211
Drumright Regional Hospital	Drumright	100%	76
Duncan Regional Hospital	Duncan	100%	249

NOTE: Hospital profiles are in alphabetical order by state, then city, then hospital within the city; Rankings are sorted by rate in descending order and exclude hospitals with less than 25 cases; (1) The number of cases is too small (n<25) for purposes of reliably predicting hospital performance; (2) Measure reflects the hospital's indication that its submission was based upon a sample of its relevant discharges; (3) Rate reflects fewer than the maximum possible quarters of data for the measure; (4) Inaccurate information submitted and suppressed for one or more quarters; (5) No data is available from the hospital for this measure; Please refer to the User's Guide for a full explanation of data

Elkview General Hospital	Hobart	100%	43
Fairfax Memorial Hospital	Fairfax	100%	34
Fairview Hospital	Fairview	100%	33
Harmon Memorial Hospital	Hollis	100%	97
Healdton Municipal Hospital	Healdton	100%	31
Holdenville General Hospital	Holdenville	100%	74
Integris Baptist Medical Center	Oklahoma City	100%	418
Integris Baptist Regional Health Center	Miami	100%	283
Integris Bass Baptist Health Center	Enid	100%	159
Integris Blackwell Regional Hospital	Blackwell	100%	155
Integris Canadian Valley Regional Hospital	Yukon	100%	190
Integris Clinton Regional Hospital	Clinton	100%	148
Integris Grove General Hospital	Grove	100%	195
Integris Marshall County Medical Center	Madill	100%	156
Integris Mayes County Medical Center	Pryor	100%	86
Integris Southwest Medical Center	Oklahoma City	100%	414
Jane Phillips Medical Center	Bartlesville	100%	309
Johnston Memorial Hospital	Tishomingo	100%	61
Kingfisher Regional	Kingfisher	100%	51
Lindsay Municipal Hospital	Lindsay	100%	32
Logan Medical Center	Guthrie	100%	57
Mary Hurley Hospital	Coalgate	100%	56
McAlester Regional Health Center	McAlester	100%	176
McCurtain Memorial Hospital	Idabel	100%	125
Medical Center of Southeastern Oklahoma	Durant	100%	299
Memorial Hospital	Frederick	100%	46
Memorial Hospital of Stillwell	Stillwell	100%	50
Mercy Health Center	Oklahoma City	100%	343
Mercy Memorial Health Center	Ardmore	100%	355
Newman Memorial Hospital	Shattuck	100%	28
Norman Regional Hospital	Norman	100%	476
O U Medical Center	Oklahoma City	100%	249
Oklahoma Heart Hospital	Oklahoma City	100%	27
Okmulgee Memorial Hospital	Okmulgee	100%	62
PHS Indian Hospital	Claremore	100%	57
Pauls Valley General Hospital	Pauls Valley	100%	91
Pawnee Municipal Hospital	Pawnee	100%	26
Perry Memorial Hospital	Perry	100%	64
Purcell Municipal Hospital	Purcell	100%	159
Pushmataha Hospital	Antlers	100%	78
Saint Anthony Hospital	Oklahoma City	100%	286
Saint Francis Hospital	Broken Arrow	100%	165
Saint Francis Hospital	Tulsa	100%	1004
Saint John Medical Center	Tulsa	100%	593
Saint Mary's Regional Medical Center	Enid	100%	193
Sayre Memorial Hospital	Sayre	100%	132
Sequoyah Memorial Hospital	Sallisaw	100%	83
Share Medical Center	Alva	100%	56
Southwestern Medical Center	Lawton	100%	175
Stillwater Medical Center	Stillwater	100%	161
Stroud Regional Medical Center	Stroud	100%	50
Unity Health Center	Shawnee	100%	286
W W Hastings Indian Hospital	Tahlequah	100%	92
Weatherford Regional Hospital	Weatherford	100%	78
Woodward Hospital and Health Center	Woodward	100%	127
Grady Memorial Hospital	Chickasha	99%	156
Great Plains Regional Medical Center	Elk City	99%	133
Henryetta Medical Center	Henryetta	99%	105
Hillcrest Medical Center	Tulsa	99%	312
Midwest Regional Medical Center	Midwest City	99%	358
Muskogee Regional Medical Center	Muskogee	99%	159
Parkview Hospital	El Reno	99%	95
Southcrest Hospital	Tulsa	99%	158
Edmond Medical Center	Edmond	98%	112
Jackson County Memorial Hospital	Altus	98%	178
Lawton Indian Hospital	Lawton	98%	40
Memorial Hospital of Texas County	Guymon	98%	101
Moore Medical Center	Moore	98%	59
Oklahoma State University Medical Center	Tulsa	98%	274
Ponca City Medical Center	Ponca City	98%	118
Saint John Sapulpa Hospital	Sapulpa	98%	94
Seminole Medical Center	Seminole	98%	49
Eastern Oklahoma Medical Center	Poteau	97%	153
Tahlequah City Hospital	Tahlequah	97%	117
Atoka Memorial Hospital	Atoka	96%	28
Valley View Regional Hospital	Ada	96%	180
Wagoner Hospital	Wagoner	96%	49
Haskell County Healthcare System	Stigler	95%	86

18. Pneumococcal Vaccine

Hospital Name	City	Rate	Cases
Medical Center of Southeastern Oklahoma	Durant	100%	153
Norman Regional Hospital	Norman	100%	259
Saint Francis Hospital	Broken Arrow	100%	107
Integris Clinton Regional Hospital	Clinton	99%	86
Integris Blackwell Regional Hospital	Blackwell	98%	91
Integris Mayes County Medical Center	Pryor	98%	43
Pauls Valley General Hospital	Pauls Valley	97%	61
Unity Health Center	Shawnee	97%	175
Duncan Regional Hospital	Duncan	96%	167
Integris Baptist Regional Health Center	Miami	96%	157
Mercy Health Center	Oklahoma City	96%	235
Craig General Hospital	Vinita	95%	64
Southcrest Hospital	Tulsa	95%	104
Bristow Medical Center	Bristow	94%	33
Integris Grove General Hospital	Grove	94%	137
Parkview Hospital	El Reno	94%	51
Grady Memorial Hospital	Chickasha	92%	89
Integris Marshall County Medical Center	Madill	92%	84
Share Medical Center	Alva	92%	38
Claremore Regional Hospital	Claremore	91%	89
Deaconess Hospital	Oklahoma City	89%	133
Jackson County Memorial Hospital	Altus	89%	111
Saint John Medical Center	Tulsa	89%	350
Sequoyah Memorial Hospital	Sallisaw	89%	44
Comanche County Memorial Hospital	Lawton	88%	184
Integris Bass Baptist Health Center	Enid	88%	98
Edmond Medical Center	Edmond	87%	67
Holdenville General Hospital	Holdenville	87%	52
Memorial Hospital	Frederick	87%	31
Perry Memorial Hospital	Perry	86%	42
Arbuckle Memorial Hospital	Sulphur	85%	27
Chickasaw Nation Health System	Ada	85%	39
McAlester Regional Health Center	McAlester	85%	119
Mercy Memorial Health Center	Ardmore	85%	220
Saint Francis Hospital	Tulsa	85%	612
Saint Mary's Regional Medical Center	Enid	85%	140
Memorial Hospital of Texas County	Guymon	84%	58
Saint Anthony Hospital	Oklahoma City	84%	155
Memorial Hospital of Stillwell	Stillwell	83%	30
Pushmataha Hospital	Antlers	83%	46
Stillwater Medical Center	Stillwater	83%	102
Integris Southwest Medical Center	Oklahoma City	82%	244
Woodward Hospital and Health Center	Woodward	81%	78
Valley View Regional Hospital	Ada	80%	102
Choctaw Memorial Hospital	Hugo	79%	48
Jane Phillips Medical Center	Bartlesville	79%	203
Logan Medical Center	Guthrie	79%	38
Ponca City Medical Center	Ponca City	79%	71
Weatherford Regional Hospital	Weatherford	79%	48
O U Medical Center	Oklahoma City	77%	73
Henryetta Medical Center	Henryetta	76%	70
Muskogee Regional Medical Center	Muskogee	76%	90
Integris Baptist Medical Center	Oklahoma City	75%	260
Great Plains Regional Medical Center	Elk City	74%	91
Wagoner Hospital	Wagoner	74%	27
Midwest Regional Medical Center	Midwest City	71%	200
Southwestern Medical Center	Lawton	69%	111
Integris Canadian Valley Regional Hospital	Yukon	68%	114
Okmulgee Memorial Hospital	Okmulgee	63%	46
McCurtain Memorial Hospital	Idabel	62%	69
W W Hastings Indian Hospital	Tahlequah	61%	31
Haskell County Healthcare System	Stigler	59%	64
Mary Hurley Hospital	Coalgate	56%	39
Tahlequah City Hospital	Tahlequah	53%	72
Oklahoma State University Medical Center	Tulsa	52%	96
Purcell Municipal Hospital	Purcell	52%	104
Saint John Sapulpa Hospital	Sapulpa	52%	46
Cushing Regional Hospital	Cushing	51%	92
Hillcrest Medical Center	Tulsa	50%	135
Sayre Memorial Hospital	Sayre	41%	58
Seminole Medical Center	Seminole	40%	25
Kingfisher Regional	Kingfisher	31%	36
Harmon Memorial Hospital	Hollis	30%	61
Johnston Memorial Hospital	Tishomingo	29%	38
Eastern Oklahoma Medical Center	Poteau	21%	92
Stroud Regional Medical Center	Stroud	19%	27
Drumright Regional Hospital	Drumright	5%	37
Fairview Hospital	Fairview	4%	25

19. Smoking Cessation Advice

Hospital Name	City	Rate	Cases
Claremore Regional Hospital	Claremore	100%	37
Integris Canadian Valley Regional Hospital	Yukon	100%	50
Integris Clinton Regional Hospital	Clinton	100%	36
Integris Grove General Hospital	Grove	100%	44
Integris Marshall County Medical Center	Madill	100%	39
Integris Mayes County Medical Center	Pryor	100%	28

NOTE: Hospital profiles are in alphabetical order by state, then city, then hospital within the city; Rankings are sorted by rate in descending order and exclude hospitals with less than 25 cases; (1) The number of cases is too small (n<25) for purposes of reliably predicting hospital performance; (2) Measure reflects the hospital's indication that its submission was based upon a sample of its relevant discharges; (3) Rate reflects fewer than the maximum possible quarters of data for the measure; (4) Inaccurate information submitted and suppressed for one or more quarters; (5) No data is available from the hospital for this measure; Please refer to the User's Guide for a full explanation of data

Valley View Regional Hospital	Ada	100%	35
Medical Center of Southeastern Oklahoma	Durant	99%	84
Deaconess Hospital	Oklahoma City	98%	50
Integris Bass Baptist Health Center	Enid	98%	44
Saint Francis Hospital	Tulsa	98%	264
Southcrest Hospital	Tulsa	98%	41
Unity Health Center	Shawnee	98%	81
Comanche County Memorial Hospital	Lawton	97%	72
Integris Baptist Regional Health Center	Miami	97%	64
Norman Regional Hospital	Norman	97%	179
Stillwater Medical Center	Stillwater	97%	32
Integris Blackwell Regional Hospital	Blackwell	96%	53
Saint John Medical Center	Tulsa	96%	148
Integris Southwest Medical Center	Oklahoma City	95%	153
Duncan Regional Hospital	Duncan	94%	51
Muskogee Regional Medical Center	Muskogee	94%	52
Saint Francis Hospital	Broken Arrow	94%	32
Southwestern Medical Center	Lawton	94%	36
Mercy Memorial Health Center	Ardmore	93%	84
Midwest Regional Medical Center	Midwest City	92%	96
Oklahoma State University Medical Center	Tulsa	92%	128
Saint Anthony Hospital	Oklahoma City	92%	98
Eastern Oklahoma Medical Center	Poteau	91%	64
Mercy Health Center	Oklahoma City	91%	79
Hillcrest Medical Center	Tulsa	89%	114
O U Medical Center	Oklahoma City	89%	97
Grady Memorial Hospital	Chickasha	87%	30
McAlester Regional Health Center	McAlester	87%	45
Jane Phillips Medical Center	Bartlesville	84%	74
Ponca City Medical Center	Ponca City	84%	31
Saint Mary's Regional Medical Center	Enid	84%	32
Chickasaw Nation Health System	Ada	83%	30
Jackson County Memorial Hospital	Altus	83%	52
McCurtain Memorial Hospital	Idabel	83%	30
Moore Medical Center	Moore	80%	25
Great Plains Regional Medical Center	Elk City	79%	33
Sequoyah Memorial Hospital	Sallisaw	76%	25
Cushing Regional Hospital	Cushing	70%	47
Integris Baptist Medical Center	Oklahoma City	69%	95
Purcell Municipal Hospital	Purcell	62%	32
Saint John Sapulpa Hospital	Sapulpa	62%	26
W W Hastings Indian Hospital	Tahlequah	58%	36
Sayre Memorial Hospital	Sayre	36%	36
Memorial Hospital of Texas County	Guymon	27%	26

Surgical Infection Prevention

20. Prophylactic Antibiotic Given

Hospital Name	City	Rate	Cases
Bone and Joint Hospital	Oklahoma City	100%	333
Oklahoma Heart Hospital	Oklahoma City	98%	184
Chickasaw Nation Health System	Ada	97%	33
Integris Grove General Hospital	Grove	97%	173
Mcbride Clinic Orthopedic Hospital	Oklahoma City	97%	138
McAlester Regional Health Center	McAlester	96%	193
Northwest Surgical Hospital	Oklahoma City	96%	228
PHS Indian Hospital	Claremore	96%	111
Saint Francis Hospital	Broken Arrow	96%	187
Integris Mayes County Medical Center	Pryor	95%	37
Saint Anthony Hospital	Oklahoma City	95%	564
Unity Health Center	Shawnee	95%	128
Grady Memorial Hospital	Chickasha	94%	68
Mercy Health Center	Oklahoma City	94%	175
Integris Canadian Valley Regional Hospital	Yukon	93%	104
Saint Francis Hospital	Tulsa	93%	1687
Community Hospital	Oklahoma City	92%	50
Duncan Regional Hospital	Duncan	92%	158
Integris Baptist Medical Center	Oklahoma City	92%	791
Jackson County Memorial Hospital	Altus	92%	119
Norman Regional Hospital	Norman	92%	677
Claremore Regional Hospital	Claremore	91%	202
Integris Bass Baptist Health Center	Enid	91%	288
Integris Southwest Medical Center	Oklahoma City	91%	497
Medical Center of Southeastern Oklahoma	Durant	91%	147
Hillcrest Medical Center	Tulsa	90%	198
Saint Mary's Regional Medical Center	Enid	90%	379
Midwest Regional Medical Center	Midwest City	89%	650
Integris Baptist Regional Health Center	Miami	88%	145
Mercy Memorial Health Center	Ardmore	88%	561
Southcrest Hospital	Tulsa	88%	378
Muskogee Regional Medical Center	Muskogee	87%	218
Valley View Regional Hospital	Ada	87%	203
Saint Francis Heart Hospital	Tulsa	86%	311
Deaconess Hospital	Oklahoma City	85%	406
Saint John Medical Center	Tulsa	85%	2555
Jane Phillips Medical Center	Bartlesville	84%	367
O U Medical Center	Oklahoma City	84%	772
Oklahoma State University Medical Center	Tulsa	83%	282
Surgical Hospital of Oklahoma	Oklahoma City	81%	114
Edmond Medical Center	Edmond	77%	115
Moore Medical Center	Moore	77%	60
Okla Ctr for Ortho & Multi-Spec Surg	Oklahoma City	77%	48
Cushing Regional Hospital	Cushing	76%	58
Stillwater Medical Center	Stillwater	75%	232
Woodward Hospital and Health Center	Woodward	71%	58
Comanche County Memorial Hospital	Lawton	65%	201
Orthopedic Hospital of Oklahoma	Tulsa	65%	139
Great Plains Regional Medical Center	Elk City	55%	85
Lawton Indian Hospital	Lawton	51%	39
Ponca City Medical Center	Ponca City	51%	86
Southwestern Medical Center	Lawton	50%	38
Southwestern Regional Medical Center	Tulsa	19%	26
Tahlequah City Hospital	Tahlequah	7%	113

21. Prophylactic Antibiotic Selection

Hospital Name	City	Rate	Cases
Bone and Joint Hospital	Oklahoma City	100%	40
Chickasaw Nation Health System	Ada	100%	33
Integris Grove General Hospital	Grove	100%	44
Mcbride Clinic Orthopedic Hospital	Oklahoma City	100%	46
Medical Center of Southeastern Oklahoma	Durant	100%	27
Oklahoma Heart Hospital	Oklahoma City	100%	44
Surgical Hospital of Oklahoma	Oklahoma City	100%	46
Unity Health Center	Shawnee	100%	49
Saint Anthony Hospital	Oklahoma City	99%	133
Integris Baptist Medical Center	Oklahoma City	98%	202
Integris Southwest Medical Center	Oklahoma City	98%	144
Jackson County Memorial Hospital	Altus	98%	53
Mercy Health Center	Oklahoma City	98%	49
Midwest Regional Medical Center	Midwest City	98%	119
Saint Francis Heart Hospital	Tulsa	98%	98
Saint Francis Hospital	Broken Arrow	98%	47
Valley View Regional Hospital	Ada	98%	91
Integris Baptist Regional Health Center	Miami	97%	39
Integris Bass Baptist Health Center	Enid	97%	73
Integris Canadian Valley Regional Hospital	Yukon	97%	30
Saint John Medical Center	Tulsa	97%	628
Cushing Regional Hospital	Cushing	96%	27
Muskogee Regional Medical Center	Muskogee	96%	69
Northwest Surgical Hospital	Oklahoma City	96%	54
Oklahoma State University Medical Center	Tulsa	96%	51
O U Medical Center	Oklahoma City	95%	175
Jane Phillips Medical Center	Bartlesville	94%	117
Southcrest Hospital	Tulsa	94%	108
Hillcrest Medical Center	Tulsa	93%	68
McAlester Regional Health Center	McAlester	93%	59
Norman Regional Hospital	Norman	93%	214
Claremore Regional Hospital	Claremore	92%	52
Deaconess Hospital	Oklahoma City	92%	132
Duncan Regional Hospital	Duncan	92%	49
Mercy Memorial Health Center	Ardmore	92%	125
Saint Mary's Regional Medical Center	Enid	92%	105
Comanche County Memorial Hospital	Lawton	91%	64
PHS Indian Hospital	Claremore	89%	37
Grady Memorial Hospital	Chickasha	88%	25
Ponca City Medical Center	Ponca City	88%	26
Saint Francis Hospital	Tulsa	88%	571
Southwestern Medical Center	Lawton	88%	33
Edmond Medical Center	Edmond	86%	49
Tahlequah City Hospital	Tahlequah	83%	46
Great Plains Regional Medical Center	Elk City	81%	26
Stillwater Medical Center	Stillwater	78%	83

22. Prophylactic Antibiotic Stopped

Hospital Name	City	Rate	Cases
Lawton Indian Hospital	Lawton	100%	36
Moore Medical Center	Moore	100%	51
Integris Grove General Hospital	Grove	99%	169
Bone and Joint Hospital	Oklahoma City	98%	327
Surgical Hospital of Oklahoma	Oklahoma City	98%	112
Woodward Hospital and Health Center	Woodward	98%	54
Chickasaw Nation Health System	Ada	97%	33
Cushing Regional Hospital	Cushing	97%	58
Mcbride Clinic Orthopedic Hospital	Oklahoma City	97%	136
Oklahoma Heart Hospital	Oklahoma City	97%	177
PHS Indian Hospital	Claremore	97%	107
Saint Francis Hospital	Broken Arrow	96%	185
Integris Baptist Medical Center	Oklahoma City	93%	766

NOTE: Hospital profiles are in alphabetical order by state, then city, then hospital within the city; Rankings are sorted by rate in descending order and exclude hospitals with less than 25 cases; (1) The number of cases is too small (n<25) for purposes of reliably predicting hospital performance; (2) Measure reflects the hospital's indication that its submission was based upon a sample of its relevant discharges; (3) Rate reflects fewer than the maximum possible quarters of data for the measure; (4) Inaccurate information submitted and suppressed for one or more quarters; (5) No data is available from the hospital for this measure; Please refer to the User's Guide for a full explanation of data

Integris Bass Baptist Health Center	Enid	92%	283
Integris Mayes County Medical Center	Pryor	92%	36
Deaconess Hospital	Oklahoma City	89%	372
O U Medical Center	Oklahoma City	88%	702
Saint Anthony Hospital	Oklahoma City	88%	507
Saint Francis Heart Hospital	Tulsa	86%	297
Saint Mary's Regional Medical Center	Enid	86%	360
Grady Memorial Hospital	Chickasha	85%	62
Saint John Medical Center	Tulsa	85%	2480
Southcrest Hospital	Tulsa	84%	353
Integris Baptist Regional Health Center	Miami	83%	140
Stillwater Medical Center	Stillwater	83%	244
Medical Center of Southeastern Oklahoma	Durant	81%	143
Northwest Surgical Hospital	Oklahoma City	81%	226
Edmond Medical Center	Edmond	80%	105
Claremore Regional Hospital	Claremore	79%	198
Integris Canadian Valley Regional Hospital	Yukon	79%	104
McAlester Regional Health Center	McAlester	79%	189
Mercy Health Center	Oklahoma City	78%	167
Mercy Memorial Health Center	Ardmore	78%	544
Saint Francis Hospital	Tulsa	76%	1634
Unity Health Center	Shawnee	76%	124
Integris Southwest Medical Center	Oklahoma City	73%	462
Orthopedic Hospital of Oklahoma	Tulsa	71%	139
Southwestern Medical Center	Lawton	71%	35
Midwest Regional Medical Center	Midwest City	70%	624
Muskogee Regional Medical Center	Muskogee	70%	203
Valley View Regional Hospital	Ada	70%	208
Comanche County Memorial Hospital	Lawton	69%	192
Jackson County Memorial Hospital	Altus	68%	113
Norman Regional Hospital	Norman	68%	650
Community Hospital	Oklahoma City	64%	50
Hillcrest Medical Center	Tulsa	64%	192
Oklahoma State University Medical Center	Tulsa	62%	266
Ponca City Medical Center	Ponca City	60%	84
Duncan Regional Hospital	Duncan	53%	152
Jane Phillips Medical Center	Bartlesville	50%	343
Great Plains Regional Medical Center	Elk City	35%	78
Tahlequah City Hospital	Tahlequah	29%	102
Okla Ctr for Ortho & Multi-Spec Surg	Oklahoma City	25%	36

Pregnancy Care

23. Inpatient Neonatal Mortality

Hospital Name	City	Rate	Cases
Lakeside Women's Hospital	Oklahoma City	0.00%	1145
Saint Anthony Hospital	Oklahoma City	0.10%	960
Southwestern Medical Center	Lawton	0.30%	339
O U Medical Center	Oklahoma City	1.94%	5100

24. Third or Fourth Degree Laceration

Hospital Name	City	Rate	Cases
O U Medical Center	Oklahoma City	2.78%	3131
Saint Anthony Hospital	Oklahoma City	3.72%	646
Lakeside Women's Hospital	Oklahoma City	5.09%	746
Southwestern Medical Center	Lawton	5.98%	184

NOTE: Hospital profiles are in alphabetical order by state, then city, then hospital within the city; Rankings are sorted by rate in descending order and exclude hospitals with less than 25 cases; (1) The number of cases is too small (n<25) for purposes of reliably predicting hospital performance; (2) Measure reflects the hospital's indication that its submission was based upon a sample of its relevant discharges; (3) Rate reflects fewer than the maximum possible quarters of data for the measure; (4) Inaccurate information submitted and suppressed for one or more quarters; (5) No data is available from the hospital for this measure; Please refer to the User's Guide for a full explanation of data

Chickasaw Nation Health System

Alternate Name: Carl Albert Indian Hospital
1001 N Country Club Road
Ada, OK 74820

Toll-Free: 800-851-9136
Phone: 580-436-3980
Fax: 580-436-7297

Ownership: Government - Local
Emergency Services: Yes

Accredited: Yes
Licensed Beds: 53

Key Personnel:
CEO. . . . . Bill Lance
Chief Medical Staff. . . . . Tini Cooper, MD

Measure	Cases	This Hospital	State Average	U.S. Average	Top Hospital
Heart Attack Care					
ACE Inhibitor or ARB for LVSD[1,3]	2	100%	79%	82%	100%
Aspirin at Arrival[1,3]	6	67%	86%	92%	100%
Aspirin at Discharge[1,3]	2	100%	85%	90%	100%
Beta Blocker at Arrival[1,3]	6	67%	78%	87%	100%
Beta Blocker at Discharge[1,3]	2	50%	78%	90%	100%
Fibrinolytic Medication Timing[3]	0	-	36%	31%	100%
PCI Within 90 Minutes of Arrival[5]	-	-	51%	54%	95%
Smoking Cessation Advice[3]	0	-	83%	88%	100%
Heart Failure Care					
ACE Inhibitor or ARB for LVSD[1]	7	71%	76%	82%	100%
Discharge Instructions[1]	17	47%	55%	61%	93%
Evaluation of LVS Function[1]	18	94%	71%	83%	99%
Smoking Cessation Advice[1]	4	50%	73%	82%	100%
Pneumonia Care					
Appropriate Initial Antibiotic	64	84%	81%	83%	94%
Blood Culture Timing	44	95%	91%	90%	100%
Influenza Vaccine[1]	23	70%	72%	70%	100%
Initial Antibiotic Timing	70	73%	82%	80%	93%
Oxygenation Assessment	91	100%	99%	99%	100%
Pneumococcal Vaccine	39	85%	68%	69%	94%
Smoking Cessation Advice	30	83%	72%	80%	100%
Surgical Infection Prevention					
Prophylactic Antibiotic Given[3]	33	97%	75%	77%	95%
Prophylactic Antibiotic Selection	33	100%	88%	90%	100%
Prophylactic Antibiotic Stopped[3]	33	97%	82%	72%	95%
Pregnancy Care					
Inpatient Neonatal Mortality	-	-	-	-	-
Third or Fourth Degree Laceration	-	-	-	3.63%	3.27%

Valley View Regional Hospital

430 N Monta Vista
Ada, OK 74820
URL: www.valleyviewregional.org
Ownership: Voluntary non-profit - Private
Emergency Services: Yes

Phone: 580-332-2323
Fax: 580-421-1386

Accredited: Yes
Licensed Beds: 180

Key Personnel:
President/CEO. . . . . Ronald Webb

Measure	Cases	This Hospital	State Average	U.S. Average	Top Hospital
Heart Attack Care					
ACE Inhibitor or ARB for LVSD[1]	2	100%	79%	82%	100%
Aspirin at Arrival	36	92%	86%	92%	100%
Aspirin at Discharge[1]	10	100%	85%	90%	100%
Beta Blocker at Arrival	26	85%	78%	87%	100%
Beta Blocker at Discharge[1]	11	82%	78%	90%	100%
Fibrinolytic Medication Timing[1]	6	17%	36%	31%	100%
PCI Within 90 Minutes of Arrival	0	-	51%	54%	95%
Smoking Cessation Advice[1]	6	83%	83%	88%	100%
Heart Failure Care					
ACE Inhibitor or ARB for LVSD	39	72%	76%	82%	100%
Discharge Instructions	120	58%	55%	61%	93%
Evaluation of LVS Function	143	90%	71%	83%	99%
Smoking Cessation Advice	27	96%	73%	82%	100%
Pneumonia Care					
Appropriate Initial Antibiotic	114	84%	81%	83%	94%
Blood Culture Timing	116	81%	91%	90%	100%
Influenza Vaccine	37	78%	72%	70%	100%
Initial Antibiotic Timing	147	80%	82%	80%	93%
Oxygenation Assessment	180	96%	99%	99%	100%
Pneumococcal Vaccine	102	80%	68%	69%	94%
Smoking Cessation Advice	35	100%	72%	80%	100%
Surgical Infection Prevention					
Prophylactic Antibiotic Given[3]	203	87%	75%	77%	95%
Prophylactic Antibiotic Selection	91	98%	88%	90%	100%
Prophylactic Antibiotic Stopped[3]	208	70%	82%	72%	95%
Pregnancy Care					
Inpatient Neonatal Mortality	-	-	-	-	-
Third or Fourth Degree Laceration	-	-	-	3.63%	3.27%

Jackson County Memorial Hospital

1200 East Pecan
Altus, OK 73521
URL: www.jcmh.com
Ownership: Govt - Hospital District or Authority
Emergency Services: Yes

Phone: 580-482-4781
Fax: 580-481-2345

Accredited: Yes
Licensed Beds: 156

Key Personnel:
President/CEO. . . . . William G Wilson
Emergency Room . . . . April Hayes
Infection Control. . . . . Dorothy Butler
ICU . . . . Becky Braddock
OB/GYN Women's Health . . . . April Hyde
Respiratory/Cardiopulmonary. . . . . Carlos Mendoza

Measure	Cases	This Hospital	State Average	U.S. Average	Top Hospital
Heart Attack Care					
ACE Inhibitor or ARB for LVSD[1]	9	100%	79%	82%	100%
Aspirin at Arrival[1]	23	91%	86%	92%	100%
Aspirin at Discharge[1]	9	89%	85%	90%	100%
Beta Blocker at Arrival	27	74%	78%	87%	100%
Beta Blocker at Discharge[1]	12	92%	78%	90%	100%
Fibrinolytic Medication Timing[1]	6	17%	36%	31%	100%
PCI Within 90 Minutes of Arrival	0	-	51%	54%	95%
Smoking Cessation Advice[1]	4	25%	83%	88%	100%
Heart Failure Care					
ACE Inhibitor or ARB for LVSD	65	89%	76%	82%	100%
Discharge Instructions	98	69%	55%	61%	93%
Evaluation of LVS Function	132	87%	71%	83%	99%
Smoking Cessation Advice	25	100%	73%	82%	100%
Pneumonia Care					
Appropriate Initial Antibiotic	116	84%	81%	83%	94%
Blood Culture Timing	70	96%	91%	90%	100%
Influenza Vaccine[1]	24	83%	72%	70%	100%
Initial Antibiotic Timing	147	93%	82%	80%	93%
Oxygenation Assessment	178	98%	99%	99%	100%
Pneumococcal Vaccine	111	89%	68%	69%	94%
Smoking Cessation Advice	52	83%	72%	80%	100%
Surgical Infection Prevention					
Prophylactic Antibiotic Given[3]	119	92%	75%	77%	95%
Prophylactic Antibiotic Selection	53	98%	88%	90%	100%
Prophylactic Antibiotic Stopped[3]	113	68%	82%	72%	95%
Pregnancy Care					
Inpatient Neonatal Mortality	-	-	-	-	-
Third or Fourth Degree Laceration	-	-	-	3.63%	3.27%

Share Medical Center

800 Share Avenue
Alva, OK 73717
URL: www.smcok.com
Ownership: Government - Local
Emergency Services: Yes

Phone: 580-327-2800
Fax: 580-430-3332

Accredited: No
Licensed Beds: 37

Key Personnel:
Administrator/CEO. . . . . Barbara Oestmann
Chief of Medical Staff. . . . . Kirtt Bierig, DO
Head of Emergency Room. . . . . Christy Williard
Emergency Room . . . . Barbara Louthan, RN
Infection Control. . . . . Cheryl Ellis, RN
Director Medical/Surgical Nursing . . . . Kim Foster
OB/GYN Womens Health. . . . . Bruce Meyer, MD
Respiratory/Cardiopulmonary. . . . . Beth Mahon

Measure	Cases	This Hospital	State Average	U.S. Average	Top Hospital
Heart Attack Care					

NOTE: Hospital profiles are in alphabetical order by state, then city, then hospital within the city; Rankings are sorted by rate in descending order and exclude hospitals with less than 25 cases; (1) The number of cases is too small (n<25) for purposes of reliably predicting hospital performance; (2) Measure reflects the hospital's indication that its submission was based upon a sample of its relevant discharges; (3) Rate reflects fewer than the maximum possible quarters of data for the measure; (4) Inaccurate information submitted and suppressed for one or more quarters; (5) No data is available from the hospital for this measure; Please refer to the User's Guide for a full explanation of data

ACE Inhibitor or ARB for LVSD[1,3]	1	0%	79%	82%	100%
Aspirin at Arrival[1,3]	3	33%	86%	92%	100%
Aspirin at Discharge[1,3]	2	50%	85%	90%	100%
Beta Blocker at Arrival[1,3]	2	50%	78%	87%	100%
Beta Blocker at Discharge[1,3]	2	50%	78%	90%	100%
Fibrinolytic Medication Timing[3]	0	-	36%	31%	100%
PCI Within 90 Minutes of Arrival	0	-	51%	54%	95%
Smoking Cessation Advice[3]	0	-	83%	88%	100%
Heart Failure Care					
ACE Inhibitor or ARB for LVSD[1]	5	60%	76%	82%	100%
Discharge Instructions[1]	23	57%	55%	61%	93%
Evaluation of LVS Function	30	90%	71%	83%	99%
Smoking Cessation Advice[1]	2	50%	73%	82%	100%
Pneumonia Care					
Appropriate Initial Antibiotic[1,3]	19	89%	81%	83%	94%
Blood Culture Timing[1]	13	100%	91%	90%	100%
Influenza Vaccine[1]	15	93%	72%	70%	100%
Initial Antibiotic Timing	48	98%	82%	80%	93%
Oxygenation Assessment	56	100%	99%	99%	100%
Pneumococcal Vaccine	38	92%	68%	69%	94%
Smoking Cessation Advice[1]	14	71%	72%	80%	100%
Surgical Infection Prevention					
Prophylactic Antibiotic Given[1,3]	1	0%	75%	77%	95%
Prophylactic Antibiotic Selection[1]	1	100%	88%	90%	100%
Prophylactic Antibiotic Stopped[1,3]	1	100%	82%	72%	95%
Pregnancy Care					
Inpatient Neonatal Mortality	-	-	-	-	-
Third or Fourth Degree Laceration	-	-	-	3.63%	3.27%

Anadarko Municipal Hospital

1002 E Central Boulevard
Anadarko, OK 73005
Phone: 405-247-2551
Fax: 405-247-9407
Ownership: Government - Local
Accredited: No
Emergency Services: Yes
Licensed Beds: 49

Key Personnel:

President/CEO . . . . Alan Riffel
Chief Medical Staff . . . . Roberta Martin

Measure	Cases	This Hospital	State Average	U.S. Average	Top Hospital
Heart Attack Care					
ACE Inhibitor or ARB for LVSD[5]	-	-	79%	82%	100%
Aspirin at Arrival[5]	-	-	86%	92%	100%
Aspirin at Discharge[5]	-	-	85%	90%	100%
Beta Blocker at Arrival[5]	-	-	78%	87%	100%
Beta Blocker at Discharge[5]	-	-	78%	90%	100%
Fibrinolytic Medication Timing[5]	-	-	36%	31%	100%
PCI Within 90 Minutes of Arrival[5]	-	-	51%	54%	95%
Smoking Cessation Advice[5]	-	-	83%	88%	100%
Heart Failure Care					
ACE Inhibitor or ARB for LVSD[1,3]	1	100%	76%	82%	100%
Discharge Instructions[1,3]	4	0%	55%	61%	93%
Evaluation of LVS Function[1,3]	4	75%	71%	83%	99%
Smoking Cessation Advice[3]	0	-	73%	82%	100%
Pneumonia Care					
Appropriate Initial Antibiotic[1,3]	9	78%	81%	83%	94%
Blood Culture Timing[3]	0	-	91%	90%	100%
Influenza Vaccine[5]	-	-	72%	70%	100%
Initial Antibiotic Timing[1,3]	4	50%	82%	80%	93%
Oxygenation Assessment[1,3]	10	100%	99%	99%	100%
Pneumococcal Vaccine[1,3]	5	0%	68%	69%	94%
Smoking Cessation Advice[1,3]	6	33%	72%	80%	100%
Surgical Infection Prevention					
Prophylactic Antibiotic Given[5]	-	-	75%	77%	95%
Prophylactic Antibiotic Selection[5]	-	-	88%	90%	100%
Prophylactic Antibiotic Stopped[5]	-	-	82%	72%	95%
Pregnancy Care					
Inpatient Neonatal Mortality	-	-	-	-	-
Third or Fourth Degree Laceration	-	-	-	3.63%	3.27%

Pushmataha Hospital

510 W Main
Box G
Antlers, OK 74523
Phone: 580-298-3344
Fax: 580-298-5736
Ownership: Govt - Hospital District or Authority
Accredited: No
Emergency Services: Yes
Licensed Beds: 49

Key Personnel:

CEO . . . . Denis Frank
Chief of Medical Staff . . . . Herbert Rowland
Director of Emergency Room . . . . Gelbert Gay
Emergency Room . . . . Nadine David
Director Infection/Disease Control . . . . Jane Bates
Director of Respiratory Therapy . . . . Richard Jackson

Measure	Cases	This Hospital	State Average	U.S. Average	Top Hospital
Heart Attack Care					
ACE Inhibitor or ARB for LVSD	0	-	79%	82%	100%
Aspirin at Arrival[1]	1	100%	86%	92%	100%
Aspirin at Discharge	0	-	85%	90%	100%
Beta Blocker at Arrival	0	-	78%	87%	100%
Beta Blocker at Discharge	0	-	78%	90%	100%
Fibrinolytic Medication Timing	0	-	36%	31%	100%
PCI Within 90 Minutes of Arrival	0	-	51%	54%	95%
Smoking Cessation Advice	0	-	83%	88%	100%
Heart Failure Care					
ACE Inhibitor or ARB for LVSD[1]	15	80%	76%	82%	100%
Discharge Instructions	40	92%	55%	61%	93%
Evaluation of LVS Function	50	86%	71%	83%	99%
Smoking Cessation Advice[1]	7	71%	73%	82%	100%
Pneumonia Care					
Appropriate Initial Antibiotic	56	91%	81%	83%	94%
Blood Culture Timing	57	81%	91%	90%	100%
Influenza Vaccine[1]	17	94%	72%	70%	100%
Initial Antibiotic Timing	63	94%	82%	80%	93%
Oxygenation Assessment	78	100%	99%	99%	100%
Pneumococcal Vaccine	46	83%	68%	69%	94%
Smoking Cessation Advice[1]	16	88%	72%	80%	100%
Surgical Infection Prevention					
Prophylactic Antibiotic Given[1,3]	4	75%	75%	77%	95%
Prophylactic Antibiotic Selection[1]	4	25%	88%	90%	100%
Prophylactic Antibiotic Stopped[1,3]	4	100%	82%	72%	95%
Pregnancy Care					
Inpatient Neonatal Mortality	-	-	-	-	-
Third or Fourth Degree Laceration	-	-	-	3.63%	3.27%

Mercy Memorial Health Center

Alternate Name: Memorial Hospital of Southern Oklahoma
1011 14th Avenue NW
Ardmore, OK 73401
Phone: 580-223-5400
Fax: 580-220-6580
Ownership: Voluntary non-profit - Other
Accredited: Yes
Emergency Services: Yes
Licensed Beds: 278

Measure	Cases	This Hospital	State Average	U.S. Average	Top Hospital
Heart Attack Care					
ACE Inhibitor or ARB for LVSD	30	87%	79%	82%	100%
Aspirin at Arrival	142	93%	86%	92%	100%
Aspirin at Discharge	131	95%	85%	90%	100%
Beta Blocker at Arrival	90	90%	78%	87%	100%
Beta Blocker at Discharge	131	95%	78%	90%	100%
Fibrinolytic Medication Timing[1]	24	46%	36%	31%	100%
PCI Within 90 Minutes of Arrival	0	-	51%	54%	95%
Smoking Cessation Advice	46	98%	83%	88%	100%
Heart Failure Care					
ACE Inhibitor or ARB for LVSD	82	85%	76%	82%	100%
Discharge Instructions	205	70%	55%	61%	93%
Evaluation of LVS Function	248	92%	71%	83%	99%
Smoking Cessation Advice	73	95%	73%	82%	100%
Pneumonia Care					
Appropriate Initial Antibiotic	228	79%	81%	83%	94%
Blood Culture Timing	126	98%	91%	90%	100%
Influenza Vaccine	67	46%	72%	70%	100%
Initial Antibiotic Timing	322	76%	82%	80%	93%

NOTE: Hospital profiles are in alphabetical order by state, then city, then hospital within the city; Rankings are sorted by rate in descending order and exclude hospitals with less than 25 cases; (1) The number of cases is too small (n<25) for purposes of reliably predicting hospital performance; (2) Measure reflects the hospital's indication that its submission was based upon a sample of its relevant discharges; (3) Rate reflects fewer than the maximum possible quarters of data for the measure; (4) Inaccurate information submitted and suppressed for one or more quarters; (5) No data is available from the hospital for this measure; Please refer to the User's Guide for a full explanation of data

Measure	Cases	This Hospital	State Average	U.S. Average	Top Hospital
Oxygenation Assessment	355	100%	99%	99%	100%
Pneumococcal Vaccine	220	85%	68%	69%	94%
Smoking Cessation Advice	84	93%	72%	80%	100%
Surgical Infection Prevention					
Prophylactic Antibiotic Given[2]	561	88%	75%	77%	95%
Prophylactic Antibiotic Selection[2]	125	92%	88%	90%	100%
Prophylactic Antibiotic Stopped[2]	544	78%	82%	72%	95%
Pregnancy Care					
Inpatient Neonatal Mortality	-	-	-	-	-
Third or Fourth Degree Laceration	-	-	-	3.63%	3.27%

Atoka Memorial Hospital

1501 South Virginia Avenue
Atoka, OK 74525
Ownership: Government - Local
Emergency Services: Yes

Phone: 580-889-3333

Accredited: No

Measure	Cases	This Hospital	State Average	U.S. Average	Top Hospital
Heart Attack Care					
ACE Inhibitor or ARB for LVSD[3]	0	-	79%	82%	100%
Aspirin at Arrival[1,3]	2	100%	86%	92%	100%
Aspirin at Discharge[1,3]	3	100%	85%	90%	100%
Beta Blocker at Arrival[1,3]	1	100%	78%	87%	100%
Beta Blocker at Discharge[1,3]	3	67%	78%	90%	100%
Fibrinolytic Medication Timing[1,3]	1	0%	36%	31%	100%
PCI Within 90 Minutes of Arrival[5]	-	-	51%	54%	95%
Smoking Cessation Advice[1,3]	1	0%	83%	88%	100%
Heart Failure Care					
ACE Inhibitor or ARB for LVSD[1]	6	17%	76%	82%	100%
Discharge Instructions[1]	10	40%	55%	61%	93%
Evaluation of LVS Function[1]	23	39%	71%	83%	99%
Smoking Cessation Advice[1]	5	60%	73%	82%	100%
Pneumonia Care					
Appropriate Initial Antibiotic	26	69%	81%	83%	94%
Blood Culture Timing[1]	5	100%	91%	90%	100%
Influenza Vaccine[4,5]	-	-	72%	70%	100%
Initial Antibiotic Timing[1]	7	71%	82%	80%	93%
Oxygenation Assessment	28	96%	99%	99%	100%
Pneumococcal Vaccine[1]	14	86%	68%	69%	94%
Smoking Cessation Advice[1]	12	75%	72%	80%	100%
Surgical Infection Prevention					
Prophylactic Antibiotic Given[5]	-	-	75%	77%	95%
Prophylactic Antibiotic Selection[5]	-	-	88%	90%	100%
Prophylactic Antibiotic Stopped[5]	-	-	82%	72%	95%
Pregnancy Care					
Inpatient Neonatal Mortality	-	-	-	-	-
Third or Fourth Degree Laceration	-	-	-	3.63%	3.27%

Jane Phillips Medical Center

3500 E Frank Phillips Boulevard
Bartlesville, OK 74006

Toll-Free: 800-824-8854
Phone: 918-333-7200
Fax: 918-331-1612

E-mail: webmaster@jpmc.org
URL: www.jpmc.org
Ownership: Voluntary non-profit - Church
Emergency Services: Yes

Accredited: Yes
Licensed Beds: 311

Key Personnel:
President/CEO. . . . . David R Stire
Chief of Medical Staff. . . . . Mark Myers

Measure	Cases	This Hospital	State Average	U.S. Average	Top Hospital
Heart Attack Care					
ACE Inhibitor or ARB for LVSD	37	95%	79%	82%	100%
Aspirin at Arrival	135	99%	86%	92%	100%
Aspirin at Discharge	161	98%	85%	90%	100%
Beta Blocker at Arrival	125	94%	78%	87%	100%
Beta Blocker at Discharge	148	97%	78%	90%	100%
Fibrinolytic Medication Timing	0	-	36%	31%	100%
PCI Within 90 Minutes of Arrival[1]	10	70%	51%	54%	95%
Smoking Cessation Advice	47	98%	83%	88%	100%
Heart Failure Care					
ACE Inhibitor or ARB for LVSD	80	89%	76%	82%	100%
Discharge Instructions	159	36%	55%	61%	93%
Evaluation of LVS Function	175	87%	71%	83%	99%
Smoking Cessation Advice	30	87%	73%	82%	100%
Pneumonia Care					
Appropriate Initial Antibiotic	257	73%	81%	83%	94%
Blood Culture Timing	175	93%	91%	90%	100%
Influenza Vaccine	61	67%	72%	70%	100%
Initial Antibiotic Timing	250	90%	82%	80%	93%
Oxygenation Assessment	309	100%	99%	99%	100%
Pneumococcal Vaccine	203	79%	68%	69%	94%
Smoking Cessation Advice	74	84%	72%	80%	100%
Surgical Infection Prevention					
Prophylactic Antibiotic Given[2,3]	367	84%	75%	77%	95%
Prophylactic Antibiotic Selection[2]	117	94%	88%	90%	100%
Prophylactic Antibiotic Stopped[2,3]	343	50%	82%	72%	95%
Pregnancy Care					
Inpatient Neonatal Mortality	-	-	-	-	-
Third or Fourth Degree Laceration	-	-	-	3.63%	3.27%

Beaver County Memorial Hospital

PO Box 640
Beaver, OK 73932
Ownership: Govt - Hospital District or Authority
Emergency Services: Yes

Phone: 580-625-4551
Fax: 580-625-4212
Accredited: No
Licensed Beds: 24

Key Personnel:
Administrator . . . . Lavern Melton
Emergency Room . . . . Deanna Brown

Measure	Cases	This Hospital	State Average	U.S. Average	Top Hospital
Heart Attack Care					
ACE Inhibitor or ARB for LVSD[3]	0	-	79%	82%	100%
Aspirin at Arrival[1,3]	1	100%	86%	92%	100%
Aspirin at Discharge[3]	0	-	85%	90%	100%
Beta Blocker at Arrival[3]	0	-	78%	87%	100%
Beta Blocker at Discharge[3]	0	-	78%	90%	100%
Fibrinolytic Medication Timing[3]	0	-	36%	31%	100%
PCI Within 90 Minutes of Arrival[5]	-	-	51%	54%	95%
Smoking Cessation Advice[3]	0	-	83%	88%	100%
Heart Failure Care					
ACE Inhibitor or ARB for LVSD[3]	0	-	76%	82%	100%
Discharge Instructions[1,3]	5	0%	55%	61%	93%
Evaluation of LVS Function[1,3]	5	0%	71%	83%	99%
Smoking Cessation Advice[3]	0	-	73%	82%	100%
Pneumonia Care					
Appropriate Initial Antibiotic[3]	0	-	81%	83%	94%
Blood Culture Timing[3]	0	-	91%	90%	100%
Influenza Vaccine[1]	1	100%	72%	70%	100%
Initial Antibiotic Timing[1,3]	10	100%	82%	80%	93%
Oxygenation Assessment[1,3]	10	100%	99%	99%	100%
Pneumococcal Vaccine[1,3]	4	25%	68%	69%	94%
Smoking Cessation Advice[1,3]	3	33%	72%	80%	100%
Surgical Infection Prevention					
Prophylactic Antibiotic Given[5]	-	-	75%	77%	95%
Prophylactic Antibiotic Selection[5]	-	-	88%	90%	100%
Prophylactic Antibiotic Stopped[5]	-	-	82%	72%	95%
Pregnancy Care					
Inpatient Neonatal Mortality	-	-	-	-	-
Third or Fourth Degree Laceration	-	-	-	3.63%	3.27%

Integris Blackwell Regional Hospital

710 S 13th Street
Blackwell, OK 74631
Ownership: Voluntary non-profit - Church
Emergency Services: Yes

Phone: 580-363-2311
Fax: 580-363-2339
Accredited: Yes
Licensed Beds: 53

Key Personnel:
CEO. . . . . James Moore
Chief Medical Staff. . . . . Dr. Paul Briggs
Infection Control. . . . . Pam Lewellyn

Measure	Cases	This Hospital	State Average	U.S. Average	Top Hospital
Heart Attack Care					
ACE Inhibitor or ARB for LVSD[1]	1	100%	79%	82%	100%

NOTE: Hospital profiles are in alphabetical order by state, then city, then hospital within the city; Rankings are sorted by rate in descending order and exclude hospitals with less than 25 cases; (1) The number of cases is too small (n<25) for purposes of reliably predicting hospital performance; (2) Measure reflects the hospital's indication that its submission was based upon a sample of its relevant discharges; (3) Rate reflects fewer than the maximum possible quarters of data for the measure; (4) Inaccurate information submitted and suppressed for one or more quarters; (5) No data is available from the hospital for this measure; Please refer to the User's Guide for a full explanation of data

Measure	Cases	This Hospital	State Average	U.S. Average	Top Hospital
Aspirin at Arrival[1]	5	80%	86%	92%	100%
Aspirin at Discharge[1]	3	67%	85%	90%	100%
Beta Blocker at Arrival[1]	2	100%	78%	87%	100%
Beta Blocker at Discharge[1]	2	100%	78%	90%	100%
Fibrinolytic Medication Timing	0	-	36%	31%	100%
PCI Within 90 Minutes of Arrival	0	-	51%	54%	95%
Smoking Cessation Advice	0	-	83%	88%	100%
Heart Failure Care					
ACE Inhibitor or ARB for LVSD[1]	16	94%	76%	82%	100%
Discharge Instructions	51	78%	55%	61%	93%
Evaluation of LVS Function	77	99%	71%	83%	99%
Smoking Cessation Advice[1]	14	100%	73%	82%	100%
Pneumonia Care					
Appropriate Initial Antibiotic	90	91%	81%	83%	94%
Blood Culture Timing	71	99%	91%	90%	100%
Influenza Vaccine	33	100%	72%	70%	100%
Initial Antibiotic Timing	141	91%	82%	80%	93%
Oxygenation Assessment	155	100%	99%	99%	100%
Pneumococcal Vaccine	91	98%	68%	69%	94%
Smoking Cessation Advice	53	96%	72%	80%	100%
Surgical Infection Prevention					
Prophylactic Antibiotic Given[1,3]	8	88%	75%	77%	95%
Prophylactic Antibiotic Selection[1]	4	75%	88%	90%	100%
Prophylactic Antibiotic Stopped[1,3]	6	67%	82%	72%	95%
Pregnancy Care					
Inpatient Neonatal Mortality	-	-	-	-	-
Third or Fourth Degree Laceration	-	-	-	3.63%	3.27%

Cimarron Memorial Hospital & Nursing Home

100 S Ellis
Boise City, OK 73933
Phone: 580-544-2501
Fax: 580-544-2517
Ownership: Voluntary non-profit - Other
Accredited: No
Emergency Services: Yes
Licensed Beds: 64

Key Personnel:

Administrator . . . . Carrell Blakely
Chief Medical Staff . . . . JL Wheeler, MD
Director Infection/Disease Control . . . . Dana Smith
Director Medical/Surgical Nursing . . . . Becki Gore, RN
Chief Radiology . . . . Mendino Beltran, MD
Director Respiratory Therapy . . . . Donna Cain

Measure	Cases	This Hospital	State Average	U.S. Average	Top Hospital
Heart Attack Care					
ACE Inhibitor or ARB for LVSD[5]	-	-	79%	82%	100%
Aspirin at Arrival[5]	-	-	86%	92%	100%
Aspirin at Discharge[5]	-	-	85%	90%	100%
Beta Blocker at Arrival[5]	-	-	78%	87%	100%
Beta Blocker at Discharge[5]	-	-	78%	90%	100%
Fibrinolytic Medication Timing[5]	-	-	36%	31%	100%
PCI Within 90 Minutes of Arrival[5]	-	-	51%	54%	95%
Smoking Cessation Advice[5]	-	-	83%	88%	100%
Heart Failure Care					
ACE Inhibitor or ARB for LVSD[3]	0	-	76%	82%	100%
Discharge Instructions[1,3]	3	33%	55%	61%	93%
Evaluation of LVS Function[1,3]	5	0%	71%	83%	99%
Smoking Cessation Advice[3]	0	-	73%	82%	100%
Pneumonia Care					
Appropriate Initial Antibiotic[1,3]	16	44%	81%	83%	94%
Blood Culture Timing[3]	0	-	91%	90%	100%
Influenza Vaccine	0	-	72%	70%	100%
Initial Antibiotic Timing[1,3]	10	80%	82%	80%	93%
Oxygenation Assessment[1,3]	16	100%	99%	99%	100%
Pneumococcal Vaccine[1,3]	11	91%	68%	69%	94%
Smoking Cessation Advice[1,3]	3	33%	72%	80%	100%
Surgical Infection Prevention					
Prophylactic Antibiotic Given[5]	-	-	75%	77%	95%
Prophylactic Antibiotic Selection[5]	-	-	88%	90%	100%
Prophylactic Antibiotic Stopped[5]	-	-	82%	72%	95%
Pregnancy Care					
Inpatient Neonatal Mortality	-	-	-	-	-
Third or Fourth Degree Laceration	-	-	-	3.63%	3.27%

Bristow Medical Center

Alternate Name: Bristow Memorial Hospital
7th and Spruce
PO Box 780
Bristow, OK 74010
Phone: 918-367-2215
Fax: 918-367-9190
E-mail: rgehrig@hillcrest.com
URL: www.hillcrest.com
Ownership: Proprietary
Accredited: No
Emergency Services: Yes
Licensed Beds: 32

Key Personnel:

President/CEO . . . . Ryan Gehrig
Chief Medical Staff . . . . Dennise Blackstad
Infection Control . . . . Tina Ordway, RN
Medical/Surgical Nursing . . . . Jim Clark, RN
Respiratory Therapy . . . . Abigail Kindell

Measure	Cases	This Hospital	State Average	U.S. Average	Top Hospital
Heart Attack Care					
ACE Inhibitor or ARB for LVSD[3]	0	-	79%	82%	100%
Aspirin at Arrival[1,3]	1	100%	86%	92%	100%
Aspirin at Discharge[1,3]	1	100%	85%	90%	100%
Beta Blocker at Arrival[1,3]	1	100%	78%	87%	100%
Beta Blocker at Discharge[1,3]	1	100%	78%	90%	100%
Fibrinolytic Medication Timing[3]	0	-	36%	31%	100%
PCI Within 90 Minutes of Arrival	0	-	51%	54%	95%
Smoking Cessation Advice[3]	0	-	83%	88%	100%
Heart Failure Care					
ACE Inhibitor or ARB for LVSD[1]	10	100%	76%	82%	100%
Discharge Instructions[1]	14	57%	55%	61%	93%
Evaluation of LVS Function[1]	19	95%	71%	83%	99%
Smoking Cessation Advice[1]	1	100%	73%	82%	100%
Pneumonia Care					
Appropriate Initial Antibiotic	37	95%	81%	83%	94%
Blood Culture Timing[1]	11	100%	91%	90%	100%
Influenza Vaccine[4,5]	-	-	72%	70%	100%
Initial Antibiotic Timing	40	92%	82%	80%	93%
Oxygenation Assessment	47	100%	99%	99%	100%
Pneumococcal Vaccine	33	94%	68%	69%	94%
Smoking Cessation Advice[1]	18	83%	72%	80%	100%
Surgical Infection Prevention					
Prophylactic Antibiotic Given[5]	-	-	75%	77%	95%
Prophylactic Antibiotic Selection[5]	-	-	88%	90%	100%
Prophylactic Antibiotic Stopped[5]	-	-	82%	72%	95%
Pregnancy Care					
Inpatient Neonatal Mortality	-	-	-	-	-
Third or Fourth Degree Laceration	-	-	-	3.63%	3.27%

Saint Francis Hospital

Alternate Name: Broken Arrow Medical Center
3000 S Elm Place
Broken Arrow, OK 74012
Phone: 918-455-3535
Fax: 918-451-5185
URL: www.sfh-ba.com
Ownership: Voluntary non-profit - Church
Accredited: Yes
Emergency Services: Yes
Licensed Beds: 71

Key Personnel:

CEO . . . . Bruce Switzer
Chief Medical Staff . . . . Colin Marouk, DO
Emergency Room . . . . Matt Warren, DO
Director Infection/Disease Control . . . . Ellen Bettinger, RN
CCU Spvg. Nurse . . . . Renita Lee, RN
Chief Radiology . . . . Thomas Harrison, DO
Director Respiratory Therapy . . . . Nancy Fennell

Measure	Cases	This Hospital	State Average	U.S. Average	Top Hospital
Heart Attack Care					
ACE Inhibitor or ARB for LVSD[1]	1	100%	79%	82%	100%
Aspirin at Arrival[1]	13	100%	86%	92%	100%
Aspirin at Discharge[1]	8	88%	85%	90%	100%
Beta Blocker at Arrival[1]	11	91%	78%	87%	100%
Beta Blocker at Discharge[1]	8	100%	78%	90%	100%
Fibrinolytic Medication Timing	0	-	36%	31%	100%
PCI Within 90 Minutes of Arrival	0	-	51%	54%	95%
Smoking Cessation Advice	0	-	83%	88%	100%

NOTE: Hospital profiles are in alphabetical order by state, then city, then hospital within the city; Rankings are sorted by rate in descending order and exclude hospitals with less than 25 cases; (1) The number of cases is too small (n<25) for purposes of reliably predicting hospital performance; (2) Measure reflects the hospital's indication that its submission was based upon a sample of its relevant discharges; (3) Rate reflects fewer than the maximum possible quarters of data for the measure; (4) Inaccurate information submitted and suppressed for one or more quarters; (5) No data is available from the hospital for this measure; Please refer to the User's Guide for a full explanation of data

Measure	Cases	This Hospital	State Average	U.S. Average	Top Hospital
Heart Failure Care					
ACE Inhibitor or ARB for LVSD[1]	19	89%	76%	82%	100%
Discharge Instructions	35	80%	55%	61%	93%
Evaluation of LVS Function	52	96%	71%	83%	99%
Smoking Cessation Advice[1]	6	100%	73%	82%	100%
Pneumonia Care					
Appropriate Initial Antibiotic	103	97%	81%	83%	94%
Blood Culture Timing	113	96%	91%	90%	100%
Influenza Vaccine	29	100%	72%	70%	100%
Initial Antibiotic Timing	129	94%	82%	80%	93%
Oxygenation Assessment	165	100%	99%	99%	100%
Pneumococcal Vaccine	107	100%	68%	69%	94%
Smoking Cessation Advice	32	94%	72%	80%	100%
Surgical Infection Prevention					
Prophylactic Antibiotic Given	187	96%	75%	77%	95%
Prophylactic Antibiotic Selection	47	98%	88%	90%	100%
Prophylactic Antibiotic Stopped	185	96%	82%	72%	95%
Pregnancy Care					
Inpatient Neonatal Mortality	-	-	-	-	-
Third or Fourth Degree Laceration	-	-	-	3.63%	3.27%

Harper County Community Hospital

N Highway 64
Buffalo, OK 73834
Ownership: Government - Local
Emergency Services: Yes

Phone: 580-735-2555
Fax: 580-735-2342
Accredited: No
Licensed Beds: 25

Key Personnel:
Administrator . . . . Jane McDowell
Chief of Medical Staff . . . . N Suthers
Head of Emergency Room . . . . Amy Yauk
Emergency Room . . . . Paula Lauer, RN
Director Medical/Surgical Nursing . . . . Paula Lauer, RN

Measure	Cases	This Hospital	State Average	U.S. Average	Top Hospital
Heart Attack Care					
ACE Inhibitor or ARB for LVSD[3]	0	-	79%	82%	100%
Aspirin at Arrival[3]	0	-	86%	92%	100%
Aspirin at Discharge[3]	0	-	85%	90%	100%
Beta Blocker at Arrival[3]	0	-	78%	87%	100%
Beta Blocker at Discharge[3]	0	-	78%	90%	100%
Fibrinolytic Medication Timing[3]	0	-	36%	31%	100%
PCI Within 90 Minutes of Arrival[5]	-	-	51%	54%	95%
Smoking Cessation Advice[3]	0	-	83%	88%	100%
Heart Failure Care					
ACE Inhibitor or ARB for LVSD[1]	1	100%	76%	82%	100%
Discharge Instructions[1]	1	100%	55%	61%	93%
Evaluation of LVS Function[1]	5	100%	71%	83%	99%
Smoking Cessation Advice[1]	2	50%	73%	82%	100%
Pneumonia Care					
Appropriate Initial Antibiotic[1]	13	100%	81%	83%	94%
Blood Culture Timing[1]	1	100%	91%	90%	100%
Influenza Vaccine[1]	3	100%	72%	70%	100%
Initial Antibiotic Timing[1]	19	89%	82%	80%	93%
Oxygenation Assessment[1]	21	100%	99%	99%	100%
Pneumococcal Vaccine[1]	15	100%	68%	69%	94%
Smoking Cessation Advice[1]	7	86%	72%	80%	100%
Surgical Infection Prevention					
Prophylactic Antibiotic Given[1,3]	1	100%	75%	77%	95%
Prophylactic Antibiotic Selection	0	-	88%	90%	100%
Prophylactic Antibiotic Stopped[1,3]	1	100%	82%	72%	95%
Pregnancy Care					
Inpatient Neonatal Mortality	-	-	-	-	-
Third or Fourth Degree Laceration	-	-	-	3.63%	3.27%

Carnegie Tri-County Municipal Hospital

PO Box 97
Carnegie, OK 73015
Ownership: Proprietary
Emergency Services: Yes

Phone: 580-654-1050
Fax: 580-654-2111
Accredited: No
Licensed Beds: 28

Key Personnel:
CEO . . . . Shane Dunning

Measure	Cases	This Hospital	State Average	U.S. Average	Top Hospital
Heart Attack Care					
ACE Inhibitor or ARB for LVSD[3]	0	-	79%	82%	100%
Aspirin at Arrival[1,3]	1	100%	86%	92%	100%
Aspirin at Discharge[3]	0	-	85%	90%	100%
Beta Blocker at Arrival[1,3]	1	100%	78%	87%	100%
Beta Blocker at Discharge[3]	0	-	78%	90%	100%
Fibrinolytic Medication Timing[3]	0	-	36%	31%	100%
PCI Within 90 Minutes of Arrival	0	-	51%	54%	95%
Smoking Cessation Advice[3]	0	-	83%	88%	100%
Heart Failure Care					
ACE Inhibitor or ARB for LVSD[1]	3	67%	76%	82%	100%
Discharge Instructions[1]	23	9%	55%	61%	93%
Evaluation of LVS Function	36	8%	71%	83%	99%
Smoking Cessation Advice[1]	4	25%	73%	82%	100%
Pneumonia Care					
Appropriate Initial Antibiotic[1]	11	100%	81%	83%	94%
Blood Culture Timing	0	-	91%	90%	100%
Influenza Vaccine[1]	5	0%	72%	70%	100%
Initial Antibiotic Timing[1]	19	79%	82%	80%	93%
Oxygenation Assessment[1]	20	100%	99%	99%	100%
Pneumococcal Vaccine[1]	18	0%	68%	69%	94%
Smoking Cessation Advice[1]	4	0%	72%	80%	100%
Surgical Infection Prevention					
Prophylactic Antibiotic Given[5]	-	-	75%	77%	95%
Prophylactic Antibiotic Selection[5]	-	-	88%	90%	100%
Prophylactic Antibiotic Stopped[5]	-	-	82%	72%	95%
Pregnancy Care					
Inpatient Neonatal Mortality	-	-	-	-	-
Third or Fourth Degree Laceration	-	-	-	3.63%	3.27%

Grady Memorial Hospital

2220 Iowa
Chickasha, OK 73018
Ownership: Govt - Hospital District or Authority
Emergency Services: Yes

Phone: 405-224-2300
Fax: 405-224-8579
Accredited: Yes
Licensed Beds: 147

Key Personnel:
Administrator/CEO . . . . Roger R Boid
Chief Medical Staff . . . . Don R Hess, MD
Emergency Room . . . . Bruce L Storms, MD
Director Infection/Disease Control . . . . Cathy Hamit, RN
CCU Spvg. Nurse . . . . Peggy Riley, RN
Director Medical/Surgical Nursing . . . . Sandra Bazemore
OB/GYN Womens Health . . . . Cary A Fisher, MD
Director Radiology . . . . Jim Wustrack
Director Respiratory Therapy . . . . Terry Handshy

Measure	Cases	This Hospital	State Average	U.S. Average	Top Hospital
Heart Attack Care					
ACE Inhibitor or ARB for LVSD	0	-	79%	82%	100%
Aspirin at Arrival[1]	4	100%	86%	92%	100%
Aspirin at Discharge[1]	5	80%	85%	90%	100%
Beta Blocker at Arrival[1]	5	80%	78%	87%	100%
Beta Blocker at Discharge[1]	5	60%	78%	90%	100%
Fibrinolytic Medication Timing	0	-	36%	31%	100%
PCI Within 90 Minutes of Arrival	0	-	51%	54%	95%
Smoking Cessation Advice	0	-	83%	88%	100%
Heart Failure Care					
ACE Inhibitor or ARB for LVSD[1]	13	69%	76%	82%	100%
Discharge Instructions	71	90%	55%	61%	93%
Evaluation of LVS Function	86	84%	71%	83%	99%
Smoking Cessation Advice[1]	20	100%	73%	82%	100%
Pneumonia Care					
Appropriate Initial Antibiotic	117	87%	81%	83%	94%
Blood Culture Timing	60	93%	91%	90%	100%
Influenza Vaccine[1]	22	95%	72%	70%	100%
Initial Antibiotic Timing	115	84%	82%	80%	93%
Oxygenation Assessment	156	99%	99%	99%	100%
Pneumococcal Vaccine	89	92%	68%	69%	94%
Smoking Cessation Advice	30	87%	72%	80%	100%
Surgical Infection Prevention					
Prophylactic Antibiotic Given[3]	68	94%	75%	77%	95%

NOTE: Hospital profiles are in alphabetical order by state, then city, then hospital within the city; Rankings are sorted by rate in descending order and exclude hospitals with less than 25 cases; (1) The number of cases is too small (n<25) for purposes of reliably predicting hospital performance; (2) Measure reflects the hospital's indication that its submission was based upon a sample of its relevant discharges; (3) Rate reflects fewer than the maximum possible quarters of data for the measure; (4) Inaccurate information submitted and suppressed for one or more quarters; (5) No data is available from the hospital for this measure; Please refer to the User's Guide for a full explanation of data

Measure	Cases	This Hospital	State Average	U.S. Average	Top Hospital
Prophylactic Antibiotic Selection	25	88%	88%	90%	100%
Prophylactic Antibiotic Stopped[3]	62	85%	82%	72%	95%
Pregnancy Care					
Inpatient Neonatal Mortality	-	-	-	-	-
Third or Fourth Degree Laceration	-	-	-	3.63%	3.27%

Claremore Regional Hospital

1202 N Muskogee Place
Claremore, OK 74017
URL: www.claremorereghospital.com
Ownership: Proprietary
Emergency Services: Yes
Phone: 918-341-2556
Accredited: Yes
Licensed Beds: 50

Key Personnel:

CEO. . . . . David Chausard
Chief Medical Staff. . . . . Cammy Brown
Chief Medical Staff. . . . . Karen Harris
Director Emergency Room. . . . . Jimmy Bible
Director of Pulmonary/Respiratory . . . . Marty Dunning

Measure	Cases	This Hospital	State Average	U.S. Average	Top Hospital
Heart Attack Care					
ACE Inhibitor or ARB for LVSD[1]	2	100%	79%	82%	100%
Aspirin at Arrival[1]	15	100%	86%	92%	100%
Aspirin at Discharge[1]	7	100%	85%	90%	100%
Beta Blocker at Arrival[1]	11	100%	78%	87%	100%
Beta Blocker at Discharge[1]	6	83%	78%	90%	100%
Fibrinolytic Medication Timing	0	-	36%	31%	100%
PCI Within 90 Minutes of Arrival	0	-	51%	54%	95%
Smoking Cessation Advice[1]	1	100%	83%	88%	100%
Heart Failure Care					
ACE Inhibitor or ARB for LVSD[1]	17	94%	76%	82%	100%
Discharge Instructions	43	86%	55%	61%	93%
Evaluation of LVS Function	66	98%	71%	83%	99%
Smoking Cessation Advice[1]	13	100%	73%	82%	100%
Pneumonia Care					
Appropriate Initial Antibiotic	87	94%	81%	83%	94%
Blood Culture Timing	90	92%	91%	90%	100%
Influenza Vaccine	34	91%	72%	70%	100%
Initial Antibiotic Timing	124	89%	82%	80%	93%
Oxygenation Assessment	149	100%	99%	99%	100%
Pneumococcal Vaccine	89	91%	68%	69%	94%
Smoking Cessation Advice	37	100%	72%	80%	100%
Surgical Infection Prevention					
Prophylactic Antibiotic Given	202	91%	75%	77%	95%
Prophylactic Antibiotic Selection	52	92%	88%	90%	100%
Prophylactic Antibiotic Stopped	198	79%	82%	72%	95%
Pregnancy Care					
Inpatient Neonatal Mortality	-	-	-	-	-
Third or Fourth Degree Laceration	-	-	-	3.63%	3.27%

PHS Indian Hospital

Alternate Name: Claremore Indian Hospital
101 S Moore
Claremore, OK 74017
Ownership: Government - Federal
Emergency Services: Yes
Phone: 918-342-6200
Fax: 918-342-6436
Accredited: Yes
Licensed Beds: 50

Key Personnel:

CEO. . . . . James Cussen
Chief Medical Staff. . . . . Paul Mobley, DO
Emergency Room . . . . Donald Bobek
Director Infection/Disease Control . . . . Patti V White
OB/GYN Womens Health. . . . . Sumathy Vannarth, MD
Chief Radiology . . . . Cathy Smith
Director Respiratory Therapy . . . . Kathy Alexander

Measure	Cases	This Hospital	State Average	U.S. Average	Top Hospital
Heart Attack Care					
ACE Inhibitor or ARB for LVSD[1,3]	1	0%	79%	82%	100%
Aspirin at Arrival[1,3]	2	100%	86%	92%	100%
Aspirin at Discharge[1,3]	1	100%	85%	90%	100%
Beta Blocker at Arrival[1,3]	2	100%	78%	87%	100%
Beta Blocker at Discharge[1,3]	1	100%	78%	90%	100%
Fibrinolytic Medication Timing[3]	0	-	36%	31%	100%
PCI Within 90 Minutes of Arrival	0	-	51%	54%	95%
Smoking Cessation Advice[1,3]	1	0%	83%	88%	100%
Heart Failure Care					
ACE Inhibitor or ARB for LVSD[1]	9	100%	76%	82%	100%
Discharge Instructions	39	74%	55%	61%	93%
Evaluation of LVS Function	40	92%	71%	83%	99%
Smoking Cessation Advice[1]	15	93%	73%	82%	100%
Pneumonia Care					
Appropriate Initial Antibiotic	46	87%	81%	83%	94%
Blood Culture Timing	38	68%	91%	90%	100%
Influenza Vaccine[1]	8	62%	72%	70%	100%
Initial Antibiotic Timing	52	83%	82%	80%	93%
Oxygenation Assessment	57	100%	99%	99%	100%
Pneumococcal Vaccine[1]	21	71%	68%	69%	94%
Smoking Cessation Advice[1]	14	86%	72%	80%	100%
Surgical Infection Prevention					
Prophylactic Antibiotic Given	111	96%	75%	77%	95%
Prophylactic Antibiotic Selection	37	89%	88%	90%	100%
Prophylactic Antibiotic Stopped	107	97%	82%	72%	95%
Pregnancy Care					
Inpatient Neonatal Mortality	-	-	-	-	-
Third or Fourth Degree Laceration	-	-	-	3.63%	3.27%

Cleveland Area Hospital

1401 West Pawnee
Cleveland, OK 74020
Ownership: Voluntary non-profit - Private
Emergency Services: Yes
Phone: 918-358-2501
Accredited: No

Measure	Cases	This Hospital	State Average	U.S. Average	Top Hospital
Heart Attack Care					
ACE Inhibitor or ARB for LVSD[3]	0	-	79%	82%	100%
Aspirin at Arrival[1,3]	2	100%	86%	92%	100%
Aspirin at Discharge[3]	0	-	85%	90%	100%
Beta Blocker at Arrival[1,3]	2	0%	78%	87%	100%
Beta Blocker at Discharge[3]	0	-	78%	90%	100%
Fibrinolytic Medication Timing[3]	0	-	36%	31%	100%
PCI Within 90 Minutes of Arrival[5]	-	-	51%	54%	95%
Smoking Cessation Advice[3]	0	-	83%	88%	100%
Heart Failure Care					
ACE Inhibitor or ARB for LVSD[1]	4	50%	76%	82%	100%
Discharge Instructions[1]	10	50%	55%	61%	93%
Evaluation of LVS Function[1]	11	82%	71%	83%	99%
Smoking Cessation Advice	0	-	73%	82%	100%
Pneumonia Care					
Appropriate Initial Antibiotic	29	83%	81%	83%	94%
Blood Culture Timing[1]	6	67%	91%	90%	100%
Influenza Vaccine[1]	11	64%	72%	70%	100%
Initial Antibiotic Timing	29	66%	82%	80%	93%
Oxygenation Assessment	34	100%	99%	99%	100%
Pneumococcal Vaccine[1]	22	45%	68%	69%	94%
Smoking Cessation Advice[1]	5	60%	72%	80%	100%
Surgical Infection Prevention					
Prophylactic Antibiotic Given[5]	-	-	75%	77%	95%
Prophylactic Antibiotic Selection[5]	-	-	88%	90%	100%
Prophylactic Antibiotic Stopped[5]	-	-	82%	72%	95%
Pregnancy Care					
Inpatient Neonatal Mortality	-	-	-	-	-
Third or Fourth Degree Laceration	-	-	-	3.63%	3.27%

Clinton Indian Hospital

Alternate Name: PHS Indian Hospital
Old Hwy 66 North
Clinton, OK 73601
Ownership: Government - Federal
Emergency Services: Yes
Phone: 580-323-2884
Fax: 580-323-2884
Accredited: Yes
Licensed Beds: 11

Key Personnel:

CEO/President. . . . . Terry Smith
Chief Medical Staff. . . . . Dolly Gardia
Emergency Room . . . . Dill Wilson

Measure	Cases	This Hospital	State Average	U.S. Average	Top Hospital

NOTE: Hospital profiles are in alphabetical order by state, then city, then hospital within the city; Rankings are sorted by rate in descending order and exclude hospitals with less than 25 cases; (1) The number of cases is too small (n<25) for purposes of reliably predicting hospital performance; (2) Measure reflects the hospital's indication that its submission was based upon a sample of its relevant discharges; (3) Rate reflects fewer than the maximum possible quarters of data for the measure; (4) Inaccurate information submitted and suppressed for one or more quarters; (5) No data is available from the hospital for this measure; Please refer to the User's Guide for a full explanation of data

Measure	Cases	This Hospital	State Average	U.S. Average	Top Hospital
Heart Attack Care					
ACE Inhibitor or ARB for LVSD[5]	-	-	79%	82%	100%
Aspirin at Arrival[5]	-	-	86%	92%	100%
Aspirin at Discharge[5]	-	-	85%	90%	100%
Beta Blocker at Arrival[5]	-	-	78%	87%	100%
Beta Blocker at Discharge[5]	-	-	78%	90%	100%
Fibrinolytic Medication Timing[5]	-	-	36%	31%	100%
PCI Within 90 Minutes of Arrival[5]	-	-	51%	54%	95%
Smoking Cessation Advice[5]	-	-	83%	88%	100%
Heart Failure Care					
ACE Inhibitor or ARB for LVSD[5]	-	-	76%	82%	100%
Discharge Instructions[5]	-	-	55%	61%	93%
Evaluation of LVS Function[5]	-	-	71%	83%	99%
Smoking Cessation Advice[5]	-	-	73%	82%	100%
Pneumonia Care					
Appropriate Initial Antibiotic[1,3]	1	0%	81%	83%	94%
Blood Culture Timing[3]	0	-	91%	90%	100%
Influenza Vaccine[5]	-	-	72%	70%	100%
Initial Antibiotic Timing[1,3]	2	50%	82%	80%	93%
Oxygenation Assessment[1,3]	3	100%	99%	99%	100%
Pneumococcal Vaccine[3]	0	-	68%	69%	94%
Smoking Cessation Advice[3]	0	-	72%	80%	100%
Surgical Infection Prevention					
Prophylactic Antibiotic Given[5]	-	-	75%	77%	95%
Prophylactic Antibiotic Selection[5]	-	-	88%	90%	100%
Prophylactic Antibiotic Stopped[5]	-	-	82%	72%	95%
Pregnancy Care					
Inpatient Neonatal Mortality	-	-	-	-	-
Third or Fourth Degree Laceration	-	-	-	3.63%	3.27%

Integris Clinton Regional Hospital

Alternate Name: Clinton Regional Hospital
PO Box 1569
Clinton, OK 73601

Toll-Free: 888-700-0277
Phone: 580-323-2363
Fax: 580-331-1463

Ownership: Government - Local
Emergency Services: Yes
Accredited: Yes
Licensed Beds: 75

Key Personnel:
Administrator . . . . Jerry D Jones
Chief Medical Staff. . . . . Amy Powell
Emergency Room . . . . Tammy Martin, RN
Director Infection/Disease Control . . . . Karol Dillard, RN
Director Respiratory Therapy . . . . Tiffany Avara, RRT

Measure	Cases	This Hospital	State Average	U.S. Average	Top Hospital
Heart Attack Care					
ACE Inhibitor or ARB for LVSD	0	-	79%	82%	100%
Aspirin at Arrival[1]	2	100%	86%	92%	100%
Aspirin at Discharge	0	-	85%	90%	100%
Beta Blocker at Arrival[1]	1	100%	78%	87%	100%
Beta Blocker at Discharge[1]	2	100%	78%	90%	100%
Fibrinolytic Medication Timing[1]	1	0%	36%	31%	100%
PCI Within 90 Minutes of Arrival	0	-	51%	54%	95%
Smoking Cessation Advice[1]	1	100%	83%	88%	100%
Heart Failure Care					
ACE Inhibitor or ARB for LVSD	50	94%	76%	82%	100%
Discharge Instructions	65	91%	55%	61%	93%
Evaluation of LVS Function	82	100%	71%	83%	99%
Smoking Cessation Advice[1]	7	100%	73%	82%	100%
Pneumonia Care					
Appropriate Initial Antibiotic	68	99%	81%	83%	94%
Blood Culture Timing	82	99%	91%	90%	100%
Influenza Vaccine	35	86%	72%	70%	100%
Initial Antibiotic Timing	132	90%	82%	80%	93%
Oxygenation Assessment	148	100%	99%	99%	100%
Pneumococcal Vaccine	86	99%	68%	69%	94%
Smoking Cessation Advice	36	100%	72%	80%	100%
Surgical Infection Prevention					
Prophylactic Antibiotic Given[1]	10	100%	75%	77%	95%
Prophylactic Antibiotic Selection[1]	6	83%	88%	90%	100%
Prophylactic Antibiotic Stopped[1]	6	100%	82%	72%	95%
Pregnancy Care					
Inpatient Neonatal Mortality	-	-	-	-	-
Third or Fourth Degree Laceration	-	-	-	3.63%	3.27%

Mary Hurley Hospital

6 N Covington Street
Coalgate, OK 74538
Ownership: Voluntary non-profit - Other
Emergency Services: Yes

Phone: 580-927-2327
Fax: 580-927-2432
Accredited: No
Licensed Beds: 20

Key Personnel:
CEO. . . . . Dean Clements
Chief of Medical Staff. . . . . R J Alton
Emergency Room . . . . Paula Brown
Emergency Room . . . . Tommie Stanberry

Measure	Cases	This Hospital	State Average	U.S. Average	Top Hospital
Heart Attack Care					
ACE Inhibitor or ARB for LVSD[5]	-	-	79%	82%	100%
Aspirin at Arrival[5]	-	-	86%	92%	100%
Aspirin at Discharge[5]	-	-	85%	90%	100%
Beta Blocker at Arrival[5]	-	-	78%	87%	100%
Beta Blocker at Discharge[5]	-	-	78%	90%	100%
Fibrinolytic Medication Timing[5]	-	-	36%	31%	100%
PCI Within 90 Minutes of Arrival[5]	-	-	51%	54%	95%
Smoking Cessation Advice[5]	-	-	83%	88%	100%
Heart Failure Care					
ACE Inhibitor or ARB for LVSD[1]	5	40%	76%	82%	100%
Discharge Instructions[1]	19	58%	55%	61%	93%
Evaluation of LVS Function	32	72%	71%	83%	99%
Smoking Cessation Advice[1]	6	33%	73%	82%	100%
Pneumonia Care					
Appropriate Initial Antibiotic	29	52%	81%	83%	94%
Blood Culture Timing[1]	6	100%	91%	90%	100%
Influenza Vaccine[1]	15	60%	72%	70%	100%
Initial Antibiotic Timing	52	60%	82%	80%	93%
Oxygenation Assessment	56	100%	99%	99%	100%
Pneumococcal Vaccine	39	56%	68%	69%	94%
Smoking Cessation Advice[1]	14	29%	72%	80%	100%
Surgical Infection Prevention					
Prophylactic Antibiotic Given[5]	-	-	75%	77%	95%
Prophylactic Antibiotic Selection[5]	-	-	88%	90%	100%
Prophylactic Antibiotic Stopped[5]	-	-	82%	72%	95%
Pregnancy Care					
Inpatient Neonatal Mortality	-	-	-	-	-
Third or Fourth Degree Laceration	-	-	-	3.63%	3.27%

Cordell Memorial Hospital

1220 N Glenn English
Cordell, OK 73632
Ownership: Govt - Hospital District or Authority
Emergency Services: Yes

Phone: 580-832-3339
Fax: 580-832-5076
Accredited: No
Licensed Beds: 35

Measure	Cases	This Hospital	State Average	U.S. Average	Top Hospital
Heart Attack Care					
ACE Inhibitor or ARB for LVSD[3]	0	-	79%	82%	100%
Aspirin at Arrival[3]	0	-	86%	92%	100%
Aspirin at Discharge[3]	0	-	85%	90%	100%
Beta Blocker at Arrival[3]	0	-	78%	87%	100%
Beta Blocker at Discharge[3]	0	-	78%	90%	100%
Fibrinolytic Medication Timing[1,3]	1	100%	36%	31%	100%
PCI Within 90 Minutes of Arrival	0	-	51%	54%	95%
Smoking Cessation Advice[3]	0	-	83%	88%	100%
Heart Failure Care					
ACE Inhibitor or ARB for LVSD[1]	1	100%	76%	82%	100%
Discharge Instructions[1]	3	33%	55%	61%	93%
Evaluation of LVS Function[1]	5	40%	71%	83%	99%
Smoking Cessation Advice	0	-	73%	82%	100%
Pneumonia Care					
Appropriate Initial Antibiotic[1]	5	100%	81%	83%	94%
Blood Culture Timing[1]	1	100%	91%	90%	100%
Influenza Vaccine[1]	1	100%	72%	70%	100%
Initial Antibiotic Timing[1]	9	89%	82%	80%	93%
Oxygenation Assessment[1]	13	100%	99%	99%	100%

NOTE: Hospital profiles are in alphabetical order by state, then city, then hospital within the city; Rankings are sorted by rate in descending order and exclude hospitals with less than 25 cases; (1) The number of cases is too small (n<25) for purposes of reliably predicting hospital performance; (2) Measure reflects the hospital's indication that its submission was based upon a sample of its relevant discharges; (3) Rate reflects fewer than the maximum possible quarters of data for the measure; (4) Inaccurate information submitted and suppressed for one or more quarters; (5) No data is available from the hospital for this measure; Please refer to the User's Guide for a full explanation of data

Measure	Cases	This Hospital	State Average	U.S. Average	Top Hospital
Pneumococcal Vaccine[1]	10	70%	68%	69%	94%
Smoking Cessation Advice[1]	2	50%	72%	80%	100%
Surgical Infection Prevention					
Prophylactic Antibiotic Given[5]	-	-	75%	77%	95%
Prophylactic Antibiotic Selection[5]	-	-	88%	90%	100%
Prophylactic Antibiotic Stopped[5]	-	-	82%	72%	95%
Pregnancy Care					
Inpatient Neonatal Mortality	-	-	-	-	-
Third or Fourth Degree Laceration	-	-	-	3.63%	3.27%

Cushing Regional Hospital

1027 E Cherry
Cushing, OK 74023
URL: www.hillcrest.com
Ownership: Proprietary
Emergency Services: Yes

Phone: 918-225-2915
Fax: 918-225-8202

Accredited: Yes
Licensed Beds: 99

Key Personnel:

Administrator/CEO . . . . Ron Cackler
Chief Medical Staff. . . . . Marylin Peck
Emergency Room . . . . Tom Dotson, MD
Director Infection/Disease Control . . . . Bernadine Allen, RN
Director of Respiratory Therapy . . . . Jim Cephart

Measure	Cases	This Hospital	State Average	U.S. Average	Top Hospital
Heart Attack Care					
ACE Inhibitor or ARB for LVSD[1]	1	100%	79%	82%	100%
Aspirin at Arrival[1]	2	50%	86%	92%	100%
Aspirin at Discharge[1]	2	100%	85%	90%	100%
Beta Blocker at Arrival[1]	4	100%	78%	87%	100%
Beta Blocker at Discharge[1]	4	100%	78%	90%	100%
Fibrinolytic Medication Timing	0	-	36%	31%	100%
PCI Within 90 Minutes of Arrival	0	-	51%	54%	95%
Smoking Cessation Advice[1]	2	50%	83%	88%	100%
Heart Failure Care					
ACE Inhibitor or ARB for LVSD[1]	16	62%	76%	82%	100%
Discharge Instructions	61	11%	55%	61%	93%
Evaluation of LVS Function	81	43%	71%	83%	99%
Smoking Cessation Advice[1]	12	92%	73%	82%	100%
Pneumonia Care					
Appropriate Initial Antibiotic	91	75%	81%	83%	94%
Blood Culture Timing	60	88%	91%	90%	100%
Influenza Vaccine	35	49%	72%	70%	100%
Initial Antibiotic Timing	113	92%	82%	80%	93%
Oxygenation Assessment	151	100%	99%	99%	100%
Pneumococcal Vaccine	92	51%	68%	69%	94%
Smoking Cessation Advice	47	70%	72%	80%	100%
Surgical Infection Prevention					
Prophylactic Antibiotic Given[3]	58	76%	75%	77%	95%
Prophylactic Antibiotic Selection	27	96%	88%	90%	100%
Prophylactic Antibiotic Stopped[3]	58	97%	82%	72%	95%
Pregnancy Care					
Inpatient Neonatal Mortality	-	-	-	-	-
Third or Fourth Degree Laceration	-	-	-	3.63%	3.27%

Drumright Regional Hospital

610 West Bypass
Drumright, OK 74030
Ownership: Proprietary
Emergency Services: Yes

Phone: 918-382-2300

Accredited: No

Measure	Cases	This Hospital	State Average	U.S. Average	Top Hospital
Heart Attack Care					
ACE Inhibitor or ARB for LVSD[3]	0	-	79%	82%	100%
Aspirin at Arrival[1,3]	1	100%	86%	92%	100%
Aspirin at Discharge[1,3]	1	100%	85%	90%	100%
Beta Blocker at Arrival[1,3]	1	100%	78%	87%	100%
Beta Blocker at Discharge[1,3]	1	100%	78%	90%	100%
Fibrinolytic Medication Timing[3]	0	-	36%	31%	100%
PCI Within 90 Minutes of Arrival[5]	-	-	51%	54%	95%
Smoking Cessation Advice[3]	0	-	83%	88%	100%
Heart Failure Care					
ACE Inhibitor or ARB for LVSD[1]	3	0%	76%	82%	100%
Discharge Instructions[1]	15	67%	55%	61%	93%
Evaluation of LVS Function[1]	17	35%	71%	83%	99%
Smoking Cessation Advice[1]	1	100%	73%	82%	100%
Pneumonia Care					
Appropriate Initial Antibiotic	55	62%	81%	83%	94%
Blood Culture Timing[1]	2	50%	91%	90%	100%
Influenza Vaccine[1]	12	0%	72%	70%	100%
Initial Antibiotic Timing	67	81%	82%	80%	93%
Oxygenation Assessment	76	100%	99%	99%	100%
Pneumococcal Vaccine	37	5%	68%	69%	94%
Smoking Cessation Advice[1]	17	82%	72%	80%	100%
Surgical Infection Prevention					
Prophylactic Antibiotic Given[1,3]	14	36%	75%	77%	95%
Prophylactic Antibiotic Selection[1]	7	0%	88%	90%	100%
Prophylactic Antibiotic Stopped[1,3]	14	100%	82%	72%	95%
Pregnancy Care					
Inpatient Neonatal Mortality	-	-	-	-	-
Third or Fourth Degree Laceration	-	-	-	3.63%	3.27%

Duncan Regional Hospital

1407 Whisenant
Duncan, OK 73533
URL: www.duncanregional.com
Ownership: Proprietary
Emergency Services: No

Phone: 580-252-5300
Fax: 580-251-8559

Accredited: Yes
Licensed Beds: 152

Key Personnel:

President/CEO. . . . . Scott Street

Measure	Cases	This Hospital	State Average	U.S. Average	Top Hospital
Heart Attack Care					
ACE Inhibitor or ARB for LVSD[1]	4	100%	79%	82%	100%
Aspirin at Arrival	38	95%	86%	92%	100%
Aspirin at Discharge[1]	20	95%	85%	90%	100%
Beta Blocker at Arrival	30	97%	78%	87%	100%
Beta Blocker at Discharge[1]	19	100%	78%	90%	100%
Fibrinolytic Medication Timing[1]	4	75%	36%	31%	100%
PCI Within 90 Minutes of Arrival	0	-	51%	54%	95%
Smoking Cessation Advice[1]	5	60%	83%	88%	100%
Heart Failure Care					
ACE Inhibitor or ARB for LVSD	34	100%	76%	82%	100%
Discharge Instructions	99	95%	55%	61%	93%
Evaluation of LVS Function	144	97%	71%	83%	99%
Smoking Cessation Advice[1]	23	100%	73%	82%	100%
Pneumonia Care					
Appropriate Initial Antibiotic	138	91%	81%	83%	94%
Blood Culture Timing	147	95%	91%	90%	100%
Influenza Vaccine	53	87%	72%	70%	100%
Initial Antibiotic Timing	196	87%	82%	80%	93%
Oxygenation Assessment	249	100%	99%	99%	100%
Pneumococcal Vaccine	167	96%	68%	69%	94%
Smoking Cessation Advice	51	94%	72%	80%	100%
Surgical Infection Prevention					
Prophylactic Antibiotic Given[3]	158	92%	75%	77%	95%
Prophylactic Antibiotic Selection	49	92%	88%	90%	100%
Prophylactic Antibiotic Stopped[3]	152	53%	82%	72%	95%
Pregnancy Care					
Inpatient Neonatal Mortality	-	-	-	-	-
Third or Fourth Degree Laceration	-	-	-	3.63%	3.27%

Medical Center of Southeastern Oklahoma

Alternate Name: Medical Center of South East Oklahoma
1800 University Boulevard
Durant, OK 74701
E-mail: info@mcsohealth.com
URL: www.mcsohealth.com
Ownership: Proprietary
Emergency Services: Yes

Phone: 580-924-3080
Fax: 580-924-0422

Accredited: Yes
Licensed Beds: 103

Key Personnel:

CEO. . . . . Jackie Harms
Chief Medical Staff. . . . . Peter Hedberg, MD
Catheterization Lab . . . . Divek Khetpal, MD
Director Emergency Room. . . . . Jeanne Pirtle, RNC
Director Surgery Department . . . . Pat Ferreri, RN

NOTE: Hospital profiles are in alphabetical order by state, then city, then hospital within the city; Rankings are sorted by rate in descending order and exclude hospitals with less than 25 cases; (1) The number of cases is too small (n<25) for purposes of reliably predicting hospital performance; (2) Measure reflects the hospital's indication that its submission was based upon a sample of its relevant discharges; (3) Rate reflects fewer than the maximum possible quarters of data for the measure; (4) Inaccurate information submitted and suppressed for one or more quarters; (5) No data is available from the hospital for this measure; Please refer to the User's Guide for a full explanation of data

Director Radiology . . . . Terry Cayton
Director Cardiopulmonary . . . . Guy Dunaway, RRT

Measure	Cases	This Hospital	State Average	U.S. Average	Top Hospital
Heart Attack Care					
ACE Inhibitor or ARB for LVSD[1]	13	100%	79%	82%	100%
Aspirin at Arrival	54	98%	86%	92%	100%
Aspirin at Discharge	35	100%	85%	90%	100%
Beta Blocker at Arrival	42	98%	78%	87%	100%
Beta Blocker at Discharge	29	100%	78%	90%	100%
Fibrinolytic Medication Timing[1]	1	0%	36%	31%	100%
PCI Within 90 Minutes of Arrival	0	-	51%	54%	95%
Smoking Cessation Advice[1]	14	100%	83%	88%	100%
Heart Failure Care					
ACE Inhibitor or ARB for LVSD	76	100%	76%	82%	100%
Discharge Instructions	190	100%	55%	61%	93%
Evaluation of LVS Function	287	100%	71%	83%	99%
Smoking Cessation Advice	62	100%	73%	82%	100%
Pneumonia Care					
Appropriate Initial Antibiotic	166	72%	81%	83%	94%
Blood Culture Timing	142	100%	91%	90%	100%
Influenza Vaccine	66	100%	72%	70%	100%
Initial Antibiotic Timing	219	97%	82%	80%	93%
Oxygenation Assessment	299	100%	99%	99%	100%
Pneumococcal Vaccine	153	100%	68%	69%	94%
Smoking Cessation Advice	84	99%	72%	80%	100%
Surgical Infection Prevention					
Prophylactic Antibiotic Given[2]	147	91%	75%	77%	95%
Prophylactic Antibiotic Selection[2]	27	100%	88%	90%	100%
Prophylactic Antibiotic Stopped[2]	143	81%	82%	72%	95%
Pregnancy Care					
Inpatient Neonatal Mortality	-	-	-	-	-
Third or Fourth Degree Laceration	-	-	-	3.63%	3.27%

Edmond Medical Center

Alternate Name: Edmond Regional Medical Center
One S Bryant Street
Edmond, OK 73034
Ownership: Proprietary
Emergency Services: Yes
Phone: 405-341-6100
Fax: 405-359-5500
Accredited: Yes
Licensed Beds: 84

Key Personnel:

Administrator/CEO . . . . Stanley D Tatum
Chief Medical Staff . . . . Gary Hill, MD
Emergency Room . . . . Teresa Griffin
Director Infection/Disease Control . . . . Barbara McConnell
Director Medical/Surgical Nursing . . . . Cynde Wilson
Chief Radiology . . . . Cleo Hunt

Measure	Cases	This Hospital	State Average	U.S. Average	Top Hospital
Heart Attack Care					
ACE Inhibitor or ARB for LVSD[1]	2	100%	79%	82%	100%
Aspirin at Arrival	34	97%	86%	92%	100%
Aspirin at Discharge[1]	21	95%	85%	90%	100%
Beta Blocker at Arrival	30	83%	78%	87%	100%
Beta Blocker at Discharge	26	85%	78%	90%	100%
Fibrinolytic Medication Timing	0	-	36%	31%	100%
PCI Within 90 Minutes of Arrival	0	-	51%	54%	95%
Smoking Cessation Advice[1]	8	100%	83%	88%	100%
Heart Failure Care					
ACE Inhibitor or ARB for LVSD	26	81%	76%	82%	100%
Discharge Instructions	55	45%	55%	61%	93%
Evaluation of LVS Function	71	80%	71%	83%	99%
Smoking Cessation Advice[1]	9	100%	73%	82%	100%
Pneumonia Care					
Appropriate Initial Antibiotic	71	73%	81%	83%	94%
Blood Culture Timing	64	94%	91%	90%	100%
Influenza Vaccine	25	88%	72%	70%	100%
Initial Antibiotic Timing	97	76%	82%	80%	93%
Oxygenation Assessment	112	98%	99%	99%	100%
Pneumococcal Vaccine	67	87%	68%	69%	94%
Smoking Cessation Advice[1]	19	100%	72%	80%	100%
Surgical Infection Prevention					
Prophylactic Antibiotic Given[2,3]	115	77%	75%	77%	95%
Prophylactic Antibiotic Selection[2]	49	86%	88%	90%	100%
Prophylactic Antibiotic Stopped[2,3]	105	80%	82%	72%	95%
Pregnancy Care					
Inpatient Neonatal Mortality	-	-	-	-	-
Third or Fourth Degree Laceration	-	-	-	3.63%	3.27%

Foundation Bariatric Hospital of Oklahoma

1800 South Renaissance Boulevard
Edmond, OK 73034
Ownership: Proprietary
Emergency Services: No
Phone: 405-359-2400
Accredited: No

Measure	Cases	This Hospital	State Average	U.S. Average	Top Hospital
Heart Attack Care					
ACE Inhibitor or ARB for LVSD[5]	-	-	79%	82%	100%
Aspirin at Arrival[5]	-	-	86%	92%	100%
Aspirin at Discharge[5]	-	-	85%	90%	100%
Beta Blocker at Arrival[5]	-	-	78%	87%	100%
Beta Blocker at Discharge[5]	-	-	78%	90%	100%
Fibrinolytic Medication Timing[5]	-	-	36%	31%	100%
PCI Within 90 Minutes of Arrival[5]	-	-	51%	54%	95%
Smoking Cessation Advice[5]	-	-	83%	88%	100%
Heart Failure Care					
ACE Inhibitor or ARB for LVSD[5]	-	-	76%	82%	100%
Discharge Instructions[5]	-	-	55%	61%	93%
Evaluation of LVS Function[5]	-	-	71%	83%	99%
Smoking Cessation Advice[5]	-	-	73%	82%	100%
Pneumonia Care					
Appropriate Initial Antibiotic[5]	-	-	81%	83%	94%
Blood Culture Timing[5]	-	-	91%	90%	100%
Influenza Vaccine[5]	-	-	72%	70%	100%
Initial Antibiotic Timing[5]	-	-	82%	80%	93%
Oxygenation Assessment[5]	-	-	99%	99%	100%
Pneumococcal Vaccine[5]	-	-	68%	69%	94%
Smoking Cessation Advice[5]	-	-	72%	80%	100%
Surgical Infection Prevention					
Prophylactic Antibiotic Given[5]	-	-	75%	77%	95%
Prophylactic Antibiotic Selection[5]	-	-	88%	90%	100%
Prophylactic Antibiotic Stopped[5]	-	-	82%	72%	95%
Pregnancy Care					
Inpatient Neonatal Mortality	-	-	-	-	-
Third or Fourth Degree Laceration	-	-	-	3.63%	3.27%

Parkview Hospital

2115 Park View Drive
El Reno, OK 73036
URL: www.parkview-hospital.com
Ownership: Govt - Hospital District or Authority
Emergency Services: Yes
Phone: 405-262-2640
Fax: 405-422-2521
Accredited: No
Licensed Beds: 54

Key Personnel:

CEO/Administrator . . . . Lex Smith
Chief Medical Staff . . . . Dr Michael Sullivan
Director Radiology . . . . Kathy Burroughs, RT(R)
Director Respiratory Therapy . . . . Randy Dudley, RRT

Measure	Cases	This Hospital	State Average	U.S. Average	Top Hospital
Heart Attack Care					
ACE Inhibitor or ARB for LVSD[1,3]	1	0%	79%	82%	100%
Aspirin at Arrival[1,3]	5	40%	86%	92%	100%
Aspirin at Discharge[1,3]	3	67%	85%	90%	100%
Beta Blocker at Arrival[1,3]	4	50%	78%	87%	100%
Beta Blocker at Discharge[1,3]	3	67%	78%	90%	100%
Fibrinolytic Medication Timing[3]	0	-	36%	31%	100%
PCI Within 90 Minutes of Arrival	0	-	51%	54%	95%
Smoking Cessation Advice[1,3]	2	50%	83%	88%	100%
Heart Failure Care					
ACE Inhibitor or ARB for LVSD[1]	1	0%	76%	82%	100%
Discharge Instructions[1]	14	29%	55%	61%	93%
Evaluation of LVS Function[1]	22	64%	71%	83%	99%
Smoking Cessation Advice[1]	2	50%	73%	82%	100%
Pneumonia Care					

NOTE: Hospital profiles are in alphabetical order by state, then city, then hospital within the city; Rankings are sorted by rate in descending order and exclude hospitals with less than 25 cases; (1) The number of cases is too small (n<25) for purposes of reliably predicting hospital performance; (2) Measure reflects the hospital's indication that its submission was based upon a sample of its relevant discharges; (3) Rate reflects fewer than the maximum possible quarters of data for the measure; (4) Inaccurate information submitted and suppressed for one or more quarters; (5) No data is available from the hospital for this measure; Please refer to the User's Guide for a full explanation of data

Measure	Cases	This Hospital	State Average	U.S. Average	Top Hospital
Appropriate Initial Antibiotic	58	76%	81%	83%	94%
Blood Culture Timing	33	85%	91%	90%	100%
Influenza Vaccine[1]	17	88%	72%	70%	100%
Initial Antibiotic Timing	76	88%	82%	80%	93%
Oxygenation Assessment	95	99%	99%	99%	100%
Pneumococcal Vaccine	51	94%	68%	69%	94%
Smoking Cessation Advice[1]	23	83%	72%	80%	100%
Surgical Infection Prevention					
Prophylactic Antibiotic Given[1]	15	93%	75%	77%	95%
Prophylactic Antibiotic Selection[1]	1	100%	88%	90%	100%
Prophylactic Antibiotic Stopped[1]	12	100%	82%	72%	95%
Pregnancy Care					
Inpatient Neonatal Mortality	-	-	-	-	-
Third or Fourth Degree Laceration	-	-	-	3.63%	3.27%

Great Plains Regional Medical Center

Alternate Name: Community Hospital
1705 West 2nd Street
PO Box 2339
Elk City, OK 73644
Phone: 580-225-2511
Fax: 580-225-9143
URL: www.gprmc-ok.com
Ownership: Voluntary non-profit - Private
Accredited: Yes
Emergency Services: Yes
Licensed Beds: 84

Key Personnel:

CEO . . . . Robin Lake
Emergency Room Manager . . . . Larry Mack, RN
Director Medical Surgery . . . . Sissy Burch
Director Women/Children . . . . Linda Dozhler
Director Surgical Services . . . . Gwen Fuchs

Measure	Cases	This Hospital	State Average	U.S. Average	Top Hospital
Heart Attack Care					
ACE Inhibitor or ARB for LVSD	0	-	79%	82%	100%
Aspirin at Arrival[1]	13	100%	86%	92%	100%
Aspirin at Discharge[1]	6	83%	85%	90%	100%
Beta Blocker at Arrival[1]	13	85%	78%	87%	100%
Beta Blocker at Discharge[1]	8	88%	78%	90%	100%
Fibrinolytic Medication Timing[1]	4	25%	36%	31%	100%
PCI Within 90 Minutes of Arrival	0	-	51%	54%	95%
Smoking Cessation Advice[1]	2	100%	83%	88%	100%
Heart Failure Care					
ACE Inhibitor or ARB for LVSD	34	88%	76%	82%	100%
Discharge Instructions	58	55%	55%	61%	93%
Evaluation of LVS Function	82	94%	71%	83%	99%
Smoking Cessation Advice[1]	7	86%	73%	82%	100%
Pneumonia Care					
Appropriate Initial Antibiotic	68	78%	81%	83%	94%
Blood Culture Timing	68	93%	91%	90%	100%
Influenza Vaccine[4,5]	-	-	72%	70%	100%
Initial Antibiotic Timing	115	78%	82%	80%	93%
Oxygenation Assessment	133	99%	99%	99%	100%
Pneumococcal Vaccine	91	74%	68%	69%	94%
Smoking Cessation Advice	33	79%	72%	80%	100%
Surgical Infection Prevention					
Prophylactic Antibiotic Given[3]	85	55%	75%	77%	95%
Prophylactic Antibiotic Selection	26	81%	88%	90%	100%
Prophylactic Antibiotic Stopped[3]	78	35%	82%	72%	95%
Pregnancy Care					
Inpatient Neonatal Mortality	-	-	-	-	-
Third or Fourth Degree Laceration	-	-	-	3.63%	3.27%

Integris Bass Baptist Health Center

Alternate Name: Bass Memorial Baptist Hospital
600 S Monroe
PO Box 3168
Enid, OK 73701
Phone: 580-233-2300
Fax: 580-233-8922
URL: www.integris-health.com/facilities
Ownership: Voluntary non-profit - Private
Accredited: Yes
Emergency Services: Yes
Licensed Beds: 253

Key Personnel:

Administrator . . . . Tom Cunningham

Measure	Cases	This Hospital	State Average	U.S. Average	Top Hospital
Heart Attack Care					
ACE Inhibitor or ARB for LVSD[1]	9	78%	79%	82%	100%
Aspirin at Arrival	69	99%	86%	92%	100%
Aspirin at Discharge	74	92%	85%	90%	100%
Beta Blocker at Arrival	60	93%	78%	87%	100%
Beta Blocker at Discharge	71	87%	78%	90%	100%
Fibrinolytic Medication Timing[1]	6	0%	36%	31%	100%
PCI Within 90 Minutes of Arrival[1]	3	100%	51%	54%	95%
Smoking Cessation Advice	35	100%	83%	88%	100%
Heart Failure Care					
ACE Inhibitor or ARB for LVSD[1]	18	89%	76%	82%	100%
Discharge Instructions	67	94%	55%	61%	93%
Evaluation of LVS Function	110	89%	71%	83%	99%
Smoking Cessation Advice[1]	15	100%	73%	82%	100%
Pneumonia Care					
Appropriate Initial Antibiotic	105	83%	81%	83%	94%
Blood Culture Timing	95	86%	91%	90%	100%
Influenza Vaccine	37	92%	72%	70%	100%
Initial Antibiotic Timing	119	92%	82%	80%	93%
Oxygenation Assessment	159	100%	99%	99%	100%
Pneumococcal Vaccine	98	88%	68%	69%	94%
Smoking Cessation Advice	44	98%	72%	80%	100%
Surgical Infection Prevention					
Prophylactic Antibiotic Given	288	91%	75%	77%	95%
Prophylactic Antibiotic Selection	73	97%	88%	90%	100%
Prophylactic Antibiotic Stopped	283	92%	82%	72%	95%
Pregnancy Care					
Inpatient Neonatal Mortality	-	-	-	-	-
Third or Fourth Degree Laceration	-	-	-	3.63%	3.27%

Saint Mary's Regional Medical Center

305 South 5th
Enid, OK 73701
Phone: 580-233-6100
Fax: 580-249-3982
URL: www.stmarysregional.com
Ownership: Proprietary
Accredited: Yes
Emergency Services: Yes
Licensed Beds: 245

Key Personnel:

CEO . . . . Rick Wallace
Director Cardio-Pulmonary Services . . . . Kent Jordan
Director Catheterization Lab . . . . Bob Brice
Intensive/Coronary Care . . . . Virginia McCall
Director Medical/Surgical Nursing . . . . Kathy Niswander
Director Maternal Care . . . . Linda Milacek
Director Surgical Services . . . . Rosalie Purdy
Surgical Materials Manager . . . . Robert Ritter
Director Radiology . . . . Robert Brice
Respiratory/Cardiopulmonary . . . . Paul Lindner

Measure	Cases	This Hospital	State Average	U.S. Average	Top Hospital
Heart Attack Care					
ACE Inhibitor or ARB for LVSD[1]	17	88%	79%	82%	100%
Aspirin at Arrival	71	93%	86%	92%	100%
Aspirin at Discharge	72	86%	85%	90%	100%
Beta Blocker at Arrival	56	77%	78%	87%	100%
Beta Blocker at Discharge	69	84%	78%	90%	100%
Fibrinolytic Medication Timing	0	-	36%	31%	100%
PCI Within 90 Minutes of Arrival[1]	4	50%	51%	54%	95%
Smoking Cessation Advice[1]	23	96%	83%	88%	100%
Heart Failure Care					
ACE Inhibitor or ARB for LVSD	55	62%	76%	82%	100%
Discharge Instructions	149	95%	55%	61%	93%
Evaluation of LVS Function	212	67%	71%	83%	99%
Smoking Cessation Advice[1]	22	100%	73%	82%	100%
Pneumonia Care					
Appropriate Initial Antibiotic	92	86%	81%	83%	94%
Blood Culture Timing	74	96%	91%	90%	100%
Influenza Vaccine	48	83%	72%	70%	100%
Initial Antibiotic Timing	162	85%	82%	80%	93%
Oxygenation Assessment	193	100%	99%	99%	100%
Pneumococcal Vaccine	140	85%	68%	69%	94%
Smoking Cessation Advice	32	84%	72%	80%	100%
Surgical Infection Prevention					
Prophylactic Antibiotic Given	379	90%	75%	77%	95%

NOTE: Hospital profiles are in alphabetical order by state, then city, then hospital within the city; Rankings are sorted by rate in descending order and exclude hospitals with less than 25 cases; (1) The number of cases is too small (n<25) for purposes of reliably predicting hospital performance; (2) Measure reflects the hospital's indication that its submission was based upon a sample of its relevant discharges; (3) Rate reflects fewer than the maximum possible quarters of data for the measure; (4) Inaccurate information submitted and suppressed for one or more quarters; (5) No data is available from the hospital for this measure; Please refer to the User's Guide for a full explanation of data

Prophylactic Antibiotic Selection	105	92%	88%	90%	100%
Prophylactic Antibiotic Stopped	360	86%	82%	72%	95%
Pregnancy Care					
Inpatient Neonatal Mortality	-	-	-	-	-
Third or Fourth Degree Laceration	-	-	-	3.63%	3.27%

Community Hospital Lakeview

One Hospital Drive
Eufaula, OK 74432
Ownership: Proprietary
Emergency Services: Yes
Phone: 918-689-2535
Fax: 918-689-7285
Accredited: No
Licensed Beds: 33

Key Personnel:
CEO. . . . . Daniel Schaecvle
Emergency Room . . . . Razzi Djevalikian, MD
Emergency Room . . . . Dorothy Merrick
Infection Control. . . . . Dorothy Merrick

Measure	Cases	This Hospital	State Average	U.S. Average	Top Hospital
Heart Attack Care					
ACE Inhibitor or ARB for LVSD[5]	-	-	79%	82%	100%
Aspirin at Arrival[5]	-	-	86%	92%	100%
Aspirin at Discharge[5]	-	-	85%	90%	100%
Beta Blocker at Arrival[5]	-	-	78%	87%	100%
Beta Blocker at Discharge[5]	-	-	78%	90%	100%
Fibrinolytic Medication Timing[5]	-	-	36%	31%	100%
PCI Within 90 Minutes of Arrival[5]	-	-	51%	54%	95%
Smoking Cessation Advice[5]	-	-	83%	88%	100%
Heart Failure Care					
ACE Inhibitor or ARB for LVSD[3]	0	-	76%	82%	100%
Discharge Instructions[1,3]	2	0%	55%	61%	93%
Evaluation of LVS Function[1,3]	5	0%	71%	83%	99%
Smoking Cessation Advice[1,3]	1	0%	73%	82%	100%
Pneumonia Care					
Appropriate Initial Antibiotic[1]	3	67%	81%	83%	94%
Blood Culture Timing	0	-	91%	90%	100%
Influenza Vaccine[1]	1	0%	72%	70%	100%
Initial Antibiotic Timing[1]	1	100%	82%	80%	93%
Oxygenation Assessment[1]	4	100%	99%	99%	100%
Pneumococcal Vaccine[1]	4	0%	68%	69%	94%
Smoking Cessation Advice[1]	2	0%	72%	80%	100%
Surgical Infection Prevention					
Prophylactic Antibiotic Given[5]	-	-	75%	77%	95%
Prophylactic Antibiotic Selection[5]	-	-	88%	90%	100%
Prophylactic Antibiotic Stopped[5]	-	-	82%	72%	95%
Pregnancy Care					
Inpatient Neonatal Mortality	-	-	-	-	-
Third or Fourth Degree Laceration	-	-	-	3.63%	3.27%

Fairfax Memorial Hospital

Highway 18 & Taft
Fairfax, OK 74637
Ownership: Proprietary
Emergency Services: Yes
Toll-Free: 877-770-8349
Phone: 918-642-3291
Fax: 918-642-5161
Accredited: No
Licensed Beds: 21

Key Personnel:
CEO. . . . . Emory Brutigan
Chief Medical Staff. . . . . James Graham

Measure	Cases	This Hospital	State Average	U.S. Average	Top Hospital
Heart Attack Care					
ACE Inhibitor or ARB for LVSD[5]	-	-	79%	82%	100%
Aspirin at Arrival[5]	-	-	86%	92%	100%
Aspirin at Discharge[5]	-	-	85%	90%	100%
Beta Blocker at Arrival[5]	-	-	78%	87%	100%
Beta Blocker at Discharge[5]	-	-	78%	90%	100%
Fibrinolytic Medication Timing[5]	-	-	36%	31%	100%
PCI Within 90 Minutes of Arrival[5]	-	-	51%	54%	95%
Smoking Cessation Advice[5]	-	-	83%	88%	100%
Heart Failure Care					
ACE Inhibitor or ARB for LVSD[1]	3	100%	76%	82%	100%
Discharge Instructions[1]	1	100%	55%	61%	93%
Evaluation of LVS Function[1]	5	100%	71%	83%	99%
Smoking Cessation Advice	0	-	73%	82%	100%
Pneumonia Care					
Appropriate Initial Antibiotic	26	92%	81%	83%	94%
Blood Culture Timing[1]	13	100%	91%	90%	100%
Influenza Vaccine[1]	9	100%	72%	70%	100%
Initial Antibiotic Timing	28	96%	82%	80%	93%
Oxygenation Assessment	34	100%	99%	99%	100%
Pneumococcal Vaccine[1]	18	89%	68%	69%	94%
Smoking Cessation Advice[1]	16	100%	72%	80%	100%
Surgical Infection Prevention					
Prophylactic Antibiotic Given[5]	-	-	75%	77%	95%
Prophylactic Antibiotic Selection[5]	-	-	88%	90%	100%
Prophylactic Antibiotic Stopped[5]	-	-	82%	72%	95%
Pregnancy Care					
Inpatient Neonatal Mortality	-	-	-	-	-
Third or Fourth Degree Laceration	-	-	-	3.63%	3.27%

Fairview Hospital

523 E State Road
Fairview, OK 73737
Ownership: Government - Local
Emergency Services: Yes
Phone: 580-227-3721
Fax: 580-227-2882
Accredited: No
Licensed Beds: 31

Key Personnel:
CEO/President. . . . . Randy Sauder
Chief of Medical Staff. . . . . Kathy Cain

Measure	Cases	This Hospital	State Average	U.S. Average	Top Hospital
Heart Attack Care					
ACE Inhibitor or ARB for LVSD[5]	-	-	79%	82%	100%
Aspirin at Arrival[5]	-	-	86%	92%	100%
Aspirin at Discharge[5]	-	-	85%	90%	100%
Beta Blocker at Arrival[5]	-	-	78%	87%	100%
Beta Blocker at Discharge[5]	-	-	78%	90%	100%
Fibrinolytic Medication Timing[5]	-	-	36%	31%	100%
PCI Within 90 Minutes of Arrival[5]	-	-	51%	54%	95%
Smoking Cessation Advice[5]	-	-	83%	88%	100%
Heart Failure Care					
ACE Inhibitor or ARB for LVSD	0	-	76%	82%	100%
Discharge Instructions[1]	7	14%	55%	61%	93%
Evaluation of LVS Function[1]	11	9%	71%	83%	99%
Smoking Cessation Advice	0	-	73%	82%	100%
Pneumonia Care					
Appropriate Initial Antibiotic[1]	22	82%	81%	83%	94%
Blood Culture Timing[1]	3	67%	91%	90%	100%
Influenza Vaccine[4,5]	-	-	72%	70%	100%
Initial Antibiotic Timing[1]	21	76%	82%	80%	93%
Oxygenation Assessment	33	100%	99%	99%	100%
Pneumococcal Vaccine	25	4%	68%	69%	94%
Smoking Cessation Advice[1]	2	0%	72%	80%	100%
Surgical Infection Prevention					
Prophylactic Antibiotic Given[5]	-	-	75%	77%	95%
Prophylactic Antibiotic Selection[5]	-	-	88%	90%	100%
Prophylactic Antibiotic Stopped[5]	-	-	82%	72%	95%
Pregnancy Care					
Inpatient Neonatal Mortality	-	-	-	-	-
Third or Fourth Degree Laceration	-	-	-	3.63%	3.27%

Memorial Hospital

319 E Josephine
Frederick, OK 73542
Ownership: Voluntary non-profit - Other
Emergency Services: Yes
Phone: 580-335-7565
Fax: 580-335-7329
Accredited: No
Licensed Beds: 48

Key Personnel:
CEO. . . . . Al Allee

Measure	Cases	This Hospital	State Average	U.S. Average	Top Hospital
Heart Attack Care					
ACE Inhibitor or ARB for LVSD[3]	0	-	79%	82%	100%
Aspirin at Arrival[1,3]	1	0%	86%	92%	100%
Aspirin at Discharge[3]	0	-	85%	90%	100%
Beta Blocker at Arrival[1,3]	1	0%	78%	87%	100%
Beta Blocker at Discharge[1,3]	1	0%	78%	90%	100%

NOTE: Hospital profiles are in alphabetical order by state, then city, then hospital within the city; Rankings are sorted by rate in descending order and exclude hospitals with less than 25 cases; (1) The number of cases is too small (n<25) for purposes of reliably predicting hospital performance; (2) Measure reflects the hospital's indication that its submission was based upon a sample of its relevant discharges; (3) Rate reflects fewer than the maximum possible quarters of data for the measure; (4) Inaccurate information submitted and suppressed for one or more quarters; (5) No data is available from the hospital for this measure; Please refer to the User's Guide for a full explanation of data

Measure	Cases	This Hospital	State Average	U.S. Average	Top Hospital
Fibrinolytic Medication Timing[3]	0	-	36%	31%	100%
PCI Within 90 Minutes of Arrival	0	-	51%	54%	95%
Smoking Cessation Advice[3]	0	-	83%	88%	100%
Heart Failure Care					
ACE Inhibitor or ARB for LVSD[1]	4	75%	76%	82%	100%
Discharge Instructions[1]	21	62%	55%	61%	93%
Evaluation of LVS Function	37	100%	71%	83%	99%
Smoking Cessation Advice[1]	8	62%	73%	82%	100%
Pneumonia Care					
Appropriate Initial Antibiotic	25	76%	81%	83%	94%
Blood Culture Timing[1]	1	100%	91%	90%	100%
Influenza Vaccine[1]	8	100%	72%	70%	100%
Initial Antibiotic Timing	31	84%	82%	80%	93%
Oxygenation Assessment	46	100%	99%	99%	100%
Pneumococcal Vaccine	31	87%	68%	69%	94%
Smoking Cessation Advice[1]	7	100%	72%	80%	100%
Surgical Infection Prevention					
Prophylactic Antibiotic Given[5]	-	-	75%	77%	95%
Prophylactic Antibiotic Selection[5]	-	-	88%	90%	100%
Prophylactic Antibiotic Stopped[5]	-	-	82%	72%	95%
Pregnancy Care					
Inpatient Neonatal Mortality	-	-	-	-	-
Third or Fourth Degree Laceration	-	-	-	3.63%	3.27%

Integris Grove General Hospital

1310 South Main Street
Grove, OK 74344
Phone: 918-786-2243
Fax: 918-787-3403
E-mail: mathje@integris-health.com
URL: www.integris-health.com
Ownership: Voluntary non-profit - Other
Accredited: Yes
Emergency Services: Yes
Licensed Beds: 72

Key Personnel:

President . . . . Greg L Martin
Chief Medical Staff . . . . James Buttler, MD
Emergency Room . . . . Diane Wilkie
Infection Control . . . . Debbie Lawson
OB/GYN Women's Health . . . . Zachary Bechtel, MD
Director Radiology . . . . John Winnie
Director Respiratory Therapy . . . . Stephanie Pigg

Measure	Cases	This Hospital	State Average	U.S. Average	Top Hospital
Heart Attack Care					
ACE Inhibitor or ARB for LVSD[1]	7	86%	79%	82%	100%
Aspirin at Arrival	37	95%	86%	92%	100%
Aspirin at Discharge	31	84%	85%	90%	100%
Beta Blocker at Arrival	32	91%	78%	87%	100%
Beta Blocker at Discharge	31	94%	78%	90%	100%
Fibrinolytic Medication Timing[1]	1	0%	36%	31%	100%
PCI Within 90 Minutes of Arrival	0	-	51%	54%	95%
Smoking Cessation Advice[1]	14	100%	83%	88%	100%
Heart Failure Care					
ACE Inhibitor or ARB for LVSD[1]	22	86%	76%	82%	100%
Discharge Instructions	70	93%	55%	61%	93%
Evaluation of LVS Function	103	91%	71%	83%	99%
Smoking Cessation Advice	26	100%	73%	82%	100%
Pneumonia Care					
Appropriate Initial Antibiotic	118	86%	81%	83%	94%
Blood Culture Timing	117	95%	91%	90%	100%
Influenza Vaccine	52	83%	72%	70%	100%
Initial Antibiotic Timing	183	91%	82%	80%	93%
Oxygenation Assessment	195	100%	99%	99%	100%
Pneumococcal Vaccine	137	94%	68%	69%	94%
Smoking Cessation Advice	44	100%	72%	80%	100%
Surgical Infection Prevention					
Prophylactic Antibiotic Given	173	97%	75%	77%	95%
Prophylactic Antibiotic Selection	44	100%	88%	90%	100%
Prophylactic Antibiotic Stopped	169	99%	82%	72%	95%
Pregnancy Care					
Inpatient Neonatal Mortality	-	-	-	-	-
Third or Fourth Degree Laceration	-	-	-	3.63%	3.27%

Logan Medical Center

200 South Academy Road
Guthrie, OK 73044
Phone: 405-282-6700
Fax: 405-282-6790
URL: www.loganhosp.com
Ownership: Govt - Hospital District or Authority
Accredited: Yes
Emergency Services: Yes

Key Personnel:

CEO . . . . Judy Freuquay
Chief Medical Staff . . . . Todd Krehbiel, MD
Emergency Room . . . . Ann Campbell, MD
Infection Control . . . . Kaye Freudenberger
Respiratory/Cardiopulmonary . . . . Mike Phillips

Measure	Cases	This Hospital	State Average	U.S. Average	Top Hospital
Heart Attack Care					
ACE Inhibitor or ARB for LVSD[1]	5	80%	79%	82%	100%
Aspirin at Arrival[1]	9	78%	86%	92%	100%
Aspirin at Discharge[1]	8	75%	85%	90%	100%
Beta Blocker at Arrival[1]	13	62%	78%	87%	100%
Beta Blocker at Discharge[1]	10	80%	78%	90%	100%
Fibrinolytic Medication Timing[1]	2	50%	36%	31%	100%
PCI Within 90 Minutes of Arrival	0	-	51%	54%	95%
Smoking Cessation Advice[1]	1	0%	83%	88%	100%
Heart Failure Care					
ACE Inhibitor or ARB for LVSD[1]	15	100%	76%	82%	100%
Discharge Instructions[1]	12	33%	55%	61%	93%
Evaluation of LVS Function	39	79%	71%	83%	99%
Smoking Cessation Advice[1]	10	50%	73%	82%	100%
Pneumonia Care					
Appropriate Initial Antibiotic	40	88%	81%	83%	94%
Blood Culture Timing	28	96%	91%	90%	100%
Influenza Vaccine[1]	10	50%	72%	70%	100%
Initial Antibiotic Timing	45	93%	82%	80%	93%
Oxygenation Assessment	57	100%	99%	99%	100%
Pneumococcal Vaccine	38	79%	68%	69%	94%
Smoking Cessation Advice[1]	16	50%	72%	80%	100%
Surgical Infection Prevention					
Prophylactic Antibiotic Given[5]	-	-	75%	77%	95%
Prophylactic Antibiotic Selection[5]	-	-	88%	90%	100%
Prophylactic Antibiotic Stopped[5]	-	-	82%	72%	95%
Pregnancy Care					
Inpatient Neonatal Mortality	-	-	-	-	-
Third or Fourth Degree Laceration	-	-	-	3.63%	3.27%

Memorial Hospital of Texas County

520 Medical Drive
Guymon, OK 73942
Phone: 580-338-3113
Fax: 580-338-5722
E-mail: mhtchr@iptsi.net
URL: www.memorialhosp.net
Ownership: Government - Local
Accredited: No
Emergency Services: Yes
Licensed Beds: 47

Key Personnel:

CEO . . . . Tim Starkey
Chief Medical Staff . . . . Kelly McNurry
Director Infection/Disease Control . . . . Julie West
Director Medical/Surgical Nursing . . . . Jane Boothby
Director Respiratory Therapy . . . . Kim Ware

Measure	Cases	This Hospital	State Average	U.S. Average	Top Hospital
Heart Attack Care					
ACE Inhibitor or ARB for LVSD[1]	2	50%	79%	82%	100%
Aspirin at Arrival[1]	7	71%	86%	92%	100%
Aspirin at Discharge[1]	5	60%	85%	90%	100%
Beta Blocker at Arrival[1]	7	86%	78%	87%	100%
Beta Blocker at Discharge[1]	8	75%	78%	90%	100%
Fibrinolytic Medication Timing[1]	2	50%	36%	31%	100%
PCI Within 90 Minutes of Arrival	0	-	51%	54%	95%
Smoking Cessation Advice[1]	4	50%	83%	88%	100%
Heart Failure Care					
ACE Inhibitor or ARB for LVSD[1]	5	100%	76%	82%	100%
Discharge Instructions[1]	19	16%	55%	61%	93%
Evaluation of LVS Function[1]	24	21%	71%	83%	99%
Smoking Cessation Advice[1]	4	75%	73%	82%	100%

NOTE: Hospital profiles are in alphabetical order by state, then city, then hospital within the city; Rankings are sorted by rate in descending order and exclude hospitals with less than 25 cases; (1) The number of cases is too small (n<25) for purposes of reliably predicting hospital performance; (2) Measure reflects the hospital's indication that its submission was based upon a sample of its relevant discharges; (3) Rate reflects fewer than the maximum possible quarters of data for the measure; (4) Inaccurate information submitted and suppressed for one or more quarters; (5) No data is available from the hospital for this measure; Please refer to the User's Guide for a full explanation of data

Measure	Cases	This Hospital	State Average	U.S. Average	Top Hospital
Pneumonia Care					
Appropriate Initial Antibiotic[2]	88	65%	81%	83%	94%
Blood Culture Timing[1,2]	11	82%	91%	90%	100%
Influenza Vaccine	28	93%	72%	70%	100%
Initial Antibiotic Timing[2]	59	64%	82%	80%	93%
Oxygenation Assessment[2]	101	98%	99%	99%	100%
Pneumococcal Vaccine[2]	58	84%	68%	69%	94%
Smoking Cessation Advice[2]	26	27%	72%	80%	100%
Surgical Infection Prevention					
Prophylactic Antibiotic Given[1,3]	19	26%	75%	77%	95%
Prophylactic Antibiotic Selection[1]	7	100%	88%	90%	100%
Prophylactic Antibiotic Stopped[1,3]	17	59%	82%	72%	95%
Pregnancy Care					
Inpatient Neonatal Mortality	-	-	-	-	-
Third or Fourth Degree Laceration	-	-	-	3.63%	3.27%

Healdton Municipal Hospital

918 SW 8th
Healdton, OK 73438
Ownership: Proprietary
Emergency Services: Yes

Phone: 580-229-0701
Fax: 580-229-0691
Accredited: No
Licensed Beds: 28

Key Personnel:
CEO. . . . . Bob Thompson
Director Infection/Disease Control . . . . Larry Lovelace

Measure	Cases	This Hospital	State Average	U.S. Average	Top Hospital
Heart Attack Care					
ACE Inhibitor or ARB for LVSD[3]	0	-	79%	82%	100%
Aspirin at Arrival[3]	0	-	86%	92%	100%
Aspirin at Discharge[3]	0	-	85%	90%	100%
Beta Blocker at Arrival[3]	0	-	78%	87%	100%
Beta Blocker at Discharge[3]	0	-	78%	90%	100%
Fibrinolytic Medication Timing[3]	0	-	36%	31%	100%
PCI Within 90 Minutes of Arrival	0	-	51%	54%	95%
Smoking Cessation Advice[3]	0	-	83%	88%	100%
Heart Failure Care					
ACE Inhibitor or ARB for LVSD[1]	2	100%	76%	82%	100%
Discharge Instructions[1]	1	0%	55%	61%	93%
Evaluation of LVS Function[1]	7	43%	71%	83%	99%
Smoking Cessation Advice	0	-	73%	82%	100%
Pneumonia Care					
Appropriate Initial Antibiotic[1]	22	86%	81%	83%	94%
Blood Culture Timing[1]	5	100%	91%	90%	100%
Influenza Vaccine[1]	4	0%	72%	70%	100%
Initial Antibiotic Timing	28	71%	82%	80%	93%
Oxygenation Assessment	31	100%	99%	99%	100%
Pneumococcal Vaccine[1]	12	58%	68%	69%	94%
Smoking Cessation Advice[1]	4	0%	72%	80%	100%
Surgical Infection Prevention					
Prophylactic Antibiotic Given[5]	-	-	75%	77%	95%
Prophylactic Antibiotic Selection[5]	-	-	88%	90%	100%
Prophylactic Antibiotic Stopped[5]	-	-	82%	72%	95%
Pregnancy Care					
Inpatient Neonatal Mortality	-	-	-	-	-
Third or Fourth Degree Laceration	-	-	-	3.63%	3.27%

Henryetta Medical Center

Dewey Bartlett & Main Streets
Henryetta, OK 74437
Ownership: Proprietary
Emergency Services: Yes

Phone: 918-652-4463
Fax: 918-652-3675
Accredited: Yes
Licensed Beds: 52

Key Personnel:
Administrator/President . . . . James P Bailey
Chief Medical Staff. . . . . Brent Davis, DO
Emergency Room . . . . Brent Davis, DO
Director Infection/Disease Control . . . . Mike Patterson
CCU Spvg. Nurse . . . . Beth Witt, RN
Director Medical/Surgical Nursing . . . . Beth Witt, RN
Chief Radiology . . . . Dennis Pennington, MD
Director Respiratory Therapy . . . . Mike Patterson

Measure	Cases	This Hospital	State Average	U.S. Average	Top Hospital
Heart Attack Care					
ACE Inhibitor or ARB for LVSD[1]	1	0%	79%	82%	100%
Aspirin at Arrival[1]	5	100%	86%	92%	100%
Aspirin at Discharge[1]	3	67%	85%	90%	100%
Beta Blocker at Arrival[1]	5	60%	78%	87%	100%
Beta Blocker at Discharge[1]	3	67%	78%	90%	100%
Fibrinolytic Medication Timing	0	-	36%	31%	100%
PCI Within 90 Minutes of Arrival	0	-	51%	54%	95%
Smoking Cessation Advice	0	-	83%	88%	100%
Heart Failure Care					
ACE Inhibitor or ARB for LVSD[1]	17	76%	76%	82%	100%
Discharge Instructions	30	67%	55%	61%	93%
Evaluation of LVS Function	41	73%	71%	83%	99%
Smoking Cessation Advice[1]	9	100%	73%	82%	100%
Pneumonia Care					
Appropriate Initial Antibiotic	56	89%	81%	83%	94%
Blood Culture Timing	71	96%	91%	90%	100%
Influenza Vaccine	31	77%	72%	70%	100%
Initial Antibiotic Timing	80	98%	82%	80%	93%
Oxygenation Assessment	105	99%	99%	99%	100%
Pneumococcal Vaccine	70	76%	68%	69%	94%
Smoking Cessation Advice[1]	22	86%	72%	80%	100%
Surgical Infection Prevention					
Prophylactic Antibiotic Given[1,3]	22	86%	75%	77%	95%
Prophylactic Antibiotic Selection[1]	6	100%	88%	90%	100%
Prophylactic Antibiotic Stopped[1,3]	22	91%	82%	72%	95%
Pregnancy Care					
Inpatient Neonatal Mortality	-	-	-	-	-
Third or Fourth Degree Laceration	-	-	-	3.63%	3.27%

Elkview General Hospital

429 W Elm
Hobart, OK 73651
E-mail: bfinch@itlnet.net
Ownership: Government - Local
Emergency Services: Yes

Phone: 580-726-3324
Fax: 580-726-6041

Accredited: No
Licensed Beds: 50

Key Personnel:
Administrator . . . . Bill Finch

Measure	Cases	This Hospital	State Average	U.S. Average	Top Hospital
Heart Attack Care					
ACE Inhibitor or ARB for LVSD[3]	0	-	79%	82%	100%
Aspirin at Arrival[1,3]	5	100%	86%	92%	100%
Aspirin at Discharge[1,3]	1	100%	85%	90%	100%
Beta Blocker at Arrival[1,3]	5	60%	78%	87%	100%
Beta Blocker at Discharge[1,3]	1	100%	78%	90%	100%
Fibrinolytic Medication Timing[1,3]	1	100%	36%	31%	100%
PCI Within 90 Minutes of Arrival	0	-	51%	54%	95%
Smoking Cessation Advice[3]	0	-	83%	88%	100%
Heart Failure Care					
ACE Inhibitor or ARB for LVSD[1,3]	10	90%	76%	82%	100%
Discharge Instructions[1,3]	19	95%	55%	61%	93%
Evaluation of LVS Function[1,3]	24	92%	71%	83%	99%
Smoking Cessation Advice[1,3]	5	100%	73%	82%	100%
Pneumonia Care					
Appropriate Initial Antibiotic	32	100%	81%	83%	94%
Blood Culture Timing[1]	2	50%	91%	90%	100%
Influenza Vaccine[1]	6	83%	72%	70%	100%
Initial Antibiotic Timing	35	91%	82%	80%	93%
Oxygenation Assessment	43	100%	99%	99%	100%
Pneumococcal Vaccine[1]	23	100%	68%	69%	94%
Smoking Cessation Advice[1]	11	91%	72%	80%	100%
Surgical Infection Prevention					
Prophylactic Antibiotic Given[1,3]	9	89%	75%	77%	95%
Prophylactic Antibiotic Selection[1]	1	100%	88%	90%	100%
Prophylactic Antibiotic Stopped[1,3]	9	89%	82%	72%	95%
Pregnancy Care					
Inpatient Neonatal Mortality	-	-	-	-	-
Third or Fourth Degree Laceration	-	-	-	3.63%	3.27%

NOTE: Hospital profiles are in alphabetical order by state, then city, then hospital within the city; Rankings are sorted by rate in descending order and exclude hospitals with less than 25 cases; (1) The number of cases is too small (n<25) for purposes of reliably predicting hospital performance; (2) Measure reflects the hospital's indication that its submission was based upon a sample of its relevant discharges; (3) Rate reflects fewer than the maximum possible quarters of data for the measure; (4) Inaccurate information submitted and suppressed for one or more quarters; (5) No data is available from the hospital for this measure; Please refer to the User's Guide for a full explanation of data

Holdenville General Hospital

100 Mcdougal Drive
Holdenville, OK 74848
Ownership: Government - Local
Emergency Services: Yes
Phone: 405-379-4200
Accredited: No

Measure	Cases	This Hospital	State Average	U.S. Average	Top Hospital
Heart Attack Care					
ACE Inhibitor or ARB for LVSD[1,3]	1	100%	79%	82%	100%
Aspirin at Arrival[1,3]	2	0%	86%	92%	100%
Aspirin at Discharge[1,3]	1	100%	85%	90%	100%
Beta Blocker at Arrival[1,3]	2	50%	78%	87%	100%
Beta Blocker at Discharge[1,3]	1	0%	78%	90%	100%
Fibrinolytic Medication Timing[3]	0	-	36%	31%	100%
PCI Within 90 Minutes of Arrival	0	-	51%	54%	95%
Smoking Cessation Advice[3]	0	-	83%	88%	100%
Heart Failure Care					
ACE Inhibitor or ARB for LVSD[1]	8	100%	76%	82%	100%
Discharge Instructions	29	66%	55%	61%	93%
Evaluation of LVS Function	40	68%	71%	83%	99%
Smoking Cessation Advice[1]	6	50%	73%	82%	100%
Pneumonia Care					
Appropriate Initial Antibiotic	35	94%	81%	83%	94%
Blood Culture Timing	42	100%	91%	90%	100%
Influenza Vaccine[1]	20	95%	72%	70%	100%
Initial Antibiotic Timing	65	95%	82%	80%	93%
Oxygenation Assessment	74	100%	99%	99%	100%
Pneumococcal Vaccine	52	87%	68%	69%	94%
Smoking Cessation Advice[1]	18	67%	72%	80%	100%
Surgical Infection Prevention					
Prophylactic Antibiotic Given[5]	-	-	75%	77%	95%
Prophylactic Antibiotic Selection[5]	-	-	88%	90%	100%
Prophylactic Antibiotic Stopped[5]	-	-	82%	72%	95%
Pregnancy Care					
Inpatient Neonatal Mortality	-	-	-	-	-
Third or Fourth Degree Laceration	-	-	-	3.63%	3.27%

Harmon Memorial Hospital

400 E Chestnut Street
Hollis, OK 73550
Ownership: Govt - Hospital District or Authority
Emergency Services: Yes
Phone: 580-688-3363
Fax: 580-688-2246
Accredited: No
Licensed Beds: 31

Key Personnel:
President/CEO. . . . . Belly Burge
Director Infection/Disease Control . . . . Sheila Lewis

Measure	Cases	This Hospital	State Average	U.S. Average	Top Hospital
Heart Attack Care					
ACE Inhibitor or ARB for LVSD	0	-	79%	82%	100%
Aspirin at Arrival[1]	7	100%	86%	92%	100%
Aspirin at Discharge[1]	3	67%	85%	90%	100%
Beta Blocker at Arrival[1]	7	71%	78%	87%	100%
Beta Blocker at Discharge[1]	3	67%	78%	90%	100%
Fibrinolytic Medication Timing[1]	4	50%	36%	31%	100%
PCI Within 90 Minutes of Arrival	0	-	51%	54%	95%
Smoking Cessation Advice	0	-	83%	88%	100%
Heart Failure Care					
ACE Inhibitor or ARB for LVSD[1]	7	29%	76%	82%	100%
Discharge Instructions[1]	18	50%	55%	61%	93%
Evaluation of LVS Function	32	22%	71%	83%	99%
Smoking Cessation Advice[1]	5	60%	73%	82%	100%
Pneumonia Care					
Appropriate Initial Antibiotic	40	60%	81%	83%	94%
Blood Culture Timing[1]	9	89%	91%	90%	100%
Influenza Vaccine[1]	8	25%	72%	70%	100%
Initial Antibiotic Timing	85	80%	82%	80%	93%
Oxygenation Assessment	97	100%	99%	99%	100%
Pneumococcal Vaccine	61	30%	68%	69%	94%
Smoking Cessation Advice[1]	16	25%	72%	80%	100%
Surgical Infection Prevention					
Prophylactic Antibiotic Given[5]	-	-	75%	77%	95%
Prophylactic Antibiotic Selection[5]	-	-	88%	90%	100%
Prophylactic Antibiotic Stopped[5]	-	-	82%	72%	95%
Pregnancy Care					
Inpatient Neonatal Mortality	-	-	-	-	-
Third or Fourth Degree Laceration	-	-	-	3.63%	3.27%

Choctaw Memorial Hospital

1405 E Kirk
Hugo, OK 74743
Ownership: Govt - Hospital District or Authority
Emergency Services: Yes
Phone: 580-326-6414
Fax: 580-326-3541
Accredited: No
Licensed Beds: 34

Key Personnel:
CEO. . . . . Emmett Sthuster
Chief Medical Staff. . . . . Ted Rowland, MD

Measure	Cases	This Hospital	State Average	U.S. Average	Top Hospital
Heart Attack Care					
ACE Inhibitor or ARB for LVSD[1,3]	1	0%	79%	82%	100%
Aspirin at Arrival[1,3]	2	100%	86%	92%	100%
Aspirin at Discharge[1,3]	1	100%	85%	90%	100%
Beta Blocker at Arrival[1,3]	2	100%	78%	87%	100%
Beta Blocker at Discharge[1,3]	1	0%	78%	90%	100%
Fibrinolytic Medication Timing[3]	0	-	36%	31%	100%
PCI Within 90 Minutes of Arrival	0	-	51%	54%	95%
Smoking Cessation Advice[3]	0	-	83%	88%	100%
Heart Failure Care					
ACE Inhibitor or ARB for LVSD[1]	5	40%	76%	82%	100%
Discharge Instructions	67	40%	55%	61%	93%
Evaluation of LVS Function	95	27%	71%	83%	99%
Smoking Cessation Advice[1]	18	100%	73%	82%	100%
Pneumonia Care					
Appropriate Initial Antibiotic	64	84%	81%	83%	94%
Blood Culture Timing	38	79%	91%	90%	100%
Influenza Vaccine[1]	16	94%	72%	70%	100%
Initial Antibiotic Timing	87	79%	82%	80%	93%
Oxygenation Assessment	97	100%	99%	99%	100%
Pneumococcal Vaccine	48	79%	68%	69%	94%
Smoking Cessation Advice[1]	23	100%	72%	80%	100%
Surgical Infection Prevention					
Prophylactic Antibiotic Given[1,3]	8	38%	75%	77%	95%
Prophylactic Antibiotic Selection[1]	2	0%	88%	90%	100%
Prophylactic Antibiotic Stopped[1,3]	8	100%	82%	72%	95%
Pregnancy Care					
Inpatient Neonatal Mortality	-	-	-	-	-
Third or Fourth Degree Laceration	-	-	-	3.63%	3.27%

McCurtain Memorial Hospital

1301 Lincoln Road
Idabel, OK 74745
Ownership: Proprietary
Emergency Services: Yes
Phone: 580-286-7623
Fax: 580-208-3199
Accredited: No
Licensed Beds: 111

Key Personnel:
CEO. . . . . Brit Messer
Chief Medical Staff. . . . . Jon Maxwell, DO
Head of Emergency Room. . . . . Margret Lappin
Emergency Room . . . . Faye Gurley
Director Infection/Disease Control . . . . Ella Ward, RN
ICU Supervising Nurse. Debbie Adams, RN
Director Medical/Surgical Nursing . . . . Debbie Adams, RN
Chief Radiology . . . . R Pritchard, MD
Head of Respiratory Care. . . . . Julie Stanspry

Measure	Cases	This Hospital	State Average	U.S. Average	Top Hospital
Heart Attack Care					
ACE Inhibitor or ARB for LVSD	0	-	79%	82%	100%
Aspirin at Arrival[1]	4	100%	86%	92%	100%
Aspirin at Discharge[1]	3	33%	85%	90%	100%
Beta Blocker at Arrival[1]	4	50%	78%	87%	100%
Beta Blocker at Discharge[1]	3	33%	78%	90%	100%
Fibrinolytic Medication Timing	0	-	36%	31%	100%
PCI Within 90 Minutes of Arrival	0	-	51%	54%	95%
Smoking Cessation Advice	0	-	83%	88%	100%
Heart Failure Care					

NOTE: Hospital profiles are in alphabetical order by state, then city, then hospital within the city; Rankings are sorted by rate in descending order and exclude hospitals with less than 25 cases; (1) The number of cases is too small (n<25) for purposes of reliably predicting hospital performance; (2) Measure reflects the hospital's indication that its submission was based upon a sample of its relevant discharges; (3) Rate reflects fewer than the maximum possible quarters of data for the measure; (4) Inaccurate information submitted and suppressed for one or more quarters; (5) No data is available from the hospital for this measure; Please refer to the User's Guide for a full explanation of data

Measure	Cases	This Hospital	State Average	U.S. Average	Top Hospital
ACE Inhibitor or ARB for LVSD[1]	9	56%	76%	82%	100%
Discharge Instructions	48	48%	55%	61%	93%
Evaluation of LVS Function	54	76%	71%	83%	99%
Smoking Cessation Advice[1]	12	83%	73%	82%	100%
Pneumonia Care					
Appropriate Initial Antibiotic	74	89%	81%	83%	94%
Blood Culture Timing	68	93%	91%	90%	100%
Influenza Vaccine	31	52%	72%	70%	100%
Initial Antibiotic Timing	99	84%	82%	80%	93%
Oxygenation Assessment	125	100%	99%	99%	100%
Pneumococcal Vaccine	69	62%	68%	69%	94%
Smoking Cessation Advice	30	83%	72%	80%	100%
Surgical Infection Prevention					
Prophylactic Antibiotic Given[1,2,3]	9	78%	75%	77%	95%
Prophylactic Antibiotic Selection[1,2]	7	100%	88%	90%	100%
Prophylactic Antibiotic Stopped[1,2,3]	9	67%	82%	72%	95%
Pregnancy Care					
Inpatient Neonatal Mortality	-	-	-	-	-
Third or Fourth Degree Laceration	-	-	-	3.63%	3.27%

Kingfisher Regional

Alternate Name: Community Hospital
PO Box 59
Kingfisher, OK 73750
E-mail: krhhosp@pldi.net
URL: www.kingfisherhospital.com
Phone: 405-375-3141
Fax: 405-375-5115
Ownership: Voluntary non-profit - Other
Emergency Services: Yes
Accredited: No
Licensed Beds: 35

Key Personnel:
Administrator/CEO . . . . Daryle Voss
Director Infection/Disease Control . . . . Debra Forman
Director Respiratory Therapy . . . . Charles Baldwin

Measure	Cases	This Hospital	State Average	U.S. Average	Top Hospital
Heart Attack Care					
ACE Inhibitor or ARB for LVSD[5]	-	-	79%	82%	100%
Aspirin at Arrival[5]	-	-	86%	92%	100%
Aspirin at Discharge[5]	-	-	85%	90%	100%
Beta Blocker at Arrival[5]	-	-	78%	87%	100%
Beta Blocker at Discharge[5]	-	-	78%	90%	100%
Fibrinolytic Medication Timing[5]	-	-	36%	31%	100%
PCI Within 90 Minutes of Arrival[5]	-	-	51%	54%	95%
Smoking Cessation Advice[5]	-	-	83%	88%	100%
Heart Failure Care					
ACE Inhibitor or ARB for LVSD[1]	12	8%	76%	82%	100%
Discharge Instructions	25	0%	55%	61%	93%
Evaluation of LVS Function	33	79%	71%	83%	99%
Smoking Cessation Advice[1]	4	0%	73%	82%	100%
Pneumonia Care					
Appropriate Initial Antibiotic	48	81%	81%	83%	94%
Blood Culture Timing[1]	2	100%	91%	90%	100%
Influenza Vaccine[1]	23	48%	72%	70%	100%
Initial Antibiotic Timing[1]	11	73%	82%	80%	93%
Oxygenation Assessment	51	100%	99%	99%	100%
Pneumococcal Vaccine	36	31%	68%	69%	94%
Smoking Cessation Advice[1]	7	29%	72%	80%	100%
Surgical Infection Prevention					
Prophylactic Antibiotic Given[5]	-	-	75%	77%	95%
Prophylactic Antibiotic Selection[5]	-	-	88%	90%	100%
Prophylactic Antibiotic Stopped[5]	-	-	82%	72%	95%
Pregnancy Care					
Inpatient Neonatal Mortality	-	-	-	-	-
Third or Fourth Degree Laceration	-	-	-	3.63%	3.27%

Comanche County Memorial Hospital

3401 N.W Gore Boulevard
Lawton, OK 73505
URL: www.memorialhealthsource.org
Phone: 580-355-8620
Fax: 580-250-5868
Ownership: Govt - Hospital District or Authority
Emergency Services: Yes
Accredited: Yes
Licensed Beds: 250

Key Personnel:
President/CEO . . . . Randall Segler
Chief Medical Staff . . . . Rick Brittingham
Emergency Room . . . . Barbara Clyde, RN
Director Medical/Surgical Nursing . . . . Marilyn Magid, RN
OB/GYN Womens Health. . . . . Robert Hillis, MD
Director of Pulmonary Care . . . . Tom Neff

Measure	Cases	This Hospital	State Average	U.S. Average	Top Hospital
Heart Attack Care					
ACE Inhibitor or ARB for LVSD	59	88%	79%	82%	100%
Aspirin at Arrival	177	97%	86%	92%	100%
Aspirin at Discharge	301	98%	85%	90%	100%
Beta Blocker at Arrival	157	96%	78%	87%	100%
Beta Blocker at Discharge	291	98%	78%	90%	100%
Fibrinolytic Medication Timing[1]	2	100%	36%	31%	100%
PCI Within 90 Minutes of Arrival[1]	12	75%	51%	54%	95%
Smoking Cessation Advice	130	99%	83%	88%	100%
Heart Failure Care					
ACE Inhibitor or ARB for LVSD	135	91%	76%	82%	100%
Discharge Instructions	278	62%	55%	61%	93%
Evaluation of LVS Function	304	96%	71%	83%	99%
Smoking Cessation Advice	76	100%	73%	82%	100%
Pneumonia Care					
Appropriate Initial Antibiotic	185	84%	81%	83%	94%
Blood Culture Timing	173	84%	91%	90%	100%
Influenza Vaccine	46	91%	72%	70%	100%
Initial Antibiotic Timing	257	76%	82%	80%	93%
Oxygenation Assessment	317	100%	99%	99%	100%
Pneumococcal Vaccine	184	88%	68%	69%	94%
Smoking Cessation Advice	72	97%	72%	80%	100%
Surgical Infection Prevention					
Prophylactic Antibiotic Given[3]	201	65%	75%	77%	95%
Prophylactic Antibiotic Selection	64	91%	88%	90%	100%
Prophylactic Antibiotic Stopped[3]	192	69%	82%	72%	95%
Pregnancy Care					
Inpatient Neonatal Mortality	-	-	-	-	-
Third or Fourth Degree Laceration	-	-	-	3.63%	3.27%

Lawton Indian Hospital

1515 Lawrie Tatum Road
Lawton, OK 73507
Toll-Free: 888-275-4886
Phone: 580-353-0350
Fax: 580-353-2914
Ownership: Government - Federal
Emergency Services: Yes
Accredited: Yes
Licensed Beds: 48

Key Personnel:
Acting CEO . . . . Hickory Starr Jr
Chief Medical Staff. . . . . Dr Boyce Poolaw, MD
Emergency Room . . . . Evaristo Tuinonis
Emergency Room . . . . Norma Condlin, MD
Director Infection/Disease Control . . . . Sue Burgess
OB/GYN Womens Health. . . . . Dr Luis Rivera
Surgical Services . . . . Dr Jaime Pilar
Chief Radiology . . . . Chin S Hoo, MD

Measure	Cases	This Hospital	State Average	U.S. Average	Top Hospital
Heart Attack Care					
ACE Inhibitor or ARB for LVSD[5]	-	-	79%	82%	100%
Aspirin at Arrival[5]	-	-	86%	92%	100%
Aspirin at Discharge[5]	-	-	85%	90%	100%
Beta Blocker at Arrival[5]	-	-	78%	87%	100%
Beta Blocker at Discharge[5]	-	-	78%	90%	100%
Fibrinolytic Medication Timing[5]	-	-	36%	31%	100%
PCI Within 90 Minutes of Arrival[5]	-	-	51%	54%	95%
Smoking Cessation Advice[5]	-	-	83%	88%	100%
Heart Failure Care					
ACE Inhibitor or ARB for LVSD[1]	10	80%	76%	82%	100%
Discharge Instructions[1]	15	20%	55%	61%	93%
Evaluation of LVS Function[1]	15	80%	71%	83%	99%
Smoking Cessation Advice[1]	4	50%	73%	82%	100%
Pneumonia Care					
Appropriate Initial Antibiotic	32	53%	81%	83%	94%
Blood Culture Timing[1]	13	77%	91%	90%	100%
Influenza Vaccine[1]	8	88%	72%	70%	100%
Initial Antibiotic Timing	37	54%	82%	80%	93%

NOTE: Hospital profiles are in alphabetical order by state, then city, then hospital within the city; Rankings are sorted by rate in descending order and exclude hospitals with less than 25 cases; (1) The number of cases is too small (n<25) for purposes of reliably predicting hospital performance; (2) Measure reflects the hospital's indication that its submission was based upon a sample of its relevant discharges; (3) Rate reflects fewer than the maximum possible quarters of data for the measure; (4) Inaccurate information submitted and suppressed for one or more quarters; (5) No data is available from the hospital for this measure; Please refer to the User's Guide for a full explanation of data

Measure	Cases	This Hospital	State Average	U.S. Average	Top Hospital
Oxygenation Assessment	40	98%	99%	99%	100%
Pneumococcal Vaccine[1]	8	50%	68%	69%	94%
Smoking Cessation Advice[1]	11	36%	72%	80%	100%
Surgical Infection Prevention					
Prophylactic Antibiotic Given[3]	39	51%	75%	77%	95%
Prophylactic Antibiotic Selection[1]	8	88%	88%	90%	100%
Prophylactic Antibiotic Stopped[3]	36	100%	82%	72%	95%
Pregnancy Care					
Inpatient Neonatal Mortality	-	-	-	-	-
Third or Fourth Degree Laceration	-	-	-	3.63%	3.27%

Southwestern Medical Center

5602 Southwest Lee Boulevard
Lawton, OK 73505
URL: www.swmconline.com
Ownership: Proprietary
Emergency Services: Yes
Phone: 580-531-4700
Fax: 580-531-4702
Accredited: Yes
Licensed Beds: 162

Key Personnel:
CEO . . . . Thomas L Rine
Chief Medical Staff . . . . Shane Ross
Emergency Room . . . . Charles Sorenson
Director Respiratory Therapy . . . . John Morris

Measure	Cases	This Hospital	State Average	U.S. Average	Top Hospital
Heart Attack Care					
ACE Inhibitor or ARB for LVSD[1]	2	100%	79%	82%	100%
Aspirin at Arrival[1]	13	77%	86%	92%	100%
Aspirin at Discharge[1]	7	57%	85%	90%	100%
Beta Blocker at Arrival[1]	5	40%	78%	87%	100%
Beta Blocker at Discharge[1]	6	83%	78%	90%	100%
Fibrinolytic Medication Timing	0	-	36%	31%	100%
PCI Within 90 Minutes of Arrival	0	-	51%	54%	95%
Smoking Cessation Advice[1]	2	100%	83%	88%	100%
Heart Failure Care					
ACE Inhibitor or ARB for LVSD	34	82%	76%	82%	100%
Discharge Instructions	86	21%	55%	61%	93%
Evaluation of LVS Function	105	76%	71%	83%	99%
Smoking Cessation Advice[1]	22	86%	73%	82%	100%
Pneumonia Care					
Appropriate Initial Antibiotic	97	88%	81%	83%	94%
Blood Culture Timing	67	91%	91%	90%	100%
Influenza Vaccine	39	69%	72%	70%	100%
Initial Antibiotic Timing	135	86%	82%	80%	93%
Oxygenation Assessment	175	100%	99%	99%	100%
Pneumococcal Vaccine	111	69%	68%	69%	94%
Smoking Cessation Advice	36	94%	72%	80%	100%
Surgical Infection Prevention					
Prophylactic Antibiotic Given[3]	38	50%	75%	77%	95%
Prophylactic Antibiotic Selection	33	88%	88%	90%	100%
Prophylactic Antibiotic Stopped[3]	35	71%	82%	72%	95%
Pregnancy Care					
Inpatient Neonatal Mortality	339	0.30%	-	-	-
Third or Fourth Degree Laceration	184	5.98%	-	3.63%	3.27%

Lindsay Municipal Hospital

Highway 19 West
Lindsay, OK 73052
Ownership: Govt - Hospital District or Authority
Emergency Services: Yes
Phone: 405-756-1404
Accredited: No

Measure	Cases	This Hospital	State Average	U.S. Average	Top Hospital
Heart Attack Care					
ACE Inhibitor or ARB for LVSD[3]	0	-	79%	82%	100%
Aspirin at Arrival[3]	0	-	86%	92%	100%
Aspirin at Discharge[3]	0	-	85%	90%	100%
Beta Blocker at Arrival[3]	0	-	78%	87%	100%
Beta Blocker at Discharge[3]	0	-	78%	90%	100%
Fibrinolytic Medication Timing[3]	0	-	36%	31%	100%
PCI Within 90 Minutes of Arrival[5]	-	-	51%	54%	95%
Smoking Cessation Advice[3]	0	-	83%	88%	100%
Heart Failure Care					
ACE Inhibitor or ARB for LVSD[1]	4	75%	76%	82%	100%
Discharge Instructions[1]	21	86%	55%	61%	93%
Evaluation of LVS Function[1]	20	25%	71%	83%	99%
Smoking Cessation Advice[1]	10	20%	73%	82%	100%
Pneumonia Care					
Appropriate Initial Antibiotic	27	81%	81%	83%	94%
Blood Culture Timing[1]	11	100%	91%	90%	100%
Influenza Vaccine[1]	12	50%	72%	70%	100%
Initial Antibiotic Timing[1]	23	78%	82%	80%	93%
Oxygenation Assessment	32	100%	99%	99%	100%
Pneumococcal Vaccine[1]	14	29%	68%	69%	94%
Smoking Cessation Advice[1]	12	17%	72%	80%	100%
Surgical Infection Prevention					
Prophylactic Antibiotic Given[3]	0	-	75%	77%	95%
Prophylactic Antibiotic Selection[1]	1	100%	88%	90%	100%
Prophylactic Antibiotic Stopped[1,3]	1	100%	82%	72%	95%
Pregnancy Care					
Inpatient Neonatal Mortality	-	-	-	-	-
Third or Fourth Degree Laceration	-	-	-	3.63%	3.27%

Integris Marshall County Medical Center

One Hospital Drive
PO Box 827
Madill, OK 73446
URL: www.integris-health.com/INTEGRIS
Ownership: Government - Federal
Emergency Services: No
Phone: 580-795-3384
Fax: 580-795-7080
Accredited: Yes

Key Personnel:
President/CEO . . . . Dave Hill
Chief of Medical Staff . . . . Bruck Zimmerman
Head of Emergency Room . . . . Carol Gay
Emergency Room . . . . Joy Henry, RN
Director Infection/Disease Control . . . . Lois Erwin
OB/GYN Womens Health . . . . William Price, MD
Chief Radiology . . . . Alan Caldwell
Director of Pulmonary/Respiratory Care . . . . Ad Jovee

Measure	Cases	This Hospital	State Average	U.S. Average	Top Hospital
Heart Attack Care					
ACE Inhibitor or ARB for LVSD	0	-	79%	82%	100%
Aspirin at Arrival[1]	8	88%	86%	92%	100%
Aspirin at Discharge[1]	5	60%	85%	90%	100%
Beta Blocker at Arrival[1]	7	57%	78%	87%	100%
Beta Blocker at Discharge[1]	6	83%	78%	90%	100%
Fibrinolytic Medication Timing	0	-	36%	31%	100%
PCI Within 90 Minutes of Arrival	0	-	51%	54%	95%
Smoking Cessation Advice	0	-	83%	88%	100%
Heart Failure Care					
ACE Inhibitor or ARB for LVSD[1]	6	50%	76%	82%	100%
Discharge Instructions	26	65%	55%	61%	93%
Evaluation of LVS Function	38	84%	71%	83%	99%
Smoking Cessation Advice[1]	6	100%	73%	82%	100%
Pneumonia Care					
Appropriate Initial Antibiotic	103	97%	81%	83%	94%
Blood Culture Timing	50	94%	91%	90%	100%
Influenza Vaccine	31	90%	72%	70%	100%
Initial Antibiotic Timing	141	86%	82%	80%	93%
Oxygenation Assessment	156	100%	99%	99%	100%
Pneumococcal Vaccine	84	92%	68%	69%	94%
Smoking Cessation Advice	39	100%	72%	80%	100%
Surgical Infection Prevention					
Prophylactic Antibiotic Given[5]	-	-	75%	77%	95%
Prophylactic Antibiotic Selection[5]	-	-	88%	90%	100%
Prophylactic Antibiotic Stopped[5]	-	-	82%	72%	95%
Pregnancy Care					
Inpatient Neonatal Mortality	-	-	-	-	-
Third or Fourth Degree Laceration	-	-	-	3.63%	3.27%

NOTE: Hospital profiles are in alphabetical order by state, then city, then hospital within the city; Rankings are sorted by rate in descending order and exclude hospitals with less than 25 cases; (1) The number of cases is too small (n<25) for purposes of reliably predicting hospital performance; (2) Measure reflects the hospital's indication that its submission was based upon a sample of its relevant discharges; (3) Rate reflects fewer than the maximum possible quarters of data for the measure; (4) Inaccurate information submitted and suppressed for one or more quarters; (5) No data is available from the hospital for this measure; Please refer to the User's Guide for a full explanation of data

Mangum City Hospital

One Wickersham Drive
Mangum, OK 73554

Toll-Free: 866-620-1000
Phone: 580-782-3353
Fax: 580-782-5944

Ownership: Proprietary
Emergency Services: Yes

Accredited: No
Licensed Beds: 40

Key Personnel:
CEO. . . . . Jim Ivey

Measure	Cases	This Hospital	State Average	U.S. Average	Top Hospital
Heart Attack Care					
ACE Inhibitor or ARB for LVSD[1,3]	1	100%	79%	82%	100%
Aspirin at Arrival[1,3]	2	100%	86%	92%	100%
Aspirin at Discharge[1,3]	3	67%	85%	90%	100%
Beta Blocker at Arrival[1,3]	2	100%	78%	87%	100%
Beta Blocker at Discharge[1,3]	3	67%	78%	90%	100%
Fibrinolytic Medication Timing[3]	0	-	36%	31%	100%
PCI Within 90 Minutes of Arrival[5]	-	-	51%	54%	95%
Smoking Cessation Advice[1,3]	2	50%	83%	88%	100%
Heart Failure Care					
ACE Inhibitor or ARB for LVSD[1]	3	67%	76%	82%	100%
Discharge Instructions[1]	11	9%	55%	61%	93%
Evaluation of LVS Function[1]	15	27%	71%	83%	99%
Smoking Cessation Advice[1]	1	0%	73%	82%	100%
Pneumonia Care					
Appropriate Initial Antibiotic[1]	18	83%	81%	83%	94%
Blood Culture Timing[1]	5	100%	91%	90%	100%
Influenza Vaccine[1]	3	100%	72%	70%	100%
Initial Antibiotic Timing[1]	15	67%	82%	80%	93%
Oxygenation Assessment[1]	24	96%	99%	99%	100%
Pneumococcal Vaccine[1]	15	73%	68%	69%	94%
Smoking Cessation Advice[1]	5	20%	72%	80%	100%
Surgical Infection Prevention					
Prophylactic Antibiotic Given[5]	-	-	75%	77%	95%
Prophylactic Antibiotic Selection[5]	-	-	88%	90%	100%
Prophylactic Antibiotic Stopped[5]	-	-	82%	72%	95%
Pregnancy Care					
Inpatient Neonatal Mortality	-	-	-	-	-
Third or Fourth Degree Laceration	-	-	-	3.63%	3.27%

Mercy Health Love County Hospital

300 Wanda Street
Marietta, OK 73448
URL: www.mercyok.net

Phone: 580-276-3347
Fax: 580-276-2182

Ownership: Proprietary
Emergency Services: Yes

Accredited: No
Licensed Beds: 30

Measure	Cases	This Hospital	State Average	U.S. Average	Top Hospital
Heart Attack Care					
ACE Inhibitor or ARB for LVSD[5]	-	-	79%	82%	100%
Aspirin at Arrival[5]	-	-	86%	92%	100%
Aspirin at Discharge[5]	-	-	85%	90%	100%
Beta Blocker at Arrival[5]	-	-	78%	87%	100%
Beta Blocker at Discharge[5]	-	-	78%	90%	100%
Fibrinolytic Medication Timing[5]	-	-	36%	31%	100%
PCI Within 90 Minutes of Arrival[5]	-	-	51%	54%	95%
Smoking Cessation Advice[5]	-	-	83%	88%	100%
Heart Failure Care					
ACE Inhibitor or ARB for LVSD[5]	-	-	76%	82%	100%
Discharge Instructions[5]	-	-	55%	61%	93%
Evaluation of LVS Function[5]	-	-	71%	83%	99%
Smoking Cessation Advice[5]	-	-	73%	82%	100%
Pneumonia Care					
Appropriate Initial Antibiotic[1,3]	3	67%	81%	83%	94%
Blood Culture Timing[1,3]	1	100%	91%	90%	100%
Influenza Vaccine[1]	5	20%	72%	70%	100%
Initial Antibiotic Timing[1,3]	7	86%	82%	80%	93%
Oxygenation Assessment[1,3]	8	88%	99%	99%	100%
Pneumococcal Vaccine[1,3]	6	17%	68%	69%	94%
Smoking Cessation Advice[1,3]	5	40%	72%	80%	100%
Surgical Infection Prevention					
Prophylactic Antibiotic Given[5]	-	-	75%	77%	95%
Prophylactic Antibiotic Selection[5]	-	-	88%	90%	100%
Prophylactic Antibiotic Stopped[5]	-	-	82%	72%	95%
Pregnancy Care					
Inpatient Neonatal Mortality	-	-	-	-	-
Third or Fourth Degree Laceration	-	-	-	3.63%	3.27%

McAlester Regional Health Center

1 E Clark Bass Blvd
McAlester, OK 74501
E-mail: nbrinlee@mrhcok.com
URL: www.mrhcok.com

Phone: 918-426-1800
Fax: 918-421-8633

Ownership: Voluntary non-profit - Other
Emergency Services: Yes

Accredited: Yes
Licensed Beds: 197

Key Personnel:
CEO. . . . . Sean Beggs
Chief of Medical Staff . . . . Milton James
Emergency Room . . . . Chris Ossenbeck
Chief Radiology . . . . Don Shuller, MD
Director Respiratory Therapy . . . . Chuck Hallbert

Measure	Cases	This Hospital	State Average	U.S. Average	Top Hospital
Heart Attack Care					
ACE Inhibitor or ARB for LVSD[1]	7	86%	79%	82%	100%
Aspirin at Arrival	42	83%	86%	92%	100%
Aspirin at Discharge[1]	23	74%	85%	90%	100%
Beta Blocker at Arrival	38	66%	78%	87%	100%
Beta Blocker at Discharge[1]	21	67%	78%	90%	100%
Fibrinolytic Medication Timing[1]	1	0%	36%	31%	100%
PCI Within 90 Minutes of Arrival	0	-	51%	54%	95%
Smoking Cessation Advice[1]	6	100%	83%	88%	100%
Heart Failure Care					
ACE Inhibitor or ARB for LVSD	58	79%	76%	82%	100%
Discharge Instructions	146	38%	55%	61%	93%
Evaluation of LVS Function	202	67%	71%	83%	99%
Smoking Cessation Advice	51	100%	73%	82%	100%
Pneumonia Care					
Appropriate Initial Antibiotic	108	69%	81%	83%	94%
Blood Culture Timing	94	93%	91%	90%	100%
Influenza Vaccine[4,5]	-	-	72%	70%	100%
Initial Antibiotic Timing	145	94%	82%	80%	93%
Oxygenation Assessment	176	100%	99%	99%	100%
Pneumococcal Vaccine	119	85%	68%	69%	94%
Smoking Cessation Advice	45	87%	72%	80%	100%
Surgical Infection Prevention					
Prophylactic Antibiotic Given[3]	193	96%	75%	77%	95%
Prophylactic Antibiotic Selection	59	93%	88%	90%	100%
Prophylactic Antibiotic Stopped[3]	189	79%	82%	72%	95%
Pregnancy Care					
Inpatient Neonatal Mortality	-	-	-	-	-
Third or Fourth Degree Laceration	-	-	-	3.63%	3.27%

Integris Baptist Regional Health Center

200 2nd Avenue SW
PO Box 1207
Miami, OK 74355
URL: www.integris-health.com

Phone: 918-542-6611
Fax: 918-540-7605

Ownership: Voluntary non-profit - Other
Emergency Services: Yes

Accredited: Yes
Licensed Beds: 124

Key Personnel:
President/CEO. . . . . Joel Hart

Measure	Cases	This Hospital	State Average	U.S. Average	Top Hospital
Heart Attack Care					
ACE Inhibitor or ARB for LVSD	0	-	79%	82%	100%
Aspirin at Arrival[1]	19	89%	86%	92%	100%
Aspirin at Discharge[1]	9	89%	85%	90%	100%
Beta Blocker at Arrival[1]	17	88%	78%	87%	100%
Beta Blocker at Discharge[1]	9	100%	78%	90%	100%
Fibrinolytic Medication Timing	0	-	36%	31%	100%
PCI Within 90 Minutes of Arrival	0	-	51%	54%	95%
Smoking Cessation Advice[1]	2	100%	83%	88%	100%
Heart Failure Care					

NOTE: Hospital profiles are in alphabetical order by state, then city, then hospital within the city; Rankings are sorted by rate in descending order and exclude hospitals with less than 25 cases; (1) The number of cases is too small (n<25) for purposes of reliably predicting hospital performance; (2) Measure reflects the hospital's indication that its submission was based upon a sample of its relevant discharges; (3) Rate reflects fewer than the maximum possible quarters of data for the measure; (4) Inaccurate information submitted and suppressed for one or more quarters; (5) No data is available from the hospital for this measure; Please refer to the User's Guide for a full explanation of data

ACE Inhibitor or ARB for LVSD	45	87%	76%	82%	100%
Discharge Instructions	129	89%	55%	61%	93%
Evaluation of LVS Function	150	100%	71%	83%	99%
Smoking Cessation Advice	27	100%	73%	82%	100%
Pneumonia Care					
Appropriate Initial Antibiotic	174	86%	81%	83%	94%
Blood Culture Timing	108	82%	91%	90%	100%
Influenza Vaccine	50	96%	72%	70%	100%
Initial Antibiotic Timing	252	88%	82%	80%	93%
Oxygenation Assessment	283	100%	99%	99%	100%
Pneumococcal Vaccine	157	96%	68%	69%	94%
Smoking Cessation Advice	64	97%	72%	80%	100%
Surgical Infection Prevention					
Prophylactic Antibiotic Given	145	88%	75%	77%	95%
Prophylactic Antibiotic Selection	39	97%	88%	90%	100%
Prophylactic Antibiotic Stopped	140	83%	82%	72%	95%
Pregnancy Care					
Inpatient Neonatal Mortality	-	-	-	-	-
Third or Fourth Degree Laceration	-	-	-	3.63%	3.27%

Midwest Regional Medical Center

2825 Parklawn Drive
Midwest City, OK 73110
URL: www.midwestregional.com
Ownership: Proprietary
Emergency Services: Yes

Phone: 405-610-4411
Fax: 405-610-1483

Accredited: Yes
Licensed Beds: 255

Key Personnel:
CEO. . . . . Doug Arnold
Director Emergency Department . . . . . . Dan Donnell, MD

Measure	Cases	This Hospital	State Average	U.S. Average	Top Hospital
Heart Attack Care					
ACE Inhibitor or ARB for LVSD	71	89%	79%	82%	100%
Aspirin at Arrival	301	95%	86%	92%	100%
Aspirin at Discharge	319	89%	85%	90%	100%
Beta Blocker at Arrival	258	81%	78%	87%	100%
Beta Blocker at Discharge	285	89%	78%	90%	100%
Fibrinolytic Medication Timing[1]	1	0%	36%	31%	100%
PCI Within 90 Minutes of Arrival[1]	20	20%	51%	54%	95%
Smoking Cessation Advice	123	92%	83%	88%	100%
Heart Failure Care					
ACE Inhibitor or ARB for LVSD	201	86%	76%	82%	100%
Discharge Instructions	400	80%	55%	61%	93%
Evaluation of LVS Function	464	94%	71%	83%	99%
Smoking Cessation Advice	97	99%	73%	82%	100%
Pneumonia Care					
Appropriate Initial Antibiotic	216	71%	81%	83%	94%
Blood Culture Timing	178	89%	91%	90%	100%
Influenza Vaccine	58	72%	72%	70%	100%
Initial Antibiotic Timing	309	74%	82%	80%	93%
Oxygenation Assessment	358	99%	99%	99%	100%
Pneumococcal Vaccine	200	71%	68%	69%	94%
Smoking Cessation Advice	96	92%	72%	80%	100%
Surgical Infection Prevention					
Prophylactic Antibiotic Given[2]	650	89%	75%	77%	95%
Prophylactic Antibiotic Selection[2]	119	98%	88%	90%	100%
Prophylactic Antibiotic Stopped[2]	624	70%	82%	72%	95%
Pregnancy Care					
Inpatient Neonatal Mortality	-	-	-	-	-
Third or Fourth Degree Laceration	-	-	-	3.63%	3.27%

Moore Medical Center

700 South Telephone Road
Moore, OK 73160
Ownership: Government - State
Emergency Services: No

Phone: 405-793-9355

Accredited: No

Measure	Cases	This Hospital	State Average	U.S. Average	Top Hospital
Heart Attack Care					
ACE Inhibitor or ARB for LVSD	0	-	79%	82%	100%
Aspirin at Arrival[1]	4	75%	86%	92%	100%
Aspirin at Discharge	0	-	85%	90%	100%
Beta Blocker at Arrival[1]	4	25%	78%	87%	100%
Beta Blocker at Discharge	0	-	78%	90%	100%
Fibrinolytic Medication Timing[1]	3	0%	36%	31%	100%
PCI Within 90 Minutes of Arrival	0	-	51%	54%	95%
Smoking Cessation Advice	0	-	83%	88%	100%
Heart Failure Care					
ACE Inhibitor or ARB for LVSD[1]	6	33%	76%	82%	100%
Discharge Instructions	28	11%	55%	61%	93%
Evaluation of LVS Function	30	90%	71%	83%	99%
Smoking Cessation Advice[1]	13	85%	73%	82%	100%
Pneumonia Care					
Appropriate Initial Antibiotic	52	71%	81%	83%	94%
Blood Culture Timing	34	91%	91%	90%	100%
Influenza Vaccine[1]	7	14%	72%	70%	100%
Initial Antibiotic Timing	43	93%	82%	80%	93%
Oxygenation Assessment	59	98%	99%	99%	100%
Pneumococcal Vaccine[1]	14	50%	68%	69%	94%
Smoking Cessation Advice	25	80%	72%	80%	100%
Surgical Infection Prevention					
Prophylactic Antibiotic Given	60	77%	75%	77%	95%
Prophylactic Antibiotic Selection[1]	22	100%	88%	90%	100%
Prophylactic Antibiotic Stopped	51	100%	82%	72%	95%
Pregnancy Care					
Inpatient Neonatal Mortality	-	-	-	-	-
Third or Fourth Degree Laceration	-	-	-	3.63%	3.27%

Muskogee Regional Medical Center

300 Rockefeller Drive
Muskogee, OK 74401
URL: www.muskogeehealth.com
Ownership: Govt - Hospital District or Authority
Emergency Services: Yes

Phone: 918-682-5501
Fax: 918-684-2552

Accredited: Yes
Licensed Beds: 366

Key Personnel:
Chief Medical Staff. . . . . Gary Lambert, DO
Cardiac Lab . . . . Joy Abbey
Catheterization Lab/ICU/CCU . . . . . . Glinda Huitt, RN
Emergency Room . . . . Berry Winn, MD
Emergency Room . . . . Sheila McMahan, RN
ICU . . . . Glinda Huitt, RN
Surgical Services . . . . Susan Julian
Respiratory/Cardiopulmonary. . . . . . . Everett Wiebe, RT

Measure	Cases	This Hospital	State Average	U.S. Average	Top Hospital
Heart Attack Care					
ACE Inhibitor or ARB for LVSD[1]	18	89%	79%	82%	100%
Aspirin at Arrival	130	96%	86%	92%	100%
Aspirin at Discharge	57	91%	85%	90%	100%
Beta Blocker at Arrival	107	98%	78%	87%	100%
Beta Blocker at Discharge	74	95%	78%	90%	100%
Fibrinolytic Medication Timing	0	-	36%	31%	100%
PCI Within 90 Minutes of Arrival	0	-	51%	54%	95%
Smoking Cessation Advice[1]	11	100%	83%	88%	100%
Heart Failure Care					
ACE Inhibitor or ARB for LVSD	83	92%	76%	82%	100%
Discharge Instructions	194	84%	55%	61%	93%
Evaluation of LVS Function	256	93%	71%	83%	99%
Smoking Cessation Advice	49	100%	73%	82%	100%
Pneumonia Care					
Appropriate Initial Antibiotic	87	91%	81%	83%	94%
Blood Culture Timing	86	88%	91%	90%	100%
Influenza Vaccine	25	80%	72%	70%	100%
Initial Antibiotic Timing	143	74%	82%	80%	93%
Oxygenation Assessment	159	99%	99%	99%	100%
Pneumococcal Vaccine	90	76%	68%	69%	94%
Smoking Cessation Advice	52	94%	72%	80%	100%
Surgical Infection Prevention					
Prophylactic Antibiotic Given	218	87%	75%	77%	95%
Prophylactic Antibiotic Selection	69	96%	88%	90%	100%
Prophylactic Antibiotic Stopped	203	70%	82%	72%	95%
Pregnancy Care					
Inpatient Neonatal Mortality	-	-	-	-	-
Third or Fourth Degree Laceration	-	-	-	3.63%	3.27%

NOTE: Hospital profiles are in alphabetical order by state, then city, then hospital within the city; Rankings are sorted by rate in descending order and exclude hospitals with less than 25 cases; (1) The number of cases is too small (n<25) for purposes of reliably predicting hospital performance; (2) Measure reflects the hospital's indication that its submission was based upon a sample of its relevant discharges; (3) Rate reflects fewer than the maximum possible quarters of data for the measure; (4) Inaccurate information submitted and suppressed for one or more quarters; (5) No data is available from the hospital for this measure; Please refer to the User's Guide for a full explanation of data

Norman Regional Hospital

901 N Porter
PO Box 1308
Norman, OK 73070
URL: www.normanregional.com
Ownership: Government - Local
Emergency Services: Yes
Phone: 405-307-1000
Fax: 405-307-1548
Accredited: Yes
Licensed Beds: 382

Key Personnel:
President/CEO . . . . David D Whitaker, FACHE

Measure	Cases	This Hospital	State Average	U.S. Average	Top Hospital
Heart Attack Care					
ACE Inhibitor or ARB for LVSD	31	94%	79%	82%	100%
Aspirin at Arrival	165	99%	86%	92%	100%
Aspirin at Discharge	170	96%	85%	90%	100%
Beta Blocker at Arrival	122	97%	78%	87%	100%
Beta Blocker at Discharge	172	99%	78%	90%	100%
Fibrinolytic Medication Timing[1]	1	0%	36%	31%	100%
PCI Within 90 Minutes of Arrival[1]	9	56%	51%	54%	95%
Smoking Cessation Advice	74	100%	83%	88%	100%
Heart Failure Care					
ACE Inhibitor or ARB for LVSD	87	93%	76%	82%	100%
Discharge Instructions	214	91%	55%	61%	93%
Evaluation of LVS Function	267	100%	71%	83%	99%
Smoking Cessation Advice	51	98%	73%	82%	100%
Pneumonia Care					
Appropriate Initial Antibiotic	219	99%	81%	83%	94%
Blood Culture Timing	303	99%	91%	90%	100%
Influenza Vaccine	98	100%	72%	70%	100%
Initial Antibiotic Timing	367	96%	82%	80%	93%
Oxygenation Assessment	476	100%	99%	99%	100%
Pneumococcal Vaccine	259	100%	68%	69%	94%
Smoking Cessation Advice	179	97%	72%	80%	100%
Surgical Infection Prevention					
Prophylactic Antibiotic Given[3]	677	92%	75%	77%	95%
Prophylactic Antibiotic Selection	214	93%	88%	90%	100%
Prophylactic Antibiotic Stopped[3]	650	68%	82%	72%	95%
Pregnancy Care					
Inpatient Neonatal Mortality	-	-	-	-	-
Third or Fourth Degree Laceration	-	-	-	3.63%	3.27%

Okeene Municipal Hospital

207 E F Street
Okeene, OK 73763
E-mail: sdunham@okeenehospital.com
URL: www.okeenehospital.com
Ownership: Voluntary non-profit - Other
Emergency Services: Yes
Phone: 580-822-4417
Fax: 580-822-3927
Accredited: No
Licensed Beds: 25

Key Personnel:
Administrator . . . . Shelly Dunham
Chief Medical Staff. . . . . Ken Parrott, MD
Director of Cardiology/Cardiac Lab. . . . . Tommy Fisher
Emergency Room . . . . A Atendido, MD
Director Infection/Disease Control . . . . Pat Lorenz, RN
Director Respiratory Therapy . . . . Tonya Huston

Measure	Cases	This Hospital	State Average	U.S. Average	Top Hospital
Heart Attack Care					
ACE Inhibitor or ARB for LVSD[3]	0	-	79%	82%	100%
Aspirin at Arrival[1,3]	3	100%	86%	92%	100%
Aspirin at Discharge[3]	0	-	85%	90%	100%
Beta Blocker at Arrival[1,3]	1	100%	78%	87%	100%
Beta Blocker at Discharge[3]	0	-	78%	90%	100%
Fibrinolytic Medication Timing[1,3]	3	67%	36%	31%	100%
PCI Within 90 Minutes of Arrival	0	-	51%	54%	95%
Smoking Cessation Advice[3]	0	-	83%	88%	100%
Heart Failure Care					
ACE Inhibitor or ARB for LVSD[1]	1	0%	76%	82%	100%
Discharge Instructions[1]	6	0%	55%	61%	93%
Evaluation of LVS Function[1]	9	56%	71%	83%	99%
Smoking Cessation Advice[1]	4	25%	73%	82%	100%
Pneumonia Care					
Appropriate Initial Antibiotic[1,3]	12	50%	81%	83%	94%
Blood Culture Timing[1,3]	1	100%	91%	90%	100%
Influenza Vaccine[1]	7	71%	72%	70%	100%
Initial Antibiotic Timing[1,3]	13	85%	82%	80%	93%
Oxygenation Assessment[1,3]	18	94%	99%	99%	100%
Pneumococcal Vaccine[1,3]	13	77%	68%	69%	94%
Smoking Cessation Advice[1,3]	4	25%	72%	80%	100%
Surgical Infection Prevention					
Prophylactic Antibiotic Given[3]	0	-	75%	77%	95%
Prophylactic Antibiotic Selection[5]	-	-	88%	90%	100%
Prophylactic Antibiotic Stopped[3]	0	-	82%	72%	95%
Pregnancy Care					
Inpatient Neonatal Mortality	-	-	-	-	-
Third or Fourth Degree Laceration	-	-	-	3.63%	3.27%

Bone and Joint Hospital

1111 North Dewey Avenue
Oklahoma City, OK 73103
Toll-Free: 888-563-5633
Phone: 405-272-9671
Fax: 405-552-9197
E-mail: cathy_mckinney@ssmhc.com
URL: www.boneandjoint.com
Ownership: Proprietary
Emergency Services: Yes
Accredited: Yes
Licensed Beds: 102

Key Personnel:
Administrator/President . . . . James A Hyde
Chief Medical Staff. . . . . Thomas P Janssen, MD
Emergency Room . . . . Brad Beatty, RN BSN
Emergency Room . . . . Warren Low, MD
Director Infection/Disease Control . . . . Patricia Vernon

Measure	Cases	This Hospital	State Average	U.S. Average	Top Hospital
Heart Attack Care					
ACE Inhibitor or ARB for LVSD[5]	-	-	79%	82%	100%
Aspirin at Arrival[5]	-	-	86%	92%	100%
Aspirin at Discharge[5]	-	-	85%	90%	100%
Beta Blocker at Arrival[5]	-	-	78%	87%	100%
Beta Blocker at Discharge[5]	-	-	78%	90%	100%
Fibrinolytic Medication Timing[5]	-	-	36%	31%	100%
PCI Within 90 Minutes of Arrival[5]	-	-	51%	54%	95%
Smoking Cessation Advice[5]	-	-	83%	88%	100%
Heart Failure Care					
ACE Inhibitor or ARB for LVSD[5]	-	-	76%	82%	100%
Discharge Instructions[5]	-	-	55%	61%	93%
Evaluation of LVS Function[5]	-	-	71%	83%	99%
Smoking Cessation Advice[5]	-	-	73%	82%	100%
Pneumonia Care					
Appropriate Initial Antibiotic[3]	0	-	81%	83%	94%
Blood Culture Timing[3]	0	-	91%	90%	100%
Influenza Vaccine[1]	1	0%	72%	70%	100%
Initial Antibiotic Timing[3]	0	-	82%	80%	93%
Oxygenation Assessment[1,3]	1	100%	99%	99%	100%
Pneumococcal Vaccine[1,3]	1	0%	68%	69%	94%
Smoking Cessation Advice[3]	0	-	72%	80%	100%
Surgical Infection Prevention					
Prophylactic Antibiotic Given	333	100%	75%	77%	95%
Prophylactic Antibiotic Selection	40	100%	88%	90%	100%
Prophylactic Antibiotic Stopped	327	98%	82%	72%	95%
Pregnancy Care					
Inpatient Neonatal Mortality	-	-	-	-	-
Third or Fourth Degree Laceration	-	-	-	3.63%	3.27%

Community Hospital

3100 Southwest 89th Street
Oklahoma City, OK 73159
Ownership: Proprietary
Emergency Services: Yes
Phone: 405-602-8100
Accredited: Yes

Measure	Cases	This Hospital	State Average	U.S. Average	Top Hospital
Heart Attack Care					
ACE Inhibitor or ARB for LVSD[5]	-	-	79%	82%	100%
Aspirin at Arrival[5]	-	-	86%	92%	100%
Aspirin at Discharge[5]	-	-	85%	90%	100%
Beta Blocker at Arrival[5]	-	-	78%	87%	100%

NOTE: Hospital profiles are in alphabetical order by state, then city, then hospital within the city; Rankings are sorted by rate in descending order and exclude hospitals with less than 25 cases; (1) The number of cases is too small (n<25) for purposes of reliably predicting hospital performance; (2) Measure reflects the hospital's indication that its submission was based upon a sample of its relevant discharges; (3) Rate reflects fewer than the maximum possible quarters of data for the measure; (4) Inaccurate information submitted and suppressed for one or more quarters; (5) No data is available from the hospital for this measure; Please refer to the User's Guide for a full explanation of data

Measure	Cases	This Hospital	State Average	U.S. Average	Top Hospital
Beta Blocker at Discharge[5]	-	-	78%	90%	100%
Fibrinolytic Medication Timing[5]	-	-	36%	31%	100%
PCI Within 90 Minutes of Arrival[5]	-	-	51%	54%	95%
Smoking Cessation Advice[5]	-	-	83%	88%	100%
Heart Failure Care					
ACE Inhibitor or ARB for LVSD[1,3]	1	100%	76%	82%	100%
Discharge Instructions[1,3]	3	0%	55%	61%	93%
Evaluation of LVS Function[1,3]	3	100%	71%	83%	99%
Smoking Cessation Advice[1,3]	2	0%	73%	82%	100%
Pneumonia Care					
Appropriate Initial Antibiotic[1]	15	53%	81%	83%	94%
Blood Culture Timing[1]	9	89%	91%	90%	100%
Influenza Vaccine[1]	4	50%	72%	70%	100%
Initial Antibiotic Timing[1]	10	70%	82%	80%	93%
Oxygenation Assessment[1]	16	100%	99%	99%	100%
Pneumococcal Vaccine[1]	7	71%	68%	69%	94%
Smoking Cessation Advice[1]	7	29%	72%	80%	100%
Surgical Infection Prevention					
Prophylactic Antibiotic Given[3]	50	92%	75%	77%	95%
Prophylactic Antibiotic Selection[1]	14	100%	88%	90%	100%
Prophylactic Antibiotic Stopped[3]	50	64%	82%	72%	95%
Pregnancy Care					
Inpatient Neonatal Mortality	-	-	-	-	-
Third or Fourth Degree Laceration	-	-	-	3.63%	3.27%

Deaconess Hospital

5501 North Portland Avenue
Oklahoma City, OK 73112
Phone: 405-604-6000
Fax: 405-604-4297
URL: www.deaconessokc.org
Ownership: Voluntary non-profit - Church
Accredited: Yes
Emergency Services: Yes
Licensed Beds: 313

Key Personnel:

President/CEO . . . . Paul Dougherty
Chief Medical Staff . . . . Ken Whittington, MD
Emergency Room . . . . Judi Merning, RN
Director Infection/Disease Control . . . . Carol Shenold, ICP
CCU Manager . . . . Michelle Engress, RN
Chief Radiology . . . . Kerri Kirchoff, MD
Director Respiratory Therapy . . . . Vicki Nations

Measure	Cases	This Hospital	State Average	U.S. Average	Top Hospital
Heart Attack Care					
ACE Inhibitor or ARB for LVSD[3]	40	88%	79%	82%	100%
Aspirin at Arrival[3]	91	93%	86%	92%	100%
Aspirin at Discharge[3]	92	95%	85%	90%	100%
Beta Blocker at Arrival[3]	44	82%	78%	87%	100%
Beta Blocker at Discharge[3]	99	97%	78%	90%	100%
Fibrinolytic Medication Timing[3]	0	-	36%	31%	100%
PCI Within 90 Minutes of Arrival[1]	3	33%	51%	54%	95%
Smoking Cessation Advice[3]	35	100%	83%	88%	100%
Heart Failure Care					
ACE Inhibitor or ARB for LVSD[3]	61	85%	76%	82%	100%
Discharge Instructions[3]	113	45%	55%	61%	93%
Evaluation of LVS Function[3]	150	91%	71%	83%	99%
Smoking Cessation Advice[3]	31	97%	73%	82%	100%
Pneumonia Care					
Appropriate Initial Antibiotic[3]	119	92%	81%	83%	94%
Blood Culture Timing	154	94%	91%	90%	100%
Influenza Vaccine	69	88%	72%	70%	100%
Initial Antibiotic Timing[3]	189	77%	82%	80%	93%
Oxygenation Assessment[3]	211	100%	99%	99%	100%
Pneumococcal Vaccine[3]	133	89%	68%	69%	94%
Smoking Cessation Advice[3]	50	98%	72%	80%	100%
Surgical Infection Prevention					
Prophylactic Antibiotic Given[3]	406	85%	75%	77%	95%
Prophylactic Antibiotic Selection	132	92%	88%	90%	100%
Prophylactic Antibiotic Stopped[3]	372	89%	82%	72%	95%
Pregnancy Care					
Inpatient Neonatal Mortality	-	-	-	-	-
Third or Fourth Degree Laceration	-	-	-	3.63%	3.27%

Integris Baptist Medical Center

Alternate Name: Baptist Medical Center of Oklahoma
3300 NW Expressway
Oklahoma City, OK 73112
Phone: 405-949-3011
Fax: 405-949-3685
URL: www.integris-health.com
Ownership: Voluntary non-profit - Private
Accredited: Yes
Emergency Services: Yes
Licensed Beds: 577

Key Personnel:

President/CEO . . . . Stanley F Hupfeld
Chief Medical Staff . . . . Brian Geister, MD
Chief Catheterization Laboratory . . . . David Vilette
Emergency Room . . . . Richard Crook, MD
Medical Director Infection/Disease . . . . V Ramgopal, MD
Director Medical/Surgical Nursing . . . . Julie Krywicki, RN
OB/GYN Womens Health . . . . David A Kallenberger, MD
Manager Surgical Services . . . . Connie Harper
Chief Radiology . . . . Georgianne Snowden, MD
Manager Pulmonary Services . . . . Harry Wetz

Measure	Cases	This Hospital	State Average	U.S. Average	Top Hospital
Heart Attack Care					
ACE Inhibitor or ARB for LVSD	100	100%	79%	82%	100%
Aspirin at Arrival	251	99%	86%	92%	100%
Aspirin at Discharge	525	100%	85%	90%	100%
Beta Blocker at Arrival	153	96%	78%	87%	100%
Beta Blocker at Discharge	474	99%	78%	90%	100%
Fibrinolytic Medication Timing	0	-	36%	31%	100%
PCI Within 90 Minutes of Arrival[1]	11	55%	51%	54%	95%
Smoking Cessation Advice	219	100%	83%	88%	100%
Heart Failure Care					
ACE Inhibitor or ARB for LVSD	310	99%	76%	82%	100%
Discharge Instructions	494	89%	55%	61%	93%
Evaluation of LVS Function	575	100%	71%	83%	99%
Smoking Cessation Advice	111	99%	73%	82%	100%
Pneumonia Care					
Appropriate Initial Antibiotic	238	89%	81%	83%	94%
Blood Culture Timing	214	95%	91%	90%	100%
Influenza Vaccine	80	79%	72%	70%	100%
Initial Antibiotic Timing	372	68%	82%	80%	93%
Oxygenation Assessment	418	100%	99%	99%	100%
Pneumococcal Vaccine	260	75%	68%	69%	94%
Smoking Cessation Advice	95	69%	72%	80%	100%
Surgical Infection Prevention					
Prophylactic Antibiotic Given	791	92%	75%	77%	95%
Prophylactic Antibiotic Selection	202	98%	88%	90%	100%
Prophylactic Antibiotic Stopped	766	93%	82%	72%	95%
Pregnancy Care					
Inpatient Neonatal Mortality	-	-	-	-	-
Third or Fourth Degree Laceration	-	-	-	3.63%	3.27%

Integris Southwest Medical Center

Alternate Name: Southwwest Medical Center of Oklahoma
4401 S Western
Oklahoma City, OK 73109
Phone: 405-636-7000
Fax: 405-636-7064
URL: www.integris-health.com
Ownership: Voluntary non-profit - Private
Accredited: Yes
Emergency Services: Yes
Licensed Beds: 369

Key Personnel:

President/CEO . . . . Bruce Lawrence
Administrator . . . . Chris Hammes
Chief Medical Staff . . . . Ralph Shadid, MD
Catheterization Lab . . . . John Rogers
Emergency Room . . . . Cyndy Ray
OB/GYN Womens Health . . . . Deanie Gustin
Director Respiratory Therapy . . . . Harry Wetz

Measure	Cases	This Hospital	State Average	U.S. Average	Top Hospital
Heart Attack Care					
ACE Inhibitor or ARB for LVSD	65	78%	79%	82%	100%
Aspirin at Arrival	228	99%	86%	92%	100%
Aspirin at Discharge	236	91%	85%	90%	100%
Beta Blocker at Arrival	181	97%	78%	87%	100%
Beta Blocker at Discharge	223	92%	78%	90%	100%

NOTE: Hospital profiles are in alphabetical order by state, then city, then hospital within the city; Rankings are sorted by rate in descending order and exclude hospitals with less than 25 cases; (1) The number of cases is too small (n<25) for purposes of reliably predicting hospital performance; (2) Measure reflects the hospital's indication that its submission was based upon a sample of its relevant discharges; (3) Rate reflects fewer than the maximum possible quarters of data for the measure; (4) Inaccurate information submitted and suppressed for one or more quarters; (5) No data is available from the hospital for this measure; Please refer to the User's Guide for a full explanation of data

Fibrinolytic Medication Timing[1]	1	0%	36%	31%	100%
PCI Within 90 Minutes of Arrival[1]	6	50%	51%	54%	95%
Smoking Cessation Advice	127	97%	83%	88%	100%
Heart Failure Care					
ACE Inhibitor or ARB for LVSD	215	84%	76%	82%	100%
Discharge Instructions	355	71%	55%	61%	93%
Evaluation of LVS Function	415	92%	71%	83%	99%
Smoking Cessation Advice	120	98%	73%	82%	100%
Pneumonia Care					
Appropriate Initial Antibiotic	249	94%	81%	83%	94%
Blood Culture Timing	267	93%	91%	90%	100%
Influenza Vaccine	76	68%	72%	70%	100%
Initial Antibiotic Timing	352	93%	82%	80%	93%
Oxygenation Assessment	414	100%	99%	99%	100%
Pneumococcal Vaccine	244	82%	68%	69%	94%
Smoking Cessation Advice	153	95%	72%	80%	100%
Surgical Infection Prevention					
Prophylactic Antibiotic Given	497	91%	75%	77%	95%
Prophylactic Antibiotic Selection	144	98%	88%	90%	100%
Prophylactic Antibiotic Stopped	462	73%	82%	72%	95%
Pregnancy Care					
Inpatient Neonatal Mortality	-	-	-	-	-
Third or Fourth Degree Laceration	-	-	-	3.63%	3.27%

Lakeside Women's Hospital

11200 North Portland Avenue
Oklahoma City, OK 73120
Ownership: Proprietary
Emergency Services: Yes

Phone: 405-936-1500
Accredited: Yes

Measure	Cases	This Hospital	State Average	U.S. Average	Top Hospital
Heart Attack Care					
ACE Inhibitor or ARB for LVSD[5]	-	-	79%	82%	100%
Aspirin at Arrival[5]	-	-	86%	92%	100%
Aspirin at Discharge[5]	-	-	85%	90%	100%
Beta Blocker at Arrival[5]	-	-	78%	87%	100%
Beta Blocker at Discharge[5]	-	-	78%	90%	100%
Fibrinolytic Medication Timing[5]	-	-	36%	31%	100%
PCI Within 90 Minutes of Arrival[5]	-	-	51%	54%	95%
Smoking Cessation Advice[5]	-	-	83%	88%	100%
Heart Failure Care					
ACE Inhibitor or ARB for LVSD[5]	-	-	76%	82%	100%
Discharge Instructions[5]	-	-	55%	61%	93%
Evaluation of LVS Function[5]	-	-	71%	83%	99%
Smoking Cessation Advice[5]	-	-	73%	82%	100%
Pneumonia Care					
Appropriate Initial Antibiotic[5]	-	-	81%	83%	94%
Blood Culture Timing[5]	-	-	91%	90%	100%
Influenza Vaccine[5]	-	-	72%	70%	100%
Initial Antibiotic Timing[5]	-	-	82%	80%	93%
Oxygenation Assessment[5]	-	-	99%	99%	100%
Pneumococcal Vaccine[5]	-	-	68%	69%	94%
Smoking Cessation Advice[5]	-	-	72%	80%	100%
Surgical Infection Prevention					
Prophylactic Antibiotic Given[1,2,3]	9	67%	75%	77%	95%
Prophylactic Antibiotic Selection[5]	-	-	88%	90%	100%
Prophylactic Antibiotic Stopped[1,2,3]	9	100%	82%	72%	95%
Pregnancy Care					
Inpatient Neonatal Mortality	1,145	0.00%	-	-	-
Third or Fourth Degree Laceration	746	5.09%	-	3.63%	3.27%

Mcbride Clinic Orthopedic Hospital

9600 North Broadway Extension
Oklahoma City, OK 73114
Ownership: Government - State
Emergency Services: No

Phone: 405-478-1717
Accredited: No

Measure	Cases	This Hospital	State Average	U.S. Average	Top Hospital
Heart Attack Care					
ACE Inhibitor or ARB for LVSD[5]	-	-	79%	82%	100%
Aspirin at Arrival[5]	-	-	86%	92%	100%
Aspirin at Discharge[5]	-	-	85%	90%	100%
Beta Blocker at Arrival[5]	-	-	78%	87%	100%
Beta Blocker at Discharge[5]	-	-	78%	90%	100%
Fibrinolytic Medication Timing[5]	-	-	36%	31%	100%
PCI Within 90 Minutes of Arrival[5]	-	-	51%	54%	95%
Smoking Cessation Advice[5]	-	-	83%	88%	100%
Heart Failure Care					
ACE Inhibitor or ARB for LVSD[5]	-	-	76%	82%	100%
Discharge Instructions[5]	-	-	55%	61%	93%
Evaluation of LVS Function[5]	-	-	71%	83%	99%
Smoking Cessation Advice[5]	-	-	73%	82%	100%
Pneumonia Care					
Appropriate Initial Antibiotic[5]	-	-	81%	83%	94%
Blood Culture Timing[5]	-	-	91%	90%	100%
Influenza Vaccine[5]	-	-	72%	70%	100%
Initial Antibiotic Timing[5]	-	-	82%	80%	93%
Oxygenation Assessment[5]	-	-	99%	99%	100%
Pneumococcal Vaccine[5]	-	-	68%	69%	94%
Smoking Cessation Advice[5]	-	-	72%	80%	100%
Surgical Infection Prevention					
Prophylactic Antibiotic Given[2,3]	138	97%	75%	77%	95%
Prophylactic Antibiotic Selection[2]	46	100%	88%	90%	100%
Prophylactic Antibiotic Stopped[2,3]	136	97%	82%	72%	95%
Pregnancy Care					
Inpatient Neonatal Mortality	-	-	-	-	-
Third or Fourth Degree Laceration	-	-	-	3.63%	3.27%

Mercy Health Center

4300 W Memorial Road
Oklahoma City, OK 73120
URL: www.mercyok.net/mhc
Ownership: Voluntary non-profit - Church
Emergency Services: Yes

Phone: 405-755-1515
Fax: 405-752-3811

Accredited: Yes
Licensed Beds: 351

Key Personnel:
President/CEO . . . . Bruce F Buchanan
Chief Medical Staff . . . . William Hughes, MD
Emergency Room . . . . Paul Orchutt, MD

Measure	Cases	This Hospital	State Average	U.S. Average	Top Hospital
Heart Attack Care					
ACE Inhibitor or ARB for LVSD[1]	1	100%	79%	82%	100%
Aspirin at Arrival[1]	14	93%	86%	92%	100%
Aspirin at Discharge[1]	16	94%	85%	90%	100%
Beta Blocker at Arrival[1]	11	73%	78%	87%	100%
Beta Blocker at Discharge[1]	12	100%	78%	90%	100%
Fibrinolytic Medication Timing	0	-	36%	31%	100%
PCI Within 90 Minutes of Arrival	0	-	51%	54%	95%
Smoking Cessation Advice[1]	4	100%	83%	88%	100%
Heart Failure Care					
ACE Inhibitor or ARB for LVSD	38	97%	76%	82%	100%
Discharge Instructions	89	73%	55%	61%	93%
Evaluation of LVS Function	128	98%	71%	83%	99%
Smoking Cessation Advice[1]	22	100%	73%	82%	100%
Pneumonia Care					
Appropriate Initial Antibiotic	143	86%	81%	83%	94%
Blood Culture Timing	163	93%	91%	90%	100%
Influenza Vaccine	73	95%	72%	70%	100%
Initial Antibiotic Timing	251	82%	82%	80%	93%
Oxygenation Assessment	343	100%	99%	99%	100%
Pneumococcal Vaccine	235	96%	68%	69%	94%
Smoking Cessation Advice	79	91%	72%	80%	100%
Surgical Infection Prevention					
Prophylactic Antibiotic Given[2]	175	94%	75%	77%	95%
Prophylactic Antibiotic Selection[2]	49	98%	88%	90%	100%
Prophylactic Antibiotic Stopped[2]	167	78%	82%	72%	95%
Pregnancy Care					
Inpatient Neonatal Mortality	-	-	-	-	-
Third or Fourth Degree Laceration	-	-	-	3.63%	3.27%

NOTE: Hospital profiles are in alphabetical order by state, then city, then hospital within the city; Rankings are sorted by rate in descending order and exclude hospitals with less than 25 cases; (1) The number of cases is too small (n<25) for purposes of reliably predicting hospital performance; (2) Measure reflects the hospital's indication that its submission was based upon a sample of its relevant discharges; (3) Rate reflects fewer than the maximum possible quarters of data for the measure; (4) Inaccurate information submitted and suppressed for one or more quarters; (5) No data is available from the hospital for this measure; Please refer to the User's Guide for a full explanation of data

Northwest Surgical Hospital

9204 North May Avenue
Oklahoma City, OK 73120
Ownership: Proprietary
Emergency Services: No

Phone: 404-848-1918

Accredited: Yes

Measure	Cases	This Hospital	State Average	U.S. Average	Top Hospital
Heart Attack Care					
ACE Inhibitor or ARB for LVSD[5]	-	-	79%	82%	100%
Aspirin at Arrival[5]	-	-	86%	92%	100%
Aspirin at Discharge[5]	-	-	85%	90%	100%
Beta Blocker at Arrival[5]	-	-	78%	87%	100%
Beta Blocker at Discharge[5]	-	-	78%	90%	100%
Fibrinolytic Medication Timing[5]	-	-	36%	31%	100%
PCI Within 90 Minutes of Arrival[5]	-	-	51%	54%	95%
Smoking Cessation Advice[5]	-	-	83%	88%	100%
Heart Failure Care					
ACE Inhibitor or ARB for LVSD[5]	-	-	76%	82%	100%
Discharge Instructions[5]	-	-	55%	61%	93%
Evaluation of LVS Function[5]	-	-	71%	83%	99%
Smoking Cessation Advice[5]	-	-	73%	82%	100%
Pneumonia Care					
Appropriate Initial Antibiotic[5]	-	-	81%	83%	94%
Blood Culture Timing[5]	-	-	91%	90%	100%
Influenza Vaccine[5]	-	-	72%	70%	100%
Initial Antibiotic Timing[5]	-	-	82%	80%	93%
Oxygenation Assessment[5]	-	-	99%	99%	100%
Pneumococcal Vaccine[5]	-	-	68%	69%	94%
Smoking Cessation Advice[5]	-	-	72%	80%	100%
Surgical Infection Prevention					
Prophylactic Antibiotic Given	228	96%	75%	77%	95%
Prophylactic Antibiotic Selection	54	96%	88%	90%	100%
Prophylactic Antibiotic Stopped	226	81%	82%	72%	95%
Pregnancy Care					
Inpatient Neonatal Mortality	-	-	-	-	-
Third or Fourth Degree Laceration	-	-	-	3.63%	3.27%

O U Medical Center

1200 Everett Drive
Oklahoma City, OK 73104
URL: www.oumedcenter.com
Ownership: Proprietary
Emergency Services: Yes

Phone: 405-271-4700
Fax: 405-271-7344

Accredited: Yes
Licensed Beds: 394

Key Personnel:

President/CEO . . . . . Cole C Eslyn
Chief Medical Staff . . . . . Timothy Coussons, MD
Chief Catheterization Laboratory . . . . . Bob Weist
Emergency Room . . . . . Gary Quick, MD
Director Infection/Disease Control . . . . . Margaret Tannehill, RN
CCU Spvg. Nurse . . . . . Cyndi Moore, RN
Chief Radiology . . . . . Bob Eaton, MD
Director Respiratory Therapy . . . . . Jeanna Lockwood

Measure	Cases	This Hospital	State Average	U.S. Average	Top Hospital
Heart Attack Care					
ACE Inhibitor or ARB for LVSD	26	96%	79%	82%	100%
Aspirin at Arrival	121	100%	86%	92%	100%
Aspirin at Discharge	152	99%	85%	90%	100%
Beta Blocker at Arrival	104	99%	78%	87%	100%
Beta Blocker at Discharge	147	97%	78%	90%	100%
Fibrinolytic Medication Timing[1]	2	50%	36%	31%	100%
PCI Within 90 Minutes of Arrival[1]	1	100%	51%	54%	95%
Smoking Cessation Advice	68	100%	83%	88%	100%
Heart Failure Care					
ACE Inhibitor or ARB for LVSD	208	90%	76%	82%	100%
Discharge Instructions	377	93%	55%	61%	93%
Evaluation of LVS Function	405	99%	71%	83%	99%
Smoking Cessation Advice	155	95%	73%	82%	100%
Pneumonia Care					
Appropriate Initial Antibiotic	128	89%	81%	83%	94%
Blood Culture Timing	156	90%	91%	90%	100%
Influenza Vaccine	33	64%	72%	70%	100%
Initial Antibiotic Timing	209	65%	82%	80%	93%
Oxygenation Assessment	249	100%	99%	99%	100%
Pneumococcal Vaccine	73	77%	68%	69%	94%
Smoking Cessation Advice	97	89%	72%	80%	100%
Surgical Infection Prevention					
Prophylactic Antibiotic Given	772	84%	75%	77%	95%
Prophylactic Antibiotic Selection	175	95%	88%	90%	100%
Prophylactic Antibiotic Stopped	702	88%	82%	72%	95%
Pregnancy Care					
Inpatient Neonatal Mortality	5,100	1.94%	-	-	-
Third or Fourth Degree Laceration	3,131	2.78%	-	3.63%	3.27%

Okla Ctr for Ortho & Multi-Spec Surg

330 Southwest 80th Street
Oklahoma City, OK 73139
Ownership: Proprietary
Emergency Services: No

Phone: 405-602-6500

Accredited: No

Measure	Cases	This Hospital	State Average	U.S. Average	Top Hospital
Heart Attack Care					
ACE Inhibitor or ARB for LVSD[5]	-	-	79%	82%	100%
Aspirin at Arrival[5]	-	-	86%	92%	100%
Aspirin at Discharge[5]	-	-	85%	90%	100%
Beta Blocker at Arrival[5]	-	-	78%	87%	100%
Beta Blocker at Discharge[5]	-	-	78%	90%	100%
Fibrinolytic Medication Timing[5]	-	-	36%	31%	100%
PCI Within 90 Minutes of Arrival[5]	-	-	51%	54%	95%
Smoking Cessation Advice[5]	-	-	83%	88%	100%
Heart Failure Care					
ACE Inhibitor or ARB for LVSD[5]	-	-	76%	82%	100%
Discharge Instructions[5]	-	-	55%	61%	93%
Evaluation of LVS Function[5]	-	-	71%	83%	99%
Smoking Cessation Advice[5]	-	-	73%	82%	100%
Pneumonia Care					
Appropriate Initial Antibiotic[5]	-	-	81%	83%	94%
Blood Culture Timing[5]	-	-	91%	90%	100%
Influenza Vaccine[5]	-	-	72%	70%	100%
Initial Antibiotic Timing[5]	-	-	82%	80%	93%
Oxygenation Assessment[5]	-	-	99%	99%	100%
Pneumococcal Vaccine[5]	-	-	68%	69%	94%
Smoking Cessation Advice[5]	-	-	72%	80%	100%
Surgical Infection Prevention					
Prophylactic Antibiotic Given[3]	48	77%	75%	77%	95%
Prophylactic Antibiotic Selection[1]	19	95%	88%	90%	100%
Prophylactic Antibiotic Stopped[3]	36	25%	82%	72%	95%
Pregnancy Care					
Inpatient Neonatal Mortality	-	-	-	-	-
Third or Fourth Degree Laceration	-	-	-	3.63%	3.27%

Oklahoma Heart Hospital

4050 W Memorial Road
Oklahoma City, OK 73120
URL: www.okheart.com
Ownership: Proprietary
Emergency Services: Yes

Phone: 405-608-3200
Fax: 405-608-3396

Accredited: Yes
Licensed Beds: 78

Key Personnel:

President/CEO . . . . . Jim Best

Measure	Cases	This Hospital	State Average	U.S. Average	Top Hospital
Heart Attack Care					
ACE Inhibitor or ARB for LVSD[2]	55	100%	79%	82%	100%
Aspirin at Arrival[2]	65	100%	86%	92%	100%
Aspirin at Discharge[2]	302	99%	85%	90%	100%
Beta Blocker at Arrival[2]	57	98%	78%	87%	100%
Beta Blocker at Discharge[2]	296	100%	78%	90%	100%
Fibrinolytic Medication Timing[2]	0	-	36%	31%	100%
PCI Within 90 Minutes of Arrival[1,2]	2	100%	51%	54%	95%
Smoking Cessation Advice[2]	120	100%	83%	88%	100%
Heart Failure Care					
ACE Inhibitor or ARB for LVSD[2]	192	99%	76%	82%	100%
Discharge Instructions[2]	295	100%	55%	61%	93%
Evaluation of LVS Function[2]	312	100%	71%	83%	99%

NOTE: Hospital profiles are in alphabetical order by state, then city, then hospital within the city; Rankings are sorted by rate in descending order and exclude hospitals with less than 25 cases; (1) The number of cases is too small (n<25) for purposes of reliably predicting hospital performance; (2) Measure reflects the hospital's indication that its submission was based upon a sample of its relevant discharges; (3) Rate reflects fewer than the maximum possible quarters of data for the measure; (4) Inaccurate information submitted and suppressed for one or more quarters; (5) No data is available from the hospital for this measure; Please refer to the User's Guide for a full explanation of data

Measure	Cases	This Hospital	State Average	U.S. Average	Top Hospital
Smoking Cessation Advice[2]	65	100%	73%	82%	100%
Pneumonia Care					
Appropriate Initial Antibiotic[1]	17	100%	81%	83%	94%
Blood Culture Timing[1]	13	100%	91%	90%	100%
Influenza Vaccine[1]	4	100%	72%	70%	100%
Initial Antibiotic Timing[1]	21	86%	82%	80%	93%
Oxygenation Assessment	27	100%	99%	99%	100%
Pneumococcal Vaccine[1]	16	88%	68%	69%	94%
Smoking Cessation Advice[1]	6	100%	72%	80%	100%
Surgical Infection Prevention					
Prophylactic Antibiotic Given[2]	184	98%	75%	77%	95%
Prophylactic Antibiotic Selection[2]	44	100%	88%	90%	100%
Prophylactic Antibiotic Stopped[2]	177	97%	82%	72%	95%
Pregnancy Care					
Inpatient Neonatal Mortality	-	-	-	-	-
Third or Fourth Degree Laceration	-	-	-	3.63%	3.27%

Oklahoma Spine Hospital

14101 Parkway Commons Drive
Oklahoma City, OK 73134
Ownership: Proprietary
Emergency Services: Yes

Phone: 405-749-2700
Accredited: Yes

Measure	Cases	This Hospital	State Average	U.S. Average	Top Hospital
Heart Attack Care					
ACE Inhibitor or ARB for LVSD[5]	-	-	79%	82%	100%
Aspirin at Arrival[5]	-	-	86%	92%	100%
Aspirin at Discharge[5]	-	-	85%	90%	100%
Beta Blocker at Arrival[5]	-	-	78%	87%	100%
Beta Blocker at Discharge[5]	-	-	78%	90%	100%
Fibrinolytic Medication Timing[5]	-	-	36%	31%	100%
PCI Within 90 Minutes of Arrival[5]	-	-	51%	54%	95%
Smoking Cessation Advice[5]	-	-	83%	88%	100%
Heart Failure Care					
ACE Inhibitor or ARB for LVSD[5]	-	-	76%	82%	100%
Discharge Instructions[5]	-	-	55%	61%	93%
Evaluation of LVS Function[5]	-	-	71%	83%	99%
Smoking Cessation Advice[5]	-	-	73%	82%	100%
Pneumonia Care					
Appropriate Initial Antibiotic[5]	-	-	81%	83%	94%
Blood Culture Timing[5]	-	-	91%	90%	100%
Influenza Vaccine[5]	-	-	72%	70%	100%
Initial Antibiotic Timing[5]	-	-	82%	80%	93%
Oxygenation Assessment[5]	-	-	99%	99%	100%
Pneumococcal Vaccine[5]	-	-	68%	69%	94%
Smoking Cessation Advice[5]	-	-	72%	80%	100%
Surgical Infection Prevention					
Prophylactic Antibiotic Given[1,2,3]	6	100%	75%	77%	95%
Prophylactic Antibiotic Selection[5]	-	-	88%	90%	100%
Prophylactic Antibiotic Stopped[1,2,3]	6	67%	82%	72%	95%
Pregnancy Care					
Inpatient Neonatal Mortality	-	-	-	-	-
Third or Fourth Degree Laceration	-	-	-	3.63%	3.27%

Orthopedic Hospital

1044 Southwest 44th Street, Suite 950
Oklahoma City, OK 73109
Ownership: Government - Federal
Emergency Services: Yes

Phone: 405-631-3085
Accredited: No

Measure	Cases	This Hospital	State Average	U.S. Average	Top Hospital
Heart Attack Care					
ACE Inhibitor or ARB for LVSD[5]	-	-	79%	82%	100%
Aspirin at Arrival[5]	-	-	86%	92%	100%
Aspirin at Discharge[5]	-	-	85%	90%	100%
Beta Blocker at Arrival[5]	-	-	78%	87%	100%
Beta Blocker at Discharge[5]	-	-	78%	90%	100%
Fibrinolytic Medication Timing[5]	-	-	36%	31%	100%
PCI Within 90 Minutes of Arrival[5]	-	-	51%	54%	95%
Smoking Cessation Advice[5]	-	-	83%	88%	100%
Heart Failure Care					
ACE Inhibitor or ARB for LVSD[5]	-	-	76%	82%	100%
Discharge Instructions[5]	-	-	55%	61%	93%
Evaluation of LVS Function[5]	-	-	71%	83%	99%
Smoking Cessation Advice[5]	-	-	73%	82%	100%
Pneumonia Care					
Appropriate Initial Antibiotic[5]	-	-	81%	83%	94%
Blood Culture Timing[5]	-	-	91%	90%	100%
Influenza Vaccine[5]	-	-	72%	70%	100%
Initial Antibiotic Timing[5]	-	-	82%	80%	93%
Oxygenation Assessment[5]	-	-	99%	99%	100%
Pneumococcal Vaccine[5]	-	-	68%	69%	94%
Smoking Cessation Advice[5]	-	-	72%	80%	100%
Surgical Infection Prevention					
Prophylactic Antibiotic Given[1,3]	1	0%	75%	77%	95%
Prophylactic Antibiotic Selection[5]	-	-	88%	90%	100%
Prophylactic Antibiotic Stopped[1,3]	1	100%	82%	72%	95%
Pregnancy Care					
Inpatient Neonatal Mortality	-	-	-	-	-
Third or Fourth Degree Laceration	-	-	-	3.63%	3.27%

Saint Anthony Hospital

1000 N Lee Street
Oklahoma City, OK 73102
URL: www.saintsok.com
Ownership: Voluntary non-profit - Church
Emergency Services: Yes

Phone: 405-272-7000
Fax: 405-272-6592
Accredited: Yes
Licensed Beds: 659

Key Personnel:

President/CEO . . . . Valinda Rutledge
Administrator/COO . . . . Valinda Rutledge
Chief Medical Staff . . . . Susan Edwards, MD
Emergency Room . . . . Jack Bair, MD
Director Infection/Disease Control . . . . Barbara Baker
Medical/Surgical Nursing . . . . Elizabeth Collier
Director Respiratory Therapy . . . . Jeff Neff

Measure	Cases	This Hospital	State Average	U.S. Average	Top Hospital
Heart Attack Care					
ACE Inhibitor or ARB for LVSD	37	92%	79%	82%	100%
Aspirin at Arrival	172	98%	86%	92%	100%
Aspirin at Discharge	223	98%	85%	90%	100%
Beta Blocker at Arrival	140	94%	78%	87%	100%
Beta Blocker at Discharge	205	98%	78%	90%	100%
Fibrinolytic Medication Timing	0	-	36%	31%	100%
PCI Within 90 Minutes of Arrival[1]	4	50%	51%	54%	95%
Smoking Cessation Advice	92	92%	83%	88%	100%
Heart Failure Care					
ACE Inhibitor or ARB for LVSD	259	85%	76%	82%	100%
Discharge Instructions	441	62%	55%	61%	93%
Evaluation of LVS Function	492	96%	71%	83%	99%
Smoking Cessation Advice	137	100%	73%	82%	100%
Pneumonia Care					
Appropriate Initial Antibiotic	182	90%	81%	83%	94%
Blood Culture Timing	195	93%	91%	90%	100%
Influenza Vaccine	57	93%	72%	70%	100%
Initial Antibiotic Timing	258	87%	82%	80%	93%
Oxygenation Assessment	286	100%	99%	99%	100%
Pneumococcal Vaccine	155	84%	68%	69%	94%
Smoking Cessation Advice	98	92%	72%	80%	100%
Surgical Infection Prevention					
Prophylactic Antibiotic Given	564	95%	75%	77%	95%
Prophylactic Antibiotic Selection	133	99%	88%	90%	100%
Prophylactic Antibiotic Stopped	507	88%	82%	72%	95%
Pregnancy Care					
Inpatient Neonatal Mortality	960	0.10%	-	-	-
Third or Fourth Degree Laceration	646	3.72%	-	3.63%	3.27%

Surgical Hospital of Oklahoma

100 Southeast 59th Street
Oklahoma City, OK 73129
Ownership: Proprietary
Emergency Services: Yes

Phone: 405-634-9300
Accredited: Yes

Measure	Cases	This Hospital	State Average	U.S. Average	Top Hospital

NOTE: Hospital profiles are in alphabetical order by state, then city, then hospital within the city; Rankings are sorted by rate in descending order and exclude hospitals with less than 25 cases; (1) The number of cases is too small (n<25) for purposes of reliably predicting hospital performance; (2) Measure reflects the hospital's indication that its submission was based upon a sample of its relevant discharges; (3) Rate reflects fewer than the maximum possible quarters of data for the measure; (4) Inaccurate information submitted and suppressed for one or more quarters; (5) No data is available from the hospital for this measure; Please refer to the User's Guide for a full explanation of data

Measure	Cases	This Hospital	State Average	U.S. Average	Top Hospital
Heart Attack Care					
ACE Inhibitor or ARB for LVSD[5]	-	-	79%	82%	100%
Aspirin at Arrival[5]	-	-	86%	92%	100%
Aspirin at Discharge[5]	-	-	85%	90%	100%
Beta Blocker at Arrival[5]	-	-	78%	87%	100%
Beta Blocker at Discharge[5]	-	-	78%	90%	100%
Fibrinolytic Medication Timing[5]	-	-	36%	31%	100%
PCI Within 90 Minutes of Arrival[5]	-	-	51%	54%	95%
Smoking Cessation Advice[5]	-	-	83%	88%	100%
Heart Failure Care					
ACE Inhibitor or ARB for LVSD[5]	-	-	76%	82%	100%
Discharge Instructions[5]	-	-	55%	61%	93%
Evaluation of LVS Function[5]	-	-	71%	83%	99%
Smoking Cessation Advice[5]	-	-	73%	82%	100%
Pneumonia Care					
Appropriate Initial Antibiotic[5]	-	-	81%	83%	94%
Blood Culture Timing[5]	-	-	91%	90%	100%
Influenza Vaccine[5]	-	-	72%	70%	100%
Initial Antibiotic Timing[5]	-	-	82%	80%	93%
Oxygenation Assessment[5]	-	-	99%	99%	100%
Pneumococcal Vaccine[5]	-	-	68%	69%	94%
Smoking Cessation Advice[5]	-	-	72%	80%	100%
Surgical Infection Prevention					
Prophylactic Antibiotic Given[3]	114	81%	75%	77%	95%
Prophylactic Antibiotic Selection	46	100%	88%	90%	100%
Prophylactic Antibiotic Stopped[3]	112	98%	82%	72%	95%
Pregnancy Care					
Inpatient Neonatal Mortality	-	-	-	-	-
Third or Fourth Degree Laceration	-	-	-	3.63%	3.27%

Okmulgee Memorial Hospital

1401 Morris Drive
PO Box 1038
Okmulgee, OK 74447
Phone: 918-756-4233
Fax: 918-756-5968
URL: www.okmulgeehospital.com

Ownership: Voluntary non-profit - Private
Accredited: Yes
Emergency Services: Yes
Licensed Beds: 66

Key Personnel:

CEO . . . . . Rex Jones
CNO . . . . . Valerie Round, RN
Chief Medical Staff . . . . . Noel Gattenby, DO
ER Manager . . . . . Janice O'Shields
Infection Control . . . . . Kahty Machetta, RN
Medical Surgical Nursing . . . . . Valerie Round, RN
Director Radiology . . . . . Charles Remer
Director Respiratory Therapy . . . . . Ioma Jones

Measure	Cases	This Hospital	State Average	U.S. Average	Top Hospital
Heart Attack Care					
ACE Inhibitor or ARB for LVSD[3]	0	-	79%	82%	100%
Aspirin at Arrival[1,3]	2	100%	86%	92%	100%
Aspirin at Discharge[1,3]	2	100%	85%	90%	100%
Beta Blocker at Arrival[1,3]	1	100%	78%	87%	100%
Beta Blocker at Discharge[1,3]	1	100%	78%	90%	100%
Fibrinolytic Medication Timing[1,3]	1	0%	36%	31%	100%
PCI Within 90 Minutes of Arrival	0	-	51%	54%	95%
Smoking Cessation Advice[3]	0	-	83%	88%	100%
Heart Failure Care					
ACE Inhibitor or ARB for LVSD[1]	3	33%	76%	82%	100%
Discharge Instructions	33	18%	55%	61%	93%
Evaluation of LVS Function	47	36%	71%	83%	99%
Smoking Cessation Advice[1]	1	0%	73%	82%	100%
Pneumonia Care					
Appropriate Initial Antibiotic	41	98%	81%	83%	94%
Blood Culture Timing	27	93%	91%	90%	100%
Influenza Vaccine[1]	13	85%	72%	70%	100%
Initial Antibiotic Timing	50	84%	82%	80%	93%
Oxygenation Assessment	62	100%	99%	99%	100%
Pneumococcal Vaccine	46	63%	68%	69%	94%
Smoking Cessation Advice[1]	18	22%	72%	80%	100%
Surgical Infection Prevention					
Prophylactic Antibiotic Given[1,3]	19	32%	75%	77%	95%
Prophylactic Antibiotic Selection[1]	6	100%	88%	90%	100%
Prophylactic Antibiotic Stopped[1,3]	19	100%	82%	72%	95%
Pregnancy Care					
Inpatient Neonatal Mortality	-	-	-	-	-
Third or Fourth Degree Laceration	-	-	-	3.63%	3.27%

Pauls Valley General Hospital

100 Valley Drive
Pauls Valley, OK 73075
Toll-Free: 800-838-5501
Phone: 405-238-5501
Fax: 405-238-5926
URL: www.telepath.com/pvgh

Ownership: Government - Local
Accredited: No
Emergency Services: Yes
Licensed Beds: 64

Key Personnel:

CEO . . . . . Charles Johnston
Chief Medical Staff . . . . . Mat Brown, MD
Chief Medical Staff . . . . . Dennis Whitehouse
Emergency Room . . . . . Merry Dudley
Director of Pulmonary . . . . . Don Gangwere

Measure	Cases	This Hospital	State Average	U.S. Average	Top Hospital
Heart Attack Care					
ACE Inhibitor or ARB for LVSD	0	-	79%	82%	100%
Aspirin at Arrival[1]	5	80%	86%	92%	100%
Aspirin at Discharge[1]	4	75%	85%	90%	100%
Beta Blocker at Arrival[1]	4	100%	78%	87%	100%
Beta Blocker at Discharge[1]	4	100%	78%	90%	100%
Fibrinolytic Medication Timing	0	-	36%	31%	100%
PCI Within 90 Minutes of Arrival	0	-	51%	54%	95%
Smoking Cessation Advice	0	-	83%	88%	100%
Heart Failure Care					
ACE Inhibitor or ARB for LVSD[1]	14	100%	76%	82%	100%
Discharge Instructions	49	88%	55%	61%	93%
Evaluation of LVS Function	67	70%	71%	83%	99%
Smoking Cessation Advice[1]	13	100%	73%	82%	100%
Pneumonia Care					
Appropriate Initial Antibiotic	64	95%	81%	83%	94%
Blood Culture Timing	41	100%	91%	90%	100%
Influenza Vaccine[1]	14	100%	72%	70%	100%
Initial Antibiotic Timing	76	89%	82%	80%	93%
Oxygenation Assessment	91	100%	99%	99%	100%
Pneumococcal Vaccine	61	97%	68%	69%	94%
Smoking Cessation Advice[1]	24	96%	72%	80%	100%
Surgical Infection Prevention					
Prophylactic Antibiotic Given[1,3]	10	80%	75%	77%	95%
Prophylactic Antibiotic Selection[1]	3	100%	88%	90%	100%
Prophylactic Antibiotic Stopped[1,3]	10	60%	82%	72%	95%
Pregnancy Care					
Inpatient Neonatal Mortality	-	-	-	-	-
Third or Fourth Degree Laceration	-	-	-	3.63%	3.27%

Pawhuska Hospital

1101 E 15th Street
Pawhuska, OK 74056
Phone: 918-287-5100
Fax: 918-287-5145

Ownership: Voluntary non-profit - Other
Accredited: No
Emergency Services: Yes
Licensed Beds: 25

Key Personnel:

Administrator . . . . . Ron Dunkle, RN
Chief Medical Staff . . . . . Mike Priest, DO
Emergency Room . . . . . Kelly Eaton, RN
Infection Control . . . . . Gertrude Greghoff

Measure	Cases	This Hospital	State Average	U.S. Average	Top Hospital
Heart Attack Care					
ACE Inhibitor or ARB for LVSD[5]	-	-	79%	82%	100%
Aspirin at Arrival[5]	-	-	86%	92%	100%
Aspirin at Discharge[5]	-	-	85%	90%	100%
Beta Blocker at Arrival[5]	-	-	78%	87%	100%
Beta Blocker at Discharge[5]	-	-	78%	90%	100%
Fibrinolytic Medication Timing[5]	-	-	36%	31%	100%
PCI Within 90 Minutes of Arrival[5]	-	-	51%	54%	95%
Smoking Cessation Advice[5]	-	-	83%	88%	100%
Heart Failure Care					

NOTE: Hospital profiles are in alphabetical order by state, then city, then hospital within the city; Rankings are sorted by rate in descending order and exclude hospitals with less than 25 cases; (1) The number of cases is too small (n<25) for purposes of reliably predicting hospital performance; (2) Measure reflects the hospital's indication that its submission was based upon a sample of its relevant discharges; (3) Rate reflects fewer than the maximum possible quarters of data for the measure; (4) Inaccurate information submitted and suppressed for one or more quarters; (5) No data is available from the hospital for this measure; Please refer to the User's Guide for a full explanation of data

ACE Inhibitor or ARB for LVSD[3]	0	-	76%	82%	100%
Discharge Instructions[1,3]	2	0%	55%	61%	93%
Evaluation of LVS Function[1,3]	2	50%	71%	83%	99%
Smoking Cessation Advice[3]	0	-	73%	82%	100%
Pneumonia Care					
Appropriate Initial Antibiotic[1]	10	90%	81%	83%	94%
Blood Culture Timing	0	-	91%	90%	100%
Influenza Vaccine[1]	3	0%	72%	70%	100%
Initial Antibiotic Timing[1]	9	100%	82%	80%	93%
Oxygenation Assessment[1]	11	82%	99%	99%	100%
Pneumococcal Vaccine[1]	8	0%	68%	69%	94%
Smoking Cessation Advice	0	-	72%	80%	100%
Surgical Infection Prevention					
Prophylactic Antibiotic Given[5]	-	-	75%	77%	95%
Prophylactic Antibiotic Selection[5]	-	-	88%	90%	100%
Prophylactic Antibiotic Stopped[5]	-	-	82%	72%	95%
Pregnancy Care					
Inpatient Neonatal Mortality	-	-	-	-	-
Third or Fourth Degree Laceration	-	-	-	3.63%	3.27%

Pawnee Municipal Hospital

1212 4th Street
Pawnee, OK 74058
Ownership: Proprietary
Emergency Services: Yes
Phone: 918-786-2431
Fax: 918-762-6346
Accredited: No
Licensed Beds: 40

Key Personnel:

Administrator . . . . . John Ketring
Chief Medical Staff. . . . . James P Riemer, DO
Director Infection/Disease Control . . . . . Dondi Pulse
Director Medical/Surgical Nursing . . . . . Tanya Mulder
Chief Radiology . . . . . Robert Cook
Director Respiratory Therapy . . . . . Mary Lasater

Measure	Cases	This Hospital	State Average	U.S. Average	Top Hospital
Heart Attack Care					
ACE Inhibitor or ARB for LVSD[1]	1	0%	79%	82%	100%
Aspirin at Arrival[1]	4	100%	86%	92%	100%
Aspirin at Discharge[1]	2	0%	85%	90%	100%
Beta Blocker at Arrival[1]	2	50%	78%	87%	100%
Beta Blocker at Discharge[1]	2	50%	78%	90%	100%
Fibrinolytic Medication Timing	0	-	36%	31%	100%
PCI Within 90 Minutes of Arrival	0	-	51%	54%	95%
Smoking Cessation Advice	0	-	83%	88%	100%
Heart Failure Care					
ACE Inhibitor or ARB for LVSD[1]	1	0%	76%	82%	100%
Discharge Instructions[1]	22	45%	55%	61%	93%
Evaluation of LVS Function	25	32%	71%	83%	99%
Smoking Cessation Advice[1]	6	67%	73%	82%	100%
Pneumonia Care					
Appropriate Initial Antibiotic[1]	20	85%	81%	83%	94%
Blood Culture Timing	0	-	91%	90%	100%
Influenza Vaccine[1]	7	71%	72%	70%	100%
Initial Antibiotic Timing[1]	24	83%	82%	80%	93%
Oxygenation Assessment	26	100%	99%	99%	100%
Pneumococcal Vaccine[1]	12	67%	68%	69%	94%
Smoking Cessation Advice[1]	6	17%	72%	80%	100%
Surgical Infection Prevention					
Prophylactic Antibiotic Given[1,3]	3	0%	75%	77%	95%
Prophylactic Antibiotic Selection[1]	3	100%	88%	90%	100%
Prophylactic Antibiotic Stopped[1,3]	3	100%	82%	72%	95%
Pregnancy Care					
Inpatient Neonatal Mortality	-	-	-	-	-
Third or Fourth Degree Laceration	-	-	-	3.63%	3.27%

Perry Memorial Hospital

501 14th Street
Perry, OK 73077
URL: www.pmh-ok.org
Ownership: Voluntary non-profit - Other
Emergency Services: Yes
Phone: 580-336-3541
Fax: 580-336-7209
Accredited: No
Licensed Beds: 28

Key Personnel:

Administrator . . . . . Joe Duerr

Measure	Cases	This Hospital	State Average	U.S. Average	Top Hospital
Heart Attack Care					
ACE Inhibitor or ARB for LVSD[3]	0	-	79%	82%	100%
Aspirin at Arrival[1,3]	2	100%	86%	92%	100%
Aspirin at Discharge[3]	0	-	85%	90%	100%
Beta Blocker at Arrival[1,3]	2	0%	78%	87%	100%
Beta Blocker at Discharge[1,3]	1	0%	78%	90%	100%
Fibrinolytic Medication Timing[1,3]	2	0%	36%	31%	100%
PCI Within 90 Minutes of Arrival[5]	-	-	51%	54%	95%
Smoking Cessation Advice[3]	0	-	83%	88%	100%
Heart Failure Care					
ACE Inhibitor or ARB for LVSD[1]	6	100%	76%	82%	100%
Discharge Instructions[1]	22	68%	55%	61%	93%
Evaluation of LVS Function	31	65%	71%	83%	99%
Smoking Cessation Advice[1]	11	100%	73%	82%	100%
Pneumonia Care					
Appropriate Initial Antibiotic	35	91%	81%	83%	94%
Blood Culture Timing[1]	11	91%	91%	90%	100%
Influenza Vaccine[1]	13	77%	72%	70%	100%
Initial Antibiotic Timing	55	96%	82%	80%	93%
Oxygenation Assessment	64	100%	99%	99%	100%
Pneumococcal Vaccine	42	86%	68%	69%	94%
Smoking Cessation Advice[1]	14	50%	72%	80%	100%
Surgical Infection Prevention					
Prophylactic Antibiotic Given[5]	-	-	75%	77%	95%
Prophylactic Antibiotic Selection[5]	-	-	88%	90%	100%
Prophylactic Antibiotic Stopped[5]	-	-	82%	72%	95%
Pregnancy Care					
Inpatient Neonatal Mortality	-	-	-	-	-
Third or Fourth Degree Laceration	-	-	-	3.63%	3.27%

Ponca City Medical Center

1900 N 14th Street
Ponca City, OK 74601
URL: www.poncamedcenter.com
Ownership: Proprietary
Emergency Services: Yes
Phone: 580-765-3321
Fax: 580-765-0341
Accredited: Yes
Licensed Beds: 140

Key Personnel:

CEO. . . . . Dennis Barts
Chief Medical Staff. . . . . Krishna Vaidya
Emergency Room . . . . . Brenda Peters
Emergency Room . . . . . Danny Cassidy, MD
Infection Control. . . . . Cheryle Hiebert
Intensive/Coronary Care . . . . . Jeanne Stara
Medical/Surgical Nursing . . . . . Judy Rexford
Respiratory/Cardiopulmonary. . . . . Merle Schroth

Measure	Cases	This Hospital	State Average	U.S. Average	Top Hospital
Heart Attack Care					
ACE Inhibitor or ARB for LVSD[1]	3	100%	79%	82%	100%
Aspirin at Arrival	47	85%	86%	92%	100%
Aspirin at Discharge[1]	16	69%	85%	90%	100%
Beta Blocker at Arrival	42	69%	78%	87%	100%
Beta Blocker at Discharge[1]	15	80%	78%	90%	100%
Fibrinolytic Medication Timing[1]	14	29%	36%	31%	100%
PCI Within 90 Minutes of Arrival	0	-	51%	54%	95%
Smoking Cessation Advice[1]	2	100%	83%	88%	100%
Heart Failure Care					
ACE Inhibitor or ARB for LVSD[1]	22	86%	76%	82%	100%
Discharge Instructions	66	92%	55%	61%	93%
Evaluation of LVS Function	81	70%	71%	83%	99%
Smoking Cessation Advice[1]	15	87%	73%	82%	100%
Pneumonia Care					
Appropriate Initial Antibiotic	92	85%	81%	83%	94%
Blood Culture Timing	60	92%	91%	90%	100%
Influenza Vaccine[1]	22	82%	72%	70%	100%
Initial Antibiotic Timing	99	81%	82%	80%	93%
Oxygenation Assessment	118	98%	99%	99%	100%
Pneumococcal Vaccine	71	79%	68%	69%	94%
Smoking Cessation Advice	31	84%	72%	80%	100%
Surgical Infection Prevention					
Prophylactic Antibiotic Given[2,3]	86	51%	75%	77%	95%

NOTE: Hospital profiles are in alphabetical order by state, then city, then hospital within the city; Rankings are sorted by rate in descending order and exclude hospitals with less than 25 cases; (1) The number of cases is too small (n<25) for purposes of reliably predicting hospital performance; (2) Measure reflects the hospital's indication that its submission was based upon a sample of its relevant discharges; (3) Rate reflects fewer than the maximum possible quarters of data for the measure; (4) Inaccurate information submitted and suppressed for one or more quarters; (5) No data is available from the hospital for this measure; Please refer to the User's Guide for a full explanation of data

Measure	Cases	This Hospital	State Average	U.S. Average	Top Hospital
Prophylactic Antibiotic Selection[2]	26	88%	88%	90%	100%
Prophylactic Antibiotic Stopped[2,3]	84	60%	82%	72%	95%
Pregnancy Care					
Inpatient Neonatal Mortality	-	-	-	-	-
Third or Fourth Degree Laceration	-	-	-	3.63%	3.27%

Eastern Oklahoma Medical Center

Alternate Name: LeFlore County Hospital Authority
105 Wall Street
Poteau, OK 74953
Phone: 918-647-8161
Fax: 918-635-3358
Ownership: Govt - Hospital District or Authority
Accredited: Yes
Emergency Services: Yes
Licensed Beds: 85

Key Personnel:

President/CEO . . . . Craig Cudworth
Emergency Room . . . . Robert Carter
CCU Spvg. Nurse . . . . Sue Hall
Supervisor Medical/Surgical . . . . Sue Hall

Measure	Cases	This Hospital	State Average	U.S. Average	Top Hospital
Heart Attack Care					
ACE Inhibitor or ARB for LVSD[1]	2	100%	79%	82%	100%
Aspirin at Arrival[1]	9	89%	86%	92%	100%
Aspirin at Discharge[1]	6	67%	85%	90%	100%
Beta Blocker at Arrival[1]	7	71%	78%	87%	100%
Beta Blocker at Discharge[1]	6	50%	78%	90%	100%
Fibrinolytic Medication Timing[1]	1	0%	36%	31%	100%
PCI Within 90 Minutes of Arrival	0	-	51%	54%	95%
Smoking Cessation Advice[1]	2	50%	83%	88%	100%
Heart Failure Care					
ACE Inhibitor or ARB for LVSD	45	62%	76%	82%	100%
Discharge Instructions	171	61%	55%	61%	93%
Evaluation of LVS Function	196	53%	71%	83%	99%
Smoking Cessation Advice	40	95%	73%	82%	100%
Pneumonia Care					
Appropriate Initial Antibiotic	107	79%	81%	83%	94%
Blood Culture Timing	48	77%	91%	90%	100%
Influenza Vaccine	26	31%	72%	70%	100%
Initial Antibiotic Timing	144	76%	82%	80%	93%
Oxygenation Assessment	153	97%	99%	99%	100%
Pneumococcal Vaccine	92	21%	68%	69%	94%
Smoking Cessation Advice	64	91%	72%	80%	100%
Surgical Infection Prevention					
Prophylactic Antibiotic Given[1,3]	12	83%	75%	77%	95%
Prophylactic Antibiotic Selection[1]	10	80%	88%	90%	100%
Prophylactic Antibiotic Stopped[1,3]	11	100%	82%	72%	95%
Pregnancy Care					
Inpatient Neonatal Mortality	-	-	-	-	-
Third or Fourth Degree Laceration	-	-	-	3.63%	3.27%

Prague Municipal Hospital

PO Drawer S
Prague, OK 74864
Phone: 405-567-4922
Fax: 405-567-4290
Ownership: Govt - Hospital District or Authority
Accredited: No
Emergency Services: Yes
Licensed Beds: 25

Key Personnel:

CEO . . . . Joan Walter
Chief Medical Staff . . . . Alexander Frank, MD
Emergency Room . . . . Dr. Alexander Frank
Manager Radiology . . . . Laura Coley

Measure	Cases	This Hospital	State Average	U.S. Average	Top Hospital
Heart Attack Care					
ACE Inhibitor or ARB for LVSD[1,3]	1	0%	79%	82%	100%
Aspirin at Arrival[3]	0	-	86%	92%	100%
Aspirin at Discharge[1,3]	1	100%	85%	90%	100%
Beta Blocker at Arrival[3]	0	-	78%	87%	100%
Beta Blocker at Discharge[3]	0	-	78%	90%	100%
Fibrinolytic Medication Timing[3]	0	-	36%	31%	100%
PCI Within 90 Minutes of Arrival[5]	-	-	51%	54%	95%
Smoking Cessation Advice[3]	0	-	83%	88%	100%
Heart Failure Care					
ACE Inhibitor or ARB for LVSD[3]	0	-	76%	82%	100%
Discharge Instructions[1,3]	3	33%	55%	61%	93%
Evaluation of LVS Function[1,3]	4	25%	71%	83%	99%
Smoking Cessation Advice[1,3]	1	0%	73%	82%	100%
Pneumonia Care					
Appropriate Initial Antibiotic[1]	6	83%	81%	83%	94%
Blood Culture Timing[1]	3	67%	91%	90%	100%
Influenza Vaccine[1]	2	100%	72%	70%	100%
Initial Antibiotic Timing[1]	8	88%	82%	80%	93%
Oxygenation Assessment[1]	10	100%	99%	99%	100%
Pneumococcal Vaccine[1]	5	100%	68%	69%	94%
Smoking Cessation Advice[1]	1	100%	72%	80%	100%
Surgical Infection Prevention					
Prophylactic Antibiotic Given[5]	-	-	75%	77%	95%
Prophylactic Antibiotic Selection[5]	-	-	88%	90%	100%
Prophylactic Antibiotic Stopped[5]	-	-	82%	72%	95%
Pregnancy Care					
Inpatient Neonatal Mortality	-	-	-	-	-
Third or Fourth Degree Laceration	-	-	-	3.63%	3.27%

Integris Mayes County Medical Center

129 North Kentucky Street
PO Box 278
Pryor, OK 74362
Phone: 918-825-1600
Fax: 918-825-7668
E-mail: white@integris-health.com
URL: www.integris-health.com
Ownership: Voluntary non-profit - Other
Accredited: Yes
Emergency Services: Yes
Licensed Beds: 73

Key Personnel:

Administrator . . . . W Charles Jordan
Chief Medical Staff . . . . Paul Battles, DO
Emergency Room . . . . Chris DeLong, DO
Director Radiology . . . . Steve Davenport

Measure	Cases	This Hospital	State Average	U.S. Average	Top Hospital
Heart Attack Care					
ACE Inhibitor or ARB for LVSD	0	-	79%	82%	100%
Aspirin at Arrival[1]	2	100%	86%	92%	100%
Aspirin at Discharge[1]	1	100%	85%	90%	100%
Beta Blocker at Arrival[1]	1	100%	78%	87%	100%
Beta Blocker at Discharge[1]	1	100%	78%	90%	100%
Fibrinolytic Medication Timing	0	-	36%	31%	100%
PCI Within 90 Minutes of Arrival	0	-	51%	54%	95%
Smoking Cessation Advice	0	-	83%	88%	100%
Heart Failure Care					
ACE Inhibitor or ARB for LVSD[1]	16	88%	76%	82%	100%
Discharge Instructions	31	97%	55%	61%	93%
Evaluation of LVS Function	52	94%	71%	83%	99%
Smoking Cessation Advice[1]	8	100%	73%	82%	100%
Pneumonia Care					
Appropriate Initial Antibiotic	67	97%	81%	83%	94%
Blood Culture Timing	56	95%	91%	90%	100%
Influenza Vaccine[1]	15	100%	72%	70%	100%
Initial Antibiotic Timing	75	93%	82%	80%	93%
Oxygenation Assessment	86	100%	99%	99%	100%
Pneumococcal Vaccine	43	98%	68%	69%	94%
Smoking Cessation Advice	28	100%	72%	80%	100%
Surgical Infection Prevention					
Prophylactic Antibiotic Given	37	95%	75%	77%	95%
Prophylactic Antibiotic Selection[1]	5	100%	88%	90%	100%
Prophylactic Antibiotic Stopped	36	92%	82%	72%	95%
Pregnancy Care					
Inpatient Neonatal Mortality	-	-	-	-	-
Third or Fourth Degree Laceration	-	-	-	3.63%	3.27%

Purcell Municipal Hospital

1500 N Green Avenue
PO Box 511
Purcell, OK 73080
Phone: 405-527-6524
Fax: 405-527-6963
Ownership: Government - Local
Accredited: No
Emergency Services: Yes
Licensed Beds: 39

Key Personnel:

Administrator . . . . Curtis Pryor
Chief Medical Staff . . . . Jill Watson, MD

NOTE: Hospital profiles are in alphabetical order by state, then city, then hospital within the city; Rankings are sorted by rate in descending order and exclude hospitals with less than 25 cases; (1) The number of cases is too small (n<25) for purposes of reliably predicting hospital performance; (2) Measure reflects the hospital's indication that its submission was based upon a sample of its relevant discharges; (3) Rate reflects fewer than the maximum possible quarters of data for the measure; (4) Inaccurate information submitted and suppressed for one or more quarters; (5) No data is available from the hospital for this measure; Please refer to the User's Guide for a full explanation of data

Emergency Room Manager . . . . Donn A Avila, RN
Infection Control . . . . Pam Kaiser, RN
Medical/Surgical Nursing . . . . Ann Goodin, RN
CEO . . . . Curtis Pryor
Respiratory Therapy Manager . . . . Karen Huckaby

Measure	Cases	This Hospital	State Average	U.S. Average	Top Hospital
Heart Attack Care					
ACE Inhibitor or ARB for LVSD	0	-	79%	82%	100%
Aspirin at Arrival[1]	10	60%	86%	92%	100%
Aspirin at Discharge[1]	6	67%	85%	90%	100%
Beta Blocker at Arrival[1]	13	38%	78%	87%	100%
Beta Blocker at Discharge[1]	7	43%	78%	90%	100%
Fibrinolytic Medication Timing	0	-	36%	31%	100%
PCI Within 90 Minutes of Arrival	0	-	51%	54%	95%
Smoking Cessation Advice[1]	1	100%	83%	88%	100%
Heart Failure Care					
ACE Inhibitor or ARB for LVSD[1]	7	57%	76%	82%	100%
Discharge Instructions	52	63%	55%	61%	93%
Evaluation of LVS Function	64	55%	71%	83%	99%
Smoking Cessation Advice[1]	10	70%	73%	82%	100%
Pneumonia Care					
Appropriate Initial Antibiotic	81	75%	81%	83%	94%
Blood Culture Timing	42	93%	91%	90%	100%
Influenza Vaccine	37	73%	72%	70%	100%
Initial Antibiotic Timing	143	79%	82%	80%	93%
Oxygenation Assessment	159	100%	99%	99%	100%
Pneumococcal Vaccine	104	52%	68%	69%	94%
Smoking Cessation Advice	32	62%	72%	80%	100%
Surgical Infection Prevention					
Prophylactic Antibiotic Given[1,3]	3	67%	75%	77%	95%
Prophylactic Antibiotic Selection	0	-	88%	90%	100%
Prophylactic Antibiotic Stopped[1,3]	3	100%	82%	72%	95%
Pregnancy Care					
Inpatient Neonatal Mortality	-	-	-	-	-
Third or Fourth Degree Laceration	-	-	-	3.63%	3.27%

Sequoyah Memorial Hospital

213 E Redwood
Sallisaw, OK 74955
Ownership: Govt - Hospital District or Authority
Emergency Services: Yes
Phone: 918-774-1150
Fax: 918-774-1155
Accredited: No
Licensed Beds: 43

Key Personnel:

CEO . . . . Charles Wade
Chief Medical Staff . . . . Jim Campbell, DO

Measure	Cases	This Hospital	State Average	U.S. Average	Top Hospital
Heart Attack Care					
ACE Inhibitor or ARB for LVSD	0	-	79%	82%	100%
Aspirin at Arrival[1]	9	56%	86%	92%	100%
Aspirin at Discharge[1]	4	75%	85%	90%	100%
Beta Blocker at Arrival[1]	4	100%	78%	87%	100%
Beta Blocker at Discharge[1]	5	60%	78%	90%	100%
Fibrinolytic Medication Timing	0	-	36%	31%	100%
PCI Within 90 Minutes of Arrival	0	-	51%	54%	95%
Smoking Cessation Advice[1]	2	100%	83%	88%	100%
Heart Failure Care					
ACE Inhibitor or ARB for LVSD[1]	4	100%	76%	82%	100%
Discharge Instructions	41	61%	55%	61%	93%
Evaluation of LVS Function	44	86%	71%	83%	99%
Smoking Cessation Advice[1]	12	75%	73%	82%	100%
Pneumonia Care					
Appropriate Initial Antibiotic	49	92%	81%	83%	94%
Blood Culture Timing	44	95%	91%	90%	100%
Influenza Vaccine[1]	9	89%	72%	70%	100%
Initial Antibiotic Timing	66	77%	82%	80%	93%
Oxygenation Assessment	83	100%	99%	99%	100%
Pneumococcal Vaccine	44	89%	68%	69%	94%
Smoking Cessation Advice	25	76%	72%	80%	100%
Surgical Infection Prevention					
Prophylactic Antibiotic Given[5]	-	-	75%	77%	95%
Prophylactic Antibiotic Selection[5]	-	-	88%	90%	100%
Prophylactic Antibiotic Stopped[5]	-	-	82%	72%	95%
Pregnancy Care					
Inpatient Neonatal Mortality	-	-	-	-	-
Third or Fourth Degree Laceration	-	-	-	3.63%	3.27%

Saint John Sapulpa Hospital

PO Box 1368
Sapulpa, OK 74067
Ownership: Voluntary non-profit - Church
Emergency Services: Yes
Phone: 918-224-4280
Fax: 918-224-4395
Accredited: No
Licensed Beds: 113

Key Personnel:

President/CEO . . . . Raymond Replogle
Chief of Medical Staff . . . . Roger Wilson
Emergency Room . . . . Beatrice Lewis, RN
Infection Control . . . . Peggy Ault
Surgical Services . . . . Kurt Lane

Measure	Cases	This Hospital	State Average	U.S. Average	Top Hospital
Heart Attack Care					
ACE Inhibitor or ARB for LVSD[5]	-	-	79%	82%	100%
Aspirin at Arrival[5]	-	-	86%	92%	100%
Aspirin at Discharge[5]	-	-	85%	90%	100%
Beta Blocker at Arrival[5]	-	-	78%	87%	100%
Beta Blocker at Discharge[5]	-	-	78%	90%	100%
Fibrinolytic Medication Timing[5]	-	-	36%	31%	100%
PCI Within 90 Minutes of Arrival[5]	-	-	51%	54%	95%
Smoking Cessation Advice[5]	-	-	83%	88%	100%
Heart Failure Care					
ACE Inhibitor or ARB for LVSD[1]	24	67%	76%	82%	100%
Discharge Instructions	46	48%	55%	61%	93%
Evaluation of LVS Function	53	62%	71%	83%	99%
Smoking Cessation Advice[1]	14	64%	73%	82%	100%
Pneumonia Care					
Appropriate Initial Antibiotic	65	85%	81%	83%	94%
Blood Culture Timing	55	87%	91%	90%	100%
Influenza Vaccine[1]	12	92%	72%	70%	100%
Initial Antibiotic Timing	83	81%	82%	80%	93%
Oxygenation Assessment	94	98%	99%	99%	100%
Pneumococcal Vaccine	46	52%	68%	69%	94%
Smoking Cessation Advice	26	62%	72%	80%	100%
Surgical Infection Prevention					
Prophylactic Antibiotic Given[5]	-	-	75%	77%	95%
Prophylactic Antibiotic Selection[5]	-	-	88%	90%	100%
Prophylactic Antibiotic Stopped[5]	-	-	82%	72%	95%
Pregnancy Care					
Inpatient Neonatal Mortality	-	-	-	-	-
Third or Fourth Degree Laceration	-	-	-	3.63%	3.27%

Sayre Memorial Hospital

PO Box 680
Sayre, OK 73662
Ownership: Voluntary non-profit - Private
Emergency Services: Yes
Phone: 580-928-5541
Fax: 580-928-3523
Accredited: No
Licensed Beds: 46

Key Personnel:

Administrator . . . . Rex Jones
Chief of Medical Staff . . . . Mel Robison
Emergency Room . . . . Kenneth Whinery, MD

Measure	Cases	This Hospital	State Average	U.S. Average	Top Hospital
Heart Attack Care					
ACE Inhibitor or ARB for LVSD[1]	1	100%	79%	82%	100%
Aspirin at Arrival[1]	12	83%	86%	92%	100%
Aspirin at Discharge[1]	9	78%	85%	90%	100%
Beta Blocker at Arrival[1]	9	22%	78%	87%	100%
Beta Blocker at Discharge[1]	8	50%	78%	90%	100%
Fibrinolytic Medication Timing[1]	1	0%	36%	31%	100%
PCI Within 90 Minutes of Arrival	0	-	51%	54%	95%
Smoking Cessation Advice[1]	1	100%	83%	88%	100%
Heart Failure Care					
ACE Inhibitor or ARB for LVSD[1]	2	50%	76%	82%	100%
Discharge Instructions	26	50%	55%	61%	93%
Evaluation of LVS Function	27	19%	71%	83%	99%

NOTE: Hospital profiles are in alphabetical order by state, then city, then hospital within the city; Rankings are sorted by rate in descending order and exclude hospitals with less than 25 cases; (1) The number of cases is too small (n<25) for purposes of reliably predicting hospital performance; (2) Measure reflects the hospital's indication that its submission was based upon a sample of its relevant discharges; (3) Rate reflects fewer than the maximum possible quarters of data for the measure; (4) Inaccurate information submitted and suppressed for one or more quarters; (5) No data is available from the hospital for this measure; Please refer to the User's Guide for a full explanation of data

Measure	Cases	This Hospital	State Average	U.S. Average	Top Hospital
Smoking Cessation Advice[1]	2	0%	73%	82%	100%
Pneumonia Care					
Appropriate Initial Antibiotic	83	95%	81%	83%	94%
Blood Culture Timing[1]	9	100%	91%	90%	100%
Influenza Vaccine	37	76%	72%	70%	100%
Initial Antibiotic Timing	120	94%	82%	80%	93%
Oxygenation Assessment	132	100%	99%	99%	100%
Pneumococcal Vaccine	58	41%	68%	69%	94%
Smoking Cessation Advice	36	36%	72%	80%	100%
Surgical Infection Prevention					
Prophylactic Antibiotic Given[5]	-	-	75%	77%	95%
Prophylactic Antibiotic Selection[5]	-	-	88%	90%	100%
Prophylactic Antibiotic Stopped[5]	-	-	82%	72%	95%
Pregnancy Care					
Inpatient Neonatal Mortality	-	-	-	-	-
Third or Fourth Degree Laceration	-	-	-	3.63%	3.27%

Seiling Municipal Hospital Authority

Alternate Name: Seiling Hospital
NE Highway 60 and 270
Seiling, OK 73663
Phone: 580-922-7361
Fax: 580-922-7718
Ownership: Government - Local
Accredited: No
Emergency Services: No
Licensed Beds: 18

Key Personnel:

CEO . . . . Deryl Gulliford, PhD

Measure	Cases	This Hospital	State Average	U.S. Average	Top Hospital
Heart Attack Care					
ACE Inhibitor or ARB for LVSD[5]	-	-	79%	82%	100%
Aspirin at Arrival[5]	-	-	86%	92%	100%
Aspirin at Discharge[5]	-	-	85%	90%	100%
Beta Blocker at Arrival[5]	-	-	78%	87%	100%
Beta Blocker at Discharge[5]	-	-	78%	90%	100%
Fibrinolytic Medication Timing[5]	-	-	36%	31%	100%
PCI Within 90 Minutes of Arrival[5]	-	-	51%	54%	95%
Smoking Cessation Advice[5]	-	-	83%	88%	100%
Heart Failure Care					
ACE Inhibitor or ARB for LVSD[1]	2	50%	76%	82%	100%
Discharge Instructions[1]	8	12%	55%	61%	93%
Evaluation of LVS Function[1]	15	20%	71%	83%	99%
Smoking Cessation Advice[1]	3	33%	73%	82%	100%
Pneumonia Care					
Appropriate Initial Antibiotic[1]	15	40%	81%	83%	94%
Blood Culture Timing[1]	4	100%	91%	90%	100%
Influenza Vaccine[1]	7	43%	72%	70%	100%
Initial Antibiotic Timing[1]	15	100%	82%	80%	93%
Oxygenation Assessment[1]	19	100%	99%	99%	100%
Pneumococcal Vaccine[1]	10	80%	68%	69%	94%
Smoking Cessation Advice[1]	6	17%	72%	80%	100%
Surgical Infection Prevention					
Prophylactic Antibiotic Given[5]	-	-	75%	77%	95%
Prophylactic Antibiotic Selection[5]	-	-	88%	90%	100%
Prophylactic Antibiotic Stopped[5]	-	-	82%	72%	95%
Pregnancy Care					
Inpatient Neonatal Mortality	-	-	-	-	-
Third or Fourth Degree Laceration	-	-	-	3.63%	3.27%

Seminole Medical Center

2401 Wrangler Boulevard
Seminole, OK 74868
Phone: 405-303-4000
Fax: 405-303-4150
URL: www.seminolemedicalcenter.com
Ownership: Proprietary
Accredited: No
Emergency Services: Yes
Licensed Beds: 32

Key Personnel:

President/CEO . . . . Mike Schuster
Hospital Administrator . . . . Roberta Kelly, RN
Chief Medical Staff . . . . Rodney McCrory
Emergency Room . . . . Mark Macklin, RN
Infection Control . . . . Troy Sainder, RN
Medical/Surgical Nursing . . . . Barbara Lewis, RN
OB/GYN Womens Health . . . . Tina Wainwright, RN
Head of Respiratory/Cardiopulmonary . . . . D Billings

Measure	Cases	This Hospital	State Average	U.S. Average	Top Hospital
Heart Attack Care					
ACE Inhibitor or ARB for LVSD[5]	-	-	79%	82%	100%
Aspirin at Arrival[5]	-	-	86%	92%	100%
Aspirin at Discharge[5]	-	-	85%	90%	100%
Beta Blocker at Arrival[5]	-	-	78%	87%	100%
Beta Blocker at Discharge[5]	-	-	78%	90%	100%
Fibrinolytic Medication Timing[5]	-	-	36%	31%	100%
PCI Within 90 Minutes of Arrival[5]	-	-	51%	54%	95%
Smoking Cessation Advice[5]	-	-	83%	88%	100%
Heart Failure Care					
ACE Inhibitor or ARB for LVSD[1,2]	4	100%	76%	82%	100%
Discharge Instructions[1,2]	17	0%	55%	61%	93%
Evaluation of LVS Function[1,2]	20	35%	71%	83%	99%
Smoking Cessation Advice[1,2]	5	20%	73%	82%	100%
Pneumonia Care					
Appropriate Initial Antibiotic[2]	40	92%	81%	83%	94%
Blood Culture Timing[1,2]	24	96%	91%	90%	100%
Influenza Vaccine[1]	9	56%	72%	70%	100%
Initial Antibiotic Timing[2]	44	89%	82%	80%	93%
Oxygenation Assessment[2]	49	98%	99%	99%	100%
Pneumococcal Vaccine[2]	25	40%	68%	69%	94%
Smoking Cessation Advice[1,2]	12	75%	72%	80%	100%
Surgical Infection Prevention					
Prophylactic Antibiotic Given[1,2,3]	1	0%	75%	77%	95%
Prophylactic Antibiotic Selection[1,2]	1	0%	88%	90%	100%
Prophylactic Antibiotic Stopped[1,2,3]	1	100%	82%	72%	95%
Pregnancy Care					
Inpatient Neonatal Mortality	-	-	-	-	-
Third or Fourth Degree Laceration	-	-	-	3.63%	3.27%

Newman Memorial Hospital

905 S Main Street
Shattuck, OK 73858
Phone: 580-938-2551
Fax: 580-938-2309
E-mail: gmitchell@newmanmemorialhospital.org
URL: www.newmanmemorialhospital.org
Ownership: Govt - Hospital District or Authority
Accredited: No
Emergency Services: Yes
Licensed Beds: 99

Key Personnel:

President/CEO . . . . Gary W Mitchell, CHE
Head of Emergency Room . . . . Jean Bartow
Infection Control . . . . Gwen Stafford, RN
Medical Surgical Nursing . . . . Jean Bartew, RN

Measure	Cases	This Hospital	State Average	U.S. Average	Top Hospital
Heart Attack Care					
ACE Inhibitor or ARB for LVSD	0	-	79%	82%	100%
Aspirin at Arrival[1]	7	86%	86%	92%	100%
Aspirin at Discharge[1]	6	50%	85%	90%	100%
Beta Blocker at Arrival[1]	6	83%	78%	87%	100%
Beta Blocker at Discharge[1]	6	100%	78%	90%	100%
Fibrinolytic Medication Timing[1]	1	100%	36%	31%	100%
PCI Within 90 Minutes of Arrival	0	-	51%	54%	95%
Smoking Cessation Advice[1]	1	100%	83%	88%	100%
Heart Failure Care					
ACE Inhibitor or ARB for LVSD[1]	2	100%	76%	82%	100%
Discharge Instructions[1]	11	64%	55%	61%	93%
Evaluation of LVS Function[1]	13	46%	71%	83%	99%
Smoking Cessation Advice[1]	1	100%	73%	82%	100%
Pneumonia Care					
Appropriate Initial Antibiotic[1]	23	74%	81%	83%	94%
Blood Culture Timing[1]	1	100%	91%	90%	100%
Influenza Vaccine[1]	7	71%	72%	70%	100%
Initial Antibiotic Timing[1]	24	88%	82%	80%	93%
Oxygenation Assessment	28	100%	99%	99%	100%
Pneumococcal Vaccine[1]	16	56%	68%	69%	94%
Smoking Cessation Advice[1]	7	86%	72%	80%	100%
Surgical Infection Prevention					
Prophylactic Antibiotic Given[1,3]	6	50%	75%	77%	95%
Prophylactic Antibiotic Selection	0	-	88%	90%	100%
Prophylactic Antibiotic Stopped[1,3]	6	83%	82%	72%	95%
Pregnancy Care					

NOTE: Hospital profiles are in alphabetical order by state, then city, then hospital within the city; Rankings are sorted by rate in descending order and exclude hospitals with less than 25 cases; (1) The number of cases is too small (n<25) for purposes of reliably predicting hospital performance; (2) Measure reflects the hospital's indication that its submission was based upon a sample of its relevant discharges; (3) Rate reflects fewer than the maximum possible quarters of data for the measure; (4) Inaccurate information submitted and suppressed for one or more quarters; (5) No data is available from the hospital for this measure; Please refer to the User's Guide for a full explanation of data

Inpatient Neonatal Mortality	-	-	-	-	-
Third or Fourth Degree Laceration	-	-	-	3.63%	3.27%

Unity Health Center

1102 W Macarthur
Shawnee, OK 74804
Ownership: Voluntary non-profit - Other
Emergency Services: Yes
Phone: 405-273-2270
Accredited: Yes

Measure	Cases	This Hospital	State Average	U.S. Average	Top Hospital
Heart Attack Care					
ACE Inhibitor or ARB for LVSD[1]	11	91%	79%	82%	100%
Aspirin at Arrival	67	94%	86%	92%	100%
Aspirin at Discharge	29	90%	85%	90%	100%
Beta Blocker at Arrival	34	97%	78%	87%	100%
Beta Blocker at Discharge	29	90%	78%	90%	100%
Fibrinolytic Medication Timing[1]	12	42%	36%	31%	100%
PCI Within 90 Minutes of Arrival	0	-	51%	54%	95%
Smoking Cessation Advice[1]	10	100%	83%	88%	100%
Heart Failure Care					
ACE Inhibitor or ARB for LVSD	72	82%	76%	82%	100%
Discharge Instructions	131	86%	55%	61%	93%
Evaluation of LVS Function	158	93%	71%	83%	99%
Smoking Cessation Advice	27	100%	73%	82%	100%
Pneumonia Care					
Appropriate Initial Antibiotic	182	86%	81%	83%	94%
Blood Culture Timing	203	97%	91%	90%	100%
Influenza Vaccine	54	98%	72%	70%	100%
Initial Antibiotic Timing	253	91%	82%	80%	93%
Oxygenation Assessment	286	100%	99%	99%	100%
Pneumococcal Vaccine	175	97%	68%	69%	94%
Smoking Cessation Advice	81	98%	72%	80%	100%
Surgical Infection Prevention					
Prophylactic Antibiotic Given[3]	128	95%	75%	77%	95%
Prophylactic Antibiotic Selection	49	100%	88%	90%	100%
Prophylactic Antibiotic Stopped[3]	124	76%	82%	72%	95%
Pregnancy Care					
Inpatient Neonatal Mortality	-	-	-	-	-
Third or Fourth Degree Laceration	-	-	-	3.63%	3.27%

Haskell County Healthcare System

Alternate Name: Haskell County Hospital
401 NW H Street
Stigler, OK 74462
Ownership: Government - Local
Emergency Services: Yes
Phone: 918-967-4682
Fax: 918-967-8694
Accredited: No
Licensed Beds: 43

Key Personnel:
Administrator/CEO . . . . Mark Harrel
Chief Medical Staff . . . . Asim Usman
Director of Emergency Room . . . . Marcie Winkentlek
Director Infection/Disease Control . . . . Joyce Johnson
Director Medical/Surgical Nursing . . . . Nancy Beal
Director of Therapy . . . . Christy Hodges
Chief Radiology . . . . Liz Snyder
Director Respiratory Therapy . . . . Gary Todd

Measure	Cases	This Hospital	State Average	U.S. Average	Top Hospital
Heart Attack Care					
ACE Inhibitor or ARB for LVSD	0	-	79%	82%	100%
Aspirin at Arrival[1]	8	50%	86%	92%	100%
Aspirin at Discharge[1]	5	40%	85%	90%	100%
Beta Blocker at Arrival[1]	7	57%	78%	87%	100%
Beta Blocker at Discharge[1]	8	62%	78%	90%	100%
Fibrinolytic Medication Timing	0	-	36%	31%	100%
PCI Within 90 Minutes of Arrival	0	-	51%	54%	95%
Smoking Cessation Advice[1]	1	100%	83%	88%	100%
Heart Failure Care					
ACE Inhibitor or ARB for LVSD[1]	5	20%	76%	82%	100%
Discharge Instructions	30	37%	55%	61%	93%
Evaluation of LVS Function	43	40%	71%	83%	99%
Smoking Cessation Advice[1]	5	40%	73%	82%	100%
Pneumonia Care					
Appropriate Initial Antibiotic	57	88%	81%	83%	94%
Blood Culture Timing[1]	12	58%	91%	90%	100%
Influenza Vaccine[4,5]	-	-	72%	70%	100%
Initial Antibiotic Timing	64	84%	82%	80%	93%
Oxygenation Assessment	86	95%	99%	99%	100%
Pneumococcal Vaccine	64	59%	68%	69%	94%
Smoking Cessation Advice[1]	22	64%	72%	80%	100%
Surgical Infection Prevention					
Prophylactic Antibiotic Given[1,3]	1	100%	75%	77%	95%
Prophylactic Antibiotic Selection	0	-	88%	90%	100%
Prophylactic Antibiotic Stopped[1,3]	1	100%	82%	72%	95%
Pregnancy Care					
Inpatient Neonatal Mortality	-	-	-	-	-
Third or Fourth Degree Laceration	-	-	-	3.63%	3.27%

Stillwater Medical Center

1323 W 6th
PO Box 2408
Stillwater, OK 74076
E-mail: susan@stillwater-medical.org
URL: www.stillwater-medical.org
Ownership: Govt - Hospital District or Authority
Emergency Services: Yes
Phone: 405-372-1480
Fax: 405-372-9552
Accredited: Yes
Licensed Beds: 133

Key Personnel:
CEO . . . . Jerry Moeller
Chief Medical Staff . . . . Randy Willis
Chief of Medical Staff . . . . Jonathan Drommond

Measure	Cases	This Hospital	State Average	U.S. Average	Top Hospital
Heart Attack Care					
ACE Inhibitor or ARB for LVSD[1]	10	100%	79%	82%	100%
Aspirin at Arrival	40	100%	86%	92%	100%
Aspirin at Discharge[1]	17	100%	85%	90%	100%
Beta Blocker at Arrival[1]	20	100%	78%	87%	100%
Beta Blocker at Discharge[1]	17	100%	78%	90%	100%
Fibrinolytic Medication Timing[1]	1	100%	36%	31%	100%
PCI Within 90 Minutes of Arrival	0	-	51%	54%	95%
Smoking Cessation Advice[1]	4	100%	83%	88%	100%
Heart Failure Care					
ACE Inhibitor or ARB for LVSD[1]	24	92%	76%	82%	100%
Discharge Instructions	66	80%	55%	61%	93%
Evaluation of LVS Function	84	93%	71%	83%	99%
Smoking Cessation Advice[1]	18	89%	73%	82%	100%
Pneumonia Care					
Appropriate Initial Antibiotic	102	90%	81%	83%	94%
Blood Culture Timing	102	98%	91%	90%	100%
Influenza Vaccine	38	84%	72%	70%	100%
Initial Antibiotic Timing	142	94%	82%	80%	93%
Oxygenation Assessment	161	100%	99%	99%	100%
Pneumococcal Vaccine	102	83%	68%	69%	94%
Smoking Cessation Advice	32	97%	72%	80%	100%
Surgical Infection Prevention					
Prophylactic Antibiotic Given[3]	232	75%	75%	77%	95%
Prophylactic Antibiotic Selection	83	78%	88%	90%	100%
Prophylactic Antibiotic Stopped[3]	244	83%	82%	72%	95%
Pregnancy Care					
Inpatient Neonatal Mortality	-	-	-	-	-
Third or Fourth Degree Laceration	-	-	-	3.63%	3.27%

Memorial Hospital of Stillwell

1401 West Locust
PO Box 272
Stillwell, OK 74960
URL: www.memorialhospital.com
Ownership: Voluntary non-profit - Private
Emergency Services: Yes
Phone: 918-696-3101
Fax: 918-696-3388
Accredited: No
Licensed Beds: 31

Key Personnel:
President . . . . Alan L Adams
Chief Radiology . . . . Phil Alexander
Pulmonary/Respiratory Care . . . . Devangh Cunningham

Measure	Cases	This Hospital	State Average	U.S. Average	Top Hospital
Heart Attack Care					

NOTE: Hospital profiles are in alphabetical order by state, then city, then hospital within the city; Rankings are sorted by rate in descending order and exclude hospitals with less than 25 cases; (1) The number of cases is too small (n<25) for purposes of reliably predicting hospital performance; (2) Measure reflects the hospital's indication that its submission was based upon a sample of its relevant discharges; (3) Rate reflects fewer than the maximum possible quarters of data for the measure; (4) Inaccurate information submitted and suppressed for one or more quarters; (5) No data is available from the hospital for this measure; Please refer to the User's Guide for a full explanation of data

Measure	Cases	This Hospital	State Average	U.S. Average	Top Hospital
ACE Inhibitor or ARB for LVSD	0	-	79%	82%	100%
Aspirin at Arrival[1]	5	60%	86%	92%	100%
Aspirin at Discharge[1]	3	100%	85%	90%	100%
Beta Blocker at Arrival[1]	4	75%	78%	87%	100%
Beta Blocker at Discharge[1]	4	100%	78%	90%	100%
Fibrinolytic Medication Timing	0	-	36%	31%	100%
PCI Within 90 Minutes of Arrival	0	-	51%	54%	95%
Smoking Cessation Advice[1]	1	100%	83%	88%	100%
Heart Failure Care					
ACE Inhibitor or ARB for LVSD	41	88%	76%	82%	100%
Discharge Instructions	72	71%	55%	61%	93%
Evaluation of LVS Function	88	92%	71%	83%	99%
Smoking Cessation Advice[1]	10	60%	73%	82%	100%
Pneumonia Care					
Appropriate Initial Antibiotic[1]	24	54%	81%	83%	94%
Blood Culture Timing[1]	22	91%	91%	90%	100%
Influenza Vaccine[1]	10	60%	72%	70%	100%
Initial Antibiotic Timing	45	82%	82%	80%	93%
Oxygenation Assessment	50	100%	99%	99%	100%
Pneumococcal Vaccine	30	83%	68%	69%	94%
Smoking Cessation Advice[1]	8	75%	72%	80%	100%
Surgical Infection Prevention					
Prophylactic Antibiotic Given[1,3]	6	50%	75%	77%	95%
Prophylactic Antibiotic Selection[1]	2	100%	88%	90%	100%
Prophylactic Antibiotic Stopped[1,3]	6	67%	82%	72%	95%
Pregnancy Care					
Inpatient Neonatal Mortality	-	-	-	-	-
Third or Fourth Degree Laceration	-	-	-	3.63%	3.27%

Stroud Regional Medical Center

2308 Highway 66 West
Stroud, OK 74079
Phone: 918-968-3571
Ownership: Proprietary
Accredited: No
Emergency Services: Yes

Measure	Cases	This Hospital	State Average	U.S. Average	Top Hospital
Heart Attack Care					
ACE Inhibitor or ARB for LVSD[3]	0	-	79%	82%	100%
Aspirin at Arrival[3]	0	-	86%	92%	100%
Aspirin at Discharge[3]	0	-	85%	90%	100%
Beta Blocker at Arrival[3]	0	-	78%	87%	100%
Beta Blocker at Discharge[3]	0	-	78%	90%	100%
Fibrinolytic Medication Timing[1,3]	1	0%	36%	31%	100%
PCI Within 90 Minutes of Arrival[5]	-	-	51%	54%	95%
Smoking Cessation Advice[3]	0	-	83%	88%	100%
Heart Failure Care					
ACE Inhibitor or ARB for LVSD[1]	7	57%	76%	82%	100%
Discharge Instructions[1]	8	62%	55%	61%	93%
Evaluation of LVS Function[1]	15	87%	71%	83%	99%
Smoking Cessation Advice[1]	2	50%	73%	82%	100%
Pneumonia Care					
Appropriate Initial Antibiotic	34	74%	81%	83%	94%
Blood Culture Timing[1]	14	93%	91%	90%	100%
Influenza Vaccine[1]	7	0%	72%	70%	100%
Initial Antibiotic Timing	36	78%	82%	80%	93%
Oxygenation Assessment	50	100%	99%	99%	100%
Pneumococcal Vaccine	27	19%	68%	69%	94%
Smoking Cessation Advice[1]	10	60%	72%	80%	100%
Surgical Infection Prevention					
Prophylactic Antibiotic Given[5]	-	-	75%	77%	95%
Prophylactic Antibiotic Selection[5]	-	-	88%	90%	100%
Prophylactic Antibiotic Stopped[5]	-	-	82%	72%	95%
Pregnancy Care					
Inpatient Neonatal Mortality	-	-	-	-	-
Third or Fourth Degree Laceration	-	-	-	3.63%	3.27%

Arbuckle Memorial Hospital

2011 W Broadway
Sulphur, OK 73086
Toll-Free: 888-557-5357
Phone: 580-622-2161
Fax: 580-622-2763
URL: www.arbucklehospital.com
Ownership: Government - Local
Accredited: No
Emergency Services: Yes
Licensed Beds: 58

Key Personnel:

Administrator . . . . Marvin Hyde
Chief Medical Staff. . . . . Atonio Lee, MD

Measure	Cases	This Hospital	State Average	U.S. Average	Top Hospital
Heart Attack Care					
ACE Inhibitor or ARB for LVSD[1,3]	1	0%	79%	82%	100%
Aspirin at Arrival[1,3]	1	0%	86%	92%	100%
Aspirin at Discharge[1,3]	1	0%	85%	90%	100%
Beta Blocker at Arrival[1,3]	1	100%	78%	87%	100%
Beta Blocker at Discharge[1,3]	1	100%	78%	90%	100%
Fibrinolytic Medication Timing[3]	0	-	36%	31%	100%
PCI Within 90 Minutes of Arrival[5]	-	-	51%	54%	95%
Smoking Cessation Advice[3]	0	-	83%	88%	100%
Heart Failure Care					
ACE Inhibitor or ARB for LVSD[1,3]	3	100%	76%	82%	100%
Discharge Instructions[1,3]	9	33%	55%	61%	93%
Evaluation of LVS Function[1,3]	21	71%	71%	83%	99%
Smoking Cessation Advice[1,3]	3	33%	73%	82%	100%
Pneumonia Care					
Appropriate Initial Antibiotic[1,3]	20	90%	81%	83%	94%
Blood Culture Timing[1]	20	80%	91%	90%	100%
Influenza Vaccine[1]	10	100%	72%	70%	100%
Initial Antibiotic Timing[3]	29	83%	82%	80%	93%
Oxygenation Assessment[3]	40	100%	99%	99%	100%
Pneumococcal Vaccine[3]	27	85%	68%	69%	94%
Smoking Cessation Advice[1,3]	9	89%	72%	80%	100%
Surgical Infection Prevention					
Prophylactic Antibiotic Given[5]	-	-	75%	77%	95%
Prophylactic Antibiotic Selection[5]	-	-	88%	90%	100%
Prophylactic Antibiotic Stopped[5]	-	-	82%	72%	95%
Pregnancy Care					
Inpatient Neonatal Mortality	-	-	-	-	-
Third or Fourth Degree Laceration	-	-	-	3.63%	3.27%

Tahlequah City Hospital

1400 E Downing
Tahlequah, OK 74465
Phone: 918-456-0641
Fax: 918-456-8886
URL: www.tahlequahcityhospital.integrity.com
Ownership: Voluntary non-profit - Other
Accredited: No
Emergency Services: Yes
Licensed Beds: 99

Key Personnel:

CEO. . . . . Gary L Jepson
Chief Medical Staff. . . . . Herbert Littleton, DO
Emergency Room . . . . John Galdamez, DO
Director Infection/Disease Control . . . . Cheri Olgesbee, RN
Director Medical/Surgical Nursing . . . . Barb Taylor, RN
OB/GYN Womens Health. . . . . Wallace Champlain, DO
Chief Radiology . . . . Charles Gosnell, MD
Director Respiratory Therapy . . . . Sandy Henry

Measure	Cases	This Hospital	State Average	U.S. Average	Top Hospital
Heart Attack Care					
ACE Inhibitor or ARB for LVSD[1]	4	75%	79%	82%	100%
Aspirin at Arrival[1]	22	95%	86%	92%	100%
Aspirin at Discharge[1]	24	92%	85%	90%	100%
Beta Blocker at Arrival[1]	18	78%	78%	87%	100%
Beta Blocker at Discharge[1]	23	91%	78%	90%	100%
Fibrinolytic Medication Timing[1]	3	0%	36%	31%	100%
PCI Within 90 Minutes of Arrival[1]	1	0%	51%	54%	95%
Smoking Cessation Advice[1]	11	36%	83%	88%	100%
Heart Failure Care					
ACE Inhibitor or ARB for LVSD	42	88%	76%	82%	100%
Discharge Instructions	68	51%	55%	61%	93%
Evaluation of LVS Function	93	87%	71%	83%	99%
Smoking Cessation Advice[1]	16	50%	73%	82%	100%

NOTE: Hospital profiles are in alphabetical order by state, then city, then hospital within the city; Rankings are sorted by rate in descending order and exclude hospitals with less than 25 cases; (1) The number of cases is too small (n<25) for purposes of reliably predicting hospital performance; (2) Measure reflects the hospital's indication that its submission was based upon a sample of its relevant discharges; (3) Rate reflects fewer than the maximum possible quarters of data for the measure; (4) Inaccurate information submitted and suppressed for one or more quarters; (5) No data is available from the hospital for this measure; Please refer to the User's Guide for a full explanation of data

Measure	Cases	This Hospital	State Average	U.S. Average	Top Hospital
Pneumonia Care					
Appropriate Initial Antibiotic	54	80%	81%	83%	94%
Blood Culture Timing	50	92%	91%	90%	100%
Influenza Vaccine[4,5]	-	-	72%	70%	100%
Initial Antibiotic Timing	88	86%	82%	80%	93%
Oxygenation Assessment	117	97%	99%	99%	100%
Pneumococcal Vaccine	72	53%	68%	69%	94%
Smoking Cessation Advice[1]	21	76%	72%	80%	100%
Surgical Infection Prevention					
Prophylactic Antibiotic Given[3]	113	7%	75%	77%	95%
Prophylactic Antibiotic Selection	46	83%	88%	90%	100%
Prophylactic Antibiotic Stopped[3]	102	29%	82%	72%	95%
Pregnancy Care					
Inpatient Neonatal Mortality	-	-	-	-	-
Third or Fourth Degree Laceration	-	-	-	3.63%	3.27%

W W Hastings Indian Hospital

100 S Bliss Avenue
Tahlequah, OK 74464
Ownership: Government - Federal
Emergency Services: Yes

Phone: 918-458-3100
Fax: 918-458-3262
Accredited: Yes
Licensed Beds: 60

Key Personnel:
CEO/President. . . . . Edwin MClemore

Measure	Cases	This Hospital	State Average	U.S. Average	Top Hospital
Heart Attack Care					
ACE Inhibitor or ARB for LVSD	0	-	79%	82%	100%
Aspirin at Arrival[1]	3	67%	86%	92%	100%
Aspirin at Discharge	0	-	85%	90%	100%
Beta Blocker at Arrival[1]	3	67%	78%	87%	100%
Beta Blocker at Discharge	0	-	78%	90%	100%
Fibrinolytic Medication Timing	0	-	36%	31%	100%
PCI Within 90 Minutes of Arrival	0	-	51%	54%	95%
Smoking Cessation Advice	0	-	83%	88%	100%
Heart Failure Care					
ACE Inhibitor or ARB for LVSD[1]	7	43%	76%	82%	100%
Discharge Instructions	33	0%	55%	61%	93%
Evaluation of LVS Function	32	78%	71%	83%	99%
Smoking Cessation Advice[1]	8	50%	73%	82%	100%
Pneumonia Care					
Appropriate Initial Antibiotic	75	87%	81%	83%	94%
Blood Culture Timing	52	87%	91%	90%	100%
Influenza Vaccine[1]	15	73%	72%	70%	100%
Initial Antibiotic Timing	80	61%	82%	80%	93%
Oxygenation Assessment	92	100%	99%	99%	100%
Pneumococcal Vaccine	31	61%	68%	69%	94%
Smoking Cessation Advice	36	58%	72%	80%	100%
Surgical Infection Prevention					
Prophylactic Antibiotic Given[1,2,3]	20	35%	75%	77%	95%
Prophylactic Antibiotic Selection[1,2]	19	84%	88%	90%	100%
Prophylactic Antibiotic Stopped[1,2,3]	18	100%	82%	72%	95%
Pregnancy Care					
Inpatient Neonatal Mortality	-	-	-	-	-
Third or Fourth Degree Laceration	-	-	-	3.63%	3.27%

Choctaw Nation Health Care Center

Alternate Name: Choctaw Nation Indian Hospital
1 Choctaw Way
Talihina, OK 74571

Toll-Free: 800-349-7026
Phone: 918-567-7000
Fax: 918-567-7026

E-mail: bblum@choctawnation.com
Ownership: Government - Federal
Emergency Services: Yes

Accredited: Yes
Licensed Beds: 39

Key Personnel:
CEO. . . . . Thomas Bonien
Chief Medical Staff. . . . . Dr. Thomas Bonien
Medical/Surgical Nursing . . . . Nancy Habick, RN
OB/GYN Womens Health. . . . . Ruby Ludlow, RN
Respiratory/Cardiopulmonary. . . . . Kevin Collins

Measure	Cases	This Hospital	State Average	U.S. Average	Top Hospital
Heart Attack Care					
ACE Inhibitor or ARB for LVSD[1,3]	1	100%	79%	82%	100%
Aspirin at Arrival[1,3]	2	100%	86%	92%	100%
Aspirin at Discharge[1,3]	1	100%	85%	90%	100%
Beta Blocker at Arrival[1,3]	1	100%	78%	87%	100%
Beta Blocker at Discharge[1,3]	1	100%	78%	90%	100%
Fibrinolytic Medication Timing[3]	0	-	36%	31%	100%
PCI Within 90 Minutes of Arrival	0	-	51%	54%	95%
Smoking Cessation Advice[3]	0	-	83%	88%	100%
Heart Failure Care					
ACE Inhibitor or ARB for LVSD[1]	5	100%	76%	82%	100%
Discharge Instructions[1]	20	15%	55%	61%	93%
Evaluation of LVS Function[1]	21	81%	71%	83%	99%
Smoking Cessation Advice[1]	5	60%	73%	82%	100%
Pneumonia Care					
Appropriate Initial Antibiotic	25	84%	81%	83%	94%
Blood Culture Timing[1]	13	77%	91%	90%	100%
Influenza Vaccine[1]	5	80%	72%	70%	100%
Initial Antibiotic Timing	27	81%	82%	80%	93%
Oxygenation Assessment	29	100%	99%	99%	100%
Pneumococcal Vaccine[1]	11	64%	68%	69%	94%
Smoking Cessation Advice[1]	8	12%	72%	80%	100%
Surgical Infection Prevention					
Prophylactic Antibiotic Given[1,3]	16	69%	75%	77%	95%
Prophylactic Antibiotic Selection[1]	4	100%	88%	90%	100%
Prophylactic Antibiotic Stopped[1,3]	14	100%	82%	72%	95%
Pregnancy Care					
Inpatient Neonatal Mortality	-	-	-	-	-
Third or Fourth Degree Laceration	-	-	-	3.63%	3.27%

Johnston Memorial Hospital

1100 Southbyrd
Tishomingo, OK 73460
E-mail: jmh@simplynet.net
Ownership: Government - Local
Emergency Services: Yes

Phone: 580-371-2327
Fax: 580-371-2127

Accredited: No
Licensed Beds: 47

Key Personnel:
Administrator . . . . Jerry Copeland
Chief Medical Staff. . . . . Richard H Tidwell, MD
Director Infection/Disease Control . . . . Carolyn Pearson, RN
OB/GYN Womens Health. . . . . Richard H Tidwell, MD

Measure	Cases	This Hospital	State Average	U.S. Average	Top Hospital
Heart Attack Care					
ACE Inhibitor or ARB for LVSD[5]	-	-	79%	82%	100%
Aspirin at Arrival[5]	-	-	86%	92%	100%
Aspirin at Discharge[5]	-	-	85%	90%	100%
Beta Blocker at Arrival[5]	-	-	78%	87%	100%
Beta Blocker at Discharge[5]	-	-	78%	90%	100%
Fibrinolytic Medication Timing[5]	-	-	36%	31%	100%
PCI Within 90 Minutes of Arrival[5]	-	-	51%	54%	95%
Smoking Cessation Advice[5]	-	-	83%	88%	100%
Heart Failure Care					
ACE Inhibitor or ARB for LVSD[1]	8	88%	76%	82%	100%
Discharge Instructions[1]	21	5%	55%	61%	93%
Evaluation of LVS Function	51	35%	71%	83%	99%
Smoking Cessation Advice[1]	9	67%	73%	82%	100%
Pneumonia Care					
Appropriate Initial Antibiotic	36	56%	81%	83%	94%
Blood Culture Timing[1]	6	100%	91%	90%	100%
Influenza Vaccine[1]	15	33%	72%	70%	100%
Initial Antibiotic Timing	51	86%	82%	80%	93%
Oxygenation Assessment	61	100%	99%	99%	100%
Pneumococcal Vaccine	38	29%	68%	69%	94%
Smoking Cessation Advice[1]	23	65%	72%	80%	100%
Surgical Infection Prevention					
Prophylactic Antibiotic Given[5]	-	-	75%	77%	95%
Prophylactic Antibiotic Selection[5]	-	-	88%	90%	100%
Prophylactic Antibiotic Stopped[5]	-	-	82%	72%	95%
Pregnancy Care					
Inpatient Neonatal Mortality	-	-	-	-	-
Third or Fourth Degree Laceration	-	-	-	3.63%	3.27%

NOTE: Hospital profiles are in alphabetical order by state, then city, then hospital within the city; Rankings are sorted by rate in descending order and exclude hospitals with less than 25 cases; (1) The number of cases is too small (n<25) for purposes of reliably predicting hospital performance; (2) Measure reflects the hospital's indication that its submission was based upon a sample of its relevant discharges; (3) Rate reflects fewer than the maximum possible quarters of data for the measure; (4) Inaccurate information submitted and suppressed for one or more quarters; (5) No data is available from the hospital for this measure; Please refer to the User's Guide for a full explanation of data

Hillcrest Medical Center

1120 S Utica Avenue
Tulsa, OK 74104
URL: www.hillcrest.com
Ownership: Voluntary non-profit - Other
Emergency Services: Yes

Phone: 918-579-1000
Fax: 918-584-6636
Accredited: Yes
Licensed Beds: 607

Key Personnel:
President/CEO. . . . . Steve Dobbs
Chief Medical Staff. . . . . D Decker, MD
Emergency Room . . . . Jeff Biddy
Emergency Room . . . . Susan Messon

Measure	Cases	This Hospital	State Average	U.S. Average	Top Hospital
Heart Attack Care					
ACE Inhibitor or ARB for LVSD	69	97%	79%	82%	100%
Aspirin at Arrival	211	99%	86%	92%	100%
Aspirin at Discharge	327	98%	85%	90%	100%
Beta Blocker at Arrival	187	97%	78%	87%	100%
Beta Blocker at Discharge	347	98%	78%	90%	100%
Fibrinolytic Medication Timing[1]	1	0%	36%	31%	100%
PCI Within 90 Minutes of Arrival[1]	4	50%	51%	54%	95%
Smoking Cessation Advice	147	94%	83%	88%	100%
Heart Failure Care					
ACE Inhibitor or ARB for LVSD	214	98%	76%	82%	100%
Discharge Instructions	527	72%	55%	61%	93%
Evaluation of LVS Function	608	94%	71%	83%	99%
Smoking Cessation Advice	153	86%	73%	82%	100%
Pneumonia Care					
Appropriate Initial Antibiotic	241	84%	81%	83%	94%
Blood Culture Timing	149	91%	91%	90%	100%
Influenza Vaccine	37	41%	72%	70%	100%
Initial Antibiotic Timing	243	81%	82%	80%	93%
Oxygenation Assessment	312	99%	99%	99%	100%
Pneumococcal Vaccine	135	50%	68%	69%	94%
Smoking Cessation Advice	114	89%	72%	80%	100%
Surgical Infection Prevention					
Prophylactic Antibiotic Given[2,3]	198	90%	75%	77%	95%
Prophylactic Antibiotic Selection[2]	68	93%	88%	90%	100%
Prophylactic Antibiotic Stopped[2,3]	192	64%	82%	72%	95%
Pregnancy Care					
Inpatient Neonatal Mortality	-	-	-	-	-
Third or Fourth Degree Laceration	-	-	-	3.63%	3.27%

Oklahoma State University Medical Center

744 W 9th Street
Tulsa, OK 74127

Toll-Free: 800-876-5664
Phone: 918-587-2561
Fax: 918-599-1750

URL: www.tulsaregional.com
Ownership: Proprietary
Emergency Services: Yes

Accredited: Yes
Licensed Beds: 415

Key Personnel:
President/CEO. . . . . Dan Fieker
Chief Medical Staff. . . . . Jenny Alexopulos, DO
Catheterization Lab . . . . Phil Langston
Emergency Room . . . . Jan Emmons
Infection Control. . . . . Janet Bacon
ICU . . . . Eric Burch

Measure	Cases	This Hospital	State Average	U.S. Average	Top Hospital
Heart Attack Care					
ACE Inhibitor or ARB for LVSD	75	83%	79%	82%	100%
Aspirin at Arrival	125	94%	86%	92%	100%
Aspirin at Discharge	206	94%	85%	90%	100%
Beta Blocker at Arrival	106	84%	78%	87%	100%
Beta Blocker at Discharge	201	93%	78%	90%	100%
Fibrinolytic Medication Timing	0	-	36%	31%	100%
PCI Within 90 Minutes of Arrival[1]	1	0%	51%	54%	95%
Smoking Cessation Advice	98	94%	83%	88%	100%
Heart Failure Care					
ACE Inhibitor or ARB for LVSD	153	86%	76%	82%	100%
Discharge Instructions	304	28%	55%	61%	93%
Evaluation of LVS Function	333	91%	71%	83%	99%
Smoking Cessation Advice	122	94%	73%	82%	100%
Pneumonia Care					
Appropriate Initial Antibiotic	151	92%	81%	83%	94%
Blood Culture Timing	131	81%	91%	90%	100%
Influenza Vaccine	52	46%	72%	70%	100%
Initial Antibiotic Timing	225	78%	82%	80%	93%
Oxygenation Assessment	274	98%	99%	99%	100%
Pneumococcal Vaccine	96	52%	68%	69%	94%
Smoking Cessation Advice	128	92%	72%	80%	100%
Surgical Infection Prevention					
Prophylactic Antibiotic Given[2]	282	83%	75%	77%	95%
Prophylactic Antibiotic Selection[2]	51	96%	88%	90%	100%
Prophylactic Antibiotic Stopped[2]	266	62%	82%	72%	95%
Pregnancy Care					
Inpatient Neonatal Mortality	-	-	-	-	-
Third or Fourth Degree Laceration	-	-	-	3.63%	3.27%

Orthopedic Hospital of Oklahoma

2408 East 81st Street, Suite 300
Tulsa, OK 74137
Ownership: Proprietary
Emergency Services: Yes

Phone: 918-477-5000
Accredited: No

Key Personnel:
General Surgery. . . . . Mark Meese, MD

Measure	Cases	This Hospital	State Average	U.S. Average	Top Hospital
Heart Attack Care					
ACE Inhibitor or ARB for LVSD[5]	-	-	79%	82%	100%
Aspirin at Arrival[5]	-	-	86%	92%	100%
Aspirin at Discharge[5]	-	-	85%	90%	100%
Beta Blocker at Arrival[5]	-	-	78%	87%	100%
Beta Blocker at Discharge[5]	-	-	78%	90%	100%
Fibrinolytic Medication Timing[5]	-	-	36%	31%	100%
PCI Within 90 Minutes of Arrival[5]	-	-	51%	54%	95%
Smoking Cessation Advice[5]	-	-	83%	88%	100%
Heart Failure Care					
ACE Inhibitor or ARB for LVSD[5]	-	-	76%	82%	100%
Discharge Instructions[5]	-	-	55%	61%	93%
Evaluation of LVS Function[5]	-	-	71%	83%	99%
Smoking Cessation Advice[5]	-	-	73%	82%	100%
Pneumonia Care					
Appropriate Initial Antibiotic[5]	-	-	81%	83%	94%
Blood Culture Timing[5]	-	-	91%	90%	100%
Influenza Vaccine[5]	-	-	72%	70%	100%
Initial Antibiotic Timing[5]	-	-	82%	80%	93%
Oxygenation Assessment[5]	-	-	99%	99%	100%
Pneumococcal Vaccine[5]	-	-	68%	69%	94%
Smoking Cessation Advice[5]	-	-	72%	80%	100%
Surgical Infection Prevention					
Prophylactic Antibiotic Given[3]	139	65%	75%	77%	95%
Prophylactic Antibiotic Selection[5]	-	-	88%	90%	100%
Prophylactic Antibiotic Stopped[3]	139	71%	82%	72%	95%
Pregnancy Care					
Inpatient Neonatal Mortality	-	-	-	-	-
Third or Fourth Degree Laceration	-	-	-	3.63%	3.27%

Saint Francis Heart Hospital

10501 East 91st Street South
Tulsa, OK 74133
Ownership: Proprietary
Emergency Services: Yes

Phone: 918-307-6000
Accredited: Yes

Measure	Cases	This Hospital	State Average	U.S. Average	Top Hospital
Heart Attack Care					
ACE Inhibitor or ARB for LVSD	109	86%	79%	82%	100%
Aspirin at Arrival	136	90%	86%	92%	100%
Aspirin at Discharge	507	98%	85%	90%	100%
Beta Blocker at Arrival	118	86%	78%	87%	100%
Beta Blocker at Discharge	510	97%	78%	90%	100%
Fibrinolytic Medication Timing[1]	1	100%	36%	31%	100%
PCI Within 90 Minutes of Arrival[1]	12	67%	51%	54%	95%
Smoking Cessation Advice	277	96%	83%	88%	100%
Heart Failure Care					

NOTE: Hospital profiles are in alphabetical order by state, then city, then hospital within the city; Rankings are sorted by rate in descending order and exclude hospitals with less than 25 cases; (1) The number of cases is too small (n<25) for purposes of reliably predicting hospital performance; (2) Measure reflects the hospital's indication that its submission was based upon a sample of its relevant discharges; (3) Rate reflects fewer than the maximum possible quarters of data for the measure; (4) Inaccurate information submitted and suppressed for one or more quarters; (5) No data is available from the hospital for this measure; Please refer to the User's Guide for a full explanation of data

ACE Inhibitor or ARB for LVSD	116	90%	76%	82%	100%
Discharge Instructions	137	79%	55%	61%	93%
Evaluation of LVS Function	93	94%	71%	83%	99%
Smoking Cessation Advice	25	96%	73%	82%	100%
Pneumonia Care					
Appropriate Initial Antibiotic[3]	0	-	81%	83%	94%
Blood Culture Timing	0	-	91%	90%	100%
Influenza Vaccine	0	-	72%	70%	100%
Initial Antibiotic Timing[3]	0	-	82%	80%	93%
Oxygenation Assessment[3]	0	-	99%	99%	100%
Pneumococcal Vaccine[3]	0	-	68%	69%	94%
Smoking Cessation Advice[3]	0	-	72%	80%	100%
Surgical Infection Prevention					
Prophylactic Antibiotic Given[3]	311	86%	75%	77%	95%
Prophylactic Antibiotic Selection	98	98%	88%	90%	100%
Prophylactic Antibiotic Stopped[3]	297	86%	82%	72%	95%
Pregnancy Care					
Inpatient Neonatal Mortality	-	-	-	-	-
Third or Fourth Degree Laceration	-	-	-	3.63%	3.27%

Saint Francis Hospital

6161 S Yale Avenue
Tulsa, OK 74136
E-mail: webadministrator@saintfrancis.com
URL: www.saintfrancis.com
Ownership: Voluntary non-profit - Other
Emergency Services: Yes

Phone: 918-494-2200
Fax: 918-494-4501
Accredited: Yes
Licensed Beds: 897

Key Personnel:
President/CEO . . . . Jake Henry, Jr
Chief Cardiac Surgery . . . . James Whiteneck, MD
Chief Catheterization Laboratory . . . . Michael Spain, MD
Emergency Room . . . . William Bickell, MD
Emergency Room . . . . Frank Mitchell, MD
Director Infection/Disease Control . . . . Dee Copeland, RN
Chief Radiology . . . . R Krieger, MD

Measure	Cases	This Hospital	State Average	U.S. Average	Top Hospital
Heart Attack Care					
ACE Inhibitor or ARB for LVSD	115	90%	79%	82%	100%
Aspirin at Arrival	472	97%	86%	92%	100%
Aspirin at Discharge	492	97%	85%	90%	100%
Beta Blocker at Arrival	316	90%	78%	87%	100%
Beta Blocker at Discharge	479	97%	78%	90%	100%
Fibrinolytic Medication Timing[1]	4	50%	36%	31%	100%
PCI Within 90 Minutes of Arrival[1]	21	29%	51%	54%	95%
Smoking Cessation Advice	208	100%	83%	88%	100%
Heart Failure Care					
ACE Inhibitor or ARB for LVSD	276	88%	76%	82%	100%
Discharge Instructions	542	54%	55%	61%	93%
Evaluation of LVS Function	646	95%	71%	83%	99%
Smoking Cessation Advice	149	99%	73%	82%	100%
Pneumonia Care					
Appropriate Initial Antibiotic	637	88%	81%	83%	94%
Blood Culture Timing	661	93%	91%	90%	100%
Influenza Vaccine	197	83%	72%	70%	100%
Initial Antibiotic Timing	754	73%	82%	80%	93%
Oxygenation Assessment	1,004	100%	99%	99%	100%
Pneumococcal Vaccine	612	85%	68%	69%	94%
Smoking Cessation Advice	264	98%	72%	80%	100%
Surgical Infection Prevention					
Prophylactic Antibiotic Given[3]	1,687	93%	75%	77%	95%
Prophylactic Antibiotic Selection	571	88%	88%	90%	100%
Prophylactic Antibiotic Stopped[3]	1,634	76%	82%	72%	95%
Pregnancy Care					
Inpatient Neonatal Mortality	-	-	-	-	-
Third or Fourth Degree Laceration	-	-	-	3.63%	3.27%

Saint John Medical Center

1923 South Utica Avenue
Tulsa, OK 74104
Ownership: Voluntary non-profit - Church
Emergency Services: Yes

Phone: 918-744-2159
Accredited: Yes

Key Personnel:
OBGYN . . . . Robert Aikman, MD
Pulmonary . . . . Ahmed Tanveer, MD
Cardiovascular . . . . Kalapura Thomachan, MD

Measure	Cases	This Hospital	State Average	U.S. Average	Top Hospital
Heart Attack Care					
ACE Inhibitor or ARB for LVSD	125	90%	79%	82%	100%
Aspirin at Arrival	415	97%	86%	92%	100%
Aspirin at Discharge	532	98%	85%	90%	100%
Beta Blocker at Arrival	350	99%	78%	87%	100%
Beta Blocker at Discharge	520	99%	78%	90%	100%
Fibrinolytic Medication Timing[1]	1	100%	36%	31%	100%
PCI Within 90 Minutes of Arrival[1]	19	63%	51%	54%	95%
Smoking Cessation Advice	214	100%	83%	88%	100%
Heart Failure Care					
ACE Inhibitor or ARB for LVSD	336	87%	76%	82%	100%
Discharge Instructions	627	74%	55%	61%	93%
Evaluation of LVS Function	725	98%	71%	83%	99%
Smoking Cessation Advice	156	97%	73%	82%	100%
Pneumonia Care					
Appropriate Initial Antibiotic	351	87%	81%	83%	94%
Blood Culture Timing	255	91%	91%	90%	100%
Influenza Vaccine	92	96%	72%	70%	100%
Initial Antibiotic Timing	425	77%	82%	80%	93%
Oxygenation Assessment	593	100%	99%	99%	100%
Pneumococcal Vaccine	350	89%	68%	69%	94%
Smoking Cessation Advice	148	96%	72%	80%	100%
Surgical Infection Prevention					
Prophylactic Antibiotic Given	2,555	85%	75%	77%	95%
Prophylactic Antibiotic Selection	628	97%	88%	90%	100%
Prophylactic Antibiotic Stopped	2,480	85%	82%	72%	95%
Pregnancy Care					
Inpatient Neonatal Mortality	-	-	-	-	-
Third or Fourth Degree Laceration	-	-	-	3.63%	3.27%

Southcrest Hospital

8801 South 101 Street
Tulsa, OK 74133
URL: www.southcresthospital.com
Ownership: Proprietary
Emergency Services: Yes

Phone: 918-294-4000
Fax: 918-294-4809
Accredited: Yes
Licensed Beds: 180

Key Personnel:
President/CEO . . . . Anthony R Young
Chief Medical Staff . . . . Stan Stacy
Director Cardiology . . . . Ernest Pickpring

Measure	Cases	This Hospital	State Average	U.S. Average	Top Hospital
Heart Attack Care					
ACE Inhibitor or ARB for LVSD[1]	24	96%	79%	82%	100%
Aspirin at Arrival	94	99%	86%	92%	100%
Aspirin at Discharge	118	100%	85%	90%	100%
Beta Blocker at Arrival	83	100%	78%	87%	100%
Beta Blocker at Discharge	114	100%	78%	90%	100%
Fibrinolytic Medication Timing	0	-	36%	31%	100%
PCI Within 90 Minutes of Arrival[1]	2	0%	51%	54%	95%
Smoking Cessation Advice	35	94%	83%	88%	100%
Heart Failure Care					
ACE Inhibitor or ARB for LVSD	98	100%	76%	82%	100%
Discharge Instructions	198	95%	55%	61%	93%
Evaluation of LVS Function	227	97%	71%	83%	99%
Smoking Cessation Advice	30	97%	73%	82%	100%
Pneumonia Care					
Appropriate Initial Antibiotic	105	90%	81%	83%	94%
Blood Culture Timing	98	96%	91%	90%	100%
Influenza Vaccine	31	87%	72%	70%	100%
Initial Antibiotic Timing	139	86%	82%	80%	93%

NOTE: Hospital profiles are in alphabetical order by state, then city, then hospital within the city; Rankings are sorted by rate in descending order and exclude hospitals with less than 25 cases; (1) The number of cases is too small (n<25) for purposes of reliably predicting hospital performance; (2) Measure reflects the hospital's indication that its submission was based upon a sample of its relevant discharges; (3) Rate reflects fewer than the maximum possible quarters of data for the measure; (4) Inaccurate information submitted and suppressed for one or more quarters; (5) No data is available from the hospital for this measure; Please refer to the User's Guide for a full explanation of data

Measure	Cases	This Hospital	State Average	U.S. Average	Top Hospital
Oxygenation Assessment	158	99%	99%	99%	100%
Pneumococcal Vaccine	104	95%	68%	69%	94%
Smoking Cessation Advice	41	98%	72%	80%	100%
Surgical Infection Prevention					
Prophylactic Antibiotic Given	378	88%	75%	77%	95%
Prophylactic Antibiotic Selection	108	94%	88%	90%	100%
Prophylactic Antibiotic Stopped	353	84%	82%	72%	95%
Pregnancy Care					
Inpatient Neonatal Mortality	-	-	-	-	-
Third or Fourth Degree Laceration	-	-	-	3.63%	3.27%

Southwestern Regional Medical Center

10109 East 79th Street South
Tulsa, OK 74133
Phone: 918-496-5000
Ownership: Proprietary
Accredited: Yes
Emergency Services: No

Measure	Cases	This Hospital	State Average	U.S. Average	Top Hospital
Heart Attack Care					
ACE Inhibitor or ARB for LVSD[3]	0	-	79%	82%	100%
Aspirin at Arrival[3]	0	-	86%	92%	100%
Aspirin at Discharge[3]	0	-	85%	90%	100%
Beta Blocker at Arrival[3]	0	-	78%	87%	100%
Beta Blocker at Discharge[3]	0	-	78%	90%	100%
Fibrinolytic Medication Timing[3]	0	-	36%	31%	100%
PCI Within 90 Minutes of Arrival	0	-	51%	54%	95%
Smoking Cessation Advice[3]	0	-	83%	88%	100%
Heart Failure Care					
ACE Inhibitor or ARB for LVSD[1,3]	2	50%	76%	82%	100%
Discharge Instructions[1,3]	4	75%	55%	61%	93%
Evaluation of LVS Function[1,3]	4	100%	71%	83%	99%
Smoking Cessation Advice[1,3]	2	50%	73%	82%	100%
Pneumonia Care					
Appropriate Initial Antibiotic	0	-	81%	83%	94%
Blood Culture Timing	0	-	91%	90%	100%
Influenza Vaccine	0	-	72%	70%	100%
Initial Antibiotic Timing[1]	6	67%	82%	80%	93%
Oxygenation Assessment[1]	9	89%	99%	99%	100%
Pneumococcal Vaccine[1]	3	0%	68%	69%	94%
Smoking Cessation Advice[1]	1	100%	72%	80%	100%
Surgical Infection Prevention					
Prophylactic Antibiotic Given[3]	26	19%	75%	77%	95%
Prophylactic Antibiotic Selection[1]	12	25%	88%	90%	100%
Prophylactic Antibiotic Stopped[1,3]	21	33%	82%	72%	95%
Pregnancy Care					
Inpatient Neonatal Mortality	-	-	-	-	-
Third or Fourth Degree Laceration	-	-	-	3.63%	3.27%

Tulsa Spine & Specialty Hospital

6901 South Olympia Avenue
Tulsa, OK 74132
Phone: 918-388-5701
Ownership: Voluntary non-profit - Private
Accredited: Yes
Emergency Services: Yes

Key Personnel:

Surgery . . . . John Frame, MD
Cardiology . . . . Simon Levitt, MD
OBGYN . . . . Darla Lofgren, MD

Measure	Cases	This Hospital	State Average	U.S. Average	Top Hospital
Heart Attack Care					
ACE Inhibitor or ARB for LVSD[5]	-	-	79%	82%	100%
Aspirin at Arrival[5]	-	-	86%	92%	100%
Aspirin at Discharge[5]	-	-	85%	90%	100%
Beta Blocker at Arrival[5]	-	-	78%	87%	100%
Beta Blocker at Discharge[5]	-	-	78%	90%	100%
Fibrinolytic Medication Timing[5]	-	-	36%	31%	100%
PCI Within 90 Minutes of Arrival[5]	-	-	51%	54%	95%
Smoking Cessation Advice[5]	-	-	83%	88%	100%
Heart Failure Care					
ACE Inhibitor or ARB for LVSD[5]	-	-	76%	82%	100%
Discharge Instructions[5]	-	-	55%	61%	93%
Evaluation of LVS Function[5]	-	-	71%	83%	99%
Smoking Cessation Advice[5]	-	-	73%	82%	100%
Pneumonia Care					
Appropriate Initial Antibiotic[5]	-	-	81%	83%	94%
Blood Culture Timing[5]	-	-	91%	90%	100%
Influenza Vaccine[5]	-	-	72%	70%	100%
Initial Antibiotic Timing[5]	-	-	82%	80%	93%
Oxygenation Assessment[5]	-	-	99%	99%	100%
Pneumococcal Vaccine[5]	-	-	68%	69%	94%
Smoking Cessation Advice[5]	-	-	72%	80%	100%
Surgical Infection Prevention					
Prophylactic Antibiotic Given[5]	-	-	75%	77%	95%
Prophylactic Antibiotic Selection[5]	-	-	88%	90%	100%
Prophylactic Antibiotic Stopped[5]	-	-	82%	72%	95%
Pregnancy Care					
Inpatient Neonatal Mortality	-	-	-	-	-
Third or Fourth Degree Laceration	-	-	-	3.63%	3.27%

Craig General Hospital

735 N Foreman
Vinita, OK 74301
Phone: 918-256-7551
Fax: 918-256-3703
Ownership: Government - Local
Accredited: No
Emergency Services: Yes
Licensed Beds: 42

Key Personnel:

Administrator . . . . B Joe Gunn
Chief Medical Staff. . . . . Lauri Bowie
Emergency Room . . . . Barbara Hodges
Director Infection/Disease Control . . . . Gwen Barbaree
Director Respiratory Therapy . . . . Debbie Abbott

Measure	Cases	This Hospital	State Average	U.S. Average	Top Hospital
Heart Attack Care					
ACE Inhibitor or ARB for LVSD	0	-	79%	82%	100%
Aspirin at Arrival[1]	4	100%	86%	92%	100%
Aspirin at Discharge[1]	3	100%	85%	90%	100%
Beta Blocker at Arrival[1]	1	0%	78%	87%	100%
Beta Blocker at Discharge[1]	2	50%	78%	90%	100%
Fibrinolytic Medication Timing	0	-	36%	31%	100%
PCI Within 90 Minutes of Arrival	0	-	51%	54%	95%
Smoking Cessation Advice[1]	1	0%	83%	88%	100%
Heart Failure Care					
ACE Inhibitor or ARB for LVSD[1]	14	93%	76%	82%	100%
Discharge Instructions	44	64%	55%	61%	93%
Evaluation of LVS Function	51	86%	71%	83%	99%
Smoking Cessation Advice[1]	11	73%	73%	82%	100%
Pneumonia Care					
Appropriate Initial Antibiotic	73	92%	81%	83%	94%
Blood Culture Timing[1]	10	80%	91%	90%	100%
Influenza Vaccine	25	96%	72%	70%	100%
Initial Antibiotic Timing	82	98%	82%	80%	93%
Oxygenation Assessment	96	100%	99%	99%	100%
Pneumococcal Vaccine	64	95%	68%	69%	94%
Smoking Cessation Advice[1]	20	70%	72%	80%	100%
Surgical Infection Prevention					
Prophylactic Antibiotic Given[1,3]	4	25%	75%	77%	95%
Prophylactic Antibiotic Selection[1]	2	50%	88%	90%	100%
Prophylactic Antibiotic Stopped[1,3]	4	75%	82%	72%	95%
Pregnancy Care					
Inpatient Neonatal Mortality	-	-	-	-	-
Third or Fourth Degree Laceration	-	-	-	3.63%	3.27%

Wagoner Hospital

Alternate Name: Wagoner Community Hospital
1200 W Cherokee
Wagoner, OK 74467
Phone: 918-485-5514
Fax: 918-485-9701
Ownership: Voluntary non-profit - Private
Accredited: No
Emergency Services: Yes
Licensed Beds: 100

Key Personnel:

CEO. . . . . John Crawford
Chief of Medical Staff. Chris Roberts

Measure	Cases	This Hospital	State Average	U.S. Average	Top Hospital
Heart Attack Care					

NOTE: Hospital profiles are in alphabetical order by state, then city, then hospital within the city; Rankings are sorted by rate in descending order and exclude hospitals with less than 25 cases; (1) The number of cases is too small (n<25) for purposes of reliably predicting hospital performance; (2) Measure reflects the hospital's indication that its submission was based upon a sample of its relevant discharges; (3) Rate reflects fewer than the maximum possible quarters of data for the measure; (4) Inaccurate information submitted and suppressed for one or more quarters; (5) No data is available from the hospital for this measure; Please refer to the User's Guide for a full explanation of data

Measure	Cases	This Hospital	State Average	U.S. Average	Top Hospital
ACE Inhibitor or ARB for LVSD[3]	0	-	79%	82%	100%
Aspirin at Arrival[3]	0	-	86%	92%	100%
Aspirin at Discharge[3]	0	-	85%	90%	100%
Beta Blocker at Arrival[3]	0	-	78%	87%	100%
Beta Blocker at Discharge[3]	0	-	78%	90%	100%
Fibrinolytic Medication Timing[3]	0	-	36%	31%	100%
PCI Within 90 Minutes of Arrival[5]	-	-	51%	54%	95%
Smoking Cessation Advice[3]	0	-	83%	88%	100%
Heart Failure Care					
ACE Inhibitor or ARB for LVSD[1,3]	5	100%	76%	82%	100%
Discharge Instructions[1,3]	21	33%	55%	61%	93%
Evaluation of LVS Function[3]	27	52%	71%	83%	99%
Smoking Cessation Advice[1,3]	7	43%	73%	82%	100%
Pneumonia Care					
Appropriate Initial Antibiotic[3]	41	78%	81%	83%	94%
Blood Culture Timing[3]	0	-	91%	90%	100%
Influenza Vaccine[5]	-	-	72%	70%	100%
Initial Antibiotic Timing[3]	36	69%	82%	80%	93%
Oxygenation Assessment[3]	49	96%	99%	99%	100%
Pneumococcal Vaccine[3]	27	74%	68%	69%	94%
Smoking Cessation Advice[1,3]	14	36%	72%	80%	100%
Surgical Infection Prevention					
Prophylactic Antibiotic Given[5]	-	-	75%	77%	95%
Prophylactic Antibiotic Selection[5]	-	-	88%	90%	100%
Prophylactic Antibiotic Stopped[5]	-	-	82%	72%	95%
Pregnancy Care					
Inpatient Neonatal Mortality	-	-	-	-	-
Third or Fourth Degree Laceration	-	-	-	3.63%	3.27%

Watonga Municipal Hospital

PO Box 370
Watonga, OK 73772
Ownership: Govt - Hospital District or Authority
Emergency Services: Yes
Phone: 580-623-7211
Fax: 580-623-7206
Accredited: No
Licensed Beds: 35

Key Personnel:
CEO. . . . . David Jordan

Measure	Cases	This Hospital	State Average	U.S. Average	Top Hospital
Heart Attack Care					
ACE Inhibitor or ARB for LVSD[1,3]	1	100%	79%	82%	100%
Aspirin at Arrival[1,3]	1	0%	86%	92%	100%
Aspirin at Discharge[1,3]	1	100%	85%	90%	100%
Beta Blocker at Arrival[1,3]	1	0%	78%	87%	100%
Beta Blocker at Discharge[1,3]	1	0%	78%	90%	100%
Fibrinolytic Medication Timing[3]	0	-	36%	31%	100%
PCI Within 90 Minutes of Arrival	0	-	51%	54%	95%
Smoking Cessation Advice[3]	0	-	83%	88%	100%
Heart Failure Care					
ACE Inhibitor or ARB for LVSD[3]	0	-	76%	82%	100%
Discharge Instructions[3]	0	-	55%	61%	93%
Evaluation of LVS Function[1,3]	4	25%	71%	83%	99%
Smoking Cessation Advice[3]	0	-	73%	82%	100%
Pneumonia Care					
Appropriate Initial Antibiotic[1,2,3]	8	88%	81%	83%	94%
Blood Culture Timing[2,3]	0	-	91%	90%	100%
Influenza Vaccine[5]	-	-	72%	70%	100%
Initial Antibiotic Timing[1,2,3]	5	80%	82%	80%	93%
Oxygenation Assessment[1,2,3]	9	100%	99%	99%	100%
Pneumococcal Vaccine[1,2,3]	5	0%	68%	69%	94%
Smoking Cessation Advice[1,2,3]	2	100%	72%	80%	100%
Surgical Infection Prevention					
Prophylactic Antibiotic Given[5]	-	-	75%	77%	95%
Prophylactic Antibiotic Selection[5]	-	-	88%	90%	100%
Prophylactic Antibiotic Stopped[5]	-	-	82%	72%	95%
Pregnancy Care					
Inpatient Neonatal Mortality	-	-	-	-	-
Third or Fourth Degree Laceration	-	-	-	3.63%	3.27%

Jefferson County Hospital

PO Box 90
Waurika, OK 73573
Ownership: Govt - Hospital District or Authority
Emergency Services: Yes
Phone: 580-228-2344
Fax: 580-228-3410
Accredited: No
Licensed Beds: 25

Key Personnel:
Administrator/CEO . . . . Buck McKinney Jr
Chief Medical Staff. . . . . Harold Start, MD
Emergency Room . . . . Steven Hwshay, DO
Director Infection/Disease Control . . . . Pam Jackson, RN
Chief Radiology . . . . David Kent
Director Respiratory Therapy . . . . Pam Jackson, RN

Measure	Cases	This Hospital	State Average	U.S. Average	Top Hospital
Heart Attack Care					
ACE Inhibitor or ARB for LVSD[5]	-	-	79%	82%	100%
Aspirin at Arrival[5]	-	-	86%	92%	100%
Aspirin at Discharge[5]	-	-	85%	90%	100%
Beta Blocker at Arrival[5]	-	-	78%	87%	100%
Beta Blocker at Discharge[5]	-	-	78%	90%	100%
Fibrinolytic Medication Timing[5]	-	-	36%	31%	100%
PCI Within 90 Minutes of Arrival[5]	-	-	51%	54%	95%
Smoking Cessation Advice[5]	-	-	83%	88%	100%
Heart Failure Care					
ACE Inhibitor or ARB for LVSD[1]	1	0%	76%	82%	100%
Discharge Instructions[1]	3	33%	55%	61%	93%
Evaluation of LVS Function[1]	4	25%	71%	83%	99%
Smoking Cessation Advice	0	-	73%	82%	100%
Pneumonia Care					
Appropriate Initial Antibiotic[1,3]	8	62%	81%	83%	94%
Blood Culture Timing[1,3]	1	100%	91%	90%	100%
Influenza Vaccine[1]	2	50%	72%	70%	100%
Initial Antibiotic Timing[1,3]	5	0%	82%	80%	93%
Oxygenation Assessment[1,3]	11	100%	99%	99%	100%
Pneumococcal Vaccine[1,3]	6	33%	68%	69%	94%
Smoking Cessation Advice[1,3]	2	50%	72%	80%	100%
Surgical Infection Prevention					
Prophylactic Antibiotic Given[5]	-	-	75%	77%	95%
Prophylactic Antibiotic Selection[5]	-	-	88%	90%	100%
Prophylactic Antibiotic Stopped[5]	-	-	82%	72%	95%
Pregnancy Care					
Inpatient Neonatal Mortality	-	-	-	-	-
Third or Fourth Degree Laceration	-	-	-	3.63%	3.27%

Weatherford Regional Hospital

Alternate Name: Southwestern Memorial Hospital
215 N Kansas Street
Weatherford, OK 73096
URL: www.weatherfordhospital.com
Ownership: Govt - Hospital District or Authority
Emergency Services: No
Phone: 580-772-5551
Fax: 580-774-4764
Accredited: No
Licensed Beds: 25

Key Personnel:
President/CEO . . . . Debbie Howe
Head of Emergency Room. . . . . Lonnie Scholl
Director Respiratory Therapy . . . . Stan Willingham

Measure	Cases	This Hospital	State Average	U.S. Average	Top Hospital
Heart Attack Care					
ACE Inhibitor or ARB for LVSD	0	-	79%	82%	100%
Aspirin at Arrival[1]	7	71%	86%	92%	100%
Aspirin at Discharge	0	-	85%	90%	100%
Beta Blocker at Arrival[1]	8	50%	78%	87%	100%
Beta Blocker at Discharge[1]	1	0%	78%	90%	100%
Fibrinolytic Medication Timing	0	-	36%	31%	100%
PCI Within 90 Minutes of Arrival	0	-	51%	54%	95%
Smoking Cessation Advice	0	-	83%	88%	100%
Heart Failure Care					
ACE Inhibitor or ARB for LVSD[1]	2	100%	76%	82%	100%
Discharge Instructions[1]	12	50%	55%	61%	93%
Evaluation of LVS Function[1]	20	60%	71%	83%	99%
Smoking Cessation Advice[1]	1	0%	73%	82%	100%
Pneumonia Care					
Appropriate Initial Antibiotic	66	55%	81%	83%	94%

NOTE: Hospital profiles are in alphabetical order by state, then city, then hospital within the city; Rankings are sorted by rate in descending order and exclude hospitals with less than 25 cases; (1) The number of cases is too small (n<25) for purposes of reliably predicting hospital performance; (2) Measure reflects the hospital's indication that its submission was based upon a sample of its relevant discharges; (3) Rate reflects fewer than the maximum possible quarters of data for the measure; (4) Inaccurate information submitted and suppressed for one or more quarters; (5) No data is available from the hospital for this measure; Please refer to the User's Guide for a full explanation of data

Measure	Cases	This Hospital	State Average	U.S. Average	Top Hospital
Blood Culture Timing[1]	5	80%	91%	90%	100%
Influenza Vaccine[4,5]	-	-	72%	70%	100%
Initial Antibiotic Timing	63	67%	82%	80%	93%
Oxygenation Assessment	78	100%	99%	99%	100%
Pneumococcal Vaccine	48	79%	68%	69%	94%
Smoking Cessation Advice[1]	12	17%	72%	80%	100%
Surgical Infection Prevention					
Prophylactic Antibiotic Given[5]	-	-	75%	77%	95%
Prophylactic Antibiotic Selection[5]	-	-	88%	90%	100%
Prophylactic Antibiotic Stopped[5]	-	-	82%	72%	95%
Pregnancy Care					
Inpatient Neonatal Mortality	-	-	-	-	-
Third or Fourth Degree Laceration	-	-	-	3.63%	3.27%

Latimer County General Hospital

806 Highway 2 N
Wilburton, OK 74578
Phone: 918-465-2391
Fax: 918-465-5169
Ownership: Govt - Hospital District or Authority
Accredited: No
Emergency Services: Yes
Licensed Beds: 33

Key Personnel:

CEO . . . . Sue Mings
Chief Medical Staff . . . . Gerald Rana
Emergency Room Director . . . . Lynda Willmoen
Director Radiology . . . . Mike Chronister
Director Respiratory Therapy . . . . Patrick Nessel

Measure	Cases	This Hospital	State Average	U.S. Average	Top Hospital
Heart Attack Care					
ACE Inhibitor or ARB for LVSD[3]	0	-	79%	82%	100%
Aspirin at Arrival[1,3]	1	100%	86%	92%	100%
Aspirin at Discharge[3]	0	-	85%	90%	100%
Beta Blocker at Arrival[1,3]	1	100%	78%	87%	100%
Beta Blocker at Discharge[3]	0	-	78%	90%	100%
Fibrinolytic Medication Timing[1,3]	2	100%	36%	31%	100%
PCI Within 90 Minutes of Arrival[5]	-	-	51%	54%	95%
Smoking Cessation Advice[3]	0	-	83%	88%	100%
Heart Failure Care					
ACE Inhibitor or ARB for LVSD	0	-	76%	82%	100%
Discharge Instructions[1]	12	83%	55%	61%	93%
Evaluation of LVS Function[1]	17	47%	71%	83%	99%
Smoking Cessation Advice[1]	3	100%	73%	82%	100%
Pneumonia Care					
Appropriate Initial Antibiotic[1]	8	75%	81%	83%	94%
Blood Culture Timing[1]	1	100%	91%	90%	100%
Influenza Vaccine[1]	2	50%	72%	70%	100%
Initial Antibiotic Timing[1]	11	82%	82%	80%	93%
Oxygenation Assessment[1]	14	100%	99%	99%	100%
Pneumococcal Vaccine[1]	7	86%	68%	69%	94%
Smoking Cessation Advice[1]	2	100%	72%	80%	100%
Surgical Infection Prevention					
Prophylactic Antibiotic Given[5]	-	-	75%	77%	95%
Prophylactic Antibiotic Selection[5]	-	-	88%	90%	100%
Prophylactic Antibiotic Stopped[5]	-	-	82%	72%	95%
Pregnancy Care					
Inpatient Neonatal Mortality	-	-	-	-	-
Third or Fourth Degree Laceration	-	-	-	3.63%	3.27%

Woodward Hospital and Health Center

900 17th Street
Woodward, OK 73801
Phone: 580-256-5511
Fax: 580-254-8431
Ownership: Proprietary
Accredited: Yes
Emergency Services: Yes
Licensed Beds: 87

Key Personnel:

CEO . . . . Troy Tauvenheim
Head of Emergency Room . . . . Lynn Sivelove
Director of Pulmonary . . . . Teresa Gold

Measure	Cases	This Hospital	State Average	U.S. Average	Top Hospital
Heart Attack Care					
ACE Inhibitor or ARB for LVSD	0	-	79%	82%	100%
Aspirin at Arrival[1]	6	83%	86%	92%	100%
Aspirin at Discharge[1]	3	100%	85%	90%	100%
Beta Blocker at Arrival[1]	7	100%	78%	87%	100%
Beta Blocker at Discharge[1]	3	100%	78%	90%	100%
Fibrinolytic Medication Timing	0	-	36%	31%	100%
PCI Within 90 Minutes of Arrival	0	-	51%	54%	95%
Smoking Cessation Advice	0	-	83%	88%	100%
Heart Failure Care					
ACE Inhibitor or ARB for LVSD[1]	18	94%	76%	82%	100%
Discharge Instructions	44	100%	55%	61%	93%
Evaluation of LVS Function	63	95%	71%	83%	99%
Smoking Cessation Advice[1]	7	86%	73%	82%	100%
Pneumonia Care					
Appropriate Initial Antibiotic	48	83%	81%	83%	94%
Blood Culture Timing	55	95%	91%	90%	100%
Influenza Vaccine	28	96%	72%	70%	100%
Initial Antibiotic Timing	101	91%	82%	80%	93%
Oxygenation Assessment	127	100%	99%	99%	100%
Pneumococcal Vaccine	78	81%	68%	69%	94%
Smoking Cessation Advice[1]	23	100%	72%	80%	100%
Surgical Infection Prevention					
Prophylactic Antibiotic Given	58	71%	75%	77%	95%
Prophylactic Antibiotic Selection[1]	17	94%	88%	90%	100%
Prophylactic Antibiotic Stopped	54	98%	82%	72%	95%
Pregnancy Care					
Inpatient Neonatal Mortality	-	-	-	-	-
Third or Fourth Degree Laceration	-	-	-	3.63%	3.27%

Integris Canadian Valley Regional Hospital

1201 Health Center Parkway
Yukon, OK 73099
Phone: 405-717-7999
Ownership: Voluntary non-profit - Other
Accredited: Yes
Emergency Services: Yes

Measure	Cases	This Hospital	State Average	U.S. Average	Top Hospital
Heart Attack Care					
ACE Inhibitor or ARB for LVSD[1]	2	100%	79%	82%	100%
Aspirin at Arrival[1]	7	100%	86%	92%	100%
Aspirin at Discharge[1]	7	100%	85%	90%	100%
Beta Blocker at Arrival[1]	7	71%	78%	87%	100%
Beta Blocker at Discharge[1]	9	44%	78%	90%	100%
Fibrinolytic Medication Timing	0	-	36%	31%	100%
PCI Within 90 Minutes of Arrival	0	-	51%	54%	95%
Smoking Cessation Advice[1]	1	100%	83%	88%	100%
Heart Failure Care					
ACE Inhibitor or ARB for LVSD[1]	23	65%	76%	82%	100%
Discharge Instructions	70	90%	55%	61%	93%
Evaluation of LVS Function	95	91%	71%	83%	99%
Smoking Cessation Advice[1]	12	92%	73%	82%	100%
Pneumonia Care					
Appropriate Initial Antibiotic	180	86%	81%	83%	94%
Blood Culture Timing	104	93%	91%	90%	100%
Influenza Vaccine[4,5]	-	-	72%	70%	100%
Initial Antibiotic Timing	163	90%	82%	80%	93%
Oxygenation Assessment	190	100%	99%	99%	100%
Pneumococcal Vaccine	114	68%	68%	69%	94%
Smoking Cessation Advice	50	100%	72%	80%	100%
Surgical Infection Prevention					
Prophylactic Antibiotic Given	104	93%	75%	77%	95%
Prophylactic Antibiotic Selection	30	97%	88%	90%	100%
Prophylactic Antibiotic Stopped	104	79%	82%	72%	95%
Pregnancy Care					
Inpatient Neonatal Mortality	-	-	-	-	-
Third or Fourth Degree Laceration	-	-	-	3.63%	3.27%

NOTE: Hospital profiles are in alphabetical order by state, then city, then hospital within the city; Rankings are sorted by rate in descending order and exclude hospitals with less than 25 cases; (1) The number of cases is too small (n<25) for purposes of reliably predicting hospital performance; (2) Measure reflects the hospital's indication that its submission was based upon a sample of its relevant discharges; (3) Rate reflects fewer than the maximum possible quarters of data for the measure; (4) Inaccurate information submitted and suppressed for one or more quarters; (5) No data is available from the hospital for this measure; Please refer to the User's Guide for a full explanation of data

Heart Attack Care

1. ACE Inhibitor or ARB for LVSD

Hospital Name	City	Rate	Cases
Avera Heart Hospital of South Dakota	Sioux Falls	96%	103
Rapid City Regional Hospital	Rapid City	93%	59
Sanford USD Medical Center	Sioux Falls	90%	59

2. Aspirin at Arrival

Hospital Name	City	Rate	Cases
Avera McKennan Hospital & Univ Hlth Ctr	Sioux Falls	100%	78
Avera Sacred Heart Hospital	Yankton	100%	26
Sanford USD Medical Center	Sioux Falls	100%	191
Avera Heart Hospital of South Dakota	Sioux Falls	99%	99
Rapid City Regional Hospital	Rapid City	99%	125
Avera Saint Luke's	Aberdeen	98%	50

3. Aspirin at Discharge

Hospital Name	City	Rate	Cases
Avera Saint Luke's	Aberdeen	100%	32
Rapid City Regional Hospital	Rapid City	100%	242
Avera Heart Hospital of South Dakota	Sioux Falls	99%	641
Avera McKennan Hospital & Univ Hlth Ctr	Sioux Falls	99%	77
Sanford USD Medical Center	Sioux Falls	99%	358

4. Beta Blocker at Arrival

Hospital Name	City	Rate	Cases
Avera Sacred Heart Hospital	Yankton	100%	26
Avera Saint Luke's	Aberdeen	100%	30
Avera Heart Hospital of South Dakota	Sioux Falls	99%	92
Avera McKennan Hospital & Univ Hlth Ctr	Sioux Falls	97%	68
Sanford USD Medical Center	Sioux Falls	96%	146
Rapid City Regional Hospital	Rapid City	95%	109

5. Beta Blocker at Discharge

Hospital Name	City	Rate	Cases
Avera Heart Hospital of South Dakota	Sioux Falls	100%	674
Avera McKennan Hospital & Univ Hlth Ctr	Sioux Falls	100%	82
Sanford USD Medical Center	Sioux Falls	99%	357
Rapid City Regional Hospital	Rapid City	97%	317
Avera Saint Luke's	Aberdeen	94%	34

8. Smoking Cessation Advice

Hospital Name	City	Rate	Cases
Avera Heart Hospital of South Dakota	Sioux Falls	100%	214
Avera McKennan Hospital & Univ Hlth Ctr	Sioux Falls	100%	29
Rapid City Regional Hospital	Rapid City	99%	130
Sanford USD Medical Center	Sioux Falls	92%	139

Heart Failure Care

9. ACE Inhibitor or ARB for LVSD

Hospital Name	City	Rate	Cases
Avera Sacred Heart Hospital	Yankton	98%	55
Avera Heart Hospital of South Dakota	Sioux Falls	96%	84
Avera McKennan Hospital & Univ Hlth Ctr	Sioux Falls	94%	64
Sanford USD Medical Center	Sioux Falls	88%	92
Rapid City Regional Hospital	Rapid City	84%	102
Prairie Lakes Hospital & Care Center	Watertown	76%	25

10. Discharge Instructions

Hospital Name	City	Rate	Cases
Avera McKennan Hospital & Univ Hlth Ctr	Sioux Falls	100%	151
Avera Sacred Heart Hospital	Yankton	99%	88
Avera Saint Luke's	Aberdeen	94%	84
Queen of Peace Hospital	Mitchell	94%	51
Avera Heart Hospital of South Dakota	Sioux Falls	93%	155
Rapid City Regional Hospital	Rapid City	88%	224
Sanford USD Medical Center	Sioux Falls	87%	196
Prairie Lakes Hospital & Care Center	Watertown	67%	58
Saint Mary's Healthcare Center	Pierre	52%	31

11. Evaluation of LVS Function

Hospital Name	City	Rate	Cases
Avera Sacred Heart Hospital	Yankton	100%	127
Avera Heart Hospital of South Dakota	Sioux Falls	99%	182
Avera McKennan Hospital & Univ Hlth Ctr	Sioux Falls	99%	215
Avera Saint Luke's	Aberdeen	99%	128
Sanford USD Medical Center	Sioux Falls	97%	262
Rapid City Regional Hospital	Rapid City	93%	290
Queen of Peace Hospital	Mitchell	92%	96
Prairie Lakes Hospital & Care Center	Watertown	82%	82
Brookings Hospital	Brookings	70%	33
Saint Mary's Healthcare Center	Pierre	64%	50

12. Smoking Cessation Advice

Hospital Name	City	Rate	Cases
Avera McKennan Hospital & Univ Hlth Ctr	Sioux Falls	100%	26
Rapid City Regional Hospital	Rapid City	98%	46
Sanford USD Medical Center	Sioux Falls	88%	41

Pneumonia Care

13. Appropriate Initial Antibiotic

Hospital Name	City	Rate	Cases
Prairie Lakes Hospital & Care Center	Watertown	96%	108
Avera McKennan Hospital & Univ Hlth Ctr	Sioux Falls	93%	100
Avera Sacred Heart Hospital	Yankton	92%	88
Queen of Peace Hospital	Mitchell	91%	103
Avera Saint Luke's	Aberdeen	89%	94
Sioux Valley Vermillian Campus	Vermillion	89%	28
Sturgis Regional Hospital	Sturgis	89%	56
Spearfish Regional Hospital	Spearfish	87%	38
Rapid City Regional Hospital	Rapid City	86%	189
Sanford USD Medical Center	Sioux Falls	86%	122
Huron Regional Medical Center	Huron	85%	71
Saint Mary's Healthcare Center	Pierre	83%	54
Gregory Health Care Center	Gregory	63%	30
Landmann-Jungman Memorial Hospital	Scotland	20%	30

14. Blood Culture Timing

Hospital Name	City	Rate	Cases
Avera Saint Luke's	Aberdeen	98%	97
Queen of Peace Hospital	Mitchell	97%	68
Avera Sacred Heart Hospital	Yankton	94%	78
Saint Mary's Healthcare Center	Pierre	94%	31
Sanford USD Medical Center	Sioux Falls	93%	70
Prairie Lakes Hospital & Care Center	Watertown	92%	72
Avera McKennan Hospital & Univ Hlth Ctr	Sioux Falls	89%	89
Rapid City Regional Hospital	Rapid City	83%	133

15. Influenza Vaccine

Hospital Name	City	Rate	Cases
Avera Sacred Heart Hospital	Yankton	100%	36
Sanford USD Medical Center	Sioux Falls	95%	37
Avera McKennan Hospital & Univ Hlth Ctr	Sioux Falls	92%	37
Prairie Lakes Hospital & Care Center	Watertown	88%	26
Queen of Peace Hospital	Mitchell	81%	37
Rapid City Regional Hospital	Rapid City	71%	48

16. Initial Antibiotic Timing

Hospital Name	City	Rate	Cases
Mobridge Regional Hospital	Mobridge	100%	25
Community Memorial Hospital	Redfield	96%	27
Avera Saint Luke's	Aberdeen	95%	129
Prairie Lakes Hospital & Care Center	Watertown	95%	154
Gregory Health Care Center	Gregory	94%	50
Queen of Peace Hospital	Mitchell	93%	149
Avera Sacred Heart Hospital	Yankton	92%	124
Brookings Hospital	Brookings	92%	60
Sturgis Regional Hospital	Sturgis	91%	57
Platte Health Center	Platte	90%	30
Sioux Valley Vermillian Campus	Vermillion	90%	31
Avera McKennan Hospital & Univ Hlth Ctr	Sioux Falls	89%	142
Spearfish Regional Hospital	Spearfish	89%	45
Rapid City Regional Hospital	Rapid City	85%	234
Landmann-Jungman Memorial Hospital	Scotland	84%	25
Saint Mary's Healthcare Center	Pierre	84%	85
Sanford USD Medical Center	Sioux Falls	84%	180
Huron Regional Medical Center	Huron	72%	80
PHS Indian Health Service Hospital	Pine Ridge	44%	27

17. Oxygenation Assessment

Hospital Name	City	Rate	Cases
Avera McKennan Hospital & Univ Hlth Ctr	Sioux Falls	100%	173
Avera Sacred Heart Hospital	Yankton	100%	175
Avera Saint Benedict Health Center	Parkston	100%	26
Avera Saint Luke's	Aberdeen	100%	183
Brookings Hospital	Brookings	100%	82
Community Memorial Hospital	Redfield	100%	38

NOTE: Hospital profiles are in alphabetical order by state, then city, then hospital within the city; Rankings are sorted by rate in descending order and exclude hospitals with less than 25 cases; (1) The number of cases is too small (n<25) for purposes of reliably predicting hospital performance; (2) Measure reflects the hospital's indication that its submission was based upon a sample of its relevant discharges; (3) Rate reflects fewer than the maximum possible quarters of data for the measure; (4) Inaccurate information submitted and suppressed for one or more quarters; (5) No data is available from the hospital for this measure; Please refer to the User's Guide for a full explanation of data

Coteau Des Prairies Hospital	Sisseton	100%	30
De Smet Memorial Hospital	De Smet	100%	30
Gregory Health Care Center	Gregory	100%	65
Huron Regional Medical Center	Huron	100%	103
Landmann-Jungman Memorial Hospital	Scotland	100%	36
Mobridge Regional Hospital	Mobridge	100%	28
Platte Health Center	Platte	100%	31
Prairie Lakes Hospital & Care Center	Watertown	100%	180
Queen of Peace Hospital	Mitchell	100%	185
Saint Mary's Healthcare Center	Pierre	100%	99
Sanford USD Medical Center	Sioux Falls	100%	256
Sioux Valley Vermillian Campus	Vermillion	100%	36
Spearfish Regional Hospital	Spearfish	100%	56
Sturgis Regional Hospital	Sturgis	100%	57
Winner Regional Healthcare Center	Winner	100%	25
Rapid City Regional Hospital	Rapid City	98%	300
PHS Indian Health Service Hospital	Pine Ridge	97%	29

18. Pneumococcal Vaccine

Hospital Name	City	Rate	Cases
Community Memorial Hospital	Redfield	100%	30
Avera Sacred Heart Hospital	Yankton	98%	125
Avera Saint Luke's	Aberdeen	98%	126
Saint Mary's Healthcare Center	Pierre	97%	72
Platte Health Center	Platte	93%	28
Queen of Peace Hospital	Mitchell	91%	130
De Smet Memorial Hospital	De Smet	89%	28
Avera McKennan Hospital & Univ Hlth Ctr	Sioux Falls	88%	131
Sanford USD Medical Center	Sioux Falls	87%	166
Rapid City Regional Hospital	Rapid City	86%	206
Spearfish Regional Hospital	Spearfish	85%	41
Brookings Hospital	Brookings	84%	58
Sturgis Regional Hospital	Sturgis	84%	43
Gregory Health Care Center	Gregory	72%	53
Prairie Lakes Hospital & Care Center	Watertown	72%	146
Huron Regional Medical Center	Huron	66%	80
Landmann-Jungman Memorial Hospital	Scotland	49%	35

19. Smoking Cessation Advice

Hospital Name	City	Rate	Cases
Avera McKennan Hospital & Univ Hlth Ctr	Sioux Falls	100%	40
Avera Sacred Heart Hospital	Yankton	100%	36
Avera Saint Luke's	Aberdeen	100%	29
Queen of Peace Hospital	Mitchell	97%	39
Rapid City Regional Hospital	Rapid City	97%	86
Sanford USD Medical Center	Sioux Falls	88%	67

Surgical Infection Prevention

20. Prophylactic Antibiotic Given

Hospital Name	City	Rate	Cases
Black Hills Surgery Center	Rapid City	99%	134
Dakota Plains Surgical Center	Aberdeen	98%	62
Avera McKennan Hospital & Univ Hlth Ctr	Sioux Falls	96%	384
Avera Sacred Heart Hospital	Yankton	96%	269
Queen of Peace Hospital	Mitchell	96%	177
Siouxland Surgery Center Lp	Dakota Dunes	96%	366
Avera Heart Hospital of South Dakota	Sioux Falls	95%	355
Huron Regional Medical Center	Huron	94%	36
Saint Mary's Healthcare Center	Pierre	94%	107
Prairie Lakes Hospital & Care Center	Watertown	93%	328
Rapid City Regional Hospital	Rapid City	91%	668
Spearfish Regional Hospital	Spearfish	91%	145
Avera Saint Luke's	Aberdeen	90%	412
Sanford USD Medical Center	Sioux Falls	90%	1128
Sioux Falls Surgical Center	Sioux Falls	79%	197
Lewis and Clark Specialty Hospital	Yankton	51%	80

21. Prophylactic Antibiotic Selection

Hospital Name	City	Rate	Cases
Avera Heart Hospital of South Dakota	Sioux Falls	100%	106
Black Hills Surgery Center	Rapid City	100%	50
Spearfish Regional Hospital	Spearfish	100%	32
Avera Sacred Heart Hospital	Yankton	99%	69
Queen of Peace Hospital	Mitchell	98%	45
Sanford USD Medical Center	Sioux Falls	98%	220
Prairie Lakes Hospital & Care Center	Watertown	96%	75
Sioux Falls Surgical Center	Sioux Falls	94%	82
Avera McKennan Hospital & Univ Hlth Ctr	Sioux Falls	93%	278
Avera Saint Luke's	Aberdeen	93%	95
Saint Mary's Healthcare Center	Pierre	92%	40
Rapid City Regional Hospital	Rapid City	91%	69
Siouxland Surgery Center Lp	Dakota Dunes	85%	94

22. Prophylactic Antibiotic Stopped

Hospital Name	City	Rate	Cases
Avera Heart Hospital of South Dakota	Sioux Falls	99%	347
Prairie Lakes Hospital & Care Center	Watertown	98%	320
Black Hills Surgery Center	Rapid City	95%	132
Lewis and Clark Specialty Hospital	Yankton	94%	79
Spearfish Regional Hospital	Spearfish	93%	141
Avera Sacred Heart Hospital	Yankton	92%	249
Sioux Falls Surgical Center	Sioux Falls	92%	197
Avera McKennan Hospital & Univ Hlth Ctr	Sioux Falls	90%	362
Saint Mary's Healthcare Center	Pierre	90%	101
Siouxland Surgery Center Lp	Dakota Dunes	90%	366
Queen of Peace Hospital	Mitchell	89%	171
Sanford USD Medical Center	Sioux Falls	88%	1060
Avera Saint Luke's	Aberdeen	87%	411
Rapid City Regional Hospital	Rapid City	86%	621
Dakota Plains Surgical Center	Aberdeen	68%	62
Huron Regional Medical Center	Huron	21%	34

Pregnancy Care

23. Inpatient Neonatal Mortality

Hospital Name	City	Rate	Cases
Saint Mary's Healthcare Center	Pierre	0.00%	477

24. Third or Fourth Degree Laceration

Hospital Name	City	Rate	Cases
Saint Mary's Healthcare Center	Pierre	5.10%	314

NOTE: Hospital profiles are in alphabetical order by state, then city, then hospital within the city; Rankings are sorted by rate in descending order and exclude hospitals with less than 25 cases; (1) The number of cases is too small (n<25) for purposes of reliably predicting hospital performance; (2) Measure reflects the hospital's indication that its submission was based upon a sample of its relevant discharges; (3) Rate reflects fewer than the maximum possible quarters of data for the measure; (4) Inaccurate information submitted and suppressed for one or more quarters; (5) No data is available from the hospital for this measure; Please refer to the User's Guide for a full explanation of data

Avera Saint Luke's

Alternate Name: Saint Luke's Midland Regional Medical Center
305 S State Street
Aberdeen, SD 57401

Toll-Free: 800-225-8537
Phone: 605-622-5000
Fax: 605-622-5041

URL: www.averastlukes.org
Ownership: Voluntary non-profit - Other
Emergency Services: Yes

Accredited: No
Licensed Beds: 137

Key Personnel:
President/CEO. . . . . Ron L Jacobson
Chief Medical Staff. . . . . Bonnie Craig
Director Infection/Disease Control . . . . Jolynn Zeller
Director Medical/Surgical Nursing . . . . Jan Patterson
Chief Radiology . . . . James McGee, MD
Director Respiratory Therapy . . . . Pam Beckering

Measure	Cases	This Hospital	State Average	U.S. Average	Top Hospital
Heart Attack Care					
ACE Inhibitor or ARB for LVSD[1]	8	62%	84%	82%	100%
Aspirin at Arrival	50	98%	94%	92%	100%
Aspirin at Discharge	32	100%	96%	90%	100%
Beta Blocker at Arrival	30	100%	90%	87%	100%
Beta Blocker at Discharge	34	94%	94%	90%	100%
Fibrinolytic Medication Timing[1]	11	18%	42%	31%	100%
PCI Within 90 Minutes of Arrival	0	-	79%	54%	95%
Smoking Cessation Advice[1]	5	100%	69%	88%	100%
Heart Failure Care					
ACE Inhibitor or ARB for LVSD[1]	24	100%	76%	82%	100%
Discharge Instructions	84	94%	51%	61%	93%
Evaluation of LVS Function	128	99%	71%	83%	99%
Smoking Cessation Advice[1]	16	100%	69%	82%	100%
Pneumonia Care					
Appropriate Initial Antibiotic	94	89%	77%	83%	94%
Blood Culture Timing	97	98%	97%	90%	100%
Influenza Vaccine[1]	24	88%	83%	70%	100%
Initial Antibiotic Timing	129	95%	86%	80%	93%
Oxygenation Assessment	183	100%	100%	99%	100%
Pneumococcal Vaccine	126	98%	73%	69%	94%
Smoking Cessation Advice	29	100%	63%	80%	100%
Surgical Infection Prevention					
Prophylactic Antibiotic Given	412	90%	85%	77%	95%
Prophylactic Antibiotic Selection	95	93%	93%	90%	100%
Prophylactic Antibiotic Stopped	411	87%	86%	72%	95%
Pregnancy Care					
Inpatient Neonatal Mortality	-	-	-	-	-
Third or Fourth Degree Laceration	-	-	-	3.63%	3.27%

Dakota Plains Surgical Center

701 8th Avenue Nw Suite C
Aberdeen, SD 57401
Ownership: Voluntary non-profit - Private
Emergency Services: No

Phone: 605-225-3300

Accredited: No

Measure	Cases	This Hospital	State Average	U.S. Average	Top Hospital
Heart Attack Care					
ACE Inhibitor or ARB for LVSD[5]	-	-	84%	82%	100%
Aspirin at Arrival[5]	-	-	94%	92%	100%
Aspirin at Discharge[5]	-	-	96%	90%	100%
Beta Blocker at Arrival[5]	-	-	90%	87%	100%
Beta Blocker at Discharge[5]	-	-	94%	90%	100%
Fibrinolytic Medication Timing[5]	-	-	42%	31%	100%
PCI Within 90 Minutes of Arrival[5]	-	-	79%	54%	95%
Smoking Cessation Advice[5]	-	-	69%	88%	100%
Heart Failure Care					
ACE Inhibitor or ARB for LVSD[5]	-	-	76%	82%	100%
Discharge Instructions[5]	-	-	51%	61%	93%
Evaluation of LVS Function[5]	-	-	71%	83%	99%
Smoking Cessation Advice[5]	-	-	69%	82%	100%
Pneumonia Care					
Appropriate Initial Antibiotic[5]	-	-	77%	83%	94%
Blood Culture Timing[5]	-	-	97%	90%	100%
Influenza Vaccine[5]	-	-	83%	70%	100%
Initial Antibiotic Timing[5]	-	-	86%	80%	93%
Oxygenation Assessment[5]	-	-	100%	99%	100%
Pneumococcal Vaccine[5]	-	-	73%	69%	94%
Smoking Cessation Advice[5]	-	-	63%	80%	100%
Surgical Infection Prevention					
Prophylactic Antibiotic Given[2,3]	62	98%	85%	77%	95%
Prophylactic Antibiotic Selection[5]	-	-	93%	90%	100%
Prophylactic Antibiotic Stopped[2,3]	62	68%	86%	72%	95%
Pregnancy Care					
Inpatient Neonatal Mortality	-	-	-	-	-
Third or Fourth Degree Laceration	-	-	-	3.63%	3.27%

Brookings Hospital

300 22nd Avenue
Brookings, SD 57006
E-mail: dbjohn@itclel.com
Ownership: Government - Local
Emergency Services: Yes

Phone: 605-696-9000
Fax: 605-697-7380

Accredited: No
Licensed Beds: 140

Key Personnel:
CEO. . . . . Dave Johnson

Measure	Cases	This Hospital	State Average	U.S. Average	Top Hospital
Heart Attack Care					
ACE Inhibitor or ARB for LVSD[1]	3	100%	84%	82%	100%
Aspirin at Arrival[1]	22	100%	94%	92%	100%
Aspirin at Discharge[1]	15	100%	96%	90%	100%
Beta Blocker at Arrival[1]	24	96%	90%	87%	100%
Beta Blocker at Discharge[1]	17	94%	94%	90%	100%
Fibrinolytic Medication Timing[3]	0	-	42%	31%	100%
PCI Within 90 Minutes of Arrival	0	-	79%	54%	95%
Smoking Cessation Advice[3]	0	-	69%	88%	100%
Heart Failure Care					
ACE Inhibitor or ARB for LVSD[1]	10	70%	76%	82%	100%
Discharge Instructions[1,3]	5	80%	51%	61%	93%
Evaluation of LVS Function	33	70%	71%	83%	99%
Smoking Cessation Advice[1,3]	1	100%	69%	82%	100%
Pneumonia Care					
Appropriate Initial Antibiotic[1,3]	10	90%	77%	83%	94%
Blood Culture Timing[1,3]	15	100%	97%	90%	100%
Influenza Vaccine[5]	-	-	83%	70%	100%
Initial Antibiotic Timing	60	92%	86%	80%	93%
Oxygenation Assessment	82	100%	100%	99%	100%
Pneumococcal Vaccine	58	84%	73%	69%	94%
Smoking Cessation Advice[1,3]	3	100%	63%	80%	100%
Surgical Infection Prevention					
Prophylactic Antibiotic Given[1,3]	17	94%	85%	77%	95%
Prophylactic Antibiotic Selection[5]	-	-	93%	90%	100%
Prophylactic Antibiotic Stopped[1,3]	15	100%	86%	72%	95%
Pregnancy Care					
Inpatient Neonatal Mortality	-	-	-	-	-
Third or Fourth Degree Laceration	-	-	-	3.63%	3.27%

Custer Regional Hospital

1039 Montgomery Street
Custer, SD 57730
Ownership: Voluntary non-profit - Private
Emergency Services: Yes

Phone: 605-673-2229
Fax: 605-673-3586
Accredited: No
Licensed Beds: 16

Key Personnel:
President/CEO. . . . . Kay Foust
Chief Medical Staff. . . . . Sarah Schryvers
Emergency Room . . . . Sarah Schryvers
Director Infection/Disease Control . . . . Wendy Honomichl
Director Medical/Surgical Nursing . . . . Sarah Schryvers
OB/GYN Womens Health. . . . . Sarah Schryvers
Chief Radiology . . . . G Robert Hanson

Measure	Cases	This Hospital	State Average	U.S. Average	Top Hospital
Heart Attack Care					
ACE Inhibitor or ARB for LVSD[1,3]	1	100%	84%	82%	100%
Aspirin at Arrival[1,3]	2	100%	94%	92%	100%
Aspirin at Discharge[1,3]	2	100%	96%	90%	100%
Beta Blocker at Arrival[1,3]	2	100%	90%	87%	100%
Beta Blocker at Discharge[1,3]	2	100%	94%	90%	100%

NOTE: Hospital profiles are in alphabetical order by state, then city, then hospital within the city; Rankings are sorted by rate in descending order and exclude hospitals with less than 25 cases; (1) The number of cases is too small (n<25) for purposes of reliably predicting hospital performance; (2) Measure reflects the hospital's indication that its submission was based upon a sample of its relevant discharges; (3) Rate reflects fewer than the maximum possible quarters of data for the measure; (4) Inaccurate information submitted and suppressed for one or more quarters; (5) No data is available from the hospital for this measure; Please refer to the User's Guide for a full explanation of data

Measure	Cases	This Hospital	State Average	U.S. Average	Top Hospital
Fibrinolytic Medication Timing[3]	0	-	42%	31%	100%
PCI Within 90 Minutes of Arrival	0	-	79%	54%	95%
Smoking Cessation Advice[3]	0	-	69%	88%	100%
Heart Failure Care					
ACE Inhibitor or ARB for LVSD[1]	4	75%	76%	82%	100%
Discharge Instructions[1]	8	75%	51%	61%	93%
Evaluation of LVS Function[1]	10	90%	71%	83%	99%
Smoking Cessation Advice	0	-	69%	82%	100%
Pneumonia Care					
Appropriate Initial Antibiotic[1]	10	90%	77%	83%	94%
Blood Culture Timing[1]	2	100%	97%	90%	100%
Influenza Vaccine	0	-	83%	70%	100%
Initial Antibiotic Timing[1]	17	76%	86%	80%	93%
Oxygenation Assessment[1]	19	100%	100%	99%	100%
Pneumococcal Vaccine[1]	11	82%	73%	69%	94%
Smoking Cessation Advice	0	-	63%	80%	100%
Surgical Infection Prevention					
Prophylactic Antibiotic Given[5]	-	-	85%	77%	95%
Prophylactic Antibiotic Selection[5]	-	-	93%	90%	100%
Prophylactic Antibiotic Stopped[5]	-	-	86%	72%	95%
Pregnancy Care					
Inpatient Neonatal Mortality	-	-	-	-	-
Third or Fourth Degree Laceration	-	-	-	3.63%	3.27%

Siouxland Surgery Center Lp

600 Sioux Point Road
Dakota Dunes, SD 57049
Ownership: Proprietary
Emergency Services: No

Phone: 605-232-3332
Accredited: No

Measure	Cases	This Hospital	State Average	U.S. Average	Top Hospital
Heart Attack Care					
ACE Inhibitor or ARB for LVSD[5]	-	-	84%	82%	100%
Aspirin at Arrival[5]	-	-	94%	92%	100%
Aspirin at Discharge[5]	-	-	96%	90%	100%
Beta Blocker at Arrival[5]	-	-	90%	87%	100%
Beta Blocker at Discharge[5]	-	-	94%	90%	100%
Fibrinolytic Medication Timing[5]	-	-	42%	31%	100%
PCI Within 90 Minutes of Arrival[5]	-	-	79%	54%	95%
Smoking Cessation Advice[5]	-	-	69%	88%	100%
Heart Failure Care					
ACE Inhibitor or ARB for LVSD[5]	-	-	76%	82%	100%
Discharge Instructions[5]	-	-	51%	61%	93%
Evaluation of LVS Function[5]	-	-	71%	83%	99%
Smoking Cessation Advice[5]	-	-	69%	82%	100%
Pneumonia Care					
Appropriate Initial Antibiotic[5]	-	-	77%	83%	94%
Blood Culture Timing[5]	-	-	97%	90%	100%
Influenza Vaccine[5]	-	-	83%	70%	100%
Initial Antibiotic Timing[5]	-	-	86%	80%	93%
Oxygenation Assessment[5]	-	-	100%	99%	100%
Pneumococcal Vaccine[5]	-	-	73%	69%	94%
Smoking Cessation Advice[5]	-	-	63%	80%	100%
Surgical Infection Prevention					
Prophylactic Antibiotic Given[2]	366	96%	85%	77%	95%
Prophylactic Antibiotic Selection[2]	94	85%	93%	90%	100%
Prophylactic Antibiotic Stopped[2]	366	90%	86%	72%	95%
Pregnancy Care					
Inpatient Neonatal Mortality	-	-	-	-	-
Third or Fourth Degree Laceration	-	-	-	3.63%	3.27%

De Smet Memorial Hospital

306 Prairie Avenue SW
PO Box 160
De Smet, SD 57231
E-mail: info@desmetmemorial.org
URL: www.desmetmemorial.org
Ownership: Voluntary non-profit - Private
Emergency Services: Yes

Phone: 605-854-3329
Fax: 605-854-3161
Accredited: No
Licensed Beds: 17

Key Personnel:
Administrator . . . . John Single
Chief Medical Staff. . . . . J Berg

Measure	Cases	This Hospital	State Average	U.S. Average	Top Hospital
Heart Attack Care					
ACE Inhibitor or ARB for LVSD[1,3]	1	100%	84%	82%	100%
Aspirin at Arrival[1,3]	1	100%	94%	92%	100%
Aspirin at Discharge[1,3]	1	100%	96%	90%	100%
Beta Blocker at Arrival[1,3]	2	100%	90%	87%	100%
Beta Blocker at Discharge[1,3]	1	100%	94%	90%	100%
Fibrinolytic Medication Timing[3]	0	-	42%	31%	100%
PCI Within 90 Minutes of Arrival	0	-	79%	54%	95%
Smoking Cessation Advice[3]	0	-	69%	88%	100%
Heart Failure Care					
ACE Inhibitor or ARB for LVSD[1]	3	67%	76%	82%	100%
Discharge Instructions[1]	4	50%	51%	61%	93%
Evaluation of LVS Function[1]	9	56%	71%	83%	99%
Smoking Cessation Advice	0	-	69%	82%	100%
Pneumonia Care					
Appropriate Initial Antibiotic[1]	16	81%	77%	83%	94%
Blood Culture Timing[1]	4	100%	97%	90%	100%
Influenza Vaccine[1]	3	100%	83%	70%	100%
Initial Antibiotic Timing[1]	21	86%	86%	80%	93%
Oxygenation Assessment	30	100%	100%	99%	100%
Pneumococcal Vaccine	28	89%	73%	69%	94%
Smoking Cessation Advice[1]	1	100%	63%	80%	100%
Surgical Infection Prevention					
Prophylactic Antibiotic Given[5]	-	-	85%	77%	95%
Prophylactic Antibiotic Selection[5]	-	-	93%	90%	100%
Prophylactic Antibiotic Stopped[5]	-	-	86%	72%	95%
Pregnancy Care					
Inpatient Neonatal Mortality	-	-	-	-	-
Third or Fourth Degree Laceration	-	-	-	3.63%	3.27%

Lead-Deadwood Regional Hospital

61 Charles Street
Deadwood, SD 57732
Ownership: Government - Local
Emergency Services: Yes

Phone: 605-722-6101
Fax: 605-719-6163
Accredited: No
Licensed Beds: 17

Key Personnel:
CEO. . . . . Sherry Bea Smith, BSN,MPA,
Chief Medical Staff. . . . . James J Holloway, MD
Infection Control. . . . . Joanne Baer, RN
Surgical Services . . . . Karen Schleenaut, MD

Measure	Cases	This Hospital	State Average	U.S. Average	Top Hospital
Heart Attack Care					
ACE Inhibitor or ARB for LVSD	0	-	84%	82%	100%
Aspirin at Arrival	0	-	94%	92%	100%
Aspirin at Discharge[3]	0	-	96%	90%	100%
Beta Blocker at Arrival	0	-	90%	87%	100%
Beta Blocker at Discharge[1]	2	50%	94%	90%	100%
Fibrinolytic Medication Timing[1]	3	67%	42%	31%	100%
PCI Within 90 Minutes of Arrival[5]	-	-	79%	54%	95%
Smoking Cessation Advice[1]	2	0%	69%	88%	100%
Heart Failure Care					
ACE Inhibitor or ARB for LVSD[1]	4	75%	76%	82%	100%
Discharge Instructions[1]	12	83%	51%	61%	93%
Evaluation of LVS Function[1]	15	73%	71%	83%	99%
Smoking Cessation Advice[1]	4	100%	69%	82%	100%
Pneumonia Care					
Appropriate Initial Antibiotic[1]	17	82%	77%	83%	94%
Blood Culture Timing[1]	6	83%	97%	90%	100%
Influenza Vaccine[1]	6	83%	83%	70%	100%
Initial Antibiotic Timing[1]	20	80%	86%	80%	93%
Oxygenation Assessment[1]	23	100%	100%	99%	100%
Pneumococcal Vaccine[1]	22	86%	73%	69%	94%
Smoking Cessation Advice[1]	1	0%	63%	80%	100%
Surgical Infection Prevention					
Prophylactic Antibiotic Given[1,2]	9	67%	85%	77%	95%
Prophylactic Antibiotic Selection[5]	-	-	93%	90%	100%
Prophylactic Antibiotic Stopped[1,2]	9	100%	86%	72%	95%
Pregnancy Care					

NOTE: Hospital profiles are in alphabetical order by state, then city, then hospital within the city; Rankings are sorted by rate in descending order and exclude hospitals with less than 25 cases; (1) The number of cases is too small (n<25) for purposes of reliably predicting hospital performance; (2) Measure reflects the hospital's indication that its submission was based upon a sample of its relevant discharges; (3) Rate reflects fewer than the maximum possible quarters of data for the measure; (4) Inaccurate information submitted and suppressed for one or more quarters; (5) No data is available from the hospital for this measure; Please refer to the User's Guide for a full explanation of data

Inpatient Neonatal Mortality	-	-	-	-	-
Third or Fourth Degree Laceration	-	-	-	3.63%	3.27%

PHS Indian Hospital

PO Box 1012
Eagle Butte, SD 57625
Ownership: Government - Federal
Emergency Services: Yes
Phone: 605-964-7724
Fax: 605-964-1169
Accredited: Yes
Licensed Beds: 27

Key Personnel:
Administrator . . . . . Donald D Annis
Chief Medical Staff . . . . . Margaret Upell
Emergency Room . . . . . Margaret Upell, MD
Director Infection/Disease Control . . . . . Margaret Zephier, RN

Measure	Cases	This Hospital	State Average	U.S. Average	Top Hospital
Heart Attack Care					
ACE Inhibitor or ARB for LVSD[5]	-	-	84%	82%	100%
Aspirin at Arrival[5]	-	-	94%	92%	100%
Aspirin at Discharge[5]	-	-	96%	90%	100%
Beta Blocker at Arrival[5]	-	-	90%	87%	100%
Beta Blocker at Discharge[5]	-	-	94%	90%	100%
Fibrinolytic Medication Timing[5]	-	-	42%	31%	100%
PCI Within 90 Minutes of Arrival[5]	-	-	79%	54%	95%
Smoking Cessation Advice[5]	-	-	69%	88%	100%
Heart Failure Care					
ACE Inhibitor or ARB for LVSD[3]	0	-	76%	82%	100%
Discharge Instructions[1,3]	2	0%	51%	61%	93%
Evaluation of LVS Function[1,3]	2	0%	71%	83%	99%
Smoking Cessation Advice[1,3]	1	0%	69%	82%	100%
Pneumonia Care					
Appropriate Initial Antibiotic[1,3]	3	0%	77%	83%	94%
Blood Culture Timing[1,3]	1	100%	97%	90%	100%
Influenza Vaccine[5]	-	-	83%	70%	100%
Initial Antibiotic Timing[1,3]	5	80%	86%	80%	93%
Oxygenation Assessment[1,3]	6	100%	100%	99%	100%
Pneumococcal Vaccine[1,3]	4	0%	73%	69%	94%
Smoking Cessation Advice[1,3]	1	0%	63%	80%	100%
Surgical Infection Prevention					
Prophylactic Antibiotic Given[5]	-	-	85%	77%	95%
Prophylactic Antibiotic Selection[5]	-	-	93%	90%	100%
Prophylactic Antibiotic Stopped[5]	-	-	86%	72%	95%
Pregnancy Care					
Inpatient Neonatal Mortality	-	-	-	-	-
Third or Fourth Degree Laceration	-	-	-	3.63%	3.27%

Gregory Health Care Center

Alternate Name: Gregory Community Hospital
400 Park Avenue
Gregory, SD 57533
Ownership: Voluntary non-profit - Church
Emergency Services: Yes
Phone: 605-835-8394
Fax: 605-835-9422
Accredited: No
Licensed Beds: 90

Key Personnel:
CEO . . . . . Carol Varland
Chief Medical Staff . . . . . R Nemer, MD

Measure	Cases	This Hospital	State Average	U.S. Average	Top Hospital
Heart Attack Care					
ACE Inhibitor or ARB for LVSD[3]	0	-	84%	82%	100%
Aspirin at Arrival[3]	0	-	94%	92%	100%
Aspirin at Discharge[3]	0	-	96%	90%	100%
Beta Blocker at Arrival[3]	0	-	90%	87%	100%
Beta Blocker at Discharge[3]	0	-	94%	90%	100%
Fibrinolytic Medication Timing[1,3]	1	100%	42%	31%	100%
PCI Within 90 Minutes of Arrival	0	-	79%	54%	95%
Smoking Cessation Advice[3]	0	-	69%	88%	100%
Heart Failure Care					
ACE Inhibitor or ARB for LVSD[1,3]	1	100%	76%	82%	100%
Discharge Instructions[1,3]	5	0%	51%	61%	93%
Evaluation of LVS Function[1,3]	11	45%	71%	83%	99%
Smoking Cessation Advice[1,3]	1	0%	69%	82%	100%
Pneumonia Care					
Appropriate Initial Antibiotic[2,3]	30	63%	77%	83%	94%
Blood Culture Timing[1,2]	1	100%	97%	90%	100%
Influenza Vaccine[1,2]	15	73%	83%	70%	100%
Initial Antibiotic Timing[2,3]	50	94%	86%	80%	93%
Oxygenation Assessment[2,3]	65	100%	100%	99%	100%
Pneumococcal Vaccine[2,3]	53	72%	73%	69%	94%
Smoking Cessation Advice[1,2,3]	12	8%	63%	80%	100%
Surgical Infection Prevention					
Prophylactic Antibiotic Given[5]	-	-	85%	77%	95%
Prophylactic Antibiotic Selection[5]	-	-	93%	90%	100%
Prophylactic Antibiotic Stopped[5]	-	-	86%	72%	95%
Pregnancy Care					
Inpatient Neonatal Mortality	-	-	-	-	-
Third or Fourth Degree Laceration	-	-	-	3.63%	3.27%

Fall River Hospital

209 N 16th St
Hot Springs, SD 57747
Ownership: Government - Local
Emergency Services: No
Phone: 605-745-3459
Accredited: No

Measure	Cases	This Hospital	State Average	U.S. Average	Top Hospital
Heart Attack Care					
ACE Inhibitor or ARB for LVSD[5]	-	-	84%	82%	100%
Aspirin at Arrival[5]	-	-	94%	92%	100%
Aspirin at Discharge[5]	-	-	96%	90%	100%
Beta Blocker at Arrival[5]	-	-	90%	87%	100%
Beta Blocker at Discharge[5]	-	-	94%	90%	100%
Fibrinolytic Medication Timing[5]	-	-	42%	31%	100%
PCI Within 90 Minutes of Arrival[5]	-	-	79%	54%	95%
Smoking Cessation Advice[5]	-	-	69%	88%	100%
Heart Failure Care					
ACE Inhibitor or ARB for LVSD[5]	-	-	76%	82%	100%
Discharge Instructions[5]	-	-	51%	61%	93%
Evaluation of LVS Function[5]	-	-	71%	83%	99%
Smoking Cessation Advice[5]	-	-	69%	82%	100%
Pneumonia Care					
Appropriate Initial Antibiotic[3]	0	-	77%	83%	94%
Blood Culture Timing[3]	0	-	97%	90%	100%
Influenza Vaccine[5]	-	-	83%	70%	100%
Initial Antibiotic Timing[3]	0	-	86%	80%	93%
Oxygenation Assessment[1,3]	1	100%	100%	99%	100%
Pneumococcal Vaccine[1,3]	1	100%	73%	69%	94%
Smoking Cessation Advice[3]	0	-	63%	80%	100%
Surgical Infection Prevention					
Prophylactic Antibiotic Given[5]	-	-	85%	77%	95%
Prophylactic Antibiotic Selection[5]	-	-	93%	90%	100%
Prophylactic Antibiotic Stopped[5]	-	-	86%	72%	95%
Pregnancy Care					
Inpatient Neonatal Mortality	-	-	-	-	-
Third or Fourth Degree Laceration	-	-	-	3.63%	3.27%

Holy Infant Hospital

512 Main Street
Hoven, SD 57450
Ownership: Government - Local
Emergency Services: Yes
Phone: 605-948-2262
Fax: 605-948-2379
Accredited: No
Licensed Beds: 27

Key Personnel:
Administrator . . . . . Jeff Marlette
Chief Medical Staff . . . . . Dion Rameriz, MD
Director Infection/Disease Control . . . . . Christi Hoffman
Director Medical/Surgical Nursing . . . . . Alexzine Miles

Measure	Cases	This Hospital	State Average	U.S. Average	Top Hospital
Heart Attack Care					
ACE Inhibitor or ARB for LVSD[5]	-	-	84%	82%	100%
Aspirin at Arrival[5]	-	-	94%	92%	100%
Aspirin at Discharge[5]	-	-	96%	90%	100%
Beta Blocker at Arrival[5]	-	-	90%	87%	100%
Beta Blocker at Discharge[5]	-	-	94%	90%	100%
Fibrinolytic Medication Timing[5]	-	-	42%	31%	100%
PCI Within 90 Minutes of Arrival[5]	-	-	79%	54%	95%
Smoking Cessation Advice[5]	-	-	69%	88%	100%

NOTE: Hospital profiles are in alphabetical order by state, then city, then hospital within the city; Rankings are sorted by rate in descending order and exclude hospitals with less than 25 cases; (1) The number of cases is too small (n<25) for purposes of reliably predicting hospital performance; (2) Measure reflects the hospital's indication that its submission was based upon a sample of its relevant discharges; (3) Rate reflects fewer than the maximum possible quarters of data for the measure; (4) Inaccurate information submitted and suppressed for one or more quarters; (5) No data is available from the hospital for this measure; Please refer to the User's Guide for a full explanation of data

Measure	Cases	This Hospital	State Average	U.S. Average	Top Hospital
Heart Failure Care					
ACE Inhibitor or ARB for LVSD[5]	-	-	76%	82%	100%
Discharge Instructions[5]	-	-	51%	61%	93%
Evaluation of LVS Function[5]	-	-	71%	83%	99%
Smoking Cessation Advice[5]	-	-	69%	82%	100%
Pneumonia Care					
Appropriate Initial Antibiotic[1,3]	1	100%	77%	83%	94%
Blood Culture Timing[3]	0	-	97%	90%	100%
Influenza Vaccine[5]	-	-	83%	70%	100%
Initial Antibiotic Timing[1]	10	90%	86%	80%	93%
Oxygenation Assessment[1]	11	100%	100%	99%	100%
Pneumococcal Vaccine[1]	9	56%	73%	69%	94%
Smoking Cessation Advice[3]	0	-	63%	80%	100%
Surgical Infection Prevention					
Prophylactic Antibiotic Given[5]	-	-	85%	77%	95%
Prophylactic Antibiotic Selection[5]	-	-	93%	90%	100%
Prophylactic Antibiotic Stopped[5]	-	-	86%	72%	95%
Pregnancy Care					
Inpatient Neonatal Mortality	-	-	-	-	-
Third or Fourth Degree Laceration	-	-	-	3.63%	3.27%

Huron Regional Medical Center

172 4th Street SE
Huron, SD 57350
URL: www.huronregional.org
Ownership: Voluntary non-profit - Private
Emergency Services: Yes
Phone: 605-353-6200
Fax: 605-353-6300
Accredited: No
Licensed Beds: 91

Key Personnel:

President/CEO . . . . John Single
Chief Medical Staff . . . . Jeff Wheeler, MD
Emergency Room . . . . Jeff Wheeler, MD
Director Infection/Disease Control . . . . Janice Farrar, RN
Surgical Services . . . . Kris Brandt, RN
Chief Radiology . . . . Rich Janes
Director Respiratory Therapy . . . . Mike Strubel

Measure	Cases	This Hospital	State Average	U.S. Average	Top Hospital
Heart Attack Care					
ACE Inhibitor or ARB for LVSD[1]	6	17%	84%	82%	100%
Aspirin at Arrival[1]	10	100%	94%	92%	100%
Aspirin at Discharge[1]	8	88%	96%	90%	100%
Beta Blocker at Arrival[1]	10	80%	90%	87%	100%
Beta Blocker at Discharge[1]	9	89%	94%	90%	100%
Fibrinolytic Medication Timing[1]	4	50%	42%	31%	100%
PCI Within 90 Minutes of Arrival[5]	-	-	79%	54%	95%
Smoking Cessation Advice[1]	1	0%	69%	88%	100%
Heart Failure Care					
ACE Inhibitor or ARB for LVSD[1]	2	50%	76%	82%	100%
Discharge Instructions[1]	9	56%	51%	61%	93%
Evaluation of LVS Function[1]	12	50%	71%	83%	99%
Smoking Cessation Advice	0	-	69%	82%	100%
Pneumonia Care					
Appropriate Initial Antibiotic	71	85%	77%	83%	94%
Blood Culture Timing[1]	7	100%	97%	90%	100%
Influenza Vaccine[1]	23	91%	83%	70%	100%
Initial Antibiotic Timing	80	72%	86%	80%	93%
Oxygenation Assessment	103	100%	100%	99%	100%
Pneumococcal Vaccine	80	66%	73%	69%	94%
Smoking Cessation Advice[1]	14	50%	63%	80%	100%
Surgical Infection Prevention					
Prophylactic Antibiotic Given[2]	36	94%	85%	77%	95%
Prophylactic Antibiotic Selection[1,2]	15	100%	93%	90%	100%
Prophylactic Antibiotic Stopped[2]	34	21%	86%	72%	95%
Pregnancy Care					
Inpatient Neonatal Mortality	-	-	-	-	-
Third or Fourth Degree Laceration	-	-	-	3.63%	3.27%

Madison Community Hospital

917 N Washington Avenue
Madison, SD 57042
Ownership: Voluntary non-profit - Private
Emergency Services: Yes
Phone: 605-256-6551
Fax: 605-256-6469
Accredited: No
Licensed Beds: 49

Key Personnel:

Administrator . . . . Tamara Miller
Chief Medical Staff . . . . RG Sample, MD
Emergency Room . . . . Donna Quade
Director Infection/Disease Control . . . . Kathy Hansen
Chief Radiology . . . . Jerri McNary
Director Respiratory Therapy . . . . Mary Hart

Measure	Cases	This Hospital	State Average	U.S. Average	Top Hospital
Heart Attack Care					
ACE Inhibitor or ARB for LVSD[3]	0	-	84%	82%	100%
Aspirin at Arrival[3]	0	-	94%	92%	100%
Aspirin at Discharge[3]	0	-	96%	90%	100%
Beta Blocker at Arrival[3]	0	-	90%	87%	100%
Beta Blocker at Discharge[3]	0	-	94%	90%	100%
Fibrinolytic Medication Timing[3]	0	-	42%	31%	100%
PCI Within 90 Minutes of Arrival[5]	-	-	79%	54%	95%
Smoking Cessation Advice[3]	0	-	69%	88%	100%
Heart Failure Care					
ACE Inhibitor or ARB for LVSD[3]	0	-	76%	82%	100%
Discharge Instructions[1,3]	1	0%	51%	61%	93%
Evaluation of LVS Function[1,3]	5	80%	71%	83%	99%
Smoking Cessation Advice[1,3]	1	100%	69%	82%	100%
Pneumonia Care					
Appropriate Initial Antibiotic[1]	10	90%	77%	83%	94%
Blood Culture Timing[1]	6	100%	97%	90%	100%
Influenza Vaccine[4,5]	-	-	83%	70%	100%
Initial Antibiotic Timing[1]	16	94%	86%	80%	93%
Oxygenation Assessment[1]	18	100%	100%	99%	100%
Pneumococcal Vaccine[1]	15	47%	73%	69%	94%
Smoking Cessation Advice[1]	1	100%	63%	80%	100%
Surgical Infection Prevention					
Prophylactic Antibiotic Given[1,3]	6	67%	85%	77%	95%
Prophylactic Antibiotic Selection[1]	3	33%	93%	90%	100%
Prophylactic Antibiotic Stopped[1,3]	6	33%	86%	72%	95%
Pregnancy Care					
Inpatient Neonatal Mortality	-	-	-	-	-
Third or Fourth Degree Laceration	-	-	-	3.63%	3.27%

Queen of Peace Hospital

525 North Foster
Mitchell, SD 57301
Ownership: Voluntary non-profit - Church
Emergency Services: Yes
Phone: 605-995-2000
Fax: 605-995-2441
Accredited: Yes
Licensed Beds: 120

Key Personnel:

CEO . . . . Tom Rasmusson
Chief Medical Staff . . . . Paul Messmussen, MD
Chief Medical Staff . . . . Jerome Howe
Emergency Room . . . . Kathy Herttinger, RN
Director Respiratory Therapy . . . . Mike Kowall

Measure	Cases	This Hospital	State Average	U.S. Average	Top Hospital
Heart Attack Care					
ACE Inhibitor or ARB for LVSD[1]	2	100%	84%	82%	100%
Aspirin at Arrival[1]	19	89%	94%	92%	100%
Aspirin at Discharge[1]	10	100%	96%	90%	100%
Beta Blocker at Arrival[1]	11	82%	90%	87%	100%
Beta Blocker at Discharge[1]	11	91%	94%	90%	100%
Fibrinolytic Medication Timing	0	-	42%	31%	100%
PCI Within 90 Minutes of Arrival	0	-	79%	54%	95%
Smoking Cessation Advice	0	-	69%	88%	100%
Heart Failure Care					
ACE Inhibitor or ARB for LVSD[1]	24	92%	76%	82%	100%
Discharge Instructions	51	94%	51%	61%	93%
Evaluation of LVS Function	96	92%	71%	83%	99%
Smoking Cessation Advice[1]	7	100%	69%	82%	100%
Pneumonia Care					
Appropriate Initial Antibiotic	103	91%	77%	83%	94%

NOTE: Hospital profiles are in alphabetical order by state, then city, then hospital within the city; Rankings are sorted by rate in descending order and exclude hospitals with less than 25 cases; (1) The number of cases is too small (n<25) for purposes of reliably predicting hospital performance; (2) Measure reflects the hospital's indication that its submission was based upon a sample of its relevant discharges; (3) Rate reflects fewer than the maximum possible quarters of data for the measure; (4) Inaccurate information submitted and suppressed for one or more quarters; (5) No data is available from the hospital for this measure; Please refer to the User's Guide for a full explanation of data

Blood Culture Timing	68	97%	97%	90%	100%
Influenza Vaccine	37	81%	83%	70%	100%
Initial Antibiotic Timing	149	93%	86%	80%	93%
Oxygenation Assessment	185	100%	100%	99%	100%
Pneumococcal Vaccine	130	91%	73%	69%	94%
Smoking Cessation Advice	39	97%	63%	80%	100%
Surgical Infection Prevention					
Prophylactic Antibiotic Given	177	96%	85%	77%	95%
Prophylactic Antibiotic Selection	45	98%	93%	90%	100%
Prophylactic Antibiotic Stopped	171	89%	86%	72%	95%
Pregnancy Care					
Inpatient Neonatal Mortality	-	-	-	-	-
Third or Fourth Degree Laceration	-	-	-	3.63%	3.27%

Mobridge Regional Hospital

Alternate Name: Mobridge Community Hospital
1401 10th Avenue W
Mobridge, SD 57601
Ownership: Voluntary non-profit - Other
Emergency Services: Yes
Phone: 605-845-3693
Fax: 605-845-8252
Accredited: No
Licensed Beds: 48

Key Personnel:

CEO. . . . . Angelia Henry

Measure	Cases	This Hospital	State Average	U.S. Average	Top Hospital
Heart Attack Care					
ACE Inhibitor or ARB for LVSD	0	-	84%	82%	100%
Aspirin at Arrival[1]	4	50%	94%	92%	100%
Aspirin at Discharge[1]	3	67%	96%	90%	100%
Beta Blocker at Arrival[1]	4	100%	90%	87%	100%
Beta Blocker at Discharge[1]	3	100%	94%	90%	100%
Fibrinolytic Medication Timing[1]	9	56%	42%	31%	100%
PCI Within 90 Minutes of Arrival	0	-	79%	54%	95%
Smoking Cessation Advice	0	-	69%	88%	100%
Heart Failure Care					
ACE Inhibitor or ARB for LVSD[1]	4	75%	76%	82%	100%
Discharge Instructions[1]	7	43%	51%	61%	93%
Evaluation of LVS Function[1]	12	67%	71%	83%	99%
Smoking Cessation Advice[1]	2	100%	69%	82%	100%
Pneumonia Care					
Appropriate Initial Antibiotic[1]	21	86%	77%	83%	94%
Blood Culture Timing[1]	3	100%	97%	90%	100%
Influenza Vaccine[1]	5	80%	83%	70%	100%
Initial Antibiotic Timing	25	100%	86%	80%	93%
Oxygenation Assessment	28	100%	100%	99%	100%
Pneumococcal Vaccine[1]	23	74%	73%	69%	94%
Smoking Cessation Advice[1]	5	20%	63%	80%	100%
Surgical Infection Prevention					
Prophylactic Antibiotic Given[5]	-	-	85%	77%	95%
Prophylactic Antibiotic Selection[5]	-	-	93%	90%	100%
Prophylactic Antibiotic Stopped[5]	-	-	86%	72%	95%
Pregnancy Care					
Inpatient Neonatal Mortality	-	-	-	-	-
Third or Fourth Degree Laceration	-	-	-	3.63%	3.27%

Avera Saint Benedict Health Center

Alternate Name: Saint Benedict Hospital
400 West Glynn Drive
Parkston, SD 57366
URL: www.averastbenedict.org
Ownership: Voluntary non-profit - Church
Emergency Services: Yes
Phone: 605-928-3311
Fax: 605-928-7368
Accredited: No
Licensed Beds: 25

Key Personnel:

Administrator . . . . Gale N Walker
Chief Medical Staff. . . . . Toni Vanderpol
Emergency Room . . . . Phillip D Barker, DO
Infection Control. . . . . Brenda Stoebner
ICU . . . . Denise Muntefering
Director Medical/Surgical Nursing . . . . Denise Muntefering, RN
Respiratory/Cardiopulmonary. . . . . Robin Radke

Measure	Cases	This Hospital	State Average	U.S. Average	Top Hospital
Heart Attack Care					
ACE Inhibitor or ARB for LVSD[1,3]	1	100%	84%	82%	100%
Aspirin at Arrival[1,3]	4	100%	94%	92%	100%
Aspirin at Discharge[1,3]	3	100%	96%	90%	100%
Beta Blocker at Arrival[1,3]	2	50%	90%	87%	100%
Beta Blocker at Discharge[1,3]	3	100%	94%	90%	100%
Fibrinolytic Medication Timing[3]	0	-	42%	31%	100%
PCI Within 90 Minutes of Arrival	0	-	79%	54%	95%
Smoking Cessation Advice[3]	0	-	69%	88%	100%
Heart Failure Care					
ACE Inhibitor or ARB for LVSD[1]	1	0%	76%	82%	100%
Discharge Instructions[1]	3	67%	51%	61%	93%
Evaluation of LVS Function[1]	10	90%	71%	83%	99%
Smoking Cessation Advice	0	-	69%	82%	100%
Pneumonia Care					
Appropriate Initial Antibiotic[1]	14	79%	77%	83%	94%
Blood Culture Timing[1]	3	100%	97%	90%	100%
Influenza Vaccine[1]	6	100%	83%	70%	100%
Initial Antibiotic Timing[1]	22	95%	86%	80%	93%
Oxygenation Assessment	26	100%	100%	99%	100%
Pneumococcal Vaccine[1]	22	100%	73%	69%	94%
Smoking Cessation Advice[1]	3	100%	63%	80%	100%
Surgical Infection Prevention					
Prophylactic Antibiotic Given[5]	-	-	85%	77%	95%
Prophylactic Antibiotic Selection[5]	-	-	93%	90%	100%
Prophylactic Antibiotic Stopped[5]	-	-	86%	72%	95%
Pregnancy Care					
Inpatient Neonatal Mortality	-	-	-	-	-
Third or Fourth Degree Laceration	-	-	-	3.63%	3.27%

Saint Mary's Healthcare Center

Alternate Name: Saint Marys Hospital
800 E Dakota Avenue
Pierre, SD 57501
Ownership: Voluntary non-profit - Church
Emergency Services: Yes
Phone: 605-224-3100
Fax: 605-224-3429
Accredited: Yes
Licensed Beds: 86

Key Personnel:

Administrator . . . . James Russell
Director Infection/Disease Control . . . . Jeanne Vogel
CCU Spvg. Nurse . . . . Teri Ellenbecker
Director Medical/Surgical Nursing . . . . Teri Ellenbecker
Director Radiology . . . . Ben Shoup
Director Respiratory Therapy . . . . Linda Hackett

Measure	Cases	This Hospital	State Average	U.S. Average	Top Hospital
Heart Attack Care					
ACE Inhibitor or ARB for LVSD[1]	1	100%	84%	82%	100%
Aspirin at Arrival[1]	7	86%	94%	92%	100%
Aspirin at Discharge[1]	4	75%	96%	90%	100%
Beta Blocker at Arrival[1]	6	83%	90%	87%	100%
Beta Blocker at Discharge[1]	4	75%	94%	90%	100%
Fibrinolytic Medication Timing[1]	11	36%	42%	31%	100%
PCI Within 90 Minutes of Arrival	0	-	79%	54%	95%
Smoking Cessation Advice[1]	1	100%	69%	88%	100%
Heart Failure Care					
ACE Inhibitor or ARB for LVSD[1]	13	54%	76%	82%	100%
Discharge Instructions	31	52%	51%	61%	93%
Evaluation of LVS Function	50	64%	71%	83%	99%
Smoking Cessation Advice[1]	8	88%	69%	82%	100%
Pneumonia Care					
Appropriate Initial Antibiotic	54	83%	77%	83%	94%
Blood Culture Timing	31	94%	97%	90%	100%
Influenza Vaccine[1]	19	89%	83%	70%	100%
Initial Antibiotic Timing	85	84%	86%	80%	93%
Oxygenation Assessment	99	100%	100%	99%	100%
Pneumococcal Vaccine	72	97%	73%	69%	94%
Smoking Cessation Advice[1]	17	88%	63%	80%	100%
Surgical Infection Prevention					
Prophylactic Antibiotic Given[3]	107	94%	85%	77%	95%
Prophylactic Antibiotic Selection	40	92%	93%	90%	100%
Prophylactic Antibiotic Stopped[3]	101	90%	86%	72%	95%
Pregnancy Care					
Inpatient Neonatal Mortality	477	0.00%	-	-	-

NOTE: Hospital profiles are in alphabetical order by state, then city, then hospital within the city; Rankings are sorted by rate in descending order and exclude hospitals with less than 25 cases; (1) The number of cases is too small (n<25) for purposes of reliably predicting hospital performance; (2) Measure reflects the hospital's indication that its submission was based upon a sample of its relevant discharges; (3) Rate reflects fewer than the maximum possible quarters of data for the measure; (4) Inaccurate information submitted and suppressed for one or more quarters; (5) No data is available from the hospital for this measure; Please refer to the User's Guide for a full explanation of data

Third or Fourth Degree Laceration	314	5.10%	-	3.63%	3.27%

PHS Indian Health Service Hospital

E Highway 18
Pine Ridge, SD 57770
Ownership: Government - Federal
Emergency Services: Yes
Phone: 605-867-5131
Fax: 605-867-3271
Accredited: Yes
Licensed Beds: 45

Key Personnel:
Administrator . . . . Vern Donnell
Chief Medical Staff . . . . Andy Hurst, MD
Infection Control . . . . Alice Sierra

Measure	Cases	This Hospital	State Average	U.S. Average	Top Hospital
Heart Attack Care					
ACE Inhibitor or ARB for LVSD[3]	0	-	84%	82%	100%
Aspirin at Arrival[3]	0	-	94%	92%	100%
Aspirin at Discharge[3]	0	-	96%	90%	100%
Beta Blocker at Arrival[3]	0	-	90%	87%	100%
Beta Blocker at Discharge[3]	0	-	94%	90%	100%
Fibrinolytic Medication Timing[5]	-	-	42%	31%	100%
PCI Within 90 Minutes of Arrival[5]	-	-	79%	54%	95%
Smoking Cessation Advice[5]	-	-	69%	88%	100%
Heart Failure Care					
ACE Inhibitor or ARB for LVSD[3]	0	-	76%	82%	100%
Discharge Instructions[1,3]	3	0%	51%	61%	93%
Evaluation of LVS Function[1,3]	16	0%	71%	83%	99%
Smoking Cessation Advice[1,3]	1	0%	69%	82%	100%
Pneumonia Care					
Appropriate Initial Antibiotic[1,3]	3	33%	77%	83%	94%
Blood Culture Timing[1,3]	1	100%	97%	90%	100%
Influenza Vaccine[5]	-	-	83%	70%	100%
Initial Antibiotic Timing[3]	27	44%	86%	80%	93%
Oxygenation Assessment[3]	29	97%	100%	99%	100%
Pneumococcal Vaccine[1,3]	14	50%	73%	69%	94%
Smoking Cessation Advice[1,3]	3	0%	63%	80%	100%
Surgical Infection Prevention					
Prophylactic Antibiotic Given[5]	-	-	85%	77%	95%
Prophylactic Antibiotic Selection[5]	-	-	93%	90%	100%
Prophylactic Antibiotic Stopped[5]	-	-	86%	72%	95%
Pregnancy Care					
Inpatient Neonatal Mortality	-	-	-	-	-
Third or Fourth Degree Laceration	-	-	-	3.63%	3.27%

Platte Health Center

Alternate Name: Avera Health-Platte Health Center
601 E 7th Street
PO Box 200
Platte, SD 57369
URL: www.phcavera.org
Ownership: Voluntary non-profit - Other
Emergency Services: No
Phone: 605-337-3364
Fax: 605-337-2670
Accredited: No
Licensed Beds: 15

Key Personnel:
CEO/President . . . . Mark Burkett
Chief Medical Staff . . . . John Bentv
Emergency Room . . . . Jerome Bentz, MD
Director Infection/Disease Control . . . . Jan Stahnke
Director Medical Surgical Nursing . . . . Jan Stahnke

Measure	Cases	This Hospital	State Average	U.S. Average	Top Hospital
Heart Attack Care					
ACE Inhibitor or ARB for LVSD[1,3]	1	100%	84%	82%	100%
Aspirin at Arrival[1,3]	2	100%	94%	92%	100%
Aspirin at Discharge[1,3]	2	100%	96%	90%	100%
Beta Blocker at Arrival[1,3]	2	100%	90%	87%	100%
Beta Blocker at Discharge[1,3]	2	100%	94%	90%	100%
Fibrinolytic Medication Timing[3]	0	-	42%	31%	100%
PCI Within 90 Minutes of Arrival	0	-	79%	54%	95%
Smoking Cessation Advice[3]	0	-	69%	88%	100%
Heart Failure Care					
ACE Inhibitor or ARB for LVSD[1]	4	100%	76%	82%	100%
Discharge Instructions[1]	2	100%	51%	61%	93%
Evaluation of LVS Function[1]	10	100%	71%	83%	99%
Smoking Cessation Advice[1]	2	100%	69%	82%	100%
Pneumonia Care					
Appropriate Initial Antibiotic[1]	9	78%	77%	83%	94%
Blood Culture Timing[1]	4	100%	97%	90%	100%
Influenza Vaccine[1]	7	86%	83%	70%	100%
Initial Antibiotic Timing	30	90%	86%	80%	93%
Oxygenation Assessment	31	100%	100%	99%	100%
Pneumococcal Vaccine	28	93%	73%	69%	94%
Smoking Cessation Advice[1]	2	50%	63%	80%	100%
Surgical Infection Prevention					
Prophylactic Antibiotic Given[5]	-	-	85%	77%	95%
Prophylactic Antibiotic Selection[5]	-	-	93%	90%	100%
Prophylactic Antibiotic Stopped[5]	-	-	86%	72%	95%
Pregnancy Care					
Inpatient Neonatal Mortality	-	-	-	-	-
Third or Fourth Degree Laceration	-	-	-	3.63%	3.27%

Black Hills Surgery Center

1868 Lombardy Drive
Rapid City, SD 57701
Ownership: Proprietary
Emergency Services: No
Phone: 605-721-4900
Accredited: No

Measure	Cases	This Hospital	State Average	U.S. Average	Top Hospital
Heart Attack Care					
ACE Inhibitor or ARB for LVSD[5]	-	-	84%	82%	100%
Aspirin at Arrival[5]	-	-	94%	92%	100%
Aspirin at Discharge[5]	-	-	96%	90%	100%
Beta Blocker at Arrival[5]	-	-	90%	87%	100%
Beta Blocker at Discharge[5]	-	-	94%	90%	100%
Fibrinolytic Medication Timing[5]	-	-	42%	31%	100%
PCI Within 90 Minutes of Arrival[5]	-	-	79%	54%	95%
Smoking Cessation Advice[5]	-	-	69%	88%	100%
Heart Failure Care					
ACE Inhibitor or ARB for LVSD[5]	-	-	76%	82%	100%
Discharge Instructions[5]	-	-	51%	61%	93%
Evaluation of LVS Function[5]	-	-	71%	83%	99%
Smoking Cessation Advice[5]	-	-	69%	82%	100%
Pneumonia Care					
Appropriate Initial Antibiotic[5]	-	-	77%	83%	94%
Blood Culture Timing[5]	-	-	97%	90%	100%
Influenza Vaccine[5]	-	-	83%	70%	100%
Initial Antibiotic Timing[5]	-	-	86%	80%	93%
Oxygenation Assessment[5]	-	-	100%	99%	100%
Pneumococcal Vaccine[5]	-	-	73%	69%	94%
Smoking Cessation Advice[5]	-	-	63%	80%	100%
Surgical Infection Prevention					
Prophylactic Antibiotic Given[2,3]	134	99%	85%	77%	95%
Prophylactic Antibiotic Selection[2]	50	100%	93%	90%	100%
Prophylactic Antibiotic Stopped[2,3]	132	95%	86%	72%	95%
Pregnancy Care					
Inpatient Neonatal Mortality	-	-	-	-	-
Third or Fourth Degree Laceration	-	-	-	3.63%	3.27%

PHS Indian Hospital

3200 Canyon Lake Drive
Rapid City, SD 57702
Ownership: Government - Federal
Emergency Services: Yes
Phone: 605-348-1900
Fax: 605-355-2504
Accredited: Yes
Licensed Beds: 32

Measure	Cases	This Hospital	State Average	U.S. Average	Top Hospital
Heart Attack Care					
ACE Inhibitor or ARB for LVSD[5]	-	-	84%	82%	100%
Aspirin at Arrival[5]	-	-	94%	92%	100%
Aspirin at Discharge[5]	-	-	96%	90%	100%
Beta Blocker at Arrival[5]	-	-	90%	87%	100%
Beta Blocker at Discharge[5]	-	-	94%	90%	100%
Fibrinolytic Medication Timing[5]	-	-	42%	31%	100%
PCI Within 90 Minutes of Arrival[5]	-	-	79%	54%	95%
Smoking Cessation Advice[5]	-	-	69%	88%	100%
Heart Failure Care					
ACE Inhibitor or ARB for LVSD[3]	0	-	76%	82%	100%

NOTE: Hospital profiles are in alphabetical order by state, then city, then hospital within the city; Rankings are sorted by rate in descending order and exclude hospitals with less than 25 cases; (1) The number of cases is too small (n<25) for purposes of reliably predicting hospital performance; (2) Measure reflects the hospital's indication that its submission was based upon a sample of its relevant discharges; (3) Rate reflects fewer than the maximum possible quarters of data for the measure; (4) Inaccurate information submitted and suppressed for one or more quarters; (5) No data is available from the hospital for this measure; Please refer to the User's Guide for a full explanation of data

Measure	Cases	This Hospital	State Average	U.S. Average	Top Hospital
Discharge Instructions[1,3]	1	0%	51%	61%	93%
Evaluation of LVS Function[1,3]	3	33%	71%	83%	99%
Smoking Cessation Advice[3]	0	-	69%	82%	100%
Pneumonia Care					
Appropriate Initial Antibiotic[1,3]	4	0%	77%	83%	94%
Blood Culture Timing[3]	0	-	97%	90%	100%
Influenza Vaccine[5]	-	-	83%	70%	100%
Initial Antibiotic Timing[1]	7	86%	86%	80%	93%
Oxygenation Assessment[1]	10	100%	100%	99%	100%
Pneumococcal Vaccine[1]	7	71%	73%	69%	94%
Smoking Cessation Advice[1,3]	2	0%	63%	80%	100%
Surgical Infection Prevention					
Prophylactic Antibiotic Given[5]	-	-	85%	77%	95%
Prophylactic Antibiotic Selection[5]	-	-	93%	90%	100%
Prophylactic Antibiotic Stopped[5]	-	-	86%	72%	95%
Pregnancy Care					
Inpatient Neonatal Mortality	-	-	-	-	-
Third or Fourth Degree Laceration	-	-	-	3.63%	3.27%

Rapid City Regional Hospital

353 Fairmont Boulevard
Rapid City, SD 57701
E-mail: humanresources@rcrh.org
URL: www.rcrh.org
Phone: 605-719-1000
Fax: 605-719-8053
Ownership: Voluntary non-profit - Private
Emergency Services: Yes
Accredited: Yes
Licensed Beds: 310

Key Personnel:
CEO . . . . Timothy Sughrue
Chief Medical Staff . . . . Charles Hart
CCU Spvg. Nurse . . . . Sherry Smith
Director Medical/Surgical Nursing . . . . Julaine Selzler
Director Respiratory Therapy . . . . Dan Cameron

Measure	Cases	This Hospital	State Average	U.S. Average	Top Hospital
Heart Attack Care					
ACE Inhibitor or ARB for LVSD	59	93%	84%	82%	100%
Aspirin at Arrival	125	99%	94%	92%	100%
Aspirin at Discharge	242	100%	96%	90%	100%
Beta Blocker at Arrival	109	95%	90%	87%	100%
Beta Blocker at Discharge	317	97%	94%	90%	100%
Fibrinolytic Medication Timing[1]	2	0%	42%	31%	100%
PCI Within 90 Minutes of Arrival[1]	11	91%	79%	54%	95%
Smoking Cessation Advice	130	99%	69%	88%	100%
Heart Failure Care					
ACE Inhibitor or ARB for LVSD	102	84%	76%	82%	100%
Discharge Instructions	224	88%	51%	61%	93%
Evaluation of LVS Function	290	93%	71%	83%	99%
Smoking Cessation Advice	46	98%	69%	82%	100%
Pneumonia Care					
Appropriate Initial Antibiotic	189	86%	77%	83%	94%
Blood Culture Timing	133	83%	97%	90%	100%
Influenza Vaccine	48	71%	83%	70%	100%
Initial Antibiotic Timing	234	85%	86%	80%	93%
Oxygenation Assessment	300	98%	100%	99%	100%
Pneumococcal Vaccine	206	86%	73%	69%	94%
Smoking Cessation Advice	86	97%	63%	80%	100%
Surgical Infection Prevention					
Prophylactic Antibiotic Given[2]	668	91%	85%	77%	95%
Prophylactic Antibiotic Selection[2]	69	91%	93%	90%	100%
Prophylactic Antibiotic Stopped[2]	621	86%	86%	72%	95%
Pregnancy Care					
Inpatient Neonatal Mortality	-	-	-	-	-
Third or Fourth Degree Laceration	-	-	-	3.63%	3.27%

Same Day Surgery Center

651 Cathedral Drive
Rapid City, SD 57701
Phone: 605-719-5000
Ownership: Proprietary
Emergency Services: No
Accredited: No

Measure	Cases	This Hospital	State Average	U.S. Average	Top Hospital
Heart Attack Care					
ACE Inhibitor or ARB for LVSD[5]	-	-	84%	82%	100%
Aspirin at Arrival[5]	-	-	94%	92%	100%
Aspirin at Discharge[5]	-	-	96%	90%	100%
Beta Blocker at Arrival[5]	-	-	90%	87%	100%
Beta Blocker at Discharge[5]	-	-	94%	90%	100%
Fibrinolytic Medication Timing[5]	-	-	42%	31%	100%
PCI Within 90 Minutes of Arrival[5]	-	-	79%	54%	95%
Smoking Cessation Advice[5]	-	-	69%	88%	100%
Heart Failure Care					
ACE Inhibitor or ARB for LVSD[5]	-	-	76%	82%	100%
Discharge Instructions[5]	-	-	51%	61%	93%
Evaluation of LVS Function[5]	-	-	71%	83%	99%
Smoking Cessation Advice[5]	-	-	69%	82%	100%
Pneumonia Care					
Appropriate Initial Antibiotic[5]	-	-	77%	83%	94%
Blood Culture Timing[5]	-	-	97%	90%	100%
Influenza Vaccine[5]	-	-	83%	70%	100%
Initial Antibiotic Timing[5]	-	-	86%	80%	93%
Oxygenation Assessment[5]	-	-	100%	99%	100%
Pneumococcal Vaccine[5]	-	-	73%	69%	94%
Smoking Cessation Advice[5]	-	-	63%	80%	100%
Surgical Infection Prevention					
Prophylactic Antibiotic Given[1,2,3]	6	83%	85%	77%	95%
Prophylactic Antibiotic Selection[5]	-	-	93%	90%	100%
Prophylactic Antibiotic Stopped[1,2,3]	6	67%	86%	72%	95%
Pregnancy Care					
Inpatient Neonatal Mortality	-	-	-	-	-
Third or Fourth Degree Laceration	-	-	-	3.63%	3.27%

Community Memorial Hospital

111 W Tenth Avenue
Redfield, SD 57469
Phone: 605-472-1110
Fax: 605-472-2661
Ownership: Government - Local
Emergency Services: Yes
Accredited: No
Licensed Beds: 32

Key Personnel:
CEO . . . . Dan Odvgaard
Emergency Room . . . . Julene Cass

Measure	Cases	This Hospital	State Average	U.S. Average	Top Hospital
Heart Attack Care					
ACE Inhibitor or ARB for LVSD[1,3]	1	0%	84%	82%	100%
Aspirin at Arrival[1,3]	2	100%	94%	92%	100%
Aspirin at Discharge[1,3]	1	100%	96%	90%	100%
Beta Blocker at Arrival[1,3]	2	100%	90%	87%	100%
Beta Blocker at Discharge[1,3]	2	100%	94%	90%	100%
Fibrinolytic Medication Timing[3]	0	-	42%	31%	100%
PCI Within 90 Minutes of Arrival[5]	-	-	79%	54%	95%
Smoking Cessation Advice[3]	0	-	69%	88%	100%
Heart Failure Care					
ACE Inhibitor or ARB for LVSD[1]	1	0%	76%	82%	100%
Discharge Instructions[1]	1	0%	51%	61%	93%
Evaluation of LVS Function[1]	5	80%	71%	83%	99%
Smoking Cessation Advice	0	-	69%	82%	100%
Pneumonia Care					
Appropriate Initial Antibiotic[1]	15	60%	77%	83%	94%
Blood Culture Timing[1]	8	100%	97%	90%	100%
Influenza Vaccine[1]	8	100%	83%	70%	100%
Initial Antibiotic Timing	27	96%	86%	80%	93%
Oxygenation Assessment	38	100%	100%	99%	100%
Pneumococcal Vaccine	30	100%	73%	69%	94%
Smoking Cessation Advice[1]	1	0%	63%	80%	100%
Surgical Infection Prevention					
Prophylactic Antibiotic Given[5]	-	-	85%	77%	95%
Prophylactic Antibiotic Selection[5]	-	-	93%	90%	100%
Prophylactic Antibiotic Stopped[5]	-	-	86%	72%	95%
Pregnancy Care					
Inpatient Neonatal Mortality	-	-	-	-	-
Third or Fourth Degree Laceration	-	-	-	3.63%	3.27%

NOTE: Hospital profiles are in alphabetical order by state, then city, then hospital within the city; Rankings are sorted by rate in descending order and exclude hospitals with less than 25 cases; (1) The number of cases is too small (n<25) for purposes of reliably predicting hospital performance; (2) Measure reflects the hospital's indication that its submission was based upon a sample of its relevant discharges; (3) Rate reflects fewer than the maximum possible quarters of data for the measure; (4) Inaccurate information submitted and suppressed for one or more quarters; (5) No data is available from the hospital for this measure; Please refer to the User's Guide for a full explanation of data

PHS Indian Hospital

Soldier Creek Road
Rosebud, SD 57570

Toll-Free: 888-299-5451
Phone: 605-747-2231
Fax: 605-747-2216

Ownership: Government - Federal
Emergency Services: Yes

Accredited: No
Licensed Beds: 35

Key Personnel:
CEO. . . . . Dr. Timothy Ryscon
Chief Medical Staff. . . . . Dr. Timothy Ryscon
Emergency Room . . . . Phyllis Provancial
Emergency Room . . . . Pam Pourier
Director of Pulmonary/Respiratory Care. . . . . . Christine Shangreaux

Measure	Cases	This Hospital	State Average	U.S. Average	Top Hospital
Heart Attack Care					
ACE Inhibitor or ARB for LVSD[5]	-	-	84%	82%	100%
Aspirin at Arrival[5]	-	-	94%	92%	100%
Aspirin at Discharge[5]	-	-	96%	90%	100%
Beta Blocker at Arrival[5]	-	-	90%	87%	100%
Beta Blocker at Discharge[5]	-	-	94%	90%	100%
Fibrinolytic Medication Timing[5]	-	-	42%	31%	100%
PCI Within 90 Minutes of Arrival[5]	-	-	79%	54%	95%
Smoking Cessation Advice[5]	-	-	69%	88%	100%
Heart Failure Care					
ACE Inhibitor or ARB for LVSD[1,3]	2	100%	76%	82%	100%
Discharge Instructions[1,3]	4	0%	51%	61%	93%
Evaluation of LVS Function[1,3]	7	86%	71%	83%	99%
Smoking Cessation Advice[1,3]	1	0%	69%	82%	100%
Pneumonia Care					
Appropriate Initial Antibiotic[1,3]	2	100%	77%	83%	94%
Blood Culture Timing[1,3]	1	100%	97%	90%	100%
Influenza Vaccine[5]	-	-	83%	70%	100%
Initial Antibiotic Timing[1]	11	64%	86%	80%	93%
Oxygenation Assessment[1]	18	100%	100%	99%	100%
Pneumococcal Vaccine[1]	11	27%	73%	69%	94%
Smoking Cessation Advice[1,3]	1	0%	63%	80%	100%
Surgical Infection Prevention					
Prophylactic Antibiotic Given[5]	-	-	85%	77%	95%
Prophylactic Antibiotic Selection[5]	-	-	93%	90%	100%
Prophylactic Antibiotic Stopped[5]	-	-	86%	72%	95%
Pregnancy Care					
Inpatient Neonatal Mortality	-	-	-	-	-
Third or Fourth Degree Laceration	-	-	-	3.63%	3.27%

Landmann-Jungman Memorial Hospital

Alternate Name: LJMH
600 Billars Street
Scotland, SD 57059
E-mail: jay.plucker@mckennan.org
URL: www.ljmh.org

Phone: 605-583-2226
Fax: 605-583-4557

Ownership: Voluntary non-profit - Private
Emergency Services: Yes

Accredited: No
Licensed Beds: 25

Key Personnel:
Administrator . . . . Jay Plucker
Chief Medical Staff. . . . . Manuel Ramos, MD

Measure	Cases	This Hospital	State Average	U.S. Average	Top Hospital
Heart Attack Care					
ACE Inhibitor or ARB for LVSD[5]	-	-	84%	82%	100%
Aspirin at Arrival[5]	-	-	94%	92%	100%
Aspirin at Discharge[5]	-	-	96%	90%	100%
Beta Blocker at Arrival[5]	-	-	90%	87%	100%
Beta Blocker at Discharge[5]	-	-	94%	90%	100%
Fibrinolytic Medication Timing[5]	-	-	42%	31%	100%
PCI Within 90 Minutes of Arrival[5]	-	-	79%	54%	95%
Smoking Cessation Advice[5]	-	-	69%	88%	100%
Heart Failure Care					
ACE Inhibitor or ARB for LVSD[1]	1	100%	76%	82%	100%
Discharge Instructions[1]	1	0%	51%	61%	93%
Evaluation of LVS Function[1]	5	60%	71%	83%	99%
Smoking Cessation Advice	0	-	69%	82%	100%
Pneumonia Care					
Appropriate Initial Antibiotic	30	20%	77%	83%	94%
Blood Culture Timing[1]	1	100%	97%	90%	100%
Influenza Vaccine[1]	10	70%	83%	70%	100%
Initial Antibiotic Timing	25	84%	86%	80%	93%
Oxygenation Assessment	36	100%	100%	99%	100%
Pneumococcal Vaccine	35	49%	73%	69%	94%
Smoking Cessation Advice[1]	1	100%	63%	80%	100%
Surgical Infection Prevention					
Prophylactic Antibiotic Given[5]	-	-	85%	77%	95%
Prophylactic Antibiotic Selection[5]	-	-	93%	90%	100%
Prophylactic Antibiotic Stopped[5]	-	-	86%	72%	95%
Pregnancy Care					
Inpatient Neonatal Mortality	-	-	-	-	-
Third or Fourth Degree Laceration	-	-	-	3.63%	3.27%

Avera Heart Hospital of South Dakota

4500 W 69th St
Sioux Falls, SD 57108

Phone: 605-977-7000

Ownership: Proprietary
Emergency Services: Yes

Accredited: Yes

Measure	Cases	This Hospital	State Average	U.S. Average	Top Hospital
Heart Attack Care					
ACE Inhibitor or ARB for LVSD	103	96%	84%	82%	100%
Aspirin at Arrival	99	99%	94%	92%	100%
Aspirin at Discharge	641	99%	96%	90%	100%
Beta Blocker at Arrival	92	99%	90%	87%	100%
Beta Blocker at Discharge	674	100%	94%	90%	100%
Fibrinolytic Medication Timing[1]	1	0%	42%	31%	100%
PCI Within 90 Minutes of Arrival[1]	1	100%	79%	54%	95%
Smoking Cessation Advice	214	100%	69%	88%	100%
Heart Failure Care					
ACE Inhibitor or ARB for LVSD	84	96%	76%	82%	100%
Discharge Instructions	155	93%	51%	61%	93%
Evaluation of LVS Function	182	99%	71%	83%	99%
Smoking Cessation Advice[1]	24	100%	69%	82%	100%
Pneumonia Care					
Appropriate Initial Antibiotic	0	-	77%	83%	94%
Blood Culture Timing[1]	2	100%	97%	90%	100%
Influenza Vaccine[1]	1	0%	83%	70%	100%
Initial Antibiotic Timing[1]	3	67%	86%	80%	93%
Oxygenation Assessment[1]	3	100%	100%	99%	100%
Pneumococcal Vaccine[1]	6	83%	73%	69%	94%
Smoking Cessation Advice	0	-	63%	80%	100%
Surgical Infection Prevention					
Prophylactic Antibiotic Given[2,3]	355	95%	85%	77%	95%
Prophylactic Antibiotic Selection[2]	106	100%	93%	90%	100%
Prophylactic Antibiotic Stopped[2,3]	347	99%	86%	72%	95%
Pregnancy Care					
Inpatient Neonatal Mortality	-	-	-	-	-
Third or Fourth Degree Laceration	-	-	-	3.63%	3.27%

Avera McKennan Hospital & Univ Hlth Ctr

800 E 21st Street
Sioux Falls, SD 57105
E-mail: info@mckennan.org
URL: www.mckennan.org

Phone: 605-322-8000
Fax: 605-322-7822

Ownership: Voluntary non-profit - Private
Emergency Services: Yes

Accredited: Yes
Licensed Beds: 490

Key Personnel:
President/CEO. . . . . Frederick W Slunecka
Emergency Room . . . . Howard Burns
Director Infection/Disease Control . . . . Don Tomac
Director Respiratory Therapy . . . . Deanna Larson

Measure	Cases	This Hospital	State Average	U.S. Average	Top Hospital
Heart Attack Care					
ACE Inhibitor or ARB for LVSD[1]	18	100%	84%	82%	100%
Aspirin at Arrival	78	100%	94%	92%	100%
Aspirin at Discharge	77	99%	96%	90%	100%
Beta Blocker at Arrival	68	97%	90%	87%	100%
Beta Blocker at Discharge	82	100%	94%	90%	100%
Fibrinolytic Medication Timing	0	-	42%	31%	100%

NOTE: Hospital profiles are in alphabetical order by state, then city, then hospital within the city; Rankings are sorted by rate in descending order and exclude hospitals with less than 25 cases; (1) The number of cases is too small (n<25) for purposes of reliably predicting hospital performance; (2) Measure reflects the hospital's indication that its submission was based upon a sample of its relevant discharges; (3) Rate reflects fewer than the maximum possible quarters of data for the measure; (4) Inaccurate information submitted and suppressed for one or more quarters; (5) No data is available from the hospital for this measure; Please refer to the User's Guide for a full explanation of data

PCI Within 90 Minutes of Arrival[1]	10	60%	79%	54%	95%
Smoking Cessation Advice	29	100%	69%	88%	100%
Heart Failure Care					
ACE Inhibitor or ARB for LVSD	64	94%	76%	82%	100%
Discharge Instructions	151	100%	51%	61%	93%
Evaluation of LVS Function	215	99%	71%	83%	99%
Smoking Cessation Advice	26	100%	69%	82%	100%
Pneumonia Care					
Appropriate Initial Antibiotic	100	93%	77%	83%	94%
Blood Culture Timing	89	89%	97%	90%	100%
Influenza Vaccine	37	92%	83%	70%	100%
Initial Antibiotic Timing	142	89%	86%	80%	93%
Oxygenation Assessment	173	100%	100%	99%	100%
Pneumococcal Vaccine	131	88%	73%	69%	94%
Smoking Cessation Advice	40	100%	63%	80%	100%
Surgical Infection Prevention					
Prophylactic Antibiotic Given[2,3]	384	96%	85%	77%	95%
Prophylactic Antibiotic Selection[2]	278	93%	93%	90%	100%
Prophylactic Antibiotic Stopped[2,3]	362	90%	86%	72%	95%
Pregnancy Care					
Inpatient Neonatal Mortality	-	-	-	-	-
Third or Fourth Degree Laceration	-	-	-	3.63%	3.27%

Sanford USD Medical Center

1305 West 18th Street
Sioux Falls, SD 57117
E-mail: info@sanfordhealth.org
URL: www.sanfordhealth.org
Ownership: Voluntary non-profit - Other
Emergency Services: Yes

Phone: 605-333-1000
Fax: 605-328-1577
Accredited: Yes
Licensed Beds: 477

Key Personnel:

President/CEO . . . . . Kelby K Krabbenhoft
Chief Medical Staff . . . . . Barbara Hall, MD
Emergency Room . . . . . Becky Nelson, MD
Director Infection/Disease Control . . . . . Lisa Docken, RN
Director Medical/Surgical Nursing . . . . . Rich Jones
OB/GYN Womens Health . . . . . Yvonne Seger, MD
Chief Radiology . . . . . Daryl Wierda, MD
Director Respiratory Therapy . . . . . Bill Roberts

Measure	Cases	This Hospital	State Average	U.S. Average	Top Hospital
Heart Attack Care					
ACE Inhibitor or ARB for LVSD	59	90%	84%	82%	100%
Aspirin at Arrival	191	100%	94%	92%	100%
Aspirin at Discharge	358	99%	96%	90%	100%
Beta Blocker at Arrival	146	96%	90%	87%	100%
Beta Blocker at Discharge	357	99%	94%	90%	100%
Fibrinolytic Medication Timing	0	-	42%	31%	100%
PCI Within 90 Minutes of Arrival[1]	6	67%	79%	54%	95%
Smoking Cessation Advice	139	92%	69%	88%	100%
Heart Failure Care					
ACE Inhibitor or ARB for LVSD	92	88%	76%	82%	100%
Discharge Instructions	196	87%	51%	61%	93%
Evaluation of LVS Function	262	97%	71%	83%	99%
Smoking Cessation Advice	41	88%	69%	82%	100%
Pneumonia Care					
Appropriate Initial Antibiotic	122	86%	77%	83%	94%
Blood Culture Timing	70	93%	97%	90%	100%
Influenza Vaccine	37	95%	83%	70%	100%
Initial Antibiotic Timing	180	84%	86%	80%	93%
Oxygenation Assessment	256	100%	100%	99%	100%
Pneumococcal Vaccine	166	87%	73%	69%	94%
Smoking Cessation Advice	67	88%	63%	80%	100%
Surgical Infection Prevention					
Prophylactic Antibiotic Given	1,128	90%	85%	77%	95%
Prophylactic Antibiotic Selection	220	98%	93%	90%	100%
Prophylactic Antibiotic Stopped	1,060	88%	86%	72%	95%
Pregnancy Care					
Inpatient Neonatal Mortality[5]	0	0.00%	-	-	-
Third or Fourth Degree Laceration[5]	0	0.00%	-	3.63%	3.27%

Sioux Falls Surgical Center

600 South Cliff Avenue
Sioux Falls, SD 57104
Ownership: Proprietary
Emergency Services: No

Phone: 605-334-6730
Accredited: No

Measure	Cases	This Hospital	State Average	U.S. Average	Top Hospital
Heart Attack Care					
ACE Inhibitor or ARB for LVSD[5]	-	-	84%	82%	100%
Aspirin at Arrival[5]	-	-	94%	92%	100%
Aspirin at Discharge[5]	-	-	96%	90%	100%
Beta Blocker at Arrival[5]	-	-	90%	87%	100%
Beta Blocker at Discharge[5]	-	-	94%	90%	100%
Fibrinolytic Medication Timing[5]	-	-	42%	31%	100%
PCI Within 90 Minutes of Arrival[5]	-	-	79%	54%	95%
Smoking Cessation Advice[5]	-	-	69%	88%	100%
Heart Failure Care					
ACE Inhibitor or ARB for LVSD[5]	-	-	76%	82%	100%
Discharge Instructions[5]	-	-	51%	61%	93%
Evaluation of LVS Function[5]	-	-	71%	83%	99%
Smoking Cessation Advice[5]	-	-	69%	82%	100%
Pneumonia Care					
Appropriate Initial Antibiotic[5]	-	-	77%	83%	94%
Blood Culture Timing[5]	-	-	97%	90%	100%
Influenza Vaccine[5]	-	-	83%	70%	100%
Initial Antibiotic Timing[5]	-	-	86%	80%	93%
Oxygenation Assessment[5]	-	-	100%	99%	100%
Pneumococcal Vaccine[5]	-	-	73%	69%	94%
Smoking Cessation Advice[5]	-	-	63%	80%	100%
Surgical Infection Prevention					
Prophylactic Antibiotic Given[2]	197	79%	85%	77%	95%
Prophylactic Antibiotic Selection[2]	82	94%	93%	90%	100%
Prophylactic Antibiotic Stopped[2]	197	92%	86%	72%	95%
Pregnancy Care					
Inpatient Neonatal Mortality	-	-	-	-	-
Third or Fourth Degree Laceration	-	-	-	3.63%	3.27%

Coteau Des Prairies Hospital

205 Orchard Drive
Sisseton, SD 57262
Ownership: Voluntary non-profit - Private
Emergency Services: Yes

Phone: 605-698-7647
Fax: 605-698-4284
Accredited: No
Licensed Beds: 31

Key Personnel:

CEO . . . . . Bill McClerrey
OB/GYN . . . . . Judy Beumer, MD

Measure	Cases	This Hospital	State Average	U.S. Average	Top Hospital
Heart Attack Care					
ACE Inhibitor or ARB for LVSD[3]	0	-	84%	82%	100%
Aspirin at Arrival[1,3]	3	67%	94%	92%	100%
Aspirin at Discharge[1,3]	2	100%	96%	90%	100%
Beta Blocker at Arrival[1,3]	4	100%	90%	87%	100%
Beta Blocker at Discharge[1,3]	5	100%	94%	90%	100%
Fibrinolytic Medication Timing[3]	0	-	42%	31%	100%
PCI Within 90 Minutes of Arrival	0	-	79%	54%	95%
Smoking Cessation Advice[3]	0	-	69%	88%	100%
Heart Failure Care					
ACE Inhibitor or ARB for LVSD[1]	5	80%	76%	82%	100%
Discharge Instructions[1,3]	3	0%	51%	61%	93%
Evaluation of LVS Function[1]	22	59%	71%	83%	99%
Smoking Cessation Advice[3]	0	-	69%	82%	100%
Pneumonia Care					
Appropriate Initial Antibiotic[1,3]	1	100%	77%	83%	94%
Blood Culture Timing[3]	0	-	97%	90%	100%
Influenza Vaccine[5]	-	-	83%	70%	100%
Initial Antibiotic Timing[1]	20	90%	86%	80%	93%
Oxygenation Assessment	30	100%	100%	99%	100%
Pneumococcal Vaccine[1]	21	48%	73%	69%	94%
Smoking Cessation Advice[3]	0	-	63%	80%	100%
Surgical Infection Prevention					
Prophylactic Antibiotic Given[1,3]	3	0%	85%	77%	95%
Prophylactic Antibiotic Selection[5]	-	-	93%	90%	100%

NOTE: Hospital profiles are in alphabetical order by state, then city, then hospital within the city; Rankings are sorted by rate in descending order and exclude hospitals with less than 25 cases; (1) The number of cases is too small (n<25) for purposes of reliably predicting hospital performance; (2) Measure reflects the hospital's indication that its submission was based upon a sample of its relevant discharges; (3) Rate reflects fewer than the maximum possible quarters of data for the measure; (4) Inaccurate information submitted and suppressed for one or more quarters; (5) No data is available from the hospital for this measure; Please refer to the User's Guide for a full explanation of data

Prophylactic Antibiotic Stopped[1,3]	2	100%	86%	72%	95%
Pregnancy Care					
Inpatient Neonatal Mortality	-	-	-	-	-
Third or Fourth Degree Laceration	-	-	-	3.63%	3.27%

PHS Indian Hospital

5 E Chestnut Street
Sisseton, SD 57262
Ownership: Government - Federal
Emergency Services: Yes

Phone: 605-698-7606
Fax: 605-698-4270
Accredited: Yes
Licensed Beds: 18

Measure	Cases	This Hospital	State Average	U.S. Average	Top Hospital
Heart Attack Care					
ACE Inhibitor or ARB for LVSD[5]	-	-	84%	82%	100%
Aspirin at Arrival[5]	-	-	94%	92%	100%
Aspirin at Discharge[5]	-	-	96%	90%	100%
Beta Blocker at Arrival[5]	-	-	90%	87%	100%
Beta Blocker at Discharge[5]	-	-	94%	90%	100%
Fibrinolytic Medication Timing[5]	-	-	42%	31%	100%
PCI Within 90 Minutes of Arrival[5]	-	-	79%	54%	95%
Smoking Cessation Advice[5]	-	-	69%	88%	100%
Heart Failure Care					
ACE Inhibitor or ARB for LVSD[5]	-	-	76%	82%	100%
Discharge Instructions[5]	-	-	51%	61%	93%
Evaluation of LVS Function[5]	-	-	71%	83%	99%
Smoking Cessation Advice[5]	-	-	69%	82%	100%
Pneumonia Care					
Appropriate Initial Antibiotic[5]	-	-	77%	83%	94%
Blood Culture Timing[5]	-	-	97%	90%	100%
Influenza Vaccine[5]	-	-	83%	70%	100%
Initial Antibiotic Timing[5]	-	-	86%	80%	93%
Oxygenation Assessment[5]	-	-	100%	99%	100%
Pneumococcal Vaccine[5]	-	-	73%	69%	94%
Smoking Cessation Advice[5]	-	-	63%	80%	100%
Surgical Infection Prevention					
Prophylactic Antibiotic Given[5]	-	-	85%	77%	95%
Prophylactic Antibiotic Selection[5]	-	-	93%	90%	100%
Prophylactic Antibiotic Stopped[5]	-	-	86%	72%	95%
Pregnancy Care					
Inpatient Neonatal Mortality	-	-	-	-	-
Third or Fourth Degree Laceration	-	-	-	3.63%	3.27%

Spearfish Regional Hospital

1440 N Main Street
Spearfish, SD 57783
URL: www.rcrh.org
Ownership: Voluntary non-profit - Private
Emergency Services: Yes

Phone: 605-644-4000
Fax: 605-644-4011
Accredited: No
Licensed Beds: 40

Key Personnel:

Administrator . . . . Larry Veitz
Cardiac Lab (non-invasive) . . . . Dawn Koehler
Emergency Room . . . . Dr. Jeff Heir
Emergency Room . . . . Kathy Culver
Infection Control. . . . . Jennifer Jones
ICU . . . . Kathyna Culver
Intensive/Coronary Care . . . . Kathy Culver
Medical/Surgical Nursing . . . . Peggy Nixon
OB/GYN Womens Health. . . . . Cindy Brady
Respiratory/Cardiopulmonary. . . . . Ann Brown

Measure	Cases	This Hospital	State Average	U.S. Average	Top Hospital
Heart Attack Care					
ACE Inhibitor or ARB for LVSD	0	-	84%	82%	100%
Aspirin at Arrival[1]	2	100%	94%	92%	100%
Aspirin at Discharge[1]	1	100%	96%	90%	100%
Beta Blocker at Arrival[1]	2	50%	90%	87%	100%
Beta Blocker at Discharge[1]	1	100%	94%	90%	100%
Fibrinolytic Medication Timing	0	-	42%	31%	100%
PCI Within 90 Minutes of Arrival	0	-	79%	54%	95%
Smoking Cessation Advice	0	-	69%	88%	100%
Heart Failure Care					
ACE Inhibitor or ARB for LVSD[1]	7	86%	76%	82%	100%
Discharge Instructions[1]	16	31%	51%	61%	93%
Evaluation of LVS Function[1]	22	73%	71%	83%	99%
Smoking Cessation Advice	0	-	69%	82%	100%
Pneumonia Care					
Appropriate Initial Antibiotic	38	87%	77%	83%	94%
Blood Culture Timing[1]	13	100%	97%	90%	100%
Influenza Vaccine[1]	20	85%	83%	70%	100%
Initial Antibiotic Timing	45	89%	86%	80%	93%
Oxygenation Assessment	56	100%	100%	99%	100%
Pneumococcal Vaccine	41	85%	73%	69%	94%
Smoking Cessation Advice[1]	7	100%	63%	80%	100%
Surgical Infection Prevention					
Prophylactic Antibiotic Given[2]	145	91%	85%	77%	95%
Prophylactic Antibiotic Selection[2]	32	100%	93%	90%	100%
Prophylactic Antibiotic Stopped[2]	141	93%	86%	72%	95%
Pregnancy Care					
Inpatient Neonatal Mortality	-	-	-	-	-
Third or Fourth Degree Laceration	-	-	-	3.63%	3.27%

Spearfish Surgery Center

1316 10th St
Spearfish, SD 57783
Ownership: Proprietary
Emergency Services: No

Phone: 605-642-3113
Accredited: No

Measure	Cases	This Hospital	State Average	U.S. Average	Top Hospital
Heart Attack Care					
ACE Inhibitor or ARB for LVSD[5]	-	-	84%	82%	100%
Aspirin at Arrival[5]	-	-	94%	92%	100%
Aspirin at Discharge[5]	-	-	96%	90%	100%
Beta Blocker at Arrival[5]	-	-	90%	87%	100%
Beta Blocker at Discharge[5]	-	-	94%	90%	100%
Fibrinolytic Medication Timing[5]	-	-	42%	31%	100%
PCI Within 90 Minutes of Arrival[5]	-	-	79%	54%	95%
Smoking Cessation Advice[5]	-	-	69%	88%	100%
Heart Failure Care					
ACE Inhibitor or ARB for LVSD[5]	-	-	76%	82%	100%
Discharge Instructions[5]	-	-	51%	61%	93%
Evaluation of LVS Function[5]	-	-	71%	83%	99%
Smoking Cessation Advice[5]	-	-	69%	82%	100%
Pneumonia Care					
Appropriate Initial Antibiotic[3]	0	-	77%	83%	94%
Blood Culture Timing[3]	0	-	97%	90%	100%
Influenza Vaccine[5]	-	-	83%	70%	100%
Initial Antibiotic Timing[1,3]	1	100%	86%	80%	93%
Oxygenation Assessment[1,3]	2	100%	100%	99%	100%
Pneumococcal Vaccine[1,3]	1	0%	73%	69%	94%
Smoking Cessation Advice[3]	0	-	63%	80%	100%
Surgical Infection Prevention					
Prophylactic Antibiotic Given[1,3]	19	89%	85%	77%	95%
Prophylactic Antibiotic Selection[5]	-	-	93%	90%	100%
Prophylactic Antibiotic Stopped[1,3]	18	100%	86%	72%	95%
Pregnancy Care					
Inpatient Neonatal Mortality	-	-	-	-	-
Third or Fourth Degree Laceration	-	-	-	3.63%	3.27%

Sturgis Regional Hospital

949 Harmon Street
Sturgis, SD 57785
URL: www.rcrh.org
Ownership: Voluntary non-profit - Other
Emergency Services: Yes

Phone: 605-720-2400
Fax: 605-720-0338
Accredited: No

Key Personnel:

CEO. . . . . Van D Hyde
Chief Medical Staff. . . . . George Tenter
Emergency Room . . . . Lynn Simons
Director Infection/Disease Control . . . . Glea Beck
Director Medical/Surgical Nursing . . . . Lynn Simon
Director Radiology . . . . Jamie Madden
Director Respiratory Therapy . . . . Steve Hoelzan

Measure	Cases	This Hospital	State Average	U.S. Average	Top Hospital

NOTE: Hospital profiles are in alphabetical order by state, then city, then hospital within the city; Rankings are sorted by rate in descending order and exclude hospitals with less than 25 cases; (1) The number of cases is too small (n<25) for purposes of reliably predicting hospital performance; (2) Measure reflects the hospital's indication that its submission was based upon a sample of its relevant discharges; (3) Rate reflects fewer than the maximum possible quarters of data for the measure; (4) Inaccurate information submitted and suppressed for one or more quarters; (5) No data is available from the hospital for this measure; Please refer to the User's Guide for a full explanation of data

Measure	Cases	This Hospital	State Average	U.S. Average	Top Hospital
Heart Attack Care					
ACE Inhibitor or ARB for LVSD[3]	0	-	84%	82%	100%
Aspirin at Arrival[1,3]	2	100%	94%	92%	100%
Aspirin at Discharge[1,3]	3	100%	96%	90%	100%
Beta Blocker at Arrival[1,3]	2	100%	90%	87%	100%
Beta Blocker at Discharge[1,3]	3	100%	94%	90%	100%
Fibrinolytic Medication Timing[1,3]	2	50%	42%	31%	100%
PCI Within 90 Minutes of Arrival	0	-	79%	54%	95%
Smoking Cessation Advice[3]	0	-	69%	88%	100%
Heart Failure Care					
ACE Inhibitor or ARB for LVSD[1]	6	100%	76%	82%	100%
Discharge Instructions[1]	7	100%	51%	61%	93%
Evaluation of LVS Function[1]	12	75%	71%	83%	99%
Smoking Cessation Advice[1]	2	100%	69%	82%	100%
Pneumonia Care					
Appropriate Initial Antibiotic	56	89%	77%	83%	94%
Blood Culture Timing[1]	11	100%	97%	90%	100%
Influenza Vaccine[1]	9	89%	83%	70%	100%
Initial Antibiotic Timing	57	91%	86%	80%	93%
Oxygenation Assessment	57	100%	100%	99%	100%
Pneumococcal Vaccine	43	84%	73%	69%	94%
Smoking Cessation Advice[1]	9	100%	63%	80%	100%
Surgical Infection Prevention					
Prophylactic Antibiotic Given[1]	6	67%	85%	77%	95%
Prophylactic Antibiotic Selection	0	-	93%	90%	100%
Prophylactic Antibiotic Stopped[1]	6	100%	86%	72%	95%
Pregnancy Care					
Inpatient Neonatal Mortality	-	-	-	-	-
Third or Fourth Degree Laceration	-	-	-	3.63%	3.27%

Sioux Valley Vermillian Campus

Alternate Name: Dakota Medical Ctr Sioux Valley Vermillian Campus
20 S Plum Phone: 605-624-2611
Vermillion, SD 57069 Fax: 605-624-4001
Ownership: Government - Federal Accredited: No
Emergency Services: Yes Licensed Beds: 36

Key Personnel:
CEO. . . . . John Paulsa
Chief Medical Staff. . . . . W Dendinger, MD
Emergency Room . . . . Beth Rust Don
Director Infection/Disease Control . . . . Tammy Spiers

Measure	Cases	This Hospital	State Average	U.S. Average	Top Hospital
Heart Attack Care					
ACE Inhibitor or ARB for LVSD[3]	0	-	84%	82%	100%
Aspirin at Arrival[1,3]	3	100%	94%	92%	100%
Aspirin at Discharge[1,3]	2	100%	96%	90%	100%
Beta Blocker at Arrival[1,3]	1	100%	90%	87%	100%
Beta Blocker at Discharge[3]	0	-	94%	90%	100%
Fibrinolytic Medication Timing[3]	0	-	42%	31%	100%
PCI Within 90 Minutes of Arrival	0	-	79%	54%	95%
Smoking Cessation Advice[1,3]	1	0%	69%	88%	100%
Heart Failure Care					
ACE Inhibitor or ARB for LVSD[1]	4	25%	76%	82%	100%
Discharge Instructions[1]	9	22%	51%	61%	93%
Evaluation of LVS Function[1]	15	33%	71%	83%	99%
Smoking Cessation Advice[1]	2	0%	69%	82%	100%
Pneumonia Care					
Appropriate Initial Antibiotic	28	89%	77%	83%	94%
Blood Culture Timing[1]	5	100%	97%	90%	100%
Influenza Vaccine[1]	8	75%	83%	70%	100%
Initial Antibiotic Timing	31	90%	86%	80%	93%
Oxygenation Assessment	36	100%	100%	99%	100%
Pneumococcal Vaccine[1]	24	83%	73%	69%	94%
Smoking Cessation Advice[1]	8	62%	63%	80%	100%
Surgical Infection Prevention					
Prophylactic Antibiotic Given[1,3]	3	100%	85%	77%	95%
Prophylactic Antibiotic Selection[1]	1	100%	93%	90%	100%
Prophylactic Antibiotic Stopped[1,3]	3	67%	86%	72%	95%
Pregnancy Care					
Inpatient Neonatal Mortality	-	-	-	-	-
Third or Fourth Degree Laceration	-	-	-	3.63%	3.27%

Prairie Lakes Hospital & Care Center

Alternate Name: Prairie Lakes Health Care Center
401 9th Avenue NW Toll-Free: 877-917-7547
PO Box 1210 Phone: 605-882-7000
Watertown, SD 57201 Fax: 605-882-7726
E-mail: info@prairielakes.com
URL: www.prairielakes.com
Ownership: Voluntary non-profit - Private Accredited: No
Emergency Services: Yes Licensed Beds: 81

Key Personnel:
President/CEO. . . . . Paul Hanson
Director Emergency Services. . . . . Jody Foster
Infection Control. . . . . Shannon Britt
Director Medical/Surgical/Pediatrics. . . . . Shelly Turbak
Director Maternal/Child Health . . . . Susan Dolen
Director Surgical Services . . . . Susan Koob
Director Radiology . . . . Tom Beaudry
Respiratory . . . . Jody Foster

Measure	Cases	This Hospital	State Average	U.S. Average	Top Hospital
Heart Attack Care					
ACE Inhibitor or ARB for LVSD[1]	2	100%	84%	82%	100%
Aspirin at Arrival[1]	16	88%	94%	92%	100%
Aspirin at Discharge[1]	13	85%	96%	90%	100%
Beta Blocker at Arrival[1]	14	64%	90%	87%	100%
Beta Blocker at Discharge[1]	11	82%	94%	90%	100%
Fibrinolytic Medication Timing	0	-	42%	31%	100%
PCI Within 90 Minutes of Arrival	0	-	79%	54%	95%
Smoking Cessation Advice[1]	1	100%	69%	88%	100%
Heart Failure Care					
ACE Inhibitor or ARB for LVSD	25	76%	76%	82%	100%
Discharge Instructions	58	67%	51%	61%	93%
Evaluation of LVS Function	82	82%	71%	83%	99%
Smoking Cessation Advice[1]	7	71%	69%	82%	100%
Pneumonia Care					
Appropriate Initial Antibiotic	108	96%	77%	83%	94%
Blood Culture Timing	72	92%	97%	90%	100%
Influenza Vaccine	26	88%	83%	70%	100%
Initial Antibiotic Timing	154	95%	86%	80%	93%
Oxygenation Assessment	180	100%	100%	99%	100%
Pneumococcal Vaccine	146	72%	73%	69%	94%
Smoking Cessation Advice[1]	24	38%	63%	80%	100%
Surgical Infection Prevention					
Prophylactic Antibiotic Given[2]	328	93%	85%	77%	95%
Prophylactic Antibiotic Selection[2]	75	96%	93%	90%	100%
Prophylactic Antibiotic Stopped[2]	320	98%	86%	72%	95%
Pregnancy Care					
Inpatient Neonatal Mortality	-	-	-	-	-
Third or Fourth Degree Laceration	-	-	-	3.63%	3.27%

Winner Regional Healthcare Center

Alternate Name: Baptist Hospital
745 E 8th Street Phone: 605-842-7100
Winner, SD 57580 Fax: 605-842-7198
E-mail: jweidner@gwtc.net
Ownership: Voluntary non-profit - Private Accredited: No
Emergency Services: No Licensed Beds: 121

Key Personnel:
CEO. . . . . Mick Penticoff
Chief Medical Staff. . . . . Tony Berg
Emergency Room . . . . Gregg Tobin, MD
Director Infection/Disease Control . . . . Wendy Heath
Director Medical/Surgical Nursing . . . . Karey Thieman
OB/GYN Womens Health. . . . . Mary Carpenter
Director Respiratory Therapy . . . . Darryl Suess

Measure	Cases	This Hospital	State Average	U.S. Average	Top Hospital
Heart Attack Care					
ACE Inhibitor or ARB for LVSD[3]	0	-	84%	82%	100%
Aspirin at Arrival[3]	0	-	94%	92%	100%
Aspirin at Discharge[3]	0	-	96%	90%	100%
Beta Blocker at Arrival[3]	0	-	90%	87%	100%
Beta Blocker at Discharge[3]	0	-	94%	90%	100%

NOTE: Hospital profiles are in alphabetical order by state, then city, then hospital within the city; Rankings are sorted by rate in descending order and exclude hospitals with less than 25 cases; (1) The number of cases is too small (n<25) for purposes of reliably predicting hospital performance; (2) Measure reflects the hospital's indication that its submission was based upon a sample of its relevant discharges; (3) Rate reflects fewer than the maximum possible quarters of data for the measure; (4) Inaccurate information submitted and suppressed for one or more quarters; (5) No data is available from the hospital for this measure; Please refer to the User's Guide for a full explanation of data

Measure	Cases	This Hospital	State Average	U.S. Average	Top Hospital
Fibrinolytic Medication Timing[3]	0	-	42%	31%	100%
PCI Within 90 Minutes of Arrival	0	-	79%	54%	95%
Smoking Cessation Advice[3]	0	-	69%	88%	100%
Heart Failure Care					
ACE Inhibitor or ARB for LVSD[1]	4	100%	76%	82%	100%
Discharge Instructions[1]	14	50%	51%	61%	93%
Evaluation of LVS Function[1]	16	75%	71%	83%	99%
Smoking Cessation Advice[1]	1	0%	69%	82%	100%
Pneumonia Care					
Appropriate Initial Antibiotic[1]	17	76%	77%	83%	94%
Blood Culture Timing[1]	5	100%	97%	90%	100%
Influenza Vaccine[1]	2	100%	83%	70%	100%
Initial Antibiotic Timing[1]	20	90%	86%	80%	93%
Oxygenation Assessment	25	100%	100%	99%	100%
Pneumococcal Vaccine[1]	20	65%	73%	69%	94%
Smoking Cessation Advice[1]	7	100%	63%	80%	100%
Surgical Infection Prevention					
Prophylactic Antibiotic Given[1]	23	100%	85%	77%	95%
Prophylactic Antibiotic Selection[1]	2	100%	93%	90%	100%
Prophylactic Antibiotic Stopped[1]	23	100%	86%	72%	95%
Pregnancy Care					
Inpatient Neonatal Mortality	-	-	-	-	-
Third or Fourth Degree Laceration	-	-	-	3.63%	3.27%

Avera Sacred Heart Hospital

Alternate Name: Sacred Heart Health Services
501 Summit Street
Yankton, SD 57078
Phone: 605-668-8000
Fax: 605-665-0170
Ownership: Voluntary non-profit - Church
Accredited: Yes
Emergency Services: Yes
Licensed Beds: 144

Key Personnel:

President/CEO . . . . Pamela Rezac, PhD
Director Surgical Nursing . . . . Diane Davis, RN
Chief Medicine . . . . Robert Neumayr, MD
OB/GYN Womens Health. . . . . David Holzworth, MD
Surgical Services . . . . Cindy Miller
Chief Surgery. . . . . Mark Brown, MD
Director Radiology . . . . Robin Berke
Director of Respiratory Therapy . . . . Laurie Mckee

Measure	Cases	This Hospital	State Average	U.S. Average	Top Hospital
Heart Attack Care					
ACE Inhibitor or ARB for LVSD[1]	11	91%	84%	82%	100%
Aspirin at Arrival	26	100%	94%	92%	100%
Aspirin at Discharge[1]	19	100%	96%	90%	100%
Beta Blocker at Arrival	26	100%	90%	87%	100%
Beta Blocker at Discharge[1]	18	100%	94%	90%	100%
Fibrinolytic Medication Timing	0	-	42%	31%	100%
PCI Within 90 Minutes of Arrival	0	-	79%	54%	95%
Smoking Cessation Advice	0	-	69%	88%	100%
Heart Failure Care					
ACE Inhibitor or ARB for LVSD	55	98%	76%	82%	100%
Discharge Instructions	88	99%	51%	61%	93%
Evaluation of LVS Function	127	100%	71%	83%	99%
Smoking Cessation Advice[1]	5	100%	69%	82%	100%
Pneumonia Care					
Appropriate Initial Antibiotic	88	92%	77%	83%	94%
Blood Culture Timing	78	94%	97%	90%	100%
Influenza Vaccine	36	100%	83%	70%	100%
Initial Antibiotic Timing	124	92%	86%	80%	93%
Oxygenation Assessment	175	100%	100%	99%	100%
Pneumococcal Vaccine	125	98%	73%	69%	94%
Smoking Cessation Advice	36	100%	63%	80%	100%
Surgical Infection Prevention					
Prophylactic Antibiotic Given	269	96%	85%	77%	95%
Prophylactic Antibiotic Selection	69	99%	93%	90%	100%
Prophylactic Antibiotic Stopped	249	92%	86%	72%	95%
Pregnancy Care					
Inpatient Neonatal Mortality	-	-	-	-	-
Third or Fourth Degree Laceration	-	-	-	3.63%	3.27%

Lewis and Clark Specialty Hospital

2601 Fox Run Parkway
Phone: 605-665-5100
Yankton, SD 57078
Ownership: Proprietary
Accredited: No
Emergency Services: No

Measure	Cases	This Hospital	State Average	U.S. Average	Top Hospital
Heart Attack Care					
ACE Inhibitor or ARB for LVSD[5]	-	-	84%	82%	100%
Aspirin at Arrival[5]	-	-	94%	92%	100%
Aspirin at Discharge[5]	-	-	96%	90%	100%
Beta Blocker at Arrival[5]	-	-	90%	87%	100%
Beta Blocker at Discharge[5]	-	-	94%	90%	100%
Fibrinolytic Medication Timing[5]	-	-	42%	31%	100%
PCI Within 90 Minutes of Arrival[5]	-	-	79%	54%	95%
Smoking Cessation Advice[5]	-	-	69%	88%	100%
Heart Failure Care					
ACE Inhibitor or ARB for LVSD[5]	-	-	76%	82%	100%
Discharge Instructions[5]	-	-	51%	61%	93%
Evaluation of LVS Function[5]	-	-	71%	83%	99%
Smoking Cessation Advice[5]	-	-	69%	82%	100%
Pneumonia Care					
Appropriate Initial Antibiotic[5]	-	-	77%	83%	94%
Blood Culture Timing[5]	-	-	97%	90%	100%
Influenza Vaccine[5]	-	-	83%	70%	100%
Initial Antibiotic Timing[5]	-	-	86%	80%	93%
Oxygenation Assessment[5]	-	-	100%	99%	100%
Pneumococcal Vaccine[5]	-	-	73%	69%	94%
Smoking Cessation Advice[5]	-	-	63%	80%	100%
Surgical Infection Prevention					
Prophylactic Antibiotic Given	80	51%	85%	77%	95%
Prophylactic Antibiotic Selection[1]	16	100%	93%	90%	100%
Prophylactic Antibiotic Stopped	79	94%	86%	72%	95%
Pregnancy Care					
Inpatient Neonatal Mortality	-	-	-	-	-
Third or Fourth Degree Laceration	-	-	-	3.63%	3.27%

NOTE: Hospital profiles are in alphabetical order by state, then city, then hospital within the city; Rankings are sorted by rate in descending order and exclude hospitals with less than 25 cases; (1) The number of cases is too small (n<25) for purposes of reliably predicting hospital performance; (2) Measure reflects the hospital's indication that its submission was based upon a sample of its relevant discharges; (3) Rate reflects fewer than the maximum possible quarters of data for the measure; (4) Inaccurate information submitted and suppressed for one or more quarters; (5) No data is available from the hospital for this measure; Please refer to the User's Guide for a full explanation of data

Heart Attack Care

1. ACE Inhibitor or ARB for LVSD

Hospital Name	City	Rate	Cases
Aspirus-Wausau Hospital	Wausau	100%	58
Gundersen Lutheran	La Crosse	100%	56
Appleton Medical Center	Appleton	99%	74
Sinai Samaritan Medical Center	Milwaukee	93%	41
Waukesha Memorial Hospital	Waukesha	93%	55
University of Wisconsin Hospital and Clinics	Madison	92%	79
Froedtert Hospital/Med College of Wisconsin	Milwaukee	91%	44
Meriter Hospital	Madison	91%	43
Saint Agnes Hospital	Fond du Lac	91%	43
Wisconsin Heart Hospital	Wauwatosa	90%	29
Saint Joseph's Hospital	Marshfield	87%	86
Aurora Saint Luke's Medical Center	Milwaukee	86%	255
Bay Area Medical Center	Marinette	84%	25
Saint Francis Hospital	Milwaukee	82%	28
Kenosha Medical Center Campus	Kenosha	81%	27
Mercy Medical Center	Oshkosh	81%	26
Saint Marys Hospital Medical Center	Madison	81%	96
Saint Vincent Hospital	Green Bay	80%	30
Saint Joseph's Hospital	Milwaukee	79%	53
Saint Elizabeth Hospital	Appleton	78%	40
Luther Midelfort Hospital	Eau Claire	75%	55
Bellin Memorial Hospital	Green Bay	68%	50
Columbia Saint Mary's Hospital Milwaukee	Milwaukee	66%	35
Community Memorial Hospital	Menomonee Falls	56%	34

2. Aspirin at Arrival

Hospital Name	City	Rate	Cases
Aspirus-Wausau Hospital	Wausau	100%	100
Aurora Baycare Medical Center	Green Bay	100%	61
Aurora Medical Center	Two Rivers	100%	34
Aurora Memorial Hospital of Burlington	Burlington	100%	25
Aurora Sheboygan Memorial Medical Center	Sheboygan	100%	41
Saint Joseph's Hospital	Marshfield	100%	175
University of Wisconsin Hospital and Clinics	Madison	100%	83
Wisconsin Heart Hospital	Wauwatosa	100%	65
Appleton Medical Center	Appleton	99%	154
Aurora Medical Center Oshkosh	Oshkosh	99%	74
Bellin Memorial Hospital	Green Bay	99%	170
Franciscan Skemp Medical Center	La Crosse	99%	74
Gundersen Lutheran	La Crosse	99%	181
Mercy Medical Center	Oshkosh	99%	74
Meriter Hospital	Madison	99%	178
Saint Elizabeth Hospital	Appleton	99%	95
WFH-All Saints Spring Street Campus	Racine	99%	169
Bay Area Medical Center	Marinette	98%	85
Columbia Saint Mary's Hospital Milwaukee	Milwaukee	98%	136
Columbia Saint Marys Ozaukee Campus	Mequon	98%	113
Community Memorial Hospital	Menomonee Falls	98%	124
Froedtert Hospital/Med College of Wisconsin	Milwaukee	98%	133
Mercy Hospital Janesville	Janesville	98%	94
Oconomowoc Memorial Hospital	Oconomowoc	98%	44
Saint Agnes Hospital	Fond du Lac	98%	122
Saint Mary's Hospital Medical Center	Green Bay	98%	98
Saint Marys Hospital Medical Center	Madison	98%	135
Sinai Samaritan Medical Center	Milwaukee	98%	111
Waukesha Memorial Hospital	Waukesha	98%	182
Aurora Saint Luke's Medical Center	Milwaukee	97%	557
Holy Family Memorial	Manitowoc	97%	78
Luther Midelfort Hospital	Eau Claire	97%	99
Saint Vincent Hospital	Green Bay	97%	121
Aurora Lakeland Medical Center	Elkhorn	96%	25
Kenosha Medical Center Campus	Kenosha	96%	143
Saint Francis Hospital	Milwaukee	96%	96
Saint Joseph's Hospital	Milwaukee	96%	179
Saint Mary's Hospital	Rhinelander	96%	25
Beloit Memorial Hospital	Beloit	95%	56
Theda Clark Medical Center	Neenah	95%	66
West Allis Memorial Hospital	Milwaukee	95%	74
Sacred Heart Hospital	Eau Claire	93%	76
Saint Nicholas Hospital	Sheboygan	91%	46

3. Aspirin at Discharge

Hospital Name	City	Rate	Cases
Aspirus-Wausau Hospital	Wausau	100%	242
Aurora Sheboygan Memorial Medical Center	Sheboygan	100%	25
Gundersen Lutheran	La Crosse	100%	291
Luther Midelfort Hospital	Eau Claire	100%	255
Mercy Medical Center	Oshkosh	100%	79
Oconomowoc Memorial Hospital	Oconomowoc	100%	43
Saint Marys Hospital Medical Center	Madison	100%	303
University of Wisconsin Hospital and Clinics	Madison	100%	181
Bellin Memorial Hospital	Green Bay	99%	350
Columbia Saint Marys Ozaukee Campus	Mequon	99%	106
Franciscan Skemp Medical Center	La Crosse	99%	99
Froedtert Hospital/Med College of Wisconsin	Milwaukee	99%	166
Sacred Heart Hospital	Eau Claire	99%	77
Saint Joseph's Hospital	Marshfield	99%	329
WFH-All Saints Spring Street Campus	Racine	99%	147
Wisconsin Heart Hospital	Wauwatosa	99%	141
Aurora Baycare Medical Center	Green Bay	98%	121
Bay Area Medical Center	Marinette	98%	48
Meriter Hospital	Madison	98%	284
Saint Elizabeth Hospital	Appleton	98%	142
Saint Francis Hospital	Milwaukee	98%	90
Saint Mary's Hospital Medical Center	Green Bay	98%	93
Sinai Samaritan Medical Center	Milwaukee	98%	102
Waukesha Memorial Hospital	Waukesha	98%	193
West Allis Memorial Hospital	Milwaukee	98%	45
Appleton Medical Center	Appleton	97%	236
Aurora Medical Center Oshkosh	Oshkosh	97%	67
Aurora Saint Luke's Medical Center	Milwaukee	97%	897
Beloit Memorial Hospital	Beloit	97%	32
Saint Vincent Hospital	Green Bay	97%	138
Theda Clark Medical Center	Neenah	97%	65
Columbia Saint Mary's Hospital Milwaukee	Milwaukee	96%	140
Holy Family Memorial	Manitowoc	96%	74
Community Memorial Hospital	Menomonee Falls	95%	112
Kenosha Medical Center Campus	Kenosha	95%	133
Saint Agnes Hospital	Fond du Lac	95%	123
Saint Joseph's Hospital	Milwaukee	93%	192
Mercy Hospital Janesville	Janesville	89%	114
Saint Nicholas Hospital	Sheboygan	59%	27

4. Beta Blocker at Arrival

Hospital Name	City	Rate	Cases
Aspirus-Wausau Hospital	Wausau	100%	69
Aurora Baycare Medical Center	Green Bay	100%	53
Bellin Memorial Hospital	Green Bay	100%	143
Franciscan Skemp Medical Center	La Crosse	100%	62
Appleton Medical Center	Appleton	99%	141
Meriter Hospital	Madison	99%	159
Saint Joseph's Hospital	Marshfield	99%	159
University of Wisconsin Hospital and Clinics	Madison	99%	70
Columbia Saint Marys Ozaukee Campus	Mequon	98%	89
Gundersen Lutheran	La Crosse	98%	141
Saint Elizabeth Hospital	Appleton	98%	90
West Allis Memorial Hospital	Milwaukee	98%	45
Wisconsin Heart Hospital	Wauwatosa	98%	44
Holy Family Memorial	Manitowoc	97%	72
WFH-All Saints Spring Street Campus	Racine	97%	147
Froedtert Hospital/Med College of Wisconsin	Milwaukee	96%	96
Mercy Medical Center	Oshkosh	96%	68
Waukesha Memorial Hospital	Waukesha	96%	152
Beloit Memorial Hospital	Beloit	95%	55
Oconomowoc Memorial Hospital	Oconomowoc	95%	40
Theda Clark Medical Center	Neenah	95%	61
Kenosha Medical Center Campus	Kenosha	94%	127
Mercy Hospital Janesville	Janesville	94%	81
Saint Agnes Hospital	Fond du Lac	94%	106
Saint Marys Hospital Medical Center	Madison	94%	103
Luther Midelfort Hospital	Eau Claire	93%	102
Columbia Saint Mary's Hospital Milwaukee	Milwaukee	92%	104
Sacred Heart Hospital	Eau Claire	92%	64
Saint Joseph's Hospital	Milwaukee	92%	104
Aurora Medical Center Oshkosh	Oshkosh	91%	57
Aurora Saint Luke's Medical Center	Milwaukee	91%	326
Bay Area Medical Center	Marinette	91%	86
Sinai Samaritan Medical Center	Milwaukee	91%	64
Saint Mary's Hospital Medical Center	Green Bay	90%	80
Saint Vincent Hospital	Green Bay	90%	105
Community Memorial Hospital	Menomonee Falls	85%	104
Saint Francis Hospital	Milwaukee	83%	53
Saint Mary's Hospital	Rhinelander	74%	27

5. Beta Blocker at Discharge

Hospital Name	City	Rate	Cases
Aurora Baycare Medical Center	Green Bay	100%	113
Aurora Sheboygan Memorial Medical Center	Sheboygan	100%	27
Franciscan Skemp Medical Center	La Crosse	100%	110
Gundersen Lutheran	La Crosse	100%	356
University of Wisconsin Hospital and Clinics	Madison	100%	235
Appleton Medical Center	Appleton	99%	279
Aspirus-Wausau Hospital	Wausau	99%	241

NOTE: Hospital profiles are in alphabetical order by state, then city, then hospital within the city; Rankings are sorted by rate in descending order and exclude hospitals with less than 25 cases; (1) The number of cases is too small (n<25) for purposes of reliably predicting hospital performance; (2) Measure reflects the hospital's indication that its submission was based upon a sample of its relevant discharges; (3) Rate reflects fewer than the maximum possible quarters of data for the measure; (4) Inaccurate information submitted and suppressed for one or more quarters; (5) No data is available from the hospital for this measure; Please refer to the User's Guide for a full explanation of data

Bellin Memorial Hospital	Green Bay	99%	362
Froedtert Hospital/Med College of Wisconsin	Milwaukee	99%	170
Luther Midelfort Hospital	Eau Claire	99%	266
Saint Joseph's Hospital	Marshfield	99%	406
Saint Marys Hospital Medical Center	Madison	99%	298
WFH-All Saints Spring Street Campus	Racine	99%	139
Waukesha Memorial Hospital	Waukesha	99%	189
Saint Mary's Hospital Medical Center	Green Bay	98%	95
Columbia Saint Mary's Hospital Milwaukee	Milwaukee	97%	152
Columbia Saint Marys Ozaukee Campus	Mequon	97%	107
Holy Family Memorial	Manitowoc	97%	72
Mercy Medical Center	Oshkosh	97%	79
Meriter Hospital	Madison	97%	266
Sacred Heart Hospital	Eau Claire	97%	93
Theda Clark Medical Center	Neenah	97%	71
Aurora Saint Luke's Medical Center	Milwaukee	96%	804
Bay Area Medical Center	Marinette	96%	50
Oconomowoc Memorial Hospital	Oconomowoc	96%	45
Saint Francis Hospital	Milwaukee	96%	84
Saint Vincent Hospital	Green Bay	96%	133
Wisconsin Heart Hospital	Wauwatosa	96%	121
Beloit Memorial Hospital	Beloit	95%	44
Saint Elizabeth Hospital	Appleton	95%	156
Saint Joseph's Hospital	Milwaukee	95%	191
Aurora Medical Center Oshkosh	Oshkosh	94%	65
Saint Agnes Hospital	Fond du Lac	94%	125
Community Memorial Hospital	Menomonee Falls	92%	129
Mercy Hospital Janesville	Janesville	92%	116
Saint Nicholas Hospital	Sheboygan	92%	26
Sinai Samaritan Medical Center	Milwaukee	92%	64
West Allis Memorial Hospital	Milwaukee	92%	49
Kenosha Medical Center Campus	Kenosha	90%	125

7. PCI Within 90 Minutes of Arrival

Hospital Name	City	Rate	Cases
Aurora Saint Luke's Medical Center	Milwaukee	82%	28

8. Smoking Cessation Advice

Hospital Name	City	Rate	Cases
Aspirus-Wausau Hospital	Wausau	100%	105
Aurora Baycare Medical Center	Green Bay	100%	35
Aurora Saint Luke's Medical Center	Milwaukee	100%	377
Franciscan Skemp Medical Center	La Crosse	100%	49
Froedtert Hospital/Med College of Wisconsin	Milwaukee	100%	68
Gundersen Lutheran	La Crosse	100%	105
Meriter Hospital	Madison	100%	84
Sacred Heart Hospital	Eau Claire	100%	30
Saint Elizabeth Hospital	Appleton	100%	53
Sinai Samaritan Medical Center	Milwaukee	100%	64
Waukesha Memorial Hospital	Waukesha	100%	63
Appleton Medical Center	Appleton	99%	92
Kenosha Medical Center Campus	Kenosha	98%	47
Saint Joseph's Hospital	Marshfield	98%	115
Wisconsin Heart Hospital	Wauwatosa	98%	49
Bellin Memorial Hospital	Green Bay	97%	116
Mercy Medical Center	Oshkosh	97%	32
Saint Francis Hospital	Milwaukee	97%	36
Saint Vincent Hospital	Green Bay	97%	36
Luther Midelfort Hospital	Eau Claire	96%	79
Saint Mary's Hospital Medical Center	Green Bay	96%	26
University of Wisconsin Hospital and Clinics	Madison	96%	103
Community Memorial Hospital	Menomonee Falls	94%	32
Saint Joseph's Hospital	Milwaukee	94%	88
Columbia Saint Marys Ozaukee Campus	Mequon	93%	30
Mercy Hospital Janesville	Janesville	93%	46
WFH-All Saints Spring Street Campus	Racine	93%	54
Columbia Saint Mary's Hospital Milwaukee	Milwaukee	91%	54
Saint Marys Hospital Medical Center	Madison	90%	135
Holy Family Memorial	Manitowoc	84%	25
Saint Agnes Hospital	Fond du Lac	78%	32

Heart Failure Care

9. ACE Inhibitor or ARB for LVSD

Hospital Name	City	Rate	Cases
Aurora Sheboygan Memorial Medical Center	Sheboygan	100%	34
Black River Memorial Hospital	Black River Falls	100%	32
Monroe Clinic and Hospital	Monroe	100%	33
Saint Mary's Hospital Medical Center	Green Bay	100%	40
Appleton Medical Center	Appleton	98%	61
Gundersen Lutheran	La Crosse	98%	59
Froedtert Hospital/Med College of Wisconsin	Milwaukee	97%	144
Holy Family Memorial	Manitowoc	97%	35
Aspirus-Wausau Hospital	Wausau	96%	78
Theda Clark Medical Center	Neenah	96%	26
Franciscan Skemp Medical Center	La Crosse	95%	38
Meriter Hospital	Madison	95%	95
Aurora Memorial Hospital of Burlington	Burlington	93%	27
Oconomowoc Memorial Hospital	Oconomowoc	93%	29
Riverview Hospital Association	Wisconsin Rapids	93%	28
Saint Joseph's Hospital	Marshfield	93%	121
Howard Young Medical Center	Woodruff	92%	26
Lakeview Medical Center of Rice Lake	Rice Lake	92%	36
West Allis Memorial Hospital	Milwaukee	92%	26
Aurora Medical Center of Washington County	Hartford	91%	33
Aurora Saint Luke's Medical Center	Milwaukee	90%	666
Elmbrook Memorial Hospital	Brookfield	90%	30
Sinai Samaritan Medical Center	Milwaukee	90%	188
Wisconsin Heart Hospital	Wauwatosa	90%	60
Bay Area Medical Center	Marinette	89%	61
Columbia Saint Mary's Hospital Milwaukee	Milwaukee	89%	160
Kenosha Medical Center Campus	Kenosha	87%	101
Saint Joseph's Hospital	Milwaukee	87%	250
Saint Mary's Hospital	Rhinelander	87%	38
Aurora Medical Center Oshkosh	Oshkosh	86%	29
Columbia Saint Marys Ozaukee Campus	Mequon	85%	59
Saint Francis Hospital	Milwaukee	85%	100
Mercy Medical Center	Oshkosh	84%	38
University of Wisconsin Hospital and Clinics	Madison	84%	141
Luther Midelfort Hospital	Eau Claire	83%	75
Beloit Memorial Hospital	Beloit	82%	73
Saint Joseph's Community Hospital of West Bend	West Bend	82%	39
Bellin Memorial Hospital	Green Bay	81%	52
Saint Agnes Hospital	Fond du Lac	80%	50
Mercy Hospital Janesville	Janesville	79%	70
Waukesha Memorial Hospital	Waukesha	77%	159
Sacred Heart Hospital	Eau Claire	76%	68
Saint Michael's Hospital	Stevens Point	76%	34
Community Memorial Hospital	Menomonee Falls	75%	79
Saint Marys Hospital Medical Center	Madison	74%	156
WFH-All Saints Spring Street Campus	Racine	74%	173
Saint Vincent Hospital	Green Bay	69%	65
Saint Elizabeth Hospital	Appleton	65%	68

10. Discharge Instructions

Hospital Name	City	Rate	Cases
Black River Memorial Hospital	Black River Falls	100%	27
Southwest Health Center	Platteville	100%	33
Theda Clark Medical Center	Neenah	100%	92
Appleton Medical Center	Appleton	99%	141
Aurora Medical Center	Kenosha	98%	54
Tomah Memorial Hospital	Tomah	98%	40
Aurora Memorial Hospital of Burlington	Burlington	97%	88
Gundersen Lutheran	La Crosse	97%	130
Aurora Sheboygan Memorial Medical Center	Sheboygan	96%	85
Aspirus-Wausau Hospital	Wausau	95%	263
Aurora Lakeland Medical Center	Elkhorn	95%	66
Red Cedar Medical Center	Menomonie	94%	47
Luther Midelfort Hospital	Eau Claire	92%	166
Meriter Hospital	Madison	91%	221
Aurora Baycare Medical Center	Green Bay	90%	48
Howard Young Medical Center	Woodruff	89%	84
Monroe Clinic and Hospital	Monroe	88%	77
Bay Area Medical Center	Marinette	87%	98
Saint Joseph's Hospital	Chippewa Falls	87%	38
Wisconsin Heart Hospital	Wauwatosa	86%	122
Saint Mary's Hospital	Rhinelander	85%	101
WFH-All Saints Spring Street Campus	Racine	85%	355
Richland Hospital	Richland Center	84%	37
Waupun Memorial Hospital	Waupun	84%	31
Aurora Medical Center	Two Rivers	83%	41
Bellin Memorial Hospital	Green Bay	82%	138
Riverview Hospital Association	Wisconsin Rapids	82%	57
Aurora Medical Center of Washington County	Hartford	81%	54
Berlin Memorial Hospital	Berlin	80%	41
Holy Family Memorial	Manitowoc	79%	85
Saint Joseph's Community Hospital of West Bend	West Bend	79%	56
Stoughton Hospital Association	Stoughton	79%	29
Memorial Medical Center	Ashland	78%	36
Saint Joseph's Hospital	Marshfield	78%	316
Saint Michael's Hospital	Stevens Point	78%	51
Amery Regional Medical Center	Amery	77%	31
Columbia Saint Mary's Hospital Milwaukee	Milwaukee	77%	303
Kenosha Medical Center Campus	Kenosha	77%	212
Fort Memorial Hospital	Fort Atkinson	76%	37
Sauk Prairie Memorial Hospital	Prairie Du Sac	76%	29
Lakeview Medical Center of Rice Lake	Rice Lake	75%	85

NOTE: Hospital profiles are in alphabetical order by state, then city, then hospital within the city; Rankings are sorted by rate in descending order and exclude hospitals with less than 25 cases; (1) The number of cases is too small (n<25) for purposes of reliably predicting hospital performance; (2) Measure reflects the hospital's indication that its submission was based upon a sample of its relevant discharges; (3) Rate reflects fewer than the maximum possible quarters of data for the measure; (4) Inaccurate information submitted and suppressed for one or more quarters; (5) No data is available from the hospital for this measure; Please refer to the User's Guide for a full explanation of data

Hospital Name	City	Rate	Cases
Langlade Memorial Hospital	Antigo	75%	28
Sacred Heart Hospital	Eau Claire	75%	141
Beloit Memorial Hospital	Beloit	74%	125
Sinai Samaritan Medical Center	Milwaukee	74%	289
Froedtert Hospital/Med College of Wisconsin	Milwaukee	71%	272
Mercy Hospital Janesville	Janesville	71%	154
Saint Agnes Hospital	Fond du Lac	71%	102
Saint Joseph's Hospital	Milwaukee	71%	456
Saint Mary's Hospital Medical Center	Green Bay	71%	103
West Allis Memorial Hospital	Milwaukee	71%	124
Saint Vincent Hospital	Green Bay	70%	171
Aurora Medical Center Oshkosh	Oshkosh	67%	52
Mercy Medical Center	Oshkosh	67%	64
Waukesha Memorial Hospital	Waukesha	67%	322
Oconomowoc Memorial Hospital	Oconomowoc	65%	72
Shawano Medical Center	Shawano	64%	45
Franciscan Skemp Medical Center	La Crosse	62%	68
Saint Francis Hospital	Milwaukee	60%	223
Columbia Saint Marys Ozaukee Campus	Mequon	59%	128
Aurora Saint Luke's Medical Center	Milwaukee	57%	1254
University of Wisconsin Hospital and Clinics	Madison	57%	224
Beaver Dam Community Hospital	Beaver Dam	56%	39
Saint Elizabeth Hospital	Appleton	56%	120
Community Memorial Hospital	Menomonee Falls	55%	147
Saint Clare's Hospital of Weston	Weston	54%	28
Elmbrook Memorial Hospital	Brookfield	53%	88
Saint Marys Hospital Medical Center	Madison	53%	271
Door County Memorial Hospital	Sturgeon Bay	47%	59
Saint Clare Hospital Health Services	Baraboo	44%	32
Watertown Memorial Hospital	Watertown	42%	48
Reedsburg Area Medical Center	Reedsburg	35%	26

11. Evaluation of LVS Function

Hospital Name	City	Rate	Cases
Aurora Baycare Medical Center	Green Bay	100%	68
Aurora Medical Center	Kenosha	100%	73
Aurora Medical Center	Two Rivers	100%	64
Aurora Medical Center of Washington County	Hartford	100%	79
Aurora Memorial Hospital of Burlington	Burlington	100%	114
Aurora Sheboygan Memorial Medical Center	Sheboygan	100%	102
Black River Memorial Hospital	Black River Falls	100%	35
Gundersen Lutheran	La Crosse	100%	166
Luther Midelfort Hospital	Eau Claire	100%	223
Mercy Medical Center	Oshkosh	100%	89
Saint Clare's Hospital of Weston	Weston	100%	36
Saint Elizabeth Hospital	Appleton	100%	160
Saint Joseph's Hospital	Marshfield	100%	386
Wisconsin Heart Hospital	Wauwatosa	100%	127
Aspirus-Wausau Hospital	Wausau	99%	312
Aurora Lakeland Medical Center	Elkhorn	99%	94
Bay Area Medical Center	Marinette	99%	136
Franciscan Skemp Medical Center	La Crosse	99%	95
Monroe Clinic and Hospital	Monroe	99%	116
Sinai Samaritan Medical Center	Milwaukee	99%	310
University of Wisconsin Hospital and Clinics	Madison	99%	275
Waukesha Memorial Hospital	Waukesha	99%	406
West Allis Memorial Hospital	Milwaukee	99%	169
Appleton Medical Center	Appleton	98%	186
Aurora Medical Center Oshkosh	Oshkosh	98%	80
Elmbrook Memorial Hospital	Brookfield	98%	96
Howard Young Medical Center	Woodruff	98%	95
Meriter Hospital	Madison	98%	288
Saint Francis Hospital	Milwaukee	98%	231
Saint Joseph's Community Hospital of West Bend	West Bend	98%	100
Saint Michael's Hospital	Stevens Point	98%	80
Tomah Memorial Hospital	Tomah	98%	54
Aurora Saint Luke's Medical Center	Milwaukee	97%	1497
Memorial Health Center	Medford	97%	30
Sacred Heart Hospital	Eau Claire	97%	193
Saint Joseph's Hospital	Milwaukee	97%	498
Bellin Memorial Hospital	Green Bay	96%	167
Community Memorial Hospital	Menomonee Falls	96%	195
Froedtert Hospital/Med College of Wisconsin	Milwaukee	96%	308
Kenosha Medical Center Campus	Kenosha	96%	274
Theda Clark Medical Center	Neenah	96%	123
WFH-All Saints Spring Street Campus	Racine	96%	424
Beaver Dam Community Hospital	Beaver Dam	95%	56
Mercy Hospital Janesville	Janesville	95%	202
Red Cedar Medical Center	Menomonie	95%	60
Our Lady of Victory Hospital	Stanley	94%	36
Lakeview Medical Center of Rice Lake	Rice Lake	93%	104
River Falls Area Hospital	River Falls	93%	28
Saint Vincent Hospital	Green Bay	93%	216
Sauk Prairie Memorial Hospital	Prairie Du Sac	93%	45
Columbia Saint Mary's Hospital Milwaukee	Milwaukee	92%	367
Saint Clare Hospital Health Services	Baraboo	91%	53
Saint Mary's Hospital	Rhinelander	90%	122
Beloit Memorial Hospital	Beloit	89%	151
Fort Memorial Hospital	Fort Atkinson	89%	70
Hayward Area Memorial Hospital	Hayward	89%	28
Saint Marys Hospital Medical Center	Madison	89%	350
Holy Family Memorial	Manitowoc	88%	125
Saint Joseph's Hospital	Chippewa Falls	88%	42
Barron Memorial Med Ctr-Mayo Health System	Barron	87%	31
Oconomowoc Memorial Hospital	Oconomowoc	87%	105
Saint Mary's Hospital Medical Center	Green Bay	86%	119
Shawano Medical Center	Shawano	86%	64
Saint Agnes Hospital	Fond du Lac	85%	164
Watertown Memorial Hospital	Watertown	85%	65
Columbia Saint Marys Ozaukee Campus	Mequon	84%	191
Reedsburg Area Medical Center	Reedsburg	84%	37
Riverview Hospital Association	Wisconsin Rapids	84%	81
Berlin Memorial Hospital	Berlin	83%	63
Memorial Medical Center	Ashland	82%	49
Good Samaritan Health Center	Merrill	81%	27
Stoughton Hospital Association	Stoughton	79%	38
Southwest Health Center	Platteville	78%	40
Door County Memorial Hospital	Sturgeon Bay	77%	81
Hudson Hospital	Hudson	76%	29
Richland Hospital	Richland Center	76%	58
Upland Hills Health	Dodgeville	75%	32
Ripon Medical Center	Ripon	72%	32
Hess Memorial Hospital	Mauston	68%	87
Langlade Memorial Hospital	Antigo	68%	38
Divine Savior Healthcare	Portage	64%	67
Waupun Memorial Hospital	Waupun	63%	49
Cumberland Memorial Hospital	Cumberland	60%	25
Amery Regional Medical Center	Amery	59%	41
Saint Nicholas Hospital	Sheboygan	55%	84
Vernon Memorial Healthcare	Viroqua	52%	27

12. Smoking Cessation Advice

Hospital Name	City	Rate	Cases
Aspirus-Wausau Hospital	Wausau	100%	38
Meriter Hospital	Madison	100%	43
Sinai Samaritan Medical Center	Milwaukee	100%	144
Aurora Saint Luke's Medical Center	Milwaukee	99%	232
Froedtert Hospital/Med College of Wisconsin	Milwaukee	99%	79
Saint Joseph's Hospital	Milwaukee	99%	163
Beloit Memorial Hospital	Beloit	97%	36
Mercy Hospital Janesville	Janesville	97%	36
Saint Francis Hospital	Milwaukee	97%	33
Bellin Memorial Hospital	Green Bay	96%	28
Saint Vincent Hospital	Green Bay	96%	26
Columbia Saint Mary's Hospital Milwaukee	Milwaukee	95%	85
Saint Joseph's Hospital	Marshfield	95%	44
Kenosha Medical Center Campus	Kenosha	94%	33
Sacred Heart Hospital	Eau Claire	94%	32
Waukesha Memorial Hospital	Waukesha	94%	49
Gundersen Lutheran	La Crosse	93%	27
Community Memorial Hospital	Menomonee Falls	90%	29
University of Wisconsin Hospital and Clinics	Madison	87%	55
WFH-All Saints Spring Street Campus	Racine	84%	80
Saint Marys Hospital Medical Center	Madison	79%	56

Pneumonia Care

13. Appropriate Initial Antibiotic

Hospital Name	City	Rate	Cases
Lakeview Medical Center of Rice Lake	Rice Lake	100%	76
Aurora Medical Center	Kenosha	99%	83
Reedsburg Area Medical Center	Reedsburg	99%	69
Aurora Medical Center Oshkosh	Oshkosh	97%	62
Aurora Memorial Hospital of Burlington	Burlington	97%	70
Froedtert Hospital/Med College of Wisconsin	Milwaukee	97%	87
River Falls Area Hospital	River Falls	97%	34
Mercy Medical Center	Oshkosh	96%	45
Saint Croix Regional Medical Center	Saint Croix Falls	96%	26
Saint Elizabeth Hospital	Appleton	96%	78
Stoughton Hospital Association	Stoughton	96%	57
Aspirus-Wausau Hospital	Wausau	95%	100
Luther Midelfort Hospital	Eau Claire	95%	131
New London Family Medical Center	New London	95%	38
Columbia Saint Marys Ozaukee Campus	Mequon	94%	140
Hayward Area Memorial Hospital	Hayward	94%	49
Baldwin Area Medical Center	Baldwin	93%	46
Berlin Memorial Hospital	Berlin	93%	42
Memorial Health Center	Medford	93%	28

NOTE: Hospital profiles are in alphabetical order by state, then city, then hospital within the city; Rankings are sorted by rate in descending order and exclude hospitals with less than 25 cases; (1) The number of cases is too small (n<25) for purposes of reliably predicting hospital performance; (2) Measure reflects the hospital's indication that its submission was based upon a sample of its relevant discharges; (3) Rate reflects fewer than the maximum possible quarters of data for the measure; (4) Inaccurate information submitted and suppressed for one or more quarters; (5) No data is available from the hospital for this measure; Please refer to the User's Guide for a full explanation of data

Hospital Name	City	Rate	Cases
Saint Joseph's Community Health Services	Hillsboro	93%	28
Saint Michael's Hospital	Stevens Point	93%	68
Sinai Samaritan Medical Center	Milwaukee	93%	148
West Allis Memorial Hospital	Milwaukee	93%	183
Aurora Baycare Medical Center	Green Bay	92%	51
Aurora Medical Center of Washington County	Hartford	92%	62
Aurora Saint Luke's Medical Center	Milwaukee	92%	559
Mercy Hospital Janesville	Janesville	92%	157
Saint Agnes Hospital	Fond du Lac	92%	90
Sauk Prairie Memorial Hospital	Prairie Du Sac	92%	49
Aurora Lakeland Medical Center	Elkhorn	91%	98
Aurora Sheboygan Memorial Medical Center	Sheboygan	91%	75
Beloit Memorial Hospital	Beloit	91%	89
Franciscan Skemp Medical Center	La Crosse	91%	100
Meriter Hospital	Madison	91%	140
Red Cedar Medical Center	Menomonie	91%	33
Saint Vincent Hospital	Green Bay	91%	91
Tomah Memorial Hospital	Tomah	91%	35
Appleton Medical Center	Appleton	90%	96
Columbia Saint Mary's Hospital Milwaukee	Milwaukee	90%	180
Monroe Clinic and Hospital	Monroe	90%	104
Saint Francis Hospital	Milwaukee	90%	153
Saint Joseph's Hospital	Marshfield	90%	94
Saint Joseph's Hospital	Milwaukee	90%	154
Saint Marys Hospital Medical Center	Madison	90%	250
Kenosha Medical Center Campus	Kenosha	89%	196
Saint Clare's Hospital of Weston	Weston	89%	35
WFH-All Saints Spring Street Campus	Racine	89%	227
Waukesha Memorial Hospital	Waukesha	89%	219
Aurora Medical Center	Two Rivers	88%	60
Beaver Dam Community Hospital	Beaver Dam	88%	67
Community Memorial Hospital	Menomonee Falls	88%	73
Door County Memorial Hospital	Sturgeon Bay	88%	58
Elmbrook Memorial Hospital	Brookfield	88%	99
Good Samaritan Health Center	Merrill	88%	25
Gundersen Lutheran	La Crosse	88%	110
Memorial Medical Center	Ashland	87%	61
Amery Regional Medical Center	Amery	86%	29
Oconomowoc Memorial Hospital	Oconomowoc	86%	128
Saint Joseph's Community Hospital of West Bend	West Bend	86%	83
Saint Mary's Hospital	Rhinelander	86%	70
Fort Memorial Hospital	Fort Atkinson	85%	55
Shawano Medical Center	Shawano	85%	86
Columbus Community Hospital	Columbus	84%	43
Holy Family Memorial	Manitowoc	84%	73
Southwest Health Center	Platteville	84%	44
Upland Hills Health	Dodgeville	84%	37
Bellin Memorial Hospital	Green Bay	83%	46
Hudson Hospital	Hudson	83%	30
Langlade Memorial Hospital	Antigo	83%	30
Vernon Memorial Healthcare	Viroqua	83%	58
Bay Area Medical Center	Marinette	82%	99
Theda Clark Medical Center	Neenah	82%	34
Watertown Memorial Hospital	Watertown	82%	38
Community Memorial Hospital	Oconto Falls	81%	26
Riverview Hospital Association	Wisconsin Rapids	81%	67
Sacred Heart Hospital	Eau Claire	80%	103
Memorial Medical Center	Neillsville	79%	28
University of Wisconsin Hospital and Clinics	Madison	79%	67
Waupun Memorial Hospital	Waupun	77%	35
Saint Clare Hospital Health Services	Baraboo	76%	33
Saint Joseph's Hospital	Chippewa Falls	75%	56
Howard Young Medical Center	Woodruff	74%	58
Richland Hospital	Richland Center	67%	30
Saint Mary's Hospital Medical Center	Green Bay	67%	104
Black River Memorial Hospital	Black River Falls	61%	38
Cumberland Memorial Hospital	Cumberland	61%	54
Spooner Health System	Sarona	41%	37

14. Blood Culture Timing

Hospital Name	City	Rate	Cases
Aurora Baycare Medical Center	Green Bay	100%	50
Aurora Sheboygan Memorial Medical Center	Sheboygan	100%	67
Bellin Memorial Hospital	Green Bay	100%	41
Berlin Memorial Hospital	Berlin	100%	41
Lakeview Medical Center of Rice Lake	Rice Lake	100%	63
Red Cedar Medical Center	Menomonie	100%	28
Saint Clare's Hospital of Weston	Weston	100%	25
Aurora Medical Center	Kenosha	99%	98
Saint Mary's Hospital Medical Center	Green Bay	99%	80
Appleton Medical Center	Appleton	98%	128
Aurora Lakeland Medical Center	Elkhorn	98%	114
Aurora Medical Center	Two Rivers	98%	58
Aurora Memorial Hospital of Burlington	Burlington	98%	66
Elmbrook Memorial Hospital	Brookfield	98%	100
Saint Joseph's Hospital	Chippewa Falls	98%	43
Saint Joseph's Hospital	Milwaukee	98%	186
Saint Vincent Hospital	Green Bay	98%	96
Waupun Memorial Hospital	Waupun	98%	41
Mercy Hospital Janesville	Janesville	97%	121
Sacred Heart Hospital	Eau Claire	97%	71
Shawano Medical Center	Shawano	97%	32
Vernon Memorial Healthcare	Viroqua	97%	29
Watertown Memorial Hospital	Watertown	97%	35
West Allis Memorial Hospital	Milwaukee	97%	230
Aurora Saint Luke's Medical Center	Milwaukee	96%	792
New London Family Medical Center	New London	96%	26
Saint Francis Hospital	Milwaukee	96%	163
Saint Mary's Hospital	Rhinelander	96%	45
Saint Michael's Hospital	Stevens Point	96%	73
Tomah Memorial Hospital	Tomah	96%	27
Upland Hills Health	Dodgeville	96%	27
Waukesha Memorial Hospital	Waukesha	96%	193
Aurora Medical Center of Washington County	Hartford	95%	73
Howard Young Medical Center	Woodruff	95%	56
Luther Midelfort Hospital	Eau Claire	95%	131
Saint Elizabeth Hospital	Appleton	95%	74
Sinai Samaritan Medical Center	Milwaukee	95%	153
Aurora Medical Center Oshkosh	Oshkosh	94%	53
Beaver Dam Community Hospital	Beaver Dam	94%	48
Community Memorial Hospital	Menomonee Falls	94%	71
Franciscan Skemp Medical Center	La Crosse	94%	108
Monroe Clinic and Hospital	Monroe	94%	96
Saint Croix Regional Medical Center	Saint Croix Falls	94%	35
Door County Memorial Hospital	Sturgeon Bay	93%	43
Gundersen Lutheran	La Crosse	93%	115
Holy Family Memorial	Manitowoc	93%	68
Memorial Medical Center	Ashland	93%	59
Saint Joseph's Community Hospital of West Bend	West Bend	93%	67
Aspirus-Wausau Hospital	Wausau	92%	103
Bay Area Medical Center	Marinette	92%	115
Kenosha Medical Center Campus	Kenosha	92%	179
Reedsburg Area Medical Center	Reedsburg	92%	25
Stoughton Hospital Association	Stoughton	92%	63
Theda Clark Medical Center	Neenah	92%	53
Mercy Medical Center	Oshkosh	91%	57
Oconomowoc Memorial Hospital	Oconomowoc	91%	78
Riverview Hospital Association	Wisconsin Rapids	91%	57
Beloit Memorial Hospital	Beloit	90%	72
Columbia Saint Mary's Hospital Milwaukee	Milwaukee	90%	177
Columbia Saint Marys Ozaukee Campus	Mequon	90%	124
Fort Memorial Hospital	Fort Atkinson	90%	51
Froedtert Hospital/Med College of Wisconsin	Milwaukee	89%	100
Saint Agnes Hospital	Fond du Lac	89%	65
Saint Marys Hospital Medical Center	Madison	89%	190
University of Wisconsin Hospital and Clinics	Madison	89%	64
Meriter Hospital	Madison	85%	80
Saint Joseph's Hospital	Marshfield	84%	101
Saint Clare Hospital Health Services	Baraboo	81%	36
Hayward Area Memorial Hospital	Hayward	79%	33
WFH-All Saints Spring Street Campus	Racine	79%	182
Hudson Hospital	Hudson	78%	27

15. Influenza Vaccine

Hospital Name	City	Rate	Cases
Kenosha Medical Center Campus	Kenosha	100%	53
West Allis Memorial Hospital	Milwaukee	100%	56
Waukesha Memorial Hospital	Waukesha	97%	71
Elmbrook Memorial Hospital	Brookfield	96%	25
Luther Midelfort Hospital	Eau Claire	96%	50
Saint Joseph's Hospital	Milwaukee	95%	41
Saint Joseph's Hospital	Marshfield	94%	34
Oconomowoc Memorial Hospital	Oconomowoc	93%	27
University of Wisconsin Hospital and Clinics	Madison	92%	25
Aurora Lakeland Medical Center	Elkhorn	91%	33
Aurora Saint Luke's Medical Center	Milwaukee	89%	174
Beaver Dam Community Hospital	Beaver Dam	87%	30
Meriter Hospital	Madison	87%	30
Monroe Clinic and Hospital	Monroe	84%	31
Franciscan Skemp Medical Center	La Crosse	82%	33
Columbia Saint Mary's Hospital Milwaukee	Milwaukee	81%	57
Saint Francis Hospital	Milwaukee	81%	47
Bay Area Medical Center	Marinette	77%	26
WFH-All Saints Spring Street Campus	Racine	75%	40
Saint Elizabeth Hospital	Appleton	72%	25
Saint Vincent Hospital	Green Bay	70%	27
Gundersen Lutheran	La Crosse	69%	29
Aspirus-Wausau Hospital	Wausau	67%	36

NOTE: Hospital profiles are in alphabetical order by state, then city, then hospital within the city; Rankings are sorted by rate in descending order and exclude hospitals with less than 25 cases; (1) The number of cases is too small (n<25) for purposes of reliably predicting hospital performance; (2) Measure reflects the hospital's indication that its submission was based upon a sample of its relevant discharges; (3) Rate reflects fewer than the maximum possible quarters of data for the measure; (4) Inaccurate information submitted and suppressed for one or more quarters; (5) No data is available from the hospital for this measure; Please refer to the User's Guide for a full explanation of data

Hospital Name	City	Rate	Cases
Saint Marys Hospital Medical Center	Madison	66%	70
Columbia Saint Marys Ozaukee Campus	Mequon	63%	41
Sacred Heart Hospital	Eau Claire	42%	33

16. Initial Antibiotic Timing

Hospital Name	City	Rate	Cases
Aurora Memorial Hospital of Burlington	Burlington	99%	92
Aurora Lakeland Medical Center	Elkhorn	97%	157
Aurora Medical Center	Kenosha	97%	113
Aurora Medical Center	Two Rivers	97%	71
Franciscan Skemp Healthcare-Sparta Campus	Sparta	97%	30
Waukesha Memorial Hospital	Waukesha	97%	301
Aurora Baycare Medical Center	Green Bay	96%	57
Aurora Medical Center of Washington County	Hartford	96%	97
Baldwin Area Medical Center	Baldwin	96%	71
Our Lady of Victory Hospital	Stanley	96%	25
Saint Joseph's Community Health Services	Hillsboro	96%	27
Sauk Prairie Memorial Hospital	Prairie Du Sac	95%	57
Shawano Medical Center	Shawano	95%	112
Calumet Memorial Hospital	Chilton	94%	33
Lakeview Medical Center of Rice Lake	Rice Lake	94%	114
Saint Clare's Hospital of Weston	Weston	94%	32
Vernon Memorial Healthcare	Viroqua	94%	93
West Allis Memorial Hospital	Milwaukee	94%	275
Aurora Medical Center Oshkosh	Oshkosh	93%	82
Aurora Sheboygan Memorial Medical Center	Sheboygan	93%	108
Gundersen Lutheran	La Crosse	93%	157
Hayward Area Memorial Hospital	Hayward	93%	68
Southwest Health Center	Platteville	93%	73
Amery Regional Medical Center	Amery	92%	38
Bay Area Medical Center	Marinette	92%	151
Reedsburg Area Medical Center	Reedsburg	92%	80
Theda Clark Medical Center	Neenah	92%	92
WFH-All Saints Spring Street Campus	Racine	92%	295
Watertown Memorial Hospital	Watertown	92%	77
Beaver Dam Community Hospital	Beaver Dam	91%	114
Community Memorial Hospital	Menomonee Falls	91%	106
Elmbrook Memorial Hospital	Brookfield	91%	144
Memorial Hospital of Lafayette County	Darlington	91%	33
Saint Francis Hospital	Milwaukee	91%	220
Saint Joseph's Hospital	Chippewa Falls	91%	79
Appleton Medical Center	Appleton	90%	186
Black River Memorial Hospital	Black River Falls	90%	40
Columbia Saint Marys Ozaukee Campus	Mequon	90%	197
Community Memorial Hospital	Oconto Falls	90%	41
Holy Family Memorial	Manitowoc	90%	115
Luther Midelfort Hospital	Eau Claire	90%	184
Ripon Medical Center	Ripon	90%	31
River Falls Area Hospital	River Falls	90%	39
Saint Mary's Hospital Medical Center	Green Bay	90%	115
Saint Vincent Hospital	Green Bay	90%	123
Sinai Samaritan Medical Center	Milwaukee	90%	205
Stoughton Hospital Association	Stoughton	90%	86
Franciscan Skemp Medical Center	La Crosse	89%	140
Oconomowoc Memorial Hospital	Oconomowoc	89%	156
Saint Joseph's Hospital	Marshfield	89%	197
Aspirus-Wausau Hospital	Wausau	88%	150
Beloit Memorial Hospital	Beloit	88%	121
Kenosha Medical Center Campus	Kenosha	88%	294
Spooner Health System	Sarona	88%	41
Upland Hills Health	Dodgeville	88%	52
Good Samaritan Health Center	Merrill	87%	38
Meriter Hospital	Madison	87%	178
Red Cedar Medical Center	Menomonie	87%	45
Wild Rose Community Memorial Hospital	Wild Rose	87%	30
Divine Savior Healthcare	Portage	86%	101
Langlade Memorial Hospital	Antigo	86%	44
Moundview Memorial Hospital & Clinics	Friendship	86%	28
Sacred Heart Hospital	Eau Claire	86%	160
Saint Croix Regional Medical Center	Saint Croix Falls	86%	36
Aurora Saint Luke's Medical Center	Milwaukee	85%	890
New London Family Medical Center	New London	85%	48
Sacred Heart Hospital	Tomahawk	85%	40
Saint Joseph's Community Hospital of West Bend	West Bend	85%	102
Saint Michael's Hospital	Stevens Point	85%	98
Columbia Saint Mary's Hospital Milwaukee	Milwaukee	84%	281
Door County Memorial Hospital	Sturgeon Bay	84%	82
Hess Memorial Hospital	Mauston	84%	74
Mercy Medical Center	Oshkosh	84%	86
Richland Hospital	Richland Center	84%	43
Saint Elizabeth Hospital	Appleton	84%	111
Fort Memorial Hospital	Fort Atkinson	83%	59
Hudson Hospital	Hudson	83%	36
Memorial Health Center	Medford	83%	29
Memorial Medical Center	Ashland	83%	88
Saint Clare Hospital Health Services	Baraboo	83%	64
Saint Nicholas Hospital	Sheboygan	83%	95
Howard Young Medical Center	Woodruff	82%	90
Saint Joseph's Hospital	Milwaukee	82%	232
Berlin Memorial Hospital	Berlin	81%	69
Cumberland Memorial Hospital	Cumberland	81%	57
Monroe Clinic and Hospital	Monroe	81%	139
Saint Mary's Hospital	Rhinelander	81%	110
Froedtert Hospital/Med College of Wisconsin	Milwaukee	80%	160
Columbus Community Hospital	Columbus	79%	52
Mercy Hospital Janesville	Janesville	78%	200
Saint Marys Hospital Medical Center	Madison	78%	306
Bellin Memorial Hospital	Green Bay	77%	56
Memorial Medical Center	Neillsville	77%	31
Tomah Memorial Hospital	Tomah	77%	52
Waupun Memorial Hospital	Waupun	76%	58
Saint Agnes Hospital	Fond du Lac	75%	122
University of Wisconsin Hospital and Clinics	Madison	75%	99
Riverview Hospital Association	Wisconsin Rapids	73%	83
Rusk County Memorial Hospital	Ladysmith	69%	26

17. Oxygenation Assessment

Hospital Name	City	Rate	Cases
Amery Regional Medical Center	Amery	100%	48
Appleton Medical Center	Appleton	100%	222
Aspirus-Wausau Hospital	Wausau	100%	204
Aurora Baycare Medical Center	Green Bay	100%	87
Aurora Lakeland Medical Center	Elkhorn	100%	190
Aurora Medical Center	Kenosha	100%	147
Aurora Medical Center	Two Rivers	100%	107
Aurora Medical Center Oshkosh	Oshkosh	100%	109
Aurora Medical Center of Washington County	Hartford	100%	114
Aurora Memorial Hospital of Burlington	Burlington	100%	125
Aurora Saint Luke's Medical Center	Milwaukee	100%	1121
Aurora Sheboygan Memorial Medical Center	Sheboygan	100%	130
Baldwin Area Medical Center	Baldwin	100%	101
Bay Area Medical Center	Marinette	100%	181
Bellin Memorial Hospital	Green Bay	100%	72
Beloit Memorial Hospital	Beloit	100%	150
Berlin Memorial Hospital	Berlin	100%	76
Black River Memorial Hospital	Black River Falls	100%	47
Calumet Memorial Hospital	Chilton	100%	42
Columbia Saint Mary's Hospital Milwaukee	Milwaukee	100%	334
Columbia Saint Marys Ozaukee Campus	Mequon	100%	246
Community Memorial Hospital	Menomonee Falls	100%	135
Community Memorial Hospital	Oconto Falls	100%	45
Divine Savior Healthcare	Portage	100%	120
Door County Memorial Hospital	Sturgeon Bay	100%	100
Elmbrook Memorial Hospital	Brookfield	100%	182
Fort Memorial Hospital	Fort Atkinson	100%	102
Franciscan Skemp Healthcare-Sparta Campus	Sparta	100%	36
Franciscan Skemp Medical Center	La Crosse	100%	199
Froedtert Hospital/Med College of Wisconsin	Milwaukee	100%	180
Good Samaritan Health Center	Merrill	100%	48
Gundersen Lutheran	La Crosse	100%	209
Hayward Area Memorial Hospital	Hayward	100%	79
Holy Family Memorial	Manitowoc	100%	139
Howard Young Medical Center	Woodruff	100%	108
Hudson Hospital	Hudson	100%	46
Indianhead Medical Center	Shell Lake	100%	27
Kenosha Medical Center Campus	Kenosha	100%	346
Lakeview Medical Center of Rice Lake	Rice Lake	100%	142
Langlade Memorial Hospital	Antigo	100%	56
Luther Midelfort Hospital	Eau Claire	100%	237
Memorial Health Center	Medford	100%	29
Memorial Hospital of Lafayette County	Darlington	100%	41
Memorial Medical Center	Ashland	100%	104
Memorial Medical Center	Neillsville	100%	39
Mercy Hospital Janesville	Janesville	100%	271
Mercy Medical Center	Oshkosh	100%	106
Meriter Hospital	Madison	100%	246
Moundview Memorial Hospital & Clinics	Friendship	100%	37
New London Family Medical Center	New London	100%	54
Oconomowoc Memorial Hospital	Oconomowoc	100%	189
Our Lady of Victory Hospital	Stanley	100%	26
Red Cedar Medical Center	Menomonie	100%	56
Reedsburg Area Medical Center	Reedsburg	100%	95
Richland Hospital	Richland Center	100%	57
Riverview Hospital Association	Wisconsin Rapids	100%	92
Rusk County Memorial Hospital	Ladysmith	100%	31
Sacred Heart Hospital	Eau Claire	100%	197
Sacred Heart Hospital	Tomahawk	100%	47
Saint Agnes Hospital	Fond du Lac	100%	160

NOTE: Hospital profiles are in alphabetical order by state, then city, then hospital within the city; Rankings are sorted by rate in descending order and exclude hospitals with less than 25 cases; (1) The number of cases is too small (n<25) for purposes of reliably predicting hospital performance; (2) Measure reflects the hospital's indication that its submission was based upon a sample of its relevant discharges; (3) Rate reflects fewer than the maximum possible quarters of data for the measure; (4) Inaccurate information submitted and suppressed for one or more quarters; (5) No data is available from the hospital for this measure; Please refer to the User's Guide for a full explanation of data

Saint Clare Hospital Health Services	Baraboo	100%	74
Saint Clare's Hospital of Weston	Weston	100%	41
Saint Croix Regional Medical Center	Saint Croix Falls	100%	49
Saint Elizabeth Hospital	Appleton	100%	140
Saint Francis Hospital	Milwaukee	100%	262
Saint Joseph's Community Health Services	Hillsboro	100%	37
Saint Joseph's Community Hospital of West Bend	West Bend	100%	140
Saint Joseph's Hospital	Chippewa Falls	100%	90
Saint Joseph's Hospital	Marshfield	100%	238
Saint Joseph's Hospital	Milwaukee	100%	303
Saint Mary's Hospital	Rhinelander	100%	124
Saint Mary's Hospital Medical Center	Green Bay	100%	144
Saint Marys Hospital Medical Center	Madison	100%	404
Saint Michael's Hospital	Stevens Point	100%	119
Saint Nicholas Hospital	Sheboygan	100%	104
Sauk Prairie Memorial Hospital	Prairie Du Sac	100%	72
Shawano Medical Center	Shawano	100%	136
Sinai Samaritan Medical Center	Milwaukee	100%	231
Southwest Health Center	Platteville	100%	77
Stoughton Hospital Association	Stoughton	100%	105
Theda Clark Medical Center	Neenah	100%	97
University of Wisconsin Hospital and Clinics	Madison	100%	151
Upland Hills Health	Dodgeville	100%	63
Vernon Memorial Healthcare	Viroqua	100%	108
WFH-All Saints Spring Street Campus	Racine	100%	365
Watertown Memorial Hospital	Watertown	100%	85
Waukesha Memorial Hospital	Waukesha	100%	383
Waupun Memorial Hospital	Waupun	100%	75
West Allis Memorial Hospital	Milwaukee	100%	356
Wild Rose Community Memorial Hospital	Wild Rose	100%	33
Beaver Dam Community Hospital	Beaver Dam	99%	137
Monroe Clinic and Hospital	Monroe	99%	169
Saint Vincent Hospital	Green Bay	99%	162
Columbus Community Hospital	Columbus	98%	66
River Falls Area Hospital	River Falls	98%	54
Spooner Health System	Sarona	98%	51
Tomah Memorial Hospital	Tomah	98%	57
Ripon Medical Center	Ripon	97%	34
Cumberland Memorial Hospital	Cumberland	96%	71
Hess Memorial Hospital	Mauston	93%	90

18. Pneumococcal Vaccine

Hospital Name	City	Rate	Cases
Aurora Medical Center	Kenosha	100%	87
Aurora Memorial Hospital of Burlington	Burlington	100%	78
Good Samaritan Health Center	Merrill	100%	29
Vernon Memorial Healthcare	Viroqua	98%	90
Aurora Medical Center	Two Rivers	97%	71
Lakeview Medical Center of Rice Lake	Rice Lake	97%	96
West Allis Memorial Hospital	Milwaukee	97%	260
Aurora Sheboygan Memorial Medical Center	Sheboygan	95%	79
Luther Midelfort Hospital	Eau Claire	95%	194
Stoughton Hospital Association	Stoughton	95%	78
Aurora Lakeland Medical Center	Elkhorn	94%	138
Southwest Health Center	Platteville	94%	47
Holy Family Memorial	Manitowoc	93%	102
Reedsburg Area Medical Center	Reedsburg	93%	69
Sacred Heart Hospital	Tomahawk	93%	41
Waukesha Memorial Hospital	Waukesha	93%	241
Aurora Baycare Medical Center	Green Bay	92%	48
Saint Joseph's Hospital	Marshfield	92%	160
Sinai Samaritan Medical Center	Milwaukee	92%	79
Saint Michael's Hospital	Stevens Point	91%	82
Aspirus-Wausau Hospital	Wausau	90%	143
Kenosha Medical Center Campus	Kenosha	90%	205
Mercy Hospital Janesville	Janesville	90%	172
Franciscan Skemp Medical Center	La Crosse	89%	156
Hayward Area Memorial Hospital	Hayward	89%	54
Monroe Clinic and Hospital	Monroe	89%	121
River Falls Area Hospital	River Falls	89%	37
Watertown Memorial Hospital	Watertown	89%	46
Baldwin Area Medical Center	Baldwin	88%	66
Red Cedar Medical Center	Menomonie	88%	42
Shawano Medical Center	Shawano	88%	86
Tomah Memorial Hospital	Tomah	88%	41
Aurora Medical Center Oshkosh	Oshkosh	87%	63
Berlin Memorial Hospital	Berlin	87%	60
Aurora Saint Luke's Medical Center	Milwaukee	86%	770
Saint Mary's Hospital	Rhinelander	86%	91
Sauk Prairie Memorial Hospital	Prairie Du Sac	86%	56
Upland Hills Health	Dodgeville	85%	53
Oconomowoc Memorial Hospital	Oconomowoc	84%	128
Saint Joseph's Hospital	Milwaukee	84%	154
Aurora Medical Center of Washington County	Hartford	83%	78
Saint Joseph's Hospital	Chippewa Falls	83%	66
Black River Memorial Hospital	Black River Falls	82%	39
Calumet Memorial Hospital	Chilton	82%	33
Columbia Saint Mary's Hospital Milwaukee	Milwaukee	82%	214
Howard Young Medical Center	Woodruff	82%	72
Cumberland Memorial Hospital	Cumberland	81%	47
Froedtert Hospital/Med College of Wisconsin	Milwaukee	81%	75
Gundersen Lutheran	La Crosse	81%	160
New London Family Medical Center	New London	81%	37
Bay Area Medical Center	Marinette	80%	117
Fort Memorial Hospital	Fort Atkinson	80%	59
Saint Elizabeth Hospital	Appleton	80%	91
Elmbrook Memorial Hospital	Brookfield	79%	130
Saint Clare Hospital Health Services	Baraboo	78%	54
Theda Clark Medical Center	Neenah	78%	72
Bellin Memorial Hospital	Green Bay	77%	43
Memorial Medical Center	Ashland	77%	77
WFH-All Saints Spring Street Campus	Racine	77%	242
Community Memorial Hospital	Oconto Falls	76%	34
Saint Vincent Hospital	Green Bay	76%	99
Mercy Medical Center	Oshkosh	75%	85
University of Wisconsin Hospital and Clinics	Madison	75%	83
Community Memorial Hospital	Menomonee Falls	74%	92
Saint Mary's Hospital Medical Center	Green Bay	74%	98
Meriter Hospital	Madison	73%	164
Saint Nicholas Hospital	Sheboygan	73%	79
Beloit Memorial Hospital	Beloit	72%	97
Columbia Saint Marys Ozaukee Campus	Mequon	70%	192
Saint Joseph's Community Hospital of West Bend	West Bend	70%	99
Saint Croix Regional Medical Center	Saint Croix Falls	68%	41
Beaver Dam Community Hospital	Beaver Dam	67%	101
Riverview Hospital Association	Wisconsin Rapids	66%	62
Saint Francis Hospital	Milwaukee	66%	164
Hess Memorial Hospital	Mauston	65%	63
Langlade Memorial Hospital	Antigo	64%	39
Ripon Medical Center	Ripon	64%	28
Spooner Health System	Sarona	62%	34
Saint Marys Hospital Medical Center	Madison	61%	299
Amery Regional Medical Center	Amery	60%	35
Appleton Medical Center	Appleton	60%	159
Richland Hospital	Richland Center	57%	35
Moundview Memorial Hospital & Clinics	Friendship	56%	25
Door County Memorial Hospital	Sturgeon Bay	55%	74
Wild Rose Community Memorial Hospital	Wild Rose	52%	25
Columbus Community Hospital	Columbus	51%	45
Divine Savior Healthcare	Portage	49%	89
Waupun Memorial Hospital	Waupun	46%	39
Memorial Hospital of Lafayette County	Darlington	45%	31
Saint Agnes Hospital	Fond du Lac	41%	118
Hudson Hospital	Hudson	38%	34
Sacred Heart Hospital	Eau Claire	33%	138

19. Smoking Cessation Advice

Hospital Name	City	Rate	Cases
Appleton Medical Center	Appleton	100%	39
Aurora Lakeland Medical Center	Elkhorn	100%	42
Aurora Medical Center	Kenosha	100%	46
Aurora Memorial Hospital of Burlington	Burlington	100%	31
Aurora Sheboygan Memorial Medical Center	Sheboygan	100%	39
Elmbrook Memorial Hospital	Brookfield	100%	36
Saint Elizabeth Hospital	Appleton	100%	37
Saint Joseph's Hospital	Milwaukee	100%	86
Sinai Samaritan Medical Center	Milwaukee	100%	103
Sacred Heart Hospital	Eau Claire	98%	50
Saint Joseph's Hospital	Marshfield	98%	65
Aurora Saint Luke's Medical Center	Milwaukee	97%	272
Froedtert Hospital/Med College of Wisconsin	Milwaukee	97%	58
Saint Vincent Hospital	Green Bay	97%	32
West Allis Memorial Hospital	Milwaukee	97%	71
Gundersen Lutheran	La Crosse	95%	63
Saint Francis Hospital	Milwaukee	94%	70
Aspirus-Wausau Hospital	Wausau	93%	42
Mercy Hospital Janesville	Janesville	93%	61
Meriter Hospital	Madison	93%	45
Saint Mary's Hospital	Rhinelander	93%	29
Oconomowoc Memorial Hospital	Oconomowoc	91%	47
Saint Joseph's Community Hospital of West Bend	West Bend	91%	32
Waukesha Memorial Hospital	Waukesha	91%	68
Luther Midelfort Hospital	Eau Claire	89%	45
WFH-All Saints Spring Street Campus	Racine	89%	81
Bay Area Medical Center	Marinette	88%	32
Beloit Memorial Hospital	Beloit	88%	41
Columbia Saint Marys Ozaukee Campus	Mequon	85%	33
Saint Mary's Hospital Medical Center	Green Bay	85%	26

NOTE: Hospital profiles are in alphabetical order by state, then city, then hospital within the city; Rankings are sorted by rate in descending order and exclude hospitals with less than 25 cases; (1) The number of cases is too small (n<25) for purposes of reliably predicting hospital performance; (2) Measure reflects the hospital's indication that its submission was based upon a sample of its relevant discharges; (3) Rate reflects fewer than the maximum possible quarters of data for the measure; (4) Inaccurate information submitted and suppressed for one or more quarters; (5) No data is available from the hospital for this measure; Please refer to the User's Guide for a full explanation of data

Hospital Name	City	Rate	Cases
Columbia Saint Mary's Hospital Milwaukee	Milwaukee	82%	78
Lakeview Medical Center of Rice Lake	Rice Lake	82%	34
Kenosha Medical Center Campus	Kenosha	81%	75
Franciscan Skemp Medical Center	La Crosse	78%	40
Saint Marys Hospital Medical Center	Madison	76%	76
Monroe Clinic and Hospital	Monroe	68%	34
University of Wisconsin Hospital and Clinics	Madison	52%	52

Surgical Infection Prevention

20. Prophylactic Antibiotic Given

Hospital Name	City	Rate	Cases
Luther Midelfort Hospital	Eau Claire	98%	882
Sinai Samaritan Medical Center	Milwaukee	97%	99
Stoughton Hospital Association	Stoughton	97%	64
Saint Croix Regional Medical Center	Saint Croix Falls	96%	73
Saint Joseph's Hospital	Chippewa Falls	96%	226
Wisconsin Heart Hospital	Wauwatosa	96%	116
Good Samaritan Health Center	Merrill	95%	77
Saint Clare Hospital Health Services	Baraboo	95%	85
Upland Hills Health	Dodgeville	95%	62
Aspirus-Wausau Hospital	Wausau	94%	544
Bellin Memorial Hospital	Green Bay	94%	417
Columbia Saint Mary's Hospital Milwaukee	Milwaukee	94%	377
Waukesha Memorial Hospital	Waukesha	94%	301
Aurora Baycare Medical Center	Green Bay	93%	126
Beaver Dam Community Hospital	Beaver Dam	93%	213
Franciscan Skemp Medical Center	La Crosse	93%	624
Saint Clare's Hospital of Weston	Weston	93%	365
Saint Joseph's Hospital	Milwaukee	93%	445
Aurora Medical Center	Two Rivers	92%	65
Bay Area Medical Center	Marinette	92%	153
Fort Memorial Hospital	Fort Atkinson	92%	234
Howard Young Medical Center	Woodruff	92%	323
Lakeview Medical Center of Rice Lake	Rice Lake	92%	330
Oconomowoc Memorial Hospital	Oconomowoc	92%	305
Red Cedar Medical Center	Menomonie	92%	64
Sauk Prairie Memorial Hospital	Prairie Du Sac	92%	318
Aurora Sheboygan Memorial Medical Center	Sheboygan	91%	96
Columbia Saint Marys Ozaukee Campus	Mequon	91%	175
Mercy Hospital Janesville	Janesville	91%	676
Saint Joseph's Community Hospital of West Bend	West Bend	91%	164
Saint Michael's Hospital	Stevens Point	91%	418
Saint Vincent Hospital	Green Bay	91%	441
Waupun Memorial Hospital	Waupun	91%	53
Aurora Medical Center Oshkosh	Oshkosh	90%	86
Aurora Memorial Hospital of Burlington	Burlington	90%	89
Meriter Hospital	Madison	90%	1209
Sacred Heart Hospital	Eau Claire	90%	209
Saint Mary's Hospital Medical Center	Green Bay	90%	518
Aurora Saint Luke's Medical Center	Milwaukee	89%	170
Theda Clark Medical Center	Neenah	89%	422
West Allis Memorial Hospital	Milwaukee	89%	95
Beloit Memorial Hospital	Beloit	88%	290
Mercy Medical Center	Oshkosh	88%	886
Saint Elizabeth Hospital	Appleton	88%	626
Saint Francis Hospital	Milwaukee	88%	328
Saint Mary's Hospital	Rhinelander	88%	382
Holy Family Memorial	Manitowoc	87%	256
Riverview Hospital Association	Wisconsin Rapids	87%	232
University of Wisconsin Hospital and Clinics	Madison	87%	420
Aurora Medical Center of Washington County	Hartford	86%	84
Berlin Memorial Hospital	Berlin	86%	186
Gundersen Lutheran	La Crosse	86%	264
Saint Marys Hospital Medical Center	Madison	86%	1541
Appleton Medical Center	Appleton	85%	1117
Memorial Hospital of Lafayette County	Darlington	85%	33
Aurora Lakeland Medical Center	Elkhorn	84%	74
Community Memorial Hospital	Menomonee Falls	84%	430
Saint Nicholas Hospital	Sheboygan	84%	64
Vernon Memorial Healthcare	Viroqua	82%	216
Hayward Area Memorial Hospital	Hayward	81%	37
Saint Joseph's Hospital	Marshfield	81%	1532
Hess Memorial Hospital	Mauston	80%	50
Calumet Memorial Hospital	Chilton	78%	27
Aurora Medical Center	Kenosha	77%	60
Saint Agnes Hospital	Fond du Lac	77%	172
Monroe Clinic and Hospital	Monroe	76%	397
Oak Leaf Surgcl Hospital	Eau Claire	76%	59
WFH-All Saints Spring Street Campus	Racine	74%	170
Froedtert Hospital/Med College of Wisconsin	Milwaukee	72%	377
Elmbrook Memorial Hospital	Brookfield	71%	311
Watertown Memorial Hospital	Watertown	66%	185
Reedsburg Area Medical Center	Reedsburg	65%	75
Door County Memorial Hospital	Sturgeon Bay	64%	70
Memorial Medical Center	Ashland	64%	163
Richland Hospital	Richland Center	63%	54
Community Memorial Hospital	Oconto Falls	62%	60
Kenosha Medical Center Campus	Kenosha	58%	130
Baldwin Area Medical Center	Baldwin	47%	74
Amery Regional Medical Center	Amery	45%	87

21. Prophylactic Antibiotic Selection

Hospital Name	City	Rate	Cases
Howard Young Medical Center	Woodruff	100%	76
Lakeview Medical Center of Rice Lake	Rice Lake	100%	71
Luther Midelfort Hospital	Eau Claire	100%	213
Saint Joseph's Hospital	Chippewa Falls	100%	47
Vernon Memorial Healthcare	Viroqua	100%	56
Aurora Baycare Medical Center	Green Bay	99%	72
Franciscan Skemp Medical Center	La Crosse	99%	142
Mercy Medical Center	Oshkosh	99%	206
Sauk Prairie Memorial Hospital	Prairie Du Sac	99%	69
Aurora Memorial Hospital of Burlington	Burlington	98%	44
Columbia Saint Marys Ozaukee Campus	Mequon	98%	57
Fort Memorial Hospital	Fort Atkinson	98%	50
Holy Family Memorial	Manitowoc	98%	43
Kenosha Medical Center Campus	Kenosha	98%	131
Saint Joseph's Community Hospital of West Bend	West Bend	98%	46
WFH-All Saints Spring Street Campus	Racine	98%	55
Watertown Memorial Hospital	Watertown	98%	44
Aurora Medical Center	Two Rivers	97%	30
Aurora Saint Luke's Medical Center	Milwaukee	97%	90
Bellin Memorial Hospital	Green Bay	97%	156
Gundersen Lutheran	La Crosse	97%	68
Saint Marys Hospital Medical Center	Madison	97%	493
Appleton Medical Center	Appleton	96%	257
Aspirus-Wausau Hospital	Wausau	96%	80
Aurora Sheboygan Memorial Medical Center	Sheboygan	96%	45
Meriter Hospital	Madison	96%	312
Riverview Hospital Association	Wisconsin Rapids	96%	76
Waukesha Memorial Hospital	Waukesha	96%	71
Columbia Saint Mary's Hospital Milwaukee	Milwaukee	95%	129
Community Memorial Hospital	Menomonee Falls	95%	83
University of Wisconsin Hospital and Clinics	Madison	95%	78
Saint Clare's Hospital of Weston	Weston	94%	78
Saint Mary's Hospital Medical Center	Green Bay	94%	129
Saint Michael's Hospital	Stevens Point	94%	117
Sinai Samaritan Medical Center	Milwaukee	94%	48
Aurora Medical Center of Washington County	Hartford	93%	42
Mercy Hospital Janesville	Janesville	93%	142
Monroe Clinic and Hospital	Monroe	93%	97
Oconomowoc Memorial Hospital	Oconomowoc	93%	44
Saint Mary's Hospital	Rhinelander	93%	96
Saint Vincent Hospital	Green Bay	93%	86
Beaver Dam Community Hospital	Beaver Dam	92%	74
Saint Clare Hospital Health Services	Baraboo	92%	26
Saint Elizabeth Hospital	Appleton	92%	129
Amery Regional Medical Center	Amery	90%	29
Theda Clark Medical Center	Neenah	90%	94
Elmbrook Memorial Hospital	Brookfield	89%	38
Memorial Medical Center	Ashland	89%	36
Saint Joseph's Hospital	Milwaukee	89%	62
Bay Area Medical Center	Marinette	88%	43
Saint Agnes Hospital	Fond du Lac	88%	65
Aurora Lakeland Medical Center	Elkhorn	87%	31
Beloit Memorial Hospital	Beloit	87%	60
Saint Francis Hospital	Milwaukee	87%	55
Saint Joseph's Hospital	Marshfield	85%	326
West Allis Memorial Hospital	Milwaukee	84%	49
Aurora Medical Center Oshkosh	Oshkosh	82%	44
Sacred Heart Hospital	Eau Claire	80%	49
Aurora Medical Center	Kenosha	79%	29
Froedtert Hospital/Med College of Wisconsin	Milwaukee	74%	208
Berlin Memorial Hospital	Berlin	30%	43

22. Prophylactic Antibiotic Stopped

Hospital Name	City	Rate	Cases
Fort Memorial Hospital	Fort Atkinson	98%	221
Saint Clare Hospital Health Services	Baraboo	98%	80
Aurora Medical Center	Two Rivers	97%	62
Waupun Memorial Hospital	Waupun	96%	52
Lakeview Medical Center of Rice Lake	Rice Lake	95%	317
Luther Midelfort Hospital	Eau Claire	95%	777
Saint Clare's Hospital of Weston	Weston	95%	363
Wisconsin Heart Hospital	Wauwatosa	95%	111
Saint Marys Hospital Medical Center	Madison	93%	1500
Vernon Memorial Healthcare	Viroqua	93%	211

NOTE: Hospital profiles are in alphabetical order by state, then city, then hospital within the city; Rankings are sorted by rate in descending order and exclude hospitals with less than 25 cases; (1) The number of cases is too small (n<25) for purposes of reliably predicting hospital performance; (2) Measure reflects the hospital's indication that its submission was based upon a sample of its relevant discharges; (3) Rate reflects fewer than the maximum possible quarters of data for the measure; (4) Inaccurate information submitted and suppressed for one or more quarters; (5) No data is available from the hospital for this measure; Please refer to the User's Guide for a full explanation of data

Saint Mary's Hospital	Rhinelander	92%	379
Aurora Medical Center of Washington County	Hartford	91%	81
Baldwin Area Medical Center	Baldwin	91%	68
Saint Michael's Hospital	Stevens Point	91%	410
Hess Memorial Hospital	Mauston	90%	49
Saint Joseph's Hospital	Milwaukee	90%	425
Good Samaritan Health Center	Merrill	89%	76
Red Cedar Medical Center	Menomonie	89%	62
Saint Joseph's Hospital	Chippewa Falls	89%	214
Amery Regional Medical Center	Amery	88%	85
Aurora Sheboygan Memorial Medical Center	Sheboygan	88%	96
Bellin Memorial Hospital	Green Bay	88%	403
Oak Leaf Surgcl Hospital	Eau Claire	88%	57
University of Wisconsin Hospital and Clinics	Madison	88%	405
Watertown Memorial Hospital	Watertown	88%	180
Aspirus-Wausau Hospital	Wausau	87%	527
Aurora Memorial Hospital of Burlington	Burlington	87%	86
Aurora Saint Luke's Medical Center	Milwaukee	87%	167
Meriter Hospital	Madison	87%	1160
West Allis Memorial Hospital	Milwaukee	87%	91
Aurora Baycare Medical Center	Green Bay	86%	113
Columbia Saint Marys Ozaukee Campus	Mequon	86%	174
Door County Memorial Hospital	Sturgeon Bay	86%	65
Gundersen Lutheran	La Crosse	86%	259
Holy Family Memorial	Manitowoc	85%	247
Saint Croix Regional Medical Center	Saint Croix Falls	85%	71
Aurora Medical Center	Kenosha	84%	56
Beaver Dam Community Hospital	Beaver Dam	84%	210
Sinai Samaritan Medical Center	Milwaukee	84%	96
Howard Young Medical Center	Woodruff	83%	319
Monroe Clinic and Hospital	Monroe	83%	387
Memorial Medical Center	Ashland	81%	156
WFH-All Saints Spring Street Campus	Racine	81%	161
Aurora Lakeland Medical Center	Elkhorn	80%	70
Bay Area Medical Center	Marinette	80%	150
Franciscan Skemp Medical Center	La Crosse	79%	603
Oconomowoc Memorial Hospital	Oconomowoc	79%	292
Saint Francis Hospital	Milwaukee	79%	318
Saint Joseph's Community Hospital of West Bend	West Bend	79%	156
Stoughton Hospital Association	Stoughton	79%	62
Theda Clark Medical Center	Neenah	79%	405
Community Memorial Hospital	Menomonee Falls	77%	429
Richland Hospital	Richland Center	77%	53
Saint Vincent Hospital	Green Bay	77%	424
Upland Hills Health	Dodgeville	77%	62
Berlin Memorial Hospital	Berlin	76%	184
Columbia Saint Mary's Hospital Milwaukee	Milwaukee	76%	372
Hayward Area Memorial Hospital	Hayward	76%	34
Sauk Prairie Memorial Hospital	Prairie Du Sac	76%	315
Community Memorial Hospital	Oconto Falls	75%	60
Riverview Hospital Association	Wisconsin Rapids	75%	231
Beloit Memorial Hospital	Beloit	74%	279
Appleton Medical Center	Appleton	71%	1087
Mercy Hospital Janesville	Janesville	71%	651
Waukesha Memorial Hospital	Waukesha	71%	282
Memorial Hospital of Lafayette County	Darlington	70%	33
Saint Joseph's Hospital	Marshfield	68%	1519
Elmbrook Memorial Hospital	Brookfield	67%	305
Reedsburg Area Medical Center	Reedsburg	66%	74
Saint Agnes Hospital	Fond du Lac	66%	158
Calumet Memorial Hospital	Chilton	65%	26
Saint Mary's Hospital Medical Center	Green Bay	63%	504
Saint Elizabeth Hospital	Appleton	62%	618
Sacred Heart Hospital	Eau Claire	61%	203
Saint Nicholas Hospital	Sheboygan	61%	64
Froedtert Hospital/Med College of Wisconsin	Milwaukee	58%	363
Aurora Medical Center Oshkosh	Oshkosh	52%	83
Kenosha Medical Center Campus	Kenosha	50%	127
Mercy Medical Center	Oshkosh	12%	879

Pregnancy Care

23. Inpatient Neonatal Mortality

Hospital Name	City	Rate	Cases
Aurora Medical Center	Two Rivers	0.00%	305
Aurora Medical Center Oshkosh	Oshkosh	0.00%	773
Divine Savior Healthcare	Portage	0.00%	309
Memorial Medical Center	Ashland	0.00%	296
Mercy Hospital Janesville	Janesville	0.00%	1190
Sacred Heart Hospital	Eau Claire	0.00%	1172
Saint Clare Hospital Health Services	Baraboo	0.00%	326
Saint Joseph's Community Hospital of West Bend	West Bend	0.15%	674
Luther Midelfort Hospital	Eau Claire	0.18%	559
Gundersen Lutheran	La Crosse	0.24%	1693
Aspirus-Wausau Hospital	Wausau	0.28%	1081
Aurora Baycare Medical Center	Green Bay	0.35%	1719
Froedtert Hospital/Med College of Wisconsin	Milwaukee	2.03%	1580

24. Third or Fourth Degree Laceration

Hospital Name	City	Rate	Cases
Memorial Medical Center	Ashland	1.84%	217
Aurora Baycare Medical Center	Green Bay	2.15%	1253
Sacred Heart Hospital	Eau Claire	2.35%	892
Aurora Medical Center	Two Rivers	3.03%	198
Aspirus-Wausau Hospital	Wausau	3.34%	958
Gundersen Lutheran	La Crosse	3.56%	1263
Froedtert Hospital/Med College of Wisconsin	Milwaukee	3.57%	1147
Aurora Medical Center Oshkosh	Oshkosh	3.72%	564
Saint Joseph's Community Hospital of West Bend	West Bend	3.85%	467
Saint Clare Hospital Health Services	Baraboo	4.12%	243
Luther Midelfort Hospital	Eau Claire	4.24%	401
Divine Savior Healthcare	Portage	4.64%	237
Mercy Hospital Janesville	Janesville	5.27%	816

NOTE: Hospital profiles are in alphabetical order by state, then city, then hospital within the city; Rankings are sorted by rate in descending order and exclude hospitals with less than 25 cases; (1) The number of cases is too small (n<25) for purposes of reliably predicting hospital performance; (2) Measure reflects the hospital's indication that its submission was based upon a sample of its relevant discharges; (3) Rate reflects fewer than the maximum possible quarters of data for the measure; (4) Inaccurate information submitted and suppressed for one or more quarters; (5) No data is available from the hospital for this measure; Please refer to the User's Guide for a full explanation of data

Amery Regional Medical Center

Alternate Name: Apple River Hospital
225 Scholl Street
Amery, WI 54001
Ownership: Voluntary non-profit - Private
Emergency Services: Yes
Phone: 715-268-8000
Fax: 715-268-1376
Accredited: No
Licensed Beds: 29

Key Personnel:
CEO. . . . . Michael Karuschak Jr
Chief Medical Staff. . . . . Craig Johnson, MD CMO
Respiratory/Cardiopulmonary. . . . . Rick Robl, RT

Measure	Cases	This Hospital	State Average	U.S. Average	Top Hospital
Heart Attack Care					
ACE Inhibitor or ARB for LVSD[5]	-	-	85%	82%	100%
Aspirin at Arrival[5]	-	-	94%	92%	100%
Aspirin at Discharge[5]	-	-	94%	90%	100%
Beta Blocker at Arrival[5]	-	-	92%	87%	100%
Beta Blocker at Discharge[5]	-	-	92%	90%	100%
Fibrinolytic Medication Timing[5]	-	-	13%	31%	100%
PCI Within 90 Minutes of Arrival[5]	-	-	75%	54%	95%
Smoking Cessation Advice[5]	-	-	91%	88%	100%
Heart Failure Care					
ACE Inhibitor or ARB for LVSD[1]	6	67%	86%	82%	100%
Discharge Instructions	31	77%	73%	61%	93%
Evaluation of LVS Function	41	59%	88%	83%	99%
Smoking Cessation Advice[1]	4	75%	80%	82%	100%
Pneumonia Care					
Appropriate Initial Antibiotic	29	86%	87%	83%	94%
Blood Culture Timing[1]	5	100%	94%	90%	100%
Influenza Vaccine[1]	5	80%	79%	70%	100%
Initial Antibiotic Timing	38	92%	87%	80%	93%
Oxygenation Assessment	48	100%	100%	99%	100%
Pneumococcal Vaccine	35	60%	78%	69%	94%
Smoking Cessation Advice[1]	7	86%	82%	80%	100%
Surgical Infection Prevention					
Prophylactic Antibiotic Given	87	45%	84%	77%	95%
Prophylactic Antibiotic Selection	29	90%	93%	90%	100%
Prophylactic Antibiotic Stopped	85	88%	80%	72%	95%
Pregnancy Care					
Inpatient Neonatal Mortality	-	-	-	-	-
Third or Fourth Degree Laceration	-	-	3.43%	3.63%	3.27%

Langlade Memorial Hospital

Alternate Name: Langlade County Memorial Hospital
112 E 5th Avenue
Antigo, WI 54409
Ownership: Voluntary non-profit - Church
Emergency Services: Yes
Phone: 715-623-2331
Fax: 715-623-9440
Accredited: Yes
Licensed Beds: 49

Key Personnel:
President . . . . Dave Schneider
Chief Medical Staff. . . . . Jay Turnbull
Emergency Room . . . . Randy Waskin
Director Infection/Disease Control . . . . Sandy Leider
Director Medical/Surgical Nursing . . . . Connie Hubatch
Chief Radiology . . . . Connie Kiesling
Director Respiratory Therapy . . . . Bob Raganyi, DDS

Measure	Cases	This Hospital	State Average	U.S. Average	Top Hospital
Heart Attack Care					
ACE Inhibitor or ARB for LVSD[5]	-	-	85%	82%	100%
Aspirin at Arrival[5]	-	-	94%	92%	100%
Aspirin at Discharge[5]	-	-	94%	90%	100%
Beta Blocker at Arrival[5]	-	-	92%	87%	100%
Beta Blocker at Discharge[5]	-	-	92%	90%	100%
Fibrinolytic Medication Timing[5]	-	-	13%	31%	100%
PCI Within 90 Minutes of Arrival[5]	-	-	75%	54%	95%
Smoking Cessation Advice[5]	-	-	91%	88%	100%
Heart Failure Care					
ACE Inhibitor or ARB for LVSD[1]	8	62%	86%	82%	100%
Discharge Instructions	28	75%	73%	61%	93%
Evaluation of LVS Function	38	68%	88%	83%	99%
Smoking Cessation Advice[1]	5	60%	80%	82%	100%
Pneumonia Care					
Appropriate Initial Antibiotic	30	83%	87%	83%	94%
Blood Culture Timing[1]	9	89%	94%	90%	100%
Influenza Vaccine[1]	10	80%	79%	70%	100%
Initial Antibiotic Timing	44	86%	87%	80%	93%
Oxygenation Assessment	56	100%	100%	99%	100%
Pneumococcal Vaccine	39	64%	78%	69%	94%
Smoking Cessation Advice[1]	10	80%	82%	80%	100%
Surgical Infection Prevention					
Prophylactic Antibiotic Given[5]	-	-	84%	77%	95%
Prophylactic Antibiotic Selection[5]	-	-	93%	90%	100%
Prophylactic Antibiotic Stopped[5]	-	-	80%	72%	95%
Pregnancy Care					
Inpatient Neonatal Mortality	-	-	-	-	-
Third or Fourth Degree Laceration	-	-	3.43%	3.63%	3.27%

Appleton Medical Center

1818 N Meade Street
Appleton, WI 54911
Toll-Free: 800-236-4101
Phone: 920-731-4101
Fax: 920-738-6319

URL: www.thedacare.org
Ownership: Voluntary non-profit - Other
Emergency Services: Yes
Accredited: Yes
Licensed Beds: 160

Key Personnel:
President/CEO. . . . . John Toussaint, MD
Chief Medical Staff. . . . . Steven E Knaus, MD
Emergency Room . . . . Chris Hugo
Coordinator Infection Control . . . . Steve DuBois
Chief OB/GYN . . . . Rami S Kaldas, MD
Manager Surgical Services . . . . Sherry Cheadle

Measure	Cases	This Hospital	State Average	U.S. Average	Top Hospital
Heart Attack Care					
ACE Inhibitor or ARB for LVSD	74	99%	85%	82%	100%
Aspirin at Arrival	154	99%	94%	92%	100%
Aspirin at Discharge	236	97%	94%	90%	100%
Beta Blocker at Arrival	141	99%	92%	87%	100%
Beta Blocker at Discharge	279	99%	92%	90%	100%
Fibrinolytic Medication Timing	0	-	13%	31%	100%
PCI Within 90 Minutes of Arrival[1]	11	100%	75%	54%	95%
Smoking Cessation Advice	92	99%	91%	88%	100%
Heart Failure Care					
ACE Inhibitor or ARB for LVSD	61	98%	86%	82%	100%
Discharge Instructions	141	99%	73%	61%	93%
Evaluation of LVS Function	186	98%	88%	83%	99%
Smoking Cessation Advice[1]	23	100%	80%	82%	100%
Pneumonia Care					
Appropriate Initial Antibiotic	96	90%	87%	83%	94%
Blood Culture Timing	128	98%	94%	90%	100%
Influenza Vaccine[1]	23	48%	79%	70%	100%
Initial Antibiotic Timing	186	90%	87%	80%	93%
Oxygenation Assessment	222	100%	100%	99%	100%
Pneumococcal Vaccine	159	60%	78%	69%	94%
Smoking Cessation Advice	39	100%	82%	80%	100%
Surgical Infection Prevention					
Prophylactic Antibiotic Given[2]	1,117	85%	84%	77%	95%
Prophylactic Antibiotic Selection[2]	257	96%	93%	90%	100%
Prophylactic Antibiotic Stopped[2]	1,087	71%	80%	72%	95%
Pregnancy Care					
Inpatient Neonatal Mortality	-	-	-	-	-
Third or Fourth Degree Laceration	-	-	3.43%	3.63%	3.27%

Saint Elizabeth Hospital

1506 S Oneida Street
Appleton, WI 54915
URL: www.affinityhealth.org
Ownership: Voluntary non-profit - Church
Emergency Services: Yes
Phone: 920-738-2000
Fax: 920-831-1324
Accredited: Yes
Licensed Beds: 352

Key Personnel:
President/CEO. . . . . Daniel E Neufelder
Emergency Room . . . . Rosemary Dvorachek, RN
Chief Medical Officer . . . . Mark Kehrberg, MD
OB/GYN Womens Health. . . . . Steve Savage, MD
Chief Radiology . . . . Robert Kinde, MD

NOTE: Hospital profiles are in alphabetical order by state, then city, then hospital within the city; Rankings are sorted by rate in descending order and exclude hospitals with less than 25 cases; (1) The number of cases is too small (n<25) for purposes of reliably predicting hospital performance; (2) Measure reflects the hospital's indication that its submission was based upon a sample of its relevant discharges; (3) Rate reflects fewer than the maximum possible quarters of data for the measure; (4) Inaccurate information submitted and suppressed for one or more quarters; (5) No data is available from the hospital for this measure; Please refer to the User's Guide for a full explanation of data

Coordinator Respiratory . . . . Lisa Degreef

Measure	Cases	This Hospital	State Average	U.S. Average	Top Hospital
Heart Attack Care					
ACE Inhibitor or ARB for LVSD	40	78%	85%	82%	100%
Aspirin at Arrival	95	99%	94%	92%	100%
Aspirin at Discharge	142	98%	94%	90%	100%
Beta Blocker at Arrival	90	98%	92%	87%	100%
Beta Blocker at Discharge	156	95%	92%	90%	100%
Fibrinolytic Medication Timing	0	-	13%	31%	100%
PCI Within 90 Minutes of Arrival[1]	5	80%	75%	54%	95%
Smoking Cessation Advice	53	100%	91%	88%	100%
Heart Failure Care					
ACE Inhibitor or ARB for LVSD	68	65%	86%	82%	100%
Discharge Instructions	120	56%	73%	61%	93%
Evaluation of LVS Function	160	100%	88%	83%	99%
Smoking Cessation Advice[1]	18	100%	80%	82%	100%
Pneumonia Care					
Appropriate Initial Antibiotic	78	96%	87%	83%	94%
Blood Culture Timing	74	95%	94%	90%	100%
Influenza Vaccine	25	72%	79%	70%	100%
Initial Antibiotic Timing	111	84%	87%	80%	93%
Oxygenation Assessment	140	100%	100%	99%	100%
Pneumococcal Vaccine	91	80%	78%	69%	94%
Smoking Cessation Advice	37	100%	82%	80%	100%
Surgical Infection Prevention					
Prophylactic Antibiotic Given	626	88%	84%	77%	95%
Prophylactic Antibiotic Selection	129	92%	93%	90%	100%
Prophylactic Antibiotic Stopped	618	62%	80%	72%	95%
Pregnancy Care					
Inpatient Neonatal Mortality	-	-	-	-	-
Third or Fourth Degree Laceration	-	-	3.43%	3.63%	3.27%

Franciscan Skemp Healthcare-Arcadia

Alternate Name: Saint Joseph's Hospital
464 South Saint Joseph Avenue
Arcadia, WI 54612
Phone: 608-323-3373
Fax: 608-323-3694
URL: www.mayohealthsystem.org
Ownership: Voluntary non-profit - Church
Accredited: Yes
Emergency Services: Yes
Licensed Beds: 25

Key Personnel:

Administrator . . . . Robert M Tracey
Chief Medical Staff . . . . Dr Burggraf
Infection Control . . . . Mary Klonecki, RN

Measure	Cases	This Hospital	State Average	U.S. Average	Top Hospital
Heart Attack Care					
ACE Inhibitor or ARB for LVSD[5]	-	-	85%	82%	100%
Aspirin at Arrival[5]	-	-	94%	92%	100%
Aspirin at Discharge[5]	-	-	94%	90%	100%
Beta Blocker at Arrival[5]	-	-	92%	87%	100%
Beta Blocker at Discharge[5]	-	-	92%	90%	100%
Fibrinolytic Medication Timing[5]	-	-	13%	31%	100%
PCI Within 90 Minutes of Arrival[5]	-	-	75%	54%	95%
Smoking Cessation Advice[5]	-	-	91%	88%	100%
Heart Failure Care					
ACE Inhibitor or ARB for LVSD[1,3]	4	50%	86%	82%	100%
Discharge Instructions[1,3]	5	80%	73%	61%	93%
Evaluation of LVS Function[1,3]	8	100%	88%	83%	99%
Smoking Cessation Advice[1,3]	3	67%	80%	82%	100%
Pneumonia Care					
Appropriate Initial Antibiotic[1]	8	100%	87%	83%	94%
Blood Culture Timing[1]	5	100%	94%	90%	100%
Influenza Vaccine[1]	3	100%	79%	70%	100%
Initial Antibiotic Timing[1]	13	92%	87%	80%	93%
Oxygenation Assessment[1]	17	100%	100%	99%	100%
Pneumococcal Vaccine[1]	9	89%	78%	69%	94%
Smoking Cessation Advice[1]	4	50%	82%	80%	100%
Surgical Infection Prevention					
Prophylactic Antibiotic Given[5]	-	-	84%	77%	95%
Prophylactic Antibiotic Selection[5]	-	-	93%	90%	100%
Prophylactic Antibiotic Stopped[5]	-	-	80%	72%	95%

Measure	Cases	This Hospital	State Average	U.S. Average	Top Hospital
Pregnancy Care					
Inpatient Neonatal Mortality	-	-	-	-	-
Third or Fourth Degree Laceration	-	-	3.43%	3.63%	3.27%

Memorial Medical Center

1615 Maple Lane
Ashland, WI 54806
Phone: 715-685-5500
Fax: 715-682-4022
URL: www.ashlandmmc.com
Ownership: Voluntary non-profit - Private
Accredited: Yes
Emergency Services: Yes
Licensed Beds: 100

Key Personnel:

President/CEO . . . . Daniel J Hymans
Chief of Medical Staff . . . . Andrew Matheus
Emergency Room . . . . Donald Patton
Manager Medical Nursing Surgical Unit . . . . Madonna Pralle, RN
Director of Pulmonary . . . . Mark Belknap

Measure	Cases	This Hospital	State Average	U.S. Average	Top Hospital
Heart Attack Care					
ACE Inhibitor or ARB for LVSD[1]	3	100%	85%	82%	100%
Aspirin at Arrival[1]	19	89%	94%	92%	100%
Aspirin at Discharge[1]	14	79%	94%	90%	100%
Beta Blocker at Arrival[1]	13	92%	92%	87%	100%
Beta Blocker at Discharge[1]	10	90%	92%	90%	100%
Fibrinolytic Medication Timing	0	-	13%	31%	100%
PCI Within 90 Minutes of Arrival	0	-	75%	54%	95%
Smoking Cessation Advice[1]	3	100%	91%	88%	100%
Heart Failure Care					
ACE Inhibitor or ARB for LVSD[1]	18	94%	86%	82%	100%
Discharge Instructions	36	78%	73%	61%	93%
Evaluation of LVS Function	49	82%	88%	83%	99%
Smoking Cessation Advice[1]	6	83%	80%	82%	100%
Pneumonia Care					
Appropriate Initial Antibiotic	61	87%	87%	83%	94%
Blood Culture Timing	59	93%	94%	90%	100%
Influenza Vaccine[1]	11	82%	79%	70%	100%
Initial Antibiotic Timing	88	83%	87%	80%	93%
Oxygenation Assessment	104	100%	100%	99%	100%
Pneumococcal Vaccine	77	77%	78%	69%	94%
Smoking Cessation Advice[1]	16	75%	82%	80%	100%
Surgical Infection Prevention					
Prophylactic Antibiotic Given	163	64%	84%	77%	95%
Prophylactic Antibiotic Selection	36	89%	93%	90%	100%
Prophylactic Antibiotic Stopped	156	81%	80%	72%	95%
Pregnancy Care					
Inpatient Neonatal Mortality	296	0.00%	-	-	-
Third or Fourth Degree Laceration	217	1.84%	3.43%	3.63%	3.27%

Baldwin Area Medical Center

Alternate Name: Baldwin Hospital
730 10th Avenue
PO Box 300
Baldwin, WI 54002
Phone: 715-684-3311
Fax: 715-684-4757
E-mail: baldhosp@baldwin-telecom.net
URL: www.baldwin-hospital.com
Ownership: Voluntary non-profit - Private
Accredited: No
Emergency Services: Yes
Licensed Beds: 33

Key Personnel:

President/CEO . . . . Greg Burns
Emergency Room . . . . Joel Stoeckeler, MD

Measure	Cases	This Hospital	State Average	U.S. Average	Top Hospital
Heart Attack Care					
ACE Inhibitor or ARB for LVSD[3]	0	-	85%	82%	100%
Aspirin at Arrival[1,3]	3	100%	94%	92%	100%
Aspirin at Discharge[1,3]	3	100%	94%	90%	100%
Beta Blocker at Arrival[1,3]	1	100%	92%	87%	100%
Beta Blocker at Discharge[1,3]	2	100%	92%	90%	100%
Fibrinolytic Medication Timing[3]	0	-	13%	31%	100%
PCI Within 90 Minutes of Arrival	0	-	75%	54%	95%
Smoking Cessation Advice[3]	0	-	91%	88%	100%
Heart Failure Care					
ACE Inhibitor or ARB for LVSD[1]	5	80%	86%	82%	100%

NOTE: Hospital profiles are in alphabetical order by state, then city, then hospital within the city; Rankings are sorted by rate in descending order and exclude hospitals with less than 25 cases; (1) The number of cases is too small (n<25) for purposes of reliably predicting hospital performance; (2) Measure reflects the hospital's indication that its submission was based upon a sample of its relevant discharges; (3) Rate reflects fewer than the maximum possible quarters of data for the measure; (4) Inaccurate information submitted and suppressed for one or more quarters; (5) No data is available from the hospital for this measure; Please refer to the User's Guide for a full explanation of data

Discharge Instructions[1]	11	45%	73%	61%	93%
Evaluation of LVS Function[1]	18	72%	88%	83%	99%
Smoking Cessation Advice[1]	2	50%	80%	82%	100%
Pneumonia Care					
Appropriate Initial Antibiotic	46	93%	87%	83%	94%
Blood Culture Timing[1]	19	89%	94%	90%	100%
Influenza Vaccine[1]	13	100%	79%	70%	100%
Initial Antibiotic Timing	71	96%	87%	80%	93%
Oxygenation Assessment	101	100%	100%	99%	100%
Pneumococcal Vaccine	66	88%	78%	69%	94%
Smoking Cessation Advice[1]	14	64%	82%	80%	100%
Surgical Infection Prevention					
Prophylactic Antibiotic Given	74	47%	84%	77%	95%
Prophylactic Antibiotic Selection[1]	9	100%	93%	90%	100%
Prophylactic Antibiotic Stopped	68	91%	80%	72%	95%
Pregnancy Care					
Inpatient Neonatal Mortality	-	-	-	-	-
Third or Fourth Degree Laceration	-	-	3.43%	3.63%	3.27%

Saint Clare Hospital Health Services

707 14th Street
Baraboo, WI 53913
URL: www.stclare.com
Ownership: Voluntary non-profit - Church
Emergency Services: Yes

Phone: 608-356-1400
Fax: 608-356-1367

Accredited: Yes
Licensed Beds: 84

Key Personnel:

President/CEO . . . . Sandra Anderson
Chief Medical Staff. . . . . Erich Herbest
Director Cardiology . . . . Al Garvan
Head Emergency Room. . . . . Theresa Weiland
Director Respiratory . . . . Bob Neilson

Measure	Cases	This Hospital	State Average	U.S. Average	Top Hospital
Heart Attack Care					
ACE Inhibitor or ARB for LVSD[1]	1	100%	85%	82%	100%
Aspirin at Arrival[1]	13	85%	94%	92%	100%
Aspirin at Discharge[1]	5	100%	94%	90%	100%
Beta Blocker at Arrival[1]	3	67%	92%	87%	100%
Beta Blocker at Discharge[1]	6	83%	92%	90%	100%
Fibrinolytic Medication Timing	0	-	13%	31%	100%
PCI Within 90 Minutes of Arrival	0	-	75%	54%	95%
Smoking Cessation Advice	0	-	91%	88%	100%
Heart Failure Care					
ACE Inhibitor or ARB for LVSD[1]	14	86%	86%	82%	100%
Discharge Instructions	32	44%	73%	61%	93%
Evaluation of LVS Function	53	91%	88%	83%	99%
Smoking Cessation Advice[1]	7	86%	80%	82%	100%
Pneumonia Care					
Appropriate Initial Antibiotic	33	76%	87%	83%	94%
Blood Culture Timing	36	81%	94%	90%	100%
Influenza Vaccine[1]	12	75%	79%	70%	100%
Initial Antibiotic Timing	64	83%	87%	80%	93%
Oxygenation Assessment	74	100%	100%	99%	100%
Pneumococcal Vaccine	54	78%	78%	69%	94%
Smoking Cessation Advice[1]	9	78%	82%	80%	100%
Surgical Infection Prevention					
Prophylactic Antibiotic Given[3]	85	95%	84%	77%	95%
Prophylactic Antibiotic Selection	26	92%	93%	90%	100%
Prophylactic Antibiotic Stopped[3]	80	98%	80%	72%	95%
Pregnancy Care					
Inpatient Neonatal Mortality	326	0.00%	-	-	-
Third or Fourth Degree Laceration	243	4.12%	3.43%	3.63%	3.27%

Barron Memorial Med Ctr-Mayo Health System

Alternate Name: Barron Medical Center
1222 E Woodland Avenue
Barron, WI 54812
URL: www.barronmedicalcenter.org
Ownership: Voluntary non-profit - Other
Emergency Services: Yes

Phone: 715-537-3186
Fax: 715-537-9023

Accredited: Yes
Licensed Beds: 29

Key Personnel:

Administrator . . . . Brad Groseth
Chief Medical Staff. . . . . Michael Damroth
Emergency Room Director. . . . . Lorna Larson, RN
Director Infection/Disease Control . . . . Kim Droege
Director Medical/Surgical Nursing . . . . Nancy Cusick, RN
Director Radiology . . . . Lori Turauski
Director Respiratory Therapy . . . . Dallas Crowe

Measure	Cases	This Hospital	State Average	U.S. Average	Top Hospital
Heart Attack Care					
ACE Inhibitor or ARB for LVSD[1,3]	1	100%	85%	82%	100%
Aspirin at Arrival[1,3]	9	89%	94%	92%	100%
Aspirin at Discharge[1,3]	8	100%	94%	90%	100%
Beta Blocker at Arrival[1,3]	6	83%	92%	87%	100%
Beta Blocker at Discharge[1,3]	6	83%	92%	90%	100%
Fibrinolytic Medication Timing[3]	0	-	13%	31%	100%
PCI Within 90 Minutes of Arrival[5]	-	-	75%	54%	95%
Smoking Cessation Advice[3]	0	-	91%	88%	100%
Heart Failure Care					
ACE Inhibitor or ARB for LVSD[1]	8	100%	86%	82%	100%
Discharge Instructions[1]	11	91%	73%	61%	93%
Evaluation of LVS Function	31	87%	88%	83%	99%
Smoking Cessation Advice[1]	3	67%	80%	82%	100%
Pneumonia Care					
Appropriate Initial Antibiotic[1]	9	100%	87%	83%	94%
Blood Culture Timing[1]	9	89%	94%	90%	100%
Influenza Vaccine[1]	6	83%	79%	70%	100%
Initial Antibiotic Timing[1]	16	94%	87%	80%	93%
Oxygenation Assessment[1]	20	100%	100%	99%	100%
Pneumococcal Vaccine[1]	14	93%	78%	69%	94%
Smoking Cessation Advice[1]	2	100%	82%	80%	100%
Surgical Infection Prevention					
Prophylactic Antibiotic Given[1,3]	6	100%	84%	77%	95%
Prophylactic Antibiotic Selection[5]	-	-	93%	90%	100%
Prophylactic Antibiotic Stopped[1,3]	6	83%	80%	72%	95%
Pregnancy Care					
Inpatient Neonatal Mortality	-	-	-	-	-
Third or Fourth Degree Laceration	-	-	3.43%	3.63%	3.27%

Beaver Dam Community Hospital

707 S University Avenue
Beaver Dam, WI 53916
Ownership: Voluntary non-profit - Private
Emergency Services: Yes

Phone: 920-887-7181
Fax: 920-887-3422
Accredited: Yes
Licensed Beds: 125

Key Personnel:

President . . . . John R Landdeck
VP . . . . Joe Bonnett
Director ICU/Medical/Surgical . . . . Judy MacDonald
Director Urgent Care & ER. . . . . Gladys Briggs
Nurse Director of Women's Health. . . . . Sue Ellen Siatos, RN
Director OR/OP/Day Surgery/OP Medical . . . . . Julie Nampel
Director of Pulmonary . . . . Sue Falton

Measure	Cases	This Hospital	State Average	U.S. Average	Top Hospital
Heart Attack Care					
ACE Inhibitor or ARB for LVSD[1]	5	100%	85%	82%	100%
Aspirin at Arrival[1]	22	95%	94%	92%	100%
Aspirin at Discharge[1]	18	78%	94%	90%	100%
Beta Blocker at Arrival[1]	20	95%	92%	87%	100%
Beta Blocker at Discharge[1]	18	83%	92%	90%	100%
Fibrinolytic Medication Timing	0	-	13%	31%	100%
PCI Within 90 Minutes of Arrival	0	-	75%	54%	95%
Smoking Cessation Advice	0	-	91%	88%	100%
Heart Failure Care					
ACE Inhibitor or ARB for LVSD[1]	16	94%	86%	82%	100%
Discharge Instructions	39	56%	73%	61%	93%
Evaluation of LVS Function	56	95%	88%	83%	99%
Smoking Cessation Advice[1]	10	40%	80%	82%	100%
Pneumonia Care					
Appropriate Initial Antibiotic	67	88%	87%	83%	94%
Blood Culture Timing	48	94%	94%	90%	100%
Influenza Vaccine	30	87%	79%	70%	100%
Initial Antibiotic Timing	114	91%	87%	80%	93%
Oxygenation Assessment	137	99%	100%	99%	100%

NOTE: Hospital profiles are in alphabetical order by state, then city, then hospital within the city; Rankings are sorted by rate in descending order and exclude hospitals with less than 25 cases; (1) The number of cases is too small (n<25) for purposes of reliably predicting hospital performance; (2) Measure reflects the hospital's indication that its submission was based upon a sample of its relevant discharges; (3) Rate reflects fewer than the maximum possible quarters of data for the measure; (4) Inaccurate information submitted and suppressed for one or more quarters; (5) No data is available from the hospital for this measure; Please refer to the User's Guide for a full explanation of data

Measure	Cases	This Hospital	State Average	U.S. Average	Top Hospital
Pneumococcal Vaccine	101	67%	78%	69%	94%
Smoking Cessation Advice[1]	23	61%	82%	80%	100%
Surgical Infection Prevention					
Prophylactic Antibiotic Given[3]	213	93%	84%	77%	95%
Prophylactic Antibiotic Selection	74	92%	93%	90%	100%
Prophylactic Antibiotic Stopped[3]	210	84%	80%	72%	95%
Pregnancy Care					
Inpatient Neonatal Mortality	-	-	-	-	-
Third or Fourth Degree Laceration	-	-	3.43%	3.63%	3.27%

Beloit Memorial Hospital

1969 W Hart Road
Beloit, WI 53511
Ownership: Voluntary non-profit - Private
Emergency Services: Yes

Phone: 608-364-5011
Fax: 608-364-5356
Accredited: Yes
Licensed Beds: 174

Key Personnel:

President/CEO . . . . Gregory K Britton
Infection Control . . . . Karen Draves
Director of Surgical Services . . . . Shirley Fischer
Director Radiology . . . . Miguel Jimenez
Director of Pulmonary . . . . Jane Hogan

Measure	Cases	This Hospital	State Average	U.S. Average	Top Hospital
Heart Attack Care					
ACE Inhibitor or ARB for LVSD[1]	12	75%	85%	82%	100%
Aspirin at Arrival	56	95%	94%	92%	100%
Aspirin at Discharge	32	97%	94%	90%	100%
Beta Blocker at Arrival	55	95%	92%	87%	100%
Beta Blocker at Discharge	44	95%	92%	90%	100%
Fibrinolytic Medication Timing[1]	8	25%	13%	31%	100%
PCI Within 90 Minutes of Arrival	0	-	75%	54%	95%
Smoking Cessation Advice[1]	12	100%	91%	88%	100%
Heart Failure Care					
ACE Inhibitor or ARB for LVSD	73	82%	86%	82%	100%
Discharge Instructions	125	74%	73%	61%	93%
Evaluation of LVS Function	151	89%	88%	83%	99%
Smoking Cessation Advice	36	97%	80%	82%	100%
Pneumonia Care					
Appropriate Initial Antibiotic	89	91%	87%	83%	94%
Blood Culture Timing	72	90%	94%	90%	100%
Influenza Vaccine[4,5]	-	-	79%	70%	100%
Initial Antibiotic Timing	121	88%	87%	80%	93%
Oxygenation Assessment	150	100%	100%	99%	100%
Pneumococcal Vaccine	97	72%	78%	69%	94%
Smoking Cessation Advice	41	88%	82%	80%	100%
Surgical Infection Prevention					
Prophylactic Antibiotic Given	290	88%	84%	77%	95%
Prophylactic Antibiotic Selection	60	87%	93%	90%	100%
Prophylactic Antibiotic Stopped	279	74%	80%	72%	95%
Pregnancy Care					
Inpatient Neonatal Mortality	-	-	-	-	-
Third or Fourth Degree Laceration	-	-	3.43%	3.63%	3.27%

Berlin Memorial Hospital

225 Memorial Drive
Berlin, WI 54923
Ownership: Voluntary non-profit - Other
Emergency Services: Yes

Phone: 920-361-1313
Fax: 920-361-5318
Accredited: Yes
Licensed Beds: 61

Key Personnel:

President/CEO . . . . Craig WC Schmidt
Chief Medical Staff . . . . Jeff Carroll, MD
Emergency Room . . . . Dan Perrault, MD
Director Infection/Disease Control . . . . Kathy Beier
CCU Spvg. Nurse . . . . Kelly Schmude
Director Medical/Surgical Nursing . . . . Marilyn Dehling
OB/GYN Womens Health . . . . Patrick Bruno, MD
Director Cardio-Pulmonary Services . . . . Cathy Pomerleau

Measure	Cases	This Hospital	State Average	U.S. Average	Top Hospital
Heart Attack Care					
ACE Inhibitor or ARB for LVSD[3]	0	-	85%	82%	100%
Aspirin at Arrival[1,3]	8	100%	94%	92%	100%
Aspirin at Discharge[1,3]	5	80%	94%	90%	100%
Beta Blocker at Arrival[1,3]	5	100%	92%	87%	100%
Beta Blocker at Discharge[1,3]	5	100%	92%	90%	100%
Fibrinolytic Medication Timing[3]	0	-	13%	31%	100%
PCI Within 90 Minutes of Arrival[5]	-	-	75%	54%	95%
Smoking Cessation Advice[3]	0	-	91%	88%	100%
Heart Failure Care					
ACE Inhibitor or ARB for LVSD[1]	14	93%	86%	82%	100%
Discharge Instructions	41	80%	73%	61%	93%
Evaluation of LVS Function	63	83%	88%	83%	99%
Smoking Cessation Advice[1]	8	100%	80%	82%	100%
Pneumonia Care					
Appropriate Initial Antibiotic	42	93%	87%	83%	94%
Blood Culture Timing	41	100%	94%	90%	100%
Influenza Vaccine[1]	8	75%	79%	70%	100%
Initial Antibiotic Timing	69	81%	87%	80%	93%
Oxygenation Assessment	76	100%	100%	99%	100%
Pneumococcal Vaccine	60	87%	78%	69%	94%
Smoking Cessation Advice[1]	9	100%	82%	80%	100%
Surgical Infection Prevention					
Prophylactic Antibiotic Given	186	86%	84%	77%	95%
Prophylactic Antibiotic Selection	43	30%	93%	90%	100%
Prophylactic Antibiotic Stopped	184	76%	80%	72%	95%
Pregnancy Care					
Inpatient Neonatal Mortality	-	-	-	-	-
Third or Fourth Degree Laceration	-	-	3.43%	3.63%	3.27%

Black River Memorial Hospital

711 W Adams Street
Black River Falls, WI 54615
URL: www.brmh.net
Ownership: Voluntary non-profit - Private
Emergency Services: Yes

Phone: 715-284-5361
Fax: 715-284-7166
Accredited: Yes
Licensed Beds: 51

Key Personnel:

CEO . . . . Stam Gaynor
Emergency Room . . . . Barb Holderman, RN
Director of Respiratory . . . . Jackie Alinson

Measure	Cases	This Hospital	State Average	U.S. Average	Top Hospital
Heart Attack Care					
ACE Inhibitor or ARB for LVSD	0	-	85%	82%	100%
Aspirin at Arrival[1]	7	100%	94%	92%	100%
Aspirin at Discharge[1]	5	100%	94%	90%	100%
Beta Blocker at Arrival[1]	7	100%	92%	87%	100%
Beta Blocker at Discharge[1]	5	100%	92%	90%	100%
Fibrinolytic Medication Timing	0	-	13%	31%	100%
PCI Within 90 Minutes of Arrival	0	-	75%	54%	95%
Smoking Cessation Advice[1]	1	100%	91%	88%	100%
Heart Failure Care					
ACE Inhibitor or ARB for LVSD	32	100%	86%	82%	100%
Discharge Instructions	27	100%	73%	61%	93%
Evaluation of LVS Function	35	100%	88%	83%	99%
Smoking Cessation Advice[1]	1	0%	80%	82%	100%
Pneumonia Care					
Appropriate Initial Antibiotic	38	61%	87%	83%	94%
Blood Culture Timing[1]	11	82%	94%	90%	100%
Influenza Vaccine[1]	9	78%	79%	70%	100%
Initial Antibiotic Timing	40	90%	87%	80%	93%
Oxygenation Assessment	47	100%	100%	99%	100%
Pneumococcal Vaccine	39	82%	78%	69%	94%
Smoking Cessation Advice[1]	6	50%	82%	80%	100%
Surgical Infection Prevention					
Prophylactic Antibiotic Given[5]	-	-	84%	77%	95%
Prophylactic Antibiotic Selection[5]	-	-	93%	90%	100%
Prophylactic Antibiotic Stopped[5]	-	-	80%	72%	95%
Pregnancy Care					
Inpatient Neonatal Mortality	-	-	-	-	-
Third or Fourth Degree Laceration	-	-	3.43%	3.63%	3.27%

NOTE: Hospital profiles are in alphabetical order by state, then city, then hospital within the city; Rankings are sorted by rate in descending order and exclude hospitals with less than 25 cases; (1) The number of cases is too small (n<25) for purposes of reliably predicting hospital performance; (2) Measure reflects the hospital's indication that its submission was based upon a sample of its relevant discharges; (3) Rate reflects fewer than the maximum possible quarters of data for the measure; (4) Inaccurate information submitted and suppressed for one or more quarters; (5) No data is available from the hospital for this measure; Please refer to the User's Guide for a full explanation of data

Bloomer Medical Center

1501 Thompson Street
Bloomer, WI 54724
E-mail: kerg.mary@mayo.edu
Ownership: Voluntary non-profit - Other
Emergency Services: Yes
Phone: 715-568-2000
Fax: 715-568-2000
Accredited: Yes
Licensed Beds: 37

Key Personnel:
CEO. . . . . John Larson, MD
Chief Medical Staff. . . . . Richard Gladitsch, MD
Director Infection/Disease Control . . . . Mel Crisp
Director Medical/Surgical Nursing . . . . Jill Hurlburt
Director Respiratory Therapy . . . . Kay Dahlka

Measure	Cases	This Hospital	State Average	U.S. Average	Top Hospital
Heart Attack Care					
ACE Inhibitor or ARB for LVSD[5]	-	-	85%	82%	100%
Aspirin at Arrival[5]	-	-	94%	92%	100%
Aspirin at Discharge[5]	-	-	94%	90%	100%
Beta Blocker at Arrival[5]	-	-	92%	87%	100%
Beta Blocker at Discharge[5]	-	-	92%	90%	100%
Fibrinolytic Medication Timing[5]	-	-	13%	31%	100%
PCI Within 90 Minutes of Arrival[5]	-	-	75%	54%	95%
Smoking Cessation Advice[5]	-	-	91%	88%	100%
Heart Failure Care					
ACE Inhibitor or ARB for LVSD	0	-	86%	82%	100%
Discharge Instructions[1]	6	100%	73%	61%	93%
Evaluation of LVS Function[1]	10	100%	88%	83%	99%
Smoking Cessation Advice	0	-	80%	82%	100%
Pneumonia Care					
Appropriate Initial Antibiotic[1]	13	92%	87%	83%	94%
Blood Culture Timing[1]	8	100%	94%	90%	100%
Influenza Vaccine[1]	3	100%	79%	70%	100%
Initial Antibiotic Timing[1]	17	100%	87%	80%	93%
Oxygenation Assessment[1]	21	100%	100%	99%	100%
Pneumococcal Vaccine[1]	18	100%	78%	69%	94%
Smoking Cessation Advice[1]	1	100%	82%	80%	100%
Surgical Infection Prevention					
Prophylactic Antibiotic Given[3]	0	-	84%	77%	95%
Prophylactic Antibiotic Selection	0	-	93%	90%	100%
Prophylactic Antibiotic Stopped[3]	0	-	80%	72%	95%
Pregnancy Care					
Inpatient Neonatal Mortality	-	-	-	-	-
Third or Fourth Degree Laceration	-	-	3.43%	3.63%	3.27%

Boscobel Area Health Care

Alternate Name: Memorial Hospital of Boscobel
205 Parker Street
Boscobel, WI 53805
URL: www.boscobelhealth.com
Ownership: Voluntary non-profit - Private
Emergency Services: Yes
Phone: 608-375-4112
Fax: 608-375-5463
Accredited: No
Licensed Beds: 123

Key Personnel:
Administrator . . . . Gary Bezucha
Chief Medical Staff. . . . . Thomas Pelz
Medical/Surgical Nursing Director . . . . Jennifer Rutkowski
Manager Radiology . . . . Rita Ferrie
Respiratory Therapy Director . . . . Deb Welsh

Measure	Cases	This Hospital	State Average	U.S. Average	Top Hospital
Heart Attack Care					
ACE Inhibitor or ARB for LVSD[1]	1	100%	85%	82%	100%
Aspirin at Arrival[1]	2	50%	94%	92%	100%
Aspirin at Discharge[1]	2	50%	94%	90%	100%
Beta Blocker at Arrival[1]	2	100%	92%	87%	100%
Beta Blocker at Discharge[1]	3	67%	92%	90%	100%
Fibrinolytic Medication Timing	0	-	13%	31%	100%
PCI Within 90 Minutes of Arrival	0	-	75%	54%	95%
Smoking Cessation Advice	0	-	91%	88%	100%
Heart Failure Care					
ACE Inhibitor or ARB for LVSD[1]	2	100%	86%	82%	100%
Discharge Instructions[1]	13	0%	73%	61%	93%
Evaluation of LVS Function[1]	16	50%	88%	83%	99%
Smoking Cessation Advice	0	-	80%	82%	100%
Pneumonia Care					
Appropriate Initial Antibiotic[1]	11	91%	87%	83%	94%
Blood Culture Timing[1]	3	100%	94%	90%	100%
Influenza Vaccine[1]	2	100%	79%	70%	100%
Initial Antibiotic Timing[1]	13	54%	87%	80%	93%
Oxygenation Assessment[1]	16	100%	100%	99%	100%
Pneumococcal Vaccine[1]	11	64%	78%	69%	94%
Smoking Cessation Advice[1]	1	100%	82%	80%	100%
Surgical Infection Prevention					
Prophylactic Antibiotic Given[5]	-	-	84%	77%	95%
Prophylactic Antibiotic Selection[5]	-	-	93%	90%	100%
Prophylactic Antibiotic Stopped[5]	-	-	80%	72%	95%
Pregnancy Care					
Inpatient Neonatal Mortality	-	-	-	-	-
Third or Fourth Degree Laceration	-	-	3.43%	3.63%	3.27%

Elmbrook Memorial Hospital

19333 W North Avenue
Brookfield, WI 53045
URL: www.elmbrookmemorial.com
Ownership: Voluntary non-profit - Church
Emergency Services: Yes
Phone: 262-785-2000
Fax: 262-785-2444
Accredited: Yes
Licensed Beds: 166

Key Personnel:
President . . . . Kimry Johnson
Director Radiology . . . . Paul Minzlaff

Measure	Cases	This Hospital	State Average	U.S. Average	Top Hospital
Heart Attack Care					
ACE Inhibitor or ARB for LVSD[1]	2	50%	85%	82%	100%
Aspirin at Arrival[1]	14	93%	94%	92%	100%
Aspirin at Discharge[1]	11	82%	94%	90%	100%
Beta Blocker at Arrival[1]	5	80%	92%	87%	100%
Beta Blocker at Discharge[1]	7	100%	92%	90%	100%
Fibrinolytic Medication Timing	0	-	13%	31%	100%
PCI Within 90 Minutes of Arrival	0	-	75%	54%	95%
Smoking Cessation Advice	0	-	91%	88%	100%
Heart Failure Care					
ACE Inhibitor or ARB for LVSD	30	90%	86%	82%	100%
Discharge Instructions	88	53%	73%	61%	93%
Evaluation of LVS Function	96	98%	88%	83%	99%
Smoking Cessation Advice[1]	11	100%	80%	82%	100%
Pneumonia Care					
Appropriate Initial Antibiotic	99	88%	87%	83%	94%
Blood Culture Timing	100	98%	94%	90%	100%
Influenza Vaccine	25	96%	79%	70%	100%
Initial Antibiotic Timing	144	91%	87%	80%	93%
Oxygenation Assessment	182	100%	100%	99%	100%
Pneumococcal Vaccine	130	79%	78%	69%	94%
Smoking Cessation Advice	36	100%	82%	80%	100%
Surgical Infection Prevention					
Prophylactic Antibiotic Given[3]	311	71%	84%	77%	95%
Prophylactic Antibiotic Selection	38	89%	93%	90%	100%
Prophylactic Antibiotic Stopped[3]	305	67%	80%	72%	95%
Pregnancy Care					
Inpatient Neonatal Mortality	-	-	-	-	-
Third or Fourth Degree Laceration	-	-	3.43%	3.63%	3.27%

Aurora Memorial Hospital of Burlington

252 McHenry Street
Burlington, WI 53105
URL: www.aurorahealthcare.org
Ownership: Voluntary non-profit - Private
Emergency Services: Yes
Phone: 262-767-6000
Fax: 262-767-6380
Accredited: Yes
Licensed Beds: 123

Key Personnel:
Administrator . . . . Ann Navera
Chief Medical Staff. . . . . Laurence Tempelis, MD
Emergency Room . . . . John Linstroth, MD
Director Infection/Disease Control . . . . Gwria McPeek
CCU Spvg. Nurse . . . . Diane Huck
Director Respiratory Therapy . . . . Terri Newbury

Measure	Cases	This Hospital	State Average	U.S. Average	Top Hospital

NOTE: Hospital profiles are in alphabetical order by state, then city, then hospital within the city; Rankings are sorted by rate in descending order and exclude hospitals with less than 25 cases; (1) The number of cases is too small (n<25) for purposes of reliably predicting hospital performance; (2) Measure reflects the hospital's indication that its submission was based upon a sample of its relevant discharges; (3) Rate reflects fewer than the maximum possible quarters of data for the measure; (4) Inaccurate information submitted and suppressed for one or more quarters; (5) No data is available from the hospital for this measure; Please refer to the User's Guide for a full explanation of data

Measure	Cases	This Hospital	State Average	U.S. Average	Top Hospital
Heart Attack Care					
ACE Inhibitor or ARB for LVSD[1]	3	100%	85%	82%	100%
Aspirin at Arrival	25	100%	94%	92%	100%
Aspirin at Discharge[1]	12	100%	94%	90%	100%
Beta Blocker at Arrival[1]	19	100%	92%	87%	100%
Beta Blocker at Discharge[1]	12	100%	92%	90%	100%
Fibrinolytic Medication Timing	0	-	13%	31%	100%
PCI Within 90 Minutes of Arrival	0	-	75%	54%	95%
Smoking Cessation Advice[1]	5	100%	91%	88%	100%
Heart Failure Care					
ACE Inhibitor or ARB for LVSD	27	93%	86%	82%	100%
Discharge Instructions	88	97%	73%	61%	93%
Evaluation of LVS Function	114	100%	88%	83%	99%
Smoking Cessation Advice[1]	14	100%	80%	82%	100%
Pneumonia Care					
Appropriate Initial Antibiotic	70	97%	87%	83%	94%
Blood Culture Timing	66	98%	94%	90%	100%
Influenza Vaccine[1]	10	100%	79%	70%	100%
Initial Antibiotic Timing	92	99%	87%	80%	93%
Oxygenation Assessment	125	100%	100%	99%	100%
Pneumococcal Vaccine	78	100%	78%	69%	94%
Smoking Cessation Advice	31	100%	82%	80%	100%
Surgical Infection Prevention					
Prophylactic Antibiotic Given[2,3]	89	90%	84%	77%	95%
Prophylactic Antibiotic Selection[2]	44	98%	93%	90%	100%
Prophylactic Antibiotic Stopped[2,3]	86	87%	80%	72%	95%
Pregnancy Care					
Inpatient Neonatal Mortality	-	-	-	-	-
Third or Fourth Degree Laceration	-	-	3.43%	3.63%	3.27%

Calumet Memorial Hospital

614 Memorial Drive
Chilton, WI 53014
Phone: 920-849-2386
Fax: 920-849-7510
URL: www.ministryhealth.org
Ownership: Voluntary non-profit - Other
Accredited: Yes
Emergency Services: Yes
Licensed Beds: 29

Key Personnel:

President/CEO . . . . Travis Anderson

Measure	Cases	This Hospital	State Average	U.S. Average	Top Hospital
Heart Attack Care					
ACE Inhibitor or ARB for LVSD[5]	-	-	85%	82%	100%
Aspirin at Arrival[5]	-	-	94%	92%	100%
Aspirin at Discharge[5]	-	-	94%	90%	100%
Beta Blocker at Arrival[5]	-	-	92%	87%	100%
Beta Blocker at Discharge[5]	-	-	92%	90%	100%
Fibrinolytic Medication Timing[5]	-	-	13%	31%	100%
PCI Within 90 Minutes of Arrival[5]	-	-	75%	54%	95%
Smoking Cessation Advice[5]	-	-	91%	88%	100%
Heart Failure Care					
ACE Inhibitor or ARB for LVSD[1]	3	100%	86%	82%	100%
Discharge Instructions[1]	11	82%	73%	61%	93%
Evaluation of LVS Function[1]	19	95%	88%	83%	99%
Smoking Cessation Advice[1]	1	100%	80%	82%	100%
Pneumonia Care					
Appropriate Initial Antibiotic[1]	21	100%	87%	83%	94%
Blood Culture Timing[1]	19	100%	94%	90%	100%
Influenza Vaccine[1]	5	80%	79%	70%	100%
Initial Antibiotic Timing	33	94%	87%	80%	93%
Oxygenation Assessment	42	100%	100%	99%	100%
Pneumococcal Vaccine	33	82%	78%	69%	94%
Smoking Cessation Advice[1]	5	60%	82%	80%	100%
Surgical Infection Prevention					
Prophylactic Antibiotic Given	27	78%	84%	77%	95%
Prophylactic Antibiotic Selection[1]	2	100%	93%	90%	100%
Prophylactic Antibiotic Stopped	26	65%	80%	72%	95%
Pregnancy Care					
Inpatient Neonatal Mortality	-	-	-	-	-
Third or Fourth Degree Laceration	-	-	3.43%	3.63%	3.27%

Saint Joseph's Hospital

2661 County Highway I
Chippewa Falls, WI 54729
Phone: 715-723-1811
Fax: 715-726-3204
URL: www.stjoeschipfalls.com
Ownership: Voluntary non-profit - Church
Accredited: Yes
Emergency Services: Yes
Licensed Beds: 193

Key Personnel:

President/CEO . . . . David Fish
Chief Medical Staff . . . . Jeffrey Brown, MD
Director of Emergency Room . . . . Maureen Pherou
Infection Control . . . . Debra Neitge
Medical/Surgical Nursing . . . . Carolyn Penk
Surgery . . . . Gary Wulff, RN
Respiratory/Cardiopulmonary . . . . Brad McNutt

Measure	Cases	This Hospital	State Average	U.S. Average	Top Hospital
Heart Attack Care					
ACE Inhibitor or ARB for LVSD[1]	1	100%	85%	82%	100%
Aspirin at Arrival[1]	17	76%	94%	92%	100%
Aspirin at Discharge[1]	16	88%	94%	90%	100%
Beta Blocker at Arrival[1]	9	89%	92%	87%	100%
Beta Blocker at Discharge[1]	13	85%	92%	90%	100%
Fibrinolytic Medication Timing	0	-	13%	31%	100%
PCI Within 90 Minutes of Arrival	0	-	75%	54%	95%
Smoking Cessation Advice[1]	2	50%	91%	88%	100%
Heart Failure Care					
ACE Inhibitor or ARB for LVSD[1]	14	93%	86%	82%	100%
Discharge Instructions	38	87%	73%	61%	93%
Evaluation of LVS Function	42	88%	88%	83%	99%
Smoking Cessation Advice[1]	2	100%	80%	82%	100%
Pneumonia Care					
Appropriate Initial Antibiotic	56	75%	87%	83%	94%
Blood Culture Timing	43	98%	94%	90%	100%
Influenza Vaccine[1]	17	88%	79%	70%	100%
Initial Antibiotic Timing	79	91%	87%	80%	93%
Oxygenation Assessment	90	100%	100%	99%	100%
Pneumococcal Vaccine	66	83%	78%	69%	94%
Smoking Cessation Advice[1]	15	100%	82%	80%	100%
Surgical Infection Prevention					
Prophylactic Antibiotic Given	226	96%	84%	77%	95%
Prophylactic Antibiotic Selection	47	100%	93%	90%	100%
Prophylactic Antibiotic Stopped	214	89%	80%	72%	95%
Pregnancy Care					
Inpatient Neonatal Mortality	-	-	-	-	-
Third or Fourth Degree Laceration	-	-	3.43%	3.63%	3.27%

Columbus Community Hospital

1515 Park Ave
Columbus, WI 53925
Phone: 920-623-2200
Ownership: Voluntary non-profit - Private
Accredited: Yes
Emergency Services: Yes

Measure	Cases	This Hospital	State Average	U.S. Average	Top Hospital
Heart Attack Care					
ACE Inhibitor or ARB for LVSD[1]	1	0%	85%	82%	100%
Aspirin at Arrival[1]	11	100%	94%	92%	100%
Aspirin at Discharge[1]	9	100%	94%	90%	100%
Beta Blocker at Arrival[1]	12	92%	92%	87%	100%
Beta Blocker at Discharge[1]	10	80%	92%	90%	100%
Fibrinolytic Medication Timing	0	-	13%	31%	100%
PCI Within 90 Minutes of Arrival	0	-	75%	54%	95%
Smoking Cessation Advice	0	-	91%	88%	100%
Heart Failure Care					
ACE Inhibitor or ARB for LVSD[1]	8	100%	86%	82%	100%
Discharge Instructions[1]	11	73%	73%	61%	93%
Evaluation of LVS Function[1]	21	67%	88%	83%	99%
Smoking Cessation Advice	0	-	80%	82%	100%
Pneumonia Care					
Appropriate Initial Antibiotic	43	84%	87%	83%	94%
Blood Culture Timing[1]	22	91%	94%	90%	100%
Influenza Vaccine[1]	8	75%	79%	70%	100%
Initial Antibiotic Timing	52	79%	87%	80%	93%

NOTE: Hospital profiles are in alphabetical order by state, then city, then hospital within the city; Rankings are sorted by rate in descending order and exclude hospitals with less than 25 cases; (1) The number of cases is too small (n<25) for purposes of reliably predicting hospital performance; (2) Measure reflects the hospital's indication that its submission was based upon a sample of its relevant discharges; (3) Rate reflects fewer than the maximum possible quarters of data for the measure; (4) Inaccurate information submitted and suppressed for one or more quarters; (5) No data is available from the hospital for this measure; Please refer to the User's Guide for a full explanation of data

Measure	Cases	This Hospital	State Average	U.S. Average	Top Hospital
Oxygenation Assessment	66	98%	100%	99%	100%
Pneumococcal Vaccine	45	51%	78%	69%	94%
Smoking Cessation Advice[1]	5	20%	82%	80%	100%
Surgical Infection Prevention					
Prophylactic Antibiotic Given[5]	-	-	84%	77%	95%
Prophylactic Antibiotic Selection[5]	-	-	93%	90%	100%
Prophylactic Antibiotic Stopped[5]	-	-	80%	72%	95%
Pregnancy Care					
Inpatient Neonatal Mortality	-	-	-	-	-
Third or Fourth Degree Laceration	-	-	3.43%	3.63%	3.27%

Cumberland Memorial Hospital

1110 7th Avenue
Cumberland, WI 54829
URL: www.cumberlandhelathcare.com
Ownership: Voluntary non-profit - Private
Emergency Services: Yes

Phone: 715-822-2741
Fax: 715-822-2740

Accredited: Yes
Licensed Beds: 40

Key Personnel:
CEO. . . . . Robert J Hansen
Chief Medical Staff. . . . . B Ankarlo, MD
Emergency Room . . . . Janet Peterson, RN
Infection Control. . . . . Toniann Knutson, RN
Medical/Surgical Nursing . . . . Mary Ann Clark
Respiratory/Cardiopulmonary. . . . . Kelly Mathison, RT

Measure	Cases	This Hospital	State Average	U.S. Average	Top Hospital
Heart Attack Care					
ACE Inhibitor or ARB for LVSD	0	-	85%	82%	100%
Aspirin at Arrival[1]	4	100%	94%	92%	100%
Aspirin at Discharge[1]	3	100%	94%	90%	100%
Beta Blocker at Arrival[1]	4	100%	92%	87%	100%
Beta Blocker at Discharge[1]	3	100%	92%	90%	100%
Fibrinolytic Medication Timing[1]	1	0%	13%	31%	100%
PCI Within 90 Minutes of Arrival	0	-	75%	54%	95%
Smoking Cessation Advice	0	-	91%	88%	100%
Heart Failure Care					
ACE Inhibitor or ARB for LVSD[1]	8	50%	86%	82%	100%
Discharge Instructions[1]	21	52%	73%	61%	93%
Evaluation of LVS Function	25	60%	88%	83%	99%
Smoking Cessation Advice[1]	4	50%	80%	82%	100%
Pneumonia Care					
Appropriate Initial Antibiotic	54	61%	87%	83%	94%
Blood Culture Timing[1]	4	100%	94%	90%	100%
Influenza Vaccine[1]	8	88%	79%	70%	100%
Initial Antibiotic Timing	57	81%	87%	80%	93%
Oxygenation Assessment	71	96%	100%	99%	100%
Pneumococcal Vaccine	47	81%	78%	69%	94%
Smoking Cessation Advice[1]	15	67%	82%	80%	100%
Surgical Infection Prevention					
Prophylactic Antibiotic Given[5]	-	-	84%	77%	95%
Prophylactic Antibiotic Selection[5]	-	-	93%	90%	100%
Prophylactic Antibiotic Stopped[5]	-	-	80%	72%	95%
Pregnancy Care					
Inpatient Neonatal Mortality	-	-	-	-	-
Third or Fourth Degree Laceration	-	-	3.43%	3.63%	3.27%

Memorial Hospital of Lafayette County

PO Box 70
Darlington, WI 53530
Ownership: Government - Local
Emergency Services: Yes

Phone: 608-776-4466
Fax: 608-776-5701
Accredited: No
Licensed Beds: 28

Key Personnel:
Administrator . . . . Sherry Kudronowicz
Chief Medical Staff. . . . . Michael Robiolio, MD
Emergency Room . . . . Bob Bernardoni
Director Infection/Disease Control . . . . Pamela Gould
OB/GYN Womens Health. . . . . Bob Bernardoni
Director Respiratory Therapy . . . . Richard Hause

Measure	Cases	This Hospital	State Average	U.S. Average	Top Hospital
Heart Attack Care					
ACE Inhibitor or ARB for LVSD	0	-	85%	82%	100%
Aspirin at Arrival[1]	10	90%	94%	92%	100%
Aspirin at Discharge[1]	6	50%	94%	90%	100%
Beta Blocker at Arrival[1]	7	100%	92%	87%	100%
Beta Blocker at Discharge[1]	7	29%	92%	90%	100%
Fibrinolytic Medication Timing	0	-	13%	31%	100%
PCI Within 90 Minutes of Arrival	0	-	75%	54%	95%
Smoking Cessation Advice	0	-	91%	88%	100%
Heart Failure Care					
ACE Inhibitor or ARB for LVSD[1]	4	50%	86%	82%	100%
Discharge Instructions[1]	18	22%	73%	61%	93%
Evaluation of LVS Function[1]	22	68%	88%	83%	99%
Smoking Cessation Advice[1]	2	0%	80%	82%	100%
Pneumonia Care					
Appropriate Initial Antibiotic[1]	22	77%	87%	83%	94%
Blood Culture Timing[1]	2	100%	94%	90%	100%
Influenza Vaccine[1]	6	67%	79%	70%	100%
Initial Antibiotic Timing	33	91%	87%	80%	93%
Oxygenation Assessment	41	100%	100%	99%	100%
Pneumococcal Vaccine	31	45%	78%	69%	94%
Smoking Cessation Advice[1]	1	0%	82%	80%	100%
Surgical Infection Prevention					
Prophylactic Antibiotic Given	33	85%	84%	77%	95%
Prophylactic Antibiotic Selection[1]	3	100%	93%	90%	100%
Prophylactic Antibiotic Stopped	33	70%	80%	72%	95%
Pregnancy Care					
Inpatient Neonatal Mortality	-	-	-	-	-
Third or Fourth Degree Laceration	-	-	3.43%	3.63%	3.27%

Upland Hills Health

800 Compassion Way
Dodgeville, WI 53533
URL: www.uplandhillshealth.org
Ownership: Voluntary non-profit - Other
Emergency Services: Yes

Phone: 608-930-8000
Fax: 608-930-7250

Accredited: Yes
Licensed Beds: 40

Key Personnel:
Administrator . . . . Ray Marmorstone
Chief Medical Staff. . . . . Phyllis Fritsch
Emergency Room . . . . Gary Grunow
Infection Control. . . . . Maria Leary
Medical/Surgical Nursing . . . . Kathy Knudson
OB/GYN Womens Health. . . . . Pamela Rice
Chief Radiology . . . . Mark Rich, MD
Director Respiratory Therapy . . . . John Mason

Measure	Cases	This Hospital	State Average	U.S. Average	Top Hospital
Heart Attack Care					
ACE Inhibitor or ARB for LVSD[1]	1	100%	85%	82%	100%
Aspirin at Arrival[1]	5	100%	94%	92%	100%
Aspirin at Discharge[1]	5	100%	94%	90%	100%
Beta Blocker at Arrival[1]	5	100%	92%	87%	100%
Beta Blocker at Discharge[1]	5	100%	92%	90%	100%
Fibrinolytic Medication Timing	0	-	13%	31%	100%
PCI Within 90 Minutes of Arrival	0	-	75%	54%	95%
Smoking Cessation Advice	0	-	91%	88%	100%
Heart Failure Care					
ACE Inhibitor or ARB for LVSD[1]	10	100%	86%	82%	100%
Discharge Instructions[1]	21	62%	73%	61%	93%
Evaluation of LVS Function	32	75%	88%	83%	99%
Smoking Cessation Advice[1]	6	67%	80%	82%	100%
Pneumonia Care					
Appropriate Initial Antibiotic	37	84%	87%	83%	94%
Blood Culture Timing	27	96%	94%	90%	100%
Influenza Vaccine[1]	9	67%	79%	70%	100%
Initial Antibiotic Timing	52	88%	87%	80%	93%
Oxygenation Assessment	63	100%	100%	99%	100%
Pneumococcal Vaccine	53	85%	78%	69%	94%
Smoking Cessation Advice[1]	6	67%	82%	80%	100%
Surgical Infection Prevention					
Prophylactic Antibiotic Given[3]	62	95%	84%	77%	95%
Prophylactic Antibiotic Selection[1]	22	95%	93%	90%	100%
Prophylactic Antibiotic Stopped[3]	62	77%	80%	72%	95%
Pregnancy Care					

NOTE: Hospital profiles are in alphabetical order by state, then city, then hospital within the city; Rankings are sorted by rate in descending order and exclude hospitals with less than 25 cases; (1) The number of cases is too small (n<25) for purposes of reliably predicting hospital performance; (2) Measure reflects the hospital's indication that its submission was based upon a sample of its relevant discharges; (3) Rate reflects fewer than the maximum possible quarters of data for the measure; (4) Inaccurate information submitted and suppressed for one or more quarters; (5) No data is available from the hospital for this measure; Please refer to the User's Guide for a full explanation of data

Inpatient Neonatal Mortality	-	-	-	-	-
Third or Fourth Degree Laceration	-	-	3.43%	3.63%	3.27%

Luther Midelfort Hospital

1221 Whipple Street
PO Box 4105
Eau Claire, WI 54702
URL: www.luthermidelfort.org
Ownership: Voluntary non-profit - Other
Emergency Services: Yes
Toll-Free: 888-838-4777
Phone: 715-838-3311
Fax: 715-838-6449
Accredited: Yes
Licensed Beds: 304

Key Personnel:
President/CEO . . . . Randall Linton, MD
Senior Vice President . . . . John Dickey

Measure	Cases	This Hospital	State Average	U.S. Average	Top Hospital
Heart Attack Care					
ACE Inhibitor or ARB for LVSD	55	75%	85%	82%	100%
Aspirin at Arrival	99	97%	94%	92%	100%
Aspirin at Discharge	255	100%	94%	90%	100%
Beta Blocker at Arrival	102	93%	92%	87%	100%
Beta Blocker at Discharge	266	99%	92%	90%	100%
Fibrinolytic Medication Timing	0	-	13%	31%	100%
PCI Within 90 Minutes of Arrival[1]	4	100%	75%	54%	95%
Smoking Cessation Advice	79	96%	91%	88%	100%
Heart Failure Care					
ACE Inhibitor or ARB for LVSD	75	83%	86%	82%	100%
Discharge Instructions	166	92%	73%	61%	93%
Evaluation of LVS Function	223	100%	88%	83%	99%
Smoking Cessation Advice[1]	23	87%	80%	82%	100%
Pneumonia Care					
Appropriate Initial Antibiotic	131	95%	87%	83%	94%
Blood Culture Timing	131	95%	94%	90%	100%
Influenza Vaccine	50	96%	79%	70%	100%
Initial Antibiotic Timing	184	90%	87%	80%	93%
Oxygenation Assessment	237	100%	100%	99%	100%
Pneumococcal Vaccine	194	95%	78%	69%	94%
Smoking Cessation Advice	45	89%	82%	80%	100%
Surgical Infection Prevention					
Prophylactic Antibiotic Given	882	98%	84%	77%	95%
Prophylactic Antibiotic Selection	213	100%	93%	90%	100%
Prophylactic Antibiotic Stopped	777	95%	80%	72%	95%
Pregnancy Care					
Inpatient Neonatal Mortality	559	0.18%	-	-	-
Third or Fourth Degree Laceration	401	4.24%	3.43%	3.63%	3.27%

Oak Leaf Surgcl Hospital

3802 Oakwood Mall Dr
Eau Claire, WI 54701
Ownership: Proprietary
Emergency Services: No
Phone: 715-831-8130
Accredited: Yes

Measure	Cases	This Hospital	State Average	U.S. Average	Top Hospital
Heart Attack Care					
ACE Inhibitor or ARB for LVSD[5]	-	-	85%	82%	100%
Aspirin at Arrival[5]	-	-	94%	92%	100%
Aspirin at Discharge[5]	-	-	94%	90%	100%
Beta Blocker at Arrival[5]	-	-	92%	87%	100%
Beta Blocker at Discharge[5]	-	-	92%	90%	100%
Fibrinolytic Medication Timing[5]	-	-	13%	31%	100%
PCI Within 90 Minutes of Arrival[5]	-	-	75%	54%	95%
Smoking Cessation Advice[5]	-	-	91%	88%	100%
Heart Failure Care					
ACE Inhibitor or ARB for LVSD[5]	-	-	86%	82%	100%
Discharge Instructions[5]	-	-	73%	61%	93%
Evaluation of LVS Function[5]	-	-	88%	83%	99%
Smoking Cessation Advice[5]	-	-	80%	82%	100%
Pneumonia Care					
Appropriate Initial Antibiotic[5]	-	-	87%	83%	94%
Blood Culture Timing[5]	-	-	94%	90%	100%
Influenza Vaccine[5]	-	-	79%	70%	100%
Initial Antibiotic Timing[5]	-	-	87%	80%	93%
Oxygenation Assessment[5]	-	-	100%	99%	100%
Pneumococcal Vaccine[5]	-	-	78%	69%	94%
Smoking Cessation Advice[5]	-	-	82%	80%	100%
Surgical Infection Prevention					
Prophylactic Antibiotic Given[2,3]	59	76%	84%	77%	95%
Prophylactic Antibiotic Selection[5]	-	-	93%	90%	100%
Prophylactic Antibiotic Stopped[2,3]	57	88%	80%	72%	95%
Pregnancy Care					
Inpatient Neonatal Mortality	-	-	-	-	-
Third or Fourth Degree Laceration	-	-	3.43%	3.63%	3.27%

Sacred Heart Hospital

900 W Clairemont Avenue
Eau Claire, WI 54701
URL: www.sacredhearthospital-ec.org
Ownership: Voluntary non-profit - Church
Emergency Services: Yes
Phone: 715-839-4121
Fax: 715-833-4976
Accredited: Yes
Licensed Beds: 344

Key Personnel:
Administrator . . . . Steve Ronstrom
Chief Medical Staff . . . . Dr. Mark Steinmatz
Medical/Surgical Nursing . . . . Laurie Voight
OB/GYN Womens Health . . . . Greg Burnett, MD
Chief Radiology . . . . Thomas Edwards, MD

Measure	Cases	This Hospital	State Average	U.S. Average	Top Hospital
Heart Attack Care					
ACE Inhibitor or ARB for LVSD[1]	21	86%	85%	82%	100%
Aspirin at Arrival	76	93%	94%	92%	100%
Aspirin at Discharge	77	99%	94%	90%	100%
Beta Blocker at Arrival	64	92%	92%	87%	100%
Beta Blocker at Discharge	93	97%	92%	90%	100%
Fibrinolytic Medication Timing	0	-	13%	31%	100%
PCI Within 90 Minutes of Arrival[1]	5	20%	75%	54%	95%
Smoking Cessation Advice	30	100%	91%	88%	100%
Heart Failure Care					
ACE Inhibitor or ARB for LVSD	68	76%	86%	82%	100%
Discharge Instructions	141	75%	73%	61%	93%
Evaluation of LVS Function	193	97%	88%	83%	99%
Smoking Cessation Advice	32	94%	80%	82%	100%
Pneumonia Care					
Appropriate Initial Antibiotic	103	80%	87%	83%	94%
Blood Culture Timing	71	97%	94%	90%	100%
Influenza Vaccine	33	42%	79%	70%	100%
Initial Antibiotic Timing	160	86%	87%	80%	93%
Oxygenation Assessment	197	100%	100%	99%	100%
Pneumococcal Vaccine	138	33%	78%	69%	94%
Smoking Cessation Advice	50	98%	82%	80%	100%
Surgical Infection Prevention					
Prophylactic Antibiotic Given[3]	209	90%	84%	77%	95%
Prophylactic Antibiotic Selection	49	80%	93%	90%	100%
Prophylactic Antibiotic Stopped[3]	203	61%	80%	72%	95%
Pregnancy Care					
Inpatient Neonatal Mortality	1,172	0.00%	-	-	-
Third or Fourth Degree Laceration	892	2.35%	3.43%	3.63%	3.27%

Edgerton Hospital and Health Services

313 Stoughton Road
Edgerton, WI 53534
Toll-Free: 800-884-3441
Phone: 608-884-3441
Fax: 608-884-1659
E-mail: mailto:mchinfo@edgertonhospital.com
URL: www.edgertonhospital.com
Ownership: Voluntary non-profit - Private
Emergency Services: Yes
Accredited: No
Licensed Beds: 86

Key Personnel:
President/CEO . . . . James Pernau
Chief Medical Staff . . . . Ron Beresky, MD
Emergency Room . . . . Shelly McGuire
Director/Infection Control . . . . Sherry Bautz
Surgical Cervices . . . . Margaret Larson
Director Radiology . . . . Roberta Nelson

Measure	Cases	This Hospital	State Average	U.S. Average	Top Hospital
Heart Attack Care					
ACE Inhibitor or ARB for LVSD[3]	0	-	85%	82%	100%

NOTE: Hospital profiles are in alphabetical order by state, then city, then hospital within the city; Rankings are sorted by rate in descending order and exclude hospitals with less than 25 cases; (1) The number of cases is too small (n<25) for purposes of reliably predicting hospital performance; (2) Measure reflects the hospital's indication that its submission was based upon a sample of its relevant discharges; (3) Rate reflects fewer than the maximum possible quarters of data for the measure; (4) Inaccurate information submitted and suppressed for one or more quarters; (5) No data is available from the hospital for this measure; Please refer to the User's Guide for a full explanation of data

Measure	Cases	This Hospital	State Average	U.S. Average	Top Hospital
Aspirin at Arrival[1,3]	4	75%	94%	92%	100%
Aspirin at Discharge[1,3]	4	75%	94%	90%	100%
Beta Blocker at Arrival[5]	-	-	92%	87%	100%
Beta Blocker at Discharge[5]	-	-	92%	90%	100%
Fibrinolytic Medication Timing[5]	-	-	13%	31%	100%
PCI Within 90 Minutes of Arrival[5]	-	-	75%	54%	95%
Smoking Cessation Advice[3]	0	-	91%	88%	100%
Heart Failure Care					
ACE Inhibitor or ARB for LVSD[1]	1	100%	86%	82%	100%
Discharge Instructions[1]	13	100%	73%	61%	93%
Evaluation of LVS Function[5]	-	-	88%	83%	99%
Smoking Cessation Advice[5]	-	-	80%	82%	100%
Pneumonia Care					
Appropriate Initial Antibiotic[1,3]	9	100%	87%	83%	94%
Blood Culture Timing[3]	0	-	94%	90%	100%
Influenza Vaccine[5]	-	-	79%	70%	100%
Initial Antibiotic Timing[1,3]	8	88%	87%	80%	93%
Oxygenation Assessment[1,3]	9	100%	100%	99%	100%
Pneumococcal Vaccine[1,3]	4	75%	78%	69%	94%
Smoking Cessation Advice[5]	-	-	82%	80%	100%
Surgical Infection Prevention					
Prophylactic Antibiotic Given[5]	-	-	84%	77%	95%
Prophylactic Antibiotic Selection[5]	-	-	93%	90%	100%
Prophylactic Antibiotic Stopped[5]	-	-	80%	72%	95%
Pregnancy Care					
Inpatient Neonatal Mortality	-	-	-	-	-
Third or Fourth Degree Laceration	-	-	3.43%	3.63%	3.27%

Aurora Lakeland Medical Center

W3985 Cty Rd Nn
Elkhorn, WI 53121
Phone: 262-741-2000
Ownership: Voluntary non-profit - Private
Accredited: Yes
Emergency Services: Yes

Measure	Cases	This Hospital	State Average	U.S. Average	Top Hospital
Heart Attack Care					
ACE Inhibitor or ARB for LVSD[1]	1	100%	85%	82%	100%
Aspirin at Arrival	25	96%	94%	92%	100%
Aspirin at Discharge[1]	12	92%	94%	90%	100%
Beta Blocker at Arrival[1]	19	100%	92%	87%	100%
Beta Blocker at Discharge[1]	11	100%	92%	90%	100%
Fibrinolytic Medication Timing	0	-	13%	31%	100%
PCI Within 90 Minutes of Arrival	0	-	75%	54%	95%
Smoking Cessation Advice[1]	3	100%	91%	88%	100%
Heart Failure Care					
ACE Inhibitor or ARB for LVSD[1]	23	96%	86%	82%	100%
Discharge Instructions	66	95%	73%	61%	93%
Evaluation of LVS Function	94	99%	88%	83%	99%
Smoking Cessation Advice[1]	14	100%	80%	82%	100%
Pneumonia Care					
Appropriate Initial Antibiotic	98	91%	87%	83%	94%
Blood Culture Timing	114	98%	94%	90%	100%
Influenza Vaccine	33	91%	79%	70%	100%
Initial Antibiotic Timing	157	97%	87%	80%	93%
Oxygenation Assessment	190	100%	100%	99%	100%
Pneumococcal Vaccine	138	94%	78%	69%	94%
Smoking Cessation Advice	42	100%	82%	80%	100%
Surgical Infection Prevention					
Prophylactic Antibiotic Given[2,3]	74	84%	84%	77%	95%
Prophylactic Antibiotic Selection[2]	31	87%	93%	90%	100%
Prophylactic Antibiotic Stopped[2,3]	70	80%	80%	72%	95%
Pregnancy Care					
Inpatient Neonatal Mortality	-	-	-	-	-
Third or Fourth Degree Laceration	-	-	3.43%	3.63%	3.27%

Saint Agnes Hospital

Alternate Name: Agnesian HealthCare

430 E Division Street
Fond du Lac, WI 54935
Phone: 920-929-2300
Fax: 920-926-4306
URL: www.agnesian.com
Ownership: Voluntary non-profit - Church
Accredited: Yes
Emergency Services: Yes
Licensed Beds: 330

Key Personnel:

President/CEO . . . . Robert A Fale
Chief Medical Staff . . . . Theodore Miller, MD
Cardiology . . . . Jim Mugan
Director Emergency Services . . . . Dorothy Garcia
Coordinator Infection Control . . . . Kayla Ericksen
Surgical/Peds Nursing . . . . Maria Zahn
Director Surgical/Pediatrics . . . . Maria Zahn

Measure	Cases	This Hospital	State Average	U.S. Average	Top Hospital
Heart Attack Care					
ACE Inhibitor or ARB for LVSD	43	91%	85%	82%	100%
Aspirin at Arrival	122	98%	94%	92%	100%
Aspirin at Discharge	123	95%	94%	90%	100%
Beta Blocker at Arrival	106	94%	92%	87%	100%
Beta Blocker at Discharge	125	94%	92%	90%	100%
Fibrinolytic Medication Timing	0	-	13%	31%	100%
PCI Within 90 Minutes of Arrival[1]	5	80%	75%	54%	95%
Smoking Cessation Advice	32	78%	91%	88%	100%
Heart Failure Care					
ACE Inhibitor or ARB for LVSD	50	80%	86%	82%	100%
Discharge Instructions	102	71%	73%	61%	93%
Evaluation of LVS Function	164	85%	88%	83%	99%
Smoking Cessation Advice[1]	23	83%	80%	82%	100%
Pneumonia Care					
Appropriate Initial Antibiotic	90	92%	87%	83%	94%
Blood Culture Timing	65	89%	94%	90%	100%
Influenza Vaccine[1]	18	61%	79%	70%	100%
Initial Antibiotic Timing	122	75%	87%	80%	93%
Oxygenation Assessment	160	100%	100%	99%	100%
Pneumococcal Vaccine	118	41%	78%	69%	94%
Smoking Cessation Advice[1]	23	83%	82%	80%	100%
Surgical Infection Prevention					
Prophylactic Antibiotic Given[3]	172	77%	84%	77%	95%
Prophylactic Antibiotic Selection	65	88%	93%	90%	100%
Prophylactic Antibiotic Stopped[3]	158	66%	80%	72%	95%
Pregnancy Care					
Inpatient Neonatal Mortality	-	-	-	-	-
Third or Fourth Degree Laceration	-	-	3.43%	3.63%	3.27%

Fort Memorial Hospital

611 Sherman Avenue E
Fort Atkinson, WI 53538
Phone: 920-568-5000
Fax: 920-568-5412
URL: www.forthealthcare.com
Ownership: Voluntary non-profit - Private
Accredited: Yes
Emergency Services: Yes
Licensed Beds: 82

Key Personnel:

President/CEO . . . . Gregory A Banaszynski
Chief Medical Staff . . . . Thomas Tackman, MD
Emergency Room . . . . Robert Sievert, DO
CCU Spvg. Nurse . . . . Pamela Kuehl, RN
Director Medical/Surgical Nursing . . . . Nancy Lawrence, RN
Chief Radiology . . . . Edward Joingco, MD
Director Respiratory Therapy . . . . Scott Deichl

Measure	Cases	This Hospital	State Average	U.S. Average	Top Hospital
Heart Attack Care					
ACE Inhibitor or ARB for LVSD[1]	4	75%	85%	82%	100%
Aspirin at Arrival[1]	17	100%	94%	92%	100%
Aspirin at Discharge[1]	13	100%	94%	90%	100%
Beta Blocker at Arrival[1]	10	70%	92%	87%	100%
Beta Blocker at Discharge[1]	11	45%	92%	90%	100%
Fibrinolytic Medication Timing[1]	3	0%	13%	31%	100%
PCI Within 90 Minutes of Arrival	0	-	75%	54%	95%
Smoking Cessation Advice	0	-	91%	88%	100%
Heart Failure Care					
ACE Inhibitor or ARB for LVSD[1]	12	92%	86%	82%	100%
Discharge Instructions	37	76%	73%	61%	93%

NOTE: Hospital profiles are in alphabetical order by state, then city, then hospital within the city; Rankings are sorted by rate in descending order and exclude hospitals with less than 25 cases; (1) The number of cases is too small (n<25) for purposes of reliably predicting hospital performance; (2) Measure reflects the hospital's indication that its submission was based upon a sample of its relevant discharges; (3) Rate reflects fewer than the maximum possible quarters of data for the measure; (4) Inaccurate information submitted and suppressed for one or more quarters; (5) No data is available from the hospital for this measure; Please refer to the User's Guide for a full explanation of data

Measure	Cases	This Hospital	State Average	U.S. Average	Top Hospital
Evaluation of LVS Function	70	89%	88%	83%	99%
Smoking Cessation Advice[1]	6	83%	80%	82%	100%
Pneumonia Care					
Appropriate Initial Antibiotic	55	85%	87%	83%	94%
Blood Culture Timing	51	90%	94%	90%	100%
Influenza Vaccine[4,5]	-	-	79%	70%	100%
Initial Antibiotic Timing	59	83%	87%	80%	93%
Oxygenation Assessment	102	100%	100%	99%	100%
Pneumococcal Vaccine	59	80%	78%	69%	94%
Smoking Cessation Advice[1]	19	68%	82%	80%	100%
Surgical Infection Prevention					
Prophylactic Antibiotic Given	234	92%	84%	77%	95%
Prophylactic Antibiotic Selection	50	98%	93%	90%	100%
Prophylactic Antibiotic Stopped	221	98%	80%	72%	95%
Pregnancy Care					
Inpatient Neonatal Mortality	-	-	-	-	-
Third or Fourth Degree Laceration	-	-	3.43%	3.63%	3.27%

Moundview Memorial Hospital & Clinics

402 W Lake Street
Friendship, WI 53934
Phone: 608-339-3331
Fax: 608-339-9385
URL: www.moundview.org
Ownership: Voluntary non-profit - Private
Accredited: No
Emergency Services: Yes
Licensed Beds: 29

Key Personnel:

Administrator . . . . Lunn Clayton
Chief Medical Staff. . . . . Martin Janssen, MD
Emergency Room . . . . M Esmaili, MD
Chief Radiology . . . . Gene Wegner, MD

Measure	Cases	This Hospital	State Average	U.S. Average	Top Hospital
Heart Attack Care					
ACE Inhibitor or ARB for LVSD[5]	-	-	85%	82%	100%
Aspirin at Arrival[5]	-	-	94%	92%	100%
Aspirin at Discharge[5]	-	-	94%	90%	100%
Beta Blocker at Arrival[5]	-	-	92%	87%	100%
Beta Blocker at Discharge[5]	-	-	92%	90%	100%
Fibrinolytic Medication Timing[5]	-	-	13%	31%	100%
PCI Within 90 Minutes of Arrival[5]	-	-	75%	54%	95%
Smoking Cessation Advice[5]	-	-	91%	88%	100%
Heart Failure Care					
ACE Inhibitor or ARB for LVSD[1]	5	100%	86%	82%	100%
Discharge Instructions[1]	15	27%	73%	61%	93%
Evaluation of LVS Function[1]	20	95%	88%	83%	99%
Smoking Cessation Advice[1]	3	0%	80%	82%	100%
Pneumonia Care					
Appropriate Initial Antibiotic[1]	21	86%	87%	83%	94%
Blood Culture Timing[1]	5	80%	94%	90%	100%
Influenza Vaccine[1]	5	80%	79%	70%	100%
Initial Antibiotic Timing	28	86%	87%	80%	93%
Oxygenation Assessment	37	100%	100%	99%	100%
Pneumococcal Vaccine	25	56%	78%	69%	94%
Smoking Cessation Advice[1]	6	50%	82%	80%	100%
Surgical Infection Prevention					
Prophylactic Antibiotic Given[5]	-	-	84%	77%	95%
Prophylactic Antibiotic Selection[5]	-	-	93%	90%	100%
Prophylactic Antibiotic Stopped[5]	-	-	80%	72%	95%
Pregnancy Care					
Inpatient Neonatal Mortality	-	-	-	-	-
Third or Fourth Degree Laceration	-	-	3.43%	3.63%	3.27%

Orthopaedic Hospital of Wisconsin

575 W River Woods Pkwy
Glendale, WI 53212
Phone: 414-961-6800
Ownership: Proprietary
Accredited: No
Emergency Services: No

Measure	Cases	This Hospital	State Average	U.S. Average	Top Hospital
Heart Attack Care					
ACE Inhibitor or ARB for LVSD[5]	-	-	85%	82%	100%
Aspirin at Arrival[5]	-	-	94%	92%	100%
Aspirin at Discharge[5]	-	-	94%	90%	100%
Beta Blocker at Arrival[5]	-	-	92%	87%	100%
Beta Blocker at Discharge[5]	-	-	92%	90%	100%
Fibrinolytic Medication Timing[5]	-	-	13%	31%	100%
PCI Within 90 Minutes of Arrival[5]	-	-	75%	54%	95%
Smoking Cessation Advice[5]	-	-	91%	88%	100%
Heart Failure Care					
ACE Inhibitor or ARB for LVSD[5]	-	-	86%	82%	100%
Discharge Instructions[5]	-	-	73%	61%	93%
Evaluation of LVS Function[5]	-	-	88%	83%	99%
Smoking Cessation Advice[5]	-	-	80%	82%	100%
Pneumonia Care					
Appropriate Initial Antibiotic[5]	-	-	87%	83%	94%
Blood Culture Timing[5]	-	-	94%	90%	100%
Influenza Vaccine[5]	-	-	79%	70%	100%
Initial Antibiotic Timing[5]	-	-	87%	80%	93%
Oxygenation Assessment[5]	-	-	100%	99%	100%
Pneumococcal Vaccine[5]	-	-	78%	69%	94%
Smoking Cessation Advice[5]	-	-	82%	80%	100%
Surgical Infection Prevention					
Prophylactic Antibiotic Given[5]	-	-	84%	77%	95%
Prophylactic Antibiotic Selection[5]	-	-	93%	90%	100%
Prophylactic Antibiotic Stopped[5]	-	-	80%	72%	95%
Pregnancy Care					
Inpatient Neonatal Mortality	-	-	-	-	-
Third or Fourth Degree Laceration	-	-	3.43%	3.63%	3.27%

Burnett Medical Center

Alternate Name: Burnett General Hospital-Burnett Medical Center
257 W Saint George Avenue
Grantsburg, WI 54840
Phone: 715-463-5353
Fax: 715-463-2423
Ownership: Voluntary non-profit - Private
Accredited: No
Emergency Services: Yes
Licensed Beds: 84

Key Personnel:

President/CEO. . . . . Tim Wick
Cardiac Rehab. . . . . Terry Giles
Infection Control. . . . . Debra Stigar
Medical/Surgical Nursing . . . . Bonnie Olson
OB/GYN/Womens Health. . . . . Delores Swenson
Respiratory/Cardiopulmonary. . . . . Terry Giles

Measure	Cases	This Hospital	State Average	U.S. Average	Top Hospital
Heart Attack Care					
ACE Inhibitor or ARB for LVSD[3]	0	-	85%	82%	100%
Aspirin at Arrival[1,3]	2	100%	94%	92%	100%
Aspirin at Discharge[1,3]	2	100%	94%	90%	100%
Beta Blocker at Arrival[1,3]	2	50%	92%	87%	100%
Beta Blocker at Discharge[1,3]	2	100%	92%	90%	100%
Fibrinolytic Medication Timing[3]	0	-	13%	31%	100%
PCI Within 90 Minutes of Arrival[5]	-	-	75%	54%	95%
Smoking Cessation Advice[3]	0	-	91%	88%	100%
Heart Failure Care					
ACE Inhibitor or ARB for LVSD	0	-	86%	82%	100%
Discharge Instructions[1]	8	62%	73%	61%	93%
Evaluation of LVS Function[1]	11	64%	88%	83%	99%
Smoking Cessation Advice[1]	1	100%	80%	82%	100%
Pneumonia Care					
Appropriate Initial Antibiotic[1]	10	60%	87%	83%	94%
Blood Culture Timing[1]	2	100%	94%	90%	100%
Influenza Vaccine[1]	5	100%	79%	70%	100%
Initial Antibiotic Timing[1]	14	86%	87%	80%	93%
Oxygenation Assessment[1]	24	100%	100%	99%	100%
Pneumococcal Vaccine[1]	14	86%	78%	69%	94%
Smoking Cessation Advice[1]	4	75%	82%	80%	100%
Surgical Infection Prevention					
Prophylactic Antibiotic Given[1]	14	57%	84%	77%	95%
Prophylactic Antibiotic Selection[1]	1	100%	93%	90%	100%
Prophylactic Antibiotic Stopped[1]	14	43%	80%	72%	95%
Pregnancy Care					
Inpatient Neonatal Mortality	-	-	-	-	-
Third or Fourth Degree Laceration	-	-	3.43%	3.63%	3.27%

NOTE: Hospital profiles are in alphabetical order by state, then city, then hospital within the city; Rankings are sorted by rate in descending order and exclude hospitals with less than 25 cases; (1) The number of cases is too small (n<25) for purposes of reliably predicting hospital performance; (2) Measure reflects the hospital's indication that its submission was based upon a sample of its relevant discharges; (3) Rate reflects fewer than the maximum possible quarters of data for the measure; (4) Inaccurate information submitted and suppressed for one or more quarters; (5) No data is available from the hospital for this measure; Please refer to the User's Guide for a full explanation of data

Aurora Baycare Medical Center

2845 Greenbrier Rd PO Box 8900
Green Bay, WI 54311
Phone: 920-288-8000
Ownership: Government - State
Accredited: No
Emergency Services: Yes

Measure	Cases	This Hospital	State Average	U.S. Average	Top Hospital
Heart Attack Care					
ACE Inhibitor or ARB for LVSD[1]	13	100%	85%	82%	100%
Aspirin at Arrival	61	100%	94%	92%	100%
Aspirin at Discharge	121	98%	94%	90%	100%
Beta Blocker at Arrival	53	100%	92%	87%	100%
Beta Blocker at Discharge	113	100%	92%	90%	100%
Fibrinolytic Medication Timing	0	-	13%	31%	100%
PCI Within 90 Minutes of Arrival[1]	3	67%	75%	54%	95%
Smoking Cessation Advice	35	100%	91%	88%	100%
Heart Failure Care					
ACE Inhibitor or ARB for LVSD[1]	21	100%	86%	82%	100%
Discharge Instructions	48	90%	73%	61%	93%
Evaluation of LVS Function	68	100%	88%	83%	99%
Smoking Cessation Advice[1]	10	100%	80%	82%	100%
Pneumonia Care					
Appropriate Initial Antibiotic	51	92%	87%	83%	94%
Blood Culture Timing	50	100%	94%	90%	100%
Influenza Vaccine[1]	9	89%	79%	70%	100%
Initial Antibiotic Timing	57	96%	87%	80%	93%
Oxygenation Assessment	87	100%	100%	99%	100%
Pneumococcal Vaccine	48	92%	78%	69%	94%
Smoking Cessation Advice[1]	24	100%	82%	80%	100%
Surgical Infection Prevention					
Prophylactic Antibiotic Given[2,3]	126	93%	84%	77%	95%
Prophylactic Antibiotic Selection[2]	72	99%	93%	90%	100%
Prophylactic Antibiotic Stopped[2,3]	113	86%	80%	72%	95%
Pregnancy Care					
Inpatient Neonatal Mortality	1,719	0.35%	-	-	-
Third or Fourth Degree Laceration	1,253	2.15%	3.43%	3.63%	3.27%

Bellin Memorial Hospital

744 South Webster Avenue
PO Box 23400
Green Bay, WI 54305
Phone: 920-433-3500
Fax: 920-433-7971
URL: www.bellin.org
Ownership: Voluntary non-profit - Church
Accredited: Yes
Emergency Services: Yes
Licensed Beds: 167

Key Personnel:

CEO. . . . . George F Kerwin
Director Medical/Surgical Nursing . . . . Dan DeGroot
Director Respiratory Therapy . . . . Dan DeGroot

Measure	Cases	This Hospital	State Average	U.S. Average	Top Hospital
Heart Attack Care					
ACE Inhibitor or ARB for LVSD	50	68%	85%	82%	100%
Aspirin at Arrival	170	99%	94%	92%	100%
Aspirin at Discharge	350	99%	94%	90%	100%
Beta Blocker at Arrival	143	100%	92%	87%	100%
Beta Blocker at Discharge	362	99%	92%	90%	100%
Fibrinolytic Medication Timing	0	-	13%	31%	100%
PCI Within 90 Minutes of Arrival[1]	10	70%	75%	54%	95%
Smoking Cessation Advice	116	97%	91%	88%	100%
Heart Failure Care					
ACE Inhibitor or ARB for LVSD	52	81%	86%	82%	100%
Discharge Instructions	138	82%	73%	61%	93%
Evaluation of LVS Function	167	96%	88%	83%	99%
Smoking Cessation Advice	28	96%	80%	82%	100%
Pneumonia Care					
Appropriate Initial Antibiotic	46	83%	87%	83%	94%
Blood Culture Timing	41	100%	94%	90%	100%
Influenza Vaccine[1]	14	86%	79%	70%	100%
Initial Antibiotic Timing	56	77%	87%	80%	93%
Oxygenation Assessment	72	100%	100%	99%	100%
Pneumococcal Vaccine	43	77%	78%	69%	94%
Smoking Cessation Advice[1]	21	86%	82%	80%	100%
Surgical Infection Prevention					
Prophylactic Antibiotic Given[2,3]	417	94%	84%	77%	95%
Prophylactic Antibiotic Selection[2]	156	97%	93%	90%	100%
Prophylactic Antibiotic Stopped[2,3]	403	88%	80%	72%	95%
Pregnancy Care					
Inpatient Neonatal Mortality	-	-	-	-	-
Third or Fourth Degree Laceration	-	-	3.43%	3.63%	3.27%

Saint Mary's Hospital Medical Center

1726 Shawano Avenue
Green Bay, WI 54303
Toll-Free: 800-666-5606
Phone: 920-498-4200
Fax: 920-498-1861
E-mail: info@stmgb.org
URL: www.stmgb.org
Ownership: Voluntary non-profit - Other
Accredited: Yes
Emergency Services: Yes
Licensed Beds: 158

Key Personnel:

President/CEO. . . . . James G Coller
Cardiology Services . . . . Daniel Doran
Emergency Room . . . . Elaine Oulette
Post Surgical Care . . . . Jennifer Nehring
OB/GYN Womens Health. . . . . Vicky Laueridge
Surgical Services . . . . Jane Beyer

Measure	Cases	This Hospital	State Average	U.S. Average	Top Hospital
Heart Attack Care					
ACE Inhibitor or ARB for LVSD[1]	20	95%	85%	82%	100%
Aspirin at Arrival	98	98%	94%	92%	100%
Aspirin at Discharge	93	98%	94%	90%	100%
Beta Blocker at Arrival	80	90%	92%	87%	100%
Beta Blocker at Discharge	95	98%	92%	90%	100%
Fibrinolytic Medication Timing	0	-	13%	31%	100%
PCI Within 90 Minutes of Arrival[1]	3	100%	75%	54%	95%
Smoking Cessation Advice	26	96%	91%	88%	100%
Heart Failure Care					
ACE Inhibitor or ARB for LVSD	40	100%	86%	82%	100%
Discharge Instructions	103	71%	73%	61%	93%
Evaluation of LVS Function	119	86%	88%	83%	99%
Smoking Cessation Advice[1]	21	90%	80%	82%	100%
Pneumonia Care					
Appropriate Initial Antibiotic	104	67%	87%	83%	94%
Blood Culture Timing	80	99%	94%	90%	100%
Influenza Vaccine[4,5]	-	-	79%	70%	100%
Initial Antibiotic Timing	115	90%	87%	80%	93%
Oxygenation Assessment	144	100%	100%	99%	100%
Pneumococcal Vaccine	98	74%	78%	69%	94%
Smoking Cessation Advice	26	85%	82%	80%	100%
Surgical Infection Prevention					
Prophylactic Antibiotic Given	518	90%	84%	77%	95%
Prophylactic Antibiotic Selection	129	94%	93%	90%	100%
Prophylactic Antibiotic Stopped	504	63%	80%	72%	95%
Pregnancy Care					
Inpatient Neonatal Mortality	-	-	-	-	-
Third or Fourth Degree Laceration	-	-	3.43%	3.63%	3.27%

Saint Vincent Hospital

835 S Van Buren Street
PO Box 1308
Green Bay, WI 54301
Phone: 920-433-0111
Fax: 920-431-3151
Ownership: Voluntary non-profit - Church
Accredited: Yes
Emergency Services: Yes
Licensed Beds: 349

Key Personnel:

Administrator . . . . Joseph Neidenbach
Chief Medical Staff. . . . . Rose Turba, MD
Emergency Room . . . . Kenneth Johnson, MD
Infection Control Nurse. . . . . Nancy Lorenzoni
OB/GYN Womens Health. . . . . Thomas Mahoney, MD
Chief Radiology . . . . Randall Kolhase, MD

Measure	Cases	This Hospital	State Average	U.S. Average	Top Hospital
Heart Attack Care					
ACE Inhibitor or ARB for LVSD	30	80%	85%	82%	100%
Aspirin at Arrival	121	97%	94%	92%	100%

NOTE: Hospital profiles are in alphabetical order by state, then city, then hospital within the city; Rankings are sorted by rate in descending order and exclude hospitals with less than 25 cases; (1) The number of cases is too small (n<25) for purposes of reliably predicting hospital performance; (2) Measure reflects the hospital's indication that its submission was based upon a sample of its relevant discharges; (3) Rate reflects fewer than the maximum possible quarters of data for the measure; (4) Inaccurate information submitted and suppressed for one or more quarters; (5) No data is available from the hospital for this measure; Please refer to the User's Guide for a full explanation of data

Measure	Cases	This Hospital	State Average	U.S. Average	Top Hospital
Aspirin at Discharge	138	97%	94%	90%	100%
Beta Blocker at Arrival	105	90%	92%	87%	100%
Beta Blocker at Discharge	133	96%	92%	90%	100%
Fibrinolytic Medication Timing	0	-	13%	31%	100%
PCI Within 90 Minutes of Arrival[1]	5	100%	75%	54%	95%
Smoking Cessation Advice	36	97%	91%	88%	100%
Heart Failure Care					
ACE Inhibitor or ARB for LVSD	65	69%	86%	82%	100%
Discharge Instructions	171	70%	73%	61%	93%
Evaluation of LVS Function	216	93%	88%	83%	99%
Smoking Cessation Advice	26	96%	80%	82%	100%
Pneumonia Care					
Appropriate Initial Antibiotic	91	91%	87%	83%	94%
Blood Culture Timing	96	98%	94%	90%	100%
Influenza Vaccine	27	70%	79%	70%	100%
Initial Antibiotic Timing	123	90%	87%	80%	93%
Oxygenation Assessment	162	99%	100%	99%	100%
Pneumococcal Vaccine	99	76%	78%	69%	94%
Smoking Cessation Advice	32	97%	82%	80%	100%
Surgical Infection Prevention					
Prophylactic Antibiotic Given[3]	441	91%	84%	77%	95%
Prophylactic Antibiotic Selection	86	93%	93%	90%	100%
Prophylactic Antibiotic Stopped[3]	424	77%	80%	72%	95%
Pregnancy Care					
Inpatient Neonatal Mortality	-	-	-	-	-
Third or Fourth Degree Laceration	-	-	3.43%	3.63%	3.27%

Aurora Medical Center of Washington County

Alternate Name: Hartford Memorial Hospital
1032 E Summer Street
Hartford, WI 53027
Phone: 262-673-2300
Fax: 262-670-7620
Ownership: Voluntary non-profit - Private
Accredited: Yes
Emergency Services: Yes
Licensed Beds: 71

Key Personnel:

President/CEO. . . . . Mark A Schwartz
Chief Medical Staff. . . . . D Erbes, MD
Emergency Room . . . . David Madenburg, DO
Director Respiratory Therapy . . . . Twyla Wadina

Measure	Cases	This Hospital	State Average	U.S. Average	Top Hospital
Heart Attack Care					
ACE Inhibitor or ARB for LVSD[1]	1	100%	85%	82%	100%
Aspirin at Arrival[1]	11	100%	94%	92%	100%
Aspirin at Discharge[1]	8	88%	94%	90%	100%
Beta Blocker at Arrival[1]	12	92%	92%	87%	100%
Beta Blocker at Discharge[1]	10	100%	92%	90%	100%
Fibrinolytic Medication Timing	0	-	13%	31%	100%
PCI Within 90 Minutes of Arrival	0	-	75%	54%	95%
Smoking Cessation Advice[1]	2	100%	91%	88%	100%
Heart Failure Care					
ACE Inhibitor or ARB for LVSD	33	91%	86%	82%	100%
Discharge Instructions	54	81%	73%	61%	93%
Evaluation of LVS Function	79	100%	88%	83%	99%
Smoking Cessation Advice[1]	7	100%	80%	82%	100%
Pneumonia Care					
Appropriate Initial Antibiotic	62	92%	87%	83%	94%
Blood Culture Timing	73	95%	94%	90%	100%
Influenza Vaccine[1]	15	87%	79%	70%	100%
Initial Antibiotic Timing	97	96%	87%	80%	93%
Oxygenation Assessment	114	100%	100%	99%	100%
Pneumococcal Vaccine	78	83%	78%	69%	94%
Smoking Cessation Advice[1]	21	95%	82%	80%	100%
Surgical Infection Prevention					
Prophylactic Antibiotic Given[2,3]	84	86%	84%	77%	95%
Prophylactic Antibiotic Selection[2]	42	93%	93%	90%	100%
Prophylactic Antibiotic Stopped[2,3]	81	91%	80%	72%	95%
Pregnancy Care					
Inpatient Neonatal Mortality	-	-	-	-	-
Third or Fourth Degree Laceration	-	-	3.43%	3.63%	3.27%

Hayward Area Memorial Hospital

11040 N State Road 77
Hayward, WI 54843
Phone: 715-634-8911
Fax: 715-934-4272
Ownership: Voluntary non-profit - Private
Accredited: No
Emergency Services: Yes
Licensed Beds: 41

Key Personnel:

CEO. . . . . Barbara Peickert
Chief Medical Staff. . . . . Ravinder Vir, MD
Director Infection/Disease Control . . . . Melody Ruehl
OB/GYN Womens Health. . . . . Anne Wallace

Measure	Cases	This Hospital	State Average	U.S. Average	Top Hospital
Heart Attack Care					
ACE Inhibitor or ARB for LVSD[1]	2	100%	85%	82%	100%
Aspirin at Arrival[1]	11	100%	94%	92%	100%
Aspirin at Discharge[1]	12	100%	94%	90%	100%
Beta Blocker at Arrival[1]	12	100%	92%	87%	100%
Beta Blocker at Discharge[1]	11	100%	92%	90%	100%
Fibrinolytic Medication Timing	0	-	13%	31%	100%
PCI Within 90 Minutes of Arrival	0	-	75%	54%	95%
Smoking Cessation Advice	0	-	91%	88%	100%
Heart Failure Care					
ACE Inhibitor or ARB for LVSD[1]	6	83%	86%	82%	100%
Discharge Instructions[1]	20	60%	73%	61%	93%
Evaluation of LVS Function	28	89%	88%	83%	99%
Smoking Cessation Advice[1]	6	67%	80%	82%	100%
Pneumonia Care					
Appropriate Initial Antibiotic	49	94%	87%	83%	94%
Blood Culture Timing	33	79%	94%	90%	100%
Influenza Vaccine[1]	14	79%	79%	70%	100%
Initial Antibiotic Timing	68	93%	87%	80%	93%
Oxygenation Assessment	79	100%	100%	99%	100%
Pneumococcal Vaccine	54	89%	78%	69%	94%
Smoking Cessation Advice[1]	17	94%	82%	80%	100%
Surgical Infection Prevention					
Prophylactic Antibiotic Given	37	81%	84%	77%	95%
Prophylactic Antibiotic Selection[1]	16	100%	93%	90%	100%
Prophylactic Antibiotic Stopped	34	76%	80%	72%	95%
Pregnancy Care					
Inpatient Neonatal Mortality	-	-	-	-	-
Third or Fourth Degree Laceration	-	-	3.43%	3.63%	3.27%

Saint Joseph's Community Health Services

Alternate Name: Saint Joseph's Memorial Hospital
400 Water Avenue
Hillsboro, WI 54634
Phone: 608-489-2211
Fax: 608-489-8181
E-mail: j.fronk.stjoseph@mut.net
Ownership: Voluntary non-profit - Private
Accredited: No
Emergency Services: Yes
Licensed Beds: 99

Key Personnel:

CEO. . . . . Bill Bruce
Chief Medical Staff. . . . . Steve Dorow, MD
Emergency Room . . . . Mary Charles, RN

Measure	Cases	This Hospital	State Average	U.S. Average	Top Hospital
Heart Attack Care					
ACE Inhibitor or ARB for LVSD[3]	0	-	85%	82%	100%
Aspirin at Arrival[1,3]	1	100%	94%	92%	100%
Aspirin at Discharge[3]	0	-	94%	90%	100%
Beta Blocker at Arrival[3]	0	-	92%	87%	100%
Beta Blocker at Discharge[3]	0	-	92%	90%	100%
Fibrinolytic Medication Timing[3]	0	-	13%	31%	100%
PCI Within 90 Minutes of Arrival	0	-	75%	54%	95%
Smoking Cessation Advice[3]	0	-	91%	88%	100%
Heart Failure Care					
ACE Inhibitor or ARB for LVSD[1]	3	33%	86%	82%	100%
Discharge Instructions[1]	11	18%	73%	61%	93%
Evaluation of LVS Function[1]	12	75%	88%	83%	99%
Smoking Cessation Advice	0	-	80%	82%	100%
Pneumonia Care					
Appropriate Initial Antibiotic	28	93%	87%	83%	94%
Blood Culture Timing[1]	7	100%	94%	90%	100%
Influenza Vaccine[1]	4	50%	79%	70%	100%

NOTE: Hospital profiles are in alphabetical order by state, then city, then hospital within the city; Rankings are sorted by rate in descending order and exclude hospitals with less than 25 cases; (1) The number of cases is too small (n<25) for purposes of reliably predicting hospital performance; (2) Measure reflects the hospital's indication that its submission was based upon a sample of its relevant discharges; (3) Rate reflects fewer than the maximum possible quarters of data for the measure; (4) Inaccurate information submitted and suppressed for one or more quarters; (5) No data is available from the hospital for this measure; Please refer to the User's Guide for a full explanation of data

Measure	Cases	This Hospital	State Average	U.S. Average	Top Hospital
Initial Antibiotic Timing	27	96%	87%	80%	93%
Oxygenation Assessment	37	100%	100%	99%	100%
Pneumococcal Vaccine[1]	17	65%	78%	69%	94%
Smoking Cessation Advice[1]	11	91%	82%	80%	100%
Surgical Infection Prevention					
Prophylactic Antibiotic Given[1,3]	3	100%	84%	77%	95%
Prophylactic Antibiotic Selection[1]	1	100%	93%	90%	100%
Prophylactic Antibiotic Stopped[1,3]	3	100%	80%	72%	95%
Pregnancy Care					
Inpatient Neonatal Mortality	-	-	-	-	-
Third or Fourth Degree Laceration	-	-	3.43%	3.63%	3.27%

Hudson Hospital

Alternate Name: Hudson Memorial Hospital
405 Stageline Road
Hudson, WI 54016
E-mail: codonovan@hudsonhospital.org
URL: www.hudsonhospital.org
Ownership: Voluntary non-profit - Other
Emergency Services: Yes

Phone: 715-531-6000
Fax: 715-531-6011

Accredited: Yes
Licensed Beds: 29

Key Personnel:
President/CEO . . . . Marian Furlong
Chief Medical Staff . . . . Gregory Young
Emergency Room . . . . Wayne Hass
Respiratory Care . . . . C Batch

Measure	Cases	This Hospital	State Average	U.S. Average	Top Hospital
Heart Attack Care					
ACE Inhibitor or ARB for LVSD[1,3]	3	67%	85%	82%	100%
Aspirin at Arrival[1,3]	7	100%	94%	92%	100%
Aspirin at Discharge[1,3]	5	100%	94%	90%	100%
Beta Blocker at Arrival[1,3]	8	62%	92%	87%	100%
Beta Blocker at Discharge[1,3]	7	71%	92%	90%	100%
Fibrinolytic Medication Timing[3]	0	-	13%	31%	100%
PCI Within 90 Minutes of Arrival	0	-	75%	54%	95%
Smoking Cessation Advice[3]	0	-	91%	88%	100%
Heart Failure Care					
ACE Inhibitor or ARB for LVSD[1]	4	75%	86%	82%	100%
Discharge Instructions[1]	13	77%	73%	61%	93%
Evaluation of LVS Function	29	76%	88%	83%	99%
Smoking Cessation Advice[1]	5	40%	80%	82%	100%
Pneumonia Care					
Appropriate Initial Antibiotic[3]	30	83%	87%	83%	94%
Blood Culture Timing	27	78%	94%	90%	100%
Influenza Vaccine[1]	8	25%	79%	70%	100%
Initial Antibiotic Timing[3]	36	83%	87%	80%	93%
Oxygenation Assessment[3]	46	100%	100%	99%	100%
Pneumococcal Vaccine[3]	34	38%	78%	69%	94%
Smoking Cessation Advice[1,3]	9	67%	82%	80%	100%
Surgical Infection Prevention					
Prophylactic Antibiotic Given[5]	-	-	84%	77%	95%
Prophylactic Antibiotic Selection[5]	-	-	93%	90%	100%
Prophylactic Antibiotic Stopped[5]	-	-	80%	72%	95%
Pregnancy Care					
Inpatient Neonatal Mortality	-	-	-	-	-
Third or Fourth Degree Laceration	-	-	3.43%	3.63%	3.27%

Mercy Hospital Janesville

1000 Mineral Point Avenue
Janesville, WI 53548

URL: www.mercyhealthsystem.org
Ownership: Voluntary non-profit - Private
Emergency Services: Yes

Toll-Free: 800-756-4147
Phone: 608-756-6000
Fax: 608-756-6168

Accredited: Yes
Licensed Beds: 275

Key Personnel:
CEO . . . . Javon R Bea
Head of Medical Staff . . . . Blaine Nowak
Head of Cardiology . . . . Lubin Kan
Director Respiratory Therapy . . . . Shelly Jones

Measure	Cases	This Hospital	State Average	U.S. Average	Top Hospital
Heart Attack Care					
ACE Inhibitor or ARB for LVSD[1]	17	100%	85%	82%	100%
Aspirin at Arrival	94	98%	94%	92%	100%
Aspirin at Discharge	114	89%	94%	90%	100%
Beta Blocker at Arrival	81	94%	92%	87%	100%
Beta Blocker at Discharge	116	92%	92%	90%	100%
Fibrinolytic Medication Timing[1]	3	0%	13%	31%	100%
PCI Within 90 Minutes of Arrival[1]	3	33%	75%	54%	95%
Smoking Cessation Advice	46	93%	91%	88%	100%
Heart Failure Care					
ACE Inhibitor or ARB for LVSD	70	79%	86%	82%	100%
Discharge Instructions	154	71%	73%	61%	93%
Evaluation of LVS Function	202	95%	88%	83%	99%
Smoking Cessation Advice	36	97%	80%	82%	100%
Pneumonia Care					
Appropriate Initial Antibiotic	157	92%	87%	83%	94%
Blood Culture Timing	121	97%	94%	90%	100%
Influenza Vaccine[4,5]	-	-	79%	70%	100%
Initial Antibiotic Timing	200	78%	87%	80%	93%
Oxygenation Assessment	271	100%	100%	99%	100%
Pneumococcal Vaccine	172	90%	78%	69%	94%
Smoking Cessation Advice	61	93%	82%	80%	100%
Surgical Infection Prevention					
Prophylactic Antibiotic Given	676	91%	84%	77%	95%
Prophylactic Antibiotic Selection	142	93%	93%	90%	100%
Prophylactic Antibiotic Stopped	651	71%	80%	72%	95%
Pregnancy Care					
Inpatient Neonatal Mortality	1,190	0.00%	-	-	-
Third or Fourth Degree Laceration	816	5.27%	3.43%	3.63%	3.27%

Aurora Medical Center

10400 South 75th Street
Kenosha, WI 53142
URL: www.aurorahealthcare.org
Ownership: Voluntary non-profit - Private
Emergency Services: Yes

Phone: 262-948-5600
Fax: 262-942-5828

Accredited: Yes
Licensed Beds: 72

Key Personnel:
Administrator . . . . Christine Olson
President/CEO . . . . G Edwin Howe

Measure	Cases	This Hospital	State Average	U.S. Average	Top Hospital
Heart Attack Care					
ACE Inhibitor or ARB for LVSD[1]	4	75%	85%	82%	100%
Aspirin at Arrival[1]	19	100%	94%	92%	100%
Aspirin at Discharge[1]	13	92%	94%	90%	100%
Beta Blocker at Arrival[1]	13	92%	92%	87%	100%
Beta Blocker at Discharge[1]	19	100%	92%	90%	100%
Fibrinolytic Medication Timing	0	-	13%	31%	100%
PCI Within 90 Minutes of Arrival	0	-	75%	54%	95%
Smoking Cessation Advice[1]	3	100%	91%	88%	100%
Heart Failure Care					
ACE Inhibitor or ARB for LVSD[1]	19	95%	86%	82%	100%
Discharge Instructions	54	98%	73%	61%	93%
Evaluation of LVS Function	73	100%	88%	83%	99%
Smoking Cessation Advice[1]	14	100%	80%	82%	100%
Pneumonia Care					
Appropriate Initial Antibiotic	83	99%	87%	83%	94%
Blood Culture Timing	98	99%	94%	90%	100%
Influenza Vaccine[1]	22	100%	79%	70%	100%
Initial Antibiotic Timing	113	97%	87%	80%	93%
Oxygenation Assessment	147	100%	100%	99%	100%
Pneumococcal Vaccine	87	100%	78%	69%	94%
Smoking Cessation Advice	46	100%	82%	80%	100%
Surgical Infection Prevention					
Prophylactic Antibiotic Given[2,3]	60	77%	84%	77%	95%
Prophylactic Antibiotic Selection[2]	29	79%	93%	90%	100%
Prophylactic Antibiotic Stopped[2,3]	56	84%	80%	72%	95%
Pregnancy Care					
Inpatient Neonatal Mortality	-	-	-	-	-
Third or Fourth Degree Laceration	-	-	3.43%	3.63%	3.27%

NOTE: Hospital profiles are in alphabetical order by state, then city, then hospital within the city; Rankings are sorted by rate in descending order and exclude hospitals with less than 25 cases; (1) The number of cases is too small (n<25) for purposes of reliably predicting hospital performance; (2) Measure reflects the hospital's indication that its submission was based upon a sample of its relevant discharges; (3) Rate reflects fewer than the maximum possible quarters of data for the measure; (4) Inaccurate information submitted and suppressed for one or more quarters; (5) No data is available from the hospital for this measure; Please refer to the User's Guide for a full explanation of data

Kenosha Medical Center Campus

6308 8th Avenue
Kenosha, WI 53143
Phone: 262-656-2011
Fax: 262-656-2124
Ownership: Voluntary non-profit - Private
Accredited: Yes
Emergency Services: Yes
Licensed Beds: 315

Key Personnel:

Coordinator Respiratory Therapy . . . . Howard Beaver

Measure	Cases	This Hospital	State Average	U.S. Average	Top Hospital
Heart Attack Care					
ACE Inhibitor or ARB for LVSD	27	81%	85%	82%	100%
Aspirin at Arrival	143	96%	94%	92%	100%
Aspirin at Discharge	133	95%	94%	90%	100%
Beta Blocker at Arrival	127	94%	92%	87%	100%
Beta Blocker at Discharge	125	90%	92%	90%	100%
Fibrinolytic Medication Timing	0	-	13%	31%	100%
PCI Within 90 Minutes of Arrival[1]	12	100%	75%	54%	95%
Smoking Cessation Advice	47	98%	91%	88%	100%
Heart Failure Care					
ACE Inhibitor or ARB for LVSD	101	87%	86%	82%	100%
Discharge Instructions	212	77%	73%	61%	93%
Evaluation of LVS Function	274	96%	88%	83%	99%
Smoking Cessation Advice	33	94%	80%	82%	100%
Pneumonia Care					
Appropriate Initial Antibiotic	196	89%	87%	83%	94%
Blood Culture Timing	179	92%	94%	90%	100%
Influenza Vaccine	53	100%	79%	70%	100%
Initial Antibiotic Timing	294	88%	87%	80%	93%
Oxygenation Assessment	346	100%	100%	99%	100%
Pneumococcal Vaccine	205	90%	78%	69%	94%
Smoking Cessation Advice	75	81%	82%	80%	100%
Surgical Infection Prevention					
Prophylactic Antibiotic Given[3]	130	58%	84%	77%	95%
Prophylactic Antibiotic Selection	131	98%	93%	90%	100%
Prophylactic Antibiotic Stopped[3]	127	50%	80%	72%	95%
Pregnancy Care					
Inpatient Neonatal Mortality	-	-	-	-	-
Third or Fourth Degree Laceration	-	-	3.43%	3.63%	3.27%

Franciscan Skemp Medical Center

Alternate Name: Saint Francis Medical Center
La Crosse Campus
700 W Avenue S
La Crosse, WI 54601
URL: www.mayohealthsytem.org
Toll-Free: 800-362-5454
Phone: 608-785-0940
Fax: 608-791-9504
Ownership: Voluntary non-profit - Church
Accredited: Yes
Emergency Services: Yes
Licensed Beds: 350

Key Personnel:

President/CEO . . . . Robert E Nesse, MD
Chief Catheterization Laboratory . . . . Betty Jorgenson
Emergency Room . . . . Sue McBride
Director Infection/Disease Control . . . . Madeline McDonald
CCU Spvg. Nurse . . . . Jacalyn Lee
OB/GYN Womens Health. . . . . M Susan Young, MD
Chief Radiology . . . . Gary Wood, MD
Director Respiratory Therapy . . . . Betty Jorgenson

Measure	Cases	This Hospital	State Average	U.S. Average	Top Hospital
Heart Attack Care					
ACE Inhibitor or ARB for LVSD[1]	23	87%	85%	82%	100%
Aspirin at Arrival	74	99%	94%	92%	100%
Aspirin at Discharge	99	99%	94%	90%	100%
Beta Blocker at Arrival	62	100%	92%	87%	100%
Beta Blocker at Discharge	110	100%	92%	90%	100%
Fibrinolytic Medication Timing	0	-	13%	31%	100%
PCI Within 90 Minutes of Arrival[1]	5	40%	75%	54%	95%
Smoking Cessation Advice	49	100%	91%	88%	100%
Heart Failure Care					
ACE Inhibitor or ARB for LVSD	38	95%	86%	82%	100%
Discharge Instructions	68	62%	73%	61%	93%
Evaluation of LVS Function	95	99%	88%	83%	99%
Smoking Cessation Advice[1]	14	93%	80%	82%	100%
Pneumonia Care					
Appropriate Initial Antibiotic	100	91%	87%	83%	94%
Blood Culture Timing	108	94%	94%	90%	100%
Influenza Vaccine	33	82%	79%	70%	100%
Initial Antibiotic Timing	140	89%	87%	80%	93%
Oxygenation Assessment	199	100%	100%	99%	100%
Pneumococcal Vaccine	156	89%	78%	69%	94%
Smoking Cessation Advice	40	78%	82%	80%	100%
Surgical Infection Prevention					
Prophylactic Antibiotic Given	624	93%	84%	77%	95%
Prophylactic Antibiotic Selection	142	99%	93%	90%	100%
Prophylactic Antibiotic Stopped	603	79%	80%	72%	95%
Pregnancy Care					
Inpatient Neonatal Mortality	-	-	-	-	-
Third or Fourth Degree Laceration	-	-	3.43%	3.63%	3.27%

Gundersen Lutheran

Alternate Name: Lutheran Hospital-La Crosse
1900 South Avenue
La Crosse, WI 54601
E-mail: careers@gundluth.org
URL: www.gundluth.org
Phone: 608-775-4743
Fax: 608-775-5594
Ownership: Voluntary non-profit - Private
Accredited: Yes
Emergency Services: Yes
Licensed Beds: 325

Key Personnel:

Emergency Room . . . . Stephanie Schwartz
Director Infection/Disease Control . . . . William Agger, MD
OB/GYN Womens Health. . . . . Charles Schauberger, MD
Chief Radiology . . . . Eugene Valentini, MD
Director Respiratory Therapy . . . . Laura Taylor

Measure	Cases	This Hospital	State Average	U.S. Average	Top Hospital
Heart Attack Care					
ACE Inhibitor or ARB for LVSD	56	100%	85%	82%	100%
Aspirin at Arrival	181	99%	94%	92%	100%
Aspirin at Discharge	291	100%	94%	90%	100%
Beta Blocker at Arrival	141	98%	92%	87%	100%
Beta Blocker at Discharge	356	100%	92%	90%	100%
Fibrinolytic Medication Timing[1]	1	0%	13%	31%	100%
PCI Within 90 Minutes of Arrival[1]	12	67%	75%	54%	95%
Smoking Cessation Advice	105	100%	91%	88%	100%
Heart Failure Care					
ACE Inhibitor or ARB for LVSD	59	98%	86%	82%	100%
Discharge Instructions	130	97%	73%	61%	93%
Evaluation of LVS Function	166	100%	88%	83%	99%
Smoking Cessation Advice	27	93%	80%	82%	100%
Pneumonia Care					
Appropriate Initial Antibiotic	110	88%	87%	83%	94%
Blood Culture Timing	115	93%	94%	90%	100%
Influenza Vaccine	29	69%	79%	70%	100%
Initial Antibiotic Timing	157	93%	87%	80%	93%
Oxygenation Assessment	209	100%	100%	99%	100%
Pneumococcal Vaccine	160	81%	78%	69%	94%
Smoking Cessation Advice	63	95%	82%	80%	100%
Surgical Infection Prevention					
Prophylactic Antibiotic Given	264	86%	84%	77%	95%
Prophylactic Antibiotic Selection	68	97%	93%	90%	100%
Prophylactic Antibiotic Stopped	259	86%	80%	72%	95%
Pregnancy Care					
Inpatient Neonatal Mortality	1,693	0.24%	-	-	-
Third or Fourth Degree Laceration	1,263	3.56%	3.43%	3.63%	3.27%

Rusk County Memorial Hospital

Alternate Name: Rusk County Memorial Hospital & Nursing Home
900 College Avenue W
Ladysmith, WI 54848
Phone: 715-532-5561
Fax: 715-532-9809
Ownership: Government - Local
Accredited: No
Emergency Services: Yes
Licensed Beds: 25

Key Personnel:

CEO. . . . . Michael Shaw
Emergency Room . . . . Mary Schneider

Measure	Cases	This Hospital	State Average	U.S. Average	Top Hospital

NOTE: Hospital profiles are in alphabetical order by state, then city, then hospital within the city; Rankings are sorted by rate in descending order and exclude hospitals with less than 25 cases; (1) The number of cases is too small (n<25) for purposes of reliably predicting hospital performance; (2) Measure reflects the hospital's indication that its submission was based upon a sample of its relevant discharges; (3) Rate reflects fewer than the maximum possible quarters of data for the measure; (4) Inaccurate information submitted and suppressed for one or more quarters; (5) No data is available from the hospital for this measure; Please refer to the User's Guide for a full explanation of data

Measure	Cases	This Hospital	State Average	U.S. Average	Top Hospital
Heart Attack Care					
ACE Inhibitor or ARB for LVSD[1,3]	1	100%	85%	82%	100%
Aspirin at Arrival[1,3]	6	100%	94%	92%	100%
Aspirin at Discharge[1,3]	4	100%	94%	90%	100%
Beta Blocker at Arrival[1,3]	6	100%	92%	87%	100%
Beta Blocker at Discharge[1,3]	5	100%	92%	90%	100%
Fibrinolytic Medication Timing[1,3]	1	0%	13%	31%	100%
PCI Within 90 Minutes of Arrival[5]	-	-	75%	54%	95%
Smoking Cessation Advice[1,3]	1	100%	91%	88%	100%
Heart Failure Care					
ACE Inhibitor or ARB for LVSD[1]	14	86%	86%	82%	100%
Discharge Instructions[1]	14	57%	73%	61%	93%
Evaluation of LVS Function[1]	22	91%	88%	83%	99%
Smoking Cessation Advice[1]	2	0%	80%	82%	100%
Pneumonia Care					
Appropriate Initial Antibiotic[1]	19	79%	87%	83%	94%
Blood Culture Timing[1]	14	86%	94%	90%	100%
Influenza Vaccine[1]	4	100%	79%	70%	100%
Initial Antibiotic Timing	26	69%	87%	80%	93%
Oxygenation Assessment	31	100%	100%	99%	100%
Pneumococcal Vaccine[1]	20	80%	78%	69%	94%
Smoking Cessation Advice[1]	1	100%	82%	80%	100%
Surgical Infection Prevention					
Prophylactic Antibiotic Given[5]	-	-	84%	77%	95%
Prophylactic Antibiotic Selection[5]	-	-	93%	90%	100%
Prophylactic Antibiotic Stopped[5]	-	-	80%	72%	95%
Pregnancy Care					
Inpatient Neonatal Mortality	-	-	-	-	-
Third or Fourth Degree Laceration	-	-	3.43%	3.63%	3.27%

Mercy Walworth Hospital & Medical Center

N2950 State Road 67
Lake Geneva, WI 53147
Phone: 262-245-2222
Ownership: Government - Federal
Accredited: No
Emergency Services: Yes

Measure	Cases	This Hospital	State Average	U.S. Average	Top Hospital
Heart Attack Care					
ACE Inhibitor or ARB for LVSD[3]	0	-	85%	82%	100%
Aspirin at Arrival[3]	0	-	94%	92%	100%
Aspirin at Discharge[3]	0	-	94%	90%	100%
Beta Blocker at Arrival[3]	0	-	92%	87%	100%
Beta Blocker at Discharge[3]	0	-	92%	90%	100%
Fibrinolytic Medication Timing[3]	0	-	13%	31%	100%
PCI Within 90 Minutes of Arrival	0	-	75%	54%	95%
Smoking Cessation Advice[3]	0	-	91%	88%	100%
Heart Failure Care					
ACE Inhibitor or ARB for LVSD[3]	0	-	86%	82%	100%
Discharge Instructions[1,3]	6	33%	73%	61%	93%
Evaluation of LVS Function[1,3]	6	100%	88%	83%	99%
Smoking Cessation Advice[1,3]	1	100%	80%	82%	100%
Pneumonia Care					
Appropriate Initial Antibiotic[1,3]	11	100%	87%	83%	94%
Blood Culture Timing[1]	15	100%	94%	90%	100%
Influenza Vaccine[1]	4	75%	79%	70%	100%
Initial Antibiotic Timing[1,3]	16	100%	87%	80%	93%
Oxygenation Assessment[1,3]	18	100%	100%	99%	100%
Pneumococcal Vaccine[1,3]	13	77%	78%	69%	94%
Smoking Cessation Advice[1,3]	2	50%	82%	80%	100%
Surgical Infection Prevention					
Prophylactic Antibiotic Given[1,3]	11	82%	84%	77%	95%
Prophylactic Antibiotic Selection[1]	1	100%	93%	90%	100%
Prophylactic Antibiotic Stopped[1,3]	11	91%	80%	72%	95%
Pregnancy Care					
Inpatient Neonatal Mortality	-	-	-	-	-
Third or Fourth Degree Laceration	-	-	3.43%	3.63%	3.27%

Meriter Hospital

202 S Park Street
Madison, WI 53715
Phone: 608-267-6000
Fax: 608-267-6568
URL: www.meriter.com
Ownership: Voluntary non-profit - Private
Accredited: Yes
Emergency Services: Yes
Licensed Beds: 448

Key Personnel:

President/CEO . . . . James L Woodward
Assistant VP Cardiovascular Services . . . . Una Alderman
Assistant VP Women's Health Services . . . . Pat Grunwald

Measure	Cases	This Hospital	State Average	U.S. Average	Top Hospital
Heart Attack Care					
ACE Inhibitor or ARB for LVSD	43	91%	85%	82%	100%
Aspirin at Arrival	178	99%	94%	92%	100%
Aspirin at Discharge	284	98%	94%	90%	100%
Beta Blocker at Arrival	159	99%	92%	87%	100%
Beta Blocker at Discharge	266	97%	92%	90%	100%
Fibrinolytic Medication Timing[1]	10	40%	13%	31%	100%
PCI Within 90 Minutes of Arrival[1]	7	57%	75%	54%	95%
Smoking Cessation Advice	84	100%	91%	88%	100%
Heart Failure Care					
ACE Inhibitor or ARB for LVSD	95	95%	86%	82%	100%
Discharge Instructions	221	91%	73%	61%	93%
Evaluation of LVS Function	288	98%	88%	83%	99%
Smoking Cessation Advice	43	100%	80%	82%	100%
Pneumonia Care					
Appropriate Initial Antibiotic	140	91%	87%	83%	94%
Blood Culture Timing	80	85%	94%	90%	100%
Influenza Vaccine	30	87%	79%	70%	100%
Initial Antibiotic Timing	178	87%	87%	80%	93%
Oxygenation Assessment	246	100%	100%	99%	100%
Pneumococcal Vaccine	164	73%	78%	69%	94%
Smoking Cessation Advice	45	93%	82%	80%	100%
Surgical Infection Prevention					
Prophylactic Antibiotic Given[2]	1,209	90%	84%	77%	95%
Prophylactic Antibiotic Selection[2]	312	96%	93%	90%	100%
Prophylactic Antibiotic Stopped[2]	1,160	87%	80%	72%	95%
Pregnancy Care					
Inpatient Neonatal Mortality	-	-	-	-	-
Third or Fourth Degree Laceration	-	-	3.43%	3.63%	3.27%

Saint Marys Hospital Medical Center

707 S Mills Street
Madison, WI 53715
Phone: 608-251-6100
Fax: 608-258-5711
URL: www.stmarysmadison.com
Ownership: Voluntary non-profit - Other
Accredited: No
Emergency Services: Yes
Licensed Beds: 440

Key Personnel:

President/CEO . . . . Gerald Lefert
Chief Medical Staff . . . . John Woodford, MD
Emergency Room . . . . Audra Thompson
Infection Control . . . . Chuck Zeisser
Intensive/Coronary Care . . . . Jody De Rosa
Respiratory/Cardiopulmonary . . . . Steve Dalebroux

Measure	Cases	This Hospital	State Average	U.S. Average	Top Hospital
Heart Attack Care					
ACE Inhibitor or ARB for LVSD	96	81%	85%	82%	100%
Aspirin at Arrival	135	98%	94%	92%	100%
Aspirin at Discharge	303	100%	94%	90%	100%
Beta Blocker at Arrival	103	94%	92%	87%	100%
Beta Blocker at Discharge	298	99%	92%	90%	100%
Fibrinolytic Medication Timing	0	-	13%	31%	100%
PCI Within 90 Minutes of Arrival[1]	9	78%	75%	54%	95%
Smoking Cessation Advice	135	90%	91%	88%	100%
Heart Failure Care					
ACE Inhibitor or ARB for LVSD	156	74%	86%	82%	100%
Discharge Instructions	271	53%	73%	61%	93%
Evaluation of LVS Function	350	89%	88%	83%	99%
Smoking Cessation Advice	56	79%	80%	82%	100%
Pneumonia Care					
Appropriate Initial Antibiotic	250	90%	87%	83%	94%

NOTE: Hospital profiles are in alphabetical order by state, then city, then hospital within the city; Rankings are sorted by rate in descending order and exclude hospitals with less than 25 cases; (1) The number of cases is too small (n<25) for purposes of reliably predicting hospital performance; (2) Measure reflects the hospital's indication that its submission was based upon a sample of its relevant discharges; (3) Rate reflects fewer than the maximum possible quarters of data for the measure; (4) Inaccurate information submitted and suppressed for one or more quarters; (5) No data is available from the hospital for this measure; Please refer to the User's Guide for a full explanation of data

Measure	Cases	This Hospital	State Average	U.S. Average	Top Hospital
Blood Culture Timing	190	89%	94%	90%	100%
Influenza Vaccine	70	66%	79%	70%	100%
Initial Antibiotic Timing	306	78%	87%	80%	93%
Oxygenation Assessment	404	100%	100%	99%	100%
Pneumococcal Vaccine	299	61%	78%	69%	94%
Smoking Cessation Advice	76	76%	82%	80%	100%
Surgical Infection Prevention					
Prophylactic Antibiotic Given[3]	1,541	86%	84%	77%	95%
Prophylactic Antibiotic Selection	493	97%	93%	90%	100%
Prophylactic Antibiotic Stopped[3]	1,500	93%	80%	72%	95%
Pregnancy Care					
Inpatient Neonatal Mortality	-	-	-	-	-
Third or Fourth Degree Laceration	-	-	3.43%	3.63%	3.27%

University of Wisconsin Hospital and Clinics

600 Highland Avenue
Madison, WI 53792
Toll-Free: 800-323-8942
Phone: 608-263-6400
Fax: 608-263-9830
URL: www.uwhospital.org
Ownership: Govt - Hospital District or Authority
Emergency Services: Yes
Accredited: Yes
Licensed Beds: 468

Key Personnel:

President/CEO . . . . Donna K Sollenberger
Chief Medical Staff . . . . Jeff Grossman, MD
Chief Catheterization Laboratory . . . . William P Miller, MD
Emergency Room . . . . Joseph Cline, MD
Director Infection/Disease Control . . . . Dennis Maki, MD
OB/GYN Womens Health . . . . Douglas Laube, MD
Chief Radiology . . . . Patrick A Turski, MD
Director Respiratory Therapy . . . . Paul Montague

Measure	Cases	This Hospital	State Average	U.S. Average	Top Hospital
Heart Attack Care					
ACE Inhibitor or ARB for LVSD[2]	79	92%	85%	82%	100%
Aspirin at Arrival[2]	83	100%	94%	92%	100%
Aspirin at Discharge[2]	181	100%	94%	90%	100%
Beta Blocker at Arrival[2]	70	99%	92%	87%	100%
Beta Blocker at Discharge[2]	235	100%	92%	90%	100%
Fibrinolytic Medication Timing[2]	0	-	13%	31%	100%
PCI Within 90 Minutes of Arrival[1,2]	4	50%	75%	54%	95%
Smoking Cessation Advice[2]	103	96%	91%	88%	100%
Heart Failure Care					
ACE Inhibitor or ARB for LVSD[2]	141	84%	86%	82%	100%
Discharge Instructions[2]	224	57%	73%	61%	93%
Evaluation of LVS Function[2]	275	99%	88%	83%	99%
Smoking Cessation Advice[2]	55	87%	80%	82%	100%
Pneumonia Care					
Appropriate Initial Antibiotic[2]	67	79%	87%	83%	94%
Blood Culture Timing[2]	64	89%	94%	90%	100%
Influenza Vaccine[2]	25	92%	79%	70%	100%
Initial Antibiotic Timing[2]	99	75%	87%	80%	93%
Oxygenation Assessment[2]	151	100%	100%	99%	100%
Pneumococcal Vaccine[2]	83	75%	78%	69%	94%
Smoking Cessation Advice[2]	52	52%	82%	80%	100%
Surgical Infection Prevention					
Prophylactic Antibiotic Given[2,3]	420	87%	84%	77%	95%
Prophylactic Antibiotic Selection[2]	78	95%	93%	90%	100%
Prophylactic Antibiotic Stopped[2,3]	405	88%	80%	72%	95%
Pregnancy Care					
Inpatient Neonatal Mortality	-	-	-	-	-
Third or Fourth Degree Laceration	-	-	3.43%	3.63%	3.27%

Holy Family Memorial

2300 Western Avenue
PO Box 1450
Manitowoc, WI 54221
Toll-Free: 800-994-3662
Phone: 920-320-20ll
Fax: 920-320-8576
URL: www.hfmhealth.org
Ownership: Voluntary non-profit - Other
Emergency Services: Yes
Accredited: Yes
Licensed Beds: 303

Key Personnel:

President/CEO . . . . Mark Herzog
Chief of Medical Staff . . . . Steven Driggers, MD
Manager Catheterization Laboratory . . . . Michael Wellner
Emergency Room . . . . Todd Nelson, MD
Director Emergency Services . . . . Mary Coenen
Director Infection/Disease Control . . . . Mike Helgesen
Director Women's Health . . . . Jodi Hibbard
Director Surgical Services . . . . Lisa Sherman

Measure	Cases	This Hospital	State Average	U.S. Average	Top Hospital
Heart Attack Care					
ACE Inhibitor or ARB for LVSD[1]	10	100%	85%	82%	100%
Aspirin at Arrival	78	97%	94%	92%	100%
Aspirin at Discharge	74	96%	94%	90%	100%
Beta Blocker at Arrival	72	97%	92%	87%	100%
Beta Blocker at Discharge	72	97%	92%	90%	100%
Fibrinolytic Medication Timing[1]	1	0%	13%	31%	100%
PCI Within 90 Minutes of Arrival[1]	2	100%	75%	54%	95%
Smoking Cessation Advice	25	84%	91%	88%	100%
Heart Failure Care					
ACE Inhibitor or ARB for LVSD	35	97%	86%	82%	100%
Discharge Instructions	85	79%	73%	61%	93%
Evaluation of LVS Function	125	88%	88%	83%	99%
Smoking Cessation Advice[1]	12	100%	80%	82%	100%
Pneumonia Care					
Appropriate Initial Antibiotic	73	84%	87%	83%	94%
Blood Culture Timing	68	93%	94%	90%	100%
Influenza Vaccine[1]	23	96%	79%	70%	100%
Initial Antibiotic Timing	115	90%	87%	80%	93%
Oxygenation Assessment	139	100%	100%	99%	100%
Pneumococcal Vaccine	102	93%	78%	69%	94%
Smoking Cessation Advice[1]	15	93%	82%	80%	100%
Surgical Infection Prevention					
Prophylactic Antibiotic Given	256	87%	84%	77%	95%
Prophylactic Antibiotic Selection	43	98%	93%	90%	100%
Prophylactic Antibiotic Stopped	247	85%	80%	72%	95%
Pregnancy Care					
Inpatient Neonatal Mortality	-	-	-	-	-
Third or Fourth Degree Laceration	-	-	3.43%	3.63%	3.27%

Bay Area Medical Center

3100 Shore Drive
Marinette, WI 54143
Phone: 715-735-6621
Fax: 715-735-6241
URL: www.bamc.org
Ownership: Voluntary non-profit - Private
Emergency Services: Yes
Accredited: Yes
Licensed Beds: 99

Key Personnel:

President/CEO . . . . David Olson

Measure	Cases	This Hospital	State Average	U.S. Average	Top Hospital
Heart Attack Care					
ACE Inhibitor or ARB for LVSD	25	84%	85%	82%	100%
Aspirin at Arrival	85	98%	94%	92%	100%
Aspirin at Discharge	48	98%	94%	90%	100%
Beta Blocker at Arrival	86	91%	92%	87%	100%
Beta Blocker at Discharge	50	96%	92%	90%	100%
Fibrinolytic Medication Timing[1]	1	0%	13%	31%	100%
PCI Within 90 Minutes of Arrival	0	-	75%	54%	95%
Smoking Cessation Advice[1]	9	100%	91%	88%	100%
Heart Failure Care					
ACE Inhibitor or ARB for LVSD	61	89%	86%	82%	100%
Discharge Instructions	98	87%	73%	61%	93%
Evaluation of LVS Function	136	99%	88%	83%	99%
Smoking Cessation Advice[1]	13	100%	80%	82%	100%
Pneumonia Care					
Appropriate Initial Antibiotic	99	82%	87%	83%	94%
Blood Culture Timing	115	92%	94%	90%	100%
Influenza Vaccine	26	77%	79%	70%	100%
Initial Antibiotic Timing	151	92%	87%	80%	93%
Oxygenation Assessment	181	100%	100%	99%	100%
Pneumococcal Vaccine	117	80%	78%	69%	94%
Smoking Cessation Advice	32	88%	82%	80%	100%
Surgical Infection Prevention					
Prophylactic Antibiotic Given[3]	153	92%	84%	77%	95%
Prophylactic Antibiotic Selection	43	88%	93%	90%	100%

NOTE: Hospital profiles are in alphabetical order by state, then city, then hospital within the city; Rankings are sorted by rate in descending order and exclude hospitals with less than 25 cases; (1) The number of cases is too small (n<25) for purposes of reliably predicting hospital performance; (2) Measure reflects the hospital's indication that its submission was based upon a sample of its relevant discharges; (3) Rate reflects fewer than the maximum possible quarters of data for the measure; (4) Inaccurate information submitted and suppressed for one or more quarters; (5) No data is available from the hospital for this measure; Please refer to the User's Guide for a full explanation of data

Prophylactic Antibiotic Stopped[3]	150	80%	80%	72%	95%
Pregnancy Care					
Inpatient Neonatal Mortality	-	-	-	-	-
Third or Fourth Degree Laceration	-	-	3.43%	3.63%	3.27%

Saint Joseph's Hospital

611 Saint Joseph Avenue
Marshfield, WI 54449
E-mail: sjhweb@stjosephs-marshfield.org
URL: www.stjosephs-marshfield.org
Ownership: Voluntary non-profit - Church
Emergency Services: Yes
Phone: 715-387-1713
Fax: 715-387-5240
Accredited: Yes
Licensed Beds: 500

Key Personnel:
President/CEO. . . . . Michael A Schmidt
Chief Medical Staff. . . . . Fredrick Wesbrook, MD
Emergency Room . . . . Peter Stamas, MD
Director Infection/Disease Control . . . . Thomas L Sell, MD
OB/GYN Womens Health. . . . . Dale Larson, MD
Chief Radiology . . . . Tim Swan, MD
Director Respiratory Therapy . . . . Rachel Boehning-Anders

Measure	Cases	This Hospital	State Average	U.S. Average	Top Hospital
Heart Attack Care					
ACE Inhibitor or ARB for LVSD	86	87%	85%	82%	100%
Aspirin at Arrival	175	100%	94%	92%	100%
Aspirin at Discharge	329	99%	94%	90%	100%
Beta Blocker at Arrival	159	99%	92%	87%	100%
Beta Blocker at Discharge	406	99%	92%	90%	100%
Fibrinolytic Medication Timing	0	-	13%	31%	100%
PCI Within 90 Minutes of Arrival[1]	4	100%	75%	54%	95%
Smoking Cessation Advice	115	98%	91%	88%	100%
Heart Failure Care					
ACE Inhibitor or ARB for LVSD	121	93%	86%	82%	100%
Discharge Instructions	316	78%	73%	61%	93%
Evaluation of LVS Function	386	100%	88%	83%	99%
Smoking Cessation Advice	44	95%	80%	82%	100%
Pneumonia Care					
Appropriate Initial Antibiotic	94	90%	87%	83%	94%
Blood Culture Timing	101	84%	94%	90%	100%
Influenza Vaccine	34	94%	79%	70%	100%
Initial Antibiotic Timing	197	89%	87%	80%	93%
Oxygenation Assessment	238	100%	100%	99%	100%
Pneumococcal Vaccine	160	92%	78%	69%	94%
Smoking Cessation Advice	65	98%	82%	80%	100%
Surgical Infection Prevention					
Prophylactic Antibiotic Given	1,532	81%	84%	77%	95%
Prophylactic Antibiotic Selection	326	85%	93%	90%	100%
Prophylactic Antibiotic Stopped	1,519	68%	80%	72%	95%
Pregnancy Care					
Inpatient Neonatal Mortality	-	-	-	-	-
Third or Fourth Degree Laceration	-	-	3.43%	3.63%	3.27%

Hess Memorial Hospital

1050 Division Street
Mauston, WI 53948
Ownership: Proprietary
Emergency Services: Yes
Toll-Free: 800-252-4377
Phone: 608-847-6161
Fax: 608-847-6017
Accredited: No
Licensed Beds: 100

Key Personnel:
CEO. . . . . San Manders

Measure	Cases	This Hospital	State Average	U.S. Average	Top Hospital
Heart Attack Care					
ACE Inhibitor or ARB for LVSD[1]	1	100%	85%	82%	100%
Aspirin at Arrival[1]	10	70%	94%	92%	100%
Aspirin at Discharge[1]	4	75%	94%	90%	100%
Beta Blocker at Arrival[1]	12	83%	92%	87%	100%
Beta Blocker at Discharge[1]	9	89%	92%	90%	100%
Fibrinolytic Medication Timing[3]	0	-	13%	31%	100%
PCI Within 90 Minutes of Arrival	0	-	75%	54%	95%
Smoking Cessation Advice[3]	0	-	91%	88%	100%
Heart Failure Care					
ACE Inhibitor or ARB for LVSD[1]	12	92%	86%	82%	100%
Discharge Instructions[1,3]	11	45%	73%	61%	93%
Evaluation of LVS Function	87	68%	88%	83%	99%
Smoking Cessation Advice[1,3]	2	50%	80%	82%	100%
Pneumonia Care					
Appropriate Initial Antibiotic[1,3]	7	86%	87%	83%	94%
Blood Culture Timing[1,3]	4	100%	94%	90%	100%
Influenza Vaccine[5]	-	-	79%	70%	100%
Initial Antibiotic Timing	74	84%	87%	80%	93%
Oxygenation Assessment	90	93%	100%	99%	100%
Pneumococcal Vaccine	63	65%	78%	69%	94%
Smoking Cessation Advice[1,3]	4	100%	82%	80%	100%
Surgical Infection Prevention					
Prophylactic Antibiotic Given[3]	50	80%	84%	77%	95%
Prophylactic Antibiotic Selection[5]	-	-	93%	90%	100%
Prophylactic Antibiotic Stopped[3]	49	90%	80%	72%	95%
Pregnancy Care					
Inpatient Neonatal Mortality	-	-	-	-	-
Third or Fourth Degree Laceration	-	-	3.43%	3.63%	3.27%

Memorial Health Center

Alternate Name: Memorial Hospital of Taylor County
135 S Gibson Street
Medford, WI 54451
URL: www.memhc.com
Ownership: Voluntary non-profit - Other
Emergency Services: Yes
Phone: 715-748-8100
Fax: 715-748-8199
Accredited: Yes
Licensed Beds: 164

Key Personnel:
Administrator/President . . . . Greg Roraff
Chief of Medical Staff. Dr Michael Haase
Director Infection/Disease Control . . . . Jane Schiszik
Director Medical/Surgical Nursing . . . . Nancy Laabs, RN
Chief Radiology . . . . Bruce Salo, MD
Respiratory/Cardiopulmonary. . . . . Dawn Fox

Measure	Cases	This Hospital	State Average	U.S. Average	Top Hospital
Heart Attack Care					
ACE Inhibitor or ARB for LVSD[5]	-	-	85%	82%	100%
Aspirin at Arrival[5]	-	-	94%	92%	100%
Aspirin at Discharge[5]	-	-	94%	90%	100%
Beta Blocker at Arrival[5]	-	-	92%	87%	100%
Beta Blocker at Discharge[5]	-	-	92%	90%	100%
Fibrinolytic Medication Timing[5]	-	-	13%	31%	100%
PCI Within 90 Minutes of Arrival[5]	-	-	75%	54%	95%
Smoking Cessation Advice[5]	-	-	91%	88%	100%
Heart Failure Care					
ACE Inhibitor or ARB for LVSD[1]	6	100%	86%	82%	100%
Discharge Instructions[1]	16	100%	73%	61%	93%
Evaluation of LVS Function	30	97%	88%	83%	99%
Smoking Cessation Advice[1]	2	50%	80%	82%	100%
Pneumonia Care					
Appropriate Initial Antibiotic	28	93%	87%	83%	94%
Blood Culture Timing[1]	9	89%	94%	90%	100%
Influenza Vaccine[1]	5	60%	79%	70%	100%
Initial Antibiotic Timing	29	83%	87%	80%	93%
Oxygenation Assessment	29	100%	100%	99%	100%
Pneumococcal Vaccine[1]	24	54%	78%	69%	94%
Smoking Cessation Advice[1]	1	0%	82%	80%	100%
Surgical Infection Prevention					
Prophylactic Antibiotic Given[1]	14	86%	84%	77%	95%
Prophylactic Antibiotic Selection[1]	3	100%	93%	90%	100%
Prophylactic Antibiotic Stopped[1]	14	100%	80%	72%	95%
Pregnancy Care					
Inpatient Neonatal Mortality	-	-	-	-	-
Third or Fourth Degree Laceration	-	-	3.43%	3.63%	3.27%

NOTE: Hospital profiles are in alphabetical order by state, then city, then hospital within the city; Rankings are sorted by rate in descending order and exclude hospitals with less than 25 cases; (1) The number of cases is too small (n<25) for purposes of reliably predicting hospital performance; (2) Measure reflects the hospital's indication that its submission was based upon a sample of its relevant discharges; (3) Rate reflects fewer than the maximum possible quarters of data for the measure; (4) Inaccurate information submitted and suppressed for one or more quarters; (5) No data is available from the hospital for this measure; Please refer to the User's Guide for a full explanation of data

Community Memorial Hospital

W180 N8085 Town Hall Road
Menomonee Falls, WI 53051
Phone: 262-251-1000
Fax: 262-253-7169
E-mail: jkohlbeck@communitymemorial.com
URL: www.communitymemorial.com
Ownership: Voluntary non-profit - Private
Accredited: Yes
Emergency Services: Yes
Licensed Beds: 237

Key Personnel:

President/CEO. . . . . William E Bestor
Chief Medical Staff. . . . . Charles Holmburg, MD
Cardiac Lab . . . . Karl Raaum
Emergency Room . . . . Dennis W Shephard, MD
Emergency Room . . . . Mary Thickens
Infection Control. . . . . Margaret Bell
ICU . . . . Deb McCann
Medical/Surgical Nursing . . . . Bobby Sanders
OB/GYN Womens Health. . . . . Sue Schuelke
Surgical Services . . . . Bobbie Sanders
Respiratory/Cardiopulmonary. . . . . Barb Fagan

Measure	Cases	This Hospital	State Average	U.S. Average	Top Hospital
Heart Attack Care					
ACE Inhibitor or ARB for LVSD	34	56%	85%	82%	100%
Aspirin at Arrival	124	98%	94%	92%	100%
Aspirin at Discharge	112	95%	94%	90%	100%
Beta Blocker at Arrival	104	85%	92%	87%	100%
Beta Blocker at Discharge	129	92%	92%	90%	100%
Fibrinolytic Medication Timing	0	-	13%	31%	100%
PCI Within 90 Minutes of Arrival[1]	12	42%	75%	54%	95%
Smoking Cessation Advice	32	94%	91%	88%	100%
Heart Failure Care					
ACE Inhibitor or ARB for LVSD	79	75%	86%	82%	100%
Discharge Instructions	147	55%	73%	61%	93%
Evaluation of LVS Function	195	96%	88%	83%	99%
Smoking Cessation Advice	29	90%	80%	82%	100%
Pneumonia Care					
Appropriate Initial Antibiotic	73	88%	87%	83%	94%
Blood Culture Timing	71	94%	94%	90%	100%
Influenza Vaccine[1]	19	84%	79%	70%	100%
Initial Antibiotic Timing	106	91%	87%	80%	93%
Oxygenation Assessment	135	100%	100%	99%	100%
Pneumococcal Vaccine	92	74%	78%	69%	94%
Smoking Cessation Advice[1]	24	92%	82%	80%	100%
Surgical Infection Prevention					
Prophylactic Antibiotic Given[2,3]	430	84%	84%	77%	95%
Prophylactic Antibiotic Selection[2]	83	95%	93%	90%	100%
Prophylactic Antibiotic Stopped[2,3]	429	77%	80%	72%	95%
Pregnancy Care					
Inpatient Neonatal Mortality	-	-	-	-	-
Third or Fourth Degree Laceration	-	-	3.43%	3.63%	3.27%

Red Cedar Medical Center

2321 Stout Road
Menomonie, WI 54751
Phone: 715-235-5531
Fax: 715-233-7645
URL: www.mayohealthsystem.org
Ownership: Voluntary non-profit - Private
Accredited: Yes
Emergency Services: Yes
Licensed Beds: 63

Key Personnel:

CEO. . . . . Tom Miller
Chief of Medical Staff. D Spendsen, MD

Measure	Cases	This Hospital	State Average	U.S. Average	Top Hospital
Heart Attack Care					
ACE Inhibitor or ARB for LVSD	0	-	85%	82%	100%
Aspirin at Arrival[1]	10	100%	94%	92%	100%
Aspirin at Discharge[1]	7	100%	94%	90%	100%
Beta Blocker at Arrival[1]	7	100%	92%	87%	100%
Beta Blocker at Discharge[1]	7	100%	92%	90%	100%
Fibrinolytic Medication Timing	0	-	13%	31%	100%
PCI Within 90 Minutes of Arrival	0	-	75%	54%	95%
Smoking Cessation Advice	0	-	91%	88%	100%
Heart Failure Care					
ACE Inhibitor or ARB for LVSD[1]	9	100%	86%	82%	100%
Discharge Instructions	47	94%	73%	61%	93%
Evaluation of LVS Function	60	95%	88%	83%	99%
Smoking Cessation Advice[1]	5	100%	80%	82%	100%
Pneumonia Care					
Appropriate Initial Antibiotic	33	91%	87%	83%	94%
Blood Culture Timing	28	100%	94%	90%	100%
Influenza Vaccine[1]	6	100%	79%	70%	100%
Initial Antibiotic Timing	45	87%	87%	80%	93%
Oxygenation Assessment	56	100%	100%	99%	100%
Pneumococcal Vaccine	42	88%	78%	69%	94%
Smoking Cessation Advice[1]	11	100%	82%	80%	100%
Surgical Infection Prevention					
Prophylactic Antibiotic Given	64	92%	84%	77%	95%
Prophylactic Antibiotic Selection[1]	9	100%	93%	90%	100%
Prophylactic Antibiotic Stopped	62	89%	80%	72%	95%
Pregnancy Care					
Inpatient Neonatal Mortality	-	-	-	-	-
Third or Fourth Degree Laceration	-	-	3.43%	3.63%	3.27%

Columbia Saint Marys Ozaukee Campus

13111 N Port Washington Rd
Mequon, WI 53097
Phone: 262-243-7300
Ownership: Voluntary non-profit - Church
Accredited: Yes
Emergency Services: Yes

Measure	Cases	This Hospital	State Average	U.S. Average	Top Hospital
Heart Attack Care					
ACE Inhibitor or ARB for LVSD[1]	13	62%	85%	82%	100%
Aspirin at Arrival	113	98%	94%	92%	100%
Aspirin at Discharge	106	99%	94%	90%	100%
Beta Blocker at Arrival	89	98%	92%	87%	100%
Beta Blocker at Discharge	107	97%	92%	90%	100%
Fibrinolytic Medication Timing	0	-	13%	31%	100%
PCI Within 90 Minutes of Arrival[1]	5	80%	75%	54%	95%
Smoking Cessation Advice	30	93%	91%	88%	100%
Heart Failure Care					
ACE Inhibitor or ARB for LVSD	59	85%	86%	82%	100%
Discharge Instructions	128	59%	73%	61%	93%
Evaluation of LVS Function	191	84%	88%	83%	99%
Smoking Cessation Advice[1]	15	87%	80%	82%	100%
Pneumonia Care					
Appropriate Initial Antibiotic	140	94%	87%	83%	94%
Blood Culture Timing	124	90%	94%	90%	100%
Influenza Vaccine	41	63%	79%	70%	100%
Initial Antibiotic Timing	197	90%	87%	80%	93%
Oxygenation Assessment	246	100%	100%	99%	100%
Pneumococcal Vaccine	192	70%	78%	69%	94%
Smoking Cessation Advice	33	85%	82%	80%	100%
Surgical Infection Prevention					
Prophylactic Antibiotic Given[2,3]	175	91%	84%	77%	95%
Prophylactic Antibiotic Selection[2]	57	98%	93%	90%	100%
Prophylactic Antibiotic Stopped[2,3]	174	86%	80%	72%	95%
Pregnancy Care					
Inpatient Neonatal Mortality	-	-	-	-	-
Third or Fourth Degree Laceration	-	-	3.43%	3.63%	3.27%

Good Samaritan Health Center

601 S Center Avenue
Merrill, WI 54452
Phone: 715-536-5511
Fax: 715-539-2170
Ownership: Voluntary non-profit - Church
Accredited: Yes
Emergency Services: Yes
Licensed Beds: 73

Key Personnel:

President/CEO. . . . . Michael Hammer
Chief Medical Staff. . . . . Ronald Krajnik
Emergency Room . . . . Jeffrey Moore, MD
Infection Control. . . . . Cheryl Jahns, RN
OB/GYN Womens Health. . . . . Gregory Gill, MD

Measure	Cases	This Hospital	State Average	U.S. Average	Top Hospital
Heart Attack Care					
ACE Inhibitor or ARB for LVSD	0	-	85%	82%	100%
Aspirin at Arrival[1]	3	67%	94%	92%	100%

NOTE: Hospital profiles are in alphabetical order by state, then city, then hospital within the city; Rankings are sorted by rate in descending order and exclude hospitals with less than 25 cases; (1) The number of cases is too small (n<25) for purposes of reliably predicting hospital performance; (2) Measure reflects the hospital's indication that its submission was based upon a sample of its relevant discharges; (3) Rate reflects fewer than the maximum possible quarters of data for the measure; (4) Inaccurate information submitted and suppressed for one or more quarters; (5) No data is available from the hospital for this measure; Please refer to the User's Guide for a full explanation of data

Measure	Cases	This Hospital	State Average	U.S. Average	Top Hospital
Aspirin at Discharge[1]	1	100%	94%	90%	100%
Beta Blocker at Arrival[1]	3	67%	92%	87%	100%
Beta Blocker at Discharge[1]	2	50%	92%	90%	100%
Fibrinolytic Medication Timing	0	-	13%	31%	100%
PCI Within 90 Minutes of Arrival[5]	-	-	75%	54%	95%
Smoking Cessation Advice[1]	1	100%	91%	88%	100%
Heart Failure Care					
ACE Inhibitor or ARB for LVSD[1]	5	100%	86%	82%	100%
Discharge Instructions[1]	17	100%	73%	61%	93%
Evaluation of LVS Function	27	81%	88%	83%	99%
Smoking Cessation Advice[1]	4	75%	80%	82%	100%
Pneumonia Care					
Appropriate Initial Antibiotic	25	88%	87%	83%	94%
Blood Culture Timing[1]	21	90%	94%	90%	100%
Influenza Vaccine[1]	3	67%	79%	70%	100%
Initial Antibiotic Timing	38	87%	87%	80%	93%
Oxygenation Assessment	48	100%	100%	99%	100%
Pneumococcal Vaccine	29	100%	78%	69%	94%
Smoking Cessation Advice[1]	10	100%	82%	80%	100%
Surgical Infection Prevention					
Prophylactic Antibiotic Given	77	95%	84%	77%	95%
Prophylactic Antibiotic Selection[1]	13	100%	93%	90%	100%
Prophylactic Antibiotic Stopped	76	89%	80%	72%	95%
Pregnancy Care					
Inpatient Neonatal Mortality	-	-	-	-	-
Third or Fourth Degree Laceration	-	-	3.43%	3.63%	3.27%

Aurora Saint Luke's Medical Center

2900 W Oklahoma Avenue
Milwaukee, WI 53215
Phone: 414-649-6000
Fax: 414-649-7982
URL: www.aurorahealthcare.org
Ownership: Voluntary non-profit - Private
Accredited: Yes
Emergency Services: Yes
Licensed Beds: 600

Key Personnel:

President/CEO. . . . . Mark Ambrosius
Chief Medical Staff. . . . . Ann Tylenda
Emergency Room . . . . Heidi J Harkins
Director Infection/Disease Control . . . . Lousie Cunningham
OB/GYN Womens Health. . . . . Jcek M Kowalski

Measure	Cases	This Hospital	State Average	U.S. Average	Top Hospital
Heart Attack Care					
ACE Inhibitor or ARB for LVSD	255	86%	85%	82%	100%
Aspirin at Arrival	557	97%	94%	92%	100%
Aspirin at Discharge	897	97%	94%	90%	100%
Beta Blocker at Arrival	326	91%	92%	87%	100%
Beta Blocker at Discharge	804	96%	92%	90%	100%
Fibrinolytic Medication Timing[1]	2	0%	13%	31%	100%
PCI Within 90 Minutes of Arrival	28	82%	75%	54%	95%
Smoking Cessation Advice	377	100%	91%	88%	100%
Heart Failure Care					
ACE Inhibitor or ARB for LVSD	666	90%	86%	82%	100%
Discharge Instructions	1,254	57%	73%	61%	93%
Evaluation of LVS Function	1,497	97%	88%	83%	99%
Smoking Cessation Advice	232	99%	80%	82%	100%
Pneumonia Care					
Appropriate Initial Antibiotic	559	92%	87%	83%	94%
Blood Culture Timing	792	96%	94%	90%	100%
Influenza Vaccine	174	89%	79%	70%	100%
Initial Antibiotic Timing	890	85%	87%	80%	93%
Oxygenation Assessment	1,121	100%	100%	99%	100%
Pneumococcal Vaccine	770	86%	78%	69%	94%
Smoking Cessation Advice	272	97%	82%	80%	100%
Surgical Infection Prevention					
Prophylactic Antibiotic Given[2,3]	170	89%	84%	77%	95%
Prophylactic Antibiotic Selection[2]	90	97%	93%	90%	100%
Prophylactic Antibiotic Stopped[2,3]	167	87%	80%	72%	95%
Pregnancy Care					
Inpatient Neonatal Mortality	-	-	-	-	-
Third or Fourth Degree Laceration	-	-	3.43%	3.63%	3.27%

Columbia Saint Mary's Hospital Columbia

2025 East Newport Avenue
Milwaukee, WI 53211
Phone: 414-961-3300
URL: www.columbia-stmarys.org
Ownership: Voluntary non-profit - Private
Accredited: No
Emergency Services: No
Licensed Beds: 82

Key Personnel:

President/CEO. . . . . Leo Brideau
Emergency Room . . . . Mike Kenny
Director Infection/Disease Control . . . . Judy Hintzman
OB/GYN Womens Health. . . . . Robert Stumpf, MD

Measure	Cases	This Hospital	State Average	U.S. Average	Top Hospital
Heart Attack Care					
ACE Inhibitor or ARB for LVSD[5]	-	-	85%	82%	100%
Aspirin at Arrival[5]	-	-	94%	92%	100%
Aspirin at Discharge[5]	-	-	94%	90%	100%
Beta Blocker at Arrival[5]	-	-	92%	87%	100%
Beta Blocker at Discharge[5]	-	-	92%	90%	100%
Fibrinolytic Medication Timing[5]	-	-	13%	31%	100%
PCI Within 90 Minutes of Arrival[5]	-	-	75%	54%	95%
Smoking Cessation Advice[5]	-	-	91%	88%	100%
Heart Failure Care					
ACE Inhibitor or ARB for LVSD[5]	-	-	86%	82%	100%
Discharge Instructions[5]	-	-	73%	61%	93%
Evaluation of LVS Function[5]	-	-	88%	83%	99%
Smoking Cessation Advice[5]	-	-	80%	82%	100%
Pneumonia Care					
Appropriate Initial Antibiotic[5]	-	-	87%	83%	94%
Blood Culture Timing[5]	-	-	94%	90%	100%
Influenza Vaccine[5]	-	-	79%	70%	100%
Initial Antibiotic Timing[5]	-	-	87%	80%	93%
Oxygenation Assessment[5]	-	-	100%	99%	100%
Pneumococcal Vaccine[5]	-	-	78%	69%	94%
Smoking Cessation Advice[5]	-	-	82%	80%	100%
Surgical Infection Prevention					
Prophylactic Antibiotic Given[5]	-	-	84%	77%	95%
Prophylactic Antibiotic Selection[5]	-	-	93%	90%	100%
Prophylactic Antibiotic Stopped[5]	-	-	80%	72%	95%
Pregnancy Care					
Inpatient Neonatal Mortality	-	-	-	-	-
Third or Fourth Degree Laceration	-	-	3.43%	3.63%	3.27%

Columbia Saint Mary's Hospital Milwaukee

2323 N Lake Drive
Milwaukee, WI 53211
Phone: 414-291-1000
Fax: 414-291-1048
URL: columbia-stmarys.com
Ownership: Voluntary non-profit - Church
Accredited: Yes
Emergency Services: Yes
Licensed Beds: 314

Key Personnel:

President/CEO. . . . . Anthony R Tersigni, EdD

Measure	Cases	This Hospital	State Average	U.S. Average	Top Hospital
Heart Attack Care					
ACE Inhibitor or ARB for LVSD	35	66%	85%	82%	100%
Aspirin at Arrival	136	98%	94%	92%	100%
Aspirin at Discharge	140	96%	94%	90%	100%
Beta Blocker at Arrival	104	92%	92%	87%	100%
Beta Blocker at Discharge	152	97%	92%	90%	100%
Fibrinolytic Medication Timing	0	-	13%	31%	100%
PCI Within 90 Minutes of Arrival[1]	5	60%	75%	54%	95%
Smoking Cessation Advice	54	91%	91%	88%	100%
Heart Failure Care					
ACE Inhibitor or ARB for LVSD	160	89%	86%	82%	100%
Discharge Instructions	303	77%	73%	61%	93%
Evaluation of LVS Function	367	92%	88%	83%	99%
Smoking Cessation Advice	85	95%	80%	82%	100%
Pneumonia Care					
Appropriate Initial Antibiotic	180	90%	87%	83%	94%
Blood Culture Timing	177	90%	94%	90%	100%
Influenza Vaccine	57	81%	79%	70%	100%
Initial Antibiotic Timing	281	84%	87%	80%	93%

NOTE: Hospital profiles are in alphabetical order by state, then city, then hospital within the city; Rankings are sorted by rate in descending order and exclude hospitals with less than 25 cases; (1) The number of cases is too small (n<25) for purposes of reliably predicting hospital performance; (2) Measure reflects the hospital's indication that its submission was based upon a sample of its relevant discharges; (3) Rate reflects fewer than the maximum possible quarters of data for the measure; (4) Inaccurate information submitted and suppressed for one or more quarters; (5) No data is available from the hospital for this measure; Please refer to the User's Guide for a full explanation of data

Measure	Cases	This Hospital	State Average	U.S. Average	Top Hospital
Oxygenation Assessment	334	100%	100%	99%	100%
Pneumococcal Vaccine	214	82%	78%	69%	94%
Smoking Cessation Advice	78	82%	82%	80%	100%
Surgical Infection Prevention					
Prophylactic Antibiotic Given[2,3]	377	94%	84%	77%	95%
Prophylactic Antibiotic Selection[2]	129	95%	93%	90%	100%
Prophylactic Antibiotic Stopped[2,3]	372	76%	80%	72%	95%
Pregnancy Care					
Inpatient Neonatal Mortality	-	-	-	-	-
Third or Fourth Degree Laceration	-	-	3.43%	3.63%	3.27%

Froedtert Hospital/Med College of Wisconsin

Alternate Name: Froedert Memorial Lutheran Hospital
9200 W Wisconsin Avenue
Milwaukee, WI 53226
Toll-Free: 800-272-3666
Phone: 414-805-3000
Fax: 414-805-7790
URL: www.froedtert.com
Ownership: Voluntary non-profit - Private
Accredited: Yes
Emergency Services: Yes
Licensed Beds: 326

Key Personnel:

President/CEO . . . . William D Petasnick
Chief Medical Staff . . . . Marcelle Neuberg, MD
Chief Medicine . . . . Richard Olds, MD
Cardiac Lab . . . . David A Rutlen, MD
Cardiac Surgery . . . . Gordon N Olinger, MD
Catheterization Lab . . . . Michael P Cinquegroni, MD
Emergency Room . . . . Stephen Hargarten, MD
Emergency Room . . . . Andrew J Norton
Infection Control . . . . Michael Frank, MD
ICU . . . . Eugene V Cheng, MD
Medical/Surgical Nursing . . . . Debra Runyan, MS
OB/GYN Womens Health . . . . Dwight P Cruikshank, MD
Director Respiratory Therapy . . . . Karl Raaum

Measure	Cases	This Hospital	State Average	U.S. Average	Top Hospital
Heart Attack Care					
ACE Inhibitor or ARB for LVSD	44	91%	85%	82%	100%
Aspirin at Arrival	133	98%	94%	92%	100%
Aspirin at Discharge	166	99%	94%	90%	100%
Beta Blocker at Arrival	96	96%	92%	87%	100%
Beta Blocker at Discharge	170	99%	92%	90%	100%
Fibrinolytic Medication Timing[1]	1	0%	13%	31%	100%
PCI Within 90 Minutes of Arrival[1]	5	100%	75%	54%	95%
Smoking Cessation Advice	68	100%	91%	88%	100%
Heart Failure Care					
ACE Inhibitor or ARB for LVSD[2]	144	97%	86%	82%	100%
Discharge Instructions[2]	272	71%	73%	61%	93%
Evaluation of LVS Function[2]	308	96%	88%	83%	99%
Smoking Cessation Advice[2]	79	99%	80%	82%	100%
Pneumonia Care					
Appropriate Initial Antibiotic[2]	87	97%	87%	83%	94%
Blood Culture Timing[2]	100	89%	94%	90%	100%
Influenza Vaccine[1,2]	21	100%	79%	70%	100%
Initial Antibiotic Timing[2]	160	80%	87%	80%	93%
Oxygenation Assessment[2]	180	100%	100%	99%	100%
Pneumococcal Vaccine[2]	75	81%	78%	69%	94%
Smoking Cessation Advice[2]	58	97%	82%	80%	100%
Surgical Infection Prevention					
Prophylactic Antibiotic Given[2,3]	377	72%	84%	77%	95%
Prophylactic Antibiotic Selection[2]	208	74%	93%	90%	100%
Prophylactic Antibiotic Stopped[2,3]	363	58%	80%	72%	95%
Pregnancy Care					
Inpatient Neonatal Mortality	1,580	2.03%	-	-	-
Third or Fourth Degree Laceration	1,147	3.57%	3.43%	3.63%	3.27%

Saint Francis Hospital

3237 South 16th Street
Milwaukee, WI 53215
Phone: 414-647-5000
Fax: 414-647-5565
URL: www.covhealth.org
Ownership: Voluntary non-profit - Church
Accredited: Yes
Emergency Services: Yes
Licensed Beds: 260

Key Personnel:

President . . . . Debra K Standridge
Chief Medical Staff . . . . Parmod Kumar, MD
Emergency Room . . . . Maureen Furno, RN
Emergency Room . . . . Dr. Craig Skold
Infection Control . . . . Pat Skonieczny, RN
ICU . . . . Debra Rickaby, RN
OB/GYN Women's Health . . . . James Hayes, MD
Chief Radiology . . . . Bruce Cardone, MD
Director Respiratory Therapy . . . . Bill Matuszak

Measure	Cases	This Hospital	State Average	U.S. Average	Top Hospital
Heart Attack Care					
ACE Inhibitor or ARB for LVSD	28	82%	85%	82%	100%
Aspirin at Arrival	96	96%	94%	92%	100%
Aspirin at Discharge	90	98%	94%	90%	100%
Beta Blocker at Arrival	53	83%	92%	87%	100%
Beta Blocker at Discharge	84	96%	92%	90%	100%
Fibrinolytic Medication Timing[1]	1	0%	13%	31%	100%
PCI Within 90 Minutes of Arrival[1]	2	50%	75%	54%	95%
Smoking Cessation Advice	36	97%	91%	88%	100%
Heart Failure Care					
ACE Inhibitor or ARB for LVSD	100	85%	86%	82%	100%
Discharge Instructions	223	60%	73%	61%	93%
Evaluation of LVS Function	231	98%	88%	83%	99%
Smoking Cessation Advice	33	97%	80%	82%	100%
Pneumonia Care					
Appropriate Initial Antibiotic	153	90%	87%	83%	94%
Blood Culture Timing	163	96%	94%	90%	100%
Influenza Vaccine	47	81%	79%	70%	100%
Initial Antibiotic Timing	220	91%	87%	80%	93%
Oxygenation Assessment	262	100%	100%	99%	100%
Pneumococcal Vaccine	164	66%	78%	69%	94%
Smoking Cessation Advice	70	94%	82%	80%	100%
Surgical Infection Prevention					
Prophylactic Antibiotic Given[3]	328	88%	84%	77%	95%
Prophylactic Antibiotic Selection	55	87%	93%	90%	100%
Prophylactic Antibiotic Stopped[3]	318	79%	80%	72%	95%
Pregnancy Care					
Inpatient Neonatal Mortality	-	-	-	-	-
Third or Fourth Degree Laceration	-	-	3.43%	3.63%	3.27%

Saint Joseph's Hospital

5000 W Chambers Street
Milwaukee, WI 53210
Phone: 414-447-2000
Fax: 414-874-4394
URL: www.wfhealthcare.org
Ownership: Voluntary non-profit - Church
Accredited: Yes
Emergency Services: Yes
Licensed Beds: 595

Key Personnel:

President . . . . Ronald Groepper
Executive Director . . . . Shelli Marquardt
Emergency Room . . . . Kathy Lord
ICU . . . . Nanci Frederich
OB/GYN Womens Health . . . . Tod Paremski, MD
Director Respiratory Therapy . . . . Janet Pangborn

Measure	Cases	This Hospital	State Average	U.S. Average	Top Hospital
Heart Attack Care					
ACE Inhibitor or ARB for LVSD	53	79%	85%	82%	100%
Aspirin at Arrival	179	96%	94%	92%	100%
Aspirin at Discharge	192	93%	94%	90%	100%
Beta Blocker at Arrival	104	92%	92%	87%	100%
Beta Blocker at Discharge	191	95%	92%	90%	100%
Fibrinolytic Medication Timing	0	-	13%	31%	100%
PCI Within 90 Minutes of Arrival[1]	7	86%	75%	54%	95%
Smoking Cessation Advice	88	94%	91%	88%	100%
Heart Failure Care					
ACE Inhibitor or ARB for LVSD	250	87%	86%	82%	100%
Discharge Instructions	456	71%	73%	61%	93%
Evaluation of LVS Function	498	97%	88%	83%	99%
Smoking Cessation Advice	163	99%	80%	82%	100%
Pneumonia Care					
Appropriate Initial Antibiotic	154	90%	87%	83%	94%
Blood Culture Timing	186	98%	94%	90%	100%
Influenza Vaccine	41	95%	79%	70%	100%

NOTE: Hospital profiles are in alphabetical order by state, then city, then hospital within the city; Rankings are sorted by rate in descending order and exclude hospitals with less than 25 cases; (1) The number of cases is too small (n<25) for purposes of reliably predicting hospital performance; (2) Measure reflects the hospital's indication that its submission was based upon a sample of its relevant discharges; (3) Rate reflects fewer than the maximum possible quarters of data for the measure; (4) Inaccurate information submitted and suppressed for one or more quarters; (5) No data is available from the hospital for this measure; Please refer to the User's Guide for a full explanation of data

Initial Antibiotic Timing	232	82%	87%	80%	93%
Oxygenation Assessment	303	100%	100%	99%	100%
Pneumococcal Vaccine	154	84%	78%	69%	94%
Smoking Cessation Advice	86	100%	82%	80%	100%
Surgical Infection Prevention					
Prophylactic Antibiotic Given[3]	445	93%	84%	77%	95%
Prophylactic Antibiotic Selection	62	89%	93%	90%	100%
Prophylactic Antibiotic Stopped[3]	425	90%	80%	72%	95%
Pregnancy Care					
Inpatient Neonatal Mortality	-	-	-	-	-
Third or Fourth Degree Laceration	-	-	3.43%	3.63%	3.27%

Sinai Samaritan Medical Center

Alternate Name: Aurora Sinai Medical Center
945 N 12th Street
Milwaukee, WI 53201
Ownership: Voluntary non-profit - Private
Emergency Services: Yes

Phone: 414-219-2000
Fax: 414-219-7402
Accredited: Yes
Licensed Beds: 454

Key Personnel:

Administrator . . . . Len Wilk
Chief Medical Staff. . . . . Debesh C Mazumdar, MD
Chief Catheterization Laboratory . . . . Tanvir Bajwa
Emergency Room . . . . Jonathan Robinson, MD
Director Infection/Disease Control . . . . Paula Jones, MD
CCU Spvg. Nurse . . . . Linda Ciezki, RN
Director Medical/Surgical Nursing . . . . Marie Golanowski, RN
OB/GYN Womens Health. . . . . LaRoyce Chambers, MD
Chief Radiology . . . . Howard H Johnson
Director Respiratory Therapy . . . . Birdie Allen

Measure	Cases	This Hospital	State Average	U.S. Average	Top Hospital
Heart Attack Care					
ACE Inhibitor or ARB for LVSD	41	93%	85%	82%	100%
Aspirin at Arrival	111	98%	94%	92%	100%
Aspirin at Discharge	102	98%	94%	90%	100%
Beta Blocker at Arrival	64	91%	92%	87%	100%
Beta Blocker at Discharge	64	92%	92%	90%	100%
Fibrinolytic Medication Timing	0	-	13%	31%	100%
PCI Within 90 Minutes of Arrival[1]	3	100%	75%	54%	95%
Smoking Cessation Advice	64	100%	91%	88%	100%
Heart Failure Care					
ACE Inhibitor or ARB for LVSD	188	90%	86%	82%	100%
Discharge Instructions	289	74%	73%	61%	93%
Evaluation of LVS Function	310	99%	88%	83%	99%
Smoking Cessation Advice	144	100%	80%	82%	100%
Pneumonia Care					
Appropriate Initial Antibiotic	148	93%	87%	83%	94%
Blood Culture Timing	153	95%	94%	90%	100%
Influenza Vaccine[1]	24	96%	79%	70%	100%
Initial Antibiotic Timing	205	90%	87%	80%	93%
Oxygenation Assessment	231	100%	100%	99%	100%
Pneumococcal Vaccine	79	92%	78%	69%	94%
Smoking Cessation Advice	103	100%	82%	80%	100%
Surgical Infection Prevention					
Prophylactic Antibiotic Given[2,3]	99	97%	84%	77%	95%
Prophylactic Antibiotic Selection[2]	48	94%	93%	90%	100%
Prophylactic Antibiotic Stopped[2,3]	96	84%	80%	72%	95%
Pregnancy Care					
Inpatient Neonatal Mortality	-	-	-	-	-
Third or Fourth Degree Laceration	-	-	3.43%	3.63%	3.27%

Monroe Clinic and Hospital

515 22nd Avenue
Monroe, WI 53566

Toll-Free: 800-338-0568
Phone: 608-324-2000
Fax: 608-324-1114

E-mail: questions@monroeclinic.org
URL: www.themonroeclinic.org
Ownership: Voluntary non-profit - Church
Emergency Services: Yes

Accredited: Yes
Licensed Beds: 221

Key Personnel:

President/CEO. . . . . Mike Sanders
Emergency Room Director. . . . . Rhonda Rodenburg
Chief Radiology . . . . Phillip Eckstrom, MD
Director Respiratory Therapy . . . . Rob Heen

Measure	Cases	This Hospital	State Average	U.S. Average	Top Hospital
Heart Attack Care					
ACE Inhibitor or ARB for LVSD[1]	1	100%	85%	82%	100%
Aspirin at Arrival[1]	15	100%	94%	92%	100%
Aspirin at Discharge[1]	6	83%	94%	90%	100%
Beta Blocker at Arrival[1]	5	100%	92%	87%	100%
Beta Blocker at Discharge[1]	9	89%	92%	90%	100%
Fibrinolytic Medication Timing[1]	1	100%	13%	31%	100%
PCI Within 90 Minutes of Arrival	0	-	75%	54%	95%
Smoking Cessation Advice[1]	1	100%	91%	88%	100%
Heart Failure Care					
ACE Inhibitor or ARB for LVSD	33	100%	86%	82%	100%
Discharge Instructions	77	88%	73%	61%	93%
Evaluation of LVS Function	116	99%	88%	83%	99%
Smoking Cessation Advice[1]	8	100%	80%	82%	100%
Pneumonia Care					
Appropriate Initial Antibiotic	104	90%	87%	83%	94%
Blood Culture Timing	96	94%	94%	90%	100%
Influenza Vaccine	31	84%	79%	70%	100%
Initial Antibiotic Timing	139	81%	87%	80%	93%
Oxygenation Assessment	169	99%	100%	99%	100%
Pneumococcal Vaccine	121	89%	78%	69%	94%
Smoking Cessation Advice	34	68%	82%	80%	100%
Surgical Infection Prevention					
Prophylactic Antibiotic Given	397	76%	84%	77%	95%
Prophylactic Antibiotic Selection	97	93%	93%	90%	100%
Prophylactic Antibiotic Stopped	387	83%	80%	72%	95%
Pregnancy Care					
Inpatient Neonatal Mortality	-	-	-	-	-
Third or Fourth Degree Laceration	-	-	3.43%	3.63%	3.27%

Theda Clark Medical Center

130 Second Street
Neenah, WI 54957

Toll-Free: 800-236-3122
Phone: 920-729-3100
Fax: 920-729-3167

URL: www.thedacare.org
Ownership: Voluntary non-profit - Private
Emergency Services: Yes

Accredited: Yes
Licensed Beds: 250

Key Personnel:

President/CEO. . . . . John Toussaint, MD
Chief Medical Staff. . . . . Steven Knaus, MD
OB/GYN Womens Health. . . . . Rami Kaldas, MD
Chief Radiology . . . . Thomas Tolly, MD

Measure	Cases	This Hospital	State Average	U.S. Average	Top Hospital
Heart Attack Care					
ACE Inhibitor or ARB for LVSD[1]	22	100%	85%	82%	100%
Aspirin at Arrival	66	95%	94%	92%	100%
Aspirin at Discharge	65	97%	94%	90%	100%
Beta Blocker at Arrival	61	95%	92%	87%	100%
Beta Blocker at Discharge	71	97%	92%	90%	100%
Fibrinolytic Medication Timing	0	-	13%	31%	100%
PCI Within 90 Minutes of Arrival[1]	1	100%	75%	54%	95%
Smoking Cessation Advice[1]	22	100%	91%	88%	100%
Heart Failure Care					
ACE Inhibitor or ARB for LVSD	26	96%	86%	82%	100%
Discharge Instructions	92	100%	73%	61%	93%
Evaluation of LVS Function	123	96%	88%	83%	99%
Smoking Cessation Advice[1]	12	100%	80%	82%	100%
Pneumonia Care					
Appropriate Initial Antibiotic	34	82%	87%	83%	94%
Blood Culture Timing	53	92%	94%	90%	100%
Influenza Vaccine[1]	12	83%	79%	70%	100%
Initial Antibiotic Timing	92	92%	87%	80%	93%
Oxygenation Assessment	97	100%	100%	99%	100%
Pneumococcal Vaccine	72	78%	78%	69%	94%
Smoking Cessation Advice[1]	24	96%	82%	80%	100%
Surgical Infection Prevention					
Prophylactic Antibiotic Given[2]	422	89%	84%	77%	95%
Prophylactic Antibiotic Selection[2]	94	90%	93%	90%	100%

NOTE: Hospital profiles are in alphabetical order by state, then city, then hospital within the city; Rankings are sorted by rate in descending order and exclude hospitals with less than 25 cases; (1) The number of cases is too small (n<25) for purposes of reliably predicting hospital performance; (2) Measure reflects the hospital's indication that its submission was based upon a sample of its relevant discharges; (3) Rate reflects fewer than the maximum possible quarters of data for the measure; (4) Inaccurate information submitted and suppressed for one or more quarters; (5) No data is available from the hospital for this measure; Please refer to the User's Guide for a full explanation of data

Measure	Cases	This Hospital	State Average	U.S. Average	Top Hospital
Prophylactic Antibiotic Stopped[2]	405	79%	80%	72%	95%
Pregnancy Care					
Inpatient Neonatal Mortality	-	-	-	-	-
Third or Fourth Degree Laceration	-	-	3.43%	3.63%	3.27%

Memorial Medical Center

Alternate Name: Memorial Hospital
216 Sunset Place
Neillsville, WI 54456
Ownership: Voluntary non-profit - Other
Emergency Services: Yes
Phone: 715-743-3101
Fax: 715-743-6245
Accredited: No
Licensed Beds: 28

Key Personnel:
CEO . . . . Glen Grady
Chief Staff . . . . Timothy Meyer, MD
Emergency Room . . . . Karen King, RN
Infection Control . . . . Ann Rust
Medical/Surgical Nursing . . . . Sarah Trunkle

Measure	Cases	This Hospital	State Average	U.S. Average	Top Hospital
Heart Attack Care					
ACE Inhibitor or ARB for LVSD	0	-	85%	82%	100%
Aspirin at Arrival[1]	3	100%	94%	92%	100%
Aspirin at Discharge[1]	3	100%	94%	90%	100%
Beta Blocker at Arrival[1]	3	100%	92%	87%	100%
Beta Blocker at Discharge[1]	3	100%	92%	90%	100%
Fibrinolytic Medication Timing	0	-	13%	31%	100%
PCI Within 90 Minutes of Arrival	0	-	75%	54%	95%
Smoking Cessation Advice	0	-	91%	88%	100%
Heart Failure Care					
ACE Inhibitor or ARB for LVSD[1,3]	5	40%	86%	82%	100%
Discharge Instructions[1,3]	9	89%	73%	61%	93%
Evaluation of LVS Function[1,3]	19	63%	88%	83%	99%
Smoking Cessation Advice[3]	0	-	80%	82%	100%
Pneumonia Care					
Appropriate Initial Antibiotic	28	79%	87%	83%	94%
Blood Culture Timing[1]	10	100%	94%	90%	100%
Influenza Vaccine[1]	5	0%	79%	70%	100%
Initial Antibiotic Timing	31	77%	87%	80%	93%
Oxygenation Assessment	39	100%	100%	99%	100%
Pneumococcal Vaccine[1]	23	30%	78%	69%	94%
Smoking Cessation Advice[1]	7	43%	82%	80%	100%
Surgical Infection Prevention					
Prophylactic Antibiotic Given[5]	-	-	84%	77%	95%
Prophylactic Antibiotic Selection[5]	-	-	93%	90%	100%
Prophylactic Antibiotic Stopped[5]	-	-	80%	72%	95%
Pregnancy Care					
Inpatient Neonatal Mortality	-	-	-	-	-
Third or Fourth Degree Laceration	-	-	3.43%	3.63%	3.27%

New London Family Medical Center

1405 Mill Street
New London, WI 54961
Toll-Free: 888-982-5330
Phone: 920-531-2000
Fax: 920-531-2098

E-mail: dmente@ahs.fv.org
Ownership: Voluntary non-profit - Private
Emergency Services: Yes
Accredited: Yes
Licensed Beds: 75

Key Personnel:
President/CEO . . . . Paul Gurgel
Emergency Room . . . . Randy Schoenrock
Director CCU . . . . Randy Shoenrock
Director Respiratory Therapy . . . . Karen Laver

Measure	Cases	This Hospital	State Average	U.S. Average	Top Hospital
Heart Attack Care					
ACE Inhibitor or ARB for LVSD[5]	-	-	85%	82%	100%
Aspirin at Arrival[5]	-	-	94%	92%	100%
Aspirin at Discharge[5]	-	-	94%	90%	100%
Beta Blocker at Arrival[5]	-	-	92%	87%	100%
Beta Blocker at Discharge[5]	-	-	92%	90%	100%
Fibrinolytic Medication Timing[5]	-	-	13%	31%	100%
PCI Within 90 Minutes of Arrival[5]	-	-	75%	54%	95%
Smoking Cessation Advice[5]	-	-	91%	88%	100%
Heart Failure Care					
ACE Inhibitor or ARB for LVSD[5]	-	-	86%	82%	100%
Discharge Instructions[5]	-	-	73%	61%	93%
Evaluation of LVS Function[5]	-	-	88%	83%	99%
Smoking Cessation Advice[5]	-	-	80%	82%	100%
Pneumonia Care					
Appropriate Initial Antibiotic	38	95%	87%	83%	94%
Blood Culture Timing	26	96%	94%	90%	100%
Influenza Vaccine[1]	5	100%	79%	70%	100%
Initial Antibiotic Timing	48	85%	87%	80%	93%
Oxygenation Assessment	54	100%	100%	99%	100%
Pneumococcal Vaccine	37	81%	78%	69%	94%
Smoking Cessation Advice[1]	11	100%	82%	80%	100%
Surgical Infection Prevention					
Prophylactic Antibiotic Given[5]	-	-	84%	77%	95%
Prophylactic Antibiotic Selection[5]	-	-	93%	90%	100%
Prophylactic Antibiotic Stopped[5]	-	-	80%	72%	95%
Pregnancy Care					
Inpatient Neonatal Mortality	-	-	-	-	-
Third or Fourth Degree Laceration	-	-	3.43%	3.63%	3.27%

Westfields Hospital

535 Hospital Road
New Richmond, WI 54017
URL: www.healthpartners.com
Ownership: Voluntary non-profit - Private
Emergency Services: Yes
Phone: 715-246-2101
Fax: 715-243-7203
Accredited: No
Licensed Beds: 40

Key Personnel:
Administrator/President . . . . Jean Needham
Chief Medical Staff . . . . David Olsen, MD
Emergency Room . . . . David De Gear, MD
Director Infection/Disease Control . . . . Charlene Mayry, RN
Director Medical/Surgical Nursing . . . . Shirley Stanek, RN
Director Respiratory Therapy . . . . Greg Gardner

Measure	Cases	This Hospital	State Average	U.S. Average	Top Hospital
Heart Attack Care					
ACE Inhibitor or ARB for LVSD	0	-	85%	82%	100%
Aspirin at Arrival[1]	4	100%	94%	92%	100%
Aspirin at Discharge[1]	4	100%	94%	90%	100%
Beta Blocker at Arrival[1]	6	100%	92%	87%	100%
Beta Blocker at Discharge[1]	5	100%	92%	90%	100%
Fibrinolytic Medication Timing[1]	1	0%	13%	31%	100%
PCI Within 90 Minutes of Arrival	0	-	75%	54%	95%
Smoking Cessation Advice[1]	1	100%	91%	88%	100%
Heart Failure Care					
ACE Inhibitor or ARB for LVSD[1]	3	67%	86%	82%	100%
Discharge Instructions[1]	11	100%	73%	61%	93%
Evaluation of LVS Function[1]	17	82%	88%	83%	99%
Smoking Cessation Advice[1]	1	100%	80%	82%	100%
Pneumonia Care					
Appropriate Initial Antibiotic[1]	20	80%	87%	83%	94%
Blood Culture Timing[1]	7	100%	94%	90%	100%
Influenza Vaccine[1]	4	75%	79%	70%	100%
Initial Antibiotic Timing[1]	12	67%	87%	80%	93%
Oxygenation Assessment[1]	22	100%	100%	99%	100%
Pneumococcal Vaccine[1]	15	87%	78%	69%	94%
Smoking Cessation Advice[1]	4	75%	82%	80%	100%
Surgical Infection Prevention					
Prophylactic Antibiotic Given[5]	-	-	84%	77%	95%
Prophylactic Antibiotic Selection[5]	-	-	93%	90%	100%
Prophylactic Antibiotic Stopped[5]	-	-	80%	72%	95%
Pregnancy Care					
Inpatient Neonatal Mortality	-	-	-	-	-
Third or Fourth Degree Laceration	-	-	3.43%	3.63%	3.27%

Oconomowoc Memorial Hospital

Alternate Name: Memorial Hospital at Oconomowoc

NOTE: Hospital profiles are in alphabetical order by state, then city, then hospital within the city; Rankings are sorted by rate in descending order and exclude hospitals with less than 25 cases; (1) The number of cases is too small (n<25) for purposes of reliably predicting hospital performance; (2) Measure reflects the hospital's indication that its submission was based upon a sample of its relevant discharges; (3) Rate reflects fewer than the maximum possible quarters of data for the measure; (4) Inaccurate information submitted and suppressed for one or more quarters; (5) No data is available from the hospital for this measure; Please refer to the User's Guide for a full explanation of data

791 Summit Avenue
Oconomowoc, WI 53066
Ownership: Voluntary non-profit - Private
Emergency Services: Yes

Phone: 262-569-9400
Fax: 262-560-4527
Accredited: Yes
Licensed Beds: 77

Key Personnel:
President/CEO . . . . John Robertstad
Chief Medical Staff . . . . Brian Lipman, MD

Measure	Cases	This Hospital	State Average	U.S. Average	Top Hospital
Heart Attack Care					
ACE Inhibitor or ARB for LVSD[1]	15	73%	85%	82%	100%
Aspirin at Arrival	44	98%	94%	92%	100%
Aspirin at Discharge	43	100%	94%	90%	100%
Beta Blocker at Arrival	40	95%	92%	87%	100%
Beta Blocker at Discharge	45	96%	92%	90%	100%
Fibrinolytic Medication Timing	0	-	13%	31%	100%
PCI Within 90 Minutes of Arrival[1]	7	29%	75%	54%	95%
Smoking Cessation Advice[1]	15	80%	91%	88%	100%
Heart Failure Care					
ACE Inhibitor or ARB for LVSD	29	93%	86%	82%	100%
Discharge Instructions	72	65%	73%	61%	93%
Evaluation of LVS Function	105	87%	88%	83%	99%
Smoking Cessation Advice[1]	17	94%	80%	82%	100%
Pneumonia Care					
Appropriate Initial Antibiotic	128	86%	87%	83%	94%
Blood Culture Timing	78	91%	94%	90%	100%
Influenza Vaccine	27	93%	79%	70%	100%
Initial Antibiotic Timing	156	89%	87%	80%	93%
Oxygenation Assessment	189	100%	100%	99%	100%
Pneumococcal Vaccine	128	84%	78%	69%	94%
Smoking Cessation Advice	47	91%	82%	80%	100%
Surgical Infection Prevention					
Prophylactic Antibiotic Given	305	92%	84%	77%	95%
Prophylactic Antibiotic Selection	44	93%	93%	90%	100%
Prophylactic Antibiotic Stopped	292	79%	80%	72%	95%
Pregnancy Care					
Inpatient Neonatal Mortality	-	-	-	-	-
Third or Fourth Degree Laceration	-	-	3.43%	3.63%	3.27%

Bond Health Center

820 Arbutus Ave-PO Box 357
Oconto, WI 54153
Ownership: Government - Federal
Emergency Services: Yes

Phone: 920-835-1100
Accredited: No

Key Personnel:
OBGYN . . . . Louise Berndt, MD
Urgent Care . . . . Bernard Kennedy, MD

Measure	Cases	This Hospital	State Average	U.S. Average	Top Hospital
Heart Attack Care					
ACE Inhibitor or ARB for LVSD[5]	-	-	85%	82%	100%
Aspirin at Arrival[5]	-	-	94%	92%	100%
Aspirin at Discharge[5]	-	-	94%	90%	100%
Beta Blocker at Arrival[5]	-	-	92%	87%	100%
Beta Blocker at Discharge[5]	-	-	92%	90%	100%
Fibrinolytic Medication Timing[5]	-	-	13%	31%	100%
PCI Within 90 Minutes of Arrival[5]	-	-	75%	54%	95%
Smoking Cessation Advice[5]	-	-	91%	88%	100%
Heart Failure Care					
ACE Inhibitor or ARB for LVSD[5]	-	-	86%	82%	100%
Discharge Instructions[5]	-	-	73%	61%	93%
Evaluation of LVS Function[5]	-	-	88%	83%	99%
Smoking Cessation Advice[5]	-	-	80%	82%	100%
Pneumonia Care					
Appropriate Initial Antibiotic[5]	-	-	87%	83%	94%
Blood Culture Timing[5]	-	-	94%	90%	100%
Influenza Vaccine[5]	-	-	79%	70%	100%
Initial Antibiotic Timing[5]	-	-	87%	80%	93%
Oxygenation Assessment[5]	-	-	100%	99%	100%
Pneumococcal Vaccine[5]	-	-	78%	69%	94%
Smoking Cessation Advice[5]	-	-	82%	80%	100%
Surgical Infection Prevention					
Prophylactic Antibiotic Given[5]	-	-	84%	77%	95%
Prophylactic Antibiotic Selection[5]	-	-	93%	90%	100%
Prophylactic Antibiotic Stopped[5]	-	-	80%	72%	95%
Pregnancy Care					
Inpatient Neonatal Mortality	-	-	-	-	-
Third or Fourth Degree Laceration	-	-	3.43%	3.63%	3.27%

Community Memorial Hospital

855 S Main Street
Oconto Falls, WI 54154
URL: www.cmhospital.org
Ownership: Voluntary non-profit - Private
Emergency Services: Yes

Phone: 920-846-3444
Fax: 920-846-4244
Accredited: No
Licensed Beds: 25

Key Personnel:
CEO . . . . Jim VanDornick
Chief Medical Staff . . . . Genadi Maltinski, MD
Emergency Room . . . . Kathy Henne
Infection Control . . . . Debbie Wesolowski
Medical/Surgical Nursing . . . . Jacky Stoll

Measure	Cases	This Hospital	State Average	U.S. Average	Top Hospital
Heart Attack Care					
ACE Inhibitor or ARB for LVSD[5]	-	-	85%	82%	100%
Aspirin at Arrival[5]	-	-	94%	92%	100%
Aspirin at Discharge[5]	-	-	94%	90%	100%
Beta Blocker at Arrival[5]	-	-	92%	87%	100%
Beta Blocker at Discharge[5]	-	-	92%	90%	100%
Fibrinolytic Medication Timing[5]	-	-	13%	31%	100%
PCI Within 90 Minutes of Arrival[5]	-	-	75%	54%	95%
Smoking Cessation Advice[5]	-	-	91%	88%	100%
Heart Failure Care					
ACE Inhibitor or ARB for LVSD[5]	-	-	86%	82%	100%
Discharge Instructions[5]	-	-	73%	61%	93%
Evaluation of LVS Function[5]	-	-	88%	83%	99%
Smoking Cessation Advice[5]	-	-	80%	82%	100%
Pneumonia Care					
Appropriate Initial Antibiotic	26	81%	87%	83%	94%
Blood Culture Timing[1]	16	94%	94%	90%	100%
Influenza Vaccine[1]	6	67%	79%	70%	100%
Initial Antibiotic Timing	41	90%	87%	80%	93%
Oxygenation Assessment	45	100%	100%	99%	100%
Pneumococcal Vaccine	34	76%	78%	69%	94%
Smoking Cessation Advice[1]	4	50%	82%	80%	100%
Surgical Infection Prevention					
Prophylactic Antibiotic Given[3]	60	62%	84%	77%	95%
Prophylactic Antibiotic Selection[1]	23	87%	93%	90%	100%
Prophylactic Antibiotic Stopped[3]	60	75%	80%	72%	95%
Pregnancy Care					
Inpatient Neonatal Mortality	-	-	-	-	-
Third or Fourth Degree Laceration	-	-	3.43%	3.63%	3.27%

Aurora Medical Center Oshkosh

855 N Westhaven Dr
Oshkosh, WI 54904
Ownership: Voluntary non-profit - Private
Emergency Services: Yes

Phone: 920-456-6000
Accredited: Yes

Key Personnel:
Director of Surgical Services . . . . Jean Cox, MD
Administrator . . . . Frances Finley, MD
OBGYN . . . . Michael Pech, MD

Measure	Cases	This Hospital	State Average	U.S. Average	Top Hospital
Heart Attack Care					
ACE Inhibitor or ARB for LVSD[1]	9	89%	85%	82%	100%
Aspirin at Arrival	74	99%	94%	92%	100%
Aspirin at Discharge	67	97%	94%	90%	100%
Beta Blocker at Arrival	57	91%	92%	87%	100%
Beta Blocker at Discharge	65	94%	92%	90%	100%
Fibrinolytic Medication Timing[1]	1	0%	13%	31%	100%
PCI Within 90 Minutes of Arrival[1]	6	67%	75%	54%	95%
Smoking Cessation Advice[1]	24	100%	91%	88%	100%
Heart Failure Care					

NOTE: Hospital profiles are in alphabetical order by state, then city, then hospital within the city; Rankings are sorted by rate in descending order and exclude hospitals with less than 25 cases; (1) The number of cases is too small (n<25) for purposes of reliably predicting hospital performance; (2) Measure reflects the hospital's indication that its submission was based upon a sample of its relevant discharges; (3) Rate reflects fewer than the maximum possible quarters of data for the measure; (4) Inaccurate information submitted and suppressed for one or more quarters; (5) No data is available from the hospital for this measure; Please refer to the User's Guide for a full explanation of data

ACE Inhibitor or ARB for LVSD	29	86%	86%	82%	100%
Discharge Instructions	52	67%	73%	61%	93%
Evaluation of LVS Function	80	98%	88%	83%	99%
Smoking Cessation Advice[1]	8	100%	80%	82%	100%
Pneumonia Care					
Appropriate Initial Antibiotic	62	97%	87%	83%	94%
Blood Culture Timing	53	94%	94%	90%	100%
Influenza Vaccine[1]	13	85%	79%	70%	100%
Initial Antibiotic Timing	82	93%	87%	80%	93%
Oxygenation Assessment	109	100%	100%	99%	100%
Pneumococcal Vaccine	63	87%	78%	69%	94%
Smoking Cessation Advice[1]	23	100%	82%	80%	100%
Surgical Infection Prevention					
Prophylactic Antibiotic Given[2,3]	86	90%	84%	77%	95%
Prophylactic Antibiotic Selection[2]	44	82%	93%	90%	100%
Prophylactic Antibiotic Stopped[2,3]	83	52%	80%	72%	95%
Pregnancy Care					
Inpatient Neonatal Mortality	773	0.00%	-	-	-
Third or Fourth Degree Laceration	564	3.72%	3.43%	3.63%	3.27%

Mercy Medical Center

500 S Oakwood Road
Oshkosh, WI 54904
URL: www.ministryhealth.org
Ownership: Voluntary non-profit - Church
Emergency Services: Yes
Phone: 920-223-2000
Fax: 920-223-0599
Accredited: Yes
Licensed Beds: 234

Key Personnel:

President/CEO . . . . Kevin Nolan
Chief Medical Staff . . . . JJ Hanusa, MD
OB/GYN Womens Health . . . . Robert Holly, MD
Chief Radiology . . . . John Aufberheid

Measure	Cases	This Hospital	State Average	U.S. Average	Top Hospital
Heart Attack Care					
ACE Inhibitor or ARB for LVSD	26	81%	85%	82%	100%
Aspirin at Arrival	74	99%	94%	92%	100%
Aspirin at Discharge	79	100%	94%	90%	100%
Beta Blocker at Arrival	68	96%	92%	87%	100%
Beta Blocker at Discharge	79	97%	92%	90%	100%
Fibrinolytic Medication Timing	0	-	13%	31%	100%
PCI Within 90 Minutes of Arrival[1]	5	60%	75%	54%	95%
Smoking Cessation Advice	32	97%	91%	88%	100%
Heart Failure Care					
ACE Inhibitor or ARB for LVSD	38	84%	86%	82%	100%
Discharge Instructions	64	67%	73%	61%	93%
Evaluation of LVS Function	89	100%	88%	83%	99%
Smoking Cessation Advice[1]	13	92%	80%	82%	100%
Pneumonia Care					
Appropriate Initial Antibiotic	45	96%	87%	83%	94%
Blood Culture Timing	57	91%	94%	90%	100%
Influenza Vaccine[1]	8	62%	79%	70%	100%
Initial Antibiotic Timing	86	84%	87%	80%	93%
Oxygenation Assessment	106	100%	100%	99%	100%
Pneumococcal Vaccine	85	75%	78%	69%	94%
Smoking Cessation Advice[1]	22	59%	82%	80%	100%
Surgical Infection Prevention					
Prophylactic Antibiotic Given[2]	886	88%	84%	77%	95%
Prophylactic Antibiotic Selection[2]	206	99%	93%	90%	100%
Prophylactic Antibiotic Stopped[2]	879	12%	80%	72%	95%
Pregnancy Care					
Inpatient Neonatal Mortality	-	-	-	-	-
Third or Fourth Degree Laceration	-	-	3.43%	3.63%	3.27%

Luther Midelfort Oakridge

Alternate Name: Osseo Area Medical Center
13025 8th Street
Osseo, WI 54758
URL: www.mayohealthsystem.org
Ownership: Voluntary non-profit - Other
Emergency Services: Yes
Phone: 715-597-3121
Fax: 715-597-6250
Accredited: Yes
Licensed Beds: 68

Key Personnel:

President/CEO . . . . Mike Ryan
Chief Medical Staff . . . . Thomas Screneck
Emergency Room . . . . Margaret Lunde, RN
Infection Control . . . . Sarah Berquist
Medical/Surgical Nursing . . . . Margaret Lunde, RN

Measure	Cases	This Hospital	State Average	U.S. Average	Top Hospital
Heart Attack Care					
ACE Inhibitor or ARB for LVSD[5]	-	-	85%	82%	100%
Aspirin at Arrival[5]	-	-	94%	92%	100%
Aspirin at Discharge[5]	-	-	94%	90%	100%
Beta Blocker at Arrival[5]	-	-	92%	87%	100%
Beta Blocker at Discharge[5]	-	-	92%	90%	100%
Fibrinolytic Medication Timing[5]	-	-	13%	31%	100%
PCI Within 90 Minutes of Arrival[5]	-	-	75%	54%	95%
Smoking Cessation Advice[5]	-	-	91%	88%	100%
Heart Failure Care					
ACE Inhibitor or ARB for LVSD[1]	2	100%	86%	82%	100%
Discharge Instructions[1]	1	100%	73%	61%	93%
Evaluation of LVS Function[1]	4	100%	88%	83%	99%
Smoking Cessation Advice[1]	1	100%	80%	82%	100%
Pneumonia Care					
Appropriate Initial Antibiotic[1]	7	100%	87%	83%	94%
Blood Culture Timing[1]	8	100%	94%	90%	100%
Influenza Vaccine[1]	3	100%	79%	70%	100%
Initial Antibiotic Timing[1]	12	75%	87%	80%	93%
Oxygenation Assessment[1]	13	100%	100%	99%	100%
Pneumococcal Vaccine[1]	8	100%	78%	69%	94%
Smoking Cessation Advice[1]	3	100%	82%	80%	100%
Surgical Infection Prevention					
Prophylactic Antibiotic Given[5]	-	-	84%	77%	95%
Prophylactic Antibiotic Selection[5]	-	-	93%	90%	100%
Prophylactic Antibiotic Stopped[5]	-	-	80%	72%	95%
Pregnancy Care					
Inpatient Neonatal Mortality	-	-	-	-	-
Third or Fourth Degree Laceration	-	-	3.43%	3.63%	3.27%

Southwest Health Center

1400 East Side Road
Platteville, WI 53818
Ownership: Voluntary non-profit - Other
Emergency Services: No
Phone: 608-348-2331
Fax: 608-342-5035
Accredited: Yes
Licensed Beds: 155

Key Personnel:

CEO . . . . Anne Klawiter
Head of Medical Staff . . . . Kevin Carr
Head of Emergency Room . . . . Cristien Duranceau
Head of Respiratory Care . . . . Becky Fhambow

Measure	Cases	This Hospital	State Average	U.S. Average	Top Hospital
Heart Attack Care					
ACE Inhibitor or ARB for LVSD	0	-	85%	82%	100%
Aspirin at Arrival[1]	14	93%	94%	92%	100%
Aspirin at Discharge[1]	8	100%	94%	90%	100%
Beta Blocker at Arrival[1]	11	91%	92%	87%	100%
Beta Blocker at Discharge[1]	9	89%	92%	90%	100%
Fibrinolytic Medication Timing	0	-	13%	31%	100%
PCI Within 90 Minutes of Arrival	0	-	75%	54%	95%
Smoking Cessation Advice	0	-	91%	88%	100%
Heart Failure Care					
ACE Inhibitor or ARB for LVSD[1]	7	86%	86%	82%	100%
Discharge Instructions	33	100%	73%	61%	93%
Evaluation of LVS Function	40	78%	88%	83%	99%
Smoking Cessation Advice[1]	3	33%	80%	82%	100%
Pneumonia Care					
Appropriate Initial Antibiotic	44	84%	87%	83%	94%
Blood Culture Timing[1]	23	100%	94%	90%	100%
Influenza Vaccine[1]	7	71%	79%	70%	100%
Initial Antibiotic Timing	73	93%	87%	80%	93%
Oxygenation Assessment	77	100%	100%	99%	100%
Pneumococcal Vaccine	47	94%	78%	69%	94%
Smoking Cessation Advice[1]	11	73%	82%	80%	100%
Surgical Infection Prevention					
Prophylactic Antibiotic Given[5]	-	-	84%	77%	95%
Prophylactic Antibiotic Selection[5]	-	-	93%	90%	100%

NOTE: Hospital profiles are in alphabetical order by state, then city, then hospital within the city; Rankings are sorted by rate in descending order and exclude hospitals with less than 25 cases; (1) The number of cases is too small (n<25) for purposes of reliably predicting hospital performance; (2) Measure reflects the hospital's indication that its submission was based upon a sample of its relevant discharges; (3) Rate reflects fewer than the maximum possible quarters of data for the measure; (4) Inaccurate information submitted and suppressed for one or more quarters; (5) No data is available from the hospital for this measure; Please refer to the User's Guide for a full explanation of data

Prophylactic Antibiotic Stopped[5]	-	-	80%	72%	95%
Pregnancy Care					
Inpatient Neonatal Mortality	-	-	-	-	-
Third or Fourth Degree Laceration	-	-	3.43%	3.63%	3.27%

Divine Savior Healthcare

Alternate Name: Divine Savior Hospital and Nursing Home
1015 W Pleasant Street
PO Box 387
Portage, WI 53901
URL: www.dshealthcare.com
Phone: 608-742-4131
Fax: 608-742-6098
Ownership: Voluntary non-profit - Church
Emergency Services: Yes
Accredited: Yes
Licensed Beds: 73

Key Personnel:
Administrator/CEO . . . . Michael T Decker
Chief of Medical Staff . . . . Susan Kreckman
Head of Emergency Room . . . . James Gariti
Emergency Room . . . . Jeffry Snyder, MD
Director Infection/Disease Control . . . . Wanda Lowry
ICU Supervising Nurse . . . . Melissa Bradbury, RN
Director Medical/Surgical Nursing . . . . Jan Bauman, RN
Director Respiratory Therapy . . . . Lynn Waldera

Measure	Cases	This Hospital	State Average	U.S. Average	Top Hospital
Heart Attack Care					
ACE Inhibitor or ARB for LVSD[1]	2	100%	85%	82%	100%
Aspirin at Arrival[1]	10	80%	94%	92%	100%
Aspirin at Discharge[1]	4	100%	94%	90%	100%
Beta Blocker at Arrival[1]	10	70%	92%	87%	100%
Beta Blocker at Discharge[1]	4	100%	92%	90%	100%
Fibrinolytic Medication Timing[3]	0	-	13%	31%	100%
PCI Within 90 Minutes of Arrival	0	-	75%	54%	95%
Smoking Cessation Advice[3]	0	-	91%	88%	100%
Heart Failure Care					
ACE Inhibitor or ARB for LVSD[1]	18	89%	86%	82%	100%
Discharge Instructions[1,3]	10	90%	73%	61%	93%
Evaluation of LVS Function	67	64%	88%	83%	99%
Smoking Cessation Advice[1,3]	1	0%	80%	82%	100%
Pneumonia Care					
Appropriate Initial Antibiotic[1,3]	10	70%	87%	83%	94%
Blood Culture Timing[1,3]	12	92%	94%	90%	100%
Influenza Vaccine[5]	-	-	79%	70%	100%
Initial Antibiotic Timing	101	86%	87%	80%	93%
Oxygenation Assessment	120	100%	100%	99%	100%
Pneumococcal Vaccine	89	49%	78%	69%	94%
Smoking Cessation Advice[1,3]	2	0%	82%	80%	100%
Surgical Infection Prevention					
Prophylactic Antibiotic Given[1,3]	23	83%	84%	77%	95%
Prophylactic Antibiotic Selection[5]	-	-	93%	90%	100%
Prophylactic Antibiotic Stopped[1,3]	23	70%	80%	72%	95%
Pregnancy Care					
Inpatient Neonatal Mortality	309	0.00%	-	-	-
Third or Fourth Degree Laceration	237	4.64%	3.43%	3.63%	3.27%

Sauk Prairie Memorial Hospital

80 1st Street
Prairie Du Sac, WI 53578
Ownership: Voluntary non-profit - Private
Emergency Services: Yes
Phone: 608-643-3311
Fax: 608-643-7151
Accredited: Yes
Licensed Beds: 36

Key Personnel:
CEO . . . . Richard Palagi
Chief Medical Staff . . . . Vicki Kilen
Emergency Room . . . . Loiz Elfen-Schlender
Emergency Room . . . . Connie Henery
Director Infection/Disease Control . . . . Sandra Schlender, RN
Director Medical/Surgical Nursing . . . . Deb Dauluf
Chief Radiology . . . . Tom Grunwald
Director Respiratory Therapy . . . . Gerry Boris

Measure	Cases	This Hospital	State Average	U.S. Average	Top Hospital
Heart Attack Care					
ACE Inhibitor or ARB for LVSD[1]	1	100%	85%	82%	100%
Aspirin at Arrival	0	-	94%	92%	100%
Aspirin at Discharge	0	-	94%	90%	100%
Beta Blocker at Arrival[1]	2	100%	92%	87%	100%
Beta Blocker at Discharge[1]	1	100%	92%	90%	100%
Fibrinolytic Medication Timing	0	-	13%	31%	100%
PCI Within 90 Minutes of Arrival	0	-	75%	54%	95%
Smoking Cessation Advice	0	-	91%	88%	100%
Heart Failure Care					
ACE Inhibitor or ARB for LVSD[1]	12	100%	86%	82%	100%
Discharge Instructions	29	76%	73%	61%	93%
Evaluation of LVS Function	45	93%	88%	83%	99%
Smoking Cessation Advice[1]	5	80%	80%	82%	100%
Pneumonia Care					
Appropriate Initial Antibiotic	49	92%	87%	83%	94%
Blood Culture Timing[1]	15	93%	94%	90%	100%
Influenza Vaccine[1]	8	100%	79%	70%	100%
Initial Antibiotic Timing	57	95%	87%	80%	93%
Oxygenation Assessment	72	100%	100%	99%	100%
Pneumococcal Vaccine	56	86%	78%	69%	94%
Smoking Cessation Advice[1]	8	50%	82%	80%	100%
Surgical Infection Prevention					
Prophylactic Antibiotic Given	318	92%	84%	77%	95%
Prophylactic Antibiotic Selection	69	99%	93%	90%	100%
Prophylactic Antibiotic Stopped	315	76%	80%	72%	95%
Pregnancy Care					
Inpatient Neonatal Mortality	-	-	-	-	-
Third or Fourth Degree Laceration	-	-	3.43%	3.63%	3.27%

WFH-All Saints Spring Street Campus

3801 Spring Street
Racine, WI 53405
URL: www.allsaintshealth.com
Phone: 262-636-4011
Fax: 262-687-2674
Ownership: Voluntary non-profit - Church
Emergency Services: Yes
Accredited: No
Licensed Beds: 226

Key Personnel:
President/CEO . . . . Kenneth Buser
Director of Emergency Room . . . . Margrett Malnory
OB/GYN Womens Health . . . . Jeffrey Musson, MD
Director Respiratory Therapy . . . . Herb Laib

Measure	Cases	This Hospital	State Average	U.S. Average	Top Hospital
Heart Attack Care					
ACE Inhibitor or ARB for LVSD[1]	21	76%	85%	82%	100%
Aspirin at Arrival	169	99%	94%	92%	100%
Aspirin at Discharge	147	99%	94%	90%	100%
Beta Blocker at Arrival	147	97%	92%	87%	100%
Beta Blocker at Discharge	139	99%	92%	90%	100%
Fibrinolytic Medication Timing[1]	2	0%	13%	31%	100%
PCI Within 90 Minutes of Arrival[1]	14	71%	75%	54%	95%
Smoking Cessation Advice	54	93%	91%	88%	100%
Heart Failure Care					
ACE Inhibitor or ARB for LVSD	173	74%	86%	82%	100%
Discharge Instructions	355	85%	73%	61%	93%
Evaluation of LVS Function	424	96%	88%	83%	99%
Smoking Cessation Advice	80	84%	80%	82%	100%
Pneumonia Care					
Appropriate Initial Antibiotic	227	89%	87%	83%	94%
Blood Culture Timing	182	79%	94%	90%	100%
Influenza Vaccine	40	75%	79%	70%	100%
Initial Antibiotic Timing	295	92%	87%	80%	93%
Oxygenation Assessment	365	100%	100%	99%	100%
Pneumococcal Vaccine	242	77%	78%	69%	94%
Smoking Cessation Advice	81	89%	82%	80%	100%
Surgical Infection Prevention					
Prophylactic Antibiotic Given[3]	170	74%	84%	77%	95%
Prophylactic Antibiotic Selection	55	98%	93%	90%	100%
Prophylactic Antibiotic Stopped[3]	161	81%	80%	72%	95%
Pregnancy Care					
Inpatient Neonatal Mortality	-	-	-	-	-
Third or Fourth Degree Laceration	-	-	3.43%	3.63%	3.27%

Reedsburg Area Medical Center

Alternate Name: Reedsburg Memorial Hospital

NOTE: Hospital profiles are in alphabetical order by state, then city, then hospital within the city; Rankings are sorted by rate in descending order and exclude hospitals with less than 25 cases; (1) The number of cases is too small (n<25) for purposes of reliably predicting hospital performance; (2) Measure reflects the hospital's indication that its submission was based upon a sample of its relevant discharges; (3) Rate reflects fewer than the maximum possible quarters of data for the measure; (4) Inaccurate information submitted and suppressed for one or more quarters; (5) No data is available from the hospital for this measure; Please refer to the User's Guide for a full explanation of data

2000 N Dewey Avenue
Reedsburg, WI 53959
URL: www.ramchealth.com
Phone: 608-524-6487
Fax: 608-524-6566
Ownership: Voluntary non-profit - Private
Emergency Services: Yes
Accredited: Yes
Licensed Beds: 53

Key Personnel:

President/CEO . . . . Mel Hahs
Chief Medical Staff . . . . K M Hoffmann, MD
Director Emergency Room . . . . Janet Bolk
Infection Control . . . . Peg Dobrovelny
ICU . . . . Janet Volk
Medical/Surgical Nursing . . . . Terri Langer, RN
OB/GYN Womens Health . . . . Diane Bindl
Respiratory Care . . . . Gail Brittan

Measure	Cases	This Hospital	State Average	U.S. Average	Top Hospital
Heart Attack Care					
ACE Inhibitor or ARB for LVSD[1]	1	0%	85%	82%	100%
Aspirin at Arrival[1]	8	88%	94%	92%	100%
Aspirin at Discharge[1]	3	100%	94%	90%	100%
Beta Blocker at Arrival[1]	8	75%	92%	87%	100%
Beta Blocker at Discharge[1]	5	100%	92%	90%	100%
Fibrinolytic Medication Timing	0	-	13%	31%	100%
PCI Within 90 Minutes of Arrival	0	-	75%	54%	95%
Smoking Cessation Advice	0	-	91%	88%	100%
Heart Failure Care					
ACE Inhibitor or ARB for LVSD[1]	11	91%	86%	82%	100%
Discharge Instructions	26	35%	73%	61%	93%
Evaluation of LVS Function	37	84%	88%	83%	99%
Smoking Cessation Advice[1]	5	40%	80%	82%	100%
Pneumonia Care					
Appropriate Initial Antibiotic	69	99%	87%	83%	94%
Blood Culture Timing	25	92%	94%	90%	100%
Influenza Vaccine[1]	18	89%	79%	70%	100%
Initial Antibiotic Timing	80	92%	87%	80%	93%
Oxygenation Assessment	95	100%	100%	99%	100%
Pneumococcal Vaccine	69	93%	78%	69%	94%
Smoking Cessation Advice[1]	15	87%	82%	80%	100%
Surgical Infection Prevention					
Prophylactic Antibiotic Given	75	65%	84%	77%	95%
Prophylactic Antibiotic Selection[1]	22	100%	93%	90%	100%
Prophylactic Antibiotic Stopped	74	66%	80%	72%	95%
Pregnancy Care					
Inpatient Neonatal Mortality	-	-	-	-	-
Third or Fourth Degree Laceration	-	-	3.43%	3.63%	3.27%

Saint Mary's Hospital

2251 North Shore Drive
Rhinelander, WI 54501
URL: www.ministryhealth.org
Phone: 715-361-2000
Fax: 715-361-2011
Ownership: Voluntary non-profit - Church
Emergency Services: Yes
Accredited: Yes
Licensed Beds: 73

Key Personnel:

CEO . . . . Kevin O'Donnell
Chief Medical Staff . . . . Judith Pagano, MD
Cardiac Lab Director . . . . Kathy Grill, RN
Catheterization Lab Director . . . . Kathy Grill
Emergency Room Manager . . . . Denise Counter
Infection Control Manager . . . . Karen Wiedeman, RN
ICU . . . . Kathy Grill
Medical Surgical Nursing . . . . Rene Iannarelli
OB/GYN/Women's Health . . . . Dorothy Skye, MD
Respiratory/Cardiopulmonary . . . . Carol Humlie

Measure	Cases	This Hospital	State Average	U.S. Average	Top Hospital
Heart Attack Care					
ACE Inhibitor or ARB for LVSD[1]	6	100%	85%	82%	100%
Aspirin at Arrival	25	96%	94%	92%	100%
Aspirin at Discharge[1]	19	95%	94%	90%	100%
Beta Blocker at Arrival	27	74%	92%	87%	100%
Beta Blocker at Discharge[1]	22	86%	92%	90%	100%
Fibrinolytic Medication Timing	0	-	13%	31%	100%
PCI Within 90 Minutes of Arrival	0	-	75%	54%	95%
Smoking Cessation Advice[1]	1	0%	91%	88%	100%
Heart Failure Care					
ACE Inhibitor or ARB for LVSD	38	87%	86%	82%	100%
Discharge Instructions	101	85%	73%	61%	93%
Evaluation of LVS Function	122	90%	88%	83%	99%
Smoking Cessation Advice[1]	12	92%	80%	82%	100%
Pneumonia Care					
Appropriate Initial Antibiotic	70	86%	87%	83%	94%
Blood Culture Timing	45	96%	94%	90%	100%
Influenza Vaccine[1]	24	92%	79%	70%	100%
Initial Antibiotic Timing	110	81%	87%	80%	93%
Oxygenation Assessment	124	100%	100%	99%	100%
Pneumococcal Vaccine	91	86%	78%	69%	94%
Smoking Cessation Advice	29	93%	82%	80%	100%
Surgical Infection Prevention					
Prophylactic Antibiotic Given	382	88%	84%	77%	95%
Prophylactic Antibiotic Selection	96	93%	93%	90%	100%
Prophylactic Antibiotic Stopped	379	92%	80%	72%	95%
Pregnancy Care					
Inpatient Neonatal Mortality	-	-	-	-	-
Third or Fourth Degree Laceration	-	-	3.43%	3.63%	3.27%

Lakeview Medical Center of Rice Lake

1100 N Main Street
Rice Lake, WI 54868
URL: www.lakeviewmedical.com
Phone: 715-234-1515
Fax: 715-234-4465
Ownership: Voluntary non-profit - Private
Emergency Services: Yes
Accredited: Yes
Licensed Beds: 75

Key Personnel:

Emergency Room . . . . Rodney G Olson, MD
Emergency Room . . . . John B Waldron, MD

Measure	Cases	This Hospital	State Average	U.S. Average	Top Hospital
Heart Attack Care					
ACE Inhibitor or ARB for LVSD[1]	4	100%	85%	82%	100%
Aspirin at Arrival[1]	21	100%	94%	92%	100%
Aspirin at Discharge[1]	16	100%	94%	90%	100%
Beta Blocker at Arrival[1]	17	100%	92%	87%	100%
Beta Blocker at Discharge[1]	19	100%	92%	90%	100%
Fibrinolytic Medication Timing	0	-	13%	31%	100%
PCI Within 90 Minutes of Arrival	0	-	75%	54%	95%
Smoking Cessation Advice[1]	5	40%	91%	88%	100%
Heart Failure Care					
ACE Inhibitor or ARB for LVSD	36	92%	86%	82%	100%
Discharge Instructions	85	75%	73%	61%	93%
Evaluation of LVS Function	104	93%	88%	83%	99%
Smoking Cessation Advice[1]	12	83%	80%	82%	100%
Pneumonia Care					
Appropriate Initial Antibiotic	76	100%	87%	83%	94%
Blood Culture Timing	63	100%	94%	90%	100%
Influenza Vaccine[1]	24	92%	79%	70%	100%
Initial Antibiotic Timing	114	94%	87%	80%	93%
Oxygenation Assessment	142	100%	100%	99%	100%
Pneumococcal Vaccine	96	97%	78%	69%	94%
Smoking Cessation Advice	34	82%	82%	80%	100%
Surgical Infection Prevention					
Prophylactic Antibiotic Given	330	92%	84%	77%	95%
Prophylactic Antibiotic Selection	71	100%	93%	90%	100%
Prophylactic Antibiotic Stopped	317	95%	80%	72%	95%
Pregnancy Care					
Inpatient Neonatal Mortality	-	-	-	-	-
Third or Fourth Degree Laceration	-	-	3.43%	3.63%	3.27%

Richland Hospital

333 E 2nd Street
Richland Center, WI 53581
E-mail: hr@richlandhospital.com
URL: www.richlandhospital.com
Phone: 608-647-6321
Fax: 608-647-6235
Ownership: Voluntary non-profit - Private
Emergency Services: Yes
Accredited: Yes
Licensed Beds: 66

Key Personnel:

CEO . . . . Harle Aber
Chief Medical Staff . . . . Thomas Richardson, MD

NOTE: Hospital profiles are in alphabetical order by state, then city, then hospital within the city; Rankings are sorted by rate in descending order and exclude hospitals with less than 25 cases; (1) The number of cases is too small (n<25) for purposes of reliably predicting hospital performance; (2) Measure reflects the hospital's indication that its submission was based upon a sample of its relevant discharges; (3) Rate reflects fewer than the maximum possible quarters of data for the measure; (4) Inaccurate information submitted and suppressed for one or more quarters; (5) No data is available from the hospital for this measure; Please refer to the User's Guide for a full explanation of data

Measure	Cases	This Hospital	State Average	U.S. Average	Top Hospital
Heart Attack Care					
ACE Inhibitor or ARB for LVSD	0	-	85%	82%	100%
Aspirin at Arrival[1]	10	100%	94%	92%	100%
Aspirin at Discharge[1]	8	100%	94%	90%	100%
Beta Blocker at Arrival[1]	9	100%	92%	87%	100%
Beta Blocker at Discharge[1]	8	100%	92%	90%	100%
Fibrinolytic Medication Timing[1]	1	0%	13%	31%	100%
PCI Within 90 Minutes of Arrival	0	-	75%	54%	95%
Smoking Cessation Advice	0	-	91%	88%	100%
Heart Failure Care					
ACE Inhibitor or ARB for LVSD[1]	15	87%	86%	82%	100%
Discharge Instructions	37	84%	73%	61%	93%
Evaluation of LVS Function	58	76%	88%	83%	99%
Smoking Cessation Advice[1]	5	80%	80%	82%	100%
Pneumonia Care					
Appropriate Initial Antibiotic	30	67%	87%	83%	94%
Blood Culture Timing[1]	21	90%	94%	90%	100%
Influenza Vaccine[1]	10	80%	79%	70%	100%
Initial Antibiotic Timing	43	84%	87%	80%	93%
Oxygenation Assessment	57	100%	100%	99%	100%
Pneumococcal Vaccine	35	57%	78%	69%	94%
Smoking Cessation Advice[1]	9	100%	82%	80%	100%
Surgical Infection Prevention					
Prophylactic Antibiotic Given	54	63%	84%	77%	95%
Prophylactic Antibiotic Selection[1]	13	92%	93%	90%	100%
Prophylactic Antibiotic Stopped	53	77%	80%	72%	95%
Pregnancy Care					
Inpatient Neonatal Mortality	-	-	-	-	-
Third or Fourth Degree Laceration	-	-	3.43%	3.63%	3.27%

Ripon Medical Center

Alternate Name: Ripon Memorial Hospital
933 Newbury Street
PO Box 390
Ripon, WI 54971
Phone: 920-748-3101
Fax: 920-748-9104
E-mail: info@riponmedicalcenter.com
URL: www.riponmedicalcenter.com
Ownership: Voluntary non-profit - Private
Emergency Services: Yes
Accredited: Yes
Licensed Beds: 25

Key Personnel:

CEO. . . . . Tommy Hobbs
Chief Medical Staff. . . . . Michael Combs, MD
Director Cardiac Rehabilitation. . . . . Sandy Schaffer
Director Emergency Room. . . . . Joann Strandell
Director Surgery Services . . . . Deb Soper
Director Respiratory Care. . . . . Lori Rhodes

Measure	Cases	This Hospital	State Average	U.S. Average	Top Hospital
Heart Attack Care					
ACE Inhibitor or ARB for LVSD[5]	-	-	85%	82%	100%
Aspirin at Arrival[5]	-	-	94%	92%	100%
Aspirin at Discharge[5]	-	-	94%	90%	100%
Beta Blocker at Arrival[5]	-	-	92%	87%	100%
Beta Blocker at Discharge[5]	-	-	92%	90%	100%
Fibrinolytic Medication Timing[5]	-	-	13%	31%	100%
PCI Within 90 Minutes of Arrival[5]	-	-	75%	54%	95%
Smoking Cessation Advice[5]	-	-	91%	88%	100%
Heart Failure Care					
ACE Inhibitor or ARB for LVSD[1]	7	71%	86%	82%	100%
Discharge Instructions[1]	12	50%	73%	61%	93%
Evaluation of LVS Function	32	72%	88%	83%	99%
Smoking Cessation Advice[1]	4	50%	80%	82%	100%
Pneumonia Care					
Appropriate Initial Antibiotic[1]	20	95%	87%	83%	94%
Blood Culture Timing[1]	9	89%	94%	90%	100%
Influenza Vaccine[1]	3	33%	79%	70%	100%
Initial Antibiotic Timing	31	90%	87%	80%	93%
Oxygenation Assessment	34	97%	100%	99%	100%
Pneumococcal Vaccine	28	64%	78%	69%	94%
Smoking Cessation Advice[1]	9	56%	82%	80%	100%
Surgical Infection Prevention					
Prophylactic Antibiotic Given[5]	-	-	84%	77%	95%
Prophylactic Antibiotic Selection[5]	-	-	93%	90%	100%
Prophylactic Antibiotic Stopped[5]	-	-	80%	72%	95%
Pregnancy Care					
Inpatient Neonatal Mortality	-	-	-	-	-
Third or Fourth Degree Laceration	-	-	3.43%	3.63%	3.27%

River Falls Area Hospital

1629 E Division Street
River Falls, WI 54022
Phone: 715-425-6155
Fax: 715-426-4555
URL: www.allina.com
Ownership: Voluntary non-profit - Private
Emergency Services: Yes
Accredited: Yes
Licensed Beds: 42

Key Personnel:

CEO. . . . . Randy Farrow
Chief Medical Staff. . . . . Dan Zimmerman
Director Infection/Disease Control . . . . Sue Nelson, RN
CCU Spvg. Nurse . . . . Tammy Ducklow, RN
Director Medical/Surgical Nursing . . . . Jane Peterson
Chief Radiology . . . . Judy Zaruba

Measure	Cases	This Hospital	State Average	U.S. Average	Top Hospital
Heart Attack Care					
ACE Inhibitor or ARB for LVSD[1]	3	67%	85%	82%	100%
Aspirin at Arrival[1]	7	100%	94%	92%	100%
Aspirin at Discharge[1]	8	100%	94%	90%	100%
Beta Blocker at Arrival[1]	5	100%	92%	87%	100%
Beta Blocker at Discharge[1]	9	89%	92%	90%	100%
Fibrinolytic Medication Timing	0	-	13%	31%	100%
PCI Within 90 Minutes of Arrival	0	-	75%	54%	95%
Smoking Cessation Advice	0	-	91%	88%	100%
Heart Failure Care					
ACE Inhibitor or ARB for LVSD[1]	12	100%	86%	82%	100%
Discharge Instructions[1]	22	82%	73%	61%	93%
Evaluation of LVS Function	28	93%	88%	83%	99%
Smoking Cessation Advice[1]	3	100%	80%	82%	100%
Pneumonia Care					
Appropriate Initial Antibiotic	34	97%	87%	83%	94%
Blood Culture Timing[1]	10	90%	94%	90%	100%
Influenza Vaccine[1]	9	78%	79%	70%	100%
Initial Antibiotic Timing	39	90%	87%	80%	93%
Oxygenation Assessment	54	98%	100%	99%	100%
Pneumococcal Vaccine	37	89%	78%	69%	94%
Smoking Cessation Advice[1]	10	90%	82%	80%	100%
Surgical Infection Prevention					
Prophylactic Antibiotic Given[5]	-	-	84%	77%	95%
Prophylactic Antibiotic Selection[5]	-	-	93%	90%	100%
Prophylactic Antibiotic Stopped[5]	-	-	80%	72%	95%
Pregnancy Care					
Inpatient Neonatal Mortality	-	-	-	-	-
Third or Fourth Degree Laceration	-	-	3.43%	3.63%	3.27%

Saint Croix Regional Medical Center

Alternate Name: Saint Croix Valley Memorial Hospital
204 S Adams Street
Saint Croix Falls, WI 54024
Toll-Free: 800-642-1336
Phone: 715-483-3261
Fax: 340-772-7398
URL: www.scrmc.org
Ownership: Proprietary
Emergency Services: Yes
Accredited: No
Licensed Beds: 92

Key Personnel:

CEO. . . . . Cindy Lundmark

Measure	Cases	This Hospital	State Average	U.S. Average	Top Hospital
Heart Attack Care					
ACE Inhibitor or ARB for LVSD[5]	-	-	85%	82%	100%
Aspirin at Arrival[5]	-	-	94%	92%	100%
Aspirin at Discharge[5]	-	-	94%	90%	100%
Beta Blocker at Arrival[5]	-	-	92%	87%	100%
Beta Blocker at Discharge[5]	-	-	92%	90%	100%
Fibrinolytic Medication Timing[5]	-	-	13%	31%	100%
PCI Within 90 Minutes of Arrival[5]	-	-	75%	54%	95%

NOTE: Hospital profiles are in alphabetical order by state, then city, then hospital within the city; Rankings are sorted by rate in descending order and exclude hospitals with less than 25 cases; (1) The number of cases is too small (n<25) for purposes of reliably predicting hospital performance; (2) Measure reflects the hospital's indication that its submission was based upon a sample of its relevant discharges; (3) Rate reflects fewer than the maximum possible quarters of data for the measure; (4) Inaccurate information submitted and suppressed for one or more quarters; (5) No data is available from the hospital for this measure; Please refer to the User's Guide for a full explanation of data

Smoking Cessation Advice[5]	-	-	91%	88%	100%
Heart Failure Care					
ACE Inhibitor or ARB for LVSD[5]	-	-	86%	82%	100%
Discharge Instructions[5]	-	-	73%	61%	93%
Evaluation of LVS Function[5]	-	-	88%	83%	99%
Smoking Cessation Advice[5]	-	-	80%	82%	100%
Pneumonia Care					
Appropriate Initial Antibiotic[3]	26	96%	87%	83%	94%
Blood Culture Timing	35	94%	94%	90%	100%
Influenza Vaccine[1]	16	100%	79%	70%	100%
Initial Antibiotic Timing[3]	36	86%	87%	80%	93%
Oxygenation Assessment[3]	49	100%	100%	99%	100%
Pneumococcal Vaccine[3]	41	68%	78%	69%	94%
Smoking Cessation Advice[1,3]	6	33%	82%	80%	100%
Surgical Infection Prevention					
Prophylactic Antibiotic Given[3]	73	96%	84%	77%	95%
Prophylactic Antibiotic Selection[1]	16	81%	93%	90%	100%
Prophylactic Antibiotic Stopped[3]	71	85%	80%	72%	95%
Pregnancy Care					
Inpatient Neonatal Mortality	-	-	-	-	-
Third or Fourth Degree Laceration	-	-	3.43%	3.63%	3.27%

Shawano Medical Center

309 North Bartlette Street
Shawano, WI 54166

Toll-Free: 800-748-2824
Phone: 715-526-2111
Fax: 715-526-7205

E-mail: smc@shawanomed.org
URL: www.shawanomed.org
Ownership: Voluntary non-profit - Other
Emergency Services: Yes
Accredited: Yes
Licensed Beds: 25

Key Personnel:

CEO/Administrator . . . . Jim Baer
Chief of Medical Staff . . . . Tod Lewis, MD
Emergency Room Manager . . . . Diane Holschbach, RN
Infection Control . . . . Pam Buppert
Manager OB/GYN/Women's Health . . . . Carol Kary, RN
Manager Radiology . . . . Jan Short
Respiratory/Cardiopulmonary . . . . Penny Block

Measure	Cases	This Hospital	State Average	U.S. Average	Top Hospital
Heart Attack Care					
ACE Inhibitor or ARB for LVSD[1]	3	100%	85%	82%	100%
Aspirin at Arrival[1]	15	87%	94%	92%	100%
Aspirin at Discharge[1]	10	80%	94%	90%	100%
Beta Blocker at Arrival[1]	14	100%	92%	87%	100%
Beta Blocker at Discharge[1]	10	100%	92%	90%	100%
Fibrinolytic Medication Timing	0	-	13%	31%	100%
PCI Within 90 Minutes of Arrival	0	-	75%	54%	95%
Smoking Cessation Advice[1]	1	0%	91%	88%	100%
Heart Failure Care					
ACE Inhibitor or ARB for LVSD[1]	17	82%	86%	82%	100%
Discharge Instructions	45	64%	73%	61%	93%
Evaluation of LVS Function	64	86%	88%	83%	99%
Smoking Cessation Advice[1]	6	83%	80%	82%	100%
Pneumonia Care					
Appropriate Initial Antibiotic	86	85%	87%	83%	94%
Blood Culture Timing	32	97%	94%	90%	100%
Influenza Vaccine[1]	20	95%	79%	70%	100%
Initial Antibiotic Timing	112	95%	87%	80%	93%
Oxygenation Assessment	136	100%	100%	99%	100%
Pneumococcal Vaccine	86	88%	78%	69%	94%
Smoking Cessation Advice[1]	23	70%	82%	80%	100%
Surgical Infection Prevention					
Prophylactic Antibiotic Given[5]	-	-	84%	77%	95%
Prophylactic Antibiotic Selection[5]	-	-	93%	90%	100%
Prophylactic Antibiotic Stopped[5]	-	-	80%	72%	95%
Pregnancy Care					
Inpatient Neonatal Mortality	-	-	-	-	-
Third or Fourth Degree Laceration	-	-	3.43%	3.63%	3.27%

Aurora Sheboygan Memorial Medical Center

2629 N 7th St
Sheboygan, WI 53083
Phone: 920-451-5000
Ownership: Voluntary non-profit - Private
Accredited: Yes
Emergency Services: Yes

Measure	Cases	This Hospital	State Average	U.S. Average	Top Hospital
Heart Attack Care					
ACE Inhibitor or ARB for LVSD[1]	8	100%	85%	82%	100%
Aspirin at Arrival	41	100%	94%	92%	100%
Aspirin at Discharge	25	100%	94%	90%	100%
Beta Blocker at Arrival[1]	22	100%	92%	87%	100%
Beta Blocker at Discharge	27	100%	92%	90%	100%
Fibrinolytic Medication Timing	0	-	13%	31%	100%
PCI Within 90 Minutes of Arrival	0	-	75%	54%	95%
Smoking Cessation Advice[1]	8	100%	91%	88%	100%
Heart Failure Care					
ACE Inhibitor or ARB for LVSD	34	100%	86%	82%	100%
Discharge Instructions	85	96%	73%	61%	93%
Evaluation of LVS Function	102	100%	88%	83%	99%
Smoking Cessation Advice[1]	14	93%	80%	82%	100%
Pneumonia Care					
Appropriate Initial Antibiotic	75	91%	87%	83%	94%
Blood Culture Timing	67	100%	94%	90%	100%
Influenza Vaccine[1]	22	95%	79%	70%	100%
Initial Antibiotic Timing	108	93%	87%	80%	93%
Oxygenation Assessment	130	100%	100%	99%	100%
Pneumococcal Vaccine	79	95%	78%	69%	94%
Smoking Cessation Advice	39	100%	82%	80%	100%
Surgical Infection Prevention					
Prophylactic Antibiotic Given[2,3]	96	91%	84%	77%	95%
Prophylactic Antibiotic Selection[2]	45	96%	93%	90%	100%
Prophylactic Antibiotic Stopped[2,3]	96	88%	80%	72%	95%
Pregnancy Care					
Inpatient Neonatal Mortality	-	-	-	-	-
Third or Fourth Degree Laceration	-	-	3.43%	3.63%	3.27%

Saint Nicholas Hospital

3100 Superior Avenue
Sheboygan, WI 53081

Toll-Free: 800-472-6710
Phone: 920-459-8300
Fax: 920-451-7280

URL: www.stnicholashospital.org
Ownership: Voluntary non-profit - Church
Emergency Services: Yes
Accredited: Yes
Licensed Beds: 185

Key Personnel:

Chief Medical Staff . . . . Philip Walker, MD
Chief Catheterization Laboratory . . . . Louie Coulis, MD
Chief Emergency Medicine . . . . Richard T Tovar, MD
Emergency Room . . . . Charles Havel, MD
Director Infection/Disease Control . . . . Sally Korff
Director Medical/Surgical Nursing . . . . Patricia Stubbe
OB/GYN Women's Health . . . . Clifford G Martin, MD
Chief Radiology . . . . Gregg Gaylord, MD
Director Respiratory Therapy . . . . Philip Detrana, MD

Measure	Cases	This Hospital	State Average	U.S. Average	Top Hospital
Heart Attack Care					
ACE Inhibitor or ARB for LVSD[1]	7	71%	85%	82%	100%
Aspirin at Arrival	46	91%	94%	92%	100%
Aspirin at Discharge	27	59%	94%	90%	100%
Beta Blocker at Arrival[1]	20	85%	92%	87%	100%
Beta Blocker at Discharge	26	92%	92%	90%	100%
Fibrinolytic Medication Timing[3]	0	-	13%	31%	100%
PCI Within 90 Minutes of Arrival	0	-	75%	54%	95%
Smoking Cessation Advice[3]	0	-	91%	88%	100%
Heart Failure Care					
ACE Inhibitor or ARB for LVSD[1]	22	86%	86%	82%	100%
Discharge Instructions[1,3]	18	44%	73%	61%	93%
Evaluation of LVS Function	84	55%	88%	83%	99%
Smoking Cessation Advice[1,3]	1	0%	80%	82%	100%
Pneumonia Care					
Appropriate Initial Antibiotic[1,3]	9	78%	87%	83%	94%
Blood Culture Timing[1,3]	11	100%	94%	90%	100%

NOTE: Hospital profiles are in alphabetical order by state, then city, then hospital within the city; Rankings are sorted by rate in descending order and exclude hospitals with less than 25 cases; (1) The number of cases is too small (n<25) for purposes of reliably predicting hospital performance; (2) Measure reflects the hospital's indication that its submission was based upon a sample of its relevant discharges; (3) Rate reflects fewer than the maximum possible quarters of data for the measure; (4) Inaccurate information submitted and suppressed for one or more quarters; (5) No data is available from the hospital for this measure; Please refer to the User's Guide for a full explanation of data

Influenza Vaccine[5]	-	-	79%	70%	100%
Initial Antibiotic Timing	95	83%	87%	80%	93%
Oxygenation Assessment	104	100%	100%	99%	100%
Pneumococcal Vaccine	79	73%	78%	69%	94%
Smoking Cessation Advice[1,3]	3	67%	82%	80%	100%
Surgical Infection Prevention					
Prophylactic Antibiotic Given[3]	64	84%	84%	77%	95%
Prophylactic Antibiotic Selection[5]	-	-	93%	90%	100%
Prophylactic Antibiotic Stopped[3]	64	61%	80%	72%	95%
Pregnancy Care					
Inpatient Neonatal Mortality	-	-	-	-	-
Third or Fourth Degree Laceration	-	-	3.43%	3.63%	3.27%

Indianhead Medical Center

113 4th Ave PO Box 300
Shell Lake, WI 54871
Phone: 715-468-7833
Ownership: Voluntary non-profit - Private
Accredited: Yes
Emergency Services: Yes

Measure	Cases	This Hospital	State Average	U.S. Average	Top Hospital
Heart Attack Care					
ACE Inhibitor or ARB for LVSD[3]	0	-	85%	82%	100%
Aspirin at Arrival[1,3]	1	100%	94%	92%	100%
Aspirin at Discharge[1,3]	1	100%	94%	90%	100%
Beta Blocker at Arrival[1,3]	1	100%	92%	87%	100%
Beta Blocker at Discharge[1,3]	1	100%	92%	90%	100%
Fibrinolytic Medication Timing[3]	0	-	13%	31%	100%
PCI Within 90 Minutes of Arrival	0	-	75%	54%	95%
Smoking Cessation Advice[3]	0	-	91%	88%	100%
Heart Failure Care					
ACE Inhibitor or ARB for LVSD[1]	4	100%	86%	82%	100%
Discharge Instructions[1]	22	59%	73%	61%	93%
Evaluation of LVS Function[1]	24	46%	88%	83%	99%
Smoking Cessation Advice[1]	1	0%	80%	82%	100%
Pneumonia Care					
Appropriate Initial Antibiotic[1]	17	82%	87%	83%	94%
Blood Culture Timing[1]	4	100%	94%	90%	100%
Influenza Vaccine[1]	4	75%	79%	70%	100%
Initial Antibiotic Timing[1]	22	100%	87%	80%	93%
Oxygenation Assessment	27	100%	100%	99%	100%
Pneumococcal Vaccine[1]	23	57%	78%	69%	94%
Smoking Cessation Advice[1]	4	75%	82%	80%	100%
Surgical Infection Prevention					
Prophylactic Antibiotic Given[5]	-	-	84%	77%	95%
Prophylactic Antibiotic Selection[5]	-	-	93%	90%	100%
Prophylactic Antibiotic Stopped[5]	-	-	80%	72%	95%
Pregnancy Care					
Inpatient Neonatal Mortality	-	-	-	-	-
Third or Fourth Degree Laceration	-	-	3.43%	3.63%	3.27%

Franciscan Skemp Healthcare-Sparta Campus

Alternate Name: Saint Mary's Hospital
310 West Main Street
Sparta, WI 54656
Phone: 608-269-2132
Fax: 608-269-4562
URL: www.mayohealthsystem.org/mhs/live/page.cfm
Ownership: Voluntary non-profit - Church
Accredited: Yes
Emergency Services: Yes
Licensed Beds: 25

Key Personnel:

President/CEO . . . . Robert E Nesse, MD
Director Medical/ Surgical Nursing . . . . Toni Eddy-Ballman

Measure	Cases	This Hospital	State Average	U.S. Average	Top Hospital
Heart Attack Care					
ACE Inhibitor or ARB for LVSD[5]	-	-	85%	82%	100%
Aspirin at Arrival[5]	-	-	94%	92%	100%
Aspirin at Discharge[5]	-	-	94%	90%	100%
Beta Blocker at Arrival[5]	-	-	92%	87%	100%
Beta Blocker at Discharge[5]	-	-	92%	90%	100%
Fibrinolytic Medication Timing[5]	-	-	13%	31%	100%
PCI Within 90 Minutes of Arrival[5]	-	-	75%	54%	95%
Smoking Cessation Advice[5]	-	-	91%	88%	100%
Heart Failure Care					
ACE Inhibitor or ARB for LVSD[1]	2	100%	86%	82%	100%
Discharge Instructions[1]	5	100%	73%	61%	93%
Evaluation of LVS Function[1]	18	78%	88%	83%	99%
Smoking Cessation Advice[1]	1	100%	80%	82%	100%
Pneumonia Care					
Appropriate Initial Antibiotic[1]	24	96%	87%	83%	94%
Blood Culture Timing[1]	18	89%	94%	90%	100%
Influenza Vaccine[1]	5	100%	79%	70%	100%
Initial Antibiotic Timing	30	97%	87%	80%	93%
Oxygenation Assessment	36	100%	100%	99%	100%
Pneumococcal Vaccine[1]	19	100%	78%	69%	94%
Smoking Cessation Advice[1]	5	100%	82%	80%	100%
Surgical Infection Prevention					
Prophylactic Antibiotic Given[5]	-	-	84%	77%	95%
Prophylactic Antibiotic Selection[5]	-	-	93%	90%	100%
Prophylactic Antibiotic Stopped[5]	-	-	80%	72%	95%
Pregnancy Care					
Inpatient Neonatal Mortality	-	-	-	-	-
Third or Fourth Degree Laceration	-	-	3.43%	3.63%	3.27%

Spooner Health System

819 Ash Street
Sarona, WI 54870
Phone: 715-635-2111
Fax: 715-635-8674
Ownership: Voluntary non-profit - Private
Accredited: No
Emergency Services: Yes
Licensed Beds: 136

Key Personnel:

Administrator . . . . Michael D Schafer
Chief Medical Staff. . . . . Laura Boelke, MD
Emergency Room . . . . Linda Trent
Director Medical/Surgical Nursing . . . . Marlynn Nordquist
Chief Radiology . . . . Craig Norheim

Measure	Cases	This Hospital	State Average	U.S. Average	Top Hospital
Heart Attack Care					
ACE Inhibitor or ARB for LVSD	0	-	85%	82%	100%
Aspirin at Arrival[1]	8	88%	94%	92%	100%
Aspirin at Discharge[1]	5	100%	94%	90%	100%
Beta Blocker at Arrival[1]	8	75%	92%	87%	100%
Beta Blocker at Discharge[1]	5	80%	92%	90%	100%
Fibrinolytic Medication Timing	0	-	13%	31%	100%
PCI Within 90 Minutes of Arrival	0	-	75%	54%	95%
Smoking Cessation Advice	0	-	91%	88%	100%
Heart Failure Care					
ACE Inhibitor or ARB for LVSD[1]	8	75%	86%	82%	100%
Discharge Instructions[1]	12	25%	73%	61%	93%
Evaluation of LVS Function[1]	22	59%	88%	83%	99%
Smoking Cessation Advice[1]	2	50%	80%	82%	100%
Pneumonia Care					
Appropriate Initial Antibiotic	37	41%	87%	83%	94%
Blood Culture Timing[1]	15	93%	94%	90%	100%
Influenza Vaccine[1]	10	20%	79%	70%	100%
Initial Antibiotic Timing	41	88%	87%	80%	93%
Oxygenation Assessment	51	98%	100%	99%	100%
Pneumococcal Vaccine	34	62%	78%	69%	94%
Smoking Cessation Advice[1]	17	82%	82%	80%	100%
Surgical Infection Prevention					
Prophylactic Antibiotic Given[5]	-	-	84%	77%	95%
Prophylactic Antibiotic Selection[5]	-	-	93%	90%	100%
Prophylactic Antibiotic Stopped[5]	-	-	80%	72%	95%
Pregnancy Care					
Inpatient Neonatal Mortality	-	-	-	-	-
Third or Fourth Degree Laceration	-	-	3.43%	3.63%	3.27%

Our Lady of Victory Hospital

1120 Pine Street
PO Box 220
Stanley, WI 54768
Phone: 715-644-5530
Fax: 715-644-6221
E-mail: papiernk@OLVH.ORG
URL: www.ministryhealth.org
Ownership: Voluntary non-profit - Private
Accredited: No
Emergency Services: Yes
Licensed Beds: 25

Key Personnel:

Administrator/CEO . . . . Cynthia Eichman

NOTE: Hospital profiles are in alphabetical order by state, then city, then hospital within the city; Rankings are sorted by rate in descending order and exclude hospitals with less than 25 cases; (1) The number of cases is too small (n<25) for purposes of reliably predicting hospital performance; (2) Measure reflects the hospital's indication that its submission was based upon a sample of its relevant discharges; (3) Rate reflects fewer than the maximum possible quarters of data for the measure; (4) Inaccurate information submitted and suppressed for one or more quarters; (5) No data is available from the hospital for this measure; Please refer to the User's Guide for a full explanation of data

Chief Medical Staff. . . . . Sharon Haywiard, MD
Emergency Room . . . . Badal Raval, MD
Director Infection/Disease Control . . . . Toni Smith, RN
Medical Surgical Nursing . . . . Debra Savina, RN
Respiratory Therapy. . . . . Mary La Rue

Measure	Cases	This Hospital	State Average	U.S. Average	Top Hospital
Heart Attack Care					
ACE Inhibitor or ARB for LVSD[1,3]	3	100%	85%	82%	100%
Aspirin at Arrival[1,3]	9	78%	94%	92%	100%
Aspirin at Discharge[1,3]	7	57%	94%	90%	100%
Beta Blocker at Arrival[1,3]	7	86%	92%	87%	100%
Beta Blocker at Discharge[1,3]	8	88%	92%	90%	100%
Fibrinolytic Medication Timing[3]	0	-	13%	31%	100%
PCI Within 90 Minutes of Arrival	0	-	75%	54%	95%
Smoking Cessation Advice[3]	0	-	91%	88%	100%
Heart Failure Care					
ACE Inhibitor or ARB for LVSD[1]	7	100%	86%	82%	100%
Discharge Instructions[1]	23	100%	73%	61%	93%
Evaluation of LVS Function	36	94%	88%	83%	99%
Smoking Cessation Advice[1]	2	50%	80%	82%	100%
Pneumonia Care					
Appropriate Initial Antibiotic[1]	17	82%	87%	83%	94%
Blood Culture Timing[1]	4	100%	94%	90%	100%
Influenza Vaccine[1]	4	75%	79%	70%	100%
Initial Antibiotic Timing	25	96%	87%	80%	93%
Oxygenation Assessment	26	100%	100%	99%	100%
Pneumococcal Vaccine[1]	18	89%	78%	69%	94%
Smoking Cessation Advice[1]	6	83%	82%	80%	100%
Surgical Infection Prevention					
Prophylactic Antibiotic Given[1]	4	0%	84%	77%	95%
Prophylactic Antibiotic Selection[1]	1	100%	93%	90%	100%
Prophylactic Antibiotic Stopped[1]	4	100%	80%	72%	95%
Pregnancy Care					
Inpatient Neonatal Mortality	-	-	-	-	-
Third or Fourth Degree Laceration	-	-	3.43%	3.63%	3.27%

Saint Michael's Hospital

900 Illinois Avenue
Stevens Point, WI 54481
Phone: 715-346-5000
Fax: 715-346-5088
Ownership: Voluntary non-profit - Church
Accredited: Yes
Emergency Services: Yes
Licensed Beds: 181

Key Personnel:

President/CEO. . . . . Jeffrey L Martin
Chief Medical Staff. . . . . Mark Fenlon, MD
Emergency Room . . . . Paulette Bessen
Director Infection/Disease Control . . . . Artie Sadlemyer
CCU Spvg. Nurse . . . . Jackie Chartier
OB/GYN Womens Health. . . . . Rick Perkins, MD
Chief Radiology . . . . RC Friedrich, MD
Director Respiratory Therapy . . . . Lynne McCloskey

Measure	Cases	This Hospital	State Average	U.S. Average	Top Hospital
Heart Attack Care					
ACE Inhibitor or ARB for LVSD[1]	5	80%	85%	82%	100%
Aspirin at Arrival[1]	24	96%	94%	92%	100%
Aspirin at Discharge[1]	17	100%	94%	90%	100%
Beta Blocker at Arrival[1]	17	94%	92%	87%	100%
Beta Blocker at Discharge[1]	17	94%	92%	90%	100%
Fibrinolytic Medication Timing	0	-	13%	31%	100%
PCI Within 90 Minutes of Arrival	0	-	75%	54%	95%
Smoking Cessation Advice[1]	2	100%	91%	88%	100%
Heart Failure Care					
ACE Inhibitor or ARB for LVSD	34	76%	86%	82%	100%
Discharge Instructions	51	78%	73%	61%	93%
Evaluation of LVS Function	80	98%	88%	83%	99%
Smoking Cessation Advice[1]	5	100%	80%	82%	100%
Pneumonia Care					
Appropriate Initial Antibiotic	68	93%	87%	83%	94%
Blood Culture Timing	73	96%	94%	90%	100%
Influenza Vaccine[1]	20	100%	79%	70%	100%
Initial Antibiotic Timing	98	85%	87%	80%	93%
Oxygenation Assessment	119	100%	100%	99%	100%
Pneumococcal Vaccine	82	91%	78%	69%	94%
Smoking Cessation Advice[1]	19	74%	82%	80%	100%
Surgical Infection Prevention					
Prophylactic Antibiotic Given	418	91%	84%	77%	95%
Prophylactic Antibiotic Selection	117	94%	93%	90%	100%
Prophylactic Antibiotic Stopped	410	91%	80%	72%	95%
Pregnancy Care					
Inpatient Neonatal Mortality	-	-	-	-	-
Third or Fourth Degree Laceration	-	-	3.43%	3.63%	3.27%

Stoughton Hospital Association

900 Ridge Street
Stoughton, WI 53589
Phone: 608-873-6611
Fax: 608-873-2234
E-mail: info@stoughtonhospital.com
URL: www.stoughtonhospital.com
Ownership: Voluntary non-profit - Private
Accredited: Yes
Emergency Services: Yes
Licensed Beds: 69

Key Personnel:

President/CEO. . . . . Terence J Brenny
Chief Medical Staff. . . . . Joyce Brehm
Emergency Room . . . . Teresa De Nucci
Infection Control. . . . . Joyce Williams
ICU . . . . Amy Hermes
Medical Surgical Nursing . . . . Amy Hermes
Respiratory/Cardiopulmonary. . . . . Teresa Denucci

Measure	Cases	This Hospital	State Average	U.S. Average	Top Hospital
Heart Attack Care					
ACE Inhibitor or ARB for LVSD[5]	-	-	85%	82%	100%
Aspirin at Arrival[5]	-	-	94%	92%	100%
Aspirin at Discharge[5]	-	-	94%	90%	100%
Beta Blocker at Arrival[5]	-	-	92%	87%	100%
Beta Blocker at Discharge[5]	-	-	92%	90%	100%
Fibrinolytic Medication Timing[5]	-	-	13%	31%	100%
PCI Within 90 Minutes of Arrival[5]	-	-	75%	54%	95%
Smoking Cessation Advice[5]	-	-	91%	88%	100%
Heart Failure Care					
ACE Inhibitor or ARB for LVSD[1]	14	86%	86%	82%	100%
Discharge Instructions	29	79%	73%	61%	93%
Evaluation of LVS Function	38	79%	88%	83%	99%
Smoking Cessation Advice[1]	4	100%	80%	82%	100%
Pneumonia Care					
Appropriate Initial Antibiotic	57	96%	87%	83%	94%
Blood Culture Timing	63	92%	94%	90%	100%
Influenza Vaccine[1]	17	100%	79%	70%	100%
Initial Antibiotic Timing	86	90%	87%	80%	93%
Oxygenation Assessment	105	100%	100%	99%	100%
Pneumococcal Vaccine	78	95%	78%	69%	94%
Smoking Cessation Advice[1]	16	75%	82%	80%	100%
Surgical Infection Prevention					
Prophylactic Antibiotic Given	64	97%	84%	77%	95%
Prophylactic Antibiotic Selection[1]	12	100%	93%	90%	100%
Prophylactic Antibiotic Stopped	62	79%	80%	72%	95%
Pregnancy Care					
Inpatient Neonatal Mortality	-	-	-	-	-
Third or Fourth Degree Laceration	-	-	3.43%	3.63%	3.27%

Door County Memorial Hospital

323 South 18th Avenue
Sturgeon Bay, WI 54235
Toll-Free: 800-522-8919
Phone: 920-743-5566
Fax: 920-743-8165
E-mail: dcmhinfo@dcmh.org
URL: www.doorcountymemorial.org
Ownership: Voluntary non-profit - Church
Accredited: Yes
Emergency Services: Yes
Licensed Beds: 89

Key Personnel:

President/CEO. . . . . Gerald M Worrick
Chief Medical Staff. . . . . James M Lewis, MD
Emergency Room . . . . Jeff Wilson, RN
Emergency Room . . . . Eugene Kastenson, MD
Infection Control. . . . . Julie Pinney, RN
ICU . . . . Sherry Christenson, RN

NOTE: Hospital profiles are in alphabetical order by state, then city, then hospital within the city; Rankings are sorted by rate in descending order and exclude hospitals with less than 25 cases; (1) The number of cases is too small (n<25) for purposes of reliably predicting hospital performance; (2) Measure reflects the hospital's indication that its submission was based upon a sample of its relevant discharges; (3) Rate reflects fewer than the maximum possible quarters of data for the measure; (4) Inaccurate information submitted and suppressed for one or more quarters; (5) No data is available from the hospital for this measure; Please refer to the User's Guide for a full explanation of data

Intensive/Coronary Care . . . . Sherri Christenson, RN
Director Medical/Surgical Nursing . . . . Sherry Christenson, RN
OB/GYN/Women's Health . . . . Dorene Dempster, MD
Director Respiratory Therapy . . . . Pam Price

Measure	Cases	This Hospital	State Average	U.S. Average	Top Hospital
Heart Attack Care					
ACE Inhibitor or ARB for LVSD	0	-	85%	82%	100%
Aspirin at Arrival[1]	4	75%	94%	92%	100%
Aspirin at Discharge[1]	3	100%	94%	90%	100%
Beta Blocker at Arrival[1]	3	100%	92%	87%	100%
Beta Blocker at Discharge[1]	4	100%	92%	90%	100%
Fibrinolytic Medication Timing	0	-	13%	31%	100%
PCI Within 90 Minutes of Arrival	0	-	75%	54%	95%
Smoking Cessation Advice	0	-	91%	88%	100%
Heart Failure Care					
ACE Inhibitor or ARB for LVSD[1]	16	62%	86%	82%	100%
Discharge Instructions	59	47%	73%	61%	93%
Evaluation of LVS Function	81	77%	88%	83%	99%
Smoking Cessation Advice[1]	5	100%	80%	82%	100%
Pneumonia Care					
Appropriate Initial Antibiotic	58	88%	87%	83%	94%
Blood Culture Timing	43	93%	94%	90%	100%
Influenza Vaccine[1]	10	40%	79%	70%	100%
Initial Antibiotic Timing	82	84%	87%	80%	93%
Oxygenation Assessment	100	100%	100%	99%	100%
Pneumococcal Vaccine	74	55%	78%	69%	94%
Smoking Cessation Advice[1]	19	89%	82%	80%	100%
Surgical Infection Prevention					
Prophylactic Antibiotic Given	70	64%	84%	77%	95%
Prophylactic Antibiotic Selection[1]	13	92%	93%	90%	100%
Prophylactic Antibiotic Stopped	65	86%	80%	72%	95%
Pregnancy Care					
Inpatient Neonatal Mortality	-	-	-	-	-
Third or Fourth Degree Laceration	-	-	3.43%	3.63%	3.27%

Tomah Memorial Hospital

321 Butts Avenue
Tomah, WI 54660
Phone: 608-372-2181
Fax: 608-374-0289
Ownership: Voluntary non-profit - Other
Emergency Services: Yes
Accredited: Yes
Licensed Beds: 25

Key Personnel:

CEO. . . . . Spil Stuart
Chief Medical Staff. . . . . Rick Erdman, MD
Emergency Room . . . . Tracy Myhre
Director Infection/Disease Control . . . . Jan Path
Medical Surgical Nursing . . . . Bev Niebuhr
Director Respiratory Therapy . . . . Alicia Blinkiewicz

Measure	Cases	This Hospital	State Average	U.S. Average	Top Hospital
Heart Attack Care					
ACE Inhibitor or ARB for LVSD[1]	2	100%	85%	82%	100%
Aspirin at Arrival[1]	17	100%	94%	92%	100%
Aspirin at Discharge[1]	14	100%	94%	90%	100%
Beta Blocker at Arrival[1]	11	100%	92%	87%	100%
Beta Blocker at Discharge[1]	14	100%	92%	90%	100%
Fibrinolytic Medication Timing	0	-	13%	31%	100%
PCI Within 90 Minutes of Arrival	0	-	75%	54%	95%
Smoking Cessation Advice[1]	3	100%	91%	88%	100%
Heart Failure Care					
ACE Inhibitor or ARB for LVSD[1]	14	86%	86%	82%	100%
Discharge Instructions	40	98%	73%	61%	93%
Evaluation of LVS Function	54	98%	88%	83%	99%
Smoking Cessation Advice[1]	6	100%	80%	82%	100%
Pneumonia Care					
Appropriate Initial Antibiotic	35	91%	87%	83%	94%
Blood Culture Timing	27	96%	94%	90%	100%
Influenza Vaccine[1]	12	100%	79%	70%	100%
Initial Antibiotic Timing	52	77%	87%	80%	93%
Oxygenation Assessment	57	98%	100%	99%	100%
Pneumococcal Vaccine	41	88%	78%	69%	94%
Smoking Cessation Advice[1]	11	100%	82%	80%	100%
Surgical Infection Prevention					
Prophylactic Antibiotic Given[5]	-	-	84%	77%	95%
Prophylactic Antibiotic Selection[5]	-	-	93%	90%	100%
Prophylactic Antibiotic Stopped[5]	-	-	80%	72%	95%
Pregnancy Care					
Inpatient Neonatal Mortality	-	-	-	-	-
Third or Fourth Degree Laceration	-	-	3.43%	3.63%	3.27%

Sacred Heart Hospital

401 West Mohawk Drive
Tomahawk, WI 54487
Toll-Free: 800-578-0840
Phone: 715-453-7700
Fax: 715-361-2006

URL: www.ministryhealth.org
Ownership: Voluntary non-profit - Church
Emergency Services: Yes
Accredited: Yes
Licensed Beds: 18

Key Personnel:

President . . . . Monica Hilt
CEO. . . . . Nick Desien
Chief Medical Staff. . . . . Ron Cortte, MD
Infection Control. . . . . Karen Wiedema, RN
Respiratory/Cardiopulmonary Manager . . . . Carol Humlie

Measure	Cases	This Hospital	State Average	U.S. Average	Top Hospital
Heart Attack Care					
ACE Inhibitor or ARB for LVSD[3]	0	-	85%	82%	100%
Aspirin at Arrival[1,3]	2	50%	94%	92%	100%
Aspirin at Discharge[1,3]	1	100%	94%	90%	100%
Beta Blocker at Arrival[1,3]	2	50%	92%	87%	100%
Beta Blocker at Discharge[1,3]	1	0%	92%	90%	100%
Fibrinolytic Medication Timing[3]	0	-	13%	31%	100%
PCI Within 90 Minutes of Arrival[5]	-	-	75%	54%	95%
Smoking Cessation Advice[1,3]	1	100%	91%	88%	100%
Heart Failure Care					
ACE Inhibitor or ARB for LVSD[1]	3	100%	86%	82%	100%
Discharge Instructions[1]	14	86%	73%	61%	93%
Evaluation of LVS Function[1]	24	96%	88%	83%	99%
Smoking Cessation Advice[1]	2	100%	80%	82%	100%
Pneumonia Care					
Appropriate Initial Antibiotic[1,3]	21	71%	87%	83%	94%
Blood Culture Timing[1,3]	10	100%	94%	90%	100%
Influenza Vaccine[1]	11	91%	79%	70%	100%
Initial Antibiotic Timing[3]	40	85%	87%	80%	93%
Oxygenation Assessment[3]	47	100%	100%	99%	100%
Pneumococcal Vaccine[3]	41	93%	78%	69%	94%
Smoking Cessation Advice[1,3]	10	100%	82%	80%	100%
Surgical Infection Prevention					
Prophylactic Antibiotic Given[5]	-	-	84%	77%	95%
Prophylactic Antibiotic Selection[5]	-	-	93%	90%	100%
Prophylactic Antibiotic Stopped[5]	-	-	80%	72%	95%
Pregnancy Care					
Inpatient Neonatal Mortality	-	-	-	-	-
Third or Fourth Degree Laceration	-	-	3.43%	3.63%	3.27%

Aurora Medical Center

Alternate Name: Two Rivers Community Hospital
5000 Memorial Drive
Two Rivers, WI 54241
Phone: 920-794-5000
Fax: 920-794-5487
URL: www.aurorahealthcare.org
Ownership: Voluntary non-profit - Private
Emergency Services: Yes
Accredited: Yes
Licensed Beds: 73

Key Personnel:

Administrator . . . . Margo Hall
Chief Medical Staff. . . . . Glenn Smith, MD
Chief Catheterization Laboratory . . . . Robert Wilson, MD
Emergency Room . . . . James Hermann, MD
Director Infection/Disease Control . . . . Vicki Grimstad
CCU Spvg. Nurse . . . . M Swoboda, RN
Director Medical/Surgical Nursing . . . . Mary Swoboda, RN
OB/GYN Womens Health. . . . . Peter VanOosten, MD
Chief Radiology . . . . Ron Kruger
Director Respiratory Therapy . . . . Jean Huempfner, RN

Measure	Cases	This Hospital	State Average	U.S. Average	Top Hospital

NOTE: Hospital profiles are in alphabetical order by state, then city, then hospital within the city; Rankings are sorted by rate in descending order and exclude hospitals with less than 25 cases; (1) The number of cases is too small (n<25) for purposes of reliably predicting hospital performance; (2) Measure reflects the hospital's indication that its submission was based upon a sample of its relevant discharges; (3) Rate reflects fewer than the maximum possible quarters of data for the measure; (4) Inaccurate information submitted and suppressed for one or more quarters; (5) No data is available from the hospital for this measure; Please refer to the User's Guide for a full explanation of data

Heart Attack Care					
ACE Inhibitor or ARB for LVSD[1]	17	71%	85%	82%	100%
Aspirin at Arrival	34	100%	94%	92%	100%
Aspirin at Discharge[1]	21	100%	94%	90%	100%
Beta Blocker at Arrival[1]	20	90%	92%	87%	100%
Beta Blocker at Discharge[1]	20	100%	92%	90%	100%
Fibrinolytic Medication Timing	0	-	13%	31%	100%
PCI Within 90 Minutes of Arrival	0	-	75%	54%	95%
Smoking Cessation Advice[1]	3	100%	91%	88%	100%
Heart Failure Care					
ACE Inhibitor or ARB for LVSD[1]	22	91%	86%	82%	100%
Discharge Instructions	41	83%	73%	61%	93%
Evaluation of LVS Function	64	100%	88%	83%	99%
Smoking Cessation Advice[1]	2	100%	80%	82%	100%
Pneumonia Care					
Appropriate Initial Antibiotic	60	88%	87%	83%	94%
Blood Culture Timing	58	98%	94%	90%	100%
Influenza Vaccine[1]	16	94%	79%	70%	100%
Initial Antibiotic Timing	71	97%	87%	80%	93%
Oxygenation Assessment	107	100%	100%	99%	100%
Pneumococcal Vaccine	71	97%	78%	69%	94%
Smoking Cessation Advice[1]	16	88%	82%	80%	100%
Surgical Infection Prevention					
Prophylactic Antibiotic Given[2,3]	65	92%	84%	77%	95%
Prophylactic Antibiotic Selection[2]	30	97%	93%	90%	100%
Prophylactic Antibiotic Stopped[2,3]	62	97%	80%	72%	95%
Pregnancy Care					
Inpatient Neonatal Mortality	305	0.00%	-	-	-
Third or Fourth Degree Laceration	198	3.03%	3.43%	3.63%	3.27%

Vernon Memorial Healthcare

507 S Main Street
Viroqua, WI 54665
E-mail: pubrel@vmh.org
URL: www.vmh.org
Ownership: Government - Federal
Emergency Services: Yes

Phone: 608-637-2101
Fax: 608-637-2141

Accredited: No
Licensed Beds: 25

Key Personnel:
CEO. . . . . Garth W Steiner
Chief Medical Staff. . . . . Mark Heberlein, MD
Emergency Room . . . . Sue Ellen Robertson
Infection Control. . . . . Romells Heisel
Medical/Surgical Nursing . . . . Sue Sullivan
Surgical Services . . . . Sue Heitman

Measure	Cases	This Hospital	State Average	U.S. Average	Top Hospital
Heart Attack Care					
ACE Inhibitor or ARB for LVSD[1]	2	100%	85%	82%	100%
Aspirin at Arrival[1]	9	100%	94%	92%	100%
Aspirin at Discharge[1]	6	100%	94%	90%	100%
Beta Blocker at Arrival[1]	10	90%	92%	87%	100%
Beta Blocker at Discharge[1]	9	89%	92%	90%	100%
Fibrinolytic Medication Timing[1]	1	100%	13%	31%	100%
PCI Within 90 Minutes of Arrival	0	-	75%	54%	95%
Smoking Cessation Advice[1]	1	100%	91%	88%	100%
Heart Failure Care					
ACE Inhibitor or ARB for LVSD[1]	3	67%	86%	82%	100%
Discharge Instructions[1]	14	86%	73%	61%	93%
Evaluation of LVS Function	27	52%	88%	83%	99%
Smoking Cessation Advice[1]	1	0%	80%	82%	100%
Pneumonia Care					
Appropriate Initial Antibiotic	58	83%	87%	83%	94%
Blood Culture Timing	29	97%	94%	90%	100%
Influenza Vaccine[1]	15	100%	79%	70%	100%
Initial Antibiotic Timing	93	94%	87%	80%	93%
Oxygenation Assessment	108	100%	100%	99%	100%
Pneumococcal Vaccine	90	98%	78%	69%	94%
Smoking Cessation Advice[1]	14	100%	82%	80%	100%
Surgical Infection Prevention					
Prophylactic Antibiotic Given	216	82%	84%	77%	95%
Prophylactic Antibiotic Selection	56	100%	93%	90%	100%
Prophylactic Antibiotic Stopped	211	93%	80%	72%	95%
Pregnancy Care					
Inpatient Neonatal Mortality	-	-	-	-	-
Third or Fourth Degree Laceration	-	-	3.43%	3.63%	3.27%

Watertown Memorial Hospital

125 Hospital Drive
Watertown, WI 53098

Toll-Free: 800-472-4210
Phone: 920-261-4210
Fax: 920-261-3940

URL: www.watertownmemorialhospital.com
Ownership: Voluntary non-profit - Private
Emergency Services: Yes

Accredited: Yes
Licensed Beds: 95

Key Personnel:
President/CEO. . . . . John Kosanovich
Chief Staff . . . . James Milford, MD
Emergency Room Manager . . . . Stacey Carlen, RN
Emergency Room . . . . Kathelene Hargarten, MD
Infection Control Nurse. . . . . Linda Gehring
ICU Director. . . . . Barb Quest, RN
Director OB/GYN/Women's Health. . . . . Lisa Harris, RN

Measure	Cases	This Hospital	State Average	U.S. Average	Top Hospital
Heart Attack Care					
ACE Inhibitor or ARB for LVSD[1]	1	0%	85%	82%	100%
Aspirin at Arrival[1]	8	88%	94%	92%	100%
Aspirin at Discharge[1]	4	100%	94%	90%	100%
Beta Blocker at Arrival[1]	5	60%	92%	87%	100%
Beta Blocker at Discharge[1]	5	80%	92%	90%	100%
Fibrinolytic Medication Timing[1]	1	0%	13%	31%	100%
PCI Within 90 Minutes of Arrival	0	-	75%	54%	95%
Smoking Cessation Advice[1]	2	50%	91%	88%	100%
Heart Failure Care					
ACE Inhibitor or ARB for LVSD[1]	18	78%	86%	82%	100%
Discharge Instructions	48	42%	73%	61%	93%
Evaluation of LVS Function	65	85%	88%	83%	99%
Smoking Cessation Advice[1]	4	100%	80%	82%	100%
Pneumonia Care					
Appropriate Initial Antibiotic	38	82%	87%	83%	94%
Blood Culture Timing	35	97%	94%	90%	100%
Influenza Vaccine[1]	14	50%	79%	70%	100%
Initial Antibiotic Timing	77	92%	87%	80%	93%
Oxygenation Assessment	85	100%	100%	99%	100%
Pneumococcal Vaccine	46	89%	78%	69%	94%
Smoking Cessation Advice[1]	13	92%	82%	80%	100%
Surgical Infection Prevention					
Prophylactic Antibiotic Given[2]	185	66%	84%	77%	95%
Prophylactic Antibiotic Selection[2]	44	98%	93%	90%	100%
Prophylactic Antibiotic Stopped[2]	180	88%	80%	72%	95%
Pregnancy Care					
Inpatient Neonatal Mortality	-	-	-	-	-
Third or Fourth Degree Laceration	-	-	3.43%	3.63%	3.27%

Waukesha Memorial Hospital

725 American Avenue
Waukesha, WI 53188

Toll-Free: 800-326-2011
Phone: 262-928-1000
Fax: 262-928-7810

URL: www.waukeshamemorial.org
Ownership: Voluntary non-profit - Private
Emergency Services: Yes

Accredited: Yes
Licensed Beds: 301

Key Personnel:
President/CEO. . . . . Ed Olson

Measure	Cases	This Hospital	State Average	U.S. Average	Top Hospital
Heart Attack Care					
ACE Inhibitor or ARB for LVSD	55	93%	85%	82%	100%
Aspirin at Arrival	182	98%	94%	92%	100%
Aspirin at Discharge	193	98%	94%	90%	100%
Beta Blocker at Arrival	152	96%	92%	87%	100%
Beta Blocker at Discharge	189	99%	92%	90%	100%
Fibrinolytic Medication Timing	0	-	13%	31%	100%
PCI Within 90 Minutes of Arrival[1]	14	79%	75%	54%	95%
Smoking Cessation Advice	63	100%	91%	88%	100%
Heart Failure Care					
ACE Inhibitor or ARB for LVSD	159	77%	86%	82%	100%

NOTE: Hospital profiles are in alphabetical order by state, then city, then hospital within the city; Rankings are sorted by rate in descending order and exclude hospitals with less than 25 cases; (1) The number of cases is too small (n<25) for purposes of reliably predicting hospital performance; (2) Measure reflects the hospital's indication that its submission was based upon a sample of its relevant discharges; (3) Rate reflects fewer than the maximum possible quarters of data for the measure; (4) Inaccurate information submitted and suppressed for one or more quarters; (5) No data is available from the hospital for this measure; Please refer to the User's Guide for a full explanation of data

Measure	Cases	This Hospital	State Average	U.S. Average	Top Hospital
Discharge Instructions	322	67%	73%	61%	93%
Evaluation of LVS Function	406	99%	88%	83%	99%
Smoking Cessation Advice	49	94%	80%	82%	100%
Pneumonia Care					
Appropriate Initial Antibiotic	219	89%	87%	83%	94%
Blood Culture Timing	193	96%	94%	90%	100%
Influenza Vaccine	71	97%	79%	70%	100%
Initial Antibiotic Timing	301	97%	87%	80%	93%
Oxygenation Assessment	383	100%	100%	99%	100%
Pneumococcal Vaccine	241	93%	78%	69%	94%
Smoking Cessation Advice	68	91%	82%	80%	100%
Surgical Infection Prevention					
Prophylactic Antibiotic Given	301	94%	84%	77%	95%
Prophylactic Antibiotic Selection	71	96%	93%	90%	100%
Prophylactic Antibiotic Stopped	282	71%	80%	72%	95%
Pregnancy Care					
Inpatient Neonatal Mortality	-	-	-	-	-
Third or Fourth Degree Laceration	-	-	3.43%	3.63%	3.27%

Waupun Memorial Hospital

620 W Brown Street
Waupun, WI 53963
URL: www.agnesian.com
Ownership: Voluntary non-profit - Church
Emergency Services: Yes

Phone: 920-324-5581
Fax: 920-324-2085

Accredited: Yes
Licensed Beds: 25

Key Personnel:
Director Infection/Disease Control . . . . Kayla Ericksen, RN
Director Medical/Surgical Nursing . . . . Cheri Goddard, RN

Measure	Cases	This Hospital	State Average	U.S. Average	Top Hospital
Heart Attack Care					
ACE Inhibitor or ARB for LVSD[5]	-	-	85%	82%	100%
Aspirin at Arrival[5]	-	-	94%	92%	100%
Aspirin at Discharge[5]	-	-	94%	90%	100%
Beta Blocker at Arrival[5]	-	-	92%	87%	100%
Beta Blocker at Discharge[5]	-	-	92%	90%	100%
Fibrinolytic Medication Timing[5]	-	-	13%	31%	100%
PCI Within 90 Minutes of Arrival[5]	-	-	75%	54%	95%
Smoking Cessation Advice[5]	-	-	91%	88%	100%
Heart Failure Care					
ACE Inhibitor or ARB for LVSD[1]	11	73%	86%	82%	100%
Discharge Instructions	31	84%	73%	61%	93%
Evaluation of LVS Function	49	63%	88%	83%	99%
Smoking Cessation Advice[1]	1	100%	80%	82%	100%
Pneumonia Care					
Appropriate Initial Antibiotic	35	77%	87%	83%	94%
Blood Culture Timing	41	98%	94%	90%	100%
Influenza Vaccine[1]	9	33%	79%	70%	100%
Initial Antibiotic Timing	58	76%	87%	80%	93%
Oxygenation Assessment	75	100%	100%	99%	100%
Pneumococcal Vaccine	39	46%	78%	69%	94%
Smoking Cessation Advice[1]	15	93%	82%	80%	100%
Surgical Infection Prevention					
Prophylactic Antibiotic Given[3]	53	91%	84%	77%	95%
Prophylactic Antibiotic Selection[1]	18	100%	93%	90%	100%
Prophylactic Antibiotic Stopped[3]	52	96%	80%	72%	95%
Pregnancy Care					
Inpatient Neonatal Mortality	-	-	-	-	-
Third or Fourth Degree Laceration	-	-	3.43%	3.63%	3.27%

Aspirus-Wausau Hospital

Alternate Name: Wausau Hospital
333 Pine Ridge Boulevard
Wausau, WI 54401

Toll-Free: 800-283-2881
Phone: 715-847-2121
Fax: 715-847-2017

URL: www.aspirus.org
Ownership: Proprietary
Emergency Services: Yes

Accredited: Yes
Licensed Beds: 321

Key Personnel:
CEO. . . . . Paul A Spaude
Chief Medical Staff. . . . . Chuck Shabirro
Director Cardiac Laboratory . . . . Scott Gavavet
Director Emergency Room. . . . . Pam Krueger
Infection Control. . . . . Jeanine Bresnahan
Director Radiology . . . . Kevin Droroct
Manager Respiratory . . . . Joe Rohling

Measure	Cases	This Hospital	State Average	U.S. Average	Top Hospital
Heart Attack Care					
ACE Inhibitor or ARB for LVSD[2]	58	100%	85%	82%	100%
Aspirin at Arrival[2]	100	100%	94%	92%	100%
Aspirin at Discharge[2]	242	100%	94%	90%	100%
Beta Blocker at Arrival[2]	69	100%	92%	87%	100%
Beta Blocker at Discharge[2]	241	99%	92%	90%	100%
Fibrinolytic Medication Timing[2]	0	-	13%	31%	100%
PCI Within 90 Minutes of Arrival[1,2]	2	100%	75%	54%	95%
Smoking Cessation Advice[2]	105	100%	91%	88%	100%
Heart Failure Care					
ACE Inhibitor or ARB for LVSD[2]	78	96%	86%	82%	100%
Discharge Instructions[2]	263	95%	73%	61%	93%
Evaluation of LVS Function[2]	312	99%	88%	83%	99%
Smoking Cessation Advice[2]	38	100%	80%	82%	100%
Pneumonia Care					
Appropriate Initial Antibiotic[2]	100	95%	87%	83%	94%
Blood Culture Timing[2]	103	92%	94%	90%	100%
Influenza Vaccine[2]	36	67%	79%	70%	100%
Initial Antibiotic Timing[2]	150	88%	87%	80%	93%
Oxygenation Assessment[2]	204	100%	100%	99%	100%
Pneumococcal Vaccine[2]	143	90%	78%	69%	94%
Smoking Cessation Advice[2]	42	93%	82%	80%	100%
Surgical Infection Prevention					
Prophylactic Antibiotic Given[2]	544	94%	84%	77%	95%
Prophylactic Antibiotic Selection[2]	80	96%	93%	90%	100%
Prophylactic Antibiotic Stopped[2]	527	87%	80%	72%	95%
Pregnancy Care					
Inpatient Neonatal Mortality[2]	1,081	0.28%	-	-	-
Third or Fourth Degree Laceration	958	3.34%	3.43%	3.63%	3.27%

Wisconsin Heart Hospital

10000 West Bluemound Road
Wauwatosa, WI 53226
URL: www.twhh.org
Ownership: Proprietary
Emergency Services: Yes

Phone: 414-778-7800
Fax: 414-266-9701

Accredited: Yes
Licensed Beds: 60

Key Personnel:
President . . . . Norma McCutcheon
President Medical Staff . . . . Jack Manley, MD/FACC

Measure	Cases	This Hospital	State Average	U.S. Average	Top Hospital
Heart Attack Care					
ACE Inhibitor or ARB for LVSD	29	90%	85%	82%	100%
Aspirin at Arrival	65	100%	94%	92%	100%
Aspirin at Discharge	141	99%	94%	90%	100%
Beta Blocker at Arrival	44	98%	92%	87%	100%
Beta Blocker at Discharge	121	96%	92%	90%	100%
Fibrinolytic Medication Timing	0	-	13%	31%	100%
PCI Within 90 Minutes of Arrival[1]	6	100%	75%	54%	95%
Smoking Cessation Advice	49	98%	91%	88%	100%
Heart Failure Care					
ACE Inhibitor or ARB for LVSD	60	90%	86%	82%	100%
Discharge Instructions	122	86%	73%	61%	93%
Evaluation of LVS Function	127	100%	88%	83%	99%
Smoking Cessation Advice[1]	19	89%	80%	82%	100%
Pneumonia Care					
Appropriate Initial Antibiotic[1]	11	100%	87%	83%	94%
Blood Culture Timing[1]	11	100%	94%	90%	100%
Influenza Vaccine[1]	2	100%	79%	70%	100%
Initial Antibiotic Timing[1]	15	87%	87%	80%	93%
Oxygenation Assessment[1]	17	100%	100%	99%	100%
Pneumococcal Vaccine[1]	12	75%	78%	69%	94%
Smoking Cessation Advice[1]	2	100%	82%	80%	100%
Surgical Infection Prevention					
Prophylactic Antibiotic Given[3]	116	96%	84%	77%	95%
Prophylactic Antibiotic Selection[1]	23	96%	93%	90%	100%
Prophylactic Antibiotic Stopped[3]	111	95%	80%	72%	95%

NOTE: Hospital profiles are in alphabetical order by state, then city, then hospital within the city; Rankings are sorted by rate in descending order and exclude hospitals with less than 25 cases; (1) The number of cases is too small (n<25) for purposes of reliably predicting hospital performance; (2) Measure reflects the hospital's indication that its submission was based upon a sample of its relevant discharges; (3) Rate reflects fewer than the maximum possible quarters of data for the measure; (4) Inaccurate information submitted and suppressed for one or more quarters; (5) No data is available from the hospital for this measure; Please refer to the User's Guide for a full explanation of data

Pregnancy Care					
Inpatient Neonatal Mortality	-	-	-	-	-
Third or Fourth Degree Laceration	-	-	3.43%	3.63%	3.27%

West Allis Memorial Hospital

8901 W Lincoln Avenue
Milwaukee, WI 53227
URL: www.aurorahealthcare.org
Ownership: Voluntary non-profit - Private
Emergency Services: Yes

Phone: 414-328-6000
Fax: 414-328-8536

Accredited: Yes
Licensed Beds: 250

Key Personnel:
CEO. . . . . Richard Kellar
Chief Medical Staff. . . . . Jeffery Showers
Chief Emergency Room. . . . . Eduardo Castrl
Emergency Room . . . . Wendy Roberts, RN
ICU . . . . Larry Conrad
OB/GYN Womens Health. . . . . James Stadler, MD

Measure	Cases	This Hospital	State Average	U.S. Average	Top Hospital
Heart Attack Care					
ACE Inhibitor or ARB for LVSD[1]	12	100%	85%	82%	100%
Aspirin at Arrival	74	95%	94%	92%	100%
Aspirin at Discharge	45	98%	94%	90%	100%
Beta Blocker at Arrival	45	98%	92%	87%	100%
Beta Blocker at Discharge	49	92%	92%	90%	100%
Fibrinolytic Medication Timing	0	-	13%	31%	100%
PCI Within 90 Minutes of Arrival	0	-	75%	54%	95%
Smoking Cessation Advice[1]	3	100%	91%	88%	100%
Heart Failure Care					
ACE Inhibitor or ARB for LVSD	26	92%	86%	82%	100%
Discharge Instructions	124	71%	73%	61%	93%
Evaluation of LVS Function	169	99%	88%	83%	99%
Smoking Cessation Advice[1]	18	100%	80%	82%	100%
Pneumonia Care					
Appropriate Initial Antibiotic	183	93%	87%	83%	94%
Blood Culture Timing	230	97%	94%	90%	100%
Influenza Vaccine	56	100%	79%	70%	100%
Initial Antibiotic Timing	275	94%	87%	80%	93%
Oxygenation Assessment	356	100%	100%	99%	100%
Pneumococcal Vaccine	260	97%	78%	69%	94%
Smoking Cessation Advice	71	97%	82%	80%	100%
Surgical Infection Prevention					
Prophylactic Antibiotic Given[2,3]	95	89%	84%	77%	95%
Prophylactic Antibiotic Selection[2]	49	84%	93%	90%	100%
Prophylactic Antibiotic Stopped[2,3]	91	87%	80%	72%	95%
Pregnancy Care					
Inpatient Neonatal Mortality	-	-	-	-	-
Third or Fourth Degree Laceration	-	-	3.43%	3.63%	3.27%

Saint Joseph's Community Hospital of West Bend

551 S Silverbrook Drive
West Bend, WI 53095
URL: www.synergyhealth.org
Ownership: Voluntary non-profit - Private
Emergency Services: Yes

Phone: 262-334-5533
Fax: 262-334-8575

Accredited: Yes
Licensed Beds: 121

Key Personnel:
President/CEO. . . . . John Reiling
Chief Medical Staff. . . . . John J Fink, MD
Director Emergency Room. . . . . Sandra Walter
Emergency Room . . . . Mary Lewis, MD
Director Infection/Disease Control . . . . Patricia Pearson
CCU Spvg. Nurse . . . . Sue McCullough
Director Medical/Surgical Nursing . . . . Marge Michael
Respiratory Therapy. . . . . Sue McCullough

Measure	Cases	This Hospital	State Average	U.S. Average	Top Hospital
Heart Attack Care					
ACE Inhibitor or ARB for LVSD[1]	2	100%	85%	82%	100%
Aspirin at Arrival[1]	15	87%	94%	92%	100%
Aspirin at Discharge[1]	11	82%	94%	90%	100%
Beta Blocker at Arrival[1]	11	73%	92%	87%	100%
Beta Blocker at Discharge[1]	9	78%	92%	90%	100%
Fibrinolytic Medication Timing[1]	1	0%	13%	31%	100%
PCI Within 90 Minutes of Arrival	0	-	75%	54%	95%
Smoking Cessation Advice	0	-	91%	88%	100%
Heart Failure Care					
ACE Inhibitor or ARB for LVSD	39	82%	86%	82%	100%
Discharge Instructions	56	79%	73%	61%	93%
Evaluation of LVS Function	100	98%	88%	83%	99%
Smoking Cessation Advice[1]	9	78%	80%	82%	100%
Pneumonia Care					
Appropriate Initial Antibiotic	83	86%	87%	83%	94%
Blood Culture Timing	67	93%	94%	90%	100%
Influenza Vaccine[1]	22	59%	79%	70%	100%
Initial Antibiotic Timing	102	85%	87%	80%	93%
Oxygenation Assessment	140	100%	100%	99%	100%
Pneumococcal Vaccine	99	70%	78%	69%	94%
Smoking Cessation Advice	32	91%	82%	80%	100%
Surgical Infection Prevention					
Prophylactic Antibiotic Given[3]	164	91%	84%	77%	95%
Prophylactic Antibiotic Selection	46	98%	93%	90%	100%
Prophylactic Antibiotic Stopped[3]	156	79%	80%	72%	95%
Pregnancy Care					
Inpatient Neonatal Mortality	674	0.15%	-	-	-
Third or Fourth Degree Laceration	467	3.85%	3.43%	3.63%	3.27%

Saint Clare's Hospital of Weston

3400 Ministry Parkway
Weston, WI 54476
Ownership: Voluntary non-profit - Private
Emergency Services: Yes

Phone: 715-393-3000

Accredited: Yes

Measure	Cases	This Hospital	State Average	U.S. Average	Top Hospital
Heart Attack Care					
ACE Inhibitor or ARB for LVSD[1,3]	1	100%	85%	82%	100%
Aspirin at Arrival[1,3]	4	100%	94%	92%	100%
Aspirin at Discharge[1,3]	4	100%	94%	90%	100%
Beta Blocker at Arrival[1,3]	1	100%	92%	87%	100%
Beta Blocker at Discharge[1,3]	2	100%	92%	90%	100%
Fibrinolytic Medication Timing[3]	0	-	13%	31%	100%
PCI Within 90 Minutes of Arrival	0	-	75%	54%	95%
Smoking Cessation Advice[3]	0	-	91%	88%	100%
Heart Failure Care					
ACE Inhibitor or ARB for LVSD[1]	4	75%	86%	82%	100%
Discharge Instructions	28	54%	73%	61%	93%
Evaluation of LVS Function	36	100%	88%	83%	99%
Smoking Cessation Advice[1]	7	100%	80%	82%	100%
Pneumonia Care					
Appropriate Initial Antibiotic	35	89%	87%	83%	94%
Blood Culture Timing	25	100%	94%	90%	100%
Influenza Vaccine[1]	3	33%	79%	70%	100%
Initial Antibiotic Timing	32	94%	87%	80%	93%
Oxygenation Assessment	41	100%	100%	99%	100%
Pneumococcal Vaccine[1]	17	94%	78%	69%	94%
Smoking Cessation Advice[1]	10	100%	82%	80%	100%
Surgical Infection Prevention					
Prophylactic Antibiotic Given	365	93%	84%	77%	95%
Prophylactic Antibiotic Selection	78	94%	93%	90%	100%
Prophylactic Antibiotic Stopped	363	95%	80%	72%	95%
Pregnancy Care					
Inpatient Neonatal Mortality	-	-	-	-	-
Third or Fourth Degree Laceration	-	-	3.43%	3.63%	3.27%

Wild Rose Community Memorial Hospital

601 Grove Avenue
PO Box 243
Wild Rose, WI 54984
URL: www.wildrosehospital.org
Ownership: Voluntary non-profit - Private
Emergency Services: Yes

Phone: 920-622-3257
Fax: 920-622-5593

Accredited: No
Licensed Beds: 27

Key Personnel:
CEO. . . . . Donald Caves
Chief Medical Staff. . . . . Dan M Fifield
Director Infection/Disease Control . . . . Helen Appleyard
Director Respiratory Therapy. . . . . Marie Dickmann

NOTE: Hospital profiles are in alphabetical order by state, then city, then hospital within the city; Rankings are sorted by rate in descending order and exclude hospitals with less than 25 cases; (1) The number of cases is too small (n<25) for purposes of reliably predicting hospital performance; (2) Measure reflects the hospital's indication that its submission was based upon a sample of its relevant discharges; (3) Rate reflects fewer than the maximum possible quarters of data for the measure; (4) Inaccurate information submitted and suppressed for one or more quarters; (5) No data is available from the hospital for this measure; Please refer to the User's Guide for a full explanation of data

Measure	Cases	This Hospital	State Average	U.S. Average	Top Hospital
Heart Attack Care					
ACE Inhibitor or ARB for LVSD[3]	0	-	85%	82%	100%
Aspirin at Arrival[3]	0	-	94%	92%	100%
Aspirin at Discharge[3]	0	-	94%	90%	100%
Beta Blocker at Arrival[3]	0	-	92%	87%	100%
Beta Blocker at Discharge[3]	0	-	92%	90%	100%
Fibrinolytic Medication Timing[3]	0	-	13%	31%	100%
PCI Within 90 Minutes of Arrival[5]	-	-	75%	54%	95%
Smoking Cessation Advice[3]	0	-	91%	88%	100%
Heart Failure Care					
ACE Inhibitor or ARB for LVSD[1]	2	50%	86%	82%	100%
Discharge Instructions[1]	15	73%	73%	61%	93%
Evaluation of LVS Function[1]	15	60%	88%	83%	99%
Smoking Cessation Advice[1]	2	100%	80%	82%	100%
Pneumonia Care					
Appropriate Initial Antibiotic[1]	24	96%	87%	83%	94%
Blood Culture Timing[1]	20	100%	94%	90%	100%
Influenza Vaccine[1]	4	50%	79%	70%	100%
Initial Antibiotic Timing	30	87%	87%	80%	93%
Oxygenation Assessment	33	100%	100%	99%	100%
Pneumococcal Vaccine	25	52%	78%	69%	94%
Smoking Cessation Advice[1]	3	67%	82%	80%	100%
Surgical Infection Prevention					
Prophylactic Antibiotic Given[5]	-	-	84%	77%	95%
Prophylactic Antibiotic Selection[5]	-	-	93%	90%	100%
Prophylactic Antibiotic Stopped[5]	-	-	80%	72%	95%
Pregnancy Care					
Inpatient Neonatal Mortality	-	-	-	-	-
Third or Fourth Degree Laceration	-	-	3.43%	3.63%	3.27%

Riverview Hospital Association

410 Dewey Street
Wisconsin Rapids, WI 54495
Ownership: Voluntary non-profit - Private
Emergency Services: Yes

Phone: 715-423-6060
Fax: 715-421-7551
Accredited: No
Licensed Beds: 99

Key Personnel:
President/CEO . . . . Celse A Berard
Chief Medical Staff. . . . . Daniel Lucas
Emergency Room . . . . Ron R Greenburg, DO
OB/GYN Womens Health. . . . . FL Dauenhauer, MD
Director Radiology . . . . David Forde
Director Respiratory Therapy . . . . Jim Mohr

Measure	Cases	This Hospital	State Average	U.S. Average	Top Hospital
Heart Attack Care					
ACE Inhibitor or ARB for LVSD[1]	7	71%	85%	82%	100%
Aspirin at Arrival[1]	24	92%	94%	92%	100%
Aspirin at Discharge[1]	15	80%	94%	90%	100%
Beta Blocker at Arrival[1]	24	96%	92%	87%	100%
Beta Blocker at Discharge[1]	20	85%	92%	90%	100%
Fibrinolytic Medication Timing	0	-	13%	31%	100%
PCI Within 90 Minutes of Arrival	0	-	75%	54%	95%
Smoking Cessation Advice[1]	2	50%	91%	88%	100%
Heart Failure Care					
ACE Inhibitor or ARB for LVSD	28	93%	86%	82%	100%
Discharge Instructions	57	82%	73%	61%	93%
Evaluation of LVS Function	81	84%	88%	83%	99%
Smoking Cessation Advice[1]	4	100%	80%	82%	100%
Pneumonia Care					
Appropriate Initial Antibiotic	67	81%	87%	83%	94%
Blood Culture Timing	57	91%	94%	90%	100%
Influenza Vaccine[1]	13	54%	79%	70%	100%
Initial Antibiotic Timing	83	73%	87%	80%	93%
Oxygenation Assessment	92	100%	100%	99%	100%
Pneumococcal Vaccine	62	66%	78%	69%	94%
Smoking Cessation Advice[1]	16	81%	82%	80%	100%
Surgical Infection Prevention					
Prophylactic Antibiotic Given[3]	232	87%	84%	77%	95%
Prophylactic Antibiotic Selection	76	96%	93%	90%	100%
Prophylactic Antibiotic Stopped[3]	231	75%	80%	72%	95%
Pregnancy Care					
Inpatient Neonatal Mortality	-	-	-	-	-
Third or Fourth Degree Laceration	-	-	3.43%	3.63%	3.27%

Howard Young Medical Center

240 Maple Street
Woodruff, WI 54568
URL: www.ministryhealth.org
Ownership: Voluntary non-profit - Church
Emergency Services: Yes

Phone: 715-356-8000
Fax: 715-356-8691
Accredited: Yes
Licensed Beds: 99

Key Personnel:
President . . . . Sheila Clough
Chief of Medical Staff. . . . . Michael Schaars, MD
Emergency Room . . . . Rick Brodhead, MD
Director/Surgical Services . . . . Kim Mears

Measure	Cases	This Hospital	State Average	U.S. Average	Top Hospital
Heart Attack Care					
ACE Inhibitor or ARB for LVSD[1]	3	100%	85%	82%	100%
Aspirin at Arrival[1]	15	100%	94%	92%	100%
Aspirin at Discharge[1]	9	89%	94%	90%	100%
Beta Blocker at Arrival[1]	15	100%	92%	87%	100%
Beta Blocker at Discharge[1]	10	100%	92%	90%	100%
Fibrinolytic Medication Timing	0	-	13%	31%	100%
PCI Within 90 Minutes of Arrival	0	-	75%	54%	95%
Smoking Cessation Advice[1]	2	100%	91%	88%	100%
Heart Failure Care					
ACE Inhibitor or ARB for LVSD	26	92%	86%	82%	100%
Discharge Instructions	84	89%	73%	61%	93%
Evaluation of LVS Function	95	98%	88%	83%	99%
Smoking Cessation Advice[1]	12	75%	80%	82%	100%
Pneumonia Care					
Appropriate Initial Antibiotic	58	74%	87%	83%	94%
Blood Culture Timing	56	95%	94%	90%	100%
Influenza Vaccine[1]	13	69%	79%	70%	100%
Initial Antibiotic Timing	90	82%	87%	80%	93%
Oxygenation Assessment	108	100%	100%	99%	100%
Pneumococcal Vaccine	72	82%	78%	69%	94%
Smoking Cessation Advice[1]	19	100%	82%	80%	100%
Surgical Infection Prevention					
Prophylactic Antibiotic Given	323	92%	84%	77%	95%
Prophylactic Antibiotic Selection	76	100%	93%	90%	100%
Prophylactic Antibiotic Stopped	319	83%	80%	72%	95%
Pregnancy Care					
Inpatient Neonatal Mortality	-	-	-	-	-
Third or Fourth Degree Laceration	-	-	3.43%	3.63%	3.27%

NOTE: Hospital profiles are in alphabetical order by state, then city, then hospital within the city; Rankings are sorted by rate in descending order and exclude hospitals with less than 25 cases; (1) The number of cases is too small (n<25) for purposes of reliably predicting hospital performance; (2) Measure reflects the hospital's indication that its submission was based upon a sample of its relevant discharges; (3) Rate reflects fewer than the maximum possible quarters of data for the measure; (4) Inaccurate information submitted and suppressed for one or more quarters; (5) No data is available from the hospital for this measure; Please refer to the User's Guide for a full explanation of data

Hospital	Heart Attack Care								Heart Failure Care				Pneumonia Care							Surgical Infection Prevention			Pregnancy Care	
	1	2	3	4	5	6	7	8	9	10	11	12	13	14	15	16	17	18	19	20	21	22	23	24
ILLINOIS																								
Abraham Lincoln Memorial Hospital, Lincoln, IL	**-** 0	**100** 4	**100** 4	**80** 5	**100** 4	**-** 0	**-** 0	**100** 1	**86** 14	**88** 26	**96** 54	**100** 7	**87** 67	**93** 55	**95** 19	**94** 77	**100** 100	**87** 69	**94** 18	**98** 52	**100** 12	**96** 47	**-** -	**-** -
Adventist GlenOaks Hospital, Glendale Heights, IL	**75** 4	**100** 22	**67** 3	**87** 15	**78** 9	**50** 2	**-** 0	**100** 1	**78** 23	**70** 43	**88** 73	**81** 16	**89** 35	**98** 63	**11** 9	**95** 76	**100** 99	**77** 57	**82** 17	**86** 37	**100** 13	**83** 35	**-** -	**-** -
Adventist LaGrange Memorial Hospital, La Grange, IL	**76** 41	**94** 134	**91** 112	**90** 104	**94** 133	**-** 0	**75** 4	**90** 39	**76** 85	**61** 293	**85** 385	**91** 33	**82** 214	**93** 231	**57** 53	**78** 307	**99** 358	**52** 228	**89** 55	**92** 151	**98** 56	**81** 146	**-** -	**-** -
Advocate Christ Med Ctr/Hope Children's, Oak Lawn, IL	**90** 83	**99** 190	**100** 214	**98** 147	**99** 239	**-** 0	**67** 6	**94** 86	**88** 154	**69** 263	**96** 340	**94** 50	**85** 85	**90** 93	**61** 23	**78** 161	**100** 171	**65** 106	**96** 24	**92** 345	**72** 88	**89** 337	**1.03** 871	**4.05** 642
Advocate Good Samaritan Hospital, Downers Grove, IL	**98** 64	**99** 215	**99** 192	**97** 190	**100** 214	**-** 0	**100** 17	**100** 59	**91** 155	**77** 298	**97** 405	**92** 37	**83** 111	**96** 131	**87** 23	**85** 171	**100** 210	**80** 142	**84** 37	**93** 339	**99** 82	**81** 323	**0.73** 1770	**3.74** 1070
Advocate Good Shephard Hospital, Barrington, IL	**86** 42	**98** 179	**99** 201	**99** 152	**98** 252	**-** 0	**80** 5	**99** 74	**98** 92	**83** 278	**99** 340	**100** 41	**81** 70	**94** 49	**50** 26	**84** 132	**100** 158	**59** 119	**63** 19	**90** 320	**92** 77	**83** 314	**0.55** 363	**3.03** 462
Advocate Illinois Masonic Medical Center, Chicago, IL	**81** 48	**100** 107	**91** 136	**96** 81	**92** 159	**-** 0	**40** 5	**83** 82	**88** 178	**68** 268	**98** 317	**90** 58	**84** 103	**84** 95	**81** 21	**72** 167	**100** 200	**59** 86	**85** 41	**90** 305	**96** 71	**70** 293	**0.61** 657	**1.41** 707
Advocate Lutheran General Children's Hospital, Park Ridge, IL	**92** 77	**100** 268	**99** 244	**99** 225	**98** 259	**-** 0	**88** 8	**98** 66	**93** 228	**79** 455	**97** 624	**87** 47	**85** 206	**95** 242	**74** 66	**86** 328	**100** 436	**81** 321	**82** 68	**94** 559	**98** 81	**65** 528	**1.09** 822	**4.76** 630
Advocate South Suburban Hospital, Hazel Crest, IL	**86** 43	**94** 188	**98** 125	**93** 149	**95** 142	**0** 1	**33** 9	**100** 51	**86** 146	**75** 296	**95** 366	**100** 65	**90** 105	**87** 86	**90** 21	**68** 164	**98** 187	**75** 118	**100** 50	**85** 236	**100** 62	**69** 225	**0.00** 255	**1.75** 343
Advocate Trinity Hospital, Chicago, IL	**77** 30	**92** 159	**80** 90	**88** 138	**82** 95	**0** 6	**-** 0	**92** 24	**82** 256	**35** 583	**90** 634	**92** 131	**84** 197	**92** 189	**14** 35	**62** 257	**99** 295	**31** 134	**89** 88	**86** 229	**100** 53	**65** 220	**0.18** 1697	**1.92** 1301
Alexian Brothers Medical Center, Elk Grove Village, IL	**90** 59	**98** 214	**98** 218	**95** 168	**97** 236	**-** 0	**73** 15	**99** 79	**83** 161	**80** 413	**96** 511	**96** 72	**84** 212	**97** 267	**-** -	**88** 312	**100** 445	**79** 305	**90** 77	**93** 592	**98** 147	**77** 554	**-** -	**-** -
Alton Memorial Hospital, Alton, IL	**92** 12	**96** 106	**95** 87	**98** 103	**100** 92	**-** 0	**-** 0	**100** 36	**100** 49	**92** 140	**96** 183	**100** 19	**84** 165	**95** 184	**89** 44	**91** 243	**100** 283	**92** 186	**98** 58	**94** 275	**99** 70	**65** 263	**0.35** 566	**3.52** 398
Anderson Hospital, Maryville, IL	**80** 15	**98** 66	**91** 35	**97** 58	**97** 33	**-** 0	**-** 0	**83** 6	**100** 53	**85** 113	**95** 152	**89** 18	**92** 181	**96** 224	**-** -	**79** 249	**100** 328	**78** 221	**91** 69	**93** 568	**95** 118	**87** 548	**-** -	**-** -
Blessing Hospital, Quincy, IL	**85** 54	**98** 206	**97** 211	**95** 152	**98** 234	**67** 6	**88** 8	**96** 90	**88** 88	**64** 226	**84** 325	**91** 54	**94** 290	**92** 449	**87** 117	**87** 519	**100** 688	**87** 479	**87** 149	**85** 226	**77** 112	**63** 214	**-** -	**-** -
Bromenn Healthcare, Normal, IL	**100** 23	**98** 132	**99** 143	**90** 99	**99** 141	**-** 0	**56** 9	**100** 49	**95** 93	**79** 151	**96** 202	**100** 25	**89** 106	**83** 145	**92** 51	**80** 182	**100** 236	**87** 167	**98** 53	**86** 1056	**97** 241	**67** 1022	**-** -	**-** -
Carle Foundation Hospital, Urbana, IL	**69** 49	**99** 158	**99** 249	**94** 140	**94** 256	**-** 0	**20** 5	**89** 93	**88** 96	**56** 205	**87** 283	**76** 33	**87** 91	**85** 95	**90** 20	**76** 116	**100** 142	**73** 108	**84** 37	**66** 215	**82** 71	**78** 205	**-** -	**-** -
Carlinville Area Hospital, Carlinville, IL	**100** 4	**100** 13	**100** 9	**93** 14	**89** 9	**0** 1	**-** 0	**0** 1	**100** 6	**65** 20	**97** 37	**0** 2	**53** 66	**100** 3	**69** 16	**61** 61	**100** 81	**58** 62	**62** 8	**-** -	**-** -	**-** -	**-** -	**-** -
Centegra Northern Illinois Medical Center, McHenry, IL	**88** 17	**95** 124	**96** 123	**91** 93	**97** 137	**100** 1	**71** 7	**100** 56	**84** 116	**71** 250	**97** 324	**89** 47	**85** 146	**94** 186	**51** 35	**87** 210	**100** 261	**63** 150	**94** 67	**81** 544	**89** 121	**79** 525	**-** -	**-** -
Central DuPage Hospital, Winfield, IL	**76** 34	**97** 180	**96** 167	**93** 146	**96** 168	**-** 0	**80** 10	**100** 53	**73** 152	**62** 309	**96** 421	**98** 55	**90** 192	**93** 226	**62** 45	**82** 277	**100** 348	**63** 225	**97** 64	**71** 297	**100** 77	**68** 289	**-** -	**-** -
CGH Medical Center, Sterling, IL	**69** 16	**96** 72	**80** 55	**93** 71	**93** 55	**-** 0	**33** 3	**100** 18	**89** 55	**97** 154	**81** 197	**100** 17	**82** 146	**93** 87	**54** 26	**84** 159	**96** 191	**56** 121	**100** 34	**93** 311	**100** 73	**70** 298	**-** -	**-** -
Clay County Hospital, Flora, IL	**-** 0	**100** 6	**100** 2	**100** 7	**100** 5	**-** 0	**-** 0	**-** 0	**93** 30	**94** 65	**98** 101	**91** 11	**87** 46	**100** 58	**100** 19	**95** 75	**100** 89	**96** 51	**100** 24	**89** 9	**100** 1	**71** 7	**-** -	**-** -
Community Hospital of Ottawa, Ottawa, IL	**100** 2	**93** 15	**100** 9	**92** 13	**90** 10	**-** 0	**-** 0	**100** 2	**81** 16	**89** 74	**91** 98	**100** 8	**88** 93	**92** 74	**76** 25	**93** 138	**99** 173	**84** 127	**86** 22	**65** 23	**-** -	**21** 19	**1.04** 288	**2.27** 220
Community Medical Center, Monmouth, IL	**-** 0	**33** 3	**100** 1	**50** 2	**100** 2	**-** 0	**-** 0	**100** 2	**83** 6	**100** 21	**72** 39	**100** 9	**84** 43	**100** 23	**67** 12	**76** 49	**100** 65	**61** 41	**100** 14	**59** 17	**100** 2	**20** 15	**-** -	**-** -
Community Memorial Hospital, Staunton, IL	**100** 1	**77** 13	**62** 8	**67** 12	**71** 7	**-** 0	**-** 0	**-** 0	**70** 10	**31** 13	**63** 27	**75** 4	**57** 21	**-** 0	**0** 10	**87** 23	**100** 32	**0** 23	**38** 8	**0** 2	**-** 0	**100** 2	**-** -	**-** -
Condell Medical Center, Libertyville, IL	**75** 63	**93** 216	**93** 191	**82** 182	**91** 217	**0** 1	**27** 15	**96** 70	**70** 129	**37** 314	**88** 406	**80** 60	**72** 161	**95** 140	**74** 34	**73** 200	**100** 264	**67** 151	**90** 58	**78** 503	**93** 82	**59** 494	**-** -	**-** -
Crawford Memorial Hospital, Robinson, IL	**50** 2	**88** 17	**85** 13	**47** 15	**58** 12	**-** 0	**-** -	**0** 4	**75** 4	**38** 21	**73** 30	**0** 5	**62** 8	**93** 15	**62** 8	**57** 30	**94** 35	**52** 25	**43** 7	**72** 67	**75** 12	**51** 63	**-** -	**-** -
Crossroads Community Hospital, Mount Vernon, IL	**100** 3	**100** 7	**100** 5	**83** 6	**67** 3	**0** 2	**-** 0	**0** 1	**88** 16	**62** 26	**78** 45	**100** 3	**75** 106	**96** 56	**96** 27	**76** 136	**100** 161	**88** 83	**88** 50	**25** 113	**97** 30	**90** 112	**-** -	**-** -
Culbertson Memorial Hospital, Rushville, IL	**-** -	**-** -	**-** -	**-** -	**-** -	**-** -	**-** -	**-** -	**71** 7	**63** 19	**94** 34	**75** 4	**92** 24	**92** 13	**100** 10	**84** 38	**100** 51	**97** 35	**100** 7	**-** -	**-** -	**-** -	**-** -	**-** -
Decatur Memorial Hospital, Decatur, IL	**88** 76	**99** 164	**99** 197	**96** 132	**99** 209	**-** 0	**43** 7	**100** 86	**89** 219	**96** 354	**99** 449	**100** 56	**83** 258	**94** 243	**95** 73	**91** 332	**100** 411	**93** 287	**99** 77	**82** 448	**93** 132	**61** 432	**0.37** 1088	**5.03** 656
Delnor Community Hospital, Geneva, IL	**83** 18	**99** 98	**99** 81	**99** 91	**98** 86	**-** 0	**33** 6	**95** 21	**87** 62	**87** 164	**97** 236	**97** 31	**92** 128	**89** 114	**100** 44	**91** 207	**100** 243	**99** 176	**78** 23	**71** 368	**79** 89	**65** 353	**0.06** 1587	**8.33** 984
Doctor John Warner Hospital, Clinton, IL	**100** 1	**71** 7	**80** 5	**80** 5	**60** 5	**-** 0	**-** 0	**0** 2	**40** 5	**0** 30	**76** 38	**0** 1	**77** 26	**100** 18	**29** 7	**78** 27	**97** 36	**38** 24	**22** 9	**-** -	**-** -	**-** -	**-** -	**-** -
Edward Hospital, Naperville, IL	**100** 58	**100** 263	**100** 268	**100** 229	**100** 264	**-** 0	**80** 15	**100** 71	**93** 215	**91** 402	**98** 517	**99** 68	**91** 271	**96** 370	**-** -	**81** 439	**100** 577	**70** 395	**91** 80	**83** 983	**99** 335	**42** 954	**0.55** 3972	**6.58** 2506
Elmhurst Memorial Hospital, Elmhurst, IL	**96** 49	**99** 225	**100** 229	**99** 189	**100** 219	**-** 0	**80** 5	**100** 52	**95** 222	**96** 453	**97** 546	**96** 73	**79** 243	**94** 204	**62** 58	**85** 334	**100** 384	**50** 266	**85** 53	**95** 659	**93** 59	**61** 628	**0.25** 1570	**3.68** 1168
Evanston Hospital, Evanston, IL	**96** 89	**99** 515	**99** 518	**99** 477	**98** 523	**0** 1	**37** 19	**94** 80	**87** 252	**55** 609	**99** 836	**83** 82	**92** 375	**92** 504	**24** 122	**92** 683	**100** 777	**34** 545	**70** 74	**89** 2015	**90** 520	**88** 1962	**0.36** 4959	**4.51** 3393
Fairfield Memorial Hospital, Fairfield, IL	**50** 2	**100** 3	**67** 3	**67** 3	**100** 3	**-** 0	**-** -	**100** 1	**75** 16	**97** 36	**78** 55	**100** 2	**74** 70	**87** 30	**-** -	**77** 82	**100** 105	**75** 69	**74** 19	**91** 11	**100** 1	**91** 11	**-** -	**-** -
Ferrell Hospital, Eldorado, IL	**0** 2	**33** 12	**50** 10	**55** 11	**18** 11	**0** 1	**-** 0	**0** 6	**25** 8	**0** 18	**66** 29	**57** 7	**42** 36	**83** 6	**50** 10	**77** 52	**96** 67	**25** 32	**54** 24	**18** 11	**50** 2	**100** 4	**-** -	**-** -
FHN Memorial Hospital, Freeport, IL	**100** 8	**97** 34	**100** 24	**94** 35	**96** 27	**50** 2	**-** 0	**100** 3	**92** 62	**84** 128	**98** 179	**100** 15	**97** 120	**99** 120	**80** 41	**89** 192	**100** 234	**84** 169	**93** 45	**95** 406	**94** 80	**80** 388	**-** -	**-** -
Galena-Stauss Hospital & Healthcare Center, Galena, IL	**-** 0	**-** 0	**-** 0	**-** 0	**-** 0	**-** 0	**-** 0	**-** 0	**100** 1	**29** 7	**50** 12	**50** 2	**90** 30	**-** 0	**100** 5	**88** 25	**100** 30	**81** 26	**25** 4	**-** -	**-** -	**-** -	**-** -	**-** -
Galesburg Cottage Hospital, Galesburg, IL	**75** 4	**81** 31	**58** 19	**70** 20	**85** 20	**-** 0	**-** 0	**100** 6	**83** 48	**81** 91	**95** 142	**84** 19	**75** 91	**91** 103	**81** 27	**81** 151	**99** 177	**84** 120	**78** 32	**85** 177	**96** 52	**79** 174	**-** -	**-** -
Gateway Regional Medical Center, Granite City, IL	**94** 18	**91** 112	**96** 91	**89** 87	**98** 87	**0** 2	**-** 0	**97** 31	**91** 81	**33** 223	**87** 269	**87** 47	**80** 142	**93** 103	**54** 28	**77** 186	**99** 198	**59** 96	**82** 67	**30** 177	**89** 47	**66** 176	**-** -	**-** -
Genesis Medical Center-Illini Campus, Silvis, IL	**79** 66	**94** 99	**86** 103	**91** 90	**89** 101	**-** 0	**40** 5	**81** 43	**80** 59	**88** 150	**88** 207	**90** 39	**72** 90	**84** 69	**62** 26	**71** 127	**100** 149	**72** 100	**70** 37	**96** 92	**99** 92	**73** 91	**0.00** 780	**3.49** 545
Gibson Community Hospital, Gibson City, IL	**-** 0	**100** 1	**-** 0	**100** 1	**-** 0	**-** 0	**-** -	**-** 0	**62** 8	**38** 8	**88** 25	**33** 3	**94** 32	**83** 23	**73** 11	**86** 42	**100** 57	**82** 33	**90** 10	**84** 31	**100** 6	**29** 31	**-** -	**-** -
Good Samaritan Regional Health Center, Mount Vernon, IL	**100** 42	**98** 98	**100** 202	**95** 77	**100** 221	**0** 1	**20** 5	**96** 92	**88** 94	**63** 238	**97** 273	**91** 46	**90** 150	**92** 151	**72** 60	**88** 238	**99** 272	**69** 188	**84** 57	**86** 442	**92** 102	**73** 426	**0.00** 739	**3.36** 476
Gottlieb Memorial Hospital, Melrose Park, IL	**97** 29	**95** 114	**95** 103	**94** 104	**97** 101	**-** 0	**0** 4	**100** 34	**97** 118	**68** 285	**96** 348	**100** 46	**88** 104	**99** 128	**88** 26	**86** 153	**100** 186	**92** 110	**100** 41	**89** 167	**82** 55	**46** 162	**-** -	**-** -
Graham Hospital, Canton, IL	**75** 4	**67** 6	**57** 7	**50** 6	**50** 6	**-** 0	**-** 0	**100** 2	**69** 42	**51** 59	**94** 96	**92** 13	**75** 61	**96** 51	**76** 21	**76** 104	**99** 126	**56** 84	**68** 28	**36** 143	**96** 53	**88** 137	**-** -	**-** -
Greenville Regional Hospital, Greenville, IL	**-** 0	**78** 9	**100** 6	**67** 6	**100** 6	**-** 0	**-** 0	**-** 0	**100** 5	**52** 29	**83** 47	**67** 3	**73** 63	**93** 60	**62** 24	**77** 98	**100** 127	**35** 85	**68** 22	**55** 22	**100** 7	**90** 20	**0.00** 130	**10.5** 76
Hamilton Memorial Hospital, McLeansboro, IL	**-** -	**-** -	**-** -	**-** -	**-** -	**-** -	**-** -	**-** -	**89** 9	**94** 32	**98** 46	**100** 4	**72** 25	**80** 5	**25** 4	**92** 38	**98** 41	**71** 21	**100** 11	**-** -	**-** -	**-** -	**-** -	**-** -

NOTE: The first number in each column (boldface) is the rate in percent, the second number is the number of patients; Please refer to the main entry for footnotes; ***Heart Attack Care:*** *1. ACE Inhibitor or ARB for LVSD; 2. Aspirin at Arrival; 3. Aspirin at Discharge; 4. Beta Blocker at Arrival; 5. Beta Blocker at Discharge; 6. Fibrinolytic Medication Timing; 7. PCI Within 90 Minutes of Arrival; 8. Smoking Cessation Advice;* ***Heart Failure Care:*** *9. ACE Inhibitor or ARB for LVSD; 10. Discharge Instructions; 11. Evaluation of LVS Function; 12. Smoking Cessation Advice;* ***Pneumonia Care:*** *13. Appropriate Initial Antibiotic; 14. Blood Culture Timing; 15. Influenza Vaccine; 16. Initial Antibiotic Timing; 17. Oxygenation Assessment; 18. Pneumococcal Vaccine; 19. Smoking Cessation Advice;* ***Surgical Infection Prevention:*** *20. Prophylactic Antibiotic Given; 21. Prophylactic Antibiotic Selection; 22. Prophylactic Antibiotic Stopped;* ***Pregnancy Care:*** *23. Inpatient Neonatal Mortality; 24. Third or Fourth Degree Laceration*

Hospital	Heart Attack Care								Heart Failure Care				Pneumonia Care							Surgical Infection Prevention			Pregnancy Care	
	1	2	3	4	5	6	7	8	9	10	11	12	13	14	15	16	17	18	19	20	21	22	23	24
Hammond-Henry Hospital, Geneseo, IL	- -	- -	- -	- -	- -	- -	- -	- -	100 5	92 13	68 19	100 2	81 26	83 12	60 5	84 19	100 32	85 20	75 4	91 35	91 11	45 33	- -	- -
Hardin County General Hospital, Rosiclare, IL	- -	- -	- -	- -	- -	- -	- -	- -	100 7	100 38	100 51	100 8	81 26	100 34	100 8	93 46	96 55	100 34	100 13	- -	- -	- -	- -	- -
Harrisburg Medical Center, Harrisburg, IL	100 2	100 11	83 6	67 9	86 7	0 1	- 0	0 1	86 29	77 88	85 119	67 18	60 87	80 49	- -	83 143	98 171	55 108	79 28	22 9	25 4	67 9	- -	- -
Heartland Regional Medical Center, Marion, IL	81 16	97 63	95 83	95 65	99 86	33 3	0 3	97 34	81 42	77 125	90 167	88 25	82 101	94 98	93 27	80 152	100 181	87 106	98 44	34 260	89 75	44 239	- -	- -
Herrin Hospital, Herrin, IL	86 7	100 16	91 11	100 18	93 15	- 0	- 0	50 2	100 28	79 141	89 173	96 23	76 116	93 107	86 29	80 168	100 210	73 134	90 50	87 170	100 41	79 151	- -	- -
Hinsdale Hospital, Hinsdale, IL	100 26	98 132	100 148	97 120	98 141	0 1	75 4	100 37	74 93	80 200	96 273	100 16	87 156	96 252	90 62	81 278	100 375	83 266	95 60	79 175	92 59	48 162	- -	- -
Holy Cross Hospital, Chicago, IL	85 33	94 200	77 118	88 152	77 117	38 8	0 3	91 35	77 123	12 265	95 313	95 82	85 142	92 150	25 24	73 218	100 233	33 93	87 61	91 170	95 38	65 153	- -	- -
Hoopeston Community Memorial Hospital, Hoopeston, IL	- 0	100 4	50 2	100 2	- 0	- 0	- 0	- 0	- 0	4 28	4 27	- 0	85 52	73 11	30 10	98 51	100 60	14 50	23 13	- -	- -	- -	- -	- -
Hopedale Medical Complex, Hopedale, IL	- -	- -	- -	- -	- -	- -	- -	- -	- -	- -	- -	- -	- -	- -	- -	- -	- -	- -	- -	- -	- -	- -	- -	- -
Illini Community Hospital, Pittsfield, IL	0 1	70 10	50 6	75 8	83 6	- 0	- 0	- 0	71 7	88 16	92 25	100 3	100 33	100 5	100 11	80 45	98 60	82 49	100 9	40 5	33 3	0 2	- -	- -
Illinois Valley Community Hospital, Peru, IL	67 3	89 9	86 7	91 11	88 8	- 0	- 0	100 1	82 28	68 74	80 113	88 16	79 101	82 98	34 35	91 160	99 178	54 131	76 25	48 184	96 46	57 181	- -	- -
Ingalls Memorial Hospital, Harvey, IL	76 46	94 175	85 177	85 157	87 189	- 0	50 2	98 53	76 90	87 271	83 303	88 58	81 123	73 99	79 24	67 183	100 203	68 98	93 57	88 407	98 81	71 404	0.55 1461	2.06 1067
Iroquois Memorial Hospital & Resident Home, Watseka, IL	100 2	98 40	100 14	83 30	93 15	12 8	- 0	100 2	88 17	56 80	84 125	92 25	81 122	92 146	- -	89 217	100 275	73 198	86 50	50 14	100 1	57 14	- -	- -
Jackson Park Hospital & Medical Center, Chicago, IL	50 2	89 18	71 7	65 20	14 7	25 4	- 0	0 3	80 71	6 200	71 217	4 90	79 66	62 16	- 0	69 52	99 67	0 16	0 20	33 3	100 2	33 3	0.40 251	1.08 186
Jersey Community Hospital, Jerseyville, IL	62 8	74 68	84 51	74 57	73 52	- 0	- 0	86 7	56 34	42 76	69 114	50 12	79 96	95 78	86 28	88 113	99 154	62 112	56 25	39 23	100 3	57 21	- -	- -
John & Mary Kirby Hospital, Monticello, IL	- -	- -	- -	- -	- -	- -	- -	- -	100 6	64 14	82 22	0 1	75 28	90 21	31 13	64 50	98 60	52 50	17 6	- -	- -	- -	- -	- -
John H Stroger Jr Hospital of Cook County, Chicago, IL	78 40	96 144	99 199	96 101	97 182	- 0	0 1	84 112	94 144	11 283	96 294	73 126	50 187	77 109	15 26	33 210	100 243	12 52	56 131	87 147	50 44	79 141	1.91 1254	1.95 768
Katherine Shaw Bethea Hospital, Dixon, IL	83 6	98 48	92 26	97 29	94 31	0 1	- 0	100 4	90 42	80 87	96 113	92 12	97 78	90 79	67 18	95 96	100 120	85 81	100 23	94 154	97 35	93 139	- -	- -
Kenneth Hall Regional Hospital, East Saint Louis, IL	100 1	100 6	100 2	88 8	100 3	- 0	- 0	100 2	81 57	44 174	60 192	68 97	57 51	96 28	0 7	70 66	91 67	17 24	54 28	20 10	80 10	20 10	- -	- -
Kewanee Hospital, Kewanee, IL	0 2	33 6	50 4	60 5	80 5	- 0	- 0	- 0	91 11	81 58	80 96	78 9	95 66	97 58	60 15	84 108	100 123	67 82	74 23	74 34	80 5	70 33	- -	- -
Kishwaukee Community Hospital, De Kalb, IL	67 3	100 17	100 8	88 8	100 7	- 0	- 0	- 0	98 51	77 111	100 130	100 8	90 107	95 83	67 24	88 145	100 175	91 113	89 38	72 157	98 62	77 149	- -	- -
Lake Forest Hospital, Lake Forest, IL	67 3	96 26	67 6	100 24	100 10	- 0	- 0	50 2	87 45	90 107	95 128	100 13	89 150	87 120	83 35	85 159	100 193	78 135	88 26	83 511	96 169	62 498	- -	- -
Lawrence County Memorial Hospital, Lawrenceville, IL	0 2	80 10	100 5	80 10	57 7	- 0	- -	100 1	100 8	97 34	94 53	86 7	89 9	83 23	92 13	90 42	100 48	64 39	75 8	- -	- -	- -	- -	- -
Lincoln Park Hospital, Chicago, IL	40 5	100 12	77 13	58 12	62 13	- 0	- 0	25 4	82 66	58 139	86 174	53 36	68 57	78 37	25 4	76 63	93 84	28 36	44 16	64 22	91 22	86 21	- -	- -
Little Company of Mary Hospital, Evergreen Park, IL	96 23	96 154	95 82	92 111	99 81	0 1	0 3	83 30	88 125	26 279	93 351	88 69	88 105	86 118	52 29	62 169	99 212	49 128	87 38	58 179	97 61	52 163	0.21 1436	2.36 932
Loretto Hospital, Chicago, IL	75 4	89 28	100 14	96 25	94 16	67 3	- 0	100 7	96 49	100 102	95 131	100 44	59 54	93 97	- -	78 119	100 129	18 44	100 37	88 8	100 3	0 8	- -	- -
Loyola University Health System, Maywood, IL	84 37	100 169	100 188	98 160	100 201	0 1	43 7	100 60	91 408	66 693	99 754	90 155	85 120	94 145	80 35	62 176	100 254	82 125	77 48	95 283	88 74	88 276	2.27 1895	2.41 997
MacNeal Hospital, Berwyn, IL	84 102	100 246	96 223	98 205	96 229	- 0	45 11	93 73	78 243	74 384	91 507	98 85	86 258	97 256	73 60	90 337	100 391	68 256	93 81	92 613	96 136	79 563	- -	- -
Marshall Browning Hospital, DuQuoin, IL	- 0	100 7	60 5	43 7	60 5	- 0	- 0	0 1	75 4	40 20	54 24	- 0	68 31	96 27	12 8	85 34	100 44	50 28	20 5	- -	- -	- -	- -	- -
Mason District Hospital, Havana, IL	100 1	100 3	100 3	100 3	100 4	- 0	- -	- 0	75 4	41 17	88 26	50 2	92 26	100 22	80 15	82 44	96 52	74 42	100 8	46 13	100 5	62 13	- -	- -
McDonough District Hospital, Macomb, IL	75 8	69 16	33 6	67 9	60 10	- 0	- 0	100 2	73 33	72 58	76 95	100 6	93 110	97 59	94 31	81 142	100 191	74 152	92 25	91 161	91 33	82 154	0.00 391	2.80 286
Memorial Hospital, Belleville, IL	69 36	99 151	98 130	93 146	98 150	- 0	75 4	98 48	84 218	90 474	99 576	100 83	80 186	90 193	- -	68 301	100 345	46 217	94 81	74 175	91 58	67 163	- -	- -
Memorial Hospital, Chester, IL	100 1	100 4	100 1	100 4	100 2	0 1	- 0	- 0	50 6	61 44	97 64	100 5	100 33	100 16	100 14	94 47	100 61	95 44	100 9	96 28	83 6	100 24	- -	- -
Memorial Hospital Carbondale, Carbondale, IL	76 70	99 87	95 175	91 75	95 219	67 3	0 2	98 101	61 113	43 215	93 242	89 54	88 67	82 79	56 18	87 114	100 152	63 100	88 34	40 226	89 72	57 218	0.21 1436	2.59 1002
Memorial Medical Center, Springfield, IL	95 128	98 295	99 507	94 255	99 539	- 0	81 16	100 201	95 207	90 400	100 504	100 84	91 261	84 331	78 81	83 433	100 561	77 358	100 144	94 1496	88 84	93 1456	- -	- -
Memorial Medical Center, Woodstock, IL	60 5	94 35	92 12	89 27	96 23	0 1	- 0	80 5	73 64	78 171	99 230	80 41	87 139	96 164	60 43	90 205	100 251	68 157	87 39	90 326	85 74	77 311	- -	- -
Mendota Community Hospital, Mendota, IL	- 0	67 3	- 0	100 3	- 0	- 0	- 0	- 0	88 8	6 17	78 32	50 4	78 18	100 8	83 6	87 31	98 44	82 40	100 4	47 17	100 2	12 16	- -	- -
Mercy Harvard Hospital, Harvard, IL	- 0	100 9	100 5	100 6	100 4	- 0	- 0	- 0	100 2	82 17	96 26	100 1	94 16	94 16	83 6	100 25	100 28	90 20	100 6	93 41	100 6	56 41	- -	- -
Mercy Hospital, Chicago, IL	86 44	91 129	93 135	95 111	98 142	20 5	20 5	91 67	88 278	85 521	98 563	94 128	82 127	81 187	34 29	63 230	100 261	35 128	79 76	93 404	98 110	80 391	- -	- -
Methodist Hospital of Chicago, Chicago, IL	50 2	100 7	60 5	75 8	40 5	- 0	- 0	100 1	30 10	100 15	79 48	35 17	67 12	76 83	23 13	77 139	93 169	8 99	62 66	57 7	100 1	100 7	- -	- -
Methodist Medical Center of Illinois, Peoria, IL	96 49	97 114	99 183	94 96	98 213	- 0	50 2	99 92	96 156	75 294	97 370	94 93	93 159	96 147	96 51	81 237	100 327	98 204	96 96	91 681	91 243	89 650	- -	- -
Michael Reese Hospital, Chicago, IL	95 20	88 48	96 54	90 41	96 53	- 0	0 2	86 22	89 167	81 242	98 313	75 79	90 31	87 52	67 15	77 82	99 94	74 39	80 35	75 96	69 26	96 93	- -	- -
Midwestern Regional Medical Center, Zion, IL	- 0	100 1	100 1	100 1	100 1	- 0	- 0	- 0	75 4	100 1	96 23	100 1	100 4	100 10	- -	60 50	100 62	22 18	100 3	73 15	- -	21 14	- -	- -
Morris Hospital, Morris, IL	89 9	98 40	100 24	82 22	91 32	- 0	100 2	100 10	90 50	90 130	99 168	100 25	89 118	89 118	52 44	90 212	100 228	57 163	100 43	79 216	95 42	61 207	- -	- -
Mount Sinai Hospital, Chicago, IL	75 24	95 125	94 111	87 110	94 109	0 2	0 3	93 43	84 189	62 340	100 374	87 127	81 69	86 83	31 16	58 130	97 136	34 44	90 48	59 177	86 49	45 156	0.71 3951	0.98 2660
Neurologic and Orthopedic Insitute of Chicago, Chicago, IL	- -	- -	- -	- -	- -	- -	- -	- -	- -	- -	- -	- -	- -	- -	- -	- -	- -	- -	- -	97 33	95 21	82 33	- -	- -
Northwest Community Hospital, Arlington Heights, IL	96 46	98 389	99 337	99 327	99 382	- 0	27 15	99 84	79 91	51 213	97 313	96 24	86 85	92 111	95 22	88 173	100 189	87 140	78 23	91 339	99 85	74 323	0.18 3398	5.29 2099
Northwestern Memorial Hospital, Chicago, IL	98 46	100 215	100 232	100 212	99 252	- 0	25 12	100 56	96 307	77 666	100 745	95 155	86 207	92 190	81 42	78 282	100 365	80 169	87 91	92 2347	98 513	88 2308	0.46 10299	6.35 7198

NOTE: The first number in each column (boldface) is the rate in percent, the second number is the number of patients; Please refer to the main entry for footnotes; ***Heart Attack Care:*** *1. ACE Inhibitor or ARB for LVSD; 2. Aspirin at Arrival; 3. Aspirin at Discharge; 4. Beta Blocker at Arrival; 5. Beta Blocker at Discharge; 6. Fibrinolytic Medication Timing; 7. PCI Within 90 Minutes of Arrival; 8. Smoking Cessation Advice;* ***Heart Failure Care:*** *9. ACE Inhibitor or ARB for LVSD; 10. Discharge Instructions; 11. Evaluation of LVS Function; 12. Smoking Cessation Advice;* ***Pneumonia Care:*** *13. Appropriate Initial Antibiotic; 14. Blood Culture Timing; 15. Influenza Vaccine; 16. Initial Antibiotic Timing; 17. Oxygenation Assessment; 18. Pneumococcal Vaccine; 19. Smoking Cessation Advice;* ***Surgical Infection Prevention:*** *20. Prophylactic Antibiotic Given; 21. Prophylactic Antibiotic Selection; 22. Prophylactic Antibiotic Stopped;* ***Pregnancy Care:*** *23. Inpatient Neonatal Mortality; 24. Third or Fourth Degree Laceration*

Hospital	Heart Attack Care								Heart Failure Care				Pneumonia Care							Surgical Infection Prevention			Pregnancy Care	
	1	2	3	4	5	6	7	8	9	10	11	12	13	14	15	16	17	18	19	20	21	22	23	24
Norwegian-American Hospital, Chicago, IL	**25** 4	**90** 42	**76** 21	**91** 35	**77** 22	**0** 4	- 0	**10** 10	**62** 76	**23** 202	**82** 242	**21** 68	**74** 61	**87** 46	- -	**78** 79	**100** 81	**37** 30	**24** 34	**50** 18	**84** 19	**28** 18	- -	- -
Oak Forest Hospital of Cook County, Oak Forest, IL	- 0	**100** 11	**100** 3	**100** 9	**100** 5	- 0	- 0	- 0	**93** 73	**80** 137	**97** 145	**99** 68	**87** 54	**96** 49	**100** 4	**71** 63	**100** 72	**100** 6	**95** 43	**82** 28	**100** 6	**36** 25	- -	- -
OSF Saint Mary Medical Center, Galesburg, IL	**60** 5	**89** 38	**100** 18	**83** 30	**88** 25	- 0	- 0	**67** 3	**86** 59	**85** 122	**96** 166	**90** 21	**86** 131	**92** 116	**94** 50	**89** 164	**100** 214	**98** 134	**98** 51	**97** 374	**95** 100	**90** 363	- -	- -
Our Lady of the Resurrection Medical Center, Chicago, IL	**88** 43	**97** 238	**96** 192	**96** 222	**96** 198	- 0	**50** 4	**96** 53	**90** 202	**71** 380	**100** 608	**96** 82	**82** 142	**88** 180	**72** 40	**85** 247	**100** 301	**68** 193	**97** 58	**63** 153	- -	**42** 133	- -	- -
Palos Community Hospital, Palos Heights, IL	**81** 32	**100** 264	**97** 213	**98** 217	**93** 211	- 0	**46** 13	**96** 68	**58** 64	**61** 211	**93** 290	**86** 29	**93** 120	**98** 127	**61** 31	**65** 153	**100** 203	**61** 142	**85** 40	**81** 221	**78** 73	**56** 213	- -	- -
Pana Community Hospital, Pana, IL	**100** 2	**100** 4	**100** 4	**75** 4	**75** 4	- 0	- -	**0** 1	**78** 9	**56** 27	**56** 41	**75** 8	**75** 20	**85** 20	**20** 5	**80** 30	**100** 37	**68** 22	**100** 3	- -	- -	- -	- -	- -
Paris Community Hospital, Paris, IL	- -	- -	- -	- -	- -	- -	- -	- -	- -	- -	- -	- -	- -	- -	- -	- -	- -	- -	- -	- -	- -	- -	- -	- -
Passavant Memorial Area Hospital, Jacksonville, IL	**100** 3	**63** 19	**82** 11	**72** 18	**83** 12	- 0	- 0	**100** 3	**82** 34	**76** 96	**95** 153	**73** 15	**91** 117	**80** 134	**90** 41	**95** 205	**100** 252	**87** 176	**83** 54	**95** 170	**95** 62	**93** 161	- -	- -
Pekin Hospital, Pekin, IL	**100** 6	**97** 29	**93** 14	**100** 31	**90** 21	**0** 1	- 0	**71** 7	**90** 50	**71** 86	**93** 128	**95** 19	**88** 99	**94** 106	**12** 33	**86** 187	**99** 224	**41** 157	**72** 50	**78** 299	**92** 77	**56** 287	- -	- -
Perry Memorial Hospital, Princeton, IL	**100** 3	**75** 16	**55** 11	**62** 16	**82** 11	- 0	- 0	- 0	**67** 9	**85** 55	**85** 88	**100** 4	**85** 46	**95** 22	**15** 13	**97** 59	**100** 81	**24** 58	**89** 9	- -	- -	- -	- -	- -
Pinckneyville Community Hospital, Pinckneyville, IL	**0** 1	**100** 5	**75** 4	**80** 5	**75** 4	- 0	- -	- 0	**62** 8	**55** 20	**79** 28	**0** 1	**78** 41	- 0	**70** 10	**94** 33	**96** 46	**70** 40	**56** 9	**0** 4	**100** 2	**25** 4	- -	- -
Proctor Hospital, Peoria, IL	**100** 27	**98** 88	**99** 93	**99** 90	**100** 111	- 0	**80** 5	**100** 29	**99** 71	**97** 145	**100** 201	**92** 24	**88** 147	**95** 181	**97** 38	**95** 214	**100** 267	**98** 205	**90** 50	**85** 634	**96** 164	**86** 623	- -	- -
Provena Covenant Medical Center, Urbana, IL	**96** 45	**97** 107	**99** 249	**89** 56	**99** 227	**50** 4	**75** 4	**97** 100	**98** 120	**83** 292	**99** 373	**85** 59	**91** 119	**97** 155	**48** 46	**70** 230	**100** 283	**56** 183	**95** 64	**82** 603	**86** 153	**66** 585	**0.32** 1236	**3.15** 890
Provena Mercy Center, Aurora, IL	**68** 41	**99** 166	**97** 184	**97** 159	**98** 183	- 0	**33** 9	**92** 12	**76** 117	**50** 32	**92** 273	**33** 3	**78** 37	**90** 59	- -	**75** 309	**100** 379	**34** 220	**4** 23	**83** 128	- -	**69** 127	**0.19** 1580	**4.60** 999
Provena Saint Joseph Hospital, Elgin, IL	**74** 31	**93** 106	**98** 95	**91** 85	**96** 111	- 0	**44** 9	**100** 11	**69** 67	**76** 17	**90** 162	**100** 9	**84** 25	**86** 29	- -	**79** 189	**100** 240	**34** 142	**67** 6	**82** 77	- -	**71** 76	**0.66** 607	**4.94** 445
Provena United Samaritans Medical Center, Danville, IL	**85** 20	**96** 74	**91** 44	**96** 73	**93** 55	- 0	- 0	**100** 19	**91** 151	**50** 359	**99** 421	**100** 63	**90** 264	**89** 246	**59** 46	**71** 385	**99** 432	**63** 220	**100** 110	**94** 270	**89** 64	**74** 249	**0.22** 896	**1.58** 634
Provident Hospital, Chicago, IL	**100** 2	**94** 53	**77** 22	**87** 54	**62** 24	- 0	- 0	**64** 11	**92** 163	**73** 402	**88** 382	**95** 185	**88** 253	**80** 231	**15** 33	**52** 292	**100** 308	**25** 69	**95** 154	**29** 17	**86** 14	**44** 16	**0.38** 526	**2.49** 401
Red Bud Regional Hospital, Red Bud, IL	- 0	**100** 1	- 0	**0** 1	- 0	- 0	- 0	- 0	**75** 8	**87** 30	**87** 61	**100** 9	**98** 42	**98** 52	**94** 17	**89** 63	**100** 88	**78** 51	**100** 14	**62** 29	**100** 4	**81** 27	- -	- -
Resurrection Medical Center, Chicago, IL	**62** 73	**97** 343	**93** 316	**89** 199	**88** 316	**0** 2	**5** 21	**90** 87	**63** 258	**45** 613	**90** 868	**73** 77	**82** 260	**96** 308	- -	**87** 422	**98** 466	**27** 322	**78** 54	**75** 60	**98** 60	**61** 51	- -	- -
Richland Memorial Hospital, Olney, IL	**50** 2	**91** 11	**62** 8	**71** 7	**100** 7	**0** 1	- 0	**0** 1	**76** 25	**54** 48	**89** 73	**33** 6	**81** 58	**98** 46	**74** 19	**88** 83	**100** 108	**51** 72	**61** 28	**86** 85	**81** 27	**57** 82	- -	- -
Riverside Medical Center, Kankakee, IL	**100** 23	**100** 93	**100** 100	**98** 53	**98** 97	**100** 2	**50** 4	**100** 43	**94** 145	**99** 305	**99** 365	**100** 66	**85** 124	**97** 177	**44** 52	**82** 262	**100** 304	**49** 202	**100** 63	**79** 402	**94** 94	**68** 380	**0.40** 1238	**2.23** 852
Rochelle Community Hospital, Rochelle, IL	- 0	**67** 3	**100** 2	**100** 3	**100** 2	- 0	- 0	- 0	**50** 4	**47** 17	**78** 23	**0** 1	**82** 22	**100** 7	- -	**79** 33	**100** 38	**37** 19	**30** 10	**100** 7	**100** 7	**100** 7	- -	- -
Rockford Memorial Hospital, Rockford, IL	**85** 54	**98** 196	**97** 272	**95** 189	**100** 284	- 0	**100** 8	**93** 98	**91** 108	**90** 239	**98** 320	**98** 62	**92** 103	**97** 158	**77** 31	**80** 192	**100** 238	**67** 159	**88** 51	**89** 506	**97** 106	**85** 498	- -	- -
Roseland Community Hospital, Chicago, IL	**100** 3	**96** 24	**91** 11	**92** 24	**91** 11	**25** 4	- 0	**60** 5	**86** 97	**86** 279	**78** 295	**70** 124	**81** 109	**64** 99	- -	**56** 154	**100** 164	**31** 48	**78** 69	**30** 10	**100** 2	**25** 8	- -	- -
Rush North Shore Medical Center, Skokie, IL	**82** 22	**96** 106	**97** 95	**92** 86	**92** 99	- 0	**33** 3	**92** 12	**79** 146	**45** 285	**96** 418	**81** 21	**80** 138	**96** 156	**60** 47	**85** 233	**100** 278	**58** 213	**60** 25	**96** 194	**100** 68	**88** 192	- -	- -
Rush Oak Park Hospital, Oak Park, IL	**67** 9	**96** 53	**89** 38	**95** 40	**92** 39	**62** 8	- 0	**100** 6	**76** 62	**65** 203	**87** 255	**90** 52	**86** 96	**94** 129	**71** 35	**81** 155	**100** 193	**70** 108	**98** 40	**80** 80	**100** 26	**36** 77	- -	- -
Rush University Medical Center, Chicago, IL	**96** 24	**100** 112	**100** 148	**100** 95	**100** 147	- 0	**50** 4	**100** 51	**96** 139	**78** 311	**100** 338	**97** 71	**93** 58	**90** 71	**67** 24	**79** 96	**100** 145	**75** 63	**95** 41	**90** 425	**98** 102	**86** 417	- -	- -
Rush-Copley Medical Center, Aurora, IL	**100** 30	**99** 154	**97** 153	**99** 118	**99** 161	**50** 2	**100** 2	**100** 52	**100** 76	**98** 189	**99** 234	**100** 48	**95** 132	**92** 91	- -	**95** 175	**100** 230	**79** 130	**100** 60	**93** 456	**94** 86	**64** 439	**0.54** 3717	**3.28** 2503
Sacred Heart Hospital, Chicago, IL	**0** 1	**100** 2	- 0	**0** 1	**0** 1	- 0	- 0	- 0	**50** 20	**4** 152	**94** 160	**25** 20	**89** 9	**33** 3	**0** 3	**33** 15	**94** 16	**0** 5	**17** 6	**0** 1	- 0	**0** 1	- -	- -
Saint Alexius Medical Center, Hoffman Estates, IL	**84** 44	**97** 152	**93** 123	**92** 106	**100** 129	- 0	**73** 11	**100** 48	**92** 120	**82** 238	**97** 315	**98** 51	**85** 156	**99** 205	**64** 47	**89** 274	**100** 315	**75** 193	**100** 62	**92** 287	**87** 61	**77** 277	- -	- -
Saint Anthony Hospital, Chicago, IL	**50** 2	**96** 28	**78** 9	**100** 14	**83** 6	**100** 1	- 0	**67** 3	**60** 60	**42** 162	**87** 179	**92** 51	**88** 69	**95** 73	**58** 12	**85** 93	**100** 115	**43** 44	**97** 39	**70** 33	**75** 16	**45** 31	- -	- -
Saint Anthony Medical Center, Rockford, IL	**94** 69	**99** 228	**99** 321	**97** 205	**97** 306	- 0	**45** 11	**98** 104	**90** 146	**88** 302	**99** 406	**96** 56	**84** 195	**94** 193	**89** 47	**79** 290	**99** 347	**80** 239	**92** 53	**92** 1107	**99** 280	**85** 1077	- -	- -
Saint Anthony's Health Center, Alton, IL	**71** 14	**91** 79	**94** 64	**86** 72	**87** 71	**50** 4	**0** 3	**89** 18	**76** 62	**69** 146	**71** 212	**78** 41	**90** 140	**98** 154	**61** 38	**82** 221	**100** 270	**76** 168	**87** 61	**63** 273	**82** 61	**45** 260	- -	- -
Saint Anthony's Memorial Hospital, Effingham, IL	**83** 6	**89** 38	**95** 20	**85** 34	**95** 19	- 0	- 0	**67** 3	**83** 30	**74** 176	**89** 202	**92** 24	**80** 176	**99** 124	- -	**85** 209	**100** 258	**76** 180	**81** 47	**81** 661	**99** 170	**87** 653	- -	- -
Saint Bernard Hospital and Health Care Center, Chicago, IL	**67** 3	**100** 32	**75** 16	**90** 30	**62** 16	- 0	- 0	**100** 3	**83** 109	**97** 275	**97** 326	**98** 129	**91** 149	**88** 183	**22** 32	**72** 232	**100** 260	**16** 86	**99** 92	**29** 21	**100** 5	**5** 20	- -	- -
Saint Elizabeth's Hospital, Belleville, IL	**82** 55	**95** 174	**96** 253	**90** 153	**96** 251	- 0	**60** 5	**89** 87	**88** 173	**63** 465	**85** 585	**78** 72	**85** 245	**91** 195	**34** 100	**80** 410	**99** 501	**28** 323	**82** 115	**81** 361	**80** 84	**72** 350	**0.00** 1255	**2.34** 942
Saint Elizabeth's Hospital, Chicago, IL	**50** 4	**92** 38	**95** 21	**86** 35	**91** 22	**33** 6	- 0	**100** 8	**84** 75	**85** 145	**95** 186	**97** 32	**72** 106	**97** 119	**50** 24	**93** 151	**100** 178	**84** 89	**100** 43	**89** 121	**92** 26	**76** 105	- -	- -
Saint Francis Hospital, Evanston, IL	**50** 20	**98** 121	**94** 110	**86** 86	**84** 96	**0** 1	**0** 4	**91** 23	**72** 163	**59** 290	**92** 401	**74** 70	**85** 261	**93** 424	**35** 99	**84** 518	**100** 622	**44** 382	**73** 103	**70** 310	**94** 111	**80** 290	- -	- -
Saint Francis Hospital, Litchfield, IL	- 0	**80** 5	**50** 4	**40** 5	**25** 4	**0** 1	- 0	- 0	**25** 20	**54** 61	**64** 91	**67** 3	**53** 98	**92** 48	**50** 24	**82** 159	**100** 176	**45** 121	**67** 15	**42** 40	**75** 12	**97** 37	- -	- -
Saint Francis Hospital & Health Center, Blue Island, IL	**79** 33	**96** 122	**93** 138	**92** 107	**96** 140	**0** 1	**25** 4	**97** 58	**78** 423	**57** 821	**90** 902	**96** 202	**87** 369	**85** 412	**62** 93	**73** 529	**100** 593	**64** 313	**93** 159	**92** 391	**92** 130	**51** 363	- -	- -
Saint Francis Medical Center, Peoria, IL	**90** 155	**98** 246	**98** 511	**95** 228	**99** 595	- 0	**38** 16	**100** 212	**88** 272	**56** 455	**91** 574	**94** 146	**92** 273	**94** 199	**85** 80	**82** 409	**100** 460	**79** 282	**97** 136	**90** 1730	**87** 406	**87** 1707	- -	- -
Saint James Hospital and Health Center, Olympia Fields, IL	**84** 56	**91** 246	**95** 197	**85** 160	**93** 198	- 0	**17** 12	**97** 79	**85** 106	**40** 292	**94** 353	**100** 59	**82** 131	**94** 131	**70** 33	**68** 221	**99** 280	**60** 146	**95** 66	**84** 379	**89** 93	**55** 365	- -	- -
Saint James OSF, Pontiac, IL	**100** 1	**100** 14	**89** 9	**92** 13	**100** 9	- 0	- 0	- 0	**76** 25	**77** 35	**97** 63	**100** 6	**84** 50	**94** 34	**100** 11	**92** 49	**100** 65	**88** 42	**64** 14	**93** 116	**100** 31	**46** 112	**0.44** 226	**3.57** 140
Saint John's Hospital, Springfield, IL	**87** 237	**99** 180	**99** 553	**98** 138	**98** 639	- 0	**79** 14	**99** 275	**78** 274	**54** 437	**98** 528	**96** 110	**90** 151	**96** 157	**43** 49	**88** 262	**100** 302	**93** 190	**85** 98	**88** 359	**90** 86	**92** 354	- -	- -
Saint Joseph Hospital, Chicago, IL	**77** 22	**98** 56	**98** 62	**100** 45	**89** 65	- 0	**50** 2	**88** 17	**80** 128	**59** 330	**94** 421	**83** 60	**87** 117	**94** 143	**58** 45	**86** 199	**100** 252	**46** 151	**82** 51	**85** 345	**94** 90	**69** 332	- -	- -
Saint Joseph Medical Center, Joliet, IL	**77** 73	**92** 280	**95** 290	**85** 255	**91** 292	**0** 1	**31** 16	**90** 101	**78** 287	**95** 663	**96** 808	**99** 77	**79** 420	**95** 74	**41** 117	**65** 609	**100** 673	**37** 399	**80** 124	**75** 989	**90** 228	**47** 959	**0.21** 1926	**4.16** 1202
Saint Joseph Medical Center, Bloomington, IL	**97** 34	**100** 90	**99** 104	**99** 81	**100** 126	- 0	**67** 6	**98** 50	**93** 72	**85** 115	**98** 156	**100** 43	**86** 92	**88** 98	**82** 28	**73** 118	**100** 156	**85** 101	**98** 43	**95** 553	**98** 121	**79** 542	- -	- -
Saint Joseph Memorial Hospital, Murphysboro, IL	**67** 3	**80** 10	**83** 6	**60** 10	**67** 6	- 0	- 0	- 0	**80** 10	**74** 50	**74** 57	**85** 13	**83** 41	**90** 29	**67** 6	**88** 50	**100** 59	**50** 40	**100** 13	- -	- -	- -	- -	- -

NOTE: The first number in each column (boldface) is the rate in percent, the second number is the number of patients; Please refer to the main entry for footnotes; ***Heart Attack Care:*** *1. ACE Inhibitor or ARB for LVSD; 2. Aspirin at Arrival; 3. Aspirin at Discharge; 4. Beta Blocker at Arrival; 5. Beta Blocker at Discharge; 6. Fibrinolytic Medication Timing; 7. PCI Within 90 Minutes of Arrival; 8. Smoking Cessation Advice;* ***Heart Failure Care:*** *9. ACE Inhibitor or ARB for LVSD; 10. Discharge Instructions; 11. Evaluation of LVS Function; 12. Smoking Cessation Advice;* ***Pneumonia Care:*** *13. Appropriate Initial Antibiotic; 14. Blood Culture Timing; 15. Influenza Vaccine; 16. Initial Antibiotic Timing; 17. Oxygenation Assessment; 18. Pneumococcal Vaccine; 19. Smoking Cessation Advice;* ***Surgical Infection Prevention:*** *20. Prophylactic Antibiotic Given; 21. Prophylactic Antibiotic Selection; 22. Prophylactic Antibiotic Stopped;* ***Pregnancy Care:*** *23. Inpatient Neonatal Mortality; 24. Third or Fourth Degree Laceration*

Hospital	Heart Attack Care								Heart Failure Care				Pneumonia Care							Surgical Infection Prevention			Pregnancy Care	
	1	2	3	4	5	6	7	8	9	10	11	12	13	14	15	16	17	18	19	20	21	22	23	24
Saint Joseph's Hospital, Highland, IL	100 1	62 8	67 6	67 6	80 5	- 0	- 0	- 0	88 8	74 31	64 50	100 4	73 41	97 38	69 13	83 71	100 81	79 57	100 13	- -	- -	- -	- -	- -
Saint Joseph's Hospital, Breese, IL	- 0	100 9	75 4	78 9	100 6	0 1	- 0	- 0	70 10	81 48	88 64	80 5	86 72	93 46	64 28	91 79	100 103	75 64	92 12	60 25	80 25	80 25	0.23 427	2.43 329
Saint Margaret's Hospital, Spring Valley, IL	0 1	100 4	100 3	86 7	83 6	33 3	- 0	- 0	91 22	68 74	93 98	82 11	77 70	94 81	71 21	91 128	100 168	32 108	68 25	89 244	98 53	31 239	- -	- -
Saint Mary's Good Samaritan, Centralia, IL	100 6	100 52	95 21	84 32	94 18	- 0	- 0	83 6	94 96	72 198	99 279	96 26	87 188	97 178	84 61	88 312	100 371	86 226	76 98	87 196	77 30	72 184	0.22 459	2.90 310
Saint Mary's Hospital, Streator, IL	100 4	92 12	86 7	100 9	100 11	- 0	- 0	100 2	93 42	80 79	94 124	94 16	91 94	91 111	87 31	92 182	100 217	83 170	100 31	75 154	100 34	73 134	0.00 215	2.47 162
Saint Mary's Hospital, Decatur, IL	88 8	91 33	84 19	84 25	100 19	0 1	- 0	100 5	86 72	87 122	97 182	93 29	82 87	92 105	97 29	85 157	99 186	97 116	98 45	89 284	96 70	76 272	0.35 567	1.45 414
Saint Mary's Hospital of Kankakee, Kankakee, IL	81 16	90 83	90 61	94 71	95 60	- 0	- 0	100 25	85 96	60 187	91 238	100 63	76 210	86 217	71 51	79 310	100 362	49 156	100 90	86 336	96 78	64 328	0.00 553	3.88 387
Saints Mary & Elizabeth Medical Center, Chicago, IL	79 24	100 63	97 99	90 61	90 99	20 5	- 0	92 40	83 117	48 307	88 336	72 68	85 158	94 142	- -	88 199	98 215	57 109	81 57	86 233	82 60	64 219	- -	- -
Salem Township Hospital, Salem, IL	- 0	88 8	88 8	86 7	75 8	- 0	- 0	- 0	67 6	80 30	34 47	83 6	77 60	85 20	0 17	77 87	90 90	3 71	80 10	25 4	100 2	100 4	- -	- -
Sarah Bush Lincoln Health Center, Mattoon, IL	100 3	100 36	100 13	100 32	100 13	- 0	- 0	100 1	100 74	82 181	99 249	100 26	88 168	80 124	82 45	94 210	100 272	94 183	94 62	93 374	71 91	63 365	- -	- -
Shelby Memorial Hospital, Shelbyville, IL	100 1	100 1	100 1	100 1	100 1	- 0	- -	- 0	100 15	56 25	91 104	67 3	72 36	100 17	- -	88 42	100 72	65 52	82 11	33 3	100 3	100 3	- -	- -
Sherman Hospital, Elgin, IL	80 46	95 199	95 232	95 188	96 234	- 0	88 17	90 81	71 127	50 289	86 366	83 59	83 146	79 136	68 41	83 224	100 262	78 121	69 59	89 696	95 174	80 681	0.34 891	2.70 667
Silver Cross Hospital, Joliet, IL	95 41	94 170	93 143	96 106	95 151	- 0	25 12	98 55	93 179	100 450	99 549	100 112	91 250	88 257	39 77	87 431	100 468	45 256	97 120	96 499	90 124	75 463	0.39 2076	2.28 1446
South Shore Hospital, Chicago, IL	62 8	81 48	79 19	79 42	88 25	0 2	- 0	50 4	79 62	64 205	92 247	82 60	73 62	82 76	15 20	74 118	95 147	3 66	71 31	20 15	67 15	100 14	- -	- -
Sparta Community Hospital, Sparta, IL	- 0	100 3	50 2	50 4	50 2	- 0	- 0	- 0	77 13	73 26	82 39	100 2	75 28	84 25	73 11	73 45	100 52	81 32	100 8	- -	- -	- -	- -	- -
Swedish American Hospital, Rockford, IL	94 80	99 234	100 290	95 135	99 327	0 1	54 13	97 146	94 209	97 367	98 470	93 88	91 174	93 142	69 35	84 226	100 275	76 169	97 75	94 1114	96 247	68 1100	0.17 2300	3.82 1572
Swedish Covenant Hospital, Chicago, IL	94 17	100 199	99 176	98 183	99 171	- 0	- 0	100 53	84 173	31 348	92 504	71 38	65 223	85 142	21 84	76 367	100 439	33 293	68 47	73 60	98 62	100 57	- -	- -
Taylorville Memorial Hospital, Taylorville, IL	75 4	78 9	100 8	100 7	67 9	- 0	- 0	67 3	91 35	98 81	91 110	70 10	82 44	95 66	88 26	93 98	100 136	95 103	96 26	66 44	82 11	80 41	- -	- -
Thomas H Boyd Memorial Hospital, Carrollton, IL	- 0	100 1	100 1	100 1	100 1	- 0	- -	- 0	- 0	50 2	0 3	- 0	67 6	100 1	100 1	92 12	100 16	47 15	0 1	- -	- -	- -	- -	- -
Thorek Hospital and Medical Center, Chicago, IL	100 4	100 22	100 15	95 21	94 18	0 2	- 0	100 3	100 27	99 100	97 118	100 29	79 48	96 57	8 13	61 125	98 141	36 69	100 36	81 59	92 13	31 58	- -	- -
Touchette Regional Hospital, Centreville, IL	100 2	80 15	80 10	81 16	90 10	- 0	- 0	0 1	84 31	36 14	66 98	67 9	100 2	100 1	- -	60 25	100 25	9 11	0 1	53 15	- -	69 13	0.31 652	1.31 459
Trinity Medical Center, Rock Island, IL	87 82	96 291	94 394	95 260	95 371	- 0	75 12	100 117	81 173	89 429	96 559	99 113	83 96	95 91	93 28	91 123	99 156	83 112	96 47	93 281	95 66	74 269	- -	- -
Union County Hospital District, Anna, IL	- 0	100 4	67 3	100 3	100 3	- 0	- -	- 0	100 7	65 34	83 42	50 2	75 40	76 29	67 9	88 73	100 85	77 48	79 24	- 0	- 0	- 0	- -	- -
University of Chicago Hospitals, Chicago, IL	91 55	96 141	98 219	91 125	96 210	- 0	33 6	90 88	89 170	46 298	98 326	83 82	76 93	76 59	60 25	69 123	100 165	54 84	76 41	85 337	65 69	75 338	- -	- -
University of Illinois at Chicago Med Ctr, Chicago, IL	79 24	100 56	95 59	96 48	92 59	- 0	25 4	61 18	92 142	24 71	96 310	74 81	79 82	76 124	- -	64 183	99 196	49 65	65 60	72 275	89 57	80 268	- -	- -
Valley West Community Hospital, Sandwich, IL	0 1	100 5	100 5	67 3	0 2	0 1	- 0	100 2	67 3	68 22	89 27	100 4	80 46	93 28	75 12	85 20	100 63	83 35	91 11	83 35	70 10	26 34	- -	- -
Vista Medical Center East, Waukegan, IL	79 24	92 137	89 112	83 123	91 115	- 0	40 5	100 43	78 123	28 269	91 347	99 82	76 156	90 235	38 64	66 398	99 428	39 225	98 89	74 263	65 72	64 259	- -	- -
Vista Medical Center West, Waukegan, IL	- -	- -	- -	- -	- -	- -	- -	- -	- -	- -	- -	- -	- -	- -	- -	- -	- -	- -	- -	- -	- -	- -	- -	- -
Wabash General Hospital, Mount Carmel, IL	100 3	67 6	80 5	75 4	75 4	- 0	- -	- 0	88 8	71 34	88 49	100 4	83 42	97 35	67 15	88 67	100 90	70 67	42 12	14 7	- 0	100 5	- -	- -
Weiss Memorial Hospital, Chicago, IL	79 29	92 85	93 71	96 76	95 78	- 0	0 1	32 34	78 100	34 180	90 250	35 68	83 63	89 82	22 18	79 131	100 166	20 98	17 29	80 228	90 62	38 209	- -	- -
West Suburban Medical Center, Oak Park, IL	72 25	97 120	83 98	96 127	81 113	36 11	100 1	98 54	78 195	80 522	98 568	98 131	82 178	94 169	- -	75 250	100 285	48 122	94 93	83 468	94 105	50 448	- -	- -
Westlake Community Hospital, Melrose Park, IL	78 18	98 80	99 68	96 70	94 65	- 0	100 2	86 21	78 92	54 221	92 288	88 57	90 58	89 73	43 23	74 124	100 153	27 81	58 31	89 197	96 49	55 185	- -	- -
INDIANA																								
Adams Memorial Hospital, Decatur, IN	100 4	86 21	86 14	67 18	100 14	- 0	- 0	0 1	86 28	72 54	72 83	40 25	85 60	100 14	82 22	86 84	97 94	77 66	62 13	43 35	91 11	32 34	- -	- -
Ball Memorial Hospital, Muncie, IN	86 114	99 297	97 386	97 254	99 352	- 0	75 12	97 132	83 201	79 372	96 515	93 76	90 283	87 248	92 61	83 339	100 429	90 242	75 118	85 1006	96 214	84 976	- -	- -
Bedford Regional Medical Center, Bedford, IN	100 4	90 20	100 11	100 14	100 13	- 0	- 0	- 0	100 34	93 57	100 77	100 6	79 57	93 58	85 20	91 78	100 102	100 68	92 24	89 65	100 20	39 61	- -	- -
Bloomington Hospital, Bloomington, IN	94 83	98 246	99 349	94 199	98 339	- 0	74 23	100 156	87 127	83 229	91 293	100 60	88 200	91 171	82 50	87 250	100 322	83 217	95 95	91 895	97 209	89 853	- -	- -
Bluffton Regional Medical Center, Bluffton, IN	100 10	94 31	97 30	96 27	100 30	- 0	- 0	100 5	98 42	100 73	99 105	100 11	91 110	98 92	100 18	97 140	100 165	99 101	100 34	98 161	96 51	99 156	0.00 274	2.96 203
Cameron Memorial Community Hospital, Angola, IN	- -	- -	- -	- -	- -	- -	- -	- -	33 3	21 29	38 39	100 1	93 59	88 49	58 12	87 70	100 85	86 56	80 20	79 39	57 7	67 39	- -	- -
Clarian North Medical Center, Carmel, IN	100 1	75 4	100 4	33 6	50 6	- 0	- 0	- 0	88 8	50 2	93 15	0 1	56 9	100 3	- -	65 17	100 26	76 17	100 2	90 39	- -	74 39	0.45 1553	5.67 970
Clarian West Medical Center, Avon, IN	33 3	93 29	85 13	76 29	64 14	- 0	- 0	100 1	73 41	88 24	97 98	100 2	67 15	75 16	- -	84 122	100 133	77 88	100 4	92 36	- -	72 32	0.11 933	4.51 621
Clark Memorial Hospital, Jeffersonville, IN	79 43	99 148	97 190	99 122	97 188	82 11	50 4	99 78	69 94	58 250	81 343	81 70	81 188	83 116	6 33	77 210	100 259	72 155	74 76	90 126	89 122	96 117	- -	- -
Columbus Regional Hospital, Columbus, IN	95 42	99 159	99 201	98 141	99 190	78 9	100 5	100 89	98 90	87 255	96 314	100 82	93 133	98 64	95 39	95 176	100 232	94 136	100 75	87 631	95 149	69 593	- -	- -
Community Health Network, Indianapolis, IN	82 38	96 127	99 111	92 75	99 102	0 4	73 11	100 54	74 136	43 213	90 306	100 75	85 191	94 172	59 39	81 271	100 317	75 186	100 64	52 79	- -	65 72	0.35 1713	6.24 2019
Community Hospital, Hammond, IN	76 33	98 171	95 147	91 110	93 164	- 0	13 15	95 19	75 310	72 139	90 800	90 21	76 46	98 52	- -	74 325	100 370	82 213	90 21	88 88	- -	47 86	0.56 2308	2.43 1441
Community Hosp of Anderson & Madison Co, Anderson, IN	100 2	100 33	100 21	100 29	100 21	83 6	- 0	100 6	92 50	91 138	97 185	100 21	96 165	96 109	- -	93 256	100 292	100 191	99 78	96 400	100 96	83 380	0.00 1008	2.65 717
Community Hospital of Bremen, Bremen, IN	- 0	100 2	100 3	100 1	100 3	- 0	- -	- 0	100 2	62 13	85 26	100 2	80 20	100 12	100 4	95 19	100 25	94 16	67 6	- -	- -	- -	- -	- -
Community Hospital South, Indianapolis, IN	90 40	99 110	99 137	98 49	100 109	- 0	82 11	100 62	76 51	54 108	91 153	100 19	88 125	89 76	54 24	83 141	100 171	84 100	100 37	93 59	- -	78 59	0.15 657	8.07 471

NOTE: The first number in each column (boldface) is the rate in percent, the second number is the number of patients; Please refer to the main entry for footnotes; ***Heart Attack Care:*** *1. ACE Inhibitor or ARB for LVSD; 2. Aspirin at Arrival; 3. Aspirin at Discharge; 4. Beta Blocker at Arrival; 5. Beta Blocker at Discharge; 6. Fibrinolytic Medication Timing; 7. PCI Within 90 Minutes of Arrival; 8. Smoking Cessation Advice;* ***Heart Failure Care:*** *9. ACE Inhibitor or ARB for LVSD; 10. Discharge Instructions; 11. Evaluation of LVS Function; 12. Smoking Cessation Advice;* ***Pneumonia Care:*** *13. Appropriate Initial Antibiotic; 14. Blood Culture Timing; 15. Influenza Vaccine; 16. Initial Antibiotic Timing; 17. Oxygenation Assessment; 18. Pneumococcal Vaccine; 19. Smoking Cessation Advice;* ***Surgical Infection Prevention:*** *20. Prophylactic Antibiotic Given; 21. Prophylactic Antibiotic Selection; 22. Prophylactic Antibiotic Stopped;* ***Pregnancy Care:*** *23. Inpatient Neonatal Mortality; 24. Third or Fourth Degree Laceration*

Hospital	Heart Attack Care								Heart Failure Care				Pneumonia Care							Surgical Infection Prevention			Pregnancy Care	
	1	2	3	4	5	6	7	8	9	10	11	12	13	14	15	16	17	18	19	20	21	22	23	24
Daviess Community Hospital, Washington, IN	**67** 9	**96** 23	**93** 15	**91** 22	**93** 14	**-** 0	**-** 0	**100** 1	**53** 34	**11** 44	**84** 62	**86** 7	**86** 142	**86** 125	**53** 32	**92** 155	**100** 206	**67** 123	**75** 40	**83** 30	**100** 30	**67** 30	**0.00** 402	**3.63** 303
Deaconess Hospital, Evansville, IN	**82** 182	**96** 394	**97** 653	**88** 332	**94** 640	**-** 0	**75** 16	**99** 273	**80** 317	**63** 631	**90** 801	**99** 182	**92** 320	**90** 318	**87** 104	**78** 479	**100** 615	**86** 404	**98** 183	**77** 1072	**95** 297	**53** 1037	**-** -	**-** -
Dearborn County Hospital, Lawrenceburg, IN	**67** 6	**100** 35	**88** 16	**100** 24	**100** 20	**33** 6	**-** 0	**100** 4	**68** 44	**39** 82	**90** 82	**90** 20	**89** 119	**87** 126	**24** 34	**79** 183	**100** 229	**67** 139	**85** 68	**95** 234	**96** 50	**74** 212	**-** -	**-** -
Decatur County Memorial Hospital, Greensburg, IN	**67** 3	**91** 11	**83** 6	**78** 9	**44** 9	**-** 0	**-** 0	**100** 1	**80** 15	**80** 40	**86** 63	**80** 10	**75** 55	**87** 23	**86** 7	**90** 63	**99** 77	**91** 44	**88** 16	**64** 66	**100** 20	**30** 64	**-** -	**-** -
Dekalb Memorial Hospital, Auburn, IN	**-** 0	**100** 9	**100** 4	**91** 11	**100** 4	**-** 0	**-** 0	**100** 1	**93** 14	**88** 40	**100** 60	**100** 7	**98** 106	**99** 78	**100** 28	**98** 118	**100** 157	**100** 100	**94** 36	**96** 46	**100** 11	**95** 43	**-** -	**-** -
Dukes Memorial Hospital, Peru, IN	**100** 1	**67** 9	**100** 7	**44** 9	**100** 7	**-** 0	**-** 0	**100** 1	**88** 8	**77** 43	**90** 63	**100** 5	**83** 47	**87** 38	**92** 13	**96** 55	**100** 65	**88** 33	**100** 21	**44** 36	**100** 3	**83** 36	**-** -	**-** -
Dunn Memorial Hospital, Bedford, IN	**94** 17	**93** 75	**95** 77	**91** 65	**99** 83	**-** 0	**33** 3	**100** 27	**83** 30	**61** 57	**94** 66	**70** 10	**60** 63	**96** 45	**85** 20	**76** 71	**98** 104	**64** 72	**76** 25	**65** 31	**33** 3	**58** 31	**-** -	**-** -
Dupont Hospital, Fort Wayne, IN	**100** 1	**71** 7	**100** 4	**78** 9	**100** 5	**-** 0	**-** 0	**100** 1	**55** 11	**58** 26	**100** 33	**100** 4	**84** 44	**100** 36	**75** 8	**88** 42	**100** 55	**97** 29	**91** 11	**79** 623	**95** 173	**74** 600	**0.09** 2296	**4.76** 1640
Elkhart General Hospital, Elkhart, IN	**98** 55	**98** 289	**98** 319	**96** 233	**99** 296	**-** 0	**75** 12	**89** 120	**78** 211	**43** 417	**82** 488	**62** 72	**89** 183	**100** 2	**50** 36	**84** 290	**98** 308	**42** 184	**62** 81	**72** 1152	**95** 277	**58** 1120	**-** -	**-** -
Fayette Memorial Hospital, Connersville, IN	**33** 3	**86** 37	**58** 26	**50** 34	**66** 29	**-** 0	**-** 0	**57** 7	**62** 29	**30** 102	**55** 143	**37** 27	**74** 62	**100** 30	**71** 14	**66** 88	**100** 104	**35** 66	**11** 18	**56** 100	**100** 14	**78** 87	**-** -	**-** -
Floyd Memorial Hospital and Health Services, New Albany, IN	**87** 60	**100** 208	**99** 226	**95** 176	**95** 211	**0** 1	**36** 11	**95** 109	**82** 118	**79** 233	**96** 312	**84** 64	**93** 199	**95** 276	**97** 74	**79** 366	**99** 471	**96** 271	**92** 130	**94** 364	**97** 109	**84** 351	**-** -	**-** -
Gibson General Hospital, Princeton, IN	**-** -	**-** -	**-** -	**-** -	**-** -	**-** -	**-** -	**-** -	**92** 13	**77** 35	**90** 61	**80** 5	**100** 24	**78** 23	**90** 10	**97** 32	**100** 45	**83** 30	**71** 14	**-** -	**-** -	**-** -	**-** -	**-** -
Good Samaritan Hospital, Vincennes, IN	**96** 50	**93** 127	**99** 152	**88** 98	**97** 152	**-** 0	**29** 7	**100** 62	**90** 109	**79** 235	**88** 307	**73** 37	**67** 99	**89** 74	**70** 33	**86** 136	**99** 187	**75** 129	**69** 42	**63** 514	**87** 164	**76** 502	**-** -	**-** -
Goshen General Hospital, Goshen, IN	**100** 7	**95** 44	**96** 27	**100** 27	**100** 26	**-** 0	**-** 0	**100** 5	**100** 45	**86** 117	**97** 158	**89** 18	**85** 109	**93** 69	**88** 24	**86** 116	**100** 146	**92** 91	**86** 28	**92** 356	**98** 82	**81** 345	**0.12** 1637	**2.81** 1316
Greene County General Hospital, Linton, IN	**-** 0	**100** 8	**67** 3	**50** 4	**67** 3	**0** 1	**-** -	**-** 0	**75** 20	**80** 35	**84** 58	**50** 4	**81** 31	**100** 26	**75** 12	**94** 52	**100** 62	**84** 45	**69** 13	**-** -	**-** -	**-** -	**-** -	**-** -
Hancock Memorial Hospital and Health Services, Greenfield, IN	**100** 3	**100** 15	**71** 7	**92** 12	**62** 8	**-** 0	**-** 0	**67** 3	**79** 33	**25** 55	**84** 90	**57** 14	**79** 190	**74** 160	**35** 46	**86** 257	**99** 286	**66** 193	**57** 63	**85** 186	**98** 41	**49** 182	**-** -	**-** -
Harrison County Hospital, Corydon, IN	**75** 4	**91** 11	**83** 6	**70** 10	**83** 6	**-** 0	**-** -	**-** 0	**73** 26	**20** 46	**100** 59	**70** 10	**64** 102	**79** 29	**64** 28	**72** 130	**100** 140	**72** 78	**45** 33	**71** 56	**83** 12	**80** 54	**-** -	**-** -
Heartland Memorial Hospital, Munster, IN	**0** 1	**86** 7	**67** 9	**14** 7	**25** 8	**-** 0	**-** 0	**-** 0	**41** 22	**22** 18	**73** 81	**0** 3	**0** 1	**-** 0	**-** -	**62** 8	**100** 12	**50** 8	**-** 0	**30** 20	**-** -	**50** 20	**-** -	**-** -
Hendricks Regional Health, Danville, IN	**78** 18	**98** 88	**94** 33	**95** 87	**97** 38	**67** 3	**-** 0	**100** 3	**77** 70	**79** 126	**94** 180	**94** 16	**86** 170	**83** 99	**92** 36	**89** 272	**100** 274	**73** 162	**85** 54	**79** 315	**92** 71	**61** 309	**-** -	**-** -
Henry County Memorial Hospital, New Castle, IN	**67** 3	**90** 10	**75** 4	**80** 5	**100** 4	**-** 0	**-** 0	**-** 0	**91** 34	**97** 59	**99** 85	**100** 6	**88** 125	**68** 76	**90** 21	**92** 168	**100** 212	**72** 123	**90** 50	**92** 176	**100** 44	**21** 169	**-** -	**-** -
Howard Regional Health System, Kokomo, IN	**80** 5	**97** 30	**96** 27	**77** 26	**96** 26	**-** 0	**50** 2	**100** 8	**80** 71	**65** 139	**91** 193	**86** 21	**86** 177	**95** 101	**81** 48	**86** 220	**99** 282	**81** 182	**93** 70	**70** 147	**93** 46	**72** 137	**-** -	**-** -
Indiana Heart Hospital, Indianapolis, IN	**98** 125	**96** 149	**100** 402	**96** 84	**99** 386	**100** 3	**77** 13	**100** 229	**100** 122	**98** 234	**99** 298	**100** 57	**67** 6	**83** 6	**-** 0	**83** 6	**100** 8	**100** 3	**100** 2	**95** 444	**100** 169	**95** 422	**-** -	**-** -
Indiana Orthopaedic Hospital, Indianapolis, IN	**-** -	**-** -	**-** -	**-** -	**-** -	**-** -	**-** -	**-** -	**-** -	**-** -	**-** -	**-** -	**-** -	**-** -	**-** -	**-** -	**-** -	**-** -	**-** -	**88** 26	**-** -	**69** 26	**-** -	**-** -
Jasper County Hospital, Rensselaer, IN	**100** 1	**33** 6	**50** 2	**75** 8	**50** 2	**-** 0	**-** -	**-** 0	**30** 20	**51** 37	**77** 56	**78** 9	**44** 63	**96** 24	**70** 10	**73** 71	**98** 84	**62** 68	**8** 12	**50** 2	**100** 2	**100** 2	**-** -	**-** -
Johnson Memorial Hospital, Franklin, IN	**100** 1	**100** 23	**100** 5	**95** 19	**100** 4	**50** 4	**-** 0	**0** 1	**79** 19	**70** 64	**95** 98	**68** 19	**91** 107	**85** 88	**92** 26	**88** 112	**100** 148	**85** 78	**91** 35	**88** 121	**100** 23	**96** 114	**-** -	**-** -
King's Daughters Hospital, Madison, IN	**100** 3	**91** 35	**90** 20	**97** 30	**88** 17	**-** 0	**-** 0	**100** 2	**94** 36	**90** 103	**99** 147	**94** 17	**88** 180	**90** 127	**-** -	**93** 194	**100** 236	**99** 148	**94** 54	**98** 133	**100** 41	**91** 130	**-** -	**-** -
Kosciusko Community Hospital, Warsaw, IN	**100** 3	**97** 38	**100** 21	**100** 24	**100** 17	**-** 0	**-** 0	**100** 2	**94** 32	**90** 68	**99** 99	**100** 7	**92** 121	**94** 121	**90** 31	**93** 141	**100** 177	**96** 108	**100** 50	**92** 239	**94** 70	**74** 238	**-** -	**-** -
Lafayette Home Hospital, Lafayette, IN	**50** 4	**100** 22	**73** 11	**73** 11	**92** 13	**-** 0	**-** 0	**100** 3	**89** 19	**50** 54	**88** 80	**88** 17	**67** 113	**94** 98	**74** 34	**80** 149	**99** 187	**61** 117	**75** 44	**87** 766	**88** 185	**60** 752	**-** -	**-** -
LaGrange Community Hospital, LaGrange, IN	**-** 0	**100** 3	**100** 3	**100** 2	**100** 2	**-** 0	**-** 0	**-** 0	**50** 2	**16** 19	**55** 22	**100** 4	**92** 64	**96** 24	**83** 18	**91** 57	**100** 70	**63** 43	**100** 19	**67** 21	**100** 3	**10** 20	**-** -	**-** -
LaPorte Hospital, La Porte, IN	**70** 20	**94** 90	**94** 93	**89** 64	**94** 94	**-** 0	**83** 6	**100** 32	**77** 102	**78** 179	**88** 243	**87** 39	**92** 108	**90** 89	**76** 25	**85** 138	**98** 164	**89** 119	**88** 40	**95** 377	**98** 92	**87** 363	**0.00** 693	**1.41** 498
Logansport Memorial Hospital, Logansport, IN	**100** 1	**94** 17	**100** 5	**81** 16	**75** 4	**-** 0	**-** 0	**-** 0	**77** 22	**73** 44	**83** 77	**46** 13	**93** 44	**93** 45	**91** 11	**78** 69	**100** 91	**82** 51	**29** 24	**82** 165	**97** 37	**87** 167	**-** -	**-** -
Lutheran Hospital of Indiana, Fort Wayne, IN	**86** 144	**96** 285	**98** 667	**91** 239	**96** 657	**-** 0	**58** 24	**99** 268	**78** 255	**58** 477	**91** 590	**99** 125	**91** 144	**94** 207	**94** 66	**86** 260	**100** 337	**93** 241	**97** 93	**72** 1709	**96** 437	**71** 1624	**0.59** 1849	**2.82** 1133
Major Hospital, Shelbyville, IN	**100** 2	**100** 13	**100** 9	**100** 11	**100** 6	**-** 0	**-** 0	**-** 0	**94** 31	**84** 67	**100** 87	**100** 10	**94** 117	**93** 106	**81** 37	**89** 183	**99** 204	**88** 137	**84** 55	**87** 92	**100** 17	**49** 89	**-** -	**-** -
Margaret Mary Community Hospital, Batesville, IN	**100** 1	**80** 10	**75** 4	**86** 7	**80** 5	**-** 0	**-** 0	**-** 0	**69** 16	**50** 34	**78** 50	**80** 5	**84** 91	**90** 68	**87** 15	**82** 131	**100** 155	**80** 111	**78** 36	**44** 126	**97** 35	**32** 124	**-** -	**-** -
Marion General Hospital, Marion, IN	**100** 8	**87** 31	**76** 17	**82** 33	**100** 19	**-** 0	**-** 0	**100** 3	**92** 62	**83** 145	**97** 196	**97** 33	**95** 111	**79** 110	**95** 22	**87** 166	**100** 198	**97** 117	**96** 51	**82** 271	**78** 88	**88** 260	**-** -	**-** -
Medical Center of Southern Indiana, Charlestown, IN	**100** 2	**67** 3	**100** 3	**67** 3	**100** 3	**-** 0	**-** 0	**100** 1	**86** 7	**87** 15	**79** 29	**100** 4	**94** 18	**25** 4	**-** -	**97** 31	**97** 32	**100** 15	**100** 6	**0** 2	**-** -	**50** 2	**-** -	**-** -
Memorial Hospital and Health Care Center, Jasper, IN	**86** 35	**94** 90	**95** 129	**93** 90	**98** 127	**100** 1	**40** 5	**100** 51	**84** 77	**55** 113	**84** 160	**100** 22	**71** 182	**97** 91	**3** 38	**74** 154	**96** 194	**81** 129	**100** 33	**56** 345	**93** 111	**74** 337	**-** -	**-** -
Memorial Hospital of South Bend, South Bend, IN	**70** 54	**97** 234	**96** 245	**91** 152	**94** 265	**-** 0	**75** 12	**82** 111	**86** 169	**78** 384	**96** 459	**86** 113	**89** 230	**88** 212	**77** 65	**73** 313	**100** 407	**89** 256	**62** 78	**82** 519	**98** 172	**86** 487	**-** -	**-** -
Methodist Hospital of Indiana, Indianapolis, IN	**86** 146	**97** 361	**96** 437	**94** 270	**97** 445	**0** 3	**68** 19	**96** 233	**80** 556	**73** 847	**98** 1026	**93** 230	**85** 106	**80** 69	**87** 15	**74** 187	**100** 248	**72** 116	**81** 73	**92** 360	**99** 67	**71** 341	**-** -	**-** -
Methodist Hospitals-North Lake Campus, Gary, IN	**79** 47	**90** 194	**82** 165	**81** 166	**86** 179	**0** 3	**11** 9	**100** 86	**78** 392	**29** 852	**79** 1070	**95** 260	**76** 202	**86** 106	**51** 63	**57** 357	**100** 432	**52** 214	**92** 111	**63** 383	**80** 127	**56** 363	**-** -	**-** -
Morgan Hospital Medical Centre, Martinsville, IN	**100** 3	**100** 15	**100** 5	**92** 13	**100** 6	**-** 0	**-** 0	**-** 0	**97** 63	**100** 28	**87** 159	**100** 8	**89** 9	**85** 20	**-** -	**95** 126	**100** 144	**68** 95	**100** 6	**50** 14	**-** -	**93** 14	**0.00** 213	**2.72** 147
Parkview Huntington Hospital, Huntington, IN	**67** 3	**75** 8	**100** 2	**75** 8	**100** 6	**-** 0	**-** 0	**0** 1	**64** 14	**82** 33	**79** 47	**100** 8	**84** 49	**92** 52	**90** 10	**83** 88	**100** 108	**84** 68	**82** 22	**89** 111	**100** 23	**91** 108	**-** -	**-** -
Parkview Memorial Hospital, Fort Wayne, IN	**92** 39	**99** 130	**100** 215	**93** 55	**99** 224	**67** 9	**73** 11	**92** 113	**89** 85	**56** 209	**92** 285	**88** 49	**92** 102	**92** 97	**68** 25	**82** 132	**100** 177	**63** 109	**81** 42	**66** 314	**97** 79	**57** 306	**-** -	**-** -
Parkview Noble Hospital, Kendallville, IN	**100** 1	**100** 6	**80** 5	**100** 3	**100** 3	**-** 0	**-** 0	**-** 0	**75** 20	**67** 67	**87** 95	**100** 17	**93** 68	**95** 62	**90** 20	**89** 85	**100** 115	**94** 65	**84** 37	**82** 78	**92** 24	**73** 75	**-** -	**-** -
Parkview Whitley Hospital, Columbia City, IN	**100** 1	**67** 6	**100** 5	**80** 5	**86** 7	**-** 0	**-** 0	**-** 0	**67** 21	**58** 33	**84** 45	**75** 8	**96** 57	**92** 49	**93** 14	**82** 65	**100** 86	**75** 53	**58** 24	**70** 61	**90** 20	**48** 58	**-** -	**-** -
Porter Memorial Health System, Valparaiso, IN	**83** 46	**96** 173	**97** 179	**88** 114	**97** 176	**-** 0	**70** 10	**100** 24	**98** 172	**94** 79	**100** 426	**100** 22	**89** 38	**92** 49	**-** -	**79** 324	**100** 379	**60** 277	**61** 23	**67** 66	**-** -	**66** 61	**0.14** 1390	**3.63** 936
Reid Hospital and Health Care Services, Richmond, IN	**98** 60	**100** 296	**99** 287	**99** 217	**99** 321	**88** 33	**100** 1	**100** 114	**100** 78	**99** 299	**99** 398	**100** 55	**94** 318	**98** 392	**98** 88	**94** 459	**100** 596	**95** 332	**100** 131	**96** 357	**96** 102	**96** 315	**-** -	**-** -
Riverview Hospital, Noblesville, IN	**96** 23	**100** 95	**100** 120	**100** 74	**99** 112	**-** 0	**100** 5	**100** 31	**100** 49	**96** 99	**99** 134	**100** 16	**87** 76	**96** 47	**96** 25	**92** 92	**100** 118	**95** 81	**100** 19	**94** 391	**79** 99	**89** 384	**-** -	**-** -

NOTE: The first number in each column (boldface) is the rate in percent, the second number is the number of patients; Please refer to the main entry for footnotes; ***Heart Attack Care:*** *1. ACE Inhibitor or ARB for LVSD; 2. Aspirin at Arrival; 3. Aspirin at Discharge; 4. Beta Blocker at Arrival; 5. Beta Blocker at Discharge; 6. Fibrinolytic Medication Timing; 7. PCI Within 90 Minutes of Arrival; 8. Smoking Cessation Advice;* ***Heart Failure Care:*** *9. ACE Inhibitor or ARB for LVSD; 10. Discharge Instructions; 11. Evaluation of LVS Function; 12. Smoking Cessation Advice;* ***Pneumonia Care:*** *13. Appropriate Initial Antibiotic; 14. Blood Culture Timing; 15. Influenza Vaccine; 16. Initial Antibiotic Timing; 17. Oxygenation Assessment; 18. Pneumococcal Vaccine; 19. Smoking Cessation Advice;* ***Surgical Infection Prevention:*** *20. Prophylactic Antibiotic Given; 21. Prophylactic Antibiotic Selection; 22. Prophylactic Antibiotic Stopped;* ***Pregnancy Care:*** *23. Inpatient Neonatal Mortality; 24. Third or Fourth Degree Laceration*

Hospital	Heart Attack Care								Heart Failure Care				Pneumonia Care							Surgical Infection Prevention			Pregnancy Care	
	1	2	3	4	5	6	7	8	9	10	11	12	13	14	15	16	17	18	19	20	21	22	23	24
Saint Anthony Medical Center, Crown Point, IN	78 32	94 155	94 126	87 127	86 134	- 0	60 5	94 48	78 116	59 272	77 355	68 37	83 224	91 143	45 33	73 209	100 268	51 171	27 41	92 583	93 131	51 573	- -	- -
Saint Anthony Memorial Health Centers, Michigan City, IN	91 22	98 109	99 88	99 98	100 86	- 0	44 9	100 36	96 68	80 167	99 205	100 35	91 180	89 95	65 26	85 187	95 220	67 126	100 49	91 284	95 91	67 278	- -	- -
Saint Catherine Hospital of East Chicago, East Chicago, IN	75 12	95 57	96 55	86 44	90 50	- 0	25 4	100 5	96 164	99 91	99 494	100 24	94 17	95 19	- -	78 148	97 162	78 74	60 10	29 63	- -	29 63	- -	- -
Saint Clare Medical Center, Crawfordsville, IN	60 5	77 13	50 8	14 14	71 7	100 1	- 0	50 2	53 30	42 64	64 104	92 12	63 102	85 27	40 20	77 108	98 121	38 80	76 25	78 138	100 33	25 137	- -	- -
Saint Elizabeth Medical Center, Lafayette, IN	74 65	99 243	98 346	94 185	95 391	100 1	62 8	90 145	68 117	76 250	81 348	70 64	71 143	97 212	71 55	87 262	99 326	64 227	70 81	86 523	80 120	58 513	- -	- -
Saint Francis at Indianapolis, Indianapolis, IN	70 27	98 113	97 172	97 115	96 176	- 0	100 15	95 96	83 48	67 90	97 108	88 26	88 41	93 30	- -	68 37	100 49	96 28	85 13	85 163	97 92	84 154	- -	- -
Saint Francis at Mooresville, Mooresville, IN	- -	- -	- -	- -	- -	- -	- -	- -	- 0	25 4	25 4	- 0	100 1	- -	- -	100 1	100 1	- 0	- 0	87 353	97 75	86 348	- -	- -
Saint Francis Beech Grove, Beech Grove, IN	80 45	88 207	98 268	87 197	97 271	- 0	- 0	91 102	78 127	50 253	88 395	62 73	89 115	89 80	87 31	83 126	100 180	83 136	72 50	79 351	91 46	79 335	- -	- -
Saint John's Health System, Anderson, IN	89 19	94 72	90 48	90 73	98 53	- 0	- 0	78 9	94 84	81 157	99 205	93 42	90 139	90 121	53 58	86 274	100 342	80 231	94 68	82 502	96 122	83 501	- -	- -
Saint Joseph Hospital, Fort Wayne, IN	100 20	98 85	99 103	93 81	95 98	0 1	38 8	100 44	83 70	96 162	96 218	100 46	85 33	91 33	83 12	83 59	100 67	92 39	94 17	72 163	100 42	71 162	- -	- -
Saint Joseph Hospital, Kokomo, IN	100 3	100 14	100 7	100 16	100 8	0 2	- 0	100 2	100 60	99 113	84 143	100 23	69 149	92 93	93 30	81 149	100 168	79 113	100 54	46 139	0 5	99 129	- -	- -
Saint Joseph Regional Med Ctr-Mishawaka, Mishawaka, IN	67 6	96 53	100 48	95 39	96 51	- 0	100 6	87 15	79 33	62 72	99 97	71 24	93 59	89 37	73 15	91 75	100 87	95 56	80 30	81 109	100 32	71 99	0.30 659	1.15 521
Saint Joseph's Regional Medical Center, South Bend, IN	86 21	97 164	99 221	98 85	96 194	- 0	73 11	96 97	87 121	85 293	97 378	95 60	90 143	97 141	89 44	83 222	100 269	83 168	75 52	91 925	99 309	92 897	1.08 1206	2.60 845
Saint Joseph's Reg Med Ctr-Plymouth Campus, Plymouth, IN	100 5	100 39	96 23	97 37	96 23	0 2	- 0	100 3	88 16	73 56	89 79	100 11	81 79	93 57	56 18	94 107	100 143	63 97	100 31	87 171	97 64	76 168	0.00 411	2.72 294
Saint Margaret Mercy Healthcare Centers, Hammond, IN	60 55	95 207	94 212	93 151	92 237	- 0	30 10	82 79	76 107	72 253	74 289	81 68	84 133	93 131	97 31	74 174	100 205	79 124	75 57	91 294	98 59	70 290	- -	- -
Saint Margaret Mercy Healthcare Centers, Dyer, IN	81 27	100 94	99 88	97 69	100 87	- 0	33 3	78 32	83 87	78 194	96 225	69 32	88 98	92 106	- -	81 134	100 168	72 95	86 42	93 198	93 60	58 195	- -	- -
Saint Mary's Medical Center, Hobart, IN	69 13	96 83	90 92	90 81	90 97	- 0	0 13	100 43	88 127	91 314	97 386	98 49	88 182	99 177	83 58	88 274	100 313	77 220	95 81	54 209	80 65	60 205	- -	- -
Saint Mary's Medical Center, Evansville, IN	79 118	98 260	97 336	95 198	99 335	0 2	38 8	99 145	87 129	97 235	93 305	100 52	87 180	89 151	77 61	68 257	99 332	72 192	90 100	66 335	96 121	71 327	- -	- -
Saint Mary's Warrick Hospital, Boonville, IN	80 5	100 16	92 12	88 17	80 15	- 0	- 0	100 1	100 8	100 25	98 48	100 4	86 64	93 58	60 10	90 69	97 91	70 64	100 22	- -	- -	- -	- -	- -
Saint Vincent Carmel Hospital, Carmel, IN	50 4	100 7	100 5	57 7	83 6	- 0	- 0	- 0	80 10	4 26	74 43	0 6	86 73	82 17	31 13	89 73	99 108	23 62	18 11	95 134	100 44	94 133	- -	- -
Saint Vincent Clay Hospital, Brazil, IN	100 2	100 3	67 3	100 3	100 3	- 0	- -	- 0	69 13	41 17	78 40	50 4	77 39	91 23	57 14	94 34	98 56	82 34	70 10	- -	- -	- -	- -	- -
Saint Vincent Frankfort Hospital, Frankfort, IN	100 2	100 4	100 4	60 5	100 5	- 0	- -	- 0	92 12	52 27	69 26	- 0	67 48	89 35	75 8	87 53	99 67	49 37	59 17	52 31	100 8	93 29	- -	- -
Saint Vincent Heart Center of Indiana, Indianapolis, IN	91 307	99 113	100 1036	97 102	100 1027	- 0	100 6	94 400	89 258	86 339	99 373	82 45	100 6	100 1	0 2	86 7	88 8	57 7	- 0	99 143	100 64	96 137	- -	- -
Saint Vincent Indianapolis Hospital, Indianapolis, IN	84 167	98 308	98 493	98 281	99 485	- 0	47 15	95 166	88 226	85 502	96 643	93 71	80 228	93 208	39 72	75 321	100 422	51 274	49 80	75 227	95 104	84 226	- -	- -
Saint Vincent Mercy Hospital, Elwood, IN	- 0	100 1	- 0	100 1	- 0	- 0	- -	- 0	80 5	60 10	57 14	0 1	78 77	96 51	93 15	84 90	99 102	67 66	76 29	- 0	- 0	- 0	- -	- -
Saint Vincent Williamsport, Williamsport, IN	25 4	60 10	71 7	55 11	75 8	- -	- -	- 0	93 15	100 35	95 55	88 8	80 40	77 13	86 7	80 50	100 66	64 36	91 22	0 1	100 1	0 1	- -	- -
Schneck Medical Center, Seymour, IN	100 4	100 17	100 9	100 17	100 9	- 0	- 0	100 1	94 31	91 74	93 98	100 15	86 128	96 100	- -	89 156	98 199	99 125	95 40	93 202	98 41	92 186	- -	- -
Scott Memorial Hospital, Scottsburg, IN	40 5	73 15	50 6	62 16	71 7	100 1	- -	100 1	71 21	84 68	61 80	40 20	81 118	82 61	55 20	81 112	100 139	63 65	68 47	- -	- -	- -	- -	- -
Starke Memorial Hospital, Knox, IN	- 0	67 9	67 3	67 6	67 3	- 0	- 0	- 0	50 10	39 38	83 48	45 11	84 99	84 55	86 21	86 125	100 133	57 69	44 39	14 7	100 1	0 7	- -	- -
Sullivan County Community Hospital, Sullivan, IN	100 2	73 15	89 9	75 16	88 8	- 0	- 0	100 2	62 13	45 33	50 48	79 14	80 59	91 44	72 18	88 78	100 84	85 53	70 20	92 24	100 9	67 24	- -	- -
Terre Haute Regional Hospital, Terre Haute, IN	81 54	97 96	97 181	86 72	98 182	- 0	0 4	100 80	72 141	68 320	86 377	100 85	79 97	97 94	77 30	80 174	100 200	72 130	100 73	87 188	85 80	43 185	- -	- -
Tipton Hospital, Tipton, IN	100 1	100 3	100 1	75 4	100 2	- 0	- 0	- 0	87 15	78 37	91 46	88 8	54 48	89 19	75 8	75 57	100 65	58 43	80 15	28 18	56 18	78 18	- -	- -
Union Hospital, Terre Haute, IN	91 86	97 228	94 259	94 177	96 293	0 2	20 5	98 103	88 145	95 332	97 405	96 47	83 199	96 148	88 48	89 284	100 339	92 203	99 98	87 854	95 212	67 809	- -	- -
Wabash County Hospital, Wabash, IN	- 0	50 2	100 2	50 2	100 2	- 0	- -	- 0	75 8	88 16	83 30	100 1	81 52	84 31	100 7	95 57	100 66	88 40	100 19	- -	- -	- -	- -	- -
West Central Community Hospital, Clinton, IN	0 1	93 15	50 10	64 14	67 9	- 0	- -	100 1	74 19	74 35	83 58	100 10	86 65	90 61	100 15	95 120	99 148	93 92	97 37	91 33	67 6	69 32	- -	- -
Westview Hospital, Indianapolis, IN	100 1	100 7	100 5	90 10	86 7	0 1	- 0	100 1	94 18	52 62	91 82	78 18	89 65	97 78	63 19	78 106	100 113	57 69	78 32	70 82	90 20	58 78	- -	- -
White County Memorial Hospital, Monticello, IN	100 1	0 4	50 2	25 4	100 2	- -	- -	0 1	73 11	78 18	78 40	62 8	76 46	90 39	62 13	87 47	94 68	70 47	79 14	81 21	100 5	80 20	- -	- -
Wishard Memorial Hospital, Indianapolis, IN	98 42	99 181	99 155	97 161	99 151	57 14	0 2	91 98	97 250	39 333	98 377	93 135	87 93	83 54	62 8	81 120	100 127	79 34	100 39	78 158	95 43	84 150	- -	- -
Witham Memorial Hospital, Lebanon, IN	100 2	95 19	100 14	76 17	92 12	- 0	- 0	100 1	83 24	95 42	74 50	100 7	66 77	80 54	44 18	89 104	99 113	77 77	100 17	62 34	100 7	88 34	- -	- -
Women's Hospital, Newburgh, IN	- -	- -	- -	- -	- -	- -	- -	- -	- -	- -	- -	- -	- -	- -	- -	- -	- -	- -	- -	96 449	96 78	88 438	0.44 3217	6.35 2001
IOWA																								
Adair County Memorial Hospital, Greenfield, IA	- -	- -	- -	- -	- -	- -	- -	- -	- 0	80 10	17 12	0 1	67 12	100 4	- -	92 12	100 18	100 15	100 3	- -	- -	- -	- -	- -
Alegent Health Community Memorial Hospital, Missouri Valley, IA	100 1	67 3	100 2	100 4	100 2	- 0	- 0	- 0	33 6	60 10	100 22	33 3	100 28	100 25	100 8	98 40	100 53	93 43	83 6	- -	- -	- -	- -	- -
Alegent Health Mercy Hospital, Corning, IA	- 0	0 1	0 2	- 0	0 1	0 1	- -	- 0	100 2	78 18	95 21	100 3	67 12	100 4	67 3	58 12	100 18	77 13	0 1	50 8	100 1	100 8	- -	- -
Allen Memorial Hospital, Waterloo, IA	83 78	98 153	99 235	94 133	97 270	0 1	67 9	98 107	79 139	67 252	92 323	92 60	95 149	89 137	89 55	88 233	100 268	94 188	95 61	96 653	100 61	96 625	0.16 619	4.73 465
Audubon County Memorial Hospital, Audubon, IA	- 0	100 4	100 4	67 3	100 3	- 0	- -	- 0	100 2	40 5	100 9	- 0	80 10	100 4	80 5	92 12	100 15	90 10	0 1	50 2	- -	50 2	- -	- -
Baum Harmon Mercy Hospital, Primghar, IA	- -	- -	- -	- -	- -	- -	- -	- -	- 0	20 5	50 8	100 2	67 3	100 1	- -	100 2	100 3	100 2	- 0	- -	- -	- -	- -	- -
Boone County Hospital, Boone, IA	- 0	100 7	67 3	100 5	67 3	- 0	- 0	- 0	86 7	60 30	42 48	62 8	77 48	97 31	88 17	86 79	100 96	84 69	50 18	- -	- -	- -	- -	- -

*NOTE: The first number in each column (boldface) is the rate in percent, the second number is the number of patients; Please refer to the main entry for footnotes; **Heart Attack Care:** 1. ACE Inhibitor or ARB for LVSD; 2. Aspirin at Arrival; 3. Aspirin at Discharge; 4. Beta Blocker at Arrival; 5. Beta Blocker at Discharge; 6. Fibrinolytic Medication Timing; 7. PCI Within 90 Minutes of Arrival; 8. Smoking Cessation Advice; **Heart Failure Care:** 9. ACE Inhibitor or ARB for LVSD; 10. Discharge Instructions; 11. Evaluation of LVS Function; 12. Smoking Cessation Advice; **Pneumonia Care:** 13. Appropriate Initial Antibiotic; 14. Blood Culture Timing; 15. Influenza Vaccine; 16. Initial Antibiotic Timing; 17. Oxygenation Assessment; 18. Pneumococcal Vaccine; 19. Smoking Cessation Advice; **Surgical Infection Prevention:** 20. Prophylactic Antibiotic Given; 21. Prophylactic Antibiotic Selection; 22. Prophylactic Antibiotic Stopped; **Pregnancy Care:** 23. Inpatient Neonatal Mortality; 24. Third or Fourth Degree Laceration*

Hospital	Heart Attack Care								Heart Failure Care				Pneumonia Care							Surgical Infection Prevention			Pregnancy Care	
	1	2	3	4	5	6	7	8	9	10	11	12	13	14	15	16	17	18	19	20	21	22	23	24
Broadlawns Medical Center, Des Moines, IA	**67** 3	**83** 12	**88** 8	**89** 9	**86** 7	- 0	- 0	**67** 3	**100** 47	**67** 75	**100** 81	**49** 41	**87** 55	**88** 43	**50** 4	**87** 60	**100** 67	**89** 9	**76** 45	**79** 52	**100** 16	**69** 49	- -	- -
Buchanan County Health Center, Independence, IA	- -	- -	- -	- -	- -	- -	- -	- -	**50** 2	**54** 13	**38** 16	- 0	**79** 24	**100** 4	**80** 5	**77** 22	**100** 34	**79** 24	**44** 9	- -	- -	- -	- -	- -
Buena Vista Regional Medical Center, Storm Lake, IA	**50** 2	**92** 13	**100** 7	**100** 6	**100** 6	- 0	- 0	- 0	**83** 6	**50** 22	**67** 46	**80** 5	**92** 24	**94** 18	**100** 11	**76** 51	**100** 79	**98** 63	**50** 10	- -	- -	- -	- -	- -
Cass County Memorial Hospital, Atlantic, IA	- 0	**57** 7	**100** 4	**67** 6	**100** 4	- 0	- -	- 0	**67** 12	**85** 13	**97** 31	**100** 5	**85** 27	**96** 27	**100** 9	**97** 39	**100** 51	**100** 38	**78** 9	**71** 14	**100** 4	**77** 13	- -	- -
Cherokee Regional Medical Center, Cherokee, IA	- -	- -	- -	- -	- -	- -	- -	- -	**100** 3	**77** 13	- -	- -	**97** 29	**91** 11	**100** 14	**91** 34	**100** 46	**91** 34	**86** 7	**100** 12	**100** 5	**92** 12	- -	- -
Clarinda Regional Health Center, Clarinda, IA	- 0	**100** 6	**100** 3	**100** 5	**100** 3	- 0	- -	- 0	- 0	**0** 1	**71** 7	**100** 1	**80** 30	**93** 15	**82** 11	**68** 37	**100** 58	**91** 45	**78** 9	- -	- -	- -	- -	- -
Clarke County Hospital, Osceola, IA	- 0	**100** 2	**100** 1	**50** 2	**100** 1	- 0	- 0	- 0	**100** 5	**0** 13	**67** 15	**100** 1	**100** 11	**100** 6	**75** 4	**82** 17	**100** 19	**91** 11	**83** 6	- -	- -	- -	- -	- -
Covenant Medical Center, Waterloo, IA	**0** 1	**100** 20	**100** 11	**94** 17	**100** 11	**0** 1	- 0	- 0	**74** 34	**88** 82	**98** 121	**95** 20	**92** 108	**89** 81	**84** 25	**80** 141	**100** 189	**85** 123	**98** 45	**93** 237	**91** 66	**49** 230	- -	- -
Crawford County Memorial Hospital, Denison, IA	- 0	**100** 6	**50** 2	**50** 6	**75** 4	- 0	- 0	- 0	**70** 10	**5** 20	**61** 41	**0** 3	**65** 31	**93** 15	**50** 16	**90** 39	**100** 51	**80** 45	**40** 5	- -	- -	- -	- -	- -
Davis County Hospital, Bloomfield, IA	- 0	- 0	- 0	**100** 1	- 0	- 0	- -	- 0	**0** 3	**37** 27	**21** 33	**67** 3	**78** 51	**100** 4	- -	**80** 41	**100** 54	**55** 33	**80** 10	- 0	- 0	- 0	- -	- -
Decatur County Hospital, Leon, IA	- -	- -	- -	- -	- -	- -	- -	- -	- 0	**100** 1	**0** 1	- 0	**50** 2	- 0	- -	**100** 2	**100** 2	**50** 2	- 0	- -	- -	- -	- -	- -
Ellsworth Municipal Hospital, Iowa Falls, IA	- 0	**0** 2	**0** 2	**100** 2	**100** 2	**0** 1	- 0	- 0	**100** 1	**88** 16	**41** 29	**50** 2	**86** 29	**100** 13	**67** 9	**90** 49	**100** 62	**92** 48	**71** 7	- -	- -	- -	- -	- -
Finley Hospital, Dubuque, IA	**83** 12	**91** 47	**97** 30	**89** 35	**91** 35	- 0	- 0	**100** 5	**79** 24	**94** 69	**87** 95	**86** 14	**85** 61	**100** 72	**90** 21	**93** 95	**100** 144	**90** 115	**90** 20	**97** 158	**94** 36	**84** 154	- -	- -
Floyd Valley Hospital, Le Mars, IA	**100** 4	**100** 11	**100** 8	**82** 11	**83** 6	- 0	- 0	- 0	**78** 9	**96** 27	**82** 49	**100** 1	**87** 15	**90** 10	**100** 7	**83** 35	**100** 41	**85** 33	**83** 6	- -	- -	- -	- -	- -
Fort Madison Community Hospital, Fort Madison, IA	**100** 5	**100** 9	**100** 5	**100** 10	**100** 5	- 0	- 0	- 0	**97** 30	**98** 54	**100** 88	**100** 8	**83** 58	**100** 58	**100** 13	**95** 85	**100** 101	**96** 78	**100** 16	**90** 105	**100** 42	**82** 100	- -	- -
Genesis Medical Center-Davenport, Davenport, IA	**81** 119	**100** 267	**98** 500	**96** 239	**96** 482	- 0	**89** 9	**99** 191	**81** 127	**59** 273	**94** 310	**81** 48	**91** 100	**91** 86	**73** 26	**86** 169	**100** 190	**86** 126	**77** 60	**87** 91	**95** 93	**88** 85	**0.08** 2372	**3.65** 1646
Genesis Medical Center-Dewitt, Dewitt, IA	- -	- -	- -	- -	- -	- -	- -	- -	**100** 1	**0** 3	**50** 4	- 0	**78** 9	**80** 15	**91** 11	**81** 26	**100** 35	**88** 24	**100** 4	- -	- -	- -	- -	- -
Great River Medical Center, West Burlington, IA	**100** 10	**100** 97	**95** 42	**98** 94	**96** 46	**58** 19	**100** 1	**100** 12	**97** 37	**93** 135	**99** 192	**100** 22	**81** 134	**94** 158	**96** 50	**84** 209	**100** 261	**94** 195	**95** 60	**83** 300	**99** 67	**82** 289	- -	- -
Greater Regional Medical Center, Creston, IA	- 0	**93** 15	**100** 9	**94** 16	**89** 9	- 0	- 0	**100** 2	**75** 4	**91** 22	**28** 32	**67** 3	**62** 40	**100** 7	**67** 12	**77** 44	**100** 65	**53** 38	**55** 11	**78** 36	**80** 5	**94** 36	- -	- -
Greene County Medical Center, Jefferson, IA	- 0	**100** 3	**100** 3	**100** 3	**100** 3	- 0	- 0	- 0	**0** 4	**93** 14	**46** 28	**67** 6	**83** 12	**100** 9	**60** 5	**100** 14	**100** 21	**93** 14	**100** 3	**50** 2	**0** 1	**50** 2	- -	- -
Grinnell Regional Medical Center, Grinnell, IA	**100** 1	**100** 7	**100** 7	**100** 5	**100** 6	**100** 1	- 0	**100** 1	**75** 8	**83** 52	**89** 93	**91** 11	**85** 75	**98** 54	**100** 18	**88** 107	**100** 126	**92** 90	**62** 16	**91** 111	**97** 31	**68** 101	- -	- -
Grundy County Memorial Hospital, Grundy Center, IA	- -	- -	- -	- -	- -	- -	- -	- -	- 0	**0** 2	**40** 5	- 0	**100** 4	- 0	- -	**100** 2	**100** 4	**100** 4	- 0	**100** 2	**100** 2	**100** 2	- -	- -
Guttenberg Municipal Hospital, Guttenberg, IA	**100** 1	**78** 9	**89** 9	**73** 11	**92** 12	**0** 2	- 0	**100** 1	**100** 2	**33** 12	**60** 20	**0** 1	**86** 7	**80** 5	**100** 3	**80** 5	**69** 13	**100** 9	- 0	**0** 1	- -	**100** 1	- -	- -
Hamilton County Public Hospital, Webster City, IA	**50** 2	**60** 5	**50** 4	**71** 7	**86** 7	- 0	- -	- 0	**100** 5	**60** 52	**97** 72	**60** 5	**80** 41	**96** 27	**90** 10	**91** 65	**100** 77	**88** 49	**78** 9	**71** 28	**100** 6	**35** 26	- -	- -
Hawarden Community Hospital, Hawarden, IA	- -	- -	- -	- -	- -	- -	- -	- -	**100** 1	**20** 5	**25** 4	- 0	**100** 6	**100** 3	**100** 3	**86** 7	**100** 8	**100** 8	**100** 2	- -	- -	- -	- -	- -
Hegg Memorial Hospital, Rock Valley, IA	- -	- -	- -	- -	- -	- -	- -	- -	**100** 1	**0** 2	**88** 8	- 0	**75** 4	- 0	**100** 1	**100** 8	**100** 9	**67** 9	**100** 1	- -	- -	- -	- -	- -
Henry County Health Center, Mount Pleasant, IA	**100** 1	**60** 15	**82** 11	**75** 16	**80** 10	- 0	- 0	**0** 1	**88** 8	**5** 19	**52** 42	**67** 3	**80** 35	**100** 4	**0** 4	**71** 31	**100** 38	**9** 22	**50** 10	**62** 8	**88** 8	**86** 7	- -	- -
Horn Memorial Hospital, Ida Grove, IA	- -	- -	- -	- -	- -	- -	- -	- -	**50** 2	**36** 11	**38** 21	**0** 3	- -	- -	- -	- -	- -	- -	- -	- -	- -	- -	- -	- -
Iowa Lutheran Hospital, Des Moines, IA	**95** 42	**99** 85	**99** 77	**87** 68	**98** 95	- 0	**75** 4	**97** 33	**91** 104	**65** 193	**95** 228	**100** 57	**91** 102	**97** 67	**76** 29	**87** 143	**100** 167	**74** 109	**89** 37	**94** 234	**97** 59	**73** 226	- -	- -
Iowa Methodist Medical Center, Des Moines, IA	**79** 124	**96** 149	**97** 273	**96** 110	**97** 286	- 0	**62** 16	**96** 91	**89** 148	**65** 235	**98** 284	**98** 41	**78** 88	**96** 52	**74** 19	**82** 114	**100** 140	**76** 108	**65** 31	**94** 332	**91** 85	**73** 324	- -	- -
Jackson County Public Hospital, Maquoketa, IA	- -	- -	- -	- -	- -	- -	- -	- -	**100** 4	**55** 11	**71** 14	**67** 3	**67** 24	**90** 10	**86** 7	**92** 26	**100** 31	**79** 24	**67** 3	- -	- -	- -	- -	- -
Jefferson County Hospital, Fairfield, IA	- 0	**50** 4	**100** 3	**50** 2	**100** 2	- 0	- 0	- 0	**100** 6	**56** 9	**89** 27	**0** 2	**82** 22	**93** 15	**100** 2	**86** 28	**97** 35	**52** 21	**25** 4	**83** 52	**100** 10	**80** 45	- -	- -
Jennie Edmundson Memorial Hospital, Council Bluffs, IA	**92** 13	**96** 76	**100** 63	**99** 74	**97** 65	**80** 5	- 0	**97** 30	**98** 65	**84** 113	**95** 143	**100** 27	**83** 113	**94** 115	**79** 43	**93** 161	**98** 201	**87** 141	**100** 33	**95** 399	**93** 98	**91** 399	- -	- -
Jones Regional Medical Center, Anamosa, IA	- -	- -	- -	- -	- -	- -	- -	- -	**0** 2	**11** 9	**81** 16	- 0	**91** 35	**95** 20	**57** 7	**78** 41	**100** 44	**75** 36	**75** 12	- -	- -	- -	- -	- -
Keokuk Area Hospital, Keokuk, IA	**100** 3	**90** 10	**100** 2	**100** 7	**100** 3	**38** 8	- 0	- 0	**92** 24	**78** 60	**95** 101	**100** 17	**70** 103	**97** 75	**92** 38	**92** 160	**100** 200	**86** 140	**84** 43	**84** 31	**92** 12	**86** 29	- -	- -
Knoxville Hospital & Clinics, Knoxville, IA	- 0	**100** 4	**100** 3	**100** 2	**100** 2	- 0	- -	- 0	**60** 5	**69** 13	**96** 25	**100** 1	**94** 17	**100** 17	**86** 7	**86** 36	**100** 43	**68** 31	**80** 5	**100** 1	**100** 2	**100** 1	- -	- -
Lakes Regional Healthcare, Spirit Lake, IA	- 0	**91** 11	**100** 8	**90** 10	**86** 7	**100** 1	- 0	- 0	**62** 8	**0** 25	**61** 38	**40** 5	**71** 45	**97** 29	**75** 8	**87** 53	**100** 69	**68** 50	**60** 10	**72** 116	**93** 28	**94** 114	- -	- -
Lucas County Health Center, Chariton, IA	- -	- -	- -	- -	- -	- -	- -	- -	- -	- -	- -	- -	- -	- -	- -	- -	- -	- -	- -	- -	- -	- -	- -	- -
Madison County Memorial Hospital, Winterset, IA	- 0	**100** 2	**100** 1	**100** 3	**0** 1	- 0	- -	- 0	**100** 2	**0** 10	**32** 19	**0** 1	**89** 55	**100** 2	**27** 11	**92** 61	**100** 78	**53** 55	**33** 15	**100** 1	- -	**100** 1	- -	- -
Manning Regional Healthcare Center, Manning, IA	- -	- -	- -	- -	- -	- -	- -	- -	- -	- -	- -	- -	**100** 3	- 0	**100** 5	**100** 10	**100** 11	**100** 11	- 0	- -	- -	- -	- -	- -
Marengo Memorial Hospital, Marengo, IA	- -	- -	- -	- -	- -	- -	- -	- -	- -	- -	- -	- -	- -	- -	- -	- -	- -	- -	- -	- -	- -	- -	- -	- -
Marshalltown Medical & Surgical Center, Marshalltown, IA	**100** 3	**96** 24	**81** 16	**100** 21	**100** 16	- 0	- 0	- 0	**100** 16	**95** 59	**93** 97	**100** 13	**89** 89	**96** 77	**96** 28	**89** 131	**100** 160	**94** 110	**92** 26	**96** 284	**95** 58	**48** 278	- -	- -
Mary Greeley Medical Center, Ames, IA	**85** 39	**95** 113	**99** 142	**96** 101	**98** 140	- 0	**80** 5	**100** 33	**97** 95	**85** 170	**98** 224	**95** 19	**91** 133	**89** 110	**96** 68	**82** 220	**98** 261	**94** 193	**87** 39	**82** 208	**99** 126	**59** 194	- -	- -
Mercy Hospital, Council Bluffs, IA	**100** 9	**100** 46	**100** 30	**100** 36	**100** 38	**67** 6	**75** 4	**100** 16	**100** 39	**98** 83	**100** 105	**100** 23	**97** 108	**99** 137	**100** 39	**98** 169	**100** 204	**100** 128	**100** 65	**95** 327	**89** 38	**94** 319	- -	- -
Mercy Hospital, Iowa City, IA	**86** 50	**98** 131	**99** 219	**92** 117	**95** 235	- 0	**22** 9	**97** 59	**83** 81	**86** 187	**93** 230	**94** 32	**81** 108	**96** 93	**79** 28	**79** 137	**99** 168	**78** 123	**85** 33	**94** 379	**99** 217	**65** 376	- -	- -
Mercy Hospital of Franciscan Sisters, Oelwein, IA	- -	- -	- -	- -	- -	- -	- -	- -	**77** 13	**93** 15	**85** 34	**80** 5	**96** 45	**98** 43	**82** 11	**86** 49	**100** 70	**96** 49	**91** 11	**80** 5	**50** 2	**20** 5	- -	- -
Mercy Medical Center, Cedar Rapids, IA	**95** 37	**100** 175	**100** 160	**99** 114	**99** 182	**0** 2	**75** 8	**99** 76	**87** 53	**91** 159	**92** 201	**95** 19	**87** 173	**97** 193	**93** 58	**88** 243	**100** 348	**84** 241	**73** 74	**91** 152	**93** 57	**63** 142	- -	- -
Mercy Medical Center, Sioux City, IA	**91** 57	**99** 190	**99** 343	**98** 186	**98** 343	- 0	**77** 13	**100** 122	**92** 100	**77** 197	**95** 242	**98** 42	**88** 132	**99** 138	**84** 43	**85** 206	**100** 258	**74** 176	**97** 66	**89** 536	**99** 70	**79** 530	- -	- -

NOTE: The first number in each column (boldface) is the rate in percent, the second number is the number of patients; Please refer to the main entry for footnotes; ***Heart Attack Care:*** *1. ACE Inhibitor or ARB for LVSD; 2. Aspirin at Arrival; 3. Aspirin at Discharge; 4. Beta Blocker at Arrival; 5. Beta Blocker at Discharge; 6. Fibrinolytic Medication Timing; 7. PCI Within 90 Minutes of Arrival; 8. Smoking Cessation Advice;* ***Heart Failure Care:*** *9. ACE Inhibitor or ARB for LVSD; 10. Discharge Instructions; 11. Evaluation of LVS Function; 12. Smoking Cessation Advice;* ***Pneumonia Care:*** *13. Appropriate Initial Antibiotic; 14. Blood Culture Timing; 15. Influenza Vaccine; 16. Initial Antibiotic Timing; 17. Oxygenation Assessment; 18. Pneumococcal Vaccine; 19. Smoking Cessation Advice;* ***Surgical Infection Prevention:*** *20. Prophylactic Antibiotic Given; 21. Prophylactic Antibiotic Selection; 22. Prophylactic Antibiotic Stopped;* ***Pregnancy Care:*** *23. Inpatient Neonatal Mortality; 24. Third or Fourth Degree Laceration*

Hospital	Heart Attack Care								Heart Failure Care				Pneumonia Care							Surgical Infection Prevention			Pregnancy Care	
	1	2	3	4	5	6	7	8	9	10	11	12	13	14	15	16	17	18	19	20	21	22	23	24
Mercy Medical Center-Centerville, Centerville, IA	100 2	100 7	100 6	100 8	100 8	- 0	- 0	- 0	88 17	70 20	95 40	67 3	58 19	88 17	100 2	97 31	100 36	73 26	75 4	73 41	86 14	67 39	- -	- -
Mercy Medical Center-Des Moines, Des Moines, IA	99 178	100 331	100 586	98 262	100 554	0 1	95 20	100 280	99 285	98 734	100 888	100 145	97 352	95 348	97 110	85 517	100 659	95 435	95 184	89 479	95 136	92 449	- -	- -
Mercy Medical Center-Dubuque, Dubuque, IA	95 59	98 190	98 289	95 172	97 267	- 0	50 10	95 85	85 75	56 162	93 189	89 19	87 108	88 97	92 26	73 175	99 214	86 166	92 26	92 455	97 94	80 447	0.11 937	2.51 677
Mercy Medical Center-Dyersville, Dyersville, IA	- -	- -	- -	- -	- -	- -	- -	- -	- 0	- 0	0 1	- 0	100 3	100 2	100 2	60 5	100 5	67 3	- 0	- -	- -	- -	- -	- -
Mercy Medical Center-North Iowa, Mason City, IA	97 61	97 172	100 270	95 148	99 268	- 0	62 16	99 86	94 139	89 249	98 332	97 36	87 142	84 140	97 39	92 168	100 216	93 162	98 43	90 703	98 235	87 694	- -	- -
Merrill Pioneer Community Hospital, Rock Rapids, IA	- -	- -	- -	- -	- -	- -	- -	- -	50 2	100 3	43 14	- 0	100 5	100 2	100 2	100 7	100 8	83 6	- 0	57 7	0 1	43 7	- -	- -
Montgomery County Memorial Hospital, Red Oak, IA	- 0	60 10	80 5	82 11	83 6	- 0	- 0	100 1	92 12	74 23	100 42	100 1	88 32	100 13	100 14	91 44	100 60	98 48	89 9	88 16	100 1	100 16	- -	- -
Northwest Iowa Health Center, Sheldon, IA	- 0	100 6	75 4	80 5	100 5	- 0	- -	- 0	82 11	85 34	70 46	100 7	98 48	100 25	79 14	100 56	100 70	68 41	85 13	- -	- -	- -	- -	- -
Orange City Area Health System, Orange City, IA	100 2	86 7	80 5	100 7	100 5	0 1	- -	- 0	100 5	40 10	72 18	- 0	65 20	100 3	100 4	77 22	100 24	95 21	67 3	0 4	- -	100 4	- -	- -
Osceola Community Hospital, Sibley, IA	- 0	100 1	0 1	100 1	100 1	- 0	- -	- 0	100 1	29 7	38 8	- 0	93 15	100 3	100 1	92 12	100 17	25 12	- 0	38 8	100 1	88 8	- -	- -
Ottumwa Regional Health Center, Ottumwa, IA	70 10	97 71	95 40	95 81	96 51	- 0	- 0	100 3	83 30	56 86	93 99	100 7	85 127	95 115	16 31	69 162	100 217	79 140	86 44	72 196	89 46	82 180	- -	- -
Palmer Lutheran Health Center, West Union, IA	- -	- -	- -	- -	- -	- -	- -	- -	100 1	100 1	100 1	- 0	100 5	86 7	100 4	94 17	100 19	100 17	0 1	- -	- -	- -	- -	- -
Pella Regional Health Center, Pella, IA	67 3	86 7	75 4	100 7	100 5	- 0	- 0	- 0	91 11	71 17	92 26	100 2	96 46	91 46	100 21	90 68	100 80	98 64	50 10	92 103	93 29	93 102	- -	- -
Regional Medical Center of Northeast Iowa, Manchester, IA	- 0	100 2	100 3	100 3	67 3	- 0	- -	100 1	100 3	84 19	79 28	- 0	92 26	95 21	75 8	86 35	100 42	94 32	60 5	- -	- -	- -	- -	- -
Ringgold County Hospital, Mount Ayr, IA	0 1	- 0	- 0	100 1	- 0	- 0	- -	- 0	- 0	14 7	50 8	100 1	100 16	80 10	100 10	90 29	100 33	94 31	67 3	- -	- -	- -	- -	- -
Saint Anthony Regional Hospital, Carroll, IA	- 0	91 11	100 5	83 6	80 5	- 0	- 0	- 0	89 9	8 12	86 59	100 1	78 9	100 6	- -	94 54	100 96	88 78	100 2	94 53	96 54	91 53	- -	- -
Saint Luke's Hospital, Cedar Rapids, IA	88 41	99 191	99 213	97 157	97 239	0 1	65 20	98 94	80 96	88 191	94 254	88 26	94 85	96 107	96 25	87 127	100 165	92 118	96 27	89 281	95 73	83 232	- -	- -
Saint Luke's Regional Medical Center, Sioux City, IA	87 15	96 53	98 43	98 42	100 38	- 0	- 0	100 12	100 38	95 81	99 118	100 17	95 175	98 131	100 52	92 220	100 280	92 183	98 66	89 670	96 151	85 651	0.14 2137	3.78 1454
Samaritan Health System, Clinton, IA	83 18	94 144	92 119	93 85	91 117	80 15	- 0	94 36	93 41	83 177	94 218	94 36	88 165	77 106	67 58	88 280	97 346	79 236	85 81	81 100	87 45	44 101	0.17 572	1.80 388
Sartori Memorial Hospital, Cedar Falls, IA	100 3	92 12	100 9	100 12	100 11	- 0	- 0	100 2	100 10	86 14	100 27	100 2	80 46	95 58	95 20	92 80	100 97	94 80	92 12	88 52	90 21	35 51	- -	- -
Shelby County Myrtue Memorial Hospital, Harlan, IA	100 1	100 1	100 2	100 1	100 2	- 0	- 0	- 0	100 17	95 20	100 64	100 4	94 49	100 54	100 24	93 84	100 98	94 79	86 7	100 10	100 2	80 10	- -	- -
Shenandoah Medical Center, Shenandoah, IA	100 1	100 5	100 3	100 4	100 3	- 0	- -	0 1	100 1	83 6	89 9	100 1	94 32	100 23	86 7	84 49	100 60	67 45	67 15	25 16	67 3	69 16	- -	- -
Sioux Center Community Hospital, Sioux Center, IA	- -	- -	- -	- -	- -	- -	- -	- -	100 1	86 7	19 16	- 0	94 33	100 7	80 5	88 25	97 36	85 27	25 4	62 13	100 4	92 12	- -	- -
Skiff Medical Center, Newton, IA	100 2	50 10	60 5	50 12	86 7	- 0	- 0	- 0	54 13	56 48	61 72	67 9	83 47	85 27	70 10	71 65	100 74	73 37	73 15	86 181	84 44	60 178	- -	- -
Spencer Hospital, Spencer, IA	100 3	100 10	100 6	100 12	100 8	- 0	- 0	100 1	86 14	86 37	86 71	67 6	91 44	97 36	85 13	93 67	100 76	98 53	90 10	95 291	78 46	88 286	- -	- -
Stewart Memorial Community Hospital, Lake City, IA	100 1	100 2	100 2	50 2	50 2	- 0	- 0	- 0	- 0	78 9	33 18	100 1	86 43	100 9	100 7	83 59	100 71	93 56	89 9	100 4	50 2	100 3	- -	- -
Trinity Regional Medical Center, Fort Dodge, IA	100 46	98 121	100 206	96 105	98 190	- 0	100 3	99 69	93 107	90 174	95 240	85 47	92 160	98 209	91 65	96 249	100 297	94 218	95 42	84 234	100 57	78 226	- -	- -
Trinity-Terrace Park Campus, Bettendorf, IA	80 5	97 32	92 36	100 27	94 35	- 0	100 1	100 10	93 27	79 47	97 58	100 14	89 53	94 48	100 15	89 66	100 90	93 59	100 17	90 157	97 34	90 154	- -	- -
Unity Hospital, Muscatine, IA	67 3	100 10	75 8	93 14	73 11	- 0	- 0	- 0	70 20	48 25	80 46	80 5	94 80	94 54	92 12	91 80	100 107	92 75	94 18	72 99	92 36	64 92	- -	- -
University of Iowa Hospitals and Clinics, Iowa City, IA	82 60	100 79	99 240	99 67	100 263	- 0	40 5	96 113	84 188	79 253	98 280	85 81	80 50	85 52	62 21	67 101	100 124	56 59	35 48	80 499	71 70	64 481	2.08 2022	5.72 1084
Van Buren County Hospital, Keosauqua, IA	- 0	100 2	100 2	100 2	100 2	- 0	- 0	100 1	89 9	60 15	71 41	100 6	89 19	87 15	100 6	91 32	100 36	83 24	86 7	- -	- -	- -	- -	- -
Veterans Memorial Hospital, Waukon, IA	- 0	100 5	100 3	100 3	67 3	- 0	- -	- 0	67 6	54 13	71 24	67 3	100 15	90 10	75 4	91 22	97 31	64 25	50 4	42 19	86 7	11 18	- -	- -
Washington County Hospital, Washington, IA	- -	- -	- -	- -	- -	- -	- -	- -	71 7	30 10	62 24	0 2	76 25	100 11	62 16	70 50	100 61	53 47	67 9	- -	- -	- -	- -	- -
Waverly Health Center, Waverly, IA	100 1	50 2	100 2	50 2	100 2	- 0	- -	- 0	100 4	38 8	67 9	100 1	75 4	67 6	- -	75 8	100 9	50 8	100 1	87 23	88 16	87 23	- -	- -
Wayne County Hospital, Corydon, IA	100 2	100 3	100 4	100 4	100 4	- 0	- -	- 0	100 3	20 10	64 14	0 1	67 12	100 2	75 4	95 19	100 25	79 19	60 5	- 0	100 2	- 0	- -	- -
Winneshiek County Memorial Hospital, Decorah, IA	100 1	100 4	100 4	100 4	100 4	- 0	- 0	- 0	94 16	77 22	94 35	100 5	82 57	91 58	100 17	96 73	100 89	94 66	67 12	- -	- -	- -	- -	- -
Wright Medical Center, Clarion, IA	- -	- -	- -	- -	- -	- -	- -	- -	- -	- -	- -	- -	- -	- -	- -	- -	- -	- -	- -	- -	- -	- -	- -	- -
KANSAS																								
Allen County Hospital, Iola, KS	- 0	100 1	100 1	100 1	100 1	- 0	- -	- 0	100 3	69 26	53 30	- 0	97 32	95 19	40 10	84 49	100 57	46 37	100 15	92 24	100 9	100 23	- -	- -
Anderson County Hospital, Garnett, KS	- 0	100 1	100 1	- 0	- 0	- 0	- -	- 0	60 5	50 8	100 16	50 2	94 17	100 6	30 10	77 22	100 26	40 15	62 8	75 4	- -	100 4	- -	- -
Ashland District Hospital, Ashland, KS	- -	- -	- -	- -	- -	- -	- -	- -	- 0	0 1	0 5	- 0	71 7	100 1	- -	80 5	100 7	67 6	- 0	- -	- -	- -	- -	- -
Atchison Hospital, Atchison, KS	- 0	80 5	100 2	100 3	0 1	- 0	- 0	- 0	54 13	18 34	58 55	33 3	83 23	100 16	100 5	76 33	100 43	74 31	50 10	72 39	86 7	54 35	- -	- -
Bob Wilson Memorial Grant Hospital, Ulysses, KS	0 2	100 3	50 2	100 4	100 2	- 0	- -	- 0	67 9	44 9	71 14	- 0	79 19	100 3	71 7	100 23	100 27	53 17	100 4	0 2	100 2	50 2	- -	- -
Central Kansas Medical Center, Great Bend, KS	- 0	93 14	100 6	62 13	70 10	- 0	- 0	- 0	57 7	18 28	62 45	75 4	94 35	100 12	50 10	91 45	100 59	43 47	75 8	22 146	94 49	11 145	0.92 433	3.62 276
Cheyenne County Hospital, Saint Francis, KS	- 0	100 4	100 4	33 3	100 3	0 1	- -	- 0	- 0	0 3	0 3	- 0	100 15	100 1	60 5	67 15	100 21	44 16	25 4	- -	- -	- -	- -	- -
Clay County Medical Center, Clay Center, KS	- 0	75 4	- 0	67 3	- 0	0 2	- -	- 0	67 3	17 6	80 15	0 2	68 63	100 10	92 12	85 65	99 75	96 56	50 8	67 3	100 1	100 3	- -	- -
Cloud County Health Center, Concordia, KS	- 0	100 3	67 3	100 3	100 3	- 0	- -	0 1	67 3	56 16	76 21	- 0	73 59	80 5	82 17	90 51	100 64	85 47	40 10	- -	- -	- -	- -	- -
Coffey County Hospital, Burlington, KS	- 0	50 2	100 1	50 2	0 1	100 3	- 0	- 0	50 6	26 34	37 52	75 4	88 43	100 1	4 26	91 67	100 75	56 54	88 16	23 22	100 3	71 17	- -	- -

NOTE: The first number in each column (boldface) is the rate in percent, the second number is the number of patients; Please refer to the main entry for footnotes; ***Heart Attack Care:*** *1. ACE Inhibitor or ARB for LVSD; 2. Aspirin at Arrival; 3. Aspirin at Discharge; 4. Beta Blocker at Arrival; 5. Beta Blocker at Discharge; 6. Fibrinolytic Medication Timing; 7. PCI Within 90 Minutes of Arrival; 8. Smoking Cessation Advice;* ***Heart Failure Care:*** *9. ACE Inhibitor or ARB for LVSD; 10. Discharge Instructions; 11. Evaluation of LVS Function; 12. Smoking Cessation Advice;* ***Pneumonia Care:*** *13. Appropriate Initial Antibiotic; 14. Blood Culture Timing; 15. Influenza Vaccine; 16. Initial Antibiotic Timing; 17. Oxygenation Assessment; 18. Pneumococcal Vaccine; 19. Smoking Cessation Advice;* ***Surgical Infection Prevention:*** *20. Prophylactic Antibiotic Given; 21. Prophylactic Antibiotic Selection; 22. Prophylactic Antibiotic Stopped;* ***Pregnancy Care:*** *23. Inpatient Neonatal Mortality; 24. Third or Fourth Degree Laceration*

Hospital	Heart Attack Care								Heart Failure Care				Pneumonia Care							Surgical Infection Prevention			Pregnancy Care	
	1	2	3	4	5	6	7	8	9	10	11	12	13	14	15	16	17	18	19	20	21	22	23	24
Coffeyville Regional Medical Center, Coffeyville, KS	57 7	89 28	83 12	61 28	54 13	0 1	- 0	50 2	55 47	68 98	72 146	50 14	73 105	94 54	53 49	79 219	100 226	47 159	67 45	78 49	35 17	88 48	- -	- -
Comanche County Hospital, Coldwater, KS	- -	- -	- -	- -	- -	- -	- -	- -	- -	- -	- -	- -	50 12	100 1	- -	91 11	100 15	17 12	100 1	- -	- -	- -	- -	- -
Community Hospital-Onaga, Onaga, KS	- 0	75 4	75 4	75 4	75 4	0 1	- 0	- 0	67 6	7 14	38 37	100 1	56 18	100 2	0 8	82 17	93 27	4 26	33 6	- -	- -	- -	- -	- -
Community Memorial Hospital, Marysville, KS	- -	- -	- -	- -	- -	- -	- -	- -	- -	- -	- -	- -	25 4	- 0	- -	80 10	100 10	20 5	25 4	- -	- -	- -	- -	- -
Cushing Memorial Hospital, Leavenworth, KS	0 1	100 7	100 2	100 5	100 2	- 0	- 0	100 1	80 15	37 38	98 52	100 11	76 63	100 34	100 11	83 71	100 75	92 38	95 21	88 17	57 7	93 14	- -	- -
Doctors Hospital, Leawood, KS	- -	- -	- -	- -	- -	- -	- -	- -	- -	- -	- -	- -	0 1	- 0	- 0	- 0	100 1	- 0	0 1	94 17	100 3	94 16	- -	- -
Ellinwood District Hospital, Ellinwood, KS	- -	- -	- -	- -	- -	- -	- -	- -	- -	- -	- -	- -	- -	- -	- -	- -	- -	- -	- -	- -	- -	- -	- -	- -
Ellsworth County Medical Center, Ellsworth, KS	0 1	80 5	25 4	86 7	20 5	- 0	- 0	- 0	20 5	5 20	51 43	- 0	79 24	100 10	62 21	80 40	100 52	55 44	100 6	- -	- -	- -	- -	- -
Emporia Surgical Hospital, Emporia, KS	- -	- -	- -	- -	- -	- -	- -	- -	- -	- -	- -	- -	- -	- -	- -	- -	- -	- -	- -	100 2	- 0	100 2	- -	- -
Fredonia Regional Hospital, Fredonia, KS	- 0	100 1	100 2	50 2	50 2	- 0	- -	0 1	0 1	0 17	26 27	0 6	53 51	0 1	4 24	88 59	100 68	2 40	5 19	- -	- -	- -	- -	- -
Galichia Heart Hospital, Wichita, KS	57 14	82 28	89 62	83 29	85 65	33 3	0 2	86 29	67 102	94 239	92 263	68 34	67 15	100 5	25 4	50 16	91 23	39 18	60 5	46 37	89 38	42 36	- -	- -
Geary Community Hospital, Junction City, KS	- 0	75 8	50 2	60 5	67 3	0 1	- 0	- 0	82 22	98 52	64 66	95 19	85 65	89 18	41 17	89 85	100 91	46 59	95 19	75 65	88 16	70 61	- -	- -
Girard Medical Center, Girard, KS	- 0	100 2	0 1	0 2	0 1	0 1	- -	- 0	25 4	69 13	41 34	100 1	83 23	100 6	57 7	73 30	100 39	36 28	62 8	47 36	100 2	31 32	- -	- -
Goodland Regional Medical Center, Goodland, KS	- 0	100 1	100 1	100 1	100 1	- 0	- 0	- 0	50 4	33 9	56 18	100 1	89 18	100 5	8 13	81 31	100 37	41 29	25 4	- -	- -	- -	- -	- -
Greeley County Hospital & LTCU, Tribune, KS	- 0	100 1	100 1	100 1	100 1	0 1	- -	- 0	50 2	0 3	36 11	0 3	60 10	100 3	50 4	- 0	100 13	44 9	0 5	- -	- -	- -	- -	- -
Greenwood County Hospital, Eureka, KS	- -	- -	- -	- -	- -	- -	- -	- -	20 5	0 9	28 32	33 3	62 69	89 19	0 30	73 22	100 93	0 56	15 20	- -	- -	- -	- -	- -
Grisell Memorial Hospital, Ransom, KS	- -	- -	- -	- -	- -	- -	- -	- -	- -	- -	- -	- -	- -	- -	- -	- -	- -	- -	- -	- -	- -	- -	- -	- -
Hamilton County Hospital, Syracuse, KS	- 0	100 1	100 1	100 1	100 1	- 0	- -	- 0	- 0	0 1	0 2	- 0	71 7	- 0	50 4	100 5	100 8	29 7	0 1	- -	- -	- -	- -	- -
Harper Hospital/District #5, Harper, KS	- 0	100 1	- 0	100 1	- 0	- 0	- -	- 0	33 3	0 5	29 17	0 1	86 22	100 2	0 10	100 22	100 24	5 20	0 4	0 1	- -	100 1	- -	- -
Hays Medical Center, Hays, KS	87 39	94 64	96 156	89 54	94 158	- 0	75 8	98 42	92 48	73 106	86 145	100 26	70 80	90 42	86 21	88 98	100 131	86 99	95 20	84 322	91 80	48 308	0.00 244	9.68 155
Heartland Surgical Specialty Hospital, Overland Park, KS	- -	- -	- -	- -	- -	- -	- -	- -	- -	- -	- -	- -	- -	- -	- -	- -	- -	- -	- -	83 58	95 20	85 54	- -	- -
Herington Municipal Hospital, Herington, KS	- 0	100 1	- 0	- 0	- 0	- 0	- -	- 0	- 0	- 0	- 0	- 0	92 12	- 0	88 8	87 15	100 16	64 11	50 2	- -	- -	- -	- -	- -
Hiawatha Community Hospital, Hiawatha, KS	0 1	100 2	100 2	100 1	100 2	- 0	- 0	- 0	90 10	5 21	71 42	14 7	85 13	100 3	80 5	90 20	100 23	71 17	0 5	61 36	100 11	91 34	- -	- -
Hillsboro Community Medical Center, Hillsboro, KS	100 1	100 1	- 0	100 2	100 2	- 0	- 0	- 0	100 1	0 2	53 15	0 1	60 5	- 0	0 2	100 5	100 9	0 5	- 0	- -	- -	- -	- -	- -
Holton Community Hospital, Holton, KS	- -	- -	- -	- -	- -	- -	- -	- -	80 5	7 14	47 17	100 1	36 11	100 1	- 0	89 9	92 13	80 5	100 2	- -	- -	- -	- -	- -
Hutchinson Hospital, Hutchinson, KS	85 55	98 178	94 214	92 149	86 198	- 0	100 10	84 70	89 64	56 156	72 206	93 28	74 148	95 74	77 44	65 211	100 277	55 178	87 61	90 803	96 182	84 787	- -	- -
Kansas City Orthopaedic Institute, Leawood, KS	- -	- -	- -	- -	- -	- -	- -	- -	- -	- -	- -	- -	- -	- -	- -	- -	- -	- -	- -	97 96	100 22	81 96	- -	- -
Kansas Heart Hospital, Wichita, KS	89 27	100 17	98 172	91 11	98 162	- 0	- 0	96 67	95 59	82 103	100 115	83 24	- 0	- 0	- 0	- 0	- 0	0 2	- 0	95 205	98 45	59 203	- -	- -
Kansas Medical Center, Andover, KS	- -	- -	- -	- -	- -	- -	- -	- -	- -	- -	- -	- -	- -	- -	- -	- -	- -	- -	- -	- -	- -	- -	- -	- -
Kansas Spine Hospital, Wichita, KS	- -	- -	- -	- -	- -	- -	- -	- -	- -	- -	- -	- -	- -	- -	- -	- -	- -	- -	- -	- 0	- 0	- 0	- -	- -
Kansas Surgery & Recovery Center, Wichita, KS	- -	- -	- -	- -	- -	- -	- -	- -	- -	- -	- -	- -	- -	- -	- -	- -	- -	- -	- -	92 198	96 51	39 198	- -	- -
Kearny County Hospital, Lakin, KS	- -	- -	- -	- -	- -	- -	- -	- -	- 0	25 8	0 11	- 0	100 5	- 0	- 0	100 6	100 6	100 3	0 1	- -	- -	- -	- -	- -
Kingman Community Hospital, Kingman, KS	100 1	75 4	100 4	83 6	100 4	- 0	- 0	- 0	71 7	20 10	52 23	33 3	79 38	100 6	- -	87 47	98 57	58 40	27 15	100 10	100 1	100 10	- -	- -
Labette County Medical Center, Parsons, KS	- 0	71 7	100 2	29 7	67 3	- 0	- 0	- 0	44 34	28 68	73 81	57 14	70 70	100 43	55 20	68 76	100 125	50 80	50 24	73 390	97 88	78 361	- -	- -
Lawrence Memorial Hospital, Lawrence, KS	100 7	100 53	100 37	100 47	100 37	0 2	0 2	94 16	100 68	87 82	98 125	100 24	89 75	87 60	77 22	92 93	100 135	96 98	100 27	82 378	98 105	77 360	- -	- -
Lindsborg Community Hospital, Lindsborg, KS	- 0	100 1	- 0	100 1	- 0	- 0	- 0	- 0	50 2	0 2	86 7	100 1	87 23	100 4	92 12	92 37	100 45	97 35	83 6	- -	- -	- -	- -	- -
Manhattan Surgical Hospital, Manhattan, KS	- -	- -	- -	- -	- -	- -	- -	- -	- -	- -	- -	- -	- -	- -	- -	- -	- -	- -	- -	61 219	98 56	96 215	- -	- -
Meade District Hospital, Meade, KS	- -	- -	- -	- -	- -	- -	- -	- -	0 1	0 7	30 10	- 0	51 41	100 1	100 17	78 51	100 75	90 58	0 11	- -	- -	- -	- -	- -
Meadowbrook Rehabilitation Hospital, Gardner, KS	- -	- -	- -	- -	- -	- -	- -	- -	- -	- -	- -	- -	- -	- -	- -	- -	- -	- -	- -	- -	- -	- -	- -	- -
Memorial Health System, Abilene, KS	100 1	86 7	80 5	100 7	100 5	- 0	- 0	- 0	67 6	18 11	44 32	100 1	81 31	86 7	- -	88 32	100 38	3 29	50 4	- -	- -	- -	- -	- -
Memorial Hospital, McPherson, KS	100 1	- 0	- 0	100 1	100 1	- 0	- -	- 0	55 11	18 34	59 54	0 4	84 50	93 30	69 16	81 70	99 90	62 66	11 9	61 31	100 6	97 29	- -	- -
Menorah Medical Center, Shawnee Mission, KS	77 13	97 62	97 75	91 46	97 66	- 0	20 5	100 27	81 42	76 98	98 132	100 20	86 86	99 74	83 23	93 111	97 140	91 109	100 22	71 246	84 116	53 235	- -	- -
Mercy Health Center, Fort Scott, KS	100 2	93 15	100 10	85 13	82 11	- 0	- 0	100 1	84 32	85 81	91 111	100 11	90 71	95 39	39 18	88 92	100 107	84 64	77 35	94 93	100 17	69 84	- -	- -
Mercy Hospital, Moundridge, KS	- 0	100 3	100 3	67 3	67 3	- 0	- 0	- 0	80 5	0 1	70 20	- 0	75 4	100 1	- -	88 17	100 23	68 22	- 0	- -	- -	- -	- -	- -
Mercy Hospital-Independence, Independence, KS	100 1	80 5	100 2	100 5	100 3	- 0	- 0	- 0	100 16	93 46	92 71	100 11	90 48	95 39	50 16	73 71	100 81	77 56	100 17	83 103	96 25	81 97	- -	- -
Mercy Regional Health Center, Manhattan, KS	50 2	100 21	91 11	93 15	91 11	- 0	- 0	100 3	84 37	27 83	89 125	53 19	93 68	100 49	86 14	81 97	100 130	76 83	58 31	74 92	95 92	78 86	- -	- -
Miami County Medical Center, Paola, KS	100 1	100 2	100 2	100 1	100 2	- 0	- -	- 0	100 3	50 8	92 13	- 0	88 33	96 25	100 12	93 41	100 58	84 32	100 20	60 52	100 17	2 50	- -	- -
Mitchell County Hospital, Beloit, KS	100 1	100 6	100 2	83 6	100 3	100 2	- -	- 0	86 7	6 31	78 54	0 1	74 38	100 30	36 14	84 62	100 88	30 69	43 7	93 29	80 5	93 28	- -	- -

NOTE: The first number in each column (boldface) is the rate in percent, the second number is the number of patients; Please refer to the main entry for footnotes; ***Heart Attack Care:*** *1. ACE Inhibitor or ARB for LVSD; 2. Aspirin at Arrival; 3. Aspirin at Discharge; 4. Beta Blocker at Arrival; 5. Beta Blocker at Discharge; 6. Fibrinolytic Medication Timing; 7. PCI Within 90 Minutes of Arrival; 8. Smoking Cessation Advice;* ***Heart Failure Care:*** *9. ACE Inhibitor or ARB for LVSD; 10. Discharge Instructions; 11. Evaluation of LVS Function; 12. Smoking Cessation Advice;* ***Pneumonia Care:*** *13. Appropriate Initial Antibiotic; 14. Blood Culture Timing; 15. Influenza Vaccine; 16. Initial Antibiotic Timing; 17. Oxygenation Assessment; 18. Pneumococcal Vaccine; 19. Smoking Cessation Advice;* ***Surgical Infection Prevention:*** *20. Prophylactic Antibiotic Given; 21. Prophylactic Antibiotic Selection; 22. Prophylactic Antibiotic Stopped;* ***Pregnancy Care:*** *23. Inpatient Neonatal Mortality; 24. Third or Fourth Degree Laceration*

Hospital	Heart Attack Care								Heart Failure Care				Pneumonia Care							Surgical Infection Prevention			Pregnancy Care	
	1	2	3	4	5	6	7	8	9	10	11	12	13	14	15	16	17	18	19	20	21	22	23	24
Morris County Hospital, Council Grove, KS	- 0	100 1	100 1	0 1	0 1	- 0	- 0	- 0	100 3	36 14	35 23	0 2	75 20	100 1	22 9	94 34	100 47	15 41	75 4	- -	- -	- -	- -	- -
Morton County Hospital, Elkhart, KS	- 0	33 3	50 2	67 3	50 2	0 1	- 0	- 0	50 4	0 5	49 37	100 1	100 3	- 0	- -	88 50	100 66	53 47	100 1	29 7	- -	100 7	- -	- -
Mount Carmel Regional Medical Center, Pittsburg, KS	91 11	100 67	95 55	95 58	94 53	50 4	100 1	100 18	91 45	58 105	97 151	89 18	80 75	99 92	83 46	91 119	100 155	83 101	60 35	83 169	81 52	66 166	- -	- -
Nemaha Valley Community Hospital, Seneca, KS	- -	- -	- -	- -	- -	- -	- -	- -	- -	- -	- -	- -	- -	- -	- -	- -	- -	- -	- -	- -	- -	- -	- -	- -
Neosho Memorial Regional Medical Center, Chanute, KS	100 1	75 8	100 6	100 8	86 7	- 0	- 0	- 0	44 18	37 41	75 68	53 15	87 61	96 49	73 26	92 75	100 102	62 65	76 29	76 76	100 13	61 64	- -	- -
Ness County Hospital District #2, Ness City, KS	- -	- -	- -	- -	- -	- -	- -	- -	- -	- -	- -	- -	- 0	- 0	- -	100 1	100 1	0 1	- 0	- -	- -	- -	- -	- -
Newman Regional Health, Emporia, KS	100 2	93 15	100 7	93 14	100 6	- 0	- 0	- 0	74 19	68 69	65 104	100 14	84 68	88 40	76 17	85 93	100 106	88 74	100 23	77 99	90 29	70 81	- -	- -
Newton Medical Center, Newton, KS	100 2	100 16	100 12	81 16	92 12	57 7	- 0	- 0	78 18	69 62	77 101	58 12	88 96	89 44	76 38	78 111	100 138	78 91	47 19	84 333	89 80	87 315	- -	- -
Olathe Medical Center, Olathe, KS	82 40	98 129	98 157	93 113	97 187	- 0	70 10	100 94	91 105	74 243	100 308	100 50	84 113	93 75	91 32	72 156	100 213	90 133	97 61	95 624	95 197	75 602	- -	- -
Osborne County Memorial Hospital, Osborne, KS	- -	- -	- -	- -	- -	- -	- -	- -	- -	- -	- -	- -	- -	- -	- -	- -	- -	- -	- -	- -	- -	- -	- -	- -
Overland Park Regional Medical Center, Overland Park, KS	84 25	98 84	95 81	92 76	99 79	- 0	80 5	100 25	88 67	72 119	94 174	74 19	88 93	89 89	52 25	85 128	100 170	62 104	87 30	89 240	95 111	73 221	0.91 2737	4.41 1657
Phillips County Hospital, Phillipsburg, KS	- 0	- 0	- 0	100 1	100 1	- 0	- -	- 0	100 6	0 5	40 15	0 1	70 10	67 3	88 8	80 10	100 18	60 15	50 2	- -	- -	- -	- -	- -
Pratt Regional Medical Center, Pratt, KS	- 0	100 2	- 0	100 2	- 0	- 0	- 0	- 0	67 3	42 26	50 30	50 8	72 36	95 19	67 12	84 58	100 61	69 49	57 7	93 112	89 35	97 110	- -	- -
Providence Medical Center, Kansas City, KS	94 66	96 153	96 172	97 118	98 180	- 0	44 9	100 71	83 209	65 394	97 476	98 131	82 148	95 152	95 39	90 191	100 246	86 134	99 93	91 478	87 143	85 428	0.13 1559	2.67 1161
Ransom Memorial Hospital, Ottawa, KS	100 1	100 5	100 4	100 3	75 4	- 0	- 0	100 1	73 15	79 33	91 44	100 3	96 69	95 55	97 34	93 97	100 116	89 83	100 32	41 27	100 7	35 26	- -	- -
Republic County Hospital, Belleville, KS	- 0	100 7	67 6	75 8	71 7	0 2	- 0	100 1	- -	- -	- -	- -	49 69	100 4	65 20	87 54	97 79	71 62	69 13	63 43	90 10	41 44	- -	- -
Sabetha Community Hospital, Sabetha, KS	- 0	100 2	100 2	0 1	100 2	- 0	- 0	- 0	75 4	0 3	73 11	- 0	100 17	100 1	67 3	95 22	100 33	68 25	50 4	75 4	- -	75 4	- -	- -
Saint Catherine's Hospital, Garden City, KS	- 0	89 9	100 3	67 9	67 3	- 0	- 0	100 1	60 10	65 31	57 42	83 6	84 74	94 48	- -	82 79	100 94	67 48	50 16	67 371	44 108	61 375	0.00 925	3.91 665
Saint Francis Health Center, Topeka, KS	86 77	99 136	95 247	95 101	96 270	0 1	33 6	99 91	91 90	78 180	99 230	91 47	91 157	92 65	94 54	82 224	100 264	92 173	91 85	83 218	97 73	87 213	0.00 925	4.76 715
Saint John Hospital, Leavenworth, KS	25 4	80 10	67 9	67 9	50 8	- 0	- 0	- 0	73 15	88 43	80 50	100 15	83 35	96 23	71 7	85 55	98 66	81 36	100 13	78 37	90 10	74 31	0.00 258	1.57 191
Saint Luke Hospital & Living Center, Marion, KS	- -	- -	- -	- -	- -	- -	- -	- -	75 4	8 13	41 27	0 2	86 14	100 1	25 8	94 16	100 28	8 25	25 4	100 1	100 1	100 1	- -	- -
Saint Luke's South, Overland Park, KS	100 4	100 43	95 42	92 40	98 41	- 0	100 3	100 17	83 41	60 70	98 89	100 7	86 66	95 43	87 23	90 78	100 94	92 64	100 10	94 211	94 81	80 206	- -	- -
Salina Regional Health Center, Salina, KS	91 35	95 120	96 194	88 115	87 192	62 13	0 3	97 73	95 60	50 137	76 186	86 28	86 120	95 110	53 53	76 173	100 211	53 147	76 55	92 623	96 143	61 604	- -	- -
Salina Surgical Hospital, Salina, KS	- -	- -	- -	- -	- -	- -	- -	- -	- -	- -	- -	- -	- -	- -	- -	- -	- -	- -	- -	93 374	99 103	76 372	- -	- -
Scott County Hospital, Scott City, KS	- -	- -	- -	- -	- -	- -	- -	- -	- -	- -	- -	- -	- -	- -	- -	- -	- -	- -	- -	- -	- -	- -	- -	- -
Shawnee Mission Medical Center, Shawnee Mission, KS	96 55	100 209	99 211	99 189	99 203	- 0	57 14	96 77	99 136	40 284	98 372	65 51	83 215	95 187	74 69	79 297	100 340	69 228	70 54	74 627	93 59	66 620	0.06 3593	4.21 2447
Smith County Memorial Hospital, Smith Center, KS	- 0	100 4	67 3	50 4	100 3	50 2	- 0	- 0	100 1	35 17	58 24	- 0	88 16	100 3	60 5	93 15	100 21	93 14	50 2	- -	- -	- -	- -	- -
South Central Kansas Regional Medical Center, Arkansas City, KS	33 3	75 12	44 9	45 11	50 8	- 0	- 0	0 1	60 5	4 26	41 44	38 8	78 58	67 3	64 25	71 58	100 71	22 49	50 18	43 49	94 16	97 36	- -	- -
Southwest Medical Center, Liberal, KS	100 1	100 11	86 7	100 8	80 5	0 1	- 0	- 0	75 8	79 28	81 37	33 3	68 28	100 14	62 13	93 46	100 68	59 34	36 14	68 98	39 23	42 97	- -	- -
Stormont-Vail Healthcare, Topeka, KS	89 37	96 184	97 233	98 171	100 229	33 3	100 14	100 74	89 118	71 216	98 298	100 48	98 166	96 204	90 72	76 250	100 331	88 221	100 102	89 431	96 67	91 411	- -	- -
Summit Surgical, Hutchinson, KS	- -	- -	- -	- -	- -	- -	- -	- -	- -	- -	- -	- -	- -	- -	- -	- -	- -	- -	- -	- -	- -	- -	- -	- -
Sumner Regional Medical Center, Wellington, KS	- 0	33 3	0 3	67 3	33 3	- 0	- 0	- 0	100 1	0 16	9 22	33 3	60 15	100 2	- -	76 21	96 25	0 19	0 4	43 7	100 3	100 7	- -	- -
Surgical and Diagnostic Center of Great Bend, Great Bend, KS	- -	- -	- -	- -	- -	- -	- -	- -	- -	- -	- -	- -	- -	- -	- -	- -	- -	- -	- -	91 23	- -	30 23	- -	- -
Susan B Allen Memorial Hospital, El Dorado, KS	- 0	100 7	100 4	100 4	100 3	- 0	- 0	100 1	100 6	92 26	73 64	100 9	85 53	100 3	88 17	88 73	100 89	88 51	88 24	81 79	96 27	63 76	0.00 292	3.68 190
Trego County-Lemke Memorial Hospital, WaKeeney, KS	- 0	100 1	100 1	100 1	100 1	- 0	- -	- 0	0 2	100 6	40 10	- 0	55 22	100 2	- -	78 23	100 24	67 21	0 3	- -	- -	- -	- -	- -
University of Kansas Medical Center, Kansas City, KS	92 61	100 110	98 245	99 106	99 242	- 0	75 8	100 111	93 165	89 261	99 295	96 81	91 134	94 142	89 35	82 202	100 265	89 90	95 99	85 342	95 74	61 330	- -	- -
Via Christi Regional Medical Center, Wichita, KS	85 153	95 581	93 715	93 531	93 691	25 4	47 15	95 301	78 360	57 707	89 842	97 159	72 197	89 81	86 28	83 184	100 262	70 161	82 77	94 790	96 136	38 763	0.34 2940	3.20 2091
Wamego City Hospital, Wamego, KS	- 0	0 1	100 1	- 0	100 1	- 0	- 0	- 0	100 2	0 10	23 13	- 0	100 4	0 1	- -	100 7	100 12	10 10	- 0	- -	- -	- -	- -	- -
Washington County Hospital, Washington, KS	- -	- -	- -	- -	- -	- -	- -	- -	- 0	20 5	50 4	- 0	78 9	- 0	100 4	100 7	100 10	100 10	0 1	- -	- -	- -	- -	- -
Wesley Medical Center, Wichita, KS	90 69	97 258	97 291	98 187	97 321	- 0	58 12	97 170	78 136	56 331	95 430	97 89	78 223	94 218	74 74	76 317	100 387	76 240	82 110	79 325	60 154	77 312	- -	- -
Western Plains Medical Company, Dodge City, KS	67 3	96 28	100 23	80 20	77 22	- 0	25 4	82 11	75 20	56 48	74 65	83 6	70 57	98 42	55 22	77 90	100 107	82 68	68 28	63 90	87 31	48 83	- -	- -
William Newton Memorial Hospital, Winfield, KS	- 0	67 3	100 1	100 3	100 2	- 0	- 0	100 1	83 6	70 20	85 26	100 1	85 26	89 19	89 18	86 35	98 46	88 40	75 4	97 62	86 22	92 62	- -	- -
Wilson County Hospital, Neodesha, KS	- -	- -	- -	- -	- -	- -	- -	- -	- -	- -	- -	- -	- -	- -	- -	- -	- -	- -	- -	- -	- -	- -	- -	- -
MICHIGAN																								
Allegan General Hospital, Allegan, MI	- 0	60 10	50 6	60 10	50 6	- 0	- 0	100 1	67 15	49 55	76 71	60 5	83 60	83 54	62 13	86 84	97 89	73 59	82 17	90 60	80 30	93 59	- -	- -
Alpena Regional Medical Center, Alpena, MI	80 5	99 69	86 36	96 52	100 48	37 19	- 0	100 11	78 81	80 176	92 223	92 24	92 165	96 149	86 36	87 205	100 255	91 181	88 51	89 419	98 110	93 406	- -	- -
Battle Creek Health System, Battle Creek, MI	77 22	93 105	90 63	93 57	93 72	- 0	- 0	97 29	84 181	55 350	97 437	97 114	87 221	86 231	- -	80 326	100 390	86 238	95 120	81 715	100 164	87 666	0.28 1067	2.80 857
Bay Regional Medical Center, Bay City, MI	82 77	93 213	97 332	88 208	93 322	- 0	71 14	99 122	74 310	94 686	97 803	99 116	91 233	91 211	60 63	86 354	100 414	76 291	98 84	91 1106	96 244	90 1065	- -	- -

NOTE: The first number in each column (boldface) is the rate in percent, the second number is the number of patients; Please refer to the main entry for footnotes; ***Heart Attack Care:*** *1. ACE Inhibitor or ARB for LVSD; 2. Aspirin at Arrival; 3. Aspirin at Discharge; 4. Beta Blocker at Arrival; 5. Beta Blocker at Discharge; 6. Fibrinolytic Medication Timing; 7. PCI Within 90 Minutes of Arrival; 8. Smoking Cessation Advice;* ***Heart Failure Care:*** *9. ACE Inhibitor or ARB for LVSD; 10. Discharge Instructions; 11. Evaluation of LVS Function; 12. Smoking Cessation Advice;* ***Pneumonia Care:*** *13. Appropriate Initial Antibiotic; 14. Blood Culture Timing; 15. Influenza Vaccine; 16. Initial Antibiotic Timing; 17. Oxygenation Assessment; 18. Pneumococcal Vaccine; 19. Smoking Cessation Advice;* ***Surgical Infection Prevention:*** *20. Prophylactic Antibiotic Given; 21. Prophylactic Antibiotic Selection; 22. Prophylactic Antibiotic Stopped;* ***Pregnancy Care:*** *23. Inpatient Neonatal Mortality; 24. Third or Fourth Degree Laceration*

Hospital	Heart Attack Care								Heart Failure Care				Pneumonia Care							Surgical Infection Prevention			Pregnancy Care	
	1	2	3	4	5	6	7	8	9	10	11	12	13	14	15	16	17	18	19	20	21	22	23	24
Bixby Medical Center, Adrian, MI	**67** 3	**92** 39	**80** 20	**96** 28	**81** 16	- 0	- 0	**100** 3	**96** 24	**74** 54	**93** 68	**100** 6	**95** 74	**89** 76	**86** 21	**78** 112	**99** 139	**91** 96	**82** 28	**64** 216	**88** 73	**83** 209	- -	- -
Bon Secours Cottage Health Services, Grosse Point, MI	**86** 21	**97** 68	**100** 48	**91** 64	**98** 57	- 0	- 0	**71** 7	**80** 190	**61** 474	**92** 549	**65** 62	**80** 247	**87** 146	**91** 44	**73** 246	**98** 300	**77** 178	**84** 74	**86** 659	**95** 233	**81** 641	- -	- -
Borgess Medical Center, Kalamazoo, MI	**78** 59	**97** 89	**98** 275	**92** 73	**96** 273	**0** 1	**43** 7	**99** 99	**82** 137	**76** 240	**98** 280	**94** 53	**90** 81	**93** 87	**86** 21	**87** 110	**100** 139	**86** 95	**86** 50	**82** 347	**89** 84	**84** 330	- -	- -
Borgess-Lee Memorial Hospital, Dowagiac, MI	**100** 1	**100** 2	**100** 1	**67** 3	**100** 1	- 0	- 0	- 0	**88** 33	**63** 65	**76** 71	**81** 16	**94** 66	**88** 57	**67** 21	**91** 79	**100** 101	**44** 52	**69** 26	**47** 15	**100** 3	**86** 14	- -	- -
Botsford General Hospital, Farmington, MI	**92** 48	**100** 249	**92** 168	**99** 231	**97** 174	- 0	**0** 7	**84** 32	**92** 200	**66** 481	**95** 622	**96** 113	**86** 243	**87** 306	- -	**81** 393	**100** 475	**59** 289	**86** 97	**89** 396	**94** 154	**84** 370	- -	- -
Brighton Hospital, Brighton, MI	- -	- -	- -	- -	- -	- -	- -	- -	- -	- -	- -	- -	- -	- -	- -	- -	- -	- -	- -	- -	- -	- -	- -	- -
Bronson Methodist Hospital, Kalamazoo, MI	**80** 124	**98** 280	**98** 388	**95** 257	**98** 428	**0** 1	**69** 13	**99** 141	**88** 190	**94** 539	**99** 664	**90** 130	**97** 222	**91** 280	**77** 71	**81** 300	**100** 426	**80** 285	**94** 104	**96** 1653	**98** 408	**90** 1605	- -	- -
Bronson Vicksburg Hospital, Vicksburg, MI	- -	- -	- -	- -	- -	- -	- -	- -	- -	- -	- -	- -	- -	- -	- -	- -	- -	- -	- -	- -	- -	- -	- -	- -
Carson City Hospital, Carson City, MI	**100** 1	**100** 9	**75** 4	**100** 5	**100** 1	- 0	- 0	**100** 3	**82** 11	**83** 30	**97** 39	**100** 5	**92** 53	**92** 26	**76** 17	**85** 54	**100** 72	**79** 43	**100** 19	**96** 176	**94** 35	**94** 172	- -	- -
Central Michigan Community Hospital, Mount Pleasant, MI	**100** 4	**97** 35	**100** 20	**86** 36	**82** 22	**50** 4	- 0	**50** 8	**88** 34	**90** 103	**94** 141	**93** 27	**87** 101	**95** 87	**86** 21	**81** 139	**100** 172	**93** 94	**96** 51	**91** 278	**97** 72	**89** 275	- -	- -
Cheboygan Memorial Hospital, Cheboygan, MI	**100** 5	**100** 16	**100** 9	**100** 14	**100** 10	**50** 2	- 0	**100** 1	**100** 23	**100** 65	**99** 79	**100** 7	**92** 64	**97** 64	**100** 21	**81** 96	**100** 114	**94** 72	**81** 16	**95** 154	**100** 40	**98** 148	**0.41** 244	**3.05** 164
Chelsea Community Hospital, Chelsea, MI	**100** 4	**100** 22	**100** 15	**90** 21	**100** 18	- 0	- 0	**100** 1	**100** 18	**87** 45	**98** 61	**100** 5	**100** 86	**94** 98	**100** 22	**92** 100	**100** 127	**99** 96	**100** 26	**99** 640	**98** 153	**96** 628	- -	- -
Chippewa County War Memorial Hospital, Sault Ste Marie, MI	**33** 3	**85** 27	**65** 17	**87** 30	**76** 21	**100** 1	- 0	**80** 5	**43** 30	**13** 85	**84** 108	**18** 11	**64** 119	**95** 78	**45** 11	**79** 132	**93** 149	**36** 90	**31** 26	**21** 107	**90** 31	**61** 99	**0.30** 333	**5.93** 236
Clinton Memorial Hospital, Saint Johns, MI	- 0	**100** 4	**100** 4	**100** 4	**100** 3	- 0	- 0	- 0	**70** 10	**43** 30	**85** 33	**100** 4	**79** 34	**95** 20	**25** 12	**84** 31	**100** 40	**72** 25	**91** 11	- -	- -	- -	- -	- -
Community Health Center of Branch County, Coldwater, MI	**100** 1	**78** 18	**67** 9	**89** 18	**56** 9	- 0	- 0	**0** 1	**67** 21	**73** 83	**65** 105	**83** 6	**85** 121	**91** 92	**62** 26	**84** 115	**100** 149	**47** 90	**71** 38	**88** 285	**88** 65	**87** 267	- -	- -
Community Hospital Watervliet, Watervliet, MI	- 0	**83** 12	**100** 5	**55** 11	**67** 3	- 0	- 0	- 0	**50** 18	**92** 12	**64** 84	**38** 8	**90** 20	**87** 15	- -	**89** 74	**99** 94	**70** 63	**70** 23	**93** 152	**98** 41	**89** 151	- -	- -
Covenant Medical Center, Saginaw, MI	**80** 145	**96** 296	**94** 338	**88** 224	**95** 454	**0** 1	**38** 8	**100** 199	**73** 360	**74** 691	**98** 808	**97** 180	**90** 290	**90** 351	**87** 68	**83** 427	**100** 541	**88** 320	**98** 148	**83** 583	**96** 143	**66** 559	- -	- -
Crittenton Hospital Medical Center, Rochester, MI	**100** 15	**98** 90	**99** 81	**91** 68	**95** 81	- 0	**67** 3	**100** 26	**88** 113	**67** 281	**98** 343	**98** 42	**88** 167	**93** 179	**50** 48	**84** 225	**100** 287	**42** 212	**95** 43	**87** 456	**97** 148	**78** 447	- -	- -
Detroit Receiving Hosp & Univ Health Ctr, Detroit, MI	**90** 42	**98** 196	**97** 169	**97** 186	**98** 161	- 0	**60** 5	**94** 86	**91** 386	**83** 672	**98** 720	**93** 323	**80** 266	**84** 210	**76** 34	**65** 322	**100** 349	**59** 76	**83** 183	**85** 96	**85** 26	**63** 81	- -	- -
Dickinson County Healthcare System, Iron Mountain, MI	**75** 4	**95** 38	**92** 26	**83** 29	**87** 30	**33** 3	- 0	**60** 5	**76** 25	**71** 83	**87** 123	**100** 6	**92** 76	**95** 74	**68** 19	**88** 103	**100** 147	**80** 103	**83** 29	**93** 255	**100** 58	**89** 247	- -	- -
Eaton Rapids Medical Center, Eaton Rapids, MI	**100** 1	**100** 7	**100** 2	**83** 6	**100** 1	- 0	- 0	- 0	**82** 11	**84** 32	**91** 34	**75** 4	**95** 20	**92** 13	**75** 4	**85** 27	**100** 31	**94** 16	**100** 9	- -	- -	- -	- -	- -
Foote Health System, Jackson, MI	**87** 38	**95** 259	**96** 137	**92** 222	**98** 168	**30** 10	**53** 17	**97** 61	**89** 138	**70** 327	**95** 401	**97** 70	**90** 128	**94** 89	**90** 30	**78** 169	**100** 202	**87** 117	**94** 54	**90** 190	**95** 60	**85** 178	- -	- -
Garden City Hospital, Garden City, MI	**96** 27	**99** 148	**95** 104	**100** 94	**98** 109	**0** 1	**100** 8	**94** 48	**94** 113	**79** 346	**96** 438	**90** 72	**93** 281	**98** 342	**74** 76	**87** 385	**100** 489	**70** 312	**73** 96	**96** 411	**99** 96	**93** 387	- -	- -
Genesys Regional Medical Center, Grand Blanc, MI	**79** 103	**98** 651	**96** 592	**95** 508	**95** 640	- 0	**36** 25	**99** 226	**80** 206	**63** 589	**91** 662	**98** 109	**93** 294	**85** 376	**38** 130	**83** 652	**100** 784	**47** 496	**95** 187	**89** 517	**97** 180	**81** 459	- -	- -
Gerber Memorial Health Services, Fremont, MI	**83** 6	**100** 17	**83** 12	**100** 9	**100** 13	- 0	- 0	**50** 2	**89** 28	**70** 80	**98** 92	**100** 13	**91** 75	**95** 80	**87** 15	**87** 95	**100** 122	**76** 87	**97** 29	**88** 228	**90** 58	**94** 218	- -	- -
Gratiot Medical Center, Alma, MI	**86** 7	**92** 51	**96** 24	**89** 36	**95** 20	**44** 9	- 0	**100** 10	**76** 51	**77** 168	**100** 232	**100** 29	**88** 109	**96** 134	**94** 32	**86** 170	**100** 219	**88** 151	**100** 35	**82** 143	**86** 49	**69** 131	**0.30** 656	**3.36** 446
Hackley Hospital, Muskegon, MI	**100** 8	**100** 62	**96** 28	**98** 61	**96** 26	- 0	- 0	**100** 2	**96** 48	**83** 121	**97** 153	**91** 22	**87** 119	**86** 94	- -	**96** 127	**100** 175	**94** 109	**95** 39	**91** 466	**97** 161	**91** 457	- -	- -
Harper University Hospital, Detroit, MI	**79** 56	**98** 83	**96** 117	**92** 72	**96** 152	- 0	**50** 2	**92** 63	**87** 388	**69** 813	**99** 872	**97** 185	**82** 90	**94** 117	**68** 38	**63** 196	**100** 222	**69** 90	**92** 53	**89** 952	**84** 203	**70** 908	**1.15** 5568	**1.18** 3893
Hayes Green Beach Memorial Hospital, Charlotte, MI	- 0	**100** 2	**100** 1	**100** 2	**100** 1	- 0	- 0	- 0	**88** 8	**60** 45	**82** 57	**73** 11	**88** 56	**90** 30	**79** 14	**78** 58	**100** 75	**37** 46	**70** 10	**62** 68	**80** 20	**69** 67	- -	- -
HealthSource Saginaw, Saginaw, MI	- -	- -	- -	- -	- -	- -	- -	- -	- -	- -	- -	- -	- -	- -	- -	- -	- -	- -	- -	- -	- -	- -	- -	- -
Henry Ford Bi-County Hospital, Warren, MI	**75** 16	**95** 88	**87** 46	**97** 58	**93** 46	- 0	- 0	**88** 16	**67** 94	**37** 268	**97** 319	**73** 45	**86** 140	**96** 157	**52** 33	**75** 207	**99** 244	**42** 128	**82** 71	**99** 253	**100** 54	**90** 241	- -	- -
Henry Ford Cottage Hospital, Detroit, MI	- -	- -	- -	- -	- -	- -	- -	- -	- -	- -	- -	- -	- -	- -	- -	**100** 1	**100** 1	- 0	- -	**80** 5	- -	**100** 5	- -	- -
Henry Ford Hospital, Detroit, MI	**96** 68	**99** 236	**99** 316	**99** 197	**99** 315	- 0	**80** 5	**97** 108	**91** 184	**48** 414	**98** 466	**90** 123	**93** 114	**87** 134	**57** 21	**77** 173	**100** 204	**59** 91	**86** 49	**93** 431	**96** 111	**89** 417	- -	- -
Henry Ford Wyandotte Hospital, Wyandotte, MI	**72** 54	**93** 273	**87** 180	**90** 290	**86** 205	**0** 1	**64** 14	**100** 53	**86** 101	**48** 227	**89** 285	**98** 40	**83** 113	**85** 124	- -	**86** 172	**100** 180	**54** 123	**98** 47	**78** 213	**86** 72	**97** 157	- -	- -
Herrick Memorial Hospital, Tecumseh, MI	**100** 1	**90** 10	**100** 5	**75** 8	**80** 5	- 0	- 0	**100** 1	**100** 6	**48** 25	**87** 31	**75** 4	**90** 50	**95** 39	**78** 9	**96** 45	**98** 64	**84** 45	**100** 10	- -	- -	- -	- -	- -
Hills & Dales General Hospital, Cass City, MI	- 0	**100** 1	**100** 1	**0** 1	**0** 1	- 0	- 0	- 0	**33** 6	**40** 30	**24** 42	**0** 1	**78** 36	**83** 29	**14** 7	**93** 44	**97** 61	**13** 38	**55** 11	**50** 8	**100** 2	**100** 8	- -	- -
Hillsdale Community Health Center, Hillsdale, MI	**100** 1	**100** 29	**100** 11	**100** 27	**100** 13	- 0	- 0	**33** 3	**98** 40	**74** 70	**87** 90	**86** 7	**87** 118	**83** 63	**71** 35	**74** 124	**100** 172	**72** 112	**83** 48	**49** 199	**79** 67	**11** 195	- -	- -
Holland Community Hospital, Holland, MI	**87** 23	**99** 128	**100** 85	**95** 96	**100** 88	- 0	**100** 6	**100** 27	**89** 70	**94** 137	**99** 180	**100** 26	**80** 178	**91** 182	**98** 50	**82** 245	**100** 287	**92** 182	**93** 69	**91** 543	**91** 139	**89** 519	**0.11** 1788	**7.07** 1231
Hurley Medical Center, Flint, MI	**88** 26	**97** 163	**98** 99	**98** 132	**95** 107	- 0	**75** 4	**98** 49	**83** 209	**81** 499	**94** 562	**87** 202	**87** 239	**90** 230	**78** 36	**72** 319	**99** 374	**73** 136	**78** 133	**84** 495	**92** 131	**82** 464	- -	- -
Huron Medical Center, Bad Axe, MI	- 0	- 0	- 0	- 0	- 0	- 0	- -	- 0	**44** 16	**7** 58	**57** 77	**0** 7	**70** 67	**58** 50	**0** 11	**92** 79	**99** 89	**3** 61	**0** 15	**45** 110	**100** 41	**79** 107	- -	- -
Huron Valley-Sinai Hospital, Commerce Twp, MI	**100** 18	**94** 100	**95** 56	**96** 76	**94** 64	- 0	- 0	**89** 9	**85** 68	**49** 225	**98** 272	**97** 32	**86** 107	**92** 107	**69** 26	**89** 148	**100** 190	**72** 100	**98** 50	**95** 625	**97** 163	**91** 607	- -	- -
Ingham Regional Medical Center, Lansing, MI	**95** 111	**99** 290	**99** 420	**95** 211	**99** 444	**100** 1	**33** 15	**100** 157	**94** 152	**98** 454	**97** 515	**100** 90	**87** 211	**69** 218	**67** 67	**83** 296	**100** 359	**54** 217	**97** 78	**92** 1642	**92** 519	**87** 1539	- -	- -
Ionia County Memorial Hospital, Ionia, MI	**100** 2	**100** 5	**100** 2	**100** 4	**100** 1	- 0	- 0	**100** 1	**88** 8	**74** 38	**90** 49	**83** 6	**91** 67	**94** 36	**25** 16	**83** 59	**100** 72	**45** 47	**87** 15	**70** 23	**100** 4	**100** 21	- -	- -
Iron County Community Hospitals, Iron River, MI	**67** 3	**71** 7	**50** 4	**100** 6	**100** 3	**0** 1	- 0	- 0	**100** 10	**68** 44	**56** 61	**33** 6	**67** 27	**89** 44	**100** 7	**79** 53	**100** 79	**64** 56	**55** 11	- -	- -	- -	- -	- -
Karmanos Cancer Center, Detroit, MI	- 0	**100** 1	**100** 1	**100** 1	**100** 1	- -	- -	- -	**50** 2	**100** 2	**67** 9	- 0	- 0	**92** 12	- -	**65** 43	**100** 49	**40** 10	**0** 1	**98** 44	**96** 46	**93** 44	- -	- -
Kelsey Memorial Hospital, Lakeview, MI	**100** 1	**100** 2	**100** 3	**100** 3	**100** 3	- 0	- 0	- 0	**100** 7	**97** 30	**100** 41	**100** 3	**90** 41	**100** 28	**100** 12	**97** 35	**100** 52	**100** 33	**100** 12	- -	- -	- -	- -	- -
Lakeland Hospital-Saint Joseph, Saint Joseph, MI	**79** 72	**96** 303	**97** 298	**96** 266	**95** 302	**0** 2	**56** 9	**98** 109	**88** 199	**82** 416	**94** 469	**99** 74	**84** 223	**94** 200	**86** 43	**81** 280	**100** 329	**74** 192	**95** 65	**70** 272	**86** 88	**60** 267	- -	- -
Lapeer Regional Medical Center, Lapeer, MI	**75** 4	**94** 85	**100** 40	**92** 80	**95** 42	**43** 14	- 0	**100** 5	**87** 70	**83** 178	**96** 212	**100** 33	**94** 159	**94** 198	**96** 49	**79** 220	**100** 254	**94** 152	**100** 73	**92** 404	**100** 107	**89** 381	- -	- -

NOTE: The first number in each column (boldface) is the rate in percent, the second number is the number of patients; Please refer to the main entry for footnotes; ***Heart Attack Care:*** *1. ACE Inhibitor or ARB for LVSD; 2. Aspirin at Arrival; 3. Aspirin at Discharge; 4. Beta Blocker at Arrival; 5. Beta Blocker at Discharge; 6. Fibrinolytic Medication Timing; 7. PCI Within 90 Minutes of Arrival; 8. Smoking Cessation Advice;* ***Heart Failure Care:*** *9. ACE Inhibitor or ARB for LVSD; 10. Discharge Instructions; 11. Evaluation of LVS Function; 12. Smoking Cessation Advice;* ***Pneumonia Care:*** *13. Appropriate Initial Antibiotic; 14. Blood Culture Timing; 15. Influenza Vaccine; 16. Initial Antibiotic Timing; 17. Oxygenation Assessment; 18. Pneumococcal Vaccine; 19. Smoking Cessation Advice;* ***Surgical Infection Prevention:*** *20. Prophylactic Antibiotic Given; 21. Prophylactic Antibiotic Selection; 22. Prophylactic Antibiotic Stopped;* ***Pregnancy Care:*** *23. Inpatient Neonatal Mortality; 24. Third or Fourth Degree Laceration*

Hospital	Heart Attack Care								Heart Failure Care				Pneumonia Care							Surgical Infection Prevention			Pregnancy Care	
	1	2	3	4	5	6	7	8	9	10	11	12	13	14	15	16	17	18	19	20	21	22	23	24
Marlette Community Hospital, Marlette, MI	- 0	67 3	- 0	0 3	- 0	- 0	- -	- 0	100 1	68 25	62 26	0 1	87 30	100 14	43 7	74 23	100 33	27 22	100 4	54 41	93 15	95 40	- -	- -
Marquette General Hospital, Marquette, MI	86 58	99 92	98 297	88 65	96 301	100 1	0 4	99 112	84 68	73 145	95 168	100 20	90 83	100 92	48 21	79 133	99 168	54 111	100 54	89 211	96 67	54 206	0.45 888	6.97 545
McKenzie Memorial Hospital, Sandusky, MI	- 0	100 2	100 2	50 2	100 2	- 0	- -	- 0	- -	- -	- -	- -	94 16	83 6	57 7	91 22	100 23	33 12	100 4	69 16	50 8	100 15	- -	- -
McLaren Regional Medical Center, Flint, MI	63 86	97 299	93 386	93 190	92 396	- 0	89 9	100 146	80 145	64 284	86 338	100 59	93 166	92 186	76 34	79 243	100 281	59 177	92 53	64 410	91 123	61 389	- -	- -
Mecosta County Medical Center, Big Rapids, MI	50 2	100 26	88 17	92 24	91 22	- 0	- 0	100 7	92 25	76 67	79 80	80 15	90 88	96 95	85 20	95 110	100 137	89 80	89 45	82 147	89 56	75 142	- -	- -
Memorial Healthcare Center, Owosso, MI	100 4	88 34	95 19	87 23	89 19	0 1	- 0	75 4	74 39	82 88	88 113	64 14	79 121	82 76	91 22	75 136	100 166	93 92	86 37	89 238	93 72	77 222	- -	- -
Memorial Medical Center West Michigan, Ludington, MI	50 2	93 15	100 6	100 6	100 7	- 0	- 0	- 0	87 45	42 79	92 98	81 16	83 60	95 79	83 12	89 89	100 110	81 81	65 23	82 160	100 60	89 148	- -	- -
Mercy General Health Partners, Muskegon, MI	94 126	100 229	100 406	99 187	99 406	- 0	27 15	100 36	91 100	77 75	98 306	100 18	100 13	100 29	- -	84 150	100 195	81 111	100 6	83 199	- -	80 193	- -	- -
Mercy Hospital, Cadillac, MI	100 5	98 66	88 26	97 62	100 27	100 1	- 0	100 2	98 40	96 79	95 99	100 14	91 116	86 102	- -	90 125	99 160	84 103	100 33	90 213	98 60	100 213	- -	- -
Mercy Hospital, Port Huron, MI	75 8	95 37	80 20	97 34	88 25	0 1	- 0	100 5	73 55	93 162	95 193	100 36	89 122	84 88	79 29	81 151	100 195	69 118	98 55	92 499	97 178	65 425	- -	- -
Mercy Hospital-Grayling, Grayling, MI	100 3	100 29	93 15	83 29	88 16	- 0	- 0	100 3	85 26	58 83	84 99	37 19	91 193	88 152	54 48	88 211	100 272	57 160	70 70	60 136	94 31	84 122	- -	- -
Mercy Memorial Hospital System, Monroe, MI	62 16	95 126	89 47	93 88	95 55	33 6	- 0	67 6	82 114	66 338	84 438	90 69	85 192	96 186	73 45	79 231	100 326	80 166	85 97	80 551	92 146	77 533	- -	- -
Metro Health Hospital, Grand Rapids, MI	100 20	100 103	100 64	99 91	100 66	- 0	90 10	100 22	100 57	96 122	97 157	100 25	97 117	96 142	87 23	92 174	100 210	95 116	100 56	79 253	94 65	83 244	- -	- -
MidMichigan Medical Center, Midland, MI	88 24	97 132	98 92	97 122	100 94	0 2	100 2	100 21	81 81	87 224	97 266	83 30	91 141	96 188	88 43	84 262	100 304	91 218	89 56	89 722	74 214	92 701	- -	- -
MidMichigan Medical Center-Clare, Clare, MI	- 0	76 17	89 9	75 16	90 10	- 0	- 0	100 3	60 20	73 116	84 126	73 26	96 112	92 124	79 33	89 159	100 182	72 122	82 44	22 64	35 17	54 63	- -	- -
MidMichigan Medical Center-Gladwin, Gladwin, MI	100 1	100 4	100 2	67 3	100 2	- 0	- 0	- 0	80 20	88 56	97 76	80 10	91 46	92 76	100 21	82 103	100 118	100 79	91 22	- -	- -	- -	- -	- -
Mount Clemens Regional Medical Center, Mount Clemens, MI	69 65	98 173	97 143	96 122	97 168	- 0	57 7	95 77	79 251	69 420	98 488	100 79	91 154	94 184	89 46	75 187	100 260	80 156	95 76	80 723	88 175	70 698	- -	- -
Munson Medical Center, Traverse City, MI	90 220	97 348	99 713	93 272	98 779	0 1	29 14	99 280	87 170	87 357	97 403	93 55	98 184	94 215	88 48	86 266	99 341	93 246	96 82	91 612	99 154	87 591	- -	- -
North Oakland Medical Center, Pontiac, MI	100 1	100 31	100 11	100 25	100 8	- 0	- 0	- 0	86 63	80 40	96 221	81 16	91 23	88 25	- -	68 162	99 193	74 93	100 7	84 67	- -	92 63	0.59 511	3.97 982
North Ottawa Community Hospital, Grand Haven, MI	100 2	60 10	71 7	86 14	88 8	- 0	- 0	50 2	70 10	71 42	85 59	100 1	87 38	90 40	88 8	84 51	100 63	78 41	57 7	81 119	98 42	93 118	- -	- -
Northern Michigan Hospital, Petoskey, MI	85 61	98 95	100 253	96 76	99 304	- 0	60 5	100 112	91 105	79 217	93 236	97 37	85 67	96 73	100 12	88 96	100 122	80 84	33 24	71 192	97 67	82 196	- -	- -
Oaklawn Hospital, Marshall, MI	- 0	100 10	89 9	100 8	90 10	- 0	- 0	100 1	94 33	87 78	97 92	100 13	96 96	96 109	93 27	94 146	99 173	93 116	93 44	93 371	99 110	95 362	- -	- -
Oakwood Annapolis Hospital, Wayne, MI	88 33	97 118	97 65	98 87	100 77	- 0	50 12	100 26	82 173	66 381	96 475	100 127	95 215	98 307	92 74	85 403	100 475	93 260	98 160	94 344	94 99	78 325	- -	- -
Oakwood Heritage Hospital, Taylor, MI	100 12	98 56	100 26	100 31	97 37	- 0	- 0	100 10	99 80	97 132	100 216	100 44	95 131	97 239	100 58	86 262	100 327	99 192	100 92	94 156	100 30	93 150	- -	- -
Oakwood Hospital & Medical Center, Dearborn, MI	92 339	95 535	98 861	97 350	98 995	0 2	47 19	99 399	90 563	71 1037	98 1236	100 270	93 432	95 515	85 94	67 642	100 803	83 472	94 231	93 1503	98 390	83 1425	- -	- -
Oakwood Southshore Medical Center, Trenton, MI	95 22	97 115	93 58	100 82	99 74	- 0	- 0	100 8	83 121	75 244	93 324	97 65	96 179	98 234	85 60	90 287	100 353	89 230	97 87	91 270	99 71	86 248	- -	- -
Otsego Memorial Hospital, Gaylord, MI	- 0	100 7	100 3	86 7	67 3	0 1	- 0	- 0	90 31	89 65	91 76	82 11	93 59	92 61	85 13	88 73	100 98	90 60	97 30	95 110	97 37	91 110	- -	- -
Pennock Hospital, Hastings, MI	100 4	89 28	94 18	96 25	88 17	- 0	- 0	100 2	94 64	70 109	98 146	93 14	86 105	99 93	88 24	87 152	100 172	94 102	88 34	95 253	96 54	94 244	- -	- -
POH Medical Center, Pontiac, MI	89 19	94 71	69 35	91 69	84 37	- 0	- 0	64 11	73 131	26 198	98 251	72 76	95 122	47 112	24 21	89 150	100 186	42 69	77 82	83 179	92 39	70 166	- -	- -
Port Huron Hospital, Port Huron, MI	85 52	95 206	97 289	91 187	98 291	- 0	40 5	96 89	89 127	81 302	95 370	97 64	93 215	93 162	76 49	83 266	100 318	79 196	100 83	83 640	97 142	86 624	- -	- -
Portage Health System, Hancock, MI	67 3	100 18	91 11	100 16	92 12	- 0	- 0	100 1	82 11	61 23	93 30	100 1	88 59	97 37	86 7	90 69	100 76	69 54	67 9	75 77	93 27	57 65	- -	- -
Providence Hospital, Southfield, MI	97 112	98 319	98 471	96 280	98 477	- 0	40 10	96 135	98 403	77 893	97 1046	87 188	94 374	85 358	74 80	90 507	100 591	65 340	89 118	95 624	98 279	89 577	- -	- -
Saint Francis Hospital, Escanaba, MI	38 8	94 32	96 24	93 30	88 25	- 0	- 0	100 2	62 34	78 86	95 102	70 10	79 104	95 113	100 21	90 156	100 194	89 125	93 29	73 138	89 36	75 120	0.00 250	5.44 147
Saint John Detroit Riverview Hospital, Detroit, MI	75 4	100 38	100 20	100 34	100 18	- 0	- 0	75 4	97 211	81 447	99 531	95 183	90 115	70 141	27 45	80 199	100 240	76 90	87 79	81 183	96 69	53 175	- -	- -
Saint John Macomb Hospital, Warren, MI	97 105	98 310	97 341	94 244	98 330	- 0	75 16	98 122	95 227	82 579	95 714	83 102	87 317	90 382	70 90	88 481	99 551	72 393	68 108	78 429	89 257	81 401	- -	- -
Saint John North Shores Hospital, Harrison Township, MI	- 0	- 0	- 0	- 0	- 0	- 0	- 0	- 0	50 2	0 2	50 14	- 0	67 3	67 3	- -	96 24	100 26	55 11	100 1	- -	- -	- -	- -	- -
Saint John Oakland Hospital, Madison Heights, MI	67 6	98 47	100 24	97 38	96 25	- 0	- 0	100 3	98 127	84 276	100 306	93 70	93 75	97 124	24 25	92 137	100 175	54 89	92 53	93 107	97 36	92 100	- -	- -
Saint John River District Hospital, East China Township, MI	89 9	100 24	91 11	96 23	91 11	- 0	- 0	100 1	98 47	93 112	94 140	70 10	86 79	81 93	71 17	83 93	97 124	94 78	92 13	92 112	100 36	84 102	- -	- -
Saint John's Hospital and Medical Center, Detroit, MI	95 147	97 342	98 508	96 259	98 570	- 0	29 17	96 217	97 294	80 642	98 729	94 203	92 394	86 419	74 85	79 575	100 666	72 327	82 192	97 1006	99 317	91 962	- -	- -
Saint Joseph Health System, Tawas City, MI	0 2	100 6	100 6	100 9	100 5	- 0	- 0	- 0	80 35	95 94	92 106	93 15	92 73	88 67	100 20	92 78	100 115	90 80	96 23	93 188	98 45	99 173	- -	- -
Saint Joseph Mercy Hospital, Ann Arbor, MI	98 163	99 415	99 642	95 314	99 640	- 0	50 18	98 263	93 330	72 745	99 917	89 142	90 301	97 370	67 104	82 512	100 655	59 466	73 152	91 374	96 91	90 357	- -	- -
Saint Joseph Mercy Livingston Hospital, Howell, MI	100 5	96 24	100 20	78 9	95 20	- 0	- 0	- 0	88 41	82 103	99 150	100 9	95 110	99 150	96 28	89 166	100 220	94 145	82 38	91 174	98 44	85 168	- -	- -
Saint Joseph Mercy Oakland, Pontiac, MI	100 97	100 280	100 409	99 248	99 398	- 0	78 9	100 136	100 261	87 585	100 685	100 105	95 186	90 303	85 72	86 380	100 469	84 293	90 124	99 1264	99 312	95 1175	- -	- -
Saint Joseph Mercy Saline Hospital, Saline, MI	- 0	100 8	100 4	80 5	80 5	- 0	- 0	- 0	100 11	82 40	95 60	100 2	90 41	96 50	85 13	94 68	100 78	85 61	92 12	91 35	100 10	89 35	- -	- -
Saint Joseph's Healthcare, Clinton Township, MI	100 54	99 323	99 308	99 278	100 305	0 1	100 13	100 95	99 158	87 530	100 693	100 75	91 292	60 301	87 68	79 386	100 447	88 298	100 104	94 1270	96 336	87 1212	- -	- -
Saint Mary Mercy Hospital, Livonia, MI	97 32	99 230	99 154	99 216	99 155	- 0	70 10	100 36	91 141	47 343	97 533	98 44	81 378	92 378	- -	81 550	100 687	49 500	92 83	85 504	93 176	78 481	0.14 711	2.22 992
Saint Mary's Health Care, Grand Rapids, MI	96 23	96 145	97 100	98 110	98 106	- 0	56 9	97 29	92 103	54 267	97 338	96 71	84 205	89 177	93 60	77 328	100 404	74 225	92 110	87 313	94 97	86 300	- -	- -
Saint Mary's of Michigan, Saginaw, MI	68 71	96 94	97 235	91 79	96 255	- 0	67 6	89 110	81 131	80 268	98 314	80 70	92 103	87 139	58 26	81 161	100 208	72 128	70 50	82 258	97 91	77 252	- -	- -

NOTE: The first number in each column (boldface) is the rate in percent, the second number is the number of patients; Please refer to the main entry for footnotes; ***Heart Attack Care:*** *1. ACE Inhibitor or ARB for LVSD; 2. Aspirin at Arrival; 3. Aspirin at Discharge; 4. Beta Blocker at Arrival; 5. Beta Blocker at Discharge; 6. Fibrinolytic Medication Timing; 7. PCI Within 90 Minutes of Arrival; 8. Smoking Cessation Advice;* ***Heart Failure Care:*** *9. ACE Inhibitor or ARB for LVSD; 10. Discharge Instructions; 11. Evaluation of LVS Function; 12. Smoking Cessation Advice;* ***Pneumonia Care:*** *13. Appropriate Initial Antibiotic; 14. Blood Culture Timing; 15. Influenza Vaccine; 16. Initial Antibiotic Timing; 17. Oxygenation Assessment; 18. Pneumococcal Vaccine; 19. Smoking Cessation Advice;* ***Surgical Infection Prevention:*** *20. Prophylactic Antibiotic Given; 21. Prophylactic Antibiotic Selection; 22. Prophylactic Antibiotic Stopped;* ***Pregnancy Care:*** *23. Inpatient Neonatal Mortality; 24. Third or Fourth Degree Laceration*

Hospital	Heart Attack Care								Heart Failure Care				Pneumonia Care							Surgical Infection Prevention			Pregnancy Care	
	1	2	3	4	5	6	7	8	9	10	11	12	13	14	15	16	17	18	19	20	21	22	23	24
Sinai-Grace Hospital, Detroit, MI	**81** 85	**95** 391	**96** 359	**93** 311	**95** 353	- 0	**33** 6	**93** 147	**84** 485	**92** 931	**99** 1083	**93** 406	**87** 206	**86** 301	**89** 57	**77** 434	**100** 519	**69** 203	**82** 146	**89** 784	**98** 198	**92** 718	- -	- -
South Haven Community Hospital, South Haven, MI	- 0	**100** 5	**50** 2	**71** 7	**67** 3	- 0	- -	- 0	**100** 10	**61** 33	**76** 38	**43** 7	**70** 71	**93** 46	**55** 11	**72** 75	**100** 87	**49** 45	**80** 20	**74** 73	**83** 30	**89** 72	**0.00** 430	**0.29** 342
Southeast Michigan Surgical Hospital, Warren, MI	- -	- -	- -	- -	- -	- -	- -	- -	- -	- -	- -	- -	- -	- -	- -	- -	- -	- -	- -	**0** 1	- -	**100** 1	- -	- -
Sparrow Hospital, Lansing, MI	**80** 112	**98** 245	**99** 408	**93** 211	**98** 410	- 0	**21** 19	**93** 145	**89** 244	**61** 493	**91** 588	**83** 87	**83** 221	**83** 221	**60** 60	**73** 328	**100** 399	**64** 249	**76** 106	**75** 1523	**88** 354	**70** 1483	- -	- -
Spectrum Health, Grand Rapids, MI	**93** 202	**100** 508	**99** 1025	**99** 414	**100** 998	**0** 1	**92** 37	**99** 380	**94** 335	**88** 826	**99** 1009	**99** 155	**97** 593	**86** 728	**91** 150	**88** 860	**100** 1061	**94** 661	**87** 271	**86** 372	**89** 119	**90** 363	**0.49** 8861	**2.15** 5726
Spectrum Health-Reed City Campus, Reed City, MI	**100** 2	**100** 7	**100** 3	**100** 7	**100** 2	- 0	- 0	**100** 1	**89** 28	**95** 59	**100** 69	**100** 14	**89** 63	**98** 66	**92** 13	**94** 94	**100** 99	**98** 62	**100** 30	**100** 38	**100** 8	**100** 38	- -	- -
Straith Hospital for Special Surgery, Southfield, MI	- -	- -	- -	- -	- -	- -	- -	- -	- -	- -	- -	- -	- -	- -	- -	- -	- -	- -	- -	- -	- -	- -	- -	- -
Sturgis Hospital, Sturgis, MI	- 0	**100** 4	**100** 5	**75** 4	**100** 4	- 0	- 0	**100** 1	**76** 25	**81** 94	**93** 119	**73** 11	**76** 67	**98** 46	**8** 13	**75** 65	**100** 81	**6** 53	**71** 17	**63** 99	**94** 36	**86** 97	**0.24** 424	**4.78** 293
Three Rivers Area Hospital, Three Rivers, MI	- 0	**73** 11	**62** 8	**73** 11	**100** 8	- 0	- 0	**100** 2	**50** 14	**65** 46	**82** 60	**83** 12	**88** 77	**86** 73	**81** 16	**84** 91	**100** 102	**72** 60	**89** 28	**24** 41	**81** 27	**100** 40	**0.00** 347	**0.00** 278
United Memorial Health Center, Greenville, MI	**100** 1	**86** 22	**100** 9	**100** 18	**100** 9	- 0	- 0	**100** 1	**100** 14	**89** 87	**99** 115	**100** 14	**89** 147	**94** 157	**100** 25	**94** 195	**100** 228	**93** 133	**95** 59	**97** 146	**100** 43	**94** 134	- -	- -
University of Michigan Medical Center, Ann Arbor, MI	**97** 70	**100** 273	**100** 396	**99** 240	**100** 386	- 0	**100** 8	**98** 125	**96** 279	**96** 569	**100** 634	**96** 120	**85** 240	**92** 357	**80** 70	**73** 397	**100** 561	**83** 293	**90** 110	**94** 1437	**97** 473	**76** 1341	- -	- -
West Branch Regional Medical Center, West Branch, MI	**100** 5	**95** 57	**95** 21	**98** 60	**100** 28	**60** 5	- 0	**100** 4	**94** 52	**69** 159	**91** 184	**92** 24	**80** 108	**94** 102	**63** 27	**70** 132	**100** 161	**51** 85	**75** 40	**65** 223	**97** 68	**45** 217	- -	- -
West Shore Medical Center, Manistee, MI	**100** 1	**75** 8	**100** 4	**44** 9	**100** 7	- 0	- 0	- 0	**50** 10	**75** 32	**72** 46	**75** 8	**95** 76	**95** 62	**6** 18	**93** 90	**100** 125	**20** 80	**86** 35	**86** 106	**97** 31	**73** 101	- -	- -
William Beaumont Hospital, Royal Oak, MI	**91** 128	**97** 356	**99** 409	**95** 298	**99** 478	- 0	**93** 14	**99** 163	**93** 225	**64** 476	**100** 592	**95** 78	**93** 242	**93** 271	**13** 61	**68** 379	**100** 501	**46** 333	**90** 93	**92** 478	**92** 119	**90** 465	- -	- -
William Beaumont Hospital, Troy, MI	**93** 90	**95** 296	**100** 252	**94** 216	**99** 273	- 0	**38** 13	**100** 85	**80** 260	**45** 543	**99** 666	**100** 62	**95** 262	**94** 295	**82** 71	**69** 381	**100** 496	**83** 320	**99** 100	**91** 712	**98** 187	**89** 662	- -	- -
Zeeland Community Hospital, Zeeland, MI	**50** 2	**100** 15	**100** 7	**85** 13	**88** 8	- 0	- 0	**100** 1	**92** 26	**94** 54	**92** 78	**100** 10	**95** 64	**97** 76	**100** 16	**95** 88	**100** 108	**97** 77	**100** 8	**92** 221	**88** 59	**91** 218	- -	- -
MINNESOTA																								
Abbott-Northwestern Hospital, Minneapolis, MN	**87** 190	**96** 245	**98** 803	**94** 220	**98** 923	**100** 1	**73** 11	**94** 348	**88** 394	**67** 681	**98** 844	**81** 135	**86** 236	**89** 201	**73** 67	**74** 341	**100** 451	**63** 287	**73** 90	**82** 173	**97** 98	**90** 166	- -	- -
Albany Area Hospital, Albany, MN	- 0	- 0	- 0	- 0	**100** 1	**0** 1	- -	- 0	- 0	**17** 6	**50** 10	**50** 2	**79** 29	**100** 3	**50** 4	**96** 27	**97** 31	**46** 24	**20** 5	**33** 3	**100** 1	**100** 2	- -	- -
Albert Lea Medical Center-Mayo Health System, Albert Lea, MN	**100** 7	**98** 43	**92** 37	**100** 43	**100** 39	- 0	- 0	**100** 9	**89** 28	**67** 52	**97** 74	**100** 6	**89** 54	**93** 59	**73** 15	**93** 83	**100** 97	**81** 78	**86** 21	**91** 206	**100** 51	**92** 194	- -	- -
Austin Medical Center, Austin, MN	**100** 9	**100** 27	**100** 14	**100** 22	**100** 11	- 0	- 0	**100** 1	**88** 26	**96** 78	**100** 113	**71** 7	**89** 84	**95** 99	**94** 31	**87** 149	**100** 172	**97** 149	**100** 14	**94** 144	**88** 26	**97** 136	- -	- -
Avera Marshall Regional Medical Center, Marshall, MN	- 0	**100** 3	**50** 2	**100** 2	**100** 2	- 0	- 0	**0** 1	**90** 10	**63** 30	**79** 42	**100** 1	**73** 44	**100** 12	**100** 5	**73** 30	**98** 49	**79** 38	**80** 5	**40** 5	**100** 5	**100** 5	- -	- -
Bigfork Valley Hospital, Bigfork, MN	- -	- -	- -	- -	- -	- -	- -	- -	**50** 2	**0** 2	**43** 7	- 0	**88** 16	**60** 5	**57** 7	**100** 18	**100** 25	**58** 19	**71** 7	- -	- -	- -	- -	- -
Buffalo Hospital, Buffalo, MN	**100** 3	**89** 9	**60** 5	**78** 9	**100** 9	- 0	- 0	- 0	**63** 27	**41** 41	**90** 59	**67** 6	**89** 74	**77** 66	**79** 19	**94** 89	**100** 123	**72** 82	**65** 26	**92** 64	**91** 35	**67** 63	- -	- -
Cambridge Medical Center, Cambridge, MN	**67** 3	**93** 15	**100** 7	**82** 11	**88** 8	- 0	- 0	- 0	**90** 20	**75** 51	**90** 77	**100** 8	**92** 80	**92** 48	**100** 20	**87** 111	**100** 149	**98** 88	**100** 30	**83** 63	**91** 35	**86** 63	- -	- -
Chippewa County Montevideo Hospital, Montevideo, MN	**100** 2	**89** 9	**100** 8	**89** 9	**86** 7	- 0	- 0	- 0	**57** 7	**0** 23	**39** 36	**0** 1	**69** 32	**100** 7	**57** 7	**88** 40	**100** 42	**30** 30	**25** 4	- -	- -	- -	- -	- -
Community Memorial Hospital, Winona, MN	**100** 4	**100** 23	**100** 16	**100** 23	**100** 17	- 0	- 0	- 0	**97** 29	**93** 15	**95** 86	**100** 2	**83** 23	**100** 24	- -	**94** 98	**100** 124	**89** 87	**86** 7	**87** 30	**37** 30	**63** 30	- -	- -
Community Memorial Hospital Association, Cloquet, MN	- 0	**100** 11	**89** 9	**100** 13	**100** 10	- 0	- 0	**0** 2	**72** 18	**15** 34	**79** 52	**43** 7	**79** 52	**77** 30	**20** 10	**75** 55	**100** 63	**74** 39	**47** 17	**55** 73	**93** 14	**96** 72	- -	- -
Deer River Healthcare Center, Deer River, MN	- 0	**83** 6	**83** 6	**86** 7	**100** 6	- 0	- -	**0** 2	**67** 3	**19** 32	**76** 38	**25** 8	**76** 29	**100** 8	**80** 5	**79** 34	**100** 38	**73** 26	**43** 7	- 0	- -	- 0	- -	- -
District One Hospital, Faribault, MN	**100** 1	**71** 7	**67** 3	**43** 7	**67** 3	- 0	- 0	**0** 1	**83** 12	**36** 36	**60** 52	**0** 1	**80** 50	**90** 42	**25** 12	**90** 68	**100** 74	**55** 51	**50** 12	**81** 75	**100** 29	**90** 71	- -	- -
Douglas County Hospital, Alexandria, MN	**100** 2	**100** 10	**100** 3	**67** 3	**100** 1	- 0	- 0	- 0	**84** 49	**75** 76	**97** 112	**100** 11	**89** 84	**96** 92	**94** 32	**93** 136	**100** 184	**95** 142	**100** 25	**91** 297	**94** 49	**89** 271	- -	- -
Fairmont Medical Center, Fairmont, MN	**100** 5	**100** 23	**100** 17	**95** 21	**100** 18	- 0	- 0	**100** 1	**100** 26	**86** 58	**94** 96	**100** 4	**96** 71	**100** 82	**96** 27	**92** 118	**100** 150	**99** 120	**100** 14	**90** 125	**97** 31	**80** 122	- -	- -
Fairview Lakes Health Services, Wyoming, MN	**100** 3	**100** 17	**100** 10	**100** 16	**100** 11	- 0	- 0	**0** 1	**96** 27	**40** 72	**100** 94	**79** 14	**89** 116	**93** 103	**100** 14	**93** 144	**100** 168	**82** 102	**72** 29	**94** 118	**100** 39	**69** 116	- -	- -
Fairview Northland Regional Health Care, Princeton, MN	**100** 3	**100** 20	**100** 10	**100** 14	**100** 11	- 0	- 0	**100** 2	**100** 20	**94** 53	**100** 72	**100** 16	**87** 61	**99** 72	**100** 12	**99** 81	**100** 101	**95** 66	**96** 28	**87** 90	**100** 22	**94** 84	- -	- -
Fairview Red Wing Hospital, Red Wing, MN	**75** 4	**92** 12	**89** 9	**91** 11	**88** 8	- 0	- 0	**0** 1	**84** 25	**74** 47	**96** 68	**78** 9	**90** 78	**97** 61	**83** 12	**90** 88	**100** 110	**88** 76	**60** 10	**93** 206	**97** 72	**85** 198	- -	- -
Fairview Ridges Hospital, Burnsville, MN	**100** 4	**100** 38	**94** 17	**100** 38	**100** 18	- 0	- 0	**100** 1	**93** 44	**91** 103	**90** 156	**58** 19	**86** 174	**97** 146	**96** 46	**80** 214	**99** 270	**86** 161	**79** 57	**88** 125	**95** 41	**83** 120	**0.19** 3088	**5.96** 2216
Fairview Southdale Hospital, Edina, MN	**98** 138	**99** 364	**100** 547	**100** 340	**100** 545	- 0	**96** 23	**100** 158	**91** 171	**92** 333	**100** 441	**100** 44	**91** 139	**98** 185	**92** 59	**82** 262	**100** 296	**93** 219	**100** 53	**96** 243	**95** 86	**91** 235	**0.00** 3643	**7.12** 2403
Falls Memorial Hospital, Int'l Falls, MN	- 0	**88** 8	**100** 3	**88** 8	**100** 3	**25** 4	- -	- 0	- 0	**11** 28	**0** 38	**100** 2	**72** 25	**100** 19	**100** 6	**66** 35	**100** 44	**64** 33	**83** 6	- -	- -	- -	- -	- -
First Care Medical Services, Fosston, MN	**100** 4	**100** 13	**100** 7	**92** 12	**100** 7	- 0	- 0	**0** 1	**100** 7	**100** 12	**89** 28	**83** 6	**75** 12	**100** 2	**100** 4	**93** 14	**100** 23	**94** 16	**100** 3	**100** 13	**100** 2	**85** 13	- -	- -
Glacial Ridge Hospital, Glenwood, MN	- -	- -	- -	- -	- -	- -	- -	- -	- -	- -	- -	- -	- -	- -	- -	- -	- -	- -	- -	- -	- -	- -	- -	- -
Glencoe Regional Health Services, Glencoe, MN	- 0	**75** 4	**67** 3	**75** 4	**100** 3	**0** 1	- 0	**0** 1	**79** 24	**31** 36	**74** 72	**0** 1	**87** 38	**100** 14	**40** 5	**83** 23	**100** 60	**69** 36	**20** 5	**65** 40	**100** 15	**79** 39	- -	- -
Grand Itasca Clinic and Hospital, Grand Rapids, MN	**100** 7	**95** 40	**84** 25	**95** 40	**97** 29	- 0	- 0	- 0	**94** 17	**27** 11	**84** 50	- 0	**87** 15	**89** 9	- -	**80** 107	**100** 123	**83** 99	**100** 4	**78** 49	- -	**90** 48	- -	- -
Hennepin County Medical Center, Minneapolis, MN	**98** 42	**99** 191	**98** 178	**99** 170	**97** 155	**0** 1	**60** 15	**96** 83	**84** 219	**47** 341	**98** 422	**70** 151	**81** 187	**75** 205	**30** 70	**61** 417	**99** 492	**19** 151	**56** 213	**72** 362	**83** 100	**74** 346	**0.52** 3080	**3.59** 2371
Hutchinson Area Health Care, Hutchinson, MN	- 0	**100** 6	**100** 5	**100** 6	**100** 4	- 0	- 0	- 0	**79** 19	**60** 43	**92** 60	**100** 8	**76** 34	**95** 37	**73** 11	**95** 58	**100** 68	**77** 48	**100** 9	**88** 138	**94** 36	**91** 134	- -	- -
Immanuel Saint Joseph's-Mayo Health System, Mankato, MN	**100** 20	**100** 105	**100** 115	**99** 98	**96** 107	**100** 1	**67** 6	**100** 30	**82** 79	**85** 138	**90** 181	**75** 12	**80** 75	**80** 66	**69** 26	**85** 81	**95** 133	**68** 109	**94** 17	**79** 135	**92** 49	**88** 129	- -	- -
Kanabec Hospital, Mora, MN	- 0	**100** 2	**100** 1	**100** 2	**100** 1	- 0	- -	- 0	**100** 9	**75** 48	**73** 63	**100** 5	**64** 50	**100** 11	**100** 14	**78** 79	**100** 81	**91** 58	**100** 14	**98** 47	**100** 17	**98** 45	- -	- -
Kittson Memorial Health Care Center, Hallock, MN	- -	- -	- -	- -	- -	- -	- -	- -	- -	- -	- -	- -	**25** 16	**100** 2	**100** 3	**100** 5	**100** 19	**33** 18	- 0	- -	- -	- -	- -	- -
Lake City Medical Center Mayo Health System, Lake City, MN	**100** 2	**75** 8	**100** 7	**88** 8	**100** 6	**33** 3	- -	**100** 1	**75** 4	**30** 10	**67** 9	- 0	**91** 11	- 0	- 0	**89** 9	**100** 15	**70** 10	**50** 2	**73** 22	**100** 6	**30** 20	- -	- -

*NOTE: The first number in each column (boldface) is the rate in percent, the second number is the number of patients; Please refer to the main entry for footnotes; **Heart Attack Care:** 1. ACE Inhibitor or ARB for LVSD; 2. Aspirin at Arrival; 3. Aspirin at Discharge; 4. Beta Blocker at Arrival; 5. Beta Blocker at Discharge; 6. Fibrinolytic Medication Timing; 7. PCI Within 90 Minutes of Arrival; 8. Smoking Cessation Advice; **Heart Failure Care:** 9. ACE Inhibitor or ARB for LVSD; 10. Discharge Instructions; 11. Evaluation of LVS Function; 12. Smoking Cessation Advice; **Pneumonia Care:** 13. Appropriate Initial Antibiotic; 14. Blood Culture Timing; 15. Influenza Vaccine; 16. Initial Antibiotic Timing; 17. Oxygenation Assessment; 18. Pneumococcal Vaccine; 19. Smoking Cessation Advice; **Surgical Infection Prevention:** 20. Prophylactic Antibiotic Given; 21. Prophylactic Antibiotic Selection; 22. Prophylactic Antibiotic Stopped; **Pregnancy Care:** 23. Inpatient Neonatal Mortality; 24. Third or Fourth Degree Laceration*

Hospital	Heart Attack Care								Heart Failure Care				Pneumonia Care							Surgical Infection Prevention			Pregnancy Care	
	1	2	3	4	5	6	7	8	9	10	11	12	13	14	15	16	17	18	19	20	21	22	23	24
Lake Region Healthcare Corporation, Fergus Falls, MN	100 5	96 27	93 15	93 28	93 14	83 12	- 0	100 2	88 34	66 71	86 120	0 5	83 48	92 51	80 10	96 82	100 102	76 76	58 12	84 179	95 83	79 174	- -	- -
Lakeside Hospital, Pine City, MN	- -	- -	- -	- -	- -	- -	- -	- -	100 1	- 0	40 5	- 0	0 2	- 0	- -	100 8	100 9	100 8	- 0	- -	- -	- -	- -	- -
Lakeview Hospital, Stillwater, MN	100 3	85 20	93 14	100 11	100 16	- 0	- 0	100 1	93 14	76 50	94 68	100 4	93 57	97 34	95 22	92 84	100 103	96 77	82 11	87 261	100 64	94 247	0.14 717	4.55 549
Lakewood Health Center, Baudette, MN	- 0	100 1	100 1	100 1	100 1	- 0	- 0	- 0	100 1	50 8	25 8	- 0	90 10	100 1	100 4	100 11	100 13	80 10	100 1	- -	- -	- -	- -	- -
Lakewood Health System Hospital, Staples, MN	- 0	100 2	100 1	100 2	100 1	- 0	- 0	0 1	100 5	4 24	47 34	17 6	61 36	100 4	29 7	91 43	100 53	19 37	22 9	92 39	100 8	76 37	- -	- -
Madison Hospital, Madison, MN	- -	- -	- -	- -	- -	- -	- -	- -	100 5	9 11	44 18	0 1	60 15	- 0	57 7	89 28	100 30	50 24	29 7	- -	- -	- -	- -	- -
Meeker County Memorial Hospital, Litchfield, MN	100 2	100 9	100 7	90 10	86 7	- 0	- 0	- 0	57 7	6 16	65 31	- 0	54 24	100 6	0 5	54 13	94 35	8 24	50 6	50 38	80 5	97 36	- -	- -
Mercy Hospital, Coon Rapids, MN	88 83	99 327	100 463	95 239	100 489	- 0	64 28	99 197	81 169	86 368	98 441	97 64	82 173	86 118	79 42	72 228	100 267	73 164	80 64	89 176	96 106	92 171	- -	- -
Mercy Hospital & Health Care Center, Moose Lake, MN	- 0	60 5	100 4	100 3	100 5	- 0	- 0	- 0	60 5	24 25	47 34	80 5	90 41	90 21	67 6	70 46	100 58	50 44	91 11	89 37	100 10	75 36	- -	- -
Methodist Hospital, Saint Louis Park, MN	96 72	100 273	99 318	96 199	99 329	- 0	85 13	95 94	90 203	72 409	99 536	85 54	90 289	92 269	73 97	83 431	100 566	79 377	79 117	97 236	89 82	91 232	0.08 3814	4.03 2801
Mille Lacs Health System, Onamia, MN	33 3	67 9	71 7	57 7	86 7	- 0	- 0	0 1	92 12	58 33	69 39	80 5	87 23	100 18	67 6	78 45	100 49	59 37	70 10	29 7	100 3	57 7	- -	- -
Miller Dwan Medical Center, Duluth, MN	- 0	- 0	100 1	- 0	100 1	- -	- -	- -	44 9	0 5	56 18	50 2	- 0	- 0	- -	100 3	100 7	73 11	100 1	89 36	- -	80 35	- -	- -
Minnesota Valley Memorial Hospital, Le Sueur, MN	- -	- -	- -	- -	- -	- -	- -	- -	- -	- -	- -	- -	86 7	100 1	100 3	100 10	100 12	75 12	- 0	- -	- -	- -	- -	- -
Monticello-Big Lake Community Hospital, Monticello, MN	- 0	75 4	100 5	50 4	60 5	- 0	- 0	- 0	92 12	24 34	80 41	56 9	87 46	83 24	42 12	72 50	89 71	46 39	41 22	86 14	100 14	43 14	0.55 550	8.68 484
Municipal Hospital and Granite Manor, Granite Falls, MN	0 1	88 8	83 6	75 4	88 8	- 0	- 0	0 2	83 6	56 9	85 13	50 2	57 21	100 3	75 4	87 31	100 38	75 20	0 7	33 3	- 0	100 2	- -	- -
New Ulm Medical Center, New Ulm, MN	75 4	83 12	67 9	92 12	83 12	- 0	- -	100 1	93 14	68 25	88 59	80 5	78 32	94 31	71 7	69 42	100 52	95 40	60 5	74 42	97 38	97 38	- -	- -
North Country Regional Hospital, Bemidji, MN	80 5	100 35	94 16	100 18	94 16	25 4	- 0	100 3	90 49	73 86	97 111	94 17	92 91	91 89	100 25	88 155	100 181	96 120	77 43	92 454	95 128	88 434	- -	- -
North Memorial Health Care, Robbinsdale, MN	87 155	99 495	98 500	96 447	98 506	100 1	92 26	97 145	85 242	58 452	91 580	68 92	87 308	91 184	77 74	90 387	100 471	64 285	85 111	62 93	98 92	79 89	- -	- -
Northfield Hospital, Northfield, MN	100 3	89 9	100 8	100 10	100 7	- 0	- 0	- 0	69 16	39 49	88 77	100 2	84 68	95 21	55 11	89 53	100 72	76 49	56 9	89 141	96 28	94 134	- -	- -
Northwest Medical Center, Thief River Falls, MN	100 1	100 10	100 5	100 9	80 5	50 2	- 0	- 0	36 11	36 36	63 52	67 3	76 25	88 8	100 2	81 32	100 42	79 28	50 6	89 147	95 38	94 142	- -	- -
Olmsted Medical Center Hospital, Rochester, MN	100 2	100 7	100 5	75 4	86 7	- 0	- 0	- 0	83 12	86 7	86 37	- 0	80 10	88 8	- -	68 47	98 62	77 39	100 4	78 40	- -	54 39	- -	- -
Ortonville Area Health Services, Ortonville, MN	50 2	92 12	88 8	75 12	82 11	0 1	- 0	- 0	100 3	18 11	50 14	33 3	33 12	- 0	0 5	100 13	86 14	0 10	0 3	- -	- -	- -	- -	- -
Owatonna Hospital, Owatonna, MN	67 3	92 12	100 10	89 9	100 9	- 0	- 0	100 2	100 15	98 51	100 62	100 4	95 84	98 62	75 16	93 81	100 94	94 78	100 13	88 78	91 47	38 73	- -	- -
Paynesville Area Health Care System, Paynesville, MN	- -	- -	- -	- -	- -	- -	- -	- -	100 4	31 13	70 20	33 3	94 16	100 3	50 2	90 20	100 22	64 14	25 4	- -	- -	- -	- -	- -
Perham Memorial Hospital and Home, Perham, MN	100 1	100 4	75 4	71 7	100 5	- 0	- 0	100 1	- 0	57 14	31 13	33 3	56 32	100 4	100 9	88 48	98 54	82 38	80 5	73 22	100 1	100 22	- -	- -
Phillips Eye Institute, Minneapolis, MN	- -	- -	- -	- -	- -	- -	- -	- -	- -	- -	- -	- -	- -	- -	- -	- -	- -	- -	- -	- -	- -	- -	- -	- -
Queen of Peace Hospital, New Prague, MN	- 0	100 2	50 2	67 3	67 3	- 0	- 0	- 0	100 5	95 20	84 31	0 1	93 15	91 11	- -	65 23	100 24	11 19	100 3	- -	- -	- -	- -	- -
Red Lake Comprehensive Health Services, Redlake, MN	- 0	0 1	- 0	0 1	- 0	- 0	- 0	- 0	100 1	0 2	86 7	- 0	100 1	100 1	- -	70 10	100 13	100 2	0 1	- -	- -	- -	- -	- -
Redwood Area Hospital, Redwood Falls, MN	100 1	67 3	100 1	75 4	100 1	- 0	- -	- 0	100 3	36 11	79 24	100 2	89 9	100 3	50 6	90 20	100 25	69 13	100 3	100 1	- -	100 1	- -	- -
Regina Medical Center, Hastings, MN	100 2	83 6	60 5	89 9	100 8	- 0	- 0	33 3	95 21	46 46	86 69	71 7	86 36	88 41	71 7	94 51	100 65	35 46	44 9	93 151	100 40	89 150	- -	- -
Regions Hospital, Saint Paul, MN	89 87	99 251	98 336	97 217	98 350	100 1	100 11	98 118	90 165	73 266	98 383	99 98	84 193	87 181	54 67	76 336	100 428	70 257	93 128	88 960	95 237	77 892	- -	- -
Rice Memorial Hospital, Willmar, MN	100 6	100 17	91 11	87 15	87 15	- 0	- 0	- 0	88 17	32 74	85 96	100 4	86 87	92 74	96 23	83 126	100 144	97 109	95 19	76 399	88 100	82 391	0.00 248	3.30 666
Ridgeview Medical Center, Waconia, MN	67 3	100 17	100 8	100 18	100 11	- 0	- 0	- 0	98 51	91 66	98 99	100 3	89 79	94 143	100 37	90 123	100 227	99 166	97 29	92 407	87 54	55 400	- -	- -
Riverview Health, Crookston, MN	50 2	89 18	75 12	79 19	75 16	- 0	- 0	- 0	56 16	56 34	48 50	17 6	79 28	100 13	50 8	85 34	100 43	75 28	83 6	88 24	100 8	65 23	- -	- -
Riverwood HealthCare Center, Aitkin, MN	100 4	100 8	100 7	100 7	83 6	0 1	- 0	- 0	100 17	66 29	82 33	33 6	0 1	100 1	- 0	- 0	100 1	100 1	- 0	- -	- -	- -	- -	- -
Rochester Methodist Hospital, Rochester, MN	- 0	100 1	100 1	100 1	100 2	- 0	- 0	- 0	79 14	53 34	98 44	100 1	89 9	100 2	100 22	61 23	98 40	92 78	92 25	96 511	98 93	87 502	0.23 444	2.58 1589
Roseau Area Hospital & Homes, Roseau, MN	100 1	100 6	100 7	67 6	100 5	100 1	- 0	- 0	83 6	22 18	45 29	100 1	88 24	86 14	78 9	76 25	98 42	79 28	75 4	- -	- -	- -	- -	- -
Saint Cloud Hospital, Saint Cloud, MN	88 113	99 211	99 570	96 168	99 604	- 0	82 11	95 213	85 256	75 430	97 556	75 73	92 209	96 226	90 63	87 314	100 390	92 287	80 87	60 436	95 86	76 418	- -	- -
Saint Elizabeth Medical Center, Wabasha, MN	- 0	100 1	100 2	100 1	100 2	- 0	- 0	- 0	- 0	100 1	20 5	- 0	100 8	100 2	- -	90 10	100 10	83 6	100 1	77 13	67 3	69 13	- -	- -
Saint Francis Medical Center, Breckenridge, MN	- 0	86 7	75 4	80 5	100 3	0 2	- -	- 0	100 4	58 19	41 37	75 4	82 33	100 1	83 6	90 41	100 57	93 45	80 10	- -	- -	- -	- -	- -
Saint Francis Regional Medical Center, Shakopee, MN	- 0	82 11	100 3	60 10	100 2	- 0	- 0	- 0	82 34	56 62	87 90	86 7	84 62	96 56	74 23	96 110	100 134	71 85	97 29	84 75	97 35	83 72	- -	- -
Saint Gabriel's Hospital, Little Falls, MN	100 1	83 6	100 4	100 4	100 7	- 0	- 0	50 2	80 5	14 14	73 26	100 1	77 43	100 30	52 21	83 72	100 85	60 67	57 14	- -	- -	- -	- -	- -
Saint James Health Services, Saint James, MN	- -	- -	- -	- -	- -	- -	- -	- -	80 5	38 8	54 13	0 2	50 10	- 0	0 1	92 12	100 14	27 11	100 2	- -	- -	- -	- -	- -
Saint John's Hospital, Maplewood, MN	80 15	100 77	93 41	98 48	96 23	- 0	- 0	50 4	84 94	82 174	96 248	85 26	81 139	90 89	93 29	91 179	100 221	90 140	44 34	77 739	95 229	77 737	0.07 3000	3.24 2343
Saint Joseph's Area Health Services, Park Rapids, MN	100 1	100 18	100 5	88 17	83 6	0 1	- 0	0 2	55 11	65 23	90 31	50 4	84 55	98 49	75 8	91 86	100 111	83 82	79 24	- -	- -	- -	- -	- -
Saint Joseph's Hospital, Saint Paul, MN	94 50	99 152	100 253	96 96	98 218	- 0	60 10	97 101	89 137	87 234	96 314	92 49	90 81	79 70	74 27	91 159	100 190	83 106	58 40	59 533	98 152	78 511	0.19 1038	2.64 910
Saint Joseph's Medical Center, Brainerd, MN	83 6	98 43	79 19	97 33	81 21	- 0	- 0	- 0	74 53	64 203	84 243	81 21	91 146	96 161	77 44	86 235	100 261	75 189	73 51	97 278	100 62	59 278	0.00 665	3.23 620
Saint Lukes Hospital, Duluth, MN	91 56	98 128	99 164	94 124	99 190	- 0	75 4	88 50	91 97	63 204	91 250	62 26	78 101	93 70	83 30	66 154	100 187	77 113	93 44	70 224	98 107	87 220	0.37 819	4.78 523

NOTE: The first number in each column (boldface) is the rate in percent, the second number is the number of patients; Please refer to the main entry for footnotes; ***Heart Attack Care:*** *1. ACE Inhibitor or ARB for LVSD; 2. Aspirin at Arrival; 3. Aspirin at Discharge; 4. Beta Blocker at Arrival; 5. Beta Blocker at Discharge; 6. Fibrinolytic Medication Timing; 7. PCI Within 90 Minutes of Arrival; 8. Smoking Cessation Advice;* ***Heart Failure Care:*** *9. ACE Inhibitor or ARB for LVSD; 10. Discharge Instructions; 11. Evaluation of LVS Function; 12. Smoking Cessation Advice;* ***Pneumonia Care:*** *13. Appropriate Initial Antibiotic; 14. Blood Culture Timing; 15. Influenza Vaccine; 16. Initial Antibiotic Timing; 17. Oxygenation Assessment; 18. Pneumococcal Vaccine; 19. Smoking Cessation Advice;* ***Surgical Infection Prevention:*** *20. Prophylactic Antibiotic Given; 21. Prophylactic Antibiotic Selection; 22. Prophylactic Antibiotic Stopped;* ***Pregnancy Care:*** *23. Inpatient Neonatal Mortality; 24. Third or Fourth Degree Laceration*

Hospital	Heart Attack Care								Heart Failure Care				Pneumonia Care							Surgical Infection Prevention			Pregnancy Care	
	1	2	3	4	5	6	7	8	9	10	11	12	13	14	15	16	17	18	19	20	21	22	23	24
Saint mary's Medical Center, Duluth, MN	94 179	100 216	99 501	98 166	99 589	- 0	69 13	98 224	87 217	62 301	93 395	88 51	88 117	94 109	77 35	80 170	100 209	84 148	81 64	89 95	92 97	93 89	- -	- -
Saint Mary's Regional Health Center, Detroit Lakes, MN	67 3	79 24	85 13	82 22	100 14	0 1	- 0	0 1	75 16	30 37	56 57	75 8	77 74	75 28	65 20	82 77	100 100	66 70	86 14	86 87	60 5	100 86	- -	- -
Saint Marys Hospital, Rochester, MN	87 62	100 124	99 233	99 103	99 269	- 0	70 10	99 75	89 135	85 247	100 329	83 30	90 73	94 72	87 23	85 124	100 167	90 134	79 19	94 494	97 105	63 483	- -	- -
Saint Michael's Hospital & Nursing Home, Sauk Centre, MN	- -	- -	- -	- -	- -	- -	- -	- -	100 1	0 4	100 6	0 1	85 13	100 6	100 1	100 19	100 20	50 14	50 2	80 10	100 2	100 10	- -	- -
Saint Peter Community Hospital, Saint Peter, MN	- 0	100 3	100 2	75 4	100 3	- 0	- -	- 0	50 8	8 13	65 26	0 5	96 23	100 14	89 9	85 27	100 35	83 24	33 3	- -	- -	- -	- -	- -
Sanford Canby Medical Center, Canby, MN	- 0	- 0	- 0	100 1	100 1	100 1	- -	- 0	100 3	33 6	69 16	0 1	50 10	100 1	80 5	84 19	100 23	57 14	100 1	0 1	- 0	100 1	- -	- -
Sanford Tracy Medical Center, Tracy, MN	- 0	100 1	100 1	100 1	100 1	- 0	- 0	- 0	67 3	25 4	75 8	- 0	100 4	100 2	- -	86 7	88 8	86 7	0 1	- -	- -	- -	- -	- -
Sioux Valley Luverne Hospital, Luverne, MN	- 0	80 5	100 4	83 6	100 3	0 1	- 0	- 0	67 3	31 13	33 21	50 2	81 27	100 2	75 8	88 41	100 49	80 41	33 3	36 22	100 3	91 22	- -	- -
Springfield Medical Center, Springfield, MN	100 1	100 2	100 1	100 2	100 2	- 0	- -	- 0	100 2	100 10	83 18	- 0	100 12	100 1	100 2	93 15	100 20	67 12	100 3	58 12	100 1	70 10	- -	- -
Stevens Community Medical Center, Morris, MN	- 0	50 2	100 1	50 2	100 1	- 0	- -	- 0	- 0	80 5	86 7	100 1	92 12	- -	- -	100 29	100 29	62 21	75 4	- -	- -	- -	- -	- -
Swift County-Benson Hospital, Benson, MN	- 0	100 3	100 3	100 3	100 3	- 0	- 0	- 0	100 6	87 15	80 25	0 1	69 29	89 9	100 12	85 34	100 44	59 34	0 10	- -	- -	- -	- -	- -
Tri-County Hospital, Wadena, MN	- 0	100 1	100 1	100 1	100 1	- 0	- -	- 0	92 13	- -	- -	- -	81 80	92 25	77 26	90 109	99 148	68 104	86 22	69 29	80 5	57 28	- -	- -
United Hospital, Saint Paul, MN	89 74	98 288	98 462	96 228	98 499	0 1	100 22	99 170	76 272	74 404	92 544	88 73	79 225	87 176	70 47	70 287	99 340	59 197	84 80	46 171	96 94	73 168	- -	- -
United Hospital District, Blue Earth, MN	100 1	80 5	75 4	100 6	67 3	- 0	- 0	- 0	85 13	68 19	75 28	0 1	86 22	100 4	100 3	88 26	100 30	65 23	0 2	67 12	100 12	100 12	- -	- -
Unity Hospital, Fridley, MN	86 7	95 62	92 39	89 45	95 43	- 0	- 0	89 9	83 76	88 207	98 272	92 38	82 176	88 140	85 47	75 239	100 280	73 191	71 52	82 94	84 49	70 94	- -	- -
University Medical Center-Mesabi, Hibbing, MN	100 4	93 28	100 13	93 30	100 18	43 7	- 0	100 6	92 60	94 115	92 160	84 25	80 102	94 83	76 33	81 167	100 191	72 115	70 37	73 117	82 17	64 111	0.52 383	2.14 234
University of Minnesota Med Ctr-Fairview, Minneapolis, MN	77 47	97 95	99 142	96 81	98 133	- 0	67 3	98 49	83 158	68 241	98 284	96 48	71 125	82 115	88 48	60 212	100 274	79 113	99 76	93 191	97 66	89 185	1.11 2873	4.53 1878
Virginia Regional Medical Center, Virginia, MN	100 3	94 16	100 10	88 17	100 10	100 2	- 0	- 0	96 24	67 54	86 115	75 8	80 49	91 47	60 25	66 82	97 100	60 73	79 14	96 55	100 21	34 53	- -	- -
Waseca Medical Center-Mayo Health System, Waseca, MN	- 0	100 4	100 2	80 5	67 3	- 0	- 0	100 1	100 7	64 14	84 25	100 1	96 26	100 12	100 7	89 28	100 36	100 26	62 8	50 2	100 1	100 2	- -	- -
Westbrook Health Center, Westbrook, MN	- -	- -	- -	- -	- -	- -	- -	- -	- 0	0 1	0 1	- 0	50 4	- 0	- -	80 5	100 5	100 2	- 0	- -	- -	- -	- -	- -
Windom Area Hospital, Windom, MN	- 0	- 0	- 0	- 0	- 0	0 1	- -	- 0	100 4	33 12	71 17	- 0	39 18	100 1	100 3	94 16	100 18	83 12	80 5	67 6	- -	100 6	- -	- -
Woodwinds Health Campus, Woodbury, MN	80 5	100 23	86 7	77 13	75 4	- 0	- 0	100 1	92 12	72 40	96 49	75 4	92 37	84 37	92 12	95 63	100 83	96 54	67 18	71 645	99 217	83 636	0.00 1508	4.49 1137
Worthington Regional Hospital, Worthington, MN	- 0	88 8	100 6	88 8	100 7	- 0	- 0	- 0	71 7	40 5	79 29	- 0	100 7	100 3	- -	84 57	100 69	92 52	50 2	86 14	100 14	86 14	- -	- -
MISSOURI																								
Advanced Healthcare Medical Center, Ellington, MO	- -	- -	- -	- -	- -	- -	- -	- -	- 0	0 13	7 15	50 4	70 23	- 0	40 5	85 26	100 31	14 14	89 9	- -	- -	- -	- -	- -
Audrain Medical Center, Mexico, MO	100 10	100 50	100 49	100 33	100 48	0 1	67 3	100 20	96 78	90 148	97 196	89 19	88 97	97 126	94 34	95 154	100 195	97 118	96 50	92 193	97 68	75 189	- -	- -
Barnes-Jewish Hospital, Saint Louis, MO	90 180	96 450	99 624	95 443	96 689	69 16	100 11	95 224	92 430	81 715	97 842	96 184	80 237	86 208	61 56	65 401	100 459	54 161	85 152	93 715	96 160	82 636	- -	- -
Barnes-Jewish Saint Peters Hospital, Saint Peters, MO	96 27	98 165	94 142	92 160	96 146	- 0	25 4	98 54	82 50	56 121	95 144	95 19	93 156	95 161	74 35	89 204	100 224	75 130	93 44	93 357	96 74	88 351	- -	- -
Barnes-Jewish West County Hospital, Saint Louis, MO	- 0	100 1	100 1	- 0	0 1	- 0	- 0	- 0	100 14	74 43	98 53	100 2	94 54	100 36	70 10	89 66	100 72	92 51	86 7	95 710	99 197	94 703	- -	- -
Barton County Memorial Hospital, Lamar, MO	- 0	100 2	0 1	100 2	100 1	- 0	- -	- 0	100 1	0 10	18 11	0 1	71 7	100 4	0 1	75 8	100 8	0 5	- 0	- -	- -	- -	- -	- -
Bates County Memorial Hospital, Butler, MO	- 0	87 15	86 7	75 12	38 8	- 0	- 0	67 3	75 4	64 81	11 109	55 11	52 66	91 44	58 19	89 80	100 89	58 55	59 22	56 39	100 17	37 38	- -	- -
Boone Hospital Center, Columbia, MO	95 152	99 186	99 498	92 178	98 523	- 0	92 12	99 206	93 339	85 498	99 573	93 76	80 143	98 124	60 45	91 186	100 236	92 166	96 45	96 804	95 164	90 757	- -	- -
Bothwell Regional Health Center, Sedalia, MO	89 9	94 65	84 25	80 61	86 29	4 26	- 0	100 3	77 108	58 139	90 182	100 29	73 134	93 97	61 33	82 221	100 243	85 163	97 59	59 237	91 81	81 230	- -	- -
Callaway Community Hospital, Fulton, MO	0 1	100 5	100 5	100 5	100 5	- 0	- 0	100 1	70 10	57 14	89 37	91 11	85 40	100 17	25 4	62 42	100 51	48 27	88 16	67 3	100 3	67 3	- -	- -
Cameron Regional Medical Center, Cameron, MO	100 1	92 12	71 7	94 16	92 12	- 0	- -	100 1	80 15	32 31	75 63	90 10	89 65	81 84	58 26	92 129	99 161	62 108	92 36	65 51	100 20	55 51	- -	- -
Capital Region Medical Center, Jefferson City, MO	100 11	100 77	99 76	98 62	99 79	0 2	100 5	97 32	98 62	88 161	98 209	95 44	92 130	92 123	84 44	91 184	100 217	92 145	93 60	87 428	92 125	86 420	- -	- -
Carroll County Memorial Hospital, Carrollton, MO	- 0	100 2	50 2	67 3	100 2	- -	- -	- -	67 3	- -	44 59	- -	- -	- -	- -	92 60	97 79	49 43	- -	- -	- -	- -	- -	- -
Cass Medical Center, Harrisonville, MO	- 0	50 4	50 4	67 6	75 4	- 0	- 0	- 0	86 7	59 22	68 28	100 4	74 61	89 28	50 6	82 55	100 61	88 42	70 20	- -	- -	- -	- -	- -
Centerpoint Medical Center of Independence, Independence, MO	80 92	93 190	97 220	90 154	96 223	- 0	82 11	96 112	80 100	64 207	84 294	89 63	87 140	93 156	59 51	88 216	99 269	61 193	91 64	87 191	89 83	31 186	- -	- -
Christian Hospital Northeast, Saint Louis, MO	90 107	98 347	94 376	91 330	96 398	40 5	67 6	99 144	85 325	70 655	93 839	99 160	83 223	90 247	81 78	80 352	100 393	72 222	99 92	92 588	82 138	85 536	- -	- -
Christian Hospital Northwest, Florissant, MO	- -	- -	- -	- -	- -	- -	- -	- -	- -	- -	- -	- -	- -	- -	- -	- -	- -	- -	- -	- -	- -	- -	- -	- -
Citizens Memorial Hospital, Bolivar, MO	100 2	100 13	92 12	88 17	85 13	- 0	- 0	- 0	93 15	55 53	83 75	78 9	76 91	93 70	67 30	74 117	100 147	62 93	88 40	81 113	97 58	52 112	- -	- -
Columbia Regional Hospital, Columbia, MO	- 0	100 3	100 4	50 2	67 3	- 0	- 0	100 1	81 36	52 46	90 58	62 21	84 38	90 21	83 6	73 30	100 48	55 29	83 18	74 177	63 65	64 162	1.37 1894	5.85 1163
Community Hospital Association, Fairfax, MO	- -	- -	- -	- -	- -	- -	- -	- -	100 2	59 17	64 25	0 3	20 35	100 1	75 8	90 39	100 56	83 47	64 11	- -	- -	- -	- -	- -
Cooper County Memorial Hospital, Boonville, MO	- 0	100 6	75 4	100 8	100 6	- 0	- 0	- 0	60 5	89 28	76 41	88 8	78 72	85 26	88 17	86 94	99 102	96 67	92 26	- -	- -	- -	- -	- -
Cox Med Ctrs-North and South & Walnut Lawn, Springfield, MO	93 100	98 412	96 542	98 366	98 559	33 12	35 17	97 234	91 140	78 306	91 407	90 87	75 457	92 363	- -	73 576	100 693	60 345	77 194	82 706	98 547	80 691	- -	- -
Cox Monett Hospital, Monett, MO	0 1	50 4	50 2	60 5	100 3	- 0	- 0	- 0	75 8	65 23	42 36	14 7	66 56	91 43	- -	70 64	100 76	63 43	63 19	76 78	100 19	50 74	- -	- -
DePaul Health Center, Bridgeton, MO	84 104	96 264	99 267	90 189	95 283	50 2	57 14	100 125	80 265	72 551	93 686	99 150	87 235	96 280	84 69	75 345	100 459	84 258	98 137	94 1224	97 312	93 1135	- -	- -

NOTE: The first number in each column (boldface) is the rate in percent, the second number is the number of patients; Please refer to the main entry for footnotes; ***Heart Attack Care:*** *1. ACE Inhibitor or ARB for LVSD; 2. Aspirin at Arrival; 3. Aspirin at Discharge; 4. Beta Blocker at Arrival; 5. Beta Blocker at Discharge; 6. Fibrinolytic Medication Timing; 7. PCI Within 90 Minutes of Arrival; 8. Smoking Cessation Advice;* ***Heart Failure Care:*** *9. ACE Inhibitor or ARB for LVSD; 10. Discharge Instructions; 11. Evaluation of LVS Function; 12. Smoking Cessation Advice;* ***Pneumonia Care:*** *13. Appropriate Initial Antibiotic; 14. Blood Culture Timing; 15. Influenza Vaccine; 16. Initial Antibiotic Timing; 17. Oxygenation Assessment; 18. Pneumococcal Vaccine; 19. Smoking Cessation Advice;* ***Surgical Infection Prevention:*** *20. Prophylactic Antibiotic Given; 21. Prophylactic Antibiotic Selection; 22. Prophylactic Antibiotic Stopped;* ***Pregnancy Care:*** *23. Inpatient Neonatal Mortality; 24. Third or Fourth Degree Laceration*

Hospital	Heart Attack Care								Heart Failure Care				Pneumonia Care							Surgical Infection Prevention			Pregnancy Care	
	1	2	3	4	5	6	7	8	9	10	11	12	13	14	15	16	17	18	19	20	21	22	23	24
Des Peres Hospital, Saint Louis, MO	98 51	99 99	98 255	98 98	97 256	0 1	50 4	99 106	90 149	88 329	94 405	99 67	86 192	93 180	- -	84 261	100 318	77 213	97 73	77 342	86 92	52 338	- -	- -
Doctors Hospital of Springfield, Springfield, MO	100 1	100 1	100 1	0 1	100 1	- 0	- 0	- 0	100 11	35 17	84 38	83 6	88 40	84 38	100 2	75 60	100 77	76 50	63 19	95 37	100 9	86 35	- -	- -
Fitzgibbon Memorial Hospital, Marshall, MO	0 1	86 7	100 3	20 5	50 2	0 1	- 0	- 0	70 23	25 56	62 89	50 4	84 90	98 43	74 23	82 125	100 137	56 82	86 35	73 88	100 22	99 88	- -	- -
Forest Park Hospital, Saint Louis, MO	81 16	96 48	91 58	100 50	95 59	0 3	- 0	65 20	84 112	42 242	88 299	49 73	51 100	96 82	62 34	68 122	100 171	59 96	62 48	61 105	89 9	79 99	- -	- -
Freeman Health System, Joplin, MO	81 64	96 209	98 364	90 143	96 296	0 1	92 13	98 165	92 105	66 209	98 246	100 48	89 298	95 300	97 98	89 409	100 476	96 281	97 132	93 337	98 114	61 321	- -	- -
Freeman Neosho Hospital, Neosho, MO	100 1	100 12	100 6	100 6	100 6	- 0	- 0	- 0	100 15	96 27	95 42	100 6	97 73	99 84	100 26	100 112	100 128	100 76	100 36	- -	- -	- -	- -	- -
General JJ Pershing Memorial Hospital, Brookfield, MO	- 0	100 2	0 2	100 2	0 2	- 0	- 0	- 0	- 0	67 18	0 46	25 4	71 70	100 17	70 23	68 77	93 88	53 59	8 13	- -	- -	- -	- -	- -
Golden Valley Memorial Hospital, Clinton, MO	0 1	79 14	88 8	50 14	44 9	- 0	- 0	100 2	66 41	59 108	77 187	74 39	84 80	90 83	- -	91 142	100 165	67 104	81 59	73 59	100 25	76 59	- -	- -
Hannibal Regional Hospital, Hannibal, MO	100 6	100 36	91 22	94 35	93 29	50 2	- 0	83 6	91 54	89 112	88 162	83 23	81 171	95 202	61 57	80 259	100 353	78 240	90 68	89 310	99 100	83 299	- -	- -
Harrison County Community Hospital, Bethany, MO	- -	- -	- -	- -	- -	- -	- -	- -	100 1	0 5	46 13	0 1	88 43	100 13	40 10	96 48	97 60	41 34	13 15	- -	- -	- -	- -	- -
Heartland Health, Saint Joseph, MO	88 84	94 261	98 261	98 163	97 318	0 2	62 8	98 125	86 220	85 469	96 569	99 89	86 322	90 311	97 95	80 412	100 511	91 318	97 159	93 323	95 250	87 312	- -	- -
Hedrick Medical Center, Chillicothe, MO	- 0	80 5	100 3	100 3	100 3	- 0	- 0	- 0	100 7	82 22	75 44	0 1	84 44	95 21	92 12	84 62	100 68	94 48	86 14	60 5	100 2	100 5	- -	- -
Hermann Area District Hospital, Hermann, MO	- -	- -	- -	- -	- -	- -	- -	- -	100 1	80 10	26 19	33 3	89 19	83 6	50 4	90 29	100 34	44 27	75 4	- -	- -	- -	- -	- -
Jefferson Memorial Hospital, Crystal City, MO	66 58	97 147	93 181	90 141	92 184	100 1	0 2	71 73	77 126	81 280	81 349	58 45	78 215	72 103	8 48	59 267	97 314	18 176	68 92	66 244	98 94	89 238	- -	- -
Lafayette Regional Health Center, Lexington, MO	50 2	100 6	80 5	71 7	75 4	- 0	- 0	100 1	81 16	97 32	82 57	86 7	73 71	91 32	70 20	81 94	100 111	57 65	95 20	17 6	100 2	50 2	- -	- -
Lake Regional Health Systems, Osage Beach, MO	84 43	95 178	96 164	82 133	90 161	- 0	62 8	99 70	79 81	86 189	77 224	89 38	89 160	92 131	95 44	91 196	100 231	83 145	89 66	76 247	77 88	61 246	- -	- -
Lee's Summit Hospital, Lee's Summit, MO	100 16	99 81	100 70	91 66	100 67	100 1	75 4	100 27	82 45	61 79	94 126	100 6	86 99	92 89	48 40	85 171	100 197	76 135	100 36	85 143	78 58	80 137	- -	- -
Liberty Hospital, Liberty, MO	87 15	98 46	90 30	91 33	97 32	- 0	- 0	100 11	64 94	63 211	90 266	97 36	82 219	94 205	57 68	89 322	100 415	90 247	100 144	80 369	95 136	84 359	- -	- -
Lincoln County Medical Center, Troy, MO	- 0	50 2	- 0	- 0	- 0	- 0	- 0	- 0	92 13	71 21	91 32	78 9	77 31	100 20	83 12	83 36	100 46	79 29	50 10	56 39	88 17	36 39	- -	- -
McCune-Brooks Hospital, Carthage, MO	50 2	55 11	83 6	50 6	67 6	- 0	- 0	- 0	86 14	45 40	78 69	80 10	92 48	93 46	75 12	89 87	100 92	66 59	79 19	70 54	100 15	29 52	- -	- -
Medical Center of Independence, Independence, MO	50 18	98 89	100 74	76 63	94 68	- 0	71 7	100 26	64 55	66 143	91 176	97 29	87 102	91 101	77 22	82 127	100 165	86 98	96 49	66 77	83 23	49 70	- -	- -
Mineral Area Regional Medical Center, Farmington, MO	75 4	70 33	60 15	68 22	50 16	- 0	- 0	100 7	83 35	27 81	85 128	90 20	82 117	89 99	- -	82 174	100 201	46 125	87 52	69 70	91 11	80 69	- -	- -
Missouri Baptist Hospital Sullivan, Sullivan, MO	- 0	100 8	100 1	100 8	100 1	- 0	- 0	- 0	96 23	87 53	99 71	100 12	97 89	98 80	100 20	93 104	100 123	95 83	100 21	95 37	67 6	100 35	- -	- -
Missouri Baptist Medical Center, Saint Louis, MO	92 96	98 179	98 367	96 160	98 375	- 0	80 5	99 131	86 293	63 551	96 701	97 71	79 312	94 317	78 96	79 476	100 560	76 404	98 119	95 773	96 167	82 723	0.07 4228	4.24 2785
Missouri Delta Medical Center, Sikeston, MO	33 3	94 31	87 15	88 16	93 14	- 0	- 0	100 2	87 85	86 188	85 234	100 63	85 115	91 107	- -	79 173	100 224	76 132	100 76	52 86	77 31	83 78	- -	- -
Missouri Southern Healthcare, Dexter, MO	100 2	96 45	93 30	91 35	91 34	- 0	- 0	100 1	67 15	6 16	44 123	67 3	60 15	93 15	- -	78 106	100 137	59 83	75 12	100 1	- -	100 1	- -	- -
Moberly Regional Medical Center, Moberly, MO	100 4	100 21	100 14	88 17	100 17	- 0	- 0	83 6	100 27	85 62	94 101	100 18	84 98	93 85	75 32	90 144	100 189	82 124	97 39	57 53	95 22	96 51	- -	- -
Nevada Regional Medical Center, Nevada, MO	100 2	83 6	83 6	67 3	100 6	- 0	- 0	100 1	80 10	56 34	82 40	80 5	75 32	94 36	100 11	96 55	100 69	86 42	100 14	86 81	83 18	52 79	- -	- -
North Kansas City Hospital, North Kansas City, MO	91 122	97 234	100 303	98 209	100 319	- 0	76 21	98 134	87 134	60 299	97 343	88 59	68 200	83 126	51 43	80 265	99 322	75 193	82 77	69 480	97 125	74 469	- -	- -
Northeast Regional Medical Center, Kirksville, MO	67 3	100 15	100 13	100 17	94 17	0 1	- 0	100 1	58 26	64 50	98 87	100 12	81 59	97 74	67 18	86 105	98 131	75 92	88 24	50 149	95 55	64 134	- -	- -
Northwest Medical Center, Albany, MO	50 2	90 10	75 8	80 10	100 8	- 0	- 0	100 1	60 5	64 25	73 41	50 6	62 32	86 7	80 5	82 44	100 50	75 24	71 14	80 5	- -	40 5	- -	- -
Ozarks Medical Center, West Plains, MO	75 8	98 53	95 40	88 48	88 41	0 4	0 1	62 8	81 48	37 89	80 140	84 25	87 115	90 120	78 32	79 163	100 204	76 118	67 58	56 156	85 54	63 131	- -	- -
Parkland Health Center, Farmington, MO	50 2	93 14	100 12	73 15	92 13	0 1	- 0	100 5	82 72	85 105	97 186	90 30	92 99	92 83	100 27	91 144	98 157	85 101	83 41	96 112	100 21	97 101	- -	- -
Pemiscot Memorial Hospital, Hayti, MO	0 1	67 6	80 5	57 7	80 5	- 0	- 0	25 4	54 28	9 150	48 179	32 22	55 42	83 18	50 8	60 43	72 47	22 18	38 13	20 5	25 4	100 4	- -	- -
Perry County Memorial Hospital, Perryville, MO	- 0	67 3	50 2	100 3	100 2	- 0	- -	- 0	100 2	100 9	89 18	100 5	92 26	86 22	100 7	88 33	100 45	97 38	88 8	82 11	100 3	91 11	0.00 144	5.08 118
Phelps County Regional Medical Center, Rolla, MO	92 13	89 91	88 56	92 78	95 73	- 0	- 0	95 21	85 68	80 133	94 187	94 34	83 193	80 175	68 47	79 266	100 284	77 175	94 81	83 106	88 103	83 101	- -	- -
Pike County Memorial Hospital, Louisiana, MO	50 2	62 8	33 3	17 6	20 5	- 0	- 0	- 0	77 13	85 26	92 53	100 6	84 38	87 52	94 16	94 79	100 93	98 59	100 24	- -	- -	- -	- -	- -
Poplar Bluff Regional Medical Center, Poplar Bluff, MO	53 15	94 95	83 98	89 96	82 100	9 11	50 2	90 52	62 119	62 252	92 308	86 65	68 261	92 171	57 61	67 281	99 383	51 243	75 102	69 597	82 102	57 577	- -	- -
Putnam County Memorial Hospital, Unionville, MO	- 0	- 0	- 0	- 0	- 0	- 0	- 0	- 0	100 1	40 5	70 10	0 1	94 17	- 0	67 6	96 23	100 27	62 21	100 6	- -	- -	- -	- -	- -
Ray County Memorial Hospital, Richmond, MO	- 0	0 2	50 2	33 3	50 2	0 1	- 0	- 0	83 6	19 31	36 55	50 2	66 32	100 7	62 8	48 33	98 41	42 24	25 4	- -	- -	- -	- -	- -
Research Belton Hospital, Belton, MO	50 2	100 9	86 7	71 7	67 6	- 0	- 0	- 0	82 17	50 6	83 63	100 1	100 4	80 5	- -	91 45	98 61	80 41	100 2	30 27	- -	50 24	- -	- -
Research Medical Center, Kansas City, MO	93 68	98 162	99 279	97 121	98 266	- 0	88 8	97 97	88 249	77 448	95 535	99 118	82 118	89 89	55 33	77 193	100 235	73 154	91 67	87 278	89 139	42 272	- -	- -
Ripley County Memorial Hospital, Doniphan, MO	- 0	67 3	100 2	67 3	100 1	- 0	- 0	- 0	20 10	59 54	49 67	73 15	70 47	100 8	31 13	80 76	100 77	24 45	86 14	- -	- -	- -	- -	- -
Sac-Osage Hospital, Osceola, MO	- 0	100 3	50 2	33 3	50 2	- 0	- -	0 1	- 0	0 30	0 38	17 12	51 43	100 8	29 7	59 39	80 44	32 28	27 15	- -	- -	- -	- -	- -
Saint Alexius Hospital, Saint Louis, MO	100 11	96 47	100 22	88 34	96 25	0 2	- 0	100 7	81 78	28 193	95 255	99 70	87 119	93 118	81 31	87 179	100 219	76 105	96 82	74 72	90 20	69 71	- -	- -
Saint Anthony's Medical Center, Saint Louis, MO	84 68	97 314	96 297	94 215	94 319	- 0	52 21	99 130	74 166	60 303	94 397	97 67	86 186	92 230	89 45	76 289	100 347	82 226	99 83	87 639	92 215	67 606	0.24 1661	5.46 1080
Saint Francis Hospital, Mountain View, MO	- 0	100 1	- 0	- 0	- 0	- 0	- -	- 0	100 2	50 10	60 25	50 2	97 33	94 36	88 16	81 57	100 74	74 54	67 12	- -	- -	- -	- -	- -
Saint Francis Hospital & Health Services, Maryville, MO	- 0	100 7	67 6	100 5	100 6	- 0	- 0	100 1	92 12	94 31	98 58	100 5	98 49	90 29	100 9	90 61	100 76	100 61	100 9	95 125	100 44	98 121	- -	- -

NOTE: The first number in each column (boldface) is the rate in percent, the second number is the number of patients; Please refer to the main entry for footnotes; ***Heart Attack Care:*** *1. ACE Inhibitor or ARB for LVSD; 2. Aspirin at Arrival; 3. Aspirin at Discharge; 4. Beta Blocker at Arrival; 5. Beta Blocker at Discharge; 6. Fibrinolytic Medication Timing; 7. PCI Within 90 Minutes of Arrival; 8. Smoking Cessation Advice;* ***Heart Failure Care:*** *9. ACE Inhibitor or ARB for LVSD; 10. Discharge Instructions; 11. Evaluation of LVS Function; 12. Smoking Cessation Advice;* ***Pneumonia Care:*** *13. Appropriate Initial Antibiotic; 14. Blood Culture Timing; 15. Influenza Vaccine; 16. Initial Antibiotic Timing; 17. Oxygenation Assessment; 18. Pneumococcal Vaccine; 19. Smoking Cessation Advice;* ***Surgical Infection Prevention:*** *20. Prophylactic Antibiotic Given; 21. Prophylactic Antibiotic Selection; 22. Prophylactic Antibiotic Stopped;* ***Pregnancy Care:*** *23. Inpatient Neonatal Mortality; 24. Third or Fourth Degree Laceration*

Hospital	Heart Attack Care								Heart Failure Care				Pneumonia Care							Surgical Infection Prevention			Pregnancy Care	
	1	2	3	4	5	6	7	8	9	10	11	12	13	14	15	16	17	18	19	20	21	22	23	24
Saint Francis Medical Center, Cape Girardeau, MO	**95** 60	**96** 176	**95** 245	**95** 130	**97** 235	- 0	**33** 12	**100** 107	**94** 119	**92** 272	**98** 341	**100** 62	**90** 102	**97** 151	**94** 47	**90** 168	**100** 234	**95** 159	**100** 45	**91** 410	**91** 205	**82** 384	- -	- -
Saint John's Hospital at Lebanon, Lebanon, MO	**75** 4	**87** 23	**81** 16	**91** 22	**94** 17	- 0	- 0	**100** 1	**89** 18	**69** 71	**73** 83	**100** 9	**74** 116	**94** 47	**96** 27	**80** 127	**100** 168	**90** 101	**97** 35	**62** 52	**94** 50	**16** 49	- -	- -
Saint John's Hospital of Aurora, Aurora, MO	- -	- -	- -	- -	- -	- -	- -	- -	**88** 8	**55** 22	**89** 36	**88** 8	**97** 69	**94** 66	**86** 21	**89** 74	**100** 93	**86** 64	**100** 23	- -	- -	- -	- -	- -
Saint John's Hospital-Caseville, Cassville, MO	- -	- -	- -	- -	- -	- -	- -	- -	**100** 1	**60** 5	**60** 5	**100** 1	**97** 34	**83** 18	**89** 9	**97** 34	**100** 43	**97** 29	**75** 12	- -	- -	- -	- -	- -
Saint John's Mercy Hospital, Washington, MO	**84** 19	**94** 85	**90** 60	**87** 55	**86** 43	**0** 1	- 0	**100** 10	**96** 79	**89** 197	**99** 231	**100** 36	**86** 183	**98** 129	**86** 58	**85** 222	**100** 294	**90** 180	**99** 71	**94** 354	**92** 36	**98** 341	- -	- -
Saint John's Mercy Medical Center, Saint Louis, MO	**92** 165	**98** 356	**98** 523	**95** 298	**98** 535	- 0	**36** 14	**100** 171	**90** 262	**80** 471	**98** 555	**100** 76	**84** 302	**93** 251	**85** 85	**82** 470	**100** 500	**89** 297	**98** 105	**94** 1001	**96** 255	**78** 958	- -	- -
Saint John's Regional Health Center, Springfield, MO	**97** 186	**98** 397	**98** 617	**94** 272	**98** 587	**100** 1	**49** 39	**100** 262	**92** 355	**82** 574	**99** 690	**100** 107	**89** 412	**97** 435	**96** 164	**86** 501	**100** 726	**95** 497	**97** 216	**91** 360	**96** 96	**89** 354	- -	- -
Saint John's Regional Medical Center, Joplin, MO	**84** 122	**96** 199	**96** 304	**88** 162	**94** 355	**64** 14	**29** 7	**94** 159	**75** 167	**57** 336	**84** 402	**80** 76	**85** 263	**88** 274	**66** 140	**88** 413	**99** 494	**57** 323	**81** 167	**86** 998	**95** 259	**69** 986	**0.33** 896	**3.79** 633
Saint Joseph Health Center, Kansas City, MO	**100** 97	**100** 221	**100** 391	**99** 180	**100** 357	- 0	**67** 9	**100** 143	**99** 160	**100** 310	**99** 385	**100** 51	**82** 203	**89** 162	**63** 41	**82** 222	**100** 278	**77** 183	**100** 49	**97** 159	**90** 71	**92** 158	**0.23** 1297	**3.79** 896
Saint Joseph Health Center-Saint Charles, Saint Charles, MO	**89** 134	**100** 222	**99** 351	**100** 222	**99** 368	**60** 5	**78** 18	**98** 128	**85** 134	**60** 264	**98** 321	**93** 58	**83** 156	**90** 203	**52** 60	**77** 260	**100** 336	**88** 236	**99** 70	**87** 724	**95** 195	**92** 701	- -	- -
Saint Joseph Hospital of Kirkwood, Saint Louis, MO	**88** 40	**98** 137	**97** 150	**99** 105	**98** 154	- 0	**50** 2	**100** 38	**96** 73	**71** 208	**97** 291	**84** 25	**81** 189	**94** 192	**77** 61	**84** 231	**100** 277	**85** 188	**90** 60	**87** 643	**95** 224	**89** 633	- -	- -
Saint Joseph Hospital West, Lake Saint Louis, MO	**88** 8	**97** 58	**87** 23	**98** 64	**93** 29	**86** 7	- 0	**88** 8	**84** 56	**57** 137	**96** 159	**93** 15	**83** 175	**95** 172	**60** 50	**87** 206	**100** 268	**72** 169	**88** 65	**90** 381	**96** 108	**84** 375	- -	- -
Saint Luke's East Lee's Summit Hospital, Lees Summit, MO	**0** 1	**100** 4	**67** 3	**67** 3	**100** 3	- 0	- 0	- 0	**73** 15	**43** 30	**92** 36	**60** 5	**74** 31	**71** 35	**50** 4	**89** 44	**100** 48	**71** 21	**56** 16	**73** 161	**89** 72	**79** 160	- -	- -
Saint Luke's Hospital, Chesterfield, MO	**90** 67	**96** 199	**97** 242	**97** 153	**94** 252	- 0	**20** 10	**98** 64	**96** 198	**96** 393	**100** 521	**97** 39	**89** 243	**94** 191	**97** 72	**83** 375	**100** 480	**95** 359	**90** 69	**73** 171	**75** 105	**60** 164	- -	- -
Saint Luke's Hospital of Kansas City, Kansas City, MO	**88** 132	**98** 175	**99** 563	**96** 135	**99** 595	**0** 1	**57** 7	**98** 250	**95** 275	**66** 421	**98** 490	**98** 119	**80** 125	**88** 115	**80** 41	**76** 206	**100** 271	**89** 171	**99** 68	**97** 763	**81** 170	**71** 737	- -	- -
Saint Luke's Northland Hospital, Kansas City, MO	**50** 2	**100** 26	**92** 13	**94** 16	**92** 12	- 0	- 0	**100** 1	**90** 21	**67** 57	**97** 72	**89** 9	**90** 82	**99** 70	**92** 26	**86** 101	**100** 121	**91** 77	**81** 36	**84** 159	**84** 51	**78** 152	- -	- -
Saint Lukes Cancer Institute, Kansas City, MO	- -	- -	- -	- -	- -	- -	- -	- -	**100** 1	**0** 3	**100** 3	**50** 2	**100** 1	**100** 7	**67** 3	**80** 5	**100** 16	**40** 5	**75** 4	**100** 19	**84** 19	**41** 17	- -	- -
Saint Mary's Health Center, Saint Louis, MO	**92** 52	**98** 201	**98** 257	**94** 173	**96** 264	- 0	**67** 9	**98** 105	**92** 250	**71** 644	**98** 775	**99** 173	**86** 241	**92** 295	**48** 54	**72** 349	**100** 433	**78** 262	**97** 115	**94** 1024	**94** 253	**87** 997	- -	- -
Saint Mary's Medical Center, Blue Springs, MO	**89** 9	**100** 54	**96** 27	**98** 48	**100** 26	- 0	- 0	**100** 3	**88** 42	**87** 94	**92** 130	**100** 20	**74** 156	**86** 118	**57** 49	**88** 189	**99** 214	**80** 132	**93** 58	**85** 86	**84** 38	**58** 74	**0.08** 1252	**5.61** 909
Saint Marys Health Center, Jefferson City, MO	**87** 15	**98** 111	**100** 105	**92** 95	**95** 110	**60** 5	**100** 8	**100** 43	**93** 75	**91** 172	**98** 217	**97** 32	**83** 131	**82** 124	**97** 39	**79** 224	**100** 243	**86** 170	**96** 47	**95** 475	**85** 96	**69** 463	- -	- -
Salem Memorial District Hospital, Salem, MO	- -	- -	- -	- -	- -	- -	- -	- -	**100** 4	**0** 7	**90** 10	**100** 2	**80** 10	**100** 5	- -	**62** 13	**100** 14	**60** 10	**100** 2	- -	- -	- -	- -	- -
Scotland County Memorial Hospital, Memphis, MO	- -	- -	- -	- -	- -	- -	- -	- -	**100** 7	**100** 5	**62** 13	**0** 3	**73** 11	- 0	- -	**50** 2	**100** 13	**62** 8	**100** 3	- -	- -	- -	- -	- -
Skaggs Community Health Center, Branson, MO	**68** 31	**99** 190	**97** 182	**94** 164	**92** 172	- 0	**73** 11	**100** 56	**78** 65	**35** 155	**95** 183	**97** 36	**67** 151	**89** 132	**87** 38	**71** 180	**100** 235	**78** 155	**88** 66	**89** 260	**92** 72	**58** 260	- -	- -
SLUCare, Saint Louis, MO	**84** 90	**96** 127	**100** 167	**95** 98	**99** 189	- 0	**75** 12	**99** 92	**84** 260	**90** 358	**98** 394	**99** 136	**91** 129	**92** 126	**57** 28	**75** 212	**100** 236	**71** 114	**93** 83	**77** 237	**93** 54	**42** 229	- -	- -
Southeast Missouri Hospital, Cape Girardeau, MO	**86** 64	**100** 126	**96** 248	**92** 91	**98** 254	- 0	**71** 7	**100** 114	**78** 105	**96** 248	**85** 302	**93** 59	**78** 152	**97** 155	- -	**69** 196	**100** 252	**60** 156	**90** 52	**79** 592	**92** 140	**65** 592	- -	- -
Ste Genevieve County Memorial Hospital, Sainte Genevieve, MO	- 0	**100** 3	**100** 1	**67** 3	**100** 1	- 0	- 0	- 0	**60** 5	**63** 35	**78** 65	**67** 3	**70** 43	**97** 35	**93** 15	**84** 58	**100** 83	**71** 52	**50** 14	**86** 42	**82** 11	**100** 41	- -	- -
Sullivan County Memorial Hospital, Milan, MO	- 0	- 0	- 0	- 0	- 0	**0** 1	- -	- 0	- 0	**0** 11	**11** 9	- 0	**79** 14	- 0	**50** 2	**90** 20	**100** 26	**25** 16	**60** 5	- -	- -	- -	- -	- -
Texas County Memorial Hospital, Houston, MO	**33** 3	**93** 14	**92** 12	**75** 16	**73** 15	**0** 1	- 0	**0** 1	**73** 11	**2** 45	**62** 66	**55** 11	**77** 95	**95** 55	**50** 18	**77** 111	**99** 139	**38** 97	**52** 31	**75** 12	**100** 5	**73** 11	- -	- -
Truman Medical Center-Lakewood, Kansas City, MO	**100** 1	**100** 3	**50** 2	**80** 5	**67** 3	- 0	- 0	**100** 1	**85** 34	**100** 11	**87** 67	**100** 4	**79** 19	**100** 11	- -	**68** 53	**100** 80	**46** 26	**82** 11	**97** 61	- -	**16** 58	- -	- -
Truman Medical Centers, Kansas City, MO	**91** 11	**97** 36	**100** 26	**89** 38	**92** 25	**0** 1	- 0	**100** 16	**90** 198	**87** 299	**97** 318	**96** 139	**88** 99	**88** 128	**68** 19	**60** 164	**100** 181	**73** 44	**92** 95	**84** 175	**92** 48	**69** 174	- -	- -
Twin Rivers Regional Medical Center, Kennett, MO	**75** 4	**83** 18	**54** 13	**67** 18	**67** 15	- 0	- 0	**100** 5	**68** 44	**100** 89	**90** 119	**100** 22	**71** 70	**75** 53	**67** 12	**74** 95	**97** 128	**71** 52	**98** 50	**95** 86	**100** 21	**89** 74	- -	- -
University of Missouri Hospital and Clinics, Columbia, MO	**100** 40	**100** 77	**100** 221	**99** 84	**100** 232	- 0	**80** 5	**97** 110	**94** 90	**86** 156	**99** 186	**94** 48	**87** 75	**91** 85	**23** 39	**69** 142	**100** 177	**58** 79	**75** 75	**84** 228	**70** 74	**76** 214	- -	- -
Washington County Memorial Hospital, Potosi, MO	- 0	**80** 5	**75** 4	**60** 5	**50** 4	- 0	- 0	- 0	**100** 1	**19** 16	**30** 20	**100** 1	**88** 68	**82** 55	**55** 11	**87** 79	**100** 100	**54** 50	**58** 26	- -	- -	- -	- -	- -
Western Missouri Medical Center, Warrensburg, MO	- 0	**100** 5	**100** 2	**67** 3	**50** 2	- 0	- 0	- 0	**65** 17	**22** 67	**52** 98	**56** 16	**82** 74	**88** 59	**29** 21	**92** 96	**98** 129	**30** 80	**63** 35	**80** 61	**96** 56	**42** 53	**0.13** 797	**2.23** 629
Wright Memorial Hospital, Trenton, MO	**50** 2	**100** 3	**100** 1	**100** 6	**100** 3	**0** 1	- -	- 0	**91** 11	**37** 27	**85** 41	**100** 5	**72** 36	**94** 18	**80** 10	**92** 48	**100** 54	**84** 38	**100** 12	**0** 1	- 0	**100** 1	- -	- -
NEBRASKA																								
Alegent Health Bergen Mercy Medical Center, Omaha, NE	**87** 46	**100** 166	**100** 197	**97** 130	**99** 203	- 0	**100** 5	**100** 71	**92** 130	**89** 276	**99** 335	**100** 49	**94** 171	**98** 191	**98** 64	**95** 242	**100** 328	**99** 216	**100** 61	**94** 814	**100** 79	**94** 785	- -	- -
Alegent Health Lakeside Hospital, Omaha, NE	**100** 10	**100** 77	**100** 61	**100** 66	**100** 66	- 0	**100** 7	**100** 20	**100** 27	**96** 55	**100** 72	**100** 9	**93** 54	**100** 53	**100** 10	**96** 71	**100** 90	**98** 57	**100** 18	**92** 146	**89** 28	**92** 142	- -	- -
Alegent Health-Midlands Hospital, Papillion, NE	**100** 16	**99** 85	**99** 74	**99** 69	**99** 71	- 0	**100** 5	**100** 37	**95** 59	**94** 113	**99** 147	**100** 36	**96** 111	**98** 105	**100** 36	**97** 133	**100** 157	**100** 100	**100** 38	**90** 112	**97** 30	**93** 107	- -	- -
Annie Jeffrey Memorial County Health Center, Osceola, NE	- -	- -	- -	- -	- -	- -	- -	- -	- -	- -	- -	- -	**100** 4	**100** 2	- -	**100** 4	**100** 6	**80** 5	**100** 1	- -	- -	- -	- -	- -
Antelope Memorial Hospital, Neligh, NE	**100** 1	**100** 2	**100** 2	**100** 2	**100** 2	- 0	- -	- 0	**0** 2	**17** 6	**21** 14	- 0	**83** 6	**100** 1	**50** 2	**90** 10	**100** 14	**50** 12	**40** 5	- -	- -	- -	- -	- -
Avera Saint Anthony's Hospital, O'Neill, NE	- -	- -	- -	- -	- -	- -	- -	- -	**100** 10	**50** 14	**75** 24	**50** 2	**97** 36	- 0	**80** 10	**88** 51	**100** 58	**62** 37	**36** 11	- -	- -	- -	- -	- -
Beatrice Community Hospital & Health Center, Beatrice, NE	- 0	**100** 1	**100** 1	- 0	**100** 1	- 0	- -	- 0	**88** 8	**86** 22	**97** 30	**60** 5	**88** 26	**78** 27	**100** 10	**89** 37	**100** 43	**97** 29	**40** 5	**88** 85	**93** 15	**44** 85	- -	- -
Beatrice State Developmental Center, Beatrice, NE	- -	- -	- -	- -	- -	- -	- -	- -	- -	- -	- -	- -	- -	- -	- -	- -	- -	- -	- -	- -	- -	- -	- -	- -
Boone County Health Center, Albion, NE	**100** 2	**86** 7	**86** 7	**90** 10	**100** 7	- 0	- 0	**100** 1	**89** 9	**8** 13	**83** 24	**0** 1	**90** 39	**100** 11	**75** 16	**93** 57	**100** 84	**80** 60	**64** 11	**57** 28	**100** 5	**96** 26	- -	- -
Box Butte General Hospital, Alliance, NE	- 0	**80** 5	**80** 5	**33** 3	**40** 5	- 0	- -	**0** 1	**75** 4	**89** 35	**45** 60	**33** 6	**95** 38	**100** 11	**13** 15	**75** 53	**100** 57	**20** 40	**18** 11	- -	- -	- -	- -	- -
Brodstone Memorial Nuckolls County Hospital, Superior, NE	- 0	**67** 3	**67** 3	**67** 3	**100** 3	- 0	- 0	**100** 1	**0** 2	**53** 15	**90** 21	- 0	**93** 15	**100** 4	**100** 6	**71** 17	**91** 23	**71** 17	**67** 3	**100** 1	- -	**100** 1	- -	- -
Brown County Hospital, Ainsworth, NE	- -	- -	- -	- -	- -	- -	- -	- -	- 0	**0** 2	**0** 2	- 0	**91** 11	**100** 1	**100** 3	**87** 15	**100** 19	**40** 15	**50** 4	- -	- -	- -	- -	- -

NOTE: The first number in each column (boldface) is the rate in percent, the second number is the number of patients; Please refer to the main entry for footnotes; ***Heart Attack Care:*** *1. ACE Inhibitor or ARB for LVSD; 2. Aspirin at Arrival; 3. Aspirin at Discharge; 4. Beta Blocker at Arrival; 5. Beta Blocker at Discharge; 6. Fibrinolytic Medication Timing; 7. PCI Within 90 Minutes of Arrival; 8. Smoking Cessation Advice;* ***Heart Failure Care:*** *9. ACE Inhibitor or ARB for LVSD; 10. Discharge Instructions; 11. Evaluation of LVS Function; 12. Smoking Cessation Advice;* ***Pneumonia Care:*** *13. Appropriate Initial Antibiotic; 14. Blood Culture Timing; 15. Influenza Vaccine; 16. Initial Antibiotic Timing; 17. Oxygenation Assessment; 18. Pneumococcal Vaccine; 19. Smoking Cessation Advice;* ***Surgical Infection Prevention:*** *20. Prophylactic Antibiotic Given; 21. Prophylactic Antibiotic Selection; 22. Prophylactic Antibiotic Stopped;* ***Pregnancy Care:*** *23. Inpatient Neonatal Mortality; 24. Third or Fourth Degree Laceration*

Hospital	Heart Attack Care								Heart Failure Care				Pneumonia Care							Surgical Infection Prevention			Pregnancy Care	
	1	2	3	4	5	6	7	8	9	10	11	12	13	14	15	16	17	18	19	20	21	22	23	24
BryanLGH Medical Center, Lincoln, NE	**81** 78	**95** 164	**97** 325	**97** 118	**95** 353	- 0	**100** 6	**92** 126	**85** 278	**84** 403	**96** 514	**94** 66	**88** 133	**95** 149	**92** 61	**84** 228	**100** 306	**92** 226	**85** 62	**93** 843	**90** 225	**84** 803	- -	- -
Butler County Health Care Center, David City, NE	- 0	- 0	- 0	- 0	- 0	**20** 5	- -	- 0	**100** 1	**100** 5	**57** 7	- 0	**69** 16	**100** 1	**83** 6	**88** 16	**100** 20	**65** 17	**67** 3	**73** 22	**75** 4	**95** 22	- -	- -
Callaway District Hospital, Callaway, NE	- -	- -	- -	- -	- -	- -	- -	- -	- 0	- 0	- 0	- 0	- 0	**100** 2	- -	**100** 4	**100** 7	**33** 6	- 0	- -	- -	- -	- -	- -
Chadron Community Hospital, Chadron, NE	- 0	- 0	- 0	- 0	- 0	**0** 1	- 0	- 0	- 0	**100** 2	**29** 7	- 0	**62** 13	**100** 2	**100** 4	**94** 17	**100** 18	**64** 14	**0** 1	- -	- -	- -	- -	- -
Chase County Hospital, Imperial, NE	- -	- -	- -	- -	- -	- -	- -	- -	- 0	**0** 1	**0** 1	- 0	**100** 11	- 0	**25** 4	**92** 13	**100** 15	**36** 11	**100** 1	- -	- -	- -	- -	- -
Cherry County Hospital, Valentine, NE	- 0	- 0	- 0	- 0	- 0	- 0	- -	- 0	- 0	**0** 1	**100** 2	- 0	**100** 6	**100** 2	**50** 4	**79** 14	**100** 17	**60** 15	**100** 1	- -	- -	- -	- -	- -
Columbus Community Hospital, Columbus, NE	**100** 2	**100** 9	**100** 6	**89** 9	**100** 7	- 0	- 0	- 0	**95** 19	**71** 28	**90** 49	**100** 6	**93** 30	**97** 35	**92** 13	**96** 50	**100** 72	**91** 54	**88** 8	**94** 205	**95** 39	**91** 198	- -	- -
Community Hospital, McCook, NE	**100** 3	**75** 4	**50** 2	**40** 5	**100** 2	- 0	- 0	- 0	**100** 1	**79** 14	**56** 16	**0** 1	**91** 45	**100** 12	**87** 15	**90** 61	**100** 75	**75** 56	**65** 17	**75** 99	**100** 27	**92** 97	- -	- -
Community Hospital, Falls City, NE	**100** 1	**100** 1	**100** 1	- 0	- 0	**67** 3	- -	- 0	**100** 4	**67** 9	**67** 21	**100** 2	**75** 12	**100** 2	**100** 6	**94** 16	**100** 25	**77** 22	**83** 6	**91** 11	**100** 1	**100** 11	- -	- -
Community Memorial Hospital, Syracuse, NE	- -	- -	- -	- -	- -	- -	- -	- -	**100** 1	**0** 3	**25** 4	- 0	**100** 1	- 0	- -	**100** 1	**100** 1	**0** 1	- 0	- -	- -	- -	- -	- -
Cozad Community Hospital, Cozad, NE	- -	- -	- -	- -	- -	- -	- -	- -	- 0	**33** 3	**60** 5	**100** 1	**64** 14	**100** 1	**100** 3	**73** 11	**100** 16	**58** 12	- 0	- -	- -	- -	- -	- -
Creighton Area Health Services, Creighton, NE	- 0	**50** 4	**67** 3	**50** 4	**100** 3	- 0	- -	- 0	- -	- -	- -	- -	**85** 34	- 0	**79** 14	**100** 43	**100** 59	**70** 50	**29** 7	- -	- -	- -	- -	- -
Creighton University Medical Center, Omaha, NE	**93** 67	**97** 101	**100** 241	**99** 100	**100** 288	- 0	**62** 8	**98** 80	**93** 149	**86** 271	**99** 303	**96** 75	**86** 70	**94** 96	**78** 18	**81** 134	**100** 158	**85** 71	**97** 61	**84** 453	**86** 86	**59** 448	- -	- -
Crete Area Medical Center, Crete, NE	- 0	- 0	- 0	- 0	- 0	- 0	- 0	- 0	**100** 2	**50** 2	**62** 8	**50** 2	**88** 8	**100** 3	**88** 8	**69** 16	**95** 20	**82** 17	**50** 4	- -	- -	- -	- -	- -
Dundy County Hospital, Benkelman, NE	- 0	**100** 1	- 0	**100** 1	- 0	- 0	- -	- 0	- 0	**33** 3	**25** 4	- 0	**50** 6	**100** 1	**100** 1	**100** 7	**100** 8	**29** 7	**0** 2	**0** 1	- -	**0** 1	- -	- -
Faith Regional Health Services-East Campus, Norfolk, NE	**88** 26	**95** 57	**99** 77	**98** 48	**100** 88	- 0	**50** 4	**100** 27	**83** 66	**71** 92	**96** 134	**95** 19	**91** 70	**100** 71	**95** 20	**91** 106	**100** 137	**98** 101	**76** 29	**90** 472	**99** 152	**89** 453	- -	- -
Fillmore County Hospital, Geneva, NE	- 0	**100** 1	**100** 1	**100** 1	**100** 2	- 0	- 0	- 0	**33** 3	**0** 1	**44** 9	**0** 1	**75** 4	- 0	**50** 2	**100** 4	**100** 10	**50** 6	**100** 2	**33** 9	**100** 4	**100** 9	- -	- -
Franklin County Memorial Hospital, Franklin, NE	- -	- -	- -	- -	- -	- -	- -	- -	- 0	**0** 3	**11** 9	- 0	**100** 8	- 0	**100** 4	**100** 11	**100** 14	**70** 10	**100** 2	- -	- -	- -	- -	- -
Fremont Area Medical Center, Fremont, NE	**100** 5	**100** 36	**100** 28	**100** 32	**100** 32	- 0	**100** 1	**78** 9	**94** 17	**82** 39	**100** 68	**88** 8	**87** 95	**98** 82	**84** 31	**91** 122	**100** 172	**70** 115	**89** 35	**97** 231	**94** 80	**88** 231	- -	- -
Garden County Hospital, Oshkosh, NE	- -	- -	- -	- -	- -	- -	- -	- -	- 0	**50** 2	**33** 3	- 0	**100** 2	- -	- -	**100** 2	**100** 2	**50** 2	- 0	- -	- -	- -	- -	- -
Good Samaritan, Kearney, NE	**82** 28	**97** 75	**99** 121	**84** 58	**98** 134	**100** 1	**50** 6	**98** 57	**88** 48	**62** 119	**89** 168	**91** 35	**93** 97	**92** 60	**58** 36	**87** 136	**100** 190	**85** 137	**92** 52	**91** 686	**97** 209	**78** 671	- -	- -
Gordon Memorial Hospital District, Gordon, NE	- -	- -	- -	- -	- -	- -	- -	- -	- -	- -	- -	- -	**96** 24	**100** 2	**92** 12	**93** 27	**100** 34	**86** 28	**50** 10	- -	- -	- -	- -	- -
Gothenburg Memorial Hospital, Gothenburg, NE	- -	- -	- -	- -	- -	- -	- -	- -	- 0	**100** 1	**50** 2	- 0	**92** 12	**100** 4	**100** 3	**93** 14	**100** 17	**87** 15	**100** 2	- -	- -	- -	- -	- -
Great Plains Regional Medical Center, North Platte, NE	**83** 6	**97** 32	**100** 19	**86** 21	**95** 19	**33** 3	- 0	**100** 4	**77** 31	**78** 91	**91** 113	**92** 26	**81** 116	**97** 76	**81** 36	**89** 158	**100** 192	**72** 130	**100** 45	**88** 170	**98** 54	**60** 167	- -	- -
Harlan County Hospital, Alma, NE	- 0	**50** 2	- 0	**0** 2	- 0	- 0	- -	- 0	- 0	**33** 3	**33** 3	**0** 1	**100** 26	**75** 4	**44** 9	**96** 28	**100** 30	**35** 23	**0** 7	- -	- -	- -	- -	- -
Henderson Health Care Services, Henderson, NE	- -	- -	- -	- -	- -	- -	- -	- -	- -	- -	- -	- -	**100** 2	- 0	- -	**100** 3	**100** 3	**100** 3	- 0	- -	- -	- -	- -	- -
Howard County Community Hospital, Saint Paul, NE	**100** 1	**80** 5	**60** 5	**100** 5	**100** 4	- 0	- 0	- 0	**80** 5	**35** 17	**100** 28	**67** 3	**86** 14	**100** 4	**80** 5	**93** 14	**100** 27	**100** 21	**100** 4	**89** 9	**100** 4	**89** 9	- -	- -
Immanuel Medical Center, Omaha, NE	**97** 35	**100** 106	**99** 160	**99** 94	**100** 181	**0** 1	**100** 7	**100** 61	**99** 84	**95** 123	**99** 181	**100** 30	**92** 101	**99** 119	**97** 34	**94** 177	**100** 206	**98** 133	**98** 58	**94** 367	**94** 65	**92** 353	- -	- -
Jefferson Community Health Center, Fairbury, NE	**100** 1	**0** 1	**0** 1	- 0	**100** 1	- 0	- -	- 0	**100** 3	**100** 5	**100** 7	- 0	**100** 21	**100** 9	**83** 12	**96** 28	**100** 33	**100** 28	**100** 2	**98** 46	**100** 8	**98** 43	- -	- -
Jennie M Melham Memorial Medical Center, Broken Bow, NE	- 0	**75** 4	**100** 2	**100** 3	**100** 2	**0** 1	- -	- 0	**75** 12	**62** 16	**83** 29	**100** 3	**91** 55	**100** 3	**85** 27	**99** 86	**100** 123	**96** 92	**77** 13	**0** 1	- -	- 0	- -	- -
Johnson County Hospital, Tecumseh, NE	- 0	**100** 1	- 0	**100** 1	- 0	- 0	- -	- 0	**100** 2	**83** 6	**82** 11	- 0	**100** 6	**100** 2	**67** 3	**100** 9	**100** 11	**88** 8	**50** 2	**100** 8	**50** 2	**62** 8	- -	- -
Kearney County Health Services, Minden, NE	- -	- -	- -	- -	- -	- -	- -	- -	- 0	- 0	**100** 1	- 0	**100** 8	**100** 1	- -	- 0	**100** 9	**83** 6	**0** 1	- -	- -	- -	- -	- -
Lincoln Surgical Hospital, Lincoln, NE	- -	- -	- -	- -	- -	- -	- -	- -	- -	- -	- -	- -	- -	- -	- -	- -	- -	- -	- -	**87** 157	**98** 54	**82** 157	- -	- -
Litzenberg Memorial County Hospital, Central City, NE	- 0	**100** 1	**100** 1	**100** 1	**100** 1	- 0	- -	- 0	**67** 3	**50** 10	**39** 18	- 0	**100** 12	**100** 5	**100** 6	**94** 32	**94** 34	**72** 25	**100** 1	**89** 9	**100** 3	**88** 8	- -	- -
Mary Lanning Memorial Hospital, Hastings, NE	**25** 4	**94** 32	**89** 19	**72** 32	**70** 20	**50** 6	- 0	**75** 8	**52** 63	**59** 95	**93** 153	**29** 7	**87** 106	**96** 104	**73** 44	**80** 172	**99** 221	**67** 159	**62** 26	**73** 324	**93** 111	**94** 310	- -	- -
Memorial Community Hospital, Blair, NE	- 0	**100** 2	**100** 1	**100** 2	**100** 1	- 0	- -	- 0	**100** 4	**83** 12	**90** 21	- 0	**72** 25	**100** 26	**91** 11	**100** 31	**100** 44	**84** 32	**78** 9	**80** 5	**100** 2	**80** 5	- -	- -
Memorial Health Center, Sidney, NE	- 0	**100** 3	**100** 1	**67** 3	**100** 1	**25** 4	- 0	- 0	**100** 4	**0** 16	**77** 22	**80** 5	**86** 21	**100** 4	**43** 7	**68** 28	**100** 32	**57** 23	**100** 6	- -	- -	- -	- -	- -
Memorial Hospital, Schuyler, NE	- 0	**100** 1	**100** 1	**0** 1	**100** 1	- 0	- -	- 0	**100** 1	**31** 13	**71** 14	- 0	**88** 17	- 0	**40** 5	**89** 27	**100** 33	**76** 25	**50** 2	- -	- -	- -	- -	- -
Memorial Hospital, Seward, NE	**100** 1	**75** 4	**100** 3	**60** 5	**67** 3	- 0	- 0	- 0	**78** 9	**0** 25	**61** 36	**0** 3	**81** 37	**100** 3	**0** 7	**92** 51	**100** 62	**7** 42	**0** 12	- -	- -	- -	- -	- -
Memorial Hospital, Aurora, NE	- 0	**100** 1	- 0	**33** 3	**67** 3	- 0	- 0	- 0	**86** 7	**75** 8	**86** 14	**0** 2	**88** 17	**100** 2	**100** 4	**79** 28	**97** 33	**95** 19	**100** 5	**100** 8	**50** 2	**88** 8	- -	- -
Methodist Hospital, Omaha, NE	**87** 46	**96** 163	**99** 170	**94** 137	**98** 188	- 0	**64** 14	**100** 49	**86** 183	**77** 296	**97** 374	**100** 46	**88** 268	**92** 243	- -	**78** 353	**99** 473	**75** 317	**91** 78	**91** 408	**100** 101	**88** 392	**0.36** 1682	**5.76** 2447
Nebraska Heart Hospital, Lincoln, NE	**92** 75	**87** 23	**98** 324	**61** 23	**97** 310	- 0	- 0	**93** 111	**88** 292	**82** 323	**99** 364	**80** 51	**100** 1	**100** 1	**50** 2	**100** 2	**100** 3	**100** 4	**100** 5	**95** 85	**100** 35	**88** 81	- -	- -
Nebraska Medical Center, Omaha, NE	**90** 58	**97** 186	**99** 244	**98** 172	**100** 249	**0** 1	**67** 9	**99** 105	**79** 177	**59** 271	**100** 327	**89** 63	**92** 61	**92** 79	**60** 15	**83** 115	**100** 149	**55** 78	**74** 35	**80** 544	**96** 75	**91** 523	**0.51** 590	**2.87** 2023
Nebraska Orthopaedic Hospital, Omaha, NE	- -	- -	- -	- -	- -	- -	- -	- -	- -	- -	- -	- -	- -	- -	- -	- -	- -	- -	- -	**94** 194	**100** 33	**88** 190	- -	- -
Nemaha County Hospital, Auburn, NE	- -	- -	- -	- -	- -	- -	- -	- -	**100** 2	**33** 6	**86** 7	**100** 1	**91** 11	**100** 3	**86** 7	**88** 26	**100** 33	**50** 20	**25** 4	**80** 5	**100** 4	**80** 5	- -	- -
Niobrara Valley Hospital, Lynch, NE	- -	- -	- -	- -	- -	- -	- -	- -	- -	- -	- -	- -	**100** 2	**100** 1	**100** 1	**67** 3	**100** 3	**33** 3	- 0	- -	- -	- -	- -	- -
Oakland Memorial Hospital, Oakland, NE	- -	- -	- -	- -	- -	- -	- -	- -	**33** 3	**86** 7	**70** 10	**25** 4	**88** 8	**100** 1	**50** 4	**70** 10	**100** 10	**71** 7	**0** 1	- -	- -	- -	- -	- -
Ogallala Community Hospital, Ogallala, NE	- 0	**100** 1	- 0	**100** 2	**100** 1	- 0	- -	**0** 1	**90** 10	**62** 16	**93** 28	**0** 2	**95** 41	**80** 5	**86** 7	**91** 35	**100** 45	**81** 26	**71** 7	**88** 8	**100** 8	**100** 8	- -	- -

NOTE: The first number in each column (boldface) is the rate in percent, the second number is the number of patients; Please refer to the main entry for footnotes; ***Heart Attack Care:*** *1. ACE Inhibitor or ARB for LVSD; 2. Aspirin at Arrival; 3. Aspirin at Discharge; 4. Beta Blocker at Arrival; 5. Beta Blocker at Discharge; 6. Fibrinolytic Medication Timing; 7. PCI Within 90 Minutes of Arrival; 8. Smoking Cessation Advice;* ***Heart Failure Care:*** *9. ACE Inhibitor or ARB for LVSD; 10. Discharge Instructions; 11. Evaluation of LVS Function; 12. Smoking Cessation Advice;* ***Pneumonia Care:*** *13. Appropriate Initial Antibiotic; 14. Blood Culture Timing; 15. Influenza Vaccine; 16. Initial Antibiotic Timing; 17. Oxygenation Assessment; 18. Pneumococcal Vaccine; 19. Smoking Cessation Advice;* ***Surgical Infection Prevention:*** *20. Prophylactic Antibiotic Given; 21. Prophylactic Antibiotic Selection; 22. Prophylactic Antibiotic Stopped;* ***Pregnancy Care:*** *23. Inpatient Neonatal Mortality; 24. Third or Fourth Degree Laceration*

Hospital	Heart Attack Care								Heart Failure Care				Pneumonia Care							Surgical Infection Prevention			Pregnancy Care	
	1	2	3	4	5	6	7	8	9	10	11	12	13	14	15	16	17	18	19	20	21	22	23	24
Osmond General Hospital, Osmond, NE	- -	- -	- -	- -	- -	- -	- -	- -	- -	- -	- -	- -	100 1	100 1	- -	100 1	0 1	- 0	- 0	- -	- -	- -	- -	- -
Pawnee County Memorial Hospital, Pawnee City, NE	- -	- -	- -	- -	- -	- -	- -	- -	67 3	40 5	57 7	100 1	100 4	100 2	67 3	100 15	100 16	71 14	100 2	- -	- -	- -	- -	- -
Pender Community Hospital, Pender, NE	- -	- -	- -	- -	- -	- -	- -	- -	- -	- -	- -	- -	67 3	- 0	- -	100 4	60 5	50 2	- 0	- -	- -	- -	- -	- -
Perkins County Health Services, Grant, NE	- 0	100 2	100 2	100 1	100 2	- 0	- -	- 0	33 3	0 5	88 8	- 0	100 17	67 3	100 13	95 21	100 26	88 25	0 2	- -	- -	- -	- -	- -
Phelps Memorial Health Center, Holdrege, NE	- 0	67 3	100 1	100 2	100 2	50 2	- 0	- 0	100 2	70 10	70 20	33 3	100 25	100 2	100 14	89 53	100 62	82 38	91 11	75 61	95 19	69 59	- -	- -
Plainview Public Hospital, Plainview, NE	- 0	100 1	100 1	100 1	100 1	- 0	- -	- 0	0 1	85 13	40 20	- 0	100 9	75 4	50 2	100 15	100 16	50 12	0 1	- -	- -	- -	- -	- -
Providence Medical Center, Wayne, NE	100 1	100 3	50 2	67 3	100 2	- 0	- 0	- 0	100 6	75 8	68 22	100 1	69 13	- 0	100 2	100 14	100 21	79 19	50 2	11 9	100 3	88 8	- -	- -
Regional West Medical Center, Scottsbluff, NE	50 4	97 32	81 21	88 24	77 13	33 3	- 0	33 3	86 21	52 62	84 88	62 16	80 66	88 57	82 34	91 97	100 121	89 80	68 28	72 381	100 116	75 375	0.00 845	2.69 668
Rock County Hospital, Bassett, NE	- -	- -	- -	- -	- -	- -	- -	- -	- -	- -	- -	- -	100 1	- 0	- -	100 2	50 2	0 1	- 0	- -	- -	- -	- -	- -
Saint Elizabeth Regional Medical Center, Lincoln, NE	84 32	99 82	99 87	97 65	98 85	- 0	80 10	97 29	88 60	91 95	96 142	64 11	93 134	90 101	88 24	86 166	100 199	89 138	69 45	86 1123	94 375	86 1090	- -	- -
Saint Francis Med Ctr/Memorial Health Center, Grand Island, NE	88 25	99 84	97 73	97 62	96 72	50 6	100 2	97 35	86 44	87 107	98 154	84 25	86 156	93 165	64 66	95 244	100 330	83 207	92 52	94 598	96 151	71 579	- -	- -
Saint Francis Memorial Hospital, West Point, NE	- 0	100 5	100 3	100 4	100 1	0 1	- -	- 0	69 13	81 21	90 41	67 3	89 19	100 3	75 4	100 26	100 32	92 26	50 4	89 47	100 8	96 45	- -	- -
Saunders Medical Center, Wahoo, NE	- 0	100 1	- 0	100 1	- 0	- 0	- -	- 0	80 5	44 9	90 20	0 2	95 21	100 10	89 9	95 38	100 44	97 35	50 2	- -	- -	- -	- -	- -
Thayer County Health Services, Hebron, NE	- 0	- 0	- 0	0 1	- 0	0 1	- -	- 0	75 4	0 9	44 18	- 0	91 11	100 2	- 0	92 26	100 32	17 12	0 1	- -	- -	- -	- -	- -
Tilden Community Hospital, Tilden, NE	- -	- -	- -	- -	- -	- -	- -	- -	- 0	0 1	100 1	- 0	80 5	100 3	0 1	100 5	100 9	80 5	50 6	- -	- -	- -	- -	- -
Tri-County Area Hospital District, Lexington, NE	- -	- -	- -	- -	- -	- -	- -	- -	100 7	50 24	81 31	33 3	92 48	100 11	69 13	91 75	99 90	87 61	79 19	89 36	86 7	49 35	- -	- -
Tri-Valley Health System, Cambridge, NE	- 0	0 1	- 0	100 1	- 0	0 1	- 0	- 0	90 10	48 23	96 28	67 3	97 32	100 2	- -	97 32	100 47	62 37	75 4	0 2	- -	100 2	- -	- -
Valley County Hospital, Ord, NE	- 0	- 0	- 0	- 0	- 0	0 1	- -	- 0	0 1	71 7	29 14	75 4	95 22	100 16	40 10	100 36	100 42	69 35	100 2	- -	- -	- -	- -	- -
Warren Memorial Hospital, Friend, NE	- -	- -	- -	- -	- -	- -	- -	- -	- 0	0 1	100 1	- 0	100 3	100 1	- -	100 3	100 4	50 4	0 1	- -	- -	- -	- -	- -
Webster County Community Hospital, Red Cloud, NE	- -	- -	- -	- -	- -	- -	- -	- -	0 1	0 3	60 5	33 3	77 13	77 13	80 10	91 22	100 40	57 30	0 4	- -	- -	- -	- -	- -
Winnebago Hospital, Winnebago, NE	- -	- -	- -	- -	- -	- -	- -	- -	0 1	40 5	60 5	0 2	- -	- -	- -	- -	- -	- -	- -	- -	- -	- -	- -	- -
York General Hospital, York, NE	- -	- -	- -	- -	- -	- -	- -	- -	- -	- -	- -	- -	81 26	92 12	100 7	88 25	100 35	96 26	100 2	98 52	100 16	98 51	- -	- -
NORTH DAKOTA																								
Altru Hospital, Grand Forks, ND	95 39	100 101	100 215	98 85	99 202	- 0	100 2	98 86	91 53	78 137	88 181	96 23	87 117	92 143	88 40	79 193	100 250	92 181	94 63	89 312	95 81	67 299	- -	- -
Carrington Health Center, Carrington, ND	100 1	100 1	100 1	100 1	100 1	- 0	- -	- 0	100 2	15 13	55 20	0 1	80 15	100 1	60 5	94 17	100 21	68 19	100 2	- -	- -	- -	- -	- -
Heart of America Medical Center, Rugby, ND	- 0	83 6	80 5	100 6	100 5	- 0	- 0	- 0	- 0	75 12	35 23	- 0	87 23	100 12	89 9	100 39	100 49	82 40	100 3	- 0	- 0	- 0	- -	- -
Hillsboro Medical Center, Hillsboro, ND	- 0	- 0	- 0	- 0	- 0	- 0	- -	- 0	- 0	- 0	75 4	- 0	81 16	86 7	100 3	100 25	100 31	97 29	75 4	- -	- -	- -	- -	- -
Innovis Health, Fargo, ND	82 39	93 81	95 190	89 66	93 182	- 0	60 5	93 68	82 44	63 107	90 133	78 18	96 56	90 51	81 16	86 66	100 87	80 64	87 15	90 167	97 60	79 159	- -	- -
Jacobson Memorial Hospital Care Center, Elgin, ND	- 0	100 3	100 2	50 2	100 1	0 1	- -	100 1	- -	- -	- -	- -	100 5	100 6	80 5	100 11	100 12	92 12	0 1	- -	- -	- -	- -	- -
Jamestown Hospital, Jamestown, ND	- 0	95 22	78 9	91 22	100 9	0 1	- 0	50 2	87 15	80 40	70 57	90 10	98 54	97 63	79 19	91 91	100 118	75 84	82 11	90 63	90 20	81 59	- -	- -
Linton Hospital, Linton, ND	100 1	0 1	0 1	0 1	50 2	- 0	- -	- 0	0 1	45 11	16 32	0 2	19 31	100 5	88 8	94 36	100 43	59 37	0 1	- -	- -	- -	- -	- -
McKenzie County Memorial Hospital, Watford City, ND	- 0	100 1	100 1	100 1	100 1	- 0	- -	- 0	100 1	0 7	47 15	- 0	75 20	50 2	0 1	100 18	100 24	6 16	33 3	- -	- -	- -	- -	- -
Medcenter One, Bismarck, ND	96 23	99 89	99 129	95 82	98 113	20 5	25 4	100 36	86 85	95 141	99 198	100 28	88 85	95 79	100 22	94 121	100 146	90 98	85 34	88 197	97 102	83 196	- -	- -
Mercy Hospital, Devils Lake, ND	100 1	91 11	83 6	80 15	86 7	0 1	- 0	- 0	43 7	77 26	67 36	100 1	77 65	100 36	54 13	81 57	100 97	48 58	52 27	86 7	100 2	57 7	0.00 310	5.00 220
Mercy Medical Center, Williston, ND	0 1	100 7	100 5	83 6	100 5	- 0	- 0	0 1	71 7	80 25	92 39	0 3	85 52	93 46	88 16	78 64	100 85	94 65	69 16	91 172	94 36	80 172	0.00 364	2.46 284
MeritCare Medical Center, Fargo, ND	97 103	99 193	99 506	98 175	100 499	- 0	83 12	98 167	73 118	77 201	99 278	70 37	89 139	93 129	77 52	80 234	100 276	84 205	74 53	93 326	87 86	88 313	- -	- -
Mountrail County Medical Center, Stanley, ND	- -	- -	- -	- -	- -	- -	- -	- -	- -	- -	- -	- -	100 13	100 2	100 2	94 18	100 20	72 18	50 4	- -	- -	- -	- -	- -
Pembina County Memorial Hospital, Cavalier, ND	- 0	- 0	- 0	- 0	- 0	- 0	- 0	- 0	50 2	100 9	38 13	100 1	72 18	- 0	- -	90 20	100 27	81 16	100 7	- -	- -	- -	- -	- -
PHS Indian Hospital at Fort Yates, Fort Yates, ND	- -	- -	- -	- -	- -	- -	- -	- -	- -	- -	- -	- -	0 1	- 0	- -	100 1	- 0	- 0	- 0	- -	- -	- -	- -	- -
Presentation Medical Center, Rolla, ND	- -	- -	- -	- -	- -	- -	- -	- -	- 0	20 5	86 7	100 1	100 7	100 8	100 3	94 18	100 20	100 18	86 7	- -	- -	- -	- -	- -
Quentin N Burdick Mem Healthcare Facility, Belcourt, ND	- -	- -	- -	- -	- -	- -	- -	- -	- 0	- 0	0 29	- 0	11 9	80 5	- -	70 50	100 58	26 31	20 5	0 2	- -	100 2	- -	- -
Saint Alexius Medical Center, Bismarck, ND	94 17	100 100	98 199	98 99	98 196	60 5	100 7	99 68	90 97	95 203	98 244	96 26	87 85	97 60	88 25	81 106	100 147	97 117	92 40	89 1204	95 263	60 1170	0.39 1290	6.05 893
Saint Andrews Health Center, Bottineau, ND	0 1	100 1	100 1	100 1	100 1	- 0	- -	- 0	0 2	57 7	78 9	0 1	100 13	100 6	0 1	89 18	100 24	55 20	0 3	- -	- -	- -	- -	- -
Saint Joseph's Hospital & Health Center, Dickinson, ND	100 3	88 32	95 21	100 22	96 25	40 5	- 0	0 1	85 13	70 53	75 85	50 8	80 30	92 38	100 12	92 53	100 67	85 48	71 14	91 165	100 40	81 167	0.00 319	3.64 220
Tioga Medical Center, Tioga, ND	- 0	100 1	100 1	100 1	100 1	- 0	- -	- 0	100 1	50 2	100 5	- 0	58 12	100 1	75 4	92 13	100 17	75 12	100 2	- -	- -	- -	- -	- -
Towner County Medical Center, Cando, ND	- 0	100 1	- 0	0 1	- 0	- 0	- -	- 0	33 3	0 3	43 7	- 0	50 2	100 3	50 2	80 5	100 11	44 9	0 1	- -	- -	- -	- -	- -
Trinity Health, Minot, ND	100 27	99 126	99 178	100 91	99 204	- 0	100 8	100 24	94 89	82 40	99 249	100 6	95 19	100 23	- -	89 192	100 238	92 172	100 5	87 134	- -	85 133	- -	- -
Union Hospital, Mayville, ND	100 1	100 7	100 4	100 11	100 8	- 0	- -	- 0	75 4	67 6	69 13	- 0	82 11	100 3	100 3	84 19	100 22	70 20	- 0	- -	- -	- -	- -	- -

NOTE: The first number in each column (boldface) is the rate in percent, the second number is the number of patients; Please refer to the main entry for footnotes; ***Heart Attack Care:*** *1. ACE Inhibitor or ARB for LVSD; 2. Aspirin at Arrival; 3. Aspirin at Discharge; 4. Beta Blocker at Arrival; 5. Beta Blocker at Discharge; 6. Fibrinolytic Medication Timing; 7. PCI Within 90 Minutes of Arrival; 8. Smoking Cessation Advice;* ***Heart Failure Care:*** *9. ACE Inhibitor or ARB for LVSD; 10. Discharge Instructions; 11. Evaluation of LVS Function; 12. Smoking Cessation Advice;* ***Pneumonia Care:*** *13. Appropriate Initial Antibiotic; 14. Blood Culture Timing; 15. Influenza Vaccine; 16. Initial Antibiotic Timing; 17. Oxygenation Assessment; 18. Pneumococcal Vaccine; 19. Smoking Cessation Advice;* ***Surgical Infection Prevention:*** *20. Prophylactic Antibiotic Given; 21. Prophylactic Antibiotic Selection; 22. Prophylactic Antibiotic Stopped;* ***Pregnancy Care:*** *23. Inpatient Neonatal Mortality; 24. Third or Fourth Degree Laceration*

Hospital	Heart Attack Care								Heart Failure Care				Pneumonia Care							Surgical Infection Prevention			Pregnancy Care	
	1	2	3	4	5	6	7	8	9	10	11	12	13	14	15	16	17	18	19	20	21	22	23	24
West River Regional Medical Center, Hettinger, ND	- 0	**92** 12	**88** 8	**89** 9	**78** 9	**67** 6	- 0	- 0	**86** 14	**67** 46	**78** 69	**100** 2	**77** 22	**100** 10	**100** 12	**98** 64	**97** 77	**85** 73	**100** 6	**82** 11	**100** 1	**90** 10	- -	- -
Wishek Community Hospital, Wishek, ND	**100** 2	**100** 7	**100** 7	**86** 7	**100** 7	**33** 3	- 0	- 0	**100** 1	**100** 6	**12** 8	- 0	**46** 13	**100** 3	**78** 9	**94** 33	**100** 40	**72** 40	**0** 2	- -	- -	- -	- -	- -
OKLAHOMA																								
Anadarko Municipal Hospital, Anadarko, OK	- -	- -	- -	- -	- -	- -	- -	- -	**100** 1	**0** 4	**75** 4	- 0	**78** 9	- 0	- -	**50** 4	**100** 10	**0** 5	**33** 6	- -	- -	- -	- -	- -
Arbuckle Memorial Hospital, Sulphur, OK	**0** 1	**0** 1	**0** 1	**100** 1	**100** 1	- 0	- -	- 0	**100** 3	**33** 9	**71** 21	**33** 3	**90** 20	**80** 20	**100** 10	**83** 29	**100** 40	**85** 27	**89** 9	- -	- -	- -	- -	- -
Atoka Memorial Hospital, Atoka, OK	- 0	**100** 2	**100** 3	**100** 1	**67** 3	**0** 1	- -	**0** 1	**17** 6	**40** 10	**39** 23	**60** 5	**69** 26	**100** 5	- -	**71** 7	**96** 28	**86** 14	**75** 12	- -	- -	- -	- -	- -
Beaver County Memorial Hospital, Beaver, OK	- 0	**100** 1	- 0	- 0	- 0	- 0	- -	- 0	- 0	**0** 5	**0** 5	- 0	- 0	- 0	**100** 1	**100** 10	**100** 10	**25** 4	**33** 3	- -	- -	- -	- -	- -
Bone and Joint Hospital, Oklahoma City, OK	- -	- -	- -	- -	- -	- -	- -	- -	- -	- -	- -	- -	- 0	- 0	**0** 1	- 0	**100** 1	**0** 1	- 0	**100** 333	**100** 40	**98** 327	- -	- -
Bristow Medical Center, Bristow, OK	- 0	**100** 1	**100** 1	**100** 1	**100** 1	- 0	- 0	- 0	**100** 10	**57** 14	**95** 19	**100** 1	**95** 37	**100** 11	- -	**92** 40	**100** 47	**94** 33	**83** 18	- -	- -	- -	- -	- -
Carnegie Tri-County Municipal Hospital, Carnegie, OK	- 0	**100** 1	- 0	**100** 1	- 0	- 0	- 0	- 0	**67** 3	**9** 23	**8** 36	**25** 4	**100** 11	- 0	**0** 5	**79** 19	**100** 20	**0** 18	**0** 4	- -	- -	- -	- -	- -
Chickasaw Nation Health System, Ada, OK	**100** 2	**67** 6	**100** 2	**67** 6	**50** 2	- 0	- -	- 0	**71** 7	**47** 17	**94** 18	**50** 4	**84** 64	**95** 44	**70** 23	**73** 70	**100** 91	**85** 39	**83** 30	**97** 33	**100** 33	**97** 33	- -	- -
Choctaw Memorial Hospital, Hugo, OK	**0** 1	**100** 2	**100** 1	**100** 2	**0** 1	- 0	- 0	- 0	**40** 5	**40** 67	**27** 95	**100** 18	**84** 64	**79** 38	**94** 16	**79** 87	**100** 97	**79** 48	**100** 23	**38** 8	**0** 2	**100** 8	- -	- -
Choctaw Nation Health Care Center, Talihina, OK	**100** 1	**100** 2	**100** 1	**100** 1	**100** 1	- 0	- 0	- 0	**100** 5	**15** 20	**81** 21	**60** 5	**84** 25	**77** 13	**80** 5	**81** 27	**100** 29	**64** 11	**12** 8	**69** 16	**100** 4	**100** 14	- -	- -
Cimarron Memorial Hospital & Nursing Home, Boise City, OK	- -	- -	- -	- -	- -	- -	- -	- -	- 0	**33** 3	**0** 5	- 0	**44** 16	- 0	- 0	**80** 10	**100** 16	**91** 11	**33** 3	- -	- -	- -	- -	- -
Claremore Regional Hospital, Claremore, OK	**100** 2	**100** 15	**100** 7	**100** 11	**83** 6	- 0	- 0	**100** 1	**94** 17	**86** 43	**98** 66	**100** 13	**94** 87	**92** 90	**91** 34	**89** 124	**100** 149	**91** 89	**100** 37	**91** 202	**92** 52	**79** 198	- -	- -
Cleveland Area Hospital, Cleveland, OK	- 0	**100** 2	- 0	**0** 2	- 0	- 0	- -	- 0	**50** 4	**50** 10	**82** 11	- 0	**83** 29	**67** 6	**64** 11	**66** 29	**100** 34	**45** 22	**60** 5	- -	- -	- -	- -	- -
Clinton Indian Hospital, Clinton, OK	- -	- -	- -	- -	- -	- -	- -	- -	- -	- -	- -	- -	**0** 1	- 0	- -	**50** 2	**100** 3	- 0	- 0	- -	- -	- -	- -	- -
Comanche County Memorial Hospital, Lawton, OK	**88** 59	**97** 177	**98** 301	**96** 157	**98** 291	**100** 2	**75** 12	**99** 130	**91** 135	**62** 278	**96** 304	**100** 76	**84** 185	**84** 173	**91** 46	**76** 257	**100** 317	**88** 184	**97** 72	**65** 201	**91** 64	**69** 192	- -	- -
Community Hospital, Oklahoma City, OK	- -	- -	- -	- -	- -	- -	- -	- -	**100** 1	**0** 3	**100** 3	**0** 2	**53** 15	**89** 9	**50** 4	**70** 10	**100** 16	**71** 7	**29** 7	**92** 50	**100** 14	**64** 50	- -	- -
Community Hospital Lakeview, Eufaula, OK	- -	- -	- -	- -	- -	- -	- -	- -	- 0	**0** 2	**0** 5	**0** 1	**67** 3	- 0	**0** 1	**100** 1	**100** 4	**0** 4	**0** 2	- -	- -	- -	- -	- -
Cordell Memorial Hospital, Cordell, OK	- 0	- 0	- 0	- 0	- 0	**100** 1	- 0	- 0	**100** 1	**33** 3	**40** 5	- 0	**100** 5	**100** 1	**100** 1	**89** 9	**100** 13	**70** 10	**50** 2	- -	- -	- -	- -	- -
Craig General Hospital, Vinita, OK	- 0	**100** 4	**100** 3	**0** 1	**50** 2	- 0	- 0	**0** 1	**93** 14	**64** 44	**86** 51	**73** 11	**92** 73	**80** 10	**96** 25	**98** 82	**100** 96	**95** 64	**70** 20	**25** 4	**50** 2	**75** 4	- -	- -
Cushing Regional Hospital, Cushing, OK	**100** 1	**50** 2	**100** 2	**100** 4	**100** 4	- 0	- 0	**50** 2	**62** 16	**11** 61	**43** 81	**92** 12	**75** 91	**88** 60	**49** 35	**92** 113	**100** 151	**51** 92	**70** 47	**76** 58	**96** 27	**97** 58	- -	- -
Deaconess Hospital, Oklahoma City, OK	**88** 40	**93** 91	**95** 92	**82** 44	**97** 99	- 0	**33** 3	**100** 35	**85** 61	**45** 113	**91** 150	**97** 31	**92** 119	**94** 154	**88** 69	**77** 189	**100** 211	**89** 133	**98** 50	**85** 406	**92** 132	**89** 372	- -	- -
Drumright Regional Hospital, Drumright, OK	- 0	**100** 1	**100** 1	**100** 1	**100** 1	- 0	- -	- 0	**0** 3	**67** 15	**35** 17	**100** 1	**62** 55	**50** 2	**0** 12	**81** 67	**100** 76	**5** 37	**82** 17	**36** 14	**0** 7	**100** 14	- -	- -
Duncan Regional Hospital, Duncan, OK	**100** 4	**95** 38	**95** 20	**97** 30	**100** 19	**75** 4	- 0	**60** 5	**100** 34	**95** 99	**97** 144	**100** 23	**91** 138	**95** 147	**87** 53	**87** 196	**100** 249	**96** 167	**94** 51	**92** 158	**92** 49	**53** 152	- -	- -
Eastern Oklahoma Medical Center, Poteau, OK	**100** 2	**89** 9	**67** 6	**71** 7	**50** 6	**0** 1	- 0	**50** 2	**62** 45	**61** 171	**53** 196	**95** 40	**79** 107	**77** 48	**31** 26	**76** 144	**97** 153	**21** 92	**91** 64	**83** 12	**80** 10	**100** 11	- -	- -
Edmond Medical Center, Edmond, OK	**100** 2	**97** 34	**95** 21	**83** 30	**85** 26	- 0	- 0	**100** 8	**81** 26	**45** 55	**80** 71	**100** 9	**73** 71	**94** 64	**88** 25	**76** 97	**98** 112	**87** 67	**100** 19	**77** 115	**86** 49	**80** 105	- -	- -
Elkview General Hospital, Hobart, OK	- 0	**100** 5	**100** 1	**60** 5	**100** 1	**100** 1	- 0	- 0	**90** 10	**95** 19	**92** 24	**100** 5	**100** 32	**50** 2	**83** 6	**91** 35	**100** 43	**100** 23	**91** 11	**89** 9	**100** 1	**89** 9	- -	- -
Fairfax Memorial Hospital, Fairfax, OK	- -	- -	- -	- -	- -	- -	- -	- -	**100** 3	**100** 1	**100** 5	- 0	**92** 26	**100** 13	**100** 9	**96** 28	**100** 34	**89** 18	**100** 16	- -	- -	- -	- -	- -
Fairview Hospital, Fairview, OK	- -	- -	- -	- -	- -	- -	- -	- -	- 0	**14** 7	**9** 11	- 0	**82** 22	**67** 3	- -	**76** 21	**100** 33	**4** 25	**0** 2	- -	- -	- -	- -	- -
Foundation Bariatric Hospital of Oklahoma, Edmond, OK	- -	- -	- -	- -	- -	- -	- -	- -	- -	- -	- -	- -	- -	- -	- -	- -	- -	- -	- -	- -	- -	- -	- -	- -
Grady Memorial Hospital, Chickasha, OK	- 0	**100** 4	**80** 5	**80** 5	**60** 5	- 0	- 0	- 0	**69** 13	**90** 71	**84** 86	**100** 20	**87** 117	**93** 60	**95** 22	**84** 115	**99** 156	**92** 89	**87** 30	**94** 68	**88** 25	**85** 62	- -	- -
Great Plains Regional Medical Center, Elk City, OK	- 0	**100** 13	**83** 6	**85** 13	**88** 8	**25** 4	- 0	**100** 2	**88** 34	**55** 58	**94** 82	**86** 7	**78** 68	**93** 68	- -	**78** 115	**99** 133	**74** 91	**79** 33	**55** 85	**81** 26	**35** 78	- -	- -
Harmon Memorial Hospital, Hollis, OK	- 0	**100** 7	**67** 3	**71** 7	**67** 3	**50** 4	- 0	- 0	**29** 7	**50** 18	**22** 32	**60** 5	**60** 40	**89** 9	**25** 8	**80** 85	**100** 97	**30** 61	**25** 16	- -	- -	- -	- -	- -
Harper County Community Hospital, Buffalo, OK	- 0	- 0	- 0	- 0	- 0	- 0	- -	- 0	**100** 1	**100** 1	**100** 5	**50** 2	**100** 13	**100** 1	**100** 3	**89** 19	**100** 21	**100** 15	**86** 7	**100** 1	- 0	**100** 1	- -	- -
Haskell County Healthcare System, Stigler, OK	- 0	**50** 8	**40** 5	**57** 7	**62** 8	- 0	- 0	**100** 1	**20** 5	**37** 30	**40** 43	**40** 5	**88** 57	**58** 12	- -	**84** 64	**95** 86	**59** 64	**64** 22	**100** 1	- 0	**100** 1	- -	- -
Healdton Municipal Hospital, Healdton, OK	- 0	- 0	- 0	- 0	- 0	- 0	- 0	- 0	**100** 2	**0** 1	**43** 7	- 0	**86** 22	**100** 5	**0** 4	**71** 28	**100** 31	**58** 12	**0** 4	- -	- -	- -	- -	- -
Henryetta Medical Center, Henryetta, OK	**0** 1	**100** 5	**67** 3	**60** 5	**67** 3	- 0	- 0	- 0	**76** 17	**67** 30	**73** 41	**100** 9	**89** 56	**96** 71	**77** 31	**98** 80	**99** 105	**76** 70	**86** 22	**86** 22	**100** 6	**91** 22	- -	- -
Hillcrest Medical Center, Tulsa, OK	**97** 69	**99** 211	**98** 327	**97** 187	**98** 347	**0** 1	**50** 4	**94** 147	**98** 214	**72** 527	**94** 608	**86** 153	**84** 241	**91** 149	**41** 37	**81** 243	**99** 312	**50** 135	**89** 114	**90** 198	**93** 68	**64** 192	- -	- -
Holdenville General Hospital, Holdenville, OK	**100** 1	**0** 2	**100** 1	**50** 2	**0** 1	- 0	- 0	- 0	**100** 8	**66** 29	**68** 40	**50** 6	**94** 35	**100** 42	**95** 20	**95** 65	**100** 74	**87** 52	**67** 18	- -	- -	- -	- -	- -
Integris Baptist Medical Center, Oklahoma City, OK	**100** 100	**99** 251	**100** 525	**96** 153	**99** 474	- 0	**55** 11	**100** 219	**99** 310	**89** 494	**100** 575	**99** 111	**89** 238	**95** 214	**79** 80	**68** 372	**100** 418	**75** 260	**69** 95	**92** 791	**98** 202	**93** 766	- -	- -
Integris Baptist Regional Health Center, Miami, OK	- 0	**89** 19	**89** 9	**88** 17	**100** 9	- 0	- 0	**100** 2	**87** 45	**89** 129	**100** 150	**100** 27	**86** 174	**82** 108	**96** 50	**88** 252	**100** 283	**96** 157	**97** 64	**88** 145	**97** 39	**83** 140	- -	- -
Integris Bass Baptist Health Center, Enid, OK	**78** 9	**99** 69	**92** 74	**93** 60	**87** 71	**0** 6	**100** 3	**100** 35	**89** 18	**94** 67	**89** 110	**100** 15	**83** 105	**86** 95	**92** 37	**92** 119	**100** 159	**88** 98	**98** 44	**91** 288	**97** 73	**92** 283	- -	- -
Integris Blackwell Regional Hospital, Blackwell, OK	**100** 1	**80** 5	**67** 3	**100** 2	**100** 2	- 0	- 0	- 0	**94** 16	**78** 51	**99** 77	**100** 14	**91** 90	**99** 71	**100** 33	**91** 141	**100** 155	**98** 91	**96** 53	**88** 8	**75** 4	**67** 6	- -	- -
Integris Canadian Valley Regional Hospital, Yukon, OK	**100** 2	**100** 7	**100** 7	**71** 7	**44** 9	- 0	- 0	**100** 1	**65** 23	**90** 70	**91** 95	**92** 12	**86** 180	**93** 104	- -	**90** 163	**100** 190	**68** 114	**100** 50	**93** 104	**97** 30	**79** 104	- -	- -
Integris Clinton Regional Hospital, Clinton, OK	- 0	**100** 2	- 0	**100** 1	**100** 2	**0** 1	- 0	**100** 1	**94** 50	**91** 65	**100** 82	**100** 7	**99** 68	**99** 82	**86** 35	**90** 132	**100** 148	**99** 86	**100** 36	**100** 10	**83** 6	**100** 6	- -	- -
Integris Grove General Hospital, Grove, OK	**86** 7	**95** 37	**84** 31	**91** 32	**94** 31	**0** 1	- 0	**100** 14	**86** 22	**93** 70	**91** 103	**100** 26	**86** 118	**95** 117	**83** 52	**91** 183	**100** 195	**94** 137	**100** 44	**97** 173	**100** 44	**99** 169	- -	- -

NOTE: The first number in each column (boldface) is the rate in percent, the second number is the number of patients; Please refer to the main entry for footnotes; ***Heart Attack Care:*** *1. ACE Inhibitor or ARB for LVSD; 2. Aspirin at Arrival; 3. Aspirin at Discharge; 4. Beta Blocker at Arrival; 5. Beta Blocker at Discharge; 6. Fibrinolytic Medication Timing; 7. PCI Within 90 Minutes of Arrival; 8. Smoking Cessation Advice;* ***Heart Failure Care:*** *9. ACE Inhibitor or ARB for LVSD; 10. Discharge Instructions; 11. Evaluation of LVS Function; 12. Smoking Cessation Advice;* ***Pneumonia Care:*** *13. Appropriate Initial Antibiotic; 14. Blood Culture Timing; 15. Influenza Vaccine; 16. Initial Antibiotic Timing; 17. Oxygenation Assessment; 18. Pneumococcal Vaccine; 19. Smoking Cessation Advice;* ***Surgical Infection Prevention:*** *20. Prophylactic Antibiotic Given; 21. Prophylactic Antibiotic Selection; 22. Prophylactic Antibiotic Stopped;* ***Pregnancy Care:*** *23. Inpatient Neonatal Mortality; 24. Third or Fourth Degree Laceration*

Hospital	Heart Attack Care								Heart Failure Care				Pneumonia Care							Surgical Infection Prevention			Pregnancy Care	
	1	2	3	4	5	6	7	8	9	10	11	12	13	14	15	16	17	18	19	20	21	22	23	24
Integris Marshall County Medical Center, Madill, OK	- 0	88 8	60 5	57 7	83 6	- 0	- 0	- 0	50 6	65 26	84 38	100 6	97 103	94 50	90 31	86 141	100 156	92 84	100 39	- -	- -	- -	- -	- -
Integris Mayes County Medical Center, Pryor, OK	- 0	100 2	100 1	100 1	100 1	- 0	- 0	- 0	88 16	97 31	94 52	100 8	97 67	95 56	100 15	93 75	100 86	98 43	100 28	95 37	100 5	92 36	- -	- -
Integris Southwest Medical Center, Oklahoma City, OK	78 65	99 228	91 236	97 181	92 223	0 1	50 6	97 127	84 215	71 355	92 415	98 120	94 249	93 267	68 76	93 352	100 414	82 244	95 153	91 497	98 144	73 462	- -	- -
Jackson County Memorial Hospital, Altus, OK	100 9	91 23	89 9	74 27	92 12	17 6	- 0	25 4	89 65	69 98	87 132	100 25	84 116	96 70	83 24	93 147	98 178	89 111	83 52	92 119	98 53	68 113	- -	- -
Jane Phillips Medical Center, Bartlesville, OK	95 37	99 135	98 161	94 125	97 148	- 0	70 10	98 47	89 80	36 159	87 175	87 30	73 257	93 175	67 61	90 250	100 309	79 203	84 74	84 367	94 117	50 343	- -	- -
Jefferson County Hospital, Waurika, OK	- -	- -	- -	- -	- -	- -	- -	- -	0 1	33 3	25 4	- 0	62 8	100 1	50 2	0 5	100 11	33 6	50 2	- -	- -	- -	- -	- -
Johnston Memorial Hospital, Tishomingo, OK	- -	- -	- -	- -	- -	- -	- -	- -	88 8	5 21	35 51	67 9	56 36	100 6	33 15	86 51	100 61	29 38	65 23	- -	- -	- -	- -	- -
Kingfisher Regional, Kingfisher, OK	- -	- -	- -	- -	- -	- -	- -	- -	8 12	0 25	79 33	0 4	81 48	100 2	48 23	73 11	100 51	31 36	29 7	- -	- -	- -	- -	- -
Lakeside Women's Hospital, Oklahoma City, OK	- -	- -	- -	- -	- -	- -	- -	- -	- -	- -	- -	- -	- -	- -	- -	- -	- -	- -	- -	67 9	- -	100 9	0.00 1145	5.09 746
Latimer County General Hospital, Wilburton, OK	- 0	100 1	- 0	100 1	- 0	100 2	- -	- 0	- 0	83 12	47 17	100 3	75 8	100 1	50 2	82 11	100 14	86 7	100 2	- -	- -	- -	- -	- -
Lawton Indian Hospital, Lawton, OK	- -	- -	- -	- -	- -	- -	- -	- -	80 10	20 15	80 15	50 4	53 32	77 13	88 8	54 37	98 40	50 8	36 11	51 39	88 8	100 36	- -	- -
Lindsay Municipal Hospital, Lindsay, OK	- 0	- 0	- 0	- 0	- 0	- 0	- -	- 0	75 4	86 21	25 20	20 10	81 27	100 11	50 12	78 23	100 32	29 14	17 12	- 0	100 1	100 1	- -	- -
Logan Medical Center, Guthrie, OK	80 5	78 9	75 8	62 13	80 10	50 2	- 0	0 1	100 15	33 12	79 39	50 10	88 40	96 28	50 10	93 45	100 57	79 38	50 16	- -	- -	- -	- -	- -
Mangum City Hospital, Mangum, OK	100 1	100 2	67 3	100 2	67 3	- 0	- -	50 2	67 3	9 11	27 15	0 1	83 18	100 5	100 3	67 15	96 24	73 15	20 5	- -	- -	- -	- -	- -
Mary Hurley Hospital, Coalgate, OK	- -	- -	- -	- -	- -	- -	- -	- -	40 5	58 19	72 32	33 6	52 29	100 6	60 15	60 52	100 56	56 39	29 14	- -	- -	- -	- -	- -
McAlester Regional Health Center, McAlester, OK	86 7	83 42	74 23	66 38	67 21	0 1	- 0	100 6	79 58	38 146	67 202	100 51	69 108	93 94	- -	94 145	100 176	85 119	87 45	96 193	93 59	79 189	- -	- -
Mcbride Clinic Orthopedic Hospital, Oklahoma City, OK	- -	- -	- -	- -	- -	- -	- -	- -	- -	- -	- -	- -	- -	- -	- -	- -	- -	- -	- -	97 138	100 46	97 136	- -	- -
McCurtain Memorial Hospital, Idabel, OK	- 0	100 4	33 3	50 4	33 3	- 0	- 0	- 0	56 9	48 48	76 54	83 12	89 74	93 68	52 31	84 99	100 125	62 69	83 30	78 9	100 7	67 9	- -	- -
Medical Center of Southeastern Oklahoma, Durant, OK	100 13	98 54	100 35	98 42	100 29	0 1	- 0	100 14	100 76	100 190	100 287	100 62	72 166	100 142	100 66	97 219	100 299	100 153	99 84	91 147	100 27	81 143	- -	- -
Memorial Hospital, Frederick, OK	- 0	0 1	- 0	0 1	0 1	- 0	- 0	- 0	75 4	62 21	100 37	62 8	76 25	100 1	100 8	84 31	100 46	87 31	100 7	- -	- -	- -	- -	- -
Memorial Hospital of Stillwell, Stillwell, OK	- 0	60 5	100 3	75 4	100 4	- 0	- 0	100 1	88 41	71 72	92 88	60 10	54 24	91 22	60 10	82 45	100 50	83 30	75 8	50 6	100 2	67 6	- -	- -
Memorial Hospital of Texas County, Guymon, OK	50 2	71 7	60 5	86 7	75 8	50 2	- 0	50 4	100 5	16 19	21 24	75 4	65 88	82 11	93 28	64 59	98 101	84 58	27 26	26 19	100 7	59 17	- -	- -
Mercy Health Center, Oklahoma City, OK	100 1	93 14	94 16	73 11	100 12	- 0	- 0	100 4	97 38	73 89	98 128	100 22	86 143	93 163	95 73	82 251	100 343	96 235	91 79	94 175	98 49	78 167	- -	- -
Mercy Health Love County Hospital, Marietta, OK	- -	- -	- -	- -	- -	- -	- -	- -	- -	- -	- -	- -	67 3	100 1	20 5	86 7	88 8	17 6	40 5	- -	- -	- -	- -	- -
Mercy Memorial Health Center, Ardmore, OK	87 30	93 142	95 131	90 90	95 131	46 24	- 0	98 46	85 82	70 205	92 248	95 73	79 228	98 126	46 67	76 322	100 355	85 220	93 84	88 561	92 125	78 544	- -	- -
Midwest Regional Medical Center, Midwest City, OK	89 71	95 301	89 319	81 258	89 285	0 1	20 20	92 123	86 201	80 400	94 464	99 97	71 216	89 178	72 58	74 309	99 358	71 200	92 96	89 650	98 119	70 624	- -	- -
Moore Medical Center, Moore, OK	- 0	75 4	- 0	25 4	- 0	0 3	- 0	- 0	33 6	11 28	90 30	85 13	71 52	91 34	14 7	93 43	98 59	50 14	80 25	77 60	100 22	100 51	- -	- -
Muskogee Regional Medical Center, Muskogee, OK	89 18	96 130	91 57	98 107	95 74	- 0	- 0	100 11	92 83	84 194	93 256	100 49	91 87	88 86	80 25	74 143	99 159	76 90	94 52	87 218	96 69	70 203	- -	- -
Newman Memorial Hospital, Shattuck, OK	- 0	86 7	50 6	83 6	100 6	100 1	- 0	100 1	100 2	64 11	46 13	100 1	74 23	100 1	71 7	88 24	100 28	56 16	86 7	50 6	- 0	83 6	- -	- -
Norman Regional Hospital, Norman, OK	94 31	99 165	96 170	97 122	99 172	0 1	56 9	100 74	93 87	91 214	100 267	98 51	99 219	99 303	100 98	96 367	100 476	100 259	97 179	92 677	93 214	68 650	- -	- -
Northwest Surgical Hospital, Oklahoma City, OK	- -	- -	- -	- -	- -	- -	- -	- -	- -	- -	- -	- -	- -	- -	- -	- -	- -	- -	- -	96 228	96 54	81 226	- -	- -
O U Medical Center, Oklahoma City, OK	96 26	100 121	99 152	99 104	97 147	50 2	100 1	100 68	90 208	93 377	99 405	95 155	89 128	90 156	64 33	65 209	100 249	77 73	89 97	84 772	95 175	88 702	1.94 5100	2.78 3131
Okeene Municipal Hospital, Okeene, OK	- 0	100 3	- 0	100 1	- 0	67 3	- 0	- 0	0 1	0 6	56 9	25 4	50 12	100 1	71 7	85 13	94 18	77 13	25 4	- 0	- -	- 0	- -	- -
Okla Ctr for Ortho & Multi-Spec Surg, Oklahoma City, OK	- -	- -	- -	- -	- -	- -	- -	- -	- -	- -	- -	- -	- -	- -	- -	- -	- -	- -	- -	77 48	95 19	25 36	- -	- -
Oklahoma Heart Hospital, Oklahoma City, OK	100 55	100 65	99 302	98 57	100 296	- 0	100 2	100 120	99 192	100 295	100 312	100 65	100 17	100 13	100 4	86 21	100 27	88 16	100 6	98 184	100 44	97 177	- -	- -
Oklahoma Spine Hospital, Oklahoma City, OK	- -	- -	- -	- -	- -	- -	- -	- -	- -	- -	- -	- -	- -	- -	- -	- -	- -	- -	- -	100 6	- -	67 6	- -	- -
Oklahoma State University Medical Center, Tulsa, OK	83 75	94 125	94 206	84 106	93 201	- 0	0 1	94 98	86 153	28 304	91 333	94 122	92 151	81 131	46 52	78 225	98 274	52 96	92 128	83 282	96 51	62 266	- -	- -
Okmulgee Memorial Hospital, Okmulgee, OK	- 0	100 2	100 2	100 1	100 1	0 1	- 0	- 0	33 3	18 33	36 47	0 1	98 41	93 27	85 13	84 50	100 62	63 46	22 18	32 19	100 6	100 19	- -	- -
Orthopedic Hospital, Oklahoma City, OK	- -	- -	- -	- -	- -	- -	- -	- -	- -	- -	- -	- -	- -	- -	- -	- -	- -	- -	- -	0 1	- -	100 1	- -	- -
Orthopedic Hospital of Oklahoma, Tulsa, OK	- -	- -	- -	- -	- -	- -	- -	- -	- -	- -	- -	- -	- -	- -	- -	- -	- -	- -	- -	65 139	- -	71 139	- -	- -
Parkview Hospital, El Reno, OK	0 1	40 5	67 3	50 4	67 3	- 0	- 0	50 2	0 1	29 14	64 22	50 2	76 58	85 33	88 17	88 76	99 95	94 51	83 23	93 15	100 1	100 12	- -	- -
Pauls Valley General Hospital, Pauls Valley, OK	- 0	80 5	75 4	100 4	100 4	- 0	- 0	- 0	100 14	88 49	70 67	100 13	95 64	100 41	100 14	89 76	100 91	97 61	96 24	80 10	100 3	60 10	- -	- -
Pawhuska Hospital, Pawhuska, OK	- -	- -	- -	- -	- -	- -	- -	- -	- 0	0 2	50 2	- 0	90 10	- 0	0 3	100 9	82 11	0 8	- 0	- -	- -	- -	- -	- -
Pawnee Municipal Hospital, Pawnee, OK	0 1	100 4	0 2	50 2	50 2	- 0	- 0	- 0	0 1	45 22	32 25	67 6	85 20	- 0	71 7	83 24	100 26	67 12	17 6	0 3	100 3	100 3	- -	- -
Perry Memorial Hospital, Perry, OK	- 0	100 2	- 0	0 2	0 1	0 2	- -	- 0	100 6	68 22	65 31	100 11	91 35	91 11	77 13	96 55	100 64	86 42	50 14	- -	- -	- -	- -	- -
PHS Indian Hospital, Claremore, OK	0 1	100 2	100 1	100 2	100 1	- 0	- 0	0 1	100 9	74 39	92 40	93 15	87 46	68 38	62 8	83 52	100 57	71 21	86 14	96 111	89 37	97 107	- -	- -
Ponca City Medical Center, Ponca City, OK	100 3	85 47	69 16	69 42	80 15	29 14	- 0	100 2	86 22	92 66	70 81	87 15	85 92	92 60	82 22	81 99	98 118	79 71	84 31	51 86	88 26	60 84	- -	- -
Prague Municipal Hospital, Prague, OK	0 1	- 0	100 1	- 0	- 0	- 0	- -	- -	- 0	33 3	25 4	0 1	83 6	67 3	100 2	88 8	100 10	100 5	100 1	- -	- -	- -	- -	- -

NOTE: The first number in each column (boldface) is the rate in percent, the second number is the number of patients; Please refer to the main entry for footnotes; ***Heart Attack Care:*** *1. ACE Inhibitor or ARB for LVSD; 2. Aspirin at Arrival; 3. Aspirin at Discharge; 4. Beta Blocker at Arrival; 5. Beta Blocker at Discharge; 6. Fibrinolytic Medication Timing; 7. PCI Within 90 Minutes of Arrival; 8. Smoking Cessation Advice;* ***Heart Failure Care:*** *9. ACE Inhibitor or ARB for LVSD; 10. Discharge Instructions; 11. Evaluation of LVS Function; 12. Smoking Cessation Advice;* ***Pneumonia Care:*** *13. Appropriate Initial Antibiotic; 14. Blood Culture Timing; 15. Influenza Vaccine; 16. Initial Antibiotic Timing; 17. Oxygenation Assessment; 18. Pneumococcal Vaccine; 19. Smoking Cessation Advice;* ***Surgical Infection Prevention:*** *20. Prophylactic Antibiotic Given; 21. Prophylactic Antibiotic Selection; 22. Prophylactic Antibiotic Stopped;* ***Pregnancy Care:*** *23. Inpatient Neonatal Mortality; 24. Third or Fourth Degree Laceration*

Hospital	Heart Attack Care								Heart Failure Care				Pneumonia Care							Surgical Infection Prevention			Pregnancy Care	
	1	2	3	4	5	6	7	8	9	10	11	12	13	14	15	16	17	18	19	20	21	22	23	24
Purcell Municipal Hospital, Purcell, OK	- 0	60 10	67 6	38 13	43 7	- 0	- 0	100 1	57 7	63 52	55 64	70 10	75 81	93 42	73 37	79 143	100 159	52 104	62 32	67 3	- 0	100 3	- -	- -
Pushmataha Hospital, Antlers, OK	- 0	100 1	- 0	- 0	- 0	- 0	- 0	- 0	80 15	92 40	86 50	71 7	91 56	81 57	94 17	94 63	100 78	83 46	88 16	75 4	25 4	100 4	- -	- -
Saint Anthony Hospital, Oklahoma City, OK	92 37	98 172	98 223	94 140	98 205	- 0	50 4	92 92	85 259	62 441	96 492	100 137	90 182	93 195	93 57	87 258	100 286	84 155	92 98	95 564	99 133	88 507	0.10 960	3.72 646
Saint Francis Heart Hospital, Tulsa, OK	86 109	90 136	98 507	86 118	97 510	100 1	67 12	96 277	90 116	79 137	94 93	96 25	- 0	- 0	- 0	- 0	- 0	- 0	- 0	86 311	98 98	86 297	- -	- -
Saint Francis Hospital, Tulsa, OK	90 115	97 472	97 492	90 316	97 479	50 4	29 21	100 208	88 276	54 542	95 646	99 149	88 637	93 661	83 197	73 754	100 1004	85 612	98 264	93 1687	88 571	76 1634	- -	- -
Saint Francis Hospital, Broken Arrow, OK	100 1	100 13	88 8	91 11	100 8	- 0	- 0	- 0	89 19	80 35	96 52	100 6	97 103	96 113	100 29	94 129	100 165	100 107	94 32	96 187	98 47	96 185	- -	- -
Saint John Medical Center, Tulsa, OK	90 125	97 415	98 532	99 350	99 520	100 1	63 19	100 214	87 336	74 627	98 725	97 156	87 351	91 255	96 92	77 425	100 593	89 350	96 148	85 2555	97 628	85 2480	- -	- -
Saint John Sapulpa Hospital, Sapulpa, OK	- -	- -	- -	- -	- -	- -	- -	- -	67 24	48 46	62 53	64 14	85 65	87 55	92 12	81 83	98 94	52 46	62 26	- -	- -	- -	- -	- -
Saint Mary's Regional Medical Center, Enid, OK	88 17	93 71	86 72	77 56	84 69	- 0	50 4	96 23	62 55	95 149	67 212	100 22	86 92	96 74	83 48	85 162	100 193	85 140	84 32	90 379	92 105	86 360	- -	- -
Sayre Memorial Hospital, Sayre, OK	100 1	83 12	78 9	22 9	50 8	0 1	- 0	100 1	50 2	50 26	19 27	0 2	95 83	100 9	76 37	94 120	100 132	41 58	36 36	- -	- -	- -	- -	- -
Seiling Municipal Hospital Authority, Seiling, OK	- -	- -	- -	- -	- -	- -	- -	- -	50 2	12 8	20 15	33 3	40 15	100 4	43 7	100 15	100 19	80 10	17 6	- -	- -	- -	- -	- -
Seminole Medical Center, Seminole, OK	- -	- -	- -	- -	- -	- -	- -	- -	100 4	0 17	35 20	20 5	92 40	96 24	56 9	89 44	98 49	40 25	75 12	0 1	0 1	100 1	- -	- -
Sequoyah Memorial Hospital, Sallisaw, OK	- 0	56 9	75 4	100 4	60 5	- 0	- 0	100 2	100 4	61 41	86 44	75 12	92 49	95 44	89 9	77 66	100 83	89 44	76 25	- -	- -	- -	- -	- -
Share Medical Center, Alva, OK	0 1	33 3	50 2	50 2	50 2	- 0	- 0	- 0	60 5	57 23	90 30	50 2	89 19	100 13	93 15	98 48	100 56	92 38	71 14	0 1	100 1	100 1	- -	- -
Southcrest Hospital, Tulsa, OK	96 24	99 94	100 118	100 83	100 114	- 0	0 2	94 35	100 98	95 198	97 227	97 30	90 105	96 98	87 31	86 139	99 158	95 104	98 41	88 378	94 108	84 353	- -	- -
Southwestern Medical Center, Lawton, OK	100 2	77 13	57 7	40 5	83 6	- 0	- 0	100 2	82 34	21 86	76 105	86 22	88 97	91 67	69 39	86 135	100 175	69 111	94 36	50 38	88 33	71 35	0.30 339	5.98 184
Southwestern Regional Medical Center, Tulsa, OK	- 0	- 0	- 0	- 0	- 0	- 0	- 0	- 0	50 2	75 4	100 4	50 2	- 0	- 0	- 0	67 6	89 9	0 3	100 1	19 26	25 12	33 21	- -	- -
Stillwater Medical Center, Stillwater, OK	100 10	100 40	100 17	100 20	100 17	100 1	- 0	100 4	92 24	80 66	93 84	89 18	90 102	98 102	84 38	94 142	100 161	83 102	97 32	75 232	78 83	83 244	- -	- -
Stroud Regional Medical Center, Stroud, OK	- 0	- 0	- 0	- 0	- 0	0 1	- -	- 0	57 7	62 8	87 15	50 2	74 34	93 14	0 7	78 36	100 50	19 27	60 10	- -	- -	- -	- -	- -
Surgical Hospital of Oklahoma, Oklahoma City, OK	- -	- -	- -	- -	- -	- -	- -	- -	- -	- -	- -	- -	- -	- -	- -	- -	- -	- -	- -	81 114	100 46	98 112	- -	- -
Tahlequah City Hospital, Tahlequah, OK	75 4	95 22	92 24	78 18	91 23	0 3	0 1	36 11	88 42	51 68	87 93	50 16	80 54	92 50	- -	86 88	97 117	53 72	76 21	7 113	83 46	29 102	- -	- -
Tulsa Spine & Specialty Hospital, Tulsa, OK	- -	- -	- -	- -	- -	- -	- -	- -	- -	- -	- -	- -	- -	- -	- -	- -	- -	- -	- -	- -	- -	- -	- -	- -
Unity Health Center, Shawnee, OK	91 11	94 67	90 29	97 34	90 29	42 12	- 0	100 10	82 72	86 131	93 158	100 27	86 182	97 203	98 54	91 253	100 286	97 175	98 81	95 128	100 49	76 124	- -	- -
Valley View Regional Hospital, Ada, OK	100 2	92 36	100 10	85 26	82 11	17 6	- 0	83 6	72 39	58 120	90 143	96 27	84 114	81 116	78 37	80 147	96 180	80 102	100 35	87 203	98 91	70 208	- -	- -
W W Hastings Indian Hospital, Tahlequah, OK	- 0	67 3	- 0	67 3	- 0	- 0	- 0	- 0	43 7	0 33	78 32	50 8	87 75	87 52	73 15	61 80	100 92	61 31	58 36	35 20	84 19	100 18	- -	- -
Wagoner Hospital, Wagoner, OK	- 0	- 0	- 0	- 0	- 0	- 0	- -	- 0	100 5	33 21	52 27	43 7	78 41	- 0	- -	69 36	96 49	74 27	36 14	- -	- -	- -	- -	- -
Watonga Municipal Hospital, Watonga, OK	100 1	0 1	100 1	0 1	0 1	- 0	- 0	- 0	- 0	- 0	25 4	- 0	88 8	- 0	- -	80 5	100 9	0 5	100 2	- -	- -	- -	- -	- -
Weatherford Regional Hospital, Weatherford, OK	- 0	71 7	- 0	50 8	0 1	- 0	- 0	- 0	100 2	50 12	60 20	0 1	55 66	80 5	- -	67 63	100 78	79 48	17 12	- -	- -	- -	- -	- -
Woodward Hospital and Health Center, Woodward, OK	- 0	83 6	100 3	100 7	100 3	- 0	- 0	- 0	94 18	100 44	95 63	86 7	83 48	95 55	96 28	91 101	100 127	81 78	100 23	71 58	94 17	98 54	- -	- -
SOUTH DAKOTA																								
Avera Heart Hospital of South Dakota, Sioux Falls, SD	96 103	99 99	99 641	99 92	100 674	0 1	100 1	100 214	96 84	93 155	99 182	100 24	- 0	100 2	0 1	67 3	100 3	83 6	- 0	95 355	100 106	99 347	- -	- -
Avera McKennan Hospital & Univ Hlth Ctr, Sioux Falls, SD	100 18	100 78	99 77	97 68	100 82	- 0	60 10	100 29	94 64	100 151	99 215	100 26	93 100	89 89	92 37	89 142	100 173	88 131	100 40	96 384	93 278	90 362	- -	- -
Avera Sacred Heart Hospital, Yankton, SD	91 11	100 26	100 19	100 26	100 18	- 0	- 0	- 0	98 55	99 88	100 127	100 5	92 88	94 78	100 36	92 124	100 175	98 125	100 36	96 269	99 69	92 249	- -	- -
Avera Saint Benedict Health Center, Parkston, SD	100 1	100 4	100 3	50 2	100 3	- 0	- 0	- 0	0 1	67 3	90 10	- 0	79 14	100 3	100 6	95 22	100 26	100 22	100 3	- -	- -	- -	- -	- -
Avera Saint Luke's, Aberdeen, SD	62 8	98 50	100 32	100 30	94 34	18 11	- 0	100 5	100 24	94 84	99 128	100 16	89 94	98 97	88 24	95 129	100 183	98 126	100 29	90 412	93 95	87 411	- -	- -
Black Hills Surgery Center, Rapid City, SD	- -	- -	- -	- -	- -	- -	- -	- -	- -	- -	- -	- -	- -	- -	- -	- -	- -	- -	- -	99 134	100 50	95 132	- -	- -
Brookings Hospital, Brookings, SD	100 3	100 22	100 15	96 24	94 17	- 0	- 0	- 0	70 10	80 5	70 33	100 1	90 10	100 15	- -	92 60	100 82	84 58	100 3	94 17	- -	100 15	- -	- -
Community Memorial Hospital, Redfield, SD	0 1	100 2	100 1	100 2	100 2	- 0	- -	- 0	0 1	0 1	80 5	- 0	60 15	100 8	100 8	96 27	100 38	100 30	0 1	- -	- -	- -	- -	- -
Coteau Des Prairies Hospital, Sisseton, SD	- 0	67 3	100 2	100 4	100 5	- 0	- 0	- 0	80 5	0 3	59 22	- 0	100 1	- 0	- -	90 20	100 30	48 21	- 0	0 3	- -	100 2	- -	- -
Custer Regional Hospital, Custer, SD	100 1	100 2	100 2	100 2	100 2	- 0	- 0	- 0	75 4	75 8	90 10	- 0	90 10	100 2	- 0	76 17	100 19	82 11	- 0	- -	- -	- -	- -	- -
Dakota Plains Surgical Center, Aberdeen, SD	- -	- -	- -	- -	- -	- -	- -	- -	- -	- -	- -	- -	- -	- -	- -	- -	- -	- -	- -	98 62	- -	68 62	- -	- -
De Smet Memorial Hospital, De Smet, SD	100 1	100 1	100 1	100 2	100 1	- 0	- 0	- 0	67 3	50 4	56 9	- 0	81 16	100 4	100 3	86 21	100 30	89 28	100 1	- -	- -	- -	- -	- -
Fall River Hospital, Hot Springs, SD	- -	- -	- -	- -	- -	- -	- -	- -	- -	- -	- -	- -	- 0	- 0	- -	- 0	100 1	100 1	- 0	- -	- -	- -	- -	- -
Gregory Health Care Center, Gregory, SD	- 0	- 0	- 0	- 0	- 0	100 1	- 0	- 0	100 1	0 5	45 11	0 1	63 30	100 1	73 15	94 50	100 65	72 53	8 12	- -	- -	- -	- -	- -
Holy Infant Hospital, Hoven, SD	- -	- -	- -	- -	- -	- -	- -	- -	- -	- -	- -	- -	100 1	- 0	- -	90 10	100 11	56 9	- 0	- -	- -	- -	- -	- -
Huron Regional Medical Center, Huron, SD	17 6	100 10	88 8	80 10	89 9	50 4	- -	0 1	50 2	56 9	50 12	- 0	85 71	100 7	91 23	72 80	100 103	66 80	50 14	94 36	100 15	21 34	- -	- -
Landmann-Jungman Memorial Hospital, Scotland, SD	- -	- -	- -	- -	- -	- -	- -	- -	100 1	0 1	60 5	- 0	20 30	100 1	70 10	84 25	100 36	49 35	100 1	- -	- -	- -	- -	- -
Lead-Deadwood Regional Hospital, Deadwood, SD	- 0	- 0	- 0	- 0	50 2	67 3	- -	0 2	75 4	83 12	73 15	100 4	82 17	83 6	83 6	80 20	100 23	86 22	0 1	67 9	- -	100 9	- -	- -

NOTE: The first number in each column (boldface) is the rate in percent, the second number is the number of patients; Please refer to the main entry for footnotes; ***Heart Attack Care:*** *1. ACE Inhibitor or ARB for LVSD; 2. Aspirin at Arrival; 3. Aspirin at Discharge; 4. Beta Blocker at Arrival; 5. Beta Blocker at Discharge; 6. Fibrinolytic Medication Timing; 7. PCI Within 90 Minutes of Arrival; 8. Smoking Cessation Advice;* ***Heart Failure Care:*** *9. ACE Inhibitor or ARB for LVSD; 10. Discharge Instructions; 11. Evaluation of LVS Function; 12. Smoking Cessation Advice;* ***Pneumonia Care:*** *13. Appropriate Initial Antibiotic; 14. Blood Culture Timing; 15. Influenza Vaccine; 16. Initial Antibiotic Timing; 17. Oxygenation Assessment; 18. Pneumococcal Vaccine; 19. Smoking Cessation Advice;* ***Surgical Infection Prevention:*** *20. Prophylactic Antibiotic Given; 21. Prophylactic Antibiotic Selection; 22. Prophylactic Antibiotic Stopped;* ***Pregnancy Care:*** *23. Inpatient Neonatal Mortality; 24. Third or Fourth Degree Laceration*

Hospital	Heart Attack Care 1	2	3	4	5	6	7	8	Heart Failure Care 9	10	11	12	Pneumonia Care 13	14	15	16	17	18	19	Surgical Infection Prevention 20	21	22	Pregnancy Care 23	24
Lewis and Clark Specialty Hospital, Yankton, SD	- -	- -	- -	- -	- -	- -	- -	- -	- -	- -	- -	- -	- -	- -	- -	- -	- -	- -	- -	**51** 80	**100** 16	**94** 79	- -	- -
Madison Community Hospital, Madison, SD	- 0	- 0	- 0	- 0	- 0	- 0	- -	- 0	- 0	**0** 1	**80** 5	**100** 1	**90** 10	**100** 6	- -	**94** 16	**100** 18	**47** 15	**100** 1	**67** 6	**33** 3	**33** 6	- -	- -
Mobridge Regional Hospital, Mobridge, SD	- 0	**50** 4	**67** 3	**100** 4	**100** 3	**56** 9	- 0	- 0	**75** 4	**43** 7	**67** 12	**100** 2	**86** 21	**100** 3	**80** 5	**100** 25	**100** 28	**74** 23	**20** 5	- -	- -	- -	- -	- -
PHS Indian Health Service Hospital, Pine Ridge, SD	- 0	- 0	- 0	- 0	- 0	- -	- -	- -	- 0	**0** 3	**0** 16	**0** 1	**33** 3	**100** 1	- -	**44** 27	**97** 29	**50** 14	**0** 3	- -	- -	- -	- -	- -
PHS Indian Hospital, Eagle Butte, SD	- -	- -	- -	- -	- -	- -	- -	- -	- 0	**0** 2	**0** 2	**0** 1	**0** 3	**100** 1	- -	**80** 5	**100** 6	**0** 4	**0** 1	- -	- -	- -	- -	- -
PHS Indian Hospital, Rapid City, SD	- -	- -	- -	- -	- -	- -	- -	- -	- 0	**0** 1	**33** 3	- 0	**0** 4	- 0	- -	**86** 7	**100** 10	**71** 7	**0** 2	- -	- -	- -	- -	- -
PHS Indian Hospital, Rosebud, SD	- -	- -	- -	- -	- -	- -	- -	- -	**100** 2	**0** 4	**86** 7	**0** 1	**100** 2	**100** 1	- -	**64** 11	**100** 18	**27** 11	**0** 1	- -	- -	- -	- -	- -
PHS Indian Hospital, Sisseton, SD	- -	- -	- -	- -	- -	- -	- -	- -	- -	- -	- -	- -	- -	- -	- -	- -	- -	- -	- -	- -	- -	- -	- -	- -
Platte Health Center, Platte, SD	**100** 1	**100** 2	**100** 2	**100** 2	**100** 2	- 0	- 0	- 0	**100** 4	**100** 2	**100** 10	**100** 2	**78** 9	**100** 4	**86** 7	**90** 30	**100** 31	**93** 28	**50** 2	- -	- -	- -	- -	- -
Prairie Lakes Hospital & Care Center, Watertown, SD	**100** 2	**88** 16	**85** 13	**64** 14	**82** 11	- 0	- 0	**100** 1	**76** 25	**67** 58	**82** 82	**71** 7	**96** 108	**92** 72	**88** 26	**95** 154	**100** 180	**72** 146	**38** 24	**93** 328	**96** 75	**98** 320	- -	- -
Queen of Peace Hospital, Mitchell, SD	**100** 2	**89** 19	**100** 10	**82** 11	**91** 11	- 0	- 0	- 0	**92** 24	**94** 51	**92** 96	**100** 7	**91** 103	**97** 68	**81** 37	**93** 149	**100** 185	**91** 130	**97** 39	**96** 177	**98** 45	**89** 171	- -	- -
Rapid City Regional Hospital, Rapid City, SD	**93** 59	**99** 125	**100** 242	**95** 109	**97** 317	**0** 2	**91** 11	**99** 130	**84** 102	**88** 224	**93** 290	**98** 46	**86** 189	**83** 133	**71** 48	**85** 234	**98** 300	**86** 206	**97** 86	**91** 668	**91** 69	**86** 621	- -	- -
Saint Mary's Healthcare Center, Pierre, SD	**100** 1	**86** 7	**75** 4	**83** 6	**75** 4	**36** 11	- 0	**100** 1	**54** 13	**52** 31	**64** 50	**88** 8	**83** 54	**94** 31	**89** 19	**84** 85	**100** 99	**97** 72	**88** 17	**94** 107	**92** 40	**90** 101	**0.00** 477	**5.10** 314
Same Day Surgery Center, Rapid City, SD	- -	- -	- -	- -	- -	- -	- -	- -	- -	- -	- -	- -	- -	- -	- -	- -	- -	- -	- -	**83** 6	- -	**67** 6	- -	- -
Sanford USD Medical Center, Sioux Falls, SD	**90** 59	**100** 191	**99** 358	**96** 146	**99** 357	- 0	**67** 6	**92** 139	**88** 92	**87** 196	**97** 262	**88** 41	**86** 122	**93** 70	**95** 37	**84** 180	**100** 256	**87** 166	**88** 67	**90** 1128	**98** 220	**88** 1060	**0.00** 0	**0.00** 0
Sioux Falls Surgical Center, Sioux Falls, SD	- -	- -	- -	- -	- -	- -	- -	- -	- -	- -	- -	- -	- -	- -	- -	- -	- -	- -	- -	**79** 197	**94** 82	**92** 197	- -	- -
Sioux Valley Vermillian Campus, Vermillion, SD	- 0	**100** 3	**100** 2	**100** 1	- 0	- 0	- 0	**0** 1	**25** 4	**22** 9	**33** 15	**0** 2	**89** 28	**100** 5	**75** 8	**90** 31	**100** 36	**83** 24	**62** 8	**100** 3	**100** 1	**67** 3	- -	- -
Siouxland Surgery Center Lp, Dakota Dunes, SD	- -	- -	- -	- -	- -	- -	- -	- -	- -	- -	- -	- -	- -	- -	- -	- -	- -	- -	- -	**96** 366	**85** 94	**90** 366	- -	- -
Spearfish Regional Hospital, Spearfish, SD	- 0	**100** 2	**100** 1	**50** 2	**100** 1	- 0	- 0	- 0	**86** 7	**31** 16	**73** 22	- 0	**87** 38	**100** 13	**85** 20	**89** 45	**100** 56	**85** 41	**100** 7	**91** 145	**100** 32	**93** 141	- -	- -
Spearfish Surgery Center, Spearfish, SD	- -	- -	- -	- -	- -	- -	- -	- -	- -	- -	- -	- -	- 0	- 0	- -	**100** 1	**100** 2	**0** 1	- 0	**89** 19	- -	**100** 18	- -	- -
Sturgis Regional Hospital, Sturgis, SD	- 0	**100** 2	**100** 3	**100** 2	**100** 3	**50** 2	- 0	- 0	**100** 6	**100** 7	**75** 12	**100** 2	**89** 56	**100** 11	**89** 9	**91** 57	**100** 57	**84** 43	**100** 9	**67** 6	- 0	**100** 6	- -	- -
Winner Regional Healthcare Center, Winner, SD	- 0	- 0	- 0	- 0	- 0	- 0	- 0	- 0	**100** 4	**50** 14	**75** 16	**0** 1	**76** 17	**100** 5	**100** 2	**90** 20	**100** 25	**65** 20	**100** 7	**100** 23	**100** 2	**100** 23	- -	- -
WISCONSIN																								
Amery Regional Medical Center, Amery, WI	- -	- -	- -	- -	- -	- -	- -	- -	**67** 6	**77** 31	**59** 41	**75** 4	**86** 29	**100** 5	**80** 5	**92** 38	**100** 48	**60** 35	**86** 7	**45** 87	**90** 29	**88** 85	- -	- -
Appleton Medical Center, Appleton, WI	**99** 74	**99** 154	**97** 236	**99** 141	**99** 279	- 0	**100** 11	**99** 92	**98** 61	**99** 141	**98** 186	**100** 23	**90** 96	**98** 128	**48** 23	**90** 186	**100** 222	**60** 159	**100** 39	**85** 1117	**96** 257	**71** 1087	- -	- -
Aspirus-Wausau Hospital, Wausau, WI	**100** 58	**100** 100	**100** 242	**100** 69	**99** 241	- 0	**100** 2	**100** 105	**96** 78	**95** 263	**99** 312	**100** 38	**95** 100	**92** 103	**67** 36	**88** 150	**100** 204	**90** 143	**93** 42	**94** 544	**96** 80	**87** 527	**0.28** 1081	**3.34** 958
Aurora Baycare Medical Center, Green Bay, WI	**100** 13	**100** 61	**98** 121	**100** 53	**100** 113	- 0	**67** 3	**100** 35	**100** 21	**90** 48	**100** 68	**100** 10	**92** 51	**100** 50	**89** 9	**96** 57	**100** 87	**92** 48	**100** 24	**93** 126	**99** 72	**86** 113	**0.35** 1719	**2.15** 1253
Aurora Lakeland Medical Center, Elkhorn, WI	**100** 1	**96** 25	**92** 12	**100** 19	**100** 11	- 0	- 0	**100** 3	**96** 23	**95** 66	**99** 94	**100** 14	**91** 98	**98** 114	**91** 33	**97** 157	**100** 190	**94** 138	**100** 42	**84** 74	**87** 31	**80** 70	- -	- -
Aurora Medical Center, Kenosha, WI	**75** 4	**100** 19	**92** 13	**92** 13	**100** 19	- 0	- 0	**100** 3	**95** 19	**98** 54	**100** 73	**100** 14	**99** 83	**99** 98	**100** 22	**97** 113	**100** 147	**100** 87	**100** 46	**77** 60	**79** 29	**84** 56	- -	- -
Aurora Medical Center, Two Rivers, WI	**71** 17	**100** 34	**100** 21	**90** 20	**100** 20	- 0	- 0	**100** 3	**91** 22	**83** 41	**100** 64	**100** 2	**88** 60	**98** 58	**94** 16	**97** 71	**100** 107	**97** 71	**88** 16	**92** 65	**97** 30	**97** 62	**0.00** 305	**3.03** 198
Aurora Medical Center of Washington County, Hartford, WI	**100** 1	**100** 11	**88** 8	**92** 12	**100** 10	- 0	- 0	**100** 2	**91** 33	**81** 54	**100** 79	**100** 7	**92** 62	**95** 73	**87** 15	**96** 97	**100** 114	**83** 78	**95** 21	**86** 84	**93** 42	**91** 81	- -	- -
Aurora Medical Center Oshkosh, Oshkosh, WI	**89** 9	**99** 74	**97** 67	**91** 57	**94** 65	**0** 1	**67** 6	**100** 24	**86** 29	**67** 52	**98** 80	**100** 8	**97** 62	**94** 53	**85** 13	**93** 82	**100** 109	**87** 63	**100** 23	**90** 86	**82** 44	**52** 83	**0.00** 773	**3.72** 564
Aurora Memorial Hospital of Burlington, Burlington, WI	**100** 3	**100** 25	**100** 12	**100** 19	**100** 12	- 0	- 0	**100** 5	**93** 27	**97** 88	**100** 114	**100** 14	**97** 70	**98** 66	**100** 10	**99** 92	**100** 125	**100** 78	**100** 31	**90** 89	**98** 44	**87** 86	- -	- -
Aurora Saint Luke's Medical Center, Milwaukee, WI	**86** 255	**97** 557	**97** 897	**91** 326	**96** 804	**0** 2	**82** 28	**100** 377	**90** 666	**57** 1254	**97** 1497	**99** 232	**92** 559	**96** 792	**89** 174	**85** 890	**100** 1121	**86** 770	**97** 272	**89** 170	**97** 90	**87** 167	- -	- -
Aurora Sheboygan Memorial Medical Center, Sheboygan, WI	**100** 8	**100** 41	**100** 25	**100** 22	**100** 27	- 0	- 0	**100** 8	**100** 34	**96** 85	**100** 102	**93** 14	**91** 75	**100** 67	**95** 22	**93** 108	**100** 130	**95** 79	**100** 39	**91** 96	**96** 45	**88** 96	- -	- -
Baldwin Area Medical Center, Baldwin, WI	- 0	**100** 3	**100** 3	**100** 1	**100** 2	- 0	- 0	- 0	**80** 5	**45** 11	**72** 18	**50** 2	**93** 46	**89** 19	**100** 13	**96** 71	**100** 101	**88** 66	**64** 14	**47** 74	**100** 9	**91** 68	- -	- -
Barron Memorial Med Ctr-Mayo Health System, Barron, WI	**100** 1	**89** 9	**100** 8	**83** 6	**83** 6	- 0	- -	- 0	**100** 8	**91** 11	**87** 31	**67** 3	**100** 9	**89** 9	**83** 6	**94** 16	**100** 20	**93** 14	**100** 2	**100** 6	- -	**83** 6	- -	- -
Bay Area Medical Center, Marinette, WI	**84** 25	**98** 85	**98** 48	**91** 86	**96** 50	**0** 1	- 0	**100** 9	**89** 61	**87** 98	**99** 136	**100** 13	**82** 99	**92** 115	**77** 26	**92** 151	**100** 181	**80** 117	**88** 32	**92** 153	**88** 43	**80** 150	- -	- -
Beaver Dam Community Hospital, Beaver Dam, WI	**100** 5	**95** 22	**78** 18	**95** 20	**83** 18	- 0	- 0	- 0	**94** 16	**56** 39	**95** 56	**40** 10	**88** 67	**94** 48	**87** 30	**91** 114	**99** 137	**67** 101	**61** 23	**93** 213	**92** 74	**84** 210	- -	- -
Bellin Memorial Hospital, Green Bay, WI	**68** 50	**99** 170	**99** 350	**100** 143	**99** 362	- 0	**70** 10	**97** 116	**81** 52	**82** 138	**96** 167	**96** 28	**83** 46	**100** 41	**86** 14	**77** 56	**100** 72	**77** 43	**86** 21	**94** 417	**97** 156	**88** 403	- -	- -
Beloit Memorial Hospital, Beloit, WI	**75** 12	**95** 56	**97** 32	**95** 55	**95** 44	**25** 8	- 0	**100** 12	**82** 73	**74** 125	**89** 151	**97** 36	**91** 89	**90** 72	- -	**88** 121	**100** 150	**72** 97	**88** 41	**88** 290	**87** 60	**74** 279	- -	- -
Berlin Memorial Hospital, Berlin, WI	- 0	**100** 8	**80** 5	**100** 5	**100** 5	- 0	- -	- 0	**93** 14	**80** 41	**83** 63	**100** 8	**93** 42	**100** 41	**75** 8	**81** 69	**100** 76	**87** 60	**100** 9	**86** 186	**30** 43	**76** 184	- -	- -
Black River Memorial Hospital, Black River Falls, WI	- 0	**100** 7	**100** 5	**100** 7	**100** 5	- 0	- 0	**100** 1	**100** 32	**100** 27	**100** 35	**0** 1	**61** 38	**82** 11	**78** 9	**90** 40	**100** 47	**82** 39	**50** 6	- -	- -	- -	- -	- -
Bloomer Medical Center, Bloomer, WI	- -	- -	- -	- -	- -	- -	- -	- -	- 0	**100** 6	**100** 10	- 0	**92** 13	**100** 8	**100** 3	**100** 17	**100** 21	**100** 18	**100** 1	- 0	- 0	- 0	- -	- -
Bond Health Center, Oconto, WI	- -	- -	- -	- -	- -	- -	- -	- -	- -	- -	- -	- -	- -	- -	- -	- -	- -	- -	- -	- -	- -	- -	- -	- -
Boscobel Area Health Care, Boscobel, WI	**100** 1	**50** 2	**50** 2	**100** 2	**67** 3	- 0	- 0	- 0	**100** 2	**0** 13	**50** 16	- 0	**91** 11	**100** 3	**100** 2	**54** 13	**100** 16	**64** 11	**100** 1	- -	- -	- -	- -	- -
Burnett Medical Center, Grantsburg, WI	- 0	**100** 2	**100** 2	**50** 2	**100** 2	- 0	- -	- 0	- 0	**62** 8	**64** 11	**100** 1	**60** 10	**100** 2	**100** 5	**86** 14	**100** 24	**86** 14	**75** 4	**57** 14	**100** 1	**43** 14	- -	- -
Calumet Memorial Hospital, Chilton, WI	- -	- -	- -	- -	- -	- -	- -	- -	**100** 3	**82** 11	**95** 19	**100** 1	**100** 21	**100** 19	**80** 5	**94** 33	**100** 42	**82** 33	**60** 5	**78** 27	**100** 2	**65** 26	- -	- -

NOTE: The first number in each column (boldface) is the rate in percent, the second number is the number of patients; Please refer to the main entry for footnotes; ***Heart Attack Care:*** *1. ACE Inhibitor or ARB for LVSD; 2. Aspirin at Arrival; 3. Aspirin at Discharge; 4. Beta Blocker at Arrival; 5. Beta Blocker at Discharge; 6. Fibrinolytic Medication Timing; 7. PCI Within 90 Minutes of Arrival; 8. Smoking Cessation Advice;* ***Heart Failure Care:*** *9. ACE Inhibitor or ARB for LVSD; 10. Discharge Instructions; 11. Evaluation of LVS Function; 12. Smoking Cessation Advice;* ***Pneumonia Care:*** *13. Appropriate Initial Antibiotic; 14. Blood Culture Timing; 15. Influenza Vaccine; 16. Initial Antibiotic Timing; 17. Oxygenation Assessment; 18. Pneumococcal Vaccine; 19. Smoking Cessation Advice;* ***Surgical Infection Prevention:*** *20. Prophylactic Antibiotic Given; 21. Prophylactic Antibiotic Selection; 22. Prophylactic Antibiotic Stopped;* ***Pregnancy Care:*** *23. Inpatient Neonatal Mortality; 24. Third or Fourth Degree Laceration*

Hospital	Heart Attack Care								Heart Failure Care				Pneumonia Care							Surgical Infection Prevention			Pregnancy Care	
	1	2	3	4	5	6	7	8	9	10	11	12	13	14	15	16	17	18	19	20	21	22	23	24
Columbia Saint Mary's Hospital Columbia, Milwaukee, WI	- -	- -	- -	- -	- -	- -	- -	- -	- -	- -	- -	- -	- -	- -	- -	- -	- -	- -	- -	- -	- -	- -	- -	- -
Columbia Saint Mary's Hospital Milwaukee, Milwaukee, WI	**66** 35	**98** 136	**96** 140	**92** 104	**97** 152	- 0	**60** 5	**91** 54	**89** 160	**77** 303	**92** 367	**95** 85	**90** 180	**90** 177	**81** 57	**84** 281	**100** 334	**82** 214	**82** 78	**94** 377	**95** 129	**76** 372	- -	- -
Columbia Saint Marys Ozaukee Campus, Mequon, WI	**62** 13	**98** 113	**99** 106	**98** 89	**97** 107	- 0	**80** 5	**93** 30	**85** 59	**59** 128	**84** 191	**87** 15	**94** 140	**90** 124	**63** 41	**90** 197	**100** 246	**70** 192	**85** 33	**91** 175	**98** 57	**86** 174	- -	- -
Columbus Community Hospital, Columbus, WI	**0** 1	**100** 11	**100** 9	**92** 12	**80** 10	- 0	- 0	- 0	**100** 8	**73** 11	**67** 21	- 0	**84** 43	**91** 22	**75** 8	**79** 52	**98** 66	**51** 45	**20** 5	- -	- -	- -	- -	- -
Community Memorial Hospital, Menomonee Falls, WI	**56** 34	**98** 124	**95** 112	**85** 104	**92** 129	- 0	**42** 12	**94** 32	**75** 79	**55** 147	**96** 195	**90** 29	**88** 73	**94** 71	**84** 19	**91** 106	**100** 135	**74** 92	**92** 24	**84** 430	**95** 83	**77** 429	- -	- -
Community Memorial Hospital, Oconto Falls, WI	- -	- -	- -	- -	- -	- -	- -	- -	- -	- -	- -	- -	**81** 26	**94** 16	**67** 6	**90** 41	**100** 45	**76** 34	**50** 4	**62** 60	**87** 23	**75** 60	- -	- -
Cumberland Memorial Hospital, Cumberland, WI	- 0	**100** 4	**100** 3	**100** 4	**100** 3	**0** 1	- 0	- 0	**50** 8	**52** 21	**60** 25	**50** 4	**61** 54	**100** 4	**88** 8	**81** 57	**96** 71	**81** 47	**67** 15	- -	- -	- -	- -	- -
Divine Savior Healthcare, Portage, WI	**100** 2	**80** 10	**100** 4	**70** 10	**100** 4	- 0	- 0	- 0	**89** 18	**90** 10	**64** 67	**0** 1	**70** 10	**92** 12	- -	**86** 101	**100** 120	**49** 89	**0** 2	**83** 23	- -	**70** 23	**0.00** 309	**4.64** 237
Door County Memorial Hospital, Sturgeon Bay, WI	- 0	**75** 4	**100** 3	**100** 3	**100** 4	- 0	- 0	- 0	**62** 16	**47** 59	**77** 81	**100** 5	**88** 58	**93** 43	**40** 10	**84** 82	**100** 100	**55** 74	**89** 19	**64** 70	**92** 13	**86** 65	- -	- -
Edgerton Hospital and Health Services, Edgerton, WI	- 0	**75** 4	**75** 4	- -	- -	- -	- -	- 0	**100** 1	**100** 13	- -	- -	**100** 9	- 0	- -	**88** 8	**100** 9	**75** 4	- -	- -	- -	- -	- -	- -
Elmbrook Memorial Hospital, Brookfield, WI	**50** 2	**93** 14	**82** 11	**80** 5	**100** 7	- 0	- 0	- 0	**90** 30	**53** 88	**98** 96	**100** 11	**88** 99	**98** 100	**96** 25	**91** 144	**100** 182	**79** 130	**100** 36	**71** 311	**89** 38	**67** 305	- -	- -
Fort Memorial Hospital, Fort Atkinson, WI	**75** 4	**100** 17	**100** 13	**70** 10	**45** 11	**0** 3	- 0	- 0	**92** 12	**76** 37	**89** 70	**83** 6	**85** 55	**90** 51	- -	**83** 59	**100** 102	**80** 59	**68** 19	**92** 234	**98** 50	**98** 221	- -	- -
Franciscan Skemp Healthcare-Arcadia, Arcadia, WI	- -	- -	- -	- -	- -	- -	- -	- -	**50** 4	**80** 5	**100** 8	**67** 3	**100** 8	**100** 5	**100** 3	**92** 13	**100** 17	**89** 9	**50** 4	- -	- -	- -	- -	- -
Franciscan Skemp Healthcare-Sparta Campus, Sparta, WI	- -	- -	- -	- -	- -	- -	- -	- -	**100** 2	**100** 5	**78** 18	**100** 1	**96** 24	**89** 18	**100** 5	**97** 30	**100** 36	**100** 19	**100** 5	- -	- -	- -	- -	- -
Franciscan Skemp Medical Center, La Crosse, WI	**87** 23	**99** 74	**99** 99	**100** 62	**100** 110	- 0	**40** 5	**100** 49	**95** 38	**62** 68	**99** 95	**93** 14	**91** 100	**94** 108	**82** 33	**89** 140	**100** 199	**89** 156	**78** 40	**93** 624	**99** 142	**79** 603	- -	- -
Froedtert Hospital/Med College of Wisconsin, Milwaukee, WI	**91** 44	**98** 133	**99** 166	**96** 96	**99** 170	**0** 1	**100** 5	**100** 68	**97** 144	**71** 272	**96** 308	**99** 79	**97** 87	**89** 100	**100** 21	**80** 160	**100** 180	**81** 75	**97** 58	**72** 377	**74** 208	**58** 363	**2.03** 1580	**3.57** 1147
Good Samaritan Health Center, Merrill, WI	- 0	**67** 3	**100** 1	**67** 3	**50** 2	- 0	- -	**100** 1	**100** 5	**100** 17	**81** 27	**75** 4	**88** 25	**90** 21	**67** 3	**87** 38	**100** 48	**100** 29	**100** 10	**95** 77	**100** 13	**89** 76	- -	- -
Gundersen Lutheran, La Crosse, WI	**100** 56	**99** 181	**100** 291	**98** 141	**100** 356	**0** 1	**67** 12	**100** 105	**98** 59	**97** 130	**100** 166	**93** 27	**88** 110	**93** 115	**69** 29	**93** 157	**100** 209	**81** 160	**95** 63	**86** 264	**97** 68	**86** 259	**0.24** 1693	**3.56** 1263
Hayward Area Memorial Hospital, Hayward, WI	**100** 2	**100** 11	**100** 12	**100** 12	**100** 11	- 0	- 0	- 0	**83** 6	**60** 20	**89** 28	**67** 6	**94** 49	**79** 33	**79** 14	**93** 68	**100** 79	**89** 54	**94** 17	**81** 37	**100** 16	**76** 34	- -	- -
Hess Memorial Hospital, Mauston, WI	**100** 1	**70** 10	**75** 4	**83** 12	**89** 9	- 0	- 0	- 0	**92** 12	**45** 11	**68** 87	**50** 2	**86** 7	**100** 4	- -	**84** 74	**93** 90	**65** 63	**100** 4	**80** 50	- -	**90** 49	- -	- -
Holy Family Memorial, Manitowoc, WI	**100** 10	**97** 78	**96** 74	**97** 72	**97** 72	**0** 1	**100** 2	**84** 25	**97** 35	**79** 85	**88** 125	**100** 12	**84** 73	**93** 68	**96** 23	**90** 115	**100** 139	**93** 102	**93** 15	**87** 256	**98** 43	**85** 247	- -	- -
Howard Young Medical Center, Woodruff, WI	**100** 3	**100** 15	**89** 9	**100** 15	**100** 10	- 0	- 0	**100** 2	**92** 26	**89** 84	**98** 95	**75** 12	**74** 58	**95** 56	**69** 13	**82** 90	**100** 108	**82** 72	**100** 19	**92** 323	**100** 76	**83** 319	- -	- -
Hudson Hospital, Hudson, WI	**67** 3	**100** 7	**100** 5	**62** 8	**71** 7	- 0	- 0	- 0	**75** 4	**77** 13	**76** 29	**40** 5	**83** 30	**78** 27	**25** 8	**83** 36	**100** 46	**38** 34	**67** 9	- -	- -	- -	- -	- -
Indianhead Medical Center, Shell Lake, WI	- 0	**100** 1	**100** 1	**100** 1	**100** 1	- 0	- 0	- 0	**100** 4	**59** 22	**46** 24	**0** 1	**82** 17	**100** 4	**75** 4	**100** 22	**100** 27	**57** 23	**75** 4	- -	- -	- -	- -	- -
Kenosha Medical Center Campus, Kenosha, WI	**81** 27	**96** 143	**95** 133	**94** 127	**90** 125	- 0	**100** 12	**98** 47	**87** 101	**77** 212	**96** 274	**94** 33	**89** 196	**92** 179	**100** 53	**88** 294	**100** 346	**90** 205	**81** 75	**58** 130	**98** 131	**50** 127	- -	- -
Lakeview Medical Center of Rice Lake, Rice Lake, WI	**100** 4	**100** 21	**100** 16	**100** 17	**100** 19	- 0	- 0	**40** 5	**92** 36	**75** 85	**93** 104	**83** 12	**100** 76	**100** 63	**92** 24	**94** 114	**100** 142	**97** 96	**82** 34	**92** 330	**100** 71	**95** 317	- -	- -
Langlade Memorial Hospital, Antigo, WI	- -	- -	- -	- -	- -	- -	- -	- -	**62** 8	**75** 28	**68** 38	**60** 5	**83** 30	**89** 9	**80** 10	**86** 44	**100** 56	**64** 39	**80** 10	- -	- -	- -	- -	- -
Luther Midelfort Hospital, Eau Claire, WI	**75** 55	**97** 99	**100** 255	**93** 102	**99** 266	- 0	**100** 4	**96** 79	**83** 75	**92** 166	**100** 223	**87** 23	**95** 131	**95** 131	**96** 50	**90** 184	**100** 237	**95** 194	**89** 45	**98** 882	**100** 213	**95** 777	**0.18** 559	**4.24** 401
Luther Midelfort Oakridge, Osseo, WI	- -	- -	- -	- -	- -	- -	- -	- -	**100** 2	**100** 1	**100** 4	**100** 1	**100** 7	**100** 8	**100** 3	**75** 12	**100** 13	**100** 8	**100** 3	- -	- -	- -	- -	- -
Memorial Health Center, Medford, WI	- -	- -	- -	- -	- -	- -	- -	- -	**100** 6	**100** 16	**97** 30	**50** 2	**93** 28	**89** 9	**60** 5	**83** 29	**100** 29	**54** 24	**0** 1	**86** 14	**100** 3	**100** 14	- -	- -
Memorial Hospital of Lafayette County, Darlington, WI	- 0	**90** 10	**50** 6	**100** 7	**29** 7	- 0	- 0	- 0	**50** 4	**22** 18	**68** 22	**0** 2	**77** 22	**100** 2	**67** 6	**91** 33	**100** 41	**45** 31	**0** 1	**85** 33	**100** 3	**70** 33	- -	- -
Memorial Medical Center, Ashland, WI	**100** 3	**89** 19	**79** 14	**92** 13	**90** 10	- 0	- 0	**100** 3	**94** 18	**78** 36	**82** 49	**83** 6	**87** 61	**93** 59	**82** 11	**83** 88	**100** 104	**77** 77	**75** 16	**64** 163	**89** 36	**81** 156	**0.00** 296	**1.84** 217
Memorial Medical Center, Neillsville, WI	- 0	**100** 3	**100** 3	**100** 3	**100** 3	- 0	- 0	- 0	**40** 5	**89** 9	**63** 19	- 0	**79** 28	**100** 10	**0** 5	**77** 31	**100** 39	**30** 23	**43** 7	- -	- -	- -	- -	- -
Mercy Hospital Janesville, Janesville, WI	**100** 17	**98** 94	**89** 114	**94** 81	**92** 116	**0** 3	**33** 3	**93** 46	**79** 70	**71** 154	**95** 202	**97** 36	**92** 157	**97** 121	- -	**78** 200	**100** 271	**90** 172	**93** 61	**91** 676	**93** 142	**71** 651	**0.00** 1190	**5.27** 816
Mercy Medical Center, Oshkosh, WI	**81** 26	**99** 74	**100** 79	**96** 68	**97** 79	- 0	**60** 5	**97** 32	**84** 38	**67** 64	**100** 89	**92** 13	**96** 45	**91** 57	**62** 8	**84** 86	**100** 106	**75** 85	**59** 22	**88** 886	**99** 206	**12** 879	- -	- -
Mercy Walworth Hospital & Medical Center, Lake Geneva, WI	- 0	- 0	- 0	- 0	- 0	- 0	- 0	- 0	- 0	**33** 6	**100** 6	**100** 1	**100** 11	**100** 15	**75** 4	**100** 16	**100** 18	**77** 13	**50** 2	**82** 11	**100** 1	**91** 11	- -	- -
Meriter Hospital, Madison, WI	**91** 43	**99** 178	**98** 284	**99** 159	**97** 266	**40** 10	**57** 7	**100** 84	**95** 95	**91** 221	**98** 288	**100** 43	**91** 140	**85** 80	**87** 30	**87** 178	**100** 246	**73** 164	**93** 45	**90** 1209	**96** 312	**87** 1160	- -	- -
Monroe Clinic and Hospital, Monroe, WI	**100** 1	**100** 15	**83** 6	**100** 5	**89** 9	**100** 1	- 0	**100** 1	**100** 33	**88** 77	**99** 116	**100** 8	**90** 104	**94** 96	**84** 31	**81** 139	**99** 169	**89** 121	**68** 34	**76** 397	**93** 97	**83** 387	- -	- -
Moundview Memorial Hospital & Clinics, Friendship, WI	- -	- -	- -	- -	- -	- -	- -	- -	**100** 5	**27** 15	**95** 20	**0** 3	**86** 21	**80** 5	**80** 5	**86** 28	**100** 37	**56** 25	**50** 6	- -	- -	- -	- -	- -
New London Family Medical Center, New London, WI	- -	- -	- -	- -	- -	- -	- -	- -	- -	- -	- -	- -	**95** 38	**96** 26	**100** 5	**85** 48	**100** 54	**81** 37	**100** 11	- -	- -	- -	- -	- -
Oak Leaf Surgcl Hospital, Eau Claire, WI	- -	- -	- -	- -	- -	- -	- -	- -	- -	- -	- -	- -	- -	- -	- -	- -	- -	- -	- -	**76** 59	- -	**88** 57	- -	- -
Oconomowoc Memorial Hospital, Oconomowoc, WI	**73** 15	**98** 44	**100** 43	**95** 40	**96** 45	- 0	**29** 7	**80** 15	**93** 29	**65** 72	**87** 105	**94** 17	**86** 128	**91** 78	**93** 27	**89** 156	**100** 189	**84** 128	**91** 47	**92** 305	**93** 44	**79** 292	- -	- -
Orthopaedic Hospital of Wisconsin, Glendale, WI	- -	- -	- -	- -	- -	- -	- -	- -	- -	- -	- -	- -	- -	- -	- -	- -	- -	- -	- -	- -	- -	- -	- -	- -
Our Lady of Victory Hospital, Stanley, WI	**100** 3	**78** 9	**57** 7	**86** 7	**88** 8	- 0	- 0	- 0	**100** 7	**100** 23	**94** 36	**50** 2	**82** 17	**100** 4	**75** 4	**96** 25	**100** 26	**89** 18	**83** 6	**0** 4	**100** 1	**100** 4	- -	- -
Red Cedar Medical Center, Menomonie, WI	- 0	**100** 10	**100** 7	**100** 7	**100** 7	- 0	- 0	- 0	**100** 9	**94** 47	**95** 60	**100** 5	**91** 33	**100** 28	**100** 6	**87** 45	**100** 56	**88** 42	**100** 11	**92** 64	**100** 9	**89** 62	- -	- -
Reedsburg Area Medical Center, Reedsburg, WI	**0** 1	**88** 8	**100** 3	**75** 8	**100** 5	- 0	- 0	- 0	**91** 11	**35** 26	**84** 37	**40** 5	**99** 69	**92** 25	**89** 18	**92** 80	**100** 95	**93** 69	**87** 15	**65** 75	**100** 22	**66** 74	- -	- -
Richland Hospital, Richland Center, WI	- 0	**100** 10	**100** 8	**100** 9	**100** 8	**0** 1	- 0	- 0	**87** 15	**84** 37	**76** 58	**80** 5	**67** 30	**90** 21	**80** 10	**84** 43	**100** 57	**57** 35	**100** 9	**63** 54	**92** 13	**77** 53	- -	- -
Ripon Medical Center, Ripon, WI	- -	- -	- -	- -	- -	- -	- -	- -	**71** 7	**50** 12	**72** 32	**50** 4	**95** 20	**89** 9	**33** 3	**90** 31	**97** 34	**64** 28	**56** 9	- -	- -	- -	- -	- -

NOTE: The first number in each column (boldface) is the rate in percent, the second number is the number of patients; Please refer to the main entry for footnotes; ***Heart Attack Care:*** *1. ACE Inhibitor or ARB for LVSD; 2. Aspirin at Arrival; 3. Aspirin at Discharge; 4. Beta Blocker at Arrival; 5. Beta Blocker at Discharge; 6. Fibrinolytic Medication Timing; 7. PCI Within 90 Minutes of Arrival; 8. Smoking Cessation Advice;* ***Heart Failure Care:*** *9. ACE Inhibitor or ARB for LVSD; 10. Discharge Instructions; 11. Evaluation of LVS Function; 12. Smoking Cessation Advice;* ***Pneumonia Care:*** *13. Appropriate Initial Antibiotic; 14. Blood Culture Timing; 15. Influenza Vaccine; 16. Initial Antibiotic Timing; 17. Oxygenation Assessment; 18. Pneumococcal Vaccine; 19. Smoking Cessation Advice;* ***Surgical Infection Prevention:*** *20. Prophylactic Antibiotic Given; 21. Prophylactic Antibiotic Selection; 22. Prophylactic Antibiotic Stopped;* ***Pregnancy Care:*** *23. Inpatient Neonatal Mortality; 24. Third or Fourth Degree Laceration*

Hospital	Heart Attack Care								Heart Failure Care				Pneumonia Care							Surgical Infection Prevention			Pregnancy Care	
	1	2	3	4	5	6	7	8	9	10	11	12	13	14	15	16	17	18	19	20	21	22	23	24
River Falls Area Hospital, River Falls, WI	**67** 3	**100** 7	**100** 8	**100** 5	**89** 9	- 0	- 0	- 0	**100** 12	**82** 22	**93** 28	**100** 3	**97** 34	**90** 10	**78** 9	**90** 39	**98** 54	**89** 37	**90** 10	- -	- -	- -	- -	- -
Riverview Hospital Association, Wisconsin Rapids, WI	**71** 7	**92** 24	**80** 15	**96** 24	**85** 20	- 0	- 0	**50** 2	**93** 28	**82** 57	**84** 81	**100** 4	**81** 67	**91** 57	**54** 13	**73** 83	**100** 92	**66** 62	**81** 16	**87** 232	**96** 76	**75** 231	- -	- -
Rusk County Memorial Hospital, Ladysmith, WI	**100** 1	**100** 6	**100** 4	**100** 6	**100** 5	**0** 1	- -	**100** 1	**86** 14	**57** 14	**91** 22	**0** 2	**79** 19	**86** 14	**100** 4	**69** 26	**100** 31	**80** 20	**100** 1	- -	- -	- -	- -	- -
Sacred Heart Hospital, Eau Claire, WI	**86** 21	**93** 76	**99** 77	**92** 64	**97** 93	- 0	**20** 5	**100** 30	**76** 68	**75** 141	**97** 193	**94** 32	**80** 103	**97** 71	**42** 33	**86** 160	**100** 197	**33** 138	**98** 50	**90** 209	**80** 49	**61** 203	**0.00** 1172	**2.35** 892
Sacred Heart Hospital, Tomahawk, WI	- 0	**50** 2	**100** 1	**50** 2	**0** 1	- 0	- -	**100** 1	**100** 3	**86** 14	**96** 24	**100** 2	**71** 21	**100** 10	**91** 11	**85** 40	**100** 47	**93** 41	**100** 10	- -	- -	- -	- -	- -
Saint Agnes Hospital, Fond du Lac, WI	**91** 43	**98** 122	**95** 123	**94** 106	**94** 125	- 0	**80** 5	**78** 32	**80** 50	**71** 102	**85** 164	**83** 23	**92** 90	**89** 65	**61** 18	**75** 122	**100** 160	**41** 118	**83** 23	**77** 172	**88** 65	**66** 158	- -	- -
Saint Clare Hospital Health Services, Baraboo, WI	**100** 1	**85** 13	**100** 5	**67** 3	**83** 6	- 0	- 0	- 0	**86** 14	**44** 32	**91** 53	**86** 7	**76** 33	**81** 36	**75** 12	**83** 64	**100** 74	**78** 54	**78** 9	**95** 85	**92** 26	**98** 80	**0.00** 326	**4.12** 243
Saint Clare's Hospital of Weston, Weston, WI	**100** 1	**100** 4	**100** 4	**100** 1	**100** 2	- 0	- 0	- 0	**75** 4	**54** 28	**100** 36	**100** 7	**89** 35	**100** 25	**33** 3	**94** 32	**100** 41	**94** 17	**100** 10	**93** 365	**94** 78	**95** 363	- -	- -
Saint Croix Regional Medical Center, Saint Croix Falls, WI	- -	- -	- -	- -	- -	- -	- -	- -	- -	- -	- -	- -	**96** 26	**94** 35	**100** 16	**86** 36	**100** 49	**68** 41	**33** 6	**96** 73	**81** 16	**85** 71	- -	- -
Saint Elizabeth Hospital, Appleton, WI	**78** 40	**99** 95	**98** 142	**98** 90	**95** 156	- 0	**80** 5	**100** 53	**65** 68	**56** 120	**100** 160	**100** 18	**96** 78	**95** 74	**72** 25	**84** 111	**100** 140	**80** 91	**100** 37	**88** 626	**92** 129	**62** 618	- -	- -
Saint Francis Hospital, Milwaukee, WI	**82** 28	**96** 96	**98** 90	**83** 53	**96** 84	**0** 1	**50** 2	**97** 36	**85** 100	**60** 223	**98** 231	**97** 33	**90** 153	**96** 163	**81** 47	**91** 220	**100** 262	**66** 164	**94** 70	**88** 328	**87** 55	**79** 318	- -	- -
Saint Joseph's Community Health Services, Hillsboro, WI	- 0	**100** 1	- 0	- 0	- 0	- 0	- 0	- 0	**33** 3	**18** 11	**75** 12	- 0	**93** 28	**100** 7	**50** 4	**96** 27	**100** 37	**65** 17	**91** 11	**100** 3	**100** 1	**100** 3	- -	- -
Saint Joseph's Community Hospital of West Bend, West Bend, WI	**100** 2	**87** 15	**82** 11	**73** 11	**78** 9	**0** 1	- 0	- 0	**82** 39	**79** 56	**98** 100	**78** 9	**86** 83	**93** 67	**59** 22	**85** 102	**100** 140	**70** 99	**91** 32	**91** 164	**98** 46	**79** 156	**0.15** 674	**3.85** 467
Saint Joseph's Hospital, Chippewa Falls, WI	**100** 1	**76** 17	**88** 16	**89** 9	**85** 13	- 0	- 0	**50** 2	**93** 14	**87** 38	**88** 42	**100** 2	**75** 56	**98** 43	**88** 17	**91** 79	**100** 90	**83** 66	**100** 15	**96** 226	**100** 47	**89** 214	- -	- -
Saint Joseph's Hospital, Marshfield, WI	**87** 86	**100** 175	**99** 329	**99** 159	**99** 406	- 0	**100** 4	**98** 115	**93** 121	**78** 316	**100** 386	**95** 44	**90** 94	**84** 101	**94** 34	**89** 197	**100** 238	**92** 160	**98** 65	**81** 1532	**85** 326	**68** 1519	- -	- -
Saint Joseph's Hospital, Milwaukee, WI	**79** 53	**96** 179	**93** 192	**92** 104	**95** 191	- 0	**86** 7	**94** 88	**87** 250	**71** 456	**97** 498	**99** 163	**90** 154	**98** 186	**95** 41	**82** 232	**100** 303	**84** 154	**100** 86	**93** 445	**89** 62	**90** 425	- -	- -
Saint Mary's Hospital, Rhinelander, WI	**100** 6	**96** 25	**95** 19	**74** 27	**86** 22	- 0	- 0	**0** 1	**87** 38	**85** 101	**90** 122	**92** 12	**86** 70	**96** 45	**92** 24	**81** 110	**100** 124	**86** 91	**93** 29	**88** 382	**93** 96	**92** 379	- -	- -
Saint Mary's Hospital Medical Center, Green Bay, WI	**95** 20	**98** 98	**98** 93	**90** 80	**98** 95	- 0	**100** 3	**96** 26	**100** 40	**71** 103	**86** 119	**90** 21	**67** 104	**99** 80	- -	**90** 115	**100** 144	**74** 98	**85** 26	**90** 518	**94** 129	**63** 504	- -	- -
Saint Marys Hospital Medical Center, Madison, WI	**81** 96	**98** 135	**100** 303	**94** 103	**99** 298	- 0	**78** 9	**90** 135	**74** 156	**53** 271	**89** 350	**79** 56	**90** 250	**89** 190	**66** 70	**78** 306	**100** 404	**61** 299	**76** 76	**86** 1541	**97** 493	**93** 1500	- -	- -
Saint Michael's Hospital, Stevens Point, WI	**80** 5	**96** 24	**100** 17	**94** 17	**94** 17	- 0	- 0	**100** 2	**76** 34	**78** 51	**98** 80	**100** 5	**93** 68	**96** 73	**100** 20	**85** 98	**100** 119	**91** 82	**74** 19	**91** 418	**94** 117	**91** 410	- -	- -
Saint Nicholas Hospital, Sheboygan, WI	**71** 7	**91** 46	**59** 27	**85** 20	**92** 26	- 0	- 0	- 0	**86** 22	**44** 18	**55** 84	**0** 1	**78** 9	**100** 11	- -	**83** 95	**100** 104	**73** 79	**67** 3	**84** 64	- -	**61** 64	- -	- -
Saint Vincent Hospital, Green Bay, WI	**80** 30	**97** 121	**97** 138	**90** 105	**96** 133	- 0	**100** 5	**97** 36	**69** 65	**70** 171	**93** 216	**96** 26	**91** 91	**98** 96	**70** 27	**90** 123	**99** 162	**76** 99	**97** 32	**91** 441	**93** 86	**77** 424	- -	- -
Sauk Prairie Memorial Hospital, Prairie Du Sac, WI	**100** 1	- 0	- 0	**100** 2	**100** 1	- 0	- 0	- 0	**100** 12	**76** 29	**93** 45	**80** 5	**92** 49	**93** 15	**100** 8	**95** 57	**100** 72	**86** 56	**50** 8	**92** 318	**99** 69	**76** 315	- -	- -
Shawano Medical Center, Shawano, WI	**100** 3	**87** 15	**80** 10	**100** 14	**100** 10	- 0	- 0	**0** 1	**82** 17	**64** 45	**86** 64	**83** 6	**85** 86	**97** 32	**95** 20	**95** 112	**100** 136	**88** 86	**70** 23	- -	- -	- -	- -	- -
Sinai Samaritan Medical Center, Milwaukee, WI	**93** 41	**98** 111	**98** 102	**91** 64	**92** 64	- 0	**100** 3	**100** 64	**90** 188	**74** 289	**99** 310	**100** 144	**93** 148	**95** 153	**96** 24	**90** 205	**100** 231	**92** 79	**100** 103	**97** 99	**94** 48	**84** 96	- -	- -
Southwest Health Center, Platteville, WI	- 0	**93** 14	**100** 8	**91** 11	**89** 9	- 0	- 0	- 0	**86** 7	**100** 33	**78** 40	**33** 3	**84** 44	**100** 23	**71** 7	**93** 73	**100** 77	**94** 47	**73** 11	- -	- -	- -	- -	- -
Spooner Health System, Sarona, WI	- 0	**88** 8	**100** 5	**75** 8	**80** 5	- 0	- 0	- 0	**75** 8	**25** 12	**59** 22	**50** 2	**41** 37	**93** 15	**20** 10	**88** 41	**98** 51	**62** 34	**82** 17	- -	- -	- -	- -	- -
Stoughton Hospital Association, Stoughton, WI	- -	- -	- -	- -	- -	- -	- -	- -	**86** 14	**79** 29	**79** 38	**100** 4	**96** 57	**92** 63	**100** 17	**90** 86	**100** 105	**95** 78	**75** 16	**97** 64	**100** 12	**79** 62	- -	- -
Theda Clark Medical Center, Neenah, WI	**100** 22	**95** 66	**97** 65	**95** 61	**97** 71	- 0	**100** 1	**100** 22	**96** 26	**100** 92	**96** 123	**100** 12	**82** 34	**92** 53	**83** 12	**92** 92	**100** 97	**78** 72	**96** 24	**89** 422	**90** 94	**79** 405	- -	- -
Tomah Memorial Hospital, Tomah, WI	**100** 2	**100** 17	**100** 14	**100** 11	**100** 14	- 0	- 0	**100** 3	**86** 14	**98** 40	**98** 54	**100** 6	**91** 35	**96** 27	**100** 12	**77** 52	**98** 57	**88** 41	**100** 11	- -	- -	- -	- -	- -
University of Wisconsin Hospital and Clinics, Madison, WI	**92** 79	**100** 83	**100** 181	**99** 70	**100** 235	- 0	**50** 4	**96** 103	**84** 141	**57** 224	**99** 275	**87** 55	**79** 67	**89** 64	**92** 25	**75** 99	**100** 151	**75** 83	**52** 52	**87** 420	**95** 78	**88** 405	- -	- -
Upland Hills Health, Dodgeville, WI	**100** 1	**100** 5	**100** 5	**100** 5	**100** 5	- 0	- 0	- 0	**100** 10	**62** 21	**75** 32	**67** 6	**84** 37	**96** 27	**67** 9	**88** 52	**100** 63	**85** 53	**67** 6	**95** 62	**95** 22	**77** 62	- -	- -
Vernon Memorial Healthcare, Viroqua, WI	**100** 2	**100** 9	**100** 6	**90** 10	**89** 9	**100** 1	- 0	**100** 1	**67** 3	**86** 14	**52** 27	**0** 1	**83** 58	**97** 29	**100** 15	**94** 93	**100** 108	**98** 90	**100** 14	**82** 216	**100** 56	**93** 211	- -	- -
Watertown Memorial Hospital, Watertown, WI	**0** 1	**88** 8	**100** 4	**60** 5	**80** 5	**0** 1	- 0	**50** 2	**78** 18	**42** 48	**85** 65	**100** 4	**82** 38	**97** 35	**50** 14	**92** 77	**100** 85	**89** 46	**92** 13	**66** 185	**98** 44	**88** 180	- -	- -
Waukesha Memorial Hospital, Waukesha, WI	**93** 55	**98** 182	**98** 193	**96** 152	**99** 189	- 0	**79** 14	**100** 63	**77** 159	**67** 322	**99** 406	**94** 49	**89** 219	**96** 193	**97** 71	**97** 301	**100** 383	**93** 241	**91** 68	**94** 301	**96** 71	**71** 282	- -	- -
Waupun Memorial Hospital, Waupun, WI	- -	- -	- -	- -	- -	- -	- -	- -	**73** 11	**84** 31	**63** 49	**100** 1	**77** 35	**98** 41	**33** 9	**76** 58	**100** 75	**46** 39	**93** 15	**91** 53	**100** 18	**96** 52	- -	- -
West Allis Memorial Hospital, Milwaukee, WI	**100** 12	**95** 74	**98** 45	**98** 45	**92** 49	- 0	- 0	**100** 3	**92** 26	**71** 124	**99** 169	**100** 18	**93** 183	**97** 230	**100** 56	**94** 275	**100** 356	**97** 260	**97** 71	**89** 95	**84** 49	**87** 91	- -	- -
Westfields Hospital, New Richmond, WI	- 0	**100** 4	**100** 4	**100** 6	**100** 5	**0** 1	- 0	**100** 1	**67** 3	**100** 11	**82** 17	**100** 1	**80** 20	**100** 7	**75** 4	**67** 12	**100** 22	**87** 15	**75** 4	- -	- -	- -	- -	- -
WFH-All Saints Spring Street Campus, Racine, WI	**76** 21	**99** 169	**99** 147	**97** 147	**99** 139	**0** 2	**71** 14	**93** 54	**74** 173	**85** 355	**96** 424	**84** 80	**89** 227	**79** 182	**75** 40	**92** 295	**100** 365	**77** 242	**89** 81	**74** 170	**98** 55	**81** 161	- -	- -
Wild Rose Community Memorial Hospital, Wild Rose, WI	- 0	- 0	- 0	- 0	- 0	- 0	- -	- 0	**50** 2	**73** 15	**60** 15	**100** 2	**96** 24	**100** 20	**50** 4	**87** 30	**100** 33	**52** 25	**67** 3	- -	- -	- -	- -	- -
Wisconsin Heart Hospital, Wauwatosa, WI	**90** 29	**100** 65	**99** 141	**98** 44	**96** 121	- 0	**100** 6	**98** 49	**90** 60	**86** 122	**100** 127	**89** 19	**100** 11	**100** 11	**100** 2	**87** 15	**100** 17	**75** 12	**100** 2	**96** 116	**96** 23	**95** 111	- -	- -

NOTE: The first number in each column (boldface) is the rate in percent, the second number is the number of patients; Please refer to the main entry for footnotes; ***Heart Attack Care:*** *1. ACE Inhibitor or ARB for LVSD; 2. Aspirin at Arrival; 3. Aspirin at Discharge; 4. Beta Blocker at Arrival; 5. Beta Blocker at Discharge; 6. Fibrinolytic Medication Timing; 7. PCI Within 90 Minutes of Arrival; 8. Smoking Cessation Advice;* ***Heart Failure Care:*** *9. ACE Inhibitor or ARB for LVSD; 10. Discharge Instructions; 11. Evaluation of LVS Function; 12. Smoking Cessation Advice;* ***Pneumonia Care:*** *13. Appropriate Initial Antibiotic; 14. Blood Culture Timing; 15. Influenza Vaccine; 16. Initial Antibiotic Timing; 17. Oxygenation Assessment; 18. Pneumococcal Vaccine; 19. Smoking Cessation Advice;* ***Surgical Infection Prevention:*** *20. Prophylactic Antibiotic Given; 21. Prophylactic Antibiotic Selection; 22. Prophylactic Antibiotic Stopped;* ***Pregnancy Care:*** *23. Inpatient Neonatal Mortality; 24. Third or Fourth Degree Laceration*

Hospitals whose Mortality Rate is Better than the U.S. National Rate

Heart Attack

Hospital	City	State	Phone	Web Site
Abbott-Northwestern Hospital	Minneapolis	Minnesota	612-863-4000	www.abbottnorthwestern.com
Advocate Lutheran General Hospital	Park Ridge	Illinois	847-723-2210	www.advocatehealth.com
Aurora Saint Lukes Medical Center	Milwaukee	Wisconsin	414-649-6000	www.aurorahealthcare.org
Avera Heart Hospital of South Dakota	Sioux Falls	South Dakota	605-977-7000	www.southdakotaheart.com
Barnes Jewish Hospital	Saint Louis	Missouri	314-747-3000	www.barnesjewish.org
Cape Cod Hospital	Hyannis	Massachusetts	508-771-1800	www.capecodhealth.org/
Evergreen Hospital Medical Center	Kirkland	Washington	425-899-1000	www.evergreenhealthcare.org
Hartford Hospital	Hartford	Connecticut	860-545-5000	www.harthosp.org
Hillcrest Hospital	Mayfield Heights	Ohio	440-312-4500	www.hillcresthospital.org
Maimonides Medical Center	Brooklyn	New York	718-283-6000	www.maimonidesmed.org
Maine Medical Center	Portland	Maine	207-871-0111	www.mmc.org
New York-Presbyterian Hospital	New York	New York	212-746-5454	www.nyp.org
Rex Hospital	Raleigh	North Carolina	919-784-3100	www.rexhealth.com
Saint Vincent Heart Center of Indiana	Indianapolis	Indiana	317-583-5000	www.theheartcenter.com
Saint Vincent's Medical Center	Bridgeport	Connecticut	203-576-6000	www.stvincents.org
Suburban Hospital Association	Bethesda	Maryland	301-896-3100	www.suburbanhospital.org
Trumbull Memorial Hospital	Warren	Ohio	330-841-9011	www.trumhosp.org

Note: Table shows hospitals whose 30-day risk-adjusted death (mortality) rate from heart attack is lower than the U.S. national rate of 16%

Heart Failure

Hospital	City	State	Phone	Web Site
Aventura Hospital & Medical Center	Aventura	Florida	305-682-7000	www.aventurahospital.com
Bay Medical Center	Panama City	Florida	850-769-1511	www.baymedical.org
Bayonne Medical Center	Bayonne	New Jersey	201-858-5000	www.bayonnemedicalcenter.org
Beth Israel Deaconess Medical Center	Boston	Massachusetts	617-667-7000	www.bidmc.harvard.edu
Beth Israel Medical Center	New York	New York	212-420-2000	www.bethisraelny.com
Brigham and Women's Hosptial	Boston	Massachusetts	617-732-5500	www.brighamandwomens.org
Christiana Hospital	Newark	Delaware	302-733-1000	www.christianacare.org
Community Hospital	Munster	Indiana	219-836-1600	www.comhs.org/community
Genesys Regional Medical Center	Grand Blanc	Michigan	810-606-5000	www.genesys.org
Glendale Memorial Hospital & Health Center	Glendale	California	818-502-1900	www.glendalememorial.com
Good Samaritan Hospital	Baltimore	Maryland	410-532-8000	www.goodsam-md.org
Hackensack University Medical Center	Hackensack	New Jersey	201-996-3760	www.humed.com
Harper University Hospital	Detroit	Michigan	313-745-8040	www.harperhospital.org
Healtheast Saint John's Hospital	Maplewood	Minnesota	651-232-7000	www.stjohnshospital-mn.org
Hillcrest Hospital	Mayfield Heights	Ohio	440-312-4500	www.hillcresthospital.org
Liberty Hospital	Liberty	Missouri	816-781-7200	www.libertyhospital.org
Loyola University Medical Center	Maywood	Illinois	708-216-9000	www.luhs.org
Maimonides Medical Center	Brooklyn	New York	718-283-6000	www.maimonidesmed.org
Marymount Hospital	Garfield Heights	Ohio	216-581-0500	www.marymount.org
Mclaren Regional Medical Center	Flint	Michigan	810-342-2000	www.mclaren.org
Memorial Hermann Healthcare System	Houston	Texas	281-929-6100	www.mhhs.org
Mercy Hospital	Miami	Florida	305-854-4400	www.mercymiami.com
Methodist Hospitals	Gary	Indiana	219-886-4000	www.methodisthospital.org
Miami Valley Hospital	Dayton	Ohio	937-208-8000	www.miamivalleyhospital.com
Mount Sinai Medical Center	Miami Beach	Florida	305-674-2121	www.msmc.com
New York-Presbyterian Hospital	New York	New York	212-746-5454	www.nyp.org
Northwestern Memorial Hospital	Chicago	Illinois	312-926-2000	www.nmh.org
Olympia Medical Center	Los Angeles	California	310-657-5900	www.olympiamedicalcenter.com
Providence Hospital	Southfield	Michigan	248-849-3000	www.stjohn.org/Providence/
Saint Agnes Hospital	Baltimore	Maryland	410-368-6000	www.stagnes.org
Sinai-Grace Hospital	Detroit	Michigan	313-966-3300	www.sinaigrace.org
Southcoast Hospital Group	Fall River	Massachusetts	508-679-3131	www.southcoast.org/charlton/
Southwest General Health Center	Middleburg Heights	Ohio	440-816-8000	www.swgeneral.com
Saint Catherine Hospital	East Chicago	Indiana	219-392-1700	www.comhs.org/stcatherine/
Western Pennsylvania Hospital Forbes Reg Campus	Monroeville	Pennsylvania	412-858-2000	www.wpahs.org
White Plains Hospital Center	White Plains	New York	914-681-0600	www.wphospital.org
William Beaumont Hospital	Royal Oak	Michigan	248-898-5000	www.beaumonthospitals.com
Willis Knighton Medical Center	Shreveport	Louisiana	318-212-4000	www.wkmc.com

Note: Table shows hospitals whose 30-day risk-adjusted death (mortality) rate from heart failure is lower than the U.S. national rate of 11%

Hospitals whose Mortality Rate is Worse than the U.S. National Rate

Heart Attack

Hospital	City	State	Phone	Web Site
Christus Saint Michael Health System	Texarkana	Texas	903-614-1000	www.christusstmichael.org/
Danville Regional Medical Center	Danville	Virginia	434-799-2100	www.danvilleregional.org
Kingman Regional Medical Center	Kingman	Arizona	928-757-2101	www.azkrmc.com
Southern Ohio Medical Center	Portsmouth	Ohio	740-356-5000	www.somc.org
Sparks Regional Medical Center	Fort Smith	Arkansas	479-441-4000	www.sparks.org
SVCMC-Catholic Medical Center of Brooklyn Queens	Jamaica	New York		
Yuma Regional Medical Center	Yuma	Arizona	928-344-2000	www.yumaregional.org

Note: Table shows hospitals whose 30-day risk-adjusted death (mortality) rate from heart attack is lower than the U.S. national rate of 16%

Heart Failure

Hospital	City	State	Phone	Web Site
Advocate Christ Hospital & Medical Center	Oak Lawn	Illinois	708-684-8000	www.advocatehealth.com
Athens Regional Medical Center	Athens	Tennessee	423-745-1411	www.athensrmc.com
Banner Thunderbird Medical Center	Glendale	Arizona	602-865-5555	www.bannerhealth.com
Baptist Memorial Hospital	Memphis	Tennessee	901-226-5000	www.baptistonline.org
Baylor All Saints Medical Center at Fort Worth	Fort Worth	Texas	817-926-2544	www.baylorhealth.com/locations/allsaints
Bromenn Healthcare	Normal	Illinois	309-454-1400	www.bromenn.org
Christus Saint Francis Cabrini Hospital	Alexandria	Louisiana	318-448-6760	www.cabrini.org
Claremore Regional Hospital	Claremore	Oklahoma	918-341-2556	www.claremorereghospital.com
Conway Regional Medical Center	Conway	Arkansas	501-329-3831	www.conwayregional.org
Corona Regional Medical Center	Corona	California	951-737-4343	www.coronaregional.com
Danville Regional Medical Center	Danville	Virginia	434-799-2100	www.danvilleregional.org
Faith Regional Health Services	Norfolk	Nebraska	402-371-3402	www.frhs.org
Forrest General Hospital	Hattiesburg	Mississippi	601-288-7000	www.forrestgeneral.com
Gnaden Huetten Memorial Hospital	Lehighton	Pennsylvania	610-377-1300	www.bluemountainhealthsystem.org
Hardin Medical Center	Savannah	Tennessee	731-926-8000	www.hardinmedicacenter.org
Hendrick Medical Center	Abilene	Texas	325-670-2000	www.hendrickhealth.org
Huguley Health System	Fort Worth	Texas	817-293-9110	www.huguley.org
Jackson Hospital & Clinic	Montgomery	Alabama	334-293-8000	www.jackson.org
Kenmore Mercy Hospital	Kenmore	New York	716-447-6100	www.chsbuffalo.org
Lodi Memorial Hospital	Lodi	California	209-334-3411	www.lodihealth.org
Manatee Memorial Hospital	Bradenton	Florida	941-745-6862	www.manateememorial.com
Massena Memorial Hospital	Massena	New York	315-769-4233	www.massenahospital.org
Medical Center of Central Georgia	Macon	Georgia	478-633-1000	www.mccg.org
Mercy Medical Center	Redding	California	530-225-6000	www.redding.mercy.org
Olympic Medical Center	Port Angeles	Washington	360-417-7000	www.olympicmedical.org
Plainview Hospital	Plainview	New York	516-719-3000	www.northshorelij.com
Port Huron Hospital	Port Huron	Michigan	810-987-5000	www.porthuronhospital.org
Providence Hospital	Mobile	Alabama	251-633-1000	www.providencehospital.org
Providence Saint Vincent Medical Center	Portland	Oregon	503-216-1234	www.providence.org
Sacred Heart Medical Center	Eugene	Oregon	541-686-7300	www.peacehealth.org
Samaritan Hospital	Troy	New York	518-271-3300	www.nehealth.com
Saint Josephs Medical Center of Stockton	Stockton	California	209-943-2000	www.stjospehscares.org
Saint Marys Hospital Medical Center	Green Bay	Wisconsin	920-498-4200	www.stmgb.org
Sutter General Hospital	Sacramento	California	916-454-2222	www.suttermedicalcenter.org
Tri-City Medical Center	Oceanside	California	760-940-5780	www.tricitymed.org

Note: Table shows hospitals whose 30-day risk-adjusted death (mortality) rate from heart failure is lower than the U.S. national rate of 11%

Hospital Mortality from Heart Attack and Heart Failure: State Summary

State	Number of Hospitals					
	Heart Attack			Heart Failure		
	Better than U.S. National Rate[1]	No Different than U.S. National Rate[2]	Worse than U.S. National Rate[3]	Better than U.S. National Rate[4]	No Different than U.S. National Rate[5]	Worse than U.S. National Rate[6]
Alabama	0	93	0	0	99	2
Alaska	0	13	0	0	20	0
Arizona	0	62	2	0	71	1
Arkansas	0	81	1	0	82	1
California	0	316	0	2	323	6
Colorado	0	61	0	0	68	0
Connecticut	2	29	0	0	32	0
Delaware	0	5	0	1	4	0
District of Columbia	0	7	0	0	7	0
Florida	0	182	0	4	180	1
Georgia	0	134	0	0	141	1
Guam	0	1	0	0	1	0
Hawaii	0	15	0	0	18	0
Idaho	0	33	0	0	37	0
Illinois	1	184	0	2	184	2
Indiana	1	117	0	3	119	0
Iowa	0	112	0	0	125	0
Kansas	0	114	0	0	132	0
Kentucky	0	100	0	0	103	0
Louisiana	0	108	0	1	117	1
Maine	1	37	0	0	39	0
Maryland	1	44	0	2	43	0
Massachusetts	1	63	0	3	62	0
Michigan	0	132	0	6	131	1
Minnesota	1	131	0	1	137	0
Mississippi	0	80	0	0	98	1
Missouri	1	117	0	1	123	0
Montana	0	41	0	0	60	0
N. Mariana Islands	0	1	0	0	1	0
Nebraska	0	74	0	0	87	1
Nevada	0	28	0	0	31	0
New Hampshire	0	26	0	0	26	0
New Jersey	0	75	0	2	73	0
New Mexico	0	38	0	0	42	0
New York	2	185	1	4	187	4
North Carolina	1	108	0	0	114	0
North Dakota	0	33	0	0	43	0
Ohio	2	155	1	4	159	0
Oklahoma	0	100	0	0	115	1
Oregon	0	57	0	0	56	2
Pennsylvania	0	170	0	1	170	1
Puerto Rico	0	47	0	0	49	0
Rhode Island	0	10	0	0	11	0
South Carolina	0	57	0	0	58	0
South Dakota	1	44	0	0	54	0
Tennessee	0	116	0	0	116	3
Texas	0	320	1	1	357	3
Utah	0	31	0	0	39	0
Vermont	0	15	0	0	16	0
Virgin Islands	0	2	0	0	2	0
Virginia	0	79	1	0	83	1
Washington	1	75	0	0	85	1
West Virginia	0	53	0	0	53	0
Wisconsin	1	118	0	0	124	1
Wyoming	0	23	0	0	26	0
U.S. and Territories	17	4453	7	38	4734	35

Note: (1) 30-day risk-adjusted death rate is lower than U.S. rate of 16%; (2) 30-day risk-adjusted death rate is about the same as U.S. rate of 16% or difference is uncertain; (3) 30-day risk-adjusted death rate is higher than U.S. rate of 16%; (4) 30-day risk-adjusted death rate is lower than U.S. rate of 11%; (2) 30-day risk-adjusted death rate is about the same as U.S. rate of 11% or difference is uncertain; (3) 30-day risk-adjusted death rate is higher than U.S. rate of 11%

What Do These Mortality Categories Show?

These categories show how hospitals' risk-adjusted 30-Day Death (mortality) rates compare to the rate across the U.S., after making adjustments for how sick patients were before they were admitted to the hospital and taking into account differences in death rates that might be due to chance.

Hospitals are shown to be Better or Worse Than U.S. National Rate only if we can be 95% certain that the difference between their risk-adjusted death (mortality) rates and the U.S. National rate is not due to chance. All others are shown in the No Different Than U.S. National Rate category.

Better than U.S. National Rate. Hospitals in the Better Than U.S. National Rate category have risk-adjusted 30-day death (mortality) rates that are lower than the U.S. National rate, and we can be 95% certain that this difference is not due to chance.

No Different than U.S. National Rate. Many hospitals in the No Different Than U.S. National Rate category have risk-adjusted 30-day death (mortality) rates that are about the same as the U.S. National rate. Other hospitals in this category have rates that are higher or lower than the U.S. National rate, but we cannot be 95% certain that these differences are not due to chance. One cannot be certain about differences when a hospital has very few relevant patients.

Worse than U.S. National Rate. Hospitals in the Worse Than U.S. National Rate category have risk-adjusted 30-day death (mortality) rates that are higher than the U.S. National rate, and we can be 95% certain that this difference is not due to chance.

Why are Death Rates for Individual Hospitals Not Shown?

Comparisons based on estimated death (mortality) rates alone can be misleading. Risk-adjusted death (mortality) rates are estimated for individual hospitals based on information taken from a particular time period (in this case, July 1, 2005 - June 30, 2006). If a slightly different time period had been chosen, chances are that each hospital's results would have been somewhat different.

Researchers almost always report a range ("confidence interval" or in this case an "interval estimate") around their estimates, to show how much variation might be due to this kind of chance. A confidence interval or interval estimate tells us we can be reasonably "confident" (in this case, 95% confident) that a hospital's death (mortality) rate fell somewhere within this specified range. The smaller the range, the more precise the estimate.

When hospitals treat a very large number of patients, chance differences will not have much effect on the overall rates. The range will be small, and the estimated death (mortality) rates will be more precise. In hospitals that treat smaller numbers of patients, however, even small chance differences could have a big impact on death (mortality) rates. The 95% confidence interval, or range, will be large, and the estimated death (mortality) rates will be much less precise.

Because the number of patients treated at U.S. hospitals varies widely, the precision of hospitals' estimated death (mortality) rates also varies.

Calculation of 30-Day Risk-Adjusted Mortality Rates

CMS calculates 30-day death (mortality) rates for heart attack and heart failure. The rates are "risk-adjusted" using Medicare claims and enrollment data in a complex statistical model. The model predicts how many patients will die within 30 days of being admitted to each hospital for heart attack or heart failure. It includes deaths whether the patients die in the hospital or after leaving, and whether or not they die for heart attack/heart failure or something else. By "risk-adjusted", we mean that the model calculates a death (mortality) rate that adjusts for the kinds of patients who go to that hospital so that hospitals that take care of sicker patients won't have a worse rate just because their patients were sicker before they arrived at the hospital.

For each hospital's rate, the model also calculates an "interval estimate" (which is like a confidence interval), which describes how much uncertainty there is around the rate-how much bigger or smaller the rate might really be. A hospital with many relevant patients will have a rate that is more precise or certain; that is, the "interval estimate" will be relatively narrow. A hospital with few relevant patients will have a rate that is less precise or certain; that is, will have a wide "interval estimate." The "risk-adjusted" hospital rate with its "interval estimate" can be compared to the U.S. National death (mortality) rate (the "national crude mortality rate"). If the interval estimate includes (overlaps with) the national crude mortality rate, the hospital's performance is considered to be "no different than U.S. National rate" and so is placed in that category. If the entire interval estimate is below the national crude mortality rate, then the hospital's performance is "worse than U.S. National rate." If the entire interval estimate is above the national crude mortality rate, the hospital's performance is "better than U.S. National rate."

Data Collection Methods

Cases Included in the Model. All Medicare beneficiaries aged 65 or older who were enrolled in Original Medicare (traditional fee-for-service Medicare) for the entire 12 months prior to their hospital admission for heart attack or heart failure, and for whom complete administrative data for that 12-month period are available, are included in the model. The model identifies (1) all short-stay acute-care hospital discharges for heart attack or heart failure in the reference year based on a principal discharge diagnosis on the Medicare beneficiary's inpatient claim, and (2) all deaths (for all causes) within 30 days of admission. Hospital stays that lasted one day or less are excluded, provided the patient was discharged alive and not against medical advice. (For the initial publication of the rates in June 2007, the reference year used for calculating mortality rates is July 2005 through June 2006. Subsequent updates to the rates are expected to use the same July/June reference year.)

Hospital mortality rates for heart attack are calculated based on all admissions for heart attack, even if an individual Medicare beneficiary was hospitalized more than once for this condition during the 12-month period. However, for purposes of calculating heart failure mortality rates, if a beneficiary had multiple admissions during the 12-month period, one admission is chosen randomly for inclusion in the model.

Use of a 30-Day Period to Assess Mortality

The model tracks deaths that occur within 30 days of a hospital admission, rather than inpatient mortality only, or mortality over some other post-discharge period. Thirty-day mortality was chosen over inpatient mortality because variability across hospitals in lengths of stay can make differences in inpatient mortality hard to interpret. For example, a heart attack patient hospitalized for 12 days may have a higher chance of dying during the hospital stay than a patient hospitalized for only 7 days, merely because the first patient's outcome is tracked for 5 days longer than the second patient's. Thirty-day mortality was chosen over longer windows (such as 90 days or one year), because mortality over longer periods may have less to do with the care received in the hospital and more to do with other complicating illnesses, patients' own behavior, or the care they received after discharge.

Use of Administrative Claims Data

Administrative claims data, rather than medical records data, are used to predict 30-day mortality. These data are widely available for Original Medicare (traditional fee-for-service) beneficiaries, are relatively inexpensive to acquire, and are timely. Using administrative data makes it possible to calculate mortality without having to do chart reviews or requiring hospitals to report additional data. Research conducted when the measures were being developed demonstrated that the administrative claims-based models perform well in predicting mortality compared with models based on chart reviews.

Risk-Adjustment and Covariates Included in the Model

Risk-Adjustment. The model adjusts for differences in patients' risks unrelated to their hospital care (risk-adjustment). The characteristics that Medicare patients bring with them when they arrive at a hospital with a heart attack or heart failure are not under the control of the hospital. However, some patient characteristics may make death more likely (increase the "risk" of death), no matter where the patient is treated or how good the care is. Moreover, some hospitals may treat people with a history of more severe disease. Therefore, when mortality rates are calculated for each hospital for a 12-month period, they are adjusted based on the unique mix of patients that hospital treated during that period. Factors included in the risk-adjustment model include age, gender, past medical history, and other diseases or conditions (comorbidities) that patients had when they arrived at the hospital that are known to increase their risk.

Past medical history and comorbidities are included in the model using CMS's hierarchical condition categories (HCCs) and a history of certain procedures. Medicare patients are assigned to one or more HCCs based on diagnoses (ICD-9 codes) obtained from the patient's discharge claim, and from the hospital inpatient, hospital outpatient, and physician Medicare claims submitted for the patient one year prior to the admission. Secondary diagnoses from the patient's hospital discharge claim that might represent complications that occurred while the patient was in the hospital, rather than conditions that were present on admission, are not included in assigning the patient's HCC. Research has shown that coding differences among providers affect HCCs only slightly. Diagnoses from unreliable sources (such as laboratory or other claims that were not based on face-to-face encounters) are not included when assigning the HCCs in the model.

To "risk-adjust" mortality rates for patient characteristics, the statistical model estimates the independent effects of age, gender, comorbidities, and a hospital-specific component of quality on mortality of patients within 30 days of hospital admission (the dependent variable). Using these estimates, the model calculates an adjusted mortality rate for each hospital that can be compared with those of other hospitals with different case mixes.

Covariates in 30-Day Mortality Risk-Adjustment Models	
Heart Attack	Heart Failure
Age-65	Age-65
Gender (male)	Gender (male)
History of PTCA	History of PTCA
History of CABG	History of CABG
History of heart failure	History of heart failure
History of MI	History of MI
AMI location (Group 1): anterior, anterolateral	
AMI location (Group 2): inferolateral, inferoposterior, inferior, other lateral, and true posterior	
Unstable angina	Unstable angina
Chronic atherosclerosis	Chronic atherosclerosis
Cardiopulmonary-respiratory failure and shock	Cardiopulmonary-respiratory failure and shock
Valvular heart disease	Valvular heart disease
Hypertension	Hypertension
Stroke	Stroke
Cerebrovascular disease	
Renal failure	Renal failure
COPD	COPD
Pneumonia	Pneumonia
Diabetes	Diabetes
Protein-calorie malnutrition	Protein-calorie malnutrition
Dementia	Dementia
Functional disability	Functional disability
Peripheral vascular disease	Peripheral vascular disease
Metastatic cancer	Metastatic cancer
Trauma in last year	Trauma in last year
Major psych disorder	Major psych disorder
Chronic liver disease	Chronic liver disease

Statistical Methods Used to Calculate Mortality Rates

Hierarchical Regression Model. The statistical model for computing 30-day risk-adjusted mortality rate measures is a "hierarchical regression model." This type of model is based on the assumption that any heart attack or heart failure patients treated at a particular hospital will experience a level of quality of care that applies to all patients treated for the same condition in that hospital. In other words, the expected risk of death for two similar heart attack or heart failure patients treated in the same hospital would be more alike than the risk of death for the same two patients treated in two different hospitals. The likelihood that an individual patient will die is therefore a combination of (1) his or her individual risk characteristics (for example, gender, comorbidities, and past medical history) and 2) the hospital's unique quality of care for all patients treated for that condition in that hospital. The model estimates the effects of both of these components on mortality.

Calculating Mortality Rates. Each hospital's "30-day risk-adjusted mortality rate" (also called the "Risk Standardized Mortality Rate" or RSMR) is computed in several steps. First, the predicted 30-day mortality for a particular hospital obtained from the hierarchical regression model is divided by the expected mortality for that hospital, which is also obtained from the regression model. Predicted mortality is the rate of deaths from heart attack or heart failure that would be anticipated in the particular hospital during the 12-month period, given the patient case mix and the hospital's unique quality of care effect on mortality. Expected mortality is the rate of deaths from heart attack or heart failure that would be expected if the same patients with the same characteristics had instead been treated at an "average" hospital, given the "average" hospital's quality of care effect on mortality for patients with that condition. This ratio is then multiplied by the national unadjusted mortality rate for the condition for all hospitals to compute a "risk-adjusted mortality rate" for the hospital. So, the higher a hospital's predicted 30-day mortality rate, relative to expected mortality for the hospital's particular case mix of patients, the higher its adjusted mortality rate will be. Hospitals with better quality will have lower rates.

(Predicted 30-day mortality/Expected mortality) * U.S. National mortality rate = RSMR

For example, suppose the model predicts that 10 percent of Hospital A's heart attack patients would die within 30 days of admission in a given year, based on their ages, gender mix, and pre-existing health conditions, and based on the estimate of the hospital's specific quality of care. Then, suppose that the expected rate of 30-day deaths for those same patients were higher – say, 15 percent – if they had instead been treated at an "average" U.S. hospital. If the actual mortality rate for the 12-month period for all heart attack patients in all hospitals in the U.S. is 12 percent, then the hospital's risk-adjusted 30-day mortality rate would be 8 percent.

(10%/15%)* 12% = RSMR for Hospital A 8%

If, instead, 9 percent of these patients would be expected to have died if treated at the average hospital, then the hospital's mortality rate would be 13.3 percent.

(10%/9%)* 12% = RSMR for Hospital A 13.3%

In the first case, the hospital performed better than the average hospital and had a relatively low risk-adjusted mortality rate (8 percent); in the second case it performed worse and had a relatively high rate (13.3 percent).

Hospitals with relatively low-risk patients whose predicted mortality rate is the same as the expected mortality rate for the average hospital for the same group of low-risk patients would have an adjusted mortality rate equal to the national rate (12 percent in this example). Similarly, hospitals with high-risk patients whose predicted mortality rate is the same as the expected mortality rate for the average hospital for the same group of high-risk patients would also have an adjusted mortality rate equal to the national rate of 12 percent. Thus, each hospital's case mix should not affect the adjusted mortality rates used to compare hospitals.

Adjusting for Small Hospitals or a Small Number of Cases. The hierarchical regression model also adjusts mortality rates results for small hospitals or hospitals with few heart attack or heart failure cases in a given year. This reduces the chance that such hospitals' performance will fluctuate wildly from year to year or that they will be wrongly classified as either a worse or better performer. For these hospitals, the model not only considers deaths among patients treated for the condition in the small sample size of cases, but pools together patients from all hospitals treated for the given condition, to make the result more reliable. In essence, the predicted mortality rate for a hospital with a small number of cases is moved toward the overall U.S. National mortality rate for all hospitals. The estimates of mortality for hospitals with few patients will rely considerably on the pooled data for all hospitals, making it less likely that small hospitals will fall into either of the outlier categories. This pooling affords a "borrowing of statistical strength" that provides more confidence in the results.

Significance Testing, Interval Estimates, and Comparing Rates Among Hospitals

Significance Testing and Interval Estimates. The model also calculates how precise the estimates of the adjusted mortality rate are, and determines upper and lower bounds (Interval Estimates) for each hospital's risk-adjusted rate. Interval estimates, which are like confidence intervals, describe how much uncertainty there is around the rate—how much bigger or smaller the rate might really be. Larger hospitals typically have more precise estimates and smaller interval estimates, since more data are available to estimate mortality. The smaller the sample size, the greater the difference in mortality rates between a hospital and the national rate must be in order for that difference to be statistically meaningful.

Comparing Mortality Rates Among Hospitals. The risk-adjusted hospital rate with its interval estimate can be compared to the U.S. National crude mortality rate. If the interval estimate includes (overlaps with) the national crude mortality rate, the hospital's performance is in the "no different than U.S. National rate" category. If the entire interval estimate is below the national crude mortality rate, then the hospital is performing "worse than U.S. National rate." If the entire interval estimate is above the national crude mortality rate, it is "better than U.S. National rate."

Glossary of Terms

Accreditation
An evaluative process in which a healthcare organization undergoes an examination of its policies, procedures and performance by an external private sector organization ("accrediting body") to ensure that it is meeting predetermined criteria. It usually involves both on- and off-site surveys. Also see the terms AOA, The Joint Commission, and Medicare-Certified Hospitals.

Acute Care Hospital
A hospital that provides inpatient medical care and other related services for surgery, acute medical conditions or injuries (usually for a short term illness or condition).

Acute Myocardial Infarction (AMI)
A condition (also called a heart attack) that occurs when the arteries leading to the heart become blocked and the blood supply is slowed or stopped. When the heart muscle can't get the oxygen and nutrients it needs, the part of the heart tissue that is affected may die.

Additional Measures
Measures included in the Hospital Quality Alliance measure set, reflecting care for discharges occurring on or after April 1, 2004 (Collection period varies by measure).

Acute Myocardial Infarction

- Fibrinolytic agent received within 30 minutes of hospital arrival
- Percutaneous Coronary Intervention (PCI) received within 90 minutes of hospital arrival (previously PCI received within 120 minutes of hospital arrival, as well as, Percutaneous Transluminal Coronary Angioplasty (PTCA) received within 90 minutes of hospital arrival)
- Smoking cessation advice/counseling
- 30-Day Risk Adjusted Heart Attack Mortality

Heart Failure

- Discharge instructions
- Smoking cessation advice/counseling
- 30-Day Risk Adjusted Heart Failure Mortality

Pneumonia

- Blood culture performed in the emergency department prior to initial antibiotic received in hospital (previously Blood culture performed prior to first antibiotic received in hospital)
- Smoking cessation advice/counseling
- Appropriate initial antibiotic selection
- Influenza vaccination status

Surgical Care Improvement/Surgical Infection Prevention

- Prophylactic antibiotic received within 1 hour prior to surgical incision
- Prophylactic antibiotic selection
- Prophylactic antibiotic discontinued within 24 hours after surgery end time

American Hospital Association (AHA)
The national organization that represents and serves all types of hospitals, health care networks, and their patients and communities. AHA takes part in national health policy development, legislative and regulatory debates, and legal matters. AHA provides education for health care leaders and is a source of information on health care issues and trends.

American Osteopathic Association (AOA)
A member association representing approximately 52,000 osteopathic physicians (D.O.s). The AOA serves as the primary certifying body for D.O.s, and is the accrediting agency for all osteopathic medical colleges and health care facilities.

The AOA writes a performance report on each hospital that it checks. You can call or write to AOA to find out a hospital's level of accreditation.

Angioplasty
In angioplasty, a catheter is used to insert a balloon that is inflated to open a blocked blood vessel. Percutaneous transluminal coronary angioplasty (PTCA) is one of several procedures used to open a blocked blood vessel, known collectively as a percutaneous coronary intervention or PCI.

Angiotensin Converting Enzyme (ACE) Inhibitor
A medicine used to treat heart attacks, heart failure, or a decreased function of the left heart. They stop production of a hormone that can narrow blood vessels. This helps reduce the pressure in the heart and lower blood pressure.

Angiotensin Receptor Blocker (ARB)
A medicine used to treat patients with heart failure and a decreased function of the left heart. ARBs block the action of a hormone that can narrow blood vessels. This helps reduce the pressure in the heart and lower blood pressure.

Antibiotic
Medicine used to fight bacteria in the body.

Atherectomy
A procedure where a blade or laser on a catheter cuts through and removes blockages in blood vessels. It is one of several procedures used to open a blocked blood vessel (known as a Percutaneous Coronary Intervention or PCI).

Beta Blocker
A type of medicine that is used to lower blood pressure, treat chest pain (angina) and heart failure, and to help prevent a heart attack. Beta blockers relieve the stress on the heart by slowing the heart rate and reducing the force with which the heart muscles contract to pump blood. They also help keep blood vessels from constricting in the heart, brain, and body.

Blood Culture
A blood test that shows if there are bacteria in the blood, and what type of bacteria it is. It helps your doctor decide which antibiotic to use to treat a bacterial infection.

Centers for Medicare & Medicaid Services (CMS)
The federal agency that runs the Medicare program for the elderly aged and disabled. In addition, CMS works with the states to run the Medicaid program for low-income individuals. CMS works to make sure that the people in these programs are able to get high quality health care. Also see the term DHHS.

Certification (Medicare-Certified)
State government agencies inspect health care providers, including hospitals, nursing homes, dialysis facilities and home health agencies, as well as other health care providers. These providers are certified if they pass inspection. Being certified is not the same as being accredited. Medicare or Medicaid only pays for care provided by certified or accredited providers.

Critical Access Hospital (CAH)
A small, generally geographically remote facility that provides outpatient and inpatient hospital services to people in rural areas. The designation was established by law, for special payments under the Medicare program. To be designated as a CAH, a hospital must be located in a rural area, provide 24-hour emergency services; have an average length-of-stay for its patients of 96 hours or less; be located more than 35 miles (or more than 15 miles in areas with mountainous terrain) from the nearest hospital or be designated by its State as a "necessary provider". Hospitals may have no more than 25 beds.

Department of Health and Human Services (DHHS)
A division of the U.S. government that administers many of the social programs at the Federal level dealing with the health and welfare of the citizens of the United States. CMS is an agency within DHHS.

Diastolic Pressure
The lowest pressure in the artery when the heart is filling with blood. In a blood pressure reading, the diastolic pressure is the second number recorded.

Do hospitals that treat sicker patients have worse death rates? (Risk-adjustment)
Hospitals that treat sicker patients do not necessarily have worse death rates. The hospital-specific 30-day death (mortality) rates used in this report have been adjusted to account for differences in patients' health before their hospital admission.

Sicker patients or patients with more health-related risks may be more likely to die than healthier patients. Moreover, patients who are sicker may be more likely to be treated at particular hospitals while patients who are healthier may be more likely to be treated at other hospitals.

To compare hospitals fairly (and to avoid penalizing those that treat sicker patients) it is therefore important to consider differences in patients' health before they were admitted to the hospital. The statistical process of accounting for differences in patients' sickness before they were admitted to the hospital is called risk-adjustment. This statistical process aims to 'level the playing field' by accounting for health risks that patients have before they enter the hospital.

Fibrinolysis, Fibrinolytic Drugs
Fibrinolytic drugs are "clot-busting" medicines that can help dissolve blood clots in blood vessels and improve blood flow to your heart. They are important for treating heart attacks. If you have a heart attack, your doctor may give you a fibrinolytic drug, perform a percutaneous coronary intervention (PCI), or both.

Hospital Quality Alliance (HQA): Improving Care Through Information
In December 2002, the American Hospital Association (AHA), Federation of American Hospitals (FAH), and Association of American Medical Colleges (AAMC) launched the Hospital Quality Alliance (HQA), a national public-private collaboration to encourage hospitals to voluntarily collect and report hospital quality performance information. This effort is intended to make important information about hospital performance accessible to the public and to inform and invigorate efforts to improve quality. CMS and the Joint Commission participate in the HQA, along with the AHA, the FAH, the AAMC, the American Medical Association, the American Nurses Association, the National Association of Children's Hospitals and Related Organizations, American Association of Retired People, American Federation of Labor and Council of Industrial Organizations, the Consumer-Purchaser Disclosure Project, the Agency for Healthcare Research and Quality, the National Quality Forum, the Blue Cross and Blue Shield Association, the National Business Coalition on Health, General Electric, and the U.S. Chamber of Commerce.

Influenza
Influenza is a serious and sometimes deadly lung infection that can spread quickly in a community. Symptoms include fever-often a high temperature of more than 102° Fahrenheit (38.9° Celsius), headache, muscle aches and pains, chills, cough and chest pain when you take a breath ("pleuritic chest pain"). Although most people recover from the illness, the Centers for Disease Control and Prevention (the CDC) estimates that in the United States more than 200,000 people are hospitalized and about 36,000 people die from the flu and its complications every year.

Influenza Vaccination ("Flu Shot")
The main way to keep from getting flu is to get a yearly flu vaccination. Scientists make a different vaccine every year because the strains of flu viruses change from year to year. Nine to 10 months before the flu season begins, they prepare a new vaccine made from inactivated (killed) flu viruses. Because the viruses have been killed, they cannot cause infection. The vaccine preparation is based on the strains of the flu viruses that are in circulation at the time.

Hospitals should check to make sure that pneumonia patients get a flu shot during flu season to protect them from another lung infection and to help prevent the spread of influenza in the community. You can also get the vaccine at your doctor's office or a local clinic, and in many communities at workplaces, supermarkets, and drugstores. You must get the vaccine every year because it changes.

Inpatient Hospital Services
Services provided to patients admitted to a hospital that include bed and board, nursing services, diagnostic or therapeutic services, and medical or surgical services.

Left Ventricular Function Assessment
A test to check how well the heart is pumping.

Long-term Care Hospital
A facility, like a nursing home, that provides a variety of services that help people with health or personal needs and activities of daily living (like walking, eating, and going to the bathroom) over a period of time. Most long-term care is custodial care, for which Medicare does not pay.

Measurement
The process of collecting data to assess performance conducted at a single point in time or repeated over time.

Medicaid
A joint federal and state program that helps with medical costs for some people with low incomes and limited resources. Medicaid programs vary from state to state, but most health care costs are covered if you qualify for both Medicare and Medicaid.

Medicare-Certified Hospital
In order to receive any payment from either the Medicare or Medicaid programs, a hospital must meet a set of basic standards for quality of care, called "conditions of participation". Medicare-certified hospitals are reviewed periodically (every three years) to assure that they are continuing to provide services of acceptable quality.

Medicare also considers or "deems" hospitals as Medicare-certified that meet the accreditation requirements of the The Joint Commission or the American Osteopathic Association. Most short-term acute care hospitals in the United States choose to be Medicare-certified, either directly or through accreditation.

Medicare Provider Number
Medicare identifies the hospitals with which it works using a unique number. These numbers were used to identify the facilities that reported data for Hospital Compare. If hospitals share a Medicare Provider Number (for example, they bill Medicare for services as a single legal entity), the performance data for those hospitals are, in effect, combined into an aggregate rate representing all of the hospitals represented by the Medicare Provider Number. If you are interested in a hospital that is part of a system or network, you may not be able to find your specific hospital.

Medigap Policy
A Medicare supplement insurance policy sold by private insurance companies to fill "gaps" in Original Medicare Plan coverage. Except in Massachusetts, Minnesota and Wisconsin, there are 10 standardized plans labeled Plan A through Plan J. Medigap policies only work with the Original Medicare Plan.

Original Medicare Plan
A pay-per-visit health plan that lets you go to any doctor, hospital, or other health care supplier who accepts Medicare and is accepting new Medicare patients. You must pay the deductible. Medicare pays its share of the Medicare-approved amount, and you pay your share (coinsurance). In some cases you may be charged more than the Medicare-approved amount. The Original Medicare Plan has two parts: Part A (Hospital Insurance) and Part B (Medical Insurance).

Osteopathic Doctor
A licensed physician who can do surgery and prescribe drugs who has training in manipulative therapy. Also called a Doctor of Osteopathy or DO.

Outcome Measures
Measures designed to reflect the results of care, rather than how frequently a specific treatment or intervention was performed.

Oxygenation Assessment
Test that measures the amount of oxygen in your blood to see if you need oxygen therapy.

Percutaneous Coronary Interventions (PCI)
The procedures called Percutaneous Coronary Interventions (PCI), such as angioplasty and atherectomy are among those that are the most effective for opening blocked blood vessels that cause heart attacks. Doctors may perform a PCI, or give medicine to open the blockage, and in some cases, may do both.

Plan of Care
A written plan of care created with your physician and hospital staff. It tells what services you will get to reach and keep your best physical, mental, and social well being. The hospital staff keeps your doctor up-to-date on how you are doing and updates your care plan as needed.

Pneumonia
An inflammation of the lungs caused by a viral or bacterial infection. This fills your lungs with mucus and lowers the oxygen level in your blood. Symptoms can include fever, fatigue, difficulty breathing, chills, a "wet" cough, and chest pain.

Pneumonia (pneumococcal) Vaccination
Vaccine given to prevent pneumonia, estimated to protect against 80% of bacteria causing pneumonia.

Process of Care Measures
Measures that show, in percentage form or as a rate, how often a health care provider gives recommended care; that is, the treatment known to give the best results for most patients with a particular condition.

Provider
A doctor, hospital, health care professional, or health care facility.

Psychiatric Hospital
A facility that provides inpatient psychiatric services for the diagnosis and treatment of mental illness on a 24-hour basis, by or under the supervision of a physician.

Quality
Quality health care is how well a doctor, hospital, health plan, or other provider of health care, keeps its members healthy or treats them when they are sick. Good quality health care means doing the right thing at the right time, in the right way, for the right person and getting the best possible results.

Quality Assurance
The process of looking at how well a medical service is provided. The process may include formally reviewing health care given to a person, or group of persons, locating the problem, correcting the problem, and then checking to see if what you did worked.

Quality Improvement Organizations (QIOs)
Groups of practicing doctors and other health care experts who are paid by the federal government to check and improve the care given to Medicare patients. They must review your complaints about the quality of care given by: inpatient hospitals, hospital outpatient departments, hospital emergency rooms, skilled nursing facilities, home health agencies, Private Fee-for-Service plans, and ambulatory surgical centers.

Rehabilitation Hospital
A hospital that specializes in improving or restoring a patient's functional ability through therapies. Sometimes called a post-acute hospital.

Risk-Adjusted 30-Day Death (Mortality) Rates
The 30-day Risk-Adjusted Death (Mortality) Rates are produced using a complex statistical model, that relies on Medicare claims and enrollment information. The model predicts patient deaths for any cause within 30 days of hospital admission for heart attack or heart failure, whether the patients die while still in the hospital or after discharge. Thirty-day mortality is used because this is the time period when deaths are most likely to be related to the care patients received in the hospital. Deaths that occur outside the hospital within 30 days are included along with deaths that occur in the hospital, because some hospitals discharge patients sooner than others.

"Starter Set" Measures

Heart Attack
- Aspirin at arrival
- Aspirin at discharge
- ACE Inhibitor or ARB for Left Ventricular Systolic Dysfunction*
- Beta Blocker at arrival
- Beta Blocker at discharge

Heart Failure
- Evaluation of Left Ventricular Systolic (LVS) Function**
- ACE Inhibitor or ARB for Left Ventricular Systolic Dysfunction*

Pneumonia
- Oxygenation Assessment
- Initial Antibiotic Timing
- Pneumococcal Vaccination Status

*Modified, effective 1Q2005 discharges. For more information, see http://www.cms.hhs.gov/HospitalQualityInits/downloads/HospitalSummaryOfMeeting1.pdf.

**Modified, effective 1Q2006 discharges.

Stent
A small wire tube inserted in a blood vessel by a catheter to hold open a blocked blood vessel. One of several procedures to open a blocked blood vessel called a percutaneous coronary intervention (PCI).

The Joint Commission
An organization that evaluates and accredits health care organizations and programs in the United States. The Joint Commission is an independent, not-for-profit organization. The Joint Commission looks at how well a hospital treats patients and how good a hospital's staff and equipment are. A hospital is accredited by The Joint Commission if it meets certain quality standards. These checks are done at least every 3 years. Most hospitals take part in these accreditations.

The Joint Commission writes a "performance report" on each hospital that it checks. You can order these reports free of charge.

Thirty-Day Mortality Model Information
See Krumholtz, H., et al. "An Administrative Claims Model Suitable for Profiling Hospital Performance Based on 30-Day Mortality Rates Among Patients with an Acute Myocardial Infarction." Circulation. Vol. 113: 1683-1692, 2006, for details on the development of the AMI model. An accompanying article in the same volume discusses the heart failure model.

Treatment
Something done to help with a health problem. For example, medicine and surgery are treatments.

Treatment Options
The choices you have when there is more than one way to treat your health problem.

Sedgwick Press
Hospital & Health Plan Directories

The Directory of Hospital Personnel, 2007

The Directory of Hospital Personnel is the best resource you can have at your fingertips when researching or marketing a product or service to the hospital market. A "Who's Who" of the hospital universe, this directory puts you in touch with over 150,000 key decision-makers. With 100% verification of data you can rest assured that you will reach the right person with just one call. Every hospital in the U.S. is profiled, listed alphabetically by city within state. Plus, three easy-to-use, cross-referenced indexes put the facts at your fingertips faster and more easily than any other directory: Hospital Name Index, Bed Size Index and Personnel Index. *The Directory of Hospital Personnel* is the only complete source for key hospital decision-makers by name. Whether you want to define or restructure sales territories... locate hospitals with the purchasing power to accept your proposals... keep track of important contacts or colleagues... or find information on which insurance plans are accepted, *The Directory of Hospital Personnel* gives you the information you need – easily, efficiently, effectively and accurately.

"Recommended for college, university and medical libraries." -ARBA

2,500 pages; Softcover ISBN 1-59237-178-7 $325.00 ◆ Online Database $545.00 ◆ Online Database & Directory Combo, $650.00

The Directory of Health Care Group Purchasing Organizations, 2006

This comprehensive directory provides the important data you need to get in touch with over 800 Group Purchasing Organizations. By providing in-depth information on this growing market and its members, *The Directory of Health Care Group Purchasing Organizations* fills a major need for the most accurate and comprehensive information on over 800 GPOs – Mailing Address, Phone & Fax Numbers, E-mail Addresses, Key Contacts, Purchasing Agents, Group Descriptions, Membership Categorization, Standard Vendor Proposal Requirements, Membership Fees & Terms, Expanded Services, Total Member Beds & Outpatient Visits represented and more. Five Indexes provide a number of ways to locate the right GPO: Alphabetical Index, Expanded Services Index, Organization Type Index, Geographic Index and Member Institution Index. With its comprehensive and detailed information on each purchasing organization, *The Directory of Health Care Group Purchasing Organizations* is the go-to source for anyone looking to target this market.

"The information is clearly arranged and easy to access...recommended for those needing this very specialized information." –ARBA

1,000 pages; Softcover ISBN 1-59237-0091-8, $325.00 ◆ Online Database, $650.00 ◆ Online Database & Directory Combo, $750.00

The HMO/PPO Directory, 2007

The HMO/PPO Directory is a comprehensive source that provides detailed information about Health Maintenance Organizations and Preferred Provider Organizations nationwide. This comprehensive directory details more information about more managed health care organizations than ever before. Over 1,100 HMOs, PPOs, Medicare Advantage Plans and affiliated companies are listed, arranged alphabetically by state. Detailed listings include Key Contact Information, Prescription Drug Benefits, Enrollment, Geographical Areas served, Affiliated Physicians & Hospitals, Federal Qualifications, Status, Year Founded, Managed Care Partners, Employer References, Fees & Payment Information and more. Plus, five years of historical information is included related to Revenues, Net Income, Medical Loss Ratios, Membership Enrollment and Number of Patient Complaints. Five easy-to-use, cross-referenced indexes will put this vast array of information at your fingertips immediately: HMO Index, PPO Index, Other Providers Index, Personnel Index and Enrollment Index. *The HMO/PPO Directory* provides the most comprehensive data on the most companies available on the market place today.

"Helpful to individuals requesting certain HMO/PPO issues such as co-payment costs, subscription costs and patient complaints. Individuals concerned (or those with questions) about their insurance may find this text to be of use to them." -ARBA

600 pages; Softcover ISBN 1-59237-158-2, $325.00 ◆ Online Database, $495.00 ◆ Online Database & Directory Combo, $600.00

To preview any of our Directories Risk-Free for 30 days, call (800) 562-2139 or fax to (518) 789-0556

Medical Device Register, 2007

The only one-stop resource of every medical supplier licensed to sell products in the US. This award-winning directory offers immediate access to over 13,000 companies - and more than 65,000 products – in two information-packed volumes. This comprehensive resource saves hours of time and trouble when searching for medical equipment and supplies and the manufacturers who provide them. Volume I: The Product Directory, provides essential information for purchasing or specifying medical supplies for every medical device, supply, and diagnostic available in the US. Listings provide FDA codes & Federal Procurement Eligibility, Contact information for every manufacturer of the product along with Prices and Product Specifications. Volume 2 - Supplier Profiles, offers the most complete and important data about Suppliers, Manufacturers and Distributors. Company Profiles detail the number of employees, ownership, method of distribution, sales volume, net income, key executives detailed contact information medical products the company supplies, plus the medical specialties they cover. Four indexes provide immediate access to this wealth of information: Keyword Index, Trade Name Index, Supplier Geographical Index and OEM (Original Equipment Manufacturer) Index. Medical Device Register, 2007 is the only one-stop source for locating suppliers and products; looking for new manufacturers or hard-to-find medical devices; comparing products and companies; know who's selling what and who to buy from cost effectively. This directory has become the standard in its field and will be a welcome addition to the reference collection of any medical library, large public library, university library along with the collections that serve the medical community.

"A wealth of information on medical devices, medical device companies... and key personnel in the industry is provide in this comprehensive reference work... A valuable reference work, one of the best hardcopy compilations available." -Doody Publishing

3,000 pages Two Volumes; Hardcover ISBN 1-59237-181-7; $325.00

The Directory of Independent Ambulatory Care Centers

This first edition of *The Directory of Independent Ambulatory Care Centers* provides access to detailed information that, before now, could only be found scattered in hundreds of different sources. This comprehensive and up-to-date directory pulls together a vast array of contact information for over 7,200 Ambulatory Surgery Centers, Ambulatory General and Urgent Care Clinics, and Diagnostic Imaging Centers that are not affiliated with a hospital or major medical center. Detailed listings include Mailing Address, Phone & Fax Numbers, E-mail and Web Site addresses, Contact Name and Phone Numbers of the Medical Director and other Key Executives and Purchasing Agents, Specialties & Services Offered, Year Founded, Numbers of Employees and Surgeons, Number of Operating Rooms, Number of Cases seen per year, Overnight Options, Contracted Services and much more. Listings are arranged by State, by Center Category and then alphabetically by Organization Name. Two indexes provide quick and easy access to this wealth of information: Entry Name Index and Specialty/Service Index. *The Directory of Independent Ambulatory Care Centers* is a must-have resource for anyone marketing a product or service to this important industry and will be an invaluable tool for those searching for a local care center that will meet their specific needs.

"Among the numerous hospital directories, no other provides information on independent ambulatory centers. A handy, well-organized resource that would be useful in medical center libraries and public libraries." –Choice

986 pages; Softcover ISBN 1-930956-90-8, $185.00 ◆ Online Database, $365.00 ◆ Online Database & Directory Combo, $450.00

Sedgwick Press
Health Directories

The Complete Directory for People with Disabilities, 2007

A wealth of information, now in one comprehensive sourcebook. Completely updated, this edition contains more information than ever before, including thousands of new entries and enhancements to existing entries and thousands of additional web sites and e-mail addresses. This up-to-date directory is the most comprehensive resource available for people with disabilities, detailing Independent Living Centers, Rehabilitation Facilities, State & Federal Agencies, Associations, Support Groups, Periodicals & Books, Assistive Devices, Employment & Education Programs, Camps and Travel Groups. Each year, more libraries, schools, colleges, hospitals, rehabilitation centers and individuals add *The Complete Directory for People with Disabilities* to their collections, making sure that this information is readily available to the families, individuals and professionals who can benefit most from the amazing wealth of resources cataloged here.

"No other reference tool exists to meet the special needs of the disabled in one convenient resource for information." –Library Journal

1,200 pages; Softcover ISBN 1-59237-147-7, $165.00 ◆ Online Database $215.00 ◆ Online Database & Directory Combo $300.00

The Complete Directory for People with Chronic Illness, 2007/08

Thousands of hours of research have gone into this completely updated 2005/06 edition – several new chapters have been added along with thousands of new entries and enhancements to existing entries. Plus, each chronic illness chapter has been reviewed by an medical expert in the field. This widely-hailed directory is structured around the 90 most prevalent chronic illnesses – from Asthma to Cancer to Wilson's Disease – and provides a comprehensive overview of the support services and information resources available for people diagnosed with a chronic illness. Each chronic illness has its own chapter and contains a brief description in layman's language, followed by important resources for National & Local Organizations, State Agencies, Newsletters, Books & Periodicals, Libraries & Research Centers, Support Groups & Hotlines, Web Sites and much more. This directory is an important resource for health care professionals, the collections of hospital and health care libraries, as well as an invaluable tool for people with a chronic illness and their support network.

"A must purchase for all hospital and health care libraries and is strongly recommended for all public library reference departments." –ARBA

1,200 pages; Softcover ISBN 1-59237-183-3, $165.00 ◆ Online Database $215.00 ◆ Online Database & Directory Combo $300.00

The Complete Learning Disabilities Directory, 2007

The Complete Learning Disabilities Directory is the most comprehensive database of Programs, Services, Curriculum Materials, Professional Meetings & Resources, Camps, Newsletters and Support Groups for teachers, students and families concerned with learning disabilities. This information-packed directory includes information about Associations & Organizations, Schools, Colleges & Testing Materials, Government Agencies, Legal Resources and much more. For quick, easy access to information, this directory contains four indexes: Entry Name Index, Subject Index and Geographic Index. With every passing year, the field of learning disabilities attracts more attention and the network of caring, committed and knowledgeable professionals grows every day. This directory is an invaluable research tool for these parents, students and professionals.

"Due to its wealth and depth of coverage, parents, teachers and others... should find this an invaluable resource." -Booklist

900 pages; Softcover ISBN 1-59237-122-1, $145.00 ◆ Online Database $195.00 ◆ Online Database & Directory Combo $280.00

The Complete Mental Health Directory, 2006/07

This is the most comprehensive resource covering the field of behavioral health, with critical information for both the layman and the mental health professional. For the layman, this directory offers understandable descriptions of 25 Mental Health Disorders as well as detailed information on Associations, Media, Support Groups and Mental Health Facilities. For the professional, *The Complete Mental Health Directory* offers critical and comprehensive information on Managed Care Organizations, Information Systems, Government Agencies and Provider Organizations. This comprehensive volume of needed information will be widely used in any reference collection.

"... the strength of this directory is that it consolidates widely dispersed information into a single volume." –Booklist

800 pages; Softcover ISBN 1-59237-124-8, $165.00 ◆ Online Database $215.00 ◆ Online & Directory Combo $300.00

Older Americans Information Directory, 2006/07

Completely updated for 2006/07, this sixth edition has been completely revised and now contains 1,000 new listings, over 8,000 updates to existing listings and over 3,000 brand new e-mail addresses and web sites. You'll find important resources for Older Americans including National, Regional, State & Local Organizations, Government Agencies, Research Centers, Libraries & Information Centers, Legal Resources, Discount Travel Information, Continuing Education Programs, Disability Aids & Assistive Devices, Health, Print Media and Electronic Media. Three indexes: Entry Index, Subject Index and Geographic Index make it easy to find just the right source of information. This comprehensive guide to resources for Older Americans will be a welcome addition to any reference collection.

"Highly recommended for academic, public, health science and consumer libraries…" –Choice

1,200 pages; Softcover ISBN 1-59237-136-1, $165.00 ◆ Online Database $215.00 ◆ Online Database & Directory Combo $300.00

The Complete Directory for Pediatric Disorders, 2007

This important directory provides parents and caregivers with information about Pediatric Conditions, Disorders, Diseases and Disabilities, including Blood Disorders, Bone & Spinal Disorders, Brain Defects & Abnormalities, Chromosomal Disorders, Congenital Heart Defects, Movement Disorders, Neuromuscular Disorders and Pediatric Tumors & Cancers. This carefully written directory offers: understandable Descriptions of 15 major bodily systems; Descriptions of more than 200 Disorders and a Resources Section, detailing National Agencies & Associations, State Associations, Online Services, Libraries & Resource Centers, Research Centers, Support Groups & Hotlines, Camps, Books and Periodicals. This resource will provide immediate access to information crucial to families and caregivers when coping with children's illnesses.

"Recommended for public and consumer health libraries." –Library Journal

1,200 pages; Softcover ISBN 1-59237-150-7 $165.00 ◆ Online Database $215.00 ◆ Online Database & Directory Combo $300.00

The Directory of Drug & Alcohol Residential Rehabilitation Facilities

This brand new directory is the first-ever resource to bring together, all in one place, data on the thousands of drug and alcohol residential rehabilitation facilities in the United States. *The Directory of Drug & Alcohol Residential Rehabilitation Facilities* covers over 1,000 facilities, with detailed contact information for each one, including mailing address, phone and fax numbers, email addresses and web sites, mission statement, type of treatment programs, cost, average length of stay, numbers of residents and counselors, accreditation, insurance plans accepted, type of environment, religious affiliation, education components and much more. It also contains a helpful chapter on General Resources that provides contact information for Associations, Print & Electronic Media, Support Groups and Conferences. Multiple indexes allow the user to pinpoint the facilities that meet very specific criteria. This time-saving tool is what so many counselors, parents and medical professionals have been asking for. *The Directory of Drug & Alcohol Residential Rehabilitation Facilities* will be a helpful tool in locating the right source for treatment for a wide range of individuals. This comprehensive directory will be an important acquisition for all reference collections: public and academic libraries, case managers, social workers, state agencies and many more.

"This is an excellent, much needed directory that fills an important gap…" –Booklist

300 pages; Softcover ISBN 1-59237-031-4, $135.00

Sedgwick Press
Education Directories

The Comparative Guide to American Elementary & Secondary Schools, 2007

The only guide of its kind, this award winning compilation offers a snapshot profile of every public school district in the United States serving 1,500 or more students – more than 5,900 districts are covered. Organized alphabetically by district within state, each chapter begins with a Statistical Overview of the state. Each district listing includes contact information (name, address, phone number and web site) plus Grades Served, the Numbers of Students and Teachers and the Number of Regular, Special Education, Alternative and Vocational Schools in the district along with statistics on Student/Classroom Teacher Ratios, Drop Out Rates, Ethnicity, the Numbers of Librarians and Guidance Counselors and District Expenditures per student. As an added bonus, *The Comparative Guide to American Elementary and Secondary Schools* provides important ranking tables, both by state and nationally, for each data element. For easy navigation through this wealth of information, this handbook contains a useful City Index that lists all districts that operate schools within a city. These important comparative statistics are necessary for anyone considering relocation or doing comparative research on their own district and would be a perfect acquisition for any public library or school district library.

"This straightforward guide is an easy way to find general information. Valuable for academic and large public library collections." –ARBA

2,400 pages; Softcover ISBN 1-59237-223-6, $125.00

Educators Resource Directory, 2007/08

Educators Resource Directory is a comprehensive resource that provides the educational professional with thousands of resources and statistical data for professional development. This directory saves hours of research time by providing immediate access to Associations & Organizations, Conferences & Trade Shows, Educational Research Centers, Employment Opportunities & Teaching Abroad, School Library Services, Scholarships, Financial Resources, Professional Consultants, Computer Software & Testing Resources and much more. Plus, this comprehensive directory also includes a section on Statistics and Rankings with over 100 tables, including statistics on Average Teacher Salaries, SAT/ACT scores, Revenues & Expenditures and more. These important statistics will allow the user to see how their school rates among others, make relocation decisions and so much more. For quick access to information, this directory contains four indexes: Entry & Publisher Index, Geographic Index, a Subject & Grade Index and Web Sites Index. *Educators Resource Directory* will be a well-used addition to the reference collection of any school district, education department or public library.

"Recommended for all collections that serve elementary and secondary school professionals." –Choice

1,000 pages; Softcover ISBN 1-59237-179-5, $145.00 ◆ Online Database $195.00 ◆ Online Database & Directory Combo $280.00

Grey House Publishing
Business Directories

The Directory of Business Information Resources, 2007

With 100% verification, over 1,000 new listings and more than 12,000 updates, this 2007 edition of *The Directory of Business Information Resources* is the most up-to-date source for contacts in over 98 business areas – from advertising and agriculture to utilities and wholesalers. This carefully researched volume details: the Associations representing each industry; the Newsletters that keep members current; the Magazines and Journals - with their "Special Issues" - that are important to the trade, the Conventions that are "must attends," Databases, Directories and Industry Web Sites that provide access to must-have marketing resources. Includes contact names, phone & fax numbers, web sites and e-mail addresses. This one-volume resource is a gold mine of information and would be a welcome addition to any reference collection.

"This is a most useful and easy-to-use addition to any researcher's library." –*The Information Professionals Institute*

2,500 pages; Softcover ISBN 1-59237-146-9, $195.00 ◆ Online Database $495.00

Nations of the World, 2007/08 A Political, Economic and Business Handbook

This completely revised edition covers all the nations of the world in an easy-to-use, single volume. Each nation is profiled in a single chapter that includes Key Facts, Political & Economic Issues, a Country Profile and Business Information. In this fast-changing world, it is extremely important to make sure that the most up-to-date information is included in your reference collection. This edition is just the answer. Each of the 200+ country chapters have been carefully reviewed by a political expert to make sure that the text reflects the most current information on Politics, Travel Advisories, Economics and more. You'll find such vital information as a Country Map, Population Characteristics, Inflation, Agricultural Production, Foreign Debt, Political History, Foreign Policy, Regional Insecurity, Economics, Trade & Tourism, Historical Profile, Political Systems, Ethnicity, Languages, Media, Climate, Hotels, Chambers of Commerce, Banking, Travel Information and more. Five Regional Chapters follow the main text and include a Regional Map, an Introductory Article, Key Indicators and Currencies for the Region. As an added bonus, an all-inclusive CD-ROM is available as a companion to the printed text. Noted for its sophisticated, up-to-date and reliable compilation of political, economic and business information, this brand new edition will be an important acquisition to any public, academic or special library reference collection.

"A useful addition to both general reference collections and business collections." –*RUSQ*

1,700 pages; Print Version Only Softcover ISBN 1-59237-177-9, $155.00

The Directory of Venture Capital & Private Equity Firms, 2007

This edition has been extensively updated and broadly expanded to offer direct access to over 2,800 Domestic and International Venture Capital Firms, including address, phone & fax numbers, e-mail addresses and web sites for both primary and branch locations. Entries include details on the firm's Mission Statement, Industry Group Preferences, Geographic Preferences, Average and Minimum Investments and Investment Criteria. You'll also find details that are available nowhere else, including the Firm's Portfolio Companies and extensive information on each of the firm's Managing Partners, such as Education, Professional Background and Directorships held, along with the Partner's E-mail Address. *The Directory of Venture Capital & Private Equity Firms* offers five important indexes: Geographic Index, Executive Name Index, Portfolio Company Index, Industry Preference Index and College & University Index. With its comprehensive coverage and detailed, extensive information on each company, *The Directory of Venture Capital & Private Equity Firms* is an important addition to any finance collection.

"The sheer number of listings, the descriptive information provided and the outstanding indexing make this directory a better value than its principal competitor, Pratt's Guide to Venture Capital Sources. Recommended for business collections in large public, academic and business libraries." –*Choice*

1,300 pages; Softcover ISBN 1-59237-176-0, $565.00/$450.00 Library ◆ Online Database (includes a free copy of the directory) $889.00

The Directory of Mail Order Catalogs, 2007

Published since 1981, the *Directory of Mail Order Catalogs* is the premier source of information on the mail order catalog industry. It is the source that business professionals and librarians have come to rely on for the thousands of catalog companies in the US. New for 2007, The Directory of Mail Order Catalogs has been combined with its companion volume, *The Directory of Business to Business Catalogs,* to offer all 13,000 catalog companies in one easy-to-use volume. Section I: Consumer Catalogs, covers over 9,000 consumer catalog companies in 44 different product chapters from Animals to Toys & Games. Section II: Business to Business Catalogs, details 5,000 business catalogs, everything from computers to laboratory supplies, building construction and much more. Listings contain detailed contact information including mailing address, phone & fax numbers, web sites, e-mail addresses and key contacts along with important business details such as product descriptions, employee size, years in business, sales volume, catalog size, number of catalogs mailed and more. Three indexes are included for easy access to information: Catalog & Company Name Index, Geographic Index and Product Index. *The Directory of Mail Order Catalogs,* now with its expanded business to business catalogs, is the largest and most comprehensive resource covering this billion-dollar industry. It is the standard in its field. This important resource is a useful tool for entrepreneurs searching for catalogs to pick up their product, vendors looking to expand their customer base in the catalog industry, market researchers, small businesses investigating new supply vendors, along with the library patron who is exploring the available catalogs in their areas of interest.

"This is a godsend for those looking for information." –Reference Book Review

1,700 pages; Softcover ISBN 1-59237-156-6 $350.00/$250.00 Library ◆ Online Database (includes a free copy of the directory) $495.00

Sports Market Place Directory, 2007

For over 20 years, this comprehensive, up-to-date directory has offered direct access to the Who, What, When & Where of the Sports Industry. With over 20,000 updates and enhancements, the *Sports Market Place Directory* is the most detailed, comprehensive and current sports business reference source available. In 1,800 information-packed pages, *Sports Market Place Directory* profiles contact information and key executives for: Single Sport Organizations, Professional Leagues, Multi-Sport Organizations, Disabled Sports, High School & Youth Sports, Military Sports, Olympic Organizations, Media, Sponsors, Sponsorship & Marketing Event Agencies, Event & Meeting Calendars, Professional Services, College Sports, Manufacturers & Retailers, Facilities and much more. *The Sports Market Place Directory* provides organization's contact information with detailed descriptions including: Key Contacts, physical, mailing, email and web addresses plus phone and fax numbers. Plus, nine important indexes make sure that you can find the information you're looking for quickly and easily: Entry Index, Single Sport Index, Media Index, Sponsor Index, Agency Index, Manufacturers Index, Brand Name Index, Facilities Index and Executive/Geographic Index. For over twenty years, *The Sports Market Place Directory* has assisted thousands of individuals in their pursuit of a career in the sports industry. Why not use "THE SOURCE" that top recruiters, headhunters and career placement centers use to find information on or about sports organizations and key hiring contacts.

1,800 pages; Softcover ISBN 1-59237-189-2, $225.00 ◆ Online Database $479.00

Food and Beverage Market Place, 2007

Food and Beverage Market Place is bigger and better than ever with thousands of new companies, thousands of updates to existing companies and two revised and enhanced product category indexes. This comprehensive directory profiles over 18,000 Food & Beverage Manufacturers, 12,000 Equipment & Supply Companies, 2,200 Transportation & Warehouse Companies, 2,000 Brokers & Wholesalers, 8,000 Importers & Exporters, 900 Industry Resources and hundreds of Mail Order Catalogs. Listings include detailed Contact Information, Sales Volumes, Key Contacts, Brand & Product Information, Packaging Details and much more. *Thomas Food and Beverage Market Place* is available as a three-volume printed set, a subscription-based Online Database via the Internet, on CD-ROM, as well as mailing lists and a licensable database.

"An essential purchase for those in the food industry but will also be useful in public libraries where needed. Much of the information will be difficult and time consuming to locate without this handy three-volume ready-reference source." –ARBA

8,500 pages, 3 Volume Set; Softcover ISBN 1-59237-152-3, $595.00 ◆ Online Database $795.00 ◆ Online Database & 3 Volume Set Combo, $995.00

The Grey House Homeland Security Directory, 2007

This updated edition features the latest contact information for government and private organizations involved with Homeland Security along with the latest product information and provides detailed profiles of nearly 1,000 Federal & State Organizations & Agencies and over 3,000 Officials and Key Executives involved with Homeland Security. These listings are incredibly detailed and include Mailing Address, Phone & Fax Numbers, Email Addresses & Web Sites, a complete Description of the Agency and a complete list of the Officials and Key Executives associated with the Agency. Next, *The Grey House Homeland Security Directory* provides the go-to source for Homeland Security Products & Services. This section features over 2,000 Companies that provide Consulting, Products or Services. With this Buyer's Guide at their fingertips, users can locate suppliers of everything from Training Materials to Access Controls, from Perimeter Security to BioTerrorism Countermeasures and everything in between – complete with contact information and product descriptions. A handy Product Locator Index is provided to quickly and easily locate suppliers of a particular product. Lastly, an Information Resources Section provides immediate access to contact information for hundreds of Associations, Newsletters, Magazines, Trade Shows, Databases and Directories that focus on Homeland Security. This comprehensive, information-packed resource will be a welcome tool for any company or agency that is in need of Homeland Security information and will be a necessary acquisition for the reference collection of all public libraries and large school districts.

"Compiles this information in one place and is discerning in content. A useful purchase for public and academic libraries." –Booklist

800 pages; Softcover ISBN 1-59237-151-5, $195.00 ◆ Online Database (includes a free copy of the directory) $385.00

The Grey House Transportation Security Directory & Handbook

This brand new title is the only reference of its kind that brings together current data on Transportation Security. With information on everything from Regulatory Authorities to Security Equipment, this top-flight database brings together the relevant information necessary for creating and maintaining a security plan for a wide range of transportation facilities. With this current, comprehensive directory at the ready you'll have immediate access to: Regulatory Authorities & Legislation; Information Resources; Sample Security Plans & Checklists; Contact Data for Major Airports, Seaports, Railroads, Trucking Companies and Oil Pipelines; Security Service Providers; Recommended Equipment & Product Information and more. Using the *Grey House Transportation Security Directory & Handbook*, managers will be able to quickly and easily assess their current security plans; develop contacts to create and maintain new security procedures; and source the products and services necessary to adequately maintain a secure environment. This valuable resource is a must for all Security Managers at Airports, Seaports, Railroads, Trucking Companies and Oil Pipelines.

800 pages; Softcover ISBN 1-59237-075-6, $195

The Grey House Safety & Security Directory, 2007

The Grey House Safety & Security Directory is the most comprehensive reference tool and buyer's guide for the safety and security industry. Arranged by safety topic, each chapter begins with OSHA regulations for the topic, followed by Training Articles written by top professionals in the field and Self-Inspection Checklists. Next, each topic contains Buyer's Guide sections that feature related products and services. Topics include Administration, Insurance, Loss Control & Consulting, Protective Equipment & Apparel, Noise & Vibration, Facilities Monitoring & Maintenance, Employee Health Maintenance & Ergonomics, Retail Food Services, Machine Guards, Process Guidelines & Tool Handling, Ordinary Materials Handling, Hazardous Materials Handling, Workplace Preparation & Maintenance, Electrical Lighting & Safety, Fire & Rescue and Security. The Buyer's Guide sections are carefully indexed within each topic area to ensure that you can find the supplies needed to meet OSHA's regulations. Six important indexes make finding information and product manufacturers quick and easy: Geographical Index of Manufacturers and Distributors, Company Profile Index, Brand Name Index, Product Index, Index of Web Sites and Index of Advertisers. This comprehensive, up-to-date reference will provide every tool necessary to make sure a business is in compliance with OSHA regulations and locate the products and services needed to meet those regulations.

"Presents industrial safety information for engineers, plant managers, risk managers, and construction site supervisors…" –Choice

1,500 pages, 2 Volume Set; Softcover ISBN 1-59237-160-4, $225.00

The Grey House Biometric Information Directory

The Biometric Information Directory is the only comprehensive source for current biometric industry information. This 2006 edition is the first published by Grey House. With 100% updated information, this latest edition offers a complete, current look, in both print and online form, of biometric companies and products – one of the fastest growing industries in today's economy. Detailed profiles of manufacturers of the latest biometric technology, including Finger, Voice, Face, Hand, Signature, Iris, Vein and Palm Identification systems. Data on the companies include key executives, company size and a detailed, indexed description of their product line. Plus, the Directory also includes valuable business resources, and current editorial make this edition the easiest way for the business community and consumers alike to access the largest, most current compilation of biometric industry information available on the market today. The new edition boasts increased numbers of companies, contact names and company data, with over 700 manufacturers and service providers. Information in the directory includes: Editorial on Advancements in Biometrics; Profiles of 700+ companies listed with contact information; Organizations, Trade & Educational Associations, Publications, Conferences, Trade Shows and Expositions Worldwide; Web Site Index; Biometric & Vendors Services Index by Types of Biometrics; and a Glossary of Biometric Terms. This resource will be an important source for anyone who is considering the use of a biometric product, investing in the development of biometric technology, support existing marketing and sales efforts and will be an important acquisition for the business reference collection for large public and business libraries.

800 pages; Softcover ISBN 1-59237-121-3, $225

The Rauch Guide to the US Adhesives & Sealants, Cosmetics & Toiletries, Ink, Paint, Plastics, Pulp & Paper and Rubber Industries

The Rauch Guides are known worldwide for their comprehensive marketing information. Acquired by Grey House Publishing in 2005, new updated and revised editions will be published throughout 2005 and 2006. Each Guide provides market facts and figures in a highly organized format, ideal for today's busy personnel, serving as ready-references for top executives as well as the industry newcomer. *The Rauch Guides* save time and money by organizing widely scattered information and providing estimates for important business decisions, some of which are available nowhere else. Each Guide is organized into several information-packed chapters. After a brief introduction, the ECONOMICS section provides data on industry shipments; long-term growth and forecasts; prices; company performance; employment, expenditures, and productivity; transportation and geographical patterns; packaging; foreign trade; and government regulations. Next, TECHNOLOGY & RAW MATERIALS provide market, technical, and raw material information for chemicals, equipment and related materials, including market size and leading suppliers, prices, end uses, and trends. PRODUCTS & MARKETS provide information for each major industry product, including market size and historical trends, leading suppliers, five-year forecasts, industry structure, and major end uses. For easy access, each *Guide* contains a chapter on INDUSTRY ACTIVITIES, ORGANIZATIONS & SOURCES OF INFORMATION with detailed information on meetings, exhibits, and trade shows, sources of statistical information, trade associations, technical and professional societies, and trade and technical periodicals. Next, the COMPANY DIRECTORY profiles major industry companies, both public and private. Generally several hundred companies are analyzed. Information includes complete contact information, web address, estimated total and domestic sales, product description, and recent mergers and acquisitions. Each Guide also contains several APPENDICES that provide a cross-reference of suppliers, subsidiaries and divisions. The Rauch Guides will prove to be an invaluable source of market information, company data, trends and forecasts that anyone in these fast-paced industries.

The Rauch Guide to the U.S. Paint Industry Softcover ISBN 1-59237-127-2 $595 ♦ The Rauch Guide to the U.S. Plastics Industry Softcover ISBN 1-59237-128-0 $595 ♦ The Rauch Guide to the U.S. Adhesives and Sealants Industry Softcover ISBN 1-59237-129-9 $595 ♦ The Rauch Guide to the U.S. Ink Industry Softcover ISBN 1-59237-126-4 $595 ♦ The Rauch Guide to the U.S. Rubber Industry Softcover ISBN 1-59237-130-2 $595 ♦ The Rauch Guide to the U.S. Pulp and Paper Industry Softcover ISBN 1-59237-131-0 $595 ♦ The Rauch Guide to the U.S. Cosmetic and Toiletries Industry Softcover ISBN 1-59237-132-9 $895

The Grey House Performing Arts Directory, 2007

The Grey House Performing Arts Directory is the most comprehensive resource covering the Performing Arts. This important directory provides current information on over 8,500 Dance Companies, Instrumental Music Programs, Opera Companies, Choral Groups, Theater Companies, Performing Arts Series and Performing Arts Facilities. Plus, this edition now contains a brand new section on Artist Management Groups. In addition to mailing address, phone & fax numbers, e-mail addresses and web sites, dozens of other fields of available information include mission statement, key contacts, facilities, seating capacity, season, attendance and more. This directory also provides an important Information Resources section that covers hundreds of Performing Arts Associations, Magazines, Newsletters, Trade Shows, Directories, Databases and Industry Web Sites. Five indexes provide immediate access to this wealth of information: Entry Name, Executive Name, Performance Facilities, Geographic and Information Resources. *The Grey House Performing Arts Directory* pulls together thousands of Performing Arts Organizations, Facilities and Information Resources into an easy-to-use source – this kind of comprehensiveness and extensive detail is not available in any resource on the market place today.

"Immensely useful and user-friendly … recommended for public, academic and certain special library reference collections." –Booklist

1,500 pages; Softcover ISBN 1-59237-138-8, $185.00 ♦ Online Database $335.00

To preview any of our Directories Risk-Free for 30 days, call (800) 562-2139 or fax to (518) 789-0556

New York State Directory, 2007/08

The New York State Directory, published annually since 1983, is a comprehensive and easy-to-use guide to accessing public officials and private sector organizations and individuals who influence public policy in the state of New York. *The New York State Directory* includes important information on all New York state legislators and congressional representatives, including biographies and key committee assignments. It also includes staff rosters for all branches of New York state government and for federal agencies and departments that impact the state policy process. Following the state government section are 25 chapters covering policy areas from agriculture through veterans' affairs. Each chapter identifies the state, local and federal agencies and officials that formulate or implement policy. In addition, each chapter contains a roster of private sector experts and advocates who influence the policy process. The directory also offers appendices that include statewide party officials; chambers of commerce; lobbying organizations; public and private universities and colleges; television, radio and print media; and local government agencies and officials.

New York State Directory - 800 pages; Softcover ISBN 1-59237-190-6; $145.00
New York State Directory with Profiles of New York – 2 volumes; 1,600 pages; Softcover ISBN 1-59237-191-4; $225

Profiles of New York ♦ Profiles of Florida ♦ Profiles of Texas ♦ Profiles of Illinois ♦ Profiles of Michigan ♦ Profiles of Ohio ♦ Profiles of New Jersey ♦ Profiles of Massachusetts ♦ Profiles of Pennsylvania ♦ Profiles of Wisconsin ♦ Profiles of Connecticut ♦ Profiles of Indiana ♦ Profiles of North Carolina ♦ Profiles of Virginia ♦ Profiles of California

Packed with over 50 pieces of data that make up a complete, user-friendly profile of each state, these directories go even further by then pulling selected data and providing it in ranking list form for even easier comparisons between the 100 largest towns and cities! The careful layout gives the user an easy-to-read snapshot of every single place and county in the state, from the biggest metropolis to the smallest unincorporated hamlet. The richness of each place or county profile is astounding in its depth, from history to weather, all packed in an easy-to-navigate, compact format. No need for piles of multiple sources with this volume on your desk. Here is a look at just a few of the data sets you'll find in each profile: History, Geography, Climate, Population, Vital Statistics, Economy, Income, Taxes, Education, Housing, Health & Environment, Public Safety, Newspapers, Transportation, Presidential Election Results, Information Contacts and Chambers of Commerce. As an added bonus, there is a section on Selected Statistics, where data from the 100 largest towns and cities is arranged into easy-to-use charts. Each of 22 different data points has its own two-page spread with the cities listed in alpha order so researchers can easily compare and rank cities. A remarkable compilation that offers overviews and insights into each corner of the state, *Profiles of New York, Profiles of Florida* and *Profiles of Texas* go beyond Census statistics, beyond metro area coverage, beyond the 100 best places to live. Drawn from official census information, other government statistics and original research, you will have at your fingertips data that's available nowhere else in one single source. Data will be published on additional states in 2006 and 2007.

Each Profiles of… title ranges from 400-800 pages, priced at $149.00 each

Research Services Directory: Commercial & Corporate Research Centers

This Ninth Edition provides access to well over 8,000 independent Commercial Research Firms, Corporate Research Centers and Laboratories offering contract services for hands-on, basic or applied research. *Research Services Directory* covers the thousands of types of research companies, including Biotechnology & Pharmaceutical Developers, Consumer Product Research, Defense Contractors, Electronics & Software Engineers, Think Tanks, Forensic Investigators, Independent Commercial Laboratories, Information Brokers, Market & Survey Research Companies, Medical Diagnostic Facilities, Product Research & Development Firms and more. Each entry provides the company's name, mailing address, phone & fax numbers, key contacts, web site, e-mail address, as well as a company description and research and technical fields served. Four indexes provide immediate access to this wealth of information: Research Firms Index, Geographic Index, Personnel Name Index and Subject Index.

"An important source for organizations in need of information about laboratories, individuals and other facilities." –ARBA

1,400 pages; Softcover ISBN 1-59237-003-9, $395.00 ♦ Online Database (includes a free copy of the directory) $850.00

International Business and Trade Directories

Completely updated, the Third Edition of *International Business and Trade Directories* now contains more than 10,000 entries, over 2,000 more than the last edition, making this directory the most comprehensive resource of the worlds business and trade directories. Entries include content descriptions, price, publisher's name and address, web site and e-mail addresses, phone and fax numbers and editorial staff. Organized by industry group, and then by region, this resource puts over 10,000 industry-specific business and trade directories at the reader's fingertips. Three indexes are included for quick access to information: Geographic Index, Publisher Index and Title Index. Public, college and corporate libraries, as well as individuals and corporations seeking critical market information will want to add this directory to their marketing collection.

"Reasonably priced for a work of this type, this directory should appeal to larger academic, public and corporate libraries with an international focus." –Library Journal

1,800 pages; Softcover ISBN 1-930956-63-0, $225.00 ♦ Online Database (includes a free copy of the directory) $450.00

To preview any of our Directories Risk-Free for 30 days, call (800) 562-2139 or fax to (518) 789-0556

Grey House Publishing Canada
Canadian Information Resources

Canadian Almanac & Directory, 2007

The Canadian Almanac & Directory contains ten directories in one – giving you all the facts and figures you will ever need about Canada. No other single source provides users with the quality and depth of up-to-date information for all types of research. This national directory and guide gives you access to statistics, images and over 45,000 names and addresses for everything from Airlines to Zoos - updated every year. It's Ten Directories in One! Each section is a directory in itself, providing robust information on business and finance, communications, government, associations, arts and culture (museums, zoos, libraries, etc.), health, transportation, law, education, and more. Government information includes federal, provincial and territorial - and includes an easy-to-use quick index to find key information. A separate municipal government section includes every municipality in Canada, with full profiles of Canada's largest urban centers. A complete legal directory lists judges and judicial officials, court locations and law firms across the country. A wealth of general information, the Canadian Almanac & Directory also includes national statistics on population, employment, imports and exports, and more. National awards and honors are presented, along with forms of address, Commonwealth information and full color photos of Canadian symbols. Postal information, weights, measures, distances and other useful charts are also incorporated. Complete almanac information includes perpetual calendars, five-year holiday planners and astronomical information. Published continuously for 160 years, The Canadian Almanac & Directory is the best single reference source for business executives, managers and assistants; government and public affairs executives; lawyers; marketing, sales and advertising executives; researchers, editors and journalists.

Hardcover ISBN 978-1-89502-149-3; 1,600 pages; $315.00

Associations Canada, 2007

The Most Powerful Fact-Finder to Business, Trade, Professional and Consumer Organizations
Associations Canada covers Canadian organizations and international groups including industry, commercial and professional associations, registered charities, special interest and common interest organizations. This annually revised compendium provides detailed listings and abstracts for nearly 20,000 regional, national and international organizations. This popular volume provides the most comprehensive picture of Canada's non-profit sector. Detailed listings enable users to identify an organization's budget, founding date, scope of activity, licensing body, sources of funding, executive information, full address and complete contact information, just to name a few. Powerful indexes help researchers find information quickly and easily. The following indexes are included: subject, acronym, geographic, budget, executive name, conferences & conventions, mailing list, defunct and unreachable associations and registered charitable organizations. In addition to annual spending of over $1 billion on transportation and conventions alone, Canadian associations account for many millions more in pursuit of membership interests. Associations Canada provides complete access to this highly lucrative market. Associations Canada is a strong source of prospects for sales and marketing executives, tourism and convention officials, researchers, government officials - anyone who wants to locate non-profit interest groups and trade associations.

Hardcover ISBN 978-1-59237-219-5; 1,600 pages; $315.00

Financial Services Canada, 2007/08

Financial Services Canada is the only master file of current contacts and information that serves the needs of the entire financial services industry in Canada. With over 18,000 organizations and hard-to-find business information, Financial Services Canada is the most up-to-date source for names and contact numbers of industry professionals, senior executives, portfolio managers, financial advisors, agency bureaucrats and elected representatives. Financial Services Canada incorporates the latest changes in the industry to provide you with the most current details on each company, including: name, title, organization, telephone and fax numbers, e-mail and web addresses. Financial Services Canada also includes private company listings never before compiled, government agencies, association and consultant services - to ensure that you'll never miss a client or a contact. Current listings include: banks and branches, non-depository institutions, stock exchanges and brokers, investment management firms, insurance companies, major accounting and law firms, government agencies and financial associations. Powerful indexes assist researchers with locating the vital financial information they need. The following indexes are included: alphabetic, geographic, executive name, corporate web site/e-mail, government quick reference and subject. Financial Services Canada is a valuable resource for financial executives, bankers, financial planners, sales and marketing professionals, lawyers and chartered accountants, government officials, investment dealers, journalists, librarians and reference specialists.

900 pages; Hardcover ISBN 978-1-59237-221-8 $315.00

To preview any of our Directories Risk-Free for 30 days, call (800) 562-2139 or fax to (518) 789-0556

Directory of Libraries in Canada, 2007/08

The Directory of Libraries in Canada brings together almost 7,000 listings including libraries and their branches, information resource centers, archives and library associations and learning centers. The directory offers complete and comprehensive information on Canadian libraries, resource centers, business information centers, professional associations, regional library systems, archives, library schools and library technical programs. The Directory of Libraries in Canada includes important features of each library and service, including library information; personnel details, including contact names and e-mail addresses; collection information; services available to users; acquisitions budgets; and computers and automated systems. Useful information on each library's electronic access is also included, such as Internet browser, connectivity and public Internet/CD-ROM/subscription database access. The directory also provides powerful indexes for subject, location, personal name and Web site/e-mail to assist researchers with locating the crucial information they need. The Directory of Libraries in Canada is a vital reference tool for publishers, advocacy groups, students, research institutions, computer hardware suppliers, and other diverse groups that provide products and services to this unique market.

850 pages; Hardcover ISBN 978-1-59237-222-5; $315.00

Canadian Environmental Directory, 2007/08

The Canadian Environmental Directory is Canada's most complete and only national listing of environmental associations and organizations, government regulators and purchasing groups, product and service companies, special libraries, and more! The extensive Products and Services section provides detailed listings enabling users to identify the company name, address, phone, fax, e-mail, Web address, firm type, contact names (and titles), product and service information, affiliations, trade information, branch and affiliate data. The Government section gives you all the contact information you need at every government level – federal, provincial and municipal. We also include descriptions of current environmental initiatives, programs and agreements, names of environment-related acts administered by each ministry or department PLUS information and tips on who to contact and how to sell to governments in Canada. The Associations section provides complete contact information and a brief description of activities. Included are Canadian environmental organizations and international groups including industry, commercial and professional associations, registered charities, special interest and common interest organizations. All the Information you need about the Canadian environmental industry: directory of products and services, special libraries and resource, conferences, seminars and tradeshows, chronology of environmental events, law firms and major Canadian companies, The Canadian Environmental Directory is ideal for business, government, engineers and anyone conducting research on the environment.

Hardcover ISBN 978-1-59237-218-8; 900 pages; $315.00

Grey House Publishing
General Reference Titles

The Value of a Dollar 1600-1859, The Colonial Era to The Civil War

Following the format of the widely acclaimed, *The Value of a Dollar, 1860-2004, The Value of a Dollar 1600-1859, The Colonial Era to The Civil War* records the actual prices of thousands of items that consumers purchased from the Colonial Era to the Civil War. Our editorial department had been flooded with requests from users of our Value of a Dollar for the same type of information, just from an earlier time period. This new volume is just the answer – with pricing data from 1600 to 1859. Arranged into five-year chapters, each 5-year chapter includes a Historical Snapshot, Consumer Expenditures, Investments, Selected Income, Income/Standard Jobs, Food Basket, Standard Prices and Miscellany. There is also a section on Trends. This informative section charts the change in price over time and provides added detail on the reasons prices changed within the time period, including industry developments, changes in consumer attitudes and important historical facts. This fascinating survey will serve a wide range of research needs and will be useful in all high school, public and academic library reference collections.

600 pages; Hardcover ISBN 1-59237-094-2, $135.00

The Value of a Dollar 1860-2004, Third Edition

A guide to practical economy, *The Value of a Dollar* records the actual prices of thousands of items that consumers purchased from the Civil War to the present, along with facts about investment options and income opportunities. This brand new Third Edition boasts a brand new addition to each five-year chapter, a section on Trends. This informative section charts the change in price over time and provides added detail on the reasons prices changed within the time period, including industry developments, changes in consumer attitudes and important historical facts. Plus, a brand new chapter for 2000-2004 has been added. Each 5-year chapter includes a Historical Snapshot, Consumer Expenditures, Investments, Selected Income, Income/Standard Jobs, Food Basket, Standard Prices and Miscellany. This interesting and useful publication will be widely used in any reference collection.

"Recommended for high school, college and public libraries." –ARBA

600 pages; Hardcover ISBN 1-59237-074-8, $135.00

Working Americans 1880-1999
Volume I: The Working Class, Volume II: The Middle Class, Volume III: The Upper Class

Each of the volumes in the *Working Americans 1880-1999* series focuses on a particular class of Americans, The Working Class, The Middle Class and The Upper Class over the last 120 years. Chapters in each volume focus on one decade and profile three to five families. Family Profiles include real data on Income & Job Descriptions, Selected Prices of the Times, Annual Income, Annual Budgets, Family Finances, Life at Work, Life at Home, Life in the Community, Working Conditions, Cost of Living, Amusements and much more. Each chapter also contains an Economic Profile with Average Wages of other Professions, a selection of Typical Pricing, Key Events & Inventions, News Profiles, Articles from Local Media and Illustrations. The *Working Americans* series captures the lifestyles of each of the classes from the last twelve decades, covers a vast array of occupations and ethnic backgrounds and travels the entire nation. These interesting and useful compilations of portraits of the American Working, Middle and Upper Classes during the last 120 years will be an important addition to any high school, public or academic library reference collection.

"These interesting, unique compilations of economic and social facts, figures and graphs will support multiple research needs. They will engage and enlighten patrons in high school, public and academic library collections." –Booklist

Volume I: The Working Class ◆ 558 pages; Hardcover ISBN 1-891482-81-5, $145.00 ◆ Volume II: The Middle Class ◆ 591 pages; Hardcover ISBN 1-891482-72-6; $145.00 ◆ Volume III: The Upper Class ◆ 567 pages; Hardcover ISBN 1-930956-38-X, $145.00

Working Americans 1880-1999 Volume IV: Their Children

This Fourth Volume in the highly successful *Working Americans 1880-1999* series focuses on American children, decade by decade from 1880 to 1999. This interesting and useful volume introduces the reader to three children in each decade, one from each of the Working, Middle and Upper classes. Like the first three volumes in the series, the individual profiles are created from interviews, diaries, statistical studies, biographies and news reports. Profiles cover a broad range of ethnic backgrounds, geographic area and lifestyles – everything from an orphan in Memphis in 1882, following the Yellow Fever epidemic of 1878 to an eleven-year-old nephew of a beer baron and owner of the New York Yankees in New York City in 1921. Chapters also contain important supplementary materials including News Features as well as information on everything from Schools to Parks, Infectious Diseases to Childhood Fears along with Entertainment, Family Life and much more to provide an informative overview of the lifestyles of children from each decade. This interesting account of what life was like for Children in the Working, Middle and Upper Classes will be a welcome addition to the reference collection of any high school, public or academic library.

600 pages; Hardcover ISBN 1-930956-35-5, $145.00

To preview any of our Directories Risk-Free for 30 days, call (800) 562-2139 or fax to (518) 789-0556

Working Americans 1880-2003 Volume V: Americans At War

Working Americans 1880-2003 Volume V: Americans At War is divided into 11 chapters, each covering a decade from 1880-2003 and examines the lives of Americans during the time of war, including declared conflicts, one-time military actions, protests, and preparations for war. Each decade includes several personal profiles, whether on the battlefield or on the homefront, that tell the stories of civilians, soldiers, and officers during the decade. The profiles examine: Life at Home; Life at Work; and Life in the Community. Each decade also includes an Economic Profile with statistical comparisons, a Historical Snapshot, News Profiles, local News Articles, and Illustrations that provide a solid historical background to the decade being examined. Profiles range widely not only geographically, but also emotionally, from that of a girl whose leg was torn off in a blast during WWI, to the boredom of being stationed in the Dakotas as the Indian Wars were drawing to a close. As in previous volumes of the *Working Americans* series, information is presented in narrative form, but hard facts and real-life situations back up each story. The basis of the profiles come from diaries, private print books, personal interviews, family histories, estate documents and magazine articles. For easy reference, *Working Americans 1880-2003 Volume V: Americans At War* includes an in-depth Subject Index. The *Working Americans* series has become an important reference for public libraries, academic libraries and high school libraries. This fifth volume will be a welcome addition to all of these types of reference collections.

600 pages; Hardcover ISBN 1-59237-024-1; $145.00
Five Volume Set (Volumes I-V), Hardcover ISBN 1-59237-034-9, $675.00

Working Americans 1880-2005 Volume VI: Women at Work

Unlike any other volume in the *Working Americans* series, this Sixth Volume, is the first to focus on a particular gender of Americans. *Volume VI: Women at Work*, traces what life was like for working women from the 1860's to the present time. Beginning with the life of a maid in 1890 and a store clerk in 1900 and ending with the life and times of the modern working women, this text captures the struggle, strengths and changing perception of the American woman at work. Each chapter focuses on one decade and profiles three to five women with real data on Income & Job Descriptions, Selected Prices of the Times, Annual Income, Annual Budgets, Family Finances, Life at Work, Life at Home, Life in the Community, Working Conditions, Cost of Living, Amusements and much more. For even broader access to the events, economics and attitude towards women throughout the past 130 years, each chapter is supplemented with News Profiles, Articles from Local Media, Illustrations, Economic Profiles, Typical Pricing, Key Events, Inventions and more. This important volume illustrates what life was like for working women over time and allows the reader to develop an understanding of the changing role of women at work. These interesting and useful compilations of portraits of women at work will be an important addition to any high school, public or academic library reference collection.

600 pages; Hardcover ISBN 1-59237-063-2; $145.00

Working Americans 1880-2005 Volume VII: Social Movements

The newest addition to the widely-successful *Working Americans* series, *Volume VII: Social Movements* explores how Americans sought and fought for change from the 1880s to the present time. Following the format of previous volumes in the Working Americans series, the text examines the lives of 34 individuals who have worked – often behind the scenes — to bring about change. Issues include topics as diverse as the Anti-smoking movement of 1901 to efforts by Native Americans to reassert their long lost rights. Along the way, the book will profile individuals brave enough to demand suffrage for Kansas women in 1912 or demand an end to lynching during a March on Washington in 1923. Each profile is enriched with real data on Income & Job Descriptions, Selected Prices of the Times, Annual Incomes & Budgets, Life at Work, Life at Home, Life in the Community, along with News Features, Key Events, and Illustrations. The depth of information contained in each profile allow the user to explore the private, financial and public lives of these subjects, deepening our understanding of how calls for change took place in our society. A must-purchase for the reference collections of high school libraries, public libraries and academic libraries.

600 pages; Hardcover ISBN 1-59237-101-9; $145.00
Seven Volume Set (Volumes I-VII), Hardcover ISBN 1-59237-133-7, $945.00

The Encyclopedia of Warrior Peoples & Fighting Groups

Many military groups throughout the world have excelled in their craft either by fortuitous circumstances, outstanding leadership, or intense training. This new second edition of The Encyclopedia of Warrior Peoples and Fighting Groups explores the origins and leadership of these outstanding combat forces, chronicles their conquests and accomplishments, examines the circumstances surrounding their decline or disbanding, and assesses their influence on the groups and methods of warfare that followed. This edition has been completely updated with information through 2005 and contains over 20 new entries. Readers will encounter ferocious tribes, charismatic leaders, and daring militias, from ancient times to the present, including Amazons, Buffalo Soldiers, Green Berets, Iron Brigade, Kamikazes, Peoples of the Sea, Polish Winged Hussars, Sacred Band of Thebes, Teutonic Knights, and Texas Rangers. With over 100 alphabetical entries, numerous cross-references and illustrations, a comprehensive bibliography, and index, the Encyclopedia of Warrior Peoples and Fighting Groups is a valuable resource for readers seeking insight into the bold history of distinguished fighting forces.

"This work is especially useful for high school students, undergraduates, and general readers with an interest in military history." –Library Journal

Pub. Date: May 2006; Hardcover ISBN 1-59237-116-7; $135.00

The Encyclopedia of Invasions & Conquests, From the Ancient Times to the Present

Throughout history, invasions and conquests have played a remarkable role in shaping our world and defining our boundaries, both physically and culturally. This second edition of the popular Encyclopedia of Invasions & Conquests, a comprehensive guide to over 150 invasions, conquests, battles and occupations from ancient times to the present, takes readers on a journey that includes the Roman conquest of Britain, the Portuguese colonization of Brazil, and the Iraqi invasion of Kuwait, to name a few. New articles will explore the late 20th and 21st centuries, with a specific focus on recent conflicts in Afghanistan, Kuwait, Iraq, Yugoslavia, Grenada and Chechnya. Categories of entries include countries, invasions and conquests, and individuals. In addition to covering the military aspects of invasions and conquests, entries cover some of the political, economic, and cultural aspects, for example, the effects of a conquest on the invade country's political and monetary system and in its language and religion. The entries on leaders – among them Sargon, Alexander the Great, William the Conqueror, and Adolf Hitler – deal with the people who sought to gain control, expand power, or exert religious or political influence over others through military means. Revised and updated for this second edition, entries are arranged alphabetically within historical periods. Each chapter provides a map to help readers locate key areas and geographical features, and bibliographical references appear at the end of each entry. Other useful features include cross-references, a cumulative bibliography and a comprehensive subject index. This authoritative, well-organized, lucidly written volume will prove invaluable for a variety of readers, including high school students, military historians, members of the armed forces, history buffs and hobbyists.

"Engaging writing, sensible organization, nice illustrations, interesting and obscure facts, and useful maps make this book a pleasure to read." –ARBA

Pub. Date: March 2006; Hardcover ISBN 1-59237-114-0; $135.00

Encyclopedia of Prisoners of War & Internment

This authoritative second edition provides a valuable overview of the history of prisoners of war and interned civilians, from earliest times to the present. Written by an international team of experts in the field of POW studies, this fascinating and thought-provoking volume includes entries on a wide range of subjects including the Crusades, Plains Indian Warfare, concentration camps, the two world wars, and famous POWs throughout history, as well as atrocities, escapes, and much more. Written in a clear and easily understandable style, this informative reference details over 350 entries, 30% larger than the first edition, that survey the history of prisoners of war and interned civilians from the earliest times to the present, with emphasis on the 19th and 20th centuries. Medical conditions, international law, exchanges of prisoners, organizations working on behalf of POWs, and trials associated with the treatment of captives are just some of the themes explored. Entries range from the Ardeatine Caves Massacre to Kurt Vonnegut. Entries are arranged alphabetically, plus illustrations and maps are provided for easy reference. The text also includes an introduction, bibliography, appendix of selected documents, and end-of-entry reading suggestions. This one-of-a-kind reference will be a helpful addition to the reference collections of all public libraries, high schools, and university libraries and will prove invaluable to historians and military enthusiasts.

"Thorough and detailed yet accessible to the lay reader. Of special interest to subject specialists and historians; recommended for public and academic libraries." - Library Journal

Pub. Date: March 2006; Hardcover ISBN 1-59237-120-5; $135.00

The Religious Right, A Reference Handbook

Timely and unbiased, this third edition updates and expands its examination of the religious right and its influence on our government, citizens, society, and politics. From the fight to outlaw the teaching of Darwin's theory of evolution to the struggle to outlaw abortion, the religious right is continually exerting an influence on public policy. This text explores the influence of religion on legislation and society, while examining the alignment of the religious right with the political right. A historical survey of the movement highlights the shift to "hands-on" approach to politics and the struggle to present a unified front. The coverage offers a critical historical survey of the religious right movement, focusing on its increased involvement in the political arena, attempts to forge coalitions, and notable successes and failures. The text offers complete coverage of biographies of the men and women who have advanced the cause and an up to date chronology illuminate the movement's goals, including their accomplishments and failures. This edition offers an extensive update to all sections along with several brand new entries. Two new sections complement this third edition, a chapter on legal issues and court decisions and a chapter on demographic statistics and electoral patterns. To aid in further research, The Religious Right, offers an entire section of annotated listings of print and non-print resources, as well as of organizations affiliated with the religious right, and those opposing it. Comprehensive in its scope, this work offers easy-to-read, pertinent information for those seeking to understand the religious right and its evolving role in American society. A must for libraries of all sizes, university religion departments, activists, high schools and for those interested in the evolving role of the religious right.

" Recommended for all public and academic libraries." - Library Journal

Pub. Date: November 2006; Hardcover ISBN 1-59237-113-2; $135.00

From Suffrage to the Senate, America's Political Women

From Suffrage to the Senate is a comprehensive and valuable compendium of biographies of leading women in U.S. politics, past and present, and an examination of the wide range of women's movements. Up to date through 2006, this dynamically illustrated reference work explores American women's path to political power and social equality from the struggle for the right to vote and the abolition of slavery to the first African American woman in the U.S. Senate and beyond. This new edition includes over 150 new entries and a brand new section on trends and demographics of women in politics. The in-depth coverage also traces the political heritage of the abolition, labor, suffrage, temperance, and reproductive rights movements. The alphabetically arranged entries include biographies of every woman from across the political spectrum who has served in the U.S. House and Senate, along with women in the Judiciary and the U.S. Cabinet and, new to this edition, biographies of activists and political consultants. Bibliographical references follow each entry. For easy reference, a handy chronology is provided detailing 150 years of women's history. This up-to-date reference will be a must-purchase for women's studies departments, high schools and public libraries and will be a handy resource for those researching the key players in women's politics, past and present.

"An engaging tool that would be useful in high school, public, and academic libraries looking for an overview of the political history of women in the US." –Booklist

Pub. Date: October 2006; Two Volume Set; Hardcover ISBN 1-59237-117-5; $195.00

An African Biographical Dictionary

This landmark second edition is the only biographical dictionary to bring together, in one volume, cultural, social and political leaders – both historical and contemporary – of the sub-Saharan region. Over 800 biographical sketches of prominent Africans, as well as foreigners who have affected the continent's history, are featured, 150 more than the previous edition. The wide spectrum of leaders includes religious figures, writers, politicians, scientists, entertainers, sports personalities and more. Access to these fascinating individuals is provided in a user-friendly format. The biographies are arranged alphabetically, cross-referenced and indexed. Entries include the country or countries in which the person was significant and the commonly accepted dates of birth and death. Each biographical sketch is chronologically written; entries for cultural personalities add an evaluation of their work. This information is followed by a selection of references often found in university and public libraries, including autobiographies and principal biographical works. Appendixes list each individual by country and by field of accomplishment – rulers, musicians, explorers, missionaries, businessmen, physicists – nearly thirty categories in all. Another convenient appendix lists heads of state since independence by country. Up-to-date and representative of African societies as a whole, An African Biographical Dictionary provides a wealth of vital information for students of African culture and is an indispensable reference guide for anyone interested in African affairs.

"An unquestionable convenience to have these concise, informative biographies gathered into one source, indexed, and analyzed by appendixes listing entrants by nation and occupational field." –Wilson Library Bulletin

Pub. Date: July 2006; Hardcover ISBN 1-59237-112-4; $125.00

American Environmental Leaders, From Colonial Times to the Present

A comprehensive and diverse award winning collection of biographies of the most important figures in American environmentalism. Few subjects arouse the passions the way the environment does. How will we feed an ever-increasing population and how can that food be made safe for consumption? Who decides how land is developed? How can environmental policies be made fair for everyone, including multiethnic groups, women, children, and the poor? American Environmental Leaders presents more than 350 biographies of men and women who have devoted their lives to studying, debating, and organizing these and other controversial issues over the last 200 years. In addition to the scientists who have analyzed how human actions affect nature, we are introduced to poets, landscape architects, presidents, painters, activists, even sanitation engineers, and others who have forever altered how we think about the environment. The easy to use A–Z format provides instant access to these fascinating individuals, and frequent cross references indicate others with whom individuals worked (and sometimes clashed). End of entry references provide users with a starting point for further research.

"Highly recommended for high school, academic, and public libraries needing environmental biographical information." –Library Journal/Starred Review

Two Volume Set; Hardcover ISBN 1-57607-385-8 $175.00

World Cultural Leaders of the Twentieth Century

An expansive two volume set that covers 450 worldwide cultural icons, World Cultural Leaders of the Twentieth Century includes each person's works, achievements, and professional careers in a thorough essay. Who was the originator of the term "documentary"? Which poet married the daughter of the famed novelist Thomas Mann in order to help her escape Nazi Germany? Which British writer served as an agent in Russia against the Bolsheviks before the 1917 revolution? These and many more questions are answered in this illuminating text. A handy two volume set that makes it easy to look up 450 worldwide cultural icons: novelists, poets, playwrights, painters, sculptors, architects, dancers, choreographers, actors, directors, filmmakers, singers, composers, and musicians. World Cultural Leaders of the Twentieth Century provides entries (many of them illustrated) covering the person's works, achievements, and professional career in a thorough essay and offers interesting facts and statistics. Entries are fully cross-referenced so that readers can learn how various individuals influenced others. A thorough general index completes the coverage.

"Fills a need for handy, concise information on a wide array of international cultural figures."-ARBA

Two Volume Set; Hardcover ISBN 1-57607-038-7 $175.00

To preview any of our Directories Risk-Free for 30 days, call (800) 562-2139 or fax to (518) 789-0556

The Asian Databook: Statistics for all US Counties & Cities with Over 10,000 Population

This is the first-ever resource that compiles statistics and rankings on the US Asian population. *The Asian Databook* presents over 20 statistical data points for each city and county, arranged alphabetically by state, then alphabetically by place name. Data reported for each place includes Population, Languages Spoken at Home, Foreign-Born, Educational Attainment, Income Figures, Poverty Status, Homeownership, Home Values & Rent, and more. Next, in the Rankings Section, the top 75 places are listed for each data element. These easy-to-access ranking tables allow the user to quickly determine trends and population characteristics. This kind of comparative data can not be found elsewhere, in print or on the web, in a format that's as easy-to-use or more concise. A useful resource for those searching for demographics data, career search and relocation information and also for market research. With data ranging from Ancestry to Education, *The Asian Databook* presents a useful compilation of information that will be a much-needed resource in the reference collection of any public or academic library along with the marketing collection of any company whose primary focus in on the Asian population.

1,000 pages; Softcover ISBN 1-59237-044-6 $150.00

The Hispanic Databook: Statistics for all US Counties & Cities with Over 10,000 Population

Previously published by Toucan Valley Publications, this second edition has been completely updated with figures from the latest census and has been broadly expanded to include dozens of new data elements and a brand new Rankings section. The Hispanic population in the United States has increased over 42% in the last 10 years and accounts for 12.5% of the total US population. For ease-of-use, *The Hispanic Databook* presents over 20 statistical data points for each city and county, arranged alphabetically by state, then alphabetically by place name. Data reported for each place includes Population, Languages Spoken at Home, Foreign-Born, Educational Attainment, Income Figures, Poverty Status, Homeownership, Home Values & Rent, and more. Next, in the Rankings Section, the top 75 places are listed for each data element. These easy-to-access ranking tables allow the user to quickly determine trends and population characteristics. This kind of comparative data can not be found elsewhere, in print or on the web, in a format that's as easy-to-use or more concise. A useful resource for those searching for demographics data, career search and relocation information and also for market research. With data ranging from Ancestry to Education, *The Hispanic Databook* presents a useful compilation of information that will be a much-needed resource in the reference collection of any public or academic library along with the marketing collection of any company whose primary focus in on the Hispanic population.

"This accurate, clearly presented volume of selected Hispanic demographics is recommended for large public libraries and research collections."-Library Journal

1,000 pages; Softcover ISBN 1-59237-008-X, $150.00

Ancestry in America: A Comparative Guide to Over 200 Ethnic Backgrounds

This brand new reference work pulls together thousands of comparative statistics on the Ethnic Backgrounds of all populated places in the United States with populations over 10,000. Never before has this kind of information been reported in a single volume. Section One, Statistics by Place, is made up of a list of over 200 ancestry and race categories arranged alphabetically by each of the 5,000 different places with populations over 10,000. The population number of the ancestry group in that city or town is provided along with the percent that group represents of the total population. This informative city-by-city section allows the user to quickly and easily explore the ethnic makeup of all major population bases in the United States. Section Two, Comparative Rankings, contains three tables for each ethnicity and race. In the first table, the top 150 populated places are ranked by population number for that particular ancestry group, regardless of population. In the second table, the top 150 populated places are ranked by the percent of the total population for that ancestry group. In the third table, those top 150 populated places with 10,000 population are ranked by population number for each ancestry group. These easy-to-navigate tables allow users to see ancestry population patterns and make city-by-city comparisons as well. Plus, as an added bonus with the purchase of *Ancestry in America*, a free companion CD-ROM is available that lists statistics and rankings for all of the 35,000 populated places in the United States. This brand new, information-packed resource will serve a wide-range or research requests for demographics, population characteristics, relocation information and much more. *Ancestry in America: A Comparative Guide to Over 200 Ethnic Backgrounds* will be an important acquisition to all reference collections.

"This compilation will serve a wide range of research requests for population characteristics … it offers much more detail than other sources." –Booklist

1,500 pages; Softcover ISBN 1-59237-029-2, $225.00

The American Tally: Statistics & Comparative Rankings for U.S. Cities with Populations over 10,000

This important statistical handbook compiles, all in one place, comparative statistics on all U.S. cities and towns with a 10,000+ population. *The American Tally* provides statistical details on over 4,000 cities and towns and profiles how they compare with one another in Population Characteristics, Education, Language & Immigration, Income & Employment and Housing. Each section begins with an alphabetical listing of cities by state, allowing for quick access to both the statistics and relative rankings of any city. Next, the highest and lowest cities are listed in each statistic. These important, informative lists provide quick reference to which cities are at both extremes of the spectrum for each statistic. Unlike any other reference, *The American Tally* provides quick, easy access to comparative statistics – a must-have for any reference collection.

"A solid library reference." -Bookwatch

500 pages; Softcover ISBN 1-930956-29-0, $125.00

The Environmental Resource Handbook, 2007/08

The Environmental Resource Handbook is the most up-to-date and comprehensive source for Environmental Resources and Statistics. Section I: Resources provides detailed contact information for thousands of information sources, including Associations & Organizations, Awards & Honors, Conferences, Foundations & Grants, Environmental Health, Government Agencies, National Parks & Wildlife Refuges, Publications, Research Centers, Educational Programs, Green Product Catalogs, Consultants and much more. Section II: Statistics, provides statistics and rankings on hundreds of important topics, including Children's Environmental Index, Municipal Finances, Toxic Chemicals, Recycling, Climate, Air & Water Quality and more. This kind of up-to-date environmental data, all in one place, is not available anywhere else on the market place today. This vast compilation of resources and statistics is a must-have for all public and academic libraries as well as any organization with a primary focus on the environment.

"…the intrinsic value of the information make it worth consideration by libraries with environmental collections and environmentally concerned users." –Booklist

1,000 pages; Softcover ISBN 1-59237-195-7, $155.00 ◆ Online Database $300.00

Weather America, A Thirty-Year Summary of Statistical Weather Data and Rankings

This valuable resource provides extensive climatological data for over 4,000 National and Cooperative Weather Stations throughout the United States. *Weather America* begins with a new Major Storms section that details major storm events of the nation and a National Rankings section that details rankings for several data elements, such as Maximum Temperature and Precipitation. The main body of *Weather America* is organized into 50 state sections. Each section provides a Data Table on each Weather Station, organized alphabetically, that provides statistics on Maximum and Minimum Temperatures, Precipitation, Snowfall, Extreme Temperatures, Foggy Days, Humidity and more. State sections contain two brand new features in this edition – a City Index and a narrative Description of the climatic conditions of the state. Each section also includes a revised Map of the State that includes not only weather stations, but cities and towns.

"Best Reference Book of the Year." –Library Journal

2,013 pages; Softcover ISBN 1-891482-29-7, $175.00

Crime in America's Top-Rated Cities

This volume includes over 20 years of crime statistics in all major crime categories: violent crimes, property crimes and total crime. *Crime in America's Top-Rated Cities* is conveniently arranged by city and covers 76 top-rated cities. *Crime in America's Top-Rated Cities* offers details that compare the number of crimes and crime rates for the city, suburbs and metro area along with national crime trends for violent, property and total crimes. Also, this handbook contains important information and statistics on Anti-Crime Programs, Crime Risk, Hate Crimes, Illegal Drugs, Law Enforcement, Correctional Facilities, Death Penalty Laws and much more. A much-needed resource for people who are relocating, business professionals, general researchers, the press, law enforcement officials and students of criminal justice.

"Data is easy to access and will save hours of searching." –Global Enforcement Review

832 pages; Softcover ISBN 1-891482-84-X, $155.00